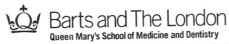

Barts and The London
Queen Mary's School of Medicine and Dentistry

WHITECHAPEL LIBRARY, TURNER STREET, LONDON E1 2AD
020 7882 7110

4 WEEK LOAN

Books are to be returned on or before the last date below,
otherwise fines may be charged.

10 JAN

Experimental and Clinical Neurotoxicology

Second Edition

Assistant Editors

John C.M. Brust, M.D.
Steven Herskovitz, M.D.
Arnold E. Merriam, M.D.
John L. O'Donoghue, V.M.D., Ph.D.
Neil L. Rosenberg, M.D.
Steven A. Sparr, M.D.

Developmental Editor

Monica Fenton, B.S.

Experimental and Clinical Neurotoxicology

SECOND EDITION

—»❯ ❮«—

Edited by
PETER S. SPENCER, Ph.D., F.R.C.Path.
Senior Scientist and Director
Center for Research on Occupational
  and Environmental Toxicology
Professor of Neurology, School of Medicine
Oregon Health Sciences University;
Research Director
Portland Environmental Hazards Research Center
Portland, Oregon, U.S.A.

HERBERT H. SCHAUMBURG, M.D.
Edwin S. Lowe Professor and Chairman of Neurology
Albert Einstein College of Medicine
Bronx, New York;
Chairman of Neurology
Montefiore Medical Center
Bronx, New York;
Attending Neurologist
Beth Israel Medical Center
New York, New York, U.S.A.

Associate Editor
ALBERT C. LUDOLPH, M.D.
Professor and Director of Neurology
University of Ulm
Ulm, Germany

NEW YORK OXFORD   OXFORD UNIVERSITY PRESS   2000

Oxford University Press

Oxford   New York
Athens   Auckland   Bangkok   Bogotá
Buenos Aires   Calcutta   Cape Town
Chennai   Dar es Salaam   Delhi   Florence   Hong Kong   Istanbul
Karachi   Kuala Lumpur   Madrid
Melbourne   Mexico City   Mumbai   Nairobi   Paris
São Paulo   Singapore   Taipei   Tokyo   Toronto   Warsaw

and associated companies in
Berlin   Ibadan

Copyright © 2000 by Oxford University Press

Published by Oxford University Press, Inc.
198 Madison Avenue, New York, New York 10016
http://www.oup.usa.org

Oxford is a registered trademark of Oxford University Press

Library of Congress Cataloging-in-Publication Data
Experimental and clinical neurotoxicology / edited by Peters S.
Spencer, Herbert H. Schaumburg ; associate editor, Albert C. Ludolph.
—2nd ed.
     p.   cm.
   Includes bibliographical references and index.
   ISBN 0-19-508477-2
   1. Neurotoxicology.   2. Nervous System—Diseases.
3. Neurotoxicology.   4. Nervous system—Diseases.   I. Spencer,
Peter S.   II. Schaumburg, Herbert H.   III. Ludolph,
Albert C.
   [DNLM: 1. Nervous system—drug effects.   2. Nervous System
Diseases—chemically induced.   3. Environmental Pollutants—
toxicity.   WL 100 E96   1999]
RC347.5.E96   1999
616.8′047—dc21
DNLM/DLC   98-18540

IMPORTANT NOTICE

Toxicology is an ever-changing science. As new experimental and clinical experience
broadens knowledge, changes in understanding of mechanism, effect, and drug treatment emerge. The editors, authors, and publisher have checked with sources believed
to be reliable in their efforts to provide information that is accurate and complete.
However, in view of the possibility of human error or changes in toxicology and in
medical and veterinary science, neither the editors nor the publisher can warrant that
the information contained herein is in every respect accurate or complete.* Readers
are encouraged to confirm the information contained herein with other reliable
sources and, for treatment of neurotoxic illness, are strongly advised to check with
textbooks of medicine and the product information provided by the pharmaceutical
company for each drug they plan to administer.

*Any legal responsibility for any errors or omissions or liability for any damages incurred as a direct or
indirect consequence of the use of the information provided in this book is therefore disclaimed.

9 8 7 6 5 4 3 2 1

Printed in the United States of America
on acid-free paper

Contents

Chapter Three
Aspects of Veterinary Neurotoxicology   83

Anthony A. Frank, Linda L. Blythe and
Peter S. Spencer

PART TWO
SUBSTANCES WITH
NEUROTOXIC POTENTIAL

NEUROTOXIC SUBSTANCES

Contributors

Edson X. Albuquerque, M.D., Ph.D.
  Professor and Chair
Department of Pharmacology and
    Experimental Therapeutics
School of Medicine
University of Maryland
Baltimore, Maryland, U.S.A.

Charles N. Allen, Ph.D.
  Scientist
Center for Research on Occupational and
    Environmental Toxicology
  Associate Professor
Department of Physiology and Pharmacology
Oregon Health Sciences University
Portland, Oregon, U.S.A.

Rainer Amann, M.D.
  Associate Professor
Department of Experimental and
    Clinical Pharmacology
Graz University
Graz, Austria

Stuart C. Apfel, M.D.
  Associate Professor
Department of Neurology and Neuroscience
Albert Einstein College of Medicine
Bronx, New York, U.S.A.

Dennis A. Aquino, Ph.D.
  Assistant Professor
Department of Neurology
Albert Einstein College of Medicine
Bronx, New York, U.S.A.

Joseph C. Arezzo, Ph.D.
  Professor
Departments of Neuroscience and Neurology
Albert Einstein College of Medicine
Bronx, New York, U.S.A.

Enrica Arnaudo, M.D.
  Assistant Professor
Department of Neurology
  Director
Electromyography Laboratory
Thomas Jefferson Medical College
Thomas Jefferson University
Philadelphia, Pennsylvania, U.S.A.

Hans Georg Baumgarten, M.D.
  Head and Chairman
Institut für Anatomie
Universitätsklinikum Benjamin Franklin
Berlin, Germany

Randall Berliner, M.D.
  Assistant Professor
Departments of Neurology and Psychiatry
Albert Einstein College of Medicine
Bronx, New York, U.S.A.

Phyllis L. Bieri, M.D.
Assistant Professor
Department of Neurology
Albert Einstein College of Medicine
Bronx, New York, U.S.A.

Dennis J. Blodgett, D.V.M., Ph.D.
Associate Professor of Toxicology
Department of Biomedical Sciences and
    Pathobiology
Virginia Tech
Blacksburg, Virginia, U.S.A.

Linda L. Blythe, D.V.M., Ph.D.
Professor of Neurology
Associate Dean of Academic and Student Affairs
College of Veterinary Medicine
Oregon State University
Corvallis, Oregon, U.S.A.

Thomas W. Bouldin, M.D.
Professor of Pathology and Ophthalmology
Departments of Pathology and Laboratory Medicine
University of North Carolina
Chapel Hill, North Carolina, U.S.A.

Frank Bretschneider, M.D.
Department of Neurology
University of Ulm
Ulm, Germany

John C.M. Brust, M.D.
Professor of Clinical Neurology
Columbia University College of Physicians and
    Surgeons
Director
Department of Neurology
Harlem Hospital Center
New York, New York, U.S.A.

George T. Bryan, M.D., Ph.D.
Professor Emeritus
Human Oncology and Medicine
    Director Emeritus
General Clinical Research Center
University of Wisconsin, U.S.A.
Madison, Wisconsin, U.S.A.

JoAnn Burkholder, Ph.D.
Professor
Department of Botany
North Carolina State University
Raleigh, North Carolina, U.S.A.

Brent T. Burton, M.D., M.P.H.
Occupational and Environmental Toxicology
Portland, Oregon, U.S.A.

Vincent P. Calabrese, M.D.
Associate Professor
Department of Neurology
Medical College of Virginia
Richmond, Virginia, U.S.A.

Donald B. Calne, D.M.
Director
Neurodegenerative Disorders Center
U.B.C. Hospital
Vancouver, B.C. Canada

Wayne W. Carmichael, Ph.D.
Professor
Department of Biological Sciences
Wright State University
Dayton, Ohio, U.S.A.

Neil R. Cashman, M.D., F.R.C.P.(C)
Professor
Department of Medicine (Neurology)
Center for Research in Neurodegenerative Diseases
University of Toronto
Toronto, Ontario, Canada

F. Cendes, M.D.
Post-Doctoral Fellow of Epilepsy Service
Departments of Neurology and Neurosurgery
Montreal Neurological Institute and Hospital
McGill University
Montreal, Quebec, Canada

Fung-Chow Chiu, M.D.
Associate Professor
Departments of Neurology and Anesthesiology
Albert Einstein College of Medicine
Bronx, New York, U.S.A.

Nai-Shin Chu, M.D.
Professor and Chairman
Department of Neurology
Chang Gung Medical College and Memorial Hospital
Taipei, Taiwan

Michael A. Collins, Ph.D.
Professor
Department of Molecular and Cellular Biochemistry
Loyola University Chicago
Stritch School of Medicine
Maywood, Illinois, U.S.A.

Deborah A. Cory-Schlecta, Ph.D.
Professor and Chair
Environmental Medicine
Director
Environmental Health Sciences Center
Professor
Departments of Pediatrics, Neurobiology and
Anatomy
University of Rochester
Rochester, New York, U.S.A.

Derek J. Cripps, M.D.
Professor
Department of Medicine
Division of Dermatology
University of Wisconsin Hospital and Clinics
Madison, Wisconsin, U.S.A.

Kevin M. Crofton, Ph.D.
Neurotoxicologist
Neurotoxicology Division
National Health Effects and Environmental
Research Laboratory
U.S. Environmental Protection Agency
Research Triangle Park, North Carolina, U.S.A.

Lourdes J. Cruz, Ph.D.
Professor
Marine Science Institute
University of the Phillipines
Quezon City, Phillipines;
Research Professor
Department of Biology
University of Utah
Salt Lake City, Utah, U.S.A.

Howard A. Crystal, M.D.
Professor
Department of Neurology
Albert Einstein College of Medicine
Bronx, New York, U.S.A.

Jeffrey I. Daniels, D.Env.
Risk Sciences Group Leader
Health and Ecological Assessment Division
Earth and Environmental Sciences Directorate
Lawrence Livermore National Laboratory
University of California
Livermore, California, U.S.A.

David A. Dankovic, Ph.D.
Toxicologist
Education and Information Division
National Institute for Occupational Safety and
Health
Centers for Disease Control and Prevention
Cincinnati, Ohio, U.S.A.

Nora Deamer-Melia, M.S.
Department of Botany
North Carolina State University
Raleigh, North Carolina, U.S.A.

Anthony P. DeCaprio, Ph.D., D.A.B.T.
Professor
Professional Education Program
School of Public Health
The University at Albany
State University of New York
Rensselaer, New York, U.S.A.

Anna Maria Di Giulio, Ph.D.
Associate Professor in Pharmacology
Pharmacological Laboratories
Department of Medicine, Surgery and Odontoiatry
University of Milan
Milan, Italy

Donato A. Di Monte, M.D.
Director, Basic Research
The Parkinson's Institute
Sunnyvale, California, U.S.A.

Donald J. Ecobichon, Ph.D.
Professor (*Retired*)
Department of Pharmacology and Toxicology
Queen's University
Kingston, Ontario, Canada

Kenneth R. Einberg, M.D.
Associate Professor
Department of Neurology
Albert Einstein College of Medicine
Bronx, New York;
Director
Neuromuscular Laboratory
Department of Neurology
Long Island Jewish Medical Center
New Hyde Park, New York, U.S.A.

Carol Eisenberg, M.B.Ch.B., Ph.D.
Assistant Professor
Department of Neurology
Albert Einstein College of Medicine
Bronx, New York, U.S.A.

Monica Fenton, B.S.
Senior Research Associate and
    Special Assistant to the Director (*Retired*)
Center for Research on Occupational and
    Environmental Toxicology
Oregon Health Sciences University
Portland, Oregon, U.S.A.

Anthony A. Frank, D.V.M., Ph.D.
Associate Professor of Clinical Pathology
Associate Dean for Research
College of Veterinary Medicine and Biomedical
    Sciences
Colorado State University
Ft. Collins, Colorado, U.S.A.

Mary Beth Genter, Ph.D.
Associate Professor
Department of Environmental Health
University of Cincinnati
Cincinnati, Ohio, U.S.A.

William H. Gerwick, Ph.D.
Professor
Medicinal and Natural Products Chemistry
College of Pharmacy
Oregon State University
Corvallis, Oregon, U.S.A.

Myron D. Ginsberg, M.D.
Scheinberg Professor of Neurology
Director
Cerebral Vascular Research Center
Department of Neurology
University of Miami School of Medicine
Miami, Florida, U.S.A.

Howard Glasgow, Ph.D.
Department of Botany
North Carolina State University
Raleigh, North Carolina, U.S.A.

Ayhan Göcmen, M.D.
Professor
Department of Pediatrics
Haceteppe University
Ankara, Turkey

Bruce G. Gold, Ph.D.
Scientist
Center for Research on Occupational and
    Environmental Toxicology
Associate Professor
Department of Cell and Developmental Biology
Oregon Health Sciences University
Portland, Oregon, U.S.A.

Mark Forest Gordon, M.D.
Assistant Professor
Department of Neurology
Albert Einstein College of Medicine
Bronx, New York;
Associate Attending
Long Island Jewish Medical Center
New Hyde Park, New York, U.S.A.

Alfredo Gorio, M.D.
Chief
Laboratories for Research on Pharmacology of
    Neurodegenerative Disorders
Pharmacological Laboratories
Department of Medicine, Surgery and Odontoiatry
University of Milan
Milan, Italy

Rainer Gothe, M.D.
Professor
Institute for Comparative Tropical Medicine and
    Parasitology
Ludwig-Maximilians University
Munich, Germany

Doyle G. Graham, M.D., Ph.D.
Professor and Chairman
Department of Pathology
Vanderbilt University School of Medicine
Nashville, Tennessee, U.S.A.

John W. Griffin, M.D.
Professor and Director of Neuroscience and
    Pathology
Department of Neurology
The Johns Hopkins University
School of Medicine
Baltimore, Maryland, U.S.A.

Zarko Grozdanovic, M.D.
Wissenschaftlichen Assistant
Institut für Anatomie
Universitätsklinikum Benjamin Franklin
Freie Universität Berlin
Berlin, Germany

Ludwig Guttman, M.D.
Hazel Ruby McQuain Professor of Neurology
Department of Neurology
Robert C. Byrd Health Sciences Center
West Virginia University
Morgantown, West Virginia, U.S.A.

Fengsheng He, M.D.
Professor
Institute of Occupational Medicine
Chinese Academy of Preventive Medicine
Beijing, People's Republic of China

Alfred Heller, M.D., Ph.D.
Professor
Department of Neurobiology,
    Pharmacology and Physiology
University of Chicago
Chicago, Illinois, U.S.A.

Steven Herskovitz, M.D.
Associate Professor
Department of Neurology
Albert Einstein College of Medicine
    Director
Neuromuscular Laboratory
Montefiore Medical Center
Bronx, New York, U.S.A.

Fred H. Hochberg, M.D.
Associate Professor
Department of Neurology
Massachusetts General Hospital
Harvard Medical School
Boston, Massachusetts, U.S.A.

Philip C. Hoffmann, Ph.D.
Professor
Department of Pharmacological and
    Physiological Sciences
University of Chicago
Chicago, Illinois, U.S.A.

Peter Holzer, Ph.D.
Professor
Department of Experimental and Clinical
    Pharmacology
Graz University
Graz, Austria

Chin-Chang Huang, M.D.
Associate Professor
Department of Neurology
Chang Gung Medical College and Memorial Hospital
Taipei, Taiwan

Jacques Hugon, M.D., Ph.D.
Professor and Chair
Department of Anatomy
Faculty of Medicine
University of Hong Kong
    Honorary Clinical Professor
Department of Medicine
Division of Neurology
Queen Mary Hospital
Hong Kong

Edward G. Hyde, Ph.D.
Lead Discovery - Biology
AstraZeneca R&D Brisbane
Mount Gravatt Research Park
Queensland, Australia

Daniel C. Javitt, M.D., Ph.D.
Director
Program in Cognitive Neuroscience and
    Schizophrenia
Associate Professor
Department of Psychiatry
New York School of Medicine
New York University
Nathan Kline Institute for Psychiatric Research
Orangeburg, New York, U.S.A.

Bernard S. Jortner, V.M.D.
Professor of Pathology
Laboratory for Neurotoxicity Studies
Departments of Biomedical Sciences and
    Pathobiology
Virginia–Maryland Regional College of
    Veterinary Medicine
Virginia Polytechnic Institute
Blacksburg, Virginia, U.S.A.

**Byron A. Kakulas, A.O., M.D.,
F.R.C.Path., F.R.C.P.A.**
Head, Department of Neuropathology
Royal Perth Hospital
    Medical Director
Australian Neuromuscular Research Institute
University of Western Australia
Perth, Australia

Michael W. Kalichman, Ph.D.
Associate Adjunct Professor
Department of Pathology
School of Medicine
University of California, San Diego
La Jolla, California, U.S.A.

Jerry G. Kaplan, M.D.
Associate Professor
Department of Neurology
Albert Einstein College of Medicine
Bronx, New York, U.S.A.

Nobufumi Kawai, M.D., Ph.D.
Department of Physiology
Jichi Medical School
Minamikawachi-machi, Tochigi-ken, Japan

William R. Kem, Ph.D.
Professor
Department of Pharmacology and Therapeutics
College of Medicine
University of Florida
Gainesville, Florida, U.S.A.

Glen Kisby, Ph.D.
Assistant Scientist
Center for Research on Occupational and
    Environmental Toxicology
Assistant Professor
Department of Physiology and Pharmacology
Oregon Health Sciences University
Portland, Oregon, U.S.A.

Hans Kolbe, M.D.
Neurologische Klinik mit
Klinischer Neurophysiologie
Medizinische Hochschule Hannover
Hannover, Germany

Paul L. Kornblith, M.D.
Adjunct Professor
University of Pittsburgh
Pittsburgh, Pennsylvania, U.S.A.

**Georg J. Krinke, M.V.Dr., C.Sc.,
Diplomate E.C.V.P.**
Novartis Crop Protection AG
Stein, Switzerland

**Thomas L. Kurt, M.D., M.P.H.,
F.A.C.P.M., F.A.C.M.T.**
Clinical Professor
Department of Internal Medicine
University of Texas Southwestern Medical Center
    at Dallas
Dallas, Texas, U.S.A.

J. William Langston, M.D.
President
The Parkinson's Institute
Sunnyvale, California, U.S.A.

George Lantos, Ph.D.
Associate Professor
Department of Radiology and Neurology
Albert Einstein College of Medicine
Bronx, New York, U.S.A.

Jorge N. Larocca, Ph.D.
Associate Professor
Department of Neurology
Albert Einstein College of Medicine
Bronx, New York, U.S.A.

Ellen J. Lehning, Ph.D.
Assistant Professor
Department of Anesthesiology
Montefiore Medical Center
Albert Einstein College of Medicine
Bronx, New York, U.S.A.

Edward D. Levin, Ph.D.
Associate Professor
Departments of Psychiatry and Pharmacology
Director
Integrated Toxicology Program
Duke University Medical Center
Durham, North Carolina, U.S.A.

Richard B. Lipton, M.D.
Professor
Department of Neurology, Psychiatry, and
Epidemiology and Social Medicine
Albert Einstein College of Medicine
Bronx, New York, U.S.A.

Richard M. LoPachin, Ph.D.
Associate Professor
Department of Anesthesiology
Montefiore Medical Center
Albert Einstein College of Medicine
Bronx, New York, U.S.A.

Marcello Lotti, M.D.
Professor
Occupational Medicine
Instituto de Medicina del Lavoro
Università di Padova
Padova, Italy

Albert C. Ludolph, M.D.
Professor and Director
Department of Neurology
University of Ulm
Ulm, Germany

Peter C. Mabie, M.D.
Assistant Professor
Department of Neurology
Albert Einstein College of Medicine
Bronx, New York, U.S.A.

Allison Mann, M.D.
Research Scientist
New York State Institute for Basic Research and
Development Disabilities
Staten Island, New York, U.S.A.

Luigi Manzo, Ph.D.
Professor
Department of Internal Medicine
University of Pavia
"S. Maugeri" Foundation Pavia Medical Center
Pavia, Italy

Joseph Maytal, M.D.
Associate Professor of Neurology and Pediatrics
Albert Einstein College of Medicine
Associate Attending
Division of Pediatric Neurology
Schneider Children's Hospital
New Hyde Park, New York, U.S.A.

Mark F. Mehler, M.D.
Professor
Department of Neurology
Albert Einstein College of Medicine
Bronx, New York, U.S.A.

William A. Meier-Ruge, M.D.
Professor
Department of Pathology
University Medical School, Basel
Basel, Switzerland

Jerry R. Mendell, M.D.
Professor and Chairman
Department of Neurology
Neuromuscular Center
Ohio State University
Columbus, Ohio, U.S.A.

Arnold E. Merriam, M.D.
Professor
Departments of Psychiatry and Neurology
Director
Division of Neuropsychiatry
Albert Einstein College of Medicine
Director of Psychiatry
Bronx Municipal Hospital Center
Bronx, New York, U.S.A.

Thomas Meyer, M.D.
Department of Neurology
University of Ulm
Ulm, Germany

Andrew P. Mizisin, Ph.D.
Associate Professor
Department of Pathology (Neuropathology)
School of Medicine
University of California San Diego
La Jolla, California, U.S.A.

Solomon L. Moshé, M.D.
Professor
Departments of Neurology, Neuroscience and
Pediatrics
Albert Einstein College of Medicine
Bronx, New York, U.S.A.

Thomas F. Murray, Ph.D.
Professor and Head
Department of Physiology and Pharmacology
College of Veterinary Medicine
The University of Georgia
Athens, Georgia, U.S.A.

Toshio Narahashi, Ph.D.
John Evans Professor of Pharmacology
Alfred Newton Richards Professor
Departments of Molecular Pharmacology and
Biological Chemistry
Northwestern University Medical School
Chicago, Illinois, U.S.A.

Edward J. Neafsey, Ph.D.
Professor
Department of Cell Biology, Neurobiology and
Anatomy
Stritch School of Medicine
Loyola University Chicago
Maywood, Illinois, U.S.A.

Martha Neff-Smith, Ph.D., M.P.H.
Associate Professor
Department of Preventive Medicine
Community Health Nursing
School of Nursing
Virginia Commonwealth University
Richmond, Virginia, U.S.A.

Lawrence C. Newman, M.D.
Associate Professor
Department of Neurology
Albert Einstein College of Medicine
Director
Bronx, New York;
Headache Institute
St. Luke's-Roosevelt Hospital
New York, New York, U.S.A.

Peter Obendorf, Ph.D.
Senior Lecturer
Department of Applied Biology and
Biotechnology
RMIT University
Melbourne, Australia

John L. O'Donoghue, V.M.D., Ph.D.
Director
Health and Environment Laboratories
Eastman Kodak Company
Rochester, New York, U.S.A.

Akio Ohnishi, M.D., D.Med.Sci.
Associate Professor
Department of Neurology
University of Occupational and Environmental Health
Kitakyushu, Japan

Baldomero M. Olivera, Ph.D.
Distinguished Professor
Department of Biology
University of Utah
Salt Lake City, Utah, U.S.A.

John W. Olney, M.D.
Professor of Psychiatry and Neuropathology
Department of Psychiatry
Washington University School of Medicine
St. Louis, Missouri, U.S.A.

George Oyler, M.D., Ph.D.
Assistant Professor
Department of Neurology
University of Maryland School of Medicine
Baltimore, Maryland, U.S.A.

Valerie Palmer, B.S.
President
Third World Medical Research Foundation
Portland, Oregon, U.S.A.

Richard G. Pellegrino, M.D., Ph.D.
President
Central Arkansas Research
Hot Springs, Arkansas, U.S.A.

Alan Pestronk, M.D.
Professor
Departments of Neurology and Pathology
Washington University School of Medicine
St. Louis, Missouri, U.S.A.

Henry A. Peters, M.D.
Professor Emeritus
Department of Neurology and Psychiatry
University of Wisconsin Medical School
Madison, Wisconsin, U.S.A.

Tom Piek, M.D.
Associate Professor (*Retired*)
Department of Pharmacology
Academic Medical Center
University of Amsterdam
Amsterdam, The Netherlands

Marianne A. Polunas, B.S.
Fellow
Neurotoxicology Laboratories
Department of Pharmacology and Toxicology
Rutgers University
Piscataway, New Jersey, U.S.A.

Alberto Portera-Sánchez, M.D., Ph.D.
Professor and Head
Department of Neurology
Hospital Universitairio "12 de Octubre"
Madrid, Spain

Manuel Posada de la Paz, M.D.
Research Coordinator of Toxic Oil Syndrome
Coordinating Center, Research Network Unit
Subdirección General de Salud
Instituto de Salud Carlos III
Madrid, Spain

Henry C. Powell, M.D., D.Sc.
Professor and Head
Division of Neuropathology
School of Medicine
University of California, San Diego
La Jolla, California, U.S.A.

Michael K. Pugsley, M.Sc., Ph.D.
Scientist
Department of Pharmacology and Toxicology
XOMA [US] LLC
Berkeley, California, U.S.A.

Kenneth R. Reuhl, Ph.D., D.A.B.T.
Professor
Neurotoxicology Laboratories
Department of Pharmacology and Toxicology
Rutgers University
Piscataway, New Jersey, U.S.A.

Matthias W. Riepe, M.D., Ph.D.
Assistant Professor
Department of Neurology
University of Ulm
Ulm, Germany

D. Gary Rischitelli, M.D., M.P.H., J.D.
Assistant Professor
Departments of Emergency Medicine, Public
Health and Preventive Medicine
Assistant Scientist
Center for Research on Occupational and
Environmental Toxicology
Oregon Health Sciences University
Portland, Oregon, U.S.A.

John D. Rogers, M.D., M.P.H.
Assistant Professor
Department of Neurology
Albert Einstein College of Medicine
Bronx, New York;
Associate Attending
Beth Israel Medical Center
New York, New York, U.S.A.

Daniel M. Rosenbaum, M.D.
Associate Professor
Department of Neurology
Albert Einstein College of Medicine
Bronx, New York, U.S.A.

Neil L. Rosenberg, M.D.
Assistant Clinical Professor
Department of Medicine
Division of Clinical Pharmacology and Medical
Toxicology
University of Colorado
School of Medicine
Denver, Colorado, U.S.A.

Hans Rosling, M.D., Ph.D.
Professor of International Health
Division of International Health
Department of Public Health Sciences
Karolinska Institutet
Stockholm, Sweden

Dwijendra N. Roy, Ph.D., D.Sc.
Staff Scientist and Associate Professor (*Retired*)
Center for Research on Occupational and
Environmental Toxicology
Oregon Health Sciences University
Portland, Oregon, U.S.A.

Mohammad I. Sabri, Ph.D.
Lecturer
Center for Research on Occupational and
Environmental Toxicology
Associate Professor
Department of Neurology
Oregon Health Sciences University
Portland, Oregon, U.S.A.

Zarife Sahenk, M.D., Ph.D.
Professor
Department of Neurology
Neuromuscular Center
Ohio State University Hospital
Columbus, Ohio, U.S.A.

Ted A. Sarafian, Ph.D.
Department of Medicine
Division of Pulmonary and Critical Care Medicine
University of California Los Angeles
Los Angeles, California, U.S.A.

Steven N. Scelsa, M.D.
Assistant Professor
Department of Neurology
Albert Einstein College of Medicine
Bronx, New York;
Director, Neuromuscular Laboratory
Department of Neurology
Beth Israel Medical Center
New York, New York, U.S.A.

Herbert H. Schaumburg, M.D.
Edwin S. Lowe Professor and Chairman
Department of Neurology
Albert Einstein College of Medicine
Bronx, New York;
Chairman
Department of Neurology
Montefiore Medical Center
Bronx, New York;
Attending Neurologist
Beth Israel Medical Center
New York, New York, U.S.A.

Donald E. Schmechel, M.D.
Associate Professor
Departments of Medicine and Neurobiology
Chief of Neurology
Durham Veterans' Affairs Medical Center
Duke University Medical Center
Durham, North Carolina, U.S.A.

J. Michael Schröder, M.D.
Professor
Institut für Neuropathologie
Medizinische Fakultät
Rheinisch-Westfälische Technische
Hochschule Aachen
Aachen, Germany

John B. Selhorst, M.D.
Souers Professor and Chairman
Department of Neurology
Saint Louis University Health Sciences Center
St. Louis, Missouri, U.S.A.

Bennett A. Shaywitz, M.D.
Professor of Pediatrics and Neurology
Co-Director
Yale Center for the Study of Learning and Attention
Yale University School of Medicine
New Haven, Connecticut, U.S.A.

Shlomo Shinnar, M.D., Ph.D.
Professor
Departments of Neurology and Pediatrics
Albert Einstein College of Medicine
Bronx, New York, U.S.A.

Mark J. Sinnett, Pharm.D.
Clinical Pharmacist
Department of Pharmacy
Montefiore Medical Center
Assistant Clinical Professor
Department of Neurology
Bronx, New York, U.S.A.

Thomas L. Slamovits, M.D.
Professor
Departments of Ophthalmology and Neurology
Albert Einstein College of Medicine
Bronx, New York, U.S.A.

William Slikker, Jr., Ph.D.
Director
Division of Neurotoxicology
National Center for Toxicological
Research
U.S. Food and Drug Administration
Jefferson, Arkansas, U.S.A.

Steven A. Sparr, M.D.
Associate Professor
Department of Neurology
Albert Einstein College of Medicine
Bronx, New York, U.S.A.

Peter S. Spencer, Ph.D., F.R.C.Path.
Director and Senior Scientist
Center for Research on Occupational
and Environmental Toxicology
Professor of Neurology
School of Medicine
Oregon Health Sciences University
Portland, Oregon;
Adjunct Professor
College of Veterinary Medicine
Oregon State University
Corvallis, Oregon, U.S.A.

Mitchell Steinschneider, Ph.D.
Associate Professor
Departments of Neurology and Pediatrics
Albert Einstein College of Medicine
Bronx, New York, U.S.A.

Richard D. Stewart, M.D., M.P.H., Ph.D.
Adjunct Professor
Department of Pharmacology and Toxicology
Medical College of Wisconsin
Milwaukee, Wisconsin, U.S.A.

Alexander Storch, M.D.
Department of Neurology
University of Ulm
Ulm, Germany

Marie Haring Sweeney, Ph.D., M.P.H.
Chief
Document Development Branch
Education and Information Division
National Institute for Occupational Safety and Health
Centers for Disease Control and Prevention
Cincinnati, Ohio, U.S.A.

John R. Taylor, M.D.
Department of Neurology
Medical College of Virginia
    Chief of Neurology
Department of Veterans' Affairs Medical Center
Richmond, Virginia, U.S.A.

Thorkild Tylleskär, M.D., Ph.D.
    Senior Lecturer
Departments of Medical Sciences and Nutrition
Uppsala University
Uppsala, Sweden

John Tor-Agbidye, D.V.M., Ph.D.
National Center for Toxicological Research
U.S. Food and Drug Administration
Jefferson, Arkansas, U.S.A.

William M. Valentine, Ph.D., D.V.M.
    Assistant Professor
Department of Pathology
Vanderbilt University School of Medicine
Nashville, Tennessee, U.S.A.

Raul Francisco Valenzuela, M.D.
    Instructor
Department of Neurology
Escuela de Medicina
Universidad Catolica de Chile
Santiago, Chile

Libor Velisek, M.D., Ph.D.
    Assistant Professor
Department of Neurology
Albert Einstein College of Medicine
Bronx, New York, U.S.A.

M. Anthony Verity, M.D.
    Professor of Neuropathology (*Retired*)
UCLA Medical Center
University of California Los Angeles
Los Angeles, California, U.S.A.

Henk P.M. Vijverberg, Ph.D.
Research Institute of Toxicology
Utrecht University
Utrecht, The Netherlands

Helge Völkel, Ph.D.
Department of Neurology
University of Ulm
Ulm, Germany

Michael J.A. Walker, Ph.D.
    Professor
Department of Pharmacology and Therapeutics
University of British Columbia
Vancouver, B.C., Canada

Steven U. Walkley, Ph.D.
    Professor
Departments of Neuroscience and Neurology
Albert Einstein College of Medicine
Bronx, New York, U.S.A.

William C. Welch, M.D., F.A.C.S.
    Associate Professor
Departments of Neurological Surgery,
        Orthopedic Surgery and Rehabilitation
        Science and Technology
    Co-Director
Spine Specialty Center
    Director
Neurological Spine Services
University of Pittsburgh School of Medicine
Pittsburgh, Pennsylvania, U.S.A.

Roy O. Weller, M.D., Ph.D., F.R.C.Path.
    Professor of Neuropathology
Department of Pathology
University of Southampton School of Medicine
Southampton University Hospitals Trust
Southampton, United Kingdom

Horst Wiethölter, M.D.
    Professor
Neurologische Klinik am
        Bürgerhospital Stuttgart
Stuttgart, Germany

Barry W. Wilson, Ph.D.
    Professor
Department of Animal Science and Environmental
        Toxicology
University of California Davis
Davis, California, U.S.A.

Anthony J. Windebank, M.D.
Dean
Mayo Medical School
Professor
Department of Neurology
Mayo Clinic and Mayo Foundation
Rochester, Minnesota, U.S.A.

Klaus Windgassen, M.D.
Professor
Department of Psychiatry
Westfälische Wilhelms-Universität
Münster, Germany

Lisa Won, Ph.D.
Associate Professor
Departments of Neurobiology,
Pharmacology and Physiology
University of Chicago
Chicago, Illinois, U.S.A.

About This Book

Experimental and Clinical Neurotoxicology has been reorganized and rewritten for this second edition. The book is now in two sections. Section A, comprising three broad chapters, provides a wide overview of the neurobiological basis for neurotoxic phenomena and a description of these phenomena in human and veterinary medicine. Section B, organized alphabetically by the name of the substance, describes the neurotoxic properties of chemicals and mixtures (including plants, venoms, etc.). Each entry includes a neurotoxicity rating (*vide infra*) that indicates the strength of association between the substance and its proposed biological action (experimental) and neurological effect (clinical).

EXPERIMENTAL
A. An accepted causal association between the entity and its reported action
B. A suspected but unproven association between the entity and its reported action
C. A proposed but unlikely association between the entity and a reported action

CLINICAL
A. A strongly supported association between the entity and the neurological condition
B. A suspected and plausible association between the entity and the neurological condition
C. A suggested but unlikely association between the entity and the neurological condition.

Preface

A science of neurotoxicology assembles knowledge on the adverse actions on nervous systems of chemicals of all types, whether synthesis of the chemical has been undertaken in nature or by humans. Understanding of a chemical's interaction with its biological receptor(s) provides a solid foundation on which to analyze the substance's clinical effects in humans and animals. We have used this philosophy in developing an encyclopedic approach to neurotoxicology that includes a wide variety of chemicals that perturb the nervous system. The individual treatment of chemicals and mixtures is simply organized in alphabetical fashion (A–Z) and comprises the bulk of the volume. This approach avoids the artificial and misleading classification of substances by their physical properties (*e.g.*, organic solvents), chemical class (*e.g.*, heavy metals), use category (*e.g.*, pesticides), location (*e.g.*, workplace chemicals), social disposition (*e.g.*, "drugs of abuse"), or therapeutic categorization (*e.g.*, antibiotics). Chemicals in this latter grouping occupy a prominent position in this volume because the neurotoxic side effects of therapeutic substances are pervasive in the West. In less developed regions of the world, the neurotoxic potential of certain food plants is a dominant theme. A new feature throughout the A–Z section is the use of a rating scheme (described on page xxxv) to assist the reader in understanding the strength of association between a substance or mixture and its purported biological actions and clinical effects. Appendix 1 alphabetically lists the A–Z entries with their respective neurotoxicity ratings, and Appendix 2 groups the entities by their clinical neurotoxic effects in humans and animals.

The book opens with an analysis of the neurobiological principles of chemical neurotoxicity and uses this approach in subsequent chapters to address clinical neurotoxic phenomena in humans and animals. The inclusion of a chapter on veterinary neurotoxicology recognizes the importance of this subdiscipline and the opportunity for discovery of cause-effect relations in animals that may also have relevance for understanding human disease. Fostering the prevention and treatment of human neurotoxic disease were also driving forces in our decision to include chemical agents designed for use in human warfare.

We are joined in this second edition by Prof. Dr. med. Albert Ludolph, who serves as Associate Editor and principal author for entries covering biological substances with neurotoxic potential. He, along with our Assistant Editors and many other distinguished colleagues, comprise the international authorship of this volume. Our Developmental Editor, Monica Fenton, shepherded the entire production from inception to completion. Valerie Palmer scrutinized chemical formulas and the Index for accuracy. Jerry Schnell, Ph.D., and Victor Miller assisted with literature research. We also acknowledge the generous assistance of Cecile Basilone, Mary Lou Hadwick, Marjorie Jeannis, Donna Platyan, Rodger Metheny, Vincentina Rubano, and Patricia Vacchelli. Berta Steiner (Bermedica Production, Ltd.) and Susan Hannan (Oxford University Press) expertly directed copyediting and manuscript development. Jeffrey House (Oxford) invested in the creation of this volume and was supportive throughout its evolution. We thank them all.

Portland, Oregon   Peter S. Spencer, Ph.D., F.R.C.Path.
Bronx, New York   Herbert H. Schaumburg, M.D.
August, 1999

Preface to the First Edition

The upsurge of interest in recent years in academia, industry and government on the effects of toxic chemicals on the nervous system has created a new discipline of neurotoxicology. The subject has fused scientists with diverse backgrounds and both basic and applied interests. This textbook attempts to provide a framework for this still amorphous field. We have tried to encompass the biologist's inquiry into the mechanism of action of neurotoxic chemicals, the clinical problem of toxic neurological disease, the issues associated with neurotoxicants of environmental significance, and the regulator's interest in developing sensitive methods for screening substances for possible neurotoxic effects. While the book has this broad purview, it is by no means encyclopedic. Indeed, in this First Edition, we have chosen to give minimal coverage to biological and neuropharmacological toxins, to pesticides, and to forensic toxicology, in order to avoid excessive duplication with other recent publications on these specialist topics (1–7).

Experimental and Clinical Neurotoxicology is divided into five sections. The first carries broad overviews of where neurotoxins act in the nervous system, the type of damage which ensues, and the relative and special vulnerabilities of different nervous system components, both during development and adult life. Section B reviews state-of-the-art experimental studies designed to determine mechanisms of toxic damage to the neuron, axon, synapse, and myelinating cell. Section C discusses, in stereotyped format, existing data for established neurotoxic substances which have received attention either because of their environmental significance or for their potential as experimental probes of nervous system dysfunction. Section D deals with applied neurotoxicology and has three principal subsections. One subsection examines the problem of screening and assessment of neurotoxic illness in man. The second is devoted to the various techniques being devised for screening chemicals for neurotoxic properties. The third subsection presents the story of the methyl *n*-butyl ketone outbreak of neurotoxicity as a paradigm for the clinical and experimental investigation of an outbreak of neurotoxicity. Finally, Section E addresses issues in neurotoxicology of public interest.

We are greatly indebted to our many contributors, to Monica Bischoff, Laurel Edwards, Elaine Garafola and Frances Spencer for manuscript preparation, and to Ruby Richardson, Diane Welch and their colleagues at The Williams and Wilkins Company for their expert management of this volume.

Bronx, New York   Peter S. Spencer, Ph.D.
1980   Herbert H. Schaumburg, M.D.

REFERENCES

1. Ceccarelli B, Clemente F: *Neurotoxins: Tools in Neurobiology, Advances in Cytopharmacology*, Vol. III, Raven Press, New York, 1979.
2. Chubb IW, Geffen LB: *Neurotoxins: Fundamental and Clinical Advances*, Adelaide University Press, Adelaide, 1979.
3. Jacoby JH, Lytle LD: *Serotonin Neurotoxins*, Vol. 305, New York Academy of Sciences, 1978.
4. Ludwig J: *Current Methods of Autopsy Practice*, W.B. Saunders, Philadelphia, 1979.
5. Narahashi T: *Neurotoxicology of Insecticides and Pheromones*, Plenum Press, New York, 1978.
6. Shankland DL, Hollingworth RM, Smyth Jr., T: *Pesticide and Venom Neurotoxicity*, Plenum Press, New York, 1978.
7. Sunshine I: *Methods in Analytical Toxicology*, CRC Press, Miami, 1978.

PART ONE

FUNDAMENTALS OF EXPERIMENTAL
AND CLINICAL NEUROTOXICOLOGY

CHAPTER ONE

Biological Principles of Chemical Neurotoxicity

Peter S. Spencer

Neurotoxicity is a direct or indirect effect of chemicals that disrupt nervous system function. Hundreds of chemicals are recognized as having systemic neurotoxic potential in humans. Many other substances are used as experimental tools to disturb or damage selected regions of the nervous system. Some act directly on neural components; others interfere with metabolic processes on which the nervous system is especially dependent. The neurotoxic properties of chemicals find expression in the deleterious alteration of nervous system function in the presence or absence of visible structural damage. Perturbations may appear and disappear rapidly, or may evolve slowly over days or weeks and regress over months or years. Neurotoxic disorders may leave scars or disappear without trace.

Chemicals that disrupt the mammalian nervous system may be synthetic substances or natural products. Naturally occurring neurotoxic agents include the noxious products of bacteria (*e.g.*, *diphtheria toxin*), algae (*anatoxin*-a), fungi (*3-nitropropionic acid*), plants (β-N-*oxalylamino*-L-*alanine*), coelenterates (*palytoxin*), insects (*apamin*), arachnids (*scorpion toxins*), molluscs (*conotoxins*), amphibia (*batrachotoxin*), reptilia (*dendrotoxins*) and of substances stored in fish (*ciguatoxin*) and certain mammals (*vitamin A*). Some agents, such as *tetrodotoxin*, are found in several disparate species. These naturally occurring substances often exhibit great target specificity, high toxic potency, discrete biological actions, and are among the best understood mechanistically. Many other less potent naturally occurring substances exhibit neurotoxic effects when encountered in large concentrations for sufficient periods of time; examples include metals (*arsenic*, *manganese*, *mercury*) and their compounds, and substances that are in a liquid (*methanol*, n-*hexane*) or gas phase (*carbon monoxide*; *ethylene oxide*) under normal ambient conditions. Some substances (*pyridoxine*, *manganese*, *selenium*) in this group, while neurotoxic in sustained heavy doses, are required in smaller amounts to support normal physiological function. Chemicals (*thiaminase*) that interfere with required substances (thiamine) have been associated with neurological illness in animals (paralysis in foxes and horses) and humans (seasonal ataxia in Nigerians). Synthetic chemicals with neurotoxic potential are most commonly encountered in the form of prescription (*2',3'-dideoxyinosine*, *ethambutol*) and over-the-counter pharmaceutical agents (*bismuth preparations*), domestic products (*pyridinethione*), fragrance raw materials (*2,6-dinitro-3-methoxy-4*-tert-*butyltoluene*), workplace chemicals (*acrylamide*), pest-control agents (*chlordane*), environmental pollutants (*tetraethyllead*), and substances (*methamphetamine*) voluntarily used to induce euphoria. Others are associated with special applications, such as chemical warfare in civilian and military settings (*sarin*).

VULNERABILITY OF THE NERVOUS SYSTEM

The nervous system's vulnerability to chemical attack depends heavily on its developmental state and the postdevelopmental organization and functional specialization of nervous tissue. The developing and mature brain is one of the organs most frequently impacted in systemic toxic states. Additionally, agents that target and damage blood and the hematopoietic system, or the liver, kidneys, or lungs, may secondarily affect neurological function. Many factors, both extrinsic and intrinsic to the neuraxis, dictate the presence, type, and severity of the effects of xenobiotics (foreign compounds) on the central nervous system (CNS) and the peripheral nervous system (PNS). Extraneural factors that influence the neurotoxic impact of chemicals are addressed first.

Extraneural Factors

Exposure, Dose, and Response

Exposure and dose are related but separate concepts. Exposure to chemicals occurs when an exposure pathway is completed. This pathway requires the presence of a chemical source, transportation of the chemical from the source to the subject, and contact between the chemical and the subject. Dose refers to that amount of chemical transferred to the exposed subject. All are exposed to substances with neurotoxic potential, but the dose is usually below the threshold needed to induce dysfunction.

Several key factors influence the dose of exogenous chemicals, the residence time and concentration of agents in the body, the substance's access to the nervous system, the nature of the chemical that reaches neural targets, and the consequences of chemical attack. These factors are of paramount importance in determining the existence, type, and duration of the neurotoxic response. Even the most potent, receptor-specific agent may fail to trigger a neurotoxic response if access to neural tissue is denied or a target receptor is developmentally regulated and has yet to be expressed.

The ability of chemicals with neurotoxic potential to induce neurological dysfunction in mature humans and animals is related to the route of administration. The different effects associated with varied routes of exposure to *aluminum* exemplify the point. Direct application to neural tissue is the most effective and damaging, as demonstrated by the induction of seizures in humans and animals following implantation of an aluminum compound in the cerebral cortex. Prolonged intravenous feeding of preterm infants with solutions contaminated with aluminum compounds is associated with impaired neurological development. Excess aluminum salts in the dialysate of human subjects undergoing renal dialysis triggers a marked and sometimes fatal encephalopathy. Introduction of aluminum chloride into the cerebrospinal fluid (CSF) of laboratory rabbits precipitates a neuronal neurofilamentous disease. In contrast, airborne exposure of adult humans and animals to aluminum has no known adverse effect on the nervous system.

Routes of chemical administration usually show decreasing efficiency in generating a toxic response in the following approximate order: direct tissue contact, intravenous, inhalation, intraperitoneal, subcutaneous, intramuscular, intradermal, oral (for monogastric species), dermal. The ability of exogenous substances to traverse the skin and lungs of mature subjects is highly variable, as exemplified by the differential respiratory absorption (retention) of the hexacarbon solvents n-*hexane* (low) and *2-hexanone* (high), which otherwise exhibit a common neurotoxic effect mediated through the metabolite *2,5-hexanedione*. Although application of chemicals to skin is often one of the least effective methods of intoxication, there are, nonetheless, several examples of neurotoxic agents which, in humans (*hexachlorophene*) and animals (*acetylethyltetramethyltetralin*), precipitate severe pathological changes in the CNS and PNS following repeated dermal application. Others, such as certain high-potency anticholinesterase agents used as chemical weapons (*VX: ethyl S-2-diisopropylaminoethyl methylphosphonothiolate*), have the capacity to induce short- and perhaps long-term effects on the nervous system after percutaneous exposure to a single drop. Oral administration of chemicals with neurotoxic potential is also an effective route of exposure, except in the case of certain proteinaceous neurotoxins, such as snake venoms, that undergo proteolysis in the target's gut and thereby lose biological activity. The toxicity of an orally administered chemical agent may also be diminished if the noxious substance is not widely dispersed in gastrointestinal fluid, thereby reducing absorption of the agent from the gut wall and its entry into the portal circulation between intestine and liver. Compounds that enter the body by this route may be modified by hepatic metabolism before passing into the systemic circulation. By contrast, a substance that traverses the skin or lungs may reach the brain (first-pass effect) before the liver or other systemic organs with metabolic capacity that can detoxify the agent.

Certain chemicals with neurotoxic potential may be sequestered in, or their effects blocked by, nonneural tissues. Blood serves an important role: examples include the binding of *bromide* and *cyanide* to erythrocytes, the sequestration of *cadmium* by metallothionine, and the binding of *anticholinesterase chemicals* to serum butyrylcholinesterase. Examples of nonhematological tissue binding of neurotoxic substances include the sequestration of *chloroquine* by the choroid layer of the eye, of *lead* and *barium* by bone, and of lipophilic substances (*chlorinated hydrocarbons, ciguatoxin*) by lipid tissues. Agents bound to nonneural tissues are not strictly stored but show a greatly reduced rate of turnover (*i.e.*, binding followed by release).

The dose of chemical received from each exposure, and

the frequency and duration of exposure, are of cardinal importance in determining the presence or absence of a neurotoxic response. Dose descriptions in experimental animal toxicology refer to *acute* (single dose given for <24 h), *subchronic* (1–3 months), and *chronic* (3 months to lifetime) exposures. Acute exposures may elicit specific neurobehavioral phenomena that are dependent both on dose and time following administration. A neurotoxic response to a single large dose of a substance often predicts neither the existence nor the type of response seen in animals repeatedly exposed to lower levels of the same agent. For example, acute exposure to *nitrous oxide* induces anesthesia; repeated exposures precipitate peripheral nerve and spinal cord damage because the substance interferes with vitamin B_{12}–dependent enzymes and triggers a disorder comparable to combined system disease. Certain chemicals may elicit distinct neurotoxic responses when administered over a range of single or repeated doses: for example, whereas therapeutic doses of the competitive muscarinic antagonist *atropine* act peripherally, larger toxic doses may cause prominent central excitation. An agent like *ciguatoxin* rapidly gains access first to peripheral nerves and only later enters the brain.

The induction of a neural response is dependent on the presence of a critical *concentration* of the chemical at the target site, and this in turn is directly related to the administered dose and the presence or absence of chemical sequestration. The relationship *in vitro* between concentration and response, and that *in vivo* between dose and response, describe the true association between a chemical and its effect. Absence of a concentration/dose–effect relationship is grounds for suspicion that an association between the chemical and the measure is other than causal.

Molecular organization and composition are key determinants of chemical neurotoxicity. The plant toxin BOAA (β-N-*oxalylamino*-L-*alanine* [synonym, β-N-*oxalylamino*-2-*diaminopropanoic acid*]) is stereospecifically neuronotoxic *in vitro*; activity is seen with the L isomer but not with the D isomer. *3-Acetylpyridine* serves as a neuronal toxin in mammals, but 2-acetylpyridine and 4-acetylpyridine both lack this property. *1,2-Diethylbenzene* damages the nervous system of rodents but 1,4-diethylbenzene does not. A similar principle operates for n-*hexane*, the only one of four isomers of hexane able to induce neurological damage in rodents exposed by inhalation. Normal alkanes with shorter or longer chain lengths are unable to induce this type of damage. The most potent toxic congeners of *polychlorinated diphenyls* on PC12 cells are those with *ortho*- or *ortho*-, *para*-chlorine substitutions.

The potency of a neurotoxic chemical refers to the range of doses over which the substance produces effects. Over a typical dose range, exogenous chemicals (*acrylamide*) elicit qualitatively uniform responses (peripheral neuropathy) with characteristic toxic effects in a dose–response pattern. Moving to another dose range may elicit a qualitatively different effect (seizures) with its own dose–response characteristics. The neurotoxic metabolites of n-*hexane* (*2-hexanol, 2-hexanone, 2,5-hexanediol, 5-hydroxy-2-hexanone* and *2,5-hexanedione*) produce a uniform chronic neurotoxic effect (distal axonopathy,) but with potencies that vary linearly with the extent of their individual biotransformation to 2,5-hexanedione, the agent actually responsible (proximate toxin) for the neurotoxic actions of these structurally and metabolically related compounds.

Exposure to two or more chemicals may have interactive biological effects that may modify the toxic potency of the agents. Effects of two substances interacting may be *additive* (*i.e.*, 1 + 1 = 2), as in the case of anticholinesterase inhibition produced by acute exposure to two *carbamate drugs*. Markedly increased toxicity of two chemicals with neurotoxic potential is *synergism* (*e.g.*, 1 + 1 = 5). A *potentiating* effect is recognized when one chemical without a specific neurotoxic effect enhances the specific neurotoxic property of a second (*e.g.*, 1 + 0 = 5). The ability of *methyl ethyl ketone* (which is unable to induce axonal degeneration) to increase the extent of peripheral neuropathy induced by n-*hexane* is an example of potentiation. The term *promotion* (instead of potentiation) has been applied to the increased severity of experimental neuropathy induced by single treatment with an *organophosphate* (OP) preceded or followed by treatment with *phenylmethanesulfonyl fluoride*. A variation of this phenomenon, *induction*, occurs when the first agent (*methyl ethyl ketone*) potentiates a subneurotoxic dose of the second substance (n-*hexane*) and induces a neurotoxic response (peripheral neuropathy). The converse of potentiation, *antagonism*, occurs when two chemicals interfere with each other's biological actions or one disrupts the action of the other chemical (*i.e.*, 1 + 1 = 1). *Dispositional antagonism* is demonstrated by the ability of *toluene* to attenuate the neuropathy-producing potential of n-*hexane* in animals and the excretion of the principal neurotoxic metabolite of *n*-hexane (*2,5-hexanedione*) in humans. *Chemical antagonism* may occur because two or more chemicals interact to form a product of reduced toxicity, as illustrated by the reduction of *heavy metal toxicity* by coadministration of *penicillamine*. *Receptor antagonism* occurs when two chemicals compete for the same receptor resulting in an effect less than would occur with either substance operating in isolation, or when one chemical abolishes the effect of the second. Examples of the latter phenomenon abound in experimental synaptic-receptor neurotoxicology (see later under Neurotransmitter Systems). *Metabolic antagonism* occurs when one agent (*ethanol*) competes with a second (*ethylene glycol*) to block formation of a toxic metabolite (*oxalate*).

Biotransformation

Principal protection from the neurotoxic effects of chemicals is provided by hepatic metabolism (detoxication) of exogenous toxic compounds. While this may occasionally result in the activation of a chemical to a primary neurotoxic agent (formation of *2,5-hexanedione* from n-*hexane*), biotransformation is broadly concerned with the conversion of lipophilic to less toxic hydrophilic metabolites (phase I) and their conjugation (phase II) prior to excretion. Biotransformation may also take place in nervous tissue. Excretion occurs principally in urine (water-soluble products), lungs (gases), and bile, but toxicants and their metabolites may also be found in CSF, sweat, tears, saliva, and milk.

Prior to excretion, substances with neurotoxic potential may be temporarily sequestered for varying periods of time in other tissues, notably plasma proteins (*dieldrin*), red blood cells (*soman*), fat deposits (*dieldrin*), choroid (*chloroquine*), bone (*lead*), kidney, and liver (*cadmium*-metallothionine). If sequestration and elimination fail (as in renal failure) to keep pace with absorption, and the free chemical gains access to the nervous system, the substance (*aluminum*) will increase in bioavailability and may reach a critical concentration at the target site. On rare occasions, as in the deliberate displacement of a sequestered heavy metal (*thallium*) by a therapeutic chelating drug, neurotoxicity may be associated with a sudden increase in circulating levels of the culpable agent. Another practical outcome of the phenomenon of sequestration is the ability to monitor the body burden of certain substances (*organochlorine pesticides*) long after exposure has ceased.

Phase I biotransformation reactions add or expose functional groups (hydroxyl, thiol, amino, carboxyl) that permit the metabolite to conjugate in phase II reactions with endogenous molecules (glucuronic acid, sulfate) that promote secretion or transfer across hepatic or renal membranes. Phase I enzymes include, among others, two oxidative enzyme systems: the microsomal cytochrome P-450 polysubstrate monooxygenase system and the mixed-function oxidase (MFO) located in the endoplasmic reticulum. Enzyme activity of the latter, which is much greater in humans than in rats, and in liver than in brain, converts tertiary amines to amine oxides, secondary amines to hydroxyl amines and nitrones, and primary amines to hydroxylamines and oximes. MFO inducers (*barbiturates, halogenated hydrocarbons*) increase phase I biotransformation; MFO inhibitors (*piperonyl butoxide*) decrease biotransfor-

mation and, thereby, may increase the neurotoxic property of certain agents (*pyrethroids*).

The P-450 monooxygenase system comprises a series of gene families, the largest of which is the P-450II family; this contains the major phenobarbital-inducible cytochromes (subfamily IIB) and the ethanol-inducible P-450 (subfamily IIE). The P-450 system promotes a series of enzymatic conversions, including the subterminal (ω-1) carbon oxidation of n-*hexane* to *2-hexanol*, aromatic hydroxylation, epoxidation (*aldrin* to *dieldrin*), N-, O-, or S-dealkylation, deamination, N-hydroxylation, sulfoxidation, desulfuration, and oxidative dehalogenation. Although the liver is the primary organ for P-450–mediated metabolism, significant activity and multiple isoforms are found in rodent brain, with immunocytochemical evidence of P-450 enzymatic activity in neuronal cell bodies and fiber tracts. Important properties of P-450–mediated biotransformation include the ability of inducers and inhibitors to increase and decrease enzyme activity, respectively, and the capacity of *carbon monoxide* to inhibit the enzymatic reaction.

Other biotransformation enzymes include epoxide hydrolase, which is distributed in many tissues, including the brain; a wide variety of esterases, including cholinesterases, which bind and are inactivated by *organophosphates* and *carbamates*; and oxidation-reduction systems for ketones and aldehydes, notably alcohol dehydrogenase, which metabolizes *ethanol, ethylene glycol,* and *methanol,* the latter to *formate,* the agent likely responsible for methanol-induced damage to optic nerves and basal ganglia.

Phase II biotransformation reactions are energy- and cofactor-dependent biosynthetic reactions that utilize uridine diphosphate glucuronosyltransferases (mostly in liver, but also in other organs including the brain) to form glucuronides that, according to the size of the aglycone moiety, are excreted in urine (small) or bile (large). Other phase II reactions include sulfation, such as the aryl sulfotransferase conjugation of *phenols;* methylation, including S-methyl transferases to convert *hydrogen sulfide* to *dimethylsulfide;* N-acetyl transferases, including the acetylation detoxication of *isoniazid* to acetyl isoniazid; amino acid conjugation, such as benzoate with glycine to form hippurate; the multigene family of glutathione-S-transferases, which is catalyzed by glutathione; and rhodanese, which is selectively responsible for conversion of *cyanide* to thiocyanate.

Species, Genotype, Gender, Nutrition, and Age

Animal species is sometimes an important factor in determining the presence of a neurotoxic response to chemical attack as well as the type and degree of the response. *Organophosphates* induce retrograde axonal degeneration of elongate CNS and PNS nerve tracts (distal axonopathy) in the hen, cat, and primate much more readily than in the rodent. Mice and rats are prone to the convulsive properties of *glutamate analogues*. Noradrenergic nerves are more vulnerable in cats than in mice or rats to the neurotoxic properties of *6-hydroxydopamine*. The molecular mechanisms underlying these phenomena are little understood.

Genetic polymorphisms may exert a dramatic effect on the hepatic biotransformation (metabolism) and potential neurotoxicity of some substances; they are likely responsible for so-called idiosyncratic reactions reported in clinical pharmacology. Use of genetically pure strains of animals in experimental neurotoxicology studies tends to obscure the role of genotype in modulating chemical neurotoxicity. Genetic polymorphism occasionally is a factor in dictating the presence or absence of a human neurotoxic response: A classic example is genetic heterogeneity in the rate of metabolic acetylation, which affects the metabolism and neurotoxic potency of drugs such as *isoniazid*. The autosomal-dominant, rapid-acetylation (detoxication) trait is more common among Orientals than Caucasians, thereby rendering members of the latter population at greater risk for isoniazid-induced peripheral neuropathy. Other types of genetic polymorphisms may predispose subjects to idiosyncratic chemical toxicity. For example, a rare mitochondrial DNA polymorphism (1555 A $\rightarrow$ G mutation in the 12S rRNA gene) results in hypersensitivity to *aminoglycoside*-induced deafness, possibly because the polymorphism increases drug access to the ribosome cleft and favors steric binding. Another example is an uncommon genetic dimorphism of the serum enzyme butyrylcholinesterase that renders individuals hypersusceptible to the effects of *succinylcholine*, a neuromuscular-depolarizing agent used to elicit muscle relaxation in anesthesia. Enzyme activity of butyrylcholinesterase is reported to show a large temporal variation over the course of a year, is higher in men than in women, and is lower in women taking oral contraceptives. Female carriers of ornithine carbamoyltransferase deficiency are hypothesized to have greatly increased susceptibility to the neurotoxic potential of N,N-*diethyl-m-toluamide*.

Gender as a determinant of biotransformation may be less important in humans than in rats, where marked differences in the metabolism and consequent functional responses to individual neuroactive chemicals (*parathion*) are recognized. Biotransformation capacity is generally greater in males than in females, and the activity in each gender can be modulated by varying the level of testosterone. Gender-specific forms of cytochrome P-450 are recognized in rats, and the expression of some forms changes with development. Total brain P-450 levels are higher in male rats than in female animals. Low cytochrome P-450 activity is found in newborn animals, but enzyme activity develops rapidly and reaches maximal activity at 30 days of age before slowly declining thereafter. Human P-450 activity, while well developed at birth, has a different isozyme pattern from that observed in adults.

Aging in humans is generally associated with an increased risk for some forms of neurotoxicity, an observation that likely stems in part from reduced hepatic and renal circulation, a decreased biotransformation capacity, and diminished renal and biliary excretion. Use of multiple medications (polypharmacy) may also be a risk factor in aged subjects. Age-related differential responses to chemicals may result from intrinsic properties of the target organ, including an accumulation of and reduced ability to handle free-radical damage. The greater neurotoxic potential in older rodents of *3-nitropropionic acid*, a suicide inhibitor of mitochondrial complex II, has been related to a reduced reserve capacity and ability to regenerate the enzyme with the advance of age. Age is also directly related to the prognosis for recovery from certain types of neurotoxic injury. Older individuals with toxic axonopathy recover slower and are left with more clinical residue than the young.

Nutritional status is another factor that may dictate the development and modulate the magnitude of the neurotoxic response to certain chemicals. For example, protein deficiency, which leads to a reduction of sulfur amino acids required for the conversion by rhodanese of *cyanide* to thiocyanate, appears to be a cardinal factor in the induction of motor-system disease (spastic paraplegia) in certain poorly nourished African groups subsisting on the tuber of the cyanogenic plant cassava (*Manihot esculenta*). The disorder is unknown in other, better nourished populations that consume significant amounts of cassava as part of a varied diet. Rats deficient in sulfur amino acids preferentially metabolize cyanide to *cyanate*, an agent that induces peripheral neuropathy in humans and rats and, at high doses, central and peripheral motor-system degeneration in macaques. Another example is the optic nerve damage in *methanol* intoxication, an event apparently mediated by the methanol metabolite *formate*; this metabolite is increased in folate-deficient nonhuman primates because a folate-dependent pathway is required to metabolize formate to carbon dioxide and water.

Factors Associated with the Nervous System
Neural Microenvironment

Extracellular and cerebrospinal fluid. The mature brain and spinal cord (CNS) are protected from some chemicals because of the formation during late development of differential filters or partial barriers to the free movement of substances. The extracellular fluid that bathes the neural tissue of the brain and spinal cord is separated from the vascular compartment by endothelial cells whose apposed surfaces contain specialized tight junctions (induced by astrocytes) that constitute a barrier to the free passage of toxicants from blood to CNS tissue. To gain access to most parts of the CNS, hematogenously derived molecules must traverse the capillary endothelium and then the plasma membranes of astrocyte foot processes that abut the outer surface of capillaries. This substantially restricts passage of ionized chemicals and agents that are bound to plasma proteins (*inorganic mercury salts*) and favors the penetration of lipid-soluble agents (*organomercurials*). Rat brain microvessels contain a number of phase I enzymes (cytochrome P-450–linked monooxygenases, epoxide hydrolase) that serve to restrict the entry of lipid-soluble chemicals into the brain.

While most parts of the brain and the entire spinal cord have specialized blood vessels that regulate passage of circulating chemicals, this *"blood-brain barrier"* is normally absent in the choroid plexus and certain discrete regions of the mature brain that are secretory (neuroendocrine) in function. These regions of the brain, known as the *circumventricular organs*, include the area postrema, hypophysis, pineal body, hypothalamic regions, subfornical organ (rat), and supraoptic crest (Fig. 1.1). Neural (CNS) tissue in these chemosensitive regions is exposed to blood-borne agents that elsewhere are excluded from the brain.

Chemical damage to the hypothalamus and neuroendocrine system can trigger a cascade of pathological events that have far-reaching effects on somatic metabolism, reproductive function, and growth. The adult obesity of rats treated postnatally with *glutamate* (which destroys the arcuate hypothalamic nucleus) is probably an example of this principle. To what extent neurons in the circumventricular organs of adult subjects succumb to injury is not well understood, since these areas are rarely examined and functional consequences may be subtle.

With the exception of the circumventricular organs, where ependymal cells have tight junctions, there is free interchange between the extracellular (interstitial) fluid of the brain and the CSF. CSF is continuously secreted by epithelial cells of the choroid plexus from a blood filtrate originating from an underlying network of permeable capillaries. Drug secretion with local toxic effects on ependymal cells has been suggested for *amoscanate*. Toxic metals (*cadmium*) may accumulate in and damage the choroid plexus. CSF circulates from the ventricles into the subarachnoid space, where it bathes the entire brain.

The pressure of the interstitial fluid is an important factor, since the brain's ability to expand is severely limited by the cranium. While neural function appears little affected by mild, chronic, diffuse elevations of intracranial pressure, some agents (*vitamin A, tetracycline, hexachlorophene*) markedly increase intracranial pressure, induce encephalopathy, and compromise optic nerves. With vitamin A and certain therapeutic drugs (*amiodarone*), interstitial edema

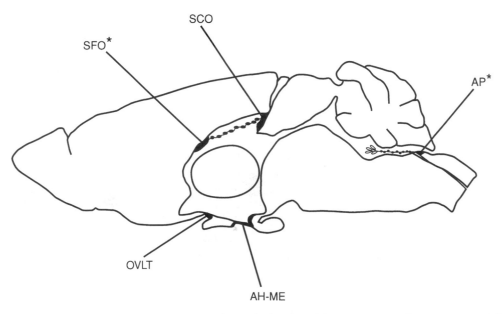

FIGURE 1.1. This diagram of a midsagittal section of rat brain indicates the location of the circumventricular organs (CVO), which are specialized brain regions abutting the ventricles. CVO include area postrema (*AP*), subcommissural organ (*SCO*), subfornical organ (*SFO*), organum vasculosum of the lamina terminalis (*OVLT*), and the arcuate-median eminence region of the hypothalamus (*AH-ME*). Asterisks indicate CVO regions most vulnerable to damage by systemically administered excitotoxins. [Reproduced with permission from John Olney.]

may increase CSF pressure and elicit headache and papilledema (pseudotumor cerebri).

Oversecretion of CSF, impaired absorption of CSF, or obstruction of CSF pathways may increase the volume of cerebral ventricles (hydrocephalus). Pregnant rats fed *tellurium* produce offspring which, at birth, display communicating (nonobstructive) hydrocephalus and, with closure of the fourth ventricle or cerebral aqueduct, may develop obstructions to CSF flow. Young mice and rats develop hydrocephalus after acute intoxication with *cadmium*.

Blood-brain barrier. The blood-brain barrier plays a major role in maintaining the microenvironment of the brain, both by excluding polar molecules and transporting required molecules. D-Glucose, the primary energy substrate of the brain, is transported by stereospecific, insulin-independent GLUT-1 glucose transporters that are enriched in brain capillary endothelium. Low glucose levels, as in starvation, stimulate the monocarboxylic acid carrier (which supplies energy requirements to the neonate) to transport ketone bodies (β-hydroxybutyrate and acetoacetate). Dicarboxylic amino acids, including *glutamate* and *aspartate* (poorly transported), and neutral and basic amino acids, are transported bidirectionally by individual, saturable, stereospecific carriers, with predominant passage into the brain. Micronutrients (vitamins, cofactors, and choline), which must be supplied to the brain, are transported by brain endothelial cells. Brain microvessels bear receptors for specific peptides, such as transferrin. Electrolyte permeability of the polar surface of the endothelium is low; chloride enters the brain by a carrier-mediated mechanism, and potassium efflux is undertaken by $Na^+/K^+-ATPase$ on the abluminal surface of the endothelial cells. Transmitters show poor penetration from blood to brain, but certain neurotransmitter precursors (L-dopa) are transported. Oxygen and other gases (*carbon dioxide, nitrous oxide*) diffuse rapidly into brain tissue. Chemicals gain access as a function of their lipid solubility. Polypeptides (*botulinum toxin, tetanus toxin*) are excluded.

The integrity of the blood-brain barrier itself may be damaged by chemicals (*shiga toxin*), and extravasation of plasma and erythrocytes may occur (*lead, monochloroacetic acid*). Certain abnormal states, whether induced (blood hyperosmolarity, anesthesia), metabolic (adrenocorticoid hypertension), pathological (meningitis), or stress-related (rats under certain conditions), promote leakage of blood-borne agents into the brain. *Mannitol* is used clinically to disrupt the blood-brain barrier and provide access for *antineoplastic agents* to suppress malignant brain tumors, a procedure with the potential for neurotoxic effects.

Blood-nerve barrier. Peripheral nerve tissue also exists within a protected microenvironment with regulated access to chemicals from extraneural tissues, notably blood. Bundles of nerve fibers (fascicles) and intervening endoneurial connective tissue are ensheathed by layers of perineurial cells; tight junctions between these cells restrict the intercellular penetration of chemicals into the intrafascicular microenvironment. Within the nerve fascicle, endoneurial capillaries are equipped with tight junctions that form a functional "*blood-nerve barrier*" restricting passage of chemicals from blood to the extracellular (endoneurial) fluid that bathes nerve fibers. This fluid is held under a positive (intrafascicular) pressure that increases in certain states (*inorganic lead intoxication*) and may render nerve fibers more susceptible to damage resulting from focal pressure differences induced by entrapment or other causes. In normal states, the blood-nerve regulatory interface is more permeable than the blood-brain barrier to small circulating proteins, more so in the cat and monkey than in the rat or mouse.

Blood-borne chemicals have ready access to certain regions of the PNS that lack blood vessels with specialized endothelial cell junctions. Many capillaries in dorsal root ganglia and autonomic ganglia have endothelial fenestrations that allow circulating chemicals to enter the interstitial fluid of the ganglia, pass between the adjacent processes of satellite cells encasing the large neurons, and thereby contact their plasmalemmae. A substance such as *doxorubicin* is detected selectively in neuronal and satellite cell nuclei of rat lumbar dorsal root ganglia within minutes of intravenous administration. Some agents, notably *cadmium* and the chloride salts of *indium, terbium, thallium,* and *mercury,* damage the capillary endothelium of peripheral sensory and autonomic ganglia of newborn or young rats.

While the peripheral sensory (dorsal root) ganglia located distally in spinal foramina are, like peripheral nerves, protected by a tough perineurial sheath, their central projections and motor nerve roots in the subarachnoid space have a thin ensheathment that allows the free exchange of materials between the CSF and endoneurium. At the distal extremities of nonencapsulated sensory terminals (muscle spindle afferents) and motor nerve terminals (neuromuscular junction), the absence of a perineurial ensheathment permits chemicals direct access to nerve fibers and their unsheathed axon endings. These nerve terminals are able to take up chemicals by endocytosis, and some biological toxins (*botulinum toxin, tetanus toxin*) have specific fragments (heavy chain) designed to promote intracellular penetration of the toxic moiety (light chain). Once inside the axon, the toxic moiety acts locally at the nerve terminal (botulinum toxin) or may be intra-axonally transported to spinal cord (tetanus toxin). The motor system is particularly vulnerable to toxins that enter muscle and are transported to the anterior horn cell. Whereas an agent like tetanus toxin (light chain) naturally exploits this route of transmission from the periphery to the CNS, other compounds may be introduced experimentally. For example, *diphtheria toxin* will cause motor neuronal degeneration after experimental intramuscular administration, although naturally infected subjects develop a predominantly demyelinating neuropathy because the toxin leaks from endoneurial vessels of peripheral nerves and selectively targets locally exposed Schwann cells, thereby activating segmental demyelination. Likewise, degeneration of anterior horn cells and dorsal root ganglia follow intramuscular injection of *doxorubicin*, whereas systemic administration of the drug selectively reaches and destroys neurons in dorsal root ganglia.

It is apparent from the foregoing observations that the structural and functional specializations of the mature PNS and CNS tissue control *access* of chemicals to the nervous system and thereby play a critically important role in dictating the presence, localization, and type of cellular damage. *Stated another way, the cellular target of a xenobiotic may be dictated as much by the agent's access to tissues as by any intrinsic property of the chemical.* Concepts such as *neuronal toxin* or *Schwann cell toxin* may reflect only the nature of the tissue response to a chemical rather than a true understanding of the molecular mechanism of neurotoxicity.

Architectural and Functional Specialization

Several additional properties of the mammalian nervous system predispose nervous tissue to chemical attack, including the following.

Blood supply and energy requirements. Mature nerve cells have an absolute dependence on a continuous supply of oxygen to generate aerobically the large amount of chemical energy needed to support ionic membrane pumps, intracellular transport mechanisms, and energy-requiring enzymes such as oxidases. The oxygen requirement of the human brain is so great that the organ utilizes 15% of total cardiac output. Chemicals that interrupt the supply of oxygen (*carbon monoxide*) or the utilization of oxygen by the brain (*azide*), or both (*cyanide*), may produce catastrophic cellular necrosis in susceptible brain regions, such as the basal ganglia. Neocortical neurons of laminae III, V, and VI; regions of the hippocampus; and cerebellar Purkinje cells also undergo degeneration in hypoxic/ischemic brain injury. Comparable brain damage may occur from the induction of hypoxic states during seizures caused by chemicals and other causes. To maintain its functional and structural integrity, therefore, CNS *tissue requires an extraordinarily large blood supply which, in turn, favors the delivery of blood-borne toxicants to the brain and spinal cord.*

The brain also requires a continuous supply of glucose to support its energy needs. Areas of high glucose consumption (as judged by the accumulation of 2-deoxy-^{14}C-glucose from blood) include the vestibular nuclei and the nuclei of the spinal tract of the trigeminal nucleus, the superior and inferior olivary nuclei, and the inferior colliculus, and also the cerebellar nuclei, some thalamic nuclei, and cells in the fourth layer of the cerebral cortex. Lesions in the distribution of some of these regions, notably brainstem nuclei, are seen in rodents treated with *6-chloro-6-deoxyglucose, metronidazole, misonidazole, 6-aminonicotinamide*, and in primates treated with *1-amino-3-chloropropanol*.

Metabolism of xenobiotics. Mammalian brain tissue is able independently to metabolize foreign chemicals; the resulting chemical transformation may *reduce* or *increase* the toxic potential of the xenobiotic. For example, the predominantly astrocytic enzyme, monoamine oxidase B, activates the proneurotoxin *1-methyl-4-phenyl-1,2,3,6-tetrahydropyridine (MPTP)*, to form the ultimate (proximate) toxin N-*methyl-4-phenylpyridinium ion (MPP$^+$)*; this is taken up selectively *via* the dopamine transporter of dopaminergic (notably nigrostriatal) neurons, where it is proposed to enter neuronal mitochondria and inhibit complex I of the electron transport chain. This reduces oxidative phosphorylation, increases toxic free radicals, promotes neuronal degeneration, perturbs extrapyramidal function, and may precipitate an irreversible parkinsonian state in the subject. Other agents (*triethylcholine, fluorocitrate, 6-aminonicotinamide*) are neurotoxic because they substitute for substrates in key anabolic (acetylcholine synthesis) or catabolic pathways (glycolysis) where, unlike their physiological analogues, they are unable to support physiological function. Cytochrome P-450 isoforms are differentially distributed in brain tissue, and between neurons and glial cells; they can be selectively and regionally induced by chemicals such as *ethanol* and *toluene*.

Regional specialization. Unlike most tissues (liver, kidney, testes), the nervous system is organized into many specialized regions serving specific functions, such as coordination, audition, balance, vision, and memory. Chemical-induced damage to discrete areas of the CNS may induce functional effects that are disproportionate to the size of the lesion. For example, small lesions in the substantia nigra (*MPTP*) may cause debilitating movement disorders; lesions in the peripheral vestibular and auditory system (*streptomycin*) may produce dramatic functional effects on the organism (vertigo, hearing loss); toxic damage to optic nerves (*meth-*

anol) may seriously impair vision; and discrete hippocampal lesions (*domoic acid*) may result in impaired retention of new memory. By contrast, small lesions in most other tissues, such as the lung or liver, have trivial effects on the function of the organ and the organism. Moreover, whereas organ repair may occur through reconstruction of damaged tissue, most neurons in the adult organism are postmitotic and therefore unable to repopulate an ablated area. Some recovery of function may be afforded through the redistribution of synaptic contacts on surviving nerve cells (neuronal plasticity). Post-injury activation and proliferation of astrocyte cells is thought to impede axonal regeneration and functional recovery. By contrast, glial cells promote the synaptic efficacy of developing retinal ganglion cells *in vitro*.

Architecture. Unlike most types of mammalian cells, mature neurons, oligodendrocytes, astrocytes, and Schwann cells possess elongated cellular processes that expose vast surface areas of membrane to chemicals present in the extracellular fluid. Additionally, each of these cell types has a segregated anabolic region (perikaryon or soma) that is responsible for supplying the metabolic needs of proportionately huge volumes of cytoplasm (axons, dendritic arbor, myelin), some of which may be distributed in small processes or compartments (synaptic bulb, adaxonal cytoplasm) at a great relative distance from the perikaryon (Fig. 1.2). Transport systems that have evolved to communicate between the perikaryon and sites of product utilization provide another important target for chemical attack. While much information is available on agents that disrupt anterograde (slow and fast) and retrograde axonal transport, less is known about the physiology and vulnerability of dendritic transport, or the transport of materials from the soma of myelinating cells (oligodendrocytes, Schwann cells) to sites of utilization in the myelin sheath. The architecture of nerve cells is stable in the mature state, although one compound (*swainsonine*) induces cortical pyramidal neurons to sprout dendrite-like growths at the axon hillock.

Cellular connectivity and mutual dependency. Neural cells are highly interconnected and dependent upon each other's presence and physiological activity for normal function. For example, the elaboration and maintenance of myelin by Schwann cells and oligodendrocytes requires the presence of intact axons to ensheath. Profound functional effects result from chemicals that induce intramyelinic edema (*hexachlorophene*) or distal axonal degeneration (*nitrofurantoin*); the former blocks electrical conductivity and

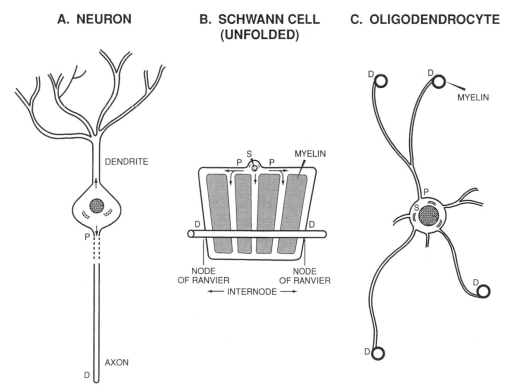

A. NEURON **B. SCHWANN CELL (UNFOLDED)** **C. OLIGODENDROCYTE**

FIGURE 1.2. Diagrammatic representations of (*A*) neuron, (*B*) Schwann cell (with myelin sheath "unrolled"), and (*C*) oligodendrocyte, to illustrate that each cell has a restricted cell soma (*S*) and elongated processes that can be divided into proximal (*P*) and distal (*D*) portions. The large processes of these cells provide a huge area for chemical attack.

the latter disconnects the nerve cell from its sensory and motor end organs. In these situations, *major functional impairment may occur without the loss of a single neural cell.*

The connectivity of neurons also provides an unparalleled opportunity for certain chemicals to migrate from cell to cell. This has physiological importance, for example, in neuronal–astrocyte interchange of metabolites regulating neurotransmitter homeostasis. In the pathological setting, cellular proximity is exploited by *tetanus toxin*, which translocates from anterior horn cells to the adjacent synapses of glycinergic neurons where it perturbs the normal inhibition of motor activity. Transsynaptic retrograde transport of *manganese* has been reported in the olfactory pathway of fish.

Electochemical communication. Cellular communication between nerve cells is dependent on the coordination of electrochemical events that are readily disrupted by a number of chemicals. Perturbed transmission of electrical impulses along axons results in functional effects for the organism, irrespective of whether electrical activity is reduced (*saxitoxin*) or increased (*pyrethroids*) by the culpable agent. Arrival of impulses at the nerve terminal activates a complex sequence of events that culminates in the release of neurotransmitter to the extracellular space, its translocation to a receptor on the neighboring neuron or target cell, and the removal of excess transmitter from the synaptic gap. These events are extraordinarily prone to chemical disruption and the consequent generation of neurotoxic phenomena (*see* later under Neurotransmitter Systems). Natural toxins (*botulinum toxin*) and venoms (β-*latrotoxin*), as well as several synthetic chemicals (*anticholinesterases*), are able to exploit this inherent vulnerability to toxic attack.

Functional reserve and aging. The nervous system appears to possess greater neuronal interconnectivity than is actually needed for the maintenance of apparently normal function. Agents that damage the nervous system have to pare down the anatomical and functional reserve before functional or clinical effects are apparent. The true extent of the functional reserve is not understood; it is also possible that techniques more sensitive than currently available will be able to detect even minor neurotoxic changes. While functions may be preserved in old age, their fidelity may be reduced, as in the case of the progressive reduction in the perception of vibration and other sensory stimuli in the extremities. This appears to be associated with pathological changes in nerve terminals (pacinian corpuscles), spinal roots (myelin bubbling), and dorsal column nuclei (axonal enlargement by tubulovesicular profiles). Such changes are reported in humans and all mammals studied. The pattern and distribution of distal nerve fiber pathology in advanced age is reminiscent of a chemically induced distal axonopathy.

Nature and Progress of the Neurotoxic Response

The nervous system has a vast repertoire of functional reactions to chemical perturbation. These responses give rise in the aggregate to a plethora of neurological and psychiatric phenomena, many of which recapitulate the clinical manifestations of diseases with other, nontoxic etiologies.

Duration and latency. Large single doses of certain substances, such as organic solvents (*ethanol, toluene*), induce functional changes in the adult organism that appear and disappear rapidly in association with the metabolism or excretion of the active agent. Other rapidly acting substances, such as *anticholinesterase nerve agents*, induce functional changes that reverse when the inhibited target protein is reactivated or replaced. Sometimes, as in the case of *methanol*, the latent period (hours) between exposure and effect is associated with the production of a metabolite (*formate*), the proximate agent responsible for cytotoxic damage. Single exposures to other compounds, such as certain heavy metals (*arsenic, mercury, thallium*), may be followed by a latent period of days or weeks before structural and functional changes become evident. *Organophosphate*-induced delayed neuropathy is another example of this phenomenon. Delayed-onset, rapidly evolving illness occurs infrequently after severe hypoxic injury, such as that seen following *carbon monoxide*–induced coma. Neurotoxic effects of some agents (*misonidazole, acrylamide, carbon disulfide*) may only become evident after repeated administration of the chemical over days, weeks, or months; this is required either to achieve a sufficiently high concentration of the agent or to develop adequate tissue damage for functional effects to surface.

Recovery and persistence. Chemicals that damage the axons of peripheral somatic or autonomic nerve fibers tend to produce functional effects that reverse as structural repair or regeneration takes place. Loss of neurons, or severe damage to peripheral nerves, spinal cord, or brain, is likely to be associated with permanent functional deficits. An example of the latter is the persistence of functional deficits in subjects one decade after an episode of severe *triorthocresyl phosphate* neuropathy when clinical evidence is seen of permanent damage to corticospinal tracts (spasticity, extensor plantar reflexes) and dorsal columns (decreased vibratory perception), and of incomplete recovery of peripheral motor (muscle atrophy and foot drop), sensory (hypesthesia below knees), and autonomic (cold, moist, cyanotic feet) function. Another example is the permanent movement disorder (dystonia) seen in children with putaminal necrosis following acute intoxication with *3-nitropropionic acid*. A third is the persistent sensory loss experienced by individuals with *pyridoxine*-induced ablation of dorsal root ganglion cells.

Progression. While neurotoxic disease commonly progresses with continuous or repeated exposure to the culpable agent (*manganese*, *toluene*), chemicals rarely, if ever, are known to produce evolving damage that appears clinically long after exposure has ceased in the form of a progressive neurological disorder. Advancing functional impairment may be found on occasion with agents that are sequestered in a tissue compartment and released over time. Retinal toxicity associated with prolonged use of *chloroquine* exemplifies this phenomenon; after binding to the pigmented layer of the choroid, the drug slowly leaches from the choroid to damage the photoreceptor layer. Subjects exposed to *methylmercury*, which slowly accumulates in brain tissue, may develop signs and symptoms of intoxication weeks after exposure. Some Japanese subjects with chronic methylmercury intoxication were reported to exhibit a gradual progression and evolution of clinical compromise over a 5- to 10-year period.

Two novel but unproven concepts merit brief mention in regard to the question of whether neurotoxic disorders can be progressive.

1. Age-related loss of neurons selectively in regions of the brain, spinal cord, and peripheral ganglia, an established biological phenomenon, is proposed to represent a mechanism by which subclinical damage from a neurotoxic event earlier in life could be unmasked and could progress with the advance of age. Interest centers on whether individuals who succumbed to subclinical nigrostriatal damage from exposure to a substance containing the neurotoxin *MPTP* are at greater risk for parkinsonism in later life. Active neuronal degeneration has been observed in the human substantia nigra more than a decade after MPTP-induced parkinsonism.
2. Nonviral environmental agents that set in motion changes that surface with progressive neurological deficits months, years, or decades after exposure are postulated but unproven. Interest is focused on certain acquired transmissible (*protease-resistant prion protein*) and nontransmissible (*genotoxins*) neurodegenerative diseases. Oral exposure in food to *cycasin*, the glucopyranoside of *methylazoxymethanol* (a potent genotoxin), is strongly correlated with the high incidence of an unusual form of amyotrophic lateral sclerosis (ALS) with parkinsonism-dementia (PD) among the indigenous Chamorro population of Guam. High-incidence ALS/PD has occurred in two other racially distinct western Pacific populations where neurotoxic cycads have been used for medicinal purposes.

VULNERABILITY OF NEURONS AND THEIR PROCESSES

This section examines agents with broad effects on neuronal functions, on excitable membranes, on neurotransmitter systems, and on axonal transport.

Somal DNA

The antineoplastic drug *doxorubicin* demonstrates selective cellular and neuronal toxicity in experimental studies. A fungal anthracycline antibiotic, the drug intercalates with DNA, interferes with DNA and RNA synthesis and with DNA topoisomerase II (which uncoils DNA), causes DNA strand breaks and sister chromatid exchange, and generates hydroxyl free radicals and hydrogen peroxide by reaction initially with cytochrome P-450 reductase. The drug binds rapidly to the cell nucleus, and chromatin fragmentation is evident within hours of exposure; this is followed by central chromatolysis and degeneration of the cell soma. Selective degeneration of primary sensory neurons is seen with systemic intoxication (doxorubicin fails to cross the blood-brain and blood-nerve barriers); sensory and motor neuronal degeneration occur after intramuscular injection and transport of the agent retrogradely to neuronal somata. Other cellular systems, such as cardiac and Schwann cells, may undergo degeneration after systemic and local exposure to doxorubicin, respectively. Rats treated experimentally with single intravenous doses of doxorubicin develop profound ataxia that reflects loss of proprioception.

Ataxia and abnormal posturing are reported in poultry exposed to *trichothecin mycotoxins* that inhibit DNA, RNA, and protein synthesis.

Podophyllotoxin, an agent that induces axonal neuropathy, inhibits topoisomerase II and thereby suppresses nucleic acid synthesis required for transcription.

Of the many drugs that have been developed to interfere with steps in DNA and nucleotide synthesis of fungi, viruses, bacteria, Protozoa, and malignant cells, some such as *5-fluorouracil*, *acyclovir*, and *vidarabine* have the potential to elicit neurotoxicity in humans, but there is no clear understanding of molecular targets and mechanisms.

Protein Synthesis and Enzyme Inhibition

Few agents have been shown selectively to disrupt the general synthesis of proteins required for neuronal integrity. Systemic intoxication with *mercury*, which inhibits thiol-dependent enzymes, disrupts protein synthesis and causes PNS and CNS neuronal degeneration. Local application of *puromycin* or *cycloheximide* blocks protein synthesis of primary sensory neurons and reduces the amount of material transported from the soma to the axon. Retrograde axonal transport of the phytotoxin *ricin* inhibits elongation of polypeptide chains in neuronal somata and causes axonal degeneration. *Diphtheria toxin* and *Pseudomonas exotoxin A* block polypeptide elongation by enzymatic inactivation of elongation factor 2.

Chemical inhibition of nervous system enzymes is a common cause of neurotoxicity. Five examples serve to illustrate the principle:

a. Inhibition of synaptic acetylcholinesterase by *organophosphate* or *carbamate* agents used in chemical warfare, pesticides, or drugs, results in the relatively prompt appearance of CNS and/or PNS manifestations associated with cholinergic toxicity.
b. Inhibition of neuropathy target esterase (NTE), a poorly defined protein with an esteratic site and unknown physiological function, is associated with delayed onset of axonal polyneuropathy. Carbamates and other substances that reversibly inhibit NTE may protect against or promote organophosphate neuropathy.
c. Inhibition of enzyme complexes associated with energy transformation in neural mitochondria may trigger neuroexcitation associated with glutamatergic overdrive and the delayed appearance of extrapyramidal signs associated with tissue necrosis in basal ganglia.
d. Inhibition of α-mannosidase activity by *swainsonine* (locoweed alkaloid) leads to lysosomal accumulation of oligosaccharides in swollen and dysfunctional neurons.
e. *Fumonisin mycotoxins* inhibit the enzymatic conversion of sphinganine to sphingosine and cause the rapid development of white matter disease in horses (equine leukoencephalomalacia).

Mitochondria and Energy State

Certain antiviral drugs (*2′,3′-dideoxyinosine* and *2′,3′-dideoxycytidine*) used in the treatment of the acquired immune deficiency syndrome (AIDS) and its prodrome may induce a painful axonal neuropathy likely to be associated with disruption of neuronal and axonal mitochondria. Mitochondrial DNA chain growth terminates because DNA polymerase γ utilizes the 5′-phosphates of these nucleoside analogues as false substrates.

Many agents reduce chemical energy in the form of adenosine triphosphate (ATP) and creatine phosphate (CP) by selectively disrupting glycolysis, Krebs cycle, or the electron transport chain, or by stimulating ATPase activity. While commonalities are evident in the pathological processes that ensue, the outcome is far from uniform. Differences in neuronal responses to ATP deficits likely result not only from the varying intrinsic properties of nerve cells but also from

factors such as the site, rate, and reversibility of disrupted energy transformation.

The *chemical site* at which energy transformation is blocked clearly determines, in part, the duration for which neuronal functions are maintained. For example, energy-dependent fast axonal transport rapidly ceases *in vitro* after desheathed peripheral nerves are treated with *cyanide* or *azide*, both of which block the terminal step of the electron transport chain; by contrast, axonal transport continues for some time after nerve fibers are bathed in *iodoacetate*, an agent that inhibits the enzyme activity of glyceraldehyde-3-phosphate dehydrogenase and blocks glycolysis but allows downstream substrates to enter mitochondria and generate ATP. Axonal transport is maintained for intermediate periods with *fluoroacetate*, which condenses with oxaloacetate to form *fluorocitrate* and thereby inhibits the tricarboxylic acid cycle.

Less clear is the importance of *the rate* at which energy blockade develops; present evidence suggests that neuronal somata with glutamate-mediated excitatory inputs are sensitive to severe, abrupt changes in energy state, whereas other neurons and their axons may be relatively refractory. Excitotoxic mechanisms (*vide infra*) leading to neuronal necrosis are unleashed in specific areas of the brain, such as the basal ganglia and hippocampus. By contrast, prolonged low-level exposure to agents known to perturb energy transformation seems to spare glutamate-vulnerable sites in the brain and other neuronal perikarya and, instead, elicit retrograde degeneration of elongate and large-diameter axons, especially in peripheral nerves. Clear demonstration of a cause-and-effect relationship between these phenomena is unavailable.

Four chemicals that act on glycolysis or the tricarboxylic acid cycle suffice to exemplify the *apparent* link between the delayed onset of axonal neuropathy and perturbation of energy transformation. *Inorganic arsenic*, which induces neuropathy in humans after a single exposure, substitutes (as pentavalent arsenate) for phosphate in the oxidation of glyceraldehyde-3-phosphate to form diphosphoglycerate and (in trivalent form) also reacts with thiols such as lipoic acid, required in the terminal step of the pyruvate dehydrogenase complex. Repeated exposure to *nitrofurantoin*, which inhibits the formation of acetyl coenzyme A (CoA) from pyruvate, may precipitate a severe axonal polyneuropathy, especially in subjects with impaired renal function. Likewise with repeated exposure of rodents to the nicotinamide analog N-*3-pyridylmethyl*-N′-p-*nitrophenylurea*, probably because nicotinamide adenine dinucleotide (NAD) and its phosphorylated form (NADP) function as coenzymes in many pathways, including steps in energy transformation in glycolysis, tricarboxylic acid cycles, and the malic enzyme shunt that generates oxaloacetate from pyruvate *via* malate. Lastly, single or multiple doses of *inorganic thallium compounds*, which form insoluble salts with riboflavin (of which the two coenzymes, flavin mononucleotide and flavin adenine dinucleotide, function in the oxidative degradation of pyruvate, fatty acids, amino acids, and in electron transport) are associated with mitochondrial damage and a painful sensory axonal neuropathy.

Agents that disrupt the mitochondrial electron transport chain have a propensity to induce basal ganglia damage. This results in large part from supraphysiological excitation of neurons equipped with glutamate receptors, failure of energy-dependent brain homeostatic mechanisms, and nerve cell (excitotoxic) degeneration. Experimental studies *in vitro* show that fast cell death (within minutes) ensues from continuous activation of ion channels coupled to glutamate receptors, intracellular influx of sodium and chloride ions, and the intracellular entry of water down the resulting osmotic gradient. Slower cell death (hours to days) is associated with Ca^{2+} entry, inappropriate activation of proteases, and the intracellular formation of toxic superoxide free radicals. Regional brain damage may result from energy compromise that is global in nature. Acute global brain energy compromise, caused by mitochondrial enzyme complex inhibitors such as *3-nitropropionic acid* (complex II) or *cyanide* (complex IV), tend to damage regions such as the putamen and globus pallidus. These areas receive major neuroexcitatory inputs in which glutamate is the proven or likely excitatory neurotransmitter. Tissue necrosis is attenuated when neurotransmitter activity is blocked by surgical disruption of glutamatergic input pathways. Regional brain damage may also ensue because agent access is restricted to the affected area. In the case of *MPTP*, the induced biochemical lesion is predominantly localized to nigrostriatal neurons. The active MPTP metabolite, *MPP*⁺, is selectively taken up by dopaminergic neurons where it inhibits NADH-ubiquinone reductase (complex I). MPP⁺-induced degeneration of nigral cells is attenuated by pharmacological blockade of glutamatergic activity and by agents that trap toxic free radicals. Pramipexole, a dopamine agonist and neuroprotective agent, attenuates oxygen radical generation and opening of the mitochondrial permeability pore, which is associated with apoptosis. Nerve cells treated with MPP⁺ in culture undergo both necrosis and apoptosis, the latter mediated by activation of a caspase-3-like protease.

Other chemicals disturb the balance between energy production and utilization by uncoupling the strict relationship between electron transport and oxidative phosphorylation. *2,4-Dinitrophenol*, which stimulates respiration far in excess of the available supply of oxygen, leads to tissue hypoxia and loss of ATP and CP throughout the brain. *6-Hydroxydopamine* uncouples mitochondrial oxidative phosphorylation and, by analogy with the selective neuronal uptake and effects of MPP⁺, elicits a pattern of neuronal degeneration restricted to catecholamine neurons. Other uncoupling agents include the fungicide, *pentachlorophenol*, and the rodenticide *bromothelin* (N-*methyl-2, 4-dinitro-*N*-[2,4,6-[tribromophenyl]-6-[trifluoromethyl]-benzeneamine*), both of which cause signs of acute neurotoxicity that include tremor, hyperexcitability, and fever. A haloperidol-derived pyridinium metabolite (*HPP*⁺), analogous to MPP⁺, potently inhibits NADH-supported mitochondrial respiration and irreversibly depletes striatal dopamine and serotonin.

Other agents interfere with oxidative phosphorylation by inhibiting the ATP-adenosine diphosphate carrier responsible for transporting the nucleotides across the mitochondrial membrane. One example is *atractyloside*, a derivative of gumniferin, a carboxyatractyloside isolated from a North African and Mediterranean thistle (*Atractylis gummifera*). Another example is *bongkrek acid,* a product of a bacterium (*Pseudomonas cocovenenans*) that may contaminate a fungus (*Rhizopus oryzae*) used in Indonesia to produce a digestable and palatable *tempeh* from coconut press cake.

Vitamin Function

Neurological function is impacted in several vitamin-deficiency states, whether of dietary or toxic origin, and in certain states of vitamin excess.

Vitamin A (as retinal) plays a key role in retinal function, and deficiency states (widespread) are associated with night blindness. Raw soybeans contain the enzyme *lipoxidase*, which oxidizes and destroys carotene. Vitamin A can act as a mammalian teratogen. In adults, *hypervitaminosis A* from consumption of vitamin A–rich foods (halibut liver) or vitamin therapy may lead to increased intracranial pressure (pseudotumor cerebri): drowsiness, irritability, headache, papilledema, and dizziness are accompanied by hepatosplenomegaly.

*Vitamin B*₁ in the form of thiamine pyrophosphate serves as a coenzyme in mitochondrial energy transformation and for transketolase, and in Na⁺ gating in neuronal membranes. The thiamine antagonist *pyrithiamine* inhibits action potentials directly and, in the diet of rodents, induces behavioral and motor changes. Antithiamine activity is found in certain bacteria (*Bacillus thiaminolyticus*), fungi (*Lentinus edodes*), bracken fern (*Pteridium aquilinum*), many higher plants (mustardseed, various edible berries, and leafy vegetables), and cold-blooded animals (certain species of crabs, mussels, herring, swordfish, and carp). So-called Chastek paralysis (*see* Chapter 3) develops in silver foxes fed raw freshwater fish harboring endogenous thiaminase.

Thiamine avitaminosis in humans (beriberi) results in thiamine-sensitive gastrointestinal symptoms, cardiac enlargement with cardiovascular insufficiency, and neurological manifestations. Adult humans consuming a diet low in thiamine develop lassitude and irritability prior to the appearance of axonal polyneuropathy. Cerebellar degeneration, with truncal ataxia, ophthalmoplegia, and confusion (Wernicke's syndrome) may occur. CNS cholinergic pathways, which are sensitive to thiamine deficiency, may be involved in memory disturbances (anterograde and retrograde amnesia) associated with chronic thiamine deficiency (Korsakoff's syndrome). Wernicke-Korsakoff syndrome, with or without polyneuropathy, is seen in association with *chronic alcoholism*, a condition associated with nutritional deficiencies. Rodents treated with *misonidazole* display a pattern of CNS and PNS neuropathology that resembles experimental thiamine deficiency. *Amprolium*, a competitive antagonist of thiamine used as a coccidiostat, is associated with polyneuropathy in poultry and, in very high doses, "polioencephalomalacia" in preruminant calves and lambs.

Riboflavin (vitamin B_2) is used in two coenzymes, flavin mononucleotide (riboflavin phosphate) and flavin adenine dinucleotide. Flavokinase, which catalyzes the phosphorylation of riboflavin, is inhibited by *chlorpromazine* and *tricyclic antidepressants*. *Quinacrine* interferes with riboflavin utilization, and *boric acid* forms a complex with riboflavin and promotes its excretion. Intoxication with boric acid is associated with gastrointestinal disorders, skin rash and desquamation, alopecia, headache, and convulsions. Riboflavin deficiency is featured by glossitis, cheilosis, dermatitis, anemia, and neuropathy.

Niacin (nicotinic acid) is used by the brain and other tissues in key coenzymes (NAD and NADP) that participate in multiple oxidation-reduction reactions. In therapeutic doses used to lower plasma cholesterol, nicotinic acid has vasodilatatory (flushing, tingling, itching) and other rare effects (amblyopia, myalgia). Human deficiency of niacin (pellagra) impacts the gastrointestinal system (diarrhea), skin (dermatitis), and brain (dementia). Cognitive changes are attended by spasticity, extensor plantar reflexes, *Gegenhalten*, and startle myoclonus. Niacin deficiency occurs in dogs (black tongue) fed *Sorghum vulgare*.

The experimental antiniacin compound, *6-aminonicotinamide* (*6-AN*), uses the synthesis pathway for NAD and NADP to form 6-AN adenine dinucleotide (6-ANAD) and the phosphorylated form 6-ANADP. These antimetabolites compete with physiological nucleotides in neurons and glial cells with cytotoxic effects: the pentose phosphate pathway is blocked by inhibition of 6-phosphogluconate dehydrogenase, and the rate of glycolysis is diminished. Tyrosine hydrolase activity is inhibited, with consequent reductions in dopamine, norepinephrine, and epinephrine. Animals develop persistent spastic paresis; lesions are found in the striatum, hippocampus, inferior olivary nucleus, and other sites.

3-Acetylpyridine (*3-AP*), another experimental antiniacin compound, produces a distribution of brain damage comparable to that seen in olivopontocerebellar atrophy. Unlike 3-AP, 2-AP does not form an antimetabolite with NADP and lacks neurotoxicity. Both 3-AP and 6-AN exhibit teratogenic effects.

N-3-Pyridylmethyl-N'-p-nitrophenylurea (*Vacor*), a niacin antagonist and insecticide, induces a niacin-sensitive impairment of fast axonal transport and distal axonal degeneration. Humans develop severe, rapid-onset, distal sensorimotor axonopathy with autonomic dysfunction and attendant acute diabetes mellitus associated with pancreatic β-cell damage.

Pantothenic acid is incorporated into Co-A which serves as a cofactor in the oxidative metabolism of carbohydrates; gluconeogenesis; fatty acid degradation; and the synthesis of porphyrins, sterols, and steroid hormones. Pantothenic acid deficiency in chicks (but not rats) is characterized by growth failure, dermatitis, "spinal cord degeneration," and poor feathering. Humans given a pantothenic acid–free diet plus ω-*methylpantothenic acid* (specific antagonist) reportedly develop a "burning sensation, muscle weakness, abdominal disorder, vasomotor instability, infection and depression." Neurotoxic effects of excess pantothenic acid are not described.

Biotin is a cofactor for enzymatic carboxylation in the metabolism of carbohydrates (pyruvate, acetyl CoA) and lipids. Biotin antagonists include *biotin sulfone*, and *desthiobiotin*. *Avidin*, a glycoprotein in egg white that binds to biotin and prevents its absorption, induces dermatitis, alopecia, and hindlimb paralysis in rats. Humans who have consumed raw eggs over a prolonged period may develop dermatitis, alopecia, hyperesthesia, muscle pain, lassitude, and anorexia. High doses of biotin have been used in the prolonged treatment of juvenile biotinidase deficiency without eliciting toxic effects.

Pyridoxine (vitamin B_6), which is concentrated in brain relative to blood, serves in the form of pyridoxal phosphate as a coenzyme in decarboxylation reactions, including the conversion of glutamate to γ-aminobutyric acid (GABA), which requires glutamic acid decarboxylase (GAD), and in transamination reactions, such as α-ketoglutarate to glutamate. *Pyridoxine megavitaminosis* causes (by an unknown mechanism) ablation of dorsal root ganglion neurons in animals and reversible sensory neuropathy or permanent sensory neuronopathy in humans.

Pyridoxine antagonists include *deoxypyridoxine* and *hydrazides*. Learning difficulty, irritability, ataxia, and seizures are associated with pyridoxine-deficiency states, the seizure intensity relating to reduced GAD activity. Tetanic convulsions are seen in animals after ingestion of the pods of *Albizia* spp., which contain a 4-methoxy derivative of pyridoxine. A widely used antituberculous drug, *isoniazid* (*isonicotinic hydrazide*), causes pyridoxine-sensitive effects in humans: acute intoxication is characterized by nausea, slurred speech, dizziness, pupillary dilatation, photophobia, and tachycardia, followed by hyperreflexia and tonic-clonic or generalized seizures. Chronic isoniazid intoxication, more common in genetic slow acetylators (*vide supra*) malnourished subjects, and those with chronic alcoholism, is characterized by sensorimotor axonal polyneuropathy. CNS glial pathology and intramyelinic edema are seen in dogs treated with convulsive and nonconvulsive doses of isoniazid. Poisoning with *crimidine* (*2-chloro-4-dimethylamino-6-methyl-pyrimidine*), a vitamin B_6 antagonist used as a rodenticide, may trigger acute convulsive seizures. Flax or linseeed (*Linum usitatissimum*) harbors the antipyridoxine peptide *linatine*, the active component of which (L-*amino-*D-*proline*) forms a hydrazone with pyridoxal phosphate.

Vitamin B_{12}, methylated cobalamin, serves as the cofactor for the conversion of homocysteine to methionine by methionine synthase; methyl groups are contributed by methyltetrahydrofolate. Deficiency of folate (chronic alcoholism) or of dietary cobalamin (vegans) leads to impaired DNA synthesis. Neurological disease in vitamin B_{12} (cyanocobalamin) deficiency is characterized by cognitive problems, gastrointestinal symptoms, long-tract spinal cord degeneration with myelin vacuolation, and sensorimotor axonal neuropathy, with or without centrocecal scotomata and optic atrophy. Clinical manifestations of this "combined system disease" are reproduced in individuals who repeatedly inhale *nitrous oxide* (which inhibits vitamin B_{12}–dependent enzymes) for its euphoric properties; nitrous oxide myeloneuropathy may occur promptly in subjects with vitamin B_{12} deficiency who are exposed to the gas during general anesthesia.

Physiological Ions

Specific cations (Na^+, K^+, Ca^{2+}, Zn^{2+}, others) serve key roles in neurotransmitter function, initiation of action potentials, axonal transport, and other key functions of neu-

rons and glial cells. Agents that perturb Na^+, K^+, and Ca^{2+} channels in excitable membranes are described later.

Zn^{2+} is of special neurotoxicological interest. Zinc, in combination with cysteine and histidine, serves as a DNA transcription factor (zinc finger) for nuclear receptors, such as those for steroid and thyroid hormones; with copper, it serves in the cuprozinc-dependent enzyme superoxide dismutase, which may protect neurons from damage by superoxide radicals. Among other physiological functions, zinc acts as a negative modulator of the N-methyl-D-aspartate (NMDA) receptor channel; as a modulator of fast axonal transport; and as a component of an enzyme (retinal dehydrogenase) required for color vision. Zinc deficiency during development has been associated with brain malformations in humans and neurobehavioral changes in animals.

The tapetum lucidum of carnivores, which has a high zinc content, is especially vulnerable to *zinc-chelating agents*. Degeneration of the tapetum lucidum, followed by retinal detachment and blindness, takes place in animals (cats, dogs) repeatedly treated with zinc-chelating agents such as *diphenylthiocarbazone*, *diethyldithiocarbamate*, and *pyridinethione*, a widely used human anti-seborrheic agent. The latter two chemicals also induce CNS-PNS distal axonal degeneration in several species, although there is no direct evidence that the pathological mechanism involves chelation of Zn^{2+} or other metals.

8-Hydroxyquinolines, such as *clioquinol*, are potent metal chelators; they have been associated with isolated cases of optic atrophy in children with the rare zinc-deficiency disorder acrodermatitis enteropathica. Prolonged oral treatment of primates with clioquinol elicits distal axonal degeneration of the optic tract and long ascending and descending pathways of the spinal cord. Humans with clioquinol neurotoxicity display a greenish iron chelate on the tongue and in the feces, but evidence that axonal degeneration is causally linked to metal chelation is lacking. The tuberculosuppressive drug *ethambutol*, which chelates zinc and other metal ions, may trigger changes in color vision, optic neuropathy and, less commonly, peripheral neuropathy.

Excessive intake of dietary *sulphur* has been linked to neurotoxicity (polioencephalomalacia) and secondary metabolic problems among ruminants (cattle, sheep). Selenium (as sodium selenate) produces massive symmetrical lesions in the anterior horns of the spinal cord of pigs.

G Proteins

Guanine nucleotide–binding (G) proteins are transmembrane proteins involved in mechanisms mediating the effects of a number of exogenous agents that affect nervous system function. The α-subunit of these heterotrimeric proteins carries the binding site for guanine nucleotides and functions by hydrolyzing guanine triphosphate (GTP). These key proteins couple a large number of receptors for extracellular mediators that activate second-messenger systems in the cell; mediators include hormones, neurotransmitters, growth factors, chemoattractants, odorants, and light. G proteins couple some neurotransmitter receptors directly to ion channels. They also control intracellular cyclic adenosine monophosphate (cAMP) levels by mediating the effects of a wide range of neurotransmitters that stimulate or inhibit adenylate cyclase activity. So-called small G proteins may mediate signal transduction in the brain (*ras*), regulate the traffic and exocytosis of synaptic vesicles (*rab3*), the assembly and function of the Golgi apparatus (adenosine diphosphate-ribosylation factor), and the assembly of cytoskeletal structures (*rho*), which is sensitive to the adenosine diphosphate–ribosylation induced by *botulinum toxin*. Other G proteins act as initiation and elongation factors in ribosomal assembly and protein elongation. *Pertussis toxin* (*Bordetella pertussis*) catalyzes the adenosine diphosphate ribosylation of certain G proteins such that they are unable to exchange guanine diphosphate for GTP following receptor activation by a range of neurotransmitters. *Cholera toxin* (*Vibrio cholerae*) catalyzes the adenosine diphosphate–ribosylation of other G proteins, including the β-subunit of retinal transducin, which is activated by photoactivated rhodopsin, a key visual pigment in rod outer-segment membranes. While cholera and pertussis toxins do not exert systemic neurotoxic effects, these agents are important tools in the armamentarium of the neuroscientist.

Excitable Membrane

A rich array of mostly naturally occurring neurotoxins targets ion channels in excitable membranes, particularly voltage-gated Na^+ channels, and also K^+, Cl^-, and Ca^{2+} channels. These channels are required for the proper functioning of neurons, axons, all types of muscle, and glial cells. Agents that alter ion channel function tend to have rapid and sometimes dramatic effects on sensory and neuromuscular function; these effects may result from either chemical-induced activation or inhibition of ion channels. The toxins in question are often complex substances manufactured by invertebrate and vertebrate species for purposes of chemical defense. Because these substances often are tailored by evolution to specific sites on individual ion channels, they are commonly employed by neurophysiologists as discrete probes of neuronal function. On occasion, they are also used to predict the three-dimensional structure

of ion channels with which they interact. Their potency as neurotoxins poses a threat to humans who usually encounter channel toxins through envenomation (snake, scorpion) or in food derived from species that bioaccumulate the noxious products (*tetrodotoxin*, *ciguatoxin*) of simple organisms. Channel agents are also found in certain plants (*veratridine*, *grayanotoxin*), and one of these (*pyrethrin*) has been exploited as the chemical basis for the widely used class of *pyrethroid* pesticides.

Sodium Ion (Na^+) Channels

Voltage-gated Na^+ channels are discrete, four-domain, transmembrane glycoprotein complexes located within the excitable plasma membrane of neurons, axons, and muscle fibers. Mammalian sodium channels consist of a transmembrane 260 kDa α-subunit bearing the Na^+ pore and a pair of 32–30 kDa β-subunits (Fig. 1.3); the three-dimensional structure has yet to be elucidated. cDNA cloning has identified three channel types in central neurons (I, II, III), a fourth (*m*1) and fifth (*h*l and I) in skeletal and cardiac muscle, respectively, and additional Na^+ channels exist in glial cells, peripheral neurons, neurosecretory cells, and epithelial cells. A selective filter on the extracellular side permits the discrete passage of Na^+, and charge-dependent conformational changes in the channel effectively open and close a "gate" on the cytoplasmic side. Rapid influx of Na^+ initiates the rising phase of the action potential leading to membrane depolarization.

Sensory nerve dysfunction (circumoral, tongue, and limb paresthesias) commonly heralds neurological dysfunction triggered by *Na^+-channel agents* acting on nerve fibers. Some agents cause significant human morbidity and mortality, including an estimated 3000 deaths in Japan between 1955 and 1975 from *tetrodotoxin* poisoning associated with the consumption of contaminated fish liver (*vide infra*), an estimated 10,000–50,000 individuals affected annually by *ciguatera intoxication* from the consumption of *ciguatoxin*-contaminated fish, and unknown numbers who develop toxicity following consumption of honey derived from plants containing *grayanotoxin* (*andromedotoxin*).

Blockade of impulse conduction occurs with agents that bind to the outer surface of the Na^+ channel and prevent Na^+ influx.

- *Tetrodotoxin.* The classic example is the potent poison *tetrodotoxin* present in several members of the suborder Tetraodontidae, notably the Japanese puffer fish (*Fugu rubripes*) and globe fish (*Spheroides rubripes*); chemically identical toxins are found in certain shellfish, starfish, newts, octopus (*Hapalochlaena maculosa*), and salaman-

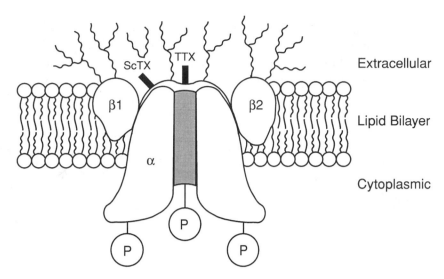

FIGURE 1.3. Structural model of a sodium channel in an excitable membrane illustrating the probable transmembrane orientation of the three subunits, oligosaccharide chains (*wavy lines*) and toxin-binding sites. *TTX*: Tetrodotoxin binding site. *ScTX*: Scorpion toxin-binding site. *P*: Sites for phosphorylation by cAMP-dependent protein kinase. [From Siegel *et al.*, 1994.]

der (*Taricha torosa*). Consumption of the puffer fish, a Japanese delicacy (*fugu*), may induce sensory abnormalities followed by rapidly progressive paralysis and death. Ingested toxin is absorbed from the gastrointestinal tract, enters the circulation, traverses endoneurial blood vessels, and binds to axolemmal Na$^+$ channels, including those concentrated at the nodes of Ranvier of myelinated nerve fibers. Agents chemically related to tetrodotoxin, namely *saxitoxin* and its structural *gonyautoxin* analogs, are found in certain marine dinoflagellates (*Gonyaulax* spp.) and are responsible for paralysis in individuals who consume contaminated shellfish. Saxitoxin and tetrodotoxin are heterocyclic molecules bearing guanidinium functions that bind externally to site 1 of the Na$^+$ channel and occlude the Na$^+$ pore.

• *Geographutoxin.* The polypeptide *μ-conotoxin* (*geographutoxin*) of the piscivorous marine snail *Conus geographus* preferentially binds to site 1 (and occludes) Na$^+$ channels of striated muscle; unlike tetrodotoxin and saxitoxin, the toxin has a relatively low affinity for Na$^+$ channels of axons. Flaccid paralysis results from block of action potentials in skeletal muscle.

• *Lipid-soluble amines.* Lipid-soluble amines (*lidocaine, procaine*) used as anesthetics represent another class of Na$^+$-channel blockers; these bind to a hydrophobic site in the channel and interfere with the gating mechanism.

Activation of Na$^+$ channels is performed by a heterogeneous collection of natural and synthetic compounds that either open Na$^+$ channels spontaneously or impede their normal closure.

Channel openers include a number of lipophilic chemicals that locate within the lipid bilayer and cause persistent activation of Na$^+$ channels. Examples include the following:

a. Plant chemicals, including *grayanotoxin*, a diterpenoid from leaves of Ericaceae such as *Rhododendron*; *veratridine* from the rhizome of *Veratrum album* (Liliaceae), *aconitine* from the monkshood (*Aconitum* spp.).

b. *Batrachotoxin*, a lipid-soluble steroid isolated from the skin of a South American frog (*Phyllobates aurotaenia*). Batrachotoxin and grayanotoxin bind to site 2 on Na$^+$ channels to block inactivation.

c. Certain organochlorine compounds, such as *DDT* [*1,1,1-trichloro-2,2-bis(p-chlorophenyl)ethane*] and *EDO* [*2,2-bis(p-ethoxyphenyl)-3,3-dimethoxyethane*] cause repetitive discharges in presynaptic fibers through prolongation of the sodium current, Na$^+$ inflow is enhanced and K$^+$ efflux is inhibited. DDT-intoxicated animals display hypersensitivity to external stimuli, tremor, and convulsions (*see also* type 1 pyrethroids, *vide infra*).

• *Ciguatoxins.* Ciguatoxins are highly potent cyclic polyethers that induce a tetrodotoxin-sensitive enhancement of Na$^+$ permeability, partial membrane depolarization, and repetitive action potentials. They inhibit binding of *brevetoxin* (from the dinoflagellate *Ptychodiscus brevis*), which binds to site 5 (domain IV) on the α-subunit and activates Na$^+$ channels. Ciguatoxins, which act on nerve cells and their terminals, and on muscle cells, are elaborated by sessile algae and dinoflagellates (particularly

Gambierdiscus toxicus) eaten by herbivorous fish which, in turn, are consumed by ever-larger carnivorous fish. Over 400 species of benthic fish are implicated in ciguatera poisoning, especially in the Caribbean Sea and islands of the Pacific Ocean. At least five toxins are held responsible, including *ciguatoxin, maitotoxin, scaritoxin,* and *palytoxin.* The magnitude of the human health threat posed by ciguatera toxicity, the potential gravity of the resulting illness, and the tendency for neuromuscular symptoms (myalgias, paresthesias) to persist for months after onset, are widely unappreciated.

- *Polypeptide toxins.* Blockade of Na⁺-channel gate inactivation is accomplished by *polypeptide toxins* isolated from certain sea anenomes, funnel-web spider (δ-*atracotoxins*) and scorpions. α-*Scorpion toxins* purified from the venom of certain African and Asian species (*Androctonus* spp., *Buthus* spp.), and U.S. species (*Centruroides sculpturatus*), bind to the external surface of the plasmalemmal protein (site 3), slow Na⁺ channel inactivation, stabilize channels in the open state, and produce a Na⁺-dependent prolongation of the action potential leading to widespread neuronal hyperexcitation. A related binding site is proposed for the peptide toxins of the sea anenomes (*Anemonia* spp.) and *Anthopleura xanthogrammatica* (*anthopleurin A, B*). β-*Scorpion toxins* (*C. sculpturatus, Tityus serrulatus*) bind to Na⁺ channels (site 4), shift the voltage dependence of Na⁺-channel activation, and cause repetitive firing. Human envenomation by *C. sculpturatus* (which contains α- *and* β-scorpion toxins), *Vejovis spinigerus,* or *Hardurus arizonensis* is associated with sharp pain on percussion of the bite site, numbness spreading from the wound throughout the affected limb, difficulty swallowing, sweating, headache, dizziness, muscle spasms of the neck, tongue fasciculation, myoclonic jerking, and respiratory paralysis.

- *Pyrethrin.* Pyrethrin, a natural organic ester insecticide from the flower of *Chrysanthemum cinerariaefolium* binds to a possible "site 6" on the Na⁺ channel, slows the inactivation of Na⁺ channels, and lethally paralyzes insects. The *synthetic pyrethroids* slow Na⁺ channel activation and inactivation, prolong the channel open time, and depolarize membranes. Human exposure to pyrethroids is associated initially with circumoral paresthesias. Pyrethroids lacking the α-cyano group (*i.e.,* type 1 pyrethroids: *permethrin, resmethrin,* and *natural pyrethrum*) cause rats to display a fine or coarse tremor, hypersensitivity to stimuli, and aggressive sparring. Animals treated with α-*cyanopyrethroids* (*i.e.,* type 2 pyrethroids: *deltamethrin, cypermethrin, fenvalerate, etc.*), which also interfere with GABA and glutamate binding, display a syndrome of choreoathetosis, salivation, tremor, and convulsions.

- *Pumiliotoxins.* Present in the skin of dendrobatid frogs (*Dendrobates pumilio*), *pumiliotoxins* activate sodium channels and have cardiotonic and myotonic activity.

Potassium Ion (K⁺) Channels

Potassium ions are primarily responsible for maintaining the resting potential of axons and, following Na⁺-induced depolarization, the voltage-dependent opening of K⁺ channels allows K⁺ ions to exit and thereby repolarize the cell. Cardiac, voluntary, and smooth muscles; secretory cells; and neuronal somata have an array of K⁺ channels, some voltage-dependent, and others modulated by Ca^{2+}, Na⁺, ATP, or increased cell volume.

At least six types of voltage-dependent K⁺ channels are recognized; these include delayed-rectifier (K_v) channels, which are activated with some delay following membrane depolarization; rapid delayed rectifier (K_{VR}), slow delayed rectifier (K_{VS}), A-channels (K_A), which are activated by depolarization after a period of hyperpolarization; inward rectifier channels (K_{IR}), which are open at resting potentials, and the sarcoplasmic reticulum channel (K_{SR}), which is strongly voltage-dependent and has low K⁺/Na⁺ selectivity.

Potassium-channel toxins with selective blocking actions have been identified in the venom of certain scorpions, bees, and snakes. Chemicals with a broad spectrum of blocking activity on several types of K⁺ channels include synthetic compounds such as *tetraethylammonium (TEA)* and *4-aminopyridine,* plant products such as *quinine,* and divalent cations such as Ba^{2+}. Acute *barium* intoxication results in gastrointestinal distress, perioral paresthesias, loss of tendon reflexes, muscle weakness, cardiac dysfunction, respiratory paralysis, and death. Monovalent ions of *thallium* (Tl^+) have a similar ionic radius to those of K⁺ ions and can restart the isolated heart after K⁺ withdrawal: *thallous salts,* once used in rodenticides, induce high-amplitude mitochondrial swelling *in vitro,* distal axonal degeneration *in vivo,* and a painful sensory neuropathy in humans (*see also* Mitochondria and Energy State, *vide supra*).

1. The synthetic autonomic ganglionic-blocking agent *TEA* blocks K_{IR}, K_A, K_{SR}, and Ca^{2+}-dependent K⁺ channels from both inside and outside the plasmalemma. Severe toxic effects include marked hypotension, syncope, paralytic ileus and constipation, bladder atony and urinary retention, and paralysis of the ciliary muscle of the eye (cycloplegia).
2. *4-Aminopyridine (4-AP),* which is used therapeutically in botulism and myasthenia gravis, binds proximate to the inner vestibule of the pore of K⁺ channels (K_v) and thereby prolongs the action potential, potentiates muscle twitch tension, and improves muscle strength. K_v channels of various

subtypes are blocked by Cs^+, Ba^{2+}, Zn^{2+}; by *tityus toxins* from the scorpion *Tityus serrulatus*; by *noxiustoxin*, a 39 amino-acid peptide from the scorpion *Centruroides noxious*, and by *α-dendrotoxin* from the venom of certain mambas (*Dendroaspis* spp.). Toxins from sea anemones, including *Anemone sulcata* (*kaliseptine, kalicludines*) and *Stichodactyla helianthus* (*stichodactyla toxin*), compete for the dendrotoxin-binding site on K^+ channels. *Stichodactyla toxin* facilitates release of acetylcholine at the avian neuromuscular junction. Sea anemone stings cause local pain with burning, itching, swelling, and erythema accompanied by fever, chills, malaise, abdominal pain, headache, and prostration.

3. *Gossypol* (*Thespia populnea*) binds to membrane phospholipids, affects K^+ transport, and induces hypokalemia with associated reversible changes in neuromuscular (flaccid paresis) and cardiac (arrhythmias) function.

4. K_A channels are blocked by *4-AP*, *TEA*, *phencyclidine*, *tetrahydroaminoacridine*, and *mast cell degranulating peptide* in venom of the bee *Apis mellifera*. Clinical signs of bee sting include local pain, erythema, urticarial reaction, and blanching, with possible anaphylaxis in those previously sensitized to venom allergens.

5. K_{VR} channels are blocked by *quinidine*. K_{IR} channels are Mg^{2+}-sensitive and blocked by *TEA*, Cs^+, Sr^+, Ba^{2+}, and *gaboon viper venom* (*Bitis gabonica*). K_{SR} channels are blocked by *4-AP*, Cs^+, and *TEA*.

6. Ca^{2+}-dependent K^+ channels. These comprise high-conductance or maxi-K channels (BK_{Ca}), intermediate-conductance channels (IK_{Ca}), small-conductance channels (SK_{Ca}), and nonspecific cation channels $K_{Na(Ca)}$.

BK_{Ca} channels in various (neural, muscle, and/or neuroendocrine) tissues are blocked by *TEA*, Ba^{2+}, *quinine*, *tubocurarine*, and scorpion peptide toxins isolated from *Buthus tamulus* (*iberiotoxin*), *Leirus quinquestriatus* (*charybdotoxin*), and *Androctonus mauretanicus* (*α-kaliotoxin*). IK_{Ca} channels are blocked by *TEA*, *quinine*, Cs^{2+}, Ba^{2+}, *calmodulin antagonists*, and *charybdotoxin*. SK_{Ca} channels are sensitive to neuromuscular blockers, such as *tubocurarine*. The 18 amino-acid peptide *apamin* (*Apis mellifera*) blocks SK_{Ca} channels in neuroblastoma, neurons, smooth muscle, and skeletal muscle. *Leuirotoxin 1* (*scyllatoxin*), a 31 amino-acid peptide toxin of the scorpion *Leuirus quinquestriatus hebraeus*, inhibits binding of apamin to rat brain membranes. $K_{Na(Ca)}$ channels are sensitive to *4-AP* and *quinine*.

Receptor-coupled K^+ channels comprise those activated by muscarine (K_M), which produce time- and voltage-dependent K^+ currents, atrial muscarine-activated channels (K_{ACh}), and 5-HT–inactivated channels (K_{5-HT}). Other K^+ channels include ATP-regulated channels (K_{ATP}); voltage-, ATP-, and Cs^{2+}-insensitive, Na^+-activated channels (K_{Na}),

and cell-volume–sensitive channels (K_{Vol}), which open when cells swell.

K_M channels are sensitive to Ba^{2+} and N-(6-aminohexyl)-5-chloro-1-naphthalene sulfonamide hydrochloride. K_{ACh} channels are blocked by Cs^{2+}, Ba^{2+}, *4-AP*, *TEA*, and *quinine*. K_{5-HT} channels are blocked by Ba^{2+} and weakly by *TEA*, *4-AP*. K_{ATP} channels, which couple cell metabolism to electrical activity, are opened by *diazoxide* and *cromakalin* and blocked by *glibenclamide*, *tolbutamide*, *lidocaine*, *quinine*, *4-AP* and Ba^{2+}. K_{Na} channels are blocked by millimolar concentrations of *TEA* and *4-AP*. K_{Vol} channels are sensitive to *quinidine* and *lidocaine*.

Chloride Ion (Cl^-) Channels

Nerve cells actively extrude Cl^- to balance the inward leakage of Cl^- by passive diffusion from higher extracellular concentrations. Increased conductance of Cl^- decreases the amplitude of the action potential, which allows nerve cells, such as primary sensory neurons, to use this mechanism to effect presynaptic inhibition.

Bromide ions (Br^-) can replace extracellular Cl^-, gain intracellular access, and exhibit a range of neurotoxic effects. Bromides were formerly (1930–1970) heavily prescribed as sedatives and antiepileptics, with marked dermatotoxic (halogen acne) and neurotoxic effects. Inorganic *bromide toxicity* (*bromism*) may arise in part because Br^- has a longer half-life than Cl^-, which is subject to preferential renal excretion. The half-life of Br^- is greatly extended (hours to months) in dogs with salt deprivation, and dehydration is universally present in subjects with chronic bromism. Mimicry of psychiatric syndromes may develop, with dullness, mood disturbances, delusions, hallucinations, restlessness, and hallucinosis. Neurological signs of bromism may include headache; tremor; ataxia; disturbances of vision, speech, swallowing, superficial sensation, and autonomic function; long-tract signs; and parkinsonism. Permanent hearing loss, a cerebellobulbar syndrome, and persistent optic neuropathy have been described with *organic bromide intoxication*.

Few chemicals that selectively bind to Cl^- channels have been identified. *Streptomyces avermitilis* produces a macrocyclic lactone disaccharide, *avermectin B_{1a}*, that binds to both ligand- and voltage-gated Cl^- channels to increase the rate of channel opening. $GABA_A$ and non–GABA-linked Cl^- channels are responsive (*vide infra*). *Abamectin*, the common name for a mixture of avermectin B_{1a} and B_{1b}, is used as an insecticide and acaricide. Avermectin has a lethal paralytic action in arthropods, and neuromuscular compromise is reported in large animals. As *ivermectin B_{1a}*, the dihydro derivative of avermectin B_{1a}, the agent is widely exploited as an antihelmintic drug in veterinary and human medicine, a use that includes prophylaxis for onchocerciasis.

Chlorotoxin is a 36 amino-acid Cl⁻ channel blocker isolated from the scorpion *Leiurus quinquestriatus*; the agent induces paralysis in crayfish and cockroaches.

Calcium Ion (Ca²⁺) Channels

Four types of Ca²⁺ channels (L, N, P, T) are recognized, and several more are likely to exist. L-type channels function in smooth muscle and cardiac muscle excitation–contraction coupling and in excitation–secretion coupling in endocrine cells and some neurons. The highest density of L-type channels in the vertebrate CNS is seen in the molecular layer of the dentate gyrus. L-type channels have been localized to dendrites and may be preferentially located at the basal region of major dendrites. N-type channels are restricted to nerve cells where they function in neurotransmitter release. High-density CNS-binding sites are found in the cerebral cortex, hippocampus (especially the stratum oriens and stratum radiatum), caudate nucleus, putamen, nucleus of the solitary tract, and the glomerular layer of the olfactory bulb. Both N- and L-type voltage-dependent Ca²⁺ channels appear to be involved in Ca²⁺ influx following *NMDA* receptor-mediated depolarization. Low-voltage-activated or T-type Ca²⁺ channels, which deactivate more slowly than L or N channels, function in repetitive spike activity in neurons and endocrine cells, and influence the sinoatrial cardiac pacemaker. P-type Ca²⁺ channels have been identified in CNS neurons, notably Purkinje cells; they mediate depolarization-induced repetitive Ca²⁺-dependent spikes.

Ca²⁺-channel blockers occur as components of certain plants, insects, spiders, snails, and snakes; synthetic Ca²⁺-channel drugs, used for the treatment of hypertension, angina, and cardiac arrhythmias, include *dihydropyridines*, *phenylalkylamines*, and *benzothiazepines*.

L-channels consist of α_1-, α_2-, β-, δ-, and γ-subunits; the α_1-subunit forms the pore and is the binding site for agonists and antagonists. L-channels are selectively blocked by *calciseptine*, a 60 amino-acid peptide toxin from the black mamba snake (*Dendroaspis polylepis polylepis*). *Calcicludine* from *Dendoaspis angusticeps* has high affinity for L-type channels but also blocks H- and P-type Ca²⁺ channels. Several drugs block L-type channels, including the phenylalkylamine *verapamil*; the benzothiazepine *diltiazem*; and the dihydropyridine drugs, *nitrendipine*, *nimodipine*, and *nifedipine*. These calcium antagonists relax vascular smooth muscle and decrease peripheral vascular resistance. Toxic side effects are usually minor: vasodilatory effects, particularly with nifedipine, include headache, facial flushing, dizziness, and peripheral edema. Calcium antagonists have also been associated with focal neurological deficits, depression, psychosis, and extrapyramidal signs.

N-type, neuron-specific channels are blocked by 24–27 amino-acid *ω-conotoxins* isolated from certain species of cone snails (*Conus* spp.) that hunt fish. These presynaptic toxins block depolarization-induced Ca²⁺ uptake *in vitro*, as well as synaptosomal uptake of radiolabeled calcium. The highly basic ω-conotoxin peptides *GVIA* (*C. geographus*) and *MVIIA* (*C. magus*) have been synthesized and studied in several species. Synthetic GVIA blocks neuromuscular transmission in fish, frogs, and birds, but not in mammals. Intracerebroventricular injection in young mice induces a tremor; motor deficits, disturbed thermoregulation, and cardiovascular changes occur in similarly treated rats. GVIA inhibition of N-type channels has also been demonstrated in rat superior cervical ganglionic neurons and rat dorsal root ganglion crossed with mouse (F11) hybrid cells. GVIA perturbs *NMDA*- or *kainate*-stimulated Ca²⁺ influx, and severely attenuates postsynaptic stimulatory potentials in hippocampal CA1 neurons. MVIIA produces a reversible Ca²⁺ block in vertebrate neurons, and tremor in mice treated *via* the intracerebroventricular route. Other ω-conotoxins active on N-type channels include the 27 amino-acid N-, P-, and Q-type polypeptide Ca²⁺ channel antagonists *MVIIC* and *MCIID* (*C. magus*), and the 24 amino-acid channel blocker *SVIA*, which paralyzes fish and is weakly active in mammals (*C. striatus*). Another N-type Ca²⁺-channel blocker composed of 36 amino acids (ω-*grammotoxin SIA*) has been isolated from the spider *Grammostola spatulata*.

ω-*Agatoxins* are a family of 48–76 amino-acid peptide toxins isolated from the North American funnel web spider (*Agelenopsis aperta*). These agents block presynaptic Ca²⁺ channels and elicit prolonged suppression of neurotransmitter release. ω-*Aga-IA* paralyzes insects but has no effect on mice receiving the drug intracranially. ω-*Aga-IIA* paralyzes insects and blocks Ca²⁺ channels in chick and rat synaptosomal membranes. ω-*Aga-IVA* and ω-*Aga-IIIA* have lower channel subtype specificity, since they block N-, and N- and P-type currents, respectively, in mammalian central and peripheral neurons. ω-Aga-IVA blocks glutamate release from rat brain synaptosomes.

P-Type Ca²⁺ channels are blocked by a 48 amino-acid ω-agatoxin, ω-*Aga-IVB*, and by a polyamine-like <5090 Da substance (FTX) also isolated from *Agelenopsis aperta*. FTX blocks Ca²⁺ action potentials in Purkinje cells and neurotransmission at the squid giant synapse; it has no effect on mammalian motoneurons.

T-Type Ca^{2+} channels are blocked nonselectively by *octanol* and *flunarizine*.

Other Ca^{2+} channel-blocking peptide toxins active on crustacean or insect neuromuscular junctions have been isolated from the spiders *Agelena opulenta* (*agelenin*), *Hololena curta* (*hololena toxin*), and *Plectreurys tristis* (*PLTX II*).

Ca^{2+}-channel activators: β-*Leptinotarsin-h*, a 57 kDa acidic protein from the hemolymph of the Colorado potato beetle (*Leptinotarsa haldemani*) appears to activate Ca^{2+} channels in mammalian brain synaptosomes and stimulates release of acetylcholine at the neuromuscular junction. *Maitotoxin* from the dinoflagellate *Gambierdiscus toxicus* enhances Ca^{2+} entry into a variety of cells, apparently by way of voltage-dependent Ca^{2+} channels. *Atrotoxin* from the western diamondback rattle snake *Crotalus atrox* increases Ca^{2+} currents in mammalian heart muscle, but its role as a Ca^{2+} channel activator is disputed.

Ionophores

Several chemically disparate agents form ionophores *de novo* in plasma membranes. The cyclododecapeptide *valinomycin* from the bacterium *Streptomyces fulvissimus* is widely used as an experimental tool to study K^+ permeability, as is the polyether *monensin*, a Na^+ ionophore from *Streptomyces cinnamonensis*. *Monensin* also alters Ca^{2+} transport, increases intracellular calcium levels, and alters myocardial contractility.

- *Palytoxin* is an extremely potent, polycyclic hemiketal neurotoxin found in a red alga (*Chondria armata*), coelenterates of the genus *Palythoa*, and species of xanthid crab (*Lophozozymus pictor*, *Demania toxica*), ingestion of which has caused fatalities in the Philippines. Palytoxin forms cation ionophores at the site of Na^+/K^+-ATPase, increases the resting Na^+ permeability, changes the current-voltage characteristics of myelinated fibers, and promotes the permeability of other cations (Li^+, Cs^+, NH_4^+). Palytoxin also depolarizes skeletal, cardiac, and smooth muscle in a Na^+-dependent manner. Intravenous administration to monkeys induces ataxia, drowsiness, limb weakness, collapse, and death, probably from cardiotoxicity.

Neurotransmitter Systems

Chemicals that perturb neurotransmitter systems are legion, and neurotoxicity may result from increased or decreased activity of these systems. Agents with neurotoxic potential target mechanisms involved in neurotransmitter synthesis, transport, presynaptic release, reuptake, the interaction between neurotransmitter and postsynaptic receptor, or the removal of neurotransmitter from the synaptic gap. In brief, any agent is a potential neurotoxin if it (a) reduces or increases presynaptic neurotransmitter release, (b) alters the concentration or residence time of the neurotransmitter in the synaptic gap, or (c) acts as an agonist or antagonist at the postsynaptic receptor.

Neurotransmitters acting through plasmalemmal receptors effect their action on target cells either through ligand-gated ion channels or through guanine nucleotide-binding (G) proteins that are coupled to intracellular effectors (*vide supra*). The latter include metabotropic glutamate receptors, γ-aminobutyric acid ($GABA_B$) receptors, β-adrenergic receptors, and muscarinic acetylcholine receptors. The superfamily of ligand-gated ion channels includes receptors for the inhibitory neurotransmitters $GABA_A$ and glycine, 5-hydroxytryptamine (5-HT_3), most of the glutamate receptors, and the nicotinic acetylcholine receptor.

Exocytosis

Exocytosis of neurotransmitter at axon terminals and of secretory products of neuroendocrine cells is triggered by an increase in the cytosolic concentration of Ca^{2+}. Docking and fusion of synaptic vesicles to the plasmalemma is followed by endocytotic membrane retrieval and recycling. Three classes of proteins participate in exocytosis in neuronal and neuroendocrine cells: (a) synapsin I, which controls the availability of synaptic vesicles, and synaptotagmin, which associates with N-type Ca^{2+} channels; (b) synaptobrevin (vesicle-associated membrane protein), syntaxin, and synaptosome-associated protein 25 (SNAP-25), all essential components of the exocytotic machinery; and (c) N-*ethyl-maleimide*-sensitive fusion protein (NSF) and soluble NSF-attachment proteins (SNAPs), which are implicated in neurotransmitter release.

- *Botulinum toxin.* *Botulinum toxin* serotypes (A, B, C_1, D, E, F, and G), from the bacterium *Clostridium botulinum*, consist of polypeptides formed into heavy (100 kDa) and light (50 kDa) chains. The heavy chain binds to the plasmalemma and facilitates entry of the light chain, a Zn-endopeptidase, into the axon terminal where it blocks synaptic transmission by cleaving synaptic-vesicle-fusion proteins required for exocytosis. SNAP-25 is cleaved at Gln197-Arg198 by *serotype A* and at Arg180-Ile181 by *serotype E*; *serotype C_1* cleaves syntaxin 1A at Lys253-Ala254 and *syntaxin 1B* at Lys252-Ala253; synaptobrevin is cleaved at Gln76-Phe77 by *serotype B*, at Lys59-Leu6 and Ala67-Asp68 by *serotype D*, at Gln58-Lys59 by *serotype F* and by *serotype G*.

Botulinum-induced blockade of depolarization-induced transmitter release at the neuromuscular junction leads to flaccid paralysis. Food-borne botulism is characterized by a symmetrical, descending paralysis with cranial nerve involvement (diplopia, dysarthria, and/or dysphagia) followed by weakness of the neck, arms, thorax, and legs. Nausea, vomiting, and abdominal pain may occur before or after onset of paralysis; dizziness, blurred vision, ptosis, dry mouth, sore throat, paralytic ileus, severe constipation, and urinary retention commonly occur. Subjects are generally alert and oriented (toxin is excluded from the brain). Secretion from neuroendocrine cells is also blocked by botulinum toxins. Feed-borne botulism affects mammals and birds.

Intramuscular injection of minute doses of botulinum toxin A is used clinically to treat movement disorders (blepharospasm, cervical dystonia) and disorders of neuromuscular transmission (myasthenia gravis, Lambert-Eaton syndrome). Most patients tolerate treatment well; adverse reactions include local pain, local weakness, dysphagia, and brachial plexopathy.

- *Tetanus toxin.* Tetanus toxin (*Clostridium tetani*) has similar-sized heavy and light chains that attach to presynaptic membranes and enter the nerve terminal, respectively. The light chain is carried retrograde by fast axonal transport to motor neurons in the spinal cord where it translocates and binds to the plasmalemma of attached spinal inhibitory neuron terminals. Here, the *tetanus light-chain fragment* cleaves synaptobrevin at Gln76-Phe77 and another protein, cellubrevin. Blockade of inhibition of motor neurons and, by a comparable process, sympathetic neurons, results in increased motor and sympathetic activity.

- α-*Latrotoxin.* α-*Latrotoxin* is a 1401 amino-acid peptide elaborated by the black widow spider (*Latrodectus* spp.) which binds to neurexin 1-α and, with the apparent participation of synaptotagmin, syntaxin and N-type Ca^{2+} channels, causes massive transmitter release at vertebrate neuromuscular junctions. This seems to be accomplished by increasing the probability of vesicle fusion with the plasmalemma and by inhibiting vesicle recycling. α-*Latrotoxin* also promotes release of GABA and amino acid neurotransmitters *in vitro*.

Acetylcholine

Acetylcholine is a neurotransmitter in the PNS; at neuromuscular junctions, autonomic ganglia, and parasympathetic effector junctions; and in the spinal cord and brain. Cholinergic neurons play a major role in the ascending reticular acting system, the loss of which is associated with learning and memory deficits. Agents that affect the cholinergic system occur as products of bacteria, plants, animals, and as synthetic chemicals; some affect both the CNS and PNS, while others are unable to cross the blood-brain barrier and confine their actions to peripheral somatic and autonomic cholinergic nerve terminals.

As with any neurotransmitter system, chemicals can disrupt the cholinergic system at many sites. One is the nerve cell body. Cholinergic nerve cells that communicate with neurons, muscle, or other target organs are themselves regulated by the sum of their excitatory and inhibitory neurotransmitter inputs. Thus, for example, the function of a cholinergic motor neuron in the spinal cord is heavily impacted by chemicals that target glutamate-mediated inputs (*vide infra*) although there is no direct action of these agents on the synthesis, transport, release, uptake, or removal of acetylcholine. Excitotoxic chemicals (*kainate*) that mimic the action of *glutamate* readily destroy cholinergic (as well as other) neurons with glutamate receptors, including the cholinergic neurons of the basal forebrain. Cholinergic nerve cell function is disrupted by agents that curtail inhibitory input, as in the case of *tetanus toxin*, which inhibits Ca^{2+}-dependent release of glycine from inhibitor interneurons that regulate motoneuron activity. Cholinergic function is also compromised by chemicals, such as *vincristine*, that nonspecifically block axonal transport and disrupt the normal anterograde transport of materials required for neurotransmitter synthesis.

Many substances are known to interfere with critical functions in the presynaptic region of cholinergic nerve terminals (Fig. 1.4). One target is the plasmalemmal Na^+-dependent high-affinity choline transport system. *Hemicholinium* {2,2'-(4,4'-biphenylylene)bis[2-hydroxy-4,4-dimethylmorpholinium]} produces neuromuscular blockade by competing with choline for the choline carrier and reversibly inhibiting choline uptake.

Choline mustard aziridinium analogues, such as *AF64A*, compete with choline for transport into the cholinergic neuron and, in high concentrations, irreversibly block choline uptake and induce retrograde axonal degeneration by an unknown mechanism. A second target of chemical attack is the synthesis of acetylcholine, specifically the enzyme choline acetyltransferase. Several substances (*naphthoquinones, halogenated cholines*) are effective enzyme inhibitors *in vitro*, and *acetyl-sec-hemicholinium-3* reduces brain acetylcholine levels *in vivo*. Acetylcholine synthesis is also disrupted by false cholinergic neurotransmitters, including cyclic choline analogs such as *triethylcholine, diethylaminoethanol*, and *3-hydroxypiperidinium*. These agents are carried by the plasmalemmal choline transporter, acetylated by choline acetyltransferase, enter synaptic vesicles, and re-

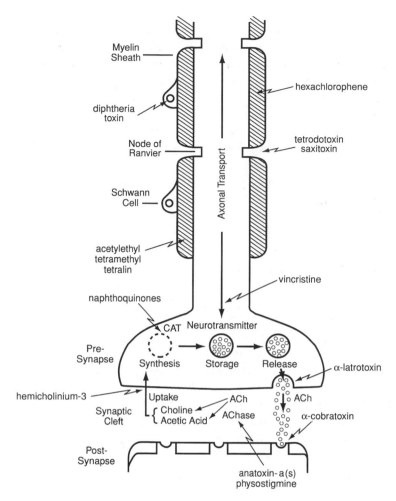

FIGURE 1.4. Targets of neurotoxic agents acting on PNS cholinergic nerve fibers (*upper portion*), terminals (*lower midportion*), and neuromuscular synapses (*lowest portion*). *ACh*: Acetylcholine. *AChase*: Acetylcholinesterase. *CAT*: choline acetyl transferase. See text for explanation.

leased synaptically where they display cholinoreceptor agonist activities that are lower than that of acetylcholine (cholinergic hypofunction). Inhibition of acetylcholine storage is yet another mechanism of presynaptic action exploited by certain agents. The experimental drug 2-(4-*phenylpiperidino*)*cyclohexanol* (*vesamicol*) induces neuromuscular blockade by selectively blocking the active transport of acetylcholine into synaptic vesicles without affecting existing vesicular stores of neurotransmitter. Another experimental drug, *cetiedil*, impacts both the vesicular uptake and the release of synaptic acetylcholine.

Several biological toxins target the presynaptic release of acetylcholine. *Botulinum toxins* (*vide supra*) impair the quantal release of acetylcholine and produce a long-lasting block of cholinergic transmission at all peripheral cholinergic synapses. Certain snake venoms contain substances (β-*bungarotoxin*, *notexin*, *taipoxin*, *crotoxin*, *mojave toxin*, *agkistrodotoxin*, *ammodytoxin A*) that interfere with the release of acetylcholine from motor nerve terminals.

These presynaptic snake toxins have a biological activity consistent with an active basic subunit with phospholipase activity coupled to one or more acidic subunits, which may function as chaperones to target the toxic subunit. These agents initially decrease spontaneous transmitter release, enhance transmission, and then gradually and irreversibly halt spontaneous and elicited release with vesicle depletion. Honeybee venom (*Apis* spp.) contains a 128 amino-acid peptide toxin, *phospholipase A$_2$*, which inhibits neurotransmitter release. α-*Latrotoxin* greatly increases presynaptic release of acetylcholine and other vesicle-bound neurotransmitters. Two other novel protein neurotoxins, *iotrochotin* and β-*leptinotarsin-h*, promote presynaptic acetylcholine release.

Acetylcholinesterase. Acetylcholinesterase, the enzyme that terminates the synaptic transmitter activity of acetycholine by its rapid hydrolysis at cholinergic synapses, is an important target of certain naturally occurring and synthetic chemicals. Acetylcholinesterase activity is located on the outer surface of the postsynaptic membrane. The enzyme monomer (from *Torpedo californica*) is an α/β-protein that contains 537 amino acids and consists of a 12-stranded mixed β-sheet surrounded by 14 α-helices. The active site lies near the bottom of a deep and narrow gorge that reaches halfway into the protein. Certain anticholinesterases (*edrophonium*) bind directly to the active center of the enzyme and act rather briefly; some others (*physostigmine, neostigmine*) carbamylate the enzyme and have longer lasting actions. *Organophosphates* interact with the anionic and/or esteratic subsites in the active center to form stable complexes, and the stability of the phosphorylated enzyme is further enhanced by the loss of one of the alkyl groups, a phenomenon known as aging. The agents may also act directly on nicotinic receptors and muscarinic receptors (*vide infra*).

Anticholinesterase agents increase the synaptic residence time of acetylcholine and thereby cause excessive stimulation of target tissue. With the inhibition of acetylcholinesterase, acetylcholine fails to undergo hydrolysis and continues to act as a neurotransmitter at cholinergic muscarinic and nicotinic receptors. Additonally, anticholinesterases inhibit the production of choline, which is proposed to serve as a GABA agonist, thereby promoting inhibitory tone. A neurotoxic syndrome (cholinergic crisis) thus develops from the prolonged stimulation of target tissue. Peripheral autonomic muscarinic toxicity is characterized by sweating, lacrimation, excessive salivation, nausea, vomiting, diarrhea, involuntary defecation and urination, bradycardia, and hypotension. Confusion, ataxia, slurred speech, reflex loss, convulsions, and central respiratory paralysis occur with agents that enter the brain. Peripheral nicotinic toxicity is reflected in the form of muscle fasciculation, easy fatigability, and global muscle weakness.

Anticholinesterase chemicals of varying potency are used as chemical warfare agents (high potency), insecticides (medium potency), and medications (low potency). Reversible carbamate enzyme inhibitors include the widely used ophthalmic medication *physostigmine* (*eserine*), originally isolated from the Calabar bean (*Physostigma venenosum*), and *pyridostigmine bromide*, a drug used both to promote neurotransmission in subjects with myasthenia gravis and as an atropine antidote enhancer to block the effects of potent acetylcholinesterase inhibitors such as *soman*. Subcutaneous injection of soman in rats produces a sustained increase of acetylcholine, seizures, and neuronal damage (predominantly in the pyriform cortex, amygdala, hippocampus, and thalamic nuclei), which is partly attenuated by atropine. Anticholinesterase agents with intermediate potencies, such as the carbamate *carbaryl* and the organophosphate *para-*

thion, are widely exploited for their insecticidal properties. The cholinergic crisis that accompanies human intoxication with anticholinesterase insecticides may trigger pathological changes in nerve terminals and adjacent muscle fibers that develop after a few days into a reversible, transjunctional myopathy. This is probably the basis for the clinical "intermediate syndrome," which features proximal weakness, compromise of the muscles of respiration, and selective cranial motor involvement. The syndrome is temporally and mechanistically distinct from the axonal polyneuropathy that may appear weeks after single or multiple exposures to certain organophosphates.

Other cholinesterase inhibitors include: *anatoxin-α(s)*, a phosphate ester of a cyclic-*N*-hydroxyguanidine elaborated by the cyanobacterium *Anabaena flos-aquae*; *onchidal*, a lipophilic acetate ester produced by certain mollusks (*Onchidella* spp.), which is toxic to fish; and *fasciculins* from the snake *Dendroaspis angusticeps*.

Nicotinic receptors. Acetylcholine receptors are traditionally divided according to their divergent responses to muscarine and nicotine.

3-(1-Methyl-2-pyrrolidinyl)pyridine (*nicotine*), an alkaloid found in a number of widely scattered plant families, including tobacco plants (*Nicotiana* spp.), increases hypothalamic corticotrophin-releasing factor, a number of hypophyseal hormones, and circulatory levels of corticosteroids and catecholamines, and alters the bioavailability of dopamine and serotonin. *Nicotine receptor antagonists* include the bis-benzylisoquinoline alkaloid D-*tubocurarine* (Menispermaceae, Loganiaceae) and the indole alkaloid *strychnine* (*Strychnos* spp.), which have neuromuscular-blocking effects. Whereas the actions of nicotinic muscle receptors (N_1) are blocked by α-snake toxins (*α-bungarotoxin* from the krait *Bungarus multicinctus*), those on neurons (N_2) in peripheral autonomic ganglia are resistant. Peripheral and CNS nicotinic receptors are multi-subunit receptors; those from the *Torpedo* electric organ are composed of two copies of the α-subunit and one each of the β-, γ-, and δ-subunits; these are assembled around a central core, the ligand-gated ion channel.

Postsynaptic acetylcholine receptors form the target of a number of biological agents found in algae (*anatoxin-a*), plants (*curare*), and animals (*α-bungarotoxins*). The majority of information is available for the nicotinic acetylcholine receptor. *Anatoxin-a* is one of two neurotoxins (*vide supra*) of blue-green algae (*Anabaena flos-aquae*): it is a potent agonist at neuromuscular, autonomic, and brain nicotinic receptors. Strains of *Anabaena* are marketed in the United States as "health foods." Anatoxin triggers a peripheral cholinergic crisis in animals that drink water containing toxic blooms. Charged ammonium compounds, such as

1,1-dimethyl-4-phenyl-piperazine, *methylarecolone*, and *methylferrugine*, serve as experimental nicotinic agonists.

Substances that act as nicotinic receptor antagonists cause muscular paralysis and may attenuate convulsions induced by strychnine and tetanus. Reversible nicotinic receptor antagonists include D-*tubocurarine*, a quaternary compound isolated from *Chondrodendron tomentosum* that contains a bis-benzylisoquinoline structure. Other curare-mimetic agents that block the binding site for acetylcholine on the α-subunits of the receptor include the peptide toxins (α-*neurotoxins*) of venoms of elapid and hydrophid snakes, including the sea snake *Laticauda semifasciata* (*erabutoxin*), the cobra *Naja naja siamensis* (α-*cobratoxin*) and the krait *Bungarus multicinctus* (α-*bungarotoxin*), an agent of remarkable toxic potency (K_M, 10^{-11}M). Since the tertiary structures of several α-*neurotoxins* have been elucidated, a detailed molecular understanding of the action of these agents at the nicotinic receptor is under development. Other curare-mimetic substances include: (a) α-*conotoxins*, peptides isolated from the molluscs *Conus geographicus* and *C. magus*; (b) *lophotoxin*, a cyclic diterpene found in several Pacific horny corals; and (c) the aconite alkaloid *methyllycaconitine* from the seed of the larkspur *Delphinium* and *dihydro-β-erythroidine* from the seed of *Erythrina* trees. Agents that inhibit acetylcholine receptor function through allosteric sites include *scopolamine* (*Datura* spp.) and the dendrobatid alkaloids *histrionicotoxin*, *pumiliotoxin*, and *gephyrotoxin*. Selective antagonists for nicotinic receptors include α-*bungarotoxin* (muscle, α7 neuronal) and *neosuragatoxin* (ganglionic, CNS neurons), a glycoside from the Japanese ivory mollusk (*Babylonia japonica*); corresponding but nonselective channel blockers include *decamethonium* and *gallamine* (muscle), and *hexamethonium* and *mecamylamine* (ganglia, CNS neurons).

Muscarinic receptors. Human muscarinic receptors (M_1–M_5) are 460–590 amino-acid receptors that transduce signals across the plasmalemma by interacting with proteins that bind and cleave guanosine nucleotides (G proteins). Named for their response to muscarine, these receptors are located on autonomic effector cells (smooth muscle, cardiac muscle, glands) innervated by postganglionic parasympathetic nerves; they are also present in brain, ganglia, and blood vessels. *Muscarine* is a product of certain fungi (*Muscaria*, *Inocybe*, *Clitocybe*); the pharmacologically related imidazole alkaloid *pilocarpine* (*Pilocarpus* spp.) has effects on the CNS (cortical arousal), eye (miosis), exocrine glands (stimulation of secretions), and cardiovascular system (hypotension, bradycardia). Muscarinic receptor antagonists include *atropine* (*Atropa belladona*, *Datura stramonium*) and *scopolamine* (*Hyoscyamus niger*), which have effects on the CNS that include initial depression and amnesia,

excitement, restlessness, hallucinations, and delirium at higher doses. Antagonists, such as the synthetic chemical warfare agent *quinuclidinyl benzilate* (*BZ*), induce dryness of the mouth, blurred vision, confusion, delirium, and coma. Selective antagonists are identified for four of the five subtypes (M_1–M_5) of muscarinic receptors: *pirenzepine* and *telenzepine* (M_1); *gallamine*, *methoctramine*, and *himbacine* (M_2); *hexahydrosiladifenidol* and p-*fluorohexahydrosiladifenidol* (M_3); and *tropicamide* (M_4). Venom from the green mamba (*Dendroaspis* spp.) contains toxins (Mtx1, Mtx2) that bind selectively to muscarinic receptors.

Glutamate/Aspartate

Glutamate is believed to mediate most excitatory synaptic traffic in the adult CNS; aspartate, another nonessential dicarboxylic diaminoacid, is also abundant in brain and may serve as an excitatory neurotransmitter. Agents that directly or indirectly increase excitatory drive, or the postsynaptic effects thereof, may cause degeneration of neurons bearing excitatory amino acid (glutamate) receptors (Fig. 1.5). Excitotoxicity, as the phenomenon is termed, may be mediated by chemicals that increase or perturb the controlled presynaptic release of neurotransmitter, reduce the normal inhibitory input to the target neuron, or compromise the cell's ability to recover from membrane depolarization by interfering with the maintenance of cellular energy or by increasing the concentration or residence time of the neurotransmitter in the synaptic gap. Glutamate released from nerve terminals is taken up by glial cells, converted to glutamine, and probably recycled back to the neuron; these steps provide other sites for chemical perturbation. In addition, various dinoflagellates and plants (certain mushrooms, seaweed, and legumes) elaborate *glutamate analogs* that enter the brain's extracellular compartment, compete with the neurotransmitter for neuronal binding sites, and act as agonists to elicit aberrant excitant effects on targeted neurons. Neurotoxic effects of certain agonists (*kainate*) may be mediated by presynaptic excitation of neurons that are stimulated to release excessive glutamate. Glutamate antagonists block the induction of excitotoxic neuronal degeneration.

CNS glutamate and aspartate must be rigorously controlled to prevent excitant neurotoxicity. Both are nonessential amino acids synthesized in the brain from glucose and other precursors; under normal conditions, circulating amino acids are excluded from the brain by the blood-brain barrier. Areas lacking this regulatory interface, such as the arcuate nucleus of the hypothalamus and retina, show acute neuronal degeneration in immature animals injected with *glutamate*. Humans are widely exposed to purified monosodium glutamate used as a taste enhancer for food. Ex-

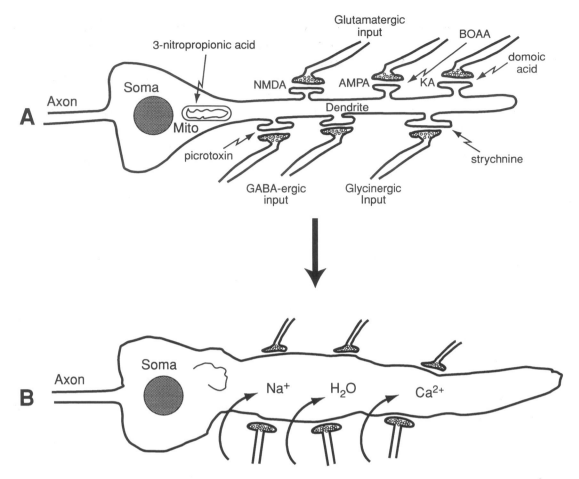

FIGURE 1.5. (A) Glutamate-mediated excitotoxicity occurs when agents act as agonists at glutamate receptors, antagonists at γ-aminobutyric acid or glycine receptors, or mitochondrial toxins. (B) Once energy stores are exhausted, there is uncontrolled influx of cations and water, dendritic and somal swelling, and calcium-stimulated nerve degeneration. *NMDA*: N-Methyl-D-aspartate receptor. *AMPA*: DL-α-Amino-3-hydroxy-5-methyl-4-isoxazole propionic acid receptor. *KA*: Kainate receptor. *Mito*: Mitochondrion. *Jagged arrows* depict sites of toxic action. *BOAA*: β-N-Oxalylamino-L-alanine.

cessive exposure by this route is associated with nausea and a burning sensation over the forearms and nape, with intense pressure over the zygoma and precordium; these manifestations constitute the Chinese restaurant syndrome, a reversible sensory condition possibly associated with PNS glutamate receptors on sensory and autonomic ganglia (which normally lack a blood-nerve barrier). Humans are also widely exposed *via* food to a dipeptide of aspartate and phenylalanine, which serves as the artificial sweetener aspartame. Human illness associated with glutamate- and aspartate-containing substances is contentious. Concern over the possibility of amino-acid excitant neurotoxicity is particularly high for infants and those who may have impaired blood-neural regulatory interfaces from illness, malnutrition, or other causes.

Large concentrations of *free aspartate* and *glutamate*, as well as other substances (notably *sesquiterpenoids*) occur in the yellow star thistle (*Centaurea* spp.), a North American

plant that induces acute-onset extrapyramidal disease in horses, with massive degeneration of the substantia nigra (probably the pars reticulata) and pallidum reminiscent of an acute excitotoxic lesion.

Receptor subtypes. The nature of the glutamate receptor subtype appears to determine in part the selective vulnerability of neurons that receive neuroexcitatory synaptic inputs. Glutamate receptors are classified by their signal transduction mechanism: (a) metabotropic glutamate receptors (mGlu₁–mGlu₈), 871–1199 amino-acid, 7-transmembrane-domain receptors formerly known as mGluRs, which operate through second-messenger systems; and (b) ionotropic glutamate receptors with ligand-gated ion channels that have a high degree of molecular and functional diversity, as demonstrated by studies of recombinant receptors expressed in *Xenopus* oocytes. Details of the structure of ionotropic glutamate receptors and channels are unknown, but three broad subtypes are evident from pharmacological and electrophysiological studies: DL-α-*amino-3-hydroxy-5-methyl-4-isoxazole propionic acid* (AMPA) receptors, *kainic acid* (KA) receptors, and NMDA receptors. Various genes encode components of the multi-subunit receptors activated by NMDA (*nmda1, nmda2A-2D*), kainate (*glu5-glu7, ka1, ka2*), or AMPA. Alternative splicing patterns increase the number of receptor subtypes.

The relationship between the regional distribution of glutamate receptors and susceptibility to neurodegeneration induced by agonists (*NMDA, AMPA, KA*) is well illustrated in the hippocampal formation: NMDA receptors are enriched in the stratum oriens and radiatum of the CA1 region, AMPA receptors are present on CA1 pyramidal cells, and kainate-sensitive regions are found in the CA3 dentate granule-cell projection zone. These agents activate mechanisms leading to acute or subacute neuronal necrosis and, possibly, to apoptotic forms of neuronal degeneration. Levels of agonist-induced excitation insufficient to induce cell degeneration may have other effects because glutamate modulates gene expression of neuronal proteins such as tau (microtubule-associated protein) and the phenomenon of long-term potentiation that may underly encoding of memory.

AMPA receptors. AMPA receptors appear to mediate fast synaptic transmission in the CNS; they are stimulated in order of potency by AMPA > glutamate > kainate. Certain *quinoxalinediones* serve as selective AMPA receptor antagonists in the experimental setting. *Quisqualic acid*, an anthelmintic principle in the fruit of *Quisqualis indica*, is a potent agonist at AMPA and glutamate metabotropic receptors (*vide infra*). Unlike NMDA, *AMPA agonists* induce degeneration of nitric oxide synthase-containing neurons and GABAergic cortical neurons. This may be relevant to the human neurotoxic effects of L-BOAA, a naturally occurring stereospecific AMPA agonist present as a *free* amino acid in the grass pea (*Lathyrus sativus*). L-BOAA induces acute neuronal degeneration in murine cortex cultures, convulsant behavior in rodents, and extensor hindlimb posturing and myoclonus in well-nourished macaques fed subconvulsive doses of the agent for prolonged periods. Humans who employ grass pea as a dietary staple develop spastic paraparesis (lathyrism) associated with pyramidal tract dysfunction. Given that BOAA traverses the blood-brain barrier poorly, that well-nourished individuals consume moderate amounts of grass pea with no adverse effects, and that lathyrism only occurs in the setting of grass pea dependency and poor nourishment, it is likely (but uninvestigated) that the human disease is associated in part by blood-brain barrier leakage (of BOAA) that may accompany malnutrition.

Kainate receptors. Kainate receptors show a different hierarchical agonist potency (kainate > glutamate > AMPA) and are associated with a different pattern of neurotoxicity. *Kainic acid* has been widely employed in neurobiology as an experimental lesioning agent, but human neurotoxicity is not recognized despite the use in the Orient of kainate-containing seaweed (*Digenea simplex*) as a vermifuge. By contrast, the systemic neurotoxicity of *domoic acid* has been studied because of an outbreak of human neurotoxicity in individuals who had consumed mussels contaminated with this algal toxin and kainate analog. Unlike L-BOAA, domoic acid enters the brain readily. Affected subjects experience headache, seizures, hemiparesis, ophthalmoplegia, and abnormalities of arousal ranging from agitation to coma. Survivors display an anterograde memory deficit with preservation of other cognitive functions. Neuropathological studies reveal severe damage to the amygdaloid nucleus and hippocampal subfields H3 and H1, which correspond to the kainate-sensitive hippocampal subfields CA3 and CA1 in rats. Mice treated with domoic acid develop head, forelimb, and whole-body tremors and convulsions associated with extensive hippocampal damage and involvement of other brain regions (amygdala, basal ganglia, thalamus, olfactory cortex, cortical mantle). Regions unprotected by the blood-brain barrier are also markedly affected. A nonneurotoxic (safe) level for human consumption of domoic acid reportedly has been established because of its presence and periodic increased concentration in certain types of seafood (*e.g.*, razor clams) along the west coast of the United States.

NMDA receptors. NMDA receptors are involved in neuronal plasticity and outgrowth as well as neuronal signaling. Glycine serves as a coagonist for the NMDA receptor–channel complex; modulation of channel opening is achieved by polyamines (spermine, spermidine), protons, redox reagents, and Zn^{2+}. The channel is blocked in a voltage-dependent manner by Mg^{2+}, a mechanism used for gating; Co^{2+}, Ni^{2+} and Mn^{2+} also block the channel. NMDA channel permeability is high for Ca^{2+} which, under normal conditions, may transiently activate a range of important intracellular enzymes, including protein kinase C, phospholipase A_2, calmodulin-dependent protein kinase II, and nitric acid synthase. Nitric oxide is proposed to serve as a synapse-specific retrograde messenger to increase neurotransmitter release.

Several NMDA receptor antagonists are known: some act at the NMDA receptor site (*2-amino-5* and *2-amino-7* derivatives of *phosphonopentanoate, 3[(±)-2-carboxypiperazin-4-yl)propyl-1-phosphate*]; others at the glycine allosteric site (D-*serine, 1-amino-cyclopropanecarboxylate; 5,7-di-*

chlorokyneurinic acid) or the polyamine site (*putresine, cadaverine*). Agents that antagonize NMDA (and glutamate) bind to the open ion channel: Exogenous voltage-dependent blockers of the NMDA ion channel include *ketamine*, (+)-*5-methyl-10,11-dihydro-5H-dibenzo[α,δ]cyclohepten-5,10-iminemaleate* (*MK801*) and *phencyclidine* (*PCP*). PCP binds to cortical and limbic NMDA receptor channels, but also impacts other neurotransmitter systems, including the nicotinic acetylcholine receptor where it acts as an allosteric antagonist. Small doses of PCP (*angel dust*) produce a sense of intoxication, staggering gait, slurred speech, nystagmus, extremity numbness, sweating, catatonic muscular rigidity, a blank stare, disorganized thoughts, drowsiness, and apathy. Intoxication with PCP of unknown purity may trigger aggression, confusion, delirium, paranoia, coma, a prolonged schizophrenic-like syndrome, convulsions, and death.

NMDA and AMPA receptors are present on most CNS neurons and may be stimulated simultaneously because they are sited together in the same postsynaptic density. Activation of both receptors increases plasmalemmal channel permeability to Na^+ and K^+; ion entry depolarizes the cell, generates current flow, and initiates an action potential. Excessive receptor stimulation results in repetitive firing that eventuates in seizures. Antagonism of AMPA receptors blocks seizure initiation; NMDA receptor antagonists reduce the intensity and duration of seizures. If Na^+ and K^+ influx is not balanced by energy-dependent cation efflux, either because of excessive receptor stimulation or failure of the plasmalemma-bound Na^+/K^+-ATPase ion pump, water will flow down the osmotic gradient and rapidly induce postsynaptic edema in dendrites and neurons bearing AMPA/NMDA receptors (Fig. 1.5). The associated uncontrolled influx of Ca^{2+}, coupled with failure of intracellular Ca^{2+}-sequestration mechanisms, will activate Ca^{2+}-dependent mechanisms (including proteases) and amplify neuronal injury or induce cell death. This is associated with failure of mitochondrial respiration and increased generation of free radicals.

Termination of excitatory neurotransmission by removal of glutamate from the synaptic gap is effected by an astroglial glutamate transport system. Perturbation of this system (*dithiocarbamate pesticides, in vitro*) should lead to an increase in concentration or residence time of synaptic glutamate, and thus potentially to excitotoxicity and neuronal degeneration. This mechanism has been proposed to participate in the pathogenesis of some forms of motor neuron disease (ALS). L-*BOAA* inhibits glutamate and aspartate transport in brain synaptosomes, a mechanism that may serve to increase the human motor neuronotoxicity (lathyrism) of this amino acid (*vide supra*).

Cellular energy state. Ionotropic glutamate receptors also play an important role in mediating neuronal cell death from energy deficits, whether ATP decrements are induced by alterations in respiratory gases (*hypoxia, hypercapnia*) or through the chemical inhibition of energy transformation. Neurotoxic agents in the latter class in particular include those that disrupt the mitochondrial electron transport chain, whether at complex I (*MPP*$^+$), complex II (*3-nitropropionic acid*), or complex IV (*carbon monoxide, cyanide*). Deprivation of energy stores in neuronal and glial cells promotes acidosis, the formation of free radicals, cell depolarization, and the release of glutamate from synaptic terminals and, possibly, larger amounts from astrocytes. Wholesale neuronal destruction may then ensue in regions receiving glutamatergic inputs, such as the hippocampus and striatum. A dramatic example of this phenomenon is the bilateral putaminal necrosis [visible by computed tomography (CT)] seen in children exhibiting profound generalized dystonia following intoxication with the mycotoxin *3-nitropropionic acid*. In experimental brain ischemia, the administration of glutamate-receptor antagonists prior to or even several hours following the insult dramatically attenuates the degree of neuronal destruction. Similarly, glutamate antagonists and agents that inhibit nitric oxide synthase attenuate or block MPTP-induced neuronal degeneration. *These observations demonstrate vividly the potential of endogenous glutamate to change from a key mediator of orderly communication within the CNS to an agent capable of widespread tissue destruction.*

Metabotropic receptors. The pharmacologically defined L-*2-amino-4-phosphonopropionic acid* (*L-AP4*) and trans-*1-amino-1,3-cyclopentanedicarboxylate* (*APDC*) metabotropic glutamate receptors are coupled through G proteins to intracellular effectors. Metabotropic receptors stimulate, in different cell types, increases in the concentration of intracellular Ca^{2+} mediated by phosphoinositide hydrolysis, phospholipase D-activated release of arachidonic acid, and changes in cAMP. Region-specific changes in excitability may follow metabotropic activation, apparently through modulation of both excitatory and inhibitory neurotransmission.

The APDC metabotropic receptor, which may serve to potentiate currents through NMDA receptors, is activated by glutamate and by the plant neurotoxins *quisqualate* and *ibotenate*. Ibotenate, together with its decarboxylation product *muscimol* (a CNS inhibitory GABA$_A$ agonist), form the active principles of fly agaric (*Amanita muscaria*), a mushroom once used as an intoxicant by tribes of the Kamchatkan peninsula of Siberia. Ingestion is followed by an initial state of excitement and myoclonus (glutamate-receptor mediated neuroexcitation?) and, subsequently, by depression and loss of consciousness (GABA-mediated CNS depression?).

β-N-*Methylamino-L-alanine* (*L-BMAA*), a minor neurotoxin of certain cycad plants (*Cycas* spp.), is an agonist at metabotropic and ionotropic receptors in the presence of physiological concentrations of bicarbonate. Oral administration of L-BMAA to macaques induces motor neuronal degeneration accompanied by behavioral changes, pyramidal and lower motor neuron dysfunction, and L-dopa–sensitive extrapyramidal signs. Another cycad toxin, *cycasin*, damages neuronal DNA and inhibits DNA repair (apurinic apyrimidinic endonuclease activity) in association with glutamate-stimulated modulation of the mRNA for tau, a microtubule-associated protein found in the paired helical filaments that accumulate in the neurofibrillary tangles of cycad-related Guam ALS/PD complex. Exposure to cycasin is thus hypothesized to alter the neuronal response to endogenous glutamate and thereby to elicit a slowly progressive neuronal degeneration (*vide supra*).

GABA

GABA, the major inhibitory neurotransmitter in mammalian brain, is synthesized from glutamic acid (*via* GAD), released from nerve terminals in a Ca^{2+}-dependent manner, removed by transport systems in presynaptic terminals and glial cells, and degraded by 4-aminobutyrate-2-oxoglutarate aminotransferase. Inhibition of GAD (*2-amino-4-pentenoic acid*) induces convulsions, and inhibition of the aminotransferase exerts an anticonvulsant action. The GABA transaminase inhibitor and anticonvulsant *vigabatrin* (*γ-vinyl-GABA*) induces arousal and behavioral disorders in treated subjects.

GABA$_A$ receptors mediate fast inhibitory postsynaptic potentials that are activated by Cl^- conductance and antagonized competitively by *bicuculline*; GABA$_B$ receptors, which are insensitive to bicuculline, are located both at presynaptic and postsynaptic sites. The GABA$_A$ receptor is a heteropentameric glycoprotein (~275 kDa) composed of multiple α-, β-, γ-, δ-, and ρ- (localized to retina) subunits, with different subunit combinations present in different neurons; together they form part of a receptor–ionophore complex with a Cl^- channel. Binding sites are present for GABA, *benzodiazepines, barbiturates, anesthetic steroids*, and *picrotoxin*. Pharmacological studies show that GABA$_A$ receptor activity is modulated by chemicals acting at (a) the competitive site as selective agonists (*isoguvacine, muscimol*) or selective antagonists (*bicuculline*), or (b) the benzodiazepine modulatory site as selective agonists (*zolpidem, flunitrazepam*), inverse agonists (*methyl-6,7-dimethoxy-4-*

ethyl-β-carboline-3-carboxylate), or selective antagonists (*flumazenil, 5-isopropoxy-4-methyl-β-carboline-3-carboxylate ethyl ester*). Other agents that antagonize GABAergic transmission at sites distinct from the amino-acid recognition site include *penicillin G, pentylenetetrazole, several bicyclophosphates*, and *picrotoxin*. Binding sites for picrotoxin and t-butylbicyclophosphorothionate appear to be closely associated with the Cl^- channel. Certain divalent metals ions, notably Zn^{2+}, but also Cd^{2+}, Ni^{2+}, Mn^{2+} and Co^{2+}, inhibit the response of neurons to GABA in some organisms.

Benzodiazepines enhance GABAergic transmission and thereby act pharmacologically as sedatives, anticonvulsants, and anxiolytics. They represent some of the most widely prescribed medications, including *diazepam* (*Valium*) and *chlordiazepoxide*. Neurotoxicity of *benzodiazepine drugs* is featured by drowsiness, somnolence, fatigue, and lethargy; muscular incoordination, hypotonia, dysarthria, dizziness, and behavioral disturbances (hyperactivity, aggression) may also occur. Another important class of CNS-depressant drugs, the anticonvulsant barbiturates, directly activate the GABA$_A$ receptor at high concentrations. Anticonvulsant barbiturates (*phenobarbital*) elicit a wide range of effects, from mild sedation to general anesthesia, while in some subjects paradoxical excitement may occur. Repeated administration results in biological tolerance and the use of increasingly large doses. Toxicity is featured by distortion of mood, judgment, and motor skills; coma; reduced breathing; loss of blood pressure; shock; hypothermia; and death.

The CNS-depressant effects of the anticonvulsant barbiturate and benzodiazepine drugs stand in marked contrast to the convulsant properties of the GABA$_A$ antagonist and polycyclic lactone picrotoxin. Isolated from a climbing shrub indigenous to Indonesia (*Anamirta cocculus*), picrotoxin consists of two compounds, *picrotin* and *picrotoxinin*; the latter powerfully stimulates the CNS and elicits widespread seizure activity. Once used as an insecticide, the incapacitating effects of picrotoxin (from bruised berries) also have been exploited to catch fish. Certain barbiturates [*1-methyl-5-(phenyl-5-propyl)-5-ethylbarbituric acid*] may interact with the picrotoxin-binding site and exert convulsant effects. The convulsant effects of *penicillin* result from its antagonistic action on GABA-mediated neurotransmission.

A number of organochlorine insecticides exert convulsant effects that are probably mediated through the picrotoxin-binding site of the GABA$_A$ receptor. These agents include the γ-*isomer of hexachlorocyclohexane* (*lindane*), *toxaphene*, and the chlorinated cyclodiene compounds *aldrin, dieldrin, endrin*, and *endosulfan*. Clinical effects of intoxication include tremor and seizures. Several mycotoxins with tremorgenic properties bind close to the chloride channel of the GABA$_A$ receptor. Type II (α-*cyanophenoxybenzyl*) pyrethroids also affect the GABA$_A$ receptor complex and induce convulsions in vertebrates, but their primary target is the Na$^+$ channel of excitable membranes (*vide supra*). *Avermectin*, an insecticidal and anthelmintic macrocyclic lactone, also binds to the GABA$_A$ receptor complex and, depending on prevailing experimental conditions, either stimulates or inhibits the binding of GABA to its receptor (*vide supra*).

GABA$_B$ (bicuculline-insensitive) receptors operate in a modulatory fashion: stimulation of presynaptic GABA$_B$ receptors influences the release of GABA and other neurotransmitters, and postsynaptic GABA$_B$ receptors (which mediate late inhibitory postsynaptic potentials) are indirectly coupled to K$^+$ channels through G proteins. Selective agonists include β-4-*chlorophenyl-GABA* (*baclofen*), a spasmolytic drug with toxic effects that include drowsiness, insomnia, dizziness, weakness, and mental confusion, with auditory and visual hallucinations following withdrawal from chronic usage. 2-*Hydroxysaclofen* is an antagonist at the GABA$_B$ receptor.

Glycine

Glycine is another CNS inhibitory amino acid neurotransmitter, notably in the brainstem and spinal cord where it is employed by interneurons to depress the firing of motoneurons regulating antagonist muscles. Glycinergic synapses are also prominent in spinal sensory, auditory, and visual pathways. Glycine is synthesized from serine, a reaction catalyzed by serine hydroxymethyltransferase, released presynaptically in a Ca^{2+}-dependent manner and, in spinal cord, removed by a high-affinity synaptosomal transport system. The postsynaptic strychnine-sensitive glycine receptor consists of a 48 kDa ligand-binding α-subunit (four identified isoforms) and a 58 kDa β-subunit (two isoforms), each of which has four transmembrane domains. Glycine binds to the α-subunit (four identified isoforms) and a 58 kDa β-subunit (two isoforms), each of which has four transmembrane domains. Glycine binding to the α-subunit induces changes in receptor conformation that lead to the opening of an ion channel for Cl$^-$. Receptor activation by endogenous agonists (glycine > β-alanine > taurine) increases Cl$^-$ conductance and hyperpolarizes the neuron.

Glycine antagonists, most of which are of neurotoxicological interest, reduce the inhibitory drive and thereby abnormally promote the activity of motor and other neurons. *Strychnine*, an indol alkaloid found in trees of the *Strychnos* genus, notably *S. nux vomica* L., binds with high affinity to the glycine receptor, blocks inhibition at glycinergic synapses, and elicits hyperreflexia; tetanic muscle contraction with opisthotonus, and alterations in tactile, auditory, vestibular, and visual function. Strychnine analogs (α-*colubrine*, 2-*aminostrychnine*) and synthetic fragments (β-*spirpyrrolidinoindolines*) retain glycine-receptor affinity and convulsant properties. The anthelmintic drug *avermectin* B$_{1a}$ noncompetitively inhibits ^{3}H-strychnine binding to the glycine receptor.

Several plant alkaloids block glycine receptors, including *gelsemine* (yellow jasmine convulsant), *hydrastine* (*Hydrastis canadensis*), *vincamine, boldine, laudanosine,* and *dendrobine. Morphine* and other alkaloids bind to the glycine receptor with low affinity. Certain muscimol analogues, such as the 5-*isoxazolols*, bind to the glycine receptor complex.

Synthetic glycine receptor antagonists and convulsants include 1,5-*diphenyl-3,7-diazaadamantan-9-ol* and 3α-*hydroxy-16-imino-5β-17-azandrostan-11-one*.

Tetanus toxin (*Clostridium tetani*) inhibits the Ca^{2+}-dependent release of neurotransmitters in the order of glycine > GABA > D-aspartate > acetylcholine. The light chain is retrogradely transported in the axons of lower motor neurons, where the toxin apparently crosses the synaptic cleft and binds to glycinergic inhibitory terminals. The toxin acts to reduce the presynaptic release of glycine, thereby serving to disinhibit α- and γ-motoneurons. Afferent stimuli arising from the periphery trigger glycine-undamped motor trains causing generalized muscle rigidity and painful muscle spasms; the latter may involve muscles of the jaw ("lockjaw"), face (*risus sardonicus*), larynx, abdomen, and back, as well as the muscles of respiration.

Catecholamines

Norepinephrine and its precursor dopamine serve as CNS neurotransmitters, and norepinephrine is the principal postganglionic sympathetic neurotransmitter in the autonomic component of the PNS. The *N*-methylated form of norepinephrine, epinephrine, is an adrenal hormone; small amounts are also found in the brain, particularly in the brainstem.

Biosynthesis of catecholamines commences with L-tyrosine which, under the catalytic influence of neuron cytosolic tyrosine hydroxylase (rate-limiting enzyme), is converted to 3,4-dihydroxy-L-phenylalanine (L-dopa). L-Dopa decarboxylase, a pyridoxine-dependent enzyme, catalyzes the removal of the carboxyl group from L-dopa to form dopamine. Dopamine β-hydrolase, which is inhibited by α-*methyldopa* and by copper chelators (*diethyldithiocarbamate*), catalyzes the conversion of dopamine to norepinephrine; these are individually packaged in synaptic vesicles and released from nerve terminals by a Ca^{2+}-dependent mechanism. Inactivation of catecholamines is the responsibility of catechol-O-methyltransferase and monoamine oxidase (MAO). MAO, a neuronal and glial enzyme that is located on the outer mitochondrial membrane and serves to cleave free cytosolic catecholamines, exists in two isoforms: MAO-A, which preferentially deaminates norepinephrine and serotonin, is selectively inhibited by *chlorgyline*; MAO-B, which has less specificity, is inhibited selectively by *deprenyl*. *Myristicin*, the active principle in nutmeg (*Myristica* spp.), inhibits MAO activity. Because chemical MAO inhibitors also depress enzyme activity of liver and gastrointestinal MAO, which serves to break down amines derived from food, subjects treated with these agents may develop hypertensive crises after ingestion of *tyramine-rich substances* (red wine, herring, blue cheese). Vasoconstrictor (pressor) amines are also found in pineapple, banana, plaintain, avocado, fava bean, wheat, oats, nuts, and tomatoes. The second catecholamine-inactivating enzyme, catechol-O-methyltransferase, catalyzes breakdown of extracellular catecholamines that have not been captured by reuptake into synaptic terminals. The reuptake system for dopamine and norepinephrine employs distinct putative 12-transmembrane Na^+/Cl^- plasmalemmal transporters. Na^+ channel openers, such as *veratridine*, and Na^+, K^+-ATPase inhibitors like *ouabain*, inhibit catecholamine transport. *Tricyclic antidepressants* and *benzoylmethylecgonine* (*i.e.*, *cocaine* from *Erythroxylon coca*) inhibit catecholamine transport, and *amphetamines* bind to the carrier and compete for transport. *Nomifensine* and *mazindol* are selective inhibitors of the dopamine transporter. *6-Hydroxydopamine* and *MPP⁺*, which destroy dopaminergic neurons, enter these cells selectively *via* the dopamine-transporter system.

Dopamine. Dopamine is the neurotransmitter stored and released by nerve terminals of several key CNS pathways. The large majority of dopamine is found in the corpus striatum (caudate nucleus and putamen) in association with terminals of axons arising from the zona compacta of the substantia nigra in the brainstem. Neurons of the nigrostriatal pathway, a key component of basal ganglia mechanisms that control the quality of motor function, undergo degeneration in Parkinson's disease and display neurofibrillary tangles in the Guam ALS/PD complex, which appears to have an environmental trigger (*vide supra*). Other dopaminergic neurons include: (a) mesocortical, originating medial to the substantia nigra and innervating frontal and cingulate cortex, septum, nucleus accumbens, and olfactory tubercle—*neuroleptic antipsychotics* may block the effects

of dopamine released by this system and induce movement disorders, and (b) tuberohypophysial, originating in the arcuate and periventricular nuclei of the hypothalamus and innervating the median eminence and pituitary, where it regulates hormonal (prolactin) release.

Human dopamine receptors form a family of at least six types of G-protein-coupled receptors. They are composed of peptides containing 387-477 amino acids and 7 transmembrane domains. The dopamine 1 receptor family, which includes receptors D_1 and D_5, are coupled to a G protein that activates adenylyl cyclase; they are expressed in cortex and hippocampus and have a low affinity for most antipsychotic drugs. The dopamine 2 receptor family includes receptors D_{2a} and D_{2b}; these are located in the caudate, have a high affinity for antipsychotics (*phenothiazines*, *butyrophenones*), and are implicated in the development of the extrapyramidal side effects of these drugs. D_3 and D_4 are found in the limbic system and cerebral cortex and, to a lesser extent, the basal ganglia. *Clozapine*, which binds to D_3 and D_4 receptors, does not cause extrapyramidal side effects.

Increased density of striatal D_2 receptors accompanies chronic administration of D_2 antagonists and striatal lesions (*denervation supersensitivity*). This phenomenon may possibly be associated with drug-induced tardive dyskinesia, one of the most debilitating and widespread of drug-induced neurotoxicities. Drug-induced GABA depletion is another of several mechanisms that has been advanced to account for this illness. First recorded 50 years ago, when antipsychotic therapy became widely available, tardive dyskinesia is featured by involuntary, repetitive lip-smacking, lip-pursing, tongue protrusion, and licking and chewing movements with or without involvement of dyskinetic movements of truncal and limb muscles. Prevalence of tardive dyskinesia with chronic neuroleptic therapy is high (20%), reversibility is variable, may be slow, and sometimes is irreversible. A possibly related persistent neuroleptic-induced disorder, tardive dystonia, is characterized by involuntary movements of cranial and/or cervical musculature, with retrocollis and incomplete opisthotonus. Dystonia with involvement of limbs (choreoathetosis, hemiballismus) is found in children with putaminal and other basal ganglia lesions following recovery from acute intoxication with sugar cane contaminated with *Arthrinium* spp. which elaborates the mitochondrial complex II toxin *3-nitropropionic acid*. Acute, tardive, reversible or persistent akathisia—a subjective sense of inner restlessness and inability to remain still—coupled with motor manifestations linked to the urge to move, is the most common movement disorder associated with *dopamine antagonists* acting either as receptor blockers or presynaptic dopamine depletors.

These drugs and *certain Ca^{2+}-channel antagonists* may also provoke the development of a slowly (weeks to months) reversible parkinsonism that may be heralded by akathisia. The neuroleptic malignant syndrome is a dangerous and unpredictable consequence of therapy characterized by extreme rigidity, fever, autonomic disturbances, and depressed or fluctuating consciousness developing over a period of days and terminating in death.

- *MPTP* depletes dopamine in the caudate and putamen, destroys neurons in the substantia nigra, and induces parkinsonism in humans and primates and motor-system dysfunction in other animals. Humans exposed to MPTP as a contaminant of a synthetic *meperidine* (opiate) analog used to induce euphoria developed parkinsonism within weeks of exposure and at a remarkably young age. Other MPTP-exposed subjects were clinically intact but showed evidence of depressed striatal fluorodopa uptake by positron emission tomography. MPTP is metabolized principally to MPP$^+$ by monoamine oxidase B (astrocytic); MPP$^+$ is transported by the dopamine transporter into the axon/neuron where it inhibits NADH:ubiquinone oxidoreductase. Depending on species, age, and dose, the following neurotoxic effects occur: reversible pharmacological dopamine deficit; retrograde nigrostriatal axonal degeneration; neuronal degeneration. Experiments with *MPTP analogues* (*see also* β-Carbolines/Isoquinolines in A–Z section) suggest the N-methyl group is essential for neurotoxicity; alkyl substitution results in a substantial reduction (ethyl) or loss (propyl) of activity.

Norepinephrine. Noradrenergic neurons, which cluster in the medulla oblongata, pons, and midbrain, form two complementary and overlapping projection systems. In rats, the ventral system originates in the dorsal medullary solitarian and lateral tegmental cell groups, where it projects to the hypothalamus, preoptic nuclei, lateral septum, and periventricular thalamus. The more extensive dorsal system is centered in the locus ceruleus and subependymal areas of the brainstem, with projections throughout the brain. The dorsal system is much more sensitive to the toxic actions of *6-hydroxydopamine*, an agent that is toxic to both noradrenergic and dopaminergic neurons.

Norepinephrine and epinephrine receptors are found in brain and peripheral tissues, and norepinephrine is the neurotransmitter of postsynaptic sympathetic axons that innervate visceral structures of the thorax, abdomen (glands and smooth muscle), head, and neck (vasomotor, pupillodilator, secretory, pilomotor). Each effector organ (eye, heart, arterioles, lung, stomach, intestine, kidney, bladder, ureter, uterus, male sex organ, skin, spleen, adrenal medulla, skeletal muscle, liver, pancreas, fat cells, salivary and lacrimal glands, pineal gland, posterior pituitary) is equipped with varied single or multiple combinations of α- and β-adrenoreceptor subtypes that differentially modulate organ function *via* G-protein-coupled activation mediated by a variety of biochemical effectors (Ca^{2+} or K$^+$ channels, phospholipases, adenylyl cyclase). Six human α-adrenoreceptors (450–466 amino acids, 7TM) coded by genes on six different chromosomes have been identified; five are found in the cerebral cortex and one (α2A), which is found in the brain and spinal cord, serves as a presynaptic autoreceptor. β-Adrenoreceptors, of which three are known, regulate function of heart, smooth muscles, hepatic glycogenolysis, and adipose lipolysis. β-*Adrenergic receptor antagonists* (β-*blockers*) are used to treat hypertension, ischemic heart disease, and certain arrhythmias. CNS effects of β-blockers include fatigue, sleep disturbances, and depression; peripheral vasoconstriction may occur, and adverse effects on cardiac (bradyarrhythmia, congestive heart failure) and pulmonary function are recognized.

Chemical-induced perturbation of adrenergic function may occur at many levels. α-*Methyltyrosine* interferes with transmitter synthesis and depletes norepinephrine. *Methyldopa* serves as a false transmitter at adrenergic synapses. *Reserpine* blocks vesicular uptake of amines and causes prolonged adrenergic blockade. *Bretylium* and *guanethidine* prevent stimulated release of norepinephrine. *Tyramine* and *amphetamine* promote transmitter release, and *clonidine* mimics the effect of the transmitter at postsynaptic receptors; all have sympathomimetic effects (*vide infra*). *Phenoxybenzamine* and *propranolol* block the action of the endogenous transmitter at postsynaptic α- and certain β-adrenergic receptors, respectively. *Pyrogallol* and *tropolone* inhibit the norepinephrine-cleavage enzyme catechol-O-methyltransferase and enhance the action of catecholamines. *Pargyline* and *tranylcypromine* inhibit MAO-induced amine cleavage and potentiate the toxic effects of tyramine.

Prolonged administration of *amphetamines* to animals produces long-lasting depression of brain norepinephrine, as well as long-lasting effects on dopaminergic and serotonergic function. Changes in cerebral blood vessels with microhemorrhages and neuronal loss are described in monkeys. Arteriolar damage and intracranial hemorrhage, hyperpyrexia, and convulsions occur in human amphetamine toxicity. *Amphetamine withdrawal* is associated with dysphoria, fatigue, anhedonia, severe depression, and anxiety disorder.

Serotonin

The indolealkylamine serotonin (5-hydroxytryptamine) serves as an effector for smooth muscle in the gastrointestinal and cardiovascular systems, an agent that promotes platelet aggregation, and a CNS neurotransmitter. The entire rat brain is supplied with serotonergic axons that originate in groups of cells in the dorsal and median raphe nuclei (and lateral extensions therefrom) and provide overlapping afferent innervation throughout the brain and spinal cord. Two main pathways project to the forebrain: the neocortex is provided with innervation from the two systems, while basal ganglia receive input predominately from dorsal raphe and hippocampus, and limbic structures from ventral raphe. Serotonergic pathways appear to have significant roles in the regulation of affect, mood, perception, and cognition. The retina also contains serotonergic fibers.

Serotonin is synthesized in the brain from L-tryptophan; increased dietary tryptophan positively modulates serotonin brain levels. Tryptophan is converted in serotonergic neurons to 5-hydroxytryptophan and, with the catalytic activity of aromatic amino acid decarboxylase (also converts dopamine to dopa), to serotonin. Initial hydroxylation is rate-limiting and irreversibly inhibited by p-*chlorophenylalanine* and p-*propyldopaectamide*. Storage of serotonin in synaptic vesicles is disrupted by *reserpine* and *tetrabenazine*. Serotonin is released by a Ca^{2+}-stimulated exocytosis mechanism at conventional synapses (neurotransmitter function) and in regions lacking synaptic specialization (neuromodulator function). Raphe neurons and terminals contain serotonin autoreceptors that regulate the somal firing rate and terminal release of serotonin, respectively. Serotonin removal from the extracellular fluid (reuptake) utilizes an energy and Na^+/Cl^--dependent transporter that is partly homologous with dopamine and norepinephrine transporters. *Fluoxetine* and *sertraline*, which compete with and inhibit serotonin uptake, serve as antidepressants. MAO converts intracellular serotonin to 5-hydroxyindoleacetaldehyde, and this is oxidized to 5-hydroxyindoleacetic acid. *Chlorgyline*, a selective inhibitor of MAO-A, raises the level of serotonin in rat brain.

Free serotonin in concentrations of 6%–10% occurs in seed of the West African legume *Griffonia simplicifolia*, used in native medicine. Serotonin toxicity in dogs and rats is said to be associated with tremor, pupillary dilatation, apparent blindness, loss of the pupillary reflex, marked hypernea, and tachycardia.

5,7-Hydroxytryptamine inhibits serotonin uptake, is transported into serotonergic neurons and causes marked damage of axons derived from both median and dorsal raphe systems. Substituted amphetamines, such as p-*chloroamphetamine*, *methylenedioxyamphetamine* (MDA), and *3,4-methylenedioxymethamphetamine* (MDMA), preferentially damage axons derived from the dorsal raphe serotonergic projection system of rodents and primates.

- *MDMA*. MDMA (*ecstasy*, *Adam*), 3,4-methylenedioxyethylamphetamine (*Eve*), 2,5-oxy-4-bromo-amphetamine and other substituted methamphetamines produce subjective effects comparable to those of *amphetamine* and *lysergic acid diethylamide* (*LSD*). Acute reactions include panic, paranoia, loss of reality, and hallucinations. Persistent adverse effects include anxiety, depression, flashbacks, irritability, panic disorder, psychosis, and memory disturbance.

- *Khat*. Khat, which is prepared from the fresh leaves of *Catha edulis*, is widely used as a stimulant in East Africa, the Middle East, and Australasia. The active agent, *cathinone* (*S-2-amino-1-phenyl-1-propanone*), has most of the CNS and peripheral actions of amphetamine and, at high doses, can induce psychosis. *Methcathinone* (*CAT*, *goob*, *crank*), primarily the S(−) enatiomer, is a synthetic street drug with actions similar to those of *cathinone*. Methcathinone has the potential to damage 5-HT and dopaminergic neurons; neurotoxicity is enatiomer- and species-dependent.

Neuropeptides

Neuropeptides released at CNS and PNS synapses function as neurotransmitters or neuromodulators. Tens of biologically active peptides are recognized. Since peptides are synthesized in the nerve cell body, packaged in secretory granules, and transported peripherally to sites of release, their normal trafficking is vulnerable to agents (*colchicine*) that block fast axonal transport. Once the peptide has arrived at the nerve terminal, it may be released into the extracellular space by exocytosis and extrusion of the secretory granule. As with other neurotransmitter systems, this is stimulated by an influx of Ca^{2+} into the nerve terminal triggered by the membrane-depolarizing effect of the arrival of a propagated action potential. Termination of neurotransmission is effected by cessation of peptide release, diffusion of the neurotransmitter from its receptor, and proteolysis by exopeptidases, which remove terminal amino acids or dipeptides, or by endopeptidases, which cleave internal peptide bonds. Neurotransmitter inactivation by reuptake of neuropeptide by the nerve terminal, or its removal by transport into a glial cell, has not been demonstrated.

Many peptides are involved in autonomic function and neurotransmission. Vasoactive intestinal peptide and neuropeptide Y, along with ATP, serve as synaptic transmitters or cotransmitters with norepinephrine. Neuropeptide Y is linked to food and water intake, central autonomic control, and regulation of mood.

Opioid peptides and orphanin-FQ. Opioid peptides are the products of three distinct proteins: preproopiomelanocortin produced by the intermediate lobe of the pituitary gland, proenkephalin, and prodynorphin. These precursors are cleaved enzymatically in peptidergic neurons to form the specific opioids used as neurotransmitters. Neurons that release opioids (β-endorphin, enkephalins, dynorphins) are found throughout the CNS. β-Endorphin-containing axons project to many areas of the brain from the arcuate nucleus of the hypothalamus and the solitarius nucleus in the medulla oblongata. Enkephalins are found in areas subserving pain perception (spinal cord lamina I and II, periaqueductal gray, periventricular gray, raphe nucleus), movement, mood and behavior (globus pallidus, stria terminalis, locus ceruleus), and the regulation of neuroendocrine function (median eminence); they also occur in nerve plexuses regulating bowel motility. Dynorphins are concentrated in the hypothalamus, posterior pituitary, amygdala, septum, spinal cord, midbrain, and striatum, with lower levels in hippocampus, thalamus, and pons.

With the exception of the enkephalins, the distribution of opioid axons and terminals correlates poorly with that of their putative receptors (μ, δ, and κ). Human opioid receptors are 400 (μ), 372 (δ) and 380 (κ) amino-acid polypeptides with 7 transmembrane domains and act through G-protein-coupled systems. Receptor subtypes have been proposed. μ-Opioid receptors are involved in *opioid*-induced supraspinal analgesia, euphoria, and chemical dependence. *Sufentanil* is a selective agonist for μ-opioid receptors, *morphine* is a partial agonist, and the opioid-receptor antagonists *naloxone* and *naltrexone* are weakly selective for μ-opioid receptors.

The functional effects of opioid peptides are essentially those of the plant alkaloid (*opium*) from which their name is derived. Opium, which is isolated from the air-dried milky exudate of *Papaver somniferum* (literally, poppy that induces sleep), induces CNS stimulation and then depression, and serves as a hypnotic and narcotic. More than 20 different alkaloids have been obtained from opium and its extracts; these include the benzylisoquinolines (*papaverine* and *noscapine*) and the phanthrenes (*morphine, codeine,* and *thebaine*). Opioid peptides modulate hormone levels and release of neurotransmitters (substance P, acetylcholine, dopamine); participate in CNS-immune system interactions; contribute to memory functions; and are involved in stress mechanisms, pain perception, temperature control, diuresis, and cardiovascular and other peripheral functions. Termination of opioid function is accomplished by extracellular cleavage of the opioid to inactive peptide fragments by the membrane-bound enzyme metalloendopeptidase. Inhibitors of this enzyme (*thiorphan, acetorphan, phosphoroamidon*) potentiate the antinociceptive effects of enkephalins.

γ-*Hydroxybutyrate* (γ-HB), a CNS depressant approved as an anesthetic in some countries but clandestinely used in the United States as a "date-rape" drug, increases brain dopamine levels and has effects through the endogenous opioid system. Acute γ-HB toxicity is associated with coma, seizures, respiratory depression, and vomiting, amnesia and hypotonia.

Morphine-binding sites are present in high concentration in the limbic system, thalamus, striatum, hypothalamus, midbrain, and spinal cord. *Morphine* and related *opioid agonists* produce analgesia, drowsiness, mood changes, mental clouding, respiratory depression, gastrointestinal spasm, and physical dependence. Toxic doses induce convulsions. All of these effects are antagonized by *naloxone* and related morphine antagonists. *Opioid withdrawal syndromes* vary in duration and intensity; administration of *naloxone* induces abrupt withdrawal from methadone in association with displacement of the opioid ligand from its receptor. Withdrawal symptoms include dysphoria, irritability, restlessness, achiness, piloerection ("cold turkey"), hot and cold flashes, muscle twitching, and lower-extremity movements ("kicking the habit").

Related in sequence homology to the cloned opioid receptors is a newly identified and widely distributed CNS receptor, the orphanin-FQ receptor, the natural ligand (orphanin-FQ) of which was previously named nociceptin for its antianalgesic properties. The receptor is also implicated in stress responses. *Etorphine* is a selective agonist.

Substance P and related neuropeptides. Substance P, an 11 amino-acid peptide, is widely distributed in the central, motor, autonomic, and enteric nervous systems, but is of special interest in relation to primary sensory neurons that (a) elaborate small-diameter afferent axons subserving pain, and (b) are sensitive to *capsaicin*, the pungent ingredient of red peppers of the genus *Capsicum*. Capsaicin consists of a vanillyl group (4-hydroxy-3-methoxy-benzyl) connected at the C-1 position *via* an acrylamide group to an alkyl chain. When applied to skin or nerves, capsaicin more or less selectively stimulates primary afferent C and Aδ fibers, which gives rise to sensations of pain (nociception) and activates avoidance reactions.

Capsaicin has selective neuronotoxic effects in mammalian dorsal root and cranial sensory ganglia (*vide infra*). In cultured sensory neurons, capsaicin activates the vanilloid receptor to open a unique, nonselective cation channel that promotes a Na^+ and Ca^{2+}-mediated inward current coupled with an efflux of K^+. Cl^- passively follows the influx of

Na^+, thereby leading to increased intracellular osmolality. Neuronal Ca^{2+} influx is largely restricted to small sensory neurons and does not occur in the larger nerve cells of dorsal root ganglia or sympathetic neurons. Ca^{2+} uptake, which stimulates the release of neuropeptide neurotransmitters, is blocked by *ruthenium red* but not by conventional Ca^{2+}*-channel inhibitors*.

The mechanism underlying the neurodegenerative action of capsaicin and its potent analog, *resiniferatoxin*, is analogous to glutamate neurotoxicity (*vide supra*). Capsaicin promotes the intracellular influx of NaCl, which has osmolar effects expressed neuropathologically in the form of cytoplasmic swelling. In addition, there is a massive influx of Ca^{2+} which, if not sequestered, activates Ca^{2+}-sensitive proteases and other cell-destructive mechanisms. Unlike glutamate excitotoxicity, which is largely mediated by synaptic ionotropic receptors and produces axon-sparing neuronal degeneration, capsaicin receptors appear to be present in both perikaryal and axonal regions of nociceptive sensory neurons. Capsaicin is therefore able to induce degeneration of both axons and somata of susceptible nerve cells.

Cannabinoid Receptors

Two types of cannabinoid (CB) receptors are recognized: human CB_1 contains 472 amino acids, CB_2, 360 amino acids; both have 7 transmembrane domains and are G-protein–coupled receptors that act to inhibit the activation of adenylate cyclase. *Arachidonyl ethanolamide* (*anandamide*) serves as the endogenous ligand. Cannabinoid receptors are present in the hippocampus, cerebellum, basal ganglia, and hypothalamus.

Cannabis sativa (Indian hemp) generates a number of bioactive substances (*cannabis*) that are very widely employed for their psychoactive properties. *Δ-9-Tetrahydrocannabinol* (*THC*) is the primary psychoactive ingredient. Cannabinoids inhibit adenylate cyclase activity and have effects on perception and memory (hippocampus), coordination (cerebellum), and craving for glucose (hypothalamus). CNS effects of cannabis include impairment of short-term memory, attention span, recall, and ability to store information, and suppression of rapid-eye-movement sleep. Muscle strength, coordination, and balance may be impaired. Dry mouth, increased heart rate, auditory and visual hallucinations, panic attacks, persecutory delusions, and depersonalization may occur. Chronic usage of cannabis has been associated with an amotivational syndrome, but causation by cannabis is unproven. Mild withdrawal symptoms may occur.

Purinoceptors and Adenosine Receptors

ATP and adenosine may serve as neurotransmitters in purinergic nerves of the gastrointestinal tract and genitourinary tract. Several types of G-protein–coupled purinoceptors (ATP-responsive) and adenosine receptors are found in the periphery and in the brain. Adenosine dilates brain blood vessels and has sedative, anxiolytic, and anticonvulsant properties. Adenosine receptors are selectively blocked by 1,3,7-trimethylxanthine (caffeine).

Caffeine and *theophylline* mimic the motor stimulation induced by dopamine receptor agonists. *8-Phenylxanthines* and *8-cycloalkylxanthines* are higher potency synthetic adenosine-receptor antagonists. Potent and selective nonxanthine adenosine-receptor antagonists have recently become available for adenosine A_{2A} receptors, stimulation of which decreases the affinity of dopamine D_2 receptor agonists for D_2 receptors in the striatum.

Caffeine, found in coffee, tea, cola, cocoa, chocolate, and hundreds of over-the-counter drugs, is perhaps the most widely used brain stimulant. *Caffeine intoxication* (caffeinism) is characterized by anxiety, sleep disturbances, mood changes, and psychophysiological complaints. Stress amplifies the effect. *Caffeine withdrawal*, which develops in 30%–50% of users within 18–24 h of drug cessation, is associated with vascular headache, drowsiness, and fatigue.

Axonal Transport

Materials required for axonal maintenance are synthesized in neuronal somata and transported distally to sites of utilization at various velocities. These axonal transport mechanisms and molecules represent important targets for several chemicals. The toxic effects of these substances vary with the function of nerve fibers in which axonal transport has been disrupted.

Rates of anterograde transport (soma to axon/terminal) vary: membrane-bound enzymes, neurotransmitter precursors, glycoproteins, lipids, and amino acids are transported at rates of 200–410 mm/day. Other materials, including mitochondrial components, are transported at lower rates (34–68 mm/day). Approximately half of the fast-transported proteins turn around and are transported retrogradely, largely as membrane-bound organelles resembling lysosomes. Retrograde fast transport (terminal/axon to soma) may also serve to ferry foreign materials (*ricin, tetanospasmin, diphtheria toxin, doxorubicin*) to neuronal somata. Retrograde transport of certain metals (*cadmium, iron, inorganic mercury, thallium,* and *manganese*) has been demonstrated in mammalian (rodents) or nonmammalian species (frog, pike).

Several neurotoxic substances interrupt the normal intra-axonal flow of materials along CNS and PNS fibers. While chemicals that perturb axonal transport mechanisms presumably affect all nerve fibers, the distal ends of the longest and largest axons are usually the first to display pathological changes, and the clinical consequences of systemic intoxication in humans usually take the form of a stocking-and-glove distribution of sensory dysfunction followed by motor weakness in a similar distribution (distal axonopathy) (Fig. 1.6C). Studies with laboratory animals confirm the special vulnerability of the distal portions of peripheral nerves and long spinal cord tracts, but also demonstrate widespread distal involvement of other neural pathways in the brains of animals treated for periods beyond that required to induce limb paralysis (*vide infra*).

Ultrastructural examination of distal nerve fibers subject to chemical-induced degeneration reveals an accumulation of organelles (synaptic-like and larger vesicles, mitochondria, dense lamellar bodies) that are normally transported retrogradely within the axon. The seemingly arrested organelles are sequestered and removed from the axon by invaginating processes of Schwann cells (PNS) or oligodendrocytes (CNS), most prominently on the distal sides of paranodes and, to a lesser extent, in internodal regions; this

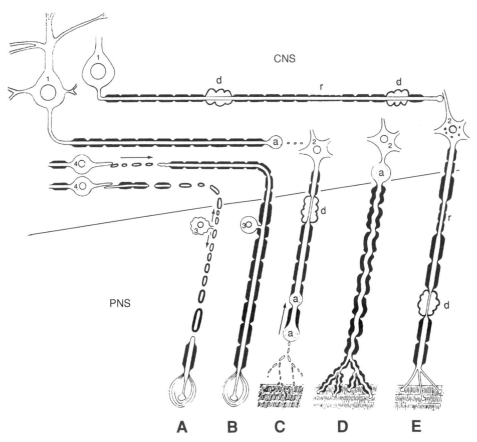

FIGURE 1.6. Cellular effects of some neurotoxic chemicals illustrated by upper (*1*) and lower (*2*) motor neurons, dorsal root ganglion cells (*3*), and second-order sensory neurons (*4*) in the gracile nucleus of the medulla oblongata. The central nervous system (*CNS*) is represented above the sloping horizontal line, the peripheral nervous system (*PNS*) below. The peripheral receptors in fibers *A* and *B* are pacinian corpuscles. Fibers *C–E* innervate extrafusal muscle fibers. (A) Neuronopathy: *Doxorubicin* irreversibly damages the neuron (*3*) resulting in a rapid anterograde (*arrows*) pattern of total axonal breakdown and myelin loss. (B) Central distal axonopathy: *Clioquinol* induces retrograde degeneration (*arrow*) of the central axonal process of the dorsal root ganglion cell (*3*) but leaves the cell and the peripheral process intact. (C) Central-peripheral distal axonopathy: *2,5-Hexanedione* induces the formation of distal neurofilament-laden axonal swellings (*a*) and retrograde axonal degeneration (*arrow*) to develop slowly in long and large central and peripheral axons. Muscle atrophy occurs unless axons regenerate and sprouts reinnervate the muscle. The anterior horn cell (*2*) is left intact and, eventually (after months to years), a secondary demyelination in the ventral root ensues (*d*). (D) β,β'-*Iminodipropionitrile* causes giant axonal swellings (*a*) to develop in the intraspinal portion of the axon; the distal axon attenuates but does not degenerate. (E) Myelinopathy: *Acetylethyltetramethyltetralin* secondarily causes myelin bubbling (*d*) focally along large-diameter central and peripheral nerve fibers. Axonal denudation is followed by remyelination (*r*): this occurs in the ventral roots and medulla oblongata when demyelination (*d*) is in progress in the peripheral nerve and elsewhere. A similar process takes place in a primary disease of the myelinating cell, except that remyelination might not occur during chemical exposure.

normal phagocytic process is greatly exaggerated in toxic (*acrylamide, tri-o-cresylphosphate, zinc pyridinethione*) and nontoxic distal axonopathies. Failure to sequester and remove calcium-laden organelles may initiate proteolytic processes that culminate in a "chemical transection" of the nerve fiber, with breakdown of the distal portion and consequent anatomical and functional disconnection between the neuron and its target organ.

Vesicles

Fast axonal transport is an energy-dependent system. Anterograde transport is promoted by a protein with ATPase activity (kinesin) and is blocked by *5'-adenylimidodiphosphate*, a nonhydrolyzable ATP analog that inhibits ATP-kinesin activity. Another protein, cytoplasmic dynein (MAP-1C), promotes retrograde fast transport. Organelles undergoing transport utilize these "motor proteins" to associate both with organelles to be transported and with microtubules, the transport guidance system. Attachment activates the ATPase, hydrolyzes ATP, and thereby generates energy to move the organelle/motor protein complex toward the positive or negative ends of microtubules (*i.e.*, anterograde and retrograde transport, respectively).

Erythro-9-[3-(2-hydroxynonyl)adenine, a structural analog of adenosine, inhibits microtubule-activated ATPase activity of MAP-1C and selectively perturbs retrograde transport in isolated lobster axons. Retrograde transport is also selectively disrupted by *p-bromophenylacetylurea* which, in systemically treated rats, induces hindlimb paralysis featured by the accumulation of tubulomembranous debris in distal axons prior to the onset of retrograde (dying-back) nerve fiber degeneration. A similar ultrastructural type of distal axonopathy develops in rodents after repeated topical application of *zinc pyridinethione* or repeated intraperitoneal injection of *2,4-dithiobiuret*. Retrograde transport is blocked in the hen sciatic nerve by an organophosphate (*di-n-butyl-2,2-dichlorovinyl phosphate*) that irreversibly inhibits neuropathy target esterase (NTE) and produces axonal neuropathy; the sulfonate *phenylmethylsulfonyl fluoride* reversibly inhibits NTE activity and fails adversely to impact axonal integrity.

Plant-derived drugs (*colchicine, vinca alkaloids*) that bind to tubulin subunits and inhibit microtubule assembly, dose-dependently block both retrograde and anterograde fast transport, disrupt microtubule integrity, and trigger axonal degeneration. Pretreatment with *taxol* blocks colchicine-induced disruption of microtubules *in vitro*. Taxol binds to β-tubulin, antagonizes disassembly of microtubules in axons and Schwann cells, increases microtubular density in axons and, in high doses, produces sensory neuropathy in

humans. *Podophyllotoxin* binds to tubulin at a site distinct from that employed by vinca alkaloids; semisynthetic principles of podophyllotoxin, *etoposide* and *teniposide*, lack the spindle-inhibiting potency of podophyllotoxin, vinca alkaloids and colchicine, form a ternary complex with topoisomerase II and DNA, and do not cause axonal neuropathy.

Cytoskeletal proteins

Whereas subcellular organelles are axonally transported bidirectionally at fast rates, cytoskeletal and soluble proteins are slowly transported anterograde from sites of synthesis in neuronal somata. Neurofilaments and microtubule proteins are transported by slow component a at rates of 0.2–0.5 mm/day in mammalian optic axons and up to 1–2 mm/day in motor axons of sciatic nerve. A wide range of polypeptides, including glycolytic enzymes and the cytoskeletal protein actin, move along axons at a faster rate (3–4 mm/day).

Doxorubicin increases the processing time for somatic protein synthesis; after intravenous administration to rats, the drug may kill sensory neurons in dorsal root ganglia and induce a proximodistal advance of degeneration (dying-forward) of sensory myelinated nerve fibers (Fig. 1.6A). Sublethal damage is featured by neuronal chromatolysis and neurofilament accumulation.

Several agents disrupt the transport of neurofilament triplet proteins along the axon. Intracisternal administration to rabbits of *aluminum chloride* or n-*butylbenzenesulfonamide* causes neurofilaments to accumulate in motor neuronal somata and even in dendrites. Direct application of other agents [β,β'-*iminodipropionitrile* (*IDPN*); *2,5-hexanedione* (*2,5-HD*)] to mammalian peripheral nerves causes a rapid loss of the normal distribution of microtubules and neurofilaments seen in cross-sections of axons; microtubules cluster in one or more groups often in the central part of the axon (through which fast transport proceeds normally), while neurofilaments lose their longitudinal orientation and are displaced peripherally. A comparable phenomenon is seen when either agent is administered systemically, but the more prominent abnormality is the accumulation of neurofilaments in focal swellings on the proximal sides of nodes of Ranvier and internodally. These neurofilamentous swellings represent a selective blockade of neurofilament transport because of chemical alteration of either neurofilament triplet peptides or of the proteins/enzymes required for their axonal transport. Focal neurofilament accumulations may develop proximally (IDPN; *1,2-diacetylbenzene*) or distally (2,5-HD); their development may be associated with atrophy (IDPN) or wallerian-like degeneration (2,5-HD) of the axon distal to the site of neurofilament blockade (Fig. 1.6C and D). Increasing the neurotoxic potency of 2,5-HD through the addition of *3-methyl* or *3,4-dimethyl* groups is associated with the development of focal swellings at intermediate and proximal regions of axons, respectively. Since the potency of these γ-diketones is associated with their propensity to form pyrroles and cross-link proteins, the spatial location (proximal vs. distal) in the axon of neurofilament arrest probably reflects the rate at which constituent or associated proteins are altered by the neurotoxic agent. Nonneurofilament protein candidates for toxic perturbation include axonally transported enzymes required for energy transformation.

VULNERABILITY OF NEUROGLIA AND MYELIN

Astrocytes and Ependymal Cells

Neuroglia of ectodermal origin include cells that (a) line the ventricles (ependymal cell), (b) form myelin (oligodendrocyte, Schwann cell), and (c) provide contact between blood vessels and neurons (astrocyte). Glial cells, notably astrocytes, may preferentially take up *metal ions* that enter the CNS. Astrocytes are connected to each other by electrical synapses; they remove certain chemical neurotransmitters (glutamate) from the extracellular space; they regulate interstitial water content and potassium ion concentration; they elaborate a glial membrane that serves as a protective covering for the CNS; and they respond to neuronal injury by proliferating, increasing production of glial fibrillary acidic protein, invading vacant space, and undergoing fibrosis. Astrocytic gliosis and microglial proliferation are nonspecific features of injured CNS tissue (*carbon monoxide*). *Ethanol* inhibits the proliferation of rat astrocytes stimulated by *muscarinic agonists*.

The circumference of cerebral capillaries is tightly invested by astrocyte foot processes that swell when extracellular osmolarity falls. Marked swelling is characteristic of *water intoxication*. Swelling of foot processes is also seen in *lead* encephalopathy; in poisoning with *methionine sulfoxamine*; in anoxic damage associated with *hypercapnia*; and after the experimental administration of *6-aminonicotinamide, isoniazid, misonidazole, ouabain,* or *monosodium glutamate* (arcuate hypothalamic nuclei). Primary astrocytic swellings in areas of high glucose consumption are seen in mice treated with *6-chloro-6-deoxyglucose*. Astrocytes increase their glycogen content in a variety of insults (*methionine sulfoxamine*), form eosinophilic intranuclear inclusion bodies in *lead intoxication*, and greatly increase the relative size of the nuclear compartment (Alzheimer type II glia) in hepatic encephalopathy (*hyperammonemia*). DL-α-*Amino adipic acid* is used experimentally as an astrocyte-specific toxin.

Ependymal cells and choroid plexus endothelium, together with other cellular elements of the CNS, are affected in several toxic conditions. *Tertiary amines* reportedly produce selective vacuolar change in the epithelium of the choroid plexus. Ependymal necrosis in the lateral ventricles adjacent to the choroid plexus is found in rats treated with *amoscanate*.

Oligodendrocytes and Schwann Cells

Oligodendrocytes, which are restricted to the CNS, are found in close association with neuronal somata (satellites), as intermediate cells with the potential to form myelin, and as interfascicular cells that elaborate lengths (internodes) of compacted plasma membrane (myelin) around a number of axons (estimated n = 30–50). The principal function of the myelin sheath is to isolate regions of electrical excitability (nodes of Ranvier) and thereby increase the velocity of nerve impulse transmission. CNS fibers maintain direct contact with extracellular fluid, which is continuous with cerebrospinal fluid. Capillaries supply the physiological needs of nerve fibers; these are equipped with tight junctions in all CNS areas (blood-brain barrier) except the circumventricular organs where blood vessels are permeable (*vide supra*). In these regions, leakage of plasma filtrate into the cerebrospinal fluid is prevented by ependymal cells with tight junctions.

Schwann cells, which are restricted to the PNS, associate with numerous small axons to form unmyelinated fibers or elaborate an internode of myelin around a single, large-diameter axon to form a myelinated fiber. Myelinated and unmyelinated peripheral nerve fibers are located within a conduit of basal lamina that borders the outer surface of the Schwann cell. Fibers are separated from each other by an extracellular (endoneurial) space containing collagen and elastin fibers, and small-diameter blood vessels equipped with tight junctions (blood-nerve barrier). Bundles of nerve fibers (fascicles) are protected from external factors by an elastic sheath of connective tissue cells (perineurium) that also have a barrier function. Myelinated and unmyelinated fibers reside in this separate physiological compartment in all regions of the PNS except (a) dorsal root and autonomic ganglia, where some blood vessels are fenestrated; (b) the terminals of motor nerve fibers and free sensory endings; and (c) the mesenteric plexus, which is bathed by fluid leaking from blood vessels in adjacent muscle layers.

Myelinating cells are presumably susceptible to agents that disrupt the synthesis, transport, and insertion of materials required to maintain cellular and myelin integrity. However, since intracellular transport systems of neuroglia are not well defined, it is only possible to identify agents with apparent primary effects on myelin and those that seem to perturb glial somatic functions. Both result in segmental demyelination with consequent disruption of nerve conduction. Remyelination and restoration of conduction occur spontaneously.

Diphtheria toxin provides the best example of an exogenous agent that induces primary demyelination in peripheral nerves as a consequence of the inhibition of protein synthesis in Schwann cells. Experimental injection of diphtheria toxin into the spinal cord also elicits oligodendrocyte demyelination. Somal disease of myelinating cells can also be induced by agents such as *ethidium bromide* and *actinomycin D*, which inhibit protein synthesis. Intracranial injection of actinomycin D induces widespread status spongiosus in the white matter of rats. Edema forms between the inner tongue and remainder of the myelin sheath, in the periaxonal space, and as intramyelinic edema due to splitting of myelin membranes at the intraperiod line. Injection of ethidium bromide induces degenerative changes in oligodendrocytes and intramyelinic edema. *Cuprizone (biscyclohexanone oxalylhydrazone)* treatment of mice also induces oligodendrocyte degeneration with intramyelinic edema.

Certain other substances (*cycloleucine*) induce reversible edematous changes in CNS and PNS myelin without apparent damage or loss of the myelin-forming cells (Fig. 1.6E). One interesting example is *acetylethyltetramethyltetralin (AETT)*, formerly used as a synthetic musk. Demyelination induced by AETT is accompanied in rats by neuronal ceroid pigmentation, irritability, and limb weakness. Dermal or oral administration to rats also causes a remarkable blue discoloration of skin, nerves, spinal cord, and brain. The chromogenic reaction, attributed to a diketo metabolite of AETT, results from interaction of this compound with amino acids, notably lysine. Chromogenic tissue reactions also occur with *1,2-diacetylbenzene* (neurotoxic) but not with non-neurotoxic 1,3-diethylbenzene. The chromogenic and neurotoxic properties of these compounds are closely related and recent work suggests demyelination may be secondary to an axonal lesion. Unstudied is whether the neurotoxic effects of chromogenic hydrocarbons are related to the widely reported (but disputed) chronic neurological effects of *mixed organic hydrocarbon solvents*.

Human neurotoxic disease has been historically associated with (a) use of the topical antiseptic *2,2'-methylenebis(3,4,6-trichlorophenol) (hexachlorophene)* and (b) exposure to a preparation of *ethyltins* sold for medicinal purposes. Animal studies show that acute *triethyltin* intoxication is associated with increased water content of the brain and spinal cord with no changes in the blood-brain barrier to proteins of high molecular weight. Edema of axons and astrocytes may precede the appearance of intramyelinic edema; inhibition of Na^+, K^+-ATPase may be the underlying mechanism. Rats fed triethyltin become anorexic, and develop hindlimb weakness, tremors, and convulsions. Brains of these animals show diffuse status spongiosus in optic nerve, basal ganglia, thalamus, corpus callosum, cerebral cortex, and elsewhere. Peripheral nerves show a proximal-to-distal gradient of decreasing myelin damage. Humans poisoned with triethyltin developed a diffuse encephalopathy with severe, persistent headache, nausea, vomiting, vertigo, visual disturbance, photophobia, transient weakness, permanent paralysis, meningeal signs, papillodema, and convulsions.

SYSTEM VULNERABILITY TO CHEMICALS

Neurotoxicology holds central the notion that chemicals perturb neurological function by interfering differentially with the structure or function of specific neural pathways, circuits, and systems. Analysis of the sites of action of chemicals on neural pathways that connect the brain with the periphery demonstrates that the most peripheral neuron in the relay system is most commonly affected, and the terminals of both afferent and efferent axons are most vulnerable. Other sites susceptible to chemical perturbation are circuits of the brain that modulate efferent output.

Special Senses

The special senses of vision, audition, balance, gustation, and olfaction depend on neural pathways that originate in peripheral receptors (eye, inner ear, mouth, nose) and terminate in the cerebral cortex or brainstem/spinal cord (vestibular system). Chemical agents that perturb the special senses most commonly interfere with the structure or function of peripheral sensory receptors. Some special receptors (cochlear hair cells) or proximal axons of special receptors (optic nerve) may be damaged secondarily by agents that cause edema because they are housed in inelastic structures. Afferent pathways for taste, smell, audition, and balance employ sensory neurons housed in ganglia that lack a blood-nerve barrier.

Olfaction

Olfaction is subserved by ciliated bipolar sensory neurons (receptors) embedded in a specialized neuroepithelium that lines the posterior nasal cavity (Fig. 1.7A). The cilia are required for odorant transduction. Cilia-bearing neurons have a limited lifespan (*circa* 30–60 days) and are continuously replaced from a basal layer of stem cells. Systemic exposure to antiproliferative drugs, such as *vincristine* and *doxorubicin*, interferes with the normal replacement of receptor cells. Intraperitoneal treatment of rats with *2-pentenenitrile* or β,β′-*iminodipropionitrile (IDPN)* damages the olfactory epithelium.

Temporal diminution of odor perception (*toluene*) is referred to as olfactory adaptation. Dysosmia (disturbed olfaction) and anosmia (loss) are associated with a number of prescription medications, drugs of abuse, and occupational chemicals. Mechanisms of action are generally poorly understood. Transient dysosmia may occur with the calcium-channel antagonists *nifedipine* and *diltiazem*. Decreased ability to smell is associated with a number of inhaled toxic chemicals, especially *organic solvents*. Snorted *cocaine* has a vasoconstrictor effect that may precipitate septal perforation with anosmia. Chronic occupational exposure to *cadmium oxide* may result in anosmia.

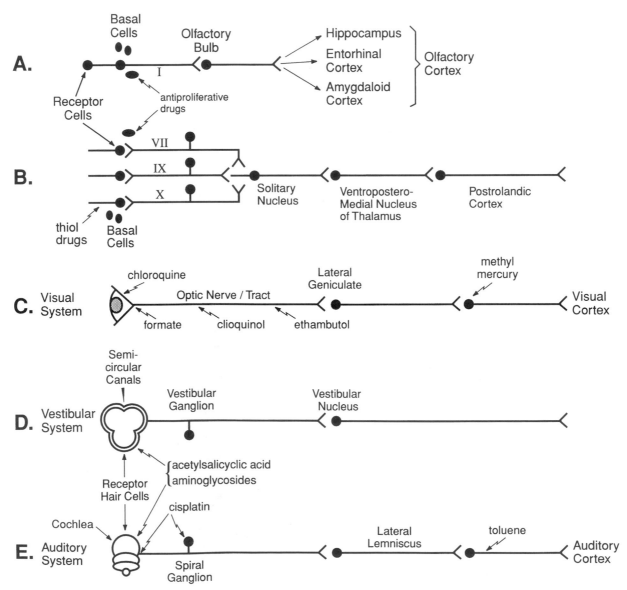

FIGURE 1.7. Agents (*jagged arrows*) that act on pathways subserving olfaction (A), gustation (B), vision (C), balance (D), or audition (E). The peripherally located receptor for each pathway is shown on the extreme left (*e.g.*, the olfactory epithelium in A and the taste receptors in B). Pathways *A–C* and *E* are shown projecting to the appropriate region of the cerebral cortex. For pathway *D*, tracts from the brainstem to the cerebral cortex are omitted. Hypoglossal nerve (*VII*); glossopharyngeal nerve (*IX*), and vagus nerve (*X*).

Receptor cells project thin unmyelinated axons along the first cranial nerve to the olfactory bulb where they synapse with interneurons and output neurons that project axons along the olfactory tract; these terminate in the olfactory cortex. The olfactory nerve thus provides a multisynaptic pathway for the passage of factors from the environment to the brain. While the *rabies virus* is known rarely to enter the brain *via* the olfactory pathway, and experimental evidence for axonal transport of *aluminum*, *manganese*, and *cadmium* transport has been offered from studies of fish and rabbits, the significance of this route for the entry of toxic substances into the brain of humans is unclear.

While olfactory neurons respond selectively to low concentrations of odorants, the nasal epithelium also contains free nerve endings of the trigeminal nerve; these respond nonselectively to a large number of volatile chemicals (*organic solvents*). Firing of free nerve endings may be perceived as nasal irritation.

Gustation

Taste perception is performed by receptor cells organized in taste buds on the surface of the tongue and pharynx. Normal tastes include sweet, bitter, sour, and salty; in humans, the latter two may be mediated by an *amiloride*-sensitive apical Na^+ channel. Receptor cells have a limited lifespan, continually undergo replacement, and are susceptible to *antiproliferative drugs* (Fig. 1.7B). Thiol drugs are linked to dysgeusia (abnormal taste): *captopril*, an inhibitor of angiotensin-converting enzyme used for the treatment of hypertension; *penicillamine* in rheumatoid arthritis, and *thiouracil*, an antithyroid drug. A metallic taste is reported in *tellurium intoxication*, and users of *smokeless tobacco* experience residual abnormal gustation.

Vision

Photoreceptors (rods and cones) are located in the outer nuclear layer of the retina; this is apposed to the melanin-containing cells that form the pigment epithelium (choroid) at the back of the eye. The choroid binds and sequesters many drugs, including the retinal toxin *chloroquine*. Temporal release of sequestered chloroquine is proposed to play a role in the drug's damaging effects on cones and rods, with consequent progressive changes in color vision (cones), night vision (rods), central vision (scotoma), and peripheral vision.

Rods and cones relay impulses laterally within the inner and outer plexiform layers of the retina (horizontal and amacrine cells) and vertically from bipolar cells to ganglion cells, the output neurons of the retina (Fig. 1.7C). Electrical activity in nonganglion retinal cells (electroretinogram) is perturbed by a large number of substances: drugs such as *cardiac glycosides* and *trimethadione* tend to induce reversible changes; others, such as *aminophenoxyalkanes* and *myristyl-γ-picolinium chloride*, elicit morphological damage. Rodents treated with *stipandrol* (*Stypandra glauca*) lose photoreceptors in the outer nuclear layer. In neonatal rats, *glutamate* destroys nerve cells in the ganglion cell layer and in the inner nuclear layer. Rods are more sensitive than cones in the rat retina to the toxic effects of *2,5-hexanedione* in combination with *light energy*. Damaged retinal ganglion cells are seen in humans and primates intoxicated with *quinine*.

Ganglion cells project axons to the optic disc where they become myelinated and together form the optic nerves, which fuse at the optic chiasm. Toxic agents may primarily damage the CNS myelin (*hexachlorophene*) or axons (*ethambutol*) of optic nerve fibers. Stipandrol causes intra-myelinic edema followed by axon degeneration. Substances that impair energy metabolism (*thallium*, *cyanide*) tend to damage proximal regions of axons projecting into the optic nerve from the papillomacular bundle ("retrobulbar neuritis"). Distal axonal degeneration, with damage in the optic tracts, is seen with agents such as *clioquinol* and *ethambutol*. Terminal axonal swelling has been noted in the lateral geniculate nucleus of rodents intoxicated with *2,5-hexanedione*. Several other substances (*acrylamide*, *carbon disulfide*) elicit both optic neuropathy and peripheral neuropathy, apparently as part of a global perturbation of axonal transport; CNS and PNS axons in these central-peripheral distal axonopathies (*vide infra*) are differentially impacted as a function of axon length and diameter.

Three parallel pathways project from the lateral geniculate nucleus to the visual cortex. Damage to neurons in the visual cortex accompanies *methylmercury* intoxication; concentric constriction of visual fields or total cortical blindness may occur in the absence of changes in the electroretinogram or morphological changes in the optic nerve, optic tract, or lateral geniculate nucleus.

Balance and Audition

Peripheral receptors of the vestibular system are located in the inner ear: the semicircular canals and otolith organs (utricle, saccule) are the two principal organs of equilibrium. Sensory receptor hair cells respond to changes in angular acceleration linearly (otoliths) and in three directions (semicircular canals). These cells are innervated by efferent axons of brainstem neurons and by afferent axons of the vestibular ganglion that project to the vestibular nucleus (Fig. 1.7D). Neurons therein are concerned with neck posture and eye movements. The vestibulocerebellum, which receives input from the vestibular nuclei, participates in the control of balance and eye movements. Disturbance of oculomotor function with disorderly eye movements (opsoclonus) is a prominent clinical feature of occupational *chlordecone* intoxication. Rats with postural deficits from treatment with *misonidazole* or *metronidazole* display lesions of vestibular nuclei and superior olives, with some involvement of cochlea and cerebellar roof nuclei. Lesions of vestibular and cochlear nuclei are also seen in rodents treated with *6-chloro-6-deoxyglucose* or *6-aminonicotinamide*, and in primates treated with *1-amino-6-chloropropane*.

Chemical-induced disorders of vestibular function may be accompanied by impairment of hearing. Human vestibular function is severely impaired by *streptomycin*, and drug-treated cats show degenerative changes of receptor cells subserving both balance and audition (Fig. 1.7E). Sound is transduced by hair cells of the organ of Corti in the cochlea. Different regions of the cochlea respond selectively to different sound frequencies. The basal outer hair cells are destroyed by *kanamycin* in guinea pigs, and humans with renal impairment may develop sudden hearing loss while under treatment with this drug. *Dihydrostreptomycin* also causes severe hearing loss, the onset of which might be delayed for several months following drug administration. Hearing loss proceeds from high to low frequencies. Other ototoxic agents include *acetylsalicylic acid*, *cis-

platin*, *carboplatin deferoxamine*, *furosemide*, *imipramine* and, in animals, a number of organic solvents. Noise may exacerbate the neurotoxic effects of some of these chemicals. Hearing, vestibular, and olfactory impairment manifest in animals treated with *IDPN*, *2-pentenenitrile* or *2-butenenitrile (2-BN)*. Acute intoxication of rats with *2-BN* or *IDPN* destroys vestibular hair cells and precipitates a syndrome characterized by circling, head-bobbing, and retropulsion; both also induce hearing loss suggestive of damage to hair cells in the cochlea. Combined administration of *ethacrynic acid* and *atoxyl* to rats causes irreversible damage to cochlear hair cells and the stria vascularis.

Sensorimotor Function

Afferent (sensory) and efferent (motor) information between the brain, spinal cord, and periphery is carried in elongate pathways that are vulnerable to a large number of chemicals (Fig. 1.8). Some (*pyrethroids*) perturb electrical activity in the excitable nerve membrane (axolemma); effects are usually rapidly reversible without the induction of nerve damage. Other agents (*hexachlorophene*, *ethidium bromide*) attack the myelin sheath or the myelinating cell of the PNS (Schwann cell) or CNS (oligodendrocyte) (*vide supra*). In these situations, nerve fibers undergo a cascade of focal demyelination and remyelination that perturbs impulse conduction and results in functional deficits. Function is restored once remyelination is effected. Other substances

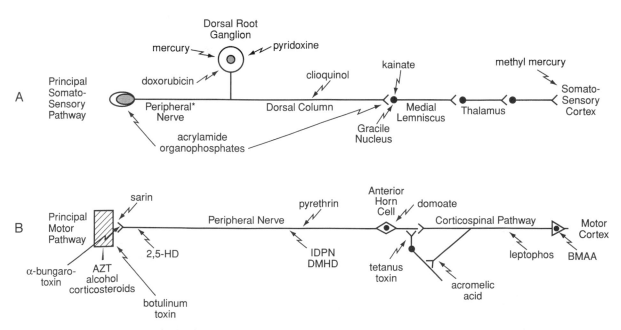

FIGURE 1.8. Agents (*jagged arrows*) acting on (A) the principal somatosensory pathway originating in a pacinian corpuscle (*extreme left*) and (B) the principal motor pathway terminating in striated muscle (*extreme left*). *AZT*: 3'-Azido-3'-deoxythymidine. *2,5-HD*: 2,5-Hexanedione. *DMHD*: 3,4-Dimethyl-2,5-hexanedione. *IDPN*: β,β'-Iminodipropionitrile. *BMAA*: β-N-Methylamino-L-alanine. Asterisk indicates also vulnerable to agents listed in B (peripheral nerve).

disrupt or destroy the perikarya of nerve cells; sensory neurons in dorsal root ganglia, which lack a blood-nerve barrier, are much more vulnerable (*methylmercury*) than the rarely affected spinal motor neurons (*domoic acid*). Loss of sensory neurons constitutes an irreversible loss of the functions subserved by these cells.

Most chemicals acting on sensorimotor function leave the perikarya of nerve cells structurally intact but unable to maintain the full length of their centrally or peripherally directed axons, which undergo distal, retrograde degeneration. Central-peripheral distal axonopathy (CPDA) or, simply, *distal axonopathy*, describes one of the most common patterns of chronic neurotoxic injury (Fig. 1.6D), a distribution of pathology that, in humans and animals, is expressed functionally as peripheral neuropathy. In these disorders, the dysfunction associated with distal axonal degeneration in long spinal cord tracts is masked by a comparable distribution of damage in peripheral nerves. However, upon regeneration and re-establishment of the connections of peripheral sensory and motor fibers, the functional consequences of severe CNS damage may become evident in the form of persistent clinical deficits (spasticity, ataxia).

Principal Sensory Pathway

Somatosensory function is disrupted by agents that alter the structure or function of primary sensory neurons. These neurons innervate peripheral receptors that transduce movement in superficial skin (Meissner's corpuscles, Merkel's cells), deep skin (pacinian corpuscles and Ruffini cells), muscle (intrafusal fibers), and tendons (Golgi organs). Mechanotransduction elicits a generator potential which, in the case of the pacinian corpuscle, is attenuated by systemic exposure to *acrylamide* (Fig. 1.8A). In normal states, the generator potential of mechanoreceptors reaches a magnitude that stimulates action potentials; these are conveyed proximally to dorsal root ganglia and centrally to dorsal column nuclei, thalamus, and somatosensory cortex. Agents such as *DDT*, *ciguatoxin*, *pyrethrin*, and *tetrodotoxin*, which interact with Na^+ channels, interfere with the excitable membrane, disrupt impulse transmission, and trigger perverse sensations in the distribution of cranial (trigeminal) and peripheral nerves.

The cell bodies of primary sensory neurons are associated with permeable (fenestrated) blood vessels (*vide supra*), which expose them continuously to substances in the circulation. Loss of nerve cells and their central and peripheral axonal projections is found in animals treated with *doxorubicin*, *methylmercury*, or *vitamin B₆*. Pyridoxine megavitaminosis, or treatment with *thalidomide* or *cisplatin*, is associated with marked distal-extremity sensory loss in adult humans. Less severe damage to primary sensory neurons is seen in CPDA-type sensorimotor polyneuropathies; toxic damage takes the form of retrograde (dying-back) degeneration of distal axons. Experimental studies demonstrate simultaneous breakdown of the distal extremities of peripheral and central axons of dorsal root ganglia during systemic intoxication with *acrylamide*, *tri-o-cresylphosphate*, or *isoniazid*. Rarely, as with *clioquinol*, distal degeneration is confined to the central projections of primary sensory neurons (Fig. 1.6C). Swollen and degenerating axons are usually encountered in the terminations of the long gracile tract (housing axons from lumbosacral regions) before similar changes are found in the cuneate nuclei.

Neurons in dorsal column nuclei and subsequent neurons in the somatosensory pathway are preserved in CPDA, probably because they are required to support relatively short axons. However, since distal axonal pathology may appear in short CNS pathways (*e.g.*, optic tracts) if intoxication is prolonged, it is likely that potential axonal vulnerability to CPDA is, in theory, global. Similarly, for agents such as β,β'-*iminodipropionitrile* (*IDPN*), which arrest anterograde axonal transport of neurofilament proteins, proximal axonal swelling with amassed neurofilaments may be apparent at multiple sites in the neuraxis and especially prominent in peripheral sensory and motor neurons.

Second-order neurons in the gracile nucleus of rats exhibit an excitotoxic pattern of pathology when *kainate* is injected into the lateral ventricle. This is characterized by intact presynaptic terminals (dorsal column input) attached to grossly edematous dendrites of toxin-targeted neurons.

Pain Pathways

Activation of nociceptive pathways leads to the perception of pain. Nociceptive receptors include those responding to cold, heat, and mechanical stimuli; these convey afferent impulses centrally in thinly myelinated Aδ fibers (thermal/mechanical nociceptors) and small, unmyelinated C fibers (polymodal nociceptors). *Tissue damage* can sensitize and activate nociceptors (hyperalgesia) through local release of blood-borne products (serotonin, bradykinin, histamine, prostaglandin, leukotrienes) and substance P from sensory endings. Substance P (as neurotransmitter) is enriched in the central ending of nociceptor afferents in the dorsal horn of the spinal cord. Nociceptive input to the dorsal horn is relayed to the brain in five ascending projection pathways, the most prominent of which is the spinothalamic tract; thalamic neurons project to the somatosensory and association cortex. Descending pathways, which inhibit nociceptive neurons in the spinal cord, originate in the periventicular and periaqueductal gray matter of the midbrain; the analgesic action of *morphine* at these sites is blocked by *naloxone*.

Chronic localized pain may be treated topically by preparations containing *capsaicin*. In animals, repeated skin application of capsaicin leads to a reversible functional desensitization that may last for hours or days. Direct application to peripheral nerves results in conduction block associated with local arrest of both anterograde axonal transport of substance P and somatostatin and retrograde transport of horseradish peroxidase, swelling of unmyelinated axons distally and proximally, loss of a proportion of unmyelinated fibers and dorsal root ganglion neurons, and prolonged or permanent loss of nociception in the corresponding area of the affected sensory nerve terminals. Systemic exposure of adult rats depletes neuropeptide stores and, in high doses, causes distal degeneration of nociceptive axons and some corresponding nerve cell bodies in sensory ganglia. Partial or total recovery (presumably by axonal regeneration of surviving neurons) occurs over a period of months.

Principal (Voluntary) Motor Pathway

Motor function is subserved by cortical motor neurons that project their axons to the spinal cord. Some of these synapse directly with anterior horn cells; others regulate the function of these lower motor neurons by synapsing with spinal interneurons—in rats, these cells are vulnerable to *acromelic acid*, a cyclic glutamate analogue (Fig. 1.8B).

The somata of motor neurons are also vulnerable to agents that behave as excitotoxins or effect excitotoxicity. Dysfunction of the motor pathway may be marked, but pathological changes are usually sparse. Primates chronically dosed with β-N-*methylamino*-L-*alanine* exhibit pyramidal dysfunction associated with chromatolysis and other changes of cortical motor neurons. Systemic intoxication with *domoic acid* perturbs anterior horn cells and precipitates weakness. *Tetanus toxin* binds glycinergic terminals in spinal cord, diminishes inhibitory modulation of motor neurons, and causes hyperexcitability and muscle spasms. *Antisense nucleotides to gene sequences coding for glutamate transporters* induce neuronal degeneration in experimental animals, presumably because cells encounter excitotoxic concentrations of extracellular glutamate.

Agents that perturb axonal transport have marked effects on anterior horn cells as on primary sensory neurons. Chemicals able to disrupt anterograde slow transport cause neurofilaments to accumulate in nerve cell bodies (*aluminum*), in the proximal regions of axons (*3,4-dimethyl-2,5-hexanedione, IDPN*), midway along their course (*3-methyl-2,5-hexanedione*), or distally (*2,5-hexanedione*). Whether

these phenomena result from changes in the properties of the transported elements or of the transport system is unknown. Other substances disrupt fast transport reversibly (*acrylamide*) or irreversibly (*organophosphates*); some cause tubulovesicular structures to accumulate terminally (*zinc pyridinethione*) and distally (*tri-o-cresyl phosphate*) before the onset of retrograde axonal degeneration (Fig. 1.6D). Comparable changes take place at the distal ends of corticospinal fibers in the pyramidal tracts of the spinal cord. Chromatolysis of anterior horn cells may develop if peripheral nerve degeneration is severe (*buckthorn intoxication*). Terminal axonal regeneration and myelination of axonal sprouts usually commence during intoxication; however, *acrylamide* arrests or retards axonal regeneration in peripheral nerves by an unknown mechanism.

Motor neurons are also vulnerable to a host of agents that perturb impulse transmission (*tetrodotoxin*) or synaptic transmission at neuromuscular junctions. Some toxins act on the presynapse to decrease (*botulinum toxin*) or increase (α-*latrotoxin*) neurotransmission; others (*carbamates*) inhibit the enzyme action of acetylcholinesterase, which normally terminates postsynaptic activation; yet others (α-*bungarotoxin*) interfere with the activation of postsynaptic acetylcholine receptors. Agents that increase synaptic transmission (*anticholinesterases*) may cause localized disruption of subjunctional muscle fibers with secondary involvement of motor nerve terminals. Drugs (*corticosteriods*) and chemicals (*alcohol*) that primarily impact striated muscle are discussed in chapter 2.

Motoneuronal function is disrupted by a number of substances that perturb the integrity of the myelin sheath (*hexachlorophene*). For unknown reasons, spinal roots are more heavily impacted than peripheral nerves. The long internodes and thick myelin sheaths of large-diameter myelinated fibers are commonly the first to undergo segmental demyelination. Schwann cells immediately occupy denuded lengths of axons, establish foreshortened axonal territories and elaborate myelin even though intoxication continues. Segmental demyelination and remyelination may occur concurrently in individual nerve fibers. Deficits are usually symmetrical; the sudden onset of asymmetrical weakness during therapy with *sodium aurothiomalate* suggests immune-mediated demyelination.

Cerebellum

More than half of the neurons in the brain are contained within the cerebellum, a structure that regulates movement and posture indirectly by influencing the output of the principal motor pathway. Damage to the cerebellum may result in erroneous planning and execution of movement. Coordination of limb movements and eye movements may be lost and balance may be impaired.

Somatic sensory information reaches the cerebellum through mossy fiber pathways, including terminations of elongate spinocerebellar tracts, which are vulnerable in experimental toxic CNS-PNS distal axonopathy (*acrylamide*) (Fig. 1.9). Granule cells and Golgi cells, which form a local circuit to taper the excitatory drive of the former on Purkinje cells, are targets in *methylmercury* intoxication (human, cat, rat) in which whole-body ataxia may be evident. Rats treated orally with L-2-chloropropionic acid develop abnormal locomotion accompanied by granule cell necrosis. Climbing fibers originating in the inferior olivary nucleus (medulla oblongata) provide the other excitatory input to Purkinje cells; rats and mice treated with *3-acetylpyridine*, which targets the inferior olivary nuclei, display ataxia, muscular incoordination, and extremity tremor. The olivocerebellar projection is also thought to mediate Purkinje cell degeneration induced by *ibogaine*. Purkinje cells, which

provide the sole (inhibitory) output of the cerebellum, are sensitive to hypoxic and related states (*acute cyanide intoxication*). These cells are reduced in number in *bismuth intoxication* and in acute *lead* encephalopathy.

Basal Ganglia

Five large subcortical nuclei constituting the basal ganglia serve to control the quality of motor function: the caudate and putamen (striatum), the globus pallidus (pallidum), the subthalamic nucleus, and the substantia nigra. Together, these nuclei regulate the motor function of the frontal cortex. Lesions of the caudate and putamen (corpus striatum) are especially associated with chorea (unpredictable, brief, jerky movements); lesions of the subthalamic nucleus with contralateral hemiballismus (flinging movements of limbs) and lesions of the pars compacta of the substantia nigra with parkinsonism (akinetic rigid syndrome).

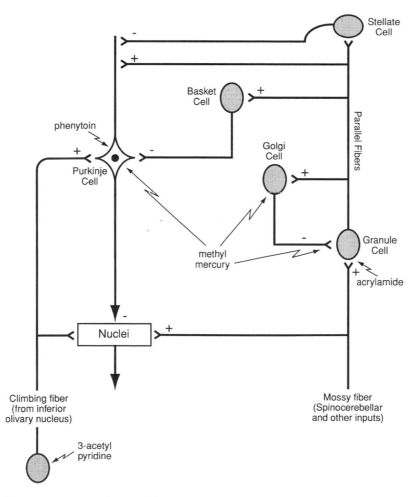

FIGURE 1.9. Agents (*jagged arrows*) acting on pathways of the cerebellum. Excitatory (+) and inhibitory (-) pathways are shown. [Modified with permission from Pansky & Allen, 1980.]

Corticostriate fibers provide the primary excitatory (glutamatergic) input to the basal ganglia. Putaminal neuronal damage and tissue necrosis can be induced by agents that block energy metabolism and promote glutamate-mediated excitotoxicity (*3-nitropropionic acid*). The pallidum and substantia nigra pars reticulata are affected in *carbon monoxide intoxication*; the putamen is especially vulnerable in *methanol intoxication*. *Manganese* intoxication may damage all subcortical nuclei of the basal ganglia save the nigrostriatal pathway. The pars compacta of the substantia nigra of humans and primates is selectively damaged by *MPTP*. Damage to the basal ganglia may result in lesion-dependent involuntary movements (tremor, chorea, hemiballismus), changes in posture and muscle tone (dystonia), and/or a poverty and slowness of movement (parkinsonism). Neurotoxic movement disorders include parkinsonism (*carbon disulfide, ethanol, manganese, mercury, MPTP*), tremor (*alcohol withdrawal, arsenic, caffeine, lead, mercury*), chorea (*alcohol withdrawal, carbon monoxide, manganese, mercury, thallium, toluene*), and dystonia (*3-nitropropionic acid*).

Functional disorders of the extrapyramidal system are seen in subjects treated with drugs widely used in medical practice. The range of movement disorders associated with the toxic (side) effects of medications includes: akathisia—restlessness, especially of legs; ballism (*phenytoin*); chorea (*amphetamines, anticonvulsants, anticholinergics*); dystonia—sustained muscle contraction with slow twisting movements (antidepressants such as *amitryptaline*); myoclonus—sudden, brief, shock-like involuntary movements (*MAO inhibitors*); parkinsonism—muscle rigidity, reduced speed and amplitude of movement (*lithium; dopamine depletors/receptor blockers*); tardive dyskinesia—delayed-onset orofacial-lingual-masticatory movements (*neuroleptics*); tremor—rhythmic oscillation of a body part, usually with fixed periodicity (*dopamine agonists, neuroleptics, tricyclic antidepressants*); tics—abrupt, stereotypic motor movement or vocalization (*L-dopa, neuroleptics, phenytoin*).

Autonomic (Involuntary) Motor System

Maintenance of internal homeostasis and rapid responses to the demands of the external environment are functions of the autonomic nervous system (enteric, parasympathetic, sympathetic). Unlike their somatic counterparts in the spinal cord, effector neurons of the autonomic nervous system are contained in peripheral ganglia with permeant blood vessels (*vide supra*). Sympathetic and parasympathetic neurons regulate the function of the pupil, lacrimal and salivary glands, airway, heart, gastrointestinal system, bladder, genitalia, blood vessels, and hair follicles. These *postganglionic* neurons are activated by *preganglionic* neurons in brainstem nuclei and spinal cord. Preganglionic neurons receive input from the hypothalamus; this brain center also regulates autonomic function hormonally *via* the endocrine system.

Acetylcholine serves as the principal neurotransmitter for all preganglionic autonomic fibers, all postganglionic parasympathetic fibers, and some postganglionic sympathetic fibers (Fig. 1.10). Drugs that selectively block nicotinic acetylcholine receptors (*curare, hexamethonium*) curtail ganglionic output. *Dimethylphenylpiperazinum* stimulates activity. Muscarinic receptors, which mediate the effects of acetylcholine at autonomic effector cells, are blocked by atropine and stimulated by *muscarinic toxins* present in certain snake venoms. Agents with anticholinesterase actions (*fasciculins, organophosphates*) stimulate sympathetic and parasympathetic activity, sometimes (*sarin*) with dramatic clinical consequences (cholinergic crisis).

Norepinephrine serves as the principal neurotransmitter for postganglionic sympathetic fibers. Neurotransmitter synthesis from tyrosine is blocked by α-*methyltyrosine*. *Guanethidine* blocks norepinephrine release. *Tyramine* and *amphetamine* promote neurotransmitter release and elicit a sympathomimetic effect. *Reserpine* blocks vesicular uptake of amines and thereby depletes synaptic transmitter. Experimental systemic administration of *6-hydroxydopamine* destroys adrenergic nerve terminals (chemical sympathectomy).

Experimental studies demonstrate that autonomic neurons synthesize, release, and respond to neurotransmitters other than acetylcholine and norepinephrine. In addition to ATP, vasoactive intestinal peptide (VIP), and the neuropeptide Y family, for which transmitter functions have been established, the list of candidate transmitters and neuromodulators includes enkephalins, somatostatin, cholecystokinin, calcitonin gene-related peptide (CGRP), and substance P. *Capsaicin* releases substance P, somatostatin, and CGRP (but not conventional neurotransmitters) from spinal cord nerve terminals and, by other mechanisms, influences cardiovascular function, endocrine control mechanisms, and thermoregulation, the latter *via* capsaicin-sensitive thermosensitive neurons in the preoptic region of the hypothalamus. Capsaicin-sensitive primary sensory neurons contain substance P, CGRP, neurokinin A, somatostatin, and VIP; these are released by capsaicin from peripheral sensory endings where they mediate local changes in blood flow, vascular permeability, and the activity of postganglionic sympathetic afferent fibers.

The autonomic nervous system is affected in several toxic neuropathies; the clinical manifestations may be mild or prominent. Because axons are smaller, autonomic nerve fi-

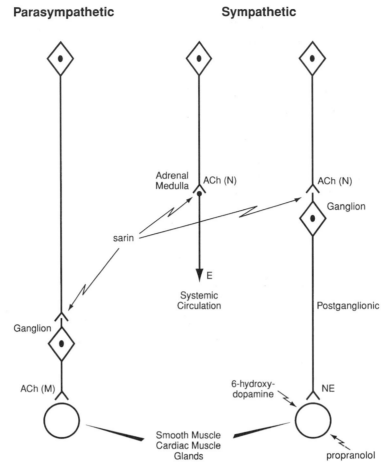

FIGURE 1.10. Agents (*jagged arrows*) acting on the autonomic motor system. Neurotransmitters/receptors. *ACh* (*N*): Acetylcholine/nicotinic. *ACh* (*M*): Acetylcholine/muscarinic. *E*: Epinephrine. *NE*: Norepinephrine. [Modified with permission from Pansky & Allen, 1980.]

bers may be less vulnerable than somatic sensorimotor fibers in toxic distal axonopathies. This is borne out by experimental studies of feline *acrylamide* intoxication: pathological changes in the vagus nerve (more affected than the splanchnic nerve) appear only when peripheral (somatic) nerves are severely affected. Impacted functions include baroreceptor reflexes of the aortic arch and vasomotor control of the mesenteric vascular bed. Abnormalities of sweating are features of chronic intoxication with *acrylamide*, *arsenic*, or *inorganic mercury*. Postural hypotension and abnormal Valsalva ratio are reported during treatment with *perhexiline maleate*. Autonomic dysfunction may develop within days of *vincristine* treatment for malignancy, possibly because unmyelinated axons are especially sensitive to this agent.

Hypothalamus, Hippocampus, and Limbic System

The hypothalamus and associated limbic structures serve to maintain internal homeostasis directly through regulation of endocrine secretion and the autonomic nervous system, and indirectly with the neocortex through the control of arousal, emotion, and motivated behavior. The hypothalamus regulates vital functions that are adversely and nonspecifically impacted by a range of chemicals: these functions include temperature, heart rate, blood pressure, blood osmolarity, circadian control, and water and food intake. Mice treated systemically in infancy with *glutamate*, *aspartate*, or *cysteic acid* display extensive damage of the arcuate hypothalamic nucleus and develop a syndrome of obesity, skeletal stunting, reproductive failure, and hypoplasia of the adenohypophysis and gonads, together with abnormally low hypothalamic, pituitary or plasma levels of growth hormone, lactogenic hormone, and prolactin. Surprisingly, no studies have explored the possibility of a relationship between human obesity and early life exposure to excitatory amino acids in food. Agents such as *reserpine*, which impact serotonergic and noradrenergic input to hypothalamic and limbic structures, trigger adverse CNS effects (depression, drowsiness, tiredness, confusion) in the human subject.

The hypothalamus receives major input from the hippocampus, which functions in the storage of declarative memory. Hippocampal neurons display long-term potentiation (a possible basis for memory) after receiving a train of excitatory stimuli. Excitatory inputs arise from the subiculum to the granule cells of the dentate gyrus; from the granule cells to the pyramidal cells of the CA3 region by way of the perforant pathway, and from CA3 neurons to pyramidal cells in CA1 by means of Schaffer collaterals. CA1 and CA3 neurons are enriched in glutamate receptors and therefore susceptible to *hypoxia* and *glutamate analogs (vide supra)*. *Domoic acid*, a kainate analog that damages the equivalent areas (H1, H3) in the human brain, disturbs memory function. Other agents that damage hippocampal neurons experimentally include systemically administered *trimethyl tin*, *trimethyl lead*, and *soman*; some of these effects may result from drug-induced seizures that generate hypoxic episodes rather than a direct neurotoxic effect of the substance. Nerve agents such as soman are proposed to damage hippocampal neurons by interfering with presynaptic cholinergic modulation of glutamatergic and GABAergic inputs.

The principal hippocampal output is an elongate myelinated pathway (fornix) that projects to the mammillary bodies and to the hypothalamus. Axonal swellings typical of hexacarbon neuropathy are evident in the mammillary bodies of cats treated with *2,5-hexanedione*. Treatment of dogs with *vigabatrin*, a GABA-transaminase inhibitor, induces intramyelinic edema in the fornix and optic tracts.

DEVELOPMENTAL NEUROTOXICITY

The dominant host factor influencing human response to exogenous chemicals is developmental state. For the fetus, the primary source of exposure to exogenous chemicals is the maternal blood supply; chemicals therein may diffuse across the placenta, enter the fetal circulation, and reach the developing nervous system. Some agents (*organic arsenicals*) accumulate in the placenta and spare the offspring from exposure. Prior to keratinization of the human fetal epidermis, beginning at 20 weeks of gestation, toxic components may diffuse from the amniotic fluid into the developing fetus. The internal environment of the postnatal organism is shielded from foreign chemicals by partial or complete barriers represented by the gastrointestinal system, lungs, and skin.

The intrinsic neural factors that determine or influence response to chemicals differ in development, at maturity, and in late life. The tissue response to chemicals during development is dictated largely by the stage of fetal growth and tissue construction. Dramatic chemical-induced changes in tissues that contain cells undergoing mitosis, migration, or differentiation are not seen when exposure to the same agent occurs prior to or following these tissue-forming events. Other developmental periods of susceptibility to chemicals are concurrent with the establishment of neuronal interconnectivity, synaptogenesis, and myelinogenesis. The normal developmental paring of excess nerve cells by programmed cell death (apoptotic and nonapoptotic) is another potential target for chemical perturbation.

Developmental state may dictate the qualitative nature of the response of humans to chemicals with neurotoxic potential. For example, infants of mothers treated with the anticonvulsant drug *sodium valproate* may display congenital malformations, including neural tube defects, whereas neurotoxicity in the adult is featured by tremor, a confusional state and, exceptionally, parkinsonism. Whereas *thalidomide* induces amelia and phocomelia present at birth, mothers using the sedative are at risk for toxic peripheral neuropathy.

Sensitive Periods of Neural Development

Although the agent, dose, and duration of exposure are the major factors that codify the response of adult humans and animals to neurotoxic chemicals, *the timing of exposure to chemicals is of overarching importance in determining the effect of exogenous agents on developing organisms*. This is dictated by the developmental stage of the organism and the critical periods of organ susceptibility to chemicals that exist within any one stage of prenatal or postnatal development. Chemicals may induce fetal death, growth retardation, premature birth, stillbirth, behavioral or functional deficits in the offspring or, for teratogenic chemicals, structural malformations of the nervous system and/or other organs that are detectable at birth (congenital) or postnatally.

Exposure to certain chemicals (*vitamin A*) during the sensitive period for brain development (gestation days 5–10 in rats) may result in marked and uncorrectable abnormalities, including anencephaly and spina bifida. By contrast, the same compound administered on gestation day 12 fails to perturb brain development. Similarly, chemical exposure of the developing human fetus during the closure of the neural tube (fourth week of gestation) may lead to defects caudally (spina bifida) or cranially (anencephaly). Once the neural tube has closed and the brain is differentiating regionally, toxic insults may cause grossly abnormal brain structures such as prosencephaly (cyclocephaly).

The proliferation, migration, and differentiation of cells that accompany the fetal stage of neural development result in a progressive increase in brain size; the most obvious effect of chemical interference is to restrict brain growth (microcephaly). This is demonstrated in rats treated on gestational days 14–16 (but not on day 17) with the potent genotoxic agent *methylazoxymethanol (MAM)*. Parenteral administration of MAM to the mother eventuates in a dose-dependent reduction in the size of the cerebral hemispheres when examined at day 28. Similar dose-dependent decreases in brain size can be induced by administration between gestational days 12 and 14 of *ethylnitrosourea (ENU)* which, like MAM, alkylates DNA with the formation of persistent adducts (O^6-alkylguanine). While the cerebral cortex of rats treated with ENU on embryonic day 14 or 15 shows differentiation into six neuronal layers, the cortex is abnormally thin and the number of neurons reduced. By contrast, minor reductions in neuronal number are seen in animals treated with ENU on gestational day 20 or 21.

The final stage of development of the human brain, especially the cerebellum, occupies the latter part of gestation and continues postnatally in many species. From gestational month 6 through 1.5 years after birth, the external granular cell layer of the cerebellum begins to release various cell types that migrate inward toward the differentiating Purkinje cell layer sequentially to form granule, basket, and stellate cells. In rodents, agents such as MAM interfere with the proliferation of external granule cells, reduce the number of cells that migrate to form the internal granule cell layer, and thereby induce a hypoplastic cerebellum with ectopic and multinucleated cells.

Postnatal development is featured by dendritic arborization, synaptogenesis, and myelination, all of which may be disrupted by foreign chemicals.

Neuronal arborization is sensitive. Defective development of dendrites and dendritic spines is found in rats made hypothyroidic, exposed to *ionizing radiation*, or deprived of food during the neonatal period. Rats treated with *MAM* during the neonatal period display Purkinje cell dendrites with postsynaptic densities on spines that lack an adjacent presynaptic element. Retarded growth and maturation of neurons/axons occur in malnutrition and in *chronic lead intoxication*.

Receptors may change with development. The α-subunit of the glycine receptor has several isoforms that are transcriptionally regulated during development, such that the adult rodent spinal-cord glycine receptor has a higher affinity for *strychnine* than the neonatal receptor.

Neurotoxic responses may differ from those in the adult Mature presynaptic and postsynaptic circuitry appears to be required for the initiation of postnatal susceptibility of the rodent striatum (day 21) and cerebellum to the glutamate analog *kainate*. The neurotoxic response of the immature rat brain to *NMDA*, which is greater than in the adult animal, is well developed much earlier (day 7). In newborn rats (1–12 days), subcutaneous injection of *capsaicin* causes a total ablation of substance P-containing and other neuropeptide-rich, small sensory neurons in dorsal root and cranial ganglia. Centrally and peripherally directed axons are thereby lost. This results in permanent deficits of nociceptive sensibility and local effector functions of these neurons, including distention-induced micturition mediated by substance P-containing neurons in the bladder wall. Other abnormalities occur in pain-avoidance reactions, thermoregulation, neuroendocrine and visceral reflexes, and satiety.

Myelination is sensitive during development. Development of glial and myelinating cells occurs in stages under the control of growth hormone. Myelin formation takes place in the late prenatal and early postnatal periods. Inhibitors of cholesterol metabolism experimentally induce degenerative changes in oligodendrocytes and CNS myelin. Animals given *triparanol* or *trans-1,4-bis*(p-*chlorobenzylaminomethyl*)*cyclohexane dihydrochloride*, agents that block steps in cholesterol biosynthesis, display oligodendrocyte degeneration, with fragmentation of the adaxonal portion of oligodendrocytes, vacuolation of myelin, demyelination, and degeneration of axons. Weanling rats given a diet containing *tellurium* develop peripheral segmental demyelination and remyelination in association with disruption of cholesterol biosynthesis. Synthesis of sterols is markedly depressed in sciatic nerve because tellurium inhibits squalene epoxidase, an enzyme involved in cholesterol biosynthesis. Newly synthesized squalene accumulates in the cytoplasm of Schwann cells. Tellurium neuropathy is not seen in older animals, presumably because cholesterol and myelin biosynthesis decreases and vulnerability to tellurium disappears. *Metallic molybdenum* fed in the diet of pregnant ewes throughout gestation to within 1 month of lambing resulted in "ataxia" of offspring associated with motor neuron damage and myelin loss.

Fetal and Newborn Toxic Syndromes

Chemicals have ready access to the developing nervous system because the CNS and PNS components thereof have yet to become segregated within the specially protected micro-environments that are "sealed" after birth (see Factors Associated with the Nervous System *vide infra*). Systemically distributed compounds such as *lead* salts, which generally do not elicit brain damage in adults, are able readily to enter the brain and cause severe encephalopathy in newborn animals and humans. The toxic effects of 6-*hydroxydopamine* are proportionately greater in newborn than in mature animals. Offspring of rodents treated with the antiseptic *hexachlorophene* may have hydrocephalus, anophthalmia, microphthalmia, and cleft palate. Chemical exposure of the fetus thus may cause structural and/or functional changes that are expressed both in the brain and in other organs.

Approximately 1300 chemicals are recognized teratogens in animals; about 20 are so recognized in humans. *Ethyl alcohol* is teratogenic in at least nine mammalian species and in humans [fetal alcohol syndrome, (FAS)]; as many as 7 per 1000 liveborns are reported to express FAS in some manner. Maternal *smoking of tobacco* has been linked to a "fetal tobacco syndrome" in the offspring. Excess vitamins A and D (cholecalciferol) are teratogenic for human and animal species, and excess vitamin D (calcitrol), vitamin E, and vitamin K are teratogenic for the mouse. *Inorganic and organic mercury compounds* are teratogenic for animals and humans. Fetal cord blood *lead* levels are dose-dependently associated with increased risk for minor anomalies, and postnatal neurobehavioral development and intelligence test scores may be compromised. Mental retardation in children has been linked to parental *lead* or *cadmium* exposure; it is proven in the case of *mercury intoxication*.

Teratogenic effects of various types are reported in laboratory animals in association with excessive exposure to metallic *boron* (brain and skeletal defects), *cadmium chloride* (hydrocephalus, eye and skeletal defects), *cesium arsenate* (multiple malformations), and *chromium chloride* (exencephaly and skeletal defects).

1. Maternal exposure to mercury compounds is an established cause of birth defects involving the nervous system. Exposure at a fetal gestation age of 6–8 months appears to be associated with the most severe outcome. Asymptomatic or symptomatic pregnant women exposed to oral organic mercurials (*methylmercuric sulfide, chloride*, or *dicyandiamide*) may bear apparently healthy offspring who develop signs of severe neurological damage in the early postnatal period. Microcephaly may be evident. Convulsions, cerebral palsy, mental retardation, motor impairment, blindness, deafness, excessive irritability, inappropriate emotional expression, and speech disorders represent the range of deficits seen in infants with methylmercury intoxication (known as Minamata disease). Methylmercuric chloride is a potent CNS teratogen in many animal species. Methylmercuric dicyandiamide administered to pregnant mice induces brain and jaw defects, cleft palate, and postnatal behavioral changes. Phenyl mercuric acetate causes CNS, eye, and tail defects in mice.
2. Maternal exposure to various substances can lead to fetal abnormalities. The most prevalent example is fetal alcohol syndrome, which impacts 10–15% of children born to mothers with *excessive chronic alcohol use*. Cognitive impairment, expressed in the form of mental retardation and learning disability, is accompanied by growth deficiency, facial dymorphism, and occasionally cardiac and skeletal abnormalities. Cognitive and behavioral (attention deficits) abnormalities in the absence of physical abnormalities affect children born to an estimated 40% of mothers who drink alcoholic beverages heavily during pregnancy.
3. Maternal use of anticonvulsants (*phenytoin, carbamazepine, primidone*, or *valproate*) is associated with development of a fetal antiepileptic drug syndrome. Anomalies involve the brain (microcephaly), cognitive or motor performance, craniofacies, limbs, and other changes.
4. Fetal exposure to maternal *cocaine* may result in microcephaly, structural abnormalities of the brain, or hemorrhagic lesions therein. Neonatal cocaine exposure syndrome is characterized by poor feeding, irritability, tremor, and abnormal sleep patterns.
5. Humans and primates exposed to *cannabis* may have offspring with decreased visual responses and increased auditory responses; these disappear within weeks to months postpartum.

Recreational illicit drugs with teratogenic potential in animals include mescaline (*Lophophora williamsii*), marijuana (*Cannabis sativa*), and cocaine (*Erythroxylum coca*). Range-plant genera with teratogenic potential for farm animals include the locoweeds *Astragalus* and *Oxytropis*, hemlock (*Conium—coniine*), jimsonweed (*Datura*), *Leucaena* (*mimosine*), *Lupinus*, tobacco (*Nicotiana*), and false hellebore (*Veratrum alkaloids*). Plants used by humans for medicinal purposes elaborate principles (*reserpine, vinca alkaloids, colchicine, atropine, hyoscyamine, scopolamine, tubocurarine, ergotamine, pilocarpine, physostigmine, ephedrine, codeine, morphine, theobromine*) with teratogenic potential in mice or rats, or both species. *Quinine* is associated with CNS abnormalities in the chinchilla, cranial nerve defects in the rabbit, inner ear defects in the guinea pig, and deafness associated with auditory nerve hypoplasia in humans. *Hypoglycin A and B* from the West Indian ackee fruit (*Blighia sapida*) are teratogenic in rats and anectodally in humans. The potato (*Solanum tuberosum*) contains an agent (*solasodine*) with teratogenic properties in the rat and hamster. In humans, the proposed link between maternal consumption of blighted potatoes and neural tube defects in the offspring is unproven.

Although most laboratory animals appear refractory, hamsters treated orally with potato sprouts containing *solanidine*, the aglycone of the *Solanum* glycoalkaloids α-*solanine* and α-*chaconine*, or with spirosolane-containing wild *Solanum* spp., have litters with craniofacial malformations including exencephaly (exposed brain), encephalocele (herniated brain), cebocephaly (nasal chamber defect), unilateral anophthalmia (single eye), and cleft palate.

Structurally, spirosolanes incorporate an oxazaspirodecane moiety onto a steroidal framework: the presence or absence of a teratogenic property appears to depend on the presence and configurational position of nitrogen in the F-ring. The teratogenic compound *solasodine*, which is present in the food plants *S. melongene* (eggplant), *S. quitoense* (Andean naranjilla), and some cultivars of *S. tuberosum* (potato), bears a nitrogen atom of the piperidine ring below the steroidal plane; *tomatidine*, by contrast, has the nitrogen atom in the β position (above the steroidal plane) and lacks a teratogenic property. (Tomatidine is the aglycone of tomatine from the tomato plant *Lycopersicon esculentum*). However, the amino nitrogen and its unshared electron pair project above the steroidal plane in α-solanine, α-chaconine, and solanidine, all three of which are teratogenic in the hamster. Since equimolar doses of both steroidal glycoalkaloids and their aglycones produce a similar incidence of malformations, the oligosaccharide component of glycoalkaloids is not required to facilitate passage of the teratogen to the fetus.

CNS AND PNS CHEMICAL ONCOGENESIS

There are no proven examples of human CNS neoplasia resulting from exogenous chemical exposure. Primary malignant tumors in adult humans mostly commonly arise from glial cells, especially astrocytes (astrocytoma). Tumors derived from neurons (gangliocytoma, neurocytoma) are rare, as are tumors with mixed neuronal and glial properties (gangliocytomas). *Cranial irradiation* is the only factor consistently associated with increased risk for malignant brain tumors in children (particularly neurilemmoma and meningioma). In adults, proposed risk factors include occupational exposure to *vinyl chloride* or *methylene chloride*. An association between *lead* exposure and risk of glioma has been suggested in humans and laboratory animals. Drinking water containing high levels (500 ppm) of *acrylonitrile* increases the number of microscopically detectable primary brain tumors in various rat strains, but epidemiological studies of acrylonitrile-exposed workers have failed to detect excess "brain cancers." Subjects with malignant disease who are treated systemically with antineoplastic agents with carcinogenic potential do not appear to be at special risk for the later development of chemical-induced primary CNS tumors.

Malignant transformation of neural cells, with the subsequent development of tumors, can be induced experimentally by topical or systemic administration of various classes of chemical carcinogen. For example, direct intracranial implantation of *methylcholanthrene* transforms normal glial and meningeal cells into highly anaplastic tumors in rodents. Systemic administration of certain compounds during development, postnatally, or adult life may induce tumor formation; active compounds include *aryldialkyltriazenes*; *alkylnitrosoureas*; and a number of other alkylating agents such as *dialkyl sulfates*, *alkylmethanesulfonates*, *propanesultone*, *propyleneimine*, *acrylonitrile*, *vinyl chloride*, *ethylene oxide*, and *bis(chloromethyl)ether*. Transplacental induction of malignant tumors of the nervous system of rats is produced by single doses of agents such as *ethylnitrosourea*, *hydrazoethane*, *azoethane*, and *azoxyethane*.

Carcinogens that form reactive species, electrophiles, or free radicals, undergo covalent reactions with most cellular macromolecules containing nucleophilic sites, including DNA. Malignant transformation is initiated by these genotoxic agents by chemical modification of DNA through covalent reactions that result in the formation of DNA adducts. DNA adducts are removed by DNA-repair enzyme systems that allow the cell to recover from the effects of the carcinogen. However, if the DNA-damaged cell enters the S phase of DNA replication prior to enzyme-induced repair, permanent genomic alterations (point mutations) may result. Newborn and young animals and humans are generally more sensitive to carcinogens, in large part because they possess higher cell replication rates. Restricted food intake, especially during development, reduces cell replication rates and the frequency of neoplasms, notably in nonneural, endocrine-sensitive organs.

Experimental treatment of rats with *ethylnitrosourea* (*ENU*), from gestational days 13–23, leads to the dose-dependent appearance in the offspring of malignant tumors of the brain, spinal cord, and cranial and peripheral nerves. Rat fetal brain tissue is approximately 50 times more sensitive than adult nervous tissue to the carcinogenic potential of ENU, and mice are proportionately much less sensitive during development and perinatally. Nonhuman primates transplacentally exposed to ENU early in gestation develop tumors in the cerebrum, brainstem, and cerebellum.

Two cardinal principles appear to underly the nervous system response to genotoxic carcinogens. One is the ability of neural cells to repair DNA damage; the second is the differential susceptibility of glial cells relative to neurons. Since most nerve cells become postmitotic and presumably refractory to neoplastic induction by genotoxic agents, it would be expected *a priori* that neuron-derived tumors would be much less common than those evolved from glial cells. This principle is upheld for neurogenic tumors induced in rats following prenatal or postnatal exposure to *nitrosamides*: while isolated cases of neoplastic transformation of neurons are reported, most CNS tumors are derived from transformed oligodendrocytes, astrocytes, or ependymal cells, and most PNS tumors from neoplastic

Schwann cells. DNA repair systems in nerve cells are perturbed by *nitrogen mustard* to a greater extent than those in astrocytes *in vitro*. The second principle relates to the relative efficacy of repair of DNA damage in the brain vs. other organs. Genotoxic alkylating agents trigger the formation of a variety of DNA adducts, some of which (*e.g.*, 7-methylguanine) are relatively innocuous because they are lost spontaneously by nonenzymic depurination; others (O^6-methylguanine), by contrast, are promutagenic because of their ability to induce point mutations following DNA synthesis. DNA damaged in this way is repaired by selective transfer of the alkyl group from the O^6 position of guanine to the cysteine moiety of a specific DNA-repair enzyme, O^6-alkylguanine transferase, which is inactivated during the repair process. While O^6-alkylguanine transferase is widely distributed in tissues, O^6-methylguanine adducts are removed much more rapidly in the liver and kidney than in the brain of young and adult animals previously treated with *methylnitrosourea* (*MNU*) or *ENU*. One-quarter of the O^6-methylguanine adducts produced by a single dose of MNU is detectable in cerebral DNA 6 months later. This suggests that rat CNS tumors are selectively triggered by alkylating agents such as *nitrosoureas* because, in contrast to the rapidly repaired DNA damage in liver and kidney cells, structural DNA alterations in glia become fixed during cell replication. However, gerbils show the same persistence of MNU-induced DNA adducts but are not susceptible to brain tumors.

The combination of these two principles implies that neural cells repair DNA damage slowly. Glial nuclear DNA is alkylated by MNU to a similar extent as neuronal nuclear DNA, but the comparable rates of DNA repair are unknown. Indeed, the question of DNA repair in postmitotic neurons has not attracted the interest of cancer biologists because these cells are largely refractory to neoplastic transformation. The long-term fate of mature nerve cells with excessive DNA damage and inadequate DNA repair is currently under investigation in relation to age-related changes and induction of neurodegenerative disease.

SELECTED BIBLIOGRAPHY

Bradley WG, Daroff RB, Fenichel GM, Marsden CD (1996) *Neurology in Clinical Practice. 2nd Ed*. Butterworth-Heinemann, Newton, MA.

Brust JCM (1993) *Neurological Aspects of Substance Abuse*. Butterworth-Heinemann, Boston.

Chang LW, Dyer RS (1995) *Handbook of Neurotoxicology*. Marcel Dekker, New York.

Dukes MNG (1997) *Meyler's Side Effects of Drugs. An Encyclopedia of Adverse Reactions and Interactions. 13th Ed*. Elsevier, Amsterdam.

Falconer IR (1993) *Algal Toxins in Seafood and Drinking Water*. Academic Press, New York.

Feldman RG (1998) *Occupational and Environmental Neurotoxicology*. Lippincott-Raven, Philadelphia.

Fowler MEF (1993) *Veterinary Zootoxicology*. CRC Press, Boca Raton, FL.

Grant MW, Schulman JS (1993) *Toxicology of the Eye. 4th Ed*. Charles C Thomas, Springfield, Il.

Hardman JG, Limbird LE (1996) *Goodman & Gilman's The Pharmacological Basis of Therapeutics. 9th Ed*. McGraw Hill, New York.

Herken H, Hucho F (1994) *Selective Neurotoxicity*. Springer-Verlag, Berlin.

Kandel ER, Schwartz JA, Jessell TM (1992) *Principles of Neural Science. 3rd Ed*. Elsevier, New York.

Kaplan HI, Sadock BJ (1995) *Comprehensive Textbook of Psychiatry. 6th Ed*. Williams & Wilkins, Baltimore.

Keeler RF, Tu AT (1983) *Handbook of Natural Toxins. Vol 1*. Marcel Dekker, New York.

Klassen CD (1996) *Casarett & Doull's Toxicology. The Basic Science of Poisons*. McGraw Hill, New York.

Niesink RJM, Jaspers RMA, Kornet LMW *et al*. (1999) *Introduction to Neurobehavioral Toxicology*. Food and Environment. CRC, Boca Raton, FL.

Schardein JL (1993) *Chemically Induced Birth Defects. 2nd Ed*. Marcel Dekker, New York.

Siegel GJ, Agranoff BW, Albers RW, Molinoff PB (1994) *Basic Neurochemistry*. Raven, New York.

Slikker W, Chang LW (1998) *Handbook of Developmental Neurotoxicology*. Academic Press, New York.

Spencer PS, Butterfield PG (1995) Environmental agents and Parkinson's disease. In: *Etiology of Parkinson's Disease*. Ellenberg JH, Koller WC, Langston JC eds. Marcel Dekker, New York p. 319.

Spencer PS, Schaumburg HH (1980) *Experimental and Clinical Neurotoxicology*. Williams & Wilkins, Baltimore.

Strobel HW, Geng J, Kawashima H, Wang H (1997) Cytochrome P-450-dependent biotransformation of drugs and other xenobiotic substrates in neural tissue. *Drug Metab Rev* 29, 1097.

Tu AT (1984–1992) *Handbook of Natural Toxins. Vols 2–7*. Marcel Dekker, New York.

Vinken PJ, Bruyn GW (1994–5) *Handbook of Clinical Neurology. Intoxications of the Nervous System. Vols 64–5*. Elsevier, New York.

Yasui M, Strong MJ, Ota K, Verity MA (1997) *Mineral and Metal Neurotoxicity*. CRC Press, Boca Raton, FL.

CHAPTER TWO

Human Neurotoxic Disease

Herbert H. Schaumburg

There are five well-recognized sources of postnatal human neurotoxic disorders*: pharmaceutical agents, either physician triggered (iatrogenic) or self-initiated; biological agents, contact with botanical, animal, or bacterial products; occupational chemical exposure, in the workplace itself; environmental chemical exposure—domestic, general; and self-administered—abuse, suicide, homicide.

Pharmaceutical neurotoxic conditions are common in North America; most are iatrogenic. It is generally easy to make a causative association when neurological disease stems from *pharmaceutical* agents. Occasionally, self-administered neurotoxic drugs or nutritional supplements cause unidentified instances of dysfunction; these rarely reach mini-epidemic proportions before other cases with the same disorder are recognized.

Biological neurotoxic agents may produce regionally specific cases or even epidemics of acute or chronic neurotoxicity.

Environmental and *occupational* neurotoxic conditions are relatively rare in North America despite the vast numbers of chemicals and agents encountered daily.

Self-administered—Neurotoxicity is associated with prolonged inhalant abuse of solvents and may accompany overdose with alcohol and street drugs. Pesticides are commonly used as suicidal agents in less-developed countries. Homicide and suicide from neurotoxic agents are rare in North America.

CAUSATION CRITERIA FOR IDENTIFICATION OF NEUROTOXICITY

Fulfillment of the following five criteria is ideal in establishing causation (the conceptual basis and amplification for these criteria are presented in the following section of this chapter).

1. Presence of the suspected agent is confirmed by history and either environmental or clinical chemical analysis.
2. Severity and temporal onset of the condition are commensurate with duration and level of exposure.
3. The condition is self-limiting, and clinical improvement follows removal from exposure.
4. Clinical features display a consistent pattern that correspond to previous cases.
5. Development of a satisfactory corresponding experimental *in vivo* or *in vitro* model is absolute proof of causation.

The single most useful instrument in acute and chronic disorders is an accurate history. Criteria 2–4 are of cardinal importance in the acute setting since the analytical laboratory rarely is available.

---

*Neurological dysfunction in children that results from *in utero* exposure to exogenous agents has been consistently associated with toluene, alcohol, and phenytoin. Neuroteratogenicity from these and other agents is discussed under the appropriate headings in the A–Z catalogue section (from p. 108).

CARDINAL TENETS OF NEUROTOXIC DISEASE

Strong Dose–Response Relationship

Most chemicals that trigger structural damage to the nervous system produce a consistent pattern of disease, commensurate with the dose and duration of exposure. Significant exposure of the nervous system to a single neurotoxic agent will invariably produce similar dysfunction in most individuals. Aside from endogenous factors that may modify the intensity of the disorder, such as age, sex, body weight, and renal/liver integrity, there are few major genetic-based variations in the human response to neurotoxic substances (*vide infra*). Few syndromes have an indirect, immunological basis.

Proximity to Exposure

Neurotoxic illness usually occurs concurrent with exposure or following a short latent period. The three most notorious exceptions, the two-to-six-week delay to neuropathy following exposure to *organophosphates*, the occasional two-month latency to onset of *cisplatin* neuropathy, and the two-month delay of onset of symptoms of *methyl mercury* intoxication, are not in the same league as the multi-year intervals characteristic of mesothelioma from asbestos exposure. Some agents may produce delayed neurotoxic effects because they are stored in non-neural tissues and released slowly (*chloroquine* in the choroid of the eye) or precipitously (*lead* in bone) during illness or chelation therapy. Other agents (*ciguatoxin*) produce repeated bouts of illness presumably because they are able to persist in the body. Some lipid-stored agents (*e.g., chlorinated hydrocarbons*) are detectable in fat biopsies years following exposure. Although this provides a valuable biological marker of previous exposure, there is no evidence that this state is associated with risk for future neurotoxic disorders, and attempts at removal or mobilization of the body burden are misguided.

Improvement Usually Follows Cessation of Exposure

Neurotoxic illness generally improves gradually after exposure to the culpable agent ceases. Improvement can occasionally be rapid (days) if biochemical or neurophysiological changes are involved in the absence of structural changes to cells or their processes. When these are present, as in a peripheral neuropathy associated with axonal degeneration, the clinical deficit may advance (coasting) before recovery commences. In the event of significant neuronal loss or irreparable damage to the brain or spinal cord, recovery may be absent or incomplete. Multi-year delayed

appearance of sensory loss following previous exposure has been reported for *inorganic mercury*; this may represent the emergence of signs secondary to age-associated neuronal loss that is superimposed upon toxin-induced degenerative changes.

Multiple Clinical Syndromes May Result from Different Exposures to a Single Toxin

Exposure to different levels of some substances may result in a dramatically different clinical picture. This fundamental principle may be overlooked in the haste to simplify a puzzling clinical problem. For example, acute massive consumption of *clioquinol* causes a toxic encephalopathy characterized by striking loss of recent memory that resembles the transient global amnesia syndrome, while prolonged exposure to lower levels may cause myelopathy in humans and laboratory animals. *Organophosphate* over-exposure may result in acute cholinergic paralysis from inhibition of acetylcholinesterase or delayed-onset distal axonopathy from unassociated mechanisms. Bizarre and apparently mysterious clinical situations may occasionally result from unusual exposures. For example, although acute, high-level exposure to acrylamide causes a toxic encephalopathy with seizures as a prominent feature, and prolonged low-level exposure produces a peripheral neuropathy of the distal axonopathy type, a puzzling syndrome of hallucinations, confusion, and cognitive disturbance, followed by distal limb sensory impairment, appeared in members of a Japanese family intoxicated with an intermediate dose of acrylamide from contaminated well water.

Some substances, such as pyridoxine, cause approximately similar types of nervous system dysfunction at high and low doses regardless of duration; a single massive intravenous dose causes a diffuse sensory neuronopathy within days, while daily oral megavitamin doses cause distal limb sensory loss after 1 year.

Asymptomatic Disease

Asymptomatic toxic disease of the nervous system occurs and, under certain circumstances, may be widespread. Unless a person performs at an unusually skilled job or requires consistent, high-level intellectual activity, a modest decline in performance may go unnoticed by the individual. An analogous phenomenon has been described in workers with subclinical toxic neuropathies who deny any disability, despite the presence of sensory dysfunction that was obvious to their spouses. A similarly unnoticed spastic paraparesis occurs in Indian farmers with a mild degree of lathyrism.

Modulation by Bystander Chemicals

An agent without known neurotoxic activity may modulate (enhance or depress) the toxicity of a known neurotoxic agent. This disquieting notion has become an emotional issue, as many fear the effects of chemical mixtures at the site of hazardous waste disposal. The phenomenon of potentiation of a neurotoxic chemical by a second, apparently innocuous agent is best exemplified by a mini-epidemic of peripheral neuropathy among Berlin youths who inhaled fumes from a paint thinner to induce euphoria. The solvent formulation initially contained the potentially neurotoxic substance n-*hexane*, but at a level that failed to produce neuropathy. However, when the solvent was reformulated by lowering the concentration of *n*-hexane and introducing methyl ethyl ketone (MEK), several developed severe peripheral neuropathy. Experimental studies subsequently demonstrated that, while MEK was unable to produce experimental neuropathy, the compound potentiated the neurotoxic property of *n*-hexane.

Chemical Formula May Not Predict Toxicity

The neurotoxic potential of a substance usually cannot reliably be predicted by its chemical formula. This has been an especially vexing issue in evaluating cases with occupational exposure to chemicals superficially similar to substances with established neurotoxic potential. Workers who handle acrylamide polymer, an innocuous substance, have been needlessly alarmed by physicians familiar only with the side effects of acrylamide monomer, a potent neurotoxin. Unpredictability prevails, in part, because the biochemical mechanisms and active metabolites of most neurotoxins are unknown. Structure-activity relationships are clear for only a few classes of substances, such as *organophosphates*, *pyrethroids*, and hydrocarbons with a common γ-diketone metabolite. Hydrocarbons with two ketone groups at slightly different spacing, may be harmless (*e.g.*, *2,5-heptanedione* is neurotoxic; *2,6-heptanedione* is not).

Age, Pre-existing Conditions or Genetic Variation in Metabolism Occasionally Modulate the Effects of a Neurotoxin

The fetal nervous system has extreme vulnerabilities to toxic exposure, especially at times of major cellular migrations. Young children or adolescents appear less vulnerable to some forms of neurotoxic exposure (*organophosphates*) and display a more robust recovery than the elderly. Several reports suggest that the aged worker is more susceptible to toxic neuropathy (n-*hexane*) and encephalopathy (*lead, organic solvents*).

Individuals with hereditary neuropathy have an enhanced vulnerability to chemotherapeutic agents associated with peripheral neuropathy; some Asian Americans have a genetic susceptibility to the ototoxicity of *aminoglycoside* antibiotics.

THE NATURE OF NEUROTOXIC DISEASE

In general, acute neurotoxic conditions, in contrast to chronic conditions, are better understood because of intense experimental investigation and laboratory models, more readily treated by *specific* therapy, less variable in presentation, easier to recognize, and less common.

Neurotoxic Clinical Syndromes (corresponds generally to Clinical Neurotoxicity Rating Scale for substances in A to Z catalogue section)

Pseudoneurotoxic Syndromes

Some agents have both a genuine neurotoxic effect and also have been erroneously identified as having other deleterious actions on the nervous system. *MEK* exemplifies this phenomenon; extreme high-level exposure can cause an acute encephalopathy; prolonged low-level exposure does not cause peripheral neuropathy. Anecdotal reports that describe cases of MEK neuropathy from exposure to solvent mixtures likely reflect the effects of another agent in the mixture, *e.g.*, *n*-hexane. Thus, MEK has a Neurotoxicity Scale Rating of A (a strong association between the substance and the condition) for acute encephalopathy and C (association is not likely to be causal) for peripheral neuropathy.

Certain other substances widely considered neurotoxic likely have little effect upon either the peripheral nervous system (PNS) or central nervous system (CNS). This misconception happens because everyday exposure to an environmental chemical or pharmaceutical agent has occurred simultaneously with an atypical or inadequately diagnosed naturally occurring condition. Two examples illustrate how these associations have been readily accepted, even when there is overwhelming experimental and clinical experience to the contrary: (a) Recent reports of occasional cases of atypical parkinsonism in workers exposed to *n*-hexane cannot be accepted as credible since parkinsonism is among the most common of neurodegenerative diseases and has never been seen in either experimental animals or humans with extreme degrees of chronic or acute *n*-hexane neuropathy, and (b) the two isolated reports of subacute motor neuropathy from trivial *dichlorophenoxyacetic acid* (2,4-D) exposure likely represent coincident occurrences of the Guillain-Barré syndrome.

Occasionally, bystander substances with genuine neurotoxic potential are uncritically and erroneously implicated as causative in unexplained pseudoneurotoxic outbreaks. For example, pyridostigmine bromide in a few oral doses of 30 mg has been considered a cause of persistent malaise among U.S. veterans of the 1991 Gulf War. Since pyridostigmine does not cross the blood-brain barrier and has been used with little consequence for decades in doses of 300 mg daily to treat myasthenia, this notion seems unreasonable at best. The rare, heavily dosed individual may develop evidence of bromism (the bromide moiety does enter the brain), and others with the a genetically based deficiency of serum butyrylcholinesterase (which may bind the drug) may display acute cholinergic signs associated with anticholinesterase actions of pyridostigmine. However, an association with the persistent cognitive and musculoskeletal complaints of some of the U.S. Gulf War veterans is most unlikely.

The phenomenon of pseudoneurotoxicity is illustrated by the recent emergence of behavioral syndromes allegedly characterized by multiorgan intolerance and self-attributed to minute amounts of environmental chemicals. These nebulous entities, variously called "idiopathic environmental intolerance," "multiple chemical sensitivity" (MCS) syndromes, or "cacosmic syndromes" (when associated with olfaction), are especially common following chronic exposure to hydrocarbon solvents or pesticide agents of any chemical type.

The conceptually simplest, least common variant of this putative disorder appears in some individuals who have experienced *genuine*, previous neurotoxic dysfunction with partial recovery. These persons re-experience similar symptoms and anxiety when casually encountering the agent or a related (sometimes an unrelated) substance in daily life. For example, patients recovered from *n*-hexane neuropathy or toluene encephalopathy may experience transient anxiety and distal numbness or headache upon smelling *gasoline fumes, perfume,* or *cigarette smoke*. In some, this is thought to reflect a conditioned reflex with stimulus generalization; these persons generally improve after deliberate repeated exposures (extinction). In others, this reaction is accompanied by high anxiety and appears to represent an atypical posttraumatic stress disorder with poor treatment outcome.

The most common variant of MCS appears in individuals with trivial initial exposure to a recognized or imagined neurotoxic substance. Re-exposure to the original agent or unrelated chemicals trigger multiorgan symptoms and psychological distress. These persons, although they do not have a recognizable medical illness, may become totally disabled by the symptoms or fear of another attack. Some feel compelled to undergo laborious detoxification or to make radical alterations in lifestyle. The protean symptoms (headache, transient confusion, lightheadedness, fatigue, joint pain, upper respiratory distress, diarrhea, bloating) of this putative disorder usually elude laboratory analysis or bedside measures. Its pathophysiology is unclear and treatment generally unsatisfactory. There has been no demonstration that symptoms of subjects with MCS segregate selectively with exposure to chemicals of concern and not with exposure to placebos. A controlled neurobehavioral study of 17 patients with symptoms of MCS suggests that these patients do not have compromised CNS functioning (4). An authoritative review states that these persons "form a heterogeneous group, including individuals who (a) have unusual sensitivities to a broad range of chemicals, although not on a strictly allergic or immunological basis; (b) amplify normal bodily sensations that they incorrectly attribute to chemical exposure; (c) amplify normal or mild irritant reactions to many environmental substances and become ill rather than only mildly somatic; (d) suffer from a primary psychiatric disorder, or (e) suffer from a psychiatric disorder secondary to MCS" (5).

Some substances associated with minor neurotoxic dysfunction have been erroneously implicated as having serious effects upon the human nervous system. For example, although *trichloroethylene, MEK,* n-*heptane,* and *styrene* may cause an acute encephalopathy following acute high-level exposure, they appear unlikely to cause the attributed peripheral neuropathy. Compounds with pseudoneurotoxic attributes are rated C on the Neurotoxicity Rating Scale.

Physical Dependence/Addiction/Abuse

Drug dependence and addiction are frequently undesired effects of drugs upon the nervous system; in the broadest sense, they could be construed to constitute neurotoxic reactions and merit considerable discussion. However, this field includes a wide range of pharmacological, political, and social issues that are beyond the scope of this text. A concise and scholarly review is available (6).

Since these terms are loosely applied in common clinical parlance, a few definitions are useful (6). *Physical dependence* is a state that becomes evident when an intense physical reaction occurs following withdrawal of the drug or administration of an antagonist.

Addiction is a state of psychic dependence; it need not always be accompanied by physical dependence. For example, abstinent tobacco smokers frequently have intense desire and craving without apparent physical findings. Conversely, many who receive opioids for pain will experience withdrawal symptoms but do not crave the drug. An addict is an individual who has a continuing social preoccation with finding drugs.

The term *abuse* is a loosely applied social or legal judgment, not a medical or biological term. One may be considered a drug abuser after a one-time inhalation of (illegal) cocaine or using a legal substance in amounts others consider excessive (alcohol).

Psychobiological Reactions

Nonspecific psychiatric symptoms such as apathy, mood fluctuations, euphoria, irritability, nightmares, and mild impairment of psychomotor performance accompany therapy with many agents used in psychiatry (antidepressants, hypnotics).

Severe anxiety and/or depression commonly accompany neurotoxic diseases; these reactions usually are psychobiological responses to the situation rather than a direct effect of a chemical upon the nervous system (*e.g.*, an effect upon catecholamines).

Certain substances consistently can, by biochemical action, induce anxiety (*amphetamines*), depression (*lead, methyldopa, reserpine*), or mania (*corticosteroids*). Some hallucinogenic pharmaceutical agents can mimic a schizophrenic psychotic reaction; however, these are *transient*, pharmacological illnesses and recovered individuals usually revert to their pre-existent psychological states. Stated otherwise, individuals who have recovered from an acute neurotoxic disease rarely display permanent, well-defined neurotic or psychotic psychiatric disorders [*Diagnostic and Statistical Manual of Mental Disorders, 4th Ed.* (DSM-IV) criteria] that reflect a biochemical effect of the agent.

Mixed behavioral syndromes of irritability, apathy, and even psychosis sometimes are early manifestations in individuals with diffuse CNS dysfunction from toxic chemicals (*carbon disulfide, manganese, bromine, toluene*). In these instances, the distinction between psychobiological reaction

and acute encephalopathy becomes arbitrary. Generally, most neurotoxic disorders do not cause psychosis without some other sign of CNS dysfunction (*e.g.*, tremor usually accompanies or closely follows manganese- or toluene-associated behavioral symptoms).

Table 2.1 lists agents associated with psychobiological reactions.

Acute Encephalopathy Syndromes (Cortical-Subcortical Neuronal Encephalopathy/Leukoencephalopathy)

The overwhelming majority of the acute toxic encephalopathies predominantly reflects cortical or subcortical (brain stem, basal nuclei) *neuronal* dysfunction; leukoencephalopathies, in which clinical manifestations reflect disease confined to *subcortical white matter*, are uncommon.

Acute cortical-subcortical neuronal encephalopathy (ACE), in common clinical use, is usually synonymous with delirium. ACE may be operationally defined as a transient (hours, days) symptomatic alteration in CNS function (disturbance of consciousness) occurring soon after an endogenous metabolic derangement or following exposure to an external agent. Sudden abstinence from some exogenous CNS cortical or brainstem depressant agents (*e.g.*, *ethanol* and *barbiturates*) can also precipitate an ACE.

Alteration in global cognitive function and levels of attention and consciousness (frequently with psychosis, confusion) are the hallmarks of ACE. Acute encephalopathies of endogenous origin are common in North American tertiary care centers; well-known causes include febrile/septic states, severe renal or hepatic dysfunction, and rapid alterations in blood glucose levels or hydrogen ion concentration. Most acute toxic encephalopathies are not characterized by CNS tissue destruction; improvement is usual.

Most ACE agents produce a nonspecific mild or severe illness, depending on dose and duration of exposure. Without an adequate history, it is difficult for emergency room personnel to determine the cause of an ACE syndrome in an acutely ill person. Only a few substances (*atropine, acetylcholine esterase inhibitors, nitrite, cocaine, phencyclidine*) induce behavioral, neurological or physical examination characteristics that allow an examiner to pinpoint the cause.

Mild, symptomatic, toxic ACEs are usually distinguished by lightheadedness and a sense of gait instability. Mild, generalized headache is occasionally present. The individual appears normal and neurological examination is usually unremarkable; occasionally, a few beats of horizontal nystagmus appear. In most instances, recovery is complete 24 h following withdrawal. This state is exemplified by the early stages of alcohol or toluene intoxication.

TABLE 2.1. Substances Associated with Psychobiological Reactions

Amanita toxins	Lysergic acid
Amphetamines	Mefloquine
Carbon disulfide	Mercury
Catha edulis	Mescaline
Corticosteroids	Methylxanthines
Datura stramonium	Phencyclidine
Indolealkylamines	Psilocybin/Psilocyn
Indomethacin	Quinacrine
Ipomoea spp.	Reserpine
Isoxazololes	Tricyclic antidepressants
L-dopa	Zolpidem

Some high-dose, acutely toxic ACEs are initially characterized by delirium that includes obvious confusion, poor judgment, and unsteady gait. Individuals appear agitated and hyperactive. If intoxication continues, disequilibrium becomes severe, consciousness diminishes to a stuporous level, and seizures may commence. In extreme cases, profound CNS depression and coma develop, accompanied by life-threatening respiratory depression. A wide range of hypnotics and tranquilizers produces this type of encephalopathy; recovery may take several days, is sometimes incomplete, and can be associated with anoxic CNS tissue destruction. Another type of ACE commences with seizures, tremors, myoclonus and ataxia before progressing to coma; *lithium* and *acyclovir* intoxications exemplify this reaction.

The "serotonin syndrome" is a recently recognized ACE with several distinguishing features (16). This condition occasionally appears in individuals who have received combined *serotonergic drugs*. Frequent drug combinations include: monoamine oxidase inhibitors (MAOIs) and selective serotonin-reuptake inhibitors, MAOIs and tricyclic antidepressants, MAOIs and tryptophan, and MAOIs and *meperidine*. The syndrome is characterized by confusion, hyperthermia, shivering, diaphoresis, ataxia and myoclonus commencing soon after the addition of a serotonergic agent. The illness is generally mild, with slight elevations of temperature; it responds within hours to drug withdrawal. If hypothermia is severe, then aggressive treatment with cooling and paralytic agents may be necessary to prevent a fatal outcome.

CNS white matter is a rare target of pharmaceutical (*cyclosporine*, *tacrolimus*, *methotrexate*) and occupational (*triethyl tin*) agents; these may cause an acute leukoencephalopathy syndrome. Some pharmaceutical agents may have predilection for occipital/parietal white matter (the posterior leukoencephalopathy syndrome); delirium is accompanied by early visual impairment and spasticity in this condition.

The encephalopathic effects of high-level exposure to some agents sometimes constitute only a small part of the clinical problem; however, the *systemic* effects of a toxin may add to the total compromise of CNS dysfunction. For example, severe pulmonary irritation and lung edema from some inhalants (*see* Tables 2.2 & 2.3) can cause cardiovascular collapse and hypoperfusion of the CNS.

TABLE 2.2. Agents Associated with Acute Encephalopathy (A Rating)

Absinthe	Dimethyl sulfate	Methyl ethyl ketone
Acetone	Domoic acid	Methyl iodide
Acetylsalicylic acid	Ergot alkaloids	Metrizamide
Acivicin	Ethanol	Metronidazole
Acyclovir	Ethchlorvynol	Misonidazole
Alanosine	Ethylene glycol	Morphine
Aluminum	Fentanyl	Mustard warfare agents
Amphetamines	Flecainide	Nalidixic acid
Atropine	Fludarabine	Nicotine
Azoles	Fluoroacetic acid	3-Nitropropionic acid
Baclofen	Fluorouracil	Nitrosoureas
Barbiturates	Gasoline	Organic solvent mixtures
Benzene	Glutethimide	Pemoline
Benzimidazole	Gold salts	Pentaborane
Benzodiazepines	Grayanotoxins	Pentazocine
Bromide	*n*-Heptane	Pertussis vaccine
2-*t*-Butylazo-2-hydroxy-	Heroin	Phencyclidine
5-methylhexane	Hydrazine	Piperazine
Cannabis	Hydrogen sulfide	Propranolol
Carbamate pesticides	Ibotenic acid	Psilocybin/psilocin
Carbamazepine	Ifosfamide	Pyriminol
Carbon monoxide	Indomethacin	Quinacrine
Carbon tetrachloride	Isopropanol	Reserpine
Carboxyatractyloside	Lead	Spirogermanium
Chloral hydrate	Lead, organic	*Stipa robusta*
Cimetidine	MDMA	Styrene
Cinnarizine	Mechlorethamine	Tetrachloroethane
Cocaine	Meperidine	Tetrachloroethylene
Cyclobenzaprine	Methadone	Toluene
Cyclopentolate	Methaqualone	Trichloroethylene
Cycloserine	Methotrexate	Trimethyltin
Cyclotrimethylenetrinitramine	Methyl bromide	Valproic acid
Cytarabine	Methyl chloride	Water
Digitalis	Methylene chloride	

MDMA: 3,4-Methylenedioxyethylamphetamine.

TABLE 2.3. Agents Associated with Acute Encephalopathy (B Rating)

Aconitine	Disulfiram	Naphthalene
Amantadine	Enflurane	Nitrobenzene
Aminocaproic acid	Ethionamide	Nitroprusside
Amyl alcohol	Flecainide	Phenol
Asparaginase	Fluoroquinolones	*Piper methysticum*
Bromocriptine	Gangciclovir	Propylene glycol
Cadmium	Griseofulvin	Quinine
Cephalosporins	Gyromitrin	*Rhodactus howesi*
Chloramphenicol	Hexamethylmelamine	Sulfonamides
Chloroquine	Interferon α	Thymidine
Clonidine	*Lupinus* spp.	Tremetone
Clozapine	Methysergide	Trihexyphenidyl
Crotolaria spp.	Misonidazole	Vidarabine
Dichloroacetylene	Mitotane	Vinca alkaloids

Tables 2.2 and 2.3 lists agents associated with acute encephalopathy.

Neuroleptic Malignant Syndrome

The neuroleptic malignant syndrome is a serious, life-threatening complication of *thioxanthine*, *phenothiazine*, and *butyrophenone* therapies; it appears within 6 months of commencement of therapy in 1% of patients receiving these dopaminergic-blockade-type neuroleptics. Many (30%) die if the disorder is not promptly recognized and treated. The prevalence of neuroleptic malignant syndrome may be greater when high doses of the more potent drugs (phenothiazines, butyrophenones) are administered parenterally.

Initial signs are catatonic rigidity and sedation, followed soon by unstable blood pressure, hyperthermia, and stupor. Severe muscle necrosis is indicated by astronomical elevations of creatine kinase (as high as 60,000 units/l; normal is < 175 units/l), and may be accompanied by myoglobinuria and renal failure. Treatment with the dopaminergic agonist, bromocriptine, or with dantrolene and drug withdrawal, are effective if done early.

The pathogenesis of this disorder is not understood; it likely does not reflect a defect in skeletal muscle calcium ion regulation as does the similar malignant hyperthermia syndrome (*vide infra*). It may reflect a febrile response in a patient with parkinsonian rigidity and a drug-induced impairment in autonomic thermoregulation.

Malignant Hyperthermia Syndrome

The malignant hyperthermia syndrome is an autosomal dominant disorder of muscle. It first appears during induction of anesthesia in unsuspected susceptible individuals who are receiving a combination of halogenated hydrocarbon inhalation anesthetics and depolarizing skeletal muscle relaxants such as *succinylcholine*. Patients experience sudden massive muscle contractions accompanied by a rise in body temperature to 42°C or higher. Circulatory collapse and death ensue unless immediate treatment with dantrolene and supportive measures are instituted.

The condition originates from a stimulus-elicited excessive release of calcium ion from the sarcoplasmic reticulum. Many individuals have a mutation in the calcium release channel, known as the *ryanodine receptor*. Because the disorder is genetically heterogeneous, preoperative pharmacological *in vitro* testing of muscle biopsies from vulnerable relatives of a known susceptible person is recommended.

Chronic Encephalopathy Syndromes

Chronic encephalopathy (CE) is an especially nebulous, unsatisfactory diagnostic entity; the term is uncommon in neurological parlance except when used to define specific ongoing metabolic derangements (*e.g.*, insidious-onset hepatic or uremic encephalopathies) or chronic drug intoxications (*e.g.*, bromism). Most appear to reflect cortical dysfunction, but the distinction between cortical and subcortical involvement in these poorly defined entities is often unclear.

Narrowly defined, the term implies CNS structural change or dysfunction (pathy) and denotes persistent alteration of CNS function, generally characterized prominently by cognitive impairment. Alteration of consciousness may be a frequent component of CE: clouding is often only prominent in initial phases of CE; it may recur at some point in the illness or gradually disappear leaving a state of mild dementia (*vide infra*). CE, thus defined, is usually distinguished from chronic dementia, a global progressive decline in intellectual function with *preserved* consciousness. The distinction is blurred in some unusual cases. For example, chronic *ethylene oxide* intoxication clearly causes chronic toxic encephalopathy (CTE), yet it is characterized by a steady decline in cognitive function without alteration of consciousness. This state persists following withdrawal.

CTE is associated with prolonged and continuous exposure to an agent. Varying degrees of improvement follow withdrawal. The term is often misused and the appellation uncritically applied to conditions that are likely psychogenic (*e.g.*, depression, malingering) (11). Clinical symptoms are persistent, vague, mild and nonspecific. When caused by occupational agents, there is initial improvement over weekends or on long holidays, but this effect disappears after several months. The most prominent symptoms are lightheadedness, poor concentration, irritability, mild lapses in memory, headache, diminished libido, and anhedonia. Many of these symptoms are seen with other illnesses (*e.g.*, the dementias) and in depression. Most studies of workers alleged to have CTE, especially studies of *organic solvent*-exposed individuals, have taken inadequate means to rule out these confounding factors. There are no physical findings, and the neurobehavioral markers are so poorly defined as to be meaningless.

CTE can be identified in a few specific scenarios encountered with some occupational and pharmaceutical agents; it also follows chronic deliberate inhalation of some substances, especially *toluene*. This is best exemplified by the mild cognitive decline and loss of initiative experienced by some individuals receiving chronic anticonvulsant medications such as *bromides*, *phenytoin*, or *phenobarbital* or subject to *chronic alcoholism*. Withdrawal from these agents is followed by partial or complete return of higher discriminative CNS function. The CTE associated with high-level, end-stage toluene abuse is a multifocal and diffuse leukoencephalopathy syndrome with clinical features of naturally occurring leukodystrophies and demyelinating diseases. These features include cerebellar ataxia and dysmetria, spasticity, visual impairment, and cognitive slowing of the subcortical dementia type (*vide infra*).

Dementia

Dementia is defined (DSM-IV) as memory disturbance plus one of four features (aphasia, apraxia, agnosia, disturbance of executive function) with preserved consciousness; the condition may be permanent or reversible. Selective impairment of one intellectual function is not considered dementia (selective decline in language is aphasia, selective

decline in memory is amnesia). Dementia as the principal manifestation of neurotoxic disease is rare.

Dementias are sometimes (controversially) categorized as "cortical" or "subcortical" types. Cortical dementias stem from diffuse neuronal dysfunction (*e.g.*, chronic excessive *bismuth* use); they are characterized by progressive decline of memory and language function with normal affect. Subcortical dementia from diffuse white matter dysfunction (*e.g.*, multiple periventricular ischemic infarcts) is characterized by profound apathy and loss of spontaneity in concert with little memory loss and preservation of language. Unfortunately, the clinical profile in a dementia rarely corresponds to anatomical loci; individuals with subcortical dementia may have profound memory loss, and language dysfunction may accompany disorders of the basal ganglia.

Seizure Disorders

Epileptic seizures are defined as the effects of an intermittent disorder of the nervous system due to the sudden, disorderly discharge of cerebral neurons. Seizures are broadly characterized as generalized or focal. Generalized seizures are bilateral, symmetrical, and have no discernible focus. The initial event is loss of consciousness, followed by a brief rigid extension of the extremities (tonic phase); this is succeeded by a period of flexor spasms of the torso and extremities (clonic phase). A series of generalized seizures without regaining consciousness is termed "status epilepticus"; it is a medical emergency. Focal (partial) seizures begin in a defined locus with initial motor or sensory phenomena; they may then become generalized.

The nature of the discharging lesion in toxin-induced seizures presumably is different in some respects from the lesion in most chronic epileptic patients; the toxin-induced seizure usually originates in previously normal neurons, while the patient with epilepsy frequently has a focus in an abnormal cortical area.

Seizures in normal individuals may accompany intoxication from many pharmaceutical agents and some occupational chemicals (especially *heavy metals*). Toxin-induced seizures are almost always generalized; focal (partial) seizures rarely occur unless the patient has a predisposition to epilepsy or an underlying focal cortical lesion. Generalized seizures may also accompany abrupt withdrawal from chronic ingestion of CNS depressant agents (*e.g.*, *barbiturates, ethanol, benzodiazepines, anticonvulsants*). Agents administered intrathecally or intravenously have greater potential for causing seizures. Most drug-induced seizures are dose-related, and conditions that augment plasma concentrations (renal failure) predispose to convulsions.

Table 2.4 lists agents associated with seizure disorders.

TABLE 2.4. Agents Associated with Seizure Disorders

Acrylonitrile	Cicutoxin	Methylxanthines
Allylglycine	Clozapine	Nalidixic acid
Amanita toxin	Cocaine	Penicillins
Aminopyridine	Cyanide	Pentaborane
Amsacrine	Cycloserine	Phenelzine & other MAOI
Anthranilic acid	Cyclotrimethylenetrinitramine	Pyrethroids
Atropine	Dichlorodiphenylethanes	Quinacrine
Baclofen	Enflurane	Sarin
Benzene hexachloride	Isoniazid	Spirogermanium
Bismuth	Lindane	Strychnine
Butyrophenones	MDMA	Tacrolimus
Carbamazepine	Mefloquine	Tetanus toxin
Cephalosporins	3-Mercaptopropionic acid	Toxaphene
Chlorinated cyclodienes	Methionine sulfoximine	Tricyclic antidepressants
Chlorpromazine & other neuroleptics		

MAOI: Monoamine oxidase inhibitor.
MDMA: Methylenedioxymethamphetamine

Headache Syndromes

Headache disorders have traditionally been divided into two broad categories, vascular and tension.

Vascular headaches are periodic, last for hours, often are familial, characterized by pulsating (throbbing) pain, and frequently accompanied by nausea. Migraine headaches are held to be vascular, and may involve both intracranial and extracranial vessels. Classic migraine is rare; its attacks are preceded by an aura and usually confined to one side of the head. Common migraine begins without warning and is generalized. The pathogenesis of these disorders is unclear. Classic migraine is held to begin as a cortical neuronal electrophysiological inhibition ("spreading depression") that triggers pain endings in pial vessels with spread to other vascular structures supplied by the trigeminal nerve. Common migraine is held to involve alterations (primarily vasodilation) in pain-sensitive extracranial vessels. Therapy is usually effective in aborting or preventing attacks; it includes vasoconstrictor agents (*ergotamine*), β-blockers (*propranolol*), or 5-hydroxytryptamine agonists (*sumatriptin*). Simple analgesics, such as aspirin and codeine, are sometimes effective in blunting the pain of an individual attack.

Tension headaches are bilateral, diffuse, last for days, and characterized as dull or aching; the pain is frequently described as "band-like." These headaches are especially common in anxious and depressed individuals. The pathogenesis was formerly held to involve contraction of scalp musculature ("muscle tension headaches"); however, several studies of scalp muscle activity during episodes have failed to confirm this notion. Mild analgesics (aspirin) are of little use; anxiolytics or antidepressants help in some instances.

Acute intoxication with many pharmaceutical and industrial agents is associated with headache, usually of the vascular type. Some agents with strong vasoactive properties have headache as a major and consistent component of their toxic syndromes; examples include *nitrites* (*dynamite, nitroglycerin, sausages*), *carbon monoxide*, solvent inhalants (*toluene*), *cocaine, aspartame, phenylethylamine* (*chocolate*), *histamine, organophosphates, lithium,* and *oral contraceptives*. It is alleged that migraineurs are more susceptible to vasoactive agents and that a single exposure to an agent such as sodium nitrate can precipitate a series of migraine episodes. In nonmigraineurs, such agents provoke a brief headache or a series of headaches lasting for only a few days.

Chronic intoxication with analgesics or vasoactive agents (*ergotamine, caffeine*) can provoke a chronic daily headache syndrome that is treated by gradual withdrawal and abstinence.

Some pharmaceutical agents (MAOI) may provoke hypertensive episodes under certain circumstances (consumption of *tyramine-containing foods*); headache is a prominent feature of this syndrome.

Anxiety and depression concerning a perceived toxic exposure is a trigger of tension headaches in susceptible persons.

Pyramidal Syndrome

The cardinal findings in pyramidal tract (corticospinal tract) disease are weakness, hyperactive tendon reflexes, and Babinski responses (dorsiflexion of the great toe following scratch of the sole of the foot). Weakness involves extensor groups of muscles in the upper limb and flexors in the lower; it may be accompanied by increased tone and resistance to stretch (spasticity) and ankle/patellar clonus. Muscle atrophy is mild and due to disuse. Gait is stiff-legged and may feature scissoring if adductor muscles are hypertonic.

Pure pyramidal syndromes are rare in neurology, since only a few degenerative diseases (*e.g.*, primary lateral sclerosis, hereditary spastic paraparesis) are confined to the upper motor neuron cell bodies or their descending corticospinal (pyramidal) tracts. Most naturally occurring neurological diseases with prominent corticospinal tract findings are characterized by focal or multifocal lesions (multiple sclerosis, encephalomalacia) that also involve sensory, cerebellar or autonomic pathways. Two toxic conditions, *konzo* and lathyrism, are characterized predominantly by pyramidal tract dysfunction (*see also* Myelopathy).

Extrapyramidal Syndromes

Toxic extrapyramidal syndromes are common following exposure to several classes of pharmaceutical agents; some drugs (especially those used in psychiatry) produce characteristic syndromes that are frequent in everyday clinical medicine (1). Certain occupational chemical exposures are followed by extrapyramidal compromise (*carbon monoxide, carbon disulfide, manganese*); these disorders are rare. There is marked individual variability in susceptibility to some types of drug-induced extrapyramidal disease, especially the acute dystonic reactions. The toxic extrapyramidal syndromes include the entire gamut of clinically recognized movement disorders; the pathophysiological mechanisms of most are unclear. They have been listed in approximate order of frequency as: parkinsonism, acute dystonias, tardive dyskinesias, akathesias, chorea, neuroleptic malignant syndrome, tics, and myoclonus (9).

Parkinsonism. A parkinsonian syndrome that closely resembles idiopathic Parkinson's disease frequently accompanies neuroleptic therapy. All of the manifestations of Parkinson's disease are present including masked facies, rapid pill-rolling tremor at rest, rigidity, and bradykinesia (slowness in initiating movements). The disorder usually appears within 2 months of commencing treatment and remits when dosage is lowered. Older individuals appear to have a higher incidence. The pathophysiology of drug-induced parkinsonism is held to stem from suppression of striatal dopamine stores, analogous to the loss of nigral cells in the naturally occurring condition.

Acute dystonias. Dystonia is a sustained contraction of a group of muscles causing an abnormal posture. Acute drug-induced dystonias are frequently confined to neck, eye, or facial muscles with resultant bizarre postures. They are especially common with *phenothiazine, butyrophenones,* and *metoclopramide;* they generally appear suddenly, usually within days of commencing treatment. While these movements readily respond to intravenous diphenhydramine, treatment is sometimes needlessly delayed because the bi-

zarre sustained postures may be erroneously attributed to another condition (*e.g.,* hysteria, tetanus).

Acute dyskinesias. Dyskinesias are forceful spasms of muscles commonly involving the lips, face, and tongue. Acute dyskinesias may accompany early L-*dopa* treatment in Parkinson's disease and are dose-related. They respond to reduction in drug. Following prolonged treatment, they may comprise a component (along with akinesia) of the "on-off" phenomenon.

Tardive dyskinesia. This distinctive disorder appears late (implied by the name) in the course of chronic antipsychotic drug therapy. The most distinctive features are constant orofacial-lingual movements usually including lip smacking, sucking, facial grimacing, and jaw opening; speech and swallowing may be disrupted. It generally occurs after at least 1 year of therapy and is estimated to appear in 50% of individuals receiving *phenothiazine* treatment. The disorder usually improves following drug withdrawal, but again emerges when therapy recommences. Occasionally, dyskinesias may reappear years following withdrawal. There is no consistently beneficial therapy. The pathophysiology is widely held to stem from hypersensitivity of dopamine receptors in the basal ganglia secondary to prolonged blockade by the antipsychotic drugs.

Akathesia. Akathesia is a state of inner restlessness characterized by a compulsion to move about, an inability to sit still. The sitting patient constantly moves and crosses the legs and then gets up to walk about in an aimless manner. This state is seen almost exclusively in *phenothiazine* therapy and can occur after only weeks of drug commencement. It usually responds to lowering of the dose.

Tics. Tics (habit spasms) are stereotyped, irresistible, habitual movements under the voluntary control of the individual. Typical tics are throat-clearing, grimacing, sniffing, twitching, protrusion of the mouth and chin, and blinking. They are common in normal individuals and more frequent during anxious spells. *Haloperidol,* heavy *cocaine* use, and *amphetamine* therapy are associated with severe, new-onset tic disorders; they disappear following drug withdrawal.

Myoclonus. Myoclonic jerks are brief, shock-like, asynchronous, asymmetrical movements of groups of muscles. They are especially common in some epileptic patients and may constitute a separate form of epilepsy; they are also associated with diffuse degenerative diseases of cortical neurons (Creutzfeldt-Jakob disease, Alzheimer's disease). *Lithium* and *bismuth* intoxications are accompanied by myoclonus, and cognitive impairment that may be mistaken for a neurodegenerative disorder.

Cerebellar Syndromes

The cardinal signs of cerebellar dysfunction are unsteady gait (disequilibrium, ataxia), hypotonia, and incoordination. Lesions of one cerebellar hemisphere or its deep nuclei cause ipsilateral limb incoordination and intention tremor (a side-to-side movement of the moving finger as it approaches and overshoots a target). Lesions confined to the cerebellar vermis cause instability and broad-based gait with little limb dysfunction. Many toxic and nutritional disorders are characterized by cerebellar dysfunction; it is usually diffuse, featured both by limb incoordination and ataxic gait (*e.g.*, *phenytoin*, alcoholic/nutritional deficiency states, *mercury intoxication*).

Hydrocephalus

Hydrocephalus is rarely caused by exogenous toxins. In common clinical parlance, hydrocephalus is divided into two distinct types. One type is *tension hydrocephalus* wherein the cerebral ventricles are dilated secondary to increased cerebrospinal fluid (CSF) pressure in conditions such as aqueductal stenosis, or the CSF absorption mechanism has become disrupted by local meningeal inflammation and fibrosis secondary to intrathecal administration of irritant pharmaceutical agents (*methotrexate*). The other type is *hydrocephalus ex vacuo* wherein the ventricles have passively enlarged secondary to axon loss consequent to neuronal degeneration and cortical atrophy in conditions such as Alzheimer's disease.

Benign Intracranial Hypertension (Pseudotumor Cerebri)

This uncommon, self-limited, idiopathic condition consists of the effects of slowly developing increased intracranial pressure. It occurs *without* evidence of hydrocephalus (enlarged lateral ventricles), demonstrable disease of brain, or abnormal CSF dynamics. Most patients with the naturally occurring condition are obese females who develop mild headache and transient visual blurring; neurological exam usually only discloses engorgement of the optic discs (papilledema). Neuroimaging reveals small or normal lateral ventricles. About one-third improve following repeated lumbar puncture; others only recover after a more protracted course and are at risk for visual loss if not managed carefully. This condition may be associated with drug therapy; offending agents include *hypervitaminosis A*, *tetracycline*, *perhexilene maleate*, and *oral contraceptives*.

Aseptic Meningitis

The syndrome of aseptic meningitis includes fever, headache, stiff neck, myalgia, and increased numbers of lymphocytes and normal glucose levels in the CSF. This is a common, self-limited disorder; most cases are associated with an enterovirus infection and recover fully within 2 weeks with symptomatic therapy. Aseptic meningitis may occur from a hypersensitivity reaction in patients with connective tissue diseases; treatment with non-steroidal anti-inflammatory agents (*ibuprofen*, *sundilac*) may provoke this reaction in these individuals.

Encephalomalacia (Stroke)

CNS focal ischemic or hemorrhagic diseases are the most common serious illnesses in North American hospital inpatient neurological practice; they rarely are secondary to exposure to neurotoxic chemicals.

Thrombotic disease of large and small vessels has been associated with oral contraceptives; cerebral embolism may occur in older men and women receiving *stilbestrol*. Intravenous substance abuse, especially *heroin* and *pentazocine*, can result in multifocal CNS small-vessel occlusive disease; this is usually attributed to injected particulate matter or to an allergic vasculitis. Abuse or overtreatment with agents with vasopressor/constrictor side effects (*ergotamine*, *amphetamine*, *phenylpropamine*, *cocaine*) can precipitate cerebral vasospasm or hemorrhage. Cocaine inhalant abuse is also alleged to cause cerebral arteritis and multifocal infarction.

Elderly individuals with preexistent vascular disease may be especially vulnerable to hypotensive effects of antihypertensive drugs, or to autonomic instability associated with biological agents (*ciguatera*) that are well tolerated by younger persons. Long term therapy with *anticoagulants*, especially when poorly monitored, is associated with increased risk for spontaneous and post-traumatic intra- and extracranial (subdural) hemorrhage in the elderly.

Tremor

Tremor is defined as a rhythmic oscillatory movement disorder; its rhythmic quality distinguishes tremor from the other movement disorders (chorea, tic, dystonia). Five broad categories of tremor are generally recognized (1): physiological tremor, resting tremor, ataxic tremor, essential (action) tremor, and asterixis.

Physiological tremor is present in all normal persons, likely is governed by muscle β-adrenergic receptors, has fine movements, has a frequency of 8–10 Hz, and is barely visible to the naked eye. It is enhanced in anxiety, exercise, hyperthyroidism, and by certain drugs (*lithium, xanthines, alcohol/sedative withdrawal*).

Resting tremor occurs with the limb in repose, has a frequency of 3–5 Hz, is most prominent in hands and fingers, and is abolished by movement; it is characteristic of Parkinson's disease (*vide supra*).

Ataxic tremor ("cerebellar intention/action tremor") occurs at the end of voluntary movements, is an irregular (often coarse) rhythmic oscillation most prominent in the distal upper limbs, interferes with skilled acts, and disappears at rest; it is characteristic of cerebellar dysfunction and is seen in intoxications affecting this structure (*phenytoin, lithium, cyclosporin A*).

Essential tremor ("benign action tremor") has a frequency of 4–8 Hz, may be familial, often resembles enhanced physiological tremor, is abolished by several agents (alcohol, primidone, clonezepam), and most likely has a cerebellar-olivary origin. Many agents induce an action-type tremor including *valproate, cimetidine, tricyclic antidepressants*, and *phenothiazine*.

Asterixis ("flapping tremor") is a movement disorder consisting of rhythmic lapses of sustained posture; patients display flapping movements of the outstretched, dorsiflexed hands. This disorder is commonly associated with hepatic and uremic encephalopathies; chemical causes include *phenytoin, valproate*, and *tocainide*.

Neural Visual System

A host of chemical-induced visual disorders can stem from effects on nonneural (lens, cornea, refractile fluid) as well as from innervated and neuroectodermal structures. This section briefly outlines a few salient features of the neurotoxicology of the visual system; Grant and Shulman's *Toxicology of the Eye, 4th Ed.*, is a generally authoritative reference (8).

Pupillary constriction (miosis) is an unusual neurotoxic effect; it may follow administration of parasympathomimetic agents (*neostigmine*), *opioids*, and *phenothiazine*. Pupillary dilatation (mydriasis) is more often chemically induced; it follows systemic administration of anticholinergics (*atropine, tricyclics*) and systemic or topical sympathomimetics (*amphetamines, neosynephrine*-containing eye drops). A severe consequence of mydriasis, in susceptible individuals, is an episode of acute angle-closure glaucoma with consequent visual compromise.

Save for nystagmus (rhythmic, jerky eye movements), disorders of extraocular motility are rarely neurotoxic in origin; some agents may precipitate acute double vision (diplopia) by breaking down a latent squint (*diazepam, tricyclic antidepressants*). Toxin-induced nystagmus is common,

usually horizontal, and reflects vestibulocerebellar dysfunction (*phenytoin, barbiturates, ototoxic antibiotics*). Opsoclonus, chaotic eye movements, is associated with *chlordecone (kepone)* toxicity.

The four principal retinal layers are pigmentary, photoreceptor, bipolar cell, and ganglion cell. Visual system toxins often affect more than one layer and produce a nonspecific pattern of visual dysfunction that has various physical findings, including central and peripheral field defects, poor central vision, and pigmentary macular degeneration. A few substances appear to have a biochemical effect primarily on one layer; they include *chloroquine* (pigmentary epithelium), *cardiac glycosides* (photoreceptors), and *methanol/formate* (retinal ganglion cells). Destruction of the retinal ganglion cells causes secondary axonal degeneration and atrophy of the optic nerve.

Primary optic nerve degeneration may occur from either a direct effect on axons or on myelin sheaths. Toxic axonopathy of the optic nerve is well recognized and occurs following systemic administration of many agents in humans and/or animals (*ethambutol, clioquinol, 2,5-hexanedione*). Demyelination of the optic nerve is common in inflammatory immunopathies (papillitis) of the CNS (multiple sclerosis); save for prolonged, deliberate inhalation use of *toluene*, primary toxic optic nerve demyelination is rare. Agents that produce widespread vacuolation in CNS myelin (*hexachlorophene*) may affect myelin and axons of the optic nerves and tracts.

Swelling of the optic nerve, papilledema, usually reflects increased intracranial pressure. Papilledema, as an isolated finding, is rarely neurotoxic. Pharmaceutical agents associated with benign intracranial hypertension (*perhexiline maleate, vitamin A*) and severe acute toxic encephalopathies associated with brain swelling (*ethylene glycol*) may be accompanied by papilledema. The essential element in the pathogenesis of papilledema is an increase in pressure upon the sheaths of the optic nerve, which communicate directly with the subarachnoid space of the brain. Papilledema from increased intracranial pressure is, surprisingly, not associated with serious visual dysfunction until late in its course. Eventually, optic atrophy and severe visual compromise appear. Lowering of raised intracranial pressure is usually followed by resolution of papilledema.

Table 2.5 lists agents associated with optic neuropathy.

Neural Auditory and Vestibular Systems (Ototoxicity)

Neurotoxic agents almost exclusively affect the cochlear and vestibular peripheral (inner ear) transducer organs or their vascular support; a primary toxic action on the ganglion cells (first-order neuron), the auditory nerve, or upon

TABLE 2.5. Agents Associated with Optic Neuropathy

Amiodarone	Ethambutol
Apamin & *Hymenoptera* spp. venoms	Methanol
Chloramphenicol	Methyl bromide
Clioquinol	Thallium

TABLE 2.6. Agents Associated with Ototoxicity

Acetylsalicylic acid	Cisplatin	Naproxen
Aminoglycoside antibiotics	Erythromycin	Quinidine
Chlorhexidine gluconate	Ethacrynic acid	Quinine
Chloroquine	Furosemide	

the CNS projections is rare. *Ototoxic antibiotics* and *diuretics* appear in high concentration in the perilymph and endolymph soon after intravenous administration and have a local toxic effect on hair cells; the mechanism of transport or secretion by the stria vascularis is unclear (13).

Decreased cochlear blood flow accompanied by transient tinnitus and hearing loss is characteristic of *salicylates* and *quinine*. Prolonged high-level exposure to such agents can cause hair cell degeneration and permanent hearing impairment.

Dysfunction, edema, and eventual degeneration of the stria vascularis, the structure responsible for endolymph production, follows intoxication with loop diuretics (*furosemide, ethacrynic acid*); hair cell loss may follow prolonged high-level exposure. Transient high-frequency hearing loss is common, permanent hearing impairment occasionally develops.

The most common neural ototoxic reaction is dysfunction and degeneration of cochlear and vestibular hair cells from aminoglycoside treatment. There are postulated effects on both the cell membrane and upon the mechanical aspects of the transducers. Some aminoglycosides are more cochleotoxic (*neomycin, kanamycin*), while others are more vestibulotoxic (*streptomycin*). Vestibulotoxicity causes imbalance, vertigo, and diminished caloric responses; vertical oscillation of the eyes is a characteristic finding. Hearing loss is initially confined to the high frequencies; eventually, severe hearing loss occurs if the drug is not withdrawn. Hearing loss is usually irreversible.

Some chemotherapeutic agents, such as *cisplatin*, also have a direct effect on hair cells, not upon the ganglion cells (in contrast to their direct neurotoxic effect on peripheral sensory ganglion cells). The *vinca alkaloids* are suggested to affect the bipolar spiral ganglion cells directly and to cause auditory nerve degeneration.

Selective dysfunction and demyelination of the distal CNS auditory projections are associated with prolonged deliberate, high-level *toluene* inhalation. Initially, there is asymptomatic loss of the terminal component of the brainstem auditory evoked potential; eventually, severe and irreversible central hearing loss ensues.

Table 2.6 lists agents associated with ototoxicity.

Olfaction and Taste

The olfactory receptor cells are actually bipolar neurons; their peripheral processes are embedded in the olfactory mucosa and the central processes converge to form the olfactory tract. Olfactory neurons have two unique features: they represent the only site in the organism where neurons are in direct contact with the environment, and they are continually generated every 30–60 days throughout the life of the individual. Toxic injury to these cells should be followed by good recovery because the mitral cells in the olfactory bulb are accustomed to receiving new synapses, even into old age.

Bilateral anosmia (loss of sense of smell) is an occasional complaint in a general neurology practice; simultaneous loss of taste (ageusia) is rare, although most anosmic individuals are also convinced that the sense of taste is impaired. This confusion reflects the importance of olfaction in detecting subtle flavors (a combination of taste and smell) through interpretation of vapor odors; qualitative testing of the basic elements (sweet, salty, bitter, sour) of taste is usually normal in these persons. "Bilateral anosmia is an increasingly common manifestation of malingering, now that it has been recognized as a compensable disability by insurance agencies in North America" (2). Since true anosmics complain of loss of taste but show normal taste, office testing of taste (oral swishes of solutions of salt, sucrose, caffeine, and citric acid) may help separate the genuine cases from malingerers. A practical *qualitative* smell identification test is available: the University of Pennsylvania Smell Identification Test. There are no reliable *quantitative* measures of taste or smell within the scope of the usual clinical examination.

Smell and taste pathways have access to neural circuits that control both emotional states of the body and certain memories. Olfactory or gustatory hallucinations are always of CNS or psychological origin; they are especially characteristic of psychomotor (partial-complex) epilepsy. Complaints of persistent unpleasant taste and odor perception appear in some psychiatric conditions; an intense aversion to certain smells (cacosmia) is a component of the MCS syndrome.

Although several chemicals with neurotoxic potential are associated with impaired sense of smell (*organic solvents, doxycycline, erythromycin, hydrogen sulfide*), the pathophysiology of this disorder is unclear. It is generally held that these agents affect chemoreceptive transduction in the olfactory mucosal bipolar receptor neurons; experimental animal studies provide some support for this proposal.

Distorted taste is reported by patients receiving a range of therapeutic drugs (*vincristine, vinblastine, griseofulvin, amitryptaline, antithyroid agents, chlorambucil, cholestyramine, gold, allopurinol*). Loss of taste (usually the perception of sweetness) accompanies therapy with L-dopa and *baclofen*. In only one instance is a specific therapy available: the administration of copper reverses the ageusia of *penicillamine* therapy. The pathophysiology of the drug-induced ageusia is unclear.

Myelopathy (Spinal Cord)

Nervous system disease confined to the spinal cord is common in general neurological practice; it is usually focal (extramedullary compression) or multifocal (demyelinating disorders). Spastic paraparesis and sensory loss in the lower limbs is the clinical syndrome associated with spinal cord disorders. *This type of focal/multifocal disorder is rarely neurotoxic.* The "spinal dorsal column sensory" and "spinal spasticity" syndromes linked with neurotoxic disease are actually due to degeneration of the distal (spinal) portions of long CNS axons of the ascending sensory tracts (*acrylamide*) or the descending motor pathways (lathyrism, *clioquinol, organophosphates*); these disorders likely reflect metabolic dysfunction in the sensory ganglion cells and/or cortical motor neurons, not focal disease of the spinal cord (*see also* Pyramidal Syndrome).

Intrathecal injection of therapeutic (chemotherapy, *corticosteroids*) or diagnostic (*myelographic contrast*) agents may be followed by arachnoiditis or spinal infarction. Massive doses of local anesthetics into the subarachnoid space can cause unwanted degeneration in the lumbar roots; locally acting neurotoxic agents (*ethanol, phenol*) are sometimes placed in the subarachnoid space in a deliberate attempt to destroy spinal roots and alleviate spinal spasticity.

There are two systemic toxic disorders that can feature focal/multifocal spinal cord lesions. One is the multifocal vascular myelopathy following intravenous drug use (*heroin* myelitis); this disorder likely reflects a hypersensitivity vasculitis (angiitis) from contaminants in the injected material. The other is thoracic demyelinating myelopathy from chronic, high-level, *nitrous oxide* intoxication; this disorder is secondary to impaired utilization of vitamin B_{12} and is a variant of combined system disease.

Peripheral Neuropathy

Distal axonopathy. Peripheral neuropathy of the distal axonopathy type is a common and thoroughly studied human neurotoxic disease. Save for sensory neuronopathy (*vide infra*), the other anatomical variants of peripheral neuropathy encountered in neurological practice (the mononeuropathy, vasculitis, demyelinating types), are rarely neurotoxic.

Mononeuropathy. Accidental injection of pharmaceutical agents (usually antibiotics) directly into peripheral nerve is an occasional event. The sciatic nerve in the buttocks of children or emaciated adults is the usual site. Severe pain is immediate and is followed by hamstring weakness and a flail foot. Severe axonal destruction and fibrosis are usual and most patients have disabling residual paralysis, sometimes accompanied by a causalgic pain syndrome.

Vasculitis/fasciitis. Two epidemics of multifocal neuropathy in concert with connective tissue and muscle disease have occurred; one followed consumption of food cooked in *adulterated rape seed oil* ("Toxic Oil"), the other from self-medication with a *tryptophan analog* (eosinophilia myalgia syndrome). Both conditions are presumably immune-mediated.

Demyelinating neuropathy. Several agents (*diphtheria toxin, arsenic*) may be associated with an acute toxic demyelinating neuropathy (presumably not inflammatory). Exposure to these agents can result in a disabling acute or subacute diffuse, predominantly motor neuropathy with areflexia and cranial nerve dysfunction. This condition resembles the Guillain-Barré syndrome, a postinfectious radiculoneuropathy caused by an immune-mediated inflammatory demyelination of spinal roots and nerves. Recovery is usually satisfactory and can be rapid in mild cases.

Subacute or chronic predominantly demyelinating neuropathy with moderate axonal degeneration is associated with therapy with *perhexiline maleate* or *amiodarone*.

Distal axonopathy (central-peripheral distal axonopathy). This common morphological reaction (retrograde axon degeneration) is encountered after chronic or subacute exposure to many pharmaceutical and occupational agents. Some cause severe systemic illness (*thallium*), others are well tolerated and patients feel well (*acrylamide, pyridoxine*). Most are associated with chronic low-level exposure. Onset is insidious, sensory symptoms are prominent, and sensory and motor signs are common. A few have a rapid onset and weakness is the dominant complaint (n-*hexane* sniffers, *dapsone, organophosphates*).

The neuropathological substrate is nonspecific degeneration of distal regions of axons in the CNS and PNS. In the PNS, degeneration appears to advance proximally toward the nerve cell body as long as exposure lasts; its reversal allows the axon slowly to regenerate along the distal

Schwann cell column to the appropriate terminal. An identical sequence usually occurs in the distal ends of long CNS axons (dorsal column, corticospinal tract), although regeneration is poor.

Nine principal clinical features correlate closely with the spatiotemporal pattern of histopathological change (14):

1. Gradual insidious onset—Chronic metabolic disease or prolonged, low-level intoxication usually produce prolonged subclinical disease with signs and symptoms gradually appearing later. Biochemical and physiological axonal abnormalities precede nerve fiber degeneration in some subclinical cases and likely account for their rapid recovery. High-level intoxications are associated with subacute onset.
2. Initial findings frequently in the lower extremities—Large and long axons are usually affected early, thus the fibers of sciatic nerve branches are especially vulnerable.
3. Stocking-glove sensory and motor loss—Axonal degeneration commences distally and slowly proceeds toward the neuron cell body, resulting in symmetrical, distal clinical signs in the legs and arms. The earliest symptoms are usually sensory: toe-tip sensations of tingling or pinprick are common initial complaints.
4. Early and symmetrical loss of ankle jerks—The axons supplying the calf muscles are of extremely large diameter and among the first affected in experimental acrylamide and hexacarbon neuropathies.
5. Normal to mildly slowed motor nerve conduction—in contrast to the demyelinating neuropathies, where the motor nerves or roots are diffusely affected. Since some motor fibers remain intact in axonal neuropathies, motor nerve conduction velocity may remain normal or only slightly slowed despite clinical signs of neuropathy. Sensory amplitudes are frequently diminished with only mild conduction slowing. *Exception*: Severe impulse slowing may accompany distal axonopathies in which the axon swells and demyelinates focally.
6. Normal CSF protein level—Since the pathological changes are usually distal and the nerve roots spared, most patients with axonal neuropathies have a normal or only slightly elevated CSF protein value.
7. Slow recovery—Since axonal regeneration (in contrast to remyelination) is a very slow process, proceeding at a rate of 2 mm/day, recovery may take many months, several years, or may never completely occur. Function is restored in reverse order to the sequence of loss.
8. Coasting—Following withdrawal from toxic exposure, symptoms and signs may intensify for weeks before recovery commences. This does not imply persistent body burden of toxin but likely reflects continued axonal degeneration and reconstitution.
9. Signs of CNS disease—This has been encountered in individuals recovering from certain toxic neuropathies. Most toxic central-peripheral distal axonopathies are characterized by tract degeneration of the distal extremities of long, large-diameter fibers in the CNS pari passu with changes in the PNS. Thus, the clinical signs of degeneration in the corticospinal and spinocerebellar pathways are usually not prominent early in the illness. However, on recovery from some severe neuropathies (*e.g.*, *n*-hexane neuropathy), the patient may manifest hyperreflexia, Babinski responses, and a stiff-legged, ataxic gait.

Tables 2.7 and 2.8 list agents associated with peripheral neuropathy.

Sensory Neuronopathy Syndrome

The term "neuronopathy" includes conditions in which the initial morphological or biochemical changes occur in the

TABLE 2.7. Agents Associated with Peripheral Neuropathy (A Rating)

Acrylamide	Ethambutol	Organophosphorus
Allyl chloride	Ethylene oxide	compounds
Amiodarone	Gold salts	Perhexiline maleate
Apamin & *Hymenoptera* spp. venoms	Hexachlorophene	Phenol
Arsenic	*n*-Hexane	Podophyllotoxin
2-*t*-Butylazo-2-hydroxy-5-methylhexane	Hydralazine	Pyridoxine
Capsaicin	Hydrazine	Pyriminol
Carbon disulfide	Isoniazid	Rabies vaccine
Chloramphenicol	*Karwinskia humboldtiana*	Suramin
Cisplatin	Lead	Tacrolimus
Colchicine	Mercury, organic	Taxoids
Cyanate	Methyl bromide	Thalidomide
Dapsone	Methyl methacrylate	Thallium
Dideoxycytidine & other nucleoside analogues	Metronidazole	L-Tryptophan (impure)
	Misonidazole	Vidarabine
Dimethylaminopropionitrile	Nitrofurantoin	Vinca alkaloids
Diphtheria toxin	Nitrous oxide	Vinyl chloride

TABLE 2.8. Agents Associated with Peripheral Neuropathy (B Rating)

Carbamate pesticides	Gangliosides	Penicillamine
Chielanthes sieberi	Germanium dioxide	Phenytoin
Chloroquine	Glutethimide	Rubella vaccine
Ciguatoxin	Hexamethylmelamine	Sarin
Cycloleucine	Lidocaine	Sulfasalazine
Cytarabine	Mercury, inorganic	Sulfonamides
Dichloroacetic acid	Methaqualone	Tetrachloroethane
Disulfiram	Methyl methacrylate	"Toxic oil"
Ethionamide	Muzolimine	Trithiozine
Euphorbia spp.	Naproxen	Zimeldine

neuron cell body. Clinical manifestations of PNS neuronopathies are restricted to segments innervated by affected nerve cell bodies. They may be focal, involving one segment (*e.g.*, herpes zoster); multifocal, involving multiple sensory or motor segments (*e.g.*, poliomyelitis); or diffuse (*e.g.*, from *pyridoxine*). They are a heterogeneous, poorly understood group of conditions and, in the broadest sense, include many disorders of motor, sensory, and autonomic neurons. They may commence prenatally or in infancy, adolescence, or adult life. Infectious neuronopathies include conditions such as poliomyelitis and herpes zoster ganglionitis.

Toxic sensory neuronopathy in humans may follow massive intravenous doses of *pyridoxine* or *cisplatin*. Toxic PNS sensory neuronopathies are readily produced in experimental animals by *doxorubicin* and *methylmercury*. There are no known human toxic motor neuronopathies.

Seven principal clinical features correlate closely with the diffuse pattern of sensory, ganglion cell loss in pyridoxine sensory neuronopathy.

1. Rapid or subacute onset following massive intravenous administration.
2. Initial sensory loss may occur anywhere—Characteristic of this disorder is the early appearance of numbness of the face coincident with diffuse sensory loss in the limbs. Presumably, this occurs because gasserian ganglion neurons are affected simultaneously with dorsal root ganglion neurons.
3. Diffuse sensory loss and ataxia with preservation of strength—The loss of sensation, sensory ataxia and dysesthesia reflect the disappearance of sensory neurons. In most subacute sensory neuronopathies, large-fiber modalities are heavily affected so that the proprioceptive deficit is greater than the loss of pain or thermal sense. Sparing of anterior horn cells accounts for preservation of strength.
4. Absent tendon reflexes—This is one of the characteristics of this condition that reflects the large-fiber sensory loss.
5. Normal motor nerve conduction, abnormal or absent sensory conduction studies—This mirrors the pattern of selective nerve cell loss.

6. Variable recovery—This reflects the death of the nerve cell body and consequent permanent loss of axons. Some cells may be only slightly impaired and transiently function poorly, but are able to reconstitute themselves without losing their axons. The phenomenon of collateral sprouting from surviving axons may account for what variable recovery occurs in these conditions.
7. No signs of CNS disease—The pure PNS sensory neuronopathy syndrome is not accompanied by CNS degeneration aside from nerve fiber loss in the central projections of the sensory neurons (dorsal columns).

Cranial Neuropathy

Dysfunction confined to isolated or multiple cranial nerves rarely has a neurotoxic etiology, save for disease of the optic and acoustic nerves. Only a handful of chemicals affects isolated cranial nerves; *dichloroacetylene* and *stilbamidine* cause trigeminal neuropathy, and *ethylene glycol* encephalopathy may involve the facial nerve. Early in the course of botulism, oculomotor and pharyngeal dysfunction may erroneously suggest a diffuse disorder of cranial nerves, such as the Guillain-Barré syndrome.

Isolated cranial nerve dysfunction is usually associated with local inflammatory (Lyme disease) or neoplastic (acoustic neuroma) conditions; multiple cranial neuropathies occur as part of diffuse peripheral neuropathies (Guillain-Barré syndrome) or diffuse inflammatory or neoplastic infiltrations of the subarachnoid space.

Ion Channel Syndromes

An acute or subacute illness is associated with sodium channel dysfunction in neurons, especially axons; in North America, most cases stem from *ciguatera* (reef fish) or *saxitoxin* (shellfish) ingestion. Puffer fish (*tetrodotoxin*) consumption in Japan remains a serious problem.

The neurological illness is heralded by abrupt onset of circumoral and oral paresthesias, notably in the tongue and gums; these rapidly progress to involve the neck and limbs. Abdominal cramps, vomiting, diarrhea, and diffuse flaccid weakness (often including respiratory paralysis) characterize most puffer fish and many shellfish intoxications. Neurological dysfunction is the initial sign of illness in saxitoxin and tetrodotoxin conditions. Nausea and diarrhea usually precede, by hours, the neurological signs in ciguatera intoxication, and the illness is usually mild; this toxin rarely causes weakness unless there has been heroic, repeated consumption of large reef fish. There are no specific antidotes for these conditions; most are self-limited, treatment is supportive.

There are naturally occurring, hereditary disorders associated with dysfunction of muscle ion channels: chloride

TABLE 2.9. Agents Associated with Axon Ion Channel Syndromes

Brevetoxins	*Kalmia latifolia*	Scorpion toxins
Buthotus hottentota	Maitotoxin	Tetrodotoxin
Ciguatoxin	Pyrethroids	Tityustoxin
Dichlorodiphenylethanes	Saxitoxin	Veratridine
Germine		

(myotonia congenita), sodium (hyperkalemic periodic paralysis), or calcium (hypokalemic periodic paralysis). Neurotoxic dysfunction of muscle ion channel is rare. Two examples are the malignant hyperthermia syndrome (calcium channel) and *conotoxin* poisoning (sodium channel).

Table 2.9 lists agents associated with axon ion channel syndromes.

Neuromuscular Transmission Syndromes

Disorders of neuromuscular transmission are conveniently clinically categorized as either pre- or postsynaptic; some toxins simultaneously affect both sites. Both types are characterized by a syndrome of progressive, symmetrical weakness with a predilection for certain muscle groups. Extraocular and other cranial nerve-innervated muscles appear especially vulnerable. Initial symptoms of double vision and difficulty speaking or swallowing often herald these disorders; these symptoms are followed by progressive, painless weakness of thoracic and limb muscles. Sensation and mentation are spared. Tendon reflexes sometimes remain present in the early phase—a helpful sign in the emergent distinction of these disorders from acute demyelinating polyneuropathy. Cholinergic signs (lacrimation, fasciculation, diarrhea, bradycardia, miosis), characteristic of some post-synaptic disorders (*e.g.*, *organophosphate* intoxication) also suggest this diagnosis. In the majority of these disorders, muscle weakness varies over time and increases with exercise. Some are serious illnesses requiring hospitalization in special-care settings; an occasional environmentally related condition (evenomations, botulism, massive organophosphate intoxication) may be fatal unless rapidly recognized and specific therapy made available. In many, dramatic responses to treatment assist in the emergent differential diagnosis. A few conditions are characterized by tight bonding of the agent to the synaptic site (botulism) and recovery may take months. Myasthenia gravis, a post-synaptic, immune mediated condition, is the only common naturally occurring disorder of neuromuscular transmission; it is readily recognized by clinical features and determination of circulating antibodies to neuromuscular junction receptors.

In general, prompt detection and treatment of neuromuscular-transmission disorders is a simple bedside procedure if two conditions prevail; there is an accurate history, and a clinician experienced in neuromuscular disease is available. Specialized electromyographic stimulationtests can help determine if dysfunction is pre- or postsynaptic. Facilitation following repetitive stimulation suggests presynaptic dysfunction; deterioration indicates a post-synaptic disorder. Pharmacological intervention varies with the site and cause of dysfunction, and drugs are best administered by skilled personnel in special-care units; endotracheal intubation and respiratory support may be necessary.

Drug-induced disorders of neuromuscular transmission are periodically seen in routine medical practice; antibiotic-related dysfunction is especially frequent in the practice of infectious disease. Drug-related disorders may pose formidable diagnostic problems. Some agents (*kanamycin*) produce an unexpected postoperative respiratory depression, others (*methoxyflurane*) provoke an unknown (subclinical) case of myasthenia gravis, while others (*penicillamine, interferon*-α) can cause an immune-mediated myasthenic syndrome.

Save for *organophosphate* intoxication (pesticides and nerve agents), environmentally caused neuromuscular dysfunction is rarely encountered in most North American medical centers. Differential diagnosis of environmentally related disease is seldom difficult, except for isolated cases of botulism.

Predominantly presynaptic agents include *botulinum neurotoxin, tick saliva,* and *black widow spider venom.* Predominantly postsynaptic agents include *anticholinesterase agents, interferon*-α, *methoxyflurane, penicillamine, tetracycline antibiotics,* and *trimethaphan.* Most toxic neuromuscular junction disorders involve both pre- and postsynaptic dysfunction; these include snake evenomations, *aminoglycoside antibiotics, anticonvulsants, polymyxin antibiotics, quinidine, lithium,* and *magnesium.*

Table 2.10 lists agents associated with neuromuscular transmission syndromes.

Myopathy

The precise incidence of toxic myopathies is unknown. In the past decade, an increasing number of substances has been identified as myotoxic, and the disorders they trigger are now frequently encountered in North American medical practice. Because they are disabling and potentially reversible, especially in the early stages, rapid recognition is important.

Proximal weakness is the hallmark of muscle disease; frequently, large limb muscle groups are heavily affected. The syndrome of progressive proximal weakness with preserved sensation strongly indicates a myopathy. Several clinical features are useful in identifying a myopathy as toxic (17):

TABLE 2.10. Agents Associated with Neuromuscular Transmission Syndromes

Aminoglycoside antibiotics	Fasciculins	Pelamitoxin
Black widow spider venom	*Hydrophiidae* toxins	Penicillamine
	Interferon-α	Polymyxin
Botulinum neurotoxin	Lincomycin	Quinine
Carbamate pesticides	Lophotoxin	Succinylcholine
Ceruleotoxin	Mamba snake toxin	Taipoxin
Cobra venom	Mandaratoxin	Tetracyclines
Crotoxin	Methyllycaconitine	Trimethaphan
Delphinium spp.	Mojavetoxin	Tubocurarine
Dendroaspis angusticeps toxins	Organophosphorus compounds	Vecuronium
Erabutoxin		

lack of pre-existing muscular symptoms; delay in onset of symptoms after exposure to a putative toxin (*e.g.,* Haff disease); lack of another cause; and some degree of resolution after the agent is withdrawn. Severe toxic myopathies may result in rhabdomyolysis and myoglobinuria sufficient to cause acute renal failure. Myoglobinuria may accompany a secondary toxic muscle disorder as well as a direct chemical insult; two prominent indirect causes are prolonged immobilization in comatose (*heroin overdose*) individuals with pressure necrosis and excessive muscle activity in seizures and delirium (*alcohol withdrawal*). Table 2.11 depicts the principal types of toxic myopathy, the responsible agents, and risk factors. The necrotizing myopathies are, by far, the most common type in this heterogeneous group; the other disorders are rare in North American clinical practice.

Necrotizing myopathy is characterized by the acute onset of localized or generalized pain (myalgia), tenderness to palpation, proximal limb weakness, and elevated serum creatine kinase (CK), a marker of muscle necrosis. The most frequent causes are *alcohol* and *cholesterol- or lipid-lowering drugs*, the "CLAM" syndrome (Cholesterol-Lowering-Agent Myopathy). If not promptly recognized and the lipid-lowering drug discontinued, myonecrosis with life-threatening rhabdomyolysis may follow. An especially virulent toxic myopathy may accompany combined *lovastatin and cyclosporine* treatment.

Corticosteroid/neuromuscular blocking agent myopathy (*vecuronium/steroid* weakness syndrome) is an entity commonly encountered in anesthesia and pulmonary medicine. Patients awaken from surgery or following treatment of an asthmatic attack with severe limb and oculomotor weakness; mild muscle necrosis and CK elevation may accompany this condition.

There are three distinct syndromes of hypokalemic myopathy. The first is a flaccid, transient, or persistent muscle weakness affecting primarily the proximal limb muscles with preserved tendon reflexes and elevated CK; few histopathological changes are detectable. The second syndrome is subacute onset of painless proximal weakness with the histopathological features of periodic hypokalemic paralysis; diffuse vacuolation and degeneration of muscle fibers. The third (rare) syndrome includes muscle necrosis and rhabdomyolysis.

Amphophilic-cation myopathy is a syndrome of slowly progressive, painless proximal weakness without significant elevation in CK. Muscle biopsy abnormalities include necrosis and cytoplasmic lamellar inclusions. The most commonly implicated agents, *chloroquine* and *amiodarone*, also cause polyneuropathy.

The fasciitis-microangiopathy syndromes associated with adulterated *rape seed oil* or *synthetic tryptophan* use are of historical and theoretical interest; these 2 entities represent almost the sole examples of possible chemical-induced, immune-mediated nerve damage.

Several agents (*i.e.,* 2,4-dichlorophenoxyacetic acid, 20,25-diazocholesterol) are associated with myotonic myopathy. Myotonia is a sustained contraction of skeletal muscle that slowly diminishes. The naturally occurring myotonic myopathies constitute a group of hereditary conditions of muscle with pathogeneses centered around dysfunction of muscle ion channels.

A delayed "myopathy/imtermediate" syndrome of paralysis of certain nicotinic neuromuscular junctions rarely may appear 24 hours or longer following *organophosphate* exposure. The clinical picture features weakness of cranial nerve innervated muscles, the diaphragm, neck, and proximal limb muscles. Most recover within two weeks if respiratory function can be maintained. Experimental studies suggest that this is a junctional myopathy (muscle damage originating in the endplate region).

Specific Syndromes and Scenarios Strongly Associated with Neurotoxins

Neurotoxic disorders rarely display pathognomonic signs (*e.g.,* the corneal Kayser-Fleischer rings that inevitably herald Wilson's disease); however, certain combinations of symptoms, physical findings and circumstances should arouse suspicion:

1. Alopecia and painful peripheral neuropathy in a wealthy person—*thallium* poisoning (by the beneficiary).
2. Ataxia, acidosis, and renal failure in a person with chronic alcoholism—*ethylene glycol* intoxication.
3. Sudden visual loss during a urological procedure—*glycine* intoxication.
4. Diarrhea and perioral numbness following a seafood meal—*ciguatera* ingestion.
5. Cardiac arrhythmia, headaches, memory loss—chronic *carbon monoxide* exposure.

TABLE 2.11. Agents Associated with Myopathy Syndromes

Type	Agent	Risk Factors
Necrotizing myopathy	1. Lovastatin, pravastatin, simvastatin	1. Cyclosporine/gemfibrozil
	2. Clofibrate, gemfibrozil	2. Renal failure
	3. ε-Aminocaproic acid	3. Therapy duration >4 weeks
	4. Alcohol abuse	
	5. Hypervitaminosis E	5. Uncontrolled self-medication
	6. Etretinate, isotretinoin?	
	7. Organophosphates	7. Accidental insecticide exposure
	8. Snake venoms	
	9. Corticosteroid myopathy: acute	9. Acute: high IV steroid dose, ventilated patients on pancuronium
Hypokalemic myopathy	Diuretics	Fasting, exercise
	Laxatives	
	Licorice, carbenoxolone	
	Amphotericin B, toluene	
	Alcohol abuse	
Amphophilic cationic drug myopathy (lysosomal storage, "lipidosis")	Chloroquine, hydroxychloroquine, quinacrine, plasmocid	Daily chloroquine dose >500 mg
	Amiodarone	
	Perhexiline maleate	
Impaired protein synthesis	Ipecac syrup, emetine	Eating disorders, >600 mg in 10 days
Antimicrotubular myopathy	Colchicine	Chronic renal failure
	Vincristine	
Inflammatory myopathy	D-penicillamine	
	Procainamide	
Fasciitis, perimyositis, microangiopathy	"Toxic oil" syndrome	Rapeseed oil (adulterated), Spain
	Eosinophilia-myalgia syndrome	Tryptophan (synthetic)
Mitochondrial myopathy	Zidovudine	
	Germanium	
Myopathy due to IM injections	Acute: IM injection of various drugs: *e.g.*, cephalothin, lidocaine, diazepam	
	Chronic: repeated IM injections: meperidine, pentazocine, intravenous drug abuse, antibiotics (in children)	Genetic factor?
Various	1. Corticosteroid myopathy; chronic anthracycline antibiotics	1. Daily prednisone >10 mg
	2. Myopathy with prominent myotonia	2. 20,25-Diazocholesterol and 2,4-D

IM: Intramuscular.
IV: Intravenous
2,4D: 2,4-Dichlorophenoxyacetic acid

[Modified from Victor and Sieb (13), with permission.]

6. Acral paresthesias in a dentist—recreational use of *nitrous oxide* for euphoric effect.
7. Sensory ataxia and numb feet in a self-conscious female—*pyridoxine* megavitaminosis.
8. Myoclonus, tremor, cognitive impairment in gastroenterology patients—heavy *bismuth* use.
9. Motor-neuron-like weakness in hands in chronic dermatologic disease—*dapsone* intoxication.

ASSESSMENT OF NEUROTOXIC DISEASE IN INDIVIDUALS

Methods and Procedures

The methods and procedures utilized in the office diagnosis of neurotoxic disorders are those of everyday neurological practice. The clinician-elicited history and a high index of suspicion are pivotal in determining a condition to be toxic; other procedures (in approximate order of usefulness) are physical examination, neuropsychological testing, specialized electrodiagnostic tests, and imaging procedures.

History

A detailed history is the cornerstone of the office evaluation of neurotoxic disease; a paramount concern is accurate information regarding the agent and the route and duration of exposure. Questioning should be directed at possible occupational exposure to fumes, volatile solvents, chemical dust, molten material, and *whether co-workers are affected.* Inquiry should also focus on possible substance abuse, food faddism, hobbies, exposure to polluted natural resources, suicidal tendency and risk of deliberate poisoning. Questions concerning health of family members or even household pets can reveal the source and magnitude of exposure. Since naturally occurring illness, such as nutritional disorders, endocrine dysfunction, and hereditary degenerative diseases, can mimic neurotoxic insult, the office history should also be directed at a wide range of medical conditions. The likelihood of traumatic nerve and spine injury should be documented, since these conditions, if bilateral, can mimic symptoms of toxic distal axonopathy. A critical portion of the history is a list of all current and recent medicines, including vitamins and nutritional supplements. In some instances, a visit to the home or workplace is indicated (11).

Physical Examination

Information obtained from the history can direct the examination to target vulnerable end points (*e.g.*, if *mercury* is the principal suspected toxin, the clinical examination should stress neurobehavioral and tremor analysis; if *acrylamide*, the focus is peripheral sensory function).

The standard office examination should begin with a brief evaluation of mental status, including level of consciousness, orientation, language, concentration, memory, mood, and affect. Should the history suggest cognitive dysfunction, quantitative neuropsychological testing is indicated. Cranial nerves are usually examined in series, with particular attention to the optic and trigeminal nerves. Motor system evaluation includes inspection for muscle atrophy, unusual movements, and tremor and gait abnormalities. Additional tests are analysis of coordination, muscle tone, and resistance to passive limb stretch and assessment of the strength of individual muscles. Sensory function, including modalities of sharpness, position, vibration, light touch, and temperature, should be determined on the distal

and proximal portion of the limbs. Tendon reflex elicitation should include the distal and proximal portion of the limbs. The plantar responses to cutaneous stimulation are usually determined last.

Neuropsychological Tests

Deficits in memory, attention, and mental and psychomotor speed have been observed following exposure to a variety of substances and provide the basis for the usual complaints of difficulty concentrating and remembering, and slowed thinking. The neuropsychological examination should include multiple tests of these functions to obtain converging evidence of impairment. In addition, the examination should include tests of premorbid and current intellectual functioning, visual perception, reasoning, and language skills to permit identification of expected patterns of performance following neurotoxic exposure. Patients with neurotoxic cognitive impairment can display mild to moderate deficits in memory or attention or rate of information processing yet display relatively preserved performance on tests of visual perception, language, and reasoning as long as they have unlimited time to view the material and respond. Similarly, current intellectual functioning estimated by untimed tests may not be lower than premorbid intellectual functioning estimated by a reading test or demographic information. Thus, identification of perceptual deficits or language impairment with relative preservation of memory and attention may reflect something other than neurotoxic impairment such as a pre-existing developmental disorder.

Computer-assisted tests that automate stimulus presentation and data acquisition are especially useful because they facilitate the measurement of reaction times that may be slowed by neurotoxic exposure. The availability of latency data time-locked to stimulus presentation provides a level of precision and sensitivity in measuring speed of information processing that is not possible with manually timed tests. Thus, for example, it is not unusual for a patient to perform within normal limits on paper-and-pencil tests of information-processing speed and to perform clearly in the defective range on computer-assisted tests. In addition, the dynamics of computer-assisted testing provides a nonthreatening challenge to patients that encourages their participation and motivation, and decreases the influence of mood and psychiatric disease on performance.

Two other issues should be addressed in the neuropsychological evaluation. Because emotional and psychiatric disturbances may develop as concomitants of neurotoxic exposure and can influence test performance, assessment of depression and personality functioning should be performed. It is also critical to ascertain the validity of the data obtained during the evaluation, since some patients may derive primary or secondary gains from malingering. This can be done by including methods for identifying malingering in the test battery and by inspecting the entire protocol to identify any illogical or unexpected patterns in performance.

Specialized Laboratory Tests

The environmental analysis is an essential feature of almost every nonpharmaceutical case. Clinical laboratory tests are of little help, since measurements of the body burden of most neurotoxins are not available save for metals, alcohol, and pharmaceuticals. *The practice of routine comprehensive screening for low levels of chemicals in blood, urine, fat, and hair, and for antibodies to presumed neurotoxic agents, is of questionable merit and should be discouraged.*

Certain specialized tests are commonly employed to augment the history and physical examination; these procedures do not specify a diagnosis of neurotoxic disease, they only detect and characterize dysfunction. Tests are directed at PNS, muscle, or CNS disease, and save for quantitative sensory testing, there is little overlap. Specialized tests of visual and auditory/vestibular function are best left to the otolaryngologist or ophthalmologist.

PNS laboratory tests. Electrophysiological studies [nerve conduction studies (NCV), needle electromyography (EMG)] are widely used quantitative neurological tools for the evaluation of peripheral nerve and muscle function. EMG may be especially helpful in identifying muscle dysfunction as a source of weakness.

Changes in sensory potential amplitudes are the most sensitive measure of axonal dysfunction. NCV studies can determine the maximal velocity of the largest diameter fibers within a nerve. The pattern of axonal dysfunction (*e.g.*, proximal *vs.* distal) may also be established by electrophysiology; this is a critical determinant for detection of neurotoxic disease. Alterations in action potential configuration (*e.g.*, temporal dispersion) and conduction velocities are sensitive measures of peripheral nerve demyelination (rarely toxic in origin), but are usually relatively unaffected in the toxic axonopathies. Even if only a small number of large-diameter fibers continues to conduct at normal velocities, the NCV can remain within normal limits. In the diagnosis of toxic neuropathies, NCV studies are principally valuable to confirm an axonopathy and help rule out alternative causes of peripheral nerve dysfunction. Mononeuropathies and nerve entrapments are especially well documented by electrodiagnosis.

Quantitative sensory function (QST) tests, described fully later, and tests of peripheral autonomic function, sweating, and heart rate variation, are occasionally useful in *monitoring* individual cases, but rarely are indicated for *diagnosis*.

Biopsy of nerve or muscle is rarely indicated or helpful in identifying toxic neuropathies and myopathies, since most eventuate in nonspecific axonal or myofibrillary degeneration, respectively.

Analyses of tremor, balance, olfaction, and taste are seldom used in evaluating individual cases.

CNS laboratory tests. The electroencephalogram (EEG) is primarily useful in evaluating and classifying seizure disorders. While the EEG is of help in monitoring patients with known acute toxic/metabolic encephalopathies, the pattern of abnormality is rarely characteristic of a specific compound. Acute encephalopathies are featured by several EEG changes, including spindle coma, burst suppression and nonspecific fast- or slow-wave activity. Hepatic coma may have prominent triphasic waves, *lithium* intoxication is associated with spike and slow-wave activity, and *phencyclidine* intoxication sometimes is distinguished by a characteristic periodic (every second) rhythmic slow-wave pattern.

Quantitative EEG (QEEG) is based on the mathematical processing of the digitally recorded EEG to highlight specific waveform components and transform the EEG into a format that elucidates specific relevant information. Topographic displays of voltage or frequency, "brain mapping," can present visually a spatial resolution of raw EEG data from different areas of the head. The term is misleading and often confused with functional cortical mapping from direct stimulation or with brain mapping by neuroimaging techniques [magnetic resonance imaging (MRI), positron emission tomography (PET)]. A critical evaluation of QEEG finds the technique of little clinical use and of major disadvantage in legal disputes because of false-positive results in normal individuals (10). "Probative value and even the test-retest reproducibility can be poor. There is great potential for abuse."

Polysomnography measures the changing patterns of EEG frequency, electrocardiography, respiration, and extraocular movements during nocturnal and, sometimes, daytime sleep. Sophisticated sleep laboratories can also monitor upper airway function, penile tumescence, and periodically sample venous blood for endocrine analyses. Acute and chronic toxic/metabolic encephalopathies may produce either insomnia or excessive sleepiness. There is no characteristic pattern of sleep disturbance associated with a specific chemical, and many neurological and psychiatric conditions are associated with abnormal sleep. Polysomnography is not useful in the diagnosis of neurotoxic disease.

Recent advances in electrophysiological procedures and microcomputer technology have led to the widespread use of evoked potentials (EPs) as an index of the integrity of sensory CNS pathways. When properly performed and interpreted, EPs can be used to monitor a sensory system from receptor to cerebral cortex. They have been particularly valuable in detecting clinically silent lesions. EPs have been extensively used in the diagnosis of neurotoxic disease, but these studies must be interpreted with caution. Many of the reported findings are subtle and subject to criticism. The clearest findings have been alterations in the short-latency auditory EPs (BAER) associated with *toluene*, visual EPs (VER) associated with *mercury*, and somatosensory EPs (SEP) associated with the central manifestation of toxic distal axonopathies.

Long-latency (P300, cognitive evoked) potentials are too variable to be of use in the diagnosis or monitoring of disease progression.

Imaging procedures. Computed tomography (CT) scans and conventional MRI help rule out naturally occurring disorders; they rarely show lesions specific for neurotoxic disease. Dynamic imaging procedures such as MRI spectroscopy, echoplanar (functional) MRI, single photon emission computerized tomography (SPECT) and PET are sensitive measures of blood flow and metabolism and may be clinical tools in the future; currently, they are principally used in research. SPECT scanning has found clinical use in longitudinal monitoring of patients with encephalomalacia; its employment as a diagnostic instrument for individual cases of neurotoxic disease is discouraged.

Illustrative Clinical Vignettes
Pseudo Neurotoxic Syndromes

CASE 1

A 30 year-old female manicurist was referred because of the 12-month gradual onset of numbness and slight weakness of the hands, followed 3 months later by similar symptoms in the feet; this was coincident with the use of solvents (acetone-toluene mixture) for removal of fingernail adhesive. She was not disabled by this condition. Examination by an experienced clinical neurotoxicologist revealed mild impairment of all sensory modalities in the distal limbs, absent Achilles reflexes, and normal strength and gait. After it was determined that these solvents were not associated with peripheral neurotoxicity, an aggressive history disclosed a 4-year, daily consumption of 100 mg pyridoxine.

The patient was glibly reassured (by the neurotoxicologist) that her condition was not occupational and would dissipate were she to stop self-administering vitamins. A perfunctory electrodiagnostic study disclosed unexpected, profound slowing of conduction in distal and proximal segments of multiple limb nerves. A subsequent lumbar puncture revealed a cerebrospinal fluid protein of 82 mg/dL, and a diagnosis of chronic inflammatory polyneuropathy (a naturally occurring, immune-mediated condition) was established.

CASE 2

A 2 month-old infant developed paralysis of the right hemidiaphragm and respiratory distress 2 weeks following commercial application of chlorpyriphos (an organophosphate in commercial use) in the nursery. During the subsequent 4 month hospitalization, he developed progressive weakness eventuating in a state of flaccid quadriplegia and respiratory paralysis. Five years later he remained unchanged; examination revealed an intact mental state, preserved sensation throughout, flaccid quadriplegia, tongue fasciculations, and total respiratory dependency. Nerve conduction studies showed no motor responses throughout, absent sensory potentials in the sural and superficial peroneal nerves, and diminished sensory amplitudes in upper limb nerves. Despite the treating pediatrician's appropriate diagnosis of a congenital disorder (spinal muscle atrophy), toxic tort litigation commenced.

Comment. These cases represent the most common scenario in North American neurotoxicology practice—the misattribution of a naturally occurring condition as neurotoxic, despite only trivial contact with a presumed or genuine neurotoxic agent. Polyneuropathy especially lends itself to this dilemma because an etiology is unestablished in about 40% of cases. Clinicians who are unfamiliar with the tenets of neurotoxic disease readily attribute these cases to chemical exposure.

The examiner in case 1 recognized the solvents as benign but ignored the commencement of symptoms in the hands, a feature incompatible with pyridoxine distal axonopathy (a condition that also has never been encountered with a daily dose of 100 mg).

In case 2, the asymmetrical onset of diaphragmmatic paralysis, while atypical in spinal muscle atrophy, has been previously described; asymmetrical, proximal onset, and progression for months following exposure is incompatible with organophosphate neuropathy. The absent sensory responses in the lower limb reflect nerve entrapments from prolonged recumbency.

Neurotoxic PNS Syndromes

CASE 1

A 25 year-old furniture stripper presented to the hospital complaining of 3 months of progressive lower limb weakness, numbness, and foot-dragging. Examination disclosed profound weakness of foot dorsiflexion, steppage gait, diminution of all sensory modalities below the mid-shin level, and absent tendon reflexes in the lower limbs. Nerve conduction tests disclosed absent sural nerve responses and profoundly slowed peroneal motor conduction. During hospitalization, he continued to worsen. Evaluation of family members for hereditary neuropathy was begun. Two weeks later, a fellow worker appeared at the outpatient clinic with an identical illness; a visit to the workplace revealed both to have been confined to a small enclosed room with an open 50-gallon drum of n-hexane; workplace measurement revealed an air level of 400 ppm n-hexane.

CASE 2

A 55 year-old female with chronic mild renal disease, not requiring hemodialysis, noted onset of numbness and weakness of lower limbs that rapidly progressed over a week. She consulted her nephrologist who noted profound weakness of foot dorsiflexion, moderately diminished touch and vibratory sensation in the feet, absent tendon reflexes throughout, and a broad-based, unsteady, steppage gait. She was admitted to the neurology intensive care unit with a presumptive diagnosis of Guillain-Barré syndrome; plasma exchange was anticipated if her gait worsened. Emergency neurophysiology studies by a neurologist experienced in neuromuscular disease detected diminished amplitudes in sural nerves and no changes in proximal nerve or roots. His insistence that this was axonal neuropathy and not Guillain-Barré syndrome triggered an aggressive history. She revealed a 3-month use of nitrofurantoin that had been prescribed for urinary tract infection by a physician unfamiliar with her chronic renal failure. Two weeks later, she was much improved.

Comment. Case 1 illustrates how clustering of a similar disorder strongly implicates an exogenous agent. Had the second patient not turned up at the same institution, the condition would have been considered spontaneous; without a workplace visit, the causative agent would not have been identified (11).

Case 2 emphasizes the prime roles of both an experienced, subspecialized neurologist and of an accurate, thorough history.

Neurotoxic CNS Syndromes

CASE 1

A 54 year-old teacher developed gradually progressive memory impairment and poor concentration over a 6-month period. He was considered depressed and had seen a psychiatrist on several occasions. There was no occupational or household contact with toxic agents, and he denied substance abuse or self-administration of pharmaceutical.

One month before admission, he developed myoclonic jerks of upper and lower limbs, and intermittent confusion. On examination, he was disheveled and emaciated. He was oriented to place, time and person, and language function was intact. He displayed impaired abstract thinking, and poor recent and remote memory. There were tremulous finger movements on intention, and frequent, nonsynchronous myoclonic jerks of all limbs. An EEG displayed mild and diffuse slowing.

A diagnosis of prion disease (spongiform encephalopathy) was entertained, and he was admitted to the hospital for evaluation and possible brain biopsy. During the preoperative evaluation period, it was noted that the patient was more lucid and myoclonic movements had decreased. Toxicology consultation suggested a urine and blood screen for bismuth; the levels returned as grossly elevated. Upon direct questioning, his wife disclosed that he had daily consumed one pint of a proprietary bismuth antacid preparation for the 2 years prior to the appearance of symptoms. Two months following the withdrawal, he was much improved.

CASE 2

A 29 year-old veterinary assistant developed gradual onset of memory loss and unsteady gait. Despite psychiatric treatment for depression, she continued to deteriorate; during the next 2 years, she became unable to remember simple tasks or drive an automobile without becoming lost. In order to carry out activities of daily life, it was necessary for her to make lists. Because of an unsteady gait and memory impairment, she was repeatedly evaluated for stigma of alcoholism; she and her husband vigorously denied substance use or self-medication, and none of her family or friends had been ill. The neurological examination disclosed mild distal sensory impairment in the lower limbs and profound impairment of recent memory with relative sparing of other cognitive functions.

Analysis of the workplace environment disclosed that she was confined, alone, in a small, poorly ventilated room and performed her job adjacent to a malfunctioning sterilizer. Analysis of the atmosphere disclosed 900 ppm of ethylene oxide. Within 6 months of removal from the workplace, her memory had improved and sensation had returned to normal.

Comment. Both cases illustrate a common clinical error, cognitive decline in a young or middle-aged person is frequently attributed to depression or excessive chronic alcohol use until a signal event occurs; a seizure in the first instance, striking memory loss in the second. The first patient denied self administration of pharmaceuticals because neither he nor his wife considered the proprietary preparation to be a drug; a belief reinforced by the absence of a label warning of the hazards of chronic bismuth use.

The second case was a formidable problem for the clinician, since the patient constituted the first linkage of disabling ethylene oxide encephalopathy to sterilizer malfunction. The association was eventually suspected after the sterilizer malfunction was documented on a routine maintenance visit. An alert and conscientious supervisor who, as a friend of long standing knew her not to be an alcoholic, requested the air analysis.

ASSESSMENT OF NEUROTOXIC DISEASE IN LARGE POPULATIONS

Before embarking on an expensive and labor-intensive epidemiological investigation of a presumed outbreak of neurotoxic disease, it is mandatory to perform a preliminary survey in the field and examine a small cohort of affected individuals. Such surveys, when done by a small multidisciplinary (*e.g.*, infectious disease, epidemiology, neurology, clinical toxicology) team of unbiased and experienced individuals, is usually of considerable value in focusing the subsequent large study on an appropriate target. For example, a careful environmental and preliminary clinical survey of African subjects with spasticity attributed to *mercury* intoxication resulted in the design of a case-control study that ruled out a neurotoxic etiology and conclusively demonstrated the causal role of human T-cell lymphotrophic virus type-1 retrovirus (12).

Study Design

The assessment of neurotoxic disease in a large population can be based on either prospective or retrospective studies. The design of accurate prospective studies requires careful consideration of the end-point measures selected, the population studied and the methods of analysis. Ideally, the design of a large population study by an epidemiologist should include input from: (a) clinicians aware of the profile of individuals exposed to the putative neurotoxic compound, (b) scientists familiar with the reliability, sensitivity, and specificity of the possible measures, and (c) environmental toxicologists capable of assessing the exposure levels within the population. Input from a statistician is also critical to estimate the power of the selected measures and the number of subjects required in the analysis. The team must balance the need to provide a broad-based screening for neurotoxic insult with the difficulty of adding too many measures and consequently diluting the findings (*i.e.*, "fishing expedition"). A cardinal consideration in study design is the adequacy of the referent population. Prospective studies for neurotoxic disease should always include a control population matched for demographic variables. A second important aspect of study design is assurance that data collection, and possibly even the analysis, is done blinded as to the status of individual subjects. Finally, the designers of prospective studies must establish, *a priori*, clear hypotheses and analysis strategies. *Post hoc* grouping of findings or sub-population analyses should be interpreted with caution; statistical significance is inevitable if enough comparisons are considered.

Retrospective studies of neurotoxic disease are more difficult to design and more open to incorrect interpretation. In these circumstances, precise information regarding exposure, adequate measures, and appropriate comparison groups are rarely available. Although retrospective studies can clearly document a correlation between measures, a causal link between exposure and clinical outcome is usually not established. In spite of these difficulties, retrospective studies are the only available tool for assessment of neurotoxic insult following some forms of acute exposure (*i.e.*, explosion at a chemical facility). The yield from retrospective studies can be greatly increased by assessment of data at multiple longitudinal points. Analysis of the progression and recovery of insult from a precise time point can strengthen causal inferences. In addition, information from well designed retrospective studies can be used to drive hypotheses and to direct future prospective studies.

Investigators confronted with an absence of exposure information have developed approaches that utilize available data. For example, studies have shown that unexplained illness among U.S. Gulf War veterans does not associate with time in the theater of operations and is proportionately similarly distributed among veterans who served exclusively at times prior to, during, or following the actual conflict period. Since these three deployment periods were associated with distinct constellations of exposures to environmental agents, vaccines and drugs, it appears unlikely that any one combination was of etiological significance and, thus, if confirmed, the illness is unlikely to be neurotoxic (15).

Methods and Procedures

The methods and procedures for field studies differ significantly from those of office assessment. Detailed clinical examinations and histories obtained by a neurologist are impractical in many field situations and must be replaced by quantitative screening tools. An ideal screening tool should be a valid index of the targeted dysfunction, rapid, reliable, standardized, quantitative, not threatening, inexpensive and capable of administration by support personnel. Some of the more useful population screening tools are: questionnaire, quantitative sensory testing, tremor analysis, computer-administered neurobehavioral testing, and biological markers. Results of QST tremor and neurobehavioral testing are to be interpreted with caution in older individuals because of age-related variability.

Questionnaire

A questionnaire is a reasonable first-line instrument to target the appropriate populations suspected of toxic disease. It is possible to obtain data on a wide range of topics; questions can be quantitative, allowing statistical analysis. Specific questions are evaluated and piloted prior to the beginning of a study. Asking about "burning" in the feet can elicit a very different response than asking about "painful cramping," yet each may reflect the same underlying condition. Autonomic symptoms relating to diarrhea, inappropriate sweating, and impotence are particularly influenced by the precise wording of the questions. Whenever possible, standardized and verified symptom questionnaires should be utilized. If an estimate of the intensity of symptoms is desired, a linear or numerical scale with adequate resolution (*i.e.*, 0–10) should be utilized.

Quantitative Sensory Testing

QST is a procedure that stems from the roots of experimental psychology and human factors testing. In the past decade, there has been a proliferation of portable, relatively inexpensive devices for the QST of vibration and thermal thresholds. Much of the impetus for these developments has been the needs of multicenter, longitudinal studies of toxic or metabolic neuropathies. Vibration thresholds are an index of the integrity of the receptors and pathways associated principally with large-diameter myelinated fibers; thermal thresholds are for the most part associated with small-diameter myelinated and unmyelinated fibers. Several psychophysical algorithms are also available and in use in field studies of peripheral neuropathy, including method of limits, scaling, signal detection, and forced-choice paradigms.

Tremor Analysis

Although tremors may be encountered in a variety of nervous system diseases, they rarely result from chemical exposure (certain drugs and heavy metals excepted). Occasionally, however, patients exposed to chemicals require evaluation of abnormal involuntary movements. Classification of movement disorders includes both the clinical circumstances under which the movement is maximal and the various physiological characteristics of the movement. Tremor can be recorded by triaxial accelerometry, which allows precise measurement of frequency and amplitude. Surface EMG recording from antagonistic muscles, although also useful in determining frequency, is of greatest use in documenting the underlying pattern of motor unit discharges. Tremor analysis is easily performed with conventional electromyographic equipment; it can be used to differentiate physiological tremor, which is present in all individuals, from resting and action tremors.

Computer-administered Neurobehavioral Testing

Computer-administered neurobehavioral tests have greatly increased the power, standardization, and ease of administration of neuropsychological procedures. Generally, a computer program trains the subject, administers the test, and records the data. The use of computers allows precise timing of data presentation and precise measurement of response latencies. Programs are available for the assessment of attention span, perceptual motor skills, memory and learning, and cognition and affect. The growing normative data base for these tests allows individual patients and groups to be compared with appropriate subpopulations with increasing accuracy.

Biological Markers

Biomarkers are classified into one of three broad categories: *susceptibility*, *exposure* or *effect*. A biomarker of *susceptibility* is an indicator of a limitation (inherent or acquired) of an organism's ability to respond to the challenge of exposure to a specific environmental factor. A biomarker of *exposure* is a xenobiotic substance (*e.g.*, *lead*) or its metabolite, or the product of an interaction between a xenobiotic agent and some target that is measured within a compartment of the organism; preferred biomarkers are the substance itself or substance-specific metabolites in readily obtainable body fluids. A biomarker of *effect* is any measurable biochemical, physiological, or other alteration within an organism that can be recognized as a potential health impairment or disease; many biomarkers of effect (*e.g.*, blood pressure, pulmonary vital capacity) are not substance-specific.

Several biomarkers of neurotoxic *susceptibility* are known. Pharmacogenetics has identified several genetic polymorphisms of enzymes involved in xenobiotic metabolism. These include members of cytochrome P450, glutathione transferase and *N*-acetyltransferase (NAT); the latter includes NAT 2 mutants with slow acetylation patterns that increase risk for neurotoxicity among 40-60% of Caucasians who are exposed to drugs such as the antituberculous agent, *isoniazid*. CYP2E1 is an inducible *ethanol*-metabolizing enzyme. *Aminoglycoside* ototoxicity has been associated with a mitochondrial DNA (mtDNA) 1555A-to-G point mutation in the 12S ribosomal RNA gene. Individuals with genetic variants of serum cholinesterase [butryl-cholinesterase (BChE)] may have an abnormal response to anticholinesterase compounds such as pyridostigmine bromide. Homozygotes with the BChE substitution represent 1 per 3500 Caucasians; heterozygotes constitute 4–5% of Caucasians and a higher percentage of African-Americans.

Valuable examples of biomarkers of neurotoxic *exposure* include *heavy metals* in blood, urine, or hair; *organochlorine pesticides* in blood, saliva, and adipose tissue, and *organophosphorus metabolites* in urine. Short-lived albumin adducts (20–25 days) and longer-lived hemoglobin adducts (4 months) provide a method to monitor exposures to certain compounds (n-*hexane*, *acrylamide*) that trigger peripheral neuropathy (7). Spectrin, an erythrocyte protein, forms dimers in the presence of the *n*-hexane metabolite *2,5-hexanedione* or *carbon disulfide*, and spectrin dimers may be detectable in rodents before the appearance of clinical or morphological evidence of axonal degeneration. Lymphocyte neuropathy target esterase activity has been used to monitor exposure to the organophosphate *chlorpyrifos*, another agent known to induce peripheral neuropathy and CNS effects in humans and animals. Erythrocyte δ-aminolevulinic acid dehydratase and zinc protoporphyrin are widely used as biomarkers of *lead* exposure.

Erythrocyte acetylcholinesterase (AChE) activity is an example of a biomarker of neurotoxic *effect*. It is widely used to monitor exposure to organophosphate chemicals employed as pesticides and chemical warfare agents. Blood AChE activity provides a crude surrogate for acetylcholinesterase that terminates neurotransmission at cholinergic synapses (7).

Data Analysis

Data analysis procedures are a critical facet of both prospective and retrospective population studies. In most cases, they determine the sensitivity of the study and the probability of "false-positive" findings. As stated above, data analysis decisions begin with consideration of population dynamics and the statistical power of the selected measures. Ideally, the method and scope of analysis should be determined prior to study onset. If multiple measures are to be grouped, simplified, or otherwise clustered, this should be determined prior to data collection rather than after a preliminary analysis. The nature of the data (*i.e.*, parametric *vs.* nonparametric) and the distribution of findings (*i.e.*, gaussian *vs.* non-gaussian) must be considered in selecting the optimal battery of statistical tests. The number of statistical comparisons must also be considered and appropriate adjustments in *p* values must be made for studies using multiple end-points.

The analysis of data in population studies generally has three goals:

1. Identification of group differences.
2. Detection of individual members of a group that differ from the population or expected norms.
3. Determination of variables that predict neurotoxic outcomes.

Subtle dysfunction may be present in a population, although no individual shows evidence of disease. In this situation, analysis of population central tendencies (means, modes, and medians) is useful. If the data are appropriately distributed, simple *t*-test or an analysis of variance is recommended. The statistical power of field studies may uncover significant dysfunction below values usually accepted as clinically abnormal in office evaluation. For example, a slowing of nerve conduction of 1.5 m/sec, meaningless in evaluating an individual patient, may be highly significant across a population of 500 subjects.

Alternatively, the majority of a population may show no effect, but a small number of subjects may demonstrate significant toxic neuropathy. In this instance, determination of the pattern of skew within the population is critical. A *chi-square* analysis comparing the expected number of outliers across population samples may be an appropriate test. If variance is not considered, a true toxic effect in a subset of the population may be masked. Separate analysis of "at-risk" samples (*e.g.*, children and older subjects) is critical when studying heterogeneous populations.

The identification of "risk factors" that significantly predict a neurotoxic outcome is particularly important in retrospective studies. Age, sex, education, and prior neurological disease are examples of factors that must be considered, alone and in combination. Linear and nonlinear regression analyses are the recommended statistical procedures for these studies, but investigators must be careful to distinguish between correlation and causation.

The interpretation of data from field studies is critically affected by the selection of a control or comparison population. Many studies have used historical control groups for comparisons and, consequently, have diminished the specificity of their findings. In the worse cases, controls have been drawn from an inappropriate group, such as medical or graduate students. Controls should be matched on as many variables as possible and should be randomly drawn from a population closely approximating the exposed or other study group.

A second overall concern for field studies is the possible biasing of population findings by the elimination of subjects with known alternative causes of nervous system disease. While identification and removal of these subjects has a certain face validity, many of the known alternative causes of nervous system disease are highly correlated with age. By removing these subjects, individuals most vulnerable for the toxic condition may be inadvertently eliminated. Furthermore, existing neurological conditions may predispose to the actions of neurotoxic chemicals. The problem is particularly vexing in peripheral nerve disease, since toxic neuropathies may be additive or may "unmask" naturally occurring conditions (*e.g.*, subclinical diabetic neuropathy).

Finally, data analysis is only as good as the data processed. No amount of clustering, transformation, or statistical treatment can overcome significant "noise" added to the measure at collection. Every effort must be made to standardize data acquisition procedures and to minimize the coefficient of variation for individual measures. Tested quality control procedures at all phases of data collection and entry are strongly recommended.

Large-Population Screening Scenarios

In assessing a large population exposed to chemicals, one of three situations usually prevails.

Situation 1

A segment of the populace is exposed to a known substance with neurotoxic potential (*acrylamide monomer* or *mercury*), and there is a need to survey for abnormalities associated with that substance (peripheral neuropathy or tremor). The approach to this situation is straightforward and the elucidation simple. The screening tools selected can be very specific and focused on the known principal effects of the agent under study. Thus, workers exposed to *acrylamide monomer* have been screened for alterations in vibration threshold, since denervation of pacinian corpuscles is an early effect of exposure in laboratory animals.

Workers exposed to mercury have principally been tested for cognitive dysfunction, tremor, and sensory loss.

Situation 2

There is exposure to chemicals not known to be neurotoxic and the populace appears to be well. There is a need to determine whether disease exists or to reassure the population and regulatory agencies that none is present.

In this situation, with neither a toxin nor disease syndrome identified, it is questionable whether the clinician has a role to play. There is a high risk of totally fruitless investigation or, even worse, of seemingly positive preliminary findings that eventually prove spurious. For this reason, these types of "fishing expeditions" are generally to be avoided.

However, exceptional cases may warrant investigation, particularly when there is great concern among the exposed population. In view of the previous discussion of subclinical or asymptomatic neurotoxicity, however, the investigator cannot responsibly give public reassurance merely on the grounds that the population is not symptomatic. In such instances, the most highly exposed individuals should be screened for symptoms and signs of nervous system dysfunction and a sizable sample (n = 30–60) of this group evaluated by a team of experienced neurologists among the medical professionals. The procedure indicated is not a rapid, highly targeted screening suitable for a large population, but rather a thorough neurological history and physical examination. Initial use of a sophisticated clinical examination is emphasized rather than screening with electrophysiological or laboratory tests. If negative findings characterize a subgroup that is sufficiently large and representative, it is unlikely that a neurotoxicological problem exists in the general population. If a possible unexplained problem is detected in the subgroup, it must be pursued further as discussed under Situation 3.

Situation 3

There is exposure to chemicals not known to be neurotoxic, but individuals clearly have neurological abnormalities. The neurotoxicologist is requested to define the illness and link it to a chemical, or to determine if it is a chance cluster of naturally occurring conditions. Situation 3 is difficult; it requires the creation of a collaborative multidisciplinary team that can maintain good relations with the patients, regulatory agencies, and industry.

There are several instances in which outbreaks of serious neurological dysfunction due to industrial agents not known to be neurotoxic were efficiently analyzed, the substance identified, and the source eliminated. Considerable publicity has attended one of these episodes: the *methyl n-butyl ketone* neuropathy epidemic in a Columbus, Ohio, factory; its elucidation stands as a paradigm of the correct approach to an outbreak of neurological disease from a chemical not previously known to be neurotoxic (3). Following initial scattered reports of peripheral neuropathy from community clinicians, attention was focused on the common feature of employment in a fabric impregnation factory. Screening electrodiagnostic tests were rapidly done on 1157 employees by clinicians experienced in neuromuscular disease; 194 were identified as suspected of having neuropathy. Meticulous clinical examinations were performed and those with naturally-occurring conditions eliminated. Examination data from the examinations were analyzed along with information about worker location and chemical concentrations in various working areas. Methyl *n*-butyl ketone was identified as the suspected agent; the creation of a corresponding experimental animal model confirmed this suspicion.

REFERENCES

1. Adams RD, Victor M, Ropper AH (1997) Disorders of motility. In: *Principles of Neurology*. McGraw Hill, New York p. 37.
2. Adams RD, Victor M, Ropper AH (1997) Disorders of smell and taste. In: *Principles of Neurology*. McGraw Hill, New York p. 231.
3. Allen N (1980) Identification of methyl *n*-butyl ketone as the causative agent. In: *Experimental and Clinical Neurotoxicology*. Spencer PS, Schaumburg HH eds. Williams & Wilkins, Baltimore p. 834.
4. Bolla K (1996) Neurobehavioral performance in multiple chemical sensitivites. *Res Toxicol Pharmacol* **24**, 352.
5. Bolla KL, Roca RP (1994) Neuropsychiatric sequelae of occupational exposure to neurotoxins. In: *Occupational Neurology and Clinical Neurotoxicology*. Bleeker M ed. Williams & Wilkins, Baltimore p. 148.
6. Brust JCM (1993) *Neurological Aspects of Substance Abuse*. Butterworth-Heineman, Boston p. 1.
7. Costa LG (1996) Biomarker research in neurotoxicology: the role of mechanistic studies to bridge the gap between the laboratory and epidemiological studies. *Environ Health Prospect* **104** (Suppl 1), 55.
8. Grant WM, Shuhman JS (1993) *Toxicology of the Eye*. Charles C Thomas, Springfield, Il.
9. Mastaglia FL (1995) Iatrogenic (drug-induced) disorders of the nervous system. In: *Neurology and General Medicine*. Aminoff MJ ed. Churchill Livingstone, New York p. 587.
10. Newer M (1997) Assessment of digital EEG, quantitative EEG, and EEG brain mapping: Report of the American Academy of Neurology and the American Clinical Neurophysiology Society. *Neurology* **49**, 284.
11. Parry GJG (1995) Neurological complications of toxin exposure in the workplace. In: *Neurology and General Medicine*. Aminoff MJ ed. Churchill Livingstone, New York p. 641.
12. Román GC, Schoenberg BS, Madden DL *et al.* (1987) Human T-lymphotrophic virus type 1 antibodies in the serum of patients with tropical spastic paraparesis in the Seychelles. *Arch Neurol* **44**, 605.
13. Rybak, LP (1993) *Ototoxicity*. WB Saunders, Philadelphia.
14. Schaumburg HH (1994) Anatomical classification of peripheral nervous system disorders. In: *Disorders of Peripheral Nerves*. Schaumburg HH, Berger A, Thomas PK eds. FA Davis, Philadelphia p. 11.
15. Spencer PS, McCauley LA, Joos SK *et al.* (1998) U.S. Gulf War veterans: Service periods in theater, differential exposures, and persistent unexplained illness. *Toxicol Lett* **102–103**, 515.
16. Sporer KA (1995) The serotonin syndrome. *Drug Safety* **13**, 94.
17. Victor M, Sieb JP (1994) Myopathies due to drugs, toxins, and nutritional deficiency. In: *Myology*. Engel A ed. McGraw Hill, New York p. 1698.

CHAPTER THREE

Aspects of Veterinary Neurotoxicology

Anthony A. Frank
Linda L. Blythe
Peter S. Spencer

Clinical veterinary neurotoxicology is concerned with the identification and treatment of the adverse effects of a wide range of chemicals with which domestic animals come into contact. These include products of fungi, plants, and certain animals; a wide range of pesticidal chemicals; feed additives; therapeutic and illicit drugs; household products; and environmental contaminants.

The direct or indirect effects of toxic factors on the nervous system of domestic mammals is the primary focus of this chapter. Because mammalian (bovine, canine, caprine, equine, feline, ovine, porcine) and other species of varying age and nutritional state are exposed under uncontrolled conditions to often-changing mixtures of chemicals in algae, plant products, animal feeds, or commercial products, understanding of the relationship between chemical structure, dose, and effect is often imprecise. Additionally, analysis and identification of etiological factors may be complicated by the presence in synthetic products of compounds (impurities, "inert" vehicles) other than the main toxicologically active agent. Furthermore, scientific investigation of suspected animal intoxications may be limited by practical and economic barriers. These limitations notwithstanding, chemical neurotoxicity in domestic animals may serve as a sentinel for human health, as in the case of *organomercurial* poisoning in domestic swine presaging comparable neurological effects in children (29).

The adverse health effects on animals of exposure to poisonous plants make up an important component of veteri-

nary neurotoxicology, and interest in these effects also extends into experimental and human medicine. For example, some poisonous plant species (*Rhododendron* spp., *Andromeda* spp., *Azalea* spp., *Kalmia* spp., *Leucothoe* spp.) harbor substances (*grayanotoxins*) that are valued probes of neuronal function (sodium channels) (see Chapter 1). Others (*Centaurea* spp.) precipitate neurological disorders in animals (equine nigropallidal encephalomalacia) that have clinical similarities to human neurological (extrapyramidal) diseases. Some (*Lathyrus* spp.) cause diseases (lathyrism) that are recognized in both animals and humans, while others (*Cycas* spp.) have neuromuscular effects in animals that support the possibility that related effects (motor neuron disease) occur in comparably exposed humans. Understanding of plant toxicity (toxicognosy) is also important for societies that employ plant products as "health foods" or self-administered medicinals.

Host Factors

Differences in behavior, anatomy, physiology, or metabolism of domestic animals impact their individual responses to chemicals (102). Horses seem to sustain more chemical-induced damage of the elongate recurrent laryngeal nerve than other species with shorter necks. Birds have an elaborate respiratory system and therefore tend to be more susceptible to toxic gases than mammals. Monogastric animals (cats, dogs, humans) react similarly to many toxic factors introduced in the diet, while ruminants (cattle, sheep, goats) respond differently. Certain disorders affect a wide range of ruminants (*Aspergillus clavatus* mycotoxicosis); others are restricted to cattle (pushing disease induced by *Matricaria nigellifolia*), to sheep (retinal/optic blindness induced by *Helichrysum* spp.), or to sheep and goats (myopathy from *Geigeria* spp.). Several intoxications are peculiar to non-ruminants, including horses (*fumonisin* B$_1$-induced leukoencephalomalacia; *yellow star thistle*-induced equine nigropallidal encephalomalacia).

Feeding habits may influence susceptibility of animals to noxious substances. Dogs rapidly consume large quantities of food without pause and with little mastication. Cats approach food cautiously, eat limited amounts, and masticate more thoroughly than canines. Ruminants regurgitate food and thoroughly expose food particles to ruminal protozoa. These distinctive behavioral characteristics of ruminant and monogastric species impact their exposure to chemical substances.

The presence or absence of an anatomical rumen is a major factor dictating the toxicological effects of chemicals in domestic mammals. A modification of the esophagus, the rumen assists with the digestion of complex carbohydrates through the activity of a large anaerobic microbial population. Most of the feed ingredients are predigested before they reach the true stomach. Ruminal microorganisms have the potential to modify ingested chemicals: on the one hand, ruminal capacity for detoxication allows ruminant species to tolerate higher levels of certain ingested toxins; on the other, toxic species may be generated in the rumen. Harmless precursors (*cyanogenic glucosides*, *nitrates*) may be converted to toxic substances (*cyanide*, *nitrite*). Cattle are therefore susceptible to nitrate poisoning, while dogs (with few intestinal microorganisms) are resistant. Large doses of nitrate may also affect horses because the posterior portion of their digestive tract harbors microorganisms that convert unabsorbed nitrate to nitrite (124). Conversely, cattle are relatively insensitive to certain *organophosphate pesticides*, such as *parathion*, because they are enzymatically converted in the rumen to nonneurotoxic products (23). Some plants (*Pinus ponderosa*) may reduce the normal protozoan population of the rumen and thereby impact nutrient utilization and detoxication of other substances.

Distinctive physiological and metabolic features also account for the varying responses of species and strains to neurotoxic substances. Some mammals (horse, rabbit, rat) are unable to vomit ingested materials with potential toxicity. Biotransformation and excretion rates may differ: *fluoroacetate* is more toxic to dogs than rats because the agent is more rapidly metabolized to *fluorocitrate* in the canine. Dogs are deficient in the acetylation of aromatic amino compounds; they also excrete *phenoxyacetic herbicides* slowly because of a poorly developed organic acid renal transport system. Cats develop fatal methemoglobinemia from a single human therapeutic dose of *acetaminophen* because of a limited ability to conjugate drugs as glucuronides.

Gender, age, dosage, nutritional state, and environmental temperature may also modify an animal's response to chemicals. Female kittens are especially vulnerable to flea and tick sprays containing a mixture of N,N-*diethyl*-m-*toluamide* (DEET) and *fenvalerate*. Ovine *molybdenum intoxication/copper deficiency* impacts neonatal animals. Protein and antioxidant (*e.g.*, *selenium*) deficiency impairs biotransformation and promotes the formation of toxic free radicals. Insecticides may be more rapidly absorbed in hot weather when greater amounts of blood are physiologically directed to skin so as to reduce the core temperature. Variations in dosing may produce distinct acute and chronic disorders: *bufadienolide*-containing plants of the Crassulaceae cause acute cardiac glycoside intoxication in sheep and goats, while small repeated doses induce a paralytic syndrome with no clinical cardiac involvement (93,94).

NONBIOLOGICAL NEUROTOXIC FACTORS

Feed, Chemicals, and Water

Feed given to livestock may contain potential toxicants in the form of additives, such as antibiotics, antiparasitic drugs, growth or performance enhancers, and metals. Of historical interest is the use of *nitrofurans* as antibiotics, a cause of opisthotonus, tremor, circling and intermittent seizures in calves (*nitrofurazone*), and ataxia and posterior weakness in swine (*furazolidone*). *Sulfonamides* have been associated with peripheral neuropathy in swine. Excessive doses of *amprolium*, an antithiamine coccidiostat, have caused polyneuropathy in poultry and polioencephalomalacia in preruminant calves and lambs. Growth and performance enhancers include the ionophore *monensin*; horses, which may be poisoned at dosages used to feed poultry, develop profuse sweating, progressive ataxia, and posterior paresis.

Nonprotein nitrogen products (*e.g.*, *urea*) added to the feed of ruminants may cause intoxication. Elevated concentrations of blood *ammonia* trigger within hours of ingestion a clinical picture that includes frothy salivation, grinding of teeth, muscle tremor, blepharospasm, incoordination, and weakness. Ammoniation of carbohydrates in a molasses feed may lead to the formation of *4-methylimidazole*, which is held responsible for a clinical disorder in cows and nursing calves ("bovine bonkers") featured by ear twitching, trembling, champing, salivation, and convulsions (36,88,153). Consumption of *raw soybeans* is associated in cattle with diarrhea, ataxia, weakness, muscle tremor, and recumbency.

Neurological disorders may result from *water* intoxication and water deprivation; the latter, a form of sodium ion intoxication seen in swine, cattle, and poultry, is characterized by thirst, constipation, intermittent convulsive seizures, circling, central nervous system (CNS) depression, blindness, and head pressing. Edema and necrosis are found in the deeper layers of the cerebral cortex and adjacent white matter. Water intoxication in calves is associated with cerebral edema (101,102).

Metals, Metalloids, and Other Elements

Metals and other elements that are both essential and potentially toxic in domestic mammals include *chromium, cobalt, copper, iron, magnesium, manganese, molybdenum, selenium, strontium,* and *zinc;* however, of these, only manganese, molybdenum, and selenium exhibit significant neurotoxicity. Metal imbalances and interactions are common. Selenium toxicity is enhanced by protein deficiency, but elevated selenium intake protects against mercury toxicosis; *lead* toxicity is enhanced by deficiencies of calcium, phosphate, iron, or zinc; and molybdenum toxicosis of cattle promotes copper excretion resulting in copper deficiency. *Sulfide/sulfate*-induced polioencephalomalacia in ruminants may result from thiamine deficiency. *Arsenic, boron, cadmium, lead, mercury,* and *thallium* are nonessential metals with neurotoxic properties.

Arsenic

Inorganic arsenic is found in certain herbicides and pesticides; the latter is a common cause of arsenic poisoning in cattle. Severe gastrointestinal abnormalities and minor CNS involvement characterize the rapidly evolving and fatal illness (124). *Phenylarsenical compounds,* present in swine and poultry feed, may cause an insidious onset of peripheral nerve disease with ataxia and paralysis of the hindquarters (50,70,114). Phenylarsenic acid derivatives are used to control swine dysentery (*Serpulina hyodysenteriae*) and as growth promoters. The two most commonly used compounds are p-*aminophenylarsonic acid* and *3-nitro-4-hydroxyphenylarsonic acid.* Feed mixing errors, inadequate water supply and decreased excretion, and feeding p-aminophenylarsonic acid at levels recommended for the less toxic 3-nitro-4-hydroxyphenylarsonic acid, are usually associated with intoxication. In experimental animal studies,

only swine are affected. Clonic seizures that can be induced by forced exercise progress to posterior paraparesis and paralysis. Some reports include signs of intracranial dysfunction, including blindness and abnormal vocalizations, although no brain lesions have been identified and electroencephalograms are normal. The typical histopathological lesion is axonal degeneration in spinal dorsal-column tracts, particularly fasciculi gracilis and cuneatus; this may reflect the presence of peripheral nervous system (PNS) axonopathy. Optic nerve demyelination occurs and may account for blindness in the absence of other CNS lesions. While the mechanism is largely unknown, the parent compounds are apparently responsible because little biotransformation occurs. Disruption of vitamin B metabolism has been suggested as the mechanism; supportive evidence is lacking.

Boron

Most reports of boron intoxication in the clinical veterinary literature deal with ingestion by ruminants of boron-based fertilizer (130,131). Variable alterations in behavior, and tremors or fasciculations followed by seizures, may occur. Few intoxications have been adequately documented, and no lesions are described. Although the mechanism of action is unknown (*see* Chapter 1), stimulation of serotonergic and dopaminergic neurons has been suggested. Use of *boric acid* as a "natural" flea control agent in homes may result in an increased number of intoxications of human-companion animals (cats, dogs), although the emetic activity of boron limits toxicity in nonruminant species.

Lead

Lead intoxication in veterinary medicine usually involves acute high-level exposure of small numbers of cattle; clinical signs are secondary to laminar cortical necrosis associated with marked cerebral capillary damage and cerebral edema. Chronic low-level exposure to dogs and cats is characterized by a variable clinical pattern. Peripheral neuropathy in horses manifests as inspiratory noise ("roaring") and inhalation pneumonia due to laryngeal and pharyngeal paralysis. Facial nerve paralysis and loss of anal sphincter tone also occur. In late-stage intoxication, horses may become ataxic, tremulous, and dysphagic (72). Exposures are often chronic and related to pasture contamination with airborne emissions from smelters. Attempts to reproduce the disease under controlled conditions have failed.

Mercurials

Inorganic and organic mercury compounds exhibit neurotoxicity (29,108,136,148); *methylmercury* in particular accumulates in the brain, especially in the cerebrum and cerebellum. Veterinary reports of methylmercury intoxication most commonly involve swine; one notable incident in 1960–1979 in Alamogordo, New Mexico, illustrates how neurotoxic responses in animals may be a sentinel for human illness (29). In this incident, pigs fed treated waste seed grain developed blindness, incoordination, and posterior paralysis; most died. Consumption of pork from slaughtered pigs was followed by the appearance in a young girl of ataxia, decreased vision, CNS depression, and coma. An elder brother and sister subsequently developed a comparable illness. The mother gave birth to an infant who displayed gross tremulous movements after birth, myoclonic jerks at 6 months of age; and hypotonia, irritability, and nystagmus at 8 months. Under controlled experimental conditions, swine fed low doses of *methylmercuric dicyandiamide* display anorexia, incoordination, aimless walking, blindness, chewing without prehension of food, paresis, voice change, tremor, paddling movements, coma, and death. The cerebral cortex is more severely affected than in other species; cerebellar granule cells less so.

Molybdenum Intoxication/Copper Deficiency

Copper deficiency or molybdenum excess causes copper absorption from the rumen; enzymes requiring copper as a cofactor fail. Disease of cerebral white matter and degeneration of motor tracts of the spinal cord result from copper deficiency. Lambs are most commonly affected (13,25,37,55,117). Neurological disease is termed "enzootic ataxia" when acquired in the neonatal period and "swayback" when acquired *in utero*. Swayback usually is associated with cavitation of cerebral white matter. Enzootic ataxia is featured by diffuse CNS demyelination; however, neuronal degeneration in specific brain nuclei suggests a primary neuraxonal disease. Goats display a cerebellar form of the disease with Purkinje and internal granular cell necrosis, most severe in the vermis. Clinical signs of enzootic ataxia are variable but generally include paresis, inability to rise, depression, and blindness. Cytochrome oxidase dysfunction is held responsible for demyelination. Copper is also a cofactor in superoxide dismutase, and oxidative injury to neurons is suggested to account for neuraxonal degeneration.

Selenium

Although, in most species, chronic low-level selenium intoxication ("alkali disease") from consumption of selenium-bearing plants results in either pulmonary edema (acute intoxication), or hair and hoof abnormalities (chronic selenosis) (156,157,159), swine develop necrosis and cavitation in lumbar ventral horns of the spinal cord (15). Caudal and cervical ventral horns are sometimes also affected, and a few studies report neuronal damage in specific brainstem nuclei (notably the facial nuclei, motor nuclei of the fifth cranial nerve and nucleus cuneatus and gracilis). The slowly developing disease is characterized by neuronal chromatolysis, neuronal loss, marked microglial infiltration, and microcavitation. Paraparesis is the sole neurological sign, and most animals remain alert and continue to eat and drink. Hindlimbs exhibit flaccid paresis, while forelimbs retain withdrawal responses. Experimental production of the lesion is rapid; onset occurs between 3 and 20 days in a dose-dependent manner. The mechanism of action is unclear, although production of similar lesions by 6-aminonicotinamide, a niacin antimetabolite, raises the possibility that selenium excess causes niacin deficiency in swine. Niacin supplementation delays onset but does not prevent disease, and tissue concentrations of niacin remain normal during selenium intoxication. Noteworthy are reports of associations between human selenium exposure and sporadic amyotrophic lateral sclerosis (60,68,87,151).

Sulfide/Sulfate-Induced Polioencephalomalacia

The term *polioencephalomalacia* (PEM), in veterinary medicine, has been associated with a wide variety of disease entities, including laminar cortical necrosis induced by *lead* and *water deprivation/sodium ion intoxication*; this lesion may result from excessive production and absorption of ruminal *hydrogen sulfide* or soluble ionic forms of sulfide (44,45,83). The initial lesion appears to be neuronal necrosis in the deep and middle cortical laminae; later, cavitation, accumulation of macrophages, and grossly apparent pseudolaminar necrosis develop. Thiamine deficiency is held responsible for four reasons: (a) Blood and tissue concentrations of thiamine are sometime decreased in PEM; (b) this lesion has been produced in sheep consuming *Marsilea drummundi*, a thiaminase-containing plant; (c) thiamine is helpful therapeutically, but this effect may be nonspecific; and (d) high-sulfate diets, which have been epidemiologically associated with PEM, are suggested to cleave thiamine into inactive forms.

Dietary sulfate-associated PEM is a common form of the disorder, and *high-sulfate diets* can induce PEM experimentally. Marked increases of ruminal sulfide concentrations coincide with onset of clinical signs. It is unclear if significant absorption of sulfide occurs in the gastrointestinal tract or from inhalation of eructated hydrogen sulfide; >60% of eructated gases are inhaled in ruminants. No alterations of thiamine concentrations of blood or cerebrospinal fluid occur.

PEM has been induced in sheep directly by intragastric administration of *sodium sulfide*. A number of factors probably affects the capacity for rumen sulfide production: (a) The state of ruminal sulfate-reducing bacteria (SRB); (b) the dietary content of metals that form insoluble precipitates with sulfide and, thus, diminish bioavailability (*e.g.*, Cu, Zn, Fe); and (c) the dietary content of readily fermentable carbohydrate that could affect SRB metabolism and ruminal hydrogen ion concentration.

Fungicides, Pesticides, Herbicides, Baits, and Repellants

Chemicals used to kill fungi (fungicides), plants (herbicides), and pests (insecticides, molluscicides, rodenticides) are causes of veterinary neurotoxic disorders. *Pentachlorophenol*, formerly used as a fungicide, herbicide, and wood preservative, uncouples oxidative phosphorylation, increases oxygen consumption, and causes fever, tremor, and weakness in swine and cattle. The triazine herbicides, which are relatively toxic to ruminants, stimulate the CNS and elicit tremor, seizures, ataxia, and weakness. Small domestic animals are commonly poisoned by insecticides: cats are generally more susceptible than dogs to *organophosphates*, *carbamates*, and *organochlorine insecticides*. Acute intoxication with organophosphate or carbamate insecticides leads to cholinesterase inhibition and signs of excessive parasympathetic and neuromuscular stimulation. Organochlorine intoxication is characterized by nervousness, agitation, tremor, hyperexcitability, incoordination, and intermittent clonic-tonic seizures. Cattle may have an abnormal posture, walk backwards, or chew or lick excessively. *Pyrethroid* toxicosis causes the rapid appearance of hypersalivation, vomiting, hyperexcitability, tremor, seizures, dyspnea, and weakness. Dogs poisoned by the topical miticide *Amitraz* (N'-(2,4-dimethyl)-N-(2,4-dimethylphenyl) [imino]methyl-N-methanimidamide) exhibit diarrhea, ataxia, disorientation, seizures, and other signs. Cats treated with citrus oil extracts at dosages suitable on dogs for the control of lice, ticks, or fleas develop ataxia, weakness, generalized paralysis, and CNS depression. Cats are also sensitive to the insect repellent *DEET*, which may cause tremor and seizures. The molluscicide *metaldehyde*, which is metabolized to *acetaldehyde*, elicits neurological dysfunction in cats, dogs, sheep, and cattle (101,102).

Rodenticide poisoning is common in small animals, especially dogs. *Metal phosphites* trigger depression, tremor, and weakness. Dogs and large domestic animals (but not poultry) are sensitive to the acute toxic effects of *strychnine*: nervousness, muscle tremors, tetanic seizures, rigidity, and myoglobinuria. Cats and dogs are much more sensitive than guinea pigs to the rodenticide *bromethalin* (*vide infra*), which uncouples oxidative phosphylation. Acute signs of fever, hyperexcitability, and muscle tremors are followed by development of posterior paresis and ascending ataxia associated with mild brain edema and spongy degeneration of white matter in brain, spinal cord, and optic nerves. *Sodium fluoroacetate*, which inhibits aconitase and blocks adenosine triphosphate (ATP) production, causes excitability, seizures, and death; the lethal doses for dogs, cats, and domestic livestock are lower than those for rodents and birds (101,102).

Other neurotoxic agents that fall under this general heading include: the bird repellant *4-amino-pyridine*; the rodenticide *α-chloralose*; *DEET* in combination with *fenvalerate* (formerly used as an insect repellant); d-*limonene*, the active component of tick and flea sprays; *metaldehyde*, a snail and slug bait; and strychnine, a ruminatoric (tartar emetic), stimulant and pesticide (102).

4-Aminopyridine

Birds that ingest repellents containing 4-aminopyridine display disorientation, distress and, occasionally, seizures (125). Use of 4-aminopyridine-containing baits is popular because flocks disperse without fatality. 4-Aminopyridine binds proximate to the inner vestibule of the pore of K^+ channels and increases neurotransmitter release, particularly acetylcholine. All mammalian species are susceptible to intoxication. Symptoms include hyperexcitability, salivation, tremors, and generalized seizures; cardiac arrhythmias, hepatic dysfunction, and metabolic acidosis also occur. The substance is used therapeutically for humans with myasthenia gravis because it prolongs the action potential, potentiates muscle twitch tension, and improves muscle strength (*see* Chapter 1).

Bromethalin

Used as an alternative to anticoagulant rodenticides, N-*methyl-2,4-dinitro-N-(2,4,6-tribromophenyl)-6-(trifluoromethyl)-benzenamine* is an uncoupler of oxidative phosphorylation that most commonly affects dogs and cats (26,31,32). ATP decline is associated with cell swelling (predominantly glial) secondary to Na^+, K^+-ATPase dysfunction. Cerebral edema and evidence of CNS anoxia may appear. Acute high-dose intoxications are followed within 1 day by the appearance of tremors, hyperthermia, hyperexcitability, and seizures. In animals that survive or ingest lower doses, CNS depression and posterior paresis appear after 5 days. Lesions range from mild intramyelinic edema to diverse spongy change in white matter.

α-Chloralose; (R)-1,2-O-(2,2,2-Trichloroethylidene)-α-D-glucofuranose

This condensation of choral (CCl₃ClO) and 5- or 6-carbon sugars was formerly used as a general indoor rodenticide (102). Birds are more susceptible than mammals, and cats more so than dogs. *α-Chloralose* is metabolized first to chloral and then to *trichloroethanol*, a CNS depressant. The agent increases the activity of cortical neurons while selectively depressing the ascending reticular formation. Cats exposed to α-chloralose initially display hyperexcitability, mild ataxia, and aggressive behavior; subsequently, in severe poisoning, there is increased sensitivity to touch and sound, posterior weakness, increased salivation, and hypothermia.

DEET plus Fenvalerate (4-Chloro-α-(1-methyl)-benzeneacetic acid cyano(3-phenoxyphenyl) methyl ester)

Although *fenvalerate* (a pyrethroid) and *DEET* (an insect repellent) are safe when used individually, combination sprays used for flea and tick control have been reported to cause intoxications in cats and dogs (30,90). Signs of hypersalivation, bradycardia, mydriasis, ataxia, tremors, depression, and seizures have suggested cholinesterase inhibition, but cholinesterase activity is uniformly unaltered. No lesions are detected. Competition for excretory pathways is suggested as the cause of intoxication. Female kittens are especially vulnerable.

Fluoroacetate

Sodium fluoroacetate (Compound 1080, C₂H₂FNaO) is used as a commercial rodent and coyote control bait. Intoxication results in species-specific disorders that include cardiac arrhythmias (leading to ventricular fibrillation) and neurological signs (20,106). Swine, sheep, and cats experience both clinical manifestations of intoxication. Cattle and horses do not develop neurological symptoms; dogs are spared cardiac dysfunction. Neurological symptoms include marked anxiety, depression and, ultimately, tetanic seizures; death is from respiratory arrest. Dogs display characteristic "running fits"; running may end when the animal collides with a barrier. Fluoroacetate reacts with acetyl-CoA to produce *fluorocitrate*, which inhibits the tricarboxylic acid cycle by inactivating aconitase. Citric and lactic acids accumulate and ATP synthesis is blocked.

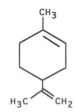

FIGURE 3.1. Limonene.

d-Limonene (1-Methyl-4-(1-methylenyl)cyclohexane)

This compound (Fig. 3.1) is present in refined citrus oil extracts that are used for the control of lice, ticks and fleas. Felines are sensitive to products containing d-*limonene*, and concentrated dip solutions are a source of excessive exposure (54,110). Clinical signs (ataxia, tremors, hypersalivation) are generally mild and rarely fatal. Symptoms usually abate without treatment within 6 hours. No morphological alterations are described, and the mechanism of action is unknown. Based on the extremely high rat LD₅₀, d-limonene is "generally regarded as safe" by the U.S. Food and Drug Administration.

Metaldehyde

This acetaldehyde polymer (C₂H₄O)ₙ is used in most snail and slug baits as a pelleted product; this is attractive to domestic species. Monogastrics and ruminants are both susceptible to intoxication; dogs are most commonly affected, and poisoning is also reported in cats, sheep, and horses (8). The acetaldehyde metabolite, which causes acidosis, is suggested to be the culpable agent. Metabolic effects of *metaldehyde* administration include decreased concentrations of γ-aminobutyric acid (GABA), norepinephrine, and serotonin. Monoamine oxidase activity is also decreased. Clinical signs in poisoned dogs and cats include anxiety, incoordination, ataxia, severe tremors, nystagmus and, in terminally ill cases, seizures, opisthotonus, and cyanosis. Tachycardia and hyperpyrexia are common. Onset of clinical signs is rapid, usually within 1–2 h of ingestion. No specific lesions are detected in rapidly fatal cases; animals surviving 2–3 days die of hepatic failure, with evidence of hepatic necrosis and neuronal degeneration in the brain.

Strychnine

Commercial preparations of this indole alkaloid are derived from seed of the southeast Asian plants *Strychnos nux-vomica* and *S. ignatii*; they are used to control rats, gophers, moles, and coyotes. *Strychnine* reversibly and selectively antagonizes the inhibitory neurotransmitter glycine in the spinal cord and medulla oblongata, thereby reducing the normal damping of sensory-motor reflexes and promoting increased activity in affected neural pathways (102). Most domestic animals (especially dogs) are affected by this highly toxic compound. Signs of intoxication appear within minutes or hours. Animals appear apprehensive, tense, and stiff. Blood pressure and heart rate rise. Violent tetanic seizures develop spontaneously or result from a sudden environmental trigger (touch, sound, light). Extensor rigidity dominates the clinical picture, with intermittent periods of relaxation that become less frequent as the disorder advances. Pupils are dilated during convulsions. Death occurs from exhaustion or anoxia. Microscopic lesions are not described.

BIOLOGICAL NEUROTOXIC FACTORS

Bacteria

Exposure to bacterial toxins may occur from the consumption of grossly contaminated food and feed. Scavenging dogs are at greatest risk for bacterial toxicosis. Sheep, goats, and cattle may succumb to *Clostridium perfringens* toxicosis in certain situations. *C. botulinum* causes botulism (*see* Chapter 1). Ruminant and monogastric species develop a neurological disorder (annual ryegrass toxicosis) from the corynetoxin-producing bacterium *Corynebacterium rathayi*.

Clostridium perfringens Type D

This anaerobic bacillus is a normal gastrointestinal tract inhabitant that, in situations of high carbohydrate loads and increased acidity, can proliferate, produce exotoxins, and cause disease. Unlike *C. perfringens* type C, which produces only enteric disease, type D also produces *epsilon toxin*, which increases capillary permeability throughout the body, including specific brain nuclei (12,42,52,84,103). Necrosis at these sites is experimentally reproducible. The primary lesion in affected areas of the brain is capillary endothelial damage in venules. Resultant edema and hemorrhage result in ischemic necrosis with eventual liquefaction and malacia. Two patterns of lesions are described in cattle. In one, dorsolateral aspects of the thalamus, the substantia nigra, the basal ganglia, and the internal capsule are affected; in the second, white matter of the frontal gyri is heavily impacted. In either pattern, the lesions are bilaterally symmetrical, and the disease is termed focal symmetrical encephalomalacia. While calves develop similar neurological lesions, affected goats display generalized cerebral edema but do not develop the characteristic lesions of focal

symmetrical encephalomalacia. The pathological changes correlate with the clinical picture of altered behavior, depression, ataxia and, occasionally, seizures and/or blindness.

Corynebacterium rathayi

Corynetoxins produced by *C. rathayi* cause annual ryegrass toxicosis in sheep, cattle and, occasionally, horses in Australia and South Africa (7,39,111). Livestock ingest the nematode-induced seedhead galls that have been infected with the toxin-producing bacterium. Clinical signs of corynetoxicity include tremors, ataxia, spasticity, nystagmus, opisthotonus, and short-duration seizures when animals are stressed or herded. Mortality of animals grazing affected pastures can approach 100%. Pathological features of microvascular damage in the CNS are edema and focal areas of perivascular neuropil degeneration.

Corynetoxins constitute a subgroup of the tunicaminyluracil antibiotics, a subclass of nucleoside antibiotics. They consist of a spectrum of fatty acids linked to a common structure composed of a C_{11} amino sugar (tunicamine), uracil, and N-acetylglucosamine (Fig. 3.2). Corynetoxins inhibit glycosylation and deplete glycoproteins in basal laminae causing increased endothelial transcytosis. Structurally related tunicaminyluracil antibiotics (*e.g.*, streptoviridin) are elaborated by different species of *Streptomyces*. Pigs consuming moldy wheat containing tunicaminyluracil antibiotics show a comparable clinical disorder of tremor, ataxia, and convulsions (21).

Blue-Green Algae

Freshwater blue-green algae (Myxophyceae) consist of nucleus-free, pigmented plant cells that form colonies, filaments, or gelatinous aggregations. Blooms of algae develop in the warm summer months, especially in bodies of freshwater with high nutrient content. They have been responsible for large-scale deaths of fish, water-fowl, companion animals, and livestock in the United States and elsewhere. Poisoning occurs when a dense bloom of toxic organisms has formed; the toxic material is concentrated in a thick green scum. Some of the poisonings are attributable to the hepatotoxic and/or neurotoxic effects of algal endotoxins;

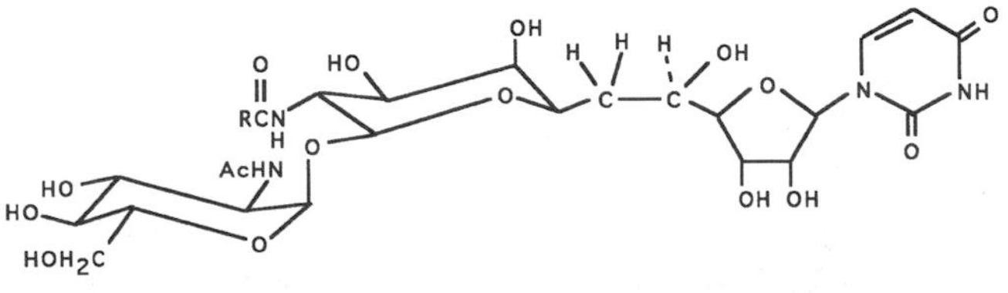

FIGURE 3.2. General structure of tunicaminyluracil antibiotics.

others to botulism, since *C. botulinum* is commonly found in decaying plankton (69).

Members of the genera *Anabaena* and *Aphanizomenon* have been linked with neurological disease. *Aphanizomenon flos-aquae* produces the sodium-channel blockers *saxitoxin* and *neosaxitoxin*. Death results from respiratory neuromuscular paralysis. *Anabaena flos-aquae* elaborates two main toxins, *anatoxin-a* and *anatoxin-a(s)* (14,79,80). Anatoxin-a(s) is an organophosphate cholinesterase inhibitor that does not cross the blood-brain barrier; it causes parasympathetic hyperactivity. Although muscarinic signs are most common, fatal cases also display signs of nicotinic activation. Seizures and death are probably from hypoxia. Anatoxin-a, formerly known as "very-fast-death factor," is a potent, postsynaptic depolarizing alkaloid. Clinical signs include rapid-onset rigidity, tremors, paralysis, and death due to respiratory failure. No pathological lesions are reported with either chemical.

Fungal Neurotoxins

Mycotoxins (secondary toxic metabolites of molds) are produced by toxigenic fungi such as *Aspergillus*, *Penicillium*, and *Fusarium*; they are most commonly isolated from cereal grains and corn. The formation of mycotoxins is closely related to environmental factors (temperature, humidity), insect infestation, and mechanical damage from harvest. Feed may become contaminated with mold-infested grain. Neurotoxic phenomena associated with mycotoxicoses range from fatal CNS lesions in horses linked to the ingestion of moldy corn to the characteristic pathophysiological effects that result from exposure to tremorgenic mycotoxins (102).

Tremorgens

Mycotoxic tremorgens are synthesized by *Acremonium* spp., *Claviceps* spp., *Aspergillus* spp., and *Penicillium* spp. This heterogeneous group of chemically related agents is responsible for a collection of neurological disorders ("staggers") of livestock. Clinical signs, which are exacerbated by excitement or exercise, include muscle tremor, incoordination, and generalized weakness resulting in paralysis. Animals recover after removal from the source of mycotoxic tremorgen. Brain lesions are not described. Convincing evidence of human neurotoxicity from these agents is lacking, although tremorgens have been repeatedly suspected in occupational illnesses of farmers and sawmill workers (74).

Six chemical classes of tremorgens are described (for chemical structures, *see* Penitrems and Other Tremorgens in the A–Z catalogue section) (141). The largest group is tryptophan-derived and features an indole-terpene moiety: they include the *penitrems*, *janthitrems*, *lolitrems*, *aflatrem*, *paxilline*, *paspaline*, *paspalicine*, *paspalinine*, and *paspalitrems A and B*. Some of these agents appear to be causally related to neurological disorders known as perennial ryegrass staggers (lolitrems) and paspalum staggers (paspalitrems). Other groups of mycotoxins include the *diketopiperazines* (verruculogen group), the *tryptoquivalines*, and the nonalkaloidal *territrems*.

The neurotoxic properties of tremorgens appear to be associated with disturbances in excitatory (glutamate, aspartate) and inhibitory (GABA) neurotransmission. Penitrem A and verruculogen increase spontaneous synaptosomal release of glutamate and aspartate (9,95). Increased concentrations of these excitatory neurotransmitters are found in the midbrain and pons of mice treated intravenously with verruculogen. Tremors may also be mediated by reduced GABA inhibitory function. Aflatrem, paxilline, paspalinine, *verruculogen*, and *verruculotoxin* bind close to the chloride channel of the $GABA_A$ receptor and inhibit receptor function (41). Lower concentrations potentiate GABA-induced chloride currents (161). In synaptosomes from sheep and rat brain (cerebrocortical and striatal), *penitrem A* increases spontaneous release of GABA. Verruculotoxin acts directly on muscles to increase twitch tension (38).

Acremonium spp. Perennial ryegrass toxicosis or staggers is a neurological condition in livestock, most commonly occurring in sheep, cattle, horses, and farmed deer grazing perennial ryegrass (*Lolium perenne*) pastures or seed straw residues in New Zealand, Australia, Britain, and in the U.S. Pacific Northwest (11,62,91,147). The Willamette Valley of Oregon, U.S.A., grows the majority of the world's ryegrass seed supply; in this locality, farmers deliberately employ varieties infected with the endophyte fungus, *Acremonium lolii*, for insect and drought resistance. This fungus also produces *lolitrem B*, a tremorgenic toxin that at approximately 2000 ppb/day produces fine head tremors, head nodding, increased muscle tone, and reluctance to move. If forced to move, the animals have a spastic gait with tetanic spasms that cause them to collapse momentarily with quick recovery. Incidence and severity of clinical signs are exacerbated by exercise. Morbidity can approach 100%; mortality is low—death is due to incapacitation. Following removal of the toxin, neurological signs reverse in less than 3 weeks, but weight loss persists. No CNS morphological lesions are detected in the acute illness; changes in chronic cases are said to include fusiform enlargements of proximal Purkinje cell axons ("torpedoes") and occasional axonal swellings scattered throughout the CNS.

A condition similar to perennial ryegrass staggers impacts South African mammals consuming *Melica ecumbens* (dronk grass). Another endophytic disorder is seen in Mexico and New Mexico, United States, in horses and other herbivores consuming *Stipa robusta* (sleepy grass). Ingestion of a moderate amount produces a profound, but not lethal, somnolent or stuporous condition lasting several days (33,133). In a bygone era, great inconvenience was occasioned to those who used poisoned horses as a principal means of transport (69). Mildly poisoned animals are dejected, inactive, and withdrawn (*vide infra*).

Aspergillus clavatus. A fatal tremorgenic syndrome of cattle in southern Africa has been associated with ingestion of moldy sorghum beer residue, sprouted maize, and a commercial ration infected with *A. clavatus* (65). The toxic agent has not been identified; it is distinct from the known *A. clavatus* tremorgens *tryptoquivaline, tryptoquivalone, nortryptoquivalone* and *tremortin A* (66). Clinical signs include constipation, hypersensitivity, tremor, incoordination, a stiff-legged gait, progressive paresis, paralysis, and death. Central chromatolysis and vacuolar neuronal degeneration are found in anterior horns of the spinal cord and in the larger neurons of numerous nuclei of the medulla oblongata, midbrain, and thalamus. Similar syndromes have been reported elsewhere in sheep and cattle dependent on feeds contaminated with *A. clavatus* (45,65,128).

Penicillium spp. Roquefortine, produced by various *Penicillium* spp. (particularly *P. roquefortii* growing on decaying organic matter), induces seizures and vomiting, and may be lethal to dogs (76,126). Mice and chickens have been similarly affected experimentally. In one study, analysis of postmortem stomach contents from dogs who were strychnine-poisoning suspects, but in which strychnine had not been detected, revealed roquefortine in 23% of samples, suggesting this condition is probably underdiagnosed (76). There are no histopathological studies.

Claviceps paspali. Various species of the *Claviceps* ascomycetous fungus parasitize the grains of cultivated and wild grasses, including cultivated rye, wheat, barley (*C. purpurea*), dalligrass, *Paspalum dilatatum* and Argentine bahia grass, *Paspalum notatum* (*C. paspali*), and tobosagrass *Hilaria mutica* (*C. cinearea*); all are known to have caused disease in the United States (69). Cattle develop a neurological disorder (paspalum staggers) when grazing on tropical or subtropical species of *Paspalum* (*e.g.*, dalligrass) infected with *Claviceps paspali*. Sheep may also be affected. *Paspalinine* and *paspalitrems* (*A–C*) are implicated; paspalitrem is most abundant (112). *C. paspali* also elaborates

the chemically related nontremorgenic substances paspaline and paspalicine (22).

Other Myconeurotoxins

Several other nontremorgenic mycotoxins have adverse effects on neurological function of domestic animals and, in the case of *ergot*, of humans. Fungal chemicals may also be responsible for prolonged somnolence in horses that have eaten sleepy grass (*see Stipa robusta*).

Claviceps purpurea (ergot). This fungus invades rye, oats, wheat, and Kentucky bluegrass (102). Two syndromes occur in cattle: a gangrenous form associated with repetitive exposure to the vasoconstrictive effects of small amounts of ergot and a convulsive form that appears to result from higher daily intake of ergot from either *C. purpurea* or *C. paspali*. Cattle display nervousness and stamping of feet after 1 week of eating hay containing *ergot alkaloids*. Animals become belligerent, develop trembling and incoordination, and may fall while running. Periods of kicking interspersed by tetanic rigidity and opisthotonus indicate severe intoxication. Besides cattle, horses and sheep, humans are susceptible to convulsive ergotism. Ergot alkaloids are derivatives of *lysergic acid* and serve as agonists at dopamine D_2 receptors.

Penicillium citreoviride. This mold elaborates the neurotoxin *citreoviridine*, one of the so-called yellow-rice toxins from moldy rice in Japan. Citreoviridine is a carbocyclic polyene that is reported to cause ascending paralysis in experimental animals, sometimes followed by convulsions and respiratory arrest. Trembling is not reported (152).

Diplodia maydis. Diplodiosis is a neurotoxic condition of cattle and sheep in southern Africa caused by ingestion of fungus-contaminated maize ears. Clinical signs appear after 2–5 days and disappear a few days later: they include reluctance to move, wide-based stance, stiff-legged high-stepping gait, repeated falling, paresis/paralysis, constipation, and salivation. Subcortical status spongiosus is reported in two animals affected for a prolonged period; these changes have not been seen in animals with experimentally induced diplodiosis (67).

Fusarium moniliforme. Originally termed moldy corn poisoning, the disease equine leukoencephalomalacia has long been associated with contamination of corn-based diets by *Fusarium moniliforme* (10,51). *Fumonisin B_1* is the toxic principle (158). Lesions of fumonisin intoxication in nonequine species include hepatocellular damage and endothelial injury, often most severe in pulmonary vasculature resulting in pulmonary edema. In equids, the vascular injury is most severe in the corona radiata. Microscopic changes include edema, hemorrhage, liquefaction, and necrosis.

Affected animals display an abrupt onset of neurological disease that has a duration ranging from hours to days. There is a wide variety of clinical signs: changes in temperament (hyperexcitability to depression), locomotor disturbances (ataxia and paresis), paralysis of the tongue, sweating, and convulsions (65). The mechanism of the endothelial damage is uncertain; alterations in lipid metabolism affecting membrane integrity have been implicated. In rats fed fumonisin, serotonin metabolism was altered, but no brain lesions were detected (109).

Rhizoctonia leguminicola. This fungus infests red clover (*Trifolium pratense*) and produces an indolizidine alkaloid (*slaframine*) related to *swainsonine* (*vide infra*), which is bioactivated to the parasympathomimetic quaternary amine ketoimine (Fig. 3.3). All species appear susceptible to slaframine intoxication ("slobbers"), although exposure patterns usually impact herbivores. Clinical signs are typical of parasympathetic stimulation (slobbering, lacrimation, diarrhea, frequent urination). No lesions are reported.

Neurotoxic Plants

Plants are complex mixtures of chemicals, one or more of which within any single species may have direct or indirect toxic effects on the nervous system. Some plant toxins have been isolated and characterized, many have not. Toxic plant chemicals may be components of the species' intermediary metabolism (nitrates are part of the nitrogen cycle), produced by the plant apparently to sequester metals (amino acids with excitant properties), or elaborated for the presumed purpose of defense against predators (cyanogenic glucosides). Ruminants may be particularly vulnerable to toxic chemicals (*methylazoxymethanol, cyanide*) stored as glucosides (*cycasin* and *dhurrin*, respectively) because the rumen contains a high concentration of β-glucosidase, which cleaves the active agent from the sugar moiety.

While toxic plants are often unpalatable (bitter), animals may resort to their consumption as a result of hunger, nutrient deficiencies that promote pica, overgrazing, or confinement of animals in unusual locations. On occasion, animals may deliberately seek out toxic plants (cycads) in a manner suggestive of addiction. The concentration of toxic principles in plants may vary with age, soil type, environmental conditions, and season. The metabolism of plant toxins in animals may be impacted by the presence of other substances, such as herbicides.

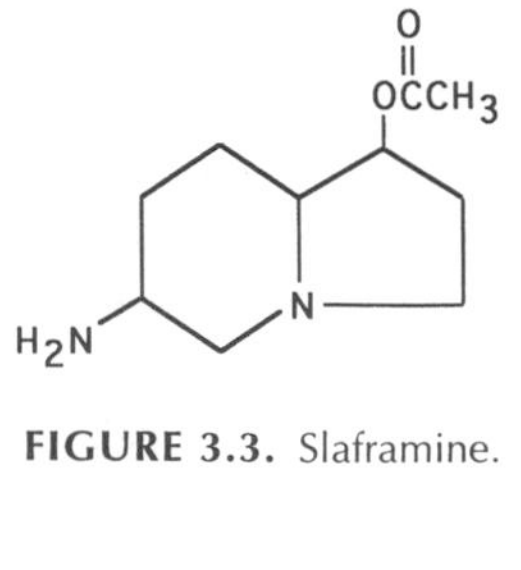

Plant compounds associated with neurotoxicity in animals include amino acids, proteins, glycosides, and alkaloids. For example, neuromuscular function may be disrupted following exposure to diterpenoid alkaloids (e.g., *methyllycaconitine*) in larkspurs, to piperidine alkaloids (e.g., *coniine*) in poison hemlock (*Conium maculatum*), or to the pyridine alkaloid (*nicotine*) of tobacco. Chemicals related to indolizidine alkaloids occur in fungi, plants (Swainsona, Solanaceae), and animals (dendrobatid frogs). Cyanogenic and cardiac glycosides are each found in hundreds of plant species. Plant nonprotein amino acids with neurotoxic potential include those that sequester metals (β-N-*oxalylamino*-L-*alanine*) or metalloids (*selenium*) derived from soil. Proteins that induce neurological signs indirectly include certain lectins (*ricin, abrin*) and *thiaminases*, which destroy vitamin B_1. Although ruminants are generally unaffected by thiaminase-containing plants (the Australian species *Marsilea drummondii* is an exception because it has an extremely high thiaminase content) because rumen microorganisms elaborate thiamine, horses ingesting bracken fern (*Pteridium aquilinum*) or horsetail (*Equisetum arvense*) in hay become ataxic and eventually collapse.[1] These animals rapidly respond to thiamine therapy.

Plants with neurotoxic properties have a wide range of effects on the nervous system. Some cause degeneration of neurons, glial cells, or their cellular processes; others disrupt the function of the autonomic or somatic components of the PNS, and many have effects on the CNS that either increase or decrease activity. Others induce disorders of

FIGURE 3.3. Slaframine.

---

[1]Originally described as Chastek paralysis, ingestion of thiaminase by carnivores results in a poorly understood injury involving the periventricular gray matter. The source of thiaminase is most commonly associated with diets rich in certain fish species, and the illness is most common in domestic mink. Affected animals initially display vague signs such as anorexia followed by ataxia, seizures, and a terminal stupor. The inferior colliculi are most consistently affected; lesions evolve from initial edema to hemorrhage. Astrocytic gliosis is common and more severe in recovered animals. Degeneration and necrosis of glia occur prior to vascular injury. Axons degenerate but neuronal cell bodies are spared (distal axonopathy). The mechanism is unknown. Because a decline in transketolase activity occurs in the same locations as the lesions and temporally precedes onset of clinical signs, disruption of this thiamine-dependent enzyme has been suggested to have a role (35,48,63,64,98,113).

skeletal or cardiac muscle. These disparate targets provide the basis for a preliminary taxonomy of plant neurotoxicoses; this will doubtless prove of limited accuracy as knowledge of these conditions accrues.

Neurodegenerative Disorders: Optic Nerve Damage

Stypandra glauca (formerly imbricata) (blindgrass). Field and experimental studies show that ingestion of *S. glauca* (Liliaceae) at certain times of the year causes an acute illness that may result in permanent blindness (59,181). The culpable agent is *stypandrol* (Fig. 3.4), a binaphthalenetetrol thought to be elaborated by the plant. Rodents consuming dried blindgrass remain alert and responsive but develop paraparesis that progresses to flaccid hindlimb paralysis and lateral recumbency. CNS intramyelinic edema is prominent, especially in the optic nerves, which subsequently undergo secondary axonal degeneration. The initial neurological signs resolve over subsequent days leaving the animals blind. Severe multifocal loss of photoreceptors is evident in the outer nuclear area (58).

Extrapyramidal and Movement Disorders

The basal ganglia of mammals are heavily impacted by agents that perturb neuronal energy metabolism, as illustrated by the development of putaminal necrosis in humans and rodents exposed to *3-nitropropionic acid* (*3-NPA*), a suicide inhibitor of the mitochondrial enzyme succinic dehydrogenase. The neurotoxic actions of 3-NPA (*Astragalus* spp.) and of other plant-derived compounds (*Centaurea solstitialis*) may give rise to dramatic and irreversible neurodegenerative disease in domestic animals. *Phalaris tuberosa* causes persistent signs of motor dysfunction that includes a movement disorder.

Astragalus spp. (*nitrotoxin*). Poisonous aliphatic nitro compounds appear in several plant families; the *Astragalus* species of the Leguminosae are most important in relation to livestock (28,61,105). The mitochondrial enzyme inhibitor 3-NPA is either present in the plant or is the lethal metabolite of another plant compound, *mimosine*, the glycoside of *3-nitro-1-propanol* (*3-NPOH*). In ruminants, rumen mi-

FIGURE 3.4. Stypandrol.

croorganisms convert mimosine to 3-NPOH; this is systemically absorbed and converted by the liver to 3-NPA. Ruminal species are more susceptible to mimosine-containing plants because the compound is converted by ruminal microorganisms to 3-NPOH; conversely, if the dose is not too high, they are less susceptible to plants containing 3-NPA because ruminal microbes degrade the compound to nontoxic metabolites. Signs of acute toxicity in livestock include agitation, ataxia, motor weakness, dyspnea, coma, and death. In chronic poisoning, weight loss and paraparesis predominate.

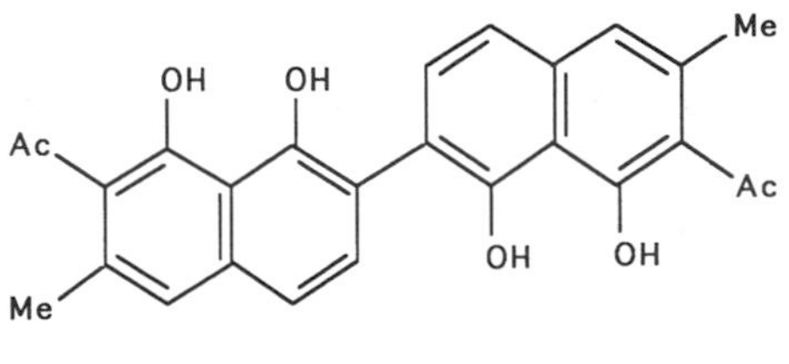

3-NPA is a suicide inhibitor of the mitochondrial enzyme succinic dehydrogenase. Enzyme inhibition decreases energy production in neurons and initiates a glutamate-mediated excitotoxic cell death (*see* Chapter 1). Human 3-NPA neurotoxicity (from consumption of mildewy sugar cane bearing the agent as a mycotoxin) is featured by an acute encephalopathic illness followed in some cases by the development of putaminal necrosis and irreversible dystonia (77). Although the gross and microscopic lesions have not been well characterized in domestic animals, the acute syndrome in sheep and cattle is associated with wallerian degeneration of the spinal cord and focal hemorrhages in the brain. In chronic intoxication of rodents, bilateral necrosis of the caudate nucleus is the most consistent lesion, with necrosis of the hippocampus, thalamus, globus pallidus, entopeduncular nucleus, rostral substantia nigra, and pars reticulata in mice.

Centaurea solstitialis (yellow star thistle) and *Acroptilon repens* (Russian knapweed). Only horses develop nigropallidal encephalomalacia ("chewing disease") after eating these plants (115,121,126,160). Clinical signs, which appear suddenly after animals have grazed on contaminated pastures for some period of time, include inability to prehend and masticate food. Swallowing is unaffected if food or water reach the back of the oropharynx. Spasticity of lips and tongue occur. Histological findings include necrosis of either or both of the substantia nigra (probably, the pars reticulata) and globus pallidus. Once clinical signs appear, treatment is without effect.

The pathophysiological mechanisms and causative agent(s) are unknown. Several polar and nonpolar agents have been isolated; none has been used in an attempt to reproduce the equine disorder. Water-soluble *C. solstitialis* fractions with excitant neuronotoxic properties in mouse cerebral cortical cultures include those with free *aspartate* (major component) and *glutamate* (122). While the presence of high concentrations of these excitatory amino acids raises the possibility of an excitotoxic CNS disorder, these plants contain other toxic factors. Lipid-soluble sesquiterpenoid agents include *solstitialin A* and *cynaropicrin*; these are toxic to cell cultures derived from substantia nigra, frontal cortex, striatum, and raphe nucleus. Three sesquiterpene toxins have been isolated from Russian knapweed by x-ray crystallography: *repin*, a compound with neurotoxic actions against chick embryo sensory neurons; *acroptilin*; and *chlororepdiolide*, a chlorinated molecule. A chick-embryo dorsal root sensory neuron assay has been used to quantify the toxicity of seven sesquiterpene lactones extracted from *A. repens* and *C. solstitialis* (115). Repin was the most toxic, and inoculation into rat brains nonselectively disrupted cellular architecture.

Phalaris tuberosa. *Phalaris* spp. and other members of Gramineae contain indole protoalkaloids and β-carbolines, including *gramine, methyltryptamine,* and *5-methoxydimethyltryptamine* (24). In addition to cardiac effects, parenteral administration of these alkaloids to sheep causes hyperexcitability, urination, pupillary dilatation, licking of lips, and head nodding. Which agents are differently responsible for the wide range of clinical phenomena in grazing animals is unclear. Possibly the β-*carbolines* are associated with abnormal movements, while cardiac, pupillary, and excitant effects are related to actions of *indole alkaloids.*

Cattle and sheep that ingest these plants may develop one of three syndromes: (a) A hyperacute syndrome characterized by sudden heart failure or recovery; (b) an acute syndrome reminiscent of rye grass staggers, from which animals frequently recover after removal from the contaminated pasture; and (c) a chronic persistent syndrome (phalaris staggers) distinguished by head nodding, ataxia, and weakness accompanied by neuropathological changes (56).

Motoneuron and Locomotor Disorders

Persistent locomotor disorders of domestic animals result from ingestion of a wide range of ancient (cycads) and modern plants. Neuropathological examination of animals with these conditions is often inadequate to specify the precise distribution, nature, and course of CNS and PNS damage. Upper motor neurons and long spinal tracts may be heavily impacted with (*Cycas* spp.) or without (*Lathyrus* spp., *Sorghum* spp.) prominent lower motorneuron involvement. The neuropathology of other plant-associated locomotor disorders (*Hypochoeris radicata, Karwinskia humboldtiana*) emphasizes damage to peripheral motor neurons, axons, and myelin.

Cycad genera. Cycadism is a locomotor disorder of cattle and sheep that graze on leaves and other components of cycads in the tropic and subtropics (49,63,162). Species of *Bowenia, Cycas,* and *Macrozamia* are held responsible in Australia; *Zamia* spp. in the Dominican Republic and Puerto Rico, and *Dioon edule* in Mexico. Feeding fresh leaves of *Cycas circinalis* produced a locomotor disorder in a cow after 85 days.

Acute effects of cycadism in animals include hepatotoxicity, enterotoxicity, and death. Rapid twitching of the eyelids, nostrils, lips, and jaw muscles, with periodic tremors of the body, are reported in sheep (155). Delayed effects of cycad consumption are characterized by a progressive and irreversible paralysis of the hindlimbs with muscle wasting. Initially, there is a staggering and weaving gait, with crossing of the legs, incoordination, and ataxia. More severe forms are characterized by posterior motor weakness, dragging of extended hindlimbs and, occasionally, a stringhalt-like action of the hocks. Function of bladder, anus, and tail is unimpaired (53). Neuropathological examination reportedly shows degeneration of descending spinal tracts, readily observed in the lumbar region, with similar involvement of the fasciculus gracilis and dorsal spinocerebellar tracts, most prominent in the cervical region (62). Brain, peripheral nerves, and muscle have not been carefully examined for neuropathological changes.

The agent responsible for the neurological syndrome in cattle and sheep is uncertain. Cycads contains azoxyglucosides (*e.g.*, cycasin), the aglycone of which is *methylazoxymethanol,* a potent hepatotoxin, experimental carcinogen, and developmental neurotoxin. Cycasin, which is neuronotoxic *in vitro* and elicits a cycadism-like disorder in large animals, is strongly correlated epidemiologically with the amyotrophic lateral sclerosis and parkinsonism-dementia complex of Guam (163), a progressive human neurodegenerative disorder that impacts indigenous people (Chamorros) who have used cycasin-containing flour from *Cycas circinalis* for food (71). *C. circinalis* also contains an excitant and neurotoxic amino acid, β-N-*methylamino-L-alanine*; repeated oral administration of large doses of this compound induces motor system and behavioral deficits in primates (139).

Sorghum spp. Pelvic limb ataxia and urinary incontinence with cystitis are reported in cattle and in horses grazing on hybrid strains of sorghum grasses; examples include a hybrid cross of *Sorghum vulgare* (sorghum) with *S. vulgare* var. Sudanese (sudan), *S. almum,* and *S. halepense* (Johnson grass) (1,85,89,149). Forced exercise may cause affected animals to stumble or fall. Animals of all ages and all breeds are affected by this irreversible neurological syndrome. Pathological features include diffuse nerve fiber degeneration in the lateral and, particularly, in the ventral funiculi of the spinal cord extending to the brainstem. *Sorghum* spp. contain the cyanogenic glucoside *dhurrin*, which yields *hydrocyanic acid* on hydrolysis (144). *Linamarin*, the principal cyanogenic glucoside in cassava (*Manihot esculenta*)—tubers and leaves of which are used by humans as a staple in the tropics and subtropics—is causally associated with irreversible subacute spastic paraparesis in protein-deficient people resident in southern Africa (34). The proximate neurotoxin is not established; however, cyanide-treated rats on a diet deficient in sulfur amino acids exhibit increased blood concentrations of *cyanate* (142,146), an agent known to elicit CNS and PNS motor system disease in chronically treated rats, primates, and humans (16,127,143).

Lathyrus sativus, L. latifolius, and other neurotoxic spp. Prolonged ingestion of these legumes causes a motoneuronal disease in several species, especially horses (stringhalt) and humans (spastic paraparesis). Although intoxication usually only occurs when a neurotoxic *Lathyrus* spp. makes up the main part of the diet, clinical signs can also occur after continuous feeding of lesser amounts. Onset of lathyrism in horses is sudden and characterized by transient paralysis of the larynx (56). Stringhalt describes an involuntary exaggerated hyperflexion of the pelvic limbs and, less commonly, the thoracic limbs (5,27,47,57,118,120,132). Pyramidal tract degeneration has been reported in cattle, sheep, and horses; the latter also shows changes in the recurrent laryngeal nerve with degeneration of laryngeal muscles (56). An excitant amino acid neurotoxin, β-N-*oxalylamino-L-alanine*, is held to be the culpable agent in lathyrism (123,138).

Hypochoeris radicata (false dandelion). A reversible stringhalt-like condition is seen in horses grazing on pastures contaminated with this weed. Although feeding trials have not been successful in reproducing the disease experimentally, and a toxin has not been isolated, epidemiological evidence points strongly to this plant or an associated soil fungal neurotoxin as the cause of the neurodegenerative disorder. European dandelion (*Taraxacum officinale*) and mallow (*Malva parviflora*) have been implicated to a lesser degree. Pathological features of horses with Australian stringhalt associated with false dandelion pastures include a peripheral distal axonopathy with secondary, neurogenic atrophy of corresponding muscles. Most commonly affected are the nerves to the pelvic limbs and the recurrent laryngeal nerve.

Xanthorrhoea spp. (grass trees). Cattle consuming young flowers of the Australian species *X. minor* or *X. preissii* develop a neurological disorder featured by loss of balance that causes the animal to fall on its side, thereby generating the sound ("wamps") used to describe the condition. Animals recover within a few weeks once removed from plant-infested areas. Pathology described as "scattered demyelination" is seen in the brainstem, spinal cord, and peripheral nerves. The culpable agent has not been identified.

Karwinskia humboldtiana (coyotillo, tullidora). A single dose of the fruit of this North American desert shrub is known experimentally to cause neuromuscular disorders in humans, other mammals, birds, reptiles, and amphibians (6,92,154). Livestock (goats, cattle, sheep, and pigs) grazing on the plant develop flaccid paraparesis following ingestion of the plant's fruit. Days, weeks, or months may intervene between ingestion and onset of clinical signs. These consist of limb weakness, incoordination, and ataxia ("limberleg"). Eventually, animals are unable to rise from the recumbent position and die. Less-affected animals recover over a period of months to years. Pathological studies of experimentally poisoned goats reveal a combination of segmental demyelination and remyelination, axonal degeneration and chromatolysis of anterior horn cells and, to a lesser extent, dorsal root ganglia. Nerve fiber regeneration occurs during the recovery period (17–19). Four groups of *bianthracene toxins* have been extracted from fruit, seed, and roots of the coyotillo; the agent(s) responsible for the induction of peripheral neuropathy is unknown (154).

Neuronal Storage Disorders

Certain plants harbor substances that are able to disrupt metabolic pathways in domestic animals and thereby cause the accumulation of intermediary metabolites in neurons and other cells. While systemic effects are present, the clinical picture is dominated by neurological dysfunction. Disease typically evolves over a period of time of continuous exposure to the culpable agent.

Swainsona, Astragalus lentiginosus, Oxytropis. Swainsonine is a trihydroxyindolizidine alkaloid in toxic plants of the genera *Astragalus* spp. and *Oxytropis* spp. in the United States, and *Swainsona* in Australia. Swainsonine inhibits the enzyme activity of α-mannosidase; this results in altered glycoprotein processing and cellular accumulation of incompletely processed oligosaccharides. Continuous feeding over weeks results in alterations of immune, gastrointestinal, and reproductive systems. Nervous system dysfunction is the most disabling component; signs include depression, blindness, intention tremors, proprioceptive deficits, ataxia, and death. This condition, "locoism," is one of the most significant toxic-plant problems for livestock in the United States. Pathological features include axonal dystrophy and vacuolar degeneration of neurons (including retinal ganglion cells), with accumulation of mannose-containing oligosaccharides in nonstaining storage vacuoles. Diagnosis can be made by measurement of either serum levels of the toxin or of α-mannosidase (140). This disease state is pathophysiologically similar to naturally occurring, genetically determined α-mannosidosis in humans and in certain breeds of cattle and Persian cats (150).

Solanum bonariensis, S. dimidiatum, S. fastigiatum and *S. kwebense.* Cattle experimentally fed *S. kwebense* develop a disorder that reproduces a neurological disease (*maldronksiekte*) described among cattle in South Africa (107). Animals appear normal unless frightened, exercised, or handled, whereupon there may be a temporary loss of balance and the appearance of transient seizures. Cerebellar atrophy is observed, with cytoplasmic vacuolar degeneration of neurons in the molecular, granular, and especially Purkinje cell layers. Identical lesions are reported in animals poisoned with species such as *S. dimidiatum* and *S. fastigiatum*. Contents of the vacuoles are unidentified; the possibility this is a storage disorder is speculative. *Solanum* spp. contain more complex *indolizidine alkaloids* than those found in *Swansona* spp. (40).

Strychnine-like and Other Convulsant Effects

This is a heterogenous collection of plant-related intoxications featured by acute, reversible changes in neuroexcitation.

Gelsemium sempervirens (yellow jessamine). This North American evergreen vine harbors *gelsemine, gelseminine,* and other *indole alkaloids* that show structural relations with strychnine (101). Poisoned cattle show weakness, incoordination, and convulsions. Birds, such as turkeys, become lethargic (56). Humans have been poisoned in South Carolina through consumption of honey made from *Gelsemium* spp. nectar (69).

Cicuta spp. (cowbane, water hemlock). These species are found in temperate climes in wetlands. The roots and stem bases contain a yellowish acrid juice that harbors a potent resinoid convulsant, *cicutoxin*. Effects in humans and livestock are similar and have been known for centuries. Symptoms, which appear within one-half hour of ingestion, are heralded by excessive salivation, tremors, and spasmodic convulsions with opisthotonus. Cattle and horses also develop a strychnine-like clinical picture with salivation, muscle twitching, violent tetanic seizures, and death from asphyxia (101). Most loss of livestock occurs in early spring

when new plant growth appears. No specific lesions are evident postmortem.

Brunfelsia calcyina var. *floribunda* and *Brunfelsia pauciflora* (yesterday-today-and-tomorrow). These ornamental evergreens of tropical and subtropical climes contain several *tropane alkaloids*; they produce clinical signs virtually indistinguishable from strychnine intoxication (75,137). No lesions are detectable at the gross or light microscopic level. The leading candidate for the specific toxic principle is *brunfelsamidine* (*pyrrole-3-carboximide*), although mechanistic studies with the purified compound have not been reported.

Cheilanthes sinnata (jimmy fern). Ingestion of this plant, a native of the southern United States, induces violent fits of trembling ("jimmies") in cattle, sheep, and goats. The disorder is exacerbated by exercise and may terminate in respiratory paralysis and death. Other species contain the enzyme *thiaminase*, which can cause the effects of thiamine deficiency in monogastric animals (*vide supra*) (56).

Corydalis spp. (fitweed) and *Dicentra* spp. (staggerweeds) The *isoquinoline alkaloids* in these common woodland plants produce rapid onset of gastrointestinal distress, tremor, ataxia, and convulsive clonic spasms, often followed by death (135). Characteristic biting movements are observed. The mechanism of seizure induction is unknown, and no lesions are visible at the gross or light microscope level. Sheep preferentially consume the fitweed and appear more sensitive than cattle to the toxins. Steers experimentally fed *Dicentra cucullaria* develop trembling. Animals run back and forth with the head held unusually high before going down. They develop a characteristic posture with the head thrown back and legs rigidly extended. Most make a complete recovery.

Cynanchum spp. Modified *pregnane glycosides* are held responsible for a syndrome among certain mammals in southern Africa featured by CNS stimulation, incoordination, tetanic seizures, and paralysis (65).

Aesculus hippocastanum and *Aesculus glabra*. Horse chestnut and buckeye, respectively, have been associated with nervous system dysfunction (tremors, hyperesthesia, paralysis, coma, convulsions, extensor rigidity) (73,78). No lesions are reported at the gross or light microscope level. The glycoside *aesculin* has been suggested as the toxin; its mechanism of action is unknown.

Albizia spp. Cattle consuming pods of these trees (*A. versicolor, A. tanganyicensis*) in southern Africa develop intermittent tetanic convulsions that are attributed to a *4-methoxy derivative of pyridoxine*, which is thought to act as a vitamin B_6 antimetabolite (65).

Effects on Cholinergic Neurotransmission: Anticholinesterase Effects

Solanum tuberosum (potato). Potato plants elaborate glycosidic steroidal alkaloids (*α-solanine, α-chaconine*) with anticholinesterase effects in blood, PNS and CNS. While the normal tuber contains insignificant amounts of these agents (Fig. 3.5), light exposure or mechanical damage induces glycoalkaloid synthesis. Ingestion of green potatoes, which are especially hazardous, occasionally causes human and animal intoxication. Animals display gastrointestinal and neurological signs, the latter including apathy, drowsiness, salivation, dyspnea, trembling, progressive weakness or paralysis, prostration, or unconsciousness (69). Humans complain of headache and abdominal pain and develop diarrhea and vomiting. Clinical signs, which reverse within a few days, include apathy, restlessness, drowsiness, mental confusion, rambling, incoherence, stupor, hallucinations, dizziness, trembling, and visual disturbances (86).

Nicotinic Receptor Blockade

Delphinium and *Aconitum*. Larkspurs (*Delphinium* spp.) indigenous to the mountains of western North America con-

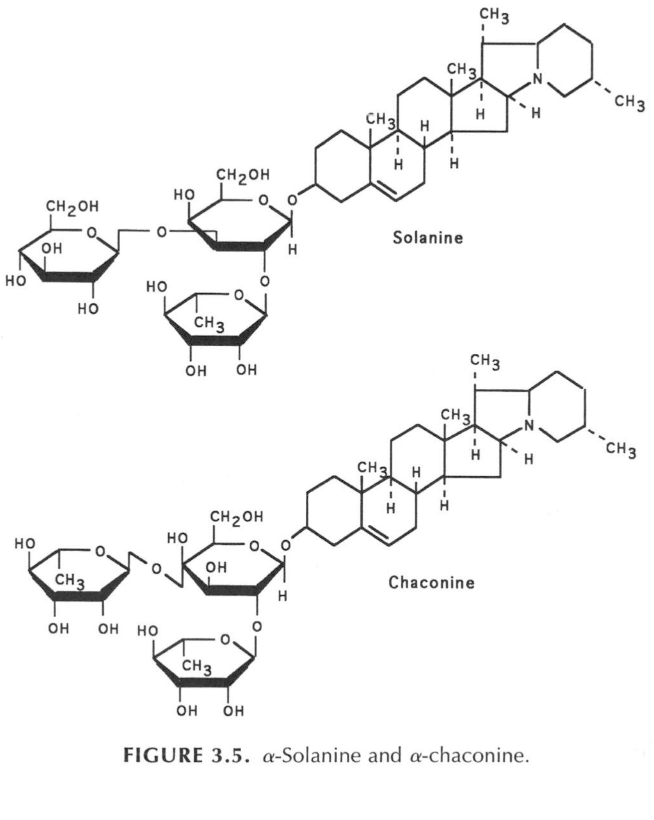

FIGURE 3.5. *α*-Solanine and *α*-chaconine.

tain more than 40 nonditerpenoid alkaloids of varying toxicity (2,3,82,99,129). Similar alkaloids occur in species of *Aconitum* (monkshood and aconite). Cattle, which are more susceptible than sheep, manifest generalized weakness, with stiffness of gait and a characteristic stance in which the hind legs are held wide apart. Involuntary muscle twitches occur in the muzzle, shoulder, flank, and hip. Periods of standing are interspersed by falling. Recovery occurs slowly, with the animal making repeated attempts to stand (69).

Methyllycaconitine, one of the common larkspur alkaloids, is a potent neuromuscular-blocking agent in cattle. However, studies of the competitive binding potency of methyllycaconitine to the nicotinic acetylcholine receptor (nAChR) have shown a higher specificity for the neuronal nAChR as compared to the muscle nAChR. The pathophysiological significance of this observation is unclear.

Nicotine-like Toxins

Conium maculatum (poison hemlock). Indigenous to Europe and introduced to North America and Asia, this large perennial herb is of historical interest for its use by the early Greeks to execute criminals and for the identification and synthesis of the first botanical alkaloid, *coniine* (2-propylpiperidine), one of several piperidine alkaloids isolated from the plant. *Conium* alkaloids have a curare-like effect on the neuromuscular junction (116). Cattle, sheep, goats, horses, and pigs have been poisoned. Clinical signs include muscular weakness, trembling, slobbering, cyanotic membranes, a rapid weak pulse, dilated pupils, knuckling at the fetlocks, and frequent eructation, urination and defecation. Humans experience an ascending muscular weakness, total paralysis of the arms and legs, loss of the power to chew, fixed pupils, respiratory paralysis, and death without convulsions or confusion (104). In human hemlock poisoning, neurotoxic manifestations may be accompanied by rhabdomyolysis and tubular necrosis (116). Teratogenic effects (skeletal malformations) are reported in livestock but not in humans exposed to poison hemlock during specific periods of gestation.

Disorders of Striated Muscle

This is another heterogenous group of plants that harbors chemicals that exert direct or indirect effects predominantly on skeletal muscles of domestic animals.

Cassia spp. These widely distributed legumes are responsible for outbreaks of a degenerative myopathy among cattle, horses, pigs, sheep, goats, and poultry in Australia and the

Americas. After a few days of ingesting *C. occidentalis*, cattle develop diarrhea, myoglobinuria, weakness, ataxia, and recumbency; they remain alert and eat until a few hours before death supervenes from myocardial failure. Postmortem studies reveal grossly pale skeletal muscle and evidence of myofiber degeneration. Mitochondrial degeneration is evident in the less-affected cardiac muscle. Biochemical studies suggest unknown toxins in *Cassia* spp. uncouple mitochondrial oxidative phosphorylation, leading to energy depletion and myofiber damage (119).

Eupatorium rugosum (white snakeroot). A member of the Compositae family found in the northern part of the United States, *E. rugosum* harbors a tremorgenic alcohol (*tremetol*) that is excreted in the milk of animals and humans (100,134,145). Toxicity decreases if the plant is dried. Nineteenth-century North American settlers in eastern states were affected by "milk sickness" caused by white snakeroot; the disorder occasionally reached epidemic proportions and was responsible for many deaths, reportedly including that of Abraham Lincoln's mother. Milk sickness in humans is characterized by gradual-onset weakness, debility, inappetence, abdominal pain, and severe repeated vomiting. Constipation, severe thirst, muscular tremors, or more general trembling is commonly observed. Acetone breath is characteristic. Delirium is followed by coma and death (69).

Significant toxicity ("trembles") from white snakeroot occurs among cattle. Experimental trembles has been produced by feeding the plant to sheep, cattle, horses, hogs, fowl, and a human being (69). Tremetol passage in the milk provides a readily recognized epidemiological scenario when nursing young of a herd are selectively affected by tremors. Muscle tremors are prominent about the face, neck, flank, and hindquarters. It is of notable veterinary interest that only the horse develops myocardial necrosis upon exposure to the plant: long-term ingestion of the plant causes myocardial degeneration and mild skeletal muscle degeneration.

Tremetol is also present in the rayless goldenrod (*Haplopappus heterophyllus*), a plant in the southwestern United States responsible for a similar syndrome of trembles in cattle (69).

Thermopsis montana. This legume has a widespread distribution in the western United States; it produces a syndrome characterized by prolonged recumbency in cattle grazing on infested pastures. Clinical recovery corresponds with the repair of damaged skeletal muscle fibers. The myocardium is unaffected.

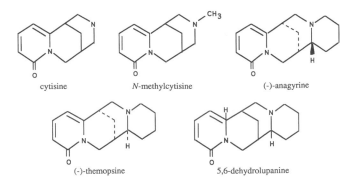

FIGURE 3.6. Quinolizidine alkaloids in *Thermopsis montana*.

Five stable quinolizidine alkaloids have been identified: *cytisine*, N-*methylcytisine*, (−)-*anagyrine*, (−)-*thermopsine*, and *5,6-dehydrolupanine* (Fig. 3.6). Animals given a purified preparation of these alkaloids develop generalized tremors, fasciculation, and irregular gait, followed by prolonged recumbency associated with hyaline degeneration of skeletal muscle fibers. The group of α-pyridone A-ring quinolizidine alkaloids may be responsible for the myopathy (4).

Laburnum anagyroides. This poisonous legume also contains *cytisine*. Clinical signs include excitement followed by incoordination, sweating and, in severe cases, convulsions, coma, and death from asphyxia (56). Heifers excrete cytisine in milk. Animals gavaged with purified *Laburnum* alkaloid extract show oral frothing, anorexia, and an irregular gait, with microscopic evidence of skeletal muscle disease (4).

Lupinus spp. (lupins). Lupins represent a large number of leguminous species, some of which serve as a fodder crop. They tolerate poor soils and drought, and have the potential to be a major source of protein for animals and humans alike. Lupins contain a number of *quinolizidines* (*lupanine*, *anagyrine*), *piperidine*, and other *alkaloids*. Seeds contain the highest concentrations, and toxicity is retained in the dry state. Acute and chronic lupin-related syndromes are recognized. Acute disease, seen among sheep in the United States, is characterized by labored breathing, hyperexcitability, convulsions, coma, and death (69). Calves gavaged with purified *Lupinus* extracts develop generalized tremor, protrusion of the nictitating ocular membranes, irregular gait, fasciculation of individual muscle groups, and temporary involuntary recumbency associated with microscopic evidence of skeletal muscle degeneration (4).

Geigeria spp. Sheep and goats intoxicated with this plant develop a syndrome characterized by necrosis of skeletal musculature and attended by muscular stiffness and paralysis. Degeneration, atrophy, and fibrosis of esophageal muscles may result in megaesophagus (93,94). The toxic agent is unknown.

Disorders of Cardiac Muscle

This group of heterogenous plants contains agents that act as cardiac glycosides or otherwise perturb cardiac as well as other functions.

Asclepias spp. The American term milkweed refers to the milky juice that exudes from broken surfaces of these plants. This material contains *cardenolides* with digitoxin-like effects and other toxic resinous substances (*galitoxin*). Toxicity may be retained in hay. Sheep, cattle, goats, horses, and domestic fowl are susceptible to intoxication. Heavy losses of sheep occurred in Colorado, U.S.A., in the early 1900s. Profound depression and weakness accompanied by staggering appear first (69). Intoxicated ruminants develop arrhythmias, hypotension, hypothermia, profuse salivation, incoordination, and violent seizures (56,101).

Experimental studies with sheep show that different plant species produce distinct combinations of clinical signs: lip tremor and intermittent extensor rigidity characterize a neurological syndrome, while a consistent respiratory grunt or groan signals a cardiovascular/gastrointestinal syndrome. Most species show effects likely associated with *cardiac glycosides*, including a lengthened P-R interval, decreased QT-corrected interval, and increased susceptibility to ventricular arrhythmias. *A. subverticillata* and *A. verticillata* show pronounced neurotoxicity in sheep (96,97). Chicks fed either species develop, within hours, profuse diarrhea followed by excitement and intermittent violent convulsions characterized by backward flips. Depression, trembling, seizures, torticollis, head pressing, and inability to stand occur later. The culpable neurotoxic agent(s) is unknown.

Cotyledon, Tylecodon, and *Kalanchoe.* These are succulent, semidesert plants eaten by animals in times of food shortage. Ingestion of relatively large quantities results in a chronic paralytic disease of stock (*krimpsiekte*) attributed to the cumulative action of *bufadienolide cardiac glycosides.* Secondary intoxication is reported in dogs and humans. Clinical signs become evident after several days of ingestion. Affected animals tire easily, stand hunched up with the feet together and the head dangling loosely, often lie down, and have difficulty in rising. They are unable to swallow or masticate. Four groups of cumulative neurotoxic bufadienolide cardiac glycosides have been identified: *cotyledoside, lanceotoxin A and B, tyledosides,* and *orbi-*

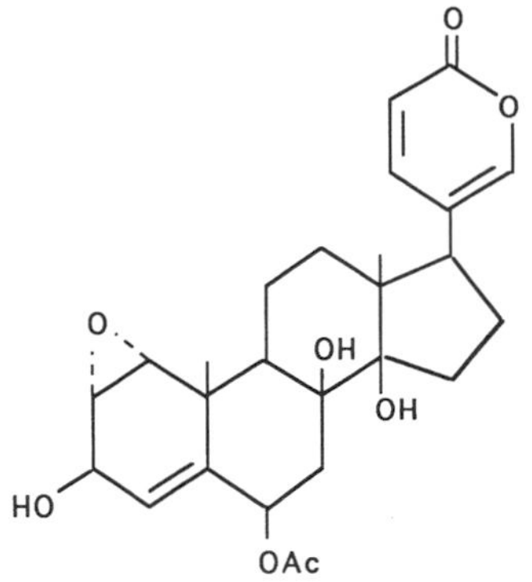

FIGURE 3.7. 1α,2α-Epoxy scillirosidin.

cusides. Scillirosidin is a noncumulative bufadienolide (Fig. 3.7) (93,94). Acute cardiac glycoside intoxication is characterized by ataxia and posterior paresis followed terminally by generalized paralysis in addition to gastrointestinal (ruminal stasis, diarrhea), respiratory (dyspnea, respiratory arrest), and cardiovascular effects (arrhythmia, ectopic rhythm, ventricular tachycardia).

Nerium oleander (oleander). This plant grows in temperate zones and contains high-potency digitoxin-like glycosides (*oleandrin, digitoxigenin,* and *nerium*). Vomiting, diarrhea, and atropine-resistant convulsions are seen in cattle and horses poisoned with a few leaves. A single leaf is considered potentially lethal to humans; fatal intoxication has even occurred after the consumption of meat that had been roasted while skewered to oleander branches. Humans develop severe gastroenteritis and cardiac toxicity with sweating, dizziness, drowsiness, dypsnea, and coma. The toxic properties of oleander are recorded by Pliny, Dioscorides, Galen, and others (69).

REFERENCES

1. Adams LG, Dollahite JW, Romane WM *et al.* (1969) Cystitis and ataxia associated with sorghum ingestion by horses. *J Amer Vet Med Assn* **155**, 518.
2. Alkondon M, Pereira EFR, Wonnacot S, Albuquerque EX (1992) Blockage of nicotinic currents in hippocampal neurons defines methyllycaconitine as a potent and specific receptor antagonist. *Mol Pharmacol* **41**, 802.
3. Bai Y, Benn MH, Majak W (1992) The alkaloids of *Delphinium nuttallianum*: the cattle-poisoning low larkspur of interior British Columbia. In: *Poisonous Plants, Proceedings of the Third International Symposium*. James LF, Keeler RF, Bailey EM Jr *et al.* eds. Iowa State University Press, Ames, Iowa p. 304.
4. Baker DC, Keeler RF (1992) Myopathy associated with *Thermopsis montana* ingestion in cattle. In: *Poisonous Plants, Proceedings of the Third International Sympo-*

sium. James LF, Keeler RF, Bailey EM Jr *et al.* eds. Iowa State University Press, Ames, Iowa p. 264.

5. Barrow MV, Simpson CF, Miller EJ (1974) Lathyrism: a review. *Quart Rev Biol* **49**, 101.

6. Bermudez MV, Gonzalez-Spencer D, Guerrero M *et al.* (1986) Experimental intoxication with fruit and purified toxins of buckthorn (*Karwinskia humboldtiana*). *Toxicon* **24**, 1091.

7. Berry PH, Howell JC, Cook RD (1987) Morphological changes in the central nervous system of sheep affected with experimental annual ryegrass (*Lolium rigidum*) toxicity. *J Comp Pathol* **90**, 603.

8. Booze TF, Oehme FW (1985) Metaldehyde toxicity: a review. *Vet Hum Toxicol* **27**, 11.

9. Bradford HF, Norris PJ, Smith CC (1990) Changes in transmitter release patterns *in vitro* induced by tremorgenic mycotoxins. *J Environ Pathol Toxicol Oncol* **10**, 17.

10. Brownie CF, Cullen J (1987) Characterization of experimentally-induced equine leukoencephalomalacia (ELEM) in ponies (*Equis caballus*): preliminary report. *Vet Hum Toxicol* **29**, 34.

11. Bryden WLK (1994) Neuromycotoxicoses in Australia. In: *Plant-Associated Toxins. Agricultural, Phytochemical and Ecological Aspects.* Colegate SM, Dorling PR eds. CAB International, Wallingford, UK p. 363.

12. Buxton D, Morgan KT (1976) Studies of lesions produced in the brains of colostrum-deprived lambs by *Clostridium welchii* (*C. perfringens*) type D toxin. *J Comp Pathol* **86**, 435.

13. Cancilla PA, Barlow RM (1966) Structural changes of central nervous system in swayback (enzootic ataxia) of lambs. *Acta Neuropathol* **6**, 251.

14. Carmichael WW, Biggs DF, Peterson MA (1979) Pharmacology of anatoxin-a, produced by the freshwater cyanophyte *Anabaena flos-aquae* NRC-44-1. *Toxicon* **17**, 229.

15. Casteel SW, Osweiler GD, Cook WO *et al.* (1985) Selenium toxicosis in swine. *J Amer Vet Med Assoc* **186**, 1084.

16. Cerami A, Allen AT, Graziano JH *et al.* (1973) Pharmacology of cyanate. 1. General effects on experimental animals. *J Phamacol Exp Ther* **185**, 653.

17. Charlton KM, Pierce KR (1970) A neuropathy in goats caused by experimental coyotillo (*Karwinskia humboldtiana*) poisoning; II. Lesions in the peripheral nervous system—teased fiber and acid phosphatase studies. *Pathol Vet* **7**, 385.

18. Charlton KM, Pierce KR (1970) A neuropathy in goats caused by experimental coyotillo (*Karwinskia humboldtiana*) poisoning; III. Distribution of lesions in peripheral nerves. *Pathol Vet* **7**, 408.

19. Charlton KM, Pierce KR (1970) A neuropathy in goats caused by experimental coyotillo (*Karwinskia humbold-*

tiana) poisoning; IV. Light and electron microscopic lesions in peripheral nerves. *Pathol Vet* **7**, 420.

20. Clarke EGC, Clarke ML (1975) Organic compounds (LL) pesticides. In: *Veterinary Toxicology.* Baillière Tindal, London p. 179.

21. Cockrum PA, Edgar JA, Payne AL, Jago MV (1992) Identification of tunicaminyluracil antibiotics in water-damaged wheat responsible for the death of pigs. In: *Poisonous Plants, Proceedings of the Third International Symposium.* James LF, Keeler RF, Bailey EM Jr *et al.* eds. Iowa State University Press, Ames, Iowa p. 615.

22. Cole RJ, Dorner JW (1986) Role of fungal tremorgens in animal disease. In: *Mycotoxins and Phycotoxins.* Steyn PS, Vleggaar R, eds. Elsevier, Amsterdam p. 501.

23. Cook JW (1957) *In vitro* destruction of some organophosphtae pesticides by bovine rumen fluid. *J Agr Food Chem* **5**, 859.

24. Corcuera LJ (1989) Indole alkaloids from *Phalaris* and other Gramineae. In: *Toxicants of Plant Origin, Vol. 1, Alkaloids.* Cheeke PR ed. CRC Press, Boca Raton, Florida p. 169.

25. Cordy DR, Knight HD (1978) California goats with a disease resembling enzootic ataxia or swayback. *Vet Pathol* **15**, 179.

26. Corman DC, Zachary JF, Buck WB (1992) Neuropathologic findings of bromethalin toxicosis in the cat. *Vet Pathol* **29**, 139.

27. Crabill, MR, Honnas DM, Taylor DS *et al.* (1994) A review of medical records used to identify 10 horses in which stringhalt developed subsequent to trauma to the dorsal metacarpus. *J Amer Vet Med Assn* **205**, 867.

28. Craig AM (1995) Detoxification of plant and fungal toxins by ruminant microbiota. In: *Ruminant Physiology: Digestion, Metabolism, Growth and Reproduction: Proceedings of the VII International Symposium on Ruminant Physiology.* Ferdinand Enke Verlag. Stuttgart, Germany p. 269.

29. Curley A, Sedlak VA, Girling ED *et al.* (1971) Organic mercury identified as the cause of poisoning in humans and hogs. *Science* **172**, 65.

30. Dorman DC, Buck WB, Trammel RD *et al.* (1990). Fenvalerate/N,N-diethyl-*m*-toluamide (DEET) toxicosis in two cats. *J Amer Vet Med Assn* **196**, 100.

31. Dorman DC, Cote LM, Buck WB (1992) Effect of an extract of *Gingko biloba* on bromethalin-induced cerebral lipid peroxidation and edema in rats. *Amer J Vet Res* **53**, 138.

32. Dorman DC, Parker AJ, Buck WB (1991) Electroencephalographic changes associated with bromethalin toxicosis in the dog. *Vet Hum Toxicol* **33**, 9.

33. Epstein W, Gerber K, Karler K (1964) The hypnotic constituent of *Stipa vasey*, sleepy grass. *Experientia* **20**, 390.

34. Essers AJA, Alsen P, Rosling H (1992) Insufficient processing of cassava induced acute intoxications and the

paralytic disease konzo in a rural area of Mozambique. *Ecol Food Nutr* **27**, 17.

35. Evans CA, Carlson WE, Green RG (1942) The pathology of Chastek paralysis in foxes. *Amer J Pathol* **18**, 79.

36. Fairbrother TE, Kerr LA, Essig HW (1987) Effects of 4-methyl imidazole in young calves. *Vet Hum Toxicol* **29**, 312.

37. Fell BF, Mills CF, Boyne RM (1965) Cytochrome oxidase deficiency in the motor neurons of copper-deficient lambs: a histochemical study. *Res Vet Sci* **6**, 170.

38. Field DJ, Bowen JM, Cole RJ (1978) Verruculotoxin potentiation of twitch tension in skeletal muscle. *Toxicol Appl Pharmacol* **46**, 529.

39. Finnie JW (1994) Pathogenesis of corynetoxin poisoning. In: *Plant-Associated Toxins. Agricultural, Phytochemical, and Ecological Aspects*. Colegate SM, Dorling PR eds. CAB International, Wallingford, UK p. 405.

40. Gaffield W, Keeler RF, Baker DC (1991) Solanum glycoalkaloids: plant toxins possessing disparate physiologically active structural entities. In: *Toxicology of Plant and Fungal Compounds, Handbook of Natural Toxins, Vol. 6*. Keeler RF, Tu AT eds. Marcel Dekker, New York p. 135.

41. Gant DB, Cole RJ, Valdes JJ *et al.* (1987) Action of tremorogenic mycotoxins on GABA$_A$ receptor. *Life Sci* **41**, 2207.

42. Gardner DE (1973) Pathology of *Clostridium welchii* type D enterotoxaemia. II. Structural and ultrastructural alterations in the tissues of lambs and mice. *J Comp Pathol* **83**, 509.

43. Gilmour JS, Inglis DM, Robb J, Maclean M (1989) A fodder mycotoxicosis of ruminants caused by contamination of a distillery by-product with *Aspergillus clavatus. Vet Rec* **124**, 133.

44. Gooneratne SR, Olkowski AA, Christensen DA (1989) Sulfur-induced polioencephalomalacia in sheep: some biochemical changes. *Can J Vet Res* **53**, 462.

45. Gould DH, McAllister MM, Savage JC, Hamar DW (1991) High sulfide concentrations in rumen fluid associated with nutritionally induced polioencephalomalacia in calves. *Amer J Vet Res* **52**, 11649.

46. Guengerich FP (1977) Activation of the parasympathomimetic alkaloid slaframine by microsomal and photochemical oxidation. *Mol Pharmacol* **13**, 185.

47. Haimanot RT, Kidane Y, Wuhib E *et al.* (1990) Lathyrism in rural northwestern Ethopia: a highly prevalent neurotoxic disorder. *Int J Epidemiol* **19**, 664.

48. Hakim AM, Pappius HM (1983) Sequence of metabolic, clinical, and histologic events in experimental thiamine deficiency. *Ann Neurol* **13**, 365.

49. Hall WTK (1987) Cycad (Zamia) poisoning Australia. *Aust Vet J* **64**, 149.

50. Harding JDJ, Lewis G, Done JT (1968) Experimental arsanillic acid poisoning in pigs. *Vet Rec* **83**, 560.

51. Harrison LR, Colvin BM, Greene JT *et al.* (1990) Pulmonary edema and hydrothorax in swine produced by fumonisin B$_1$, a toxic metabolite of *Fusarium moniliforme. J Vet Diagn Invest* **2**, 217.

52. Hartley WJ (1956) A focal symmetrical encephalomalacia of lambs. *N Z Vet J* **4**, 129.

53. Hooper PT (1983) Cycad poisoning. In: *Handbook of Natural Toxins. Pt. 1. Plant and Fungal Toxins*. Keeler RF, Tu AT eds. Marcel Dekker, New York p. 463.

54. Hooser SB, Beasley VR, Everitt J (1986) Effects of an insecticidal dip containing *d*-limonene in the cat. *J Amer Med Assoc* **189**, 905.

55. Howell JMcC, Davidson AN, Oxberry J (1969) Observations on the lesions in the white matter of the spinal cord of swayback sheep. *Acta Neuropathol* **12**, 33.

56. Humphreys DJ (1988) *Veterinary Toxicology. 3rd Ed*. Ballière Tindall, London.

57. Huntington PJ, Jeffcott LB, Friend SC *et al.* (1989) Australian stringhalt—epidemiological, clinical and neurological investigations. *Equine Vet J* **21**, 266.

58. Huxtable CR, Colegate SM, Dorling PR (1989) Stypandrol and *Stypandra* toxicosis. In: *Toxicants of Plant Origin. Vol. IV. Phenolics*. Cheeke PR ed. CRC Press, Boca Raton, Florida p. 83.

59. Huxtable CR, Dorling PR, Slatter DH (1980) Myelin oedema, optic neuropathy, and retinopathy in experimental *Stypandra imbricata* toxicosis. *Neuropathol Appl Neurobiol* **6**, 221.

60. Ince PG, Shaw PJ, Candy JM *et al.* (1994) Iron, selenium and glutathione peroxidase activity are elevated in sporadic motor neuron disease. *Neurosci Lett* **182**, 87.

61. James LF, Hartley WJ, Williams MC, Van Kampen KR (1980) Field and experimental studies in cattle and sheep poisoned by nitro-bearing *Astragalus* or their toxins. *Amer J Vet Res* **4**, 377.

62. Jubb KV, Kennedy PC, Palmer N (1992) *Pathology of Domestic Animals*. Academic Press, San Diego.

63. Jubb KVF, Huxtable CR (1993) The nervous system. In: *Pathology of the Domestic Animals. 4th Ed. Vol 1*. Jubb KVF, Kennedy PC, Palmer N eds. Academic Press, San Diego, California p. 267.

64. Jubb KVF, Saunders LZ, Coates HV (1956) Thiamine deficiency encephalopathy in cats. *J Comp Pathol* **66**, 217.

65. Kellerman TS, Coetzer JAW, Naude TW (1992) Plant poisonings and mycotoxicoses of livestock in Southern Africa. In: *Poisonous Plants, Proceedings of the Third International Symposium*. James LF, Keeler RF, Bailey EM Jr *et al.* eds. Iowa State University Press, Ames, Iowa p. 43.

66. Kellerman TS, Pienaar JG, van der Westhuizen GCA *et al.* (1984) A highly fatal tremorgenic mycotoxicosis of cattle caused by *Aspergillus clavatus. Onderstepoort J Vet Res* **51**, 271.

67. Kellerman TS, Rabie, CJ, van der Westhuizen GCA *et al.* (1985) Induction of diplodiosis, a neuromycotoxicosis in domestic ruminants with cultures of indigenous and exotic isolates of *Diplodia maydis. Onderstepoort J Vet Res* **52**, 35.

68. Kilness AW, Hochberg FH (1977) Amyotrophic lateral sclerosis in a high selenium environment. *J Amer Med Assn* **237**, 2843.

69. Kingsbury JM (1964) *Poisonous Plants of United States and Canada.* Prentice Hall, Englewood Cliffs, NJ.

70. Kennedy S, Rice DA, Cush PF (1986) Neuropathology of experimental 3-nitro-4-hydroxyphenylarsonic acid toxicosis in pigs. *Vet Pathol* **23**, 454.

71. Kisby GE, Ellison M, Spencer PS (1992) Content of the neurotoxins cycasin (methylazoxymethanol-D-glucoside) and BMAA (β-N-methylamino-L-alanine) in cycad flour prepared by Guam Chamorros. *Neurology* **42**, 1336.

72. Knight HD, Buraw RG (1973) Chronic lead poisoning in horses. *J Amer Vet Med Assn* **162**, 781.

73. Kornheiser KM (1983) Buckeye poisoning in cattle. *Vet Med Small Anim Clin* **769**.

74. Land CJ, Hult K, Fuchs R *et al.* (1987) Tremorgenic mycotoxins from *Aspergillus fumigatus* as a possible occupational health problem in sawmills. *Appl Environ Microbiol* **53**, 787.

75. Lloyd HA, Fales HM, Goldman ME *et al.* (1985) Brunfelsamidine: a novel convulsant from the medicinal plant *Brunfelsia grandiflora. Tetrahedron Lett* **26**, 2623.

76. Lowes N (1992) Roquefortine identified as a major differential diagnosis in suspected strychnine poisoning in dogs. *Can Vet J* **33**, 193.

77. Ludolph AC, He F, Spencer PS *et al.* (1991) 3-Nitropropionic acid—exogenous animal neurotoxin and possible striatal toxin. *Can J Neurol Sci* **18**, 492.

78. Magnusson RA, Whittier WD, Veit HP *et al.* (1983) Yellow buckeye (*Aesculus octandra* Marsh) toxicity in calves. *Bov Practice* **18**, 195.

79. Mahmood NA, Carmichael WW (1986) The pharmacology of anatoxin-a(s), a neurotoxin produced by the cyanobacterium *Anabaena flos-aquae* NRC-525-17. *Toxicon* **24**, 425.

80. Mahmood NA, Carmichael WW (1987) Anatoxin-a(s), an anticholinesterase from the cyanobacterium *Anabaena flos-aquae* NRC-525-17. *Toxicon* **25**, 1221.

81. Main DC, Slatter DH, Huxtable CR *et al.* (1981) *Stypandra imbricta* (blindgrass) toxicosis in goats and sheep—clinical and pathologic findings in four field cases. *Aust Vet J* **57**, 132.

82. Manners, GD, Panter KE, Ralphs MH *et al.* (1994) The toxic evaluation of nonditerpenoid alkaloids in three tall larkspur (*Delphinium*) species. In: *Plant-Associated Toxins. Agricultural, Phytochemical and Ecological Aspects.* Colegate SM, Dorling PR eds. CAB International, Wallingford, UK p. 178.

83. McAllister MM, Gould DH, Hamar DW (1992) Sulfide-induced polioencephalomalacia in lambs. *J Comp Pathol* **106**, 267.

84. McDonel JL (1980) *Clostridium perfringens* toxins (type A, B, C, D, E). *Pharmacol Ther* **10**, 617.

85. McKenzie RA, McMicking LI (1977) Ataxia and urinary incontinence in cattle grazing sorghum. *Aust Vet J* **53**, 496.

86. McMillan M, Thompson JG (1979) Outbreak of suspected solanine poisoning in schoolboys—examination of criteria of solanine poisoning. *Quart J Med* **48**, 227.

87. Mitchell JD, East BW, Harris IA, Pentland B (1991) Manganese, selenium and other trace elements in spinal cord, liver and bone in motor neurone disease. *Eur Neurol* **31**, 7.

88. Morgan SE, Edwards WC (1986) Bovine bonkers: new terminology for an old problem. A review of toxicity problems associated with ammoniated feeds. *Vet Hum Toxicol* **28**, 16.

89. Morgan SE, Johnson B, Brewer B (1990) Sorghum cystitis ataxia syndrome in horses. *Vet Hum Toxicol* **32**, 582.

90. Mount ME, Moller G, Cook J *et al.* (1991) Clinical illness associated with a commercial tick and flea product in dogs and cats. *Vet Hum Toxicol* **33**, 19.

91. Munday BL, Mason RW (1967) Lesions in ryegrass staggers in sheep. *Aust Vet J* **43**, 598.

92. Munoz-Martinez EJ, Cuera J, Joseph-Nathan P (1983) Denervation caused by tullidora (*Karwinskia humboldtiana*). *Neuropathol Appl Neurobiol* **9**, 121.

93. Naude TW, Anderson LAP, Schultz RA *et al.* (1992) A chronic paralytic syndrome of small stock caused by cumulative bufadienolide cardiac glycosides. In: *Poisonous Plants, Proceedings of the Third International Symposium.* James LF, Keeler RF, Bailey EM Jr *et al.* eds. Iowa State University Press, Ames, Iowa p. 392.

94. Naude TW, Coetzer JAW, Kellerman TS (1992) Variation in animal species' response to plant poisonings and mycotoxicoses in southern Africa. In: *Poisonous Plants, Proceedings of the Third International Symposium.* James LF, Keeler RF, Bailey EM Jr *et al.* eds. Iowa State University Press, Ames, Iowa p. 11.

95. Norris PJ, Smith CCT, De Bellewoche J *et al.* (1980) Actions of tremorgenic fungal toxins on neurotransmitter release. *J Neurochem* **34**, 33.

96. Ogden L, Burrows GE, Tyrl RJ, Ely RW (1992) Experimental intoxication in sheep by *Asclepias*. In: *Poisonous Plants, Proceedings of the Third International Symposium.* James LF, Keeler RF, Bailey EM Jr *et al.* eds. Iowa State University Press, Ames, Iowa p. 495.

97. Ogden L, Burrows GE, Tyrl RJ, Gormham SL (1992) Comparison of *Asclepias* species based on their toxic effects in chickens. In: *Poisonous Plants, Proceedings of the*

Third International Symposium. James LF, Keeler RF, Bailey EM Jr *et al.* eds. Iowa State University Press, Ames, Iowa p. 500.

98. Okada HM, Chihaya Y, Matsukawa K (1987) Thiamine deficiency encephalopathy in foxes and mink. *Vet Pathol* **24**, 180.

99. Olsen JD, Manners GD (1989) Toxicology of diterpenoid alkaloids in rangeland larkspur (*Delphinium* spp.). In: *Toxicants of Plant Origin. Vol. 1, Alkaloids.* Cheeke PR ed. CRC Press, Boca Raton, Florida p. 291.

100. Olson CT, Keller WC, Gerken DF, Reed SM (1984) Suspected tremetol poisoning in horses. *J Amer Vet Med Assoc* **185**, 1001.

101. Osweiler G (1996) *Toxicology, National Veterinary Medical Series.* Williams & Wilkins, Philadelphia.

102. Osweiller GD, Carson TL, Buck WB, Van Gelder GA (1985) *Clinical and Diagnostic Veterinary Toxicology. 3rd Ed.* Kendall Hunt, Dubuque, Iowa.

103. Oxer DT (1956) Enterotoxaemia in goats. *Aust Vet J* **32**, 62.

104. Panter KE, Keeler RF (1989) Piperidine alkaloids of posion hemlock. In: *Toxicants of Plant Origin. Vol. 1, Alkaloids.* Cheeke PR ed. CRC Press, Boca Raton, FL p. 109.

105. Pass MA (1994) Toxicity of plant-derived aliphatic nitrotoxins. In: *Plant-Associated Toxins. Agricultural, Phytochemical and Ecological Aspects.* Colegate SM, Dorling PR eds. CAB International, Wallingford, UK p. 541.

106. Peters R (1954) Biochemical light upon an ancient poison: a lethal synthesis. *Endeavor* **13**, 147.

107. Pienaar JG, Kellerman TS, Basson PA *et al.* (1976) Maldronksiekte in cattle: a neuronopathy caused by *Solanum kwebense* N. E. Br. *Onderstepoort J Vet Res* **43**, 67.

108. Pierce PE, Thompson JF, Likowsky WH *et al.* (1972) Alkyl mercury poisoning in humans. *J Amer Med Assn* **220**, 1439.

109. Porter JK, Voss KA, Bacon CW, Norred WP (1990) Effects of *Fusarium moniliforme* and corn associated with equine leukoencephalomalacia on rat neurotransmittors and metabolites. *Proc Soc Exp Biol Med* **194**, 265.

110. Powers KA, Hooser SB, Sundberg JP, Beasley VR (1988) An evaluation of the acute toxicity of an insecticidal spray containing linalool, *d*-limonene, and piperonyl butoxide applied topically to domestic cats. *Vet Hum Toxicol* **30**, 206.

111. Purcell DA (1985) Annual ryegrass toxicity: a review. In: *Plant Toxicology.* Seawright AA, Hegarty MP, James LF *et al.* eds. Yeerongpilly, Queensland, Queensland Poisonous Plants Committee.

112. Raisbeck MF, Rottinghaus GE, Kendall JD (1991) Effects of naturally occurring mycotoxins on ruminants. In: *Mycotoxins and Animal Foods.* Smith JE, Henderson RS eds. CRC Press, Boca Raton, FL p. 647.

113. Read DH, Harrington DD (1981) Experimentally-induced thiamine deficiency in beagle dogs: clinical observations. *Amer J Vet Res* **42**, 984.

114. Rice DA, Kennedy S, McMurray CH, Blanchflower WJ (1985) Experimental 3-nitro-4-hydroxyphenylarsonic acid toxicosis in pigs. *Res Vet Sci* **39**, 47.

115. Riopelle RJ, Boegman RJ, Little PB, Stevens KL (1992) Neurotoxicity of sesquiterpene lactones. In: *Poisonous Plants.* Proceedings of the Third International Symposium. James LF, Keeler RF, Bailey EM Jr *et al.* eds. Iowa State University Press, Ames, Iowa p. 298.

116. Rizzi D, Basile C, Di Maggio A *et al.* (1991) Clinical spectrum of accidental hemlock poisoning: neurotoxic manifestations, rhabdomyolysis and acute tubular necrosis. *Nephrol Dial Transplant* **6**, 939.

117. Roberts HE, Williams BM, Harvard A (1966) Cerebral oedema in lambs associated with hypocuprosis and its relationship to swayback. *J Comp Pathol* **76**, 279.

118. Robertson-Smith RG, Jeffcott LB, Friend SCE *et al.* (1985) An unusual incidence of neurological disease affecting horses during a drought. *Aust Vet J* **62**, 6.

119. Rowe LD (1991) Cassia-induced myopathy. In: *Toxicology of Plant and Fungal Compounds. Handbook of Natural Toxins, Vol. 6.* Keeler RF, Tu AT eds. Marcel Dekker, New York p. 335.

120. Roy DN (1981) Toxic amino acids and proteins from *Lathyrus* plants and other leguminous species: a literature review. *Commonwealth Bureau of Nutrition: Nutrit Abstr Rev—Series A.* **51**, 691.

121. Roy DN, Craig AM, Blythe LL (1993) Equine nigropallidal encephalomalacia and *Centaurea solstitialis* (yellow star thistle): partial isolation and identification of neurotoxins. *Neurodegeneration* **2**, 51.

122. Roy DN, Peyton DH, Spencer PS (1995) Isolation and identification of two potent neurotoxins, aspartic acid and glutamic acid, from yellow star thistle (*Centaurea solstitialis*). *Nat Toxins* **3**, 174.

123. Roy DN, Spencer PS (1989) Lathyrogens. In: *Toxicants of Plant Origin, Vol III. Proteins and Amino Acids.* Cheeke PR ed. CRC Press, Boca Raton, FL p. 169.

124. Rumbeiha WK, Oehme FW (1993) Veterinary toxicology. In: *General and Applied Toxicology, Vol. 2.* Ballantyne B, Marrs T, Turner P eds. Stockton Press, New York p. 1287.

125. Schafer EW, Burtong RB, Cunningham DJ (1973) A summary of the acute toxicity of 4-aminopyridine to birds and mammals. *Toxicol Appl Pharmacol* **26**, 532.

126. Scott PM (1984) Roquefortine. In: *Mycotoxins—Production, Isolation, Separation and Purification.* Bertina V ed. Elsevier, Amsterdam p. 463.

127. Shaw C-M, Papayannopoulou T, Stamatoyannopoulous G (1974) Neuropathology of cyanate toxicity in rhesus monkeys. *Pharmacology* **12**, 166.

128. Shlosberg A, Zadikov I, Perl S *et al.* (1992) A lethal mass neurotoxicosis in sheep caused by *Aspergillus clavatus*-contaminated feed. In: *Poisonous Plants, Proceedings of the Third International Symposium.* James LF, Keeler RF, Bailey EM Jr *et al.* eds. Iowa State University Press, Ames, Iowa p. 397.

129. Siemion RS, Raisbeck MF, Waggoner JW, Tidwell MA (1992) *In-vitro* ruminal metabolism of larkspur alkaloids. *Vet Hum Toxicol* **34**, 206.

130. Sisk DB, Colvin BM, Bridges CR (1988) Acute, fatal illness in cattle exposed to boron fertilizer. *J Amer Vet Med Assn* **193**, 943.

131. Sisk DB, Colvin BM, Merrill A *et al.* (1990) Experimental acute inorganic boron toxicosis in the goat: effects on serum chemistry and CSF biogenic amines. *Vet Hum Toxicol* **32**, 205.

132. Slocombe RF, Huntington PJ, Friend SC *et al.* (1992) Pathological aspects of Australian stringhalt. *Equine Vet J* **24**, 174.

133. Smalley HE, Crookshank HR (1976) Toxicity studies on sleepy grass, *Stipa robusta* (Vasey). *Southwest Vet* **29**, 35.

134. Smetzer DL, Coppock RW, Ely RW *et al.* (1983) Cardiac effects of white snakeroot intoxication in horses. *Equine Pract* **5**, 26.

135. Smith RA, Lewis D (1990) Apparent *Corydalis aurea* intoxication of cattle. *Vet Hum Toxicol* **32**, 63.

136. Snyder RD (1971) Congenital mercury poisoning. *N Engl J Med* **284**, 1014.

137. Spainhour CB Jr, Fiske RA, Flory W, Reagor JC (1990) A toxicological investigation of the garden shrub *Brunfelsia calcyina* var. *floribunda* (yesterday-today-and-tomorrow) in three species. *J Vet Diagn Invest* **2**, 3.

138. Spencer PS (1995) Lathyrism. In: *Handbook of Clinical Neurology, Pt. 2. Vol. 21.* Vinken PJ, Bruyn GW, Klawans HL eds. Elsevier, Amsterdam p. 1.

139. Spencer PS, Nunn PB, Hugon J *et al.* (1987) Guam amyotrophic lateral sclerosis–parkinsonism-dementia linked to a plant excitant neurotoxin. *Science* **237**, 517.

140. Stegelmeier BL, James LF, Panter KE, Molyneux RJ (1995) Serum swainsonine concentration and α-mannosidase activity in cattle and sheep ingesting *Oxytropis sericea* and *Astragalus lentiginosus* (locoweeds). *Amer J Vet Res* **56**, 149.

141. Steyn PS, Vleggar R (1985) Tremorgenic mycotoxins. *Fortschr Chem Org Naturst* **48**, 1.

142. Swenne I, Eriksson U, Christoffersson R *et al.* (1996) Cyanide detoxification in rats exposed to acetonitrile and fed a low protein diet. *Fund Appl Toxicol* **31**, 66.

143. Tellez-Nagel I, Korthals JK, Vlassara HV, Cerami A (1977) An ultrastructural study of chronic sodium-cyanate neuropathy. *J Neuropathol Exp Neurol* **36**, 351.

144. Tewe OO, Iyayi EA (1989) Cyanogenic glycosides. In: *Toxicants of Plant Origin, Vol. II, Glycosides.* Cheeke PR ed. CRC Press, Boca Raton, FL p. 43.

145. Thompson W (1989) Depression and choke in a horse: probable white snakeroot toxicosis. *Vet Hum Toxicol* **31**, 321.

146. Tor-Agbidye J (1997) Cyanide metabolism in sulfur amino acid deficiency: relevance to understanding cassava-related neurodegenerative diseases. Ph.D. Thesis. Oregon State University, Corvallis, Oregon.

147. Tor-Agbidye J, Blythe LL, Craig AM (1994) Correlation of quantities of ergovaline and lolitrem B toxins to clinical cases of tall fescue toxicosis and perennial ryegrass staggers. In: *Plant-Associated Toxins. Agricultural, Phytochemical and Ecological Aspects.* Colegate SM, Dorling PR eds. CAB International, Wallingford, UK p. 369.

148. Tryphonas L, Nielsen NO (1973) Pathology of chronic alkylmercurial poisoning in swine. *Amer J Vet Res* **34**, 379.

149. Van Kampern KR (1970) Sudan grass and sorghum poisoning of horses: a possible lathyrogenic disease. *J Amer Vet Med Assn* **156**, 629.

150. Vandevelde M, Fankhauser R, Bichsel P *et al.* (1982) Hereditary neurovisceral mannosidosis associated with α-mannosidase deficiency in a family of Persian cats. *Acta Neuropathol* **58**, 64.

151. Vinceti M, Guidetti D, Pinotti M *et al.* (1996) Amyotrophic lateral sclerosis after long-term exposure to drinking water with high selenium content. *Epidemiology* **7**, 529.

152. Wannemacher RW Jr, Bunner DL, Neufleld HA (1991) Toxicity of trichothecenes and other related mycotoxins in laboratory animals. In: *Mycotoxins and Animal Foods.* Smith HJE, Henderson RS eds. CRC Press, Boca Raton, FL p. 499.

153. Weis WP, Conrad HR, Martin CM (1986) Etiology of ammoniated hay toxicosis. *J Anim Sci* **63**, 525.

154. Weller RO, Mitchell J, Doyle Daves G Jr (1980) Buckthorn (*Karwinskia humboldtiana*) toxins. In: *Experimental and Clinical Neurotoxicology.* Spencer PS, Schaumburg HH eds. Williams & Wilkins, Baltimore, MD p. 336.

155. Whiting MG (1963) Toxicity of cycads. *Econ Bot* **17**, 271.

156. Wilson TM, Cramer PG, Owen RL *et al.* (1989) Porcine focal symmetrical poliomyelomalacia: test for an interaction between dietary selenium and niacin. *Can J Vet Res* **53**, 454.

157. Wilson TM, Hammerstedt RH, Palmer IS, DeLahunta A (1988) Porcine focal symmetrical poliomyelomalacia: experimental reproduction with oral doses of encapsulated sodium selenite. *Can J Vet Res* **52**, 83.

158. Wilson TM, Ross PF, Rice LG *et al.* (1990) Fumonisin B$_1$ levels associated with an epizootic of equine leukoencephalomalacia. *J Vet Diagn Invest* **2**, 213.

159. Wilson TR, Scholz RW, Drake TR (1983) Selenium toxicity and porcine focal symmetrical poliomyelomalacia:

description of a field outbreak and experimental reproduction. *Can J Comp Med* **47**, 412.

160. Wong RY (1992) Application of x-ray crystallography to the determination of molecular structure and conformation of poisonous plant constituents. In: *Poisonous Plants, Proceedings of the Third International Symposium.* James LF, Keeler RF, Bailey Jr EM *et al.* eds. Iowa State University Press, Ames, Iowa p. 542.

161. Yao Y, Peter AB, Baur R, Sigel E (1989) The tremorgen aflatrem is a positive allosteric modulator of the gamma aminobutyric acid A receptor channel expressed in *Xenopus* oocytes. *Mol Pharmacol* **35**, 319.

162. Yasuda N, Kono I, Shimizu T (1985) Pathological studies on cycad poisoning of cattle experimentally caused by feeding with leaves of cycad, *Cycas revoluta Thunb. Gakujutsu-Hokoko-Bull-Fac-Agric-Kagoshima-Univ. Kagoshima* **35**, 171.

163. Zhang ZX, Anderson DW, Mantel N, Román GC (1996) Motor neuron disease on Guam: geographic and familial occurrence, 1956–85. *Acta Neurol Scand* **94**, 51.

PART TWO

SUBSTANCES WITH
NEUROTOXIC POTENTIAL

Neurotoxic Substances

Criteria for Neurotoxicity Ratings

Alphabetical listing of substances linked to neurotoxic phenomena in humans and animals. The strength of association is indicated by a neurotoxicity rating. The letter A indicates a strong association between the substance and the condition; B denotes a suspected and plausible but unproven association; C suggests the proposed association is not likely to be causal.

Absinthe (Wormwood)

Albert C. Ludolph
Herbert H. Schaumburg

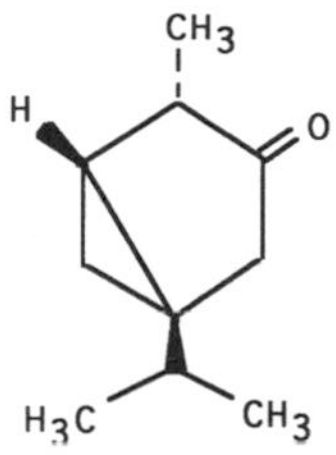

THUJONE
$C_{10}H_{16}O$

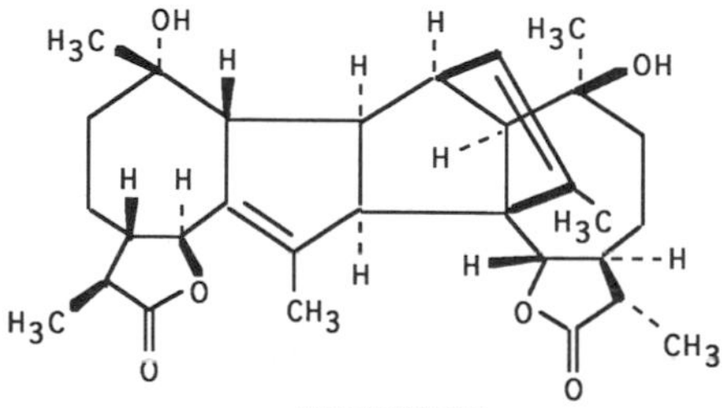

ABSINTHIN
$C_{30}H_{40}O_6$

Thujone. 4-Methyl-1-(1-methylethyl)bicyclo[3.1.0]-hexane-3-one; 3-Thujanone.

Absinthin. [3S-(3α,$3a\alpha$,6β,$6a\alpha$,$6b\beta$,7α,$7a\beta$,8α,$10a\beta$,11β,-$13a\alpha$,$13b\alpha$,$13c\beta$,$14b\beta$)]-3,3a,4,5,6,6a,6b,7,7a,8,9,10,10a,-13a,13c,14b-Hexadecahydro-6,8-dihydroxy-3,6,8,11,14,15-hexamethyl-2H-7,13b-ethenopentaleno[1″,2″:6,7;5″,4″: 6′,7′]dicyclohepta[1,2-b:1′,2′-b′]difuran-2,12(11H)-dione.

NEUROTOXICITY RATING

Clinical

A   Acute encephalopathy (seizures)

B   Psychobiological reaction (insomnia, agitation, hallucinations, bizarre behavior)

B   Chronic encephalopathy (seizures, tremor, cognitive dysfunction)

Experimental

B   Seizure disorder

Oil of wormwood, the neurotoxic component of absinthe, is an extract of the leaves, stem, and flowers of the bushy weed *Artemisia absinthium*. The oil has been employed as an anthelmintic since the Middle Ages; it is still used in very small amounts to flavor vermouth and as a fragrance in some liniments. Absinthe is a highly intoxicating (70% alcohol) French liqueur developed in the early nineteenth century by Henri Louis Pernod. The commercial beverage was a distilled combination of oil of wormwood, alcohol, herbs, and seeds. The striking blue-green aperitif was too strong and bitter to drink straight. Consumption was a ritual wherein cold water was poured over a sugar cube poised on a slotted spoon over a glass of undiluted absinthe; the resulting milky fluid was then slowly imbibed (1). Absinthe consumption became widespread in France following the Franco-Prussian War. Especially popular in Paris, its consumption was depicted and sometimes endorsed by artists (Edouard Manet, Henri de Toulouse-Lautrec) and literary figures (Charles Baudelaire, Oscar Wilde). Vincent van Gogh, an absinthe addict, is said to have sliced off his own ear and mailed it to a lady friend while intoxicated (4,5). Pablo Picasso, responding to the French legislative attempts to ban it, constructed a sculpture consisting of six abstract glasses of metal and ceramic topped with absinthe spoons. Production ceased in 1915 in France when it was blamed for increased instances of psychosis and suicide. Absinthe liqueur is illegal in North America, but its ingredients are readily available. It has had a revival as a popular drink in the Czech Republic (6).

Experimental administration of oil of wormwood to dogs, guinea pigs, and rabbits was shown by nineteenth century investigators to cause generalized seizures. A terpene hydrocarbon constituent of wormwood, thujone, has been implicated as the epileptogenic component of absinthe (2). Parenteral administration of 40 mg/kg of thujone to rats causes generalized seizures. Since thujone and tetrahydrocannabinol (THC) have similar molecular geometries and functional groups, it has been suggested that thujone exerts its psychomimetic effects by reacting with CNS tetrahyrocannabinol receptors (3).

Neurological dysfunction in human absinthism is associated with long-term ingestion of the liqueur and appeared, to French physicians, to be distinct from effects of the co-existent alcohol. The syndrome is poorly delineated in the older literature and dose–response relationships are unclear. Classic manifestations of absinthism include insom-

nia, bizarre behavior, auditory and visual hallucinations, cognitive decline and, eventually, generalized seizures (1).

A well-documented recent report describes the abrupt onset of generalized seizures with secondary rhabdomyolysis and renal failure in a 31-year-old healthy man (7). Seizures appeared within hours of ingesting, for the first time, a 10-ml bolus of oil of wormwood in the mistaken belief that it was absinthe. The oil of wormwood contained neither alcohol nor other adulterants. He had an uneventful recovery.

REFERENCES

1. Arnold WN (1989) Absinthe. *Sci Amer* **260**, 112.
2. Bonkovsky HL, Cable EE, Cable JW *et al.* (1992) Porphyrogenic properties of the terpenes camphorpinene, and thujone (with a note on historic implications for absinthe and the illness of Vincent van Gogh). *Biochem Pharmacol* **43**, 2359.
3. del Castillo J, Anderson M, Rubottom GM (1974) Marijuana, absinthe and the central nervous system. *Nature* **253**, 365.
4. Loftus LS, Arnold WN (1991) Vincent van Gogh's illness: acute intermittent porphyria? *Brit Med J* **303**, 1589.
5. Morrant JC (1993) The wing of madness: the illness of Vincent van Gogh. *Can J Psychiat* **38**, 480.
6. Steinmetz G (1996) In Prague, absinthe makes heart fonder, and head cloudier. *Wall St J* December 24.
7. Weisbord SD, Soule JB, Kimmel PL (1997) Poison on line —acute renal failure caused by oil of wormwood purchased through the Internet. *N Engl J Med* **337**, 825.

Acacia berlandieri Benth.

Albert C. Ludolph

NEUROTOXICITY RATING

Clinical

B   Ataxia (goats, sheep)

About 800 species of *Acacia* are known, and they are distributed in savannas and arid regions of Australia, Africa, India, and the Americas. *Acacia* spp. are robust, drought-resistant, protein-rich legumes that harbor cyanogenic glycosides and other potentially toxic compounds. Human contact possibly occurs only during famine, but cases of intoxication have not been reliably reported.

A. berlandieri is a perennial shrub distributed in southwestern Texas and into Mexico. Plant materials contain the sympathomimetic amine N-methyl-phenylethylamine (2)

and the related compounds N-methyltyramine, and hordenine (1). Extraction methods are published (4).

Sheep and goats that graze heavily on the plant develop an undefined neurological disorder known colloquially as *limberleg* or *guajillo wobbles*. Neurological dysfunction develops after long-term (6–9 months) grazing or prolonged (months) experimental feeding of *A. berlandieri* (3). The disorder is said to commence with "ataxia" of the hindlimbs and, occasionally, the forelimbs are involved. Significant lesions have not been described. N-Methyl-phenylethylamine is claimed to be the neurotoxic principle, but neither this nor the three "toxic amines" noted above have been subjected to experimental scrutiny. Other *Acacia* spp. contain fluoroacetic acid (*A. georginae*).

REFERENCES

1. Adams HR, Camp BJ (1966) The isolation and identification of three alkaloids from *Acacia berlandieri*. *Toxicon* 4, 85.
2. Camp BJ, Lyman CM (1956) The isolation of N-methyl-β-phenethylamine from *Acacia berlandieri*. *J Amer Pharmacol Assoc* 11, 719.
3. Kingsbury JM (1964) *Poisonous Plants of the United States and Canada*. Prentice Hall, Englewood Cliffs, NJ p. 305.
4. Pemberton IJ, Smith GR, Forbes TDA, Hensarling CM (1993) Technical note: An improved method for extraction and quantification of toxic phenethylamines from *Acacia berlandieri*. *Amer Assoc Anim Sci* 71, 467.

Acetone

Herbert H. Schaumburg

$$CH_3COCH_3$$

ACETONE

$$C_3H_6O$$

Dimethyl ketone; 2-Propanone

NEUROTOXICITY RATING

Clinical

A Acute encephalopathy (CNS depression)

A Headache

Experimental

A CNS depression

Acetone, dimethyl ketone, is widely used as an industrial solvent; it is also a naturally occurring constituent of blood and urine. Acetone is a volatile liquid at room temperature and has a distinctive sweet pungent odor. It is considered to be a low hazard because few adverse health effects are reported despite its wide use. It is an eye and mucous membrane irritant at levels of 500 ppm; at very high concentrations (12,000 ppm), it causes CNS depression. The U.S. 1991 time-wieghted Threshold Limit Value is 750 ppm.

The minimal lethal concentration for rats is 16,000 ppm for 4 h, and 46,000 ppm for mice at 1 h. Rats exposed to 10,000 ppm for 4 h/day for 10 days show slowed behavior, but no changes are detectable on histopathological examination (4). The anesthetic concentration for mice is 99 mg/ml. It is alleged that acetone can potentiate the toxic effect of other substances; reported effects include enhancement of the ethanol-induced loss of righting reflex in mice by reducing the rate of elimination of alcohol; and potentiation of acrylonitrile toxicity by altering the rate of cyanide generation (1,3,4). It is also claimed that acetone can potentiate the neurotoxicity of *n*-hexane by altering the toxicokinetics of its 2,5-hexanedione metabolite (5).

Humans receiving a single, short-term, high-level inhalation exposure rapidly exhale the inspired acetone; there is almost no plasma retention 2 h later. Large single doses are predominantly excreted unchanged in expired air; smaller repeated doses are metabolized to carbon dioxide. Repeated controlled exposures for 4 h/day for 5 days cause retention of acetone and persistent detectable levels 16 h later. These results suggest that repeated exposures during the work week may lead to bioaccumulation (6).

Several meticulous, controlled, human studies of inhalation at levels of 250 ppm for 4 h over a 4-day period and 500 ppm for 6 h daily for 6 days indicate that acetone may cause mild neurobehavioral effects at these levels. Effects include increased visual reaction time and poor auditory tone perception; these effects were not seen in the same group exposed to similar levels of methyl ethyl ketone (2).

Uncontrolled exposure to 1000 ppm for 3 h daily for 7 years is reported to cause headache, light headedness, fatigue, and respiratory tract irritation. High-level exposures (12,000 ppm for 3 h) in the occupational setting are associated with light headedness, headache, somnolence, and malaise (7). Ingestion of 200 ml of acetone produced stupor and respiratory depression in a 42 year-old male; he recovered.

REFERENCES

1. Cunningham J, Sharkawi M, Plaa G (1989) Pharmacological and metabolic interactions between ethanol and methyl *n*-butyl ketone, methyl isobutyl ketone, methyl ethyl ketone, or acetone in mice. *Fund Appl Toxicol* 13, 102.
2. Dick RB, Setzer JV, Taylor BJ *et al.* (1989) Neurobehavioural effects of short duration exposures to acetone and methyl ethyl ketone. *Brit J Ind Med* 46, 111.
3. Freeman JJ, Hayes EP (1988) Microsomal metabolism of acetonitrile to cyanide: Effects of acetone and other compounds. *Biochem Pharmacol* 37, 1153.

4. Krasavage WJ, O'Donoghue JL, DiVincenzo GD (1982) Ketones. In: *Patty's Industrial Hygiene and Toxicology. Vol 11C*. Clayton GD, Clayton FE eds. John Wiley, New York p. 4709.
5. Ladefofoged O, Perbellini L (1987) Acetone-induced changes in the toxicokinetics of 2,5-hexanedione in rabbits. *Scand J Work Environ Health* 12, 627.
6. Parmeggiani L, Sassi C (1954) Occupational poisoning with acetone—clinical disturbances, investigations in workrooms and physiopathological research. *Med Lav* 45, 431.
7. Ross DS (1973) Short communications—acute acetone intoxication involving eight male workers. *Ann Occup Hyg* 16, 73.

Acetyl Ethyl Tetramethyl Tetralin

Peter S. Spencer

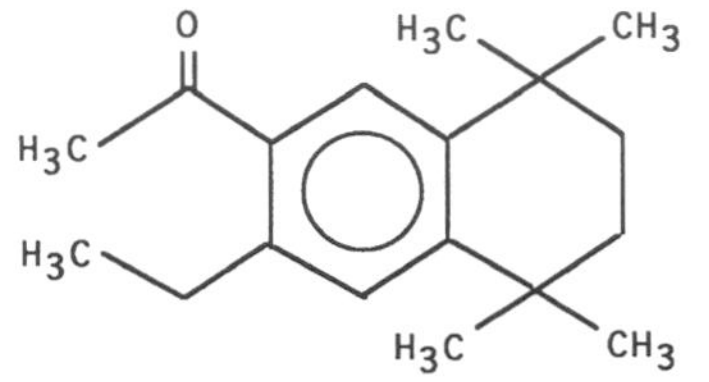

ACETYL ETHYL TETRAMETHYL TETRALIN
$C_{18}H_{26}O$

1,1,4,4-Tetramethyl-6-ethyl-7-acetyl-1,2,3,4-tetrahydronaphthalene; Musk tetralin; Polycyclic musk

NEUROTOXICITY RATING

Experimental

A Neuronal ceroid lipofuscinosis
A Sensorimotor neuropathy

Acetyl ethyl tetramethyl tetralin (AETT) is a tetralin musk that was widely used between 1955 and 1977 as a musky fixative in soap perfumes; as an ingredient of colognes, creams, aftershave lotions, perfumes, and detergents; and as an odor-masking agent in so-called unscented products. Industry-estimated concentrations of AETT in commercial products ranged from 0.002%–0.05%; one fragrance product contained 0.95% AETT. The Council of Europe (8) also sanctioned AETT as an artificial flavoring substance that could be added temporarily to foodstuffs without hazard to human health. Worldwide production in 1977 by U.S., Swiss, and Japanese manufacturers was estimated at 0.75 million lb, placing the compound among the "large-volume"-selling musks (1). Approximately 100,000 lb/year of AETT were used in the United States prior to 1977. The experimental chromogenic and neurotoxic properties of AETT, discovered in 1975, are described in the first edition of this text (18). Chromogenicity refers to the blue discoloration of tissues (including brain, spinal cord, and peripheral nerves) found in animals treated with single or repeated doses of AETT or a number of chemically related compounds (*see* Diethylbenzene, Table 9) (18).

General Toxicology

AETT can be manufactured from ethylbenzene and 2,5-dichloro-2,3-dimethylhexane (18). It is a white, crystalline compound with a MW of 258.41, a MP of 43°C, and a BP of 130°C. It is practically insoluble in water, 55% soluble in alcohol, 10% in vegetable oil, and 62% in diethyl phthalate. The odor of AETT is described as sweet and distinctly musky; it is chemically unrelated to natural and most synthetic (nitro) musks (18).

Judged by the appearance of blue tissue coloration after repeated dosing, AETT is apparently absorbed from the skin and gut of rats, and from the skin of mice, hamsters, and guinea pigs (18). A blue discoloration apparently is not produced by the application of AETT to the shaven skin of rabbits; this cannot be interpreted as due to lack of penetration, since the chromogenic metabolite of AETT may not be generated in this species. Application of ^{14}C-AETT to human skin resulted in the appearance of radioactive label in urine, and skin application, ingestion, or inhalation of tetralin or tetralin-containing materials caused green-colored urine to be excreted (4,5,17).

A single unpublished study examined the pharmacokinetics of ^{14}C-AETT (18). This reportedly demonstrated that label from AETT, given intraperitoneally or intravenously to rats, is rapidly distributed to tissues including the CNS, and later redistributed primarily *via* the liver to the gastrointestinal tract. Excretion after a single intravenous dose was slow and primarily *via* the feces. About 50% of the administered dose was excreted by 48 h and approximately 62% by 120 h. Of the total eliminated, only 15%–20% was routed *via* urine. AETT and the chomogenic metabolite of AETT were reportedly identified in brain and liver tissue, but most of the radiolabel was found in more polar, unidentified metabolites. Whole-body autoradiography with ^{14}C-AETT reportedly showed a wide distribution of label with concentration in lipid-rich areas. Cerebrum, cerebellum, pons, medulla oblongata, Vth cranial nerve, and spinal cord contained label (18).

AETT is one of several monocyclic and dicyclic hydrocarbons with chromogenic potential (see Diethylbenzene, Table 9). This remarkable phenomenon appears to be directly related to the neurotoxic properties of the two chromogenic agents (AETT and 1,2-diethylbenzene) that have been subjected to experimental scrutiny (12,13,18). Both are metabolized to more active 1,2-diacetyl derivatives that form blue pigments on contact with biological tissue. The 1,2-diacetyl derivative of AETT forms a blue color with amino acids, peptides, some proteins, and tissue (18); apparently, the pigment displays a yellow color at a pH >7.5 (2). Structure-activity considerations suggested the possibility that the 1,2-diacetyl moiety forms "ninhydrin-like" triketoindane compounds that react with amino groups to form Ruhemann's purple (18). However, the recent demonstration that 1,2-diacetylbenzene induces proximal giant axonal swellings filled with neurofilaments suggests that the compound reacts with amino acids in a manner equivalent to aliphatic γ-diketones that form 2,5-dimethylpyrrole adducts with neurofilament and other proteins (see n-Hexane, Metabolites and Derivatives). Contrary to earlier reports, this would indicate that a primary axonal lesion is responsible for the prominent demyelination seen in AETT-treated animals.

AETT is a derivative of tetralin (tetrahydronaphthalene), a colorless liquid used in various industrial solvent applications. Sparse information is available on the metabolism of tetralin in humans, but data are published for several laboratory animals. One species, the rabbit, is relatively refractory to the generation of blue pigment following exposure to tetralin or AETT. Adult doe albino rabbits, treated by gavage with 3.4 mmol/kg ^{14}C-tetralin, excreted a number of conjugated metabolites (10). The major metabolite, 1,2,3,4-tetrahydro-1-naphthol (α-tetralol), accounted for approximately 50% of the administered dose; other conjugated metabolites included 1,2,3,4-tetrahydro-2-naphthol (β-tetralol, 25%), 4-hydroxy-α-tetralone (6%), cis-tetralin-1,2-diol (0.4%) and trans-tetralin-1,2-diol (0.6%). Sulfate conjugates comprised 12% of the dose. Approximately 90% of the dose was excreted in urine within 2 days; another 0.6%–1.8% was found in feces, and <0.2% was identified in expired breath (10). 4-Hydroxytetralone was found as one intermediate metabolite (10). A woman who deliberately ingested 250 ml of a material containing tetralin (31.5%), paraffin oil (52.7%), acetone (15.7%), and copper oleate (0.03%) excreted green-gray urine during the 24-h period after hospital admission: nonconjugated α-tetralol, tetralin, and an unidentified metabolite were found in urine together with glucuronides of 1,2,3,4-tetrahydro-1-naphthol and β-tetralol (10).

Animal Studies

Blue discoloration of tissues is produced in rats following intraperitoneal (i.p.) injection of AETT (30 mg/kg, body weight); in rabbits, daily doses up to 500 mg/kg by the same route were ineffective. Blue-colored urine (but not blue tissue coloration) was seen in a monkey receiving 50 mg/kg/day orally for 16 days, a dose sufficient to turn organs of a susceptible species blue within 3 days (18).

The acute oral LD_{50} for AETT in the mouse is 800 mg/kg body weight. For AETT in ethanol (10% w/v), the LD_{50} for the female rat is 316 mg/kg (oral), 126 mg/kg (i.p.) and 584 mg/kg (unoccluded percutaneous). Characteristically, signs of acute toxicity are manifested by hyperexcitability, depression, and progressive tremors, in that order. Around the LD_{50}, death is usually delayed between 2 and 7 days after treatment. However, the typical blue coloration of the CNS and other internal organs can be detected in rats within 24 h of a single LD_{50} dose. Based on a comparison of intraperitoneal LD_{50} doses, species differences representing increased sensitivity to AETT exist as follows: rats > mouse = hamster > guinea pig > rabbit > monkey (18).

AETT is a cumulative neurotoxin in rats; it produces a characteristic panoply of functional and neuropathological changes that develop as a function of dose (18–20). Female rats are more susceptible than males; the rat fetus reportedly fails to develop blue discoloration although maternal tissues turn blue (18). Hyperirritability with biting—also reported in guinea pigs treated with 2-(N,N-dipropyl)-amino-5,6-dihydroxytetralin (7)—is the first sign of neurotoxicity in the adult rat. This was reported in female rats receiving products containing topical doses of AETT as low as 0.1 mg/kg/day, 5 days/week for periods up to 26 weeks. Blue coloration of organs, including the brain, spinal and peripheral nerves, is seen in female rats treated with topical doses of AETT of 1.8 mg/kg/day, 5 days/week for periods up to 26 weeks. With increasing dosage, the blue coloration intensifies; it is consistently observed at doses above 3 mg/kg/day. Gray matter is more discolored than white matter; regions such as spinal ganglia (densely colored) stand out in relief against adjacent tissues. Neuropathological changes appear in rats receiving topical applications in excess of 3 mg/kg/day; these changes consist of abnormally pigmented neurons located in the hypoglossal nucleus (19,20). Concurrent with the appearance of neuronal lipopigmentation, animals develop a peculiar, intermittent back arching. A learning disability is reported in AETT-treated rats (11). Treatment with higher levels of AETT results in gait abnormalities which, with time, progress to ataxia, limb weakness, foot-drop, and eversion of the hindfeet. These neurological signs appear to correspond to the onset of extensive CNS and PNS nerve fiber changes and prominent degeneration of Purkinje cells (1,19,20). Extending the duration of AETT treatment causes little additional functional deficit, probably because denuded axon segments become remyelinated while other fibers undergo demyelination (20). However, the color of nervous tissues changes from blue to green-gray. The coloration of tissue slowly dissipates on cessation of intoxication, but functional and neuropathological changes persist at least for several months.

AETT promotes the formation of lipopigments in neurons and glial cells (prior to demyelination). Neuronal pigments are similar to those encountered in human ceroid lipofuscinosis (15). The most widespread type of neuronal lipopigment granule, occurring early in the AETT-induced disorder and increasing in number with time, stains light brown with hematoxylin and eosin, pinkish red with Schmorl's reagent, and dark blue in epoxy sections stained with toluidine blue. These cytosomes are also periodic acid-Schiff–positive, strongly acid-fast, and display primary autofluorescence at 460 nm. They are found in most neurons but are exceptionally prominent in pyramidal cells of the entorhinal cortex, especially the olfactory tubercles, hypoglossal nuclei, anterior horns of the spinal cord, and sensory neurons of dorsal root ganglia. Ultrastructurally, the cytosomes are surrounded by a single membrane and display a dense matrix containing lamellar profiles. A second type of abnormal neuronal inclusion is large and sometimes occupies much of the cytoplasmic area. These stain bright red with hematoxylin and eosin; they appear to be located not only in intact neurons but also in proximity to degenerating neurons or free in the tissue. Ultrastructurally, the inclusions are composed of dense, granular material, lacking a limiting membrane and punctuated by small, clear areas of cytoplasm. Clumps of dense material, found free in the cytoplasm adjacent to nodular protrusions of the dense, central mass, may fuse with the latter (18–20). Comparable electron-dense masses have been reported in human motor neuron diseases, where they are known as Bunina bodies (14).

Demyelination commences with splitting of the myelin sheath at the intraperiod line and is followed by the accumulation of edema fluid, which causes the formation of myelin "bubbles." In the spinal cord and medulla oblongata, myelin bubbling is symmetrical and develops first in large-diameter fibers in a ventral locus and spreads to other areas with time. In the PNS, myelin bubbling first affects large-diameter fibers in ventral roots where it is consistently restricted to one side of the root fascicle. Later, peripheral nerves develop similar changes. Examination of single myelinated fibers demonstrated that myelin bubbling is segmental (internodal) and scattered multifocally. Phagocytes crowd blood vessels and strip myelin from damaged internodes leaving shrunken axon segments. After the phagocytes have removed parts of the myelin sheath, the denuded axons become associated with Schwann cells and undergo remyelination with the formation of thin, foreshortened stretches of myelin (18,19). The ability of Schwann cells to form columns after nerve-fiber degeneration and to elaborate new myelin sheaths around demyelinated and regenerating axons indicates these functions are not substantially affected by AETT (21).

In Vitro Studies

Percutaneous absorption studies performed *in vitro* with fuzzy rat skin demonstrated that ^{14}C-AETT was metabolized at 2.5 pmol/min/mg protein; 1.9% of the absorbed metabolite was found in two peaks of unknown identity (3).

The purified chromogenic metabolite of AETT (presumably, the 1,2-diacetyl derivative) turned rat and rabbit brain dark blue *in vitro* at levels as low as 0.1% (w/v). Both AETT and its chromogenic metabolite uncouple oxidative phosphorylation in rat liver and brain mitochondria (6). Neither compound inhibits the enzyme activity of carbonic anhydrase in rat brain homogenates (6).

Human Studies

Despite the former widespread use of AETT in soaps and cosmetics, there are no known reports of tissue discoloration or neurological disease in association with exposure to AETT in these products. However, human exposure to the parent compound, tetralin, a primary skin irritant, has been associated both with excretion of green-colored urine and symptoms in part referable to the nervous system. A man excreted green urine after ingestion of 5.7 g of a pigment called di-tetralin (17). A woman excreted green-gray urine within approximately 1 day of ingesting approximately 250 ml of an ectoparasiticide containing 31.5% tetralin (9). Hospitalized patients on a ward with a floor that had been waxed with a tetralin-based polish experienced eye irritation, headache, nausea, diarrhea, and green urine (3,16). Two painters using tetralin-containing varnishes under conditions of poor ventilation had characteristic "tetralin urine"; these workers experienced mucous membrane irritation, profuse lacrimation, headache, and stupor (3,16).

Toxic Mechanisms

The chromogenic properties of AETT and its ability upon repeated exposure to induce ceroid-like lipofuscinosis appear to be closely related properties. Substitution of one ethyl group for a methyl group on the benzene ring of AETT abolishes both the chromogenic and neurotoxic actions (18).

The proposal that the chromogenic and neurotoxic properties of AETT result from biotransformation to an active 1,2-diacetyl metabolite receives substantial support from the observation that 1,2-diacetylbenzene is both a direct-acting chromogen and a cumulative neurotoxin that induces a sensorimotor and cranial neuropathy in rats (12,13) (see Diethylbenzene).

The prominent demyelination of central and peripheral axons in AETT-treated animals may be secondary to axonal disease. The ability of Schwann cells to form columns after nerve-fiber degeneration and to elaborate new myelin sheaths around demyelinated and regenerating axons indicate these functions are not substantially affected by AETT (21).

REFERENCES

1. Akasaki Y, Takeuchi S, Miyoshi K (1990) Cerebellar degeneration induced by acetyl-ethyl-tetramethyl-tetralin (AETT) *Acta Neuropathol* **80**, 129.
2. Arctander S (1969) No. 3080 Versalide. In: *Perfume and Flavor Chemicals (Aroma Chemicals)*, edited and published by Arctander S, Montclair, NJ.
3. Bronaugh RL, Stewart RF, Storm JF (1989) Extent of cutaneous metabolism during percutaneous absorption of xenobiotics. *Toxicol Appl Pharmacol* **99**, 524.
4. Browning E (1965) Aromatic hydrocarbons. II Tetralin. In: *Toxicity and Metabolism of Industrial Solvents*. Elsevier, New York p. 119.
5. Browning E (1965) *Toxic Solvents*. Edward Arnold, London p. 44.
6. Cammer W (1980) Toxic demyelination: biochemical studies and hypothetical mechanisms. In: *Experimental and Clinical Neurotoxicology*. Spencer PS, Schaumburg HH eds. Williams & Wilkins, Baltimore p. 239.
7. Costall B, DeSouza CX, Naylor RJ (1980) Topographical analysis of the actions of 2-(N,N-dipropyl)amino-5,6-dihydroxy-tetralin to cause biting behavior and locomotor hyperactivity from the striatum of the guinea-pig. *Neuropharmacology* **19**, 623.
8. Council of Europe (1974) Natural flavoring substances. Partial agreement in the social and public health field. *Council of Europe*. Strasbourg, List 2, No. 2320, p. 328.
9. Drayer DE, Reidenberg MM (1979) Metabolism of tetralin and toxicity of Cuprex in man. *Drug Metab Disposition* **1**, 577.
10. Elliott TH, Hanam J (1968) The metabolism of tetralin. *Biochem J* **108**, 551.
11. Furuhashi A, Akasaki Y, Sato M, Miyoshi K (1994) Effects of AETT-induced neuronal ceroid lipofuscinosis on learning ability in rats. *Jpn J Psychiat Neurol* **48**, 645.
12. Gagnaire F, Becker MN, Marignac B *et al.* (1992) Diethylbenzene inhalation-induced electrophysiological deficits in peripheral nerves and changes in brainstem auditory potentials in rats. *J Appl Toxicol* **12**, 335.
13. Gagnaire F, Ensminger A, Marignac B, De Ceaurriz J (1991) Possible involvement of 1,2-diacetylbenzene in diethylbenzene-induced neuropathy in rats. *J Appl Toxicol* **11**, 262.
14. Hart MN, Cancilla PA, Frommes S, Hirano A (1977) Anterior horn cell degeneration and Bunina-type inclusions associated with dementia. *Acta Neuropathol* **38**, 225.
15. Horoupian DS, Ross RT (1977) Pigment variant of neuronal ceroid lipofuscinosis (Kuf's disease). *Can J Neurol Sci* **4**, 67.
16. Longacre SL (1987) Tetralin. In: *Ethel Browning's Toxicity and Metabolism of Industrial Solvents. 2nd Ed. Vol 1. Hydrocarbons.* Snyder R ed. Elsevier, Amsterdam p. 143.
17. Pohl J, Rawicz M (1919) The fate of tetrahydronaphthalene (tetralin) in the animal body. *Z Physiol Chem* **104**, 95. [Cited in *Chem Abst* **13**, 2089].
18. Spencer PS, Foster V, Sterman AB, Horoupian D (1980) Acetyl ethyl tetramethyl tetralin. In: *Experimental and Clinical Neurotoxicology.* Spencer PS, Schaumburg HH eds. Williams and Wilkins, Baltimore p. 296.
19. Spencer PS, Sterman AB, Horoupian D *et al.* (1979) Neurotoxic changes in rats exposed to the fragrance compound acetyl ethyl tetramethyl tetralin. *Neurotoxicology* **1**, 221.
20. Spencer PS, Sterman AB, Horoupian D, Foulds MM (1979) Neurotoxic fragrance produces ceroid and myelin disease. *Science* **204**, 633.
21. Sterman AB, Spencer PS (1981) The pathogenesis of primary internodal demyelination produced by acetyl ethyl tetramethyl tetralin: Evidence for preserved Schwann cell somal function. *J Neuropathol Exp Neurol* **40**, 112.

3-Acetylpyridine

Hans Kolbe

3-ACETYLPYRIDINE
C₇H₇NO

Methyl pyridyl ketone; 1-(3-Pyridinyl)ethanone

NEUROTOXICITY RATING

Experimental

A   Seizure disorder

A   Multisystem neuronal degeneration

A   Anti-NADH agent

3-Acetylpyridine (3-AP) is a colorless liquid freely soluble in acids. After intraperitoneal or subcutaneous injection, it is readily absorbed and metabolized; there is no urinary excretion of 3-AP (4). *In vivo*, pyridine-3-methylcarbinol is formed by 3-AP reduction; this pharmacologically active metabolite of 3-AP is readily glucuronized (1). Another important 3-AP biotransformation is oxidation to nicotinic acid, which is excreted in the urine as N^1-methylnicotinamide, nicotinic acid, and nicotinamide (4). Studies with ^{14}C-labeled 3-AP showed that 30% of the label is eliminated as $^{14}CO_2$ and 44% is excreted in urine (4).

3-AP causes a distinctive pattern of lesions in the adrenal glands and neuraxis, with a high vulnerability of cells in the inferior olive and hippocampal CA3 and CA4 cells (2). Unlike 6-aminonicotinamide, another antagonist and nicotinamide, the primary target of 3-AP is the neuron; glial changes are secondary.

Wistar rats, treated with 65 mg/kg 3-AP intraperitoneally, develop a characteristic picture of intoxication within 24 h. This includes tremor, an unsteady and awkward gait with considerable swaying, hyperkinetic movements, a strange rolling behavior, and myoclonic jerks of the head and trunk. Fifty percent of the animals died between 3 and 7 days. Remaining animals recovered gradually (10); they presented with a conspicuous appearance: there were ataxia with a broad-based gait, hyperkinesis, and paroxysmal cramp-like events with hypertonia. Rats showed abnormal behavior, tremors, and seizures, with spikes and waves in the electroencephalogram (12).

As early as 6 h after 3-AP application, there is a characteristic pattern of brain lesions (3). Marked degeneration is found in the inferior olive, with near-total loss of climb-ing fibers normally projecting from this structure into the cerebellum. Caudal parts of the olive remain relatively undamaged. Marked degenerative changes are seen in the substantia nigra, pars compacta, and, occasionally, in the pars reticulata and the ventral tegmental area. The damage to nigral neurons is most prominent medially in pars compacta; remaining neurons are shrunken and spindle-shaped even 1 year after the intoxication. In the caudate-putamen, degeneration is seen 24 h after 3-AP, without any damage to neuronal perikarya. A few cells degenerate in the neighboring entopeduncular nucleus. In hippocampal and entorhinal cortex, degeneration in the granular layer of the dentate gyrus starts 6 h after 3-AP injection. In the following hours, a distinctive pattern of degeneration develops along the septotemporal axis of the dentate gyrus, with the greatest proportion of damaged granular cells ventrally (3). Degenerating CA3-4 cells have been reported previously after injection of 3-AP (13). In several other brain regions, cell death occurs selectively after 3-AP. There is damage to the cholinergic neurons of the hypoglossal nucleus, but also in nucleus ambiguus, dorsal motor nucleus, nucleus intercalatus, nucleus dorsalis raphe, interpeduncular nucleus, and entopeduncular nucleus. A few degenerating neurons are observed in the nucleii of the basal forebrain and, inconsistently, in the hypothalamus (3).

These data show a consistent pattern of degeneration 6–48 h after injection of 3-AP. Thus, 3-AP causes much more than just selective chemical "olivectomy," as previously proposed (17). The consequences are more widespread. Clinical phenomenology and morphological pattern of cell lesions with loss of climbing fiber input to the cerebellum and degeneration of the nigrostriatal dopamine system suggest that 3-AP intoxication may provide a useful model for olivopontocerebellar atrophy. Both have many functional and morphological features in common (11,16). That some of the effects of 3-AP can be abolished by the subsequent injection of nicotinamide (17) led to the suggestion that the 3-AP–induced CNS lesions represent an accelerated picture of nicotinamide deficiency.

The antagonistic action of 3-AP on nicotinamide is caused by production of the abnormal compounds 3-acetylpyridine-adenine-dinucleotide (3-APAD) and 3-acetylpyridine-adenine-dinucleotide phosphate (3-APADP) (8). Of the two, 3-APAD is toxicologically less important because it does not lose its ability to act as a hydrogen receptor donor in nicotinamide-adenine dinucleotide (NAD)-dependent dehydrogenase reactions. Inhibition of metabolic pathways is therefore unlikely by this false cofactor (7). Higher concentrations of 3-APADP, reflecting an effective exchange of nicotinamide and 3-AP, were found in brain regions with high activity of nicotinamide-adenine-dinucleotide phosphate (NADP)-glycohydrolase [E.C. 3.2.2.5] and led to marked neuronal degeneration. In distant cell populations, the proportion of 3-AP–containing dinucleotide is 50% of the total dinucleotide content (20). This could be of considerable functional consequence because the K_m value for 3-APADP in NADP-dependent oxidoreductase is one order of magnitude higher than the K_m for NADP. Because of the widespread functional involvement of NADP-dependent oxidoreductases in many important metabolic processes, the physiological consequences are remarkable and widespread (6).

A decreased reaction velocity of NADP-dependent dehydrogenases in the presence of the NADP analogue, 3-APADP, could lead to functional disturbances in susceptible neurons. Metabolic turnover is slowed at the isocitrate dehydrogenase step of the Krebs cycle in the presence of 3-APADP. The K_m of 3-AP at this enzyme step is 2×10^{-4} as compared to 2×10^{-5} with the natural coenzyme NADP (9). This could explain the lower levels of amino acid neurotransmitters (aspartate and homocystic acid, mainly) in the presence of 3-AP. A diminished precursor pool of aspartate was discussed by one group (18). Aspartate is probably the neurotransmitter released from synaptic terminals of the olivocerebellar climbing fibers to the Purkinje cells. 3-AP treatment reduces the stimulated release of aspartate by 40% in slices of cerebellar hemispheres (19).

The conversion of hydrofolic acid to tetrahydrofolic acid by NADH-dependent dihydrofolate reductase [E.C. 1.5.1.3] is decreased by 50% if NADPH is replaced by 3-APADP (9). The first two steps of one of the two main metabolic pathways of glucose are NADP-dependent. In the pentose phosphate pathway, glucose-6-phosphate dehydrogenase and 6-phosphogluconate-dehydrogenase are not only dependent on the coenzyme NADP, they are also important providers of NADPH for synthetic processes. 3-AP reduces the metabolic flow through this pathway to one-sixth of normal values (9), with many consequences to other metabolic processes. The decreased hydrogen transfer of these dehydrogenases in the presence of 3-APADP lowers the efficacy of reductases in general (4). A marked decrease of glutathione reductase [E.C. 1.6.4.2] has been observed (9). As a consequence of this specific inhibition of dehydrogenases, glucose metabolism is heavily disturbed in brain regions of inferior olive, hippocampus, and basal ganglia with high metabolic activity (5,14).

Despite its widespread systemic metabolic effects, 3-AP is remarkably selective in inducing a distinct pattern of brain damage similar to multisystem atrophy (olivoponto-cerebellar type) (11). Main targets of toxicity are the inferior olive; the nigrostriatal system; and cell populations in basal forebrain, hypothalamus, and the brain stem (2).

Most interesting is the damaging action of 3-AP on nigrostriatal cells. It is mainly directed toward dopaminergic cells projecting to the dorsolateral ("motor") striatum, comparable to the pattern of damage caused by another pyridine neurotoxin, 1-methyl-4-phenyl-1,2,3,6-tetrahydro-pyridine.

The selective vulnerability of these brain areas toward 3-AP results from local peculiarities: A high activity of glucohydrolase leads to a specially effective synthesis of the false coenzyme 3-APADP. A high metabolic activity (i.e., carbohydrate metabolism) reveals the functional impairment of NADP-dependent dehydrogenases in the presence of 3-APADP. Because of the widespread functional involvement of these enzymes and the importance of reduced pyridine dinucleotide phosphate for synthetic processes (15), functional impairment, up to cell death, occurs readily and early in these active cell populations. Transmitter functions closely related to carbohydrate metabolism are especially disturbed.

REFERENCES

1. Anderson BM, Ciotti CJ, Kaplan NO (1958) Chemical properties of 3-substituted pyridine nucleotide. *J Biol Chem* 234, 1219.
2. Anderson WA, Flumerfelt BA (1980) A light and electron microscopic study of the effects of 3-acetylpyridine intoxication on the inferior olivary complex and cerebellar cortex. *J Comp Neurol* 190, 157.
3. Balaban CD (1985) Central neurotoxic effects of intraperitoneally administered 3-acetyl-pyridine, harmaline and niacinamide in Sprague-Dawley and Long-Evans rats: A critical review of central 3-acetylpyridine neurotoxicity. *Brain Res Rev* 9, 21.
4. Beher WT, Baker GD, Madoff M (1959) Studies of antimetabolites. V. Metabolism *in vivo* of 3-acetylpyridine. *J Biol Chem* 234, 2388.
5. Bernard JF, Buisseret-Delmas C, Laplante S (1984) Inferior olivary neurons: 3-Acetylpyridine effects on glucose consumption, axonal transport, electrical activity and harmaline-induced tremor. *Brain Res* 322, 382.
6. Brunneman A, Coper H (1964) Die aktivität NAD- und NADP-abhängiger Enzyme in verschiedenen Teilen des Rattengehirns. *Naunyn-Schmied Arch Exp Pathol Pharmakol* 246, 223.
7. Brunneman A, Coper H, Herken H (1963) Biosynthese von 3-Acetyl-pyridinadenindinucleotidphosphat (3-APADP) aus Nicotinamidadenindinucleotidphosphat. *Naunyn-Schmied Arch Exp Pathol Pharmakol* 245, 541.
8. Coper H, Herken H (1963) Schädigung des Zentralnervensystems durch Antimetabolite der Nikotinsäureamide.

Ein Beitrag zur Molekularpathologie der Pyridinnukleotide. *Deut Med Wochenschr* 88, 2025.

9. Coper H, Neubert D (1964) Einfluβ von NADP-Analogen auf die Reactionsgeschwindigkeit einiger NADP-bedürftiger Oxidoreduktasen. *Biochem Biophys Acta* 89, 23.

10. Denk H, Haider M, Kovac W, Syudynka G (1968) Verhaltensänderung und neuropathologie bei der 3-acetylpyridinvergiftung der Ratte. *Acta Neuropathol* 10, 34.

11. Deutch AY, Rosin DL, Goldstein M, Roth RH (1989) 3-Acetylpyridine-induced degeneration of the nigrostriatal dopamine system: an animal model of olivopontocerebellar atrophy-associated parkinsonism. *Exp Neurol* 105, 1.

12. Herken H (1968) Functional disorder of the brain induced by synthesis of nucleotides containing 3-acetylpyridine. *Z Klin Chem Klin Biochem* 6, 357.

13. Hicks SP (1955) Pathologic effects of antimetabolites. I. Acute lesions in the hypothalamus, peripheral ganglia and adrenal medulla caused by 3-acetylpyridine and prevented by nicotinamide. *Amer J Pathol* 31, 189.

14. Hotta SS (1962) Glucose metabolism in brain tissue. The hexose-monophosphate shunt and its role in glutathione reduction. *J Neurochem* 9, 43.

15. Kaplan NO, Ciotti MM (1956) Chemistry and properties of 3-acetylpyridine analog of diphosphopyridine nucleotide. *J Biol Chem* 221, 823.

16. Koeppen AH, Barron KD (1984) The neuropathology of olivopontocerebellar atrophy. In: *The Olivopontocerebellar Atrophies*. Duvoisin RC, Plaitakis A eds. Raven Press, New York p. 13.

17. Llinas R, Walton K, Hillman DE (1975) Inferior olive: Its role in motor learning. *Science* 190, 1230.

18. Nadi NS, Kanter D, McBride WJ, Aprison MH (1977) Effects of 3-acetylpyridine on several putative neurotransmitter amino acids in the cerebellum and the medulla of the rat. *J Neurochem* 28, 661.

19. Vollenweider FX, Cuenod M, Do KQ (1990) Effect of climbing fiber deprivation on release of endogenous aspartate, glutamate, and homocysteate in slices of cat cerebellar hemispheres and vermis. *J Neurochem* 54, 1533.

20. Willing H, Neuhoff V, Herken H (1964) Der Austausch von 3-Acetylpyridin gegen Nikotinsaureamid in den Pyridinnukleotiden verschiedener Hirnregionen. *Naunyn-Schmied Arch Exp Pathol Pharmakol* 247, 254.

Acetylsalicylic Acid

Peter C. Mabie

ACETYLSALICYLIC ACID
$C_9H_8O_4$

Aspirin; Salicylic acid acetate

NEUROTOXICITY RATING

Clinical

A   Acute encephalopathy (seizures, hallucinations)

A   Ototoxicity (tinnitus, hearing loss)

A   Teratogenicity (neonatal intracranial hemorrhage)

Experimental

A   Uncouples oxidative phosphorylation

Acetylsalicylic acid (aspirin), the synthetic derivative of salicylic acid, is one of the most widely used medications; it is the prototypical nonopioid analgesic, antipyretic, and anti-inflammatory agent. Inhibition of the prostaglandin biosynthetic enzyme cyclooxygenase is thought to be the primary therapeutic mechanism (10,22). Aspirin is supplied in numerous oral formulations, including buffered, effervescent, enteric-coated, and in combination with opioid analgesics, antihistamines, cough suppressants, and other medications; rectal preparations are also available. Salicylic acid is used topically to treat skin disorders such as warts and psoriasis. Aspirin toxicity is common from deliberate self-poisoning and accidental excessive administration (3,14,17,19). Severe aspirin toxicity has been likened to a pseudosepsis syndrome with multisystem failure (12). The neurological manifestations are encephalopathy, tinnitus, hearing loss, and neurogenic hyperventilation (3,10,14,17,19). Although intentional overdose of aspirin occurs most commonly, the morbidity and mortality of unintentional overdose probably exceed that of intentional overdose (3).

Orally administered aspirin is rapidly absorbed from the stomach and upper small intestine, with plasma salicylate levels peaking 1–3 h after a single therapeutic dose, depending on dosage form, gastric contents, gastric-emptying time, and gastric pH (1,6,10). After a large oral overdose, blood levels may continue to rise for 24 h (8). Rectal absorption is slower and less reliable than that from oral administration. Significant transdermal absorption may occur following extensive cutaneous application (5). Aspirin is hydrolyzed in the gastrointestinal mucosa and liver to salicylate, which binds to plasma proteins such as albumin, and is distributed throughout most body tissues and fluids, including cerebrospinal fluid. The half-life of aspirin in plasma is about 15 min, and the half-life of salicylate ranges from 2 h for low doses to up to 30 h for high doses (1,6,10). Systemic distribution of salicylate depends primarily on passive, pH-dependent processes; cerebrospinal salicylate elimination, in contrast, occurs *via* low-capacity, saturable active transport by the choroid plexus (1,6,10). Salicylate is primarily metabolized by the liver to salicyluric acid; salicyl phenolic glucuronide and salicyl acyl glucuronide are also formed, as are gentisic acid, gentisuric acid, 2,3-dihyroxybenzoic acid, and 2,3,5-trihyroxybenzoic acid. Salicylate and its hepatic metabolites are excreted in the urine in a dose- and pH-dependent manner. In humans with normal renal function, a single therapeutic dose is typically excreted within 72 h (1). Recommended therapeutic doses range from 80 mg to 8 g daily (10). Therapeutic concentrations range from below 60 mg/l to 300 mg/l for maximal anti-inflammatory effects (10).

There are multiple target sites for aspirin. The analgesic effect is likely mediated by inhibition of prostaglandin sensitization of peripheral pain receptors (16). An additional mechanism within the hypothalamus is suggested (1). The antipyretic effect is also thought to be due to inhibition of cyclooxygenase prostaglandin synthesis in the hypothalamus (1,10). As an antithrombotic agent, aspirin acts by reducing platelet aggregation by inhibiting the production of thromboxane A_2 (10). High doses of aspirin have been used to increase urinary excretion of uric acid.

In addition to its intended therapeutic effects, aspirin has physiological effects that become increasingly pronounced as salicylate plasma concentrations rise. Gastrointestinal effects are common, including nausea, dyspepsia, and gastric mucosal irritation and bleeding. The effects of aspirin on acid-base balance are complex, often resulting in mixed acid-base disorders. Aspirin directly stimulates the medullary respiratory center, resulting in neurogenic hyperventilation with respiratory alkalosis. Aspirin uncouples oxidative phosphorylation, resulting in increased carbon dioxide production in skeletal muscle, and compensatory increase in renal bicarbonate excretion (10). Metabolic acidosis (increased organic and inorganic acids) occurs secondary to salicylate interference with normal carbohydrate and amino acid metabolism coupled with renal dysfunction (1,14); in severe toxicity, there is life-threatening metabolic acidosis and respiratory depression with respiratory acidosis. Hyperpyrexia, pulmonary edema, hepatotoxicity, and renal failure occur with increasing salicylate levels (10). Tinnitus and hearing loss probably result from increased labyrinthine pressure (23) or a toxic effect on cochlear hair cells (14). Hearing loss usually occurs with plasma salicylate levels >200 mg/l and is reversible in almost all cases (1,15). The association between salicylate use during pregnancy and congenital abnormalities and/or fetal death remains unsubstantiated (1,4). A significant association has been found between maternal aspirin use and neonatal intracranial hemorrhage (18). The encephalopathy of aspirin toxicity has been postulated to be related to increased intracranial pressure (7). Reduced brain glucose with normal plasma glucose has been reported in a patient with salicylate poisoning (21). There is no evidence that aspirin has any direct toxic effect on the PNS.

Possible embryolethal and teratogenic effects of salicylate have been studied with rat whole-embryo cultures. Rat embryos cultured with 100–300 mg/l salicylate demonstrated decreased viability, diminished size, and severe dysmorphogenesis (11,20). Significant cell death within the developing neural tube has been reported (11).

Toxic exposure in humans occurs both following deliberate self-poisoning and as a result of repeated administration of therapeutic doses (3,14,17). Toxicity is common after a single dose of 100 mg/kg in children and 10 g in adults (2). In general, severity of toxicity correlates with the plasma salicylate level 6 h after ingestion: mild (300–500 mg/l), moderate (500–750 mg/l), and severe (>750 mg/l) (14). In cases of toxicity due to multiple doses, tinnitus and hearing loss are the most common symptoms (10). Additional manifestations, depending on severity, include visual complaints, headache, gastrointestinal upset, pulmonary edema, hyperpyrexia, and various signs of encephalopathy: confusion, agitation, lethargy, slurred speech, hallucinations, asterixis, electroencephalogram abnormalities, generalized seizures, and coma (1,3,14,17). Focal neurological deficits are rare (3). Acidosis increases salicylate levels in the cerebrospinal fluid (1,6). CNS salicylate concentration correlates with severity of encephalopathy and mortality (1). Young children are more susceptible to severe metabolic acidosis (17). Death may occur due to progression of multisystem abnormalities and development of vasomotor and respiratory depression (3,14,17). Toxicity following deliberate single-dose self-poisoning manifests with similar symptoms and signs that evolve more rapidly (3). There are similarities between salicylate toxicity and sepsis (12).

Reye's syndrome, consisting of toxic encephalopathy, hyperammonemia, and liver failure, is associated with aspirin use in children with varicella or influenza-like illnesses (1,10). Although the association between aspirin ingestion and Reye's syndrome is strong, the occasional incidence of

Reye's syndrome without aspirin ingestion suggests that aspirin does *not* cause Reye's syndrome (1).

The incidence of adult aspirin intoxication has declined over the past several decades as acetaminophen and alternative nonsteroidal anti-inflammatory agents have become more available. In children, accidental poisoning has also declined due to mandated child-resistant packages (14). Rare cases of toxicity have been reported following transdermal absorption of salicylate (5) and ingestion of candy containing methyl salicylate (9). Accidental salicylate intoxication is associated with increased age and underlying age-related medical conditions; diagnosis is often delayed, neurological abnormalities are common, and prognosis is guarded (3).

Optimal management of aspirin toxicity requires early diagnosis, preventing further absorption, correcting fluid, electrolyte, and acid-base derangements, and when moderate or severe, increasing elimination of salicylate. Rapid diagnosis requires a high index of suspicion, and should be suggested when a patient presents with encephalopathy, tachypnea, or acid-base abnormalities (3). To prevent additional aspirin absorption, gastric aspiration may be helpful up to 24 h after a large oral ingestion (13). Multiple doses of activated charcoal (50–100 g) may prevent absorption if given soon after ingestion, especially if enteric-coated or sustained-release formulations have been ingested (1). Fluid and electrolyte abnormalities, particularly hypokalemia, should be corrected. Bicarbonate, saline, and calcium should be administered judiciously as required. In patients without significant underlying cardiac or renal disease, forced alkaline diuresis, with a urine pH of 8.0–8.5, accelerates renal salicylate excretion; other fluid and electrolyte abnormalities should always be corrected first. Hemodialysis is indicated for patients with severe CNS toxicity or metabolic acidosis that does not improve with initial therapy (14,24).

REFERENCES

1. American Hospital Formulary Service Drug Information (1996) *Non-steroidal Anti-inflammatory Agents.* McEvoy GK ed. Amer Soc Health-Sys Pharmacol, Bethesda p. 1361.

2. American Medical Association (AMA) Drug Evaluations (1986) *General Analgesics. 6th Ed.* Lampe KE ed. AMA, Chicago p. 53.

3. Anderson RJ, Potts DE, Gabow PA *et al.* (1976) Unrecognized adult salicylate intoxication. *Ann Intern Med* **85**, 745.

4. Buchan PC, Macdonald HN (1979) Aspirin in pregnancy. *Lancet* **2**, 147.

5. Davies MG, Briffa D, Greaves MW (1979) Systemic toxicity from topically applied salicylic acid. *Brit Med J* **1**, 661.

6. Davison C (1971) Salicylate metabolism in man. *Ann N Y Acad Sci* **179**, 249.

7. Dove DJ, Jones T (1982) Delayed coma associated with salicylate intoxication. *J Pediatr* **100**, 493.

8. Ferguson RK, Boutros AR (1970) Death following self-poisoning with aspirin. *J Amer Med Assn* **213**, 1186.

9. Howrie DL, Moriarty R, Breit R (1985) Candy flavouring as a source of salicylate poisoning. *Pediatrics* **75**, 869.

10. Insel PA (1990) Analgesic-antipyretics and antiinflammatory agents; drugs employed in the treatment of rheumatoid arthritis and gout. In: *The Pharmacological Basis of Therapeutics. 8th Ed.* Gilman AG, Rall TW, Nies AS, Taylor P eds. Pergamon Press, New York p. 638.

11. Joschko MA, Dreosti IE, Tulsi RS (1993) The teratogenic effects of salicylic acid on the developing nervous sytem in rats *in vitro. Teratology* **48**, 105.

12. Leatherman JW, Schmitz PG (1991) Fever, hyperdynamic shock, and multiple-system failure. A pseudo-sepsis syndrome associated with chronic salicylate intoxication. *Chest* **100**, 1391.

13. Matthew H, Mackintosh TF, Tompsett SL, Cameron JC (1966) Gastric aspiration and lavage in acute poisoning. *Brit Med J* **1**, 1333.

14. Meredith TJ, Vale JA (1986) Non-narcotic analgesics. Problems of overdosage. *Drugs* **32**, 177.

15. Myers EN, Bernstein JM, Fostiropolous G (1965) Salicylate ototoxicity: A clinical study. *N Engl J Med* **273**, 587.

16. Perl ER (1976) Sensitization of nociceptors and its relation to sensation. In: *Advances in Pain Research and Therapy. Vol 1.* Bonica JJ, Albe-Fersard D eds. Raven Press, New York p. 17.

17. Proudfoot AT (1983) Toxicity of salicylates. *Amer J Med* **75** Suppl, 99.

18. Rumack CM, Guggenheim MA, Rumack BH *et al.* (1980) Neonatal intracranial hemmorhage and maternal use of aspirin. *Obstet Gynecol* **58**, 52S.

19. Ryder HW, Shaver M, Ferris EB (1945) Salicylism accompanied by respiratory alkalosis and toxic encephalopathy. *N Engl J Med* **232**, 617.

20. Spezia F, Fournex R, Vannier B (1992) Action of allopurinol and aspirin on rat whole-embryo cultures. *Toxicology* **72**, 239.

21. Thurston JH, Pollock PG, Warren SK, Jones EM (1970) Reduced brain glucose with normal plasma glucose in salicylate poisoning. *J Clin Invest* **49**, 2139.

22. Vane JR, Botting R (1987) Inflammation and the mechanism of action of anti-inflammatory drugs. *FASEB J* **1**, 89.

23. Waltner JG (1955) The effect of salicylates on the inner ear. *Ann Otol Rhinol Laryngol* **64**, 617.

24. Yip L, Dart RC, Gabow PA (1994) Concepts and controversies in salicylate toxicity. *Emerg Med Clin N Amer* **12**, 351.

Acivicin

Herbert H. Schaumburg

NEUROTOXICITY RATING

Clinical

A Acute encephalopathy (confusion, hallucinations)

Acivicin, a substituted isoxazole derived from fermentation of *Streptomyces sviceus*, is a glutamine antagonist that has been suggested as an antimetabolite cancer chemotherapy agent. The antitumor effect of acivicin is believed to be exerted by inhibition of glutamine-dependent synthetic enzymes and is associated with profound changes in intracellular glutathione metabolism; it also inhibits many key enzymes in pyrimidine biosynthesis. In preliminary clinical trials, it has not demonstrated striking advantages over existing agents, and there has been considerable myelosuppression and neurotoxicity.

Acivicin is rapidly absorbed and widely distributed following oral, subcutaneous, or intraperitoneal administration (6). It is probably transported across the blood-brain barrier by the large neutral amino acid carrier (1). Peak cerebrospinal levels occur 2 h following administration of an intravenous bolus. Metabolites have not been identified, and the mechanism of excretion is unclear. In the mouse, 53–83% is excreted by the kidney, and renal excretion exceeds creatinine clearance.

Myelosuppression is the most serious systemic undesired side effect. It is mild on single-dose schedules, more pronounced following a 72-h infusion, and dose-limiting when the drug is administered daily for 5 days. Both neutropenia and thrombocytopenia occur, and severity is proportional to the administered dose. Mild gastrointestinal distress also accompanies the 72-h infusion.

Acivicin administered to higher mammalian species (cat, dog, monkey) diffuses rapidly into the cerebrospinal fluid and is followed by behavioral changes, ataxia, and somnolence, held to be equivalent to the human neurotoxic reaction to this agent. A single intraperitoneal dose of 60 mg/kg in the cat causes ataxia within 1 h, followed by sedation for 2 days. Coadministration of an amino acid mixture lowers the level of acivicin in the spinal fluid to one-fifth of the usual post-acivicin level and prevents ataxia and somnolence (6). It is suggested that a similar strategy may prevent neurotoxicity in humans.

Human neurotoxicity occurs with all regimens, and severity is proportional to the plasma levels of acivicin; patients with plasma levels >2.5 μg/ml are particularly at risk (2,3,5–9). The response to a single dose is a reversible encephalopathy. At low doses (<75 mg/m^2), nightmares, confusion, and headaches occur; high doses are additionally accompanied by paranoia, vertigo, hallucinations, and ataxia. Administration by a 72-h infusion produces a similar constellation of symptoms; however, they are less intense and occur only at high doses. Concomitant intravenous infusion of a mixture of 16 amino acids reduces drug-induced neurotoxicity and allows the dose of acivicin to be escalated two-fold over previously tolerable doses (4).

REFERENCES

1. Chikhale EG, Chikhale PJ, Borchardt RT (1995) Carrier-mediated transport of the antitumor agent acivicin across the blood-brain barrier. *Biochem Pharmacol* 49, 941.
2. Earhart RH, Koeller JM, Davis TE *et al.* (1983) Phase I trial and pharmacokinetics of acivicin administered by 72-hour infusion. *Cancer Treatment Rep* 67, 683.
3. Falkson G, Cnaan A, Simson IW *et al.* (1990) A randomized phase II study of acivicin and 4'-deoxydoxorubicin in patients with hepatocellular carcinoma in an Eastern cooperative oncology group study. *Amer J Clin Oncol* 13, 510.
4. Hidalgo M, Rodriguez G, Kuhn JG *et al.* (1998) A Phase I and pharmacological study of the glutamine antagonist acivicin with the amino acid solution aminosyn in patients with advanced solid malignancies. *Clin Cancer Res* 4, 2763.
5. Maroun JA, Stewart DJ, Verma S *et al.* (1990) Phase I study of acivicin and cisplatin in non-small-cell lung cancer. A National Cancer Institute of Canada study. *Amer J Clin Oncol* 13, 401.
6. O'Dwyer PJ, Alonso MT, Leyland-Jones B (1984) Acivicin: A new glutamine antagonist in clinical trials. *J Clin Oncol* 2, 1064.
7. Taylor SA, Crowley J, Pollock TW *et al.* (1991) Objective antitumor activity of acivicin in patients with recurrent CNS malignancies: A Southwest Oncology Group trial. *J Clin Oncol* 9, 1476.
8. Williams MG, Earhart RH, Bailey H *et al.* (1990) Prevention of central nervous system toxicity of the antitumor antibiotic acivicin by concomitant infusion of an amino acid mixture. *Cancer Res* 50, 5475.
9. Willson JK, Fischer PH, Tutsch K *et al.* (1988) Phase I clinical trial of a combination of dipyridamole and acivicin based upon inhibition of nucleoside salvage. *Cancer Res* 48, 5585.

Aconitine

Peter S. Spencer

ACONITINE
$C_{34}H_{47}NO_{11}$

($1\alpha,3\alpha,6\alpha,14\alpha,15\alpha,16\beta$)-20-Ethyl-1,6,16-trimethoxy-4-(methoxymethyl)aconitane-3,8,13,14,15-pentol 8-acetate 14-benzoate

NEUROTOXICITY RATING

Clinical

A Ion channel syndrome (voltage-sensitive Na^+ channels)

B Acute encephalopathy (dystonia, confusion, death)

The family Ranunculaceae contains a number of exceptionally toxic herbaceous perennials, such as *Aconitum napellus* L. (monkshood), *A. vulparia* Reichb. ex Spreng (wolf's bane), and *Delphinium elatum* L. (larkspur) (3). The aconite plants contain C-19 and C-20 diterpene alkaloids that fall into two broad classes: the first has a common 4-ring system, with carbon atoms C-19 and C-20 forming a cyclic amine; the second has a 7-membered ring as the backbone, with carbon atoms C-17 and C-19 forming a heterocycle by connection to an amine. The majority of aconite alkaloids has the latter ring system, and the most important representative is aconitine (6).

Aconitum spp. have a long history of medicinal and homicidal use in Europe (5). The specific diterpene alkaloid pattern of more than 30 *Aconitum* spp. is available because of the widespread involvement of this genus in Chinese traditional and folk medicine (6). Commonly used for this purpose are the dried roots of *A. carmichaeli* Debx. and *A. kusnezoffii* Reichb., which contain aconitine in addition to four or five other diterpene alkaloids. Approximately 0.1% aconitine is found in *A. napellus* L., a cause of toxicity among humans and grazing animals in the western United States. The taste of this species is sweet at first, but is followed by tingling and numbness (4).

The mouse LD_{50} for aconitine is 0.22 mg/g (intravenously) (6). The high potency of aconitine and its analogs correlates with the presence of both an acetyl and a benzoyl group (9). Rats treated with aconite root extract at daily doses of 1.1 g/kg die within 3–6 days. Aconitine binds to site 2 of the Na^+ channels and suppresses their inactivation (1). Cardiotoxicity is also evident in rodents treated with aconitine, and arrhythmia in both mice and rats is associated with the presence of a benzoyl ester group (9). Anti-inflammatory and analgesic activity of aconitine alkaloids are also recognized (6).

Aconite is a potent, quick-acting poison in mammals (7); death may occur in humans and animals within hours after only a few milligrams. Most cases result from ingestion, but the toxin is also well absorbed through the skin and mucous nembranes. Humans exposed to a toxic dose orally develop burning and tingling sensations in the mouth and distal extremities, sweating, and a chilly sensation. Paresthesias spread to involve the whole body, the sensation in the mouth being that of numbness and coldness (anesthesia dolorosa). Nausea, vomiting, diarrhea, skeletal muscle paralysis, and intense pain may ensue (3). Changes in speech, visual impairment, anxiety, and chest pain are also reported (4). Abnormal electrocardiographic signs include arrhythmia, ventricular tremor, atrioventricular block, and myocardial damage (8). Death takes place through cardiac or respiratory failure; consciousness is maintained until expiration occurs.

Specific treatment for aconite poisoning is unavailable, and the prognosis is poor. Treatment is focused on removing the poison from the stomach by way of induced vomiting, gastric lavage, and activated charcoal. Cardiac and respiratory support may be needed (3).

Three groups of Aconitum alkaloids are recognized. Members of one group, which is characterized by two ester bonds at the diterpene skeleton, activate voltage-dependent Na^+ channels and inhibit noradrenaline uptake. Members of the second group of less potent monoesters block voltage-dependent sodium channels and have antinociceptive, antiarrhythmic and antiepileptiform properties. A third group reportedly has antiarrhythmic actions but is inactive on neurons (1).

REFERENCES

1. Ameri A (1998) The effects of Aconitum alkaloids on the central nervous system. *Prog Neurobiol* **56**, 211.
2. Druckrey H (1943/44) Todliche medizinale Aconitin-Vergiftung. *Samml Vergiftungsfallen* **13**, 21.
3. Frohne D, Pfander HJ. *A Color Atlas of Poisonous Plants. A Handbook for Pharmacists, Doctors, Toxicologists, and Biologists.* Wolfe, London p. 178.

4. Kingsbury JM (1964) *Poisonous Plants of the United States and Canada.* Prentice Hall, Englewood Cliffs, NJ p. 127.
5. Le Strange R (1977) *A History of Herbal Plants.* Angus and Robertson, UK.
6. Tang W, Eisenbrand G (1992) *Aconitum* spp. In: *Chinese Drugs of Plant Origin. Chemistry, Pharmacology and Uses in Traditional and Modern Medicine.* Springer-Verlag, Berlin p. 19.
7. Trease GE, Evans WC (1978) *Pharmacognosy. 11th Ed.* Cassell & Collier Macmillan, London p. 617.
8. Yang OH (1985) Poisoning of *Aconitum* species and its prevention and treatment. *Chin J Integr Trad West Med* 5, 511.
9. Zhou YP, Liu WH, Zeng GY *et al.* (1984) Toxicity of aconitine and its analogs and their effects on cardiac contractile function. *Acta Pharmacol Sin* 19, 641.

CASE REPORT

Druckrey (2) provides the following graphic description of a case of aconitine poisoning:

A few minutes after taking the powder, the patient became violently ill; agonizing vomiting was soon followed by diarrhea . . . 10 minutes after taking the powder the patient complained of severe pains in the head, neck, and back, and especially that "his heart was painful", and also that his eyesight had gone. The pains were so severe that the patient's cries could be heard through the whole house. When the woman was telephoning the doctor, the latter heard the screaming through the telephone even though it was situated on another floor . . . two hours after taking the powder, the patient died in hospital.

Acromelic Acid

Albert C. Ludolph

NEUROTOXICITY RATING

Experimental

A   Neuronopathy (spinal cord interneurons)

A   Seizure disorder

A   Excitotoxin

Acromelic acid A and B (ACRO-A and ACRO-B) are naturally occuring cyclic amino acids and depolarizing kainate analogues derived from the mushroom *Clitocybe acromelalga* (1,2). Despite pharmacological similarities, administration of the A isomer to experimental animals causes a neurological illness unlike that of kainate. When administered systemically (5 mg/kg body weight), rats initially display tonic extension, and cramps of hindlimbs followed by generalized seizures. If animals survive these convulsions, they may develop initially flaccid and, eventually, spastic paraparesis accompanied by increased muscle tone (4). Animals dying during seizures do not exhibit any CNS pathology. Surviving rats have selective lesions of small interneurons in the lumbosacral spinal cord with sparing of anterior horn cells; in contrast, reactive astrocytes are detected in the hippocampal CA4 region and stratum moleculare/lacunare (4). The spinal cord changes clearly indicate that the pattern of vulnerability induced by this glutamate analog differs from damage induced by kainate, although biochemical studies show that ACRO-A binds to two kainate-binding sites in the rat brain (5). The neuro-toxic action of acromelic acid on spinal neurons is attenuated by concomitant administration of 6-cyano-7-nitroquinoxaline-2,3-dione, an antagonist at N-methyl-D-aspartate receptors (3,6). Cases of human toxicity induced by *C. acromelalga* are not known.

REFERENCES

1. Konno K, Hashimoto K, Ohfune Y *et al.* (1988) Acromelic acids A and B. Potent neuroexcitatory amino acids isolated from *Clitocybe acromelalga. J Amer Chem Soc* 110, 4807.
2. Konno K, Shirahama H, Matsumoto T (1983) Isolation and structure of acromelic A and B, new kainoids of *Clitocybe acromelalga. Tetrahed Lett* 24, 939.
3. Kwak S, Nakamura R (1995) Selective degeneration of inhibitory interneurons in the rat spinal cord induced by intrathecal infusion of acromelic acid. *Brain Res* 702, 61.
4. Shin K, Hitoshi A, Michiko I, Haruhiko S (1992) Acromelic acid, a novel kainate analogue, induces long-lasting paraparesis with selective degeneration of interneurons in the rat spinal cord. *Exp Neurol* 116, 145.
5. Smith AL, McIlhinney RA (1992) Effects of acromelic acid A on the binding of ³H-kainic acid and ³H-AMPA to rat brain synaptic plasma membranes. *Brit J Pharmacol* 105, 83.
6. Tsuji K, Nakamura Y, Ogata T *et al.* (1995) Neurotoxicity of acromelic acid in cultured neurons from rat spinal cord. *Neuroscience* 68, 585.

Acrylamide

Bruce G. Gold
Herbert H. Schaumburg

$$H - \overset{\overset{\displaystyle H}{|}}{C} = \overset{\overset{\displaystyle H}{|}}{C} - \overset{\overset{\displaystyle O}{||}}{C} - \overset{\overset{\displaystyle H}{|}}{N} - H$$

ACRYLAMIDE
C_3H_5NO

2-Propenamide

NEUROTOXICITY RATING

Clinical

A Peripheral neuropathy

Experimental

A Peripheral neuropathy

A Cerebellar neuronopathy

Acrylamide monomer is a man-made compound synthesized by the hydration of acrylonitrile with sulfuric acid monohydrate. Acrylamide is an odorless, colorless-to-white, crystalline solid. Flake-like white crystals form upon purification with benzene. It has a MW of 71.08, density of 1.122 g/cm^3 at 30°C, MP of 84.5°C, and BP of 125°C at 24 mm Hg (6). Acrylamide is highly soluble in both water (2.15 g/ml at 30°C) and polar organic solvents (*e.g.*, 1.55 g/ml in methanol; 0.68 g/ml in ethanol at 30°C). It readily polymerizes at the melting point and under ultraviolet light, and should be stored in a cool, dark place (6).

Acrylamide is a vinyl monomer with a high chemical reactivity. Although it does not readily undergo spontaneous polymerization, under appropriate conditions polymerization can occur. The C-C double-bound form is highly reactive with thiols, hydroxy, and amino groups. Polymerization is formed by nucleophilic attack at the electrophilic vinyl group. Commercial polymerization of the neurotoxic monomer into nontoxic polymers began in the early 1950s. The polymers are used (a) as flocculents to separate solids from aqueous solutions in the treatment of wastewater, (b) as a grouting agent (to make the soil waterproof) in mining and in the construction of dams, tunnels, and swimming pools, (c) as a strengthener of paper and cardboard; and (d) in electrophoresis chromatography (80,90). In the United States alone, production of acrylamide increased from 50 million pounds in 1972 (as reported in the first edition of this book) to 86.2 million pounds in 1983 (13). It is no longer produced as a commercial product in North America.

Acrylamide monomer has neurotoxic potential and, in the past, was responsible for many instances of peripheral neuropathy. Acrylamide neuropathy is now rarely encountered in North America; its principal interest to neuroscientists is as a reliable and convenient means of producing distal axonopathy in experimental animals.

General Toxicology

Acrylamide is readily absorbed by all tissues, including skin, and is distributed throughout body water within minutes; it disappears rapidly from the serum, with minute amounts persisting in nervous tissue for more than 14 days (32). The LD$_{50}$ in mice and rats by intraperitoneal injection is 170 mg/kg and 120 mg/kg, respectively (80,90). Its neurotoxic effects are the same regardless of the route of exposure (*i.e.*, intraperitoneal [i.p.], intravenous, subcutaneous, intramuscular, oral, or dermal).

The neurotoxicity of acrylamide appears to require metabolism to an active form of the compound. The agent undergoes oxidization at the double bond, which is required for neurotoxicity (33), to the epoxide glycidamide (2,3-epoxy-1-propenamide) by cytochrome P-450 (4,8). However, this metabolic pathway remains controversial (1,12); there are conflicting reports (33,82) concerning the ability of cytochrome P-450 inducers (such as phenobarbital) to enhance, as predicted by this model, acrylamide neurotoxicity. Detoxification is *via* epoxide hydratase to 2,3-dihydroxy propenamide (87). Elimination is rapid and exponential (t = 2 h) *via* glutathione conjugation (54), although significant amounts have been noted to persist in the rat 14 days after injection. Attempts to monitor acrylamide exposure in workers by urine measurements have been unsuccessful.

Upon systemic exposure, its major target is the nervous system; there is little general human toxicity from acrylamide, aside from fatigue and weight loss. Besides its neurotoxicity, acrylamide has also been found to be carcinogenic and genotoxic in rats and mice (7,16,40). It is capable of binding to DNA *in vitro* (76), and DNA damage in Chinese hamster cells is observed with concentrations as low as 5 mM (91). Large systemic doses (100 mg/kg/day, i.p. for 3 weeks) causes DNA breakage in male germ cells (76) and produces dominant-lethal mutations in male mice (69,70). Whether any of the neurotoxicity produced by acrylamide results from similar damage to DNA in postmitotic neurons is unknown. The finding of increased CNS glial tumors (40) has not been substantiated (16).

Animal Studies

The first experimental report of acrylamide neurotoxicity in laboratory animals appeared in 1956 (28). This was followed in 1958 by a study (43) demonstrating the cumulative nature of the toxicity.

Repeated exposures are necessary to produce peripheral neuropathy of the distal axonopathy type. Studies of acrylamide axonopathy generally have utilized either short-term (up to 14 days), high-level daily administration (25–90 mg/kg) or prolonged (6 weeks to 3 years), low-level (0.5–10 mg/kg) dosing. Similar patterns of distal, retrograde (dying-back) degeneration have been produced in rats, dogs, cats, and primates. Each of these two regimens results in distinct spatiotemporal patterns of dysfunction and fiber degeneration, especially in the CNS; failure to appreciate this phenomenon has led to confusion in some reports of acrylamide neurotoxicity.

Low Doses

The initial ultrastructural change is an accumulation of 10 nm neurofilaments, most marked at distal ends of peripheral nerves (61,68,80,81). Nerve terminals may become grossly enlarged by accumulations of neurofilaments. Paranodal accumulations of neurofilaments may cause axonal swelling and subsequent retraction of myelin; this may result in the appearance of paranodal demyelination. Study of the spatiotemporal evolution of distal axonal changes in rats, cats, and monkeys indicates that the earliest detectable morphological changes occur in large myelinated axons of the tibial nerve branches to calf muscles, large myelinated axons in branches of the peroneal nerve to anterior compartment muscles, nerve terminals of pacinian corpuscles in cat toe pads, and primary annulospiral endings of muscle spindles in hind-foot lumbrical muscles (68,80). In general, neurofilaments initially accumulate at multiple paranodal sites in the distal regions of long and large-diameter axons. The early changes in pacinian corpuscles and annulospiral endings correlate with the profound loss of vibratory sense and depressed tendon reflexes that characterize the human neuropathy. Recent work has demonstrated that, in acrylamide-intoxicated animals, motor nerve terminals of hindlimb neuromuscular junctions exhibit degenerative alterations prior to changes in preterminal axons (14). Degenerating fibers observed at the midthoracic level of the canine vagus nerve may be a factor in acrylamide-induced megaesophagus.

Unmyelinated fibers in somatic nerves and in sympathetic nerve trunks degenerate in advanced stages of acrylamide intoxication.

Evidence of axonal regeneration during low-level intoxication is a feature of acrylamide neuropathy and several other toxic axonopathies; this occurs in rats, cats, and humans.

Widespread, tract-oriented distal axonal degeneration in the CNS accompanies the peripheral nerve changes. Axonal degeneration in the gracile nuclei appears to develop at the same time that changes occur in the most vulnerable areas of the PNS. Preterminal degeneration has been observed in one study that utilized unusually low-level dosing for an extreme interval (67). Other vulnerable areas are the rostral regions of the dorsal spinocerebellar tracts and caudal regions of the long descending motor pathways in the lumbar spinal cord. In rats and monkeys with more prolonged intoxication, shorter tracts, such as the visual pathways, are affected, and axonal swellings appear in the lateral geniculate body.

High Doses

Administration of 30 mg/kg daily produces chromatolytic change in dorsal root ganglion cells (at a time when distal axonal degeneration is not yet apparent) and degeneration of Purkinje cells within 1 week. Within 14 days, widespread and simultaneous swellings of peripheral motor and sensory nerve endings appear, as well as widespread terminal and preterminal swelling in spinal cord, brainstem, and cerebellum.

When a focal nerve crush is followed by high-level acrylamide dosing, acrylamide does not prevent initiation of regeneration at the rat neuromuscular junction but eventually causes degeneration of maturing sprouts (14). Several studies describe impaired axonal regeneration in rats dosed with high levels of acrylamide; one, an ultrastructural study of axon sprouts, described abundant neurofilaments and axonal organelles in growth cones, implying that anterograde transport of these materials is not impeded by acrylamide (27). Nerve ligation together with acrylamide dosing causes retrograde axonal degeneration from the point of ligation, even in proximal loci of the nerve. These proximal sites are normally spared in distal axonopathy, suggesting that acrylamide impairs or misdirects the normal axon repair process (9).

A single dose of 75 mg/kg causes proximal (dorsal and ventral root) axonal swelling, presumably secondary to impaired transport of all slow-component proteins (not just neurofilaments) from neuronal cell bodies (21). Repeated doses of 30 mg/kg cause diffuse proximal axonal atrophy that progresses in a distal direction (somatofugal atrophy) with continued intoxication at a time when there is little distal change, suggesting that this regimen produces an axotomy-like reaction in axon and nerve cell body.

Specific alterations in cytoplasmic organization are noted in sensory ganglia, autonomic ganglia, and Purkinje cell bodies of animals treated with 30–50 mg/kg for 5 days (10,83,84). The subcellular reorganization occurs prior to acrylamide-induced axonal degeneration and involves changes in nuclear position, Nissl bodies, granular endoplasmic reticulum, and mitochondrial number. Unusual changes in Purkinje cells include clusters of microtubules that appear to migrate to the plasmalemma where protrusions form under overlying synaptic attachments. Based on the early onset and distinctive pattern of change in Purkinje cells, it has been suggested that this cellular remodeling represents a direct toxic effect of high-level acrylamide (10).

There have been many electrophysiological studies of experimental acrylamide-intoxicated animals. Early reports describe slowed peripheral nerve conduction in rats, cats, and primates (18,86). Single sensory nerve fiber conduction studies demonstrate the earliest change to be a failure of response of muscle stretch receptors. Studies of the responses of primary and secondary endings of muscle spindles reveal that the earliest abnormalities are elevated threshold and diminished response of spindle endings (86). It is suggested that the attenuated dynamic response of primary muscle spindles may be the basis for depressed tendon reflexes in the human neuropathy. It also seems likely that disordered peripheral sensory mechanisms, acting in concert with dysfunction in the cerebellum, may contribute to the severe gait ataxia that characterizes chronic neurotoxicity in humans. The spinal cord component of the monosynaptic stretch reflex is also clearly abnormal.

Experimental studies demonstrate involvement of the sympathetic and parasympathetic nervous systems, including megaesophagus, urinary bladder dysfunction, poor breathing pattern, and impairment of baroreceptor and cough reflexes (59,60). Electrophysiological studies of the autonomic system reveal no changes of unmyelinated fiber conduction but slowed conduction in myelinated sympathetic nerve fibers (59). One study demonstrated impairment of neural control of the mesenteric vascular bed in severely affected animals, and it was concluded that both preganglionic myelinated and postganglionic unmyelinated fibers are damaged by acrylamide (60).

Several studies support the view that physiological changes antedate nerve fiber degeneration and behavioral dysfunction. One such study of pacinian corpuscles in the mesentery of cats treated with acrylamide demonstrated loss of detectable generator potentials prior to appearance of terminal axon changes as monitored by electron microscopic examination of chemically fixed or freeze-fractured,

physiologically tested corpuscles (78). Studies of somatosensory evoked potentials from the lower extremities of intoxicated primates revealed changes in short-latency (gracile) components at a time when peripheral conduction and behavior were normal and clinical signs of neuropathy were absent (67). No morphological changes were detected in the PNS or CNS of these monkeys. The potentials returned to normal within 2 months of cessation of intoxication. Some monkeys, dosed at levels of 1.0, 2.0, and 3.0 mg/kg/day (below the reported no-effect level), displayed onset of dysfunction only after very prolonged intoxication (940 days). This finding suggests the current permissible levels of human exposure to toxins of this type should be reassessed.

Human Studies

The neurotoxicity of acrylamide was recognized in the 1950s after only 5 months of commercial manufacture; the earliest report of acrylamide neuropathy involved workers synthesizing acrylamide during this period (18). They first noticed tingling and numbness of their fingers and, subsequently, lower limb ataxia. Upon discontinuation of exposure, symptoms markedly improved within 1 week. Most subsequent reported exposures, such as in Japan in the late 1950s (17), occurred in factory workers handling monomeric acrylamide, with dermal contact (as opposed to inhalation) being the likely route of absorption. At least one instance, unrelated to work, appears to have arisen from contaminated drinking water (38).

By 1992, 67 documented cases of acrylamide poisoning had been reported worldwide, excluding China (34,89); this includes an outbreak in 1985 consisting of five cases from a plant in South Africa (58). In addition, a report from the People's Republic of China (34) indicates that at least 90 cases of acrylamide intoxication occurred in that country in the mid-1980s. Historically, most cases come to light upon active investigation of factories (19,42), and it is likely that many mild and subclinical cases still go unrecognized. Two occurrences in South Africa and China prompted more aggressive investigative studies of chemical plants in these countries. These studies revealed a 67%–73% prevalence of acrylamide-induced abnormalities in exposed workers (58).

The nature of neurological dysfunction varies with dose and rate of intoxication. Extremely high exposures, in suicide attempts, are associated with generalized seizures. Moderately high exposures, as in a Japanese family whose drinking water was contaminated with 40 ppm acrylamide, can cause an encephalopathy characterized by confusion, disorientation, memory loss, and hallucinations (38). Of the five cases reported in South Africa (*vide infra*), one had cerebellar and ocular involvement; all demonstrated full clinical recovery (58). In cases involving severe intoxication, signs of cerebellar dysfunction always preceed peripheral neuropathy.

Symmetrical, distal sensory-motor neuropathy is the most common clinical feature of chronic, low-level acrylamide intoxication. Common initial complaints are numbness and excessive sweating of the hands and feet, and an unsteady gait. Excessive sweating is frequently accompanied by skin peeling and other signs of exfoliative dermatitis. Difficulty in walking is usually disproportionate to the mild initial weakness (19).

Objective signs are present in all symptomatic individuals and reflect distal peripheral motor and sensory dysfunction and, possibly, CNS cerebellar dysfunction.

Repetitive exposure to toxic doses of acrylamide results in weakness of the hands and feet combined with an unusually diffuse loss of tendon reflexes. Sensory change inevitably includes depression of vibration sense; paresthesias and other positive sensory phenomena are unusual. Muscle tenderness occasionally has been described, but the condition is not painful (19). Clumsiness and occasional intention tremor may be present in the upper extremities, and a broad-based swaying gait is a common early finding. Cranial nerve palsy and autonomic dysfunction (aside from increased sweating and cold extremities) are not features of this condition. There have been neither postmortem studies in acrylamide neuropathy nor nerve biopsies during the active phase of illness. Sural nerve biopsy specimens from two patients recovering from acrylamide neuropathy displayed diminished numbers of large-diameter fibers.

Most individuals with acrylamide neuropathy show only slight reduction of motor and sensory nerve conduction velocity. The amplitudes of sensory nerve action potentials usually are markedly reduced in upper and lower extremities; this has been suggested as a sensitive electrophysiological test (45).

Removal from acrylamide exposure in the early stages of neuropathy results in gradual and, eventually, complete functional recovery. Careful examination may reveal persistent depression of vibration sense as the sole abnormality. In more severely affected individuals, improvement usually continues for many months, but frequently there is residual distal weakness, gait ataxia, and impaired vibration sense. Persistent sensory dysfunction may stem from degeneration of axons in dorsal columns and ataxia from changes in cerebellar efferent and afferent fibers.

There is considerable interest in detecting subclinical acrylamide neuropathy in exposed workers. Estimation of sensory nerve action potential amplitude appears to be a sensitive electrophysiological measurement (2). Quantitative assessment of distal-extremity vibratory sense is also a useful clinical measure, an idea supported by a study of vibratory sense in acrylamide-dosed monkeys (52). Routine diagnostic clinical laboratory tests, including cerebrospinal fluid examination, are usually unremarkable.

Recognition of the clinical features of acrylamide intoxication is more important than laboratory tests for diagnosis. The diagnosis is not difficult in an individual with proven industrial or occupational exposure. The presence of gait ataxia, moist peeling hands, and peripheral neuropathy in such individuals leaves little room for doubt. A detailed occupational history is probably the most important diagnostic procedure because acrylamide neurotoxicity almost never stems from unrecognized environmental sources.

There is no known treatment for the neuropathy associated with acrylamide exposure. Neurotrophins have been considered to prevent experimental acrylamide neuropathy. A recent report describes the ability of 4-methyl catechol (4-MC), a derivative of catecholamine that induces the level of nerve growth factor (NGF) and possibly additional neurotrophins in the sciatic nerve (29), to reduce the changes in motor nerve conduction velocity in acrylamide-treated rats (66). However, a failure to substantiate this observation morphologically (B.G. Gold, unpublished observation) makes the reason for the electrophysiological findings unclear. Moreover, any clinical use of 4-MC is doubtful given its reported carcinogenicity (3).

Toxic Mechanisms

Initial studies on the mechanism by which acrylamide produces its neurotoxicity focused upon the role of energy metabolism. Repeated exposures are known to impair glycolytic (37) and oxidative (35,73) metabolism; both in vitro and in vivo, acrylamide selectively inhibits the sulfhydryl-containing enzymes enolase, glyceraldehyde-3-phosphate dehydrogenase, and phosphofructokinase. Support for the role of an inhibition in glycolysis in acrylamide neurotoxicity can be found in the demonstration that coadministration of pyruvate retards the onset of acrylamide axonopathy (64). However, subsequent studies reporting the failure of acrylamide to inhibit adenosine triphosphate (ATP) production in vitro (71) or to impair brain mitochondrial respiration in vivo (53) do not support the energy defect hypothesis (79). While inhibition of energy metabolism does not appear to be pathogenetic in acrylamide-induced axonal degeneration, it remains possible that such a mechanism underlies the changes in Purkinje cells, which have a high metabolic requirement (9).

The major debate, as yet unresolved, is whether acrylamide produces axonal degeneration through an effect at the level of the neuronal cell body or axon. Evidence exists in support of both of these putative targets (10,41,68,83,84). In terms of the neuronal cell body, the atypical alterations observed in rat cerebellar Purkinje cells following high-level intoxication (30–50 mg/kg/day) are alleged to support a direct effect of acrylamide on the cell bodies (10). Damage to cerebellar Purkinje cells is a possible correlate of the profound ataxia observed in some exposed humans; the other correlates are degeneration of muscle spindle afferents and spinocerebellar axons. However, it has not been convincingly demonstrated that the unusual alterations produced in cerebellar neurons are specific to acrylamide. Changes in dorsal root ganglion (DRG) and autonomic nerve cell bodies have been described following high-level exposure (41,83,84). These appear to be largely indistinguishable from those produced by direct mechanical transection of the nerve (axotomy) and are suggested to arise from a loss of retrogradely transported trophic factor (*e.g.*, NGF) due to the ability of acrylamide to disrupt retrograde axonal transport (*vide infra*) prior to axonal degeneration (55,56; for further discussion *see* 20,24).

Acrylamide axonopathy is associated with an impairment in both fast (39,55,56,65) and slow (21,75) axonal transport systems. The impairment in slow transport observed following a single injection most likely underlies the pathogenesis of the formation of neurofilamentous axonal swellings (61,68,80). Changes in slow axonal transport following repeated exposures, in contrast, reproduce those following axotomy (21,75) and are likely to arise secondary to axonal injury and/or defect in delivery to the nerve cell body's response to a lost trophic support (*vide supra*). These include (a) increased expression of the proto-oncogene *c-jun* (15) and (b) aberrant expression of phosphorylated neurofilaments in the neuronal cell body (23,36) by calcium/calmodulin-dependent kinases (62,63).

The earliest known physiological alteration produced by acrylamide is impairment in fast axonal transport; the accumulation of tubulovesicular structures (11) most likely represents the morphological correlate of a defect in fast transport (77). This reduction in both retrograde (55,56) and anterograde (31,85) transport systems can be observed in animals within hours following a single intraperitoneal injection of acrylamide. Furthermore, acrylamide has been found selectively to impair the fast anterograde transport of glycoproteins (25,31). The proposal (79) that acrylamide could inhibit fast anterograde transport secondary to a reduction in energy metabolism (*vide supra*) is inconsistent with the production of a selective defect in the movement of axonally transported membrane-bound organelles rich in glycoproteins. Moreover, a preliminary report (50) showed that, unlike the metabolic poison cyanide, acrylamide does not alter the maximal rate of intracellular vesicular movement in cultured neurons.

An alternative mechanism by which acrylamide might preferentially impair the movement of a select group of membrane-bound organelles along microtubules is by inhibiting the function of the fast anterograde transport motor, kinesin. Recent studies indicate that acrylamide inhibits the ability of kinesin to interact with microtubules (72), rather than having a direct effect on kinesin activity (51). The functional correlate of this alteration is a reduction in the number of anterogradely moving vesicles, as observed in cultured rat embryonic neurons (30). Together, these findings suggest a model whereby acrylamide preferentially impairs the microtubules' association with a kinesin isoform (perhaps specific for large myelinated axons) responsible for transport of membrane-bound organelles rich in glycoproteins.

Acrylamide blocks retrogradely moving vesicles in embryonic neurons *in vitro* (30). This suggests that acrylamide, in a fashion analogous to kinesin (72), may similarly impair dynein-microtubule interactions. Such a mechanism could underlie the early reduction in retrograde axonal transport by acrylamide (55,56). Moreover, the finding that glycidamide exhibits a fourfold greater potency in its ability to impair bidirectional vesicular transport (31) provides support (at a physiological level) for the hypothesis that this compound is the active toxic metabolite of acrylamide.

Direct support for the ability of acrylamide to impair the function of microtubule-based movement can be found in the recent demonstration that acrylamide disrupts another microtubule-based system, *i.e.*, mitosis in human fibrosarcoma cells (74). Taken together with the neuronal studies described above, these findings suggest microtubule-based systems as the target for acrylamide toxicity in general (13,90) and that microtubule-based fast anterograde transport system is the specific neuronal target underlying development of acrylamide-induced axonal degeneration. The proposition that the microtubule system is the likely target for acrylamide neurotoxicity *in vivo* appears to be supported by the increased susceptibility of the axon to acrylamide-induced axonal degeneration in rats pretreated with β,β-iminodipropionitrile, an agent that produces microtubule-neurofilament segregation (22). In this context, acrylamide has been shown to bind to neurofilaments and microtubule proteins *in vitro* (44). While binding to neurofilaments could lead to neurofilamentous axonal swellings, the formation of neurofilament accumulations *per se* is not sufficient to produce axonal degeneration (*see* Iminodipropionitrile, this volume). However, axonal degeneration of CNS fibers in acrylamide neuropathy appears to depend upon the presence of neurofilaments, as revealed by the failure of acrylamide to produce axonal degeneration in the neurofilament-deficient quail (88). Taken together, these studies indicate that neurofilamentous swellings play a role in the pathogenesis of acrylamide-induced axonal degeneration.

It is unclear how the axon undergoes degeneration in acrylamide neuropathy. Electron microprobe x-ray studies suggest that ion regulation in distal paranodal axon regions is compromised by diminished axolemmal Na^+/K^+-ATPase activity (46–48). It is alleged that decreased Na^+/K^+-ATPase activity is a consequence of aberrant cell body processing and/or deficient axonal transport. Reduced Na^+ pump activity promotes membrane depolarization in conjunction with axoplasmic accumulation of Na^+ and loss of K^+. Thermodynamically, this favors the reverse influx of Ca^{2+}, which eventually overwhelms buffering mechanisms and leads to distal axonal degeneration. Distal axons are predisposed to regulatory failure of this type due to a dependency on cell body output and the unique differential distribution of enzymes, ion channels, and exchangers among nodal and internodal regions. This model is not specific for acrylamide; it could also account for axon degeneration occurring as a result of exposure to other chemical neurotoxicants and following axotomy and mechanical injury (48). In sum, the changes in elemental composition appear to reflect secondary or compensatory responses to injury.

Besides producing axonal degeneration, systemic acrylamide intoxication impairs axonal regeneration (27,57). Direct subepineurial injections demonstrate that acrylamide retards axonal regeneration directly at the level of the axon (20), despite the ability of the neuronal cell body to remodel into a regenerative program (6,23). However, the axotomy response in the nerve cell body appears to be suppressed (5), which may contribute to the defect in regeneration. Recent evidence (B.G. Gold, unpublished observation) indicates that acrylamide inhibits the injury-induced induction of the FK506-binding protein (FKBP), a receptor protein for the immunosuppressant FK506, which plays a role in axonal regeneration (25,26,49). Deciphering the origin of this defect in FKBP expression may provide insight into the defect in axonal regeneration in acrylamide neuropathy.

REFERENCES

1. Abou-Donia MB, Ibrahim SM, Corcoran JJ et al. (1993) Neurotoxicity of glycidamide, an acrylamide metabolite, following intraperitoneal injections in rats. *J Toxicol Environ Health* **39**, 447.
2. Arezzo JC, Schaumburg HH, Petersen CA (1983) Rapid screening for peripheral neuropathy: A field study with the Optacon. *Neurology* **33**, 626.
3. Asakawa E, Hinose M, Hagiwara A et al. (1994) Carcinogenicity of 4-methoxyphenol and 4-methylcatechol in F344 rats. *Int J Cancer* **56**, 146.
4. Bergmark E, Calleman CJ, Costa LG (1991) Formation of hemoglobin adducts of acrylamide and its epoxide metabolite glycidamide in the rat. *Toxicol Appl Pharmacol* **111**, 352.
5. Bisby MA, Redshaw JD (1987) Acrylamide neuropathy: Changes in the composition of proteins of fast axonal transport resemble those observed in regenerating axons. *J Neurochem* **48**, 924.
6. Budavari S, O'Neil MJ, Smith A, Heckleman PE (1989) *The Merck Index: An Encyclopedia of Chemicals, Drugs, and Biologicals. 11th Ed.* Merck & Co, Rahway, NJ.
7. Bull RJ, Robinson M, Laurie RD et al. (1984) Carcinogenic effects of acrylamide in Sencar and A/J mice. *Cancer Res* **44**, 107.
8. Calleman CJ, Bergmark E, Costa LG (1990) Acrylamide is metabolized to glycidamide in the rat: Evidence from hemoglobin adduct formation. *Chem Res Toxicol* **3**, 406.
9. Cavanagh JB (1982) The pathokinetics of acrylamide intoxication: A reappraisal of the problem. *Neuropathol Appl Neurobiol* **8**, 315.
10. Cavanagh JB, Gysbers MF (1983) Ultrastructural features of the Purkinje cell damage caused by acrylamide in the rat: A new phenomenon in cellular neuropathology. *J Neurocytol* **12**, 413.
11. Chretien M, Patey G, Souyri F, Droz B (1981) "Acrylamide-induced" neuropathy and impairment of axonal transport of proteins. II. Abnormal accumulations of smooth endoplasmic reticulum as sites of focal retention of fast transported proteins: Electron microscopic radioautographic study. *Brain Res* **205**, 15.
12. Costa LG, Deng H, Calleman CJ, Bergmark E (1995) Evaluation of the neurotoxicity of glycidamide, an epoxide metabolite of acrylamide: Behavioral, neurochemical and morphological studies. *Toxicology* **98**, 151.
13. Dearfield KL, Abernathy CO, Ottley MS et al. (1988) Acrylamide: Its metabolism, developmental and reproductive effects, genotoxicity, and carcinogenicity. *Mutat Res* **195**, 45.
14. DeGrandchamp RL, Lowndes HE (1990) Early degeneration and sprouting at the rat neuromuscular junction following acrylamide administration. *Neuropathol Appl Neurobiol* **16**, 239.
15. Endo H, Sabri MI, Stephens JM et al. (1993) Acrylamide induced immediate-early gene expression in rat brain. *Brain Res* **609**, 231.
16. Friedman MA, Dulak LH, Stedham MA (1995) A lifetime oncogenicity study in rats with acrylamide. *Fund Appl Toxicol* **27**, 95.
17. Fujita A, Shibata M, Kato H et al. (1960) Clinical observations on acrylamide poisoning. *Nippon Iji Shimpo* **1869**, 27.

18. Fullerton PM, Barnes JM (1966) Peripheral neuropathy in rats produced by acrylamide. *Brit J Ind Med* **23**, 210.

19. Garland TO, Paterson MWH (1967) Six cases of acrylamide poisoning. *Brit Med J* **4**, 134.

20. Gold BG, Austin DR, Griffin JW (1991) Regulation of aberrant neurofilament phosphorylation in neuronal perikarya. II. Correlation with continued axonal elongation following axotomy. *J Neuropathol Exp Neurol* **50**, 627.

21. Gold BG, Griffin JW, Price DL (1985) Slow axonal transport in acrylamide neuropathy: Different abnormalities produced by single-dose and continuous administration. *J Neurosci* **5**, 1755.

22. Gold BG, Halleck MM (1989) Axonal degeneration and axonal caliber alterations following combined β,β'-iminodipropionitrile (IDPN) and acrylamide administration. *J Neuropathol Exp Neurol* **48**, 653.

23. Gold BG, Price DL, Griffin JW et al. (1988) Neurofilament antigens in acrylamide neuropathy. *J Neuropathol Exp Neurol* **47**, 145.

24. Gold BG, Spencer PS (1993) Neurotrophic function in normal nerve and in peripheral neuropathies. In: *Neuroregeneration.* Gorio A ed. Raven Press, New York p. 101.

25. Gold BG, Storm-Dickerson T, Austin DR (1994) The immunosuppressant FK506 increases functional recovery and nerve regeneration following peripheral nerve injury. *Restor Neurol Neurosci* **6**, 287.

26. Gold BG, Storm-Dickerson T, Katoh K, Austin DR (1995) The immunosuppressant FK506 increases the rate of axonal regeneration in rat sciatic nerve. *J Neurosci* **15**, 7509.

27. Griffin JW, Price DL, Drachman DB (1977) Impaired axonal regeneration in acrylamide intoxication. *J Neurobiol* **8**, 355.

28. Hamblin DO (1956) The toxicity of acrylamide. A preliminary report. In: *Hommage au Doyen René Fabre S.E.D.E.S.*, Paris p. 159.

29. Hanaoke Y, Takekazu O, Furukawa S et al. (1994) The therapeutic effects of 4-methylcatechol, a stimulator of endogenous nerve growth factor synthesis, on experimental diabetic neuropathy in rats. *J Neurol Sci* **122**, 28.

30. Harris CH, Gulati AK, Freidman MA, Sickles DW (1994) Toxic neurofilamentous axonopathies and fast axonal transport. V. Reduced bi-directional vesicle transport in cultured neurons by acrylamide and glycidamide. *J Toxicol Environ Health* **42**, 343.

31. Harry GJ, Morell P, Bouldin TW (1992) Acrylamide exposure preferentially impairs axonal transport of glycoproteins in myelinated axons. *J Neurosci Res* **31**, 554.

32. Hashimoto K, Aldridge WN (1970) Biochemical studies on acrylamide: A neurotoxic agent. *Biochem Pharmacol* **19**, 2592.

33. Hashimoto K, Sakamoto J, Tanil H (1981) Neurotoxicity of acrylamide and related compounds and their effects on male gonads in mice. *Arch Toxicol* **47**, 179.

34. He F, Zhang S, Wang H et al. (1989) Neurological and electroneuromyographic assessment of the adverse effects of acrylamide on occupationally exposed workers. *Scand J Work Environ Health* **15**, 125.

35. Howland RD (1981) The etiology of acrylamide neuropathy. Enolase, phosphofructokinase and glyceraldehyde-3-phosphate dehydrogenase activities in peripheral nerves, spinal cord, brain and skeletal muscles of acrylamide-intoxicated cats. *Toxicol Appl Pharmacol* **60**, 324.

36. Howland RD, Alli P (1986) Altered phosphorylaton of rat neuronal cytoskeletal proteins in acrylamide-induced neuropathy. *Brain Res* **363**, 333.

37. Howland RD, Vyas IL, Lowndes HE (1980) The etiology of acrylamide neuropathy: Possible involvement of neuron specific enolase. *Brain Res* **190**, 529.

38. Igisu H, Goto I, Kawamura Y et al. (1975) Acrylamide encephalopathy due to well water pollution. *J Neurol Neurosurg Psychiat* **38**, 581.

39. Jakobsen J, Sidenius P (1983) Early and dose-dependent decrease of retrograde axonal transport in acrylamide-intoxicated rats. *J Neurochem* **40**, 447.

40. Johnson K, Gorzinski S, Bodner K et al. (1986) Chronic toxicity and oncogenicity study on acrylamide incorporated in the drinking water of Fischer 344 rats. *Toxicol Appl Pharmacol* **85**, 154.

41. Jones HB, Cavanagh JB (1984) The evolution of intracellular responses to acrylamide in rat spinal ganglion neurons. *Neuropathol Appl Neurobiol* **10**, 101.

42. Kesson CM, Lawson DH, Baird AW (1977) Acrylamide poisoning. *Postgrad Med J* **4**, 134.

43. Kuperman AS (1958) Effects of acrylamide on the central nervous system in the cat. *J Pharmacol Exp Ther* **123**, 180.

44. Lapadula DM, Bowe M, Carrington CD et al. (1989) *In vitro* binding of [^{14}C] acrylamide to neurofilament and microtubule proteins of rats. *Brain Res* **481**, 157.

45. LeQuesne PM (1978) Neurophysiological investigation of subclinical and minimal toxic neuropathies. *Muscle Nerve* **1**, 392.

46. LoPachin RM, Castiglia CM, Saubermann AJ (1992) Acrylamide disrupts elemental composition and water content of rat tibial nerve. I. Myelinated axons. *Toxicol Appl Pharmacol* **115**, 21.

47. LoPachin RM, Castiglia CM, Saubermann AJ (1992) Acrylamide disrupts elemental composition and water content of rat tibial nerve. II. Schwann cells and myelin. *Toxicol Appl Pharmacol* **115**, 35.

48. LoPachin RM, Lehning EJ (1994) Acrylamide induced distal axon degeneration: A proposed mechanism of action. *Neurotoxicology* **15**, 247.

49. Lyons WE, Steiner JP, Snyder SH, Dawson TM (1995) Neuronal regeneration enhances the expression of the immunophilin FKBP-12. *J Neurosci* **15**, 2985.

50. Martenson CH, Anthony DC, Sheetz MP, Graham DG (1992) A quantitation of fast axonal transport in cultured

chick dorsal root ganglion (DRG) explants following exposure to acrylamide (ACR), methacrylamide (M-ACR) and cyanide. *Toxicologist* **12**, 191.

51. Martenson CH, Sheetz MP, Graham DG (1993) Effect of acrylamide on the activity of purified dynein and kinesin. *Toxicologist* **13**, 125.

52. Maurissen JP, Weiss B, Cox C (1990) Vibration sensitivity recovery after a second course of acrylamide intoxication. *Fund Appl Toxicol* **15**, 93.

53. Medrano CJ, LoPachin RM (1989) Effects of acrylamide and 2,5-hexanedione on brain mitochondrial respiration. *Neurotoxicology* **10**, 249.

54. Miller DB (1982) Neurotoxicity of pesticidal carbamates. *Neurobehav Toxicol Teratol* **4**, 779.

55. Miller MS, Miller MJ, Burks TF, Sipes IG (1983) Altered retrograde axonal transport of nerve growth factor after single and repeated doses of acrylamide in the rat. *Toxicol Appl Pharmacol* **69**, 96.

56. Miller MS, Spencer PS (1984) Single doses of acrylamide reduce retrograde transport velocity. *J Neurochem* **43**, 1401.

57. Morgan-Hughes JA, Sinclair S, Durston JHJ (1974) The pattern of peripheral nerve regeneration induced by crush in rats with severe acrylamide neuropathy. *Brain* **97**, 235.

58. Myers JE (1991) Acrylamide neuropathy in a South African factory: An epidemiologic investigation. *Amer J Ind Med* **19**, 487.

59. Post EJ, McLeod JG (1977) Acrylamide autonomic neuropathy in the cat. Part I. Neurophysiological and histological studies. *J Neurol Sci* **33**, 353.

60. Post EJ, McLeod JG (1977) Acrylamide autonomic neuropathy in the cat. Part II. Effects on mesenteric vascular control. *J Neurol Sci* **33**, 375.

61. Prineas J (1969) The pathogenesis of dying-back polyneuropathies. Part II. An ultrastructural study of experimental acrylamide intoxication in the cat. *J Neuropathol Exp Neurol* **28**, 598.

62. Reagan KE, Wilmarth KR, Friedman M, Abou-Donia MB (1994) Acrylamide increases *in vitro* calcium and calmodulin-dependent kinase-mediated phosphorylation of rat brain and spinal cord neurofilament proteins. *Neurochem Int* **25**, 133.

63. Reagan KE, Wilmarth KR, Friedman MA, Abou-Donia MB (1995) *In vitro* calcium and calmodulin-dependent kinase-mediated phosphorylation of rat brain and spinal cord neurofilament proteins is increased by glycidamide administration. *Brain Res* **671**, 12.

64. Sabri MI, Dairman W, Fenton M *et al.* (1989) Effect of exogenous pyruvate on acrylamide neuropathy in rats. *Brain Res* **483**, 1.

65. Sahenk Z, Mendell JR (1981) Acrylamide and 2,5-hexanedione neuropathies: Abnormal bidirectional transport rate in distal axons. *Brain Res* **219**, 397.

66. Saita K, Ohi T, Hanaoka Y *et al.* (1995) Effects of 4-methylcatechol, a stimulator of endogenous nerve growth factor synthesis, on experimental acrylamide-induced neuropathy in rats. *Neurotoxicology* **16**, 403.

67. Schaumburg HH, Arezzo JC, Spencer PS (1989) Delayed onset of distal axonal neuropathy in primates after prolonged low-level administration of a neurotoxin. *Ann Neurol* **26**, 576.

68. Schaumburg HH, Wiśniewski HM, Spencer PS (1974) Ultrastructural studies of the dying-back process. I. Peripheral nerve terminal and axon degeneration in systemic acrylamide intoxication. *J Neuropathol Exp Neurol* **33**, 260.

69. Sega GA, Generoso EE, Brimer PA (1990) Acrylamide exposure induces a delayed unscheduled DNA synthesis in germ cells of male mice that is correlated with the temporal pattern of adduct formation in testis DNA. *Environ Mol Mutagen* **16**, 137.

70. Shelby MD, Cain KT, Hughes LA *et al.* (1986) Dominant lethal effects of acrylamide in male mice. *Mutat Res* **173**, 35.

71. Sickles DW, Fowler SR, Testino AR (1990) Effects of neurofilamentous axonopathy-producing neurotoxicants on *in vitro* production of ATP by brain mitochondria. *Brain Res* **528**, 25.

72. Sickles DW, Friedman MA (1994) Acrylamide reduces ATP-dependent release of kinesin from microtubules. *Toxicologist* **14**, 206.

73. Sickles DW, Goldstein BD (1986) Acrylamide produces a direct, dose-dependent and specific inhibition of oxidative metabolism in motoneurons. *Neurotoxicology* **7**, 187.

74. Sickles DW, Welter DA (1995) Acrylamide arrests mitosis and prevents chromosome migration in the absence of changes in spindle microtubules. *J Toxicol Environ Health* **44**, 73.

75. Sidenius P, Jakobsen J (1983) Anterograde axonal transport in rats during intoxication with acrylamide. *J Neurochem* **40**, 697.

76. Solomon JJ, Fedyk J, Mukai F, Segal A (1985) Direct alkylation of 2′-deoxynucleosides and DNA following *in vitro* reaction with acrylamide. *Cancer Res* **45**, 3465.

77. Souyri F, Chretien M, Droz B (1981) 'Acrylamide-induced' neuropathy and impairment of axonal transport of proteins. I. Multifocal retention of fast transported proteins at the periphery of axons as revealed by light microscope radioautography. *Brain Res* **205**, 1.

78. Spencer PS, Hanna R, Pappas GD (1977) Inactivation of Pacinian corpuscle mechano-sensitivity by acrylamide. *J Gen Physiol* **70**, 17a.

79. Spencer PS, Sabri MI, Schaumburg HH, Moore CL (1979) Does a defect of energy metabolism in the nerve fiber underlie axonal degeneration in polyneuropathies? *Ann Neurol* **5**, 501.

80. Spencer PS, Schaumburg HH (1974) A review of acrylamide neurotoxicity. Part I. Properties, uses and human exposure. *Can J Neurol Sci* **1**, 143.

81. Spencer PS, Schaumburg HH (1974) Ultrastructural studies of the dying-back process. III. The evolution of experimental peripheral giant axonal degeneration. *J Neuropathol Exp Neurol* **36**, 276.

82. Srivastava SP, Seth PK, Das M, Mukhtar H (1985) Effects of mixed-function oxidase modifiers on neurotoxicity of acrylamide in rats. *Biochem Pharmacol* **34**, 1099.

83. Sterman AB (1983) Altered sensory ganglia in acrylamide neuropathy. Quantitative evidence of neuronal reorganization. *J Neuropathol Exp Neurol* **42**, 166.

84. Sterman AB (1984) Acrylamide-induced remodeling of perikarya in rat superior cervical ganglia. *Neuropathol Appl Neurobiol* **10**, 221.

85. Storm-Dickerson T, Spencer PS, Gold BG (1992) Early and selective impairment in the fast anterograde transport (FAT) of glycoproteins in acrylamide (AC) neuropathy. *Soc Neurosci Abstr* **18**, 1084.

86. Sumner AJ, Asbury AK (1975) Physiological studies of the dying-back phenomenon: Muscle stretch afferents in acrylamide neuropathy. *Brain* **98**, 91.

87. Sumner SCJ, MacNeela JP, Fennell TR (1992) Characterization and quantitation of urinary metabolites of [1,2,3-^{13}C] acrylamide in rats and mice using ^{13}C nuclear magnetic resonance spectroscopy. *Chem Res Toxicol* **5**, 81.

88. Takahashi A, Mizutani M, Agr B, Itakura C (1994) Acrylamide-induced neurotoxicity in the central nervous system of Japanese quails: Comparative studies of normal and neurofilament-deficient quails. *J Neuropathol Exp Neurol* **53**, 276.

89. Takahashi M, Ohara T, Hashimoto K (1971) Electrophysiological study of nerve injuries in workers handling acrylamide. *Int Arch Arbeitsmed* **28**, 1.

90. Tilson HA (1981) The neurotoxicity of acrylamide: An overview. *Neurobehav Toxicol Teratol* **3**, 445.

91. Tsuda H, Shimizu CS, Taketomi MK *et al.* (1993) Acrylamide: Induction of DNA damage, chromosomal aberrations and cell transformation without gene mutations. *Mutagenesis* **8**, 23.

CASE REPORT

A 45 year-old male grouter received daily high-level skin exposure to acrylamide monomer, the principal component of the grouting compound. After 3 months, he complained of fatigue and a 7 lb weight loss, and also noticed that his hands were red and his skin peeling. By 4 months, he felt slightly unstable while walking and would occasionally lose balance when turning corners. Numbness of the feet and an aching pain in the calves developed by 5 months. He continued to work for another 2 weeks until his hands became numb and his gait so unsteady that he was accused of drinking on the job. He had no urinary bladder dysfunction or impotence.

Upon examination, his palms were red, moist, and peeling. Vital signs and general physical examination were normal. Neurological examination revealed no abnormalities of cranial nerves or mental status. His speech was unremarkable, and no nystagmus was present. Strength in the proximal upper extremities was normal, but there was weakness, without wasting, of the intrinsic muscles of the hands and weakness of the wrist extensors (4/5 MRC scale). Neck, trunk, abdominal, and proximal lower-extremity muscles were of normal strength. There was weakness of dorsiflexion at the ankles (4/5 MRC scale). The tendon reflexes in the arms were sluggish, and there was loss of knee and ankle jerks, and absent plantar responses. A mild loss of pinprick sense was evident below the wrist and knees (glove-and-stocking distribution). Position sense was normal throughout. There was a striking loss of vibration sense (256 cps) over ankle, knee, and wrist. Coordinated movements in the upper extremities were unaffected. There was no past-pointing or loss of check of rapid movement, but truncal ataxia was evident. Heel-to-knee-to-shin maneuvers were unsteady and poorly performed. His gait was broad-based and, on sudden turns, he reached for support. He was unable to stand with his feet together and eyes open without falling to either side. Motor nerve conduction in the medial and ulnar nerves was 55 m/sec (normal), and 35 m/sec (mild slowing) in the common peroneal nerve. Lumbar puncture revealed clear, acellular fluid with a normal protein value.

Six months later, motor and sensory examinations were normal except for a moderate impairment of vibration sensation in the lower extremities. The tendon reflexes were 2 throughout except for an absent Achilles reflex. His gait was narrow-based without staggering except when requested to make sudden turns. He could stand with the feet together, and Romberg's sign was not present.

This patient illustrates many of the cardinal features usually associated with a mild to moderate degree of toxic axonal neuropathy: insidious onset, gradual progression, symmetrical distal (stocking-and-glove) motor and sensory loss, normal cerebrospinal fluid protein level, and mild impairment in motor nerve conduction. Unusual features of this illness included the truncal and gait ataxia, and the severe loss of vibration sensation. Early, severe loss of vibration sense, disproportionate to impairment of other sensory modalities or weakness, and early gait ataxia are consistent features of human acrylamide intoxication.

Acrylonitrile

Kevin M. Crofton
Mary Beth Genter

$$CH_2 = CH - CN$$

ACRYLONITRILE
C_3H_3N

2-Propenenitrile; Vinyl cyanide; Cyanoethylene

NEUROTOXICITY RATING

Clinical

A   Seizure disorder

Experimental

A   Glial neoplasm

Acrylonitrile is an industrial chemical used in a wide range of commercial applications. Estimated domestic production ranges from $0.8-1.2 \times 10^9$ kg/year (4,25), and worldwide production is approximately 4×10^9 kg/year (4). The U.S. National Institutes for Occupational Safety and Health (18) estimated that 125,000 persons have been occupationally exposed to acrylonitrile in the United States. Acrylonitrile is a colorless, highly reactive, explosive, and flammable chemical; it decomposes to cyanide during pyrolysis and is heavier than air, which presents a significant hazard during fires (4). Acrylonitrile is employed as an intermediate in the production of pharmaceuticals, dyes, synthetic fibers, and plastics. Its major use is as a monomer in the production of acrylic and modacrylic fibers and acrylonitrile-styrene-butadiene and styrene-acrylonitrile resins (4,19,25). It is also used in the production of other known neurotoxicants, including acrylamide (4,25) and dimethylaminopropionitrile (13). Use of acrylonitrile as an agricultural fumigant has been discontinued (15).

Acrylonitrile is regulated as a probable human carcinogen (26,35). The permissible exposure limit (PEL) in the occupational setting is 2 ppm (4.3 mg/m^3) as an 8-h time-weighted average (1). There is currently no drinking water standard in place, but the U.S. Environmental Protection Agency has set the Maximum Contaminant Level Goal (MCLG) for acrylonitrile at zero because the agent is classified as a probable human carcinogen (27). There is no current established reference dose (RfD) for acrylonitrile. The reference concentration (RfC), based on the compound's property of inducing degeneration and inflammation of respiratory epithelium, is 2×10^{-3} mg/m^3 (26).

Acrylonitrile is a direct-acting mutagen in some strains of *Escherichia coli*, but requires activation to exhibit mutagenic activity in the Ames assay (5,16,29). Several DNA adducts resulting from the *in vitro* reaction between 2-cyanoethylene oxide (CEO) (*vide infra*) and DNA have

been characterized (33,34); however, the mutation(s) resulting in acrylonitrile-induced carcinogenesis has not been determined.

Acrylonitrile is absorbed after oral, dermal, and inhalation exposure. Two major pathways are believed to be important in the metabolism of acrylonitrile, one involving direct, nonenzymatic conjugation with glutathione (GSH), and the other mediated by cytochrome P-450 oxidation (Fig. 1). The oxidative pathway is considered to be a route of bioactivating acrylonitrile, as acrylonitrile is metabolized in the liver and the lung to the direct-acting mutagen CEO; (11,21,28). CEO, but not acrylonitrile, readily binds to DNA *in vitro* (11). CEO distributes widely through the body and can be detected in rodent blood and brain 5–10 minutes after an oral dose of acrylonitrile (12). Under GSH-depleting conditions, a greater proportion of acrylonitrile is metabolized *via* an oxidative pathway (20). P-450–mediated oxidation of [^{14}C]-acrylonitrile to [^{14}C]-CEO doubles upon administration of glutathione-depleting agents and is associated with increased binding of radiolabel to proteins and target-tissue nucleic acids (20).

There are few well-conducted experimental animal studies on the short-term effects of acrylonitrile on the nervous system. Symptoms observed after single exposures at very high doses include tremors, urination, defecation, salivation, and convulsions (2,10). These signs of toxicity have

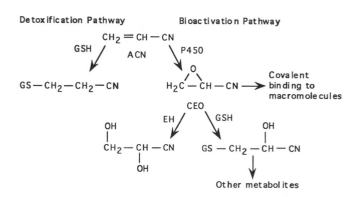

FIGURE 1. Putative pathways for the metabolism of acrylonitrile. Nonenzymatic conjugation with glutathione (GSH) is the major metabolic pathway, serving as a means of detoxifying acrylonitrile. A small fraction of an administered dose is oxidized to 2-cyanoethylene oxide (CEO) by cytochrome P-450 enzymes; because CEO can bind to proteins and nucleic acids, causing tissue damage and/or mutations, this is a bioactivation pathway. CEO can be detoxified by epoxide hydrolase (EH) or reaction with GSH. [Adapted from Roberts *et al.*, 1989, with permission.]

been attributed to metabolic liberation of cyanide (31) and a cholinergic action (2,7,9). Indeed, atropine has been shown to attenuate cholinergic signs induced by acrylonitrile administration (9).

Acrylonitrile is carcinogenic in the rat. Chronic bioassays in rats have consistently shown excess tumors in the brain, stomach, and Zymbal's glands following either inhalation or oral routes of exposure (3,8,14). The nervous system tumors are characterized as astrocytomas or gliomas (3).

Clinical signs of neurotoxicity are reported in only one chronic rat bioassay: Bigner and associates (3) stated that a dose-related increase in paralysis, head-tilt, circling, and seizures was observed within the 18 month study. These effects were seen at doses that also produced weight loss, mortality, and brain tumors. Dudley and colleagues (6) reported for the same species that 8 weeks of inhalation exposure produced hindlimb weakness. There have been no formal assessments of neurotoxicity in long-term studies of the chronic effects of acrylonitrile.

Developmental toxicity tests, performed using gavage and inhalation routes of exposure, reveal that acrylonitrile is fetotoxic and appears to be weakly teratogenic in rats at doses associated with maternal toxicity (17,22,31). *In vitro* studies with cultured whole-rat embryos demonstrate that glutathione depletion enhances the teratogenic potential of acrylonitrile (23). Administration of sodium thiosulfate exerts a protective effect against both the systemic toxicity and the teratogenicity of acrylonitrile, suggesting that HCN is the teratogenic metabolite (32).

Acrylonitrile is associated with testicular toxicity in mice. Daily oral administration of 10 mg/kg for 60 days resulted in degeneration of the seminiferous tubules and decreased sperm count (24).

Short-term exposure in humans results in eye irritation, headache, fatigue, weakness, and nausea (31). Acrylonitrile reportedly also causes impaired judgment and convulsions (25). Epidemiological studies of occupationally exposed humans reveal an increased incidence of malignant tumors of the lung, stomach, bladder, and prostate (for review, *see* 30). Excess brain cancer deaths have not been observed in any of the epidemiology studies (30).

REFERENCES

1. ACGIH (1994) American Conference of Governmental Industrial Hygienists, Threshold Limit Values, Cincinnati, Ohio.
2. Benz FW, Nerland DE, Pierce WM, Babink C (1990) Acute acrylonitrile toxicity: Studies on the mechanism of the antidotal effect of D- and L-cysteine and their *N*-acetyl derivatives. *Toxicol Appl Pharmacol* 102, 142.
3. Bigner DD, Bigner SH, Burger PC *et al.* (1986) Primary brain tumors in Fischer 344 rats chronically exposed to acrylonitrile in their drinking water. *Food Chem Toxicol* 24, 129.
4. Bradzil JF (1991) Acrylonitrile. In: *Kirk-Othmer Encyclopedia of Chemical Technology, Fourth Ed. Vol 1. A to Alkaloids*. How-Grant M ed. Wiley-Interscience, New York p. 352.
5. deMeester C, Poncelet F, Roberfroid M, Mercier M (1978) Mutagenic activity of acrylonitrile. A preliminary study. *Arch Int Physiol Biochim* 86, 418.
6. Dudley HC, Sweeney TR, Miller JW (1942) Toxicology of acrylonitrile (vinyl cyanide). II. Studies of the effects of daily inhalation. *J Ind Hyg Toxicol* 24, 255.
7. Fanini D, Trieff NM, Ramanujam VMS *et al.* (1985) Effects of acute acrylonitrile exposure on metrazol induced seizures in the rat. *Neurotoxicology* 6, 29.
8. Gallagher GT, Maull EA, Kovacs K, Szabo S (1988) Neoplasms in rats ingesting acrylonitrile for two years. *J Amer Coll Toxicol* 7, 603.
9. Ghanayem BI, Farooqui MY, Elshabrawy O *et al.* (1991) Assessment of the acute acrylonitrile-induced neurotoxicity in rats. *Neurotoxicol Teratol* 13, 499.
10. Graham JDP (1965) Hydroxycobalamin as an antidote to acrylonitrile. *Toxicol Appl Pharmacol* 7, 367.
11. Guengerich FP, Geiger LE, Hogy LL, Wright PL (1981) *In vitro* metabolism of acrylonitrile to 2-cyanoethylene oxide, reaction with glutathione, and irreversible binding to proteins and nucleic acids. *Cancer Res* 41, 4925.
12. Kedderis GL, Batra R, Held SD *et al.* (1993) Rodent tissue distribution of 2-cyanoethylene oxide, the epoxide metabolite of acrylonitrile. *Toxicol Lett* 69, 25.
13. Keogh JP (1983) Classical syndromes in occupational medicine: dimethylaminopropionitrile. *Amer J Ind Med* 4, 479.
14. Maltoni C, Ciliberti A, Cotti G, Perino G (1977) Carcinogenicity bioassays on rats of acrylonitrile administered by inhalation and ingestion. *Med Lav* 68, 401.
15. Meister RT (1994) *Farm Chemicals Handbook*. Meister Publishing Co, Willoughby, Ohio p. C8.
16. Milvy P, Wolff M (1977) Mutagenic studies with acrylonitrile. *Mutat Res* 48, 271.
17. Murray FJ, Schwetz BA, Nischke KD *et al.* (1979) Teratogenicity of acrylonitrile given to rats by gavage or by inhalation. *Food Cosmet Toxicol* 16, 547.
18. NIOSH (1977) *Acrylonitrile. Current Intelligence Bulletin No. 18*. National Institute for Occupational Safety and Health, Cincinnati, Ohio.
19. O'Donoghue J (1985) Cyanide, nitriles and isocyanates. In: *Neurotoxicity of Industrial and Commercial Chemicals. Vol II*. O'Donoghue JL ed. CRC Press, Boca Raton, Florida p. 25.
20. Pilon D, Roberts AE, Rickert DE (1988) Effect of glutathione depletion on the irreversible association of acrylonitrile with tissue macromolecules after oral administration to rats. *Toxicol Appl Pharmacol* 95, 311.

21. Roberts AE, Lacy SA, Pilon D *et al.* (1989) Metabolism of acrylonitrile to 2-cyanoethylene oxide in F-344 rat liver microsomes, lung microsomes, and lung cells. *Drug Metab Disposition* **17**, 481.

22. Saillenfait AM, Bonnet P, Guenier, deCeaurriz J (1993) Relative developmental toxicites of inhaled aliphatic mononitriles in rats. *Fund Appl Toxicol* **20**, 365.

23. Saillenfait AM, Payan JP, Langonne I *et al.* (1993) Modulation of acrylonitrile-induced embryotoxicity *in vitro* by glutathione depletion. *Arch Toxicol* **67**, 164.

24. Tandon R, Saxena DK, Chandra SV *et al.* (1988) Testicular effects of acrylonitrile in mice. *Toxicol Lett* **42**, 55.

25. US EPA (1984) *Health Assessment Document for Acrylonitrile: Final Report.* EPA-600/S8-82-007F, United States Environmental Protection Agency, Washington, DC.

26. US EPA (1995) Acrylonitrile. In: *Integrated Risk Informations System (IRIS).* Office of Health and Environmental Assessment, Environmental Criteria and Assessment Office, United States Environmental Protection Agency, Cincinnati, Ohio.

27. US EPA (1995) *Drinking Water Regulations and Health Advisories.* Office of Water, United States Environmental Protection Agency, Washington, DC.

28. van Bladeren PJ, Delbressome LPC, Hoogeterp JJ *et al.* (1981) Formation of mercapturic acids from acrylonitrile, crotononitrile, and cinnamonitrile by direct conjugation and *via* an intermediate oxidation process. *Drug Metab Disposition* **9**, 246.

29. Venitt S, Bushnell CT, Osborne M (1977) Mutagenicity of acrylonitrile (cyanoethylene) in *Escherichia coli. Mutat Res* **45**, 283.

30. Ward CE, Starr TB (1993) Comparison of cancer risks projected from animal bioassays to epidemiological studies of acrylonitrile-exposed workers. *Regul Toxicol Pharmacol* **18**, 2142.

31. Willhite CC (1982) Toxicology Update: Acrylonitrile. *J Appl Toxicol* **2**, 54.

32. Willhite CC, Fern VH, Smith RP (1981) Teratogenic effects of aliphatic nitriles. *Teratology* **23**, 317.

33. Yates JM, Fennell TR, Turner MJ *et al.* (1994) Characterization of phosphodiester adducts produced by the reaction of cyanoethylene oxide with nucleotides. *Carcinogenesis* **15**, 277.

34. Yates JM, Sumner SC, Turner MJ *et al.* (1994) Characterization of an adduct and its degradation product produced by the reaction of cyanoethylene oxide with deoxythymidine and DNA. *Carcinogenesis* **14**, 1363.

35. Woutersen RA (1998) Toxicologic profile of acrylonitrile. *Scand J Work Environ Health* **24** Suppl 2, 5.

Acyclovir

Herbet H. Schaumburg

ACYCLOVIR
$C_8H_{11}N_3O_3$

2-Amino-1,9-dihydro-9-[(2-hydroxyethoxy)methyl]-6*H*-purin-6-one

NEUROTOXICITY RATING

Clinical

A Acute encephalopathy (confusion, hallucinations)

Acyclovir is a synthetic purine nucleoside analog widely used in the treatment of *Herpes simplex* and *Varicella zoster* virus infections. It blocks replication by inhibiting viral DNA synthesis. Before inhibition can occur, acyclovir must be phosphorylated by viral thymidine kinase; the affinity for viral thymidine kinase is 200 times greater than that for the corresponding mammalian enzyme.

The drug is usually administered parenterally in doses of 5–9 mg/kg for systemic injection; oral and topical administration dramatically reduce bioavailability. Acyclovir is rapidly distributed throughout the body and eliminated mostly unchanged by glomerular filtration and renal tubular secretion. Renal insufficiency may be associated with neurotoxicity (6).

There is little systemic toxicity; local irritation at the infusion site and rare instances of obstructive nephropathy are described.

A reversible encephalopathy is estimated to appear in <1% of patients treated with conventional dosages (1–7). Disorientation and confusion develop initially, followed by a florid delirium with hallucinations, dysarthria, restlessness, and tremor. In severe cases, there are both myoclonic jerks and generalized seizures. Two conditions predispose to encephalopathy: one occurs when drug is administered to bone marrow-transplant recipients; the other when it is given to patients with renal compromise. Individuals subject to bone marrow transplantation may be predisposed because they are leukemic, receive intrathecal methotrexate and, sometimes, α-interferon (7). Patients with renal compromise experience prolonged, elevated plasma levels that are reduced only by hemodialysis; peritoneal dialysis is ineffective (2).

One individual receiving an oral dose of 600 mg daily for 4 months experienced mild encephalopathy (depression, fatigue, irritability, lethargy) (5). Clinical manifestations persisted after reducing the dose to 400 mg but cleared completely within 3 days of drug withdrawal. Acyclovir was recommended at a level of 200 mg daily without adverse effects.

REFERENCES

1. Bean B, Aeppli D (1985) Adverse effects of high-dose intravenous acyclovir in ambulatory patients with acute herpes zoster. *J Infect Dis* **151**, 362.
2. Davenport A, Goel S, Jackenzie JC (1992) Neurotoxicity of acyclovir in patients with end-stage renal failure treated with continuous ambulatory peritoneal dialysis. *Amer J Kidney Dis* **20**, 647.
3. Ernst ME, Franey RJ (1998) Acyclovir- and ganciclovir-induced neurotoxicity. *Ann Pharmacother* **32**, 111.
4. Feldman S, Rodman J, Gregory B (1988) Excessive serum concentration of acyclovir and neurotoxicity. *J Infect Dis* **157**, 385.
5. Krigel RL (1986) Reversible neurotoxicity due to oral acyclovir in a patient with chronic lymphocytic leukemia. *J Infect Dis* **154**, 189.
6. Matsumoto R, Yoshida T, Tabata K *et al.* (1996) A patient with thyroid carcinoma who developed consciousness disturbance during acyclovir administration for herpes zoster. *Rinsho Shinkeigaku* **36**, 590.
7. Wade JC, Meyers JD (1983) Neurologic symptoms associated with parenteral acyclovir treatment after marrow transplantation. *Ann Intern Med* **98**, 921.

Agaritine

Peter S. Spencer

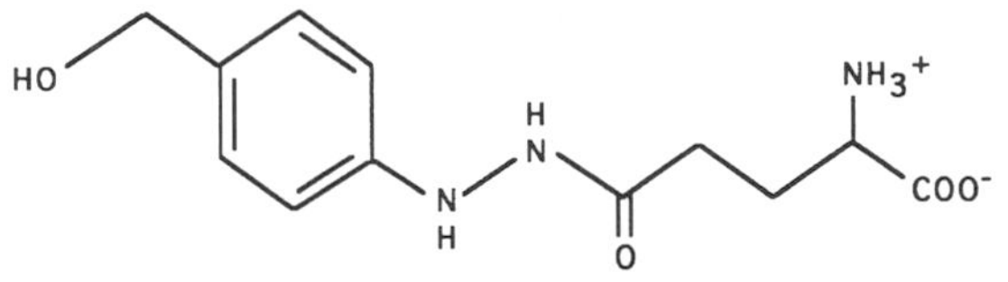

L-Glutamic acid-5-[2-[4-(hydroxymethyl)-phenyl]hydrazide; β-N-[γ-L(+)-Glutamyl]-4-hydroxymethylphenylhydrazine

NEUROTOXICITY RATING

Experimental

A   Seizure disorder

Agaritine is a naturally occurring hydrazine present in fresh, dried, and processed samples of the common edible mushroom (*Agaricus bisporus*). Concentration in fresh plant material is given as 100–250 mg/kg (3) or approximately 0.03% (1). N2-[L-(+)-Glutamyl]-4-(hydroxymethylphenyl)-hydrazine is a major murine metabolite (5). When agaritine was injected into Swiss mice at 25–400 mg/kg body weight, high doses caused excitation, convulsions, and death (4). Several agaritine derivatives have been shown to produce tumors in laboratory animals (2).

REFERENCES

1. LaRue TA (1977) Naturally occurring compounds containing a nitrogen-nitrogen bond. *Lloydia* **40**, 307.
2. Price RJ, Walters DG, Hoff C *et al.* (1996) Metabolism of [ring-U^{14}-C] agaritine by precision-cut rat, mouse and human liver and lung slices. *Food Chem Toxicol* **34**, 603.
3. Sharman M, Patey AL, Gilbert J (1990) A survey of the occurrence of agaritine in U.K. cultivated mushrooms and processed mushroom products. *Food Addit Contam* **7**, 649.
4. Toth B, Nagel D, Shimizu H *et al.* (1975) Tumorigenicity of *n*-propyl, *n*-amyl, and alkyl-hydrazines. Toxicity of agaritine. *Proc Amer Assn Cancer Res* **16**, 61.
5. Walton K, Coombs MM, Catterall FS *et al.* (1997) Bioactivation of the mushroom hydrazine, agaritine, to intermediates that bind covalently to proteins and induce mutations in the Ames test. *Carcinogenesis* **18**, 1603.

Agatoxins

Albert C. Ludolph

NEUROTOXICITY RATING

Experimental

A   Glutamate (NMDA) antagonists (α-agatoxins)

A   Voltage-dependent Na$^+$ channel activation (μ-agatoxins)

A   Ca^{2+} channel blockade (ω-agatoxins)

The venom of the American funnel web spider *Agelenopsis aperta* (family Agelenidae) contains several classes of naturally occurring insecticides. *α-Agatoxins* are low-molecular-weight acylpolyamines that reversibly paralyze insects by postsynaptic blockade of glutamatergic transmission. It has been shown *in vitro* that α-agatoxins are reversible, selective, and noncompetitive antagonists of the N-methyl-D-aspartate (NMDA) glutamate receptor subtype in the mammalian brain (9). Their potency is comparable with the standard noncompetitive NMDA antagonist MK-801 (9). This channel-blocking effect may functionally mask the stimulatory effect of α-agatoxins at the polyamine site of the receptor (13).

Six *μ-agatoxins* from the funnel web spider are currently known (I–VI). These peptides are presynaptic activators of voltage-dependent Na$^+$ channels. They cause repetitive firing and excessive spontaneous transmitter release at insect neuromuscular junctions, with paralysis, tremor, and excitation (2,11), an effect likely to be insect-specific.

In contrast, *ω-agatoxins* are antagonists at presynaptic and synaptosomal calcium channels; they also paralyze injected insects (5). The effect of these peptides is species-dependent; some of these compounds are also neurotoxic in mice. At least eight subtypes of ω-agatoxins (IA, IB, IC, IIA, IIB, IIIA, IIIB, IVa) can be distinguished. Molecular size, amino acid sequence, and electrophysiological and biochemical characteristics permit this subclassification (1,3,4,6,10,12). ω-Agatoxins are used as pharmacological tools to characterize and subclassify calcium channels of vertebrates and invertebrates; they share with other ion-channel toxins from spiders, cone shells, and certain plants and fungi, a common structural motif consisting of a cystine knot and a triple-stranded, antiparallel beta sheet (7). Binding sites of ω-agatoxin IVA, which are widely distributed in the mammalian CNS, are found in the cerebellum on the somata and dendrites of Purkinje cells, granule cells and interneurons, and in the hippocampus, on the somata of pyramidal cells of the CA1–CA4 region and on the somata of granule cells in the dentate gyrus (6).

REFERENCES

1. Adams ME, Bindokas VP, Hasegawa L, Venema VJ (1990) Omega-agatoxins: Novel calcium channel antagonists of two subtypes from funnel web spider (*Agelenopsis aperta*) venom. *J Biol Chem* **265**, 861.

2. Adams ME, Herold EE, Venema VJ (1989) Two classes of channel-specific toxins from funnel web spider venom. *J Comp Physiol A* **164**, 333.

3. Bindokas VP, Venema VJ, Adams ME (1991) Differential antagonism of transmitter release by subtypes of omega-agatoxins. *J Neurophysiol* **66**, 590.

4. Mintz IM, Venema VJ, Adams ME, Bean BP (1991) Inhibition of L-type and N-type ion channels by the spider venom toxin omega-Aga-IIIa. *Proc Nat Acad Sci USA* **88**, 6628.

5. Mintz IM, Venema VJ, Swiderek KM *et al.* (1992) P-type calcium channels blocked by the spider toxin omega-Aga-IVa. *Nature* **355**, 827.

6. Nakanishi S, Fujii A, Kimura T *et al.* (1995) Spatial distribution of omega-agatoxin IVA binding sites in mouse brain slices. *Neurosci Res* **41**, 532.

7. Norton RS, Pallaghy PK (1998) The cystine knot structure of ion channel toxins and related polypeptides. *Toxicon* **36**, 1573.

8. Ohizumi Y (1997) Application of physiologically active substances isolated from natural resources to pharmacological studies. *Jpn J Pharmacol* **73**, 263.

9. Parks TN, Müller AL, Artman LD *et al.* (1991) Arylamine toxins from funnel-web spider (*Agenelopsis aperta*) venom antagonize N-methyl-D-aspartate receptor function in mammalian brain. *J Biol Chem* **266**, 21523.

10. Pocock JM, Venema VJ, Adams ME (1992) Omega-agatoxins differentially block calcium channels in locust, chick and rat synaptosomes. *Neurochem Int* **20**, 263.

11. Skinner WS, Adams ME, Quistad GB *et al.* (1989) Purification and characterization of two classes of neurotoxins from the funnel web spider, *Agelenopsis aperta*. *J Biol Chem* **264**, 21590.

12. Venema VJ, Swiderek KM, Lee TD *et al.* (1992) Antagonism of synaptosomal calcium channels by subtypes of omega-agatoxins. *J Biol Chem* **267**, 2610.

13. Williams K (1993) Effects of *Agelenopsis aperta* toxins on the N-methyl-D-aspartate receptor: Polyamine-like and high-affinity antagonist actions. *J Pharmacol Exp Ther* **266**, 231.

L-Alanosine A

Albert C. Ludolph

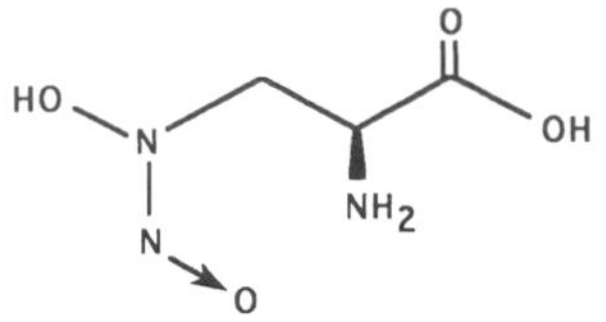

L-ALANOSINE A
$C_3H_7N_3O_4$

3-(Hydroxynitrosoamino)-L-alanine

NEUROTOXICITY RATING

Clinical

A   Acute encephalopathy (headache, confusion)

Experimental

A   Excitotoxicity

L-Alanosine is an analogue of L-aspartic acid isolated from the fungus *Streptomyces alanosinicus* (1,5). The compound has immunosuppressive, antitumor, antimicrobial, and antiviral properties (1,5). In the 1980s, clinical interest centered on the antineoplastic activity of alanosine A; however, therapeutic expectations were not met. L-Alanosine disrupts *de novo* purine synthesis at the level of adenylosuccinate lyase and synthetase. Because of its structural similarities to aspartate, glutamine, and glutamate, it also interferes with their respective uptake mechanisms, and their anabolic and catabolic pathways. Its function as a copper chelator likely does not contribute to its neurotoxic and antineoplastic properties.

Experimental studies in adult mice failed to demonstrate neurotoxicity (6). However, glutamate-like lesions of the arcuate nucleus of the hypothalamus, subfornical organ, and area postrema of young mice were observed after intraperitoneal injection of L-alanosine (4). Dogs dose-relatedly de-veloped repetitive lip-licking, hyperexcitability, tonic muscle spasms, flaccid paralysis of hindlimbs, mydriasis, and laryngospasm at reported doses ranging from 100–800 mg/kg body weight (5).

There are few observations of potential human neurotoxicity. After an intravenous high-dosage bolus, two patients developed renal failure accompanied by headache, confusion, and disorientation (2). Peripheral neuropathies developed when alanosine A was combined with vinblastine, acivicin, and aminothiadiazole (3); however, the absence of neuropathies in other combinations make it unlikely that alanosine A is a peripheral neurotoxin.

REFERENCES

1. Ahluwalia GS, Grem JL, Hao Z, Cooney DA (1990) Metabolism and action of amino acid analog anti-cancer agents. *Pharmacol Ther* **46**, 243.
2. Creagan ET, Schutt AJ, Ingle JN, Fallon JR (1983) Phase II clinical trial of L-alanosine in advanced upper aerodigestive cancer. *Cancer Treatment Rep* **67**, 1047.
3. Elson PJ, Kvols LK, Vogl SE *et al.* (1988) Phase II trials of 5-day vinblastine infusion (NSC 49842), L-alanosine (NSC 153353), activin (NSC 163501), and aminothiadiazole (NSC 4278) in patients with recurrent or metastatic renal cell carcinoma. *Invest New Drugs* **6**, 97.
4. Olney JW, Fuller T, de Gubareff T (1977) Alanosine—an antileukemic agent with glutamate-like neurotoxic properties. *J Neuropathol Exp Neurol* **36**, 619.
5. Tiyagi AG, Cooney DA (1984) Biochemical pharmacology, metabolism, and mechanism of action of L-alanosine, a novel natural antitumor agent. *Adv Pharmacol Chemother* **20**, 69.
6. Tiyagi AG, Thake DC, McGee E, Cooney DA (1981) Determinations of the toxicity of L-alanosine to various organs of the mouse. *Toxicology* **21**, 59.

Allyl Chloride

Fengsheng He

$$CH_2 = CHCH_2Cl$$

ALLYL CHLORIDE
C_3H_5Cl

Chlorallylene; 3-Chloro-1-propene; 3-Chloropropylene

NEUROTOXICITY RATING
Clinical
A Peripheral neuropathy
Experimental
A Peripheral neuropathy

Allyl chloride is a colorless or yellow chlorinated liquid with an irritating and unpleasant odor. It is volatile, highly reactive, and flammable. It is utilized primarily as an intermediate in the manufacture of epichlorohydrin and glycerin. The agent is also used in the synthesis of allyl compounds, such as sodium allyl sulfonate. The time-weighted Threshold Limit Value of allyl chloride is 1 ppm in the United States, United Kingdom, Australia, and Germany; its Maximal Allowable Concentration is 2 mg/m^3 (0.66 ppm) in China.

The pharmacokinetic fate of allyl chloride is dose- and route-dependent following oral or inhalation exposure. Allyl chloride causes marked depletion of nonprotein sulfhydryls (NPSH) in the liver, kidney, and lung in rats exposed at 1000 or 2000 ppm for a single 6 h exposure. A slight decrease in NPSH was found in rats exposed at 100 ppm for a comparable period, and no diminution of NPSH was seen in rats exposed to 10 ppm allyl chloride vapor (1).

In animal studies, topical application of allyl chloride causes dermal irritation, but one drop in a rabbit's eye caused only mild transient injury due to the low boiling point and rapid evaporation of the chemical. The oral LD$_{50}$ levels of allyl chloride in mouse and rat are 425 mg/kg and 460 mg/kg, respectively (5). The 2 h LC$_{50}$ levels in mouse, rat, guinea pig, rabbit, and cat are 11.5, 11.0, 5.8, 22.5, and 10.5 mg/l, respectively. In short-term mouse inhalation studies, initial signs of irritation (scratching the nose, lacrimation, and salivation) were followed by hypoactivity, hypopnea, and paralysis of hindlimbs. Drowsiness, unconsciousness, tremor, and convulsion were noted in all animals. There was also marked pulmonary congestion, hemorrhages and edema, focal necrosis in renal glomerular epithelium, and cloudy swelling of hepatocytes (1).

Inhalation studies using an allyl chloride concentration of 68.6 ppm (206 mg/m^3), 6 h/day, 6 days/week for 3 months have been conducted in rabbits (5). In the second

month of exposure, dosed animals showed denervation potentials by electromyography and developed unsteady gait and flaccid paralysis followed by muscular atrophy and emaciation. Histopathological studies disclosed wallerian degeneration of sciatic nerve fibers (3).

Hindlimb weakness appeared in mice dosed with 500 mg/kg allyl chloride *per os*, three times weekly, for periods of 2–17 weeks (2). Functional disability was more frequent in male mice than in females. Histopathological study disclosed nerve fiber degeneration in many peripheral nerves and in spinal roots. Motor nerves were more affected than sensory nerves, and evidence of degeneration was more marked distally. Dorsal, ventral, and lateral columns of the spinal cord contained degenerated fibers. An early axonal change was multifocal accumulations of 10 nm neurofilaments. Other axons were found to contain aggregations of organelles, often of degenerated mitochondria. Abnormalities of Schwann cell cytoplasm independent of axonal change suggested a direct effect of allyl chloride upon these cells. Later stages of nerve fiber degeneration were also evident, with breakdown of myelin sheaths and the presence of macrophages containing myelin debris. No neuronal death was observed, but occasional anterior horn cells showed swelling of the Golgi apparatus. Vacuolar changes in astrocytes and their processes were present in the ventral horn in cervical and lumbar regions of spinal cord. In sum, murine allyl chloride neuropathy appears to be a central–peripheral distal type of axonopathy (*see* Chapter 1).

Two outbreaks of neuropathy in allyl chloride workers were first reported in China in the early 1970s, one in a factory producing sodium allyl sulfonate and the other in a plant manufacturing epichlorohydrin (2–4). Twenty-six subjects in one factory were exposed to allyl chloride at levels of 2.6–6650 mg/m^3 (0.86–2217 ppm) for 2.5 months to 6 years; in another factory, 27 subjects were exposed at 0.2–25.13 mg/m^3 (0.06–8.37 ppm) for periods of 1–4.5 years. Most workers in the first factory had weakness, paresthesias, and numbness in extremities, with sensory impairment in a glove-and-stocking distribution, as well as reduced ankle reflexes. Electroneuromyography showed neurogenic abnormalities in 10 of the 19 subjects examined; the prevalence of neuropathy, therefore, was 56.2%. Workers in the second factory were less severely affected; there were few abnormal neurological signs, but electroneuromyographic abnormalities consistent with mild neuropathy were found in 13 of the 27 subjects. Insomnia, dizziness, and anorexia were uncommon. No significant abnormalities of other organs were noted.

Chronic allyl chloride intoxication causes an insidious onset of symptoms (3). Patients may complain of lacrimation and sneezing during initial exposure. Most develop weakness in the legs and hands; they have difficulty in walking fast and gripping small objects with fingers. Tingling and numbness in hands and feet are frequently reported. Pain is either absent or minimal, and usually limited to mild cramping. Evidence of symmetrical, distal, motor, and sensory dysfunction are the prominent findings. Sensory deficits include loss of pinprick, light touch, and vibration sensation; they are marked in the distal parts of the extremities and may progress to the level of elbows and knees in severe cases. Position sense is relatively intact. Weakness is distal and often mild; severe cases may display paresis in legs. Ankle reflexes are absent in advanced cases. Diminution of temperature sense and hyperhydrosis in hands and feet are rare. Cranial nerves are not involved. Electrodiagnostic findings include spontaneous fibrillation and positive sharp waves, and increased distal latencies with modest changes in conduction velocity. Electromyographic evidence of denervation potentials appears more frequently in patients with severe chronic allyl chloride poisoning.

Diagnosis of chronic allyl chloride poisoning can be established on the basis of verified exposure to allyl chloride, and symptoms, signs, and electrodiagnostic evidence of polyneuropathy. Other causes of neuropathy must be excluded in isolated cases.

Improvement commences after exposure ceases. Treatment is symptomatic and supportive. Recovery from sensory, reflex, and neurophysiological dysfunction is usually not noted until the 9th to 11th month of treatment. Loss of ankle reflexes may persist (3).

The mechanism underlying allyl chloride neurotoxicity is unknown. The accumulation of neurofilaments induced by allyl chloride does not seem to share a common mechanism with the 2,5-hexanedione axonopathy, which is associated with cross-linking of neurofilament proteins *in vitro* and *in vivo* (6).

REFERENCES

1. American Conference of Governmental Industrial Hygienists (1991) Allyl chloride. In: *Documentation of the Threshold Limit Values and Biological Exposure Indices. 6th Ed.* ACGIH, Cincinnati, OH p. 36.
2. He F, Jacobs JM, Scaravilli F (1981) The pathology of allyl chloride neurotoxicity in mice. *Acta Neuropathol* 55, 125.
3. He F, Lu B, Zhang S *et al.* (1985) Chronic allyl chloride poisoning. An epidemiological, clinical, toxicological and neuropathological study. *Med Lav* 7, 5.
4. He F, Zhang S (1985) Effects of allyl chloride on occupationally exposed subjects. *Scand J Work Environ Health* 43, 11.
5. Lu B, Dong S, Yu A, Xian Y (1982) Studies on the toxicity of allyl chloride. *Ecotoxicol Environ Safety* 6, 19.
6. Nagano M, Yamamoto H, Harada K *et al.* (1993) Comparative study of modification and degradation of neurofilament proteins in rats subchronically treated with allyl chloride, acrylamide, or 2,5-hexanedione. *Environ Res* 63, 229.

Allylglycine

Albert C. Ludolph

$$CH_3(CH_2)_2CH(NH_2)COOH$$

ALLYLGLYCINE
$C_5H_{11}NO_2$

2-Aminopentenoic acid; Norvaline; 2-Aminovaleric acid

NEUROTOXICITY RATING
Clinical
A   Seizure disorder
Experimental
A   Seizure disorder
A   Inhibition of GABA synthesis

Allylglycine is used experimentally to induce convulsions and status epilepticus in rodents and nonhuman primates (1,2). This is the effect of its metabolite, 2-keto-4-pentenoic acid, which disrupts the synthesis of γ-aminobutyric acid (GABA) by inhibition of glutamic acid decarboxylase *in vivo* and *in vitro* (5). Generalized seizures lasting 1–3 min are induced after systemic application of allylglycine and a latent period of 0.5–4 h; they may be repetitive and merge into status epilepticus (2). In rhesus monkeys and baboons, generalized seizures reportedly commence with horizontal nystagmus, conjugate deviation of the eyes, and turning the head to one side, and are accompanied by rhythmic spikes in the electroencephalogram of the contralateral posterior hemisphere (2). In baboons, hypoglycemia was observed in recurrent seizures associated with hippocampal damage (3). Neurochemical alterations induced by administration of allylglycine to rats have been described (4). In the photosensitive Senegalese baboon, *Papio papio*, allylglycine reduces cerebrospinal fluid levels of GABA and, to a lesser degree, alanine but not glutamine (6). These biochemical effects are apparently independent of seizure activity (6).

REFERENCES

1. De-Deyn PP, D'Hooge R, Marescau B, Pei YQ (1992) Chemical models of epilepsy with some reference to their applicability in the development of anticonvulsants. *Epilepsy Res* 12, 87.
2. Meldrum BS (1975) Epilepsy and gamma-butyric acid-mediated inhibition. *Int Rev Neurobiol* 17, 1.
3. Meldrum BS, Horton RW, Brierley JB (1974) Epileptic brain damage in adolescent baboons following seizures induced by allylglycine. *Brain* 97, 407.
4. Meldrum BS, Swan JH, Otterson OP, Storm-Matthisen J (1987) Redistribution of transmitter amino acids in rat hippocampus and cerebellum during seizures induced by L-allylglycine and bicuilline: an immunocytochemical study with antisera against conjugated GABA, glutamate and aspartate. *Neuroscience* 22, 17.
5. Orlowski M, Reingold DF, Stanley ME (1977) D- and L-Stereoisomers of allylglycine: convulsive action and inhibition of brain L-glutamate decarboxylase. *J Neurochem* 28, 349.
6. Valin A, Voltz C, Naquet R, Lloyd KG (1991) Effects of pharmacological manipulation on neurotransmitter and other amino acid transmitter levels in the CSF of the Senegalese baboon *Papio papio*. *Brain Res* 538, 15.

Almitrine Bimesilate

Herbert H. Schaumburg

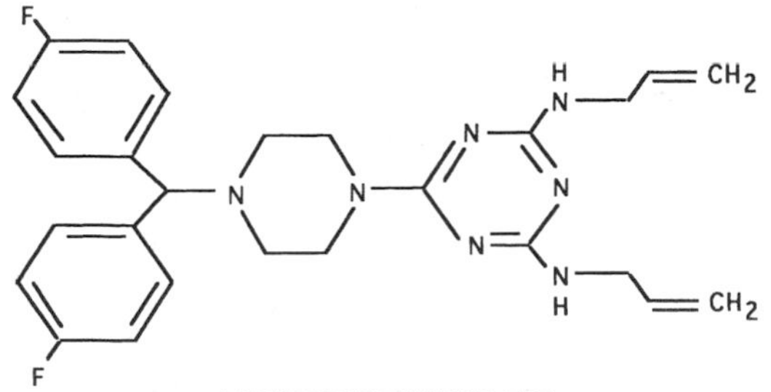

ALMITRINE BIMESILATE
$C_{26}H_{29}F_2N_7$

6-[4-[Bis(4-fluorophenyl)methyl]-1-piperazinyl]-*N*,*N'*-di-2-propenyl-1,3,5-triazine-2,4-diamine

NEUROTOXICITY RATING

Clinical

C   Peripheral neuropathy

Almitrine bimesilate is a peripheral chemoreceptor agonist used as a respiratory stimulant. There are several anecdotal reports of sensory neuropathy occasionally accompanying its use (1–4). All patients lost weight and experienced distal limb paresthesias. None of the reports contains credible electrophysiological or histopathological data.

Rats treated for prolonged periods with difluorobenzhydrylpiperadine, a detriazinyl metabolite of almitrine, reportedly developed an ataxic or spastic gait. Lamellated and crystalloid bodies were found in sensory neurons, satellite cells, Schwann cells, and endothelial cells of thoracic and lumbar dorsal root ganglia, and in hindlimb muscles and muscle spindles (5,6).

REFERENCES

1. Bardsley PA, Howard P, DeBacker W *et al.* (1991) Two years treatment with almitrine bismesylate in patients with hypoxic chronic obstructive airway disease. *Eur Resp J* 4, 308.
2. Gherardi R, Belec L, Louarn F (1989) Almitrine-induced peripheral neuropathy and weight loss. *J Neurol* 236, 374.
3. Watanabe S, Kanner RE, Curtillo AG *et al.* (1989) Long-term effect of almitrine bismesylate in patients with hypoxemic chronic obstructive pulmonary disease. *Amer Rev Resp Dis* 140, 1269.
4. Weitzenblum E, Arnaud F, Bignon J *et al.* (1992) Sequential administration of a reduced dose of almitrine to patients with chronic obstructive bronchopneumopathies. A controlled multicenter study. *Rev Mal Resp* 9, 455.
5. Yamanaka Y, Sakamoto E, Sakuma Y *et al.* (1995) Lipidosis of the dorsal root ganglia in rats treated with an almitrine metabolite. *Arch Toxicol* 69, 391.
6. Yamanaka Y, Shimada T, Mochizuki R *et al.* (1997) Neuronal and muscular inclusions in rats with hindlimb dysfunction after treating with difluorobenzhydrylpiperadine. *Toxicol Pathol* 25, 150.

Aluminum and Its Compounds

Peter S. Spencer

The natural abundance and widespread use of aluminum (Al) account for the metal's ubiquitous presence in air, food, and water. Al is found in the body of apparently normal humans, although there is no known physiological function for the metal. The neurotoxic potential of Al and its compounds is a complex and controversial subject. There is solid clinical evidence that Al overload in subjects with chronic renal dysfunction has the potential to cause fatal acute and chronic encephalopathic states. The risk posed by the combination of renal compromise and Al exposure has also raised important questions about the mental development of preterm infants on prolonged intravenous feeding with solutions containing Al compounds. There is also a body of epidemiological and experimental animal data that has sought—so far unconvincingly—to relate Al exposure in food and water to the etiology of sporadic Alzheimer's disease and the western Pacific amyotrophic lateral sclerosis and Parkinsonism–dementia complex (ALS/PDC). Al has also been singled out as a possible etiological factor in an unconfirmed condition ("potroom palsy") described in workers employed at an aluminum smelter.

Elemental Al is a tin-white, malleable, ductile solid metal with a MP of 600°C and BP of 2327°C. It is the most abundant metal in the earth's crust (~8.8% w/w), where it is found predominantly as aluminosilicates and clay minerals. In aqueous solution in acid soils (pH < 5.5), the charged trivalent Al species exists as an octahedral hexahydrate, $Al(H_2O_6)_6^{3+}$, a species held responsible for the metal's potential toxic effects on plants (34). Lowering the hydrogen ion concentration results in successive deprotonations until, at neutral pH, Al precipitates as $Al(OH)_3$ or redissolves in the form of tetrahedral aluminate, $Al(OH)_4^{-}$, the primary soluble Al(III) species at pH >6.2 (55).

Metallic Al, produced by electrolysis of alumina prepared from bauxite, finds heavy use in the construction and automobile industries, and in consumer appliances, durables, containers, canning, cookware, and signage. Al compounds are employed in water purification (Al sulfates), food processing (Na-Al sulfate and silicate), and medicines, including antacids (Al hydroxide). Between 1944 and 1979, a finely powdered form of metallic Al and an Al oxide, known as McIntyre's powder, was administered by inhalation to Canadian gold miners as a prophylaxis for occupational silicosis (73). From 1970 onward, orally administered Al compounds were routinely given to patients with uremia to control serum phosphorus levels and thereby prevent metastatic calcification and secondary hyperparathyroidism (2,39). Use of these phosphate binders increases oral intake of Al from 2–15 mg/day in the diet to quantities measured in grams (2,101). Patients with renal disease under treatment with dialysis are also exposed to water containing Al from natural sources and added flocculants. The Al content of dialysate is carefully controlled in the United States to minimize the potential for osteo-, hemato-, and neurotoxicity.

General Toxicology

Al exists only in the trivalent (Al^{3+}) oxidation state in biological systems. Its chemistry predicts that Al^{3+} binds strongly to oxygen, carboxylate, and deprotonated hydroxy and phosphate groups (55). The ionic radius of Al^{3+} is similar to that of Fe^{3+} and Mg^{2+} with which it is most likely to compete (55). Substitution of Al^{3+} for Mg^{2+} or Ca^{2+} in metal-ion cofactor-dependent enzyme systems is likely to interfere with enzyme activity because Al^{3+} has a much slower ligand exchange rate (55). In blood, approximately 90% of Al^{3+} binds to transferrin (largely inert form) and 10% to citrate; by contrast, in cerebrospinal fluid (CSF), where the citrate/transferrin ratio is two to three orders of magnitude greater, Al^{3+} is likely bound principally to the more bioavailable citrate form. Free $[Al^{3+}]$ in blood and CSF are similar ($<10^{-14}$ M); however, the precise speciation of Al in biological fluids is uncertain (33,55). Free Al^{3+} binds strongly to amines and nucleoside diphosphates and triphosphates; amino acids, nucleic acids, and calmodulin bind Al^{3+} weakly. Al^{3+} apparently is able to cross-link proteins, and proteins and nucleic acids (55).

Absorption of aluminum by animals and humans after oral administration of various Al species containing ^{27}Al and ^{26}Al reportedly is low (<1%) (104); however, other estimates range from 0.06%–1% in animals and from 0.005%–24% in humans (98). The amount absorbed is said to be heavily dependent on intraluminal Al speciation, presence of competing (Fe^{3+}, Ca^{2+}) or complexing substances (citrate, ascorbic acid), and intraluminal hydrogen ion concentration. Absorption is facilitated by citrate, ascorbate, and calcium deficiency; silicon and fluoride may reduce absorption (104).

Transfer of Al from lung to blood in Al workers—likely a function of Al particle composition and size—appears to be in the range of 1%–2%, with higher rates of absorption at lower airborne concentrations (104). Percutaneous absorption of certain Al compounds is suggested by animal studies in which application of low aqueous concentrations of Al chlorohydrate (the active ingredient of antiperspirants) to the shaven dorsal skin of mice raised Al concentrations in serum, brain (especially hippocampus), and urine (6). Patients with skin burns may be at risk for parenteral absorption of Al from bath water (43).

Animal studies suggest the possibility that environmental Al may enter the brain directly *via* a nasal olfactory pathway (70); Al(III) was found in the cerebral cortex, hippocampus, entorhinal area, olfactory bulb, and cerebellar Purkinje cells of rats which for 2 weeks had inhaled Al acetylacetonate, a neutral, hydrolytically stable and lipophilic compound (105).

The human body burden of Al ranges from 50–150 mg; daily intake is 10–100 mg. Plasma levels of Al are <3 mg/ml (2); the half-life is >40 h (98). Absorbed Al accumulates mainly in bone, muscle, liver, and kidneys; lowest concentrations are found in the brain in cases of Al overload (*vide infra*) (93). Al is excreted mainly in urine: one study of 50 healthy volunteers reported urinary Al excretion of 12.2 ± 8.6 mg/24 h (97). Al welders have been reported to have raised levels of blood Al, but not as high as those seen in patients undergoing renal dialysis without clinical signs of encephalopathy (84). Occupational exposure for about 20 years was associated with urine Al concentrations two orders of magnitude higher than those in nonexposed workers (83). The half-life of urinary Al reportedly was 6 months or longer after long-term occupational exposure to the metal (81).

Al traverses the blood-brain regulatory interface and increases the permeability of certain other substances (7,17). Brain Al concentrations sufficient to induce acute or chronic encephalopathy in humans have occurred in patients with renal disease after exposure to Al-containing pharmaceuticals, after parenteral exposure to Al from contaminated media for hemo- and peritoneal dialysis (2), and after intravesical irrigation of the urinary bladder with alum solution for treatment of hemorrhagic cystitis (69). Long-term parenteral nutrition with Al-contaminated products is another method of potential iatrogenic Al intoxication (42). Postmortem analyses of brain tissue from patients who died of dialysis encephalopathy (*vide infra*) show that Al is primarily deposited in gray matter (4).

Animal Studies

The neurotoxic properties of Al in animals have been recognized for over 100 years (20). In 1937, a neurological syndrome characterized by motor malfunction and convulsions was described in animals given a single CNS injection of an Al salt (75). Experiments conducted in the 1940s demonstrated that several Al compounds induced recurrent convulsive seizures when applied directly to the cerebral cortex (46). From the 1960s onward, interest focused on the observation that Al-treated animals displayed neurofibrillary degeneration that bore a superficial resemblance to the neuropathology of Alzheimer's disease and western Pacific ALS/PDC (41,88,99). Ultrastructural examination, however, showed the Al-induced neuronal changes to consist of dense perikaryal masses of normal 10 nm neurofilaments (78,88), indistinguishable from those that accumulate in toxic states induced by a range of unrelated chemicals.

Al-treated rabbits showed a reduced rate of slow axonal transport of neurofilament subunits in sciatic and hypoglossal nerves (10,91), and normal fast axonal transport in sciatic nerve (51). Brain 200 kDa neurofilament subunit protein and microtubule-associated protein-2 were heavily phosphorylated in rats treated orally with Al (38). Immunological reactivity to phosphorylated neurofilaments (a marker of neuronal pathology) was present in cortical layers III and V, basal forebrain, ventral hippocampus, nucleus raphe dorsalis, and locus ceruleus (47).

Cynomolgus monkeys fed a low-calcium, high-Al diet remained behaviorally and clinically normal but showed central chromatolysis and accumulations of neurofilaments in motor neurons of spinal cord, brainstem, and cerebral cortex (28,102). Loss of synaptic density was reported in the brains of rabbits after prolonged treatment (200 days) with Al tartrate administered by intraperitoneal injection (92). Changes in synaptic activity, transmitters, receptors, and related enzyme systems have been reviewed (59). Al inhibits choline transport in rat brain, reduces neural choline acetyltransferase activity, and inhibits uptake of choline, glutamate, norepinephrine, and serotonin into rat synaptosomes (2,49). Learning and memory deficits are present in Al-treated animals (rats, rabbits, cats) (13,50,71,72,103).

Injection of Al powder into the CSF of adult rabbits induces a slowly progressive encephalomyelopathy with cerebellar degeneration characterized at first by postural alterations and, then, by myoclonic jerks and muscle weakness. Initially, giant axonal swellings filled with neurofilaments were numerous in the gray matter and particularly prominent in the most proximal axonal segments of anterior horn cells. Neurofibrillary degeneration decreased and neuronophagia of lower motor neurons increased in the second and third months when animals also showed evidence of paranodal swelling, myelin retraction, nerve fiber degeneration, and neurogenic atrophy of associated muscles (11).

In Vitro Studies

There is an extensive literature on the cellular and biochemical effects of Al (2,59). Erythrocytes show a marked decrease in membrane fluidity and an increase in membrane fragility (106). Al non-uniquely induces the formation of tetrodotoxin-insensitive Na^+-permeable plasmalemmal ionic channels in neuroblastoma cells (68). These cells utilize plasma-membrane transferrin receptors to take up Al into the intracellular compartment, where it may be found in extraordinarily high concentrations (up to 10–20 mM) (79). Al accumulates in the chromatin of neural cells *in vivo* and may change the accessibility of chromatin to exogenous nucleases *in vitro* (16,94). Al displaces ethidium bromide binding to DNA, forms complexes with DNA, and increases the association between linker histones and DNA (40,53). Al decreases ribosomal RNA content and increases protein synthesis in neuroblastoma cells (62). Activity of rat brain mitochondrial hexokinase—one of the rate-limiting enzymes of glycolysis—is inhibited by Al (27,49).

Human Studies

Brain function of individuals with *normal* kidney function is, with few exceptions, not known to be overtly affected by aluminum. Occupational exposure to Al-containing materials, while associated in some reports with pulmonary disease and certain malignancies, has very rarely been linked with clear-cut neurological disease. Neuropsychological deficits reported in long-term Al-exposed workers have been challenged and require further study. Proposed associations between lifetime exposure to Al in water and food and the development of progressive neurodegenerative disorders, including sporadic Alzheimer's disease, are heavily touted hypotheses.

Acute and chronic encephalopathic states from Al overload occur in adults and children with *impaired* kidney function who are treated with oral phosphate-binding agents that contain Al and/or Al-contaminated dialysates (5,31,66). Dialysis encephalopathy was recognized in 0.4% (*n* = 229) of treated patients in 1980 and 0.1% (*n* = 129) in 1990 (2). Chelation and removal of Al can reverse the course of this otherwise progressive and fatal neurotoxic disorder (1).

Intravenously fed preterm infants, whose renal function is frequently compromised during their initial postnatal course, also appear to be at risk for Al toxicity from long-term exposure to contaminated intravenous feeding solutions (45,76). Developmental attainment on the Bayley Mental Development index at a corrected post-term age of 18 months was reduced in preterm infants treated for prolonged periods with intravenous solutions delivering Al doses of approximately 20 mg/kg/day as compared with 3 mg/kg/day. The indices of brain function were not statistically different, but a dose-related effect was suggested (9).

Aluminum Neurotoxicity in Uremic Subjects

Chronic and fulminant forms of Al toxicity and neurotoxicity are recognized in uremic patients (2). Acute neurotoxicity, with plasma Al levels > 500 mg/ml (18.5 mmol/l), may (a) manifest as *grand mal* seizures during dialysis with heavily Al-contaminated solutions, (b) appear within days of treatment with deferoxamine[†] (DFO) chelation therapy to displace sequestered Al from bone and other compartments, or (c) surface after weeks or months of oral administration of a combination of citrate and Al compounds (2). Onset is sudden in adults, with agitation, confusion, seizures, myoclonic jerking, coma, and death within days to weeks. Children may have a more insidious onset of disease featured by intellectual impairment, seizures, and regression of verbal and motor skills (77). Electroencephalographic (EEG) changes are similar to those seen in the chronic form of the disease.

Chronic Al neurotoxicity in uremic patients is commonly associated with fracturing osteomalacia and microcytic hypochromic anemia.[‡] Dialysis encephalopathy is seen in patients with Al plasma levels of 100–200 mg/l after years of parenteral Al exposure from an Al-contaminated dialysate (4,23). Patients develop insidiously a syndrome heralded by intermittent speech disturbance characterized by stuttering and stammering. EEG abnormalities, present in states of wakefulness and sleep, precede (4–6 months) and accompany clinical symptoms; they are featured by paroxysmal high-voltage delta activity on a largely normal background rhythm.

Personality changes, disorientation, seizures, and visual and auditory hallucinations accompany the speech impairment. Dementia evolves gradually over the course of the disease; first to appear is disturbed concentration, lack of

---

[†]*N'*-[5-[[4-[[5-(Acetylhydroxyamino)pentylamino]-1,4-dioxobutyl]-hydroxyamino]pentyl]-*N*-(5-aminopentyl)-*N*-hydroxybutanediamide. Some reports refer to the methanesulfonate derivative, desferrioxamine.

[‡]"Proximal myopathy" is also described in these subjects (2) but not in heavily Al-intoxicated animals, which feature an extreme proximal motor axonopathy (11) that conceivably could masquerade clinically as proximal muscle weakness.

attention, and disorientation; memory deterioration develops, and then confusion appears. Paranoia and suicidal ideation may manifest. Asterixis and myoclonus appear and, 7–9 months after onset, the patient becomes mute, globally demented, and dies (2). Histological examination of brains of 12 patients who had died of dialysis encephalopathy revealed mild spongiform pathology in the cerebral cortex and nonspecific neuronal changes (12). Gray-matter Al levels of 12 mg/kg dry weight were three times higher in patients with dialysis encephalopathy relative to those who had been comparably dialyzed but who were free of neurological disease; in both, Al levels were markedly higher than those in controls (1 mg/kg dry weight) (80).

Plasma Al levels are used to monitor dialysis patients and other subjects at risk for iatrogenic Al toxicity. Al levels of <10 mg/l are considered normal; 60 mg/l suggests the possibility of an increased body Al burden; >100 mg/l indicates potential toxicity and need for increased monitoring; >200 mg/l is often associated with overt Al toxicity, and >500 mg/l is indicative of acute Al intoxication. Body burden of Al may be estimated by bone biopsy or a DFO chelation challenge; the latter releases Al roughly in proportion to bone Al content (63,93). Prevention of Al toxicity in renal patients has been achieved through use of dialysis fluids containing low Al concentrations (<10 mg/l), calcium-based instead of Al-based phosphate binders, regular plasma Al monitoring and, if indicated, once-weekly intramuscular administration of DFO (0.5–1.0 g/12 h) prior to dialysis, with removal of the chelate at the time of dialysis (3,18,93).

Removal of parenteral and oral sources of Al is the first line of treatment. Patients with plasma Al level >150–200 mg/l after DFO challenge, or with increased bone Al levels with osteomalacia, are candidates for DFO chelation (2). Those with marked overload are at risk for acute DFO-induced Al neurotoxicity (2). Efficacious treatment of chronic Al neurotoxicity requires repeated administration of small weekly doses of DFO (5–10 mg/kg body weight during the last 30 min of a dialysis session) over a period of 10–12 months, monitoring of plasma Al and EEG, and reduction of therapy if plasma Al levels rise excessively (2,93). Chelation therapy has not prevented a fatal outcome in adults with acute Al toxicity, and children treated for this condition have been left with severe motor and learning disabilities (77). Diazepam has been used as an effective prophylaxis for dialysis-related seizures in subjects with Al overload (2).

Seizures are a consistent feature of acute and chronic Al encephalopathy in uremic patients, of rare cases of Al intoxication in the occupational setting (*vide infra*), and of mammals treated experimentally with Al compounds. The neurophysiological bases of this phenomenon and of the dementia seen in chronic Al encephalopathy are unknown.

Controlled Exposures in the Mining Industry

Some information on the chronic effects of Al exposure among individuals with presumed normal renal function can be gleaned from studies of Canadian gold and uranium miners who were exposed under controlled conditions to McIntyre's powder (reportedly 15% elemental Al and 85% Al oxide) for the prevention of human silicosis[†] (73).

Beginning in 1936, Canadian scientists undertook a series of animal studies in which rabbits inhaled for periods up to 6 months concentrations of quartz dust in the presence or absence of <1% metallic aluminum. These studies reportedly demonstrated that animals dusted with quartz alone developed silicosis in 5–7 months, whereas those additionally treated with Al showed no evidence of silicosis for 17 months. To be effective in blocking silicosis, the Al powder required a certain particle diameter, an absence of surface contamination, and administration as a uniform mixture with fine silica particles in a concentration of 1% of the quartz by weight. This appeared to optimize conditions for the conversion of silica to silica hydride using nascent hydrogen generated by reaction of metallic Al with the aqueous surface of the airway system. The authors of this research, an industry-sponsored group, claimed that "inhalation and retention of aluminum in large quantities over long periods showed no adverse effects on the general health of animals and no evidence of toxicity or damage to the lungs or any other tissues."

These experimental studies prompted the precious-metals mining industry in Ontario, Canada, to engage an independent medical team to assess the possible use of Al for the prevention of human silicosis among gold and uranium miners. Pilot studies showed that 55% of 34 miners who completed 200–300 5–30 min daily inhalation treatments showed a reduction or disappearance of dyspnea, cough, chest pain and fatigue, and one-third showed improvement on repeat testing of respiratory function. The balance remained clinically stationary while, in contrast, 66% of a control, Al-untreated group showed clinical progression. Further studies reportedly demonstrated that Al treatment offered the possibility of symptomatic improvement in acute and subacute silicosis, but not in the well-established chronic disease (19). Thereafter, gold mines in Ontario,

---

[†]Silicosis is a fibrotic lung disease caused by prolonged inhalation and retention of silicon dioxide (silica, quartz) and manifest by dyspnea, cough, chest tightness, and reduced capacity to work. A fibrotic lung disease has also been documented in workers exposed to powdered Al metal (26).

Canada, used McIntyre Al powder for group prophylaxis against silicosis. Recommended exposure was for 10 min to an Al dust concentration of 20,000–34,000 ppm air in the miners' changing rooms before each underground shift. Estimated annual alveolar Al burden accumulated by Al-treated miners was approximately 375 mg (73).

The prophylaxis program was stopped in 1979 on the recommendation of a scientific task force, which found (a) that a fall in mortality from silicotic lung diseases had coincided with the term of the program, (b) that mining practices had reduced silica dust levels such that there was no evidence of a benefit from continued exposure of miners to aluminum, and (c) that McIntyre powder did not produce apparent adverse effects (cf. 64,65). Assessment of the cognitive function of 631 Al-exposed miners vs. 722 Al-unexposed miners revealed that cognitive measures assessing perceptual accuracy, information processing, and abstract reasoning were poorer in the first group (73). However, this study did not adjust for pre-exposure cognitive capacity by years of schooling.

Occupational Exposures

Excess cancers have been reported in Al-reduction plant workers who may be occupationally exposed to a number of chemicals other than aluminum (44). Notable among these are known carcinogens, including benzo[a]pyrene and other polycyclic aromatic hydrocarbons found in the air of the potroom and carbon-plant components of Al-reduction plants. The largest of these studies, performed for the U.S. Aluminum Association, analyzed 3320 deaths in a population of over 23,000 Al workers. Excess mortality was found in relation to lung cancer, leukemia, lymphoma, hypertensive diseases, and motor-vehicle accidents, with a borderline excess of nervous system tumors (21). With the exception of motor-vehicle accidents and hypertensive disease, comparable findings were obtained in a study of U.S. Al-reduction plant workers (61). Maximum standardized mortality ratios (SMRs) in this study were reached between 15 and 19 years of employment, with lower SMRs before and after. Another study of 21,829 workers with 5 or more years of cumulative employment in one or more of 14 Al-reduction plants showed no excess deaths from lung cancer but demonstrated a higher-than-expected mortality from lymphohematopoietic cancers, genitourinary cancers, pancreatic cancer, nonmalignant respiratory disease, and benign and unspecified neoplasms (74). The incidence of bladder cancer also has been reported to be elevated in Al smelter workers (89).

A comprehensive picture of mortality in the Al-reduction industry was carried out among 5406 male Canadian workers who were employed at an Al smelter from 1950 onward (29). Death certificates were analyzed for approximately 90% of the 28.5% of subjects who had died. Subjects died of the following causes at approximately the same rate as, or less frequently than, men of similar age in the Province of Quebec: tuberculosis; circulatory disease; hypertensive heart disease; trauma; leukemia; and malignant diseases of the pancreas, genital organs, brain, intestine, rectum and other abdominal areas. Several conditions were more frequently encountered: respiratory disease, pneumonia and bronchitis, malignant neoplasms (all sites), Hodgkin's disease, and other hypertensive disease. Mortality from malignant neoplasms of the bladder and lung were described as meaningfully related to years of exposure and to the number of years exposed to condensed pitch volatiles (i.e., carcinogens) produced by the burning of the anode in the electrolytic cell during the Al-reduction process. There were no recorded deaths from Alzheimer's disease in this cohort or a second, smaller cohort employed at another Al-reduction plant that showed an excess of lung cancer.

A Yugoslavian team studied 87 Al-foundry workers with >6 years of employment and evidence of elevated body burdens of Al following DFO challenge. Relative to age-matched controls, formal neuropsychological testing revealed slower psychomotor reaction and more "dissociation of oculomotor coordination," and some impairment of performance on Wechsler's tests for memory coding, picture completion, and object assembling (36). Evidence of a relationship between degree of neuropsychological deficit and body burden of Al was not provided.

Neuropsychiatric symptoms were assessed by administering a questionnaire to 73 male Swedish metal welders with 10 or more years of exposure to fumes from Al welding (82). Male railroad-track welders exposed to Al, lead, manganese, chromium, and/or nickel were used as a referent group; this was poorly matched for age and number of years of exposure to welding fumes. Al welders were found to be more likely to indicate problems with concentration and depression. No objective clinical neuropsychological examination was undertaken, and the validity of studies based exclusively on an analysis of self-reported symptoms is open to question.

Neuropsychological deficits were also sought in a study of Norwegian workers with occupational exposure for at least 10 years either in the potroom or foundry of a primary Al production plant (8). Those with diseases or a history of trauma that might affect brain function were excluded. Controls consisted of blue-collar workers employed for at least 10 years in manual work and with no work history in the potroom or foundry. Data were obtained from 38 workers (22 exposed plus 16 control) with a mean age of

63.1 years. Al levels in serum were normal; those in urine were moderately elevated in potroom workers. Formal neuropsychological testing revealed no differences among groups in memory tests or reaction time. Potroom workers scored poorly on one of two tests of motor function, a result that was interpreted as evidence of a "subclinical tremor," the significance of which is unknown.

There are two reports of single individuals who developed neurological disease consistent with Al overexposure. A metal worker developed jerking movements, impaired coordination, and seizures (86). Another worker with pulmonary fibrosis inhaled Al dust and developed focal epilepsy and dementia (58, *vide infra*).

CASE REPORT

This individual developed the disorder at age 49 after 13.5 years as a ball-mill operator in an Al-flake powder factory. He developed repeated episodes of clonic jerking of the left leg and left arm, together with memory and speech difficulties. Neurological examination revealed slurred speech, deterioration of memory for recent events, *a mild spastic left-sided weakness, increased tendon reflexes and, eventually, extensor plantar reflexes. His* mental state deteriorated *and the epileptic fits* progressed to generalized seizures, coma, and death. *Postmortem analysis of lungs and brain revealed Al concentrations 20 times in excess of normal, and lungs showed histological evidence of fibrosis. The brain showed no histological evidence to support a diagnosis of Pick's disease or Alzheimer's disease. None of the other employees, including those who had worked for longer periods of time on the same or related jobs, displayed evidence of lung fibrosis; neurological examinations on the subjects were not performed.*

A seemingly related disorder affected a 29-year-old male who developed focal and generalized ingravescent epilepsy, with mental decline comparable to epileptic dementia, 15 years after accidental explosive intracranial implantation of metallic Al. Neurofibrillary pathology was absent on postmortem histological examination of the brain (24).

A condition, "potroom palsy," has been described among Al-smelter potroom workers where chemical exposures include: particulate alumina, fluorides, hydrogen sulfide, sulfur oxides, carbon monoxide, carbon dioxide, cyanide, lithium, and polycyclic aromatic hydrocarbons. Three subjects with work histories of >12 years in the same potroom of a U.S. Al-smelting plant were reported to have neurological disorders characterized by incoordination and tremor, cognitive deficits and, in one, spastic paraparesis. Bone revealed *normal* levels of Al and elevated levels of fluorine (52); joint

pain associated with early osteofluorosis has been reported among workers engaged in Al production (35). A subsequent report from these investigators described findings in 25 workers with a mean of 18.7 years of employment in the same Al-smelting plant (96). More than half used alcohol and most were depressed at the time of examination. Loss of balance, memory loss, and joint pain were major complaints. Tremor, "dyssynergy" of upper extremity movements, or ataxia of gait were reportedly present to some degree in 21. Two were said to have a diagnosis consistent with multiple sclerosis. Neuropsychological examination reportedly revealed substantial deficits in memory, abstract reasoning, and sustained concentration (52). Overt manifestations of Al encephalopathy—namely, speech disorder, myoclonus, and seizures—were *absent*. An etiological link between this disorder and Al is unproven.

Environmental Exposures

Several epidemiological studies have investigated the possibility of a link between the concentration of Al in drinking water and the prevalence of Alzheimer's disease. A British study found a slightly elevated relative risk for probable Alzheimer's disease when water levels of Al were 0.02 mg/l or greater; however, there was no increased incidence with increasing Al concentrations (56). A French study reported an increased risk for probable Alzheimer's disease and an inverse association for other dementias for water concentrations exceeding 0.04 mg/l (60). Similar results were reported from Canada (25,67), and significant correlations between water Al concentration and dementia prior to death were reported from Norway (22). Other studies have shown no overall relationship between water content of Al and mental impairment or Alzheimer's disease (95,100), including an investigation that expanded the earlier French study (37).

At least four studies have sought a relationship between Alzheimer's disease and use of Al-containing medicaments, which include antacids, enteric coated tablets, and antiperspirants. One found no relationship with prolonged use of antacids or Al-containing antacids. A weak positive association was present for use of Al-containing antiperspirants for 1 year or longer (30).

Other studies have suggested that Al accumulates in the brains of patients with Alzheimer's disease. Initial reports of brain Al levels found to be encephalopathic in susceptible mammalian species (13,14) could not be confirmed (54,57,90). Analysis of a wide range of neurological disorders found elevated brain Al in some cases, but this was not a consistent finding within a given disorder (90).

Exposure to Al in food and water also has been advanced as part of a complex explanation for the environmental etiology of another progressive neurodegenerative disorder, western Pacific ALS/PDC. Clinical, epidemiological, and elemental studies that gave rise to this proposal have been reviewed (87). ALS/PDC, which features Alzheimer-like neurofibrillary tangles that sometimes contain Al, iron, and other elements, has been highly prevalent among the indigenous (Chamorro) population of Guam. Clinically similar isolates have been reported among residents in foci of Japan (Kii peninsula, Honshu Island) and New Guinea (Irian Jaya, Indonesia). The disorder has declined or disappeared in all three areas of high incidence, including Irian Jaya where the sessile population continues to employ the same source of drinking water and consumes food from vegetation grown on the same soil (85). Although Al is detectable in the brains of Guam Chamorros with neurodegenerative disease, there is no significant association between the age-adjusted incidence of motor neuron disease on Guam and the geographical distribution of Al in the island's water sources (107). By contrast, there is a very strong and highly significant correlation between the age-adjusted disease incidence and the geographical concentration of cycasin (methylazoxymethanol-β-glucoside) in food derived from the cycad plant, a cause of neuromuscular disease in grazing animals and a traditional source of medicine and/or food in all three high-incidence foci (85) (see Cycasin, this volume). The etiologic role of specific environmental factors in the etiology of western Pacific ALS/PDC has yet to be established.

In summary, while an association between neurodegenerative disease, ALS/PDC, Alzheimer disease, potroom palsy, and environmental exposure to Al cannot be ruled out, convincing data to support the proposed associations are lacking. It bears emphasizing that mammals with Al neurotoxicity do not display the neuropathological hallmarks of Alzheimer's disease or ALS/PDC, and occupational Al encephalopathy (vide supra) and Al-associated dialysis encephalopathy (vide infra) exhibit clinical and neuropathological hallmarks distinct from those associated with these idiopathic neurodegenerative disorders. These facts notwithstanding, one report noted Alzheimer-like changes in tau protein processing in brains of renal dialysis patients (32), and another reported improvement of Alzheimer's disease following DFO chelation (15).

REFERENCES

1. Ackrill P, Day PP (1993) The use of desferrioxamine in dialysis-associated disease. In: Moving Points in Nephrology. Mallick NP, Polak VE eds. Contrib Nephrol, Karger, Basel p. 125.
2. Alfrey AC (1997) Dialysis encephalopathy. In: Mineral and Metal Neurotoxicity. Yasui M, Strong MJ, Ota K, Verity MA eds. CRC Press, Boca Raton, Florida p. 127.
3. Alfrey AC, Froment DC (1990) Dialysis encephalopathy. In: Aluminum and Renal Failure, Developments in Nephrology. Vol 26. De Broe ME, Coburn JE eds. Kluwer, Dordrecht p. 249.
4. Alfrey AC, LeGendre GR, Kaehny WD (1976) The dialysis encephalopathy syndrome. Possible aluminum intoxication. N Engl J Med 294, 184.
5. American Academy of Pediatrics Committee on Nutrition (1986) Aluminum toxicity in infants and children. Pediatrics 78, 1150.
6. Anane R, Bonini M, Grafeille J-M, Creppy EE (1995) Bioaccumulation of water soluble aluminum chloride in the hippocampus after transdermal uptake in mice. Arch Toxicol 69, 568.
7. Banks WA, Kastin AJ (1983) Aluminium increases permeability of the blood brain barrier to labelled DSIP and β-endorphin: Possible implications for senile and dialysis dementia. Lancet ii, 1227.
8. Bast-Pattersen R, Drablos PA, Goffeng LO et al. (1994) Neuropsychological deficit among elderly workers in aluminum production. Amer J Indust Med 25, 649.
9. Bishop NJ, Morley R, Day JP, Lucas A (1997) Aluminum neurotoxicity in preterm infants receiving intravenous-feeding solutions. N Engl J Med 336, 1557.
10. Bizzi A, Crane CD, Gambetti LA, Gambetti P (1984) Aluminum effect on slow axonal transport: A novel impairment of slow axonal transport. J Neurosci 4, 722.
11. Bugiani O, Ghetti B (1982) Progressing encephalomyelopathy with muscular atrophy, induced by aluminum powder. Neurobiol Aging 3, 209.
12. Burks JS, Alfrey AC, Huddlestone J et al. (1976) A fatal encephalopathy in chronic hemodialysis patients. Lancet i, 764.
13. Crapper DR, Dalton AJ (1973) Aluminium induced neurofibrillary degeneration, brain electrical activity and alterations in acquisition and retention. Physiol Behav 10, 935.
14. Crapper DS, Krishnan SS, Quittkat S (1976) Aluminum, neurofibrillary degeneration and Alzheimer's disease. Science 180, 511.
15. Crapper McLachlan DR, Dalton AJ, Kruck TPA et al. (1991) Intramuscular desferrioxamine in patients with Alzheimer's disease. Lancet 337, 1304.
16. DeBoni U, Scott J, Crapper DR (1974) Intracellular aluminium binding: A histochemical study. Histochemie 40, 31.
17. Deloncle R, Pages N (1997) Aluminum: On both sides of the blood-brain barrier. In: Mineral and Metal Neurotoxicity. Yasui M, Strong MJ, Ota K, Verity MA eds. CRC Press, Boca Raton, Florida p. 91.
18. DeWolff FA, van der Voet (1986) Biological monitoring of aluminium in renal patients. Clin Chim Acta 160, 183.

19. Dix WB (1975) *Brief to the Royal Commission of the Health and Safety of Workers in Mines in Ontario.* McIntyre Foundation, Ottawa.

20. Dollken P (1897) Ueber die Wirkung des Aluminum mit besonderer Berucksichtigung der durch das aluminum verursachten Lasionen im Zentralenerven system. *Naunyn-Schmied Arch Exp Pathol Pharmacol* **40**, 58.

21. Equitable Environmental Health Inc. (1977) *Mortality of Aluminum Workers—Final Report.* Prepared for the US Aluminum Association.

22. Flaten TP (1992) Geographical associations between aluminum in drinking water, Parkinson's disease and amyotrophic lateral sclerosis in Norway. *Environ Geochem Health* **12**, 152.

23. Flendrig JA, Kruis H, Das HA (1976) Aluminium and dialysis dementia. *Lancet* **i**, 1235.

24. Foncin JF, El Hachimi KH (1986) 'Neurofibrillary degeneration' in Alzheimer's disease: A discussion with a contribution to aluminum pathology in man. In: *Senile Dementia: Early Detection, Current Problems in Senile Dementia. No. 1.* Bes A, Cahn S, Hoyer J *et al.* eds. John Libbey Eurotext, London p. 191.

25. Frecker MF (1991) Dementia in Newfoundland: Identification of a geographic isolate? *J Epidemiol Comm Health* **45**, 307.

26. Friberg L, Norberg GF, Vouk HB (1979) *Handbook on the Toxicology of Metals.* Elsevier, New York.

27. Furumo NC, Viola RE (1989) Aluminium-adenine nucleotides as alternate substrates for creatine kinase. *Arch Biochem Biophys* **275**, 33.

28. Garruto RM, Shankar SK, Tanagihara *et al.* (1989) Low-calcium, high aluminium diet-induced motor neuron pathology in cynomolgus monkeys. *Acta Neuropathol* **78**, 210.

29. Gibbs GW (1985) Mortality of aluminum reduction plant workers, 1950–1977. *J Occup Med* **27**, 761.

30. Graves AB, White E, Koepsell TD *et al.* (1990) The association between aluminum-containing products and Alzheimer's disease. *J Clin Epidemiol* **43**, 35.

31. Gruskin AB (1988) Aluminum: A pediatric overview. *Adv Pediat* **35**, 281.

32. Harrington CR, Wischik CM, McArthur FK *et al.* (1994) Alzheimer's disease-like changes in tau protein processing: Association with aluminium accumulation in brains of renal dialysis patients. *Lancet* **343**, 993.

33. Harris WR, Berthon G, Day JP *et al.* (1996) Speciation of aluminum in biological systems. *J Toxicol Environ Health* **48**, 543.

34. Haug AR, Vitorello V (1997) Cellular aspects of aluminum toxicity in plants. In: *Mineral and Metal Neurotoxicity.* Yasui M, Strong MJ, Ota K, Verity MA eds. CRC Press, Boca Raton, Florida p. 85.

35. Hodge HC, Smith FA (1977) Occupational fluoride exposure. *J Occup Med* **19**, 12.

36. Hosovski E, Mastelica Z, Sunderic D, Radulovic D (1990) Mental abilities of workers exposed to aluminum. *Med Lav* **81**, 119.

37. Jacqmin H, Commenges D (1992) *Aluminum—Maladie d'Alzheimer: Rapport du Recherche.* Université de Bordeaux II. Départment d'Informations médicale. Bordeaux, France.

38. Johnson GVW, Jope RS (1988) Phosphorylation of rat brain cytoskeletal proteins is increased after orally administered aluminum. *Brain Res* **456**, 95.

39. Kaehny WD, Hegg AP, Alfrey AC (1977) Gastrointestinal absorption of aluminum from aluminum-containing antacids. *N Engl J Med* **296**, 1389.

40. Karlik SJ, Eichhorn GL, Lewis PN, Crapper DR (1980) The interaction of aluminium with deoxyribonucleic acid. *Biochemisty* **19**, 5991.

41. Klatzo I, Wiśniewski HM, Streicher E (1965) Experimental production of neurofibrillary degeneration. *J Neuropathol Exp Neurol* **24**, 187.

42. Klein GL (1995) Aluminum in parenteral solutions revisited—again. *Amer J Clin Nutr* **61**, 449.

43. Klein GL, Herndon DN, Rutan TC *et al.* (1994) Risk of aluminum accumulation in patients with burns and ways to reduce it. *J Burn Care Rehab* **15**, 354.

44. Konstantivov FG, Kuz'minykh AL (1973) Tarry substances and 3-4 BAP in the air in electrolytic shops of aluminum workers and their carcinogenic significance. *Gig Sanit* **2**, 190.

45. Koo WW, Krug-Wispe SK, Succop P *et al.* (1992) Sequential serum aluminium and urine aluminum: creatinine ratio and tissue aluminum loading in infants with fractures/rickets. *Pediatrics* **89**, 877.

46. Kopeloff LM, Barrera SE, Kopeloff N (1942) Recurrent convulsive seizures in animals produced by immunologic and chemical means. *Amer J Psychiat* **98**, 881.

47. Kowall NW, Pendelbury WW, Kessler JB *et al.* (1989) Aluminium induced neurofibrillary degeneration affects a subset of neurons in rabbit cerebral cortex, basal forebrain and upper brainstem. *Neuroscience* **29**, 329.

48. Lai JCK, Blass JP (1984) Inhibition of brain glycolysis by aluminum. *J Neurochem* **42**, 438.

49. Lai JCK, Lim L, Davison AN (1982) Effects of Ca^{2+}, Mn^{2+} and Al^{3+} on rat brain synaptosomal uptake of noradrenaline and serotonin. *J Inorg Biochem* **17**, 215.

50. Lipman JJH, Colowick SP, Lawrence PL, Abumrad NN (1988) Aluminium-induced encephalopathy in the rat. *Life Sci* **42**, 863.

51. Liwnicz BH, Kristensson K, Wiśniewski HM *et al.* (1974) Observations on axoplasmic transport in rabbits with aluminum-induced neurofibrillary tangles. *Brain Res* **80**, 413.

52. Longstreth WT Jr, Rosenstock K, Heyer NJ (1985) Potroom palsy? Neurologic disorder in three aluminum workers. *Arch Intern Med* **145**, 1972.

53. Lukiw WJ, Kruck TP, McLachlan DR (1989) Linker histone-DNA complexes: Enhanced stability in the presence of aluminium lactate and implications for Alzheimer's disease. *FEBS Lett* **253**, 59.

54. Markesberry WR, Ehmann WD, Hossain TIM (1981) Instrumental neutron activation analysis of brain aluminum in Alzheimer's disease and aging. *Ann Neurol* **10**, 511.

55. Martin RB (1997) Chemistry of aluminum in the central nervous system. In: *Mineral and Metal Neurotoxicity*. Yasui M, Strong MJ, Ota K, Verity MA eds. CRC Press, Boca Raton, Florida p. 75.

56. Martyn CN, Osmond C, Edwardson JA *et al.* (1989) Geographic relation between Alzheimer's disease and aluminum in drinking water. *Lancet* **i**, 59.

57. McDermott JR, Smith AI, Iqbal K, Wiśniewski HM (1979) Brain aluminum in aging and Alzheimer's disease. *Neurology* **29**, 809.

58. McLaughlin AIG, Kazantzos G, King E *et al.* (1962) Pulmonary fibrosis and encephalopathy associated with inhalation of aluminum dust. *Brit J Indust Med* **19**, 253.

59. Meiri H, Banin E, Roll M, Rousseau A (1993) Toxic effects of aluminum on nerve cells and synaptic transmission. *Prog Neurobiol* **40**, 89.

60. Michel P, Commenges D, Dartigues JF *et al.* (1991) Study of the relationship between aluminum concentrations in drinking water and risk of Alzheimer's disease. In: *Alzheimer's Disease: Basic Mechanisms, Diagnosis and Therapeutic Strategies*. Iqbal K, McLachlan DRC, Winblad B, Wiśniewski HM eds. John Wiley, Chichester p. 887.

61. Milham S (1979) Mortality in aluminum reduction plant workers. *J Occup Med* **21**, 475.

62. Miller CA, Levine EM (1974) Effects of aluminum salts on cultured neuroblastoma cells. *J Neurochem* **22**, 751.

63. Milliner DS, Nebeker HG, Ott SM *et al.* (1984) Use of deferoxamine infusion test in the diagnosis of aluminum-related osteodystrophy. *Ann Intern Med* **101**, 775.

64. Muller J, Kusiak RA, Suranyi G, Ritchie AC (1986) *Study of Mortality of Ontario Gold Miners 1955–1997*. Ontario Ministry of Labor, Ottawa.

65. Muller J, Kusiak RA, Suranyi G, Ritchie AC (1987) *Study of Mortality of Ontario Gold Miners 1955–1997*. Addendum. Ontario Ministry of Labor, Ottawa.

66. Nathan E, Pedersen SE (1980) Dialysis encephalopathy in a non-dialysed uraemic boy treated with aluminium hydroxide orally. *Acta Pediatr Scand* **69**, 793.

67. Neri LC, Hewitt D (1991) Aluminium, Alzheimer's disease, and drinking water. *Lancet* **i**, 338.

68. Oortigiesen M, van Kleef RGDG, Vuverberg HPM (1990) Novel type of ion channel activated by Pb^{2+}, Cd^{2+} and Al^{3+} in cultured mouse neuroblastoma cells. *J Membr Biol* **113**, 261.

69. Perazella M, Brown E (1993) Acute aluminum toxicity and alum bladder irrigation in patients with renal failure. *Amer J Kidney Dis* **21**, 44.

70. Perl DP, Good FF (1987) Uptake of aluminum into the central nervous system along nasal-olfactory pathways. *Lancet* **i**, 1028.

71. Petit TL, Biederman GB, Jonas P, Le Boutillier JC (1985) Neurobehavioral development following aluminium administration in infant rabbits. *Exp Neurol* **88**, 640.

72. Rabe A, Lee MH, Shek, Wiśniewski HM (1982) Learning deficit in immature rabbits with aluminum induced neurofibrillary changes. *Exp Neurol* **76**, 441.

73. Rifat SL, Eastwood MR, McLachlan DR, Corey DN (1990) Effects of exposure of miners to aluminium powder. *Lancet* **336**, 1162.

74. Rockette HE, Arena VC (1983) Mortality studies of aluminum reduction plant workers: Potroom and carbon department. *J Occup Med* **25**, 549.

75. Scherp HW, Church CF (1937) Neurotoxic action of aluminium salts. *Proc Soc Exp Biol Med* **36**, 851.

76. Sedman AB, Klein GL, Merritt RJ *et al.* (1985) Evidence of aluminum loading in infants receiving intravenous therapy. *N Engl J Med* **312**, 1337.

77. Sedman AB, Wilkening GN, Warady BA *et al.* (1984) Encephalopathy in childhood secondary to aluminum toxicity. *J Pediat* **105**, 836.

78. Selkoe DJ, Liem RKH, Yen SH, Shelanski ML (1979) Biochemical and immunological characterization of neurofilaments in experimental neurofibrillary degeneration induced by aluminum. *Brain Res* **163**, 235.

79. Shi B, Haug A (1989) Aluminum uptake by neuroblastoma cells. *J Neurochem* **55**, 551.

80. Sideman S, Manor D (1982) The dialysis dementia syndrome and aluminum intoxication. *Nephron* **31**, 1.

81. Sjögren B, Elinder CG, Lidums V, Chang G (1988) Uptake and urinary excretion of aluminum among welders. *Int Arch Occup Environ Health* **60**, 77.

82. Sjögren B, Gustavsson P, Hogstedt C (1990) Neuropsychiatric symptoms among welders exposed to neurotoxic metals. *Brit J Indust Med* **47**, 704.

83. Sjögren B, Lidums V, Hakansson M, Hedstrom L (1985) Exposure and urinary excretion of aluminium during welding. *Scand J Work Environ Health* **11**, 39.

84. Sjögren B, Lundberg I, Liduma V (1983) Aluminium in the blood and urine of industrially exposed workers. *Brit J Indust Med* **40**, 301.

85. Spencer PS, Kisby GE (1992) Slow toxins and Western Pacific amyotrophic lateral sclerosis. In: *Handbook of Amyotrophic Lateral Sclerosis*. Smith A ed. Marcel Dekker, New York p. 575.

86. Spofforth J (1921) Case of aluminium poisoning. *Lancet* **i**, 1301.

87. Strong MJ, Garruto RM (1997) Motor neuron disease. In: *Mineral and Metal Neurotoxicity*. Yasui M, Strong MJ, Ota K, Verity MA eds. CRC Press, Boca Raton, Florida p. 107.

88. Terry RD, Peña C (1965) Experimental production of

neurofibrillary degeneration. 2. Electron microscopy, microscopy, histochemistry and electron microprobe analysis. *J Neuropathol Exp Neurol* **24**, 200.

89. Theriault G, Cordier S, Tremblay C, Gingras S (1984) Bladder cancer in the aluminium industry. *Lancet* **i**, 947.

90. Traub RD, Rains TC Garrutto RM *et al.* (1981) Brain destruction alone does not elevate brain aluminum. *Neurology* **31**, 986.

91. Troncoso JC, Hoffman PN, Griffin JW *et al.* (1985) Aluminum intoxication: A disorder of neurofilament transport in motor neurons. *Brain Res* **342**, 172.

92. Uemura E, Ireland WP (1984) Synaptic density in chronic animals with experimental neurofibrillary changes. *Exp Neurol* **85**, 1.

93. Van der Voet GB, De Wolff FA (1994) Neurotoxicity of aluminum. In: *Handbook of Clinical Neurology. Vol 20 (64). Intoxications of the Nervous System. Pt 1.* De Wolff FA ed. Elsevier, Amsterdam p. 273.

94. Walker PW, LeBlanc J, Sikorska M (1989) Effects of aluminium and other cations on the structure of brain and liver chromatin. *Biochemistry* **28**, 3911.

95. Wettstein A, Aeppli J, Gautachi K, Peters M (1991) Failure to find a relationship between mnestic skills of octogenarians and aluminium in drinking water. *Arch Occup Environ Health* **63**, 97.

96. White DM, Longstreth WT, Rosenstock L *et al.* (1992) Neurologic syndrome in 25 workers from an aluminum smelting plant. *Arch Intern Med* **152**, 1443.

97. Wilhelm M, Hohr D, Abel J, Ohnesorge FK (1989) Renal aluminum excretion. *Biol Trace Elem Res* **21**, 241.

98. Wilhelm M, Jager DE, Ohnesorge FK (1990) Aluminium toxicokinetics. *Pharmacol Toxicol* **66**, 4.

99. Wiśniewski H, Karsczewski W, Wiśniewska K (1966) Neurofibrillary degeneration of nerve cells after injection of aluminium cream. *Acta Neuropathol* **6**, 211.

100. Wood DJ, Cooper C, Stevens J, Edwardson J (1988) Bone mass and dementia in hip fracture patients from areas with different aluminum concentrations in water supplies. *Age Ageing* **17**, 415.

101. World Health Organization (WHO) (1989) Evaluation of Certain Food Additives and Contaminants. Thirty-third Report of the Joint FAO/WHO Expert Committee on Food Additives. *WHO Technical Report Series* **776**, 27.

102. Yano I, Yoshida S, Uebayashi Y *et al.* (1987) Degenerative changes in the central nervous system of Japanese monkeys induced by oral administration of aluminum salt. *Biomed Res* **10**, 33.

103. Yokel RA (1989) Aluminum produces age-related behavioral toxicity in the rabbit. *Neurotoxicol Teratol* **11**, 237.

104. Yokel RA (1997) The metabolism and toxicokinetics of aluminum relevant to neurotoxicity. In: *Mineral and Metal Neurotoxicity.* Yasui M, Strong MJ, Ota K, Verity MA eds. CRC Press, Boca Raton, Florida p. 81.

105. Zatta P, Favarato M, Nicolini M (1993) Deposition of aluminum in brain tissues of rats exposed to inhalation of aluminum acetylacetonate. *Neuroreport* **4**, 1119.

106. Zatta P, Perazzolo M, Corain B (1989) Tris acetylacetonate aluminum induces osmotic fragility and acanthocyte formation in suspended erythrocytes. *Toxicol Lett* **45**, 15.

107. Zhang ZX, Anderson DW, Mantel N, Román G (1996) Motor neuron disease on Guam. *Acta Neurol Scand* **94**, 51.

Amanita Toxins

Albert C. Ludolph

MUSCAZONE
$C_5H_6N_2O_4$

Muscazone
α-Amino-2,3-dihydro-2-oxo-5-oxazoleacetic acid;
α-Amino-2-oxo-4-oxazoline-5-acetic acid

NEUROTOXICITY RATING

Clinical

A   Psychobiological reaction

A   Seizure disorder

Experimental

A   Glutamate agonist (ibotenic acid)

A   GABA agonist (muscimol)

Poisoning by mushrooms belonging to the genus Amanita is associated with two distinct clinical syndromes, the *Amanita phalloides* syndrome and the *Amanita muscaria* (or *pantherina*) syndrome. Neurological signs and symptoms of the former are secondary to renal and hepatic damage; the latter causes a psychobiological reaction often accompanied by seizures and myoclonic jerks. Use of the psychotropic effects associated with *A. muscaria* is a cultural tradition in northeast Asia (10); deliberate intake occurs in North America and Europe. A recent review is available (11).

Amanita phalloides poisoning is the principal cause of mushroom-induced deaths in humans. Although neurological signs and symptoms may appear during the late phase of poisoning, available evidence does not support a direct neurotoxic effect of these mushrooms. The occurrence, characterization, methods of analysis, chemistry, and mechanisms of toxicity of *Amanita phalloides* toxins have been described in detail elsewhere (12,13). The clinical syndrome of *Amanita phalloides* poisoning is caused by amatoxins (13) and divided into three phases: During the early phase (6–24 h after intake), a severe gastrointestinal syndrome associated with diarrhea, nausea, and vomiting that results in exsiccosis, hypotonia, and tachycardia is observed. Coagulation factors may be reduced during this phase (13). Treatment mainly consists of fluid and electrolyte replacement. After a second latency and—sometimes—apparent remission, the third phase of the disease surfaces on days 3–5; a severe hepatorenal syndrome and encephalopathy are responsible for most deaths occuring during this phase of poisoning. Spontaneous intracerebral hemorrhage may occur. Gastric lavage is the best treatment within 36 h of mushroom ingestion. To reduce serum concentrations of amatoxins, forced diuresis, hemoperfusion, hemofiltration, hemodialysis, or plasmapheresis can be considered. Pharmacological treatment remains pragmatic. Some authors recommend therapy with high doses of antibiotics (penicillin or ceftazidime) and silibinin (1,13), although evidence from controlled studies is lacking. Liver transplantation may prove a successful therapeutic approach (4-6,8,9). The mechanism of poisoning is closely related to the inhibitory effect of amatoxins on RNA polymerase II (13).

Other *Amanita* spp. (in particular *A. muscaria, A. regalis,* and *A. pantherina*) contain several pharmacologically active compounds. The major causes of the clinical syndrome are the isoxazole amino acid ibotenic acid (*see* Ibotenic Acid, this volume), a glutamate receptor agonist, its decarboxylation product, the γ-aminobutyric acid agonist muscimol, and muscazone (3). Each of these compounds is resistant to cooking and readily absorbed by the gastrointestinal tract. Because of its low concentration (0.003%), muscarine is not responsible for neurotoxic effects. Muscazone is a colorless crystal with a MW of 158.11 that decomposes above 190°C.

The *muscaria* syndrome most frequently occurs following accidental ingestion, but deliberate intake may occur (2,7). In men, symptoms commence 30–180 min after oral intake, usually without gastroenteritic prodromi. They form a psychobiological syndrome with early restlessness and irritability followed by illusions, visual hallucinations, delirium, euphoria, and ataxia. In particular, intoxication by *A. pantherina* is accompanied by myoclonic jerks (7). After a terminal sleep, recovery occurs in most cases. A "fatigue" syndrome and memory deficits may be long-term sequelae (7). Generalized seizures and coma may also occur, but death is rare (2,7). Gastric lavage is recommended. Administration of atropine is contraindicated since it exacerbates the psychobiological syndrome.

REFERENCES

1. Beer JH (1993) Der falsche Pilz. Diagnose und Therapie der Pilzvergiftungen, speziell der Knollenblätterpilzvergiftung. *Schweiz Med Wochenschr* **123**, 892.
2. Benjamin DR (1992) Mushroom poisoning in infants and children: the *Amanita pantharina/muscaria* group. *Clin Toxicol* **30**, 13.
3. Eugster CH (1969) Chemie der Wirkstoffe aus dem Fliegenpilz (*Amanita muscaria*). *Fortschr Chem Org Naturst* **27**, 262.
4. Galler GW, Weisenberg E, Brasitus TA (1992) Mushroom poisoning: the role of orthotopic liver transplantation. *J Clin Gastroenterol* **15**, 229.
5. Jaeger A, Jehl F, Flesch F *et al.* (1993) Kinetics of amatoxins in human poisoning: therapeutic implications. *Clin Toxicol* **31**, 63.
6. Klein AS, Hart J, Brems JJ *et al.* (1989) *Amanita* poisoning: treatment and the role of liver transplantation. *Amer J Med* **86**, 187.
7. Leonhardt W (1949) Über Rauschzustände bei Pantherpilzvergiftungen. *Nervenarzt* **20**, 181.
8. Pinson CW, Daya MR, Benner KG *et al.* (1990) Liver transplantation for severe *Amanita phalloides* mushroom poisoning. *Amer J Surg* **159**, 493.
9. Pouyet M, Caillon P, Ducerf C *et al.* (1991) Orthotopic liver transplantation for dangerous *Amanita phalloides* poisoning. *Presse Méd* **20**, 2095.
10. Saar M (1991) Ethnomycological data from Siberia and North-East Asia on the effect of *Amanita muscaria*. *J Ethnopharmacol* **31**, 157.
11. Vetter J (1998) Toxins of *Amanita phalloides*. *Toxicon* **36**, 123.
12. Wieland T (1983) The toxic peptides from *Amanita* mushrooms. *Int J Pept Protein Res* **22**, 257.
13. Wieland T, Faulstich H (1983) Peptide toxins from *Amanita*. In: *Handbook of Natural Toxins, Part I. Plant and Fungal Toxins.* Keeler RF, Tu A eds. Marcel Dekker, Basel p. 585.

Amantadine

John D. Rogers

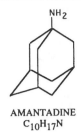

AMANTADINE
$C_{10}H_{17}N$

Tricyclo[3.3.1.1³,⁷]decan-1-amine

NEUROTOXICOLOGY RATING

Clinical

B   Acute encephalopathy (confusion, hallucinations)

Amantadine hydrochloride, a tricyclic amine, was initially used as an antiviral agent for prophylaxis against influenza A infection (3). The mechanism of action is thought to be due to interference with normal ion channel function of the influenza A M2 integral membrane protein (5). It is now used principally for treatment of Parkinson's disease (2) and drug-induced parkinsonism (1,4). Frequently used as a first-line drug for patients with early Parkinson's disease, amantadine can be effective for tremor and rigidity as well as bradykinesia. Its mechanism of action is suggested to be due to dopamine-reuptake inhibition or as a dopamine agonist; it has also been shown to have action at the *N*-methyl-D-aspartate (NMDA) receptor (8). Amantadine reduces NMDA toxicity as measured by lactate dehydrogenase release in a neuron-enriched cerebrocortical culture (7).

Side effects include confusion, visual hallucinations, urinary retention, and hesitancy; these are reversible and usually dose dependent. Rarely, a dermatologic condition, *livedo reticularis*, occurs; this manifests as edema and skin changes in the legs (6).

Amantidine is teratogenic in animals (9).

REFERENCES

1. Borison RL (1983) Amantadine in the management of extrapyramidal side effects. *Clin Neuropharmacol* **6**, S57.
2. Calne DB (1993) Treatment of Parkinson's disease. *N Engl J Med* **329**, 1021.
3. Douglas RG (1990) Drug therapy. Prophylaxis and treatment of influenza. *N Engl J Med* **322**, 443.
4. Greenblatt DJ, DiMascio A, Harmatz JS *et al.* (1977) Pharmacokinetics and clinical effects of amantadine in drug-induced extrapyramidal syndromes. *J Clin Pharmacol* **17**, 704.
5. Hay AJ (1992) The action of adamantanamines against influenza A viruses: Inhibition of the M2 ion channel protein. *Semin Virol* **3**, 21.
6. Huzulakova I, Dukes MNG (1984) Drugs affecting autonomic functions of the extrapyramidal system. In: *Meyler's Side Effects of Drugs. 10th Ed*. Dukes MNG ed. Elsevier, New York p. 232.
7. Lustig HS, Ahern KV, Greenberg DA (1992) Antiparkinsonian drugs and *in vitro* excitotoxicity. *Brain Res* **597**, 148.
8. Stoof JC, Booij J, Drukarch B (1992) Amantadine as *N*-methyl-D-aspartic acid receptor agonist: New possibilities for therapeutic applications. *Clin Neurol Neurosurg* **94**, S4.
9. Vernier DG (1986) Amantadine: Pharmacology and toxicology. *Toxicol Appl Pharmacol* **15**, 642.

α-Aminoadipic Acid

Albert C. Ludolph

$$HO_2CCH(NH_2)CH_2CH_2CH_2CO_2H$$

α-AMINOADIPIC ACID
$C_6H_{11}NO_4$

2-Aminohexanedioic acid

NEUROTOXICITY RATING

Experimental

A   Astrocyte toxicity

DL-α-Aminoadipic acid (DL-αAA), a 6-carbon chemical analog of the excitatory amino acid glutamate, is an astrocyte-specific toxin used experimentally to induce functional or morphological impairment of this cell type *in vivo* and *in vitro* (2–4). Selectivity is likely to be determined by astroglial uptake (1). The D-isomer (D-αAA) is experimentally used as a competitive antagonist at the *N*-methyl-D-aspartate glutamate receptor (2). The L-isomer (L-αAA) is neurotoxic and gliotoxic (3). Human toxicity is not described.

REFERENCES

1. Huck S, Grass F, Hortnagl H (1984) The glutamate ana-logue α-aminoadipic acid is taken up by astrocytes before exerting its gliotoxic effect *in vitro*. *J Neurosci* **4**, 2650.
2. Mc Bean GJ (1990) Intrastriatal injection of DL-aminoadipate reduces kainate toxicity *in vitro*. *Neuroscience* **34**, 225.
3. Olney JW, De Gubareff T, Collins JF (1980) Stereospecif-icity of the gliotoxic and antineurotoxic actions of α-aminoadipate. *Neurosci Lett* **19**, 277.
4. Takada M, Li ZK, Hattori T (1990) Astroglial ablation pre-vents MPTP-induced nigrostriatal neuronal death. *Brain Res* **509**, 55.

ε-Aminocaproic Acid

Daniel M. Rosenbaum

$$H_2N(CH_2)_5COOH$$
ε-AMINOCAPROIC ACID
$C_6H_{13}NO_2$

6-Aminohexanoic acid; Amicar

NEUROTOXICOLOGY RATING
Clinical

A   Myopathy (myonecrosis)
B   Acute encephalopathy (delirium)
C   Seizure disorder

Amicar is one of a group of agents that acts to inhibit fi-brinolysis. An analog of lysine, it binds to lysine-binding sites on plasminogen and plasmin, thus blocking the bind-ing of plasmin to fibrin. As a potent inhibitor of fibrinolysis, it has been used to treat a number of bleeding conditions. However, its efficacy is not clearly established because thrombi that form during treatment with Amicar are not lysed. It has been used to reduce bleeding after procedures such as prostate surgery or tooth extraction in hemophili-acs. It has also been widely used to prevent rebleeding after aneurysmal subarachnoid hemorrhage, but initial enthusi-asm for its use in this setting waned because of an increase in thrombotic complications (2).

Amicar is well absorbed after oral administration. Peak plasma levels occur at 2 h. Approximately 50% of the drug is excreted unchanged in the urine after 12 h. A single in-travenous dose has a duration of action <3 h (12). After prolonged administration, Amicar distributes throughout both the extravascular and intravascular compartments and readily penetrates red blood cells and other tissues.

A simply designed animal study demonstrated significant effects on the electroencephalogram, cerebral blood flow, and intracranial pressure (21). Attempts to induce Amicar myopathy in the rat have been unsuccessful (9).

Well-controlled studies utilizing Amicar in a limited num-ber of patients revealed no serious toxicity (11). Minor ef-fects include nasal congestion, conjunctival suffusion, nau-sea, vomiting, diarrhea, maculopapular or morbilliform rashes, and transient hypotension (3,4). These are probably, in part, allergic reactions. Extracranial thrombotic compli-cations are also described; these include urinary obstruction in both hemophiliacs (17,18) and nonhemophiliacs (7), in-trapleural clot formation (13,14), and the occurrence of both acute right heart failure and renal failure secondary to glomerular capillary thrombosis. Intracranial thrombosis has been reported in a 42-year-old woman who developed superior sagittal and left transverse sinus thrombosis asso-ciated with prolonged Amicar therapy for menorrhagia (1).

The most common, albeit still rare, neurotoxicity asso-ciated with Amicar is painful muscle necrosis with myo-globinuria. This may occur up to several weeks after the infusion of a high dose (30 g/day) of Amicar (5,16). The first case report was published in 1969; it described a pa-tient with hereditary angioneurotic edema treated with Amicar at a dose of 30 g/day for 5 weeks (10). Symptoms resolved after discontinuation of the drug but recurred upon reinstitution of therapy. In an especially convincing case report (8), a patient treated for myelodysplasia after treatment for ovarian carcinoma developed myonecrosis approximately 8 weeks after Amicar therapy at a dose of 24 g/day. Symptoms and biochemical abnormalities re-solved after discontinuation of therapy. Recently, there ap-peared a similar case report of a 12-year-old girl who de-veloped a myopathy subsequent to treatment with Amicar (20).

There has been one report of a patient known to have iodine hypersensitivity who developed an acute delirium with auditory, visual, and kinesthetic hallucinations after an intravenous dose of 2 g of Amicar (19). The episode lasted 8 min; there were no residual neurological deficits. There have been two case reports of Amicar-induced seizures; however, in one, Amicar was administered with glycine; the other involved a patient with severe liver disease (4,15).

Symptoms of Amicar-associated myonecrosis are similar to carnitine deficiency–associated myopathy (6). Lysine is required for carnitine production and Amicar is structurally similar to lysine. Amicar may act as a competitive analog to lysine and result in a "carnitine deficiency"–like state.

REFERENCES

1. Achiron A, Gornish M, Melamed E (1990) Cerebral sinus thrombosis as a potential hazard of antifibrinolytic treatment in menorrhagia. *Stroke* **21**, 817.

2. Adams HA, Love BB (1995) Medical management of aneurysmal subarachnoid hemorrhage. In: *Stroke: Pathophysiology, Diagnosis and Management. 2nd Ed.* Barnett HJM, Mohr JP, Stein BM, Yatsu FM eds. Churchill Livingstone, New York p. 1041.

3. Chakrabarti A, Colleft KA (1980) Purpuric rash due to epsilon-aminocaproic acid. *Brit Med J* **281**, 197.

4. Feffer SE, Parray HR, Westring DW (1978) Seizure after infusion of aminocaproic acid. *J Amer Med Assn* **240**, 2468.

5. Frank MM, Sergent JS, Kine MA *et al.* (1972) Epsilon-aminocaproic acid therapy of hereditary angioneurotic edema. *N Engl J Med* **286**, 808.

6. Gilbert EF (1985) Carnitine deficiency. *Pathology* **17**, 161.

7. Goggins JT, Allen TD (1972) Insoluble fibrin clots within the urinary tract as a consequence of epsilon aminocaproic acid therapy. *J Urol* **107**, 647.

8. Kane MJ, Silverman LR, Rand JH *et al.* (1988) Myonecrosis as a complication of the use of epsilon aminocaproic acid: A case report and review of the literature. *Amer J Med* **85**, 861.

9. Kennard C, Swash M, Henson RA (1980) Myopathy due to epsilon amino-caproic acid. *Muscle Nerve* **3**, 202.

10. Korsan-Bengtsenk, Ysander L, Blohme G, Tibbin E (1969) Extensive muscle necrosis after long term treatment with EACA in a case of hereditary periodic edema. *Acta Med Scand* **185**, 341.

11. Loeliger EA, Broekmans AW (1988) Drugs affecting blood clotting. In: *Meyler's Side Effects of Drugs*. Duke MNG ed. Elsevier, Amsterdam p. 733.

12. Majerus PW, Broze GI Jr, Miletich JP, Tollefsen DM (1995) Anticoagulant; thrombotic and antiplatelet drugs. In: *The Pharmacological Basis of Therapeutics. 9th Ed.* Hardman JG, Limbird LE eds. McGraw-Hill, New York p. 1353.

13. McNicol GP (1962) Disordered fibrinolytic activity and its control. *Scot Med J* **7**, 26.

14. McNicol GP, Fletcher AP, Allejaersig N, Sterry S (1961) The use of epsilon aminocaproic acid, a potent inhibitor of fibrinolytic activity, in the management of postoperative hematuria. *J Urol* **86**, 829.

15. Rabinovici R, Heyma A, Khuger Y, Shinar E (1989) Convulsions induced by aminocaproic acid infusion. *DICP Ann Pharmacother* **23**, 780.

16. Rizza RA, Schlonick S, Contey RL (1976) Myoglobinuria following aminocaproic acid administration. *J Amer Med Assn* **236**, 1845.

17. Stark SN, White JG, Langer L *et al.* (1965) Epsilon aminocaproic acid therapy as a cause of intrarenal obstruction in hematuria of hemophiliacs. *Scand J Haematol* **22**, 99.

18. Van Itterbeek H, Vermylen J, Verstraete M (1968) High obstruction of urine flow as complication of treatment with fibrinolysis inhibitors of hematuria. *Acta Haematol* **39**, 237.

19. Wijsenbeck AJ, Sella A, Vardi M, Yesurun D (1978) Acute delirious state after aminocaproic acid. *Lancet* **1**, 221.

20. Winter SS, Chaffee S, Kahter SG, Graham ML (1995) Epsilon-aminocaproic acid-associated myopathy in a child. *J Pediat Hematol Oncol* **17**, 53.

21. Yamaura A, Nakamura T, Makino H, Hagihara Y (1980) Cerebral complication of antifibrinolytic therapy in the treatment of ruptured intracranial aneurysm. Animal experiment and a review of literature. *Eur Neurol* **19**, 77.

1-Amino-3-Chloro-2-Propanol

Peter S. Spencer

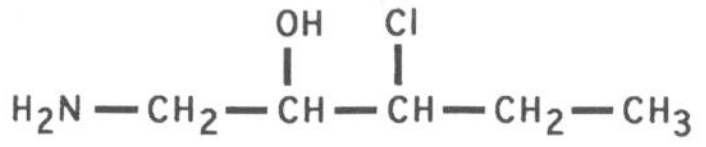

1-AMINO-3-CHLORO-2-PROPANOL
$C_5H_{12}NOCl$

NEUROTOXICITY RATING

Experimental

A   CNS microvacuolation

1-Amino-3-chloro-2-propanol (ACP) is an analog of α-chlorohydrin (3-chloro-1,2-propanediol); both are orally active male antifertility agents, and ACP has neurotoxic effects in primates (1). Young adult male rhesus monkeys fed gelatine capsules containing the agent experienced vomiting, inappetance and weight loss (ACP dosage of 150–300 mg/kg/day), poor coordination and inability to balance (300 mg/kg/day for 2–3 weeks), and marked hindlimb weakness (250 mg/kg/day for 20 weeks). At 13 weeks of dosing, neuropathological changes were present in the medulla oblongata of animals treated with 50–300 mg/kg/day; these were described as consisting of focal vacuolar edema (location unknown) with minimal myelin loss, coupled with occasional degeneration of neurons and axons accompanied by modest glial proliferation. By week 20, lesions were characterized by small areas of gliosis surrounded by vacuoles. Animals treated with larger ACP doses (8 × 500 mg over 4 days) showed, at 14 days, comparable neuropathological changes in the corpus pontobulbare and vestibular nuclei. Unlike α-chlorohydrin, ACP did not suppress bone marrow function in these animals (1).

REFERENCES

1. Heywood R, Sortwell RJ, Prentice DE (1978) The toxicity of 1-amino-3-chloro-2-propanol hydrochloride (CL88,236) in the rhesus monkey. *Toxicology* 9, 219.

Aminoglycoside Antibiotics (Streptomycin)

Herbert H. Schaumburg

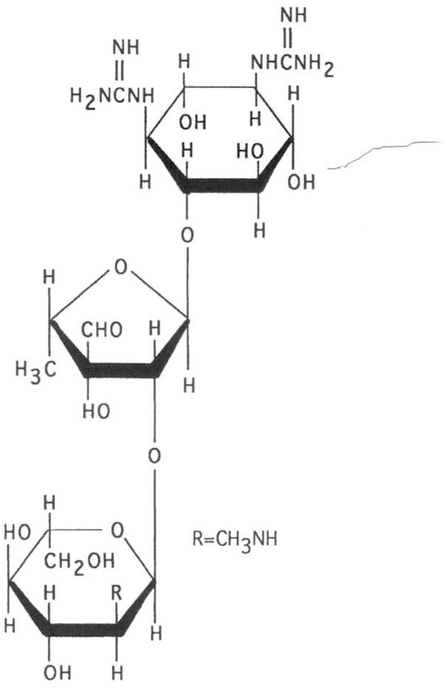

STREPTOMYCIN
$C_{21}H_{39}N_7O_{12}$

O-2-Deoxy-2-(methylamino)-α-L-glucopyranosyl-(1→2)-O-5-deoxy-3-C-formyl-α-L-lyxofuranosyl-(1→4)-N,N'-bis(aminoiminomethyl)-D-streptamine

NEUROTOXICITY RATING

Clinical

A   Ototoxicity

A   Neuromuscular transmission syndrome

Experimental

A   Ototoxicity

A   Ion channel dysfunction (pre- and postsynaptic neuromuscular blockade)

The aminoglycoside antibiotics include gentamycin, tobramycin, amikacin, netilmycin, kanamycin, neomycin and streptomycin. All contain aminosugars linked to an aminocyclitol ring by glycosidic bonds. The aminoglycoside families are distinguished by the aminosugars attached to the aminocyclitol; for example, the neomycin family has three aminosugars attached to a central 2-deoxystreptamine, while the kanamycin and gentamycin families have only two. The aminoglycoside antibiotics are used primarily to treat infections from aerobic gram-negative bacteria. They are bactericidal and act by interfering with protein synthesis in susceptible organisms. Resistance to the bactericidal effect results from acquisition of plasmids containing genes that encode aminoglycoside-metabolizing enzymes. Ototoxicity is a major limit to their use; they are administered with caution for this reason. Acute neuromuscular blockade is occasionally associated with aminoglycoside therapy, especially when the drugs are administered in concert with general anesthesia. Aminoglycosides are available only by prescription in North America.

General Toxicology

As polar cations, the aminoglycosides are poorly absorbed from the gastrointestinal tract and are excreted unchanged in the feces (9). Neomycin, the most potent ototoxin, can be administered orally without fear of complications; it is used as an intestinal antiseptic (6). All are absorbed rapidly following intramuscular injection; peak plasma levels are achieved within 90 min. Because of their strong polar nature, they do not reach the eye or nervous system and are excluded from many cells; aminoglycosides appear and persist in only the endolymph/perilymph of the inner ear and the renal cortex, presumably contributing to toxicity at those sites (11,13). Contrary to former reports, large doses of aminoglycosides with high plasma levels do not result in progressive drug accumulation in endolymph and perilymph; rather, inner ear concentrations remain at low levels (25). More critical to ototoxicity is the long otic half-life (5 times plasma half-life) of aminoglycosides, rapid otic uptake, and saturation (31). The plasma half-life is 2–3 h and almost all is excreted unchanged by the kidney. Patients with impaired renal function are at a greater risk for ototoxicity.

Nephrotoxicity is the only serious (nonneural) side effect; it reflects the strong retention of aminoglycoside in the proximal tubule. Transient renal dysfunction occurs in up to 25% of patients receiving standard doses; permanent dysfunction may develop if there is pre-existent renal disease or massive doses of the drug are administered. The most important consequence of nephrotoxicity may be reduced excretion, leading to ototoxicity.

Animal Studies
Ototoxicity

The type, incidence, and extent of ototoxicity vary among the aminoglycosides. The incidence in experimental animals is 18% for gentamycin, and only 2% for netilmycin (34). Some affect primarily the cochlear system (neomycin, kanamycin, amikacin), while others are primarily vestibulotoxic (dibekacin) or damage both organs equally (gentamycin, tobramycin). Streptomycin and dihydrostreptomycin provide striking examples of structure–toxicity relationships; although differing by only one hydroxyl group, the former is preferentially vestibulotoxic while the latter is more likely to injure the cochlea.

Short-term high-level systemic or topical application of aminoglycosides produces acute reversible dysfunction in cochlear hair cells by disrupting transduction mechanisms; prolonged administration is associated with delayed irreversible degeneration of cochlear and vestibular hair cells.

Short-term systemic administration (10 mg/kg gentamycin in rats), suppresses the microphonic potential (44). A physiological study of bullfrog hair cells demonstrated that streptomycin maintains mechanosensory channels in their open position; the authors state these results are best explained by assuming that streptomycin interferes with mechanoadaptation by blocking the entry of calcium ions through the transduction channels (12). These reversible effects on the electrical properties of hair cells following short-term administration may be analogous to the aminoglycoside-induced, acute, calcium-reversible, neuromuscular junction dysfunction (*vide infra*).

Prolonged administration of aminoglycosides produces cochlear and vestibular hair cell degeneration in most mammalian species, including rats, guinea pigs, cats, and monkeys (7). Within hours of systemic administration, gentamycin enters cochlear tissues and can be detected in hair cells; evidence of toxicity appears only after weeks of daily dosing (31). A similar phenomenon can be shown in tissue culture; isolated outer hair cells, the most vulnerable elements, remain viable in the presence of gentamycin (14). These phenomena suggest the toxicity of gentamycin is attributable to a metabolic product thereof (10,43). Tissue culture studies indicate that the toxic metabolite can be rendered inactive by a glutathione-dependent reaction (23).

Administration of 100 mg/kg of neomycin to guinea pigs for more than 3 weeks produces consistent changes in cochlear hair cells. Loss of these cells commences in the innermost row of basal turns and progresses to the outer rows (22). Eventually, apical outer hair cells and inner hair cells originating from the base may be affected. Early ultrastructural changes include vesiculation of mitochondrial cristae, clumping of nuclear chromatin, nuclear swelling, and loss of ribosomes. Early changes in hair cells are accompanied by shrinkage of marginal cells in the striae vascularis. Similar degenerative events in hair cells occur after short-term topical application of aminoglycosides through a tympanic window or following single transtympanic injection (4). Measurement of auditory function in experimental animals given aminoglycosides discloses progressive high-frequency hearing loss in monkeys and loss of the pinna reflex in rodents. Alteration in cochlear microphonic potentials and in cochlear whole-nerve action potentials occurs first in the high frequencies and later in the lower (3). Aminoglycosides that affect vestibular hair cells produce early alterations in short-latency vestibular-evoked responses and the vestibular cochlear reflex (15).

Pretreatment of guinea pigs with poly-1-aspartic acid, an agent that prevents aminoglycoside-induced nephrotoxicity in rats, is claimed to prevent loss of high-frequency perception following 21 days of gentamicin dosing (30).

Neuromuscular Blockade

All aminoglycoside antibiotics can cause neuromuscular blockade (NMB) secondary to both presynaptic and post-synaptic actions; the balance between pre- and postsynaptic effects varies among agents. The order of decreasing potency of NMB is neomycin, kanamycin, amikacin, gentamycin, and tobramycin (40). Aminoglycoside-induced NMB is transient, almost totally antagonized experimentally by calcium and partially antagonized by neostigmine (21,39). The presynaptic inhibition of acetylcholine release by neomycin is so predictable that it has been used to reverse experimental organophosphorous-anticholinesterase–induced NMB (5). Most studies have been performed in isolated rat diaphragm–phrenic nerve or the costocutaneous nerve–muscle preparation of the garter snake (18,19).

All aminoglycoside antibiotics significantly inhibit presynaptic acetylcholine release. Intracellular recordings of neurons treated with gentamycin indicate that aminoglycosides act extracellularly to block preterminal influx of calcium (8). NMB is promptly reversed by adding calcium to the preparations. Aminoglycosides may act at the same presynaptic site as ω-conotoxin GVIA (ω-conotoxin) (33). Neomycin is the most potent in producing presynaptic NMB; 100 μmol reduces the amplitude of end-plate currents by >90%.

There are striking differences in the degree of postsynaptic neuromuscular transmission blockade among the aminoglycosides, and there may be two distinct mechanisms. Streptomycin and neomycin have been most carefully studied (18,19). Streptomycin displays only a slight postsynaptic effect, is little affected by neostigmine, and appears to act by blocking the receptor. Neomycin displays considerable postsynaptic inhibition (partially reversible by neostigmine) and appears to interact with the ionic channels of the receptor in their open configuration.

In Vitro Studies
Ototoxicity

The effect of aminoglycosides on inner ear tissue cultures varies with the developmental stage of the preparation.

Normal embryogenesis continues for several days when mouse inner ears are explanted late in development and then exposed (1). In contrast, explantation after gestation day 16 results in morphological changes after 24 h of drug treatment; these include inhibition of hair cell development with fusion and, eventually, complete destruction of these cells (2). Cochlear cultures from postnatal mice develop membrane blebs in the apical surfaces of the hair cells (36). Isolated hair cells do *not* display degenerative change even after exposure to high levels of gentamycin. This suggests that drug/tissue interactions and metabolism are critical for toxicity. Further support for this notion comes from experiments in which outer hair cells are exposed to gentamicin that has been incubated with a drug-metabolizing enzyme fraction from liver. In contrast to the gentamycin, the resulting metabolite is toxic. Incubation of the toxic metabolite with glutathione renders it inactive against hair cells (10,14,23,43). This likely explains the observation that lowered hepatic glutathione levels potentiate the combined toxicity of ethacrynic acid and kanamycin (27).

One of the most studied biochemical mechanisms of ototoxicity is the binding of aminoglycosides to polyphosphoinositides. Studies in isolated cochlea, lipid bilayers, and artificial membranes indicate that the affinity of aminoglycosides for phosphatidylinositol-4,5-biphosphate is highly specific, and the metabolism of this lipid in the inner ear is inhibited by long-term drug treatment (37,41). This could affect both the generation of second messengers and also alter membrane permeability. The high correlation between *in vitro* measures of membrane disturbance and the ototoxicity of 8-aminoglycosides in the intact animal supports a relationship between ototoxicity and phosphoinositides.

Human Studies
Ototoxicity

The reported incidence of ototoxicity has varied and depends upon the aminoglycoside used, the underlying disease, and the sensitivity of the monitoring device. In addition, a maternally transmitted genetic susceptibility to aminoglycoside-induced hearing loss has been identified in some Chinese groups (29); this is associated with a mitochondrial DNA point mutation in the 12s ribosomal RNA gene at nucleotide position 1555 (35). A small proportion of individuals at risk for spontaneous (nonfamilial) aminoglycoside ototoxicity also harbors this specific mutation (20).

Clinically recognizable hearing loss and vestibular damage are reported in about 4% of aminoglycoside-treated patients, but screening with high-frequency pure-tone audiograms shows significant subclinical hearing loss in 26% (17). Elderly patients with septicemia or renal failure, or both, are especially vulnerable (16). Hearing loss or vestibular dysfunction may appear after one or two doses of an aminoglycoside; it is usually reversible within 3 days of drug withdrawal (24). The usual pattern of ototoxicity is an insidious onset of dysfunction following 2 or 3 weeks of treatment at a therapeutic dosage. For example, vestibular damage may be clinically apparent after administration of 5–30 g streptomycin at a 1-g daily level; after 4 months, vestibular damage is present in 30%. Clinicians carefully monitor peak and trough plasma levels of aminoglycosides and perform repeated tests of cochlear or vestibular function in patients requiring prolonged therapy.

The first sign of cochlear dysfunction is high-frequency tone loss detected on an audiogram; the first symptom, usually 1 week later, is high-pitched tinnitus, followed within days by hearing impairment obvious to the patient. If the drug is stopped at this stage, full or partial recovery is the rule; further dosing eventuates in low-frequency hearing loss and conversation becomes impaired. Vestibular dysfunction is frequently heralded by headache, followed by the sudden appearance of nausea, disequilibrium, and vertigo (32). The acute phase lasts 1 or 2 weeks and is replaced by a 2-month illness resembling chronic labyrinthitis with severe positional disequilibrium and vertigo. Withdrawal of drug is followed by a compensatory stage during which labyrinthine function is replaced by use of visual and deep proprioceptive clues. Recovery may take a year; many are left with some residual dysfunction.

The vestibulotoxic properties of streptomycin are so predictable and consistent that this agent has been used to perform a chemical labyrinthotomy in patients with end-stage Ménière's disease (38).

Neuromuscular Blockade

Aminoglycoside-induced NMB in humans has occurred most commonly with the coadministration of nondepolarizing agents active at the neuromuscular junction (*d*-tubocurarine, succinylcholine), or with the coexistence of neuromuscular diseases (myasthenia gravis); occasional instances occur without a predisposing factor. With wide recognition of this toxicity, aminoglycoside-induced NMB is rare in North America (28,40).

Other modifying factors include:

1. Total dose and route—intravenous, intrapleural, and intraperitoneal are especially risk-prone.
2. Excretion—renal impairment is a predisposing factor.
3. Other disease states—gram-negative septicemia is highly associated.

The dose of aminoglycoside need not be great and duration is variable. As little streptomycin as 1 g daily for 3 days and 3 doses of 45 mg of gentamycin given over a 48-h period, have caused flaccid quadriplegia. The time between the last dose and onset is also variable; it has occurred within 1 h or after as long as 26 h. The onset of paralysis is rapid and often evolves from weakness of grip and foot dorsiflexion to quadriplegia and respiratory paralysis within 4–8 h. Recovery is rapid following withdrawal of drug and drop in plasma aminoglycoside levels; hemodialysis may be necessary in cases with impaired renal function.

Calcium chloride and neostigmine are sometimes administered in an attempt to reverse NMB. These agents are most often used by anesthesiologists, with variable success, in emergent postoperative situations while waiting for the plasma levels of drug to decline (40).

Intrathecal Toxicity

It is widely held that intraventricular or intrathecal administration of aminoglycosides is safe. Neither ototoxicity nor NMB is reported to follow intrathecal administration. However, assessment of these patients is often inadequate because they are usually critically ill.

Polyradiculitis has been reported following intrathecal administration of gentamycin, kanamycin, or streptomycin. It is unclear if this was due to the aminoglycoside or to a diluent, since all used intravenous preparations containing preservatives such as phenol and benzyl alcohol. Optic neuropathy rarely may accompany intrathecal streptomycin administration; its significance is uncertain, since reversible optic neuropathy and anosmia are rare complications of prolonged systemic streptomycin treatment (42).

An autopsy of one individual who received intrathecal administration of gentamycin disclosed multifocal lesions in the myelinated fibers of the pons and mesencephalon (46). Intracisternal administration of preservative-free gentamycin produces similar lesions in rabbits (46). These lesions are most prominent in deep white matter tracts, not in subpial areas with the greatest contact with cerebrospinal fluid. The lesions are minute and multiple, resembling a spongy degeneration of the white matter. Axonal and myelin degeneration are present in these foci. An experimental ultrastructural study following intracisternal administration in the rabbit suggests that the pathogenesis stems from an initially high sensitivity of astroglial cells and, later, to the sensitivity of the myelinated fibers to gentamycin-induced injury (26). A study of the effect of gentamycin injected into the lumbar subarachnoid space of the rat disclosed that paralysis and electrophysiological changes are confined to the hindlimbs (45).

Toxic Mechanisms

The acute, reversible ototoxicity and neuromuscular blockade appear to stem from calcium antagonism at the external cell membrane channels of the corresponding anatomical sites (18). The delayed ototoxicity, which is associated with hair cell degeneration, most likely is due to local effects of a yet-uncharacterized aminoglycoside metabolite. The biochemical mechanisms underlying the acute and chronic effects are unknown; it is suggested that the chronic effect may stem, in part, from an interaction of aminoglycosides and phosphoinositide lipids (37).

REFERENCES

1. Anniko M, Nordemar H (1979) Embryogenesis of the inner ear. I. Development and differentiation of the mammalian insta ampullaris *in vivo* and *in vitro*. *Arch Otorhinolaryngol* **224**, 285.

2. Anniko M, Takada A, Schacht J (1982) Comparative ototoxicities of gentamicin and netilmicin in three model systems. *Amer J Otolaryngol* **3**, 422.

3. Arpini A, Cornacchia L, Albiero L et al. (1979) Auditory function in guinea pigs treated with netilmicin and other aminoglycoside antibiotics. *Arch Otorhinolaryngol* **224**, 137.

4. Bareggi R, Grill V, Narducci P et al. (1990) Gentamicin ototoxicity: Histological and ultrastructural alterations after transtympanic administration. *Pharmacol Res Commun* **22**, 635.

5. Bradley RJ (1986) Reversal of organophosphate-induced muscle block by neomycin. *Brain Res* **381**, 397.

6. Breen KJ, Bryant RE, Levinson JD et al. (1972) Neomycin absorption in man. *Ann Intern Med* **76**, 211.

7. Brummett R (1983) Animal models of aminoglycoside antibiotic ototoxicity. *Rev Infect Dis* **5**(Suppl 2), S294.

8. Carlson CG, Dettbarn W-D (1985) The aminoglycoside antibiotic, gentamicin, fails to block increases in miniature endplate potential frequency induced by the sulfhydryl reagent, N-ethylmaleimide, in low calcium solutions. *Brain Res* **30**, 349.

9. Cox CD (1970) Gentamicin. *Med Clin North Amer* **54**, 1305.

10. Crann SA, Huang MY, McLaren JD et al. (1992) Formation of a toxic metabolite from gentamicin by a hepatic cytosolic fraction. *Biochem Pharmacol* **43**, 1835.

11. Davies RR, Brummett RE, Bendrick TW, Himes DL (1984) Dissociation of maximum concentration of kanamycin in plasma and perilymph from ototoxic effect. *J Antimicrob Chemother* **14**, 291.

12. Denk W, Keolian RM, Webb WW (1992) Mechanical response of frog saccular hair bundles to the aminoglycoside block of mechanoelectrical transduction. *J Neurophysiol* **68**, 927.

13. Desrochers CS, Schacht J (1982) Neomycin concentrations in inner ear tissues and other organs of the guinea pig after chronic drug administration. *Acta Otolaryngol* **93**, 233.

14. Dulon D, Zajic G, Aran JM et al. (1989) Aminoglycoside antibiotics impair calcium entry but not viability and motility in isolated cochlear outer hair cells. *J Neurosci Res* **24**, 338.

15. Elidan J, Lin J, Honrubia V (1987) Vestibular ototoxicity of gentamicin assessed by the recording of a short-latency vestibular-evoked response in cats. *Laryngoscope* **97**, 865.

16. Esterhal JL, Bednar J, Kimmelman CP (1986) Gentamicin-induced ototoxicity complicating treatment of chronic osteomyelitis. *Clin Orthop Related Res* **209**, 186.

17. Fausti SA, Henry JA, Schaffer HI et al. (1992) High-frequency audiometric monitoring for early detection of aminoglycoside ototoxicity. *J Infect Dis* **165**, 1026.

18. Fiekers JF (1983) Effects of the aminoglycoside antibiotics, streptomycin and neomycin, on neuromuscular transmission. I. Pre-synaptic considerations. *J Pharmacol Exp Ther* **225**, 487.

19. Fiekers JF (1983) Effects of the aminoglycoside antibiotics, streptomycin and neomycin, on neuromuscular transmission. II. Post-synaptic considerations. *J Pharmacol Exp Ther* **225**, 496.

20. Fischel-Ghodsian N, Prezant TR, Bu X et al. (1993) Mitochondrial ribosomal RNA gene mutation in a patient with sporadic aminoglycoside ototoxicity. *Amer J Otolaryngol* **14**, 399.

21. Foldes FF, Bikhazi GB (1989) The influence of temperature and calcium concentration on the myoneural effect of antibiotics. *Acta Physiol Pharmacol Latinoam* **39**, 343.

22. Forge A (1985) Outer hair cell loss and supporting cell expansion following chronic gentamicin treatment. *Hear Res* **35**, 39.

23. Garetz S, Schacht J (1992) Sulfhydryl compounds reduce gentamicin-induced outer hair cell damage *in vitro*. *Abs Assoc Res Otolaryngol* **15**, 110.

24. Hain TC, Zee DS (1991) Abolition of optokinetic nystagmus by aminoglycoside ototoxicity. *Ann Otol Rhinol Laryngol* **100**, 580.

25. Henley CM, Schacht J (1988) Pharmacokinetics of aminoglycoside antibiotics in blood, inner-ear fluids and tissues and their relationship to ototoxicity. *Audiology* **27**, 137.

26. Hodges GR, Watanabe I (1980) Chemical injury of the spinal cord of the rabbit after intracisternal injection of gentamicin. An ultrastructural study. *J Neuropathol Exp Neurol* **39**, 452.

27. Hoffman DW, Whitworth CA, Jones KL et al. (1987) Nutritional status, glutathione levels, and ototoxicity of loop diuretics and aminoglycoside antibiotics. *Hear Res* **31**, 217.

28. Holtzman JL (1976) Gentamicin neuromuscular blockade. *Ann Intern Med* **84**, 55.

29. Hu DN, Qui WQ, Wu BT *et al.* (1991) Genetic aspects of antibiotic-induced deafness: Mitochondrial inheritance. *J Med Genet* **28**, 79.

30. Hulka GF, Prazma J, Brownlee RE *et al.* (1993) Use of poly-1-aspartic acid to inhibit aminoglycoside cochlear ototoxicity. *Amer J Otolaryngol* **14**, 352.

31. Huy PTB, Bernard P, Schacht J (1986) Kinetics of gentamicin uptake and release in the rat: Comparison of inner ear tissues and fluids and other organs. *J Clin Invest* **77**, 1492.

32. Jongkees LBW, Hulk J (1950) The action of streptomycin on vestibular function. *Acta Otolaryngol* **38**, 225.

33. Keith RA, LaMonte D, Salama AI (1990) Neomycin and omega-conotoxin GVIA interact at a common neuronal site in peripheral tissues. *J Autonom Pharmacol* **10**, 139.

34. Moore RD, Smith CR, Lipsky JJ *et al.* (1984) Risk factors for nephrotoxicity in patients wth aminoglycosides. *Ann Intern Med* **100**, 352.

35. Prezant TR, Agapian JV, Bohlman MC *et al.* (1993) Mitochondrial ribosomal RNA mutation associated with both antibiotic-induced and non-syndromic deafness. *Nature Genet* **4**, 289.35.

36. Richardson GP, Russell IJ (1991) Cochlear cultures as a model system for studying aminoglycoside-induced ototoxicity. *Hear Res* **53**, 293.

37. Schacht J, Weiner N (1986) Aminoglycoside-induced hearing loss: A molecular hypothesis. *ORL-J Oto-rhino-laryngol* **48**, 116.

38. Silverstein H (1984) Streptomycin treatment for Ménière's disease. *Ann Otol Rhinol Laryngol* **93**, 44.

39. Singh YN, Harvey AL, Marshall IG (1978) Antibiotic-induced paralysis of the mouse phrenic nerve-hemidiaphragm preparation, and reversibility by calcium and neostigimine. *Anesthesiology* **84**, 418.

40. Sokoll MD, Gergis SD (1981) Antibiotics and neuromuscular function. *Anesthesiology* **55**, 148.

41. Stockhorst E, Schacht J (1977) Radioactive labeling of phospholipids and proteins by cochlear perfusion in the guinea pig and the effects of neomycin. *Acta Otolaryngol* **83**, 401.

42. Sykowsk P (1952) Streptomycin in miliary choroidal tuberculosis. *Amer J Ophthamol* **35**, 414.

43. Takada A, Bledsoe S, Schacht J (1985) An energy-dependent step in aminoglycoside ototoxicity: Prevention of gentamicin ototoxicity during reduced endolymphatic potential. *Hear Res* **19**, 245.

44. Takada A, Schacht J (1982) Calcium antagonism and reversibility of gentamicin-induced loss of cochlear microphonics in the guinea pig. *Hear Res* **8**, 179.

45. Tolliver JM, Warnick JE (1985) Aminoglycoside-induced biphasic hindlimb paralysis in the rat: A histological and electrophysiological assessment. *Fund Appl Toxicol* **5**, 933.

46. Watanabe I, Hodges GR, Dworzac DL *et al.* (1978) Neurotoxicity of intrathecal gentamicin: A case report and experimental study. *Ann Neurol* **4**, 564.

6-Aminonicotinamide

Hans Kolbe

6-AMINONICOTINIC ACID
$C_6H_6N_2O_2$

6-Amino-3-pyridinecarboxylic acid

NEUROTOXICITY RATING

Experimental

A Gliotoxicity

A Antinicotinamide agent

6-Aminonicotinamide (6-AN) appears to be the most potent antagonist of nicotinamide known. Introduction of an amino group to position 6 of the pyridine ring leads to remarkable pharmacological and toxicological properties.

Following reports on the inhibitory activity of 6-AN against several experimental tumors, intensive toxicological studies were undertaken for the possible clinical use of this substance as an anticancer agent (9,23).

The toxic potency of 6-AN in rabbits was observed in studies of the inhibition of sulfonamide acetylation (11). There was a delayed onset of toxic effects, with a loss of control of the hindlimbs being the first sign. It was suggested (11) that this delayed onset of action is due to the transformation of 6-AN to an ineffective analogue of the pyridine nucleotides. The LD_{50} for mice was found to be 35 mg/kg; this was increased by simultaneous administration of nicotinamide.

6-AN was also given to cats; three animals received 7, 5, 15, and 30 mg/kg of 6-AN, respectively (24), and 5 h later, dysmetria of the hindlimbs was observed. Within 72 h, all 4 limbs were paralyzed; knee jerks and placing reaction remained intact. By day 10, there was wasting in the hindlimb muscles of an animal that received 30 mg/kg 6-AN. Cats receiving smaller doses displayed maximal postural disturbances at 72 h but recovered steadily afterwards. In one animal treated with 15 mg/kg 6-AN, some dysmetria was present 4 months later.

One of five dogs given daily doses of 4 mg/kg 6-AN for a maximum of 10 days tolerated this very well with no functional impairment. A second dog died on day 8 after displaying hyperexcitement, hyperthermia with incoordinated movements, and twitching of ears and cheeks on day 7. After 10 days of 6-AN treatment, a third dog developed bobbing of the head that was suppressed by purposeful movements, followed by twitching of the ears and lips and incoordination of the hindlimbs. The animal died on day 18. The remaining two dogs, paralyzed after 1 week of 6-AN application, retained normal reflexes and hyperexcitability. They swallowed with difficulty and salivated excessively. On pathological examination, lesions were evident in the anterior horn of the spinal cord and in brainstem nuclei (24).

A dose of 8 mg/kg 6-AN was given to 47 rats (24). Of these, 19 were killed for examination, and 18 died spontaneously, mainly on the second or third day. The remaining 19 rats developed a characteristic course of functional decline: incoordination of the hindlimbs developed within 24 h, followed by paralysis on day 2. On day 3, all extremities were involved. By day 10, wasting of the hindlimb muscles was present. Five paralyzed animals recovered and were normal after some weeks. The spinal cords and brains of the surviving ten animals were examined histologically and showed marked tissue destruction in the spinal cord anterior horn and in some nuclei of the brainstem.

Impairment of placement reaction and stiffness of legs as early as 6 h after 8 mg/kg 6-AN was shown in rats (26). With dosages of 16–64 mg/kg 6-AN, animals became sluggish and developed weakness in the hind limbs. They grew more and more lethargic and hypoactive, became reluctant to move, lost their righting responses and finally lay on their sides with their hindlimbs extended, exhibiting intermittently rapid rhythmic movements of limbs and head. Swallowing was also impaired. Animals were sacrificed at 1, 3, 6, 9, and 24 h and on days 2, 3, 4, 8, and 10. The spinal cord was consistently affected, the anterior horns being predominantly involved. Nuclei of medulla, pons, midbrain, and of the roof of the cerebellum were severely affected, as were the geniculate bodies, thalamus, and corpus striatum. In a detailed study (21) on the time course of morphological changes following 6-AN administration, it was shown that the alterations started in neuroglia leaving neurons in the affected areas unchanged. Within 36 h after administration

of 6-AN, astrocytes and oligodendrocytes showed progressive vacuolation and destruction of the rough endoplasmic reticulum, dilatation of perinuclear cisterns, and necrosis. Involvement of neurons appeared to be a secondary event. The structural changes induced by 6-AN were dose dependent: 5 mg/kg produced a transient paresis clinically and only attenuated glial swelling; 10 mg/kg led to permanent paresis with glial necrosis in the anterior horn. Swelling and vacuolation of glial cells became manifest 12 h after application of the toxin. At this time, destruction of the rough endoplasmic reticulum occurred with the ribosomes disappearing, followed by distention of tubular and cisternal structures. These were most prominent around the nucleus leading to a half-moon–shaped deformation of the organelle. Mitochondria appeared well preserved. After 36 h, glial perikarya were necrotic; 2–4 days after 6-AN the neuropil was completely destroyed in the anterior horn. Following the loss of glial cells, there was extension of the extracellular space with fairly isolated neurons and only some synapses preserved. During the following 12 months, an astrocytic scar filled the lesioned areas; there was a complete loss of neuropil and disappearance of most neurons (21). Simultaneous changes in oligodendroglia led to splitting of the intraperiod lines of myelin sheaths and eventually to progressive fragmentation. Secondary changes in neurons affected mainly the tubular system and the dendrites. At later stages, there was involvement of nerve endings with a loss of vesicles (21).

A similar course of events was decribed in rat optic nerve (20). In newborn mice, lesions comparable to those seen in human pellagra were observed after a single dose of 6-AN. The mice displayed ataxia, developed paresis of the hindlimbs, and became hydrocephalic. Hydrocephalus was seen in the offspring of rats treated with 6-AN during pregnancy (3).

All reports emphasized the striking similarity of localization and histopathology of 6-AN–induced changes and those in experimental thiamine deficiency and other disorders such as hepatocerebral encephalopathy, metachromatic leukodystrophy, Leigh's disease, Wernicke's encephalopathy, and metronidazol intoxication. This led to the concept of *glia syndrome* or gliopathy (22).

There is only one report on effects of 6-AN in humans (9): after 6-AN had shown promise against a number of experimental neoplasms, a study was set up to evaluate the toxicity of 6-AN in humans. Sixty patients with advanced malignant disease were treated with doses of 6-AN ranging from 0.2 mg/kg to 1.5 mg/kg (9). No serious toxicity was noticed during the first 4 weeks of 0.2 mg/kg of 6-AN. Blepharitis, conjunctivitis, excessive tearing, and photophobia were seen in some of the patients. Eighth nerve damage leading to bilateral deafness occurred in one patient who received a total dose of 691 mg 6-AN. At a dose level of 0.4 mg/kg daily, CNS toxicity emerged earlier, with ocular and oral symptoms like lethargy, tinnitus, and deafness starting later. At doses between 0.6 and 1.5 mg/kg of 6-AN, toxic symptoms occurred almost immediately after application with nausea, vomiting, and headache, followed by stomatitis, buccal ulcerations, cheilosis, and glossitis at day 4 (1). A week after 6-AN application, marked disorientation was observed, followed by tinnitus and progressive hearing loss. One patient became severely ataxic on day 6. Therapy was discontinued in all cases; toxic manifestations reversed only in those symptoms related to nicotinamide deficiency. The authors of this study postulated two toxic mechanisms induced by 6-AN: a pellagra-like syndrome that is promptly reversed by giving nicotinamide, and a direct action on the CNS, leading to irreversible damage to vulnerable regions.

The biochemical mechanism by which 6-AN acts on the nervous system is well understood. A rather nonspecific catalytic activity of the glycohydrolase [E.C. 3.2.2.6] of the endoplasmic reticulum (14) incorporates 6-AN into the cofactors nicotinamide-adenine-dinucleotide (NAD) and nicotinamide-adenine-dinucleotide-phosphate (NADP) leading to the 6-AN analogues 6-ANAD or 6-ANADP (4,8). These two compounds are competitive inhibitors of NAD- or NADP-linked enzymes due to their inability to act as hydrogen carriers. NADP-linked 6-phosphogluconate-dehydrogenase [E.C. 1.1.1.44] is the enzyme most affected, resulting in a 200-fold increase of its substrate, 6-phosphogluconate. The accumulation of 6-phosphogluconate is a marker for the extent of 6-ANADP synthesis; the highest concentrations are found in brain regions with marked morphological alterations (16,21) (i.e., in basal ganglia, midbrain, pons, medulla oblongata, and medulla spinalis).

The accumulation of 6-phosphogluconate (up to 10^{-3} M) causes an inhibition of the enzyme activity of phoshoglucose-isomerase [E.C. 5.3.1.9] with a K_i of 5×10^{-6} (8,13). This competitive inhibition of phosphoglucose isomerase by 6-phosphogluconate accumulation causes changes in intermediary metabolism, especially in glucose metabolism:

1. The ratio of metabolite concentration at the phosphoglucose isomerase changes from 3.9 in controls to 16.3 in the brains of 6-AN–treated rats (16).
2. Lactate and pyruvate concentrations are lowered probably as a consequence of reduced metabolic flow through glycolysis (16).
3. Krebs cycle substrate concentrations (citrate, malate, 2-oxoglutarate) are decreased significantly (2,7).
4. Fatty acid synthesis is inhibited even at low doses of 6-AN; cholesterol synthesis is unaffected (10). Metabolic compartmentation could be the reason for the different behavior of the two lipogenic processes that are both NADP-dependent.
5. Free glucose is elevated in brains of 6-AN–treated animals.

A graded effect of 6-AN on the pattern of glucose utilization emerges from measurements of $^{14}CO_2$ yields from differently labeled ^{14}C-glucose (5,10). Even at very low doses of 6-AN, there is marked inhibition of the pentose-phosphate pathway (18). Lactate formation is decreased by 28%, signaling a reduced metabolic flow in glycolysis. At higher dosages, 6-AN causes inhibition both of the Krebs cycle and of the glutamate–γ-aminobutyric acid (GABA) shunt.

There is controversy with regard to the extent of the reduction of glycolytic flux rates, whereas unanimity prevails concerning the marked blockade of the pentose phosphate pathway (6,8,10). It is worth remembering the morphological studies on 6-AN that show a distinct pattern of vulnerability in brain and spinal cord (24,26) and a more pronounced effect on glial cells (21). The preferential damage to neuroglia is so conspicuous that the term "acute 6-AN gliopathy" was coined (21). The selective vulnerability of astrocytes and oligodendrocytes towards 6-AN was confirmed by studies on clonal cells of neuronal and glial origin (17). The accumulation of 6-phosphogluconate was much greater in glial than in neuronal cells. This differential effect can be explained by a more effective dephosphorylation in neuronal cells leading to higher gluconate excretion by these cells. Glycolytic flux and adenosine triphosphate (ATP) content are markedly more diminished by 6-AN in cells of glial origin. Gluconate itself is no inhibitor of phosphoglucose isomerase. The more pronounced inhibition of the glutamate-GABA shunt, compared to the glycolytic and Krebs cycle flow rates, is readily explained by the importance of this pathway for glial cells. They are highly involved in glutamate uptake from glutamatergic neurotransmission by recycling this important transmitter as glutamine to the nerve endings. To provide this important supportive function to neurons, astroglia are well equipped with an active glutamate shunt with very high turnover rates coupled to a very active Krebs cycle (25). GABA production and glutamate recycling or synthesis are obviously important functions of glia. Some of the early effects of 6-AN intoxicaton could be caused by disturbances of GABAergic and glutamatergic neurotransmission.

Some neurological sequelae after low doses of 6-AN are better explained by a decrease of dopamine content in the striatum (15). Moreover, 6-AN intoxication interferes with the use of the remaining dopamine. Electromyographic analysis of the persistently elevated muscle tone in the hindlimbs of 6-AN–treated rats showed rigidity, easily abolished by low doses of lisuride or levodopa (19). Normally, a 37% decrease of dopamine content in the striatum could not explain parkinsonian symptoms. It was demonstrated, however, that the dopamine cells were unable to release dopamine adequately (15). Being unable to find any change in catecholamine synthesis, the authors were inclined to think that dopaminergic transmission is directly disrupted by 6-AN.

Studies on pheochromocytoma cells (PC-12 clone) treated with 6-AN showed a decrease of intracellular tetrahydrobiopterin correlating with the diminished dopamine synthesis (12). Adding $NADH_2$ to the culture medium restored dopa production without normalizing biopterin levels, thus clearly indicating a 6-AN influence on the first step of biopterin synthesis or on the recycling of the oxidized cofactor (12). Tetrahydrobiopterin is an important cofactor of tyrosine hydroxylase, occurring only at subsaturating concentrations and thus playing a role in dopamine synthesis regulation. Tyrosine hydrolase is the rate-limiting enzyme in catecholamine synthesis that is interestingly found at subnormal levels in parkinsonian brains.

In summary, high doses of 6-AN, a potent antimetabolite of nicotinamide, produces widespread necrosis of glial cells within 36 h of application and the eventual death of the animal. Lower doses of 6-AN, however, lead to a more sustained course of toxicity in the brain with a distinct pattern of selective vulnerability mainly due to reduced neurotransmitter synthesis.

REFERENCES

1. Aikawa H, Suzuki K (1986) Lesions in the skin, intestine and central nervous system induced by an antimetabolite of niacin. *Amer J Pathol* **122**, 335.
2. Bielecki L, Krieglstein J (1976) Decreased GABA and glutamate concentration in rat brain after treatment with 6-aminonicotinamide. *Naunyn-Schmied Arch Pharmacol* **294**, 157.
3. Chamberlain JG (1972) 6-Aminonicotinamide (6-AN)-induced abnormalities of the developing ependyma and choroid plexus as seen with the scanning electron microscope. *Teratology* **6**, 281.
4. Dietrich LS, Friedland IM, Kaplan LA (1958) Pyridine nucleotide metabolism: Mechanism of action of the niacin antagonist, 6-aminonicotinamide. *J Biol Chem* **233**, 964.
5. Gaitonde MK, Evison E, Evans GM (1983) The rate of utilization of glucose *via* hexose monophosphate shunt in brain. *J Neurochem* **41**, 1253.
6. Gaitonde MK, Jones J, Evans G (1987) Metabolism of glucose into glutamine *via* the hexose monophosphate shunt and its inhibition by 6-aminonicotinamide in rat brain in vivo. *Proc R Soc Lond (Biol)* **231**, 71.

7. Gaitonde MK, Murray E, Cunningham VI (1989) Effect of 6-phosphogluconate on phosphoglucose-isomerase in rat brain *in vitro* and *in vivo*. *J Neurochem* **52**, 1348.
8. Herken H, Lange K, Kolbe H (1969) Brain disorders induced by pharmacological blockade of pentose phosphate pathway. *Biochem Biophys Res Commun* **36**, 93.
9. Herter FP, Weissman SG, Thompson HG *et al.* (1961) Clinical experience with 6-aminonicotinamide. *Cancer Res* **21**, 31.
10. Hothersall JS, Zabairu S, McLean P, Greenbaum AL (1981) Alternative pathways of glucose utilization in brain; changes in the pattern of glucose utilization in brain resulting from treatment of rats with 6-aminonicotinamide. *J Neurochem* **37**, 1484.
11. Johnson WJ, McColl JD (1955) 6-Aminonicotinamide—a potent nicotinamide antagonist. *Science* **122**, 834.
12. Jung W, Herken H (1989) Inhibition of biopterin synthesis and DOPA production in PC-12 pheochromocytoma cells induced by aminonicotinamide. *Naunyn-Schmied Arch Pharmacol* **339**, 424.
13. Kahana SE, Lowry OH, Schulz DW *et al.* (1960) The kinetics of phosphoglucoisomerase. *J Biol Chem* **235**, 2178.
14. Kaplan NO, Ciotti MM (1956) Chemistry and properties of 3-acetylpyridine analog of diphosphopyridine nucleotide. *J Biol Chem* **221**, 823.
15. Kehr W, Halbhübner K, Loos D, Herken H (1978) Impaired dopamine function and muscular rigidity induced by 6-aminonicotinamide in rats. *Naunyn-Schmied Arch Pharmacol* **304**, 317.
16. Keller K, Kolbe H, Lange K, Herken H (1972) Behaviour of the glycolytic system of rat brain and kidney *in vivo* after inhibition of the glucose phosphate isomerase: I. Kinetic studies on rat brain glucose phosphate isomerase. *Hoppe Seylers Z Physiol Chem* **353**, 1389.
17. Kolbe H, Keller K, Lange K, Herken H (1976) Metabolic consequences of drug-induced inhibition of the pentose-phosphate pathway in neuroblastoma and glioma cells. *Biochem Biophys Res Commun* **73**, 378.
18. Lange K, Kolbe H, Keller K, Herken H (1970) Der Kohlenhydratstoffwechsel des Gehirns nach Blockade des Pentose-Phosphat-Weges durch 6-Aminonicotinsäureamid. *Hoppe Seylers Z Physiol Chem* **351**, 1241.
19. Loos D, Halbhübner K, Herken H (1977) Lisuride, a potent drug in the treatment of muscular rigidity in rats. *Naunyn-Schmied Arch Pharmacol* **300**, 195.
20. Meyer-König E (1973) Ultrastruktur der Glia- und Axonschädigung durch 6-Aminonicotin-amid (6-AN) am Sehnerv der Ratte. *Acta Neuropathol* **26**, 115.
21. Schneider H, Cervous-Navarro I (1974) Acute gliopathy in spinal cord and brain stem induced by 6-aminonicotinamide. *Acta Neuropathol* **27**, 11.
22. Seitelberger F (1970) General neuropathology of central neuroglia: The concept of glial syndromes. *VI Congr Internat Neuropathol Masson*, Paris p. 392.

23. Shapiro DM, Dietrich LS, Shils ME (1957) Quantitative biochemical differences between tumor and host as a basis for cancer chemotherapy. V. Niacin and 6-aminonicotinamide. *Cancer Res* **17**, 600.
24. Sternberg SS, Philips FS (1958) 6-Aminonicotinamide and acute degenerative changes in the central nervous system. *Science* **127**, 644.
25. Van den Berg CJ, Krzlic L, Mela P, Waelsch H (1969) Compartmentation of glutamate metabolism in brain: Evidence for the existence of two different tricarboxylic acid cycles in brain. *Biochem J* **113**, 281.
26. Wolf A, Cowen D (1959) Pathological changes in the central nervous system produced by 6-aminonicotinamide. *Bull N Y Acad Med* **35**, 814.

α-Aminopyridine

Albert C. Ludolph

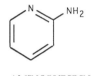

α-AMINOPYRIDINE
$C_5H_6N_2$

2-Pyridinamine

NEUROTOXICITY RATING

Clinical

A   Seizure disorder

Experimental

A   Ion channel dysfunction (voltage-dependent K^+ channels)

Aminopyridines block voltage-activated potassium channels, thereby increasing action potential duration (6) and neurotransmitter release. They have been used with moderate success in the treatment of multiple sclerosis (4,17) and Lambert-Eaton myasthenic syndrome (15). The most serious side effects are generalized seizures (4). Cardiac arrhythmias (5) and gastrointestinal symptoms also occur (1).

4-Aminopyridine is an organic base and exists in both charged and uncharged forms in aqueous solution (12). 3,4-Diaminopyridine has approximately 40 times the blocking potency of 4-aminopyridine (16); however, 4-aminopyridine is more lipid-soluble than 3,4-diaminopyridine and, therefore, more readily crosses the blood-brain barrier (14). High-performance liquid chromatography methods for determination of 4-aminopyridine in tissue samples and plasma are available (7,20).

Treatment of rats *in vivo* with 5 mg/kg of 4-aminopyridine induces generalized convulsions in 74% of the animals and death in 13% (11). Epileptiform discharges upon application of 4-aminopyridine occur in hippocampal slice preparations (2).

Due to the higher lipophilicity, human CNS toxicity is more pronounced for 4-aminopyridine. Treatment with 4-aminopyridine can cause seizures (4,19). Other CNS side effects are dizziness, gait instability, and confusion (4,17). Upon treatment with 3,4-diaminopyridine, mild PNS dysfunction (acral paresthesias, abdominal pain) appear (4,17). Side effects are more pronounced after intravenous infusion and they are accompanied by pain in the infusion arm (21).

Aminopyridines are open-channel blockers of voltage-activated potassium channels (8,18,22). The block occurs at the intracellular mouth of the pore (13). Aminopyridines facilitate action potential propagation and neurotransmitter release. 3,4-Diaminopyridine produces a dose- and time-dependent accumulation of inositol phosphates that is maximal at a dosage of 1 mM 3,4-diaminopyridine (10). Besides their action on neuronal potassium channels, block of transient potassium outward current is also observed in astrocytes (9) and Schwann cells (3).

REFERENCES

1. Aisen ML, Sevilla D, Gibson G *et al.* (1995) 3,4-Diaminopyridine as a treatment for amyotrophic lateral sclerosis. *J Neurol Sci* **129**, 21.
2. Albowitz B, Kuhnt U, Ehrenreich L (1990) Optical recording of epileptiform voltage changes in the neocortical slice. *Exp Brain Res* **81**, 241.
3. Baker M, Howe JR, Ritchie JM (1993) Two types of 4-aminopyridine-sensitive potassium current in rabbit Schwann cells. *J Physiol* **464**, 321.
4. Bever CJ (1994) The current status of studies of aminopyridines in patients with multiple sclerosis. *Ann Neurol* **36**, S118.
5. Boerma CE, Rommes JH, van Leeuwen RB, Bakker J (1995) Cardiac arrest following an iatrogenic 3,4-diaminopyridine intoxication in a patient with Lambert-Eaton myasthenic syndrome. *J Toxicol-Clin Toxicol* **33**, 249.
6. Bostock H, Sherratt RM, Sears TA (1980) Overcoming conduction failure in demyelinated nerve by prolonging action potentials. *Nature* **274**, 385.
7. Casteel SW, Thomas BR (1990) A high-performance liquid

chromatography method for determination of 4-amino-pyridine in tissues and urine. *J Vet Diagn Invest* **2**, 132.

8. Castle NA, Fadous S, Logothetis DE, Wang GK (1994) Aminopyridine block of Kv1.1 potassium channels expressed in mammalian cells and *Xenopus* oocytes. *Mol Pharmacol* **45**, 1242.

9. Clark BA, Mobbs P (1994) Voltage-gated currents in rabbit retinal astrocytes. *Eur J Neurosci* **6**, 1406.

10. Dong Z, Zhu PH (1995) 3,4-Diaminopyridine-induced hydrolysis of phosphoinositide in cultured neurons from embryo chick forebrain. *Neuropharmacology* **34**, 297.

11. Fragoso-Veloz J, Massieu L, Alvarado R, Tapia R (1990) Seizures and wet-dog shakes induced by 4-aminopyridine, and their potentiation by nifedipine. *Eur J Pharmacol* **178**, 275.

12. Howe JR, Ritchie JM (1991) On the active form of 4-aminopyridine: Block of K⁺ currents in rabbit Schwann cells. *J Physiol* **433**, 183.

13. Kirsch GE, Shieh CC, Drewe JA *et al.* (1993) Segmental exchanges define 4-aminopyridine binding and the inner mouth of K⁺ pores. *Neuron* **11**, 503.

14. Lemeignan M, Millant H, Lamiable D (1984) Evaluation of 4-aminopyridine and 3,4-diaminopyridine on mammalian neuromuscular transmission and the effect of pH changes. *Brain Res* **304**, 166.

15. Lundh H, Nilsson O, Rosen I (1990) Current therapy of the Lambert-Eaton myasthenic syndrome. *Prog Brain Res* **84**, 163.

16. Molgo J, Lundh H, Thesleff F (1980) Potency of 3,4-diaminopyridine and 4-aminopyridine on mammalian neuromuscular transmission and the effect of pH changes. *Eur J Pharmacol* **61**, 25.

17. Polman CH, Bertelsmann FW, de Waal R *et al.* (1994) 4-Aminopyridine is superior to 3,4-diaminopyridine in the treatment of patients with multiple sclerosis. *Arch Neurol* **51**, 1136.

18. Russell SN, Publicover NG, Hart PJ *et al.* (1994) Block by 4-aminopyridine of a Kv1.2 delayed rectifier K⁺ current expressed in *Xenopus*. *J Physiol* **481**, 571.

19. Stork CM, Hoffman RS (1994) Characterization of 4-aminopyridine in overdose. *J Toxicol-Clin Toxicol* **32**, 583.

20. van der Horst A, de Goede PN, van Diemen HA *et al.* (1992) Determination of 4-amino-pyridine in serum by solid-phase extraction and high-performance. *J Chromatogr* **574**, 166.

21. Van Diemen HA, Polman CH, Koetsier JC *et al.* (1993) 4-Aminopyridine in patients with multiple sclerosis: dosage and serum level related to efficacy and safety. *Clin Neuropharmacol* **16**, 195.

22. Yamane T, Furukawa T, Hiraoka M (1995) 4-Aminopyridine block of the noninactivating cloned K⁺ channel Kv1.5 expressed in *Xenopus* oocytes. *Amer J Physiol* **269**, H556.

Amiodarone

Steven Herskovitz

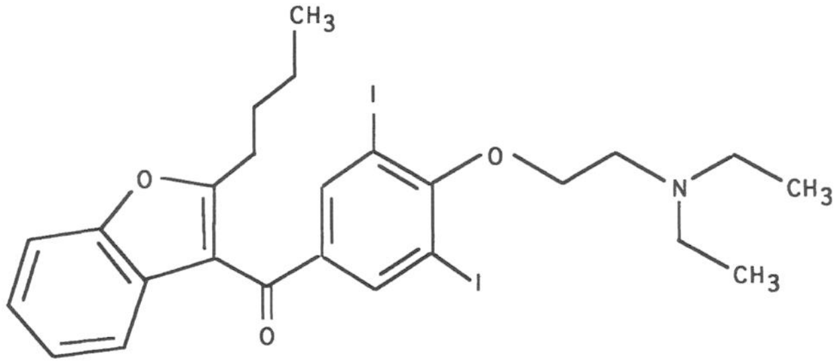

AMIODARONE
C₂₅H₂₉I₂NO₃

2-Butyl-3-[3,5-diiodo-4-(β-diethylaminoethoxy)benzoyl]benzofuran

NEUROTOXICITY RATING
Clinical
A Peripheral neuropathy
A Myopathy

A Optic neuropathy
B Cerebellar syndrome (tremor)
B Extrapyramidal syndrome (parkinsonism)
B Benign intracranial hypertension
Experimental
A Myopathy
A Peripheral neuropathy (local administration)

Amiodarone, a diiodinated benzofuran derivative, was initially developed as an antianginal agent and later as a highly efficacious cardiac antiarrhythmic agent in the management of supraventricular and ventricular arrhythmias. Because of frequent and serious side effects, it is approved in the United States only for the treatment of refractory, life-threatening ventricular arrhythmias. Like the other class III antiarrhythmic drugs, bretylium and sotalol, it shares the capacity to prolong the duration of action potentials and refractoriness of Purkinje and ventricular muscle (4). The principal neurotoxic effects of amiodarone are a sensorimotor polyneuropathy, tremor, and ataxia. Isolated case reports describe myopathy, optic neuropathy, basal ganglia dysfunction, encephalopathy, and pseudotumor cerebri.

Oral amiodarone is poorly and slowly absorbed; bioavailability ranges from 22% to 86% (3,4,17). As it is highly lipophilic, distribution is extensive into tissues, but it does not cross the blood-brain or blood-nerve barriers. Peak plasma concentrations occur about 5–6 h after an oral dose. Metabolism occurs slowly in the liver; <1% is excreted unchanged in the urine. The plasma half-life is estimated to be about 25–60 days, but may be as long as 100 days. The only metabolite is desethylamiodarone, which accumulates during long-term treatment with a plasma concentration that may exceed that of the parent compound; its pharmacological activity is not well known. Long-term therapeutic effectiveness for arrhythmias is associated with an amiodarone plasma concentration of 1.0–2.5 μg/ml. Treatment is generally initiated with an oral loading dose of 800–1600 mg/day for 1–3 weeks, followed by daily doses of 600–800 mg for 4 weeks before maintenance daily doses of 200–600 mg. Amiodarone increases the plasma concentration of phenytoin. Side effects with amiodarone are poorly correlated with serum levels. Some reports vary, but clearly suggest a relationship between toxicity and the dose and duration of treatment (17,30). Because of the drug's long elimination half-life, recovery can be very slow following its discontinuation.

Almost all patients on chronic amiodarone therapy will eventually develop side effects; many are mild and do not require drug discontinuation, others are life threatening. Virtually every organ system may be involved (3,30). These include respiratory (interstitial pneumonitis or alveolitis), cardiac (prolonged QT interval causing dysrhythmias, conduction disturbances), endocrine (hyperthyroidism or hypothyroidism in up to 6%, altered serum lipids), gastrointestinal (hepatotoxicity), and skin (photosensitivity, bluish pigmentation). Up to 100% of patients develop a reversible, usually asymptomatic keratopathy, with whorl-like corneal microdeposits similar to those caused by other amphiphilic drugs such as perhexilene maleate.

Several animal studies document nervous system dysfunction. Rats and mice fed large doses of amiodarone for up to 90 days develop dose-related loss of weight, decreased motor activity, weakness, and tremor (11). Cytoplasmic lysosomal lipid inclusions are found in autonomic and dorsal root ganglia, myenteric plexus and centrally in the area postrema, choroid plexus, ocular tissues, and pituitary. Increased blood-nerve permeability induced by sciatic nerve crush results in short-lived appearance of inclusions but

does not affect the rate of axonal regeneration. In another study, rats treated with amiodarone intraperitoneally at 20 mg/kg/day for up to 6 weeks developed motor incoordination and increased pain thresholds (26). Amiodarone injected endoneurially into rat tibial nerve at low concentrations (25 μg/ml) produces electrophysiological evidence of demyelination with conduction block and pathological evidence of segmental demyelination (29). Higher concentrations result in increasingly severe axonal degeneration. It is suggested that the different pathological changes noted in the human neuropathy may be related to variable blood-nerve barrier efficacy leading to different drug concentrations in the nerve.

Chronic administration of amiodarone in mice produces a myopathy with autophagic vacuolation and phospholipid inclusions; denervation induces necrosis of mainly type 2 fibers and a significant increase in amiodarone and desethylamiodarone concentrations in the muscle (10). Cytoplasmic lipid inclusions, similar to those in humans, can be reproduced experimentally in retinal cells of rats with local application or oral administration of amiodarone (5). Desethylamiodarone alone, as well as its parent compound, can induce lipidosis in rat alveolar macrophages, suggesting that it too is active (28).

Suicidal oral self-administration of 8 g of amiodarone induced profuse sweating, prolonged QT interval, and sinus bradycardia, but no untoward effects over 3 months of follow-up (3).

Neurological dysfunction appeared in 5%–74% of patients in a large series (30). Tremor, with or usually without neuropathy, is the most frequent neurotoxic effect reported, occuring in 43% and 39% of patients in two large series (8,24), and appearing early in the course of therapy. It is a 6–10 Hz action tremor, bilateral and asymmetrical, and clinically indistinguishable from essential tremor (8). Unsteady gait is also common, occuring in 7% and 37% of cases in these same series (8,24). It is not always explainable on the basis of neuropathy, and occasionally is associated with limb ataxia and other findings clearly suggesting cerebellar dysfunction (1,8). There have been no neuropathological correlates of tremor and ataxia.

Peripheral neuropathy is next most common; it correlates poorly with daily dose, total dose, or treatment duration. Most have received moderate to large doses for months to years, but symptoms occur with as little as 200 mg/day and with durations of 1 month; this suggests interindividual variability of amiodarone metabolism (25). Symmetrical sensorimotor polyneuropathy has a distal predominance; some reports note proximal weakness, and occasionally the neuropathy is predominantly motor (1,2,8,13,14,18,21,22,25). There is a glove-and-stocking loss of some or all sensory modalities, depressed reflexes, and an ataxic gait. There is one report of autonomic neuropathy (19). Whether mild or severe, neuropathy usually improves if the drug is discontinued or the dosage is lowered (21).

The cerebrospinal fluid shows normal or mildly elevated protein, without pleocytosis (25). Nerve conduction and needle electromyographic (EMG) studies describe both a predominant axonopathy with reduced amplitudes and distal denervation and demyelination. Changes include conduction slowing (2,14,15,21,22,25). Sural nerve biopsy specimens similarly show either predominant axonal degeneration affecting fibers of all sizes (22), predominant or almost pure demyelination (15), or a mixture. Numerous lysosomal inclusions are present in Schwann cells, axoplasm, fibroblasts, capillary endothelial and perithelial cells, and perineural cells (1,15,18,22,25). Concentrations of amiodarone and desethylamiodarone in a sural nerve biopsy were 80 times higher than in serum in one instance (14).

A few patients have developed myopathy, with or without neuropathy. The EMG contained myopathic potentials and muscle biopsy showed vacuolar changes, lipid inclusions, and marked accumulation of amiodarone and desethylamiodarone (7,9,13,22).

Scattered reports document convincing, usually reversible, parkinsonian features, including resting tremor, bradykinesia, or rigidity (31). Other infrequently reported manifestations of basal ganglia dysfunction include myoclonus, hemiballismus and dyskinesias (24, 31). A report of reversible acute encephalopathy with electroencephalographic slowing is unconvincing (24).

Optic neuropathy is a well-recognized rare complication (12,23,20). Histopathological examination of retrobulbar optic nerve revealed intracytoplasmic lamellar inclusions in large axons in one patient (20). Amiodarone has been implicated in isolated, reversible cases of pseudotumor cerebri (6).

The mechanism of amiodarone tissue toxicity is uncertain. Like other amphiphilic drugs such as perhexilene maleate, amiodarone forms intralysosomal lipid complexes leading to the observed inclusions in multiple tissues. An immunological mechanism may explain observations, such as early-onset toxicity, possible steroid responsiveness in pulmonary toxicity, and immune perturbations (30). Studies of rat brain synaptosomes have suggested that neurotoxicity might be mediated by effects on ATPase activity or Ca^{2+} homeostasis (16,27).

REFERENCES

1. Abarbanel JM, Osiman A, Frisher S, Herishanu Y (1987) Peripheral neuropathy and cerebellar syndrome associated with amiodarone therapy. *Isr J Med Sci* **23**, 893.

2. Anderson NE, Lynch NM, O'Brien KP (1985) Disabling neurological complications of amiodarone. *Aust N Z J Med* **15**, 300.

3. Aronson JK (1992) Positive inotropic drugs and drugs used in dysrhythmias. In: *Meyler's Side Effects of Drugs. 12th Ed.* Dukes MNG ed. Elsevier, Amsterdam p. 385.

4. Bigger JT, Hoffman BJ (1990) Anti-arrhythmic drugs. In: *The Pharmacological Basis of Therapeutics. 8th Ed.* Gilman AG, Rall TR, Nies AS, Taylor P eds. Pergamon, New York p. 866.

5. Bockhardt H, Drenckhahn D, Lüllmann-Rauch R (1978) Amiodarone-induced lipidosis-like alterations in ocular tissues of rats. *Albrecht Von Graefes Arch Klin Exp Ophthalmol* **207**, 91.

6. Borruat FX, Regli F (1993) Pseudotumor cerebri as a complication of amiodarone therapy. *Amer J Ophthalmol* **116**, 776.

7. Carella F, Riva E, Morandi L *et al.* (1987) Myopathy during amiodarone treatment: A case report. *Ital J Neurol Sci* **8**, 605.

8. Charness ME, Morady F, Scheinman MM (1984) Frequent neurologic toxicity associated with amiodarone therapy. *Neurology* **34**, 669.

9. Clouston PD, Donnely PE (1989) Acute necrotising myopathy associated with amiodarone therapy. *Aust N Z J Med* **19**, 483.

10. Costa-Jussa FR, Guevara A, Brook GA *et al.* (1988) Changes in denervated skeletal muscle of amiodarone-fed mice. *Muscle Nerve*, **11**, 627.

11. Costa-Jussa FR, Jacobs JM (1985) The pathology of amiodarone neurotoxicity. I. Experimental studies with reference to changes in other tissues. *Brain* **108**, 735.

12. Feiner LA, Younge BR, Kazmier FJ *et al.* (1987) Optic neuropathy and amiodarone therapy. *Mayo Clin Proc* **62**, 702.

13. Fernando Roth R, Itabashi H, Louie J *et al.* (1990) Amiodarone toxicity: Myopathy and neuropathy. *Amer Heart J* **119**, 1223.

14. Fraser AG, McQueen INF, Watt AH, Stephens MR (1985) Peripheral neuropathy during longterm high-dose amiodarone therapy. *J Neurol Neurosurg Psychiat* **48**, 576.

15. Jacobs JM, Costa-Jussa FR (1985) The pathology of amiodarone neurotoxicity. II. Peripheral neuropathy in man. *Brain* **108**, 753.

16. Kodavanti PRS, Pentlyala SN, Yallapragada, Desaiah D (1992) Amiodarone and desethylamiodarone increase intrasynaptosomal free calcium through receptor mediated channel. *Naunyn-Schmied Arch Pharmacol* **345**, 213.

17. Latini R, Tognoni G, Kates RE (1984) Clinical pharmacokinetics of amiodarone. *Clin Pharmacokinet* **9**, 136.

18. Lemaire JF, Autret A, Biziere K *et al.* (1982) Amiodarone neuropathy: Further arguments for human drug-induced neurolipidosis. *Eur Neurol* **21**, 65.

19. Manolis AS, Tordjman T, Mack KD, Estes NA 3rd (1987)

Atypical pulmonary and neurologic complications of amiodarone in the same patient. Report of a case and review of the literature. *Arch Intern Med* **147**, 1805.

20. Mansour AM, Puklin JE, O'Grady R (1988) Optic nerve ultrastructure following amiodarone therapy. *J Clin Neuro-Ophthalmol* **8**, 231.

21. Martinez-Arizala A, Sobol SM, McCarty GE *et al.* (1983) Amiodarone neuropathy. *Neurology* **33**, 643.

22. Meier C, Kauer B, Muller U, Ludin HP (1979) Neuro-myopathy during chronic amiodarone treatment. A case report. *J Neurol* **220**, 231.

23. Nazarian SM, Jay WM (1988) Bilateral optic neuropathy associated with amiodarone therapy. *J Clin Neuro-Ophthalmol* **8**, 25.

24. Palakurthy PR, Iyer V, Meckler RJ (1987) Unusual neurotoxicity associated with amiodarone therapy. *Arch Intern Med* **147**, 881.

25. Pellissier JF, Pouget J, Cros D *et al.* (1984) Peripheral neuropathy induced by amiodarone chlorhydrate. *J Neurol Sci* **63**, 251.

26. Rao KSP, Fernando JC, Ho IK, Mehendale HM (1986) Neurotoxicity in rats following subchronic amiodarone treatment. *Res Commun Chem Pathol Pharmacol* **52**, 217.

27. Rao KSP, Rao SB, Camus PH, Mehendale HM (1986) Effect of amiodarone on Na$^+$, K$^+$-ATPase and Mg^{2+}-ATPase activities in rat brain synaptosomes. *Cell Biochem Funct* **4**, 143.

28. Reasor MJ, Ogle CL, Walker ER, Kacew S (1988) Amiodarone-induced phospholipidosis in rat alveolar macrophages. *Amer Rev Resp Dis* **137**, 510.

29. Santoro L, Barbieri F, Nucciotti R *et al.* (1992) Amiodarone-induced experimental acute neuropathy in rats. *Muscle Nerve* **15**, 788.

30. Vrobel TR, Miller PE, Mostow ND, Rakita L (1989) A general overview of amiodarone toxicity: Its prevention, detection, and management. *Prog Cardiovasc Dis* **31**, 393.

31. Werner EG, Olanow CW (1989) Parkinsonism and amiodarone therapy. *Neurology* **25**, 630.

Amoscanate

Georg J. Krinke

AMOSCANATE
C$_{13}$H$_9$N$_3$O$_2$S

4-Isothiocyanato-4'-nitrodiphenylamine; C 9333-Go; CGP-4540

NEUROTOXICITY RATING

Experimental

A Periventricular necrosis

A Retinopathy

The antiparasitic agent amoscanate was originally designed for treatment of hookworm infection in the gastrointestinal tract; it was not intended for absorption (2). To obtain an absorbable form, the original formulation was micronized; this construct proved highly effective against *Schistosoma mansoni* and *S. japonicum* in infected experimental animals. The toxicology data presented here are only applicable to the absorbable formulation with a median particle size of not more than 2 μm (1).

Amoscanate causes a moderate, reversible hyperbilirubinemia in rats. This and other isothiocyanates produce biliary tract lesions, ameliorated by coadministration of erythromycin, indicating a role of intestinal flora in this effect. A ^{14}C-labeled distribution study suggests a small quantity of the labeled drug or a metabolite appears in the brain (1).

High oral doses produced impaired motor activity in cats, dogs, and rats. Neuropathological examination revealed cerebral and retinal lesions only in rats. Primates were refractory to amoscanate toxicity (1). Young adult rats given amoscanate at doses of either 250 or 500 mg/kg/day *per os* for 28 days developed periventricular necrotic lesions in the medial striatum. Microscopic features included extracellular edema, calcified microgranular deposits, neuronal loss, reactive astrocytes, and microglia cells. Myelinated fibers traversing the necrotic area were usually intact.

During the first few hours following drug administration, there was a transient decrease in exploratory and locomotor activity (1). Animals that developed severe periventricular necrosis displayed abnormal rigid posturing for long periods (4).

A dose–effect relationship was sought in young adult Sprague-Dawley rats of either sex by oral administration of 25, 125, or 500 mg/kg in one, three, or ten daily consecutive doses. About half the animals were examined the day after the last dose and the remaining rats at the end of a 20-day treatment-free period. At least three consecutive doses of 125 or 500 mg/kg were needed to induce a brain lesion. The early change was ependymal necrosis in the lateral ventricles adjacent to the choroid plexus; this suggested that intoxication may have occurred locally *via* the cerebrospinal fluid (3,4).

Retinopathy appeared in concert with cerebral lesions in rats treated with daily doses of 125 or 500 mg/kg amoscanate for 3 or 10 subsequent days. Retinal lesions primarily were in the photoreceptor layer; they persisted after a 3-week recovery period. Flash-evoked potentials and electroretinograms were recorded in rats exposed to ten daily oral doses of 125 mg/kg; both showed decreased amplitudes and prolonged latencies. The electroretinogram also disclosed an increased threshold. All of these changes were associated with damage to the outer photoreceptor layer (6). Decreased amplitude of the electroretinogram (especially b-wave) and degeneration of retina have been observed in a similar study of rats treated with 40 or 125 mg/kg *per os* for 3 or 10 days, while no retinopathy occurred in rats exposed to 10 mg/kg (5).

To evaluate the tolerance and safety in humans of the 5% aqueous suspension of 2 μm particles, two prospective, randomized, double-blind, placebo-controlled studies were carried out in healthy male volunteers. In the first study, three of four men who received 3.5 mg/kg developed mild, reversible hepatotoxicity. In the second study, individuals receiving 1 mg/kg amoscanate, 1 of 12 drug recipients developed transient liver chemistry changes. There was no clinical evidence in either study of neurological, cardiovascular, or ocular toxicity (7).

The location of the lesion in rat brain indicates a probable accumulation of the drug or its metabolite in the periventricular area. This might indicate a role for drug secretion by the choroid plexus (1), or might reflect some other factor leading to accumulation in the cerebrospinal fluid specific for the rat brain (3).

REFERENCES
1. Clark AW, Kiel SM, Parhad IN (1982) Neuropathology of the antischistosomal agent amoscanate administered in high oral doses to rats. *Neurotoxicology* **3**, 1.
2. Doshi JC, Vaidya AS, Himansu GS *et al.* (1977) Clinical trials of a new anthelmintic, 4-isothiocyanato-4'-nitrodiphenylamine (C9333-Go/CGP4540), for the cure of hookworm infection. *Amer J Trop Med Hyg* **26**, 636.
3. Krinke G, Gaepel P, Krueger L, Thomann P (1983) Early effects of high-dose absorbable amoscanate on rat brain. *Toxicol Lett* **19**, 261.
4. Krinke GJ (1988) Neurotoxic effects of amoscanate, rat. In: *ILSI Monographs on Pathology of Laboratory Animals, Nervous System.* Jones TC, Nohr U, Hunt RD eds. Springer-Verlag, Berlin p. 84.
5. Maertins T, Kroetlinger F, Sander E *et al.* (1993) Electroretinographic assessment of early retinopathy in rats. *Arch Toxicol* **67**, 120.
6. Schaeppi U, Krinke G, Fitzgerald RE, Ziel R (1987) Retinotoxicity of amoscanate in the albino rat. *Concepts Toxicol* **4**, 179.
7. Shapiro TA, Were JB, Talalay P *et al.* (1986) Clinical evaluation of amoscanate in healthy male volunteers. *Amer J Trop Med Hyg* **35**, 945.

Amphetamines and Related Compounds

Alfred Heller
Lisa Won
Philip C. Hoffmann

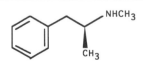

METHAMPHETAMINE
$C_{10}H_{15}N$

Methamphetamine
(S)-*N,α*-Dimethylbenzeneethanamine

NEUROTOXICITY RATING

Clinical

A   Acute encephalopathy

A   Physical dependence and withdrawal

A   Psychobiological reaction (anxiety)

B   Teratogenicity

C   Psychobiological reaction (chronic psychosis)

Experimental

A   Dopaminergic axonopathy

In the past, amphetamines have been used to treat depression, fatigue, hyperkinetic behavior disturbances of children, postencephalitic parkinsonism, enuresis, nausea of pregnancy, and obesity. At present, methamphetamine is available for the treatment of attention-deficit hyperactivity disorder (52,182). Many amphetamine derivatives have neurotoxic potential. This chapter is restricted to those amphetamine derivatives used as therapeutic agents or drugs of abuse that represent major neurotoxic hazards to the human population.

Methamphetamine hydrochloride is a water-soluble, white, odorless, crystalline powder. The hydrochloride salt of the dextrorotatory isomer of methamphetamine (Desoxyn) is available in both tablet and parenteral form. In the United States, methamphetamine is a Schedule II drug under the Controlled Substances Act. Schedule II drugs have a high potential for abuse with severe likelihood of causing psychic or physical dependence (52).

General Toxicology

Methamphetamine is rapidly absorbed following oral, subcutaneous, or intravenous administration. It readily passes the blood-brain barrier (103). The drug has been abused by both oral and parenteral routes. A common form of administration is inhalation of methamphetamine following volatilization. In human volunteers, the pulmonary route results in a very rapid rise in plasma levels of the drug compared to the oral route. The plasma concentrations then plateau over the first 3–4 h before beginning an exponential decline. Using a noncompartmental approach, an elimination half-life of about 12 h is obtained (range, 8–17 h). The observed plateau and long half-life of methamphetamine contribute to accumulation of the drug with repeated self-administration, even with long dosing intervals (32).

Plasma levels of methamphetamine peak at 35–38 ng/ml 3 h after an oral dose of approximately 18 mg (0.25 mg/kg). Similar plasma concentrations are obtained 1 h after inhalation of 21 mg of methamphetamine. The subjective effects are two to three times greater in subjects smoking the drug than in individuals taking it orally, despite the similarity in peak plasma concentrations. The difference in subjective effects may be explained by the more rapid rate of rise in plasma methamphetamine concentration with smoking than with oral ingestion (32).

Following oral administration of methamphetamine to humans, the main compound excreted in urine is the unchanged drug. Other major metabolites excreted are 4-hydroxymethamphetamine and amphetamine, which are formed by ring hydroxylation and N-demethylation, respectively (20). Studies in rats have demonstrated that pretreatment with methamphetamine itself can inhibit both ring hydroxylation and demethylation of methamphetamine (198). As is typical for weak bases such as methamphetamine, its urinary excretion is enhanced by acidification of urine (13).

Acute intoxication from amphetamine-like drugs in the naïve drug user causes dizziness, tremor, irritability, confusion, hallucinations, chest pain, palpitations, hypertension, sweating, and cardiac arrhythmias. Increased body temperature, convulsions, and shock may occur and may result in death. Acute methamphetamine intoxication can be treated with diazepam to control seizures and with chlorpromazine to antagonize drug-mediated elevations in blood pressure (52).

A risk of hemorrhagic or ischemic stroke within 3 days after drug use has also been reported in abusers who inhaled methamphetamine (199). Hemorrhagic stroke has also occurred with oral or intravenous administration of methamphetamine (36).

Various pathological findings in the cardiopulmonary system and CNS after deaths attributed to methamphetamine have been reported (35,111,159). These include hemorrhagic pulmonary edema, contraction-band necrosis of the myocardium, ruptured berry aneurysm, aortic dissection, intracranial hemorrhage, vasculitis, massive subarachnoid hemorrhage, and hematoma of the corpus callosum. Cerebral edema and intracerebral hemorrhage, probably secondary to a sudden rise in blood pressure from methamphetamine administration, have also been reported; so has necrosis of blood vessels.

Animal Studies

Studies of methamphetamine's effects on both central dopaminergic and serotonergic neurons in rodents and nonhuman primates have established its severe neurotoxic potential. An extensive literature describes the neurotoxic effects of methamphetamine at the biochemical and morphological levels using both *in vivo* and *in vitro* techniques (26). Male rats are somewhat more susceptible than females to methamphetamine neurotoxicity (188).

The ability of methamphetamine to cause persistent decreases in dopamine levels and in the activity of tyrosine hydroxylase in the CNS has been known since the 1970s (79,154). In general, the major effects of methamphetamine in the CNS are on dopaminergic axonal projections. Serotonergic axons are also affected by high doses of methamphetamine; the ring-substituted methamphetamine derivatives (see later under MDMA and MDA and elsewhere in this volume) tend to be selective for serotonergic neurons. Early studies on the dopaminergic system demonstrated that prolonged exposure to methamphetamine reduces both neostriatal dopamine and its metabolites dihydroxyphenylacetic acid (DOPAC) and homovanillic acid (HVA), the deaminated o-methyoxylated derivative of dopamine, and the enyzme responsible for the rate-limiting step in cate-cholamine biosynthesis, tyrosine hydroxylase (79,146).

Extensive studies have described the long-lasting effects of methamphetamine on monoaminergic systems. Repeated administration of methamphetamine produces long-term effects on dopaminergic neurons as evidenced by significant reductions in striatal dopamine content in rats and guinea pigs 2 weeks after the last drug injection (187). In the rhesus monkey, decreases in caudate levels of dopamine resulting from methamphetamine can persist for up to 3 years (195). In concert with lasting reductions in neurotransmitter content are reports of decreased striatal tyrosine hydroxylase activity 30 days following methamphetamine treatment (65). Reductions in the number of striatal dopamine-uptake sites (185) and D_1 receptors in the substantia nigra (96) of rats have also been observed 3 weeks after methamphetamine administration. In addition to producing enduring effects on the dopaminergic system, methamphetamine is neurotoxic to serotonergic neurons as evidenced by decreases in rat striatal tryptophan hydroxylase activity as well as striatal serotonin and 5-hydroxyindoleacetic acid (5-HIAA) levels; these changes persist for at least 110 days following drug treatment (10). While there are clearly long-lasting effects of methamphetamine on dopaminergic and serotonergic neurons, noradrenergic, cholinergic, and γ-aminobutyric acid (GABA)-ergic systems do not appear to be altered by methamphetamine (67,185).

Morphological studies, both *in vivo* and *in vitro* (*vide infra*), suggest the drug's dopaminergic actions are restricted to nerve terminals and axons, with sparing of the parent neurons (132). Fluorescent histochemistry has shown that methamphetamine-induced decreases in dopamine are associated with damage to the dopaminergic terminals in the rat as demonstrated by the presence of swollen nerve fibers in the striatum (90). Evidence for axonal degeneration has been provided by a number of techniques including classical silver staining methods that selectively impregnate degenerating axons (132). By means of tyrosine hydroxylase immunocytochemistry of the striatum, it is possible to show the neurodegenerative effects are confined to the dopaminergic nerve endings. Degeneration and disappearance of tyrosine hydroxylase–containing synaptic endings is observed in striatum with preservation of longer, varicose branching fibers, which are probably preterminal axons (62). Observations at the electron microscopic level demonstrate that tyrosine hydroxylase–positive synaptic boutons in the rat are diminished by chronic treatment with methamphetamine. These reductions in dopaminergic boutons are selective for those lacking mitochondria (70). In contrast to the effects of methylenedioxy analogs of amphetamine (MDA, MDMA) on serotonergic axons, it is as

yet unclear whether methamphetamine produces selective effects on morphological subtypes of dopaminergic neurons. Calbindin D-28k (calcium binding protein)–containing axons, which are known to be resistant to the effects of the neurotoxin, 1-methyl-4-phenyl-1,2,3,6-tetrahydropyridine (see later under MPTP) (69), are also spared in idiopathic Parkinson's disease (196). In contrast, in the case of methamphetamine, it would appear that calbindin D-28k–containing neurons (*i.e.*, those arising from dopaminergic cell bodies in pars compacta) are not spared by this agent (for review, *see* 9).

Rats chronically treated with methamphetamine show a decrement in both ^{3}H-mazindol-labeled dopamine-uptake sites and tissue dopamine content in the striatum. These decreases are regionally heterogeneous, with the ventral striatum exhibiting the largest decrease in both ^{3}H-mazindol binding and dopamine content, while the neighboring nucleus accumbens and the dorsal caudate putamen remain relatively unaffected (42). In addition, methamphetamine does not produce a uniform loss of dopamine histofluorescence in the striatum itself, at least at short survival times. While there is a marked reduction in striatal dopamine fluorescence 90 min after a 10 mg/kg dose in the rat, patches of fluorescence remain that are associated with blood vessels. It would appear, therefore, that there are differential effects both with respect to regional levels of dopamine and dopamine nerve-terminal susceptibility to this neurotoxin (49). Heterogeneity in striatal dopamine loss over longer survival times of 7–14 days following methamphetamine has also been observed in Swiss-Webster mice; there is a positive correlation between the amount of dopamine in various subdivisions of caudate putamen and the extent of methamphetamine-induced dopamine depletion. This is in contrast to the effects of MPTP, where depletion of dopamine is correlated with the number of dopamine-uptake sites (94).

High doses of methamphetamine can also produce degeneration in nondopaminergic neurons. Following one 100 mg/kg dose of methamphetamine, there is a loss of a subpopulation of somatosensory cortical neurons (30). While this area of brain receives a monoaminergic innervation, it does not contain catecholaminergic or serotonergic cell bodies. However, silver impregnation methods reveal degenerating cell bodies. The affected pyramidal cells have darkly stained, shrunken perikarya and fragmented, argyrophylic dendrites located in lamina II and III of the somatosensory cortex. Ultrastructural studies show degeneration of axon terminals and neurons 3 days after the last drug treatment (2 × 35 mg/kg). Two types of pyramidal cells in the frontal cortex are affected. One is nonargyrophylic and shows an abnormal electron-dense cytoplasm and nucleoplasm, but survives methamphetamine treatment. The other is argyrophylic and appears to be actually degenerating as evidenced by fragmented cytoplasm and disintegrating organelles. The drug-induced morphological changes observed in both types of affected neurons are blocked when haloperidol is given in conjunction with methamphetamine (189).

Methamphetamine neurotoxicity is enhanced by cocaine pretreatment in terms of the dose required and extent of dopamine loss; this may be of social importance given the use of multiple drugs by abusers (78).

Many experimental studies have examined the consequences of methamphetamine neurotoxicity on animal behavior. Minor behavioral effects secondary to dopaminergic damage are known to occur both in human parkinsonism and in animal models in which extensive destruction of this system is produced by either 6-hydroxydopamine, a specific dopaminergic neurotoxin, or by MPTP, a meperidine derivative and established cause of human parkinsonism (84). In the case of methamphetamine, it has been difficult to obtain clear evidence for behavioral consequences of neurotoxic damage. An extensive study involving partial monoamine depletion with methamphetamine failed to show changes in locomotor activity, food and water intake, or scheduled control behaviors following doses that halved dopamine levels (158). In the rhesus monkey, doses of methamphetamine that produce a 32% depletion of dopamine were not observed to produce effects on performance of fine motor control tasks (3).

Rodent studies have revealed correlations between methamphetamine administration, resultant dopaminergic loss, and functional deficits. In rats trained to depress and release a lever for water reinforcement, control animals show a gradual increase in reaction-time speed over a test period of some 9 weeks. Methamphetamine-treated animals, however, although capable of performing the task assigned, are incapable of increasing their reaction-time speed over a similar extended period (136). These findings suggest that damage secondary to this drug results in loss and efficiency of motor control. A study of the effect of methamphetamine on other motor skills was conducted in rats that received four injections of the drug (12 mg/kg every 2 h) resulting in 45% and 36% reductions in striatal dopamine and serotonin, respectively (190). Prior to drug treatment, rats were trained to perform the following motor tasks: (a) active avoidance, in which the animals learned to avoid footshock preceded by a conditioned stimulus (i.e., auditory tone of 2500 Hz); (b) inhibitory avoidance, whereby rats learned to avoid crossing over to the "shock" side of the test chamber in the absence of a conditioned stimulus; (c) balance-beam performance, in which rats traversed a beam

of 2 cm width; and (d) rotarod performance, during which the animals had to maintain themselves on a rotating rod. Treatment with methamphetamine reduced active avoidance performance and the ability of the rats to balance on the beam. Other types of behaviors, such as inhibitory avoidance or rotarod performance, were unaffected.

The levels of reduction in transmitter produced by methamphetamine may not, in themselves, be sufficient to produce marked behavioral changes (135). In human parkinsonism, clinical symptoms may be minor even in the face of fairly extensive decreases in brain dopamine. In primates suffering MPTP-induced nigrostriatal damage, essentially complete depletions of striatal dopamine are required before a Parkinson-like syndrome is seen (150; for discussion of the relation between symptoms and lesion size in the nigrostriatal system, see 203). In addition, there is clear evidence that compensatory changes following damage to dopaminergic neurons occur, such as an increase in dopamine metabolism by the surviving neurons and increases in dopamine receptor numbers (1,33,204), which could overcome the dopamine deficiency produced by methamphetamine toxicity. There is certainly evidence that following methamphetamine-induced damage to dopaminergic systems, the surviving dopaminergic axons are capable of adapting to injury. One study using in vivo dialysis methods, in which it is possible to measure extracellular concentrations of dopamine and metabolites in freely moving animals, showed that extracellular concentrations of striatal dopamine were the same in methamphetamine-treated and saline-treated control animals despite substantial depletions of this transmitter in the striatal tissue (137). In fact, the methamphetamine-damaged rat was capable of increasing its extracellular dopamine level to the same extent as controls in response to a challenge dose of (+)-amphetamine. It may well be, as the authors suggest, that such adaptive responses may mitigate the development of behavioral deficits in animals subjected to neurotoxic doses of methamphetamine.

An additional variable may be the nature of the behavioral test selected in particular situations. Since dopamine depletion is associated with extrapyramidal dysfunction, behavioral tests that do not involve assessment of such deficits may not reveal functional problems. There is also species susceptibility to methamphetamine. [Rodents are, in fact, less susceptible to behavioral deficits induced by MPTP as compared to primates (23,83,84).] Despite the failure to readily observe behavioral changes in experimental animals, one should not conclude that methamphetamine neurotoxicity in humans is without functional consequences.

Methamphetamine readily crosses the sheep placenta, producing significant and persistent maternal and fetal cardiovascular effects, which may have long-term consequences, especially if the drug is administered repetitively (172). Since repetitive methamphetamine self-administration occurs regularly in pregnant drug abusers, exposure of human fetuses to methamphetamine *in utero* is a significant medical and social problem. The results of limited studies of the effect of prenatal exposure to amphetamines on postnatal brain neurochemistry in rodents have been contradictory. When methamphetamine is administered to pregnant rats in their drinking water (80 mg/l) throughout gestation, increases in serotonin, 5-HIAA, dopamine, and norepinephrine levels are observed in several forebrain regions of their offspring 9 months following drug treatment (180,181). Others have reported a reduction in dopamine levels and serotonin-receptor binding in the frontal cortex of 5 week-old offspring of dams treated daily throughout gestation with 2 mg/kg methamphetamine (142). No effect on brain levels of dopamine and norepinephrine has been observed in 3–4 month-old offspring of rats receiving 0.5 mg/kg of amphetamine daily during the 3 weeks of pregnancy (112). Administration of amphetamine (3 mg/kg twice daily, b.i.d.) to rats during a restricted period of gestation (gestational day 5 until term) has been reported to decrease brain levels of norepinephrine in 1-month-old offspring, whereas at later ages (84 days old), there is an increase in brain norepinephrine levels and a reduction in dopamine levels as compared to saline-treated controls (64). Treatment of mice with amphetamine (5 mg/kg) during the last 6–7 days of pregnancy has been shown to increase brain levels of norepinephrine in their 1-month-old offspring (107). Studies of other neurochemical parameters have indicated that low doses (2–5 mg/kg, b.i.d.) of methamphetamine throughout pregnancy result in reduction in striatal dopamine and serotonin-uptake sites in 1.5-month-old rats (191). In contrast, higher doses (10 mg/kg, b.i.d.) of this drug increase dopamine- and serotonin-uptake sites (191). There are also indications that intrauterine exposure to amphetamine (2 mg/kg) from gestational day 7 until birth may have long-term effects on other, nonmonoaminergic neurotransmitter systems (such as GABA) in the exposed offspring (15). The discrepancies observed in these studies are most probably a function of the use of a variety of dosage regimens or periods of gestational exposure.

Several studies have attempted to correlate monoaminergic indices with behavioral alterations observed in offspring exposed to amphetamines *in utero*. Offspring of rats treated daily with amphetamine (2 mg/kg from gestational day 7 until birth) demonstrate increased locomotor activity at 8 and 15 days of postnatal age; however, no alterations in brain concentrations of dopamine, serotonin or norepinephrine are observed in these animals (15). Twenty-one-day-old mice treated daily during the last 6–7 days *in utero* with 5 mg/kg amphetamine show heightened locomotor, rearing and grooming activity, but no changes in brain levels of dopamine or norepinephrine (107). Despite the lack of correlation between neurotransmitter concentrations and effects on behavior in most studies, one report described a correlation between an increase in the number of midbrain dopamine-uptake sites and open-field activity in 6-week-old offspring exposed throughout pregnancy to a high dose (10 mg/kg, b.i.d.) of methamphetamine (191). Offspring exposed to a low dose (2 mg/kg, b.i.d.) of drug showed a reduction in the number of striatal dopamine uptake sites, but this did not relate in any way to the behaviors assessed. Increases or decreases in the number of serotonin-uptake sites in several brain regions correlated with open-field activity.

There is little information on the effect of this drug on the early postnatal brain. In general, studies *in vivo* (91,142,186,191) suggest that methamphetamine is less effective in causing persistent transmitter depletion in the early postnatal brain, at least with respect to dopaminergic neurons. This difference in sensitivity may be related to the relative immaturity in the early neonatal brain of dopaminergic axonal arbors, the site of methamphetamine toxicity.

Anatomical studies with respect to methamphetamine-induced neurotoxicity in postnatal brain are also few. One light and electron microscopic study of the acute neurotoxic effects of methamphetamine in developing male gerbils (1–24 months of age) demonstrated that the drug's selectivity for specific brain regions is dependent upon developmental age. Animals were sacrificed 3 days following a single, intermediate or large dose of methamphetamine and processed for histological analysis of neurotoxicity using silver-staining techniques. Degenerating axon terminals and accumulation of axonal terminal lysosomes of prefrontal cortex and/or striatum were found. Occasionally, darkly stained neurons with shrunken cell bodies were observed in the striatum. Treatment of juvenile animals (1–2 months old) with methamphetamine (25–60 mg/kg) resulted in argyrophilic labeling of prefrontal cortex. Administered to young adults (2–6 months old), methamphetamine (16–21 mg/kg) induced changes in prefrontal cortex and/or striatum. Adult animals (8–24 months old) treated with methamphetamine (6–12 mg/kg) showed labeling exclusively in the striatum (179).

In Vitro Studies

In vitro experiments suggest that concentrations of methamphetamine in the range of 10^{-5} to 10^{-4} M damage monoaminergic neurons (14,34,80,81,194). Dopaminergic and serotonergic cells *in vivo* are, in fact, exposed to such concentrations of drug following systemic administration of behaviorally active doses of methylenedioxyamphetamine, a congener of methamphetamine (201). Such concentrations are attained in brain and are probably even higher in monoaminergic axon terminals due to selective uptake of methamphetamine.

Several *in vitro* systems have been used to examine neuronal toxicity. One approach has been the use of rotation-mediated three-dimensional reaggregate cultures in which embryonic cells from specific brain regions are dissociated and placed into flasks in rotatory culture. Brain cells adhere to each other and form aggregates—small roughly spherical cell clusters 300–400 μm in diameter. When dopaminergic neurons are coaggregated with their target cells of the corpus striatum, there is a reconstitution of a functional nigrostriatal projection. In such reaggregate cultures, the nigrostriatal system mimics the development, specific connectivity (synapse formation with DARPP-32-containing cells of the striatum), function, and pharmacology of the dopaminergic system in the intact brain for periods of up to 1 year (for review, *see* 27,60).

Using the three-dimensional reaggregate approach and computer-assisted cell-counting techniques (183), it has been possible to demonstrate substantial reductions in endogenous dopamine levels in cultures equivalent in age to a 2-week postnatal mouse following 7 days of treatment with 10^{-4} M methamphetamine, without any reduction in dopaminergic cell numbers (81). This demonstrates that neonatal dopamine neurons, like their adult counterparts (132), can survive massive injury probably because the neurotoxic effects of methamphetamine are restricted to the cell processes with sparing of the cell bodies. Cell survival following exposure to methamphetamine has been directly demonstrated in monolayer cultures of ventral midbrain, where dopamine neurons are grown in two dimensions on a plate of cortical astrocytes so that the individual neurons and their processes can be visualized by tyrosine hydroxylase immunoreactivity. Even with 6 days of exposure to concentrations of 5×10^{-4} M methamphetamine, tyrosine hydroxylase–positive cell bodies were present, but only remnants of processes could be seen (34). Although some cell loss occurs following exposure to 10^{-4} M methamphetamine for 5 days in cells from fetal mesencephalon cultured in wells, the much greater reduction (−80%) in dopamine uptake suggests that damage to axons and terminals dominates the anatomical expression of methamphetamine neurotoxicity (14).

The three-dimensional reaggregate system has proved particularly useful for monitoring the effects of methamphetamine on neonatal cells and their capacity for recovery.

Since dopaminergic neurons can be maintained for long periods of time in culture, their morphological and neurochemical status can be monitored over time by sampling aggregates from individual flasks or by analysis of monoamine metabolites in the culture media (for review, *see* 60). In 15- to 22-day-old aggregate cultures, a period equivalent to 1–2 weeks of postnatal age, exposure for 7 days to methamphetamine (10^{-4} M) produced marked reductions in dopamine (−71%) and serotonin (−67%) (194). Monoamine levels in both the control and methamphetamine-treated groups increased during the drug-free recovery period (days 22–42 of culture). Damaged monoaminergic neurons never recovered from the initial injury, and the absolute loss in injured neurons was maintained throughout the 3-week recovery period. Serotonergic neurons in this system were affected by methamphetamine as much as dopaminergic neurons and showed similar deficits in transmitter level and recovery pattern (194). The prolonged loss of dopamine and serotonin *in vitro* suggests that methamphetamine-induced injury in the developing brain is irreversible during critical periods of maturation when monoaminergic systems play an essential role in normal development. Interruption in monoaminergic function during early life may well be the cause of developmental deficits reported in children exposed to methamphetamine *in utero*.

Human Studies

Amphetamine-induced euphoria, sustained mood elevation, and psychic stimulation is frequently followed by dysphoria and depression. These drugs also increase physical energy and decrease need for sleep, effects that have led to their widespread abuse. In the 1960s, "speed" was the street name for amphetamine and methamphetamine, and abusers were known as "speed freaks" (108). Individuals who used these stimulants repeatedly became tolerant to the drug's effects and then depended on serial injections of escalating doses, over several days and weeks, to achieve the same level of euphoria and stimulation. Compulsive subjects use methamphetamine frequently (eight to ten times a day) in high doses (0.3–1.0 g/day) for a 3–10 day period (82).

Over the past 10–15 years, several waves of widespread and severe methamphetamine abuse have impacted most of the technologically advanced countries, including the United States, Japan, and Sweden (108). A variety of substances variously described as "crystal, crank, go-fast, zip, or crysty" contains methamphetamine. The drug is widely abused in the United States, and it has been documented as the most widely abused drug in Japan (50). Methamphetamine use had a major resurgence in the United States in the 1990s, particularly in a volatile form, "ice," which is inhalable when heated. Its stimulatory effects frequently cannot be distinguished by the addict from those of cocaine, a more expensive street drug. A recent overview of the current status of the problem of methamphetamine abuse is available (5).

Despite the extensive and worldwide abuse of methamphetamine, no direct evidence of monoaminergic neuronal injury in humans is available. The only controlled study conducted in humans examined the pharmacokinetics and bioavailability of methamphetamine (see earlier under General Toxicology) (32). The most convincing evidence that abusers suffer such damage is the occurrence of methamphetamine-induced psychosis, which has been extensively studied both in Japan and the West. The Japanese experience suggests that the onset of such psychotic episodes is the result of progressive brain damage following months or years of chronic methamphetamine abuse. The current epidemic of methamphetamine abuse, which began in Japan in 1970, peaked in 1984 and is now in somewhat of a decline (50). Methamphetamine psychosis is of particular interest from a neurotoxicological viewpoint, since the material supplied to abusers is approximately 99% pure methamphetamine (82). Methamphetamine users in this population, in contrast to other abusers, apparently restrict their usage to the pure drug so the psychotic episodes are presumably not the result of concurrent use of other common drugs such as cocaine (141).

The psychotic symptomatology induced by methamphetamine is complex, but it is essentially composed of a highly paranoid psychotic state with auditory and visual hallucinations. While this syndrome may be difficult to distinguish from acute or chronic schizophrenia, some reports (particularly from the United States) indicate that cases of acute methamphetamine psychosis differ from paranoid schizophrenia in terms of the state of consciousness. Similarly, in some of the early Japanese studies of this syndrome, individuals hospitalized for methamphetamine-induced psychosis were reported to be able to maintain good relationships with others despite their obvious, highly fearful paranoid symptoms (177).

Of particular pertinence to the issue of chronic neurotoxicity are reports in the Japanese literature of increased vulnerability to psychotic episodes among individuals who have been hospitalized due to an initial episode of methamphetamine-induced psychosis. Such individuals can suffer a relapse in symptoms (43%–49% of cases of hospital admission for methamphetamine-induced psychosis) identical to the first episode. Relapses have been observed following rcinitiation of methamphetamine abuse after long periods of abstinence (months to years), following alcohol ingestion, even in the absence of documented substance abuse.

The issue of increased vulnerability to psychosis following a documented methamphetamine-induced psychotic episode has been challenged by Western observers whose experience suggests first, that methamphetamine-induced psychosis is an acute event distinct from paranoid schizophrenia and related closely to drug ingestion and clearance (4) and, second, that where long-term recurrence of psychosis occurs in such abusers, it is the result of a preexisting psychotic state. Detailed critical discussions of this issue are provided (4,82,141). The possibility should not be excluded, however, that both views are correct, and the divergent experience relates either to the quality or content of drug being provided or the differing genetic backgrounds of the two populations involved. The latter issue is of particular interest, since genetic background clearly affects neurotoxic responses to amphetamine (116,128).

Up to one-third of substance abusers are of childbearing age, and many abusers continue drug use during pregnancy (118). Despite the obvious health implications of methamphetamine abuse during pregnancy, there are only minimal concrete data on the effects of methamphetamine on the human fetus. One study compared pregnancy and fetal outcomes in a group of 52 self-reporting methamphetamine abusers and nonabusing mothers (89). While there are many complexities in interpreting such studies, it is clear that the neonates exposed to methamphetamines had somewhat lower body weights (−10%), birth lengths (−3.4%), and head circumference (−2%). Similarly, reductions in occipital head circumferences have been found in a group of 46 infants exposed to either cocaine or methamphetamine (119). Follow-up studies on such infants are, at best, difficult and limited; some data suggest "*in utero*" methamphetamine exposure can result in "lethargy, poor feeding, poor alertness, and severe lassitude" (119). In addition, follow-up after a benign neonatal course revealed subsequent cases of "oculomotor apraxia, a parkinsonian dystonia, a severe tactile dystonia, pronounced intention tremor, severe active hypotonia and hemiparesis." Examination of the brains of neonates exposed to methamphetamine during gestation has been conducted using echoencephalography (ECHO) (38). One-third (31.5%) of methamphetamine-exposed neonates had abnormal ECHO findings "suggestive of acute or past CNS injury" as compared to 5.3% in the control group. In a combined cocaine/methamphetamine group, there were significantly more ECHO findings suggestive of prior hemorrhage or ischemia, white matter cavitation, and intraventricular, subependymal, or subarachnoid hemorrhage. Whether such changes impact learning skills has yet to be determined (38).

Toxic Mechanisms

Methamphetamine is thought to release dopamine from the cytoplasmic pool, and dopamine itself may be a key element in dopaminergic axonal damage. Experimental manipulations that decrease the size of the transmitter pool (*i.e.*, inhibition of dopamine synthesis by α-methyltyrosine) attenuate methamphetamine-induced dopaminergic neurotoxicity (184), while manipulations that increase the size of the transmitter pool (*i.e.*, reserpine) with the opposite effect increase methamphetamine-induced dopaminergic neurotoxicity (152). The neurotoxic effects of methamphetamine also depend on a functional dopaminergic-uptake system; administration of amfonelic acid, a dopamine-uptake inhibitor, blocks methamphetamine-induced decreases in striatal tyrosine hydroxylase activity (143) and prevents depletions of striatal dopamine in rats (93). In addition, dopamine receptor antagonists block striatal depletions of tyrosine hydroxylase activity, dopamine, DOPAC, and HVA concentrations produced by methamphetamine (66,95,163).

Proposed mechanisms of methamphetamine neurotoxicity to monoaminergic neurons include the conversion of neurotransmitters released by methamphetamine to known neurotoxic compounds; the formation of superoxides; the induction of hyperthermia, and the possibility of neurotoxicity secondary to stimulation of glutamate receptors or inhibition of GABAergic systems.

The neurotoxic effects of methamphetamine on monoaminergic terminals are most likely related to its capacity to release monoamines. Dopamine released from the cytoplasmic pool can certainly on theoretical grounds undergo enzymatic (monoamine oxidase) or nonenzymatic oxidation. This can result in the formation of superoxides, hydrogen peroxide, and hydroxyl free radicals. The formation of hydroxyl free radicals ("oxidative stress") is probably the main cause of cellular damage secondary to oxidation. In addition, it has been shown that in the presence of hydroxyl radicals, dopamine can be converted to 6-hydroxydopamine (29,54,161), a well-known dopaminergic neurotoxin (156).

Two interrelated concepts of methamphetamine-induced damage to dopaminergic axons are centered on oxidative mechanisms. The more intriguing is the idea that methamphetamine-induced release of dopamine leads to the formation of 6-hydroxydopamine *in vivo*, and that this agent is the primary neurotoxic moiety. A similar mechanism would obtain in the case of serotonergic axons with the formation of a specific serotonergic neurotoxin, 5,7-dihydroxytryptamine. Formation of neurotoxins following methamphetamine exposure is an appealing hypothesis, since it would explain many of the neurotoxic effects of the drug. 6-Hydroxydopamine has been detected in rat brain following methamphetamine administration (157).

The involvement of oxidative stress (formation of hydroxyl radicals) in the mediation of methamphetamine neurotoxicity is supported by findings that antioxidants attenuate the effect of methamphetamine (37). Oxidative stress has been demonstrated to occur at the cellular level following methamphetamine treatment of neuronal monolayer cultures from the ventral tegmental area, a brain region containing dopaminergic neurons (34). When these neurons are exposed to 10^{-5} M methamphetamine in the presence of 2,7-dichlorofluorescin—a compound that becomes fluorescent in the presence of hydroxyperoxides or hydroxyl radicals—such neurons show swelling, particularly in varicosities, many of which become fluorescent indicating localized oxidative stress. The most convincing evidence that oxidative stress is involved in methamphetamine neurotoxicity comes from studies of transgenic mice that overexpress copper/zinc, superoxide dismutase (CuZn SOD), an enzyme that removes oxygen-based radicals (125). High doses (25 mg/kg) of methamphetamine, which produce marked reductions in striatal dopamine in control mice, are without significant effect on transmitter levels in the transgenic CuZn SOD mouse, suggesting that the transgenic mice have a greater capacity for scavenging oxygen radicals.

In addition to the production of oxidative stress, methamphetamine is clearly capable of producing hyperthermia when administered at ambient temperatures. This compound is capable of raising rectal temperatures 1°–2°C by 30 min after injection of 5–10 mg/kg of methamphetamine in the mouse (73). Similar hyperthermic effects can be elicited in the rat. The effect of methamphetamine on body temperature and monoamine depletion can be attenuated by administering the drug while maintaining animals in an environmental temperature of 4°C (17). The effect of hyperthermia clearly involves an interaction with other neurotoxic factors: while a decline in striatal dopamine correlates well with maximal body temperatures produced by methamphetamine, hyperthermia alone, produced by elevations in environmental temperature, does not produce a reduction in striatal dopamine. Reduction of methamphetamine-induced hyperthermia by co-administration of a noncompetitive *N*-methyl-D-aspartate (NMDA) receptor antagonist dizocilpine (MK-801), which results in hypothermia, also protects against methamphetamine-induced striatal dopamine depletions and depletions of hippocampal serotonin (44). Additional evidence of the importance of body temperature on methamphetamine neurotoxicity are the findings that the protective effects of agents such as MK-801 and haloperidol are blocked by environmental elevations in body temperature (16).

The excitatory amino acids may also contribute to methamphetamine's toxicity to dopaminergic neurons either through effects on dopamine release or *via* oxidative stress. Striatal infusion of NMDA prior to methamphetamine treatment enhances striatal dopamine depletion (165). Noncompetitive and competitive antagonists of NMDA prevent methamphetamine-induced depletions in striatal dopamine content and tyrosine hydroxylase activity in mice (164,165). It has been postulated that noncompetitive NMDA receptor antagonists, such as MK-801, are capable of attenuating striatal dopamine depletions (and therefore, dopamine neurotoxicity) produced by methamphetamine due to the ability of these agents to reduce methamphetamine-stimulated dopamine overflow, possibly by blocking NMDA receptors on dopamine axon terminals (95). Not all NMDA receptor antagonists are capable of protecting against neurotoxicity produced by methamphetamine (85,178); this suggests that the mechanism(s) by which methamphetamine exerts its toxic actions on dopaminergic neurons is probably not the same as that mediating gluta-

mate excitotoxicity. In addition, the type of cellular damage inflicted by each of these agents differs in that methamphetamine causes injury to axon terminals whereas glutamate is toxic to cell bodies.

The neurotoxic action of methamphetamine on striatal dopaminergic axon terminals can also be antagonized by various agents that potentiate GABA, an inhibitory transmitter that modulates dopaminergic neuronal activity. Chlormethiazole, an agonist at the $GABA_A$ receptor, has been demonstrated to block methamphetamine-induced loss of tyrosine hydroxylase activity and to attenuate the loss of dopamine in rats (55). Concurrent administration of GABA transaminase inhibitors such as aminooxyacetic acid, α-acetylene GABA, and ethanolamine-O-sulfate, which block the metabolism of GABA, also prevent methamphetamine-induced decreases in striatal tyrosine hydroxylase activity (66,155).

3,4-METHYLENEDIOXYAMPHETAMINE
$C_{10}H_{13}NO_2$

3,4-METHYLENEDIOXYMETHAMPHETAMINE
$C_{11}H_{15}NO_2$

3,4-Methylenedioxyamphetamine, MDA
3,4-Methylenedioxymethamphetamine, MDMA

NEUROTOXICITY RATING

Clinical

A   Acute encephalopathy

A   Autonomic syndrome (hyperthermia)

A   Seizure disorder

B   Chronic encephalopathy

C   Psychobiological reaction (chronic psychosis)

Experimental

A   Seizure disorder

A   Autonomic dysfunction (hyperthermia)

A   Serotonergic axonopathy

Methylenedioxymethamphetamine (MDMA) (Ecstasy) and methylenedioxyamphetamine (MDA) are methylenedioxy ring-substituted amphetamines that have been of considerable interest both as purported aids to psychotherapy and as widely used drugs of abuse. While possessing the central stimulant properties of amphetamine, these agents, additionally, have unique psychological effects. The actions of MDMA and MDA are very similar. The primary focus of this section is on MDMA, which is a major drug of abuse. For both MDMA and MDA, the S-(+) enantiomer has greater CNS activity than the R-(−) enantiomer. Ingestion

of MDMA results in a complex altered state of consciousness with increased ability to relate to others and to communicate more easily. MDMA's subjective effects include a decrease in defensiveness and aggression, an alteration in perception of time, as well as feelings of warmth and openness with sensual overtones, despite decreased sexual activity. All of these psychological effects produce a state of consciousness that facilitates interpersonal interactions (101). These psychological properties led to the introduction in the 1970s of MDMA as an aid to communication in the psychotherapeutic setting. Although MDMA was subsequently classified as a Schedule I substance by the U.S. Drug Enforcement Agency due to its central neurotoxic potential, MDMA has continued to be a popular drug of abuse, particularly among younger individuals. Given the combination of psychomotor stimulation and an increase in the ability to relate to others, MDMA has become part of a phenomenon, initially begun in the United Kingdom, of all-night dance parties involving electronically generated music and lights and referred to as "raves" (99,101,144,162).

General Toxicology

No pharmacokinetic information is available in the human for the methylenedioxy ring-substituted amphetamines, MDMA and MDA. In the rat, pharmacokinetic studies reveal that there are stereochemical differences in the loss of MDMA from the plasma, with the $(+)$ and $(-)$ isomer having half-lives of 74 min and 100 min, respectively (24).

N-Demethylation of MDMA, with conversion to MDA, occurs in the rodent (21,24,47) with levels of MDA formed being three times greater for the $(+)$ isomer as compared to the $(-)$ isomer. Cleavage of the methylenedioxy bridge also occurs to form catechols both *in vitro* and *in vivo*, and these metabolic products have been observed in human urine (87,88) (for a detailed discussion of the metabolism of the methylenedioxy derivatives, *see* 25). Such cleavage of the methylenedioxy bridge (demethylenation) is of interest with respect to the neurotoxic potential of this compound, which can lead to the formation of the catechol, dihydroxymethamphetamine and, in the presence of superoxide, can produce the potentially neurotoxic o-quinone (63). In a similar fashion, MDMA can first undergo aromatic hydroxylation at the 2-position on the ring and subsequent demethylenation to form trihydroxymethamphetamine, an analog of 6-hydroxydopamine, a compound with known neurotoxic action at least on dopaminergic neurons.

Information on the general toxicity of MDMA is limited. Convulsions can be induced in the dog and monkey by high doses of either MDMA or MDA (58). In the rat, no gross or autopsy findings were observed following 28 days of oral MDMA at doses that produced hyperactivity and excitability (48). In the dog, a similar dosage schedule resulted in reduction in testicular size and prostatic enlargement in a few animals.

While the oral LD_{50} of MDMA in the mouse appears to be approximately 80–150 mg/kg (58), ingestion of MDMA in humans at much lower doses has been associated with a significant number of deaths. While some caution is justified in attributing all of the effects in humans to MDMA, given the illicit source of the drug and the possibility of contamination, nevertheless it seems prudent to consider MDMA unsafe, particularly under certain circumstances. MDMA has gained increasing popularity as a recreational drug in social settings in both the United Kingdom and the United States. A 1987 survey of undergraduate students at Stanford University, California, indicated that 39% of those questioned had used the drug at least once (121), and the drug has enjoyed considerable popularity as an adjunct to "rave" dance parties. While the amounts of MDMA ingested by humans (1–4 mg/kg) is clearly below the LD_{50} in the mouse (80–150 mg/kg), ingestion in the human has been associated with adverse reactions as well as a number of deaths in the United Kingdom (for a review of the use of this drug in the U.K. and the U.S., *see* 127).

Although no extensive published reports of severe reactions have appeared in the United States, a wide variety of severe complications can follow ingestion of MDMA including "convulsion, collapse, hyperpyrexia, disseminated intravascular coagulation, rhabdomyolysis and acute renal failure" (61). The drug has also been associated with the induction of arrhythmias (41), and there have been increasing reports of MDMA as a source of unexplained jaundice or hepatomegaly in younger individuals.

The most severe problem encountered to date with MDMA is secondary to the hyperthermia produced by this drug, particularly in settings with high ambient temperature, poor ventilation, and low fluid intake such as those encountered in British night clubs, which were the sites of "rave" dance parties. Fifteen deaths in young individuals have been attributed to such conditions during the 1990s with patients exhibiting body temperatures as high as 110°F and deaths occurring within 2–60 h after hospital admission with severe hyperthermia, renal failure, and disseminated intravascular coagulation (61,127). These deaths caused the British government to mandate adequate water supplies at night clubs, and this has apparently solved the problem of fatalities (101).

Animal Studies

MDMA, like other amphetamine derivatives, produces acute stimulatory effects on the sympathetic nervous system resulting in mydriasis and piloerection, as well as elevated heart rates and a marked increase in metabolism (58). MDMA produces striking elevation of autonomic thermal regulatory responses in the rat at 30 mg/kg that are temperature dependent and include an elevated metabolic rate, evaporative water loss, and strikingly rapid increases in body temperature (53). Internal body temperature can rise rapidly to well over 42°C, with resultant death. The increase in body temperature is probably secondary to serotonin release in the hypothalamus and is obviously pertinent to the "heat shock" deaths attributed to MDMA in humans.

Mice are less sensitive than rats to neurotoxic damage by MDMA (171,175). MDMA administration in the rat produces a dose-dependent elevation in locomotor activity (167) and a so-called serotonin motor syndrome that includes, among other signs, a "Straub tail" (a tail maintained at a 90-degree angle to the body), splayed hindlimbs, and forepaw treading involving a pivoting motion due to lateral side-to-side forepaw stepping with relatively stationary hindlimbs (160,167). This complex effect on locomotor activity declines over time with successive doses of MDMA, presumably due to the serotonin-depleting effects of the drug (for review of the behavioral effects, *see* 170). Several authors have speculated on the possible relationship of the effects of MDMA on activity to use of this drug in humans as part of dance parties (101,162). MDMA is primarily a stimulant with little or no hallucinogenic activity. Both baboons and rhesus monkeys will self-administer MDMA (12), and the drug lowers the threshold for intracranial stimulation in rats (68), effects consistent with its abuse in the human population. Several animal studies suggest the drug may have properties that distinguish it from other stimulants and hallucinogens, consistent with its unique psychological properties in humans.

The primary selective neurochemical effect of MDMA is a biphasic depletion of brain serotonin (for complete review, see 170). A single, 10 mg/kg subcutaneous injection of MDMA in the rat will produce a rapid (3 h), marked (84%) reduction in cortical serotonin that returns to normal levels by 24 h. This is followed by a slower decline in serotonin levels, with reduction to 74% of control by 1 week, and is accompanied by a reduction in the uptake of ^{3}H-serotonin by whole-brain synaptosomes (143). Long-term depletion in serotonin shows stereochemical specificity. (+)-MDMA produces serotonin depletion and reduction in uptake by 1 week, but the (−)-isomer is without effect (143). The longer term effects on serotonin depletion are related to the neurotoxic effects of the drug. Dopamine levels can, however, be reduced by higher and multiple drug doses in the rat (31,115).

The long-term depletion of serotonin, tryptophan hydroxylase activity, and serotonin-uptake sites following treatment with the methylenedioxy analogs of amphetamine are secondary to a loss of serotonergic axonal processes (for review, see 147,170). The initial concerns regarding the toxicity of these agents arose in part from studies with (±) MDA. This agent was found to produce relatively long-term (2-week) reductions in serotonin levels and uptake sites, and there was evidence of degenerating serotonergic nerve terminals in hippocampus and striatum as indicated by silver impregnation (129). It was on the basis of this study that MDMA was designated as a Schedule I drug. The anatomic nature of the effects of MDA and MDMA on serotonergic neurons has been studied in great detail using immunocytochemical methods that permit visualization of serotonergic neurons and their processes in the CNS. MDA and MDMA, like the effects of methamphetamine on dopaminergic neurons, spare serotonergic cell bodies and produce a widespread long-term loss of fine serotonin axon terminals throughout the brain with a sparing of dopaminergic endings (117). The serotonergic axons affected arise primarily from the dorsal raphe nucleus (92). Some regional sparing of serotonin processes can be observed in hippocampus and lateral hypothalamus, among other areas, but these are primarily fibers of passage and beaded axons characterized by large spherical varicosities arising from the median raphe group of serotonergic neurons.

MDMA produces dose-dependent depletions of serotonin in the somatosensory cortex of the monkey, even at doses as low as 2.5 mg/kg (eight doses over 4 days), producing a 44% depletion of serotonin levels in this subdivision of the brain (131). Morphological analysis in the monkey, 2 weeks following eight doses of 5 mg/kg, reveals cytopathological changes restricted to the dorsal raphe serotonergic neurons without loss of such cells and a complete sparing of median raphe serotonergic neurons. A marked reduction in serotonergic fine axons in the cerebral cortex is also observed. These findings are of particular concern, since the monkey is approximately eight times more sensitive to MDMA than the rodent and these effects in the monkey are seen with doses approximating those used by human drug abusers. Since it is generally thought that humans may be even more sensitive to toxic drug action than nonhuman primates (71,131), there is considerable reason for concern regarding neuronal damage in human drug abusers.

Significant evidence for recovery from the effects of MDMA exists in the rodent, including return of cortical serotonin-uptake sites by 1 year, serotonin levels by 32 weeks, and a slow reinnervation as assessed on morphological grounds that varies from area to area but does not reach control levels in neocortex even after 8 weeks (11). Studies in the monkey demonstrated that marked reductions in serotonin are present in most areas of the brain even up to 18 months after MDMA (for review of reinnervation, see 9,133). In squirrel monkeys treated with MDMA at 5 mg/kg b.i.d. for 4 days and examined 72 weeks later, profound reductions were observed in serotonin-uptake sites in forebrain, including areas such as the neocortex, hippocampus, striatum, and many thalamic nuclei (46). However, these studies also demonstrated marked increases in serotonin-uptake sites in areas such as the hypothalamus. The changes in serotonin-uptake sites were accompanied by equivalent changes in the density of serotonergic axons in these areas. While serotonergic axonal sprouting after MDMA may occur, the reinnervation pattern may be highly abnormal, resulting in continued denervation of distant target sites such as neocortex, while more proximal target areas such as the hypothalamus become reinnervated or even hyperinnervated by sprouting axons. These findings have led to the suggestion that MDMA injury "can lead to lasting reorganization of the ascending serotonin axon projections" and that "such lasting changes in brain innervation in MDMA-treated animals may have implications for humans using MDMA recreationally." Thus, not only might such effects lead to possible long-term cognitive changes, but also derangements of neuroendocrine or other functions by hyperinnervation (46).

Only one rat study has been conducted on the effects of MDMA on development. In this case, pregnant mothers were gavaged with up to 10 mg/kg with MDMA on alternate days between 6 and 18 days of gestation (174). No neurochemical effect on brain levels of serotonin, its metabolite, 5-hydroxyindoleacetic acid (5-HIAA), or serotonin-uptake sites was observed despite the fact that dose-dependent decreases in these parameters were seen in the mothers. Only minor behavioral effects were noted in the pups at periods up to 11 days postnatal. This is clearly an area that needs further investigation, given the fact that MDMA is a widely abused recreational drug and there is a high possibility of exposure in human pregnant females. Given the profound effects of this drug in damaging the serotonergic system, it is clear that additional studies on development following exposure to this drug *in utero* are necessary before it is concluded that administration of this drug to pregnant human females is without substantial risk to the offspring.

Human Studies

No direct neurochemical or morphological evidence for MDMA's neurotoxicity in humans is available. A number of suggestive results have been reported. It is the case that L-tryptophan increases serum prolactin concentration in control subjects, which is apparently not seen in MDMA users. The peak change in the area under the curve of the serum prolactin response also seemed to be depressed in the MDMA users, but since the difference from control did not attain statistical significance, the results are only suggestive and clearly more definitive studies are needed (124). Suggestive results regarding persistent effects of MDMA in the human have been obtained by examining the sleep patterns in some 23 MDMA users compared to age- and sex-matched controls. MDMA users showed significantly less total sleep (19 min) and less non–rapid-eye-movement (REM) sleep than controls. Changes in non-REM sleep were due to an average of 37 min less stage-II sleep with stages I, III, and IV being unaffected. Although these studies do not provide direct evidence for serotonin axonal neurotoxicity, they do suggest that MDMA usage can lead to long-term changes in brain areas involved in human sleep generation (2). A direct approach to assessing possible MDMA-induced serotonin neurotoxicity has focused on 5-HIAA levels, the major metabolite of serotonin in lumbar cerebrospinal fluid (CSF) of MDMA users (130). The results of these studies are conflicting, since in one of the studies there were reductions in cerebrospinal fluid 5-HIAA

(132), while in an earlier study (122) no changes were observed between control and MDMA users.

There are several reports of persistent neuropsychiatric difficulties in MDMA users. These include chronic psychosis, memory disturbances, major depressive disorders, and panic disorders. Such effects can persist for months, long after the drug has been metabolized (for review, *see* 99).

Toxic Mechanisms

Despite fairly extensive studies, no definitive mechanism for MDMA selective toxicity to serotonergic neurons is available (for review, *see* 18). Direct intracerebral injection of MDMA or MDA has no effect on serotonergic neurons or serotonergic axons in the area injected (110). The injection of (+)-MDMA in the vicinity of the serotonergic cell bodies of the dorsal and median raphe has no effect on serotonergic cell bodies or monoamines or metabolite concentrations in the hippocampus or striatum (120). For this reason, studies have been undertaken to determine whether the toxic effects of MDMA or MDA may be secondary to the peripheral production of neurotoxic metabolites of these compounds. Blockade of metabolism does not, however, affect the serotonin-depleting effects of MDMA (148,169). Intracerebroventricular injection of two major metabolites of MDA, α-methyldopamine and 3-O-methyl-α-methyldopamine, does not produce a long-term depletion of brain serotonin (98). Two MDMA metabolites that do have an effect are 2,4,5-trihydroxymethamphetamine and 2,4,5-trihydroxyamphetamine—derivatives of 6-hydroxydopamine (43,74,88,202). However, these compounds also damage dopaminergic axons, and it seems unlikely that their formation could be the mechanism by which MDMA selectively destroys serotonergic axons.

Particularly interesting are findings on the effect of the selective neurotoxicity of MDMA and MDA suggesting that this toxicity is dependent on central dopaminergic stores. MDMA does not deplete dopamine levels in the striatum, but direct measurement of dopamine release in the awake behaving rat using voltammetry measurements show that MDMA causes dopamine release, an effect that persists for as long as 3 h after intraperitoneal injection of the drug (113,197). Removal of central dopaminergic stores essentially blocks the effects of MDMA on serotonergic neurons (145,176). Consistent with the notion that dopamine plays an important role in the neurotoxicity of MDMA is the fact that inhibitors of 5-HT_2 serotonin receptors prevent the MDMA-induced elevation of dopamine concentration and antagonize long-term depletions of serotonin in the cortex and hippocampus (149). These effects can be reversed by administration of the dopamine precursor, L-dopa. MDMA acutely increases striatal dopamine synthesis, which is dependent upon the activation of 5-HT$_2$ receptors (114). The ability of 5-HT$_2$ antagonists to block MDMA-induced deficits in the serotonergic nervous system is thought to be due to interference with MDMA's activation of nigrostriatal dopamine synthesis and release, actions that are necessary for lasting serotonin depletion. Other mechanisms have been proposed (170).

(dl)-FENFLURAMINE
C$_{12}$H$_{16}$F$_3$N

(dl)-Fenfluramine
N-Ethyl-α-methyl-3-(trifluoromethyl)benzeneethanamine

NEUROTOXICITY RATING

Experimental

A   Serotonergic axonopathy

Fenfluramine is a structural analog of amphetamine that has been used as (a) a pharmacological adjuvant to weight reduction and is thought to act through serotonergic systems in the hypothalamus (51), and (b) as potential therapy for infantile autism (8,22). Fenfluramine differs from other appetite suppressants in that it is more likely to produce CNS depression than CNS stimulation (182). Racemic fenfluramine was frequently given in combination with phentermine, another amphetamine derivative and appetite suppressant. Combined administration of fenfluramine and phentermine (Phen/Fen) enhances the toxicity of these agents on serotonergic neurons (86). In September 1997, fenfluramine was withdrawn from the market following reports of valvular heart disease in women who had been treated with fenfluramine and phentermine. The histopathological features were similar to those in carcinoid or ergotamine-induced valvular heart disease, other serotonin-related syndromes (5a,31a). Fenfluramine was not recommended as an appetite suppressant in children under 12 years of age (182). Fenfluramine is a controlled substance in the United States and is listed on Schedule IV (drugs of low abuse potential).

General Toxicology

Fenfluramine is well absorbed from the gastrointestinal tract. Its maximal therapeutic effect is obtained within 2–4 h. De-ethylation of fenfluramine results in norfenflura-

mine, which is pharmacologically active. Norfenfluramine is, in turn, metabolized to m-trifluoromethylbenzoic acid. The latter is conjugated to glycine and excreted in the urine as m-trifluoromethyhippuric acid, which represents 60%–90% of the urinary excretion products. Fenfluramine, itself, and norfenfluramine are also excreted in the urine (123,138). As a weak base, the rate of fenfluramine excretion is pH-dependent, and acidification of the urine increases the amount of fenfluramine excreted. The half-life of fenfluramine is approximately 20 h; this can be cut in half if urinary acidity is kept below pH 5.0 and fluids are forced (20). Fenfluramine is lipid soluble and crosses the blood-brain barrier. In monkeys, fenfluramine and norfenfluramine readily cross the placenta (123).

The most common adverse effects of fenfluramine are drowsiness, diarrhea, and dry mouth. Tolerance to many of these side effects appears to develop within a few weeks (134). Cases of pulmonary hypertension associated with fenfluramine use have been reported (40,102) as have cases of valvular heart disese in women treated with fenfluramine and phentermine (5a,31a). In adults, 80–100 times the usual therapeutic dose (i.e., 60–100 mg/day) is toxic but usually not fatal (123). Acute intoxication can include hyperpyrexia, shivering, agitation, convulsions, confusion, mydriasis, nystagmus, altered reflexes, and cardiac arrest. There has been one case reported where a woman died from pyrexia after ingestion of over 1 g of fenfluramine (140).

Animal Studies

Studies in animals have shown that the anorectic action of fenfluramine is mainly due to the d-isomer (106). Its primary metabolite, d-norfenfluramine, has been shown to have even greater potency as an anorectic (104). It has been demonstrated in the rat that there is a significant correlation between the total amount of weight lost and brain exposure to fenfluramine or norfenfluramine (200). The anorectic activity of fenfluramine and norfenfluramine is attributed to their pharmacological effect on central serotonergic neurons. Fenfluramine appears to inhibit serotonin uptake preferentially, whereas norfenfluramine releases serotonin from the nonvesicular transmitter pool. For both compounds, the d-isomer shows greater potency than the l-isomer with respect to pharmacological action on serotonergic neurons (105). When rats are treated with dl-fenfluramine at doses >4 mg/kg, there are dose-dependent decreases in forebrain levels of serotonin and 5-HIAA, as well as reductions in the density of serotonin-uptake sites (200). In addition, there appears to be a significant negative correlation between the density of such uptake sites and the total concentration of fenfluramine in brain.

In addition to its anorectic activity, studies in several species have demonstrated that *dl*-fenfluramine and *d*-fenfluramine are potentially neurotoxic to central serotonergic neurons. When administered to adult rats in a single high dose (15–60 mg/kg) or in repeated doses (6.25–24 mg/kg), *dl*-fenfluramine produces long-lasting reductions in brain serotonin levels (28,59,77,151,173), serotonin-uptake sites (7,28,151,200), as well as tryptophan hydroxylase activity, the rate-limiting enzyme in serotonin biosynthesis (173). *d*-Fenfluramine is more potent than racemic fenfluramine in producing long-term depletion of brain serotonin concentrations in the rat (77). Repeated administration of *dl*-fenfluramine to guinea pigs (6.25–12.5 mg/kg) and rhesus monkeys (10 mg/kg) results in decreased brain levels of serotonin lasting for at least 2 and 8 weeks, respectively, following the last drug treatment (151). Mice, rats, and squirrel monkeys treated with multiple doses of *d*-fenfluramine (5–10 mg/kg) also demonstrate persistent decrements of brain serotonin, lasting as long as 17 months following drug treatment in the case of squirrel monkeys (97). While there is clearly a long-term reduction in serotonin level following fenfluramine treatment, no lasting alteration of catecholaminergic markers has been observed with either the racemic mixture or *d*-fenfluramine (76,77,200).

The sustained reduction in serotonergic neurochemical markers, long after the drug has been metabolized, suggests that fenfluramine is neurotoxic to these neurons. Morphological studies also provide evidence of fenfluramine neurotoxicity that is selective for serotonergic neurons. Repeated administration of *dl*-fenfluramine to rats, either orally (5 mg/kg), intraperitoneally (26.8 mg/kg), or subcutaneously (5–24 mg/kg), results in a significant decrease in the density of serotonin-immunoreactive axons in several forebrain regions (6,109,166). Remaining serotonergic fibers have morphological characteristics suggestive of degeneration; they are thickened and irregularly shaped with fragmented axonal segments and uneven, swollen varicosities (6,109,166). Similar reductions in the density of serotonin-immunoreactive axons in the forebrain of squirrel monkeys have been reported following multiple subcutaneous injections (5 mg/kg, b.i.d. for 4 days) of *d*-fenfluramine (99,134). As seen with MDMA, fenfluramine preferentially affects fine-caliber serotonergic axons while sparing the thicker, beaded axons [see earlier under 3,4-Methylenedioxymethamphetamine].

Fenfluramine is similar to other structural analogs of amphetamine (methamphetamine, MDA, MDMA) in that it appears to damage serotonergic axons while sparing their cell bodies (6,109). The drug-induced loss of serotonergic axons is corroborated by autoradiographic studies that demonstrate a reduction in serotonin-uptake sites labeled with ^{3}H-paroxetine (7). In addition, reduced ^{3}H-paroxetine binding in rats treated with fenfluramine is accompanied by decreases in the maximal uptake and synaptosomal loading of ^{14}C-serotonin; this provides further evidence for the view that fenfluramine damages serotonergic nerve terminals (192). The axonal damage produced by fenfluramine is selective for serotonergic neurons, since the integrity of catecholaminergic axons, assessed using tyrosine hydroxylase immunocytochemical techniques as well as ^{3}H-mazindol binding and autoradiography, appears unaffected (6,7,200).

Although the fenfluramine-induced deficit in serotonergic neuronal markers is long lasting, there is evidence, at least in the rat, to suggest that serotonergic neurons are capable of a slow, partial recovery from the neurotoxic damage produced by this compound. Rats treated with *dl*-fenfluramine (80 mg/kg for 2 days) suffer destruction of 80% of their serotonergic nerve terminals, as measured by a decrease in ^{3}H-paroxetine binding to serotonin-uptake sites on synaptic membranes, as well as a reduction in the rate of serotonin uptake into synaptosomes. However, 25 weeks later, these biochemical markers for serotonergic nerve terminals are restored to 72% of control. Maximal loading of synaptosomes with serotonin is also found to recover to 79% of the control value. These data suggest regeneration of serotonin-containing nerve endings after fenfluramine treatment has ended (193). Examination of the density of serotonin-immunoreactive axons in rat hippocampus following a single high dose of *dl*-fenfluramine (26.8 mg/kg) reveals a gradual increase in fiber density, but still an incomplete restoration of the normal pattern of innervation by 40 days following drug treatment (166). The long duration of the regeneration of axon terminals most likely accounts for the persistent reduction in brain serotonin levels observed following fenfluramine treatment.

The anorectic action of fenfluramine can be demonstrated in laboratory animals as well as the development of long-lasting tolerance to this action. The potential relationship of such tolerance to long-term depletions of brain serotonin induced by fenfluramine has been evaluated using milk intake as an index of tolerance to the anorectic effect of fenfluramine in rats (76). Rats that previously had been allowed to drink sweetened condensed milk were treated for 4 days with saline or *dl*-fenfluramine (6.25 mg/kg, b.i.d.). Two and 8 weeks following this dosage regimen, the animals were challenged with single injections of fenfluramine (1.25–12.5 mg/kg) and were tested for milk intake. At both time points, rats that had been treated for 4 days previously with fenfluramine required higher doses of the drug than saline-control animals to suppress milk intake, indicating that they had become tolerant to fenfluramine's anorectic effect. Rats tested 2 weeks following the initial drug regimen demonstrated greater tolerance to the suppression of milk intake by acute fenfluramine than animals that had 8 weeks to recover. Correspondingly, there was a greater depletion of brain serotonin in the 2-week *vs.* the 8-week animals. Thus, it appears from this study that the degree of tolerance produced by fenfluramine is correlated with the extent of brain serotonin depletion. It is not known whether a similar reduction in brain serotonin level occurs when humans become tolerant to the appetite suppressant effects of this agent.

The finding that fenfluramine produces long-term neurotoxicity to central serotonergic neurons across a variety of animal species raises concern in relation to human use of this agent. The dose of fenfluramine required to produce neurotoxicity is not in gross excess of the dose used to suppress appetite. For example, in the rat, 5 mg/kg of *dl*-fenfluramine given subcutaneously reduces food intake by 50%, and long-lasting reductions in brain serotonin levels are observed with doses as low as 6.25 mg/kg (151). In the baboon, there is an approximate two-fold difference between the effective dose for suppression of food intake and the dose producing serotonin neurotoxicity (153). In these two species, there is a relatively narrow margin of safety between effective and toxic doses of *dl*-fenfluramine.

Human Studies

For a number of years, racemic (*dl*)-fenfluramine was used in the management of obesity in conjunction with caloric restriction, exercise, and behavior modification. This appetite suppressant was only recommended for short-term use (a few weeks) with a maximal daily dose of 120 mg (182). Clinical studies showed that doses higher than 120 mg/day did not have any greater effect on weight loss and, in fact, increased the incidence of adverse side effects (reviewed in 123). Intermittent use of *dl*-fenfluramine was not as effective as continuous use and was contraindicated because of the higher incidence of side effects (123). Tolerance to racemic fenfluramine occurred after 6 months. Further treatment (>6 months) reportedly only maintained the weight level (39). Reviews of the efficacy of *dl*-fenfluramine in therapeutic trials indicated drug-induced weight loss was modest (6.6–7 lb) over a 12-week period (168), and similar weight loss was achieved by caloric restriction alone (123) or by behavior modification (39). Follow-up studies showed that many patients rapidly regained the weight lost under drug therapy upon withdrawal of *dl*-fenfluramine (reviewed in 39).

d-Fenfluramine is effective at half the dose of racemic fenfluramine and, thus, patients usually received only 30 mg daily. Similar to *dl*-fenfluramine, *d*-fenfluramine was pur-

ported to have low abuse potential (57) with few side effects, at least with short-term use (45). A one-year international clinical trial consisting of 822 obese patients on a calorie-restricted diet showed that patients treated with *d*-fenfluramine had a higher cumulative mean weight loss than patients treated with placebo (56). However, by the end of the 12-month trial, there was only a small difference in body weight loss (<6 lb) between the drug and placebo group. Both *d*-fenfluramine and placebo-treated patients lost the greatest amount of body weight within the first 6 months. Thereafter, there was no further reduction in body weight in either group, suggesting that tolerance had occurred.

Fenfluramine and phentermine (another amphetamine derivative) were individually approved by the U.S. Food and Drug Administration (FDA) for use as appetite suppressants. Although the drug combination had not been approved by the FDA, in 1996 the total number of prescriptions in the United States for fenfluramine and phentermine exceeded 18 million (31a). Fenfluramine was withdrawn in September 1997 because of reports of valvular heart disease in women who had taken fenfluramine and phentermine. Patients presented with cardiovascular symptoms or a heart murmur; some had evidence of newly documented pulmonary hypertension. Histopathology revealed plaque-like encasement of heart-valve leaflets and chordal structures with intact valve architecture. Similar changes are seen in other serotonin-related valvular syndromes, notably carcinoid or ergotamine-induced heart valve disease (5a,31a).

Toxic Mechanisms

d-Norfenfluramine, the primary, active metabolite of *d*-fenfluramine, is responsible for serotonergic neurotoxicity because, in the rat, this metabolite is more effective than the parent compound in reducing hippocampal and cortical levels of serotonin and 5-HIAA as well as decreasing ^{3}H-paroxetine binding to serotonin-uptake sites (75). Direct intracerebral infusion of *d*-norfenfluramine (500 μg/h) for 2 h in rats has also been shown to produce reductions in forebrain levels of serotonin lasting for at least 1 week following drug administration (72). The notion that *d*-norfenfluramine is the primary causative agent in producing fenfluramine-induced neurotoxicity is disputed by findings in the mouse demonstrating that fenfluramine produces long-term reductions of brain serotonin levels in the presence of little *d*-norfenfluramine (97). Furthermore, pretreatment of rats with SKF-525A, an agent that inhibits the conversion of fenfluramine to norfenfluramine, does not appreciably attenuate the neurotoxic action of *d*-fcnfluramine (19).

Unlike methamphetamine, the serotonergic neurotoxicity produced by fenfluramine does not appear to be mediated by activation of glutamate receptors or by a hyperthermic mechanism (44,139). Fenfluramine produces hypothermia in rats as opposed to the hyperthermia known to result from administration of methamphetamine or MDMA.

The anorectic action of fenfluramine can be dissociated from serotonergic neurotoxicity. When the serotonergic-uptake blocker fluoxetine is administered to rats concurrently with d-fenfluramine, the long-lasting deficit in brain serotonin is prevented, but fenfluramine's action on food intake is not affected (100). In addition, it has been demonstrated in microdialysis studies in rat hypothalamus that fluoxetine prevents fenfluramine-induced serotonin release, but its action on food intake is not altered (126). The anorexic action of fenfluramine can, however, be blocked with metergoline, a $5-HT_1/5-HT_2$ serotonin antagonist; this suggests the involvement of serotonin receptors in mediating appetite suppression.

REFERENCES

1. Agid Y, Javoy F, Glowinski J (1973) Hyperactivity of the remaining dopaminergic neurons after partial destruction of the nigrostriatal dopaminergic system in the rat. *Nature New Biol* **245**, 150.

2. Allen RP, McCann UD, Ricaurte GA (1993) Persistent effects of (+/−)-3,4-methylene-dioxymethamphetamine (MDMA, "ecstasy") on human sleep. *Sleep* **16**, 560.

3. Ando K, Johanson CE, Seiden LS, Schuster CR (1985) Sensitivity changes to dopaminergic agents in fine motor control of rhesus monkeys after repeated methamphetamine administration. *Pharmacol Biochem Behav* **22**, 737.

4. Angrist B (1994) Amphetamine psychosis: Clinical variations of the syndrome. In: *Amphetamine and Its Analogs: Psychopharmacology, Toxicology and Abuse*. Cho AK, Segal DS eds. Academic Press, San Diego p. 387.

5. Anon (1997) *Proceedings of the National Consensus Meeting on the Use, Abuse and Sequelae of Abuse of Methamphetamines with Implications for Treatment and Research*. U.S. Department of Health and Human Services, Publication No. (SMA 96-8013).

5a. Anon (1997) Cardiac valvulopathy associated with exposure to fenfluramine or dexfenfluramine: U.S. Department of Health and Human Services interim public health recommendations, November 1997. *Morb Mortal Wkly Rep* **46**, 1061.

6. Appel NM, Contrera JF, De Souza EB (1989) Fenfluramine selectively and differentially decreases the density of serotonergic nerve terminals in rat brain: Evidence from immunocytochemical studies. *J Pharmacol Exp Ther* **249**, 928.

7. Appel NM, Mitchell WM, Contrera JF *et al.* (1990) Effects of high-dose fenfluramine treatment on monoamine uptake sites in rat brain: Assessment using quantitative autoradiography. *Synapse* **6**, 33.

8. August GJ, Raz N, Papinacolaou AC *et al.* (1984) Fenfluramine treatment in infantile autism. Neurochemical, electrophysiological, and behavioral effects. *J Nerv Ment Dis* **172**, 604.

9. Axt KJ, Mamounas LA, Molliver ME (1994) Structural features of amphetamine neurotoxicity. In: *Amphetamine and Its Analogs: Psychopharmacology, Toxicology and Abuse*. Cho AK, Segal DS eds. Academic Press, San Diego p. 315.

10. Bakhit C, Morgan ME, Peat MA, Gibb JW (1981) Long-term effects of methamphetamine on the synthesis and metabolism of 5-hydroxytryptamine in various regions of the rat brain. *Neuropharmacology* **20**, 1135.

11. Battaglia G, Yeh SY, De Souza EB (1988) MDMA-induced neurotoxicity: Parameters of degeneration and recovery of brain serotonin neurons. *Pharmacol Biochem Behav* **29**, 269.

12. Beardsley PM, Balster RL, Harris LS (1986) Self-administration of methylenedioxymethamphetamine (MDMA) by rhesus monkeys. *Drug Alcohol Dependence* **18**, 149.

13. Beckett AH, Rowland M (1965) Urinary excretion kinetics of methylamphetamine in man. *J Pharm Pharmacol* **17**, 109S.

14. Bennett BA, Hyde CE, Pecora JR (1993) Differing neurotoxic potencies of methamphetamine, mazindol and cocaine in mesencephalic cultures. *J Neurochem* **60**, 1444.

15. Bigl V, Dalitz E, Kunert E *et al.* (1982) The effect of d-amphetamine and amitriptyline administered to pregnant rats on the locomotor activity and neurotransmitters of the offspring. *Psychopharmacology* **77**, 371.

16. Bowyer JF, Davies DL, Schmued L *et al.* (1994) Further studies of the role of hyperthermia in methamphetamine neurotoxicity. *J Pharmacol Exp Ther* **268**, 1571.

17. Bowyer JF, Tank AW, Newport GD *et al.* (1992) The influence of environmental temperature on the transient effects of methamphetamine on dopamine levels and dopamine release in rat striatum. *J Pharmacol Exp Ther* **260**, 817.

18. Brodkin J, Malyala A, Nash JF (1993) Effect of acute monoamine depletion on 3,4-methylenedioxymethamphetamine-induced neurotoxicity. *Pharmacol Biochem Behav* **45**, 647.

19. Caccia S, Anelli M, Ferrarese A *et al.* (1993) The role of d-norfenfluramine in the indole-depleting effect of d-fenfluramine in the rat. *Eur J Pharmacol* **233**, 71.

20. Caccia S, Conforti I, Duchier J (1985) Pharmacokinetics of fenfluramine and norfenfluramine in volunteers given D- and DL-fenfluramine for 15 days. *Eur J Clin Pharmacol* **29**, 221.

21. Caldwell J, Dring LG, Williams RT (1972) Metabolism of ^{14}C-methamphetamine in man, the guinea and the rat. *Biochem J* **129**, 11.

22. Campbell M (1988) Fenfluramine treatment of autism. *J Child Psychol Psychiat* **29**, 1.

23. Chiueh CC, Markey SP, Burns RS *et al.* (1983) *N*-Methyl-4-phenyl-1,2,3,6-tetrahydropyridine, a parkinsonian syndrome causing agent in man and monkey, produces different effects in guinea pig and rat. *Pharmacologist* **25**, 131.

24. Cho AK, Hiramatsu M, Distefano E *et al.* (1990) Stereochemical differences in the metabolism of 3,4-methylenedioxymethamphetamine *in vivo* and *in vitro*: A pharmacokinetic analysis. *Drug Metab Disposition* **18**, 686.

25. Cho AK, Kumagai Y (1994) Metabolism of amphetamine and other arylisopropylamines. In: *Amphetamine and Its Analogs: Psychopharmacology, Toxicology and Abuse.* Cho AK, Segal DS eds. Academic Press, San Diego p. 43.

26. Cho AK, Segal DS (1994) *Amphetamine and Its Analogs: Psychopharmacology, Toxicology and Abuse.* Academic Press, San Diego.

27. Choi HK, Won L, Heller A (1993) Dopaminergic neurons grown in three-dimensional reaggregate culture for periods of up to one year. *J Neurosci Meth* **46**, 233.

28. Clineschmidt BV, Zacchei AG, Totaro JA *et al.* (1978) Fenfluramine and brain serotonin. *Ann N Y Acad Sci* **308**, 222.

29. Cohen G (1984) Oxy-radical toxicity in catecholamine neurons. *Neurotoxicology* **5**, 77–82.

30. Commins DL, Seiden LS (1986) α-Methyltyrosine blocks methylamphetamine-induced degeneration in the rat somatosensory cortex. *Brain Res* **365**, 15.

31. Commins DL, Vosmer G, Virus RM *et al.* (1987) Biochemical and histological evidence that methylenedioxymethylamphetamine (MDMA) is toxic to neurons in the rat brain. *J Pharmacol Exp Ther* **241**, 338.

31a. Connolly HM, Crary JL, McGoon MD *et al.* (1997) Valvular heart disease associated with fenfluramine-phentermine. *N Engl J Med* **337**, 581.

32. Cook CE (1991) Pyrolytic characteristics, pharmacokinetics, and bioavailability of smoked heroin, cocaine, phencyclidine, and methamphetamine. *U.S. Natl Inst Drug Abuse (NIDA) Res Monogr* **115**, 6.

33. Creese I, Burt DR, Snyder SH (1977) Dopamine receptor binding enhancement accompanies lesion-induced behavioral supersensitivity. *Science* **197**, 596.

34. Cubells JF, Rayport S, Rajendran G (1994) Methamphetamine neurotoxicity involves vacuolization of endocytic organelles and dopamine-dependent oxidative stress. *J Neurosci* **14**, 2260.

35. Davis GG, Swalwell CI (1994) Acute aortic dissections and ruptured berry aneurysms associated with methamphetamine abuse. *J Forensic Sci* **39**, 1481.

36. Delaney P, Estes M (1980) Intracranial hemorrhage with amphetamine abuse. *Neurology* **30**, 1125.

37. DeVito MJ, Wagner GC (1989) Methamphetamine-induced neuronal damage: A possible role for free radicals. *Neuropharmacology* **28**, 1145.

38. Dixon SD, Bejar R (1989) Echoencephalographic findings in neonates associated with maternal cocaine and methamphetamine use: Incidence and clinical correlates. *J Pediat* **115**, 770.

39. Douglas JG, Munro JF (1982) Drug treatment and obesity. *Pharmacol Ther* **18**, 351.

40. Douglas JG, Munro JF, Kitchin AH *et al.* (1981) Pulmonary hypertension and fenfluramine. *Brit Med J* **283**, 881.

41. Dowling GP, McDonough ET, Bost RO (1987) "Eve" and "Ecstasy". A report of five deaths associated with the use of MDEA and MDMA. *J Amer Med Assn* **257**, 1615.

42. Eisch AJ, Gaffney M, Weihmuller FB *et al.* (1992) Striatal subregions are differentially vulnerable to the neurotoxic effects of methamphetamine. *Brain Res* **598**, 321.

43. Elayan I, Gibb JW, Hanson GR *et al.* (1992) Long-term alteration in the central monoaminergic systems of the rat by 2,4,5-trihydroxyamphetamine but not by 2-hydroxy-4,5-methylenedioxymethamphetamine or 2-hydroxy-4,5-methylenedioxyamphetamine. *Eur J Pharmacol* **221**, 281.

44. Farfel GM, Seiden LS (1995) Role of hypothermia in the mechanism of protection against serotonergic toxicity. II. Experiments with methamphetamine, *p*-chloroamphetamine, fenfluramine, dizocilpine and dextromethorphan. *J Pharmacol Exp Ther* **272**, 868.

45. Finer N, Craddock D, Lavielle R, Keen H (1988) Effect of 6 months therapy with dexfenfluramine in obese patients: Studies in the United Kingdom. *Clin Neuropharmacol* **2**, S179.

46. Fischer C, Hatzidimitriou G, Wlos J *et al.* (1995) Reorganization of ascending 5-HT axon projections in animals previously exposed to the recreational drug (±) 3,4-methylenedioxy-methamphetamine (MDMA, "Estasy"). *J Neurosci* **15**, 5476.

47. Fitzgerald RL, Blanke RV, Rosecrans JA, Glennon RA (1989) Stereochemistry of the metabolism of MDMA to MDA. *Life Sci* **45**, 295.

48. Frith CH, Chang LW, Lattin DL (1987) Toxicity of methylenedioxymethamphetamine (MDMA) in the dog and the rat. *Fund Appl Toxicol* **9**, 110.

49. Fukui K, Kariyama H, Kashiba A (1986) Further confirmation of heterogeneity of the rat striatum: Different mosaic patterns of dopamine fibers after administration of methamphetamine or reserpine. *Brain Res* **382**, 81.

50. Fukui S, Wada K, Iyo M (1994) Epidemiology of amphetamine abuse in Japan and its social implications. In: *Amphetamine and Its Analogs: Psychopharmacology, Toxicology and Abuse.* Cho AK, Segal DS eds. Academic Press, San Diego p. 459.

51. Garattini S, Buczko W, Jori A (1975) On the mechanism of action of fenfluramine. *Postgrad Med J* **51**, 27.

52. Gilman GA, Rall TW, Nies AS, Taylor P (1990) *Goodman and Gilman's The Pharmacological Basis of Therapeutics*: Pergamon Press, New York.

53. Gordon CJ, Watkinson WP, O'Callaghan JP (1991) Effects of 3,4-methylenedioxymethyl-amphetamine on autonomic thermoregulatory responses of the rat. *Pharmacol Biochem Behav* **38**, 339.

54. Graham DG, Tiffany SM, Bell WR *et al.* (1978) Autooxidation versus covalent binding of quinones as the mechanism of toxicity of dopamine, 6-hydroxydopamine, and related compounds toward C1300 neuroblastoma cells *in vitro*. *Mol Pharmacol* **14**, 644.

55. Green AR, De Souza RJ, Williams JL *et al.* (1992) The neurotoxic effects of methamphetamine on 5-hydroxytryptamine and dopamine in brain: Evidence for the protective effect of chlormethiazole. *Neuropharmacology* **31**, 315.

56. Guy-Grand B, Apfelbaum M, Crepaldi G *et al.* (1989) International trial of long-term dexfenfluramine in obesity. *Lancet* **i**, 1142.

57. Guy-Grand BJP (1988) Place of dexfenfluramine in the management of obesity. *Clin Neuropharmacol* **2**, S216.

58. Hardman HF, Haavik CO, Seevers MH (1973) Relationship of the structure of mescaline and seven analogs to toxicity and behavior in five species of laboratory animals. *Toxicol Appl Pharmacol* **25**, 299.

59. Harvey JA, McMaster SE (1975) Fenfluramine: Evidence for a neurotoxic action on midbrain and a long-term depletion of serotonin. *Psychopharmacol Commun* **1**, 217.

60. Heller A, Won L, Choi H (1993) Reaggregate cultures. In: *In Vitro Biological Systems: Preparation and Maintenance, Methods in Toxicology*. Vol 1. Tyson CA, Frazier JM eds. Academic Press, New York p. 27.

61. Henry JA (1992) Ecstasy and the dance of death. *Brit Med J* **305**, 5.

62. Hess A, Desiderio C, McAuliffe WG (1990) Acute neuropathological changes in the caudate nucleus caused by MPTP and methamphetamine: Immunohistochemical studies. *J Neurocytol* **19**, 338.

63. Hiramatsu M, Kumagai Y, Unger SE, Cho AK (1990) Metabolism of methylenedioxymethamphetamine: formation of dihydroxymethamphetamine and a quinone identified as its glutathione adduct. *J Pharmacol Exp Ther* **254**, 521.

64. Hitzemann BA, Hitzemann RJ, Brase DA (1976) Influence of prenatal *d*-amphetamine administration on development and behavior of rats. *Life Sci* **18**, 605.

65. Hotchkiss AJ, Gibb JW (1980) Long-term effects of multiple doses of methamphetamine on tryptophan hydroxylase and tyrosine hydroxylase activity in rat brain. *J Pharmacol Exp Ther* **214**, 257.

66. Hotchkiss AJ, Gibb JW (1980) Blockade of methamphetamine-induced depression of tyrosine hydroxylase by GABA transaminase inhibitors. *Eur J Pharmacol* **66**, 201.

67. Hotchkiss AJ, Morgan ME, Gibb JW (1979) The long-term effects of multiple doses of methamphetamine on neostriatal tryptophan hydroxylase, tyrosine hydroxylase, choline acetyltransferase and glutamate decarboxylase activities. *Life Sci* **25**, 1373.

68. Hubner CB, Bird M, Rassnick S, Kornetsky C (1988) The threshold lowering effects of MDMA (ecstasy) on brain-stimulation reward. *Psychopharmacology* **95**, 49.

69. Iacopino A, Christakos S, German D *et al.* (1992) Calbindin-D_{28K}-containing neurons in animal models of neurodegeneration: Possible protection from excitotoxicity. *Mol Brain Res* **13**, 251.

70. Ihara Y, Sato M, Otsuki S *et al.* (1986) Morphological changes in rat striatal boutons after chronic methamphetamine and haloperidol treatment. *Neurosci Res* **3**, 403.

71. Insel TR, Battaglia G, Johanssen JN *et al.* (1989) 3,4-Methylenedioxymethamphetamine ("Ectasy") selectively destroys brain serotonin terminals in rhesus monkeys. *J Pharmacol Exp Ther* **249**, 713.

72. Invernizzi R, Fracasso C, Caccia S *et al.* (1991) Effects of intracerebroventricular administration of *d*-fenfluramine and *d*-norfenfluramine, as a single injection or 2-h infusion, on serotonin in brain: Relationship to concentrations of drugs in brain. *Neuropharmacology* **30**, 119.

73. Itoh Y, Oishi R, Nishibori M, Saeki K (1986) Comparison of effects of phencyclidine and methamphetamine on body temperature in mice: A possible role for histamine neurons in thermoregulation. *Naunyn-Schmied Arch Pharmacol* **332**, 293.

74. Johnson M, Elayan I, Hanson GR *et al.* (1992) Effects of 3,4-dihydroxymethamphetamine and 2,4,5-trihydroxymethamphetamine, two metabolites of 3,4-methylenedioxymethamphetamine, on central serotonergic and dopaminergic systems. *J Pharmacol Exp Ther* **261**, 447.

75. Johnson MP, Nichols DE (1990) Comparative serotonin neurotoxicity of the stereoisomers of fenfluramine and norfenfluramine. *Pharmacol Biochem Behav* **36**, 105.

76. Kleven MS, Schuster CR, Seiden LS (1988) Effect of depletion of brain serotonin by repeated fenfluramine on neurochemical and anorectic effects of acute fenfluramine. *J Pharmacol Exp Ther* **246**, 822.

77. Kleven MS, Seiden LS (1989) D-, L-, and DL-Fenfluramine cause long-lasting depletions of serotonin in rat brain. *Brain Res* **505**, 351.

78. Kleven MS, Seiden LS (1991) Repeated injection of cocaine potentiates methamphetamine-induced toxicity to dopamine-containing neurons in rat striatum. *Brain Res* **557**, 340.

79. Koda LY, Gibb JW (1973) Adrenal and striatal tyrosine hydroxylase activity after methamphetamine. *J Pharmacol Exp Ther* **185**, 42.

80. Kontur PJ, Hoffmann PC, Heller A (1987) Neurotoxic effects of methamphetamine assessed in three-dimensional reaggregate tissue cultures. *Develop Brain Res* **31**, 7.

81. Kontur PJ, Won LA, Hoffmann PC, Heller A (1991) Survival of developing dopaminergic neurons in reaggregate tissue culture following treatment with methamphetamine. *Neurosci Lett* **129**, 254.

82. Konuma K (1994) Use and abuse of amphetamines in Japan. In: *Amphetamine and Its Analogs: Psychopharmacology, Toxicology and Abuse*. Cho AK, Segal DS eds. Academic Press, San Diego p. 415.

83. Langston JW (1985) MPTP and Parkinson's disease. *Trends Neurosci* **8**, 79.

84. Langston JW, Ballard P, Irwin I (1983) Chronic parkinsonism in humans due to a product of meperidine-analog synthesis. *Science* **219**, 979.

85. Layer RT, Bland LR, Skolnick P (1993) MK-801, but not drugs acting at strychnine-insensitive glycine receptors, attenuate methamphetamine nigrostriatal toxicity. *Brain Res* **625**, 38.

86. Lew R, Weisenberg G, Vosmer G, Seiden LS (1997) Combined phentermine/fenfluramine administration enhances depletion of serotonin from central terminal fields. *Synapse* **26**, 36.

87. Lim HK, Foltz RL (1988) *In vivo* and *in vitro* metabolism of 3,4-(methylenedioxy)methamphetamine in the rat: Identification of metabolites using an ion trap detector. *Chem Res Toxicol* **1**, 370.

88. Lim HK, Foltz RL (1991) Ion trap tandem mass spectrometric evidence for the metabolism of 3,4-(methylenedioxy)methamphetamine to the potent neurotoxins 2,4,5-trihydroxymethamphetamine and 2,4,5-trihydroxyamphetamine. *Chem Res Toxicol* **4**, 626.

89. Little BB, Snell LM, Gilstrap LC III (1988) Methamphetamine abuse during pregnancy: Outcome and fetal effects. *Obstet Gynecol* **72**, 541.

90. Lorez H (1981) Fluorescence histochemistry indicates damage of striatal dopamine nerve terminals in rats after multiple doses of methamphetamine. *Life Sci* **28**, 911.

91. Lucot JB, Wagner GC, Schuster CR (1982) Decreased sensitivity of rat pups to long-lasting dopamine and serotonin depletions produced by methylamphetamine. *Brain Res* **247**, 181.

92. Mamounas LA, Mullen CA, O'Hearn E, Molliver ME (1991) Dual serotoninergic projections to forebrain in the rat: Morphologically distinct 5-HT axon terminals exhibit differential vulnerability to neurotoxic amphetamine derivatives. *J Comp Neurol* **314**, 558.

93. Marek GJ, Vosmer G, Seiden LS (1990) Dopamine uptake inhibitors block long-term neurotoxic effects of methamphetamine upon dopaminergic neurons. *Brain Res* **513**, 274.

94. Marshall JF, Navarrete RJ (1990) Contrasting tissue factors predict heterogenous striatal dopamine neurotoxicity after MPTP or methamphetamine treatment. *Brain Res* **534**, 348.

95. Marshall JF, O'Dell SJ, Weihmuller FB (1993) Dopamine-glutamate interactions in methamphetamine-induced neurotoxicity. *J Neural Transm-Gen Sect* **91**, 241.

96. McCabe RT, Hanson GR, Dawson TM *et al.* (1987) Methamphetamine-induced reduction in D_1 and D_2 dopamine receptors as evidenced by autoradiography: Comparison with tyrosine hydroxylase activity. *Neuroscience* **23**, 253.

97. McCann UD, Hatzidimitriou G, Ridenour A *et al.* (1994) Dexfenfluramine and serotonin neurotoxicity: Further preclinical evidence that clinical caution is indicated. *J Pharmacol Exp Ther* **269**, 792.

98. McCann UD, Ricaurte GA (1991) Major metabolites of (±)-3,4-methylenedioxyamphetamine (MDA) do not mediate its toxic effects on brain serotonin neurons. *Brain Res* **545**, 279.

99. McCann UD, Ricaurte GA (1994) Use and abuse of ring-substituted amphetamines. In: *Amphetamine and Its Analogs: Psychopharmacology, Toxicology and Abuse*. Cho AK, Segal DS eds. Academic Press, San Diego p. 371.

100. McCann UD, Yuan J, Ricaurte GA (1995) Fenfluramine's appetite suppression and serotonin neurotoxicity are separable. *Eur J Pharmacol* **283**, R5.

101. McDowell DM, Kleber HD (1994) MDMA: Its history and pharmacology. *Psychiat Ann* **24**, 127.

102. McMurray J, Bloomfield P, Miller HC (1986) Irreversible pulmonary hypertension after treatment with fenfluramine. *Brit Med J* **292**, 239.

103. Melega WP, Williams AE, Schmitz DA *et al.* (1995) Pharmacokinetic and pharmacodynamic analysis of the actions of *d*-amphetamine and *d*-methamphetamine on the dopamine terminal. *J Pharmacol Exp Ther* **274**, 90.

104. Mennini T, Bizzi A, Caccia S *et al.* (1991) Comparative studies on the anorectic activity of *d*-fenfluramine in mice, rats, and guinea pigs. *Naunyn-Schmied Arch Pharmacol* **343**, 483.

105. Mennini T, Garattini S, Caccia S (1985) Anorectic effect of fenfluramine isomers and metabolites: Relationship between brain levels and *in vitro* potencies on serotonergic mechanisms. *Psychopharmacology* **85**, 111.

106. Mennini T, Gobbi M, Taddei C (1988) Characterization of high affinity and stereospecific ^{3}H-*d*-fenfluramine binding rat brain. *Neurochem Int* **13**, 345.

107. Middaugh LD, Blackwell LA, Santos CA III (1974) Effects of *d*-amphetamine sulfate given to pregnant mice on activity and on catecholamines in the brains of offspring. *Develop Psychobiol* **7**, 429.

108. Miller MA, Hughes AL (1994) Epidemiology of amphetamine use in the United States. In: *Amphetamine and Its Analogs: Psychopharmacology, Toxicology and Abuse*. Cho AK, Segal DS eds. Academic Press, San Diego p. 439.

109. Molliver DC, Molliver ME (1990) Anatomic evidence for a neurotoxic effect of (±)-fenfluramine upon serotonergic projections in the rat. *Brain Res* **511**, 165.

110. Molliver ME, O'Hearn E, Battaglia G, De Souza EB (1986) Direct intracerebral administration of MDA and MDMA does not produce serotonin neurotoxicity. *Soc Neurosci Abstr* **12**, 1234.

111. Mori A, Suzuki H, Ishiyama I (1992) Three cases of acute methamphetamine intoxication—analysis of optically active methamphetamine. *Jpn J Legal Med* **46**, 266.

112. Nasello AG, Ramirez OA (1978) Brain catecholamines metabolism in offspring of amphetamine treated rats. *Pharmacol Biochem Behav* **9**, 17.

113. Nash JF (1990) Ketanserin pretreatment attenuates MDMA-induced dopamine release in the striatum as measured by *in vivo* microdialysis. *Life Sci* **47**, 2401.

114. Nash JF, Meltzer HY, Gudelsky G (1990) Effect of 3,4-methylenedioxymethamphetamine on 3,4-dihydroxyphenylalanine accumulation in the striatum and nucleus accumbens. *J Neurochem* **54**, 1062.

115. Nichols DE (1994) Medicinal chemistry and structure-activity relationships. In: *Amphetamine and Its Analogs: Psychopharmacology, Toxicology and Abuse*. Cho AK, Segal DS eds. Academic Press, San Diego p. 3.

116. Nurnberger J, Gershon E, Jimerson D *et al.* (1981) Pharmacogenetics of *d*-amphetamine in man. In: *Genetic Research Strategies for Psychobiology and Psychiatry*. Gershon ES, Matthysse S, Breakfield XO, Ciranello RD eds. Boxwood Press, Pacific Grove p. 257.

117. O'Hearn E, Battaglia G, De Souza EB *et al.* (1988) Methylenedioxyamphetamine (MDA) and methylenedioxymethamphetamine (MDMA) cause selective ablation of serotonergic axon terminals in forebrain: Immunocytochemical evidence for neurotoxicity. *J Neurosci* **8**, 2788.

118. O'Malley PM, Bachman JG, Johnston LD (1988) Period, age, and cohort effects on substance use among young Americans: A decade of change, 1976–86. *Amer J Public Health* **78**, 1315.

119. Oro AS, Dixon SD (1987) Perinatal cocaine and methamphetamine exposure: Maternal and neonatal correlates. *J Pediat* **111**, 571.

120. Paris JM, Cunningham KA (1991) Lack of serotonin neurotoxicity after intraraphe microinjection of (+)-3,4-methylenedioxymethamphetamine (MDMA). *Brain Res Bull* **28**, 115.

121. Peroutka SJ (1987) Incidence of recreational use of 3,4 methylenedioxymethamphetamine (MDMA, "ecstasy") on an undergraduate campus. *N Engl J Med* **317**, 1542.

122. Peroutka SJ, Pasco N, Faull KF (1987) Monoamine metabolites in the cerebrospinal fluid of recreational users of 3,4-methylenedioxymethamphetamine (MDMA; "Ecstasy"). *Res Commun Subst Abuse* **8**, 125.

123. Pinder RM, Brogde RN, Sawyer PR *et al.* (1975) Fenfluramine: A review of its pharmacological properties and therapeutic efficacy in obesity. *Drugs* **10**, 241.

124. Price LH, Ricaurte GA, Krystal JH (1989) Neuroendocrine and mood responses to intravenous L-tryptophan in 3,4-methylenedioxymethamphetamine (MDMA) users. *Arch Gen Psychiat* **46**, 20.

125. Przedborski S, Kostic V, Jackson-Lewis V *et al.* (1992) Transgenic mice with increased Cu/Zn-superoxide dismutase activity are resistant to N-methyl-4-phenyl-1,2,3,6-tetrahydropyridine-induced neurotoxicity. *J Neurosci* **12**, 1658.

126. Raiteri M, Giambattista G, Vallebuona F (1995) *In vitro* and *in vivo* effects of *d*-fenfluramine: No apparent relation between 5-hydroxytryptamine release and hypophagia. *J Pharmacol Exp Ther* **273**, 643.

127. Randall T (1992) Ecstasy-fueled 'rave' parties become dances of death for English youths. *J Amer Med Assn* **268**, 1505.

128. Reis DJ, Baker H, Fink JS *et al.* (1979) A genetic control of central dopamine neurons in relation to brain organization, drug responses and behavior. In: *Catecholamines: Basic and Clinical Frontiers*. Pergamon Press, New York p. 23.

129. Ricaurte GA, Bryan G, Strauss L *et al.* (1985) Hallucinogenic amphetamine selectively destroys brain serotonin nerve terminals. *Science* **229**, 986.

130. Ricaurte GA, Finnegan KT, Irwin I (1990) Aminergic metabolites in cerebrospinal fluid of humans previously exposed to MDMA: Preliminary observations. *Ann N Y Acad Sci* **600**, 699.

131. Ricaurte GA, Forno LS, Wilson MA *et al.* (1988) (±) 3,4-Methylenedioxymethamphetamine selectively damages central serotonergic neurons in nonhuman primates. *J Amer Med Assn* **260**, 51.

132. Ricaurte GA, Guillery RW, Seiden LS *et al.* (1982) Dopamine nerve terminal degeneration produced by high doses of methylamphetamine in the rat brain. *Brain Res* **235**, 93.

133. Ricaurte GA, Katz JL, Martello MB (1992) Lasting effects of (±)-3,4-methylenedioxymethamphetamine (MDMA) on central serotonergic neurons in nonhuman primates: Neurochemical observations. *J Pharmacol Exp Ther* **261**, 616.

134. Ricaurte GA, Molliver ME, Martello MB *et al.* (1991) Dexfenfluramine neurotoxicity in brains of non-human primates. *Lancet* **338**, 1487.

135. Ricaurte GA, Sabol KE, Seiden L (1994) Functional consequences of neurotoxic amphetamine exposure. In: *Amphetamine and Its Analogs: Psychopharmacology, Toxicology and Abuse*. Cho AK, Segal DS eds. Academic Press, San Diego p. 297.

136. Richards JB, Baggott MJ, Sabol KE (1993) A high-dose methamphetamine regimen results in long-lasting deficits on performance of a reaction-time task. *Brain Res* **627**, 254.

137. Robinson TE, Yew J, Paulson PE (1990) The long-term effects of neurotoxic doses of methamphetamine in the

extracellular concentration of dopamine measured with microdialysis in striatum. *Neurosci Lett* **110**, 193.

138. Rowland NE, Carlton J (1986) Neurobiology of an anorectic drug: Fenfluramine. *Prog Neurobiol* **27**, 13.

139. Sabol KE, Richards JB, Seiden LS (1992) Fenfluramine-induced increases in extracellular hippocampal serotonin are progressively attenuated *in vivo* during a four-day fenfluramine regimen in rats. *Brain Res* **571**, 64.

140. Santer N (1969) Fenfluramine overdosage. *Lancet* **ii**, 322.

141. Sato M (1992) A lasting vulnerability to psychosis in patients with previous methamphetamine psychosis. *Ann N Y Acad Sci* **654**, 160.

142. Sato M, Fujiwara Y (1986) Behavioral and neurochemical changes in pups prenatally exposed to methamphetamine. *Brain Dev* **8**, 390.

143. Schmidt CJ (1987) Neurotoxicity of the psychedelic amphetamine, methylenedioxymethamphetamine. *J Pharmacol Exp Ther* **240**, 1.

144. Schmidt CJ (1994) Neurochemistry of ring-substituted amphetamine analogs. In: *Amphetamine and Its Analogs: Psychopharmacology, Toxicology and Abuse.* Cho AK, Segal DS eds. Academic Press, San Diego p. 151.

145. Schmidt CJ, Black CK, Taylor VL (1990) Antagonism of the neurotoxicity due to a single administration of methylenedioxymethamphetamine. *Eur J Pharmacol* **181**, 59.

146. Schmidt CJ, Gibb JW (1985) Role of the dopamine uptake carrier in the neurochemical response to methamphetamine: Effects of amfonelic acid. *Eur J Pharmacol* **109**, 73.

147. Schmidt CJ, Kehne JH (1990) Neurotoxicity of MDMA: Neurochemical effects. *Ann N Y Acad Sci* **600**, 665.

148. Schmidt CJ, Taylor VL (1987) Depression of rat brain tryptophan hydroxylase activity following the acute administration of methylenedioxymethamphetamine. *Biochem Pharmacol* **36**, 4095.

149. Schmidt CJ, Taylor VL, Abbate GM, Nieduzak TR (1991) 5-HT$_2$ antagonists stereoselectively prevent the neurotoxicity of 3,4-methylenedioxymethamphetamine by blocking the acute stimulation of dopamine synthesis: Reversal by L-dopa. *J Pharmacol Exp Ther* **256**, 230.

150. Schneider J, Pope A, Simpson A *et al.* (1992) Recovery from experimental parkinsonism with GM1 ganglioside treatment. *Science* **256**, 843.

151. Schuster CR, Lewis M, Seiden LS (1986) Fenfluramine: neurotoxicity. *Psychopharmacol Bull* **22**, 148.

152. Seiden LS (1991) Neurotoxicity of methamphetamine: Mechanisms of action and issues related to aging. *U.S. Natl Inst Drug Abuse (NIDA) Res Monogr* **115**, 24.

153. Seiden LS (1995) *Neurotoxicity and Efficacy of Fenfluramine.* U.S. Food and Drug Administration Advisory Panel, Sept 28, 1995.

154. Seiden LS, Fischman MW, Schuster CR (1975/76) Long-term methamphetamine-induced changes in brain cate-

cholamines in tolerant rhesus monkeys. *Drug Alcohol Dependence* **1**, 215.

155. Seiden LS, Sabol KE (1995) Neurotoxicity of methamphetamine-related drugs and cocaine. In: *Handbook of Neurotoxicology.* Chang LW, Dyer RS eds. Marcel Dekker, New York p. 825.

156. Seiden LS, Sabol KE, Ricaurte GA (1993) Amphetamine: Effects on catecholamine systems and behavior. *Annu Rev Pharmacol Toxicol* **32**, 639.

157. Seiden LS, Vosmer G (1984) Formation of 6-hydroxydopamine in caudate nucleus of the rat brain after a single large dose of methylamphetamine. *Pharmacol Biochem Behav* **21**, 29.

158. Seiden LS, Woolverton WL, Lorens SA *et al.* (1993) Behavioral consequences of partial monoamine depletion in the CNS after methamphetamine-like drugs: The conflict between pharmacology and toxicology. *U.S. Natl Inst Drug Abuse (NIDA) Res Monogr* **136**, 34.

159. Shibata S, Mori K, Sekine I *et al.* (1991) Subarachnoid and intracerebral hemorrhage associated with necrotizing angiitis due to methamphetamine abuse. *Neurol Med Chir (Tokyo)* **31**, 49.

160. Slikker W, Holson RR, Ali SF *et al.* (1989) Behavioral and neurochemical effects of orally administered MDMA in the rodent and nonhuman primate. *Neurotoxicology* **10**, 529.

161. Slivka A, Cohen G (1985) Hydroxyl radical attack on dopamine. *J Biol Chem* **260**, 15466.

162. Solowij N, Hall W, Lee N (1992) Recreational MDMA use in Sydney: A profile of 'Ecstasy' users and their experiences with the drug. *Brit J Addict* **87**, 1161.

163. Sonsalla PK, Gibb JW, Hanson GR (1986) Roles of D$_1$ and D$_2$ dopamine receptor subtypes in mediating the methamphetamine-induced changes in monoamine systems. *J Pharmacol Exp Ther* **238**, 932.

164. Sonsalla PK, Nicklas WJ, Heikkila RE (1989) Role for excitatory amino acids in methamphetamine-induced nigrostriatal dopaminergic toxicity. *Science* **243**, 398.

165. Sonsalla PK, Riordan DE, Heikkila RE (1991) Competitive and noncompetitive antagonists at N-methyl-D-aspartate receptors protect against methamphetamine-induced dopaminergic damage in mice. *J Pharmacol Exp Ther* **256**, 506.

166. Sotelo C (1991) Immunohistochemical study of short- and long-term effects of DL-fenfluramine on the serotonergic innervation of the rat hippocampal formation. *Brain Res* **541**, 309.

167. Spanos LJ, Yamamoto BK (1989) Acute and subchronic effects of methylenedioxymethamphetamine [(±)MDMA] on locomotion and serotonin syndrome behavior in the rat. *Pharmacol Biochem Behav* **32**, 835.

168. Stahl K, Imperiale TF (1993) An overview of the efficacy and safety of fenfluramine and mazindol in the treatment of obesity. *Arch Fam Med* **2**, 1033.

169. Steele TD, Brewster WK, Johnson MP et al. (1991) Assessment of the role of alpha-methylepinine in the neurotoxicity of MDMA. *Pharmacol Biochem Behav* **39**, 345.

170. Steele TD, McCann UA, Ricaurte GA (1994) 3,4-Methylenedioxymethamphetamine (MDMA, "Ecstasy"): Pharmacology and toxicology in animals and humans. *Addiction* **89**, 539.

171. Steele TD, Nichols DE, Yim GKW (1987) Stereochemical effects of 3,4-methylenedioxymethamphetamine (MDMA) and related amphetamine derivatives on inhibition of uptake of ³H-monoamines into synaptosomes from different regions of rat brain. *Biochem Pharmacol* **36**, 2297.

172. Stek AM, Fisher BK, Baker RS et al. (1993) Maternal and fetal cardiovascular responses to methamphetamine in the pregnant sheep. *Amer J Obstet Gynecol* **169** (4), 888.

173. Steranka LR, Sanders-Bush E (1979) Long-term effects of fenfluramine on central serotonergic mechanisms. *Neuropharmacology* **18**, 895.

174. St. Omer VE, Ali SF, Holson RR (1991) Behavioral and neurochemical effects of prenatal methylenedioxymethamphetamine (MDMA) exposure in rats. *Neurotoxicol Teratol* **13**, 13.

175. Stone DM, Hanson GR, Gibb JW (1987) Differences in the central serotonergic effects of methylenedioxymethamphetamine (MDMA) in mice and rats. *Neuropharmacology* **26**, 1657.

176. Stone DM, Johnson M, Hanson GR (1988) Role of endogenous dopamine in the central serotonergic deficits induced by 3,4-methylenedioxymethamphetamine. *J Pharmacol Exp Ther* **247**, 79.

177. Tatetsu S (1972) Methamphetamine psychosis. In: *Current Concept on Amphetamine Abuse*. Ellinwood EH, Cohen S eds. DHEW Publication No. (HSM) 72-9085, U.S. Government Printing Office, Washington, DC p. 159.

178. Terleckyj I, Sonsalla PK (1994) The *sigma* receptor ligand (±)-BMY 14802 prevents methamphetamine-induced dopaminergic neurotoxicity *via* interactions at dopamine receptors. *J Pharmacol Exp Ther* **269**, 44.

179. Teuchert-Noodt G, Dawirs RR (1991) Age-related toxicity in prefrontal cortex and caudate-putamen complex of gerbils (*Meriones unguiculatus*) after a single dose of methamphetamine. *Neuropharmacology* **30**, 733.

180. Tonge SR (1973) Permanent alterations in 5-hydroxyindole concentrations in discrete areas of rat brain produced by pre- and neonatal administration of methylamphetamine and chlorpromazine. *J Neurochem* **20**, 625.

181. Tonge SR (1973) Permanent alterations in catecholamine concentrations in discrete areas of brain in the offspring of rats treated with methylamphetamine and chlorpromazine. *Brit J Pharmacol* **47**, 425.

182. USP DI (1995) *Drug Information for the Health Care Professional. Vol 1. 5th Ed.* Rand McNally, Taunton, Massachusetts.

183. Vidal L, Heller B, Won L, Heller A (1995) Quantitation of dopaminergic neurons in 3-dimensional reaggregate tissue culture by computer-assisted image analysis. *J Neurosci Meth* **56**, 89.

184. Wagner GC, Lucot JB, Schuster CR (1983) L-Methyltyrosine attenuates and reserpine increases methamphetamine-induced neuronal changes. *Brain Res* **270**, 285.

185. Wagner GC, Ricaurte GA, Seiden LS et al. (1980) Long-lasting depletions of striatal dopamine and loss of dopamine uptake sites following repeated administration of methamphetamine. *Brain Res* **181**, 151.

186. Wagner GC, Schuster CR, Seiden LS (1981) Neurochemical consequences following administration of CNS stimulants to the neonatal rat. *Pharmacol Biochem Behav* **14**, 117.

187. Wagner GC, Seiden LS, Schuster CR (1979) Methamphetamine-induced changes in brain catecholamines in rats and guinea pigs. *Drug Alcohol Dependence* **4**, 435.

188. Wagner GC, Tekirian TL, Cheo CT (1993) Sexual differences in sensitivity to methamphetamine toxicity. *J Neural Transm* **93**, 67.

189. Wahnschaffe U, Esslen J (1985) Structural evidence for the neurotoxicity of methylamphetamine in the frontal cortex of gerbils (*Meriones unguiculatus*): A light and electron microscopical study. *Brain Res* **337**, 299.

190. Walsh SL, Wagner GC (1992) Motor impairments after methamphetamine-induced neurotoxicity in the rat. *J Pharmacol Exp Ther* **263**, 617.

191. Weissman AD, Caldecott-Hazard S (1993) *In utero* methamphetamine effects: I. Behavior and monoamine uptake sites in adult offspring. *Synapse* **13**, 241.

192. Westphalen RI, Dodd RR (1993) New evidence for a loss of serotonergic nerve terminals in rats treated with d,l-fenfluramine. *Pharmacol Toxicol* **72**, 249.

193. Westphalen RI, Dodd PR (1993) The regeneration of d,l-fenfluramine-destroyed serotonergic nerve terminals. *Eur J Pharmacol* **238**, 399.

194. Won LA, Kontur PJ, Choi HR et al. (1992) Acute and persistent effects of methamphetamine on developing monoaminergic neurons in reaggregate tissue culture. *Brain Res* **575**, 6.

195. Woolverton WL, Ricaurte GA, Forno LS (1989) Long-term effects of chronic methamphetamine administration in rhesus monkeys. *Brain Res* **486**, 73.

196. Yamada T, McGeer PL, Baimbridge KG et al. (1990) Relative sparing in Parkinson's disease of substantia nigra dopamine neurons containing calbindin-D$_{28K}$. *Brain Res* **526**, 303.

197. Yamamoto BK, Spanos LJ (1988) The acute effects of methylenedioxymethamphetamine on dopamine release in the awake-behaving rat. *Eur J Pharmacol* **148**, 195.

198. Yamamoto T, Takano R, Egashira T et al. (1984) Metabolism of methamphetamine, amphetamine and *p*-hydroxymethamphetamine by rat-liver microsomal preparations *in vitro*. *Xenobiotica* 14, 867.

199. Yen DJ, Wang SJ, Ju TH et al. (1994) Stroke associated with methamphetamine inhalation. *Eur Neurol* 34, 16.

200. Zaczek R, Battaglia G, Culp S et al. (1990) Effects of repeated fenfluramine administration on indices of monoamine function in rat brain: Pharmacokinetic, dose response, regional specificity and time course data. *J Pharmacol Exp Ther* 253, 104.

201. Zaczek R, Hurt S, Culp S et al. (1989) Characterization of brain interactions with methylene-dioxyamphetamine and methylenedioxymethamphetamine. *U.S. Natl Inst Drug Abuse (NIDA) Res Monogr* 94, 223.

202. Zhao ZY, Castagnoli N Jr, Ricaurte GA et al. (1992) Synthesis and neurotoxicological evaluation of putative metabolites of the serotonergic neurotoxin 2-(methylamino)-1-[3,4-(methylenedioxy)phenyl] propane [(methylenedioxy)methamphetamine]. *Chem Res Toxicol* 5, 89.

203. Zigmond MJ, Hastings TG, Abercrombie ED (1992) Neurochemical responses to 6-hydroxydopamine and L-dopa therapy: implications for Parkinson's disease. *Ann N Y Acad Sci* 648, 71.

204. Zigmond MJ, Stricker EM (1974) Ingestive behavior following damage to central dopamine neurons: Implications for homeostasis and recovery of function. In: *Neuropsychopharmacology of Monoamines and Regulatory Enzymes*. Raven Press, New York p. 385.

Amphotericin B

Herbert H. Schaumburg

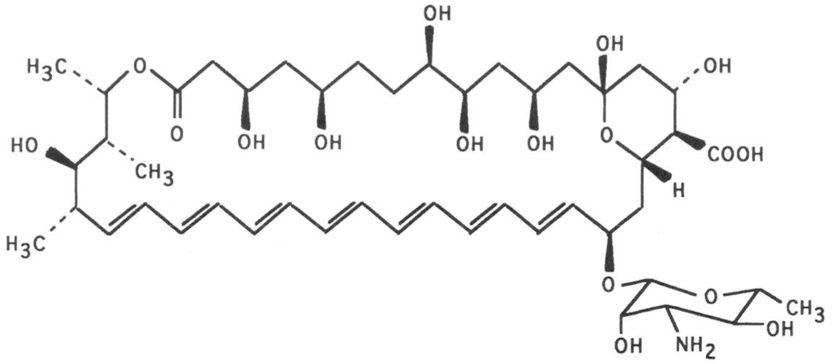

AMPHOTERICIN B
$C_{47}H_{73}NO_{17}$

Amphozone; Fungizone

NEUROTOXICITY RATING
Clinical

A   Myelopathy (local administration)

Amphotericin B, a fungistatic polyene antibiotic produced by *Streptomyces nodosus*, is a primary drug in the treatment of disseminated cryptococcoses.

Formidable systemic toxicity is associated with intravenous administration, including fever, chills, azotemia, and hypokalemia. Neurotoxicity has not been clearly associated with intravenous administration, since there is little penetration into the cerebrospinal fluid. Reports of neurological illness (seizures, tremors, paresis) associated with intravenous administration of amphotericin likely represent CNS manifestations of the underlying infectious disease. Intrathecal administration is frequently accompanied by severe local pain and transient signs of generalized meningeal reaction. Persistent focal myelopathy and disseminated radiculopathy are reported; they are attributed to meningovascular reactions to local accumulations of the drug (1).

In Wistar rats, amphotericin B produced local and systemic effects characterized by neuronal degeneration and myelin damage after intracisternal and intravenous injection, respectively. The monomethyl ester derivative of amphotericin B exhibited a lower neurotoxic potency (2).

REFERENCE
1. Carnevale NT, Calgiani N, Stevens DZ (1980) Amphotericin B induced myelopathy. *Arch Intern Med* 140, 1189.
2. Reuhl KR, Vapiwala M, Ryzlak MT, Schaffner CP (1993) Comparative neurotoxicities of amphotericin B and its mono-methyl ester derivative in rats. *Antimicrob Agents Chemother* 37, 419.

Amsacrine

Albert C. Ludolph

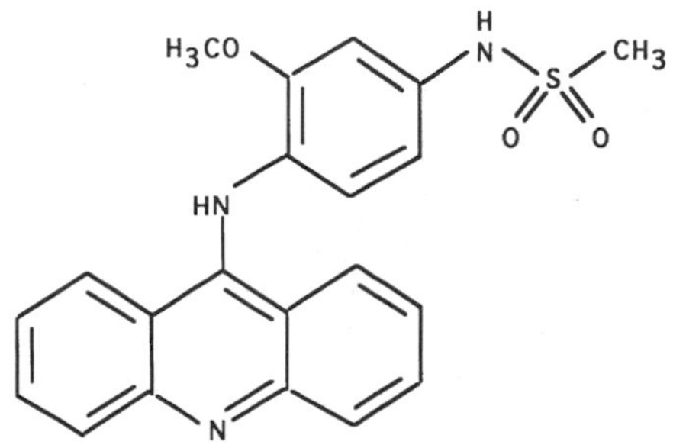

AMSACRINE
$C_{21}H_{19}N_3O_3S$

N-[4-(9-Acridinylamino)-3-methoxyphenyl]
methanesulfonamide; AMSA

NEUROTOXICITY RATING

Clinical

A   Seizure disorder (local administration)

The synthetic aminoacridine, amsacrine (AMSA, *m*-AMSA), is used as an antitumor agent, since it intercalates into DNA and inhibits nuclear and mitochondrial topoisomerase II in mammals (8). The enzyme is inhibited because amsacrine induces a covalent attachment of topoisomerase to both strands of the double helix by stabilizing the cleavable complex, a reaction intermediate. *m*-AMSA, like cisplatin and mitomycin C, inhibits ubiquitin-adenosine triphosphate (ATP)-dependent proteolysis (4). The related compound *o*-AMSA is ineffective as a cancer treatment.

The blood-brain barrier severely limits the entry of intravenously administered *m*-AMSA into cerebrospinal fluid (CSF) (1). After direct intraventricular administration, *m*-AMSA had a CSF half-life of only 115 min and clinical neurotoxic effects were not observed. Histopathological studies were not performed. Generalized seizures accompanied treatment with amsacrine in a few patients (6,7,9). Single lethal doses of *m*-AMSA cause ataxia and seizures in dogs and monkeys (3). Other observations on neurological manifestations, such as peripheral neuropathy (2,5), are likely unrelated to *m*-AMSA.

REFERENCES

1. Gormley P, Riccardi R, O'Neill D, Poplack D (1984) Intrathecally administered *m*-AMSA in the rhesus monkey. *Cancer Drug Deliv* 1, 101.
2. Grove WR, Fortner CL, Wiemik PH (1982) Review of amsacrine, an investigational antineoplastic drug. *Clin Pharm* 1, 320.
3. Henry MC, Port CD, Guarino AM *et al.* (1976) Preclinical toxicologic evaluation of 4'-(9-acridinylamino)-methanesulphon-*m*-anisidide (AMSA) therapy. Report no. IITRI-Tox 2499922-76-2. Bethesda, MD: U.S. National Cancer Institute, NIH.
4. Isoe T, Naito M, Hirai R, Tsuruo T (1991) Inhibition of ubiquitin-ATP-dependent proteolysis and ubiquitination by cisplatin. *Anticancer Res* 11, 1905.
5. Jehn U, Heinemann V (1991) New drugs in the treatment of acute and chronic leukemia with some emphasis on *m*-AMSA. *Anticancer Res* 11, 705.
6. Legha SS, Latreille J, McCredie KB, Bodey GP (1979) Neurologic and cardiac rhythm abnormalities associated with 4'-(9-acridinylamino)-methanesulfon-*m*-anisidide (AMSA) therapy. *Cancer Treatment Rep* 63, 2001.
7. Legha SS, Keating MJ, McCredie KB *et al.* (1982) Evaluation of AMSA in previously treated patients with acute leukemia: Results of therapy in 109 adults. *Blood* 60, 484.
8. Lin JH, Castora FJ (1991) DNA topoisomerase II from mammalian mitochondria is inhibited by the antitumor drugs, *m*-AMSA and VM-26. *Biochem Biophys Res Commun* 176, 690.
9. Mittelman A, Arlin MA (1983) AMSA-induced seizures in patients with hypokalemia. *Cancer Treatment Rep* 67, 102.

A-MTX

Albert C. Ludolph

Wasp toxin

NEUROTOXICITY RATING
Experimental
A Ion channel dysfunction?

A-MTX is a high-molecular-weight (43,700) neurotoxin venom of the braconid wasp, *Microbracon hebetor* (3). The compound inhibits presynaptic excitatory neuromuscular transmission in insects (2). γ-Aminobutyric acidergic and cholinergic neurotransmission seem to be unaffected (2). Differential sensitivity can be observed in insects of different orders (1), and A-MTX is likely inactive in non-insects (2). B-MTX, a second neurotoxin (MW 56,700) in *M. hebetor* venom, also blocks excitatory neuromuscular transmission in insects (2).

REFERENCES

1. Piek T (1982) Solitary wasp venoms and toxins as tools for the study of neuromuscular transmission in insects. In: *Neuropharmacology of Insects. Ciba Found Symp* 88. Pitman, London p. 275.
2. Piek T (1984) Pharmacology of *Hymenoptera* venoms. In: *Handbook of Natural Toxins. Vol 2. Insect Poisons, Allergens and Other Invertebrate Venoms.* Tu AT ed. Marcel Dekker, New York p. 135.
3. Visser BJ, Labruyere WT, Spanjer W, Piek T (1983) Characterization of two paralysing protein toxins (A-MTX and B-MTX), isolated from a homogenate of the wasp *Microbracon hebetor* (Say). *Comp Biochem Physiol Pt B* **75B**, 523.

Amyl Alcohols

Herbert H. Schaumburg

$$CH_3CH_2CH_2CH(OH)CH_3$$

1-PENTANOL
$C_5H_{12}O$

1-Pentanol; *n*-Amyl alcohol

NEUROTOXICITY RATING
Clinical
B Acute encephalopathy (vertigo, delerium)

The amyl alcohols are a group of eight structural isomers of saturated 5-carbon aliphatic alcohols widely used as industrial solvents. The metabolism and toxicology of only *n*-amyl alcohol (1-pentanol) is well characterized. A Threshold Limit Value has not been established.

n-Amyl alcohol is well absorbed following ingestion or inhalation and readily enters the brain. At the murine acute oral LD_{50} level, 3.03 g/kg, there is gastrointestinal irritation and CNS depression. *n*-Amyl alcohol is severely irritating to the skin and mucous membranes of experimental animals and humans.

Human industrial or accidental inhalation exposures to high levels of pure amyl alcohol mixtures have not been described; all instances have involved mixtures containing other aliphatic or aromatic hydrocarbons. Signs attributed to high-level exposure to amyl alcohols include corneal irritation, cough, dyspnea, headache, vertigo, double vision, delirium, stupor, and coma (1). Nonindustrial cases from drinking fusel oil have additionally displayed glycosuria.

REFERENCE

1. Lington AW, Bevan C (1994) Amyl alcohols. In: *Patty's Industrial Hygiene and Toxicology. Vol ll.* Clayton G, Clayton F eds. Wiley Neuroscience, New York p. 2652.

Anabasine

Albert C. Ludolph

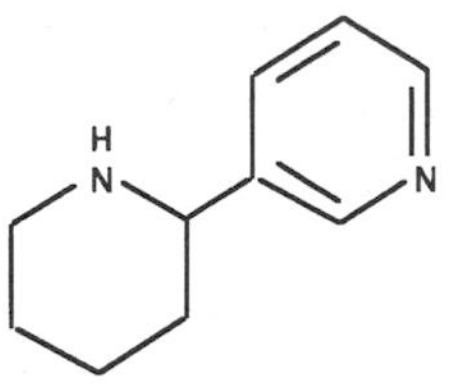

ANABASINE
$C_{10}H_{14}N_2$

2-(3-Pyridyl)piperidine

NEUROTOXICITY RATING

Experimental

A Ataxia

Anabasine is a low-molecular-weight component of cigarette smoke and an alkaloid produced by *Nicotiana* spp., in particular *N. acaulis*, *N. glauca* (wild tree tobacco), *N. petuniodes*, and *N. solanifolia* (2). Anatabine, 2-(3-pyridyl)-1,2,3,6-tetrahydropyridine, resembles anabasine chemically. The other two major alkaloids in *Nicotiana* spp. are nicotin and nornicotin. The chemically related compound anabasine is the major toxin of the Pacific hoplonemertine *Paranemertes peregrina*, which presumably uses the alkaloid for defense or to paralyze its prey (7). Anabasine is also a natural product of the species *Amphiporus angulatus*, *Amphiporus lactifloreus*, and *Zygonemertes virescens*. (7). No cases of human poisoning by these species are reported. The toxin anabasine is also produced by *Aphaenogaster* spp. (11).

Application of anabasine or dried plant material to pregnant sows induced arthrogryposis and cleft palates in the offspring (6); a dosage of 2.6 mg/kg body weight anabasine caused tremors, gait disturbances, and recumbency in the pregnant animals. In sheep (5), *N. glauca* plants containing anabasine acutely caused excessive salivation, irregular gait, wobbling while walking or standing, and death. In goats, (10) anabasine induced ataxia, incoordination, muscular weakness, prostration, and eventual death. The toxic effects of *Nicotiana* spp. on livestock have been recently reviewed (9).

Similar to nicotine, but less potently, anabasine activates Na^+ and K^+ channels in mouse brain synaptosomes (8). The compound inhibits acetylcholinesterase *in vitro* (4). Experiments in mice showed that chronic anabasine treatment (like nicotine) increases the number of brain nicotine receptors (1).

A few cases of human toxicity dominated by nicotine-like effects have been reported. One possible human case of fatal poisoning by ingestion of leaves of *N. glauca* has occurred (3). Anabasine, the major toxin of this plant, was detected by chemical analysis in all body specimens examined.

REFERENCES

1. Bhat RV, Turner SL, Selvaag SR *et al.* (1991) Regulation of brain nicotinic receptors by chronic agonist infusion. *J Neurochem* **56**, 1932.
2. Bush LP, Crowe MW (1989) *Nicotiana* alkaloids. In: *Toxicants of Plant Origin*. Cheeke PR ed. CRC Press, Boca Raton, Florida p. 87.
3. Castorena JL, Garriott JC, Bernhardt FE, Shaw RF (1987) A fatal poisoning from *Nicotiana glauca*. *J Toxicol-Clin Toxicol* **25**, 429.
4. Karadsheh N, Kussie P, Linthicum DS (1991) Inhibition of acetylcholinesterase by caffeine, anabasine, and methyl pyrrolidine and their derivatives. *Toxicol Lett* **55**, 335.
5. Keeler RF, Crowe MW (1984) Teratogenicity and toxicity of wild tree tobacco, *Nicotiana glauca* in sheep. *Cornell Vet* **74**, 50.
6. Keeler RF, Crowe MW, Lambert EA (1984) Teratogenicity in swine of the tobacco alkaloid anabasine isolated from *Nicotiana glauca*. *Teratology* **30**, 61.
7. Kem WR (1988) Worm toxins. In: *Handbook of Natural Toxins. Vol 3. Marine Toxins and Venoms*. Tu AT ed. Marcel Dekker, New York p. 388.
8. Marks MJ, Farnham DA, Grady SR, Collins AC (1993) Nicotinic receptor function determined by stimulation of rubidium efflux from mouse brain synaptosomes. *J Pharmacol Exp Ther* **264**, 542.
9. Panter KE, James LF, Gardner DR (1999) Lupines, poison-hemlock and *Nicotiana* spp: toxicity and teratogenicity in livestock. *Nat Toxins* **8**, 117.
10. Panter KE, Keeler RF, Bunch TD, Callan RJ (1990) Congenital skeletal malformations and cleft palate induced in goats by ingestion of *Lupinus*, *Conium*, and *Nicotiana* species. *Toxicon* **28**, 1377.
11. Wheeler JW, Olubajo O, Storm CB, Duffield RM (1981) Anabasine: Venom alkaloid of *Aphaenogaster* ants. *Science* **211**, 1051.

Anatoxins

Wayne W. Carmichael
Edward G. Hyde

ANATOXIN-A
$C_{10}H_{15}NO$

ANATOXIN-A(S)
$C_7H_{17}N_4O_4P$

Anatoxin-a; (2-acetyl-9-azabi*cyclo* [4.2.1] non-2-ene)

NEUROTOXICITY RATING

Experimental

A   Neuromuscular transmission dysfunction

A   Nicotinic receptor agonist

Anatoxin-a(s)

NEUROTOXICITY RATING

Experimental

A   Flaccid paralysis

A   Neuromuscular transmission dysfunction (cholinesterase inhibition)

Anatoxin-a is a bicyclic secondary amine isolated from at least three genera of freshwater cyanobacteria (blue-green algae) including *Anabaena*, *Aphanizomenon*, and *Oscillatoria*. Certain strains of *Oscillatoria rubescens* also produce a methylene homologue of anatoxin-a called homoanatoxin-a (4). The structure of anatoxin-a was determined by x-ray crystallography, and synthetic routes to the structure were explored. Originally extracted from cells of these organisms by a variety of techniques—mainly high-performance liquid chromatography and thin-layer chromatography (11,26)—anatoxin-a was synthesized prior to 1984 in optically pure form, from either cocaine or 1-methylpyrrole (2,3).

Neither of these synthetic strategies allowed significant chemical modification of anatoxin-a for detailed structure–activity studies. Optically pure (+)-anatoxin-a, along with the inactive (−)-isomer, can now be obtained from L-glutamic acid in gram quantities (18,25,28). With the synthesis of anatoxin-a simplified, analogs with chemical modification of the nitrogen or the carbonyl side chain, and fused-ring analogs could be synthesized in yields sufficient to perform structure-activity studies (14,15,27). Biosynthesis of anatoxin-a has been proposed from ornithine/arginine *via* putrescine. Putrescine is oxidized to pyrroline,

a precursor of anatoxin-a (9). Other research using ^{13}C nuclear magnetic resonance shows that anatoxin-a biosynthesis from glutamic acid takes place in a way that does not support a pathway related to tropane alkaloids (13).

The activities of 15 derivatives of anatoxin-a, including the active and inactive optical isomers, have been investigated in a variety of systems. Several assays were used, including (a) binding assays with PNS and CNS nicotinic receptors exploring competitive and noncompetitive (channel-blocking properties) interactions, (b) functional assays of evoked twitch response from isolated nerve-muscle preparations, and (c) electrophysiological effects on resting membrane potentials and action potentials. Pharmacologically, anatoxin-a is a potent agonist at nicotinic receptors and is more potent than the natural ligand, acetylcholine. The toxic potential of anatoxin-a was first observed in cases of wild and domestic animal poisonings and the *in vivo* evaluation of algal extracts in laboratory animals (5,10).

In isolated skeletal muscle preparations, anatoxin-a added to the bathing solution in concentrations of 2.5 mmol or greater produces reversible blockade of the directly elicited muscle twitch and long-lasting depression of the indirectly elicited twitch (30). Electrophysiological analysis of the actions of anatoxin-a at the acetylcholine receptor shows a rapid depolarization of the membrane potential followed by desensitization of the receptor. Anatoxin-a fails to inhibit the receptor by blocking the cation channel (30). The agent is thus similar to the natural agonist, acetylcholine, producing a depolarizing blockade of the acetylcholine receptor.

Preliminary structure–activity studies compared anatoxin-a to other rigid or rotationally constrained nicotinic agonists. The focus of this early work was on the secondary amine of anatoxin-a. Compounds with a tertiary or quaternary amine [such as (−)-ferrugiine, arecolone, and 3-acetylpyridoine methiodide] were compared with anatoxin-a for their ability to activate frog rectus abdominus muscle. Anatoxin-a was shown to be the most potent; the (+)-isomer was 1000 times more potent than the (−)-isomer, showing that the nicotinic receptor is sensitive to stereochemistry (29). Additional studies were undertaken to define the role of stereochemistry in the greater potency of anatoxin-a relative to acetylcholine. Anatoxin-a was shown to bind to the nicotinic receptor with higher affinity than that of acetylcholine and to desensitize the receptor to a lesser extent. The high affinity of anatoxin-a for the nicotinic receptor may be due in part to the rigid nature of the compound and protonation of the amine at physiological pH (31).

The structures that lead to potent agonists based on anatoxin-a were further defined as were the modifications that produced selectivity for peripheral *vs.* central nicotinic receptors (33,35). Anatoxin-a was modified on the carbonyl side chain into three broad groups: (a) the carbon adjacent to the carbonyl was replaced with a hydrogen, methyl ester, a primary alcohol, or the double bond was reduced on the ring; (b) the carbonyl was reduced to an alcohol, with or without a methyl group on the carbonyl carbon, or (c) the carbon adjacent to the carbonyl was replaced with an amide. Modification of the nitrogen generates less potent agonists and was not pursued in these studies (7,32). All analogs were at least tenfold less potent than anatoxin-a in their ability to induce contraction of the frog rectus abdominus muscle, and they were comparably less potent in displacing ^{125}I-α-bungarotoxin from nicotinic receptors. However, in rat brain P2 membranes that contain nicotinic receptors with a high affinity for nicotine- and bungarotoxin-binding proteins of anatoxin-a, anatoxinic acid isoxaxolidide, anatoxinic acid methoxyamide, and anatoxinal had selectivity for neuronal nicotinic receptors labeled with nicotine but not for bungarotoxin-binding proteins or muscle nicotinic receptors. Stereochemical selectivity was also evident for neuronal nicotinic receptors.

Increasing the side chain length by one carbon produces the compound homoanatoxin, which is only slightly less potent than anatoxin-a. This suggests that one can increase the side-chain length and create affinity ligands for purification of nicotinic receptors (16,36).

Anatoxin-a has been used as a probe for dissecting out specific nicotinic receptor subtypes in brain homogenates and on cultured neurons (1,24,34). Structural modification of anatoxin-a has led to analogues that can differentiate between peripheral and central nicotinic receptors. Further characterization of neuronal nicotinic receptors with these analogues may add to the number of known α-subunit subtypes. Thus, the semirigid nicotinic agonist anatoxin-a and its analogues provide a strong basis for studies of nicotinic molecular pharmacology, particularly in the brain where many nicotinic receptor subtypes are present but little is known about their physiology or pharmacology.

Anatoxin-a(s)

Anatoxin-a(s) is a naturally produced organophosphate isolated from *Anabaena flos-aquae* strains different from the strain that produces anatoxin-a (8,19). Responsible for animal poisonings in various water supplies (6,21), the structure was determined by ^{1}H–nuclear magnetic resonance to be a guanidine methyl phosphate ester (22). Intraperitoneal injection of anatoxin-a(s) to rats produced signs of cholinergic overstimulation, including salivation, lacrimation, urinary incontinence, defecation, convulsions, fasciculation and, finally, respiratory arrest. *In vitro* experiments with isolated nerve-muscle preparations showed no direct agonist effects of anatoxin-a(s) but, instead, augmentation of the acetylcholine response to antagonize the action of *d*-tubocurarine (19). Anatoxin-a(s) is a potent, irreversible inhibitor of acetylcholinesterase from rat blood and electric eel and butyrylcholinesterase from horse serum (20). The inhibitory kinetics of anatoxin-a(s) support the *in vivo* pharmacological profile for an anticholinesterase agent. Anatoxin-a(s) intoxication can be reversed by treatment for cholinesterase poisoning, including the use of oxime reactivators, carbamates, and atropine (17). Anatoxin-a(s) biosynthesis studies have shown that all the carbons are derived from amino acids. Three methyl carbons arise from L-methionine while L-arginine accounts for C-2, C-4, and C-6 (23). The biosynthetic intermediate from L-arginine is (2S,4S)-4-hydroxyarginine (12).

REFERENCES

1. Alkondon M, Albuquerque EX (1993) Diversity of nicotinic acetylcholine receptors in rat hippocampal neurons. I. Pharmacological and functional evidence for distinct structural subtypes. *J Pharmacol Exp Ther* **265**, 1455.

2. Bates HA, Rapoport H (1979) Synthesis of anatoxin-a via intramolecular cyclization of iminium salts. *J Amer Chem Soc* **101**, 1259.

3. Campbell HF, Edwards OE, Kolt R (1977) Synthesis of nor-anatoxin-a and anatoxin-a. *Can J Chem* **55**, 1372.

4. Carmichael WW (1992) Cyanobacteria secondary metabolites—The cyanotoxins. *J Appl Bacteriol* **72**, 445.

5. Carmichael WW, Biggs DF, Gorham PR (1975) Toxicology and pharmacological action of *Anabaena flos-aquae* toxin. *Science* **187**, 542.

6. Cook WO, Beasley VR, Lovell RA et al. (1989) Consistent inhibition of peripheral cholinesterases by neurotoxins from the freshwater cyanobacterium *Anabaena flos-aquae*: studies of ducks, swine, mice, and a steer. *Environ Toxicol Chem* **8**, 915.

7. Costa AC, Swanson KL, Aracava Y et al. (1990) Molecular effects of dimethylanatoxin on the peripheral nicotinic acetylcholine receptor. *J Pharmacol Exp Ther* **252**, 507.

8. Devlin JP, Edwards OE, Gorham PR et al. (1977) Anatoxin-a, a toxic alkaloid from *Anabaena flos-aquae* NRC-44h. *Can J Chem* **55**, 1367.

9. Gallon JR, Kittakopp P, Brown EG (1994) Biosynthesis of anatoxin-a by *Anabaena flos-aquae*: examination of primary enzymic steps. *Phytochemistry* **35**, 1195.

10. Gorham PR, McLachlan J, Hammer UT, Kim WK (1964) Isolation and culture of toxic strains of *Anabaena*

flos-aquae (Lyngb.) de Breb. *Verh Int Verein Limnol* **15**, 793.

11. Harada KI, Kimura Y, Ogawa K *et al*. (1989) A new procedure for the analysis and purification of naturally occurring anatoxin-a from the blue-green alga *Anabaena flos-aquae*. *Toxicon* **27**, 1289.

12. Hemscheidt T, Burgoyne DL, Moore RE (1995) Biosynthesis of anatoxin-a(s), (2S, 4S)-4-hydroxy arginine as an intermediate. *J Chem Soc Chem Commun* 205.

13. Hemscheidt T, Papala J, Sivonen K, Skulberg OM (1995) Biosynthesis of anatoxin-a in *Anabaena flos-aquae* and homoanatoxin-a in *Oscillatoria formosa*. *J Chem Soc Chem Commun* 1361.

14. Hernandez A, Rapoport H (1994) Conformationally constrained analogues of anatoxin. Chirospecific synthesis of s-*trans* carbonyl ring-fused analogues. *J Org Chem* **59**, 1058.

15. Howard MH, Sardina FJ, Rapoport H (1990) Chirospecific syntheses of nitrogen and side-chain modified anatoxin analogues. Synthesis of (1R)-anatoxinal and (1R)-anatoxinic acid derivatives. *J Org Chem* **55**, 2829.

16. Huby NJ, Thompson P, Wonnacott S, Gallagher T (1991) Structural modification of anatoxin-a. Synthesis of model affinity ligands for the nicotinic acetylcholine receptor. *J Chem Soc Chem Commun* 243.

17. Hyde EG, Carmichael WW (1991) Anatoxin-a(s), a naturally occurring organophosphate is an irreversible active site-directed inhibitor of acetylcholinesterase (E.C. 3.1.1.7) *J Biochem Toxicol* 195.

18. Koskinen AM, Rapoport H (1985) Synthesis and conformational studies on anatoxin-a: A potent acetylcholine agonist. *J Med Chem* **28**, 1301.

19. Mahmood NA, Carmichael WW (1986) The pharmacology of anatoxin-a(s), a neurotoxin produced by the freshwater cyanobacterium *Anabaena flos-aquae* NRC 525-17. *Toxicon* **24**, 425.

20. Mahmood NA, Carmichael WW (1987) Anatoxin-a(s), an anticholinesterase from the cyanobacterium *Anabaena flos-aquae* NRC-525-17. *Toxicon* **25**, 1221.

21. Mahmood NA, Carmichael WW, Pfahler D (1988) Anticholinesterase poisonings in dogs from a cyanobacterial (blue-green algae) bloom dominated by *Anabaena flos-aquae*. *Amer J Vet Res* **49**, 300.

22. Matsunaga S, Moore RE, Niemczura WP, Carmichael WW (1989) Anatoxin-a(s), a potent anticholinesterase from *Anabaena flos-aquae*. *J Amer Chem Soc* **111**, 8021.

23. Moore BS, Ohtani I, deKoning CB *et al*. (1992) Biosynthesis of anatoxin-a(s). Origin of the carbons. *Tetrahedron Lett* **33**, 6595.

24. Pereira EF, Reinhardt-Maelicke S, Schrattenholz A *et al*. (1993) Identification and functional characterization of a new agonist site on nicotinic acetylcholine receptors of cultured hippocampal neurons. *J Pharmacol Exp Ther* **265**, 1474.

25. Peterson JS (1984) Chirospecific syntheses of (+)- and (−)-anatoxin-a. *J Amer Chem Soc* **106**, 4539.

26. Rapala J, Sivonen K, Luukkainen R, Niemelä SI (1993) Anatoxin-a concentration in *Anabaena* and *Aphanizomenon* under different environmental conditions and comparison of growth by toxic and non-toxic *Anabaena* strains—a laboratory study. *J Appl Phycol* **5**, 581.

27. Sardina FJ, Howard MH, Koskinen AM, Rapoport H (1989) Chirospecific synthesis of nitrogen and side chain modified analogues of (+)-anatoxin. *J Org Chem* **54**, 4654.

28. Sardina FJ, Howard MH, Moringstar M, Rapoport H (1990) Enantiodivergent synthesis of (+)- and (−)-anatoxin from L-glutamic acid. *J Org Chem* **55**, 5025.

29. Spivak CE, Waters J, Witkop B, Albuquerque EX (1982) Potencies and channel properties induced by semirigid agonists at frog nicotinic acetylcholine receptors. *Mol Pharmacol* **23**, 337.

30. Spivak CE, Witkop B, Albuquerque EX (1980) Anatoxin-a: A novel, potent agonist at the nicotinic receptor. *Mol Pharmacol* **18**, 384.

31. Swanson KL, Allen CN, Aronstam RS *et al*. (1986) Molecular mechanisms of the potent and stereospecific nicotinic receptor agonist (+)-anatoxin-a. *Mol Pharmacol* **29** 250.

32. Swanson KL, Aracava Y, Sardina FJ *et al*. (1989) N-Methylanatoxinol isomers: derivatives of the agonist (+)-anatoxin-a block the nicotinic acetylcholine receptor ion channel. *Mol Pharmacol* **35**, 223.

33. Swanson KL, Aronstam RS, Wonnacott S *et al*. (1991) Nicotinic pharmacology of anatoxin analogs. 1. Side chain structure-activity relationships at peripheral agonist and noncompetitive antagonist sites. *J Pharmacol Exp Ther* **259**, 377.

34. Thomas P, Stephens M, Wilkie G *et al*. (1993) (+)-Anatoxin-a is a potent agonist at neuronal nicotinic acetylcholine receptors. *J Neurochem* **60**, 2308.

35. Wonnacott S, Jackman S, Swanson KL *et al*. (1991) Nicotinic pharmacology of anatoxin analogs. II. Side chain structure-activity relationships at neuronal nicotinic ligand binding sites. *J Pharmacol Exp Ther* **259**, 387.

36. Wonnacott S, Swanson KL, Albuquerque EX *et al*. (1992) Homoanatoxin: A potent analogue of anatoxin-a. *Biochem Pharmacol* **43**, 419.

Anisatin

Peter S. Spencer

NEUROTOXICITY RATING

Experimental

A GABA antagonist

Anisatin and related sesquiterpene lactones (veranisatins A,B,C) are convulsants isolated from star anise (*Illicium anisatum*) and other *Illicium* spp. (6). The plants are used as medicinal herbs in China, Japan, and North and Central America. Human poisoning from ingestion of a tea prepared from *I. verum* is reported from Mexico (5).

Over 60 compounds have been identified in the essential oil of the pericarp of *I. modestum* A.C. Smith (1). Other sesquiterpene lactones with an anisatin-like carbon skeleton (8,9-*seco*-prezizaane skeleton) are reported in *I. floridanum* Ellis (American star thistle) (7).

Veranisatins induced convulsions and lethal toxicity in mice given 3 mg/kg *per os* and hypothermia at lower dosages (6). Anisatin and veranisatin decreased locomotion enhanced by methamphetamine at oral doses of 0.03 and 0.1 mg/kg, respectively.

Anisatin is a picrotoxin-like, noncompetitive γ-aminobutyric acid (GABA) antagonist (2,4). At physiological temperatures, anisatin may modulate benzodiazepine-GABA receptor coupling through barbiturate-picrotoxin-sensitive sites (3).

REFERENCES

1. Huang J, Wang J, Yang C et al. (1996) GC-MS analysis of essential oil from the pericarp of *Illicium modestum* A.C. Smith. *Chung Kuo Chung Yao Tsa Chih* **21**, 168. [In Chinese].
2. Kudo Y, Oka JI, Yamada K (1981) Anisatin, a GABA antagonist, isolated from *Illicium anisatum*. *Neurosci Lett* **7**, 25.
3. Matsumoto K, Fukuda H (1982) Anisatin modulation of GABA- and pentobarbital-induced enhancement of diazepam binding in rat brain. *Neurosci Lett* **32**, 175.
4. Matsumoto K, Fukuda H (1983) Anisatin modulation of temperature-dependent inhibition [³H]muscimol binding by chloride ion. *Brain Res* **270**, 103.
5. Montoya-Cabrera MA (1990) Poisoning by star anise (*Illicium anise*) tea. *Gac Med Mex* **126**, 341. [In Spanish].
6. Nakamura Y, Okuyama E, Yamazaki M (1996) Neurotropic components from star anise. *Chem Pharm Bull (Tokyo)* **44**, 1908.
7. Schmidt TJ, Schmidt HM, Muller E et al. (1998) New sesquiterpene lactones from *Illicium floridanum*. *J Nat Prod* **61**, 230.

Anthranilic Acid and Derivatives

Albert C. Ludolph

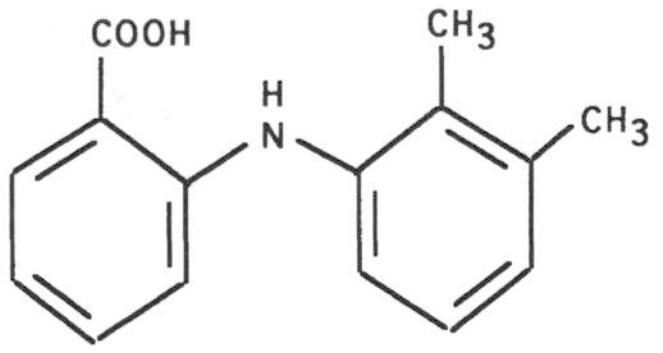

MEFENAMIC ACID
$C_{15}H_{15}NO_2$

Mefenamic acid; 2-[(2,3-Dimethylphenyl)amino]benzoic acid

NEUROTOXICITY RATING

Clinical

A Seizure disorder

Anthranilic acid and its derivatives (fenamates) are nonsteroidal anti-inflammatory drugs that include the substances antrafenine, etofenamate, floctafenine, flufenamic acid, gla- fenine, meclofenamate, mefenamic acid, niflumic acid, talinflumate, and tolfenamic acid (3). The analgesic, anti-inflammatory, and antipyretic effect of this group of compounds is thought to be due to inhibition of cyclooxygenase; some substances, particularly mefenamic acid, also seem to antagonize effects of prostaglandins. Plasma concentrations of mefenamic acid, meclofenamic acid, glafenine, and tolfenamic acid peak 90–120 min after oral ingestion, while flufenamic acid absorption seems to be slower (3).

Overdosage of mefenamic acid precipitated generalized muscle twitching and generalized seizures in 15 of 54 patients (1). Seizure occurrence correlates with plasma concentrations of the compound, and the clinical picture is similar to the profile of neurotoxicity seen in experimental animals (5). Similarly, in a single 13-year-old patient, coma followed by *grand mal* convulsions was reported after oral ingestion of mefenamic acid (4). Since most other anthranilic acid derivatives are infrequently prescribed, it is unclear whether the development of convulsions in mefenamic acid overdosage is specific for this compound. Mefenamic acid obviously decreases the seizure threshold; patients with epilepsy should not receive the drug (6). Headache has been ascribed to practically all of the anthranilic acid derivatives, and rhabdomyolysis was observed after administration of niflumic acid (2) and glafenine in three cases (6). Anthranilic acid derivatives are no longer used, since the benefits are less than other nonsteroidal anti-inflammatory analgesics.

REFERENCES

1. Balali-Mood M, Critchley JAJH, Proudfoot AT, Prescott LF (1981) Mefenamic acid overdosage. *Lancet* **i**, 1354.

2. Biscarini L (1992) Anti-inflammatory analgesics and drugs used in gout. In: *Meyler's Side Effects of Drugs*. Dukes MNG ed. Elsevier, Amsterdam p. 181.

3. Brogden RN (1986) Non-steroidal antiinflammatory analgesics other than salicylates. *Drugs* **32**, 27.

4. Goessinger H, Hruby K, Haubenstock A *et al.* (1982) Coma in mefenamic acid poisoning. *Lancet* **ii**, 384.

5. Kaump DH (1966) Pharmacology of the fenemates. Experimental observations on flufenamic, mefenamic, and meclofenamic acid. II. Toxicology in animals. *Ann Phys Med* 16.

6. Prescott LF, Balali-Mood M, Critchley JAJH, Proudfoot AT (1981) Avoidance of mefenamic acid in epilepsy. *Lancet* **ii**, 418.

Antillatoxin

William H. Gerwick
Thomas F. Murray

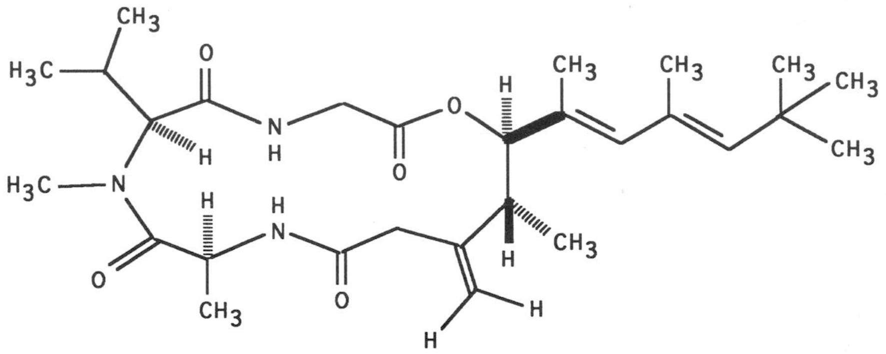

ANTILLATOXIN
$C_{28}H_{45}N_3O_5$

NEUROTOXICITY RATING

Experimental

A   Acutely neurotoxic (excitotoxic)

Antillatoxin is a complex cyclic lipopeptide ichthyotoxin obtained from a Curaçao collection of the tropical marine cyanobacterium (blue-green alga) *Lyngbya majuscula*. It was isolated through a fish toxicity-directed fractionation scheme, and shows an LD_{50} of 50 ng/ml to the common goldfish. The structure of antillatoxin was originally assigned by two-dimensional nuclear magnetic resonance studies in concert with chemical degradations (1). Revision of the stereochemistry at C4 from S to R followed from total-synthesis studies on antillatoxin and its stereoisomers (2,3). Antillatoxin's neurotoxicity to a primary culture of rat cerebellar granule neurons was produced acutely and concentration-dependently (LC_{50}, 20.1 nM). Its cytotoxicity is prevented by the noncompetitive N-methyl-D-aspartate receptor antagonists dextrorphan and dizocilpine (MK-801) (FW Bernan, WH Gerwick and TF Murray, *Toxicon*, in press).

REFERENCES

1. Orjala J, Nagle DG, Hsu V, Gerwick WH (1995) Antillatoxin, an exceptionally ichthyotoxic cyclic lipopeptide from the tropical cyanobacterium *Lyngbya majuscula*. *J Am Chem Soc* **117**, 8281.

2. Yokokawa F, Shioiri T (1998) Total synthesis of antillatoxin, an ichthyotoxic cyclic lipopeptide, having the proposed structure. What is the real structure of antillatoxin? *J Org Chem* **63**, 8638.

3. Yokokawa F, Fujiwara H, Shioiri T (1999) Total synthesis and revision of absolute configuration of antillatoxin, an ichthyotoxic cyclic lipopeptide of marine origin. *Tetrahedron Lett* (in press).

Apamin and Hymenoptera Venoms

Zarife Sahenk
Jerry R. Mendell

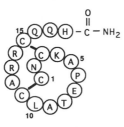

APAMIN
$C_{79}H_{131}N_{31}O_{24}S_4$

NEUROTOXICITY RATING

Clinical

A Peripheral neuropathy

A Optic neuropathy (hypersensitivity)

A Myopathy (necrotizing)

Experimental

A Peripheral neuropathy (local administration)

Members of the order Hymenoptera (bees, wasps, hornets, and fire ants) are potentially dangerous, venomous insects and, in many parts of the world, their stings are among the most frequent causes of insect-associated accidents. In the United States, the most common hymenopterous stings are from honey bees (*Apis mellifera*), yellow jackets (*Vespa pennsylvanica*), and paper wasps (*Polistes annularis*). Honey bee and European wasp stings (*Paravaspula vulgaris* and *P. germanica*) are the most common throughout Europe.

Both CNS and PNS complications may result from the stings of these insects. Anaphylactic reactions are seen most often and present with a variety of nonspecific signs and symptoms including headache, dizziness, nausea, vomiting, irritability, tremor, restlessness, confusion, disorientation, somnolence, and even loss of consciousness. Generalized seizures may occur. Anaphylactic reactions can have profound cardiovascular effects resulting in hypotension and neurological manifestations of global and, less often, focal ischemia (4,6,7,17).

Infrequently, patients develop neurological disorders thought to be immune-mediated (1,8,12–15,22,23). These disorders are delayed in onset by 2–14 days (Table 1) and may represent a delayed or Arthus-type hypersensitivity. It

TABLE 1. Delayed-Onset Neurological Manifestations of Hymenoptera Stings

Reference	Age/Sex	Sting Site	Delay
Guillain-Barré Syndrome			
Bachman *et al.* (1)			
Case 1	51/F	Fire ant, foot	7 days
Case 2	37/M	Bees, multiple	7 days
Case 3	44/M	Bee, inner thigh	5 days
Case 4	8/M	Bee, not stated	5 days
Wallace & Ludwig (23)	46/M	Hornet and bees back, neck, ear	2 days
Light *et al.* (13)			
Case 1	37/M	Bees, multiple	10 days
Miller-Fisher variant			
Case 2	8/M	Bees, not stated	3 days
Marks *et al.* (14)	8/M	Bees, multiple over eye and extremities	2 days
Plexitis			
Ross (18)	34/M	Bees, multiple, arms and chest	2 days
Goldstein *et al.* (7,8)	46/M	Hornet, hand	7 days
Myeloradiculopathy			
Jellinger & Spunda (12)	70/M	Hornet, leg	14 days
Means *et al.* (15)	52/F	Yellow jacket, shoulder	over 1 day
Van Antwerpen (22)	12/F	Wasp, hand	7 days
Optic Neuritis			
Berrios & Serrano (3)	11/M	Bee, left brow	14 days
*Song & Wray (21)	38/M	Bee, in the eye	hours
Singh & Chaudhray (20)	36/F	Wasp, multiple on face, head and neck, hands	2 days

*Unilateral optic neuritis.

has been postulated that certain patients harbor a latent hypersensitivity to nerve antigen that reactivates or is enhanced following the hymenopteran sting (1). The venom may act as an adjuvant, accelerating the immune response resulting in an overt neurological condition. Specific complications that have been described include Guillain Barré syndrome (GBS) including the Miller-Fisher variant, brachial plexitis, and myeloradiculopathy. In some cases, a direct toxic effect of the venom has been postulated. For example, one patient developed weakness in the upper extremity very rapidly following a bee sting in the posterior triangle of the neck (20). The neurological deficit was transient, resolving within approximately 1 h of the insult. The toxic effects of the venom could be mediated by pharmacologically active components including enzymes with necrotizing properties (hyaluronidase and phospholipase A_2), as well as a range of small protein and peptide toxins (apamin, mellitin, and mast cell degranulating peptide) (9–11). Of interest, the experimental injection of honey bee venom in sciatic nerves of rats induces severe wallerian degeneration and specific myelin changes (honeycomb appearance) (19). Transient effects of bee venom could be related to apamin-induced inhibition of calcium-dependent K^+ channels (20).

The toxic effects of venom on skeletal muscle have also been illustrated by cases of rhabdomyolysis associated with acute renal failure following the aggressive, swarming behavior of africanized or "killer" bees (16). This is a particular problem in Central America, including Mexico, where the insect species is well established. Although the quantity of venom per insect is less in the africanized bees, the swarming activity can lead to serious consequences. Some neurological complications result from local (toxic) effects, others may be immune mediated; ocular complications fall into this category. Bee and wasp stings to the eye and periocular tissue are a well known cause of acute ocular inflammation. However, the optic nerve and retina are spared unless there is an immune-mediated reaction. Unilateral and bilateral optic neuritis after bee stings have been reported (3,20,21). Based on detailed visual evoked potential studies and electroretinograms done on a case of unilateral optic neuritis, optic neuritis is believed to result from focal demyelination caused by an allergic reaction to the bee venom (21).

In the United States, only ants in the genus *Solenopsis* and genus *Pogonomyrmex* have been documented to cause anaphylaxis and other medical sequelae. Two species, *Solenopsis invicta*, Buren and *S. richteri*, Forel, collectively termed imported fire ants (IFA), were introduced into the United States from South America and currently inhabit the southeast and south central states. *Solenopsis* spp. live in large colonies, display aggressive behavior, and attack in swarms.

Neurological manifestations secondary to IFA sting are rare. Anaphylaxis, generalized seizures, and focal motor seizures in the absence of systemic hypotension have been reported (5). A case of GBS has been associated with IFA sting (1). Approximately 90% of IFA venom is composed of piperadine alkaloids, which are known to have hemolytic, insecticidal, and cytotoxic properties (2).

REFERENCES

1. Bachman DS, Paulson GW, Mendell JR (1982) Acute inflammatory polyradiculoneuropathy following Hymenoptera stings. *J Amer Med Assn* **247**, 1443.
2. Baer H, Liu T-Y, Anderson MC *et al.* (1979) Protein components of fire ant venom (*Solenopsis invicta*). *Toxicology* **17**, 397.
3. Berrios RR, Serrano LA (1994) Bilateral optic neuritis after a bee sting. *Amer J Ophthalmol* **117**, 677.
4. Day JM (1962) Death to cerebral infarction after wasp stings. *Arch Neurol* **7**, 184.
5. Fox RW, Lockley RF, Bukantz SC (1982) Neurologic sequelae following the imported fire ant sting. *J Allerg Clin Immunol* **70**, 120.
6. Gale AN (1982) Insect-sting encephalopathy. *Brit Med J* **284**, 20.
7. Goldstein NP, Rucker CW, Klass DW (1964) Encephalopathy and papilledema after bee sting. *J Amer Med Assn* **188**, 1083.
8. Goldstein NP, Rucker W, Woltman HW (1960) Neuritis occurring after insect stings. *J Amer Med Assn* **173**, 1727.
9. Habermann E (1972) Bee and wasp venoms. *Science* **177**, 315.
10. Hay SM, Hay FA, Austwick DH (1992) Bee sting brachial block. *Arch Emerg Med* **9**, 369.
11. Hider RC (1988) Honeybee venom: A rich source of pharmacologically active peptides. *Endeavour* **12**, 60.
12. Jellinger K, Spunda C (1961) Aufsteigende neuritis nachinsectenstich. *Wien Klin Wochenschr* **73**, 81.
13. Light WC, Reisman RE, Shimizu M, Arbesman CE (1977) Unusual reactions following insect stings. *J Allerg Clin Immunol* **59**, 391.
14. Marks HG, Augustyn P, Allen RS (1977) Fisher's syndrome in children. *Pediatrics* **60**, 726.
15. Means ED, Barron KD, Van Dyne BJ (1973) Nervous system lesions after sting by yellow jacket: a case report. *Neurology* **23**, 881.
16. Mejia G, Arbelaez M, Henao J *et al.* (1986) Acute renal failure due to multiple stings by Africanized bees. *Ann Intern Med* **104**, 210.
17. Meszaros I (1986) Transient ischemic attack caused by Hymenoptera stings: The brain as an anaphylactic shock organ. *Eur Neurol* **25**, 268.

18. Ross AT (1939) Peripheral neuritis: Allergy to honeybee stings. *Allergy* **10**, 382.
19. Saida K, Mendell JR, Sahenk Z (1977) Peripheral nerve changes induced by local application of bee venom. *J Neuropathol Exp Neurol* **36**, 783.
20. Singh I, Chaudhray U (1986) Bilateral optic neuritis following multiple wasp stings. *J Ind Med Assn* **84**, 251.
21. Song HS, Wray SH (1991) Bee sting optic neuritis. *J Clin Neuro-Ophthalmol* **11**, 45.
22. Van Antwerpen CL (1988) Myeloradiculopathy associated with wasp sting. *Pediat Neurol* **4**, 379.
23. Wallace TW, Ludwig RN (1970) Hornet sting neuritis. *Cleveland Clin Quart* **37**, 117.

CASE REPORT

A 37-year-old man received multiple bee stings to his limbs and trunk 10 days prior to the onset of progressive weakness and paresthesias. He was treated initially in the emergency room with diphenhydramine hydrochloride. No systemic reaction was observed. Ten days later he developed weakness and paresthesias in the upper extremities. The condition progressed rapidly leading to lower-extremity involvement, respiratory distress, and dysphagia. He developed bilateral facial nerve palsies. Muscle stretch reflexes were absent. There was a loss of proprioception, vibration, and touch in the legs, accompanied by pin-like sensations. Laboratory assessment revealed very high serum IgG and IgE antibody titers against bee and yellow jacket venom and phospholipase A. Cerebrospinal fluid protein was 166 mg/dl without cells with a normal glucose concentration. Electrophysiological studies suggested a demyelinating neuropathy that was confirmed by sural nerve biopsy. Approximately 6 weeks after the onset, he started to show recovery and became ambulatory after 2 months. (Abstracted from Case 2, reference 1)

Arsenic

Anthony J. Windebank

NEUROTOXICITY RATING
Clinical

A   Peripheral neuropathy

Arsenic is a group Vb metal. Elemental arsenic is uncommon in nature and rarely a source of industrial, occupational, or accidental human exposure. The element exists more commonly as organic or inorganic compounds. Large numbers of people in Bangladesh and West Bengal, India, drink well water contaminated with high levels of arsenic derived from arsenic-rich iron oxyhydroxides in the alluvial aquifers of the Ganges delta (24,30).

Organic arsenicals were used in the treatment of syphilis following Ehrlich's description of their effectiveness against trypanosomes. They were also used as diuretics before the introduction of the thiazides, but they have not been in therapeutic use since 1950 and are no longer available in most countries. Arsenic salts are metabolized into arsenates by shellfish. These compounds, which are essentially nontoxic in consumers of shellfish, may confuse diagnostic studies that depend upon measurement of elemental arsenic.

Inorganic salts are produced as by-products of copper and lead smelting. Calcium arsenate and copper acetoarsenate were used as pesticides until about 1960; toxicity resulting from accidental exposure occasionally occurs during cleaning or destruction of old farm buildings. The inorganic salts are indefinitely stable and remain hazardous for 50 years. Arsenic compounds are also used for preservation of wood, especially for marine applications. Arsenic trioxide, which is formed when treated wood is burned, has been a source of accidental human exposure to arsenic (34). Other uses of arsenic have included glass manufacture, cattle and sheep dips, leather manufacture, paper dyes, and chemical-warfare agent [lewisite, Agent L, dichloro-(2-chlorovinyl)-arsine (39)]. Arsenic-containing buffers (cacodylate) are used in histology laboratories. Accidental arsenical contamination of food and beverages occurred in the past and is now very rare. In North America, the most common form of human arsenic toxicity results from intentional overdose for the purposes of murder or suicide.

Inorganic arsenic salts are generally white, crystalline compounds that are soluble in water. Many have a sweetish flavor, a property that has allowed their use as poisons in beverages. Salts vary in toxic potency but are generally lethal if >0.5 g is ingested by an adult human.

There are no legitimate pharmaceutical or food uses for arsenic. Industrial and agricultural use is regulated in the United States by appropriate Occupational Safety and Health Administration guidelines. Material Safety Data Sheets are available for laboratory and industrial compounds.

General Toxicology

Arsenic is generally ingested by mouth either as a solution or in contaminated dust. It can be absorbed through lungs and skin at a low rate so that there is potential for toxicity from chronic environmental exposure. This has not been well documented for humans. Arsenic salts are rapidly absorbed from the gastrointestinal tract. Peak serum levels are reached 30–60 min after a single oral dose. Arsenic distributes through total body water and is rapidly cleared by the kidneys. Inorganic arsenic is enzymatically methylated to methylarsonic acid and dimethylarsinic acid; large individual variations are evident among human populations, suggesting the possibility of methyltransferase polymorphism (39). Kidney excretion occurs in three phases with half times of 2 h, 8 h, and 8 days (25). Arsenic compounds probably do not cross the blood-brain barrier readily (46). They are usually charged, and massive doses result only in transient CNS impairment without permanent residua. Primary target organs are the gastrointestinal tract, skin, bone marrow, kidneys, and PNS. Gastrointestinal symptoms occur soon after ingestion and are probably due to direct, local gut irritation. Vomiting and diarrhea, which may be bloody, are severe and can result in rapid systemic collapse. Renal damage occurs rapidly as arsenic is excreted. Bone marrow depression with anemia and pancytopenia may be seen with severe and chronic exposure (20). Dermatological changes include a gray discoloration of the skin, especially on the flanks; small, tear-drop–shaped areas of depigmentation; hyperkeratosis, redness, and sloughing of palms and soles; and Mees' lines; these horizontal areas of depigmentation in the fingernails correspond temporally to episodes of acute exposure. Similar transverse lines occur with acute lead and thallium poisoning; they should not be confused with leukonychia accompanying acute systemic illnesses, such as liver, cardiac, or renal failure. Isolated reports have suggested that long-term chronic exposure to arsenicals may result in carcinogenesis (16).

There is evidence that tolerance for arsenic and resistance to its toxic effects may be induced in humans. The "arsenic eaters of the Tyrol" were a group of villagers who used an arsenic-containing tonic to promote well-being. This "tonic" was extremely toxic to nonhabituated outsiders. Similarly, the apocryphal tale of Rasputin recounted that he had been poisoned so many times that he was immune to the effects of arsenicals.

Animal Studies

There is no reasonable experimental animal model of arsenic neuropathy because severe nephropathy, gastrointestinal disturbance, and death supervene before neuropathy appears. Accidental and experimental phenyl arsenic acid intoxication of swine induced paraparesis and morphological changes in dorsal columns suggesting degeneration of peripheral sensory axons (18). Animal pharmacokinetic studies have provided information about tissue distribution and clearance. Studies have examined the rate of absorption from the gastrointestinal tract in the rat (13), interactions between elements in the diet (11,23), and the form in which arsenic is ingested (13). For example, arsenic in soil has a tenfold lower bioavailability than orally administered solution (13,32). Phosphate in the diet inhibits the absorption of arsenic (11) presumably because of competitive uptake mechanisms. Potential therapeutic approaches have also been studied in animals (19). Animals have also been used to determine the best indicators of low-level dietary exposure (29).

In Vitro Studies

Insights into mechanisms of resistance and neurotoxicity have been gained from *in vitro* studies. Many bacterial strains become resistant due to expression of an adenosine triphosphate (ATP)-dependent membrane pump that removes arsenic from the cell by way of an anion pump (1,35,36,45). This resistance is encoded by a set of genes carried on a plasmid and is thus similar to antibiotic resistance. A similar pump exists in eukaryotic cells; it is encoded by the multidrug resistance (mdr) gene; the gene product is an ATP-dependent pump related to the cystic fibrosis chloride channel. There is some indirect evidence that eukaryotic cell resistance may be conferred by induction of P glycoprotein (31). However, direct studies in arsenic-resistant Chinese hamster ovary cells (CHO-SA7) suggest that up-regulation of glutathione-S-transferase π is responsible for resistance (41).

Human Studies

There have been few controlled exposures of human subjects to arsenic. In one study, radiolabeled arsenic compounds were intravenously injected to study tissue distribution and excretion (25). Almost all other information has come from accidental or intentional human exposures. The effects of both acute and chronic exposure are well described in the general medical literature.

Chronic exposure occurs in industry. Arsenic is used in the smelting industry, where inhalation exposure is common (21). Accidental exposure has occurred through industrial ground water (8,14) and food (4) contamination. Rarely, chronic exposure has resulted from the handling or burning of marine wood treated with arsenic-containing protectants (10,28,33). Chronic exposure, producing peripheral neuropathy, is rare (15,17,21). Patients experience gradual onset of lower-limb distal paresthesias with a slow progressive loss of large-fiber sensory function and ataxia. In reported cases, this has inevitably been accompanied by other manifestations of arsenic exposure, including skin discoloration and anemia. Chronic arsenic intoxication as a cause of distal symmetrical neuropathy has rarely been reported.

Acute exposure to arsenic often occurs as the result of accidental or intentional ingestion (42). Acute toxicity occurs when >0.5 g of an arsenic salt is ingested. Systemic manifestations include nausea, vomiting, diarrhea, confusion, delirium, coma, circulatory collapse, and death within 24 h. If the individual survives, chronic manifestations of acute toxicity appear within 7–10 days. These include anemia, gray discoloration of the skin, Mees lines, and peripheral neuropathy. The peripheral neuropathy is stereotypical and subacute in onset (2,4,6,7,9,22,42,43). Initial symptoms include distal paresthesias followed rapidly over days by ascending sensory loss and weakness, which may progress to respiratory failure in severe cases (12,44). Progression may occur for up to 6 weeks after a single acute exposure (22). Stabilization occurs in 1–2 months of onset and is followed by prolonged gradual recovery that may be incomplete (7,44).

Differential diagnosis of acute arsenic intoxication includes acute inflammatory demyelinating polyradiculoneuropathy (AIDP; Guillain-Barré syndrome), acute intermittent porphyria, and other neurotoxic disorders including those associated with certain marine toxins and other metals, especially thallium. The clinical features of all of these disorders are dominated by an acute gastrointestinal illness followed by a rapidly progressive neuropathy. Skin or nail changes, anemia, confusion, and renal impairment should alert the clinician to the possibility of a metal intoxication. Since intoxication usually results from intentional homicide or suicide attempts, the source of exposure may not be volunteered.

Electrophysiological features of acute arsenic neuropathy typically suggest a distal, motor and sensory axonopathy (22,44). Rarely, electrophysiological features suggest proximal demyelination with characteristics of AIDP (5).

Diagnosis depends upon demonstration of excessive arsenic exposure. A single intravenous injection of arsenic is excreted in the urine in three different phases with half times of 2 h, 8 h, and 8 days (25). Urine levels may, therefore, be elevated for weeks following a single massive dose. Plasma levels are of little clinical diagnostic value. Urine heavy metal screens are often used in the diagnosis of chronic neuropathy. Urine arsenic should not exceed 25 μg/

24 h in unexposed subjects. Values in the range of 25–1000 μg/24 h are occasionally encountered in these screening tests. This almost always represents excretion of nontoxic arsenates present in seafood. Reference laboratories can distinguish between nontoxic organic and toxic inorganic arsenic excretion products (27). This additional measurement is costly. Since arsenic does not usually cause chronic neuropathy, indiscriminate urine screening is inappropriate. If the clinical suspicion of arsenic toxicity is high and urine measurements are equivocal, other tissues may be studied. Hair and nail arsenic measurements provide evidence of past exposure; levels of >1 μg/g are regarded as evidence of intoxication. For forensic purposes, care should be taken to ensure that hair and nails are collected from the patient and that substitutions do not occur (42,44).

Treatment should be directed at removing the patient from the source of exposure, maintaining circulatory and renal function, and promoting excretion of arsenic. Cathartics and emetics are of little benefit because arsenic solutions are absorbed very rapidly. Several series of case reports suggest that neuropathy may be prevented or lessened by rapid early enhancement of arsenic excretion (3,26,43). Several agents have been used to increase arsenic excretion. The chelating agent, British antilewisite (BAL; dimercaprol) (37,38), is given by deep intramuscular injection as a 100 mg/ml solution in peanut oil. The dose for mild poisoning is 2.5 mg/kg, four times a day for 2 days, twice on the third day, and daily thereafter. For severe poisoning, 3 mg/kg is given every 4 h for 2 days, four times on the third day, and twice daily thereafter. Once oral intake is possible, penicillamine is effective in increasing urine excretion. Dosages are similar to those used to treat Wilson's disease. Treatment should be continued until urine arsenic falls below 25 μg/24 h.

Marrow depression is common after acute exposure but usually recovers without additional treatment. Repeated or chronic exposure to arsenic may lead to the development of malignancies, especially of skin and bone marrow.

Toxic Mechanisms

In isolated cell and enzyme systems, arsenic is a potent uncoupler of oxidative phosphorylation. Arsenate (+5 oxidation state) substitutes for inorganic phosphate and forms arsenic analogs of high-energy phosphates. They are unstable and break down regenerating inorganic arsenic (39). The less toxic arsenates resemble phosphates but are generally less stable. Because they do not form bonds with thiol groups, arsenates are not incorporated into hair or nails.

Arsenite compounds (+3 oxidation state) react directly with sulfhydryl groups in proteins; this reaction is probably responsible for the systemic toxic effects; presumably, the neurotoxicity has a related pathogenesis but the mechanism is unclear. Arsenite (3+) may react with a single sulfhydryl group producing an arsenic-thiol mercaptide or with 2 sulfhydryls forming a stable ring. Such ring formation is thought to be important in the arsenic-mediated inhibition of various enzyme systems including pyruvate dehydrogenase. Arsenite (3+) may also bind to lipoic acid, forming a stable lipoate arsenate ring that inhibits the conversion of pyruvate to acetyl coenzyme A. BAL was developed during World War II as an antidote to potential chemical-warfare agents containing arsenic (38). It is a dithiol that forms a stable ring with arsenic. This relatively nontoxic compound is then excreted in the urine (42).

REFERENCES

1. Cervantes C, Ji G, Ramírez JL, Silver S (1994) Resistance to arsenic compounds in microorganisms. *FEMS Microbiol Rev* **15**, 355.

2. Danan M, Conso F, Dally S et al. (1985) Arsenous anhydride poisoning. Peripheral neuropathy and changes in cognitive functions. *Ann Med Intern* **136**, 479.

3. DiNapoli J, Hall AH, Drake R, Rumack BH (1989) Cyanide and arsenic poisoning by intravenous injection. *Ann Emerg Med* **18**, 308.

4. Dong HQ, Wang KL, Ma YJ et al. (1993) A clinical analysis of 117 cases of acute arsenic poisoning. *Chung Hua Nei Ko Tsa Chih* **32**, 813.

5. Donofrio PD, Wilbourn AJ, Albers JW et al. (1987) Acute arsenic intoxication presenting as Guillain-Barré-like syndrome. *Muscle Nerve* **10**, 114.

6. Dyck PJ, Gutrecht JA, Bastron JA et al. (1968) Histologic and teased-fiber measurements of sural nerve in disorders of lower motor and primary sensory neurons. *Mayo Clin Proc* **43**, 81.

7. Fincher R-M, Koerker RM (1987) Long-term survival in acute arsenic encephalopathy. Follow-up using newer measures of electrophysiologic parameters. *Amer J Med* **82**, 549.

8. Franzblau A, Lilis R (1989) Acute arsenic intoxication from environmental arsenic exposure. *Arch Environ Health* **44**, 385.

9. Ghariani M, Adrien ML, Raucoules M et al. (1991) Subacute arsenic poisoning. *Ann Fr Anesth Reanim* **10**, 304.

10. Gidseg G (1985) Toxic effects of marine plywood. *J Amer Med Assn* **253**, 980.

11. Gonzalez MJ, Aguilar MV, Martinez-Para MC (1995) Gastrointestinal absorption of inorganic arsenic (V): The effect of concentration and interactions with phosphate and dichromate. *Vet Human Toxicol* **37**, 131.

12. Greenberg C, Davies S, McGowan T et al. (1979) Acute respiratory failure following severe arsenic poisoning. *Chest* **76**, 596.

13. Groen K, Vaessen HA, Kliest JJ et al. (1994) Bioavailability of inorganic arsenic from bog ore-containing soil in the dog. *Environ Health Perspect* **102**, 182.

14. Guha Mazumder DN, Das Gupta J, Chakraborty AK et al. (1992) Environmental pollution and chronic arsenicosis in South Calcutta. *Bull WHO* **70**, 481.

15. Heaven R, Duncan M, Vukelja SJ (1994) Arsenic intoxication presenting with macrocytosis and peripheral neuropathy, without anemia. *Acta Haematol* **92**, 142.

16. Kasper ML, Schoenfield L, Strom RL, Theologides A (1984) Hepatic angiosarcoma and bronchioloalveolar carcinoma induced by Fowler's solution. *J Amer Med Assn* **252**, 3407.

17. Kelafant GA, Kasarskis EJ, Horstman SW et al. (1993) Arsenic poisoning in central Kentucky: A case report. *Amer J Ind Med* **24**, 723.

18. Kennedy S, Rice DA, Cush PF (1986) Neuropathology of experimental 3-nitro-4-hydroxyphenyl arsenic acid toxicosis in pigs. *Vet Pathol* **23**, 454.

19. Kreppel H, Paepcke U, Thiermann H et al. (1993) Therapeutic efficacy of dimercaptosuccinic acid (DMSA) analogues in acute arsenic trioxide poisoning in mice. *Arch Toxicol* **67**, 580.

20. Kyle RA, Pease GL (1965) Hematologic aspects of arsenic intoxication. *N Engl J Med* **273**, 18.

21. Lagerkvist BJ, Zetterlund B (1994) Assessment of exposure to arsenic among smelter workers: A five-year follow-up. *Amer J Ind Med* **25**, 477.

22. Le Quesne PM, McLeod JG (1977) Peripheral neuropathy following a single exposure to arsenic. Clinical course in four patients with electrophysiological and histological studies. *J Neurol Sci* **32**, 437.

23. Mahaffey KR, Capar SG, Gladen BC, Fowler BA (1981) Concurrent exposure to lead, cadmium and arsenic. Effects on toxicity and tissue metal concentrations in the rat. *J Lab Clin Med* **98**, 463.

24. Nickson R, McArthur J, Burgess Q et al. (1998) Arsenic poisoning of Bangladesh groundwater. *Nature* **395**, 338.

25. Mealey J Jr., Brownell GL, Sweet WH (1959) Radioarsenic in plasma, urine, normal tissues, and intracranial neoplasms; distribution and turnover after intravenous injection in man. *Arch Neurol Psychiat* **81**, 310.

26. Moore DF, O'Callaghan CA, Berlyne G et al. (1994) Acute arsenic poisoning: Absence of polyneuropathy after treatment with 2,3-dimercaptopropanesulphonate (DMPS). *J Neurol Neurosurg Psychiat* **57**, 1133.

27. Moyer TP (1993) Testing for arsenic. *Mayo Clin Proc* **68**, 1210.

28. Nakawatase TV, Nakatsuka CH (1993) Arsenic toxicity in Hawaii: A case report and review. *Hawaii Med J* **52**, 258.

29. Neiger RD, Osweiler GD (1992) Arsenic concentrations in tissues and body fluids of dogs on chronic low-level dietary sodium arsenite. *J Vet Diagn Invest* **4**, 334.

30. Mandal BK, Chowdhury TR, Samanta G *et al.* (1998) Impact of safe water for drinking and cooking on five arsenic-affected families for 2 years in West Bengal, India. *Sci Total Environ* **218**, 185.

31. Ouellette M, Borst P (1991) Drug resistance and P-glycoprotein gene amplification in the protozoan parasite *Leishmania. Res Microbiol* **142**, 737.

32. Pascoe GA, Blanchet RJ, Linder G (1994) Bioavailability of metals and arsenic to small mammals at a mining waste-contained wetland. *Arch Environ Contam Toxicol* **27**, 44.

33. Peters HA, Croft WA, Darcey BA, Olson MA (1983) Seasonal arsenic poisoning from burning treated wood—a newly recognized health hazard. *Neurology* **33**, 192.

34. Peters HA, Croft WA, Woolson EA *et al.* (1984) Seasonal arsenic exposure from burning chromium-copper-arsenate-treated wood. *J Amer Med Assn* **251**, 2393.

35. Rosen BP, Weigel U, Monticello RA, Edwards BPF (1991) Molecular analysis of an anion pump: Purification of the ArsC protein. *Arch Biochem Biophys* **284**, 381.

36. Rosenstein R, Nikoleit K, Götz F (1994) Binding of ArsR, the repressor of the *Staphylococcus xylosus* (pSX267) arsenic resistance operon to a sequence with dyad symmetry within the *ars* promoter. *Mol Gen Genet* **242**, 566.

37. Stocken LA, Thompson RHS (1946) British anti-lewisite: I. Arsenic derivatives of thiol proteins. *Biochem J* **40**, 529.

38. Stocken LA, Thompson RHS (1946) British anti-lewisite: II. Dithiol compounds as antidotes for arsenic. *Biochem J* **40**, 535.

39. Vahter M (1999) Methylation of inorganic arsenic in different mammalian species and population groups. *Sci Prog* **82**, 69.

40. Vallee BL, Ulmer DD, Wacker WEC (1960) Arsenic toxicology and biochemistry. *Arch Ind Health* **21**, 56.

41. Wang H-F, Lee T-C (1993) Glutathione S-transferase pi facilitates the excretion of arsenic from arsenic-resistant Chinese hamster ovary cells. *Biochem Biophys Res Commun* **192**, 1093.

42. Windebank AJ (1987) Peripheral neuropathy due to chemical and industrial exposure. In: *Handbook of Clinical Neurology.* Vinken PJ, Bruyn GW, Klawans HL eds. Elsevier Science Publishers, Amsterdam p. 263.

43. Windebank AJ (1993) Metal neuropathy. In: *Peripheral Neuropathy. 3rd Ed.* Dyck PJ, Thomas PK, Low PA *et al.* eds. WB Saunders, Philadelphia p. 1549.

44. Windebank AJ, McCall JT, Dyck PJ (1984) Metal neuropathy. In: *Peripheral Neuropathy. 2nd Ed.* Dyck PJ, Thomas PK, Lambert EH, Bunge RP eds. WB Saunders, Philadelphia p. 2133.

45. Wu J, Rosen BP (1993) The *arsD* gene encodes a second *trans*-acting regulatory protein of the plasmid-encoded arsenical resistance operon. *Mol Microbiol* **8**, 615.

46. Zheng W, Perry DF, Nelson DL, Aposhian HV (1991) Choroid plexus protects cerebrospinal fluid against toxic metals. *FASEB J* **5**, 2188.

1-Aryl-3,3-Dialkyltriazenes

Peter S. Spencer

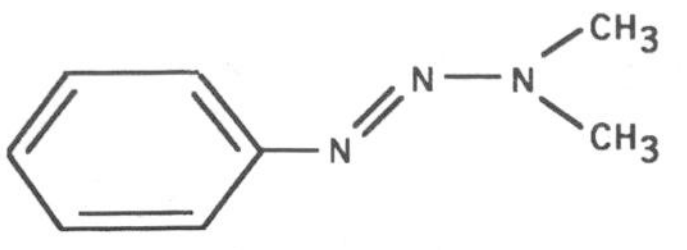

1-PHENYL-3,3-DIMETHYLTRIAZENE
$C_8H_{11}N_3$

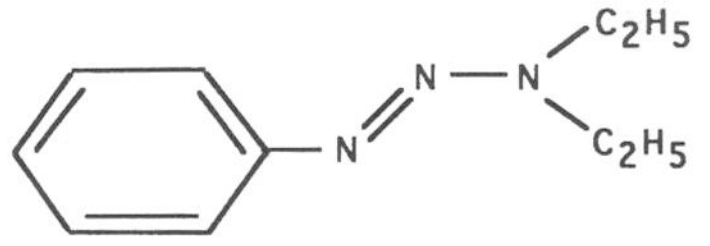

1-PHENYL-3,3-DIETHYLTRIAZENE
$C_{10}H_{15}N_3$

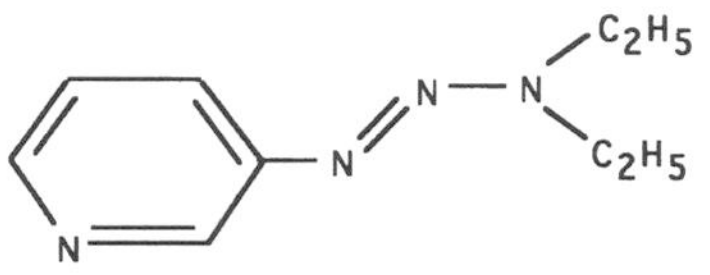

1-PYRIDYL-3,3-DIETHYLTRIAZENE
$C_9H_{14}N_4$

NEUROTOXICITY RATING

Experimental

A   Neurogenic tumors

1-Aryl-3,3-dialkyltriazenes are alkylating carcinogens that, irrespective of their route of administration, more or less selectively produce brain tumors in rats. The proximate carcinogen is derived from a monoalkyl metabolite (3). It is suggested that a six-membered ring with hydrogen bridging is formed following α-hydroxylation in the *cis* position to the first nitrogen atom. Degradation of the ring is proposed to yield formaldehyde and monomethyltriazene, which by protonation decomposes to form aniline and methyldiazonium ion; the latter alkylates guanine in nucleic acids of brain, liver, and kidney (1,2). The ultimate biochemical action of the 1-aryl-3,3-dialkyltriazenes therefore appears to be closely related to that of methylazoxymethanol (*see* Cycasin), although there is no explanation for the selective neurotropic carcinogenicity of the triazene compounds (1).

Pregnant rats treated on day 15 with a single subcutaneous dose of 110 mg/kg of 1-phenyl-3,3-triazene or a single intravenous dose of 1-pyridyl-3,3-diethyltriazene developed neurogenic tumors in 11 of 12 and 18 of 20 of the offspring, respectively. No tumors were seen in similarly treated animals given 75 mg/kg 1-phenyl-3,3-dimethyltriazene on day 15; however, this dosage was effective in producing 12 neurogenic, 4 renal and 1 hepatic tumors when administered subcutaneously on day 23 of gestation (1,4). Ten mostly malignant neurinomas were found in 9 of 39 offspring of animals treated with 5-(3,3-dimethyl-1-triazeno)-imidazole-4-carboxamide (5). Oral or subcutaneous administration of 1-phenyl-3,3-dimethyltriazene produced tumors in brain, spinal cord, and/or peripheral nerves of adult rats (5).

REFERENCES

1. Druckrey H (1973) Chemical structure and action in transplacental carcinogenesis and teratogenesis. In: *Transplacental Carcinogenesis*. Tomatis L, Mohr I eds. International Agency for Research on Cancer (IARC) Scientific Publications No. 4, IARC, Lyon p. 45.
2. Krüger FW, Preussmann R, Niepelt H (1971) Mechanisms of carcinogenesis with 1-aryl-3,3-dialkyltriazenes. III. *In vivo* methylation of RNA and DNA with 1-phenyl-3-3-^{14}C-dimethyltriazene. *Biochem Pharmacol* 20, 529.
3. Preussmann R, Druckrey H, Ivankovic S, von Hodenberg A (1969) Chemical structure and carcinogenicity of aliphatic hydrazo, azo, and azoxy compounds and triazenes, potential *in vivo* alkylating agents. *Ann N Y Acad Sci* 163, 697.
4. Zeller WJ (1980) Pränatal karsinogene Wirkung von 5-(3,3-Dimethyl-1-triazene)-imidazol-4-carboxamid (DTIC) bei den Nachkommen von BD IX-Ratten. *Arch Geschwulstforsch* 50, 306.
5. Zeller WJ (1992) Neurotropic carcinogenesis. In: *Selective Neurotoxicity*. Herken H, Hucho F eds. Springer-Verlag, Berlin p. 207.

L-Asparaginase

Herbert H. Schaumburg

L-Asparagine amidohydrolase

NEUROTOXICITY RATING

Clinical

A   Encephalomalacia

B   Acute encephalopathy (confusion, somnolence)

L-Asparaginase is an enzyme that hydrolyzes asparagine to aspartic acid and ammonia; it causes a cytotoxic cellular deficiency of L-asparagine in populations of neoplastic cells unable to synthesize additional L-asparagine. Its principal use is as an antineoplastic agent in the treatment of acute lymphoblastic leukemia. L-Asparaginase can induce remission when given as a single agent, but duration of remission is longer when used in combination with other antileukemic agents. It is administered intravenously or intramuscularly. The usual intravenous doses of L-asparaginase are 6,000 IU/m^2 every other day for 3 weeks or daily doses of 1000–20,000 IU/m^2 for 10–20 days. The half-life after intravenous administration is 8–30 h; plasma levels of L-asparagine fall to immeasurable levels immediately following administration. The volume of distribution for L-asparaginase is greater than the plasma volume and it appears to be sequestered within organs. L-Asparaginase does not enter the CNS, and neurotoxicity is secondary to indirect effects of the drug.

Most of the systemic toxic effects of L-asparaginase therapy are secondary to hypersensitivity reactions or inhibition of protein synthesis. Hypersensitivity phenomena appear in one-quarter of patients; they include urticaria, dyspnea, fever, hypotension, and epigastric pain. Diminished synthesis of hemostatic factors accounts for the most serious side effects of L-asparaginase therapy and can cause either thrombosis or hemorrhage, depending upon the balance of decrease in procoagulant and anticoagulant proteins. Reduced levels of fibrinogen and other clotting factors and fibrinolytic enzymes are common, but systemic bleeding occurs in only 1% of patients. The agent is not cytotoxic to bone marrow stem cells, gastrointestinal mucosa, or hair follicles.

Reversible signs of L-asparaginase–induced CNS dysfunction (confusion, somnolence, memory loss) appear in about 15% of cases; they were recognized shortly following introduction of the drug (6). Initially attributed to secondary metabolic derangements (hyperammonemia, hepatic dysfunction), it now appears likely that many instances represent diffuse CNS ischemia attributable to disturbances in hemostasis (2,3,5).

Clinically obvious instances of cerebral hemorrhage and infarction are the most serious neurological side effects of L-asparaginase treatment and occur in about 1% of patients receiving the drug (1,5). One review discovered 38 reports of cerebrovascular complications of therapy in children without evidence of CNS leukemia (1). Thrombosis of cerebral veins or sinuses is especially common; onset of severe headache or neurological deficit is an indication to obtain prompt magnetic resonance imaging to detect early venous lesions (4). Most instances of cerebrovascular disease appear after 21 days of therapy, and cerebrovascular lesions from higher doses are more likely to be hemorrhagic. The prognosis of cerebrovascular complications is remarkably good; most have made a satisfactory recovery. This likely reflects the youth of most patients. Therapy depends upon the coagulation status of an individual case; it includes replacement of depleted plasma proteins with fresh-frozen plasma and treatment directed at the specific cerebrovascular lesion. Risk of recurrence with further L-asparaginase therapy is low, but prophylactic pretreatment with fresh-frozen plasma is suggested (1).

REFERENCES

1. Feinberg WM, Swenson MR (1988) Cerebrovascular complications of L-asparaginase therapy. *Neurology* 38, 127.
2. Ott N, Ramsay NKC (1988) Sequelae of thrombotic or hemorrhagic complications following L-asparaginase therapy for childhood lymphoblastic leukemia. *J Pediat Hematol Oncol* 10, 191.
3. Priest JR, Ramsay NKC, Steinherz PG *et al.* (1982) A syndrome of thrombosis and hemorrhage complicating L-asparaginase therapy for childhood acute lymphoblastic leukemia. *J Pediat* 100, 984.
4. Schick RM, Jolesz F, Barnes PD, Macklis JD (1989) MR diagnosis of dural venous sinus thrombosis complicating L-asparaginase therapy. *Comput Med Imaging Graph* 13, 319.
5. White L, Fishman LS, Shore NA (1981) Strokes and the neurotoxicity of L-asparaginase. *J Pediat* 99, 168.
6. Whitecar JP, Bodey GP, Harris JE, Freireich EJ (1970) Current concepts, L-asparaginase. *N Engl J Med* 282, 732.

Aspartame

Bennett A. Shaywitz

ASPARTAME
$C_{14}H_{18}N_2O_5$

N-L-α-Aspartyl-L-phenylalanine 1-methyl ester

NEUROTOXICITY RATING
Clinical
C Chronic encephalopathy

Aspartame (APM) is a dipeptide of aspartic acid and phenylalanine that is 180–200 times sweeter than sucrose in solution. Approximately 200 safety and metabolism studies have been conducted on APM and its degradation products, *in vitro*, in animals and in humans; these studies have been summarized in various monographs and reviews (1,7,8,10,13,19). Metabolic studies have demonstrated that APM is metabolized in the gastrointestinal tract to its three components: aspartic acid (ASP), phenylalanine (PHE), and methanol (19,20). A no-observed-effect level (NOEL) of >2000–4000 mg/kg body weight was established for APM in animals after a comprehensive battery of toxicology and pharmacology studies. The safety and metabolism of APM, as well as the pharmacokinetics of its components, have been extensively studied in humans as well. The results of clinical studies indicate that APM exposures at doses 50 to 100 times the reported daily consumption levels (90th percentile 14-day averages) are not associated with adverse health effects.

APM was initially approved as a food additive by the U.S. Food and Drug Administration (FDA) in 1974. Approval was temporarily rescinded when issues were raised concerning possible neurotoxicity of APM constituents and the diketopiperazine breakdown product. Some also suggested that APM or its products may predispose to brain tumor development. The results of lifetime carcinogenicity studies in rodents and available data from other animal research indicated this was unlikely. After evaluation of these issues, the FDA reinstated the food additive approval of APM in 1981 and, in 1983, expanded approval to include use in carbonated soft drinks.

Regulatory bodies typically assign an Acceptable Daily Intake (ADI) for a food additive prior to approval. The ADI is the consumption level that is considered to be safe on a continuing basis; occasionally exceeding the ADI is not considered harmful (22). The ADI (expressed in milligrams of additive per kilogram body weight) is usually the NOEL from animal toxicology studies divided by a safety factor of 100. The Scientific Committee for Foods of the European Economic Community and the Joint Expert Committee for Food Additives of the Food and Agriculture Organization/World Health Organization thus established an ADI for APM of 40 mg/kg/day. In the United States, the FDA established an ADI for APM of 50 mg/kg/day based additionally on data available from humans. Intake of APM at or near either of these ADIs is unlikely either as a single bolus consumption or on a consistent basis (2,3,22).

Methanol is formed by the hydrolysis of the phenylalanine methyl ester moiety of APM. It has been speculated that such APM-derived methanol may be potentially toxic to the brain and retina. However, the amounts of methanol released from APM are well below those encountered from normal dietary exposures in fruits, vegetables, and juices (10,19).

ASP, along with glutamate (GLU), comprises about 20%–25% of dietary protein. Large doses of nonprotein GLU or ASP administered orally by bolus are capable of causing excitatory damage to the arcuate nucleus in neonatal rodents (reviewed in 13). Excitotoxic damage after administration of these two dietary amino acids occurs in neonatal rodents only when plasma ASP concentrations exceed 1100 μmole/l, or plasma GLU concentrations exceed 750 μmole/l, or the combined plasma concentrations of ASP plus GLU exceed 1280 μmole/l (13,19). In the human adult, fasting plasma concentrations are around 20–25 μM for GLU and are 1–5 μM for ASP (13). Plasma concentrations of both ASP and GLU in humans remain within postprandial ranges even after large doses of APM. High-dose APM (34 mg/kg) produced no change in fasting plasma ASP levels in healthy adults (19). Acute bolus dosing of APM in healthy adults (up to 200 mg/kg), 1-year-old infants (up to 100 mg/kg) and phenylketonuria (PKU) heterozygotes (up to 100 mg/kg) produced no significant changes in plasma ASP concentrations when APM dosages were <100 mg/kg. Small increases in plasma ASP concentrations occurred when APM dosages were 100 mg/kg or greater but remained within normal postprandial ranges. Chronic administration of high doses of APM (75 mg/kg/day for 24 weeks) did not change mean fasting plasma ASP concentrations (11).

PHE is an essential amino acid comprising approximately 5% of dietary protein. PHE is converted in the liver to tyrosine by the enzyme phenylalanine hydroxylase. Tyrosine, in turn, is utilized in protein synthesis as well as being the precursor of CNS catecholamine neurotransmitters and norepinephrine and epinephrine in the adrenal medulla. At reported consumption levels (2), the PHE component of APM provides approximately 1% of a 4-year-old child's daily dietary intake of PHE *vs.* approximately 2% of an adult's. Acute, repeated and long-term studies have been done in healthy adults to evaluate the safety of the PHE component of APM. After a 34-mg/kg bolus dose of APM in adults, peak plasma PHE concentrations were approximately 120 μmole/l but remained within normal postprandial range (90–150 μmole/l). After 200 mg/kg of APM in healthy adults, plasma PHE concentrations achieved a peak of approximately 490 μmole/l and rapidly declined towards baseline over several hours (19).

PHE is one of a group of large neutral amino acids (LNAA) that competes for entry into the brain through a carrier transport system. The rate of entry of PHE into the brain is predicted by the ratio of the plasma concentration of PHE to the sum of the plasma concentrations of the other LNAA (reviewed in 10,12). Fluctuations in the ratio of PHE to other LNAA occur as the result of dietary manipulations and the normal variability of the diet. Since APM is a source of PHE without the competing amino acids, it has been suggested that APM may lead to increases in the PHE/LNAA ratio, and thus, brain PHE concentrations. It has been further speculated that such changes in brain PHE concentrations would result in changes in brain neurotransmitters, brain function, seizures, behavioral changes, or cognitive function (12,14). While isolated effects of APM on brain neurotransmitter or metabolite concentrations have been noted in a few animal studies, it is clear these effects are neither consistent nor reproducible (10). Studies evaluating the receptor kinetics or release of brain neurotransmitters, which are considered more reliable than steady-state concentrations when evaluating changes in neurotransmission, fail to show a treatment effect of large doses of APM or PHE (reviewed in 10). Similarly, animal studies evaluating seizure susceptibility, behavior, and CNS development have shown no reproducible effects following acute or chronic administration of high doses of APM (recent reviews include 1,8,19).

The widespread use of a food additive such as APM makes it inevitable that adverse health events will be associated coincidentally with the consumption of products containing that food additive (22). Anecdotal reports of adverse experiences following APM consumption have been monitored and reviewed by epidemiologists at the U.S. Centers for Disease Control and Prevention (CDC) and the FDA. These investigators concluded that (a) the complaints are generally mild and common in the general population, (b) there is no consistent pattern of symptoms that can causally be related to APM, and (c) only through focused clinical studies can these allegations be thoroughly studied (3,22). APM tolerance studies have been done in healthy adults, children, and adolescents; individuals heterozygous for phenylketonuria (PKU) who have a somewhat impaired ability to metabolize PHE; and individuals who may be heavy users of APM, such as obese individuals and diabetics. In addition, studies have evaluated the tolerance of APM by individuals who have altered amino acid and protein metabolism (*e.g.*, those with liver and renal disease). These results have demonstrated that even large doses of APM in excess of the ADI are not associated with adverse effects in either healthy adults and children or in various subpopulations (1,5,6,7,11,19).

The results of double-blind, placebo-controlled studies show that in normal healthy humans there is no alteration in cognition, mood, behavior, or electrophysiology that can be attributed to consumption of APM, even when doses are sufficient to raise the plasma PHE/LNAA ratio. APM has been shown to have no effects on behavior or cognition in pilots (21), normal or hyperactive children, although some of these studies were designed to evaluate the effect of sugar on behavior and aspartame was used as the placebo (26). Studies have been conducted specifically in potentially vulnerable populations, such as in individuals with headache (9,16,24), seizures (4,15,17), affective disorders (25), attention deficit disorder (18,26), and individuals heterozygous for PKU (23). In general, these studies support an absence of effects following APM administration. One study suggested that ingestion of APM by migraineurs causes an increase in headache frequency for some subjects (9) although, in a population of individuals reporting headaches after consuming products containing APM in a controlled double-blind setting, APM was no more likely to produce headache than placebo (16). Two studies in potentially vulnerable populations provided suggestive results, one concerning the effects of APM on adults with depression (25) and the other reporting neurophysiological alterations in the electroencephalograms of children with absence epilepsy (4). In both studies, however, interpretation of the results is confounded on the bases of statistical design limitations and inadequately controlled experimental paradigms. In the large majority of studies that evaluated normal individuals, adults and children with seizures (including absence seizures), children with attention deficit disorder or children considered sugar-reactive, and PKU heterozygous adults, there was no evidence of effects from APM administration.

REFERENCES

1. Butchko HH, Kotsonis FN (1989) Aspartame: review of recent research. *Comment Toxicol* **3**, 253.

2. Butchko HH, Kotsonis FN (1991) Acceptable daily intake *vs.* actual intake: The aspartame example. *J Amer Coll Nutr* **10**, 258.

3. Butchko HH, Tschanz C, Kotsonis FN (1994) Postmarketing surveillance of food additive. *Regul Toxicol Pharmacol* **20**, 105.

4. Camfield PR, Camfield CS, Dooley JM *et al.* (1992) Aspartame exacerbates EEG spike-wave discharge in children with generalized absence epilepsy: A double-blind controlled study. *Neurology* **42**, 1000.

5. Gupta V, Cochran C, Parker TF *et al.* (1989) Effect of aspartame on plasma amino acid profiles of diabetic patients with chronic renal failure. *Amer J Clin Nutr* **49**, 1302.

6. Hertelendy ZI, Mendenhall CL, Rouster SD *et al.* (1993) Biochemical and clinical effects of aspartame in patients with chronic, stable alcoholic liver disease. *Amer J Gastroenterol* **88**, 737.

7. Janssen PJCM, van der Heijden CA (1988) Aspartame: Review of recent experimental and observational data. *Toxicology* **50**, 1.

8. Jobe PC, Dailey JW (1993) Aspartame and seizures. *Amino Acids* **4**, 197.

9. Koehler SM, Glaros A (1988) The effect of aspartame on migraine headache. *Headache* **28**, 10.

10. Lajtha A, Reilly MA, Dunlop DS (1994) Aspartame consumption: Lack of effects on neural function. *J Nutr Biochem* **5**, 266.

11. Leon AS, Hunninghake DB, Bell C *et al.* (1989) Safety of long-term large doses of aspartame. *Arch Intern Med* **149**, 2318.

12. Maher TJ, Wurtman RJ (1987) Possible neurologic effects of aspartame, a widely used food additive. *Environ Health Perspect* **75**, 53.

13. Meldrum B (1993) Amino acids as dietary excitotoxins: A contribution to understanding neurodegenerative disorders. *Brain Res* **18**, 293.

14. Pardridge WM (1986) Potential effects of the dipeptide sweetener aspartame on the brain. In: *Nutrition and the Brain. Vol. 7* Wurtman RJ, Wurtman JJ eds. Raven Press, New York p. 199.

15. Rowan AJ, Shaywitz BA, Tuchman L *et al.* (1995) Aspartame and seizure susceptibility: Results of a clinical study in reportedly sensitive individuals. *Epilepsia* **36**, 270.

16. Schiffman SS, Buckley CE, Sampson HA *et al.* (1987) Aspartame and susceptibility to headache. *N Engl J Med* **317**, 1181.

17. Shaywitz BA, Anderson GM, Novotny EJ *et al.* (1994) Aspartame has no effect on seizures or epileptiform discharges in epileptic children. *Ann Neurol* **35**, 98.

18. Shaywitz BA, Sullivan CM, Anderson GM *et al.* (1994) Aspartame, behavior, and cognitive function in children with attention deficit disorder. *Pediatrics* **93**, 70.

19. Stegink LD, Filer LJ Jr (1984) *Aspartame: Physiology and Biochemistry*. Marcel Dekker, New York.

20. Stegink LD, Filer LJ Jr, Bell EF *et al.* (1989) Effect of repeated ingestion of aspartame-sweetened beverage on plasma amino acid, blood methanol, and blood formate concentrations in normal adults. *Metabolism* **38**, 357.

21. Stokes AF, Belger A, Banich MT, Bernadine E (1994) Effects of alcohol and chronic aspartame ingestion upon performance in aviation relevant cognitive tasks. *Aviat Space Environ Med* **65**, 7.

22. Tollefson L, Barnard RJ (1992) An analysis of FDA passive surveillance reports of seizures associated with consumption of aspartame. *J Amer Diet Assn* **92**, 596.

23. Trefz F, de Sonneville L, Matthis P *et al.* (1994) Neuropsychological and biochemical investigations in heterozygotes for phenylketonuria during ingestion of high dose aspartame (a sweetener containing phenylalanine). *Hum Genet* **93**, 369.

24. Van Den Eeden SK, Koepsell TD, Longstreth WT Jr *et al.* (1994) Aspartame ingestion and headaches: a randomized crossover trial. *Neurology* **44**, 1787.

25. Walton RG, Hudak R, Green-Waite RJ (1993) Adverse reactions to aspartame: Double-blind challenge in patient from a vulnerable population. *Biol Psychiat* **34**, 13.

26. Wolraich ML, Lindgren SD, Stumbo PJ *et al.* (1994) Effects of diets high in sucrose or aspartame on the behavior and cognitive performance of children. *N Engl J Med* **330**, 301.

Atropine

Brent T. Burton

ATROPINE
$C_{17}H_{23}NO_3$

endo-($\pm$)-α-(Hydroxymethyl)benzeneacetic acid 8-methyl-8-azabicyclo[3.2.1]oct-3-yl ester

NEUROTOXICITY RATING

Clinical

A Acute encephalopathy (confusion, hallucinations)

A Seizure disorder

Experimental

A Muscarinic receptor antagonist

Atropine is one of several naturally occurring belladonna alkaloids found in deadly nightshade (*Atropa belladonna*) and Jimson weed (*Datura stramonium*), as well as other common plants (8). The chemical structure of atropine is an organic ester composed of tropic acid and tropine. The asymmetrical molecule yields a racemic mixture of both *d*- and *l*-isomers, though pharmacological activity is almost exclusively limited to the *l* form (9).

Atropine and other naturally occurring belladonna alkaloids (*e.g.*, scopolamine) have been replaced with numerous synthetic and semisynthetic therapeutic antimuscarinic agents with properties that make them more desirable than atropine. For example, the extremely long duration of action of atropine in the eye makes the use of other anticholinergic agents with shorter effects more desirable. Nonetheless, atropine continues to be a valuable drug in the emergency treatment of bradydysrhythmias and cardiac arrest. It is also used in anesthesia to inhibit excessive salivation and avoid the muscarinic effects of neostigmine during reversal of paralysis by nondepolarizing neuromuscular-blocking agents (5). Atropine is recommended as an antidote in cases of poisoning by cholinesterase inhibitors, such as organophosphate compounds or certain mushrooms. Although atropine has been previously used as a gastrointestinal and ureteral antispasmodic, antiasthmatic, and in the treatment of peptic ulcer disease, newer, more specific and effective therapies have largely made its use obsolete for these conditions.

Atropine is a parasympatholytic agent that exhibits its effects by competition for acetylcholine receptors at muscarinic sites of exocrine glands, cardiac muscle, and postganglionic nerves; hence, atropine is considered an anticholinergic substance. Although usually administered parenterally for therapeutic purposes, atropine is rapidly absorbed from the gastrointestinal tract following ingestion and is also well absorbed from mucosal surfaces. Following absorption, atropine is approximately 50% protein bound; 94% of the atropine dose is excreted in the urine (4). Atropine crosses the placenta but does not cause a clinically significant decrease in fetal heart rate (1). Atropine is a lipid-soluble tertiary amine that easily crosses the blood-brain barrier. In contrast, quaternary ammonium derivatives of atropine are more potent than the parent compound and have less CNS activity due to poor penetration of the blood-brain barrier (6).

Much of the pharmacological and toxicological literature is derived from clinical experience and pertains to humans. However, there are some important species differences in responses to atropine. For example, dogs do not experience hyperthermia with atropine poisoning, apparently because they do not rely upon sweating to control body temperature (10). Some species, such as the rabbit and other rodents, have endogenous atropine esterase, which allows them to tolerate large doses of atropine without the development of toxicity (10).

Because atropine has been used extensively as a pharmacological agent, there is a wealth of knowledge about its pharmacological and toxicological effects. Therapeutic doses of atropine usually result in negligible CNS effects, while larger doses of atropine may lead to sedation, confusion, hallucinations, or delirium, with subsequent coma and convulsions. In some cases, administration of atropine in therapeutic doses has resulted in symptoms characterized as the "central anticholinergic syndrome" manifested by restlessness, and hallucinations, somnolence, or unconsciousness (3). The central anticholinergic syndrome is presumed to be due to central blockade of muscarinic cholinergic receptors. Atropine applied topically or absorbed systemically blocks the iris sphincter muscle and the ciliary muscle of the lens producing mydriasis and paralysis of accommodation for up to 10 days. Secretions from mucous membranes are inhibited, resulting in drying of the nose, mouth, pharynx, and respiratory tract. Administration of atropine causes bronchodilation and reduction of bronchial secretions, reducing the incidence of laryngospasm during general anesthesia (7). The effect of atropine on the heart is primarily upon rate. Small parenteral doses (0.4–0.6 mg) may produce paroxysmal vagal stimulation and a decrease in heart rate, particularly if atropine is infused slowly (2). However, larger doses cause a progressive increase in tachycardia due to blockade of vagal innervation of the sinoatrial node (8). This effect makes atropine a valuable modality in the treatment of bradydysrhythmias and cardiac arrest. Atropine has little direct effect upon blood pressure, but overdosage may produce hypotension from dilatation of cutaneous blood vessels with the production of a characteristic flushed appearance to the skin. Sweating is also inhibited, resulting in the appearance of warm, red, dry skin leading to an increase in body temperature. Gastrointestinal effects of atropine produce marked decreases in motility of the stomach and of small and large intestines.

Intentional or accidental overdosage of atropine or other anticholinergic drugs produces rapid development of symptoms and clinical findings of the anticholinergic toxic syndrome. This syndrome is characterized by dry skin, flushing, hyperthermia, mydriasis, tachycardia, urinary retention, delirium, hallucinations, and respiratory insufficiency.

REFERENCES

1. Abboud T, Raya J, Sadri S *et al.* (1983) Fetal and maternal cardiovascular effects of atropine and glycopyrrolate. *Anesth Analg* **62**, 426.

2. Chamberlain DA, Turner P, Sneddon JM (1967) Effects of atropine on heart rate in healthy man. *Lancet* **ii**, 12.

3. Duvoisin RC, Katz RL (1968) Reversal of central anticholinergic syndrome in man by physostigmine. *J Amer Med Assn* **2106**, 1963.

4. Kalser SC (1971) The fate of atropine in man. *Ann N Y Acad Sci* **179**, 667.

5. Mirakhur RK (1988) Anticholinergic drugs and anesthesia. *Can J Anaesth* **35**, 433.

6. Proakis AG, Harris GB (1978) Comparative penetration of glycopyrrolate and atropine across the blood brain and placental barriers in anesthetized dogs. *Anesthesiology* **48**, 339.

7. Rosen M (1960) Atropine in the treatment of laryngeal spasm. *Brit J Anaesth* **32**, 190.

8. Shutt LE, Bowes JB (1979) Atropine and hyoscine. *Anaesthesia* **34**, 476.

9. Stoelting RK (1991) Anticholinergic drugs. In: *Pharmacology and Physiology in Anesthetic Practice*. JB Lippincott Co, Philadelphia, p. 242.

10. Weiner N (1980) Atropine, scopolamine, and related antimuscarinic drugs. In: *Goodman and Gilman's The Pharmacological Basis of Therapeutics. 6th Ed.* Gilman AG, Goodman LS, Gilman A eds. Macmillan Publishing Co, New York p. 120.

Avermectins

Albert C. Ludolph

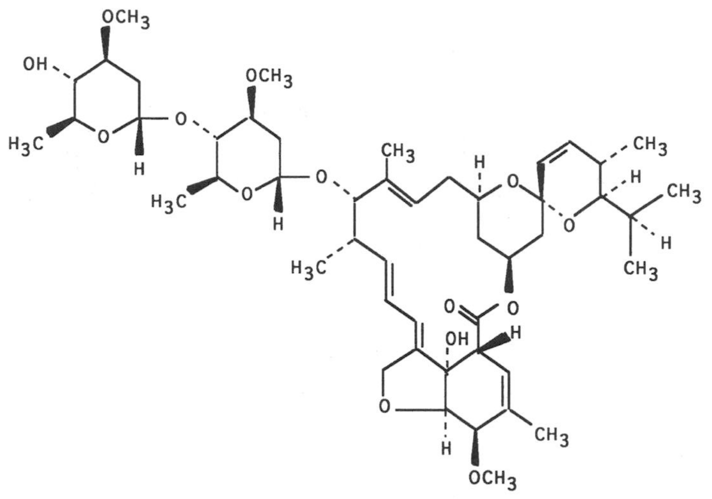

AVERMECTIN A$_{1a}$
C$_{49}$H$_{74}$O$_{14}$

NEUROTOXICITY RATING

Experimental

A Ataxia

A Mydriasis

B Ion channel syndrome (chloride channel agonist)

Avermectins, a group of macrocyclic lactones, are the products of the soil microorganism *Streptomyces avermitilis* (3). Two series of compounds exist (A and B), both of which have two structural subsets, 1 and 2 (6). The most important compound is avermectin B$_{1a}$ because of its outstanding potency against a number of endo- and ectoparasites. Avermectin B$_{1a}$ serves as a starter for the semisynthetic 22,23-dihydroavermectin B$_{1a}$, the main component of the widely used antiparasitic drug ivermectin. Milbemycins are structurally related to avermectins but lack the C-13 disaccharide component. This is a semisynthetic derivative of avermectins and contains at least 80% 22,23-dihydroavermectin B$_{1a}$ and not more than 20% 22,23-dihydroavermectin B$_{1b}$. Ivermectin is a white powder, highly lipophilic like all avermectins, and soluble in organic solvents such as methylene chloride, alcohols, and dimethylsulfoxide. A mixture of avermectin B$_{1a}$ and B$_{1b}$ (abamectin) is used as a miticide and insecticide in agriculture.

In humans, ivermectin is absorbed after oral ingestion, parenteral or—comparatively poorly—cutaneous application (5). Peak serum concentrations are reached 3–5 h after oral intake, and the compound is primarily distributed into liver and fat. Ivermectin is almost totally excreted in the feces; only 2% is detected in urine. Residual tissue concentrations are highest in liver and fat (4). Although the elimination half-life of ivermectin is comparatively short, for unknown reasons its biological (microfilaricidal) activity persists in rodents for at least 30 days (1). Abamectin is degraded when exposed to sunlight in water and has a half-life of about 12 h. Whether the widespread use of ivermectin has negative effects on cattle dung decomposition is discussed (11).

Avermectins are extensively used in veterinary medicine as endo- and ectoantiparasiticides. Their principal mode of action is a potent paralyzing effect on arthropods and nematodes. In humans, ivermectin is used as an antihelmintic in the treatment and prophylaxis of onchocerciasis (river blindness) in Africa, Yemen, and Latin America (12). While the disease caused by *Onchocerca volvulus* can be controlled by this compound, there are questions regarding long-term effects of ivermectin, particularly on posterior segment disease (12). Reported ocular side effects include transient limbitis, iridocyclitis, flare, altered retinal perfusion, papillitis, and choroidoretinal infiltration (12).

Despite intensive study, the molecular mode of action of avermectins is unclear (for reviews, *see* 2,13). Avermectins apparently bind to several chloride-channel proteins and increase ion permeability; however, their binding site is distinct from other known effector proteins of these channels. When the binding site of avermectins is defined, their differential effects on chloride-channel opening and conductance in different species will likely be explained. Results of these studies will also impact understanding of the neurotoxicity of avermectins.

The spectrum of side effects of avermectins includes syndromes of neurotoxicity (8). The toxicological syndrome induced by abamectin and ivermectin is similar; however, ivermectin seems to be somewhat less toxic. Since avermectins are large molecules, under normal circumstances they do not cross the blood-brain barrier of mammals, and no major side effects are expected in mature animals with an intact blood-brain barrier. Neonatal animals, in which the blood-brain barrier is likely to be less developed, are more susceptible to neurotoxic effects. Motor-system deficits are also reported in repeatedly exposed animals of certain species.

Controlled studies on the neurological side effects of avermectins in a variety of species are reported (8,9). In general, rodents are more sensitive to the neurotoxic potential of these agents; dosages of 0.2 mg/kg in mice and rats have produced tremors and ataxia. After oral administration of tenfold the recommended dose of ivermectin (2.0 mg/kg) for 2 days, 5 of 11 horses reportedly developed impairment of vision, depression, and ataxia (9); after a single dose of 12.0 mg/kg, horses showed signs of acute toxicity such as "depression, ataxia, mydriasis, lower-lip drop and depressed respiration." Two foals developed forelimb lameness after 3 doses of 0.6–1.0 mg/kg at 2-week intervals; however, this was not thought to be related to ivermectin neurotoxicity since there was apparently no consistent dose–response relationship (9). In cattle, acute toxicity after subcutaneous administration of 8.0 mg/kg ivermectin was characterized by "ataxia, general motor depression, muscular fasciculation, extensor rigidity of the limbs, increased respiration, and mydriasis" (9). Serum iron levels decreased after administration of these high doses; histology was unremarkable. After oral or subcutaneous administration of 4.0 mg/kg, cattle showed CNS dysfunction which included listlessness and depression, progressing to recumbency and death; a contributory effect of the vehicle (propylene glycol) was suspected (9). A slightly different picture was observed after injection of avermectin B₁ into cattle. Early signs of toxicosis, such as depression and ataxia, were seen after single doses as little as 727 μg/kg (calves) to 1 mg/kg body weight. In sheep and goats, a syndrome of acute toxicity has not been identified. Swine developed such a syndrome at 300 μg/kg, but comparable toxicity is not reported in sheep and goats (9). Beagles receiving single doses of 2–10 mg/kg also displayed depression and ataxia. Collies showed extreme sensitivity to the ivermectin formulated for horses, sheep, cattle, and swine; an oral dose of 200 mg/kg ivermectin reportedly induced "ataxia, dysmetria, depression, tremors, mydriasis, and recumbency" (9). Unusually high CNS concentrations of ivermectin were found in the animals that died.

Uncontrolled studies of neurological side effects of lower doses of avermectins are few; however, they are of interest in relation to the extremely widespread use of this class of compounds and their possible pathogenetic mechanisms. The most intriguing observation relates to Murray Grey cattle in Australia in 1985 (10). Three steers weighing 120–200 μg/kg developed signs of motor-system disease 2–3 days after injection of avermectin B₁; muscle fasciculation, lingual paralysis, knuckling of fetlocks, swaying gait, incoordination, and drooping of the ears accompanied by apparent blindness were observed. A fourth animal developed signs after 20 days: fasciculation, a wide-base stance, and an apparent paresis of neck muscles were evident. "When forced to move it was mildly ataxic and dragged the hooves of both forefeet" (10). A field trial was performed thereafter, and one animal developed neurological signs similar to that seen in the previous four animals. Neuropathological examination reportedly did not reveal any significant changes. However, high-performance liquid chromatography analysis detected a five- to tenfold increase of avermectin B₁ in the CNS of affected animals compared with that in a control. The result of the field trial and the absence of other factors "suggests avermectin B₁ to be responsible for the condition" (10). The authors state "the neurological signs seen in these cattle treated with avermectin B₁ at about 200 μg/kg were similar to signs seen in other cattle treated at a dose rate greater than 1000 μg/kg" and refer to unpublished data (10). It is evident that the hypothesis that animals suffering from impairment of blood-brain barrier function are at risk for motor-system disease after administration of avermectin B₁ must be seriously examined.

Data on human exposures to avermectins are limited. After single doses of 200 μg/kg, neurotoxicity was not observed. Reversible mydriasis and somnolence was seen in a child who accidentally ingested 7–8 mg/kg (2). Myalgia was reported in another person (7). No antidote exists, and γ-aminobutyric acidergic drugs should be avoided during an acute intoxication.

REFERENCES

1. Bennett JL, Williams JF, Dave V (1988) Pharmacology of ivermectin. *Parasitol Today* **4**, 226.
2. Campbell WC (1989) *Ivermectin and Abamectin.* Springer Verlag, New York.
3. Campbell WC, Fisher MH, Stapley EO *et al.* (1983) Ivermectin: A potent new antiparasitic drug. *Science* **221**, 823.
4. Chiu S-HL, Lu AYH (1989) Metabolism and tissue residues. In: *Ivermectin and Abamectin.* Campbell WC ed. Springer Verlag, New York p. 131.
5. Edwards G, Breckenridge AM (1985) Clinical pharmacokinetics of anthelmintic drugs. *Clin Pharmacokinet* **15**, 67.
6. Fisher MH, Mrozik H (1989) Chemistry. In: *Ivermectin*

and Abamectin. Campbell WC ed. Springer Verlag, New York p. 1.

7. Kumaraswami V, Ottesen EA, Vijayasekaran V *et al.* (1988) Ivermectin for the treatment of *Wucheria bancrofti* filariasis. *J Amer Med Assn* **259**, 3150.

8. Lankas GR, Gordon LR (1989). Toxicology. In: *Ivermectin and Abamectin.* Campbell WC ed. Springer Verlag, New York p. 90.

9. Pulliam JD, Preston JM (1989) Safety of ivermectin in target animals. In: *Ivermectin and Abamectin.* Campbell WC ed. Springer-Verlag, New York p. 149.

10. Seaman JT, Eagleson JS, Carrigan MJ, Webb RF (1987) Avermectin B1 toxicity in a herd of Murray Grey cattle. *Aust Vet J* **64**, 284.

11. Wall R, Strong L (1987) Environmental consequences of treating cattle with the antiparasitic drug ivermectin. *Nature* **327**, 418.

12. Whitworth JAG, Gilbert CE, Mabey DM *et al.* (1991) Effects of repeated doses of ivermectin on ocular onchicerciasis: Community-based trial in Sierra Leone. *Lancet* **338**, 1100.

13. Wright DJ (1986) Biological activity and mode of action of avermectins. In: *Neuropharmacology and Pesticide Action.* Ford MG, Lunt GG, Reay RC, Usherwood PNR eds. Harwood, UK p. 174.

Azacitidine

Herbert H. Schaumburg

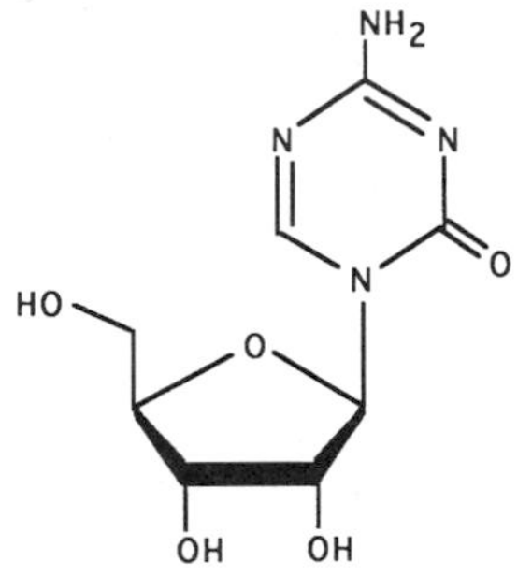

AZACITIDINE
$C_8H_{12}N_4O_5$

4-Amino-1-β-D-ribofuranosyl-1,3,5-triazin-2(1H)-one; Ladakamycin; 5-Azacytidine

NEUROTOXICITY RATING

Experimental

A   CNS teratogen

5-Azacytidine is an analogue of the naturally occurring pyrimidine, cytidine. The drug differs from the naturally occurring nucleoside in the substitution of nitrogen for carbon at the 5 position on the pyrimidine ring. 5-Azacytidine competes with cytidine triphosphate for incorporation into RNA resulting in polyribosomal degradation and defective protein synthesis, causing cell death. It is also incorporated into DNA and inhibits DNA methylation, an important step in regulation of gene expression. The apoptotic potency of 5-azacytidine reflects both RNA and DNA effects; the differences in cell cycle specificity vary with concentration of the drug (4).

5-Azacytidine is used in the treatment of acute lymphocytic leukemia (7). The principal toxicity of the drug is myelosuppression. There are no reports of experimental animal or human neurotoxicity. 5-Azacytidine has been repeatedly administered intrathecally to primates without ill effect (2).

5-Azacytidine has been widely used in experimental neuroteratology. The drug is administered to pregnant mice at various stages of gestation and has caused limb-bud maldevelopment (1), cleft palate (6), and disruption of gliogenesis in the rat optic nerve (5). Gross morphological studies of the mouse pups born of mothers treated late in pregnancy describe reduction of size of hippocampal and cingulate cortices (3). Behavioral study of these pups disclosed that the basic patterns of parenteral behavior were spared.

REFERENCES

1. Branch S, Francis BM, Brownie CF, Chernoff N (1996) Teratogenic effects of the demethylating agent 5-aza-2'-deoxycytidine in the Swiss Webster mouse. *Toxicology* **11**, 37.

2. Heideman RL, McCully C, Balis FM, Poplack DG (1993) Cerebrospinal fluid pharmacokinetics and toxicology of intraventricular and intrathecal arabinosyl-5-azacytosine (fazarabine, NSC 281272) in the nonhuman primate. *Invest New Drug* **11**, 135.

3. Londei T, Misto R, Vismara C, Leone VG (1995) Congenital brain damage spares the basic patterns of parental behavior in affected mice. *Brain Res* **677**, 61.

4. Murakami T, Li X, Gong J *et al.* (1995) Induction of

apoptosis by 5-azacytidine: Drug concentration-dependent differences in cell cycle specificity. *Cancer Res* 55, 3093.

5. Ransom BR, Yamate CL, Black JS, Waxman SG (1985) Rat optic nerve: Disruption of gliogenesis with 5-azacytidine during early postnatal development. *Brain Res* 337, 41.

6. Rogers JM, Francis BM, Sulik KK *et al.* (1994) Cell death and cell cycle perturbation in the developmental toxicity of the demethylating agent. *Teratology* 50, 332.

7. Wijermans PW, Krulder JW, Huijgens PC, Neve P (1997) Continuous infusion of low-dose 5-aza-2'-deoxycytidine in elderly patients with high-risk myelodysplastic syndrome. *Leukemia* 11, 1.

Azoles

Herbert H. Schaumburg

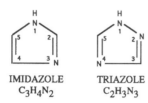

IMIDAZOLE
$C_3H_4N_2$

TRIAZOLE
$C_2H_3N_3$

Imidazole; 1,3-Diazole
1*H*-1,2,4-Triazole; Pyrrodiazole

NEUROTOXICITY RATING
Clinical

A   Acute encephalopathy (confusion, hallucinations)

The azole antifungal agents include the imidazoles (clotrimazole, ketoconazole, miconazole) and the triazoles (fluconazole, terconazole). The major effect on fungi is inhibition of sterol 14-α-demethylase, a microsomal cytochrome P-450–dependent enzyme system. Azoles thus impair the biosynthesis of ergosterol for cytoplasmic membranes and inhibit growth. They are widely used in topical preparations with few adverse reactions; some (fluconazole, ketoconazole) are used systemically and have been widely employed in combating infections in immunocompromised patients. High-level systemic dosage is associated with hepatotoxicity, hyponatremia from inappropriate antidiuretic hormone secretion, and endocrine abnormalities (likely secondary to dysfunctional steroid synthesis).

Systemic administration is accompanied by headache and somnolence in 10% of cases. Acute toxic psychosis with confusion, hallucinations, and delusions is rarely described with each agent (1,2). Intrathecal administration is associated with arachnoiditis, without ischemic myelopathy (3).

REFERENCES
1. Cohen J (1980) Antifungal chemotherapy. *Lancet* ii, 532.
2. Robinson PA, Knirsch AK, Joseph JA (1990) Fluconazole for life-threatening fungal infections in patients who cannot be treated with conventional antifungal agents. *Rev Infect Dis* 12, S349.
3. Stevens DA (1977) Miconazole in the treatment of systemic fungal infections. *Amer Rev Resp Dis* 116, 801.

Baclofen

Herbert H. Schaumburg

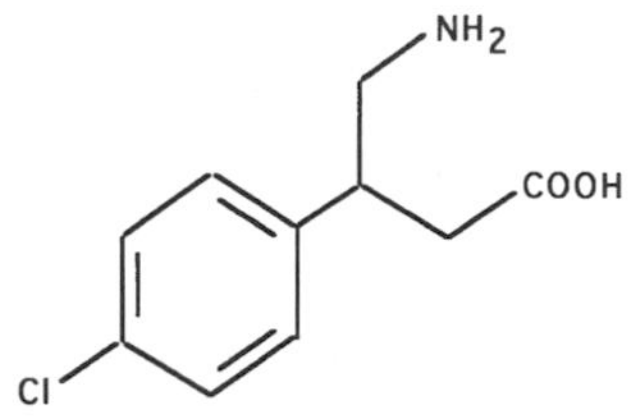

BACLOFEN
$C_{10}H_{12}ClNO_2$

β-(Aminomethyl)-4-chlorobenzenepropanoic acid

NEUROTOXICITY RATING

Clinical

A Seizure disorder

A Acute encephalopathy (sedation, stupor)

Baclofen, a structural analog of γ-aminobutyric acid, is used in the treatment of spinal spasticity. Its antispastic effect stems from a depressant action on monosynaptic and polysynaptic transmission in the spinal cord. The drug reduces excitatory postsynaptic potentials in ventral horn motor neurons. Orally administered baclofen is rapidly absorbed, has a plasma half-life of 4 h, and is excreted unchanged in the kidney. Determination of individual dosage requires gradual, cautious titration to reach a level that reduces muscle spasm and rigidity without causing severe weakness or drowsiness. The initial dose is 5 mg every 12 h, increasing to a level near 80 mg daily. Chronic administration of baclofen *via* an intrathecal pump has proven effective and safe; it is used in patients who become somnolent at therapeutic oral doses or if spasticity is resistant to high oral doses of the drug (3).

Baclofen has few persistent neurotoxic consequences at usual doses in individuals with normal renal function. Drowsiness and fatigue are common; most accommodate to these effects if dosage is gradually increased. Stupor, hypotension, respiratory depression, and coma are rare and usually respond to prompt administration of physostigmine (4). Generalized seizures have appeared in individuals with underlying focal brain lesions or pre-existent epilepsy and in normal persons following abrupt withdrawal of drug (2). Isolated case reports of psychiatric disorders in the course of baclofen therapy are likely to be idiosyncratic reactions; one prospective study indicates few adverse psychological effects (1).

REFERENCES

1. Jamous A, Kennedy P, Psychol C, Grey N (1994) Psychological and emotional effects of the use of oral baclofen: A preliminary study. *Paraplegia* **32**, 349.
2. Kofler M, Kronenberg MF, Rifici C *et al.* (1994) Epileptic seizures associated with intrathecal baclofen application. *Neurology* **44**, 25.
3. Penn RD (1992) Intrathecal baclofen for spasticity of spinal origin: Seven years of experience. *J Neurosurg* **77**, 236.
4. Teddy P, Jamous A, Gardner B *et al.* (1992) Complications of intrathecal baclofen. *Brit J Neurosurg* **6**, 115.

Barbiturates

Joseph Maytal
Shlomo Shinnar

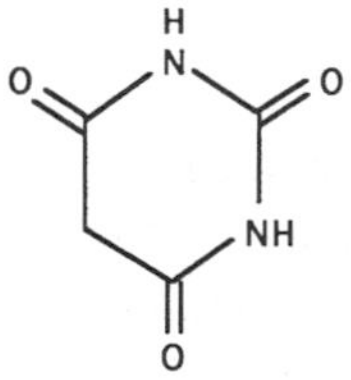

BARBITURIC ACID
$C_4H_4N_2O_3$

Barbituric acid; 2,4,6-Trioxohexahydropyrimidine

NEUROTOXICITY RATING

Clinical

A Acute encephalopathy (sedation, coma)

B Chronic encephalopathy

B Teratogenicity

Experimental

A GABA facilitation

A CNS depression

A CNS teratogen

The barbiturates are nonselective CNS depressants used as sedative-hypnotics and, in subhypnotic doses, as anticonvulsants.

Barbituric acid has no CNS depressant activity, but the substitution of alkyl or aryl groups at position C5 confers sedative-hypnotic activity. Anticonvulsant properties diminish if the alkyl side chains in the C5 position are long. A phenyl group at C5 or N3 confers selective anticonvulsant activity on a barbiturate. Compounds available in the United States are shown in Table 2 (40). With few exceptions, substitutions on the structural nucleus influence the duration of action. For example, the substitution of the oxygen at C2 by sulfur produces thiobarbiturates, which are more liposoluble than the corresponding oxybarbiturates and are classified as ultra-short-acting barbiturates. Alternatively, substitution of a phenyl group at R3 produces compounds that are classified as long-acting (14).

Phenobarbital, 5-ethyl-5-phenyl butyric acid, is one of the most widely used barbiturates. Phenobarbital is a white, odorless, crystalline powder that is very slightly soluble in water and soluble in organic solvents such as ether and ethanol.

The mechanism of sedative/hypnotic action of the barbiturates and benzodiazepines is similar. Both drugs bind to the chloride channel molecule that functions as the γ-aminobutyric acid (GABA) receptor. GABA is the major inhibitory neurotransmitter in the brain, and the barbiturates facilitate the action of GABA at multiple sites in the CNS. In contrast to benzodiazepines, barbiturates appear to increase the duration of the GABA-gated channel opening (51). At high concentrations, the barbiturates may also be GABA-mimetic—directly activating chloride channels (50). Barbiturates are less selective in their action than benzodi-azepines, and the multiplicity of sites of action of barbiturates may be the basis for their ability to induce surgical anesthesia and for their prolonged central depressant effects.

The use of barbiturates as sedative-hypnotic drugs has declined enormously because of a nonspecific effect in the CNS and a lower therapeutic index than that of benzodiazepines. In addition, tolerance occurs more frequently than for the benzodiazepines. Liability for abuse is greater, and the number of drug interactions is considerable. Although the use of barbiturates as sedative-hypnotics has largely been replaced by benzodiazepines, phenobarbital and butalbital are still commercially available as "sedatives" in combined preparations used to treat a variety of medical conditions. They are also sometimes used to antagonize unwarranted CNS stimulant effects of various drugs, such as ephedrine, theophilline, and dextroamphetamines.

Phenobarbital was one of the first effective treatments for epilepsy and, for many years, was a mainstay antiepileptic treatment. In a significant percentage of patients, it reduces the incidence of seizures at doses that do not produce CNS depression. The drug is currently mostly used for generalized, tonic-clonic, and partial seizures in children and in neonatal seizures (36). In developing countries, phenobarbital remains a first-line antiepileptic drug in all age groups because of its wide availability and low cost. The ultra-short-acting barbiturates, such as thiopental sodium, are used extensively in the induction of surgical anesthesia.

The barbiturates and their sodium salts are addictive; some are substances of abuse. They are subject to control under the U.S. Federal Controlled Substances Act; phenobarbital is a Schedule IV drug, secobarbital is Schedule II (high abuse potential).

Barbiturates are absorbed in varying degrees following oral or parenteral administration. The salts are more rapidly absorbed than the acids. The rate of absorption is increased if the sodium salt is ingested as a dilute solution or taken on empty stomach (38). The onset of effect varies from 10–60 min, depending upon the agent and the formulation. When necessary, intramuscular injections of sodium salt solutions are placed deep into large muscles. With some agents, special preparations are available for rectal administration. The intravenous route is normally reserved for the treatment of status epilepticus (phenobarbital sodium) and for induction and maintenance of general anesthesia (e.g., thiopental, methohexital) (40).

Following absorption, barbiturates are rapidly distributed to all tissues and fluids, and high concentrations are found in the brain, liver, and kidney; they readily cross the placenta. The more lipid-soluble the barbiturate, the more rapidly its tissue penetration (38). Binding to plasma pro-

TABLE 2. Barbiturates Currently Available in the United States

Barbiturate	R_{5a}	R_{5b}
Amobarbital	Ethyl	Isopentyl
Aprobarbital	Allyl	Isopropyl
Butabarbital	Ethyl	Sec-butyl
Butalbital	Allyl	Isobutyl
Mephobarbital*	Ethyl	Phenyl
Metharbital*	Ethyl	Ethyl
Methohexital*	Allyl	1-Methyl-2-pentynyl
Pentobarbital	Ethyl	1-Methylbutyl
Phenobarbital	Ethyl	Phenyl
Secobarbital	Allyl	1-Methylbutyl
Thiopental†	Ethyl	1-Methylbutyl

*R_3 = H, except in mephobarbital, metharbital, and methohexital, where it is replaced by CH_3.

†O, except in thiopental, where it is replaced by S.

[Modified from Hardman JG, Limbird LE (1996) *Goodman and Gilman's The Pharmacological Basis of Therapeutics. 9th Ed.* McGraw-Hill, New York.]

tein is a function of lipid solubility and is greatest for thiopental, which is 65% bound. The highly lipid-soluble barbiturates, led by those used to induce anesthesia, undergo redistribution after intravenous injection. Uptake into less vascularized areas, especially muscle and fat, leads to a decline in the concentration of barbiturate in plasma and brain (40).

Barbiturates are metabolized primarily by the hepatic microsomal system; the metabolic products are excreted in the urine and, less commonly, in the feces. About 25% of phenobarbital and nearly all of aprobarbital (long-acting barbiturates) are excreted unchanged in the urine. All the other barbiturates are nearly completely metabolized and/or conjugation precedes renal excretion. The oxidation of radicals at C5 is the most important biotransformation responsible for termination of biological activity. Oxidation results in the formation of alcohols, ketones, phenols, or carboxylic acids, which may appear in the urine as such or as glucuronic acid conjugates (40).

The best known effects of barbiturates on the liver are those on the microsomal drug-metabolizing system. The barbiturates combine with cytochrome P-450 and competitively interfere with the biotransformation of endogenous substrates such as steroids, as well as a number of other drugs. Thus, adverse drug interactions and potential endocrine imbalances are a serious hazard (40).

Neurological, psychological, and systemic adverse effects occur with long-term use of phenobarbital when the drug is used as an anticonvulsant, even at the usual serum concentrations of the drug in the broad therapeutic range of 15–40 μg/ml.

Studies of the effects of barbiturates on animal behavior started 30 years ago with the demonstration of behavioral changes and learning deficits in adult rats prenatally exposed to phenobarbital (3). A decade later, another study revealed learning deficits as well as other behavioral deficits in rats prenatally exposed to barbiturates (34). Since 1975, there has been increasing interest in the effects of exposure to barbiturates on the developing animal. Some rodent studies of chronic prenatal and neonatal exposure to phenobarbital demonstrated reductions in brain weight and protein synthesis (17,37,57,60). It was also shown that early exposure to phenobarbital induced a reduction of brain weight that persisted into adulthood (6).

Prenatal exposure to barbiturate resulted in 30% fewer prenatally-forming cerebellar Purkinje cells and 15% fewer hippocampal pyramidal cells (6,22). Long-term abnormalities also were found in various layers in the cerebellum, hippocampus, olfactory bulbs, and cortex (56). The number of dendritic spines per millimeter of the surviving neurons in the neonatally exposed animals was reduced (59). An ultrastructural study of the cerebellar cortex demonstrated extensive degenerating processes and mitochondrial abnormalities (20). Biochemical studies revealed short- and long-term alterations in the activity of several neurotransmitter systems, especially the dopaminergic system (46,58).

Adult mice displayed seizures during withdrawal from chronic phenobarbital consumption (4). Other studies suggest that mice exposed to phenobarbital neonatally are significantly more susceptible to audiogenic and electroshock-induced seizures than controls (34,57).

Chronic treatment of mouse spinal cord cultures with phenobarbital resulted in decrements in both the number of large neurons and activity of choline acetyltransferase (5,44). In addition, neurons surviving long-term phenobarbital exposure showed simplified patterns of dendritic branching (45). Other studies demonstrated abnormalities in mouse cerebral cortex cultures after chronic treatment with phenytoin and phenobarbital (35), indicating that chronic treatment of cerebral cortical cells with phenobarbital may result in neurotoxic effects on formed, yet still developing neurons. Although *in vivo* and *in vitro* experiments may not be directly applicable in human infants, there is concern since phenobarbital is currently the preferred antiepileptic drug for neonatal seizures and is widely administered to pregnant women with seizures.

Long-term use of phenobarbital as an anticonvulsant, even at doses that produce serum concentrations within the therapeutic range of 15–40 μg/ml, may cause adverse changes in behavior, cognitive function, and affect (47). High serum concentrations cause nystagmus, dysarthria, incoordination, and ataxia (31).

Sedation is the hallmark of barbiturate toxicity. Complaints of fatigue, listlessness, and loss of interest in social activities are common (31). Sedation occurs primarily during the first days of treatment and usually clears rapidly as tolerance develops (10,11,26). Development of tolerance is evidenced by decrease in symptoms despite increasing phenobarbital concentrations from 18 μg/ml at 2 weeks to 24 μg/ml at 12 weeks (31).

A paradoxical behavioral effect of phenobarbital occurs in children and in the elderly; it produces insomnia and hyperactivity, even with a serum concentration of <15 μg/ml (18,55). There does not appear to be a relationship between the plasma concentration of phenobarbital and behavioral side effects (55). One study found no differences in hyperactivity between a group of 35 toddlers given phenobarbital and a control group given placebo. However, dose-related irritability and erratic sleep, without frank hyperactivity, were common in the phenobarbital group (13).

Alteration of affect, particularly depression, can be produced even at therapeutic plasma levels of phenobarbital

(31). It may be difficult to determine whether such mood changes are a direct neurotoxic effect of phenobarbital, a reaction to an addition of another drug to treat seizures, or a newly diagnosed illness (9,42). A higher incidence of depression and suicidal behavior was found in adolescents with epilepsy receiving phenobarbital relative to those receiving carbamazepine; the increased risk was limited to those adolescents with a family history of major affective disorders (9). The effect would appear to be real and probably represents an idiosyncratic reaction in susceptible individuals. Treatment with an alternative antiepileptic drug, such as carbamazepine, often results in amelioration of the depressive symptomatology (9).

Cognitive disturbances with poor school performance and compromised work may develop independent of sedation and hypnotic activity in children receiving phenobarbital (32). In early reports, institutionalized epileptic patients showed some improvement in intelligence testing after treatment with antiepileptic drugs (30,48). Studies that compared patients on phenobarbital either to patients on other antiepileptic drugs (12,42,53) or to patients on placebo (13,19) show that phenobarbital impairs learning ability (19,53) or depresses cognitive performance. Other studies have found no difference in intelligence scores between placebo groups and phenobarbital-treated groups (1,13,23,54). Barbiturates can impair performance on vigilance tests (33), tests requiring sustained effort or attention (26,29), and perceptual-motor tests (26). Memory impairment is a common complaint of epileptic patients. Phenobarbital was found to have deleterious effects on short-term memory with test performance related to dose (15).

Barbiturate overdose, with a phenobarbital level exceeding $50-60$ μg/ml, causes neurological dysfunction and depression of consciousness. Excessively high doses first produce ataxia, dysarthria, nystagmus, incoordination, and uncontrolled sleepiness (31). As serum levels climb, stupor and coma ensue, and eventually, there is cardiorespiratory arrest. Lethal blood levels are $100-200$ μg/ml. The toxic oral dose of barbiturate varies but, in general, 1 g of most barbiturates produces serious poisoning in an adult. Death commonly occurs after $2-10$ g of ingested barbiturates. The phenobarbital toxic dose and its lethal serum level are lower in cases of acute poisoning in individuals without prior exposure to the drug. Serum levels of $20-40$ μg/ml, which would be considered within the therapeutic range in treatment of seizure disorders, may produce fatal respiratory depression if achieved acutely in a previously untreated subject. Adults are more susceptible than children to the acute respiratory depression induced by phenobarbital.

Physical dependence may occur with prolonged use of phenobarbital. Drug dependence results from repeated continuous administration of a barbiturate, generally in amounts exceeding therapeutic dose levels. The characteristics of barbiturate dependence include a strong desire to continue taking the drug, tendency to increase the dose, and psychic and physical dependence on the effects of the drug. Daily administration in excess of 400 mg of phenobarbital or secobarbital for approximately 90 days is likely to produce some degree of physical dependence. As tolerance to barbiturates develops, the amount needed to maintain the same level of intoxication increases. The symptoms of barbiturate withdrawal can be severe and may be fatal. Withdrawal symptoms include anxiety, emotional lability, insomnia, tremors, diaphoresis, confusion, and seizures (16,25,27). The withdrawal symptoms can be reversed in early stages by reinstituting the drug. To end phenobarbital therapy, the drug should be tapered slowly to avoid seizures that may occur during withdrawal, even in individuals with no prior history of seizures. As phenobarbital readily crosses the placenta, a neonatal withdrawal syndrome has occurred in infants born to epileptic mothers treated with phenobarbital; hyperexcitability, tremors, irritability, and gastrointestinal symptoms may continue for days to several months (7,16).

Understanding the teratogenicity of phenobarbital is confounded by its common use in combination with antiepileptic drugs, such as phenytoin, that have been implicated in the induction of fetal anomalies ("fetal hydantoin syndrome") (49). Two children exposed to phenobarbital and primidone *in utero* displayed facial dysmorphism, prenatal and postnatal growth deficiency, developmental delay, and minor anomalies (43). The specific dysmorphic features— short nose, broad nasal bridge, hypertelorism, epicanthal folds, ptosis, low-set ears—were noted to be similar to children with hydantoin and fetal alcohol syndromes. Craniofacial abnormalities are also described in children with intrauterine exposure to primidone. Hirsute foreheads, thick nasal roots, anteverted nostrils, long philtrum, and hypoplastic nails were noted. The children were also small for their gestational age and had psychomotor retardation (21). One study describes decreased fetal head growth associated with maternal use of phenobarbital and hydantoin and suggested that phenytoin alone is not associated with small head circumference, but phenytoin and phenobarbital together are (24). Other reports support the notion that phenobarbital therapy during pregnancy may be associated with impaired intellect in the offspring (2,49,52). Despite these risks, phenobarbital is considered, by some, a reasonably safe drug of choice during pregnancy (28).

Most neurotoxic side effects of phenobarbital subside with a single reduction in dosage. Improvement is gradual because of slow elimination of the drug. Recommendation for change in treatment in a case of toxicity varies according to the severity. The management of phenobarbital overdose includes protecting the airway and support of ventilation and blood pressure. Absorption of drugs from the gastrointestinal tract may be decreased by giving charcoal in addition to, or instead of, gastric emptying. Alkalinization and induction of forced diuresis hasten phenobarbital excretion, but dialysis and hemoperfusion have been found to be more effective and cause less troublesome alterations in electrolyte equilibrium.

The mechanism of phenobarbital neuronal toxicity is unknown. It has been suggested that phenobarbital blocks the action of trophic substances critical to neuronal survival (44). Blockade of electrical activity reduces the survival of neurons in cultures (5), and this may represent another mechanism detrimental to neuronal survival. In immature neurons, growth-cone elongation may be dependent upon an influx of Ca^{2+} (8); phenobarbital has been shown to inhibit depolarization-dependent Ca^{2+} uptake by synaptosomes (39). This may be the result of chronic phenobarbital exposure with long-term phenobarbital-dependent reduction in gross terminal Ca^{2+} influx.

Other Barbiturates
Primidone

Primidone is an effective agent for treatment of all types of epilepsy, except absence seizures. Primidone may be viewed as a congener of phenobarbital in which the carbonyl oxygen of the urea moiety is replaced by two hydrogen atoms. The anticonvulsive effects of primidone, which resemble those of phenobarbital, are attributed to both the drug and its active metabolites, principally phenobarbital (41). Primidone is converted to two active metabolites, phenobarbital and phenylethylmalonic acid (PEMA). Approximately 40% of the unconjugated drug is excreted in the urine; PEMA, and to a lesser extent phenobarbital and its metabolites, constitute the remainder. Sedation, vertigo, dizziness, nausea, ataxia, and nystagmus are common. Patients may also experience an acute sense of intoxication immediately following administration of primidone. There is no clear relationship between the concentration of primidone or its other metabolites in plasma, and the drug's therapeutic effect.

Mephobarbital

Mephobarbital is an *N*-methyl phenobarbital. Most of its activity during long-term therapy can be attributed to the accumulation of its metabolite, phenobarbital. The pharmacological properties, toxicity, and clinical uses are as for phenobarbital. Oral absorption is poor and the dose is approximately twice that of phenobarbital (41).

REFERENCES

1. Aldridge Smith J, Wallace SJ (1982) Intellectual progress related to recurrence of fits and to anticonvulsant therapy. *Arch Dis Child* 57, 104.

2. Annegers JF, Elvback LR, Hauser WA *et al.* (1974) Do anticonvulsants have a teratogenic effect? *Arch Neurol* 31, 364.

3. Armitage SG (1952) The effects of barbiturates on the behavior of rat offspring as measured in learning and reasoning situations. *J Comp Physiol Psychol* 45, 146.

4. Belknap JK, Waddingham S, Ondrusck G (1973) Barbiturate dependence in mice induced by a simple short-term oral procedure. *Physiol Psychol* 1, 394.

5. Bergey GK, Swaiman KF, Schrier BK *et al.* (1981) Adverse effects of phenobarbital on morphological and biochemical development of fetal mouse spinal cord neurons in culture. *Ann Neurol* 9, 584.

6. Bergman A, Russelli-Austin L, Yedwab G, Yanai J (1980) Neuronal deficits in mice following phenobarbital exposure during various periods in fetal development. *Acta Anat* 108, 227.

7. Bleyer WA, Marshal RE (1972) Barbiturate withdrawal syndrome in a passively addicted infant. *J Amer Med Assn* 221, 185.

8. Bolsover SR, Spector I (1986) Measurements of calcium transients in the soma, neurite, and growth cone of single cultured neurons. *J Neurosci* 6, 1934.

9. Brent DA, Crumrine PK, Varma R *et al.* (1990) Phenobarbital treatment and major depressive disorder in children with epilepsy: A naturalistic follow up. *Pediatrics* 85, 1086.

10. Buchthal F, Svensmark O, Simonsen H (1968) Relation of EEG and seizures to phenobarbital in serum. *Arch Neurol* 19, 567.

11. Butler TC, Mahafee C, Waddell WJ (1954) Studies of elimination, accumulation, tolerance, and dosage schedules. *J Pharmacol Exp Ther* 111, 425.

12. Calandre EP, Dominguez-Granados R, Gomez-Rubio M *et al.* (1990) Cognitive effects of long term treatment with phenobarbital and valproic acid in school children. *Acta Neurol Scand* 81, 504.

13. Camfield CS, Chaplin S, Doyle AB *et al.* (1979) Side effects of phenobarbital in toddlers; behavior and cognitive aspects. *J Pediat* 95, 361.

14. Dailey JW (1989) Sedative-hypnotic and anxiolytic drugs. In: *Modern Pharmacology. 4th Ed.* Craig CR, Stitzel RE eds. Little Brown, Boston p. 369.

15. Delaney RC, Rosen AJ, Mattson RH, Novelly RA (1980) Memory function in focal epilepsy: A comparison of non-surgical, unilateral temporal lobe and frontal lobe samples. *Cortex* 16, 103.

16. Desmond MM, Schwanecke RP, Wilson G *et al.* (1972) Maternal barbiturate utilization and neonatal withdrawal symptomatology. *J Pediat* **80**, 190.

17. Diaz J, Schain RJ (1978) Phenobarbital: Effects of long term administration on behavior and brain of artificially reared rats. *Science* **199**, 90.

18. Domizio S, Verroti A, Ramenghi LA *et al.* (1993) Antiepileptic therapy and behavior disturbances in children. *Child Nerv Syst* **9**, 272.

19. Farrwell JR, Lee YJ, Hirtz DG *et al.* (1990) Phenobarbital for febrile seizures—effects on intelligence and on seizure recurrence. *N Engl J Med* **322**, 364.

20. Fishman RHB, Ornoy A, Yanai J (1983) Ultrastructural evidence of long-lasting cerebellar degeneration after early exposure to phenobarbital in mice. *Exp Neurol* **79**, 212.

21. Gustavson EE, Chen H (1985) Goldenhar syndrome. Enteroencephalocele and aqueductal stenosis following fetal primidone exposure. *Teratology* **32**, 13.

22. Hannah RS, Roth SH, Spira AW (1982) The effect of chlorpromazine and phenobarbital on cerebellar Purkinje cells. *Teratology* **26**, 21.

23. Hellstrom B, Barlach-Christofferson M (1980) Influence of phenobarbital on the psychomotor development and behavior in pre-school children with convulsions. *Neuropediatrie* **11**, 151.

24. Hiilesmaa VK, Teramo K, Granstrom ML (1981) Fetal head growth retardation associated with maternal antiepileptic drugs. *Lancet* **2**, 161.

25. Hollister LE (1965) Nervous system reactions to drugs. *Ann N Y Acad Sci* **123**, 342.

26. Hutt SJ, Jackson PM, Belsham A, Higgins G (1968) Perceptual motor behavior in relation to blood phenobarbitone level: A preliminary report. *Develop Med Child Neurol* **10**, 626.

27. Isbell H, Fraser HF (1950) Addiction to analgesics and barbiturates. *Pharmacol Rev* **2**, 355.

28. Janz D (1975) The teratogenic risk of antiepileptic drugs. *Epilepsia* **16**, 159.

29. Kortensky C, Orzack MH (1964) A research note on some of the critical factors on the dissimilar effects of chlorpromazine and secobarbital on the digit symbol substitution and continuous performance tests. *Psychopharmacology* **6**, 79.

30. Lennox WG (1942) Brain injury, drugs, and environment as causes of mental decay in epilepsy. *Amer J Psychiat* **99**, 174.

31. Mattson RH, Cramer JA (1989) Phenobarbital toxicity. In: *Antiepileptic Drugs. 3rd Ed*. Levy R, Mattson R, Meldrum J *et al.* eds. Raven Press, New York p. 341.

32. Mattson RH, Cramer JA, McCutchen CB, VA Epilepsy Cooperative Study Group (1989) Barbiturate related connective tissue disorders. *Arch Intern Med* **149**, 911.

33. Mirsky AF, Kornetsky C (1964) On the dissimilar effects of drugs on the digit symbol substitution and continuous performance tests: A review and preliminary integration

34. Murai N (1966) Effect of maternal medication during pregnancy upon behavioral development of offspring. *Tohoku J Exp Med* **89**, 265.

35. Neale EA, Sher PK, Graubard BI *et al.* (1985) Differential toxicity of chronic exposure to phenytoin, phenobarbital, or carbamazepine in cerebral cortical cell cultures. *Pediat Neurol* **1**, 143.

36. Painter MJ (1989) Phenobarbital, clinical use. In: *Antiepileptic Drugs. 3rd Ed*. Levy R, Mattson R, Meldrum J *et al.* eds. Raven Press, New York p. 329.

37. Pastalos PN, Wiggins RC (1982) Brain maturation following administration of phenobarbital, phenytoin, and sodium valproate to developing rats or to their dams: Effects on synthesis of brain myelin and other subcellular membrane proteins. *J Neurochem* **39**, 915.

38. *Physician's Desk Reference 48th Ed*. (1994) Montvale: Medical Economics, 1255 pages.

39. Prichard JW (1982) Phenobarbital: Mechanisms of action. In: *Antiepileptic Drugs*. Woodbury DM, Penry JK, Pippenger CE eds. Raven Press, New York p. 1365.

40. Rall TW (1990) Hypnotic and sedatives; ethanol. In: *The Pharmacological Basis of Therapeutics. 8th Ed*. Gilman AG, Rall TW, Nies AS, Taylor P eds. Pergamon Press, New York p. 358.

41. Rall TW, Schleifer LS (1990) Drugs effective in the therapies of the epilepsies. In: *The Pharmacological Basis of Therapeutics. 8th Ed*. Gilman AG, Rall TW, Nies AS, Taylor P eds. Pergamon Press, New York p. 445.

42. Schain RJ, Ward JW, Guthrie D (1977) Carbamazepine as an anticonvulsant in children. *Neurology* **27**, 476.

43. Seip M (1976) Growth retardation, dysmorphic facies and minor malformations following massive exposure to phenobarbitone *in utero*. *Acta Paediat* **65**, 617.

44. Serrano EE, Kunis DM, Ranson BR (1988) Effects of chronic phenobarbital exposure on cultured mouse spinal cord neurons. *Ann Neurol* **24**, 429.

45. Serrano EE, Ranson BR (1983) Effects of chronic exposure to phenobarbital on cultured mammalian central neurons. *Soc Neurosci* **9**, 1238.

46. Shaywitz SE, Cohen DJ, Shaywitz BE (1978) Biochemical basis of minimal brain dysfunction. *J Pediat* **92**, 179.

47. Shinnar S, Kang H (1994) Idiosyncratic phenobarbital toxicity mimicking a neurodegenerative disorder. *J Epilepsy* **7**, 34.

48. Sommerfeld-Ziskind E, Ziskind E (1940) Effect of phenobarbital on the mentality of epileptic patients. *Arch Neurol Psychol* **43**, 70.

49. Spiegel BD, Meadow SR (1972) Maternal epilepsy and abnormalities of the fetus and newborn. *Lancet* **ii**, 839.

50. Trevor AJ, Way WL (1995) Sedative-hypnotic drugs. In: *Basic and Clinical Pharmacology. 6th Ed*. Katzung BG ed. Appleton & Lange, Norwalk, Connecticut p. 333.

51. Twyman RE, Rogers CJ, Macdonald RL (1989) Differ-

ential regulation of GABA receptor channels by diazepam and phenobarbital. *Ann Neurol* 25, 213.

52. Van der Pol MC, Hadders-Algra M, Huisjes HS, Touwen BCL (1991) Antiepileptic medication in pregnancy: Late effects on the children's central nervous system development. *Amer J Obstet Gynecol* 164, 121.

53. Vining EPG, Mellits ED, Dorsen MM *et al.* (1987) Psychologic and behavioral effects of antiepileptic drugs in children: A double-blind comparison between phenobarbital and valproic acid. *Pediatrics* 80, 165.

54. Wapner L, Thurston DL, Holowach J (1962) Phenobarbital: Its effect on learning in epileptic children. *J Amer Med Assn* 182, 937.

55. Wolf S, Forsythe A (1978) Behavior disturbance, phenobarbital, and febrile seizures. *Pediatrics* 61, 728.

56. Yanai J (1984) An animal model for the effect of barbiturate on the development of the central nervous system. *Neurobehav Teratol* 5, 111.

57. Yanai J, Bergman A (1981) Neuronal deficits after neonatal exposure to phenobarbital. *Exp Neurol* 73, 199.

58. Yanai J, Fares F, Gavish M *et al.* (1989) Neural and behavioral alterations after early exposure to phenobarbital. *Neurotoxicology* 10, 543.

59. Yanai J, Iser C (1981) Stereologic study on Purkinje cells in mice following early exposure to barbiturate. *Psychopharmacology* 64, 707.

60. Yanai J, Rosseli-Austin L, Tabakoff B (1979) Neuronal deficits in mice following prenatal exposure to phenobarbital. *Exp Neurol* 64, 237.

Barium

Steven Herskovitz

NEUROTOXICITY RATING

Clinical

A Myopathy (hypokalemic paralysis)

Experimental

A Myopathy

Barium is a divalent alkaline earth metal with an atomic number of 56. The insoluble salt, barium sulfate, is radiopaque and used as a suspension in contrast radiography. The soluble salts (acetate, carbonate, chloride, hydroxide, nitrate, and sulfide) have many applications in industry, such as in pesticides and depilatory agents, and are highly toxic. Barium neurotoxicity consists of a syndrome of hypokalemia and acute paralysis that mimics periodic paralysis (4).

Barium sulfate meals or enemas for radiological examination are systemically nontoxic; constipation and abdominal pain may appear (2). There are risks of barium fecoliths, perforation following barium enema, and barium lung embolism from accidental venous intravasation. Inhalation of insoluble barium compounds, occurring chiefly in workers involved in processing barium ores, may result in baritosis, a benign pneumoconiosis (3).

Barium salts are rapidly absorbed from the small intestine and excreted principally in the feces (3,10). Barium carbonate is converted by gastric acid to its absorbable form, barium chloride; peak serum levels occur in 2 h and the elimination half-life is 3.6 days. A large proportion of absorbed barium is sequestered in bone. An oral toxic dose in humans is approximately 200 mg; the adult lethal dose is reported to be between 1 and 15 g.

Acute barium poisoning in dogs results in paralysis, diarrhea, and cardiac dysrhythmias that are reversible with potassium (15). An intracellular potassium shift, resulting in hypokalemia, has been demonstrated in canine erythrocytes. In frog sartorius muscle, barium reduces potassium efflux (19). In the rat, paralysis is induced within minutes at doses of 16–25 mg/kg at a rate of 0.5 mg/min; this correlates with the development of hypokalemia (16).

Ingestion causes human cases of barium salt poisoning; these instances represent suicidal/homicidal attempts or accidental contamination of foodstuffs. Occasional cases occur in industrial inhalation accidents (17) or from large surface burns with molten barium chloride (18). Several large epidemic poisonings provide the majority of cases. In the Szechuan province of China, repeated outbreaks from 1930 onward (Pa Ping, or Kiating paralysis) were eventually attributed to contamination of table salt with barium chloride (1,9). In 1945, 85 British soldiers in Persia were poisoned when barium carbonate rodenticide (average dose, 10.5 g) was accidentally substituted for flour (13). Over 100 people were poisoned in Israel in 1963 when barium carbonate was accidentally substituted for potato meal in the preparation of sausages (6,12).

The only example of long-term human barium exposure may be in cases from Pa Ping where, in addition to the acute syndrome, some patients experienced recurrent nocturnal paralytic episodes strikingly similar to periodic paralysis (1,9). Acute toxicity begins within minutes to hours following ingestion, with a prodrome of nausea, vomiting, diarrhea, abdominal pain, xerostomia, and perioral (occasionally acral) paresthesias (1,6,8–10,12,13,17). Flaccid areflexic quadriparesis, with or without respiratory and cranial nerve involvement, evolves over several hours. There may be prominent neck and respiratory muscle weakness. Relative preservation of reflexes despite severe weakness may occur (6). Weakness ranges from involvement of one limb to quadriplegia. Sensory exam and mental status are usually normal. Additional clinical features may include testicular tenderness, muscle twitching, headaches, diaphoresis, salivation, hypertension, ventricular tachyarrhythmias, and reversible acute renal insufficiency (17,20). Fatalities are related to respiratory paralysis or arrhythmia. A single case report describes co-occurrence of an extrapyramidal syndrome with basal ganglia and thalamic hyperintensity on magnetic resonance imaging in a person with severe barium-induced paralysis (7).

Hypokalemia is commonly profound, with levels as low as 0.8 mEq/l (3,5), and is reflected by T-wave abnormalities and prominent U waves in the electrocardiogram. Rhabdomyolysis is rare (10). There have been few electrodiagnostic investigations and muscle biopsies. In one case, initially inexcitable muscles were followed in the recovery period by myopathic motor units and normal motor conduction velocities (14). Sensory and mixed nerve potentials were elicited; repetitive stimulation generated normal responses. Muscle biopsy showed only mild, nonspecific type IIb atrophy. Autopsy of one case reported in 1943 showed congestion of nerve roots and chromatolysis of neurons in Clarke's column (1).

Following potassium repletion, recovery is rapid over hours to days. Oral sulfates are recommended to convert any remaining intestinal barium to the nontoxic sulfate. Intravenous administration of sodium or magnesium sulfate is best avoided, as renal failure may occur from precipitated barium sulfate in renal calyces.

Barium poisoning can simulate other neuromuscular conditions with overlapping clinical features, and diagnosis is difficult unless the clinical history clearly relates the illness to barium consumption. The differential diagnosis includes neurotoxic fish poisoning (ciguatera and others), Guillain-Barré syndrome, tick paralysis, botulism, diphtheria, and periodic paralysis.

Experimental studies suggest the paralysis of barium toxicity is related to a shift of extracellular potassium ions into muscle (15,16,19). Barium ions competitively block passive cellular potassium ion efflux, and it is postulated that continued activity of the sodium-potassium ion pump results in intracellular potassium accumulation and extracellular hypokalemia (11). Hypertension, gastrointestinal hypermotility, and muscle twitching (15) may reflect a direct stimulation of skeletal and smooth muscle.

REFERENCES

1. Allen AS (1943) Pa Ping or Kiating paralysis. *Chin Med J* **61**, 296.
2. Ansell G (1992) Radiological contrast media and radiopharmaceuticals. In: *Meyler's Side Effects of Drugs. 12th Ed*. Dukes MNG ed. Elsevier, Amsterdam p. 1165.
3. Baselt RC (1982) *Disposition of Toxic Drugs and Chemicals in Man. 2nd Ed*. Biomedical Publications, Davis, California.
4. Berning J (1975) Hypokalemia of barium poisoning. *Lancet* i, 110.
5. Deng JF, Jan IS, Cheng HS (1991) The essential role of a poison center in handling an outbreak of barium carbonate poisoning. *Vet Hum Toxicol* **33**, 173.
6. Diengott D, Rozsa O, Levy N, Muammar S (1964) Hypokalemia in barium poisoning. *Lancet* ii, 343.
7. Fogliani J, Giraud E, Henriquet D (1993) Intoxication voluntaire par le baryum. *Ann Fr Anesth Reanim* **12**, 508.
8. Gould DB, Sorrell MR, Lupariello AD (1973) Barium sulfide poisoning. Some factors contributing to survival. *Arch Intern Med* **132**, 891.
9. Huang KW (1943) Pa Ping (transient paralysis simulating family periodic paralysis). *Chin Med J* **51**, 305.
10. Johnson CH, VanTassell VJ (1991) Acute barium poisoning with respiratory failure and rhabdomyolysis. *Ann Emerg Med* **20**, 1138.
11. Layzer RB (1982) Periodic paralysis and the sodium-potassium pump. *Ann Neurol* **11**, 547.
12. Lewi Z, Bar-Khayim Y (1964) Food poisoning from barium carbonate. *Lancet* ii, 342.
13. Morton W (1945) Poisoning by barium carbonate. *Lancet* ii, 738.
14. Phelan DM, Hagley SR, Guerin MD (1984) Is hypokalemia the cause of paralysis in barium poisoning? *Brit Med J* **289**, 882.
15. Roza O, Berman LB (1971) The pathophysiology of barium: Hypokalemic and cardiovascular effects. *J Pharmacol Exp Ther* **177**, 433.
16. Schott GD, McArdle B (1974) Barium-induced skeletal muscle paralysis in the rat, and its relationship to human familial periodic paralysis. *J Neurol Neurosurg Psychiat* **37**, 32.
17. Shankle R, Keane JR (1988) Acute paralysis from inhaled barium carbonate. *Arch Neurol* **45**, 579.
18. Steward DW, Hummel RP (1984) Acute poisoning by a barium chloride burn. *J Trauma* **24**, 768.
19. Volle RL (1970) Blockade by barium of potassium fluxes in frog sartorius muscle. *Life Sci* **9**, 175.
20. Wetherill SF, Guarino MJ, Cox RW (1981) Acute renal failure associated with barium chloride poisoning. *Ann Intern Med* **95**, 187.

Batrachotoxin and Related Compounds

Peter S. Spencer

BATRACHOTOXIN
$C_{31}H_{42}N_2O_6$

Batrachotoxinin A 20-(2,4-dimethyl-1H-pyrrole-3-carboxylate); 3α,9α-Epoxy-14β,18β-(epoxyethano-N-methylimino)-5β-pregna-7,16-diene-3β,11α,20α-triol 20α-ester with 2,4-dimethylpyrrole-3-carboxylic acid.

Batrachotoxinin A: $C_{24}H_{35}NO_5$

Homobatrachotoxin: $C_{32}H_{44}N_2O_6$

NEUROTOXICITY RATING

Experimental

A   Ion channel agent (Na$^+$ channel)

Batrachotoxin (BTX) is a potent steroidal alkaloid (MW 539) isolated from secretions of the granular skin glands of the Colombian dendrobatid poison dart frog (*Phyllobates aurotaenia*) (1,5). Other cardiotoxic and neurotoxic alkaloids in the frog's skin secretions include batrachotoxinin A (BTX-A, MW 417) and homobatrachotoxin (MW 552) (1); the latter compound is also found in the feathers and skin of the hooded pitohui bird of New Guinea. Skin secretions from these small, brightly colored amphibians have been used by Indians of the Choco rain forests of Colombia to prepare deadly darts for their blowguns (1). BTX is used by neurophysiologists as an experimental tool to study ion transport in electrogenic and synaptosomal membranes.

BTX acts at the Na$^+$ channel receptor site 2; an important component of the BTX-binding site is the S6 transmembrane region of domain I of the Na$^+$ channel α subunit (10,11). Application of BTX to excitable membranes prolongs the Na$^+$-channel open time and, thereby, the sodium current recorded from the whole cell or the axon (6,7). BTX uncouples the fast inactivation of Na$^+$ currents from the immobilization of Na$^+$-gating charge in the squid giant axon (9). The single-channel gating kinetics of BTX-modified Na$^+$ channels have been characterized (2).

The LD$_{50}$ of BTX subcutaneously injected into mice is 2 mg/kg. Intravenous administration of >0.1 mg/kg BTX induces cardiac arrhythmias that terminate in ventricular fibrillation and death. BTX blocks neuromuscular transmission irreversibly; it first blocks the twitch response of muscle fibers to indirect stimulation of the nerve, while the response to direct stimulation declines during a slowly developing contracture. The final block is irreversible and results from blockade of neurotransmitter release; this is associated with swelling of nerve terminals and enlargement and derangement of presynaptic mitochondria (1).

Synthetic BTX derivatives obtained from 7,8-dihydrobatrachotoxinin A (DBTX-A) have been developed and their actions on Na$^+$ currents studied. Replacement of a methylene by a carbonyl group in the homomorpholine ring near the tertiary nitrogen atom abolishes DBTX activity; this suggests a requirement for tertiary nitrogen protonation for BTX to interact with the channel receptor (8). BTX-A benzoate binds with high affinity to voltage-sensitive Na$^+$ channels in synaptosomes from guinea pig cerebral cortex; binding is competitively antagonized by local anesthetics and noncompetitively and irreversibly antagonized by procaine isothiocyanate (3). (+/−)-Kavain, an anticonvulsant kava pyrone from *Piper methysticum* (*see Piper methysticum*), concentration-dependently suppresses binding of BTX (K$_i$ 72 mmol/l) in 4-aminopyridine–stimulated synaptosomes, a model of repetitively firing neurons (4).

REFERENCES

1. Albuquerque EX, Daly JW, Witkop B (1971) Batrachotoxin: Chemistry and pharmacology. *Science* **172**, 995.
2. Correa AM, Bezanilla F, Latorre R (1992) Gating kinetics of batrachotoxin-modified Na$^+$ channels in the squid giant axon. Voltage and temperature effects. *Biophys J* **61**, 1332.
3. Creveling CR, Bell ME, Burke TR Jr (1990) Procaine isothiocyanate: An irreversible inhibitor of the specific binding of [^{3}H]batrachotoxinin-A benzoate to sodium channels. *Neurochem Res* **14**, 441.
4. Gleitz J, Friese J, Beile A *et al.* (1996) Anticonvulsive action of (+/−)-kavain estimated from its properties on stimulated synaptosomes and Na$^+$ channel receptor sites. *Eur J Pharmacol* **315**, 89.
5. Myers K, Daly JW (1983) Dart-poison frogs. *Sci Amer* **248**, 120.

6. Quandt FN, Narahashi T (1982) Modification of single Na⁺ channels by batrachotoxin. *Proc Nat Acad Sci* USA **79**, 6732.

7. Khodorov BI (1985) Batrachotoxin as a tool to study voltage-sensitive sodium channels of excitable membranes. *Prog Biophys Mol Biol* **45**, 57.

8. Khodorov BI, Yelin EA, Zaborovskaya LD *et al.* (1992) Comparative analysis of the effects of synthetic derivatives of batrachotoxin on sodium currents in frog node of Ranvier. *Cell Mol Neurobiol* **12**, 59.

9. Tanguy J, Yeh JZ (1988) Batrachotoxin uncouples gating charge immobilization from fast Na inactivation in squid giant axons. *Biophys J* **54**, 719.

10. Trainer VL, Brown GB, Caterall WA (1996) Site of covalent labeling of a photoreactive batrachotoxin derivative near transmembrane segment IS6 of the sodium channel alpha unit. *J Biol Chem* **271**, 11261.

11. Wang SY, Wang GK (1998) Point mutations in segment I-S6 render voltage-gated Na⁺ channels resistant to batrachotoxin. *Proc Natl Acad Sci* USA **95**, 2653.

Benzalkonium Chloride

Peter S. Spencer

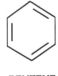

BENZALKONIUM CHLORIDE

R = mixture of alkyls from C_8H_{17} to $C_{18}H_{37}$

NEUROTOXICITY RATING

Experimental

A   Topical neurotoxin

Benzalkonium chloride (BTC), a mixture of alkyldimethylbenzylammonium chlorides, has been used topically as an experimental neurotoxin to explore the effects of ganglionectomy on the function of the gastrointestinal tract. Application to the lower esophagus of the rat resulted in proximal dilatation and distal narrowing, a picture comparable to that seen in clinical achalasia (1). The disinfectant and detergent properties of BTC are used in some injectable betamethasone preparations; in sheep, large spinal intrathecal doses have been linked to arachnoiditis (2).

REFERENCES

1. Goto S, Grosfeld JL (1989) The effect of a neurotoxin (benzalkonium chloride) on the lower esophagus. *J Surg Res* **47**, 117.

2. Latham JM, Fraser RD, Blumbergs P, Bogduk N (1997) The pathologic effects of intrathecal betamethasone. *Spine* **14**, 1558.

Benzene

Herbert H. Schaumburg

BENZENE
C_6H_6

Benzol; Cyclohexatriene

NEUROTOXICITY RATING

Clinical

A   Acute encephalopathy (sedation, stupor)

C   Optic neuropathy

Benzene, the simplest aromatic compound, is a common industrial substance and a minor (2%) component of gasoline; it is annually produced in billion-gallon quantities. Its wide use reflects ready availability and low cost. Benzene is an intermediate in the production of styrene, phenol, *cyclo*hexane, and other organic chemicals; it is also used in the manufacture of detergents, pesticides, and solvents. High-level exposure causes CNS depression; chronic low-level exposure depresses the hematopoietic system and is associated with leukemia. Because of the potentially severe systemic toxicity, North American products containing more than 0.1% benzene must carry a consumer warning.

The time-weighted Threshold Limit Value is 0.1 ppm (0.3 mg/m³).

Inhalation exposure to this volatile substance is now the most common route. Acute human exposures occur mainly from accidental spills in confined poorly ventilated enclosures. The absorption, circulation, and metabolism are similar in man and murine species. Inhaled benzene is rapidly detected in all organs and readily enters the CNS. The metabolism of benzene is complex, yielding glucuronide and sulfate conjugates of phenol, quinol, and catechol. Tests for urine levels of phenol are used as an index of benzene exposure. Exposure to benzene may induce the microsomal mixed function oxidase, cytochrome P-450 IIE1, which is likely responsible for the oxygenation of benzene, but also generates oxygen radicals; this is held as a major factor in benzene's oncological potential and its hematological toxicity (5). Although benzene has been associated with many types of genetic damage, it has been classified as a non-mutagen by the Ames test, and attempts to detect genotoxic effects in blood of exposed individuals have failed (4). Depression of bone marrow function occurs after months or years of low-level exposure. It is initially manifest as stimulation of all three principal bone marrow elements and soon is followed by progressive anemia and thrombocytopenia. In the early stages, bone marrow depression is reversible; continued exposure has led to fatal aplastic anemia. Acute high-level inhalation exposure through deliberate sniffing has caused sudden death in adolescents; this is attributed to cardiac irritability and ventricular fibrillation (3). Oral ingestion of 9–12 g of benzene causes staggering gait, vomiting, delirium, tachycardia, hypotension, coma, and (occasionally) death.

The depressant effects of acute exposure on the CNS depend upon level and duration of exposure. In fact, benzene-induced CNS depression is so reliable at high levels of exposure that an attempt was made to use the substance as a general anesthetic. Responses to airborne levels are as follows: 25 ppm, no effect regardless of duration; 50–150 ppm, headache and lassitude; 500 ppm, sleepiness after 3–4 h; 3000 ppm, sleep within 30 min, then progressive stupor; 7000 ppm, stupor within 30 min.

Anecdotal reports of isolated incidents of optic neuritis (2) or transverse myelitis (1) are unconvincing.

REFERENCES

1. Herregods P, Chappel R, Mortier G (1984) Benzene poisoning as a possible cause of transverse myelitis. *Paraplegia* **22**, 305.
2. Renard B, Cavigneaux C (1950) Do changes in the fundus of the eye follow changes in the blood in benzene poisoning? *Arch Mal Prof* **11**, 38.
3. Winek CL, Collom WD, Wecht CH (1967) Fatal benzene exposure by glue-sniffing. *Lancet* **i**, 683.
4. Yardley-Jones A, Anderson D, Jenkinson PC *et al.* (1988) Genotoxic effects in peripheral blood and urine of workers exposed to low level benzene. *Brit J Ind Med* **45**, 694.
5. Yardley-Jones A, Anderson D, Parke DV (1991) The toxicity of benzene and its metabolism and molecular pathology in human risk assessment. *Brit J Ind Med* **48**, 437.

Benzene Hexachloride

Herbert H. Sahaumburg

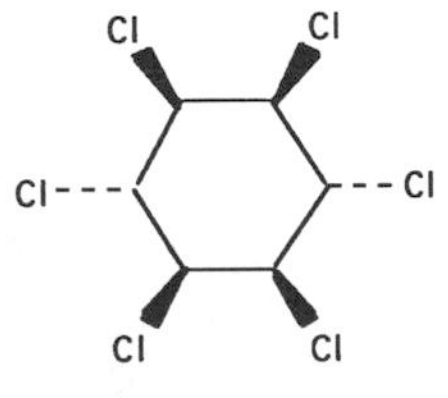

LINDANE
$C_6H_6Cl_6$

Lindane
(1α,2α,3β,4α,5α,6β)1,2,3,4,5,6-Hexachlorocyclohexane

NEUROTOXICITY RATING

Clinical

A   Seizure disorder

Experimental

A   Seizure disorder

A   Inhibition of GABA synapses

Lindane is the γ-isomer of six structural isomers of benzene hexachloride. A 1.0% topical solution of lindane is the standard treatment of scabies infestations caused by the arachnid mite *Sarcoptes scabiei* (Acari: Sarcoptidae). It is also available as a shampoo. The 1.0% solution is applied once, in a thin film, over the entire body below the neck; the solution, once dried, is allowed to remain for 12 h and then washed away. Serious adverse reactions are not associated with correct use of topical lindane in adults or large children. Special care and more dilute solutions are advocated for infants.

The benzene hexachlorides are absorbed through the gastrointestinal tract and from dermal application. Lindane has the most rapid excretion and the shortest half-life of the benzene hexachlorides; its whole-body elimination in rats is 37 days.

Rats and rabbits given systemic doses of 190 mg/kg develop loss of balance and generalized seizures. Rabbits are especially susceptible to dermal lindane and exhibit seizures following topical applications of 60 mg/kg. Seizures in mice are attenuated by pretreatment with excitatory amino acid antagonists (2).

There are numerous reports of generalized seizures in humans following accidental ingestion of lindane. The lowest threshold for seizures from a single oral dose is approximately 50 mg/kg. In one incident, 11 persons drank coffee that had accidental substitution of lindane for sugar. Each person received approximately 0.6 g or about 86 mg/kg of lindane. Within 4 h, they described sensations of malaise and dizziness that were soon followed by several generalized seizures. They recovered consciousness within 4 h and were discharged from hospital within 2 days without residual neurological findings (1).

Lindane acts on the CNS in a manner similar to picrotoxin (*see* Picrotoxin, this volume) (3,4).

REFERENCES

1. Bambov C, Chomakov M, Dimitrova N (1966) Group intoxication with lindane. *Suvrem Med* 17, 477.
2. Blaszczak P, Turski WA (1998) Excitatory amino acid antagonists alleviate convulsive and toxic properties of lindane in mice. *Pharmacol Toxicol* 82, 137.
3. Joy RM, Walby WF, Stark LG, Albertson TE (1995) Lindane blocks GABA$_A$-mediated inhibition and modulates pyramidal cell excitability in the rat hippocampal slice. *NeuroToxicology* 16, 217.
4. Nagata K, Narahashi T (1995) Differential effects of hexachlorocyclohexane isomers on the GABA receptor-chloride channel complex in rat dorsal root ganglion neurons. *Brain Res* 704, 85.

Benzimidazole

Herbert H. Schaumburg

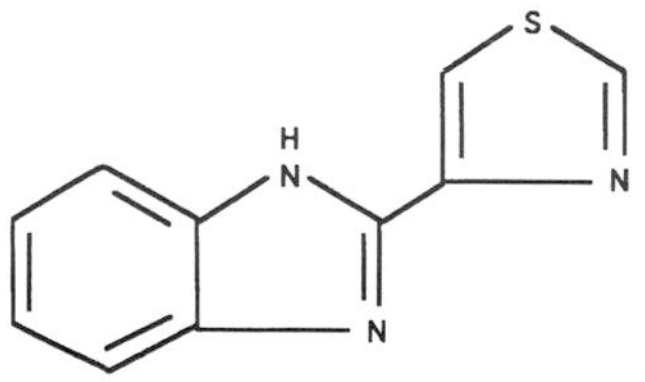

THIOBENDAZOLE
$C_{10}H_7N_3S$

Thiabendazole; 2-(4-Thiazolyl)-1*H*-benzimidazole

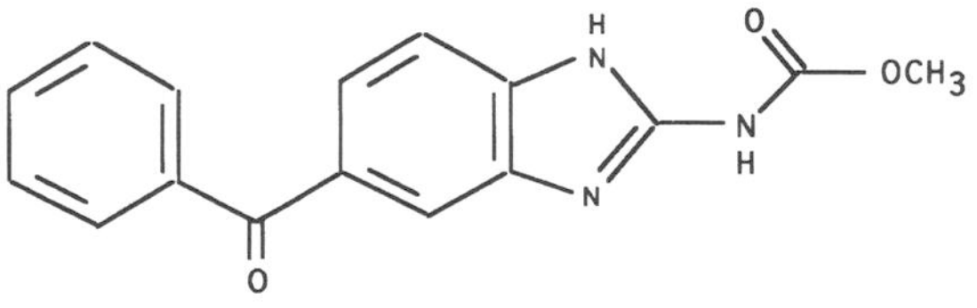

MEBENDAZOLE
$C_{16}H_{13}N_3O_3$

Mebendazole; (5-Benzoyl-1*H*-benzimidazol-2-yl) carbamic acid methyl ester

NEUROTOXICITY RATING
Clinical

A   Acute encephalopathy (confusion, hallucinations, seizures)
B   Headache

Two substituted 1,3-benzodiazoles (benzimidazoles), thiabendazole and mebendazole, serve as broad-spectrum anthelmintics. Niridazole, formerly a treatment for schistosomiasis, has been supplanted by more effective agents. The benzimidazoles inhibit cellular enzyme systems (*e.g.*, mitochondrial fumarase reductase) essential for helminth survival and also suppress the assembly of microtubules. They have few serious adverse effects aside from gastrointestinal distress and occasional hepatic dysfunction (2).

Drowsiness, fatigue, malaise, and headache are common; most individuals accommodate to these symptoms and therapy can continue (2). Rarely, a disabling acute encephalopathy develops with disorientation, hallucinations, and generalized seizures (1). This has been fatal, and epileptic individuals should use these agents with caution.

REFERENCES

1. Tchao P, Templeton T (1983) Thiabendazole-associated grand mal seizures in a patient with Down syndrome. *J Pediat* 102, 317.
2. Van den Bosche H, Rochette F, Horig C (1982) Mebendazole and related antihelminthics. *Adv Pharmacol Chemother* 19, 67.

Benzodiazepines

Howard A. Crystal
Herbert H. Schaumburg

DIAZEPAM
$C_{16}H_{13}ClN_2O$

Diazepam; 7-Chloro-1,3-dihydro-1-methyl-5-phenyl-2H-1,4-benzodiazepin-2-one

NEUROTOXICITY RATING
Clinical
A Acute encephalopathy (sedation, coma)
B Chronic encephalopathy (cognitive impairment)
Experimental
A GABA$_A$ receptor binding
A CNS depression (sedation)

Benzodiazepines (BZDs) were first synthesized in 1957 and, shortly thereafter, were found to have sleep-inducing and antianxiety activity (54,55). In 1960, chlordiazepoxide (Librium) became the first BZD marketed in the United States. Before the introduction of BZDs, barbiturates were the mainstays of the pharmacological treatment of anxiety and insomnia. Because BZDs cause little respiratory depression and are much less likely to cause fatal overdose than barbiturates, BZDs have become extraordinarily popular medications and are among the most widely used prescription drugs in North America and Europe.

The name benzodiazepines was coined because the drugs are formed by the fusion of a benzene ring with a seven-membered diazepam ring.

The clinical usefulness of benzodiazepines probably results from their modulation of the plasma membrane γ-aminobutyric acid A (GABA$_A$) receptor. Differences in clinical activity result from at least three factors: (a) the binding constant for the specific BZD agonist and the BZD receptor, (b) the lipid solubility of the BZD, and (c) the path of metabolism of the BZD (6,16). There is a rank-order correlation between the avidity of receptor binding and clinical potency (16).

General Toxicology

BZDs are rapidly and completely absorbed from the stomach. The time from single oral dose to maximal blood level is 0.5–8 h (6). Ethanol may enhance the rate of BZD absorption in the stomach (19).

All BZDs are lipid soluble, and there is rapid uptake from the blood by highly perfused organs such as the brain (6,16). BZD blood levels then undergo rapid decline as the drug is redistributed in fat in less well-perfused tissues. As BZD leaves fat stores, blood levels decrease more slowly.

2-Keto benzodiazepines such as diazepam undergo hepatic microsomal oxidation *via* N-dealkylation or aliphatic hydroxylation. Age (15,40,52), liver disease (17,63), or concomitant medications such as cimetidine (28) or oral contraceptives (1) influence microsomal oxidation and slow metabolism. The benzodiazepines that undergo oxidation generally have a long half-life, and the oxidized products are biologically active. The 3-OH-benzodiazepines (including oxazepam, lorazepam, and temazepam) undergo glucuronide conjugation in the liver (63) and have short to intermediate half-lives. Glucuronide conjugation is less likely than microsomal oxidation to be affected by age, disease, or concomitant medications (16).

BZDs interact additively, but not synergistically, with other drugs that modulate the GABA receptor (6,9). The combined use of BZDs with other drugs that modulate the GABA receptor, such as ethanol or barbiturate, can lead to marked (sometimes fatal) CNS depression.

Until 1980, most prescribed BZDs had an intermediate or long duration of action (33). Advantages of long-duration drugs are that fewer doses are required, there is less fluctuation if a dose is missed, and there is less rebound on withdrawal. Their primary disadvantage is that toxic levels can accumulate more easily than with shorter-duration drugs. This problem is of special concern in elderly and medically ill patients (61).

Bolus injection of intravenous diazepam is the therapy of choice for the initial treatment of generalized status epilepticus because it usually stops a seizure within 1–5 min (10). Because of its rapid redistribution, blood levels of diazepam associated with antiseizure efficacy are maintained for only 10–15 min.

BZDs are superior to placebo for the treatment of insomnia (3,16,26,27,37). Tolerance does develop to the soporific effects of BZDs, and their effectiveness may wane after 2 weeks of continued use.

Animal Studies

In experimental animals, low doses of BZDs are anxiolytic; this effect is blocked by verapamil and is independent of GABA (*vide infra*). High dosages are anticonvulsant and appear to act through GABA; massive doses cause muscle relaxation and sedation. Animals will self-administer BZDs, but less vigorously than barbiturates.

Experimental animal studies have provided considerable insight into the molecular pharmacology of BZDs. Benzodiazepines bind to two classes of cellular receptors—plasma membrane GABA$_A$ receptors and receptors on the outer mitochondrial membrane (8,9,48,60). The GABA$_A$ receptor is a chloride ionophore complex. When GABA is occupying the GABA-binding site of this complex, concomitant binding of a BZD to the BZD-binding site leads to an increased frequency of openings of the chloride ionophore, thus leading to increased chloride ion conductance, and hyperpolarization. The hyperpolarized cell is harder to depolarize and less likely to generate its own action potential. BZDs only modulate the action of GABA on the GABA receptor. In the absence of GABA, BZDs have no effect on the receptor.

GABA receptors with BZD-binding sites are found on neurons throughout the brain, with highest concentrations in the limbic system and the neocortex (35,57).

In animal models, within 1 week of initiating benzodiazepine administration, there is down-regulation of GABA$_A$ receptors (34). Upon withdrawal of the benzodiazepine, the animal becomes hyperactive, and there is up-regulation of GABA$_A$ receptors (34).

β-Carbolines, such as β-carboline-3-carboxylic acid ethyl ester methyl amide (9), and endogenous compounds called diazepam-binding inhibitors (DBIs) (5), bind to the BZD receptor site but are associated with decreased chloride ion permeability. These substances are called inverse agonists to distinguish them from direct agonists (such as diazepam).

Flumazenil represents a third class of drugs that bind to the BZD receptor site (48). These drugs, called antagonists, block the BZD receptor and prevent endogenous or exogenous agonists or inverse agonist from acting on the BZD receptor. The GABA$_A$ receptor then functions in its unmodulated state.

BZDs bind to a receptor on the outer mitochondrial membrane and enhance movement of cholesterol from cytoplasm across the outer mitochondrial membrane to the inner mitochondrial membrane (60). Within mitochondria, cholesterol is converted into steroid hormones. Consistent with this function, levels of peripheral BZD receptors are highest in adrenal cortex, testes, and ovaries. Mitochondrial BZD receptors are also located with CNS glia (60).

Two classes of endogenous substances with BZD-like activity have been identified—DBIs and endozepines (5,31). Endozepines are 300–500 daltons, protease resistant, and react with antibodies raised to diazepam. DBIs are endogenous 10- to 15-kDa proteins that interfere with the binding of ^{3}H-diazepam to BZD receptors. DBIs are not immunoreactive with antibodies to clinically useful BZDs.

The functions of endozepines or DBIs in brain are not known. The effects of training on levels of endogenous BZD-like substances have been studied (23); stressful avoidance-learning paradigms were associated with a 60%–90% decrease in BZD-like immunoreactivity in amygdala, medial septum, and cortex, but not in cerebellum. Nonstressful learning was associated with smaller decreases.

Human Studies

Subjects given a single dose of benzodiazepines frequently experience cognitive dysfunction, especially impairment of anterograde memory (7). Other frequent manifestations include ataxia, impaired motor control, and sleepiness (14,16,17,21,53). The mechanism of the acute sedative effect of a 1-mg dose of BZDs is secondary to stimulation of the GABAergic system.

An effect of benzodiazepines on long-term storage of items in newly learned verbal memory has been demonstrated (15). Subjects administered a selective-reminding test 1.5 h after a single dose of triazolam showed impairment of newly acquired memories that had entered remote memory. Control subjects recalled 13.3 (out of 16 words) per trial; subjects who received 0.25 mg of drug recalled 11.1 words per trial. Twenty-four hours later, the effects of that single dose of drug on retrieval from long-term storage were even more dramatic. Recall of subjects who received placebo, 0.125 mg of triazolam, or 0.25 mg of triazolam were 10.2, 6.0, and 2.0 words, respectively.

The effects of benzodiazepines on anterograde memory must be interpreted in light of several mitigating factors. First, anxiety undeniably interferes with learning and memory. Frequently, the influence of anxiety on performance follows a U-shaped curve. Performance can be better with low levels of anxiety than with no anxiety at all. However, high levels of anxiety interfere with performance. Several studies have shown that BZDs improve performance on cognitive tests in very anxious patients. Second, insomnia is also associated with impaired memory, and insomniacs complain of poor memory much more than patients without sleep problems. Insomniac patients treated with BZDs score better on memory tests than insomniacs treated with placebo. Third, testing a patient's memory in a neuropsychological laboratory gives only an approximation of what the subjective memory function is like in everyday life. Both a patient's performance in the laboratory and his/her complaints of memory problems must be evaluated. Most anxious patients treated with BZDs complain little of memory impairment.

BZDs do not interfere with retrieval of facts held in very-long-term storage nor do they interfere with learning of implicit or procedural memory (21).

BZDs are risk factor for falls in the elderly (43,51). BZD use can markedly impair driving ability. In one study, the morning after test subjects had taken 20 mg of flurazepam for two consecutive nights, they drove as poorly as if they had a blood alcohol level of 100 μg/dl—the legal limit in most states (36).

There are numerous anecdotal reports of an association between BZD therapy and dyscontrol and disinhibition (*i.e.*, inability to function) (46). Manifestations of dyscontrol included episodes of destruction of personal property, physical violence (including homicide), and suicide attempts (18,36,50,56). These episodes have been reported with all BZDs and may be dose dependent. Such reports are difficult to interpret because the patients had underlying psychiatric disorders and were frequently taking other prescribed and/or illicit drugs. Several reports suggest that patients who have taken BZDs for many years have cognitive deficits that persist for years after the BZDs are stopped (7,21,29,30). No longitudinal study has tested neuropsychological function in patients before, during, immediately after, and long after chronic BZD treatment. These studies are suggestive but not convincing.

One study (58) compared neuropsychological function during and after BZD treatment, but data on level of performance before treatment were not available. At baseline (while on drug), the BZD patients score significantly worse on the Logical Memory and Paired Associates test, the Digit Symbol test of the Wechsler Adult Intelligence Scale, and the Trail-Making test. When tested immediately after withdrawal, subjects' scores changed little. Six months later, their scores had improved from baseline but remained significantly worse than those of the controls.

Another study (49) compared neuropsychological test scores among older BZD-dependent patients, alcohol-dependent patients, and controls before and immediately after gradual drug withdrawal. After withdrawal from the benzodiazepines, patients still scored worse than controls on tests of auditory learning. Patients on chronic BZD therapy scored worse than controls on tests of visual perception and sustained attention (13), and a similar study found that neuropsychological scores of patients who had taken benzo-

diazepines chronically were worse than those of a matched control group (39). Subjects were repeatedly retested over 64 days during withdrawal from the benzodiazepines. Scores of the benzodiazepine group improved, but were still significantly below the controls. An important variable to consider in interpreting these data is the effect of anxiety on performance; these studies compared anxious patients with nonanxious controls (13,49,58). Only one study compared performance between anxious patients on and off BZDs and anxious patients who had never taken BZDs (30). Scores of patients on drug did not differ from controls.

BZD-like activity is elevated in brain (22) in some animal models of hepatic encephalopathy (25), but interpretation of these data is difficult (24,42,62). Endogenous BZD activity is increased in frontal cortex among some patients dying from hepatic encephalopathy (2). The efficacy of the BZD antagonist flumazenil in the treatment of hepatic encephalopathy (24,32,41) is under trial.

High levels of substances with BZD-like immunoreactivity have been found at the time of stupor in the serum of some patients with idiopathic recurring stupor (47,59). When the patients were awake and alert, levels returned to normal.

Sudden withdrawal of benzodiazepine from patients maintained on this therapy for as little as a week has been associated with anxiety, sleeplessness, tremor, confusion, seizures, depression, and psychosis (4,20,45). Slow drug withdrawal is mandatory.

REFERENCES

1. Abernethy DR, Greenblatt DJ, Divoll M *et al.* (1982) Impairment of diazepam metabolism by low-dose estrogen-containing oral-contraceptive steroids. *N Engl J Med* 306, 791.

2. Basile AS, Hughes PM *et al.* (1991) Elevated brain concentrations of 1,4-benzodiazepines in fulminant hepatic failure. *N Engl J Med* 325, 473.

3. Bliwise D, Seidel W, Greenblatt DJ, Dement W (1984) Nighttime and daytime efficacy of flurazepam and oxazepam in chronic insomnia. *Amer J Psychiat* 151, 19.

4. Cairns C (1992) Toxicologic problems. Benzodiazepine overdose and withdrawal. In: *Principles and Practice of Emergency Management. Part 6.* Schartz GR ed. Lea & Febiger, Philadelphia p. 2684.

5. Costa E, Guidotti A (1991) Diazepam binding inhibitor (DBI): A peptide with multiple biological actions. *Life Sci* 49, 325.

6. Cowley DS, Roy-Byrne PP, Greenblatt DJ (1991) Benzodiazepines: Pharmacokinetics and pharmacodynamics. In: *Benzodiazepines in Clinical Practice: Risks and Benefits.* Roy-Byrne PP, Cowley DS eds. American Psychiatric Press, Washington, DC p. 19.

7. Curran H (1986) Tranquilizing memories: A review of the effects of benzodiazepines on human memory. *Biol Psychol* **23**, 179.

8. Doble A, Martin IL (1992) Multiple benzodiazepine receptors: No reason for anxiety. *Trends Pharmacol Sci* **13**, 76.

9. Drugan R, Holmes PV (1990) Central and peripheral benzodiazepine receptors: Involvement in an organism's response to physical and psychological stress. *Neurosci Biobehav* **15**, 277.

10. Engel J (1989) Antiepileptic drugs. In: *Seizures and Epilepsy*. Plum F, Gilman S, Martin JB eds. FA Davis, Philadelphia p. 410.

11. Feighner JP, Aden GC, Fabre LF *et al.* (1983) Comparison of alprazolam, imipramine, and placebo in the treatment of depression. *J Amer Med Assn* **249**, 3057.

12. Flugy A, Gagliano M, Cannizzaro C *et al.* (1992) Antidepressant and anxiolytic effects of alprazolam versus the conventional antidepressant desipramine and the anxiolytic diazepam in the forced swim test in rats. *Eur J Pharmacol* **214**, 233.

13. Golombok S, Moodley P, Lader M (1988) Cognitive impairment in long-term benzodiazepine users. *Psychol Med* **18**, 375.

14. Greenblatt DJ (1992) Pharmacology of benzodiazepine hypnotics. *J Clin Psychiat* **53**, 7.

15. Greenblatt DJ, Harmatz JS, Shapiro L *et al.* (1991) Sensitivity to triazolam in the elderly. *N Engl J Med* **324**, 1691.

16. Greenblatt DJ, Shader RI, Abernethy DR (1983) Current status of benzodiazepines. *N Engl J Med* **309**, 354.

17. Gudex C (1991) Adverse effects of benzodiazepines. *Soc Sci Med* **33**, 587.

18. Hall RC, Joffe JR (1972) Aberrant response to diazepam: A new syndrome. *Amer J Psychiat* **129**, 738.

19. Hayes SL, Pablo G, Radomski T, Palmer RF (1977) Ethanol and diazepam absorption. *N Engl J Med* **296**, 186.

20. Hollister LE, Motzenbecker FP, Degan RO (1961) Withdrawal reactions from chlordiazepoxide. *Psychopharmacology* **2**, 63.

21. Hommer DW (1991) Benzodiazepines: Cognitive and psychomotor effects. In: *Benzodiazepines In Clinical Practice; Risks and Benefits*. Roy-Byrne PP, Cowley DS eds. American Psychiatric Press, Washington, DC p. 111.

22. Izquierdo I, Da Silva C, Silva MB *et al.* (1993) Memory expression of habituation and of inhibitory avoidance is blocked by CNQX infused into the entorhinal cortex. *Behav Neural Biol* **60**, 5.

23. Izquierdo I, Medina JH (1991) GABA$_A$ receptor modulation of memory: The role of endogenous benzodiazepines. *Trends Pharmacol Sci* **12**, 260.

24. Jones EA, Basile AS, Mullen KD *et al.* (1990) Flumazenil: Potential implications for hepatic encephalopathy. *Pharmacol Ther* **45**, 331.

25. Jones EA, Basile AS, Yurdaydin C, Skolnich P (1993) Do benzodiazepine ligands contribute to hepatic encephalopathy. *Adv Exp Med Biol* **341**, 57.

26. Kales A, Kales J (1983) Sleep laboratory studies of the hypnotic drugs: Efficacy and withdrawal effects. *J Clin Psychopharmacol* **3**, 140.

27. Kales A, Kales J, Soldatos CR (1982) Insomnia and other sleep disorders. *Med Clin N Amer* **66**, 971.

28. Klotz U, Reimann I (1980) Delayed clearance of diazepam due to cimetidine. *N Engl J Med* **302**, 1012.

29. Lister RG (1991) The effects of benzodiazepines and 5-HT1A agonists on learning and memory. In: *5-HT1a Agonists, 5-HT3 Antagonists and Benzodiazepines: Their Comparative Behavioral Pharmacology*. Rodgers RJ, Cooper SJ eds. John Wiley & Sons, New York p. 267.

30. Lucki I, Rickels K, Giler AM (1986) Chronic use of benzodiazepines and psychomotor and cognitive test performance. *Psychopharmacology* **88**, 426.

31. Medina JH, Pena C, Piva M *et al.* (1992) Benzodiazepines in the brain—their origin and possible biological roles. *Mol Neurobiol* **6**, 377.

32. Meier R, Gyr K, Scholer A (1991) Persisting benzodiazepine metabolites responsible for the reaction of the benzodiazepine antagonist flumazenil in patients with hepatic encephalopathy. *Gastroenterology* **101**, 274.

33. Mendelson WB (1992) Clinical distinctions between long-acting and short-acting benzodiazepines. *J Clin Psychiat* **53**, 4.

34. Miller LG (1991) Chronic benzodiazepine administration: From the patient to the gene. *J Clin Pharmacol* **31**, 492.

35. Mohler H, Okada T (1977) Benzodiazepine receptor: Demonstration in the central nervous system. *Science* **198**, 849.

36. O'Hanlon JF, Vokerts ER (1986) Hypnotics and actual driving performance. *Acta Psychiat Scand* **74**, 95.

37. Pascualy R (1991) Benzodiazepines and sleep. In: *Benzodiazepines In Clinical Practice; Risks and Benefits*. Roy-Byrne PP, Cowley DS eds. American Psychiatric Press, Washington, DC p. 91.

38. Pattern SB, Love EJ (1994) Drug-induced depression. Incidence, avoidance and management. *Drug Safety* **10**, 203.

39. Petursson H, Gudjonsson GH, Lader MH (1983) Psychometric performance during withdrawal from long-term benzodiazepine treatment. *Psychopharmacology* **81**, 345.

40. Pomara N, Stanley B, Block R *et al.* (1985) Increased sensitivity of the elderly to the central nervous system depressant effects of diazepam. *J Clin Psychiat* **46**, 185.

41. Pomier-Layrargues G, Giguere JF, Lavoie J *et al.* (1994) Flumazenil in cirrhotic patients in hepatic coma: A randomized double-blind placebo-controlled crossover trial. *Hepatology* **19**, 32.

42. Puspok A, Herneth A, Steindl P, Ferenci P (1993) Hepatic encephalopathy in rats with thioacetamide-induced acute

liver failure is not mediated by endogenous benzodiazepines. *Gastroenterology* **105**, 851.

43. Ray W, Griffin MR, Schaffner W *et al.* (1987) Psychotro-
    pic drug use and the risk of hip fracture. *N Engl J Med*
    316, 363.

44. Rickels K, Feighner JP, Smith WT (1985) Alprazolam, am-
    itriptyline, doxepin and placebo in treatment of depres-
    sion. *Arch Gen Psychiat* **42**, 134.

45. Roth T, Roehrs TA (1992) Issues in the use of benzodi-
    azepine therapy. *J Clin Psychiat* **53**, 14.

46. Rothschild AJ (1992) Disinhibition, amnestic reactions,
    and other adverse reactions secondary to triazolam: A re-
    view of the literature. *J Clin Psychiat* **53**, 69.

47. Rothstein JD, Guidotti A, Tinuper P *et al.* (1992) Endog-
    enous benzodiazepine receptor ligands in idiopathic recur-
    ring stupor. *Lancet* **340**, 1002.

48. Roy-Byrne PP, Nutt DJ (1991) Benzodiazepines: Biological
    mechanisms. In: *Benzodiazepines in Clinical Practice;
    Risks and Benefits.* Roy-Byrne PP, Cowley DS eds. Amer-
    ican Psychiatric Press, Washington, DC p. 3.

49. Rummans TA, Davis LJ, Morse RM, Ivnik RJ (1993)
    Learning and memory impairment in older, detoxified,
    benzodiazepine-dependent patients. *Mayo Clin Proc* **68**,
    731.

50. Ryan HF, Merril B, Scott GE *et al.* (1968) Increase in su-
    icidal thoughts and tendencies. Association with diazepam
    therapy. *J Amer Med Assn* **203**, 1137.

51. Ryynanen OP, Kivela SL, Honkanen R *et al.* (1993) Med-
    ications and chronic diseases as risk factors for falling in-
    juries in the elderly. *Scand J Soc Med* **21**, 264.

52. Salzman C, Shader RI, Harmatz J, Robertson L (1975)
    Psychopharmacologic investigations in elderly volunteers:
    Effect of diazepam in males. *J Amer Geriat Soc* **23**, 451.

53. Salzman C (1993) Issues and controversies regarding ben-
    zodiazepine use. *Natl Inst Drug Abuse Res Monograph
    Ser* **131**, 68.

54. Shader RI, Greenblatt DJ (1993) Use of benzodiazepines
    in anxiety disorders. *N Engl J Med* **328**, 1398.

55. Shader RI, Greenblatt DJ (1993) Use of benzodiazepines
    in anxiety disorders. Comment. *N Engl J Med* **329**, 1500.

56. Smith BD, Salzman C (1991) Do benzodiazepines cause
    depression? *Hosp Comm Psychiat* **42**, 1101.

57. Squires RF, Braestrup C (1977) Benzodiazepine receptors
    in rat brain. *Nature* **266**, 732.

58. Tata PR, Rollins J, Collins M *et al.* (1994) Lack of cog-
    nitive recovery following withdrawal from long-term ben-
    zodiazepine use. *Psychol Med* **24**, 203.

59. Tinuper P, Montagna PM, Corelli P *et al.* (1992) Idio-
    pathic recurring stupor: a case with possible involvement
    of the gamma-aminobutyric (GABA)ergic system. *Ann
    Neurol* **31**, 503.

60. Verma A, Synder SH (1989) Peripheral type benzodiaze-
    pine receptors. *Ann Rev Pharmacol Toxicol* **29**, 307.

61. Vogel G (1992) Clinical uses and advantages of low doses
    of benzodiazepine hypnotics. *J Clin Psychiat* **53**, 19.

62. Widler P, Fisch HU, Schoch P *et al.* (1993) Increased ben-
    zodiazepine-like activity is neither necessary nor sufficient
    to explain acute hepatic encephalopathy in the thioace-
    tamide-treated rat. *Hepatology* **18**, 1459.

63. Zito JM (1994) *Psychotherapeutic Drug Manual, 3rd Ed.*
    John Wiley & Sons, New York.

Bicuculline

Albert C. Ludolph

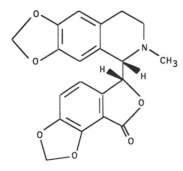

BICUCULLINE
C$_{20}$H$_{17}$NO$_6$

[R-(R*,S*)]-6-(5,6,7,8-Tetrahydro-6-methyl-1,3-dioxolo[4,5-
g]isoquinolin-5-yl)furo[3,4-e]-1,3-benzodioxol-8(6H)-one

NEUROTOXICITY RATING

Experimental

A   Ion channel dysfunction (GABA chloride-channel agonist)

A   Seizure disorder (acute administration)

Bicuculline is a naturally occuring convulsant phthalide isoquinoline alkaloid from Dutchman's breeches (*Dicentra cucullaria*), *Adlumia fungosa*, Fumariaceae, and *Corydalis*
spp. The substance acts as a stereospecific competitive antagonist of the γ-aminobutyric acid (GABA)$_A$-activated
chloride channel (4,7). At physiological pH, bicuculline—
but not its quaternary salts—is rapidly hydrolyzed to bi-
cucune, an inactive metabolite. Immediately after intravenous injection (minimal convulsive dose 0.2–0.4 mg/kg) to

experimental rats, cats, monkeys, or baboons, bicuculline induces generalized seizures that may have a long clonic phase (5). Young rats may show increased susceptibility to the epileptogenic effect (5). After topical application to rats, the compound also induces focal epileptic seizures (2). Focal and secondary generalized seizures can be induced after low-dose application of bicuculline to the deep prepyriform cortex of the rat (8,9).

The morphological lesion associated with status epilepticus induced by bicuculline in the rat is characterized as neuronal changes and astroglial swelling (1) and does not include cortical dendritic changes (10)—a profile distinct from the lesion induced by excitatory neurotransmitters such as glutamate. Changes of cerebral blood flow and energy metabolism are also described in this model system (3,6).

REFERENCES
1. Atillo A, Soderfeldt B, Kalimo H *et al.* (1983) Pathogenesis of brain lesions caused by experimental epilepsy. Light- and electron-microscopic changes in the rat hippocampus following bicuculline-induced status epilepticus. *Acta Neuropathol* **59**, 11.
2. Campbell AM, Holmes O (1984) Bicuculline epileptogenesis in the rat. *Brain Res* **323**, 239.
3. Folbergrova J, Ingvar M, Siesjoe BK (1981) Metabolic changes in cerebral cortex, hippocampus, and cerebellum during sustained bicuculline-induced seizures. *J Neurochem* **37**, 1228.
4. Johnston GAR (1976) Physiologic pharmacology of GABA and its antagonists in vertebrate nervous system. In: *GABA in Nervous System Function.* Roberts E, Chase TN, Tower DB eds. Raven Press, New York p. 395.
5. Meldrum BS (1975) Epilepsy and gamma-aminobutyric acid-mediated inhibition. *Int Rev Neurobiol* **17**, 1.
6. Meldrum BS, Nilsson B (1976) Cerebral blood flow and metabolic rate early and late in prolonged epileptic seizures induced in rats by bicuculline. *Brain* **99**, 523.
7. Nowak LM, Young AB, MacDonald RL (1982) GABA and bicuculline actions on mouse spinal cord cortical neurones in cell culture. *Brain Res* **244**, 155.
8. Piredda S, Gale K (1985) A crucial epileptogenic site in the deep prepyriform cortex. *Nature* **317**, 623.
9. Piredda S, Lim CR, Gale K (1985) Intracerebral site of convulsant action of bicuculline. *Life Sci* **36**, 1295.
10. Soderfeldt B, Kalimo H, Olsson Y, Siesjoe BK (1983) Transient and persistent cell changes in rat cerebral cortex in the early recovery period. *Acta Neuropathol* **62**, 87.

Bismuth

Mark Forest Gordon

NEUROTOXICITY RATING

Clinical

A Ataxia

A Chronic encephalopathy

A Seizure disorder (myoclonus)

A Seizure disorder

Bismuth (Bi), derived from the German *Weisse Masse* (white mass), is a grayish-white, crystalline heavy metal classified in group V of the periodic table, atomic number 83, and atomic weight 208.98. Its MP is 271.4°C and its BP is 1564 ± 5°C. The only stable valency is 3^+. Bi is brittle, superficially oxidized by air and frequently becomes irridescent. Bi is a poor conductor of electricity, but, of all the metals, it is the most diamagnetic and has the greatest Hall effect (2). The element occurs in the earth's crust (0.2 ppm); it is a by-product in refining of lead, copper, tin, silver, and gold ores.

Bi is used in fusible alloys and boiler plugs, electric fuses, low-melting solders, temperature bathing for steel, silvering mirrors, dental techniques, and as a radiographic contrast medium (2). Several Bi salts are used therapeutically. In veterinary medicine, Bi preparations are used to treat lesions, buccal warts, and gastrointestinal ulcerations. Organic Bi preparations, such as the tartrate and the salicylate, were used to treat syphilis until the 1940s. Bi subsalicylate is a commonly used over-the-counter drug for indigestion, nausea, and diarrhea. Inorganic compounds, such as Bi subnitrate, subcarbonate, and subgallate, treat various gastrointestinal complaints, including ulcers. Colloid Bi subcitrate (CBS) is used therapeutically for gastrointestinal and duodenal ulcers and *Helicobacter* (*Campylobacter*) *pylori*–associated gastritis. Bi iodoform paraffin paste (BIPP), which contains iodoform and Bi subnitrate or carbonate in liquid paraffin, has medical, dental, and surgical uses. Bi subgallate is a topical antiseptic.

The solubility of most Bi salts in water is very low. Bi can be absorbed from the gastrointestinal tract after intake of Bi-containing medication, but the bioavailability is <1%. The site and mechanism of Bi absorption and its chemical form in blood are unknown. Elemental distribution is independent of the particular compound or route of administration. Bi concentrations are usually highest in the kidneys. Plasma concentrations rise with prolonged therapy. Small amounts of the metal pass the blood-brain barrier and Bi appears diffusely in the brain (19). The half-life of Bi is 20–30 days in blood, with slow turnover in multiple compartments, such as kidney, lung, spleen, liver, brain, muscle, and the enterohepatic circulation (10). Elimination half-life from the cerebrospinal fluid (CSF) is estimated to be 16 days (1). Bi is eliminated by urinary and fecal routes. The steady-state concentration of Bi is higher in renal failure.

Large intraperitoneal doses of Bi subnitrate produce neurobehavioral signs in adult female Swiss-Webster mice; highest Bi levels are found in the olfactory bulb, hypothalamus, septum, and brainstem (16). Bi causes dose-dependent renal damage in female Wistar rats (19). Injected into the gluteal arteries of experimental animals, Bi compounds cause sudden arterial constriction, including that of the aorta, and transient paraplegia.

Continuous application of 3 μg of Bi to rat hippocampus cultures causes degeneration of CA1 pyramidal cells; at higher concentrations, the majority of hippocampal neurons degenerates (15).

The mechanism of Bi toxicity in humans is unknown. The main target organs are kidney, bone, and brain. Different compounds cause different adverse effects. Insoluble inorganic compounds cause neurotoxicity, while organic compounds often cause kidney and bone disease. Occupational exposure to Bi is limited and of unknown significance (19). Although large amounts of Bi-containing medications are consumed worldwide in often uncontrolled situations, the risk for Bi-related neurotoxicity seems very low (19).

General adverse effects of Bi compounds include stomatitis, gingivitis, a diffuse or blackish-blue discoloration of the mucosa and gingiva, dermatitis, jaundice, and constipation or impaction. A grayish-black stool discoloration should not be confused with melena. Use of Bi subsalicylate and other nonacetylsalicylic acid salicylates has not been associated with development of Reye's syndrome, but it is prudent to avoid ingestion of Bi salicylates during outbreaks of varicella or influenza. Certain Bi salts may have special toxicity because of their chemical composition. Bi subsalicylate, widely used in oral preparations, can break down and cause salicylate poisoning. Thus, aspirin should not be used with Bi salicylates.

Various Bi compounds, including bi-, tri-, and thioglycollamate and bidiallylacetate, and overdoses of CBS have caused renal failure (19). Bone lesions after Bi therapy for syphilis are located in the pelvis, femur, and vertebrae, occasionally with osteoporosis. Patients with Bi encephalopathy sometimes have fractures of the thoracic vertebrae and demineralization of the humeral head leading to necrosis, osteolysis, and fractures of the proximal humerus (19).

Repeated intramuscular Bi for the treatment of syphilis produced bilateral reversible flaccid paraplegia, generalized sensory deficit below the groin, urinary retention, and violet-colored legs. Bi neurotoxicity typically presents subacutely and gradually after prolonged oral administration (5–20 g/day of Bi salts for 2 months to 6 years) with mental changes (memory loss, confusion, delirium, psychosis, depression, excitation, insomnia, coma), ataxia, dysarthria, tremors, myoclonus, and seizures (3–5,7). It is usually reversible over several weeks or months when Bi intake is stopped. Most patients recover completely, however, residual phenomena such as intellectual impairment, affective disorder, headache, tremor, insomnia, and osteoarthropathy may remain (3). Bi subsalicylate intoxication may be fatal (17). A few patients develop encephalopathy after receiving intraoral, intranasal, or extradural application of BIPP (18), possibly due to the iodoform.

The cause of death of those who die with Bi toxicity is often not registered. One patient had laminar necrosis of cerebral and cerebellar cortex, nuclear dentatus, and putamen (6). Loss of cerebellar Purkinje cells and cerebral cortex neurons (7,11) is considered to result from anoxia.

In 1973, 28 Australian patients with a colostomy or ileostomy treated with Bi subgallate (about 700 mg/day) developed a reversible encephalopathy (14). High-dose Bi preparations were commonly used in Australia and France; 1040 cases of Bi intoxication were reported between 1973 and 1977 (3–5,7). All Bi-containing preparations at the time were associated with encephalopathy. In 1980, 72 of 942 French cases of Bi encephalopathy ended in death, although it has never been proven that these deaths were directly related to Bi intake (13). Comparison of subjects with encephalopathy and a healthy control group of Bi consumers showed no difference in age profile, sex, quantity of drug consumed, duration of intake, use of other medications, or diet (13). Sporadic cases of Bi encephalopathy are still reported (8,9).

Elevated blood levels of Bi and reversibility of symptoms are needed to diagnose Bi encephalopathy (19). Electroencephalogram (EEG), brain computed tomography (CT) scan, neurophysiological testing, and abdominal x-ray may provide supportive evidence.

Bi levels may be assessed in blood, plasma, serum, CSF, or urine. The metal should be undetectable in blood or serum of persons not recently taking Bi preparations. In 618 patients with encephalopathy, blood concentrations of Bi were 10–4600 μg/l (12). No relationship was found between blood Bi level and symptom severity (12). The decline in blood Bi concentration correlated with clinical recovery. There was no clear relationship between metal concentration in the blood and urine or in the blood and CSF. The EEG in 31 of 45 Bi-intoxicated patients showed monomorphic 4–6 cps activity in bilateral temporofronto-rolandic regions that was unaffected by eye opening and photostimulation, and an absence of alpha rhythm over the occipital regions. Comatose patients had bursts of frontal delta and theta slowing. Although convulsions were described in many patients, no EEG epileptiform activity was noted (21). Brain CT may show increased density in the cerebral and cerebellar cortex and basal ganglia, or the CT may be normal. Spinal fluid is normal in most patients with Bi intoxication (19). A radiopaque substance is apparent in x-rays of the large intestines.

The differential diagnosis of Bi neurotoxicity is broad and depends on the salient clinical features. The progessive delirium, dementia, myoclonus, and ataxia may suggest Creutzfeldt-Jakob disease. Multifocal myoclonus also may be due to Alzheimer's disease, myoclonic epilepsy, progressive myoclonic ataxia (Ramsay-Hunt), postanoxic myoclonus, viral encephalopathies including herpes and subacute sclerosing panencephalitis, metabolic abnormalities including renal and hepatic dysfunction, hyponatremia, hypoglycemia, nonketotic hyperglycemia, poisoning with heavy metals, methyl bromide and dichlorodiphenyltrichloroethane, and medication overdoses.

Bi intake should be stopped once encephalopathy is suspected. The element should be evacuated by gastrointestinal lavage followed by high-dose charcoal and laxatives. Absorption of the metal is very low, but the continued presence of Bi in the intestine may increase or sustain the body load. Other measures may be needed, such as artificial respiration, benzodiazepines, or anticonvulsants, to suppress myoclonus. Hemodialysis and D-penicillamine in a patient with renal failure after a CBS overdose was not useful. Experimental study of various chelators for the treatment of Bi toxicity in an *in vivo* model of Bi-loaded rats showed that dimercaprol (BAL), *meso*-2,3-dimercaptosuccinic acid (DMSA), or D,L-2,3-dimercapto-propane-1-sulfonic acid (DMPS) reduced the Bi concentrations in most organs, especially the kidney and liver, and increased the urinary elimination of the metal (DMPS, BAL). BAL was the only chelator that effectively lowered the brain Bi concentration, and ethylenediaminetetraacetic acid (EDTA) actually increased brain levels (20). The most effective and safe therapy for Bi poisoning is DMSA (or DMPS) administered orally until symptom resolution. BAL, which elicits pain upon intramuscular administration and has a high toxic potential, should be reserved for patients with life-threatening

nephrotoxicity or severe Bi encephalopathy due to its strong toxic potential and its painful intramuscular administration. EDTA is contraindicated because of the risk of redistribution of the body Bi load to the brain.

The mechanism of Bi neurotoxicity is unknown. Renal impairment, enhanced Bi absorption, or the formation of an unknown Bi species with specific entry into the brain or a specific neurotoxicity, may play a role (19).

REFERENCES

1. Allain P, Chaleil D, Emile J (1980) L'élévation des concentrations de bismuth dans les tissues des malades intoxiqués. *Thérapie* **35**, 303.
2. Budaveri S (1989) *The Merck Index. 11th Ed.* Merck and Co, Rahway, NJ.
3. Buge A, Rancurel G, Dechy H (1977) Encéphalopathies mycloniques bismuthiques. Formes évolutives, complications tardives, durables ou définitives. *Rev Neurol* **133**, 401.
4. Buge A, Rancurel G, Dechy H (1978) Encéphalopathies bismuthiques. Donnees etiologiques et epidemiologiques. *Nouv Presse Med* **739**, 3531.
5. Buge A, Rancurel G, Poisson M, Dechy H (1974) Encéphalopathies mycloniques par les sels de bismuth. *Nouv Presse Med* **3**, 2315.
6. Buge A, Supino-Viterbo V, Rancurel G *et al.* (1979) Corrélations évolutives: Cliniques électro-encéphalographiques, tomodensitométriques et toxicologiques, dans cinq cas d'encéphalopathies bismutiques. *Semin Hôp Paris* **55**, 1466.
7. Burns R, Thomas D, Barron VJ (1974) Reversible encephalopathy possibly associated with bismuth subgallate ingestion. *Brit Med J* **1**, 220.
8. Gordon MF, Abrams RI, Rubin DB *et al.* (1995) Bismuth subsalicylate toxicity as a cause of prolonged encephalopathy with myoclonus (brief report). *Movement Disord* **10**, 220.
9. Jungreis AC, Schaumburg HH (1993) Encephalopathy from abuse of bismuth subsalicylate (Pepto-Bismol). *Neurology* **43**, 1265.
10. Lambert JR (1991) Pharmacology of bismuth-containing compounds. *Rev Infect Dis* **8**, S691.
11. Liessens JL, Monstrey J, Vanden Eeckhout E *et al.* (1978) Bismuth encephalopathy: A clinical and anatomopathological report of one case. *Acta Neurol Belg* **78**, 301.
12. Martin-Bouyer G, Barin C, Beugnet A *et al.* (1978) Intoxications par les sels de bismuth administrés par voie orale. *Gastroenterol Clin Biol* **2**, 349.
13. Martin-Bouyer G, Foulon B, Guerbois H, Barin C (1981) Epidemiological study of encephalopathies following bismuth administration *per os*: Characteristics of intoxicated subjects: Comparison with a control group. *Clin Toxicol* **18**, 1277.

14. Morrow AW (1973) Request for reports: Adverse reactions with bismuth subgallate. *Med J Australia* **1**, 192.

15. Muller M, Rietschin L, Grogg F *et al.* (1994) Selective degeneration of CA1 pyramidal cells by chronic application of bismuth. *Hippocampus* **4**, 204.

16. Ross JF, Broadwell RD, Poston MR, Lawhorn GT (1994) Highest brain bismuth levels and neuropathology are adjacent to fenestrated blood vessels in mouse brain after intraperitoneal dosing of bismuth subnitrate. *Toxicol Appl Pharmacol* **124**, 191.

17. Sainsbury SJ (1991) Fatal salicylate toxicity from bismuth subsalicylate. *West J Med* **155**, 637.

18. Sharma RR, Cast IP, Redfern RM, O'Brien C (1994) Extradural application of bismuth iodoform paraffin paste causing relapsing bismuth encephalopathy: A case report with CT and MRI studies. *J Neurol Neurosurg Psychiat* **57**, 990.

19. Slikkerveer A, de Wolff FA (1994) Bismuth: Biokinetics and neurotoxicity. In: *Handbook of Clinical Neurology. Intoxications of the Nervous System. Part I.* Vinken PJ, Bruyn GW eds. Elsevier, Amsterdam p. 331.

20. Slikkerveer A, Jong HB, Helmich RB, de Wolff FA (1992) Development of therapeutic procedure for bismuth intoxication with chelating agents. *J Lab Clin Med* **120**, 529.

21. Supino-Viterbo V, Sicard C, Risvegliato M *et al.* (1977) Toxic encephalopathy due to ingestion of bismuth salts: Clinical and EEG studies in 45 patients. *J Neurol Neurosurg Psychiat* **40**, 748.

Black Widow Spider Venom

Alfredo Gorio
Anna Maria Di Giulio

NEUROTOXICITY RATING

Clinical

A Neuromuscular transmission syndrome

Experimental

A Ion channel dysfunction (presynaptic blockade of peripheral neurotransmission—systemic administration)

A Ion channel dysfunction (presynaptic blockade of central neurotransmission—*in vitro*)

Venom of the black widow spider (BWSV; *Latrodectus* spp.) is a mixture of proteins with potent neurotoxic activity. Aqueous extracts of spider salivary glands yielded a number of fractions (11). Fraction B purified to a single peak, B5 (MW, >130 kDa; isoelectric point of pH 5.2–5.5) or α-latrotoxin (44); this agent shows selective effects on vertebrate neuromuscular synapses with a potency five times greater than crude BWSV. Fractions B5, A and B have no effect on the crayfish stretch receptor, the cockroach heart, or houseflies. Fraction E selectively activates the crayfish stretch receptor and is effective at the lobster neuromuscular junction (10); activity resides in a subfraction E2 (MW, ~65 kDa) (11). Subfraction C3 (MW, <130 kDa) is toxic for cockroach heart and houseflies (11).

Fraction B5 is composed of two polypeptides; there are no sugar moieties and the mixture lacks proteolytic and lipolytic activity The larger peptide, which corresponds to α-latrotoxin, has a molecular weight of 156,885 and is composed of 1401 amino acids with ankyrin-like repeats (23, 25). The low-molecular-weight peptide is composed of 70 amino acids (MW, 8 kDa).

The action of systemic α-latrotoxin is restricted to peripheral neuromuscular and autonomic synapses; the agent does not affect nerve excitability and does not cross the blood-brain barrier (5,12,18). *In-vitro* studies of CNS synapses indicate that BWSV causes blockade of all types of central neurotransmission as well. Binding of α-latrotoxin to the *Torpedo* electric organ causes a potent activation of transmitter release with loss of synaptic vesicles (26). Immunoelectron microscopy reveals toxin binding to the entire presynaptic plasma membrane, with no discrimination between neurotransmitter-release sites and sites of Schwann cell apposition (26).

Affinity of the toxin for its receptor is high (K_d 10^{-10} M). Partially purified α-latrotoxin receptor has a molecular weight of approximately 200 kDa (40). Pure receptor was isolated from bovine brain membrane proteins by affinity chromatography on immobilized α-latrotoxin using a two-stage KCl gradient (34); early attempts to isolate the toxin–receptor complex by cross-linking were unsuccessful (29). α-Latrotoxin receptor is a 160–200 kDa protein named neurexin 1 (46). Interaction of the toxin with its receptor is thought to activate a presynaptic structure, composed of neurexin 1, synaptotogamin, syntaxin, and N-type calcium channels, that regulates neurotransmitter release. Transmitter release is followed by depletion of neurotransmitter and blockade of conduction.

General Toxicity

Most experimental studies have employed salivary gland extracts of three species of black widow spider: *Latrodectus tredecimguttatus* (temperate areas of Europe and North Africa), *Latrodectus mactans* (warm area of North, Central and South America), and *Latrodectus geometricus* (tropical Americas).

BWSV acts presynaptically to cause a massive release of transmitter at vertebrate and invertebrate synapses; neurotransmitter stores are depleted and synaptic transmission is blocked (20). At peak excitation, application of spider antivenin promptly restores normal synaptic activity at vertebrate and invertebrate neuromuscular junctions (22,27). Similarly, antivenin restores resting membrane potential and cell functions when spider antivenin is applied to crayfish stretch receptors or cockroach giant neurons that are fully depolarized and inactivated by BWSV (18,30).

Postsynaptic function is usually preserved; ultrastructure, membrane potential, and receptor sensitivity for neurotransmitter are unchanged (20). However, BWSV depolarizes giant neurons of the cockroach *Periplaneta americana* and the cell body of the crayfish stretch receptor; their respective axons retain the ability to conduct impulses (5,18).

BWSV reverses blockade of synaptic transmission induced by botulinum toxin, an agent that acts presynaptically to induce muscle paralysis (20,21,41). In addition, intramuscular injection of BWSV causes degeneration of botulinum-blocked presynaptic axons; these regenerate and restore functional neuromuscular junctions within 3–5 days (7).

BWSV and purified α-latrotoxin also promote neurotransmitter release from CNS synapses *in vitro*. In rat cerebral cortex slices, BWSV causes a concentration-dependent release not only of acetylcholine (ACh) but also of norepinephrine and γ-aminobutyric acid (GABA); neurotransmitter release is accompanied by depletion of synaptic vesicles (44). BWSV-induced promotion of GABA release also occured in Na$^+$- and Ca^{2+}-free media (43). α-Latrotoxin promoted the release of amino acid neurotransmitters from cerebellar primary cultures (17). BWSV venom therefore seems to show no synapse-type selectivity.

At the neuromuscular junction *in vitro*, BWSV induces a massive presynaptic release of ACh and an enormous increase in the frequency of miniature end-plate potentials (MEPP) (12). Within minutes of BWSV addition to the recording chamber, ACh release and MEPP frequency rises several hundred-fold and individual potentials are obscured by the intense discharge; this level of synaptic activity is maintained for 10–30 min before it subsides and further neuromuscular transmission is blocked (27). Whereas ap-

plication of 25 mM K$^+$ prior to BWSV increases the rate of ACh release, there is no effect after 60 min of BWSV treatment (12). At this time, ultrastructural examination reveals swollen presynaptic nerve terminals depleted of synaptic vesicles (4,12). Freeze-fracture studies demonstrate fusion of vesicle membranes with the presynaptic membrane and derangement of active zones (3,35). The action of BWSV at the neuromuscular junction is blocked by concanavalin A, an inhibition that is overcome by coincubation with colchicine (37). In sum, therefore, BWSV appears to promote docking and fusion of synaptic vesicles with the plasma membrane and to inhibit membrane recycling to form new synaptic vesicles (15). The extent of ACh loss promoted by BWSV is comparable to that seen with high potassium concentrations in the presence of the ACh-synthesis inhibitor hemicholinium-3 (12).

Some of the presynaptic effects of BWSV are due to causes other than fusion of synaptic vesicle membrane with the plasmalemma. Terminal swelling seems to be an osmolar effect triggered by increased cation flux across the presynaptic membrane. Whereas incubation of frog muscle with BWSV in medium free of Na$^+$ and Ca^{2+} induces a massive release of neurotransmitter, vesicle depletion, and vacuolar swelling of presynaptic terminals, addition of Ca^{2+} (but not Mg^{2+}) prevents synaptic vesicle depletion, causing vesicles to clump in dense amorphous structures, and inducing large-amplitude swelling of mitochondria. Vesicle clumping apparently induced by calcium also occurred in normal Ringer's solution (42). Substitution of Na$^+$ by glucosamine—a molecule impermeant to BWSV-induced cationic channels in lipid bilayers and presynaptic membranes of the frog neuromuscular junction—prevents presynaptic swelling in the presence of high extracellular concentrations of BWSV. These data suggest that influx of excess Na$^+$ is primarily responsible for BWSV-induced presynaptic swelling.

Massive influx of sodium might also mediate BWSV-induced blockade of membrane recycling, as the following experiments suggest. When BWSV was applied for 1 h in Na$^+$-free glucosamine-containing medium, the venom exhibited its full toxic effect. Removal of venom and application of antivenin in glucosamine medium for 15 min, followed by a return to a normal cationic medium, resulted in recovery of normal neuromuscular transmission with no return of BWSV sensitivity within 1–2 h (13).

BWSV-induced promotion of ACh release *in vitro* is not strictly and absolutely dependent on the presence of monovalent or divalent cations in the bathing medium (14). Changes in MEPP frequency are not usually not seen when BWSV is applied to muscle soaked in 1 mM ethylene glycol tetra-acetic acid in the absence of added Mg^{2+} (33). If, however, the temperature is raised above 30°–31°C or the solution made hyperosmolar, BWSV induces a massive release of neurotransmitter with a corresponding enormous rise in MEPP frequency despite the absence of divalent cations (13,14). Additionally, if sodium is replaced by glucosamine in the divalent-free medium, BWSV also depletes synaptic vesicles at the mouse neuromuscular junction.

Single channels of conductance of $<10^{-11}$ Ohm are formed when purified α-latrotoxin is applied to artificial lecithin:cholesterol membranes (1:2 molar ratio) bathed in solutions containing 100 mM KCl and 5 mM Tris-HCl at pH 7.5. When membrane potential is clamped at 100 mV, the channels remain open and show discrete current steps of uniform size (3.6×10^{-11} amp; 220 pS). Channels are cationic, equally permeable to Na^+ and K^+, slightly less to Ca^{2+} and Mg^{2+}, and impermeable to glucosamine (9,36). A different type of channel seems to form in PC-12 cells treated with α-latrotoxin; although the cation selectivity is maintained, the conductance is smaller ($\sim$15 pS) (16). Preincubation of α-latrotoxin with antibody against the 14-amino-acid C-terminal peptide of the venom inhibits Ca^{2+} influx, while neurotransmitter release is maintained (19). Toxin treatment of *Xenopus* oocytes injected with brain mRNA induces cation-selective channels that show cooperative burst activity, the single-channel conductance ranging from 3–200 pS (8).

BWSV triggers phosphoinositide metabolism, but this may not play an important role in the presynaptic activity of α-latrotoxin (2). The effect may be secondary to the activation of synaptotagmin—an inositol polyphosphate-binding protein (31)—by neurexin after α-latrotoxin binding has taken place.

Human Studies

BWSV is absorbed from the site of the bite and distributed throughout the body; its molecular size prevents passage across the blood-brain and blood-nerve barriers. In the early stages of BWSV envenomation, clinical manifestations are principally associated with hyperactivation of motor, sensory, and autonomic sympathetic nerves (1,38). Motor manifestations include tremor, dysarthria, spasmodic movement of legs, and clonic muscle contractions followed by paralysis. Sensory dysfunction, characterized by intense generalized pain and hyperesthesia, is accompanied by increased salivation, lacrimation, priapism, sweating, and tachycardia (1,38) Abdominal pain and rigidity may be so profound as to mimic an abdominal catastrophe (perpetual gastric ulcer, renal stone).

Black widow spider bite, despite its dramatic clinical syndrome, is rarely fatal. Death from cardiovascular arrest may occur in young children or elderly and hypertensive individuals. Effects of untreated spider bites usually subside within 48–72 h. Prompt administration of antiserum raised against an extract of the spider's salivary gland can rapidly reverse the effects of spider bites (6). The specific antivenin neutralizes the venom of all *Latrodectus* spp. Because the antivenin is equine, horse-serum sensitivity testing is essential before the antivenin is administered. Parenteral opioids and benzodiazepines may relieve pain in individuals who are allergic to antivenin.

Toxic Mechanism

BWSV binds selectively to presynaptic receptors, induces a massive quantal release of neurotransmitter, prevents recycling of vesicle membrane, and induces synaptic blockade. Since the culpable peptide neurotoxin, α-latrotoxin, fails to cross the blood-brain barrier, clinically significant effects are restricted to somatic and autonomic PNS cholinergic synapses, notably neuromuscular junctions.

REFERENCES

1. Bettini S, Cantore GP (1959) Quadro clinico del latrodectismo. *Riv Parasitol* **20**, 49.
2. Cattaneo A, Grasso A (1986) A functional domain on the α-latrotoxin molecule, distinct from binding site, involved in catecholamine secretion from PC12 cells: Identification with monoclonal antibodies. *Biochemistry* **25**, 2730.
3. Ceccarelli B, Grohovaz F, Hurlbut WP (1979) Freeze-fracture studies of frog neuromuscular junctions during intense release of transmitter. I. Effects of black widow spider venom and Ca^{2+}-free solutions on the structure of the active zone. *J Cell Biol* **81**, 163.
4. Clark AW, Mauro A, Longenecker HE Jr, Hurlbut WP (1970) Effects on the fine structure of frog neuromuscular junction. *Nature* **225**, 703.
5. D'Ajello VF, Magni F, Bettini S (1971) The effect of the venom of the black widow spider, *Latrodectus mactans tredecimguttatus*, on the giant neurons of *Periplaneta americana*. *Toxicon* **9**, 103.
6. D'Amour EF, Becker FE, Van Riper W (1936) The black widow spider. *Quart Rev Biol* **11**, 123.
7. Duchen W, Gomez S, Queiroz LS (1981) The neuromuscular junction of the mouse after black widow spider venom. *J Physiol* **316**, 279.
8. Filippov AK, Tertishnikova SM, Alekseev AE *et al.* (1994) Mechanism of α-latrotoxin action as revealed by patch-clamp experiments on *Xenopus* oocytes injected with rat brain messenger RNA. *Neuroscience* **61**, 179.
9. Finkelstein A, Rubin LL, Tzeng M-C (1976) Black widow spider venom: Effect of the purified toxin on lipid bilayer membranes. *Science* **193**, 1009.

10. Fritz LC, Tzeng M-C, Mauro A (1980) Different components of black widow spider venom mediate transmitter release at vertebrate and lobster neuromuscular junctions. *Nature* **283**, 486.

11. Frontali N, Ceccarelli B, Gorio A *et al.* (1976) Purification from black widow spider venom of a protein factor causing the depletion of synaptic vesicles at neuromuscular junctions. *J Cell Biol* **68**, 462.

12. Gorio A, Hurlbut WP, Ceccarelli B (1978) Acetylcholine compartments in mouse diaphragm. Comparison of the effects of black widow spider venom, electrical stimulation and high concentration of potassium. *J Cell Biol* **78**, 716.

13. Gorio A, Mauro A (1979) Black widow spider venom mode of action. In: *Advances in Cytopharmacology. Vol 3.* Ceccarelli B, Clementi F eds. Raven Press, New York p. 129.

14. Gorio A, Mauro A (1979) Reversibility and mode of action of black widow spider venom on the vertebrate neuromuscular junction. *J Gen Physiol* **73**, 245.

15. Gorio A, Rubin LL, Mauro A (1978) Double mode of action of black widow spider venom on frog neuromuscular junction. *J Neurocytol* **7**, 193.

16. Grasso A, Alema S, Rufini S, Senni MI (1980) Black widow spider toxin-induced calcium fluxes and transmitter release in a neurosecretory cell line. *Nature* **283**, 774.

17. Grasso A, Mercanti-Ciotti MT (1993) The secretion of aminoacid transmitters from cerebellar primary cultures probed by α-latrotoxin. *Neuroscience* **54**, 595.

18. Grasso A, Paggi P (1967) Effect of *Latrodectus mactans tredecimguttatus* venom on the crayfish stretch receptor neuron. *Toxicon* **5**, 1.

19. Grishin EV, Himmelreich NH, Pluzhnikov KA *et al.* (1993) Modulation of functional activities of the neurotoxin from black widow spider venom. *FEBS Lett* **336**, 205.

20. Hurlbut WP, Ceccarelli B (1979) Use of black widow spider venom to study the release of neurotransmitter. In: *Advances in Cytopharmacology. Vol 3.* Ceccarelli B, Clementi F eds. Raven Press, New York p. 87.

21. Kao I, Drachman DB, Price DL (1976) Botulinum toxin: Mechanism of presynaptic blockade. *Science* **193**, 1256.

22. Kawai NA, Mauro A, Grundfest H (1972) Effect of black widow spider venom on the lobster neuromuscular junctions. *J Gen Physiol* **60**, 650.

23. Kiyatkin N, Dulubova I, Chekhovskaya I, Grishin E (1990) Cloning and structure of cDNA encoding α-latrotoxin from black widow spider venom. *FEBS Lett* **270**, 127.

24. Kiyatkin N, Dulubova I, Chekhovskaya I *et al.* (1992) Structure of the low molecular weight protein copurified with α-latrotoxin. *Toxicon* **7**, 771.

25. Kiyatkin N, Dulubova I, Grishin E (1993) Cloning and structural analysis of α-latroinsectotoxin cDNA. Abundance of ankyrin-like repeats. *Eur J Biochem* **213**, 121.

26. Linial M, Ilouz N, Feinstein N (1995) Alpha-latrotoxin is a potent inducer of neurotransmitter release in torpedo electric organ. Functional and morphological characterization. *Eur J Neurosci* **7**, 742.

27. Longenecker HE Jr, Hurlbut WP, Mauro A, Clark AW (1970) Effects of black widow spider venom on frog neuromuscular junction. *Nature* **225**, 701.

28. Mallart A, Haimann C (1985) Different effects of alpha-latrotoxin on mouse nerve endings and fibers. *Muscle Nerve* **8**, 151.

29. Merdolesi J (1984) The receptor for α-latrotoxin; studies in pre-synaptic membranes and membrane extracts. In: *Investigation of Membrane Located Receptors.* Ried E, Cook GMW, Moore DJ eds. Plenum Press, New York p. 469.

30. Neri L, Bettini S, Frack M (1965) The effect of *Latrodectus mactans tredecimguttatus* venom on the endogenous activity of *Periplaneta americana* nerve cord. *Toxicon* **3**, 95.

31. Niinobe M, Yamaguchi Y, Fukuda M, Mokoshiba K (1994) Synaptotagmin is an inositol polyphosphate binding protein: Isolation and characterization as an inositol 1,3,4,5-tetraphosphate binding protein. *Biochem Biophys Res Commun* **205**, 1036.

32. O'Connor VM, Shamotienko O, Grishin E, Betz H (1993) On the structure of the 'synaptosecretosome'. Evidence for a neurexin/synaptotagmin/syntaxin/Ca^{2+} channel complex. *FEBS Lett* **326**, 255.

33. Ornberg RL (1977) The divalent cation dependence of spontaneous quantal release. *Soc Neurosci Abstr* **3**, 375.

34. Petrenko AG, Perin MS, Davletov BA *et al.* (1991) Binding of synaptotagmin to the α-latrotoxin receptor implicates both in synaptic vesicle exocytosis. *Nature* **353**, 65.

35. Pumplin DW, Reese TS (1977) Action of brown widow spider venom and botulinum toxin on the frog neuromuscular junction examined with freeze-fracture technique. *J Physiol-London* **273**, 443.

36. Robello R, Rolandi R, Alemà S, Grasso A (1984) Transbilayer orientation and voltage dependence of α-latrotoxin induced channels. *Proc Roy Soc London Ser B* **220**, 477.

37. Rubin LL, Gorio A, Mauro A (1978) Effect of concanavalin A on black widow spider venom activity at the neuromuscular junction: Implications for mechanisms of venom action. *Brain Res* **143**, 107.

38. Sampayo RRL (1944) Pharmacological action of the venom of *Latrodectus mactans* and other *Latrodectus* spiders. *J Pharmacol Exp Ther* **80**, 309.

39. Scalzone JM, Wells SL (1994) *Latrodectus mactans* (black widow spider) envenomation: An unusual cause for abdominal pain in pregnancy. *Obstet Gynecol* **83**, 830.

40. Scheer H (1985) Purification of the putative α-latrotoxin receptor from bovine synaptosomal membranes in an active binding form. *EMBO J* **4**, 323.

41. Simpson L (1986) Molecular pharmacology of botulinum toxin and tetanus toxin. *Annu Rev Pharmacol Toxicol* **26**, 427.

42. Smith JE, Clark AW, Kuster TA (1977) Suppression by elevated calcium of black widow spider venom activity at frog neuromuscular junctions. *J Neurocytol* **6**, 519.

43. Storchak LG, Pashkov VN, Pozdnyakova NG *et al.* (1994) α-Latrotoxin-stimulated GABA release can occur in Ca^{2+}-free, Na$^+$-free medium. *FEBS Lett* **351**, 267.

44. Tzeng M-C, Siekevitz P (1979) Action of α-latrotoxin from BWSV on a cerebral cortex preparation: Release of neurotransmitters, depletion of synaptic vesicles and binding to membrane. In: *Advances in Cytopharmacology. Vol 3.* Ceccarelli B, Clementi F eds. Raven Press, New York p. 117.

45. Ushkaryov YA, Grishin EV (1986) Black widow spider neurotoxin and its interaction with rat brain receptors. *Bioorg Khim* **12**, 71.

46. Ushkaryov YA, Petrenko AG, Geppert M, Sudhof TC (1992) Neurexins: Synaptic cell surface proteins related to the α-latrotoxin receptor and laminin. *Science* **257**, 50.

Botulinum Neurotoxin

Phyllis L. Bieri

NEUROTOXICITY RATING

Clinical

A   Neuromuscular transmission syndrome (diffuse; focal—local injection)

Experimental

A   Neuromuscular transmission dysfunction (blockade of acetylcholine release)

Botulinum neurotoxin (BoNT) is the most potent biological neurotoxin known. Intoxication with BoNT causes botulism, a potentially fatal neuroparalytic illness. Named from the Latin word for sausage (*botulus*), botulism was known in nineteenth century Europe to be associated with poorly preserved foods, especially blood sausages. Botulism and the organism that produces BoNT were first described in 1897 by van Ermengem, a professor of bacteriology at the University of Ghent Medical School in Belgium. He analyzed an outbreak of botulism among 24 musicians who participated in a wake and feasted on partially preserved raw ham. Investigation revealed that the offending ham had been at the bottom of the barrel, submerged in insufficiently concentrated brine, thus providing ideal anaerobic conditions for the novel bacteria. He termed the gram-positive, spore-forming bacteria *Bacillus botulinus*, and correctly deduced that botulism is a specific intoxication caused by a heat-labile, highly potent toxin produced by bacteria frequently found in partially preserved food products. The organism was later renamed *Clostridium botulinum* (81). Its natural habitat is soil, where it has been found on every continent examined. *C. botulinum* spores, carried by dust, are commonly present on vegetables, fresh fruits, fish, and other agricultural products (*e.g.* honey) (67).

At least seven immunologically distinct botulinum neurotoxins (types A–G) are synthesized by *Clostridium botulinum*. Toxigenic strains of BoNT are also produced by *C. baratii* (BoNT/F) and *C. butyricum* (BoNT/E) (27,47,78). The cDNA-deduced amino acid sequences of strains A–F have been described and show homology with tetanus, particularly in the light chain, which contains a Zn^{2+}-binding motif (8,25,35,46,52,77,78,82). BoNTs are synthesized by toxigenic clostridia as single-chain, inactive progenitor toxins and cleaved to generate toxins with two chains joined by a disulfide bond. The heavy chain (100 kDa) is responsible for specific binding of BoNT to neuronal cells and for penetration of the light (L) chain (50 kDa) into the cell. The L chain is the active portion of the neurotoxin and is responsible for preventing release of acetylcholine at the neuromuscular junction (64). In BoNT poisoning, cholinergic vesicles at presynaptic terminal release sites fail to fuse with the presynaptic membrane and undergo exocytosis. The resulting neuromuscular blockade causes clinical manifestations of botulism, or leads to focal muscle paralysis when BoNT is locally injected in pharmacological doses.

C. botulinum organisms are divided into four distinct culture groups, based on growth temperature, proteolytic activity, and lipolytic action (Table 3). Group I cultures are proteolytic strains that produce toxins A, B, or F. In this group, endogenous enzymes cleave the single chain ("nicking"), thus activating the toxin. Group II cultures are nonproteolytic strains that produce toxins B, E, or F, and require exogenous enzymes, such as trypsin, for activation. Group III cultures are weakly proteolytic or nonproteolytic strains that produce toxins C or D. Group IV cultures produce BoNT/G toxin, are proteolytic, and are the only lipase-negative strains. This group has also been referred to as *C. argentinense* (72). BoNT/G is the only BoNT strain with genes linked to a plasmid (26). In contrast, the genes

TABLE 3. Characteristics of *C. botulinum* Culture Groups*

Group	Toxin(s)	Proteolytic Status	Spore Heat Resistance	Lipase	Botulism Features
I	A, B, F	Proteolytic	High	+	Humans, severe disease
II	B, E, F	Nonproteolytic	Low	+	Humans, less severe disease
III	C, D	Nonproteolytic, or weakly proteolytic	Intermediate	+	Animals, especially birds
IV	G	Proteolytic	Unknown	−	Unknown

*Based on data from Simpson *et al.* (65).

that encode all other BoNT serotypes are found on chromosomal DNA (88). Groups I and II cause the vast majority of human botulism cases. Complicating this classification is the finding that strains of the same genotype often produce different toxins (*e.g.*, some saccharolytic strains can produce BoNT/B, BoNT/E, or BoNT/F) (36). Conversely, different genotypes can produce the same toxin (*e.g.*, BoNT/B is produced by saccharolytic and proteolytic genotypes).

General Toxicology

BoNT has a mouse intraperitoneal (i.p.) LD_{50} of 0.00625 ng (74). Using the molecular weight of approximately 150 kDa and Avogadro's constant, this calculates to 5×10^6 molecules in one mouse LD_{50}. Humans can develop botulism from 7 mouse i.p. LD_{50} units when given parenterally, and from 7000 mouse LD_{50} units if ingested (40). Vegetative cells of *C. botulinum* contain 100-fold higher concentrations of BoNT than do the spores. As a cytoplasmic protein, BoNT is released upon lysis of the cell. *C. botulinum* spores are heat resistant and require a pH > 4.6. Low salt and sugar concentrations are necessary for growth, whereas strict anaerobic conditions are not. *C. botulinum* is unable to compete well against other microbes and is frequently implicated in illness associated with ingestion of partially preserved home-canned products.

Mechanisms of Cellular Toxicity

BoNT and tetanus neurotoxin belong to a family of zinc-dependent metalloendopeptidases that require reduction of the interchain disulfide bond to become activated (22,54,55,57). These clostridial neurotoxins are potent inhibitors of synaptic vesicle exocytosis at nerve terminals. The protease activity of all seven BoNT serotypes is located on the L chain and specifically cleaves synaptic target proteins, including synaptobrevin, synaptosomal-associated protein-25 (SNAP-25), and syntaxin. Synaptobrevin was first identified in the *Torpedo* electric organ and is a highly conserved, 13-kDa integral membrane protein exposed on the surface of synaptic vesicles most likely responsible for

vesicle docking (68,79). BoNT/B, BoNT/D, BoNT/F, and BoNT/G are specific for synaptobrevin, whereas BoNT/A and BoNT/E cleave SNAP-25 at a single site in synaptosomes (7,10,45,56,59,63,84,85). BoNT/A specifically removes nine amino acids from the C-terminus of SNAP-25, resulting in a truncated SNAP-25. The SNAP-25 fragment does not inhibit formation or disassembly of the synaptosomal fusion complex; it most likely blocks exocytosis by disrupting the process of membrane fusion itself (50). BoNT/C cleaves syntaxin, an integral membrane protein present on the presynaptic membrane and implicated in the docking of synaptic vesicles at presynaptic active zones (Table 4) (11,58). BoNT/C is the only serotype that binds two zinc atoms per toxin molecule, in contrast to all other BoNT serotypes, which contain one zinc atom. Zinc chelation results in a striking reduction in the intracellular potency of all seven BoNT serotypes, as well as that of tetanus toxin 9 (65). A single mutation in the Zn^{2+}-binding motif of BoNT/A completely prevents SNAP-25 cleavage and the resulting neuroparalytic action of BoNT/A (87) *in vitro* and *in vivo*.

Animal Studies

Neuromuscular blockade in rats was shown to be significantly more potent and prolonged following BoNT/A than BoNT/B injection (61). BoNT/E was similarly less potent and shorter acting than BoNT/A. Although acetylcholine release is blocked by BoNT, nerve terminals and neuromuscular junctions do not degenerate (23,24). The inactivated nerve terminals incorporate new acetylcholine receptors into their membranes (86), and motor axon sprouting causes new neuromuscular junctions to form (32). This marked motor nerve outgrowth following BoNT intoxication results in an increase in total nerve terminal length, which is due to both an increase in the number of terminal branches and in average branch length. Weakness resolves when sufficient numbers of newly formed neuromuscular junctions appear, and when the initially asynchronous quantal transmitter release following nerve stimulation becomes synchronous (20).

TABLE 4. BoNT Serotype Target Sites*

Serotype	Target	Cleavage Site	Intracellular Location
BoNT/A	SNAP-25	Gln^{197}-Arg^{198}	Presynaptic plasma membrane
BoNT/B	Synaptobrevin	Gln^{76}-Phe^{77}	Synaptic vesicle
BoNT/C	Syntaxin 1A	Lys^{253}-Ala^{254}	Presynaptic plasma membrane
	Syntaxin 1B	Lys^{252}-Ala^{253}	Presynaptic plasma membrane
BoNT/D	Synaptobrevin	Lys^{59}-Leu^{60}	Synaptic vesicle
	Synaptobrevin	Ala^{67}-Asp^{68}	Synaptic vesicle
	Cellubrevin	?	Endocytotic vesicles
BoNT/E	SNAP-25	Arg^{180}-Ile^{181}	Presynaptic plasma membrane
BoNT/F	Synaptobrevin	Gln^{58}-Lys^{59}	Synaptic vesicle
	Cellubrevin	?	Endocytotic vesicles
BoNT/G	Synaptobrevin	Ala^{81}-Ala^{82}	Synaptic vesicle

*Based on data from Huttner (37).

BoNT/A injection in rats has been associated with myopathic changes up to 30 weeks following injection. The changes include extensive vacuolation of the sarcoplasm and degeneration of junctional folds, suggesting a myotoxic effect of BoNT (31). Since intrafusal muscle fibers are also blocked by BoNT/A, activation of muscle spindle afferents is also affected (53). Local BoNT/A injection for dystonias may be effective not only by preventing extrafusal fiber activation, but also by modifying the γ efferent system. These findings have important implications in the chronic use of BoNT/A for treatment of focal dystonias and other movement disorders.

In Vitro Studies

Rat brain synaptosomal preparations have documented the specific proteolytic activity of BoNT serotypes. Selective proteolysis of synaptic target proteins blocked glutamate release in the following manner: BoNT/D and BoNT/F cleaved synaptobrevin; BoNT/A and BoNT/E cleaved SNAP-25; and BoNT/C cleaved syntaxin (9).

BoNT is slow acting, both *in vivo* and *in vitro*. When applied directly to intact *in vitro* preparations, BoNT takes minutes to hours to affect transmission. This is explained by binding and internalization of the toxin, as well as its enzymatic action. BoNT/A and BoNT/B inhibit the release of a wide variety of transmitters from *in vitro* preparations, demonstrating that the mechanism of action is common to vesicle exocytotic function (42).

The observation that local injection of BoNT preferentially weakens hyperactive muscles was first noted in rat diaphragm preparations, in which paralysis was faster when nerve-ending activity was greatest (34). These and other studies that show ephaptic transmission is blocked by BoNT suggest that those muscle fibers involved in focal muscle spasms are most likely to be affected by local injec-

tion of BoNT (30). *In-vitro* rat diaphragm preparations have also been used to investigate potential therapeutic effects of BoNT antagonists. The potassium-channel inhibitor 3,4-diaminopyridine rapidly reversed BoNT/A-induced muscle paralysis for at least 8 h (1).

The mechanism of BoNT-induced sprouting of motor axons seen in many whole-animal systems was explored in a nerve-muscle *in vitro* preparation using chick embryo ciliary ganglion motor neurons cocultured with chick leg muscle cells. BoNT/A caused increased neurite branching when neurons and myocytes were physically separated, and in the presence of curare-induced postsynaptic blockade. The neurite-branching effects of BoNT are therefore presynaptically mediated and are independent of simple synaptic blockade (12).

Injured cell membranes rapidly reseal following injury *via* a mechanism that is inhibited by BoNT/A and BoNT/B. This suggests that SNAP-25 and synaptobrevin participate in membrane resealing, with the implication that mechanisms for cell membrane resealing may involve synaptic vesicle delivery, docking, and fusion, similar to neurotransmitter release *via* exocytosis (71).

Human Studies

Food-borne botulism is caused by ingestion of food that contains preformed BoNT. BoNT is absorbed in the upper small intestine, then passes *via* lymphatics to the bloodstream. BoNT binds rapidly and irreversibly to acetylcholine receptors at the neuromuscular junction, autonomic ganglia, and postganglionic parasympathetic endings (74). Two other mechanisms of entry have been described for BoNT. Wound botulism occurs when *C. botulinum* spores germinate, causing production of BoNT in contaminated wounds. Infant botulism is caused by ingestion of spores that germinate and produce BoNT in the gastrointestinal tract. A fourth type of botulism, termed "unclassified," occurs in patients older than 1 year in whom no source of infection can be identified. Most cases occur in adults with gastrointestinal disease, including a history of abdominal surgery, or in the presence of broad-spectrum antibiotic coverage. Intoxication is presumed to arise from germination of spores in the intestinal tract, similar to infant botulism (17).

BoNT/A, BoNT/B, and BoNT/E cause the majority of human botulism cases. *C. botulinum* strains that produce these serotypes have distinctive regional distributions. In the United States, BoNT/A predominates west of the Rocky Mountains, while proteolytic strains of BoNT/B are more common in the Middle Atlantic seaboard states (67). Nonproteolytic BoNT/B strains are less lethal and are found in northern Europe, where they cause the majority of botulism cases. BoNT/E has a marine distribution; it is found in Alaska, along the Great Lakes, in Canada, and in Japan. *C. botulinum* spores are ubiquitous, and their frequency of isolation in soil samples approaches 20%. The number of BoNT/A spores in soil was found to vary from 10–200 spores/g of soil. Areas in which the organism occurs most frequently have the highest incidences of food-borne botulism (66,67). BoNT/C and BoNT/D cause disease in animals, particularly in birds. BoNT/G has been isolated from soil and was described in association with sudden infant death syndrome (SIDS) as well as sudden death in adults (69,70). BoNT/A produces the most severe illness, requiring mechanical ventilation more frequently than with BoNT/B or BoNT/E, whereas BoNT/E is associated with the shortest incubation period. These clinical findings have been substantiated by animal studies measuring onset and severity of paralysis by different serotypes (83).

In food-borne botulism, gastrointestinal symptoms often occur shortly after ingestion of contaminated food and include nausea, vomiting, abdominal distention, and diarrhea, followed by constipation or ileus in severe cases. Local toxic effects on myenteric autonomic ganglia are presumed responsible for the "stubborn constipation" initially described by van Ermengem. A short incubation period manifests with early neurological signs and prognosticates a more severe illness with protracted recovery times (75). Neurological symptoms typically begin with cranial nerve dysfunction, and include diplopia, blurred vision, dysarthria, and dysphagia. Dizziness, described as "light headedness," is a frequent early symptom, and true vertigo can also be present. Sore throat with extreme dryness of mouth and tongue, coupled with findings of a hyperemic swollen pharynx, are common and have led to a mistaken diagnosis of streptococcal or viral pharyngitis (39). Clinically there may be ptosis, extraocular muscle palsies, diminished gag

reflex, and tongue weakness. Autonomic nervous system dysfunction has been reported more commonly in BoNT/B and BoNT/E than in BoNT/A intoxication; this may manifest as dilated or unreactive pupils, dryness of eyes and mouth, postural hypotension, and urinary retention. Pupillary abnormalities are frequently absent early in the illness (15); prominent early pupillary dilatation was associated with increased risk of respiratory failure (76). The pattern of muscle weakness is typically symmetrical, but may be asymmetrical, and respiratory insufficiency may occur prior to significant arm and leg weakness. Deep tendon reflexes may be normal, hypoactive, or absent; rarely they are hyperactive. Paresthesias were reported by 14% of patients in one series and do not exclude the diagnosis (34).

Treatment of botulism is mainly supportive. Trivalent equine antitoxin (anti-BoNT/A, -BoNT/B, and -BoNT/E) is available from the U.S. Centers for Disease Control and Prevention (CDC) and should be given as early as possible by intravenous and intramuscular routes to attempt to halt clinical progression (14). Antitoxin can only neutralize circulating BoNT, since BoNT binds irreversibly to nerve terminals. Hypersensitivity reactions should be tested for prior to administration of antitoxin. In food-borne botulism, enemas can be administered (if no ileus is present) in an attempt to remove unabsorbed BoNT from the gastrointestinal tract. Use of aminoglycoside and polymyxin antibiotics is contraindicated because of their toxic effects at the neuromuscular junction (3). Botulism fatality rates have greatly diminished in the past several decades because of advances in intensive care; most fatalities are now due to nosocomial infections or respirator malfunction.

The differential diagnosis of botulism includes Guillain-Barré syndrome, especially the Miller-Fisher variant, other bacterial food poisonings (*e.g.*, enterotoxic staphylococcal food poisoning), organophosphate poisoning, atropine poisoning, tick paralysis, diphtheria, myasthenia gravis, and the Lambert-Eaton myasthenic syndrome (13).

Data from electrophysiological studies can be useful in supporting the early diagnosis of botulism, before laboratory confirmation of disease. Motor conduction velocities are normal, as are sensory amplitudes and latencies. In clinically affected muscles, the compound muscle action potentials show low amplitudes; however, motor amplitudes can be normal in 15% of patients (15). Posttetanic (or postexercise) facilitation is the hallmark of presynaptic neuromuscular junction dysfunction; this phenomenon tends to be less severe in botulism than in Lambert-Eaton syndrome. Nearly 40% of botulism cases fail to show facilitation and, when present, the degree of facilitation ranges from 30–100%. In contrast, the degree of facilitation in Lambert-Eaton syndrome can be twofold or higher (16). Facilitation is seen more frequently (84% of patients) in BoNT/B intoxication (34). At slow rates of stimulation, the decremental response in botulism is minimal (<8%) or absent. Needle electromyography (EMG) in clinically affected muscles reveals myopathic motor units, with low-amplitude, short-duration, polyphasic potentials (16). Single-fiber EMG studies reveal abnormal jitter, with or without blocking, which improves with higher motor-unit firing rates, in contrast to myasthenia gravis where jitter increases with higher firing rates (13).

From 1975 through 1992, there were 257 outbreaks of food-borne botulism in the United States, involving 543 individual cases (33). The majority of cases was in western or Rocky Mountain states. This may be partially explained by high-altitude cooking, where the boiling temperature of water is insufficient to destroy *C. botulinum* spores, which require temperatures of 120°C for 30 min to be inactivated. It is therefore recommended that pressure cookers be used for canning at high altitudes, with ½ lb added to the pressure gauge for each additional 1000 feet above sea level (15).

Infant botulism was first described in 1976 and occurs when ingested *C. botulinum* spores germinate, multiply, and produce BoNT in the intestinal lumen of infants (51). From 1975 through 1992, there were 1134 cases of infant botulism reported to the CDC, with BoNT/B more common than BoNT/A, and rare cases due to BoNT/C, BoNT/E, and BoNT/F (33,48). Infant botulism has therefore become the predominant form of botulism seen in the United States. The disease occurs almost exclusively between the ages of 2 weeks and 6 months, with a mean age of onset of 10 weeks. This restricted age distribution may be partly explained by studies that showed that 7–13-day-old mice were readily colonized by BoNT, whereas younger and older mice were resistant to oral intoxication. Germ-free mice were especially susceptible to infection (73). The particular susceptibility of this age group in mice corresponds to that in humans when adjusted for species lifespan, and presumably results from age-related changes in intestinal flora. Ingestion of honey prior to onset of illness was found in 44% of BoNT/B cases *vs.* 9% of controls (5,18). In California, the risk of acquiring BoNT/B illness increased almost eightfold if there was a history of previous honey ingestion. It has therefore been recommended by several U.S. public health agencies that infants not be fed honey, especially if under 6 months of age (4). Breast-feeding was found to be protective against the fulminant form of infant botulism resembling SIDS. In contrast, it was associated with an increased incidence of infant botulism cases requiring hospitalization. Breast-feeding may thus provide a window of time necessary for hospitalization in the more severe, fulminant cases of infant botulism (4).

The earliest manifestations of infant botulism are constipation, followed by impaired ability to suck and swallow. As in classic food-borne botulism, the flaccid paralysis typically begins in cranial nerve-innervated muscles and descends; however, in infants, ptosis and ophthalmoparesis can be mild and easily overlooked. Once muscle weakness and hypotonia become generalized, the infant becomes overtly floppy (3). Symptom severity can vary greatly, from lethargy, mild weakness, and decreased appetite, to fulminant, generalized weakness with respiratory arrest. Stool cultures demonstrate *C. botulinum* and BoNT, whereas assays of the serum are usually negative. Nerve conduction studies can corroborate the diagnosis, showing typical facilitation of compound muscle response to rapid stimulation rates. Electromyography may reveal abundant, low-amplitude motor units. With proper supportive treatment the disease is self-limited, even without antiserum treatment, and mortality rates are low (3%). However, a fulminant type of infant botulism has been associated with cases previously classified as SIDS, presumably by causing paroxysmal dyspnea (5). Use of antimicrobial agents is not recommended in infant botulism because of concern that *C. botulinum* lysis may release additional toxin (6).

Wound botulism is rare. First described in 1943, there have been 47 cases in the United States through 1992, with 22 of those occurring in California. BoNT/A was more frequent than BoNT/B, with 32 cases *vs.* 13, respectively. Two cases were caused by BoNT/F due to *C. baratii* (33). Wound botulism is both an infection and an intoxication; the organism gains entrance *via* traumatized subcutaneous tissues, usually in lacerations or compound fractures contaminated by soil. The wounds can appear surprisingly benign, however, with gas or suppuration appearing in less than half the cases in one series (43). Two cases have been reported in injection drug users (41). Once infection is established, BoNT is elaborated by *C. botulinum*, and clinical signs appear after a longer incubation period of 4–18 days. Fever may occur if the wound is grossly infected. Nausea, vomiting, and diarrhea or constipation are characteristically absent in wound botulism, presumably due to a lack of local effects of BoNT on myenteric autonomic ganglia.

Ultrastructural studies of human motor end-plate regions in botulism show postsynaptic regions denuded of their nerve terminals. In addition, there is a decrease in total nerve-terminal area as well as an increase in postsynaptic membrane length compared to the presynaptic length (80). In all cases, clinical recovery occurs with synthesis of new synaptic end plates. The observed course of clinical recovery is therefore relatively slow following BoNT intoxication.

Therapeutic use of BoNT/A for a wide variety of neurological, ophthalmic, and other disorders manifest by excessive or inappropriate muscle contraction has become increasingly common (21). Treatment is safe and effective, with clinical side effects rare. However, distant effects on neuromuscular transmission have been associated with local injections of BoNT/A, seen as increased jitter in single-fiber EMG studies and increased mean fiber density (28,49). Gastrointestinal autonomic pathways were affected following BoNT/A injection for blepharospasm, evidenced by gallbladder hypomotility following each injection, causing recurrent biliary colic (60). Five to 10% of patients receiving chronic BoNT/A injections develop anti-BoNT/A antibodies and fail to respond to further treatment. Risk factors for acquiring BoNT/A antibodies include higher mean dose per treatment, more frequent injections, and younger age at onset of treatment (29,38). BoNT/F has been shown effective in patients refractory to BoNT/A, although BoNT/F has a shorter duration of action, most likely due to relatively diminished toxicity (44,62).

Toxic Mechanisms

Multiple lines of evidence suggest that clostridial neurotoxins have evolved from an ancestral protease responsible for blocking the exocytotic fusion and docking machinery of synaptic vesicles. Select BoNT serotypes target individual members of the membrane fusion complex at unique sites, resulting in failure of neuroexocytosis and release of acetylcholine (7). Clostridial neurotoxins have become powerful tools in the investigation of events occurring during vesicle exocytosis in neuronal, endocrine, and nonneuronal cells. Although all clostridial neurotoxins attack synaptic-vesicle-fusion proteins *via* their light chains, the biological difference between BoNT serotypes lies in the heavy chains, which are responsible for different transport routes carrying the light chains to the final place of action (2).

The therapeutic implications regarding recent advances in the understanding of zinc-dependent proteases are substantial. A zinc endopeptidase able to cross the neuronal plasmalemma would antagonize the action of BoNT. Eventually, agents that not only antagonize BoNT but reverse its effects by restoring vesicle fusion and docking machinery might become available (19).

REFERENCES

1. Adler M, Scovill J, Parker G et al. (1995) Antagonism of botulinum toxin-induced muscle weakness by 3,4-diaminopyridine in rat phrenic nerve-hemidiaphragm preparations. *Toxicon* 33, 527.

2. Ahnert-Hilger G, Bigalke H (1995) Molecular aspects of tetanus and botulinum neurotoxin poisoning. *Prog Neurobiol* 46, 83.

3. Arnon SS, Chin J (1979) The clinical spectrum of infant botulism. *Rev Infect Dis* 1, 614.

4. Arnon SS, Damus K, Chin J (1981) Infant botulism: Epidemiology and relation to sudden infant death syndrome. *Epidemiol Rev* 3, 45.

5. Arnon SS, Midura TF, Damus K et al. (1979) Honey and other environmental risk factors for infant botulism. *J Pediat* 94, 331.

6. Bartlett JC (1986) Infant botulism in adults. *N Engl J Med* 315, 254.

7. Binz T, Blasi J, Yamasaki S et al. (1994) Proteolysis of SNAP-25 by types E and A botulinal neurotoxins. *J Biol Chem* 269, 1617.

8. Binz T, Kurazono H, Wille M et al. (1990) The complete sequence of botulinum neurotoxin type A and comparison with other clostridial neurotoxins. *J Biol Chem* 265, 9153.

9. Blasi J, Binz T, Yamasaki S et al. (1994) Inhibition of neurotransmitter release by clostridial neurotoxins correlates with specific proteolysis of synaptosomal proteins. *J Physiol-Paris* 88, 235.

10. Blasi J, Chapman ER, Link E et al. (1993) Botulinum neurotoxin A selectively cleaves the synaptic protein SNAP-25. *Nature* 365, 160.

11. Blasi J, Chapman ER, Yamasaki S et al. (1993) Botulinum neurotoxin C1 blocks neurotransmitter release by means of cleaving HPC-1/syntaxin. *EMBO J* 12, 4821.

12. Bonner PH, Friedli AF, Baker RS (1994) Botulinum A toxin stimulates neurite branching in nerve-muscle cocultures. *Brain Res Develop Brain Res* 79, 39.

13. Bradley WG, Ferucci JT Jr, Shahani BT (1980) Case records of the Massachusetts General Hospital: Case 48-1980. *N Engl J Med* 303, 1347.

14. Centers for Disease Control (1979) *Botulism in the United States, 1899-1977: Handbook for Epidemiologists, Clinicians and Laboratory Workers.* CDC, Atlanta, Georgia.

15. Cherington M (1974) Botulism. Ten-year experience. *Arch Neurol* 30, 432.

16. Cherington M (1982) Electrophysiologic methods as an aid in diagnosis of botulism: A review. *Muscle Nerve* 5, S28.

17. Chia JK, Clark JB, Ryan CA et al. (1986) Botulism in an adult associated with food-borne intestinal infection with *Clostridium botulinum. N Engl J Med* 315, 239.

18. Chin J, Arnon SS, Midura TF (1979) Food and environmental aspects of infant botulism in California. *Rev Infect Dis* 1, 693.

19. Coffield JA, Considine RV, Simpson LL (1994) Clostridial neurotoxins in the age of molecular medicine. *Trends Microbiol* 2, 67.

20. Comella JX, Molgo J, Faille L (1993) Sprouting of mammalian motor nerve terminals induced by *in vivo* injection of botulinum type-D toxin and the functional recovery of paralyzed neuromuscular junctions. *Neurosci Lett* **153**, 61.

21. Denislic M, Pirtosek Z, Vodusek DB *et al.* (1994) Botulinum toxin in the treatment of neurological disorders. *Ann N Y Acad Sci* **710**, 76.

22. de Paiva A, Ashton AC, Foran P *et al.* (1993) Botulinum A like type B and tetanus toxins fulfills criteria for being a zinc-dependent protease. *J Neurochem* **61**, 2338.

23. Duchen LW (1971) An electron microscopic study of the changes induced by botulinum toxin in the motor endplates of slow and fast skeletal muscle fibres of the mouse. *J Neurol Sci* **14**, 47.

24. Duchen LW, Strich SJ (1968) The effects of botulinum toxin on the pattern of innervation of skeletal muscle in the mouse. *Quart J Exp Physiol* **53**, 84.

25. East AK, Richardson PT, Allaway D *et al.* (1992) Sequence of the gene encoding type F neurotoxin of *Clostridium botulinum*. *FEMS Microbiol Lett* **75**, 225.

26. Eklund MW, Poysky FT, Mseitif LM *et al.* (1988) Evidence for plasmid-mediated toxin and bacteriocin production in *Clostridium botulinum* type G. *Appl Environ Microbiol* **54**, 1405.

27. Giménez JA, Sugiyama H (1988) Comparison of toxins of *Clostridium butyricum* and *Clostridium botulinum* type E. *Infect Immunity* **56**, 926.

28. Girlanda P, Vita G, Nicolosi C *et al.* (1992) Botulinum toxin therapy: Distant effects on neuromuscular transmission and autonomic nervous system. *J Neurol Neurosurg Psychiat* **55**, 844.

29. Greene P, Fahn S, Diamond B (1994) Development of resistance to botulinum toxin type A in patients with torticollis. *Movement Disord* **9**, 213.

30. Hallett M, Glocker FX, Deuschl G (1994) Mechanism of action of botulinum toxin. *Ann Neurol* **36**, 449.

31. Hassan SM, Jennekens FGI, Veldman H (1995) Botulinum toxin-induced myopathy in the rat. *Brain* **118**, 533.

32. Hassan SM, Jennekens FGI, Wieneke G *et al.* (1994) Elimination of superfluous neuromuscular junctions in rat calf muscles recovering from botulinum toxin-induced paralysis. *Muscle Nerve* **17**, 623.

33. Hatheway CL (1995) Private communication, Botulism Laboratory, Division for Bacterial and Mycotic Disease, National Center for Infectious Diseases, U.S. Centers for Disease Control and Prevention, Atlanta, Georgia.

34. Hughes JM, Blumenthal JR, Merson MH *et al.* (1981) Clinical features of types A and B food-borne botulism. *Ann Intern Med* **95**, 442.

35. Hutson RA, Collins MD, East AK *et al.* (1994) Nucleotide sequence of the gene coding for non-proteolytic *Clostridium botulinum* type B neurotoxin: Comparison with other clostridial neurotoxins. *Curr Microbiol* **28**, 101.

36. Hutson RA, Thompson DE, Collins MD (1993) Genetic interrelationships of saccharolytic *Clostridium botulinum* types B, E and F and related clostridia as revealed by small-subunit rRNA gene sequences. *FEMS Microbiol Lett* **108**, 103.

37. Huttner WB (1993) Snappy exocytoxins. *Nature* **365**, 104.

38. Jankovic J, Schwartz K (1995) Response and immunoresistance to botulinum toxin injections. *Neurology* **45**, 1743.

39. Koenig MG, Spickard A, Cardella MA *et al.* (1964) Clinical and laboratory observations on type E botulism in man. *Medicine* **43**, 517.

40. Lamanna C, Hart ER (1967) Potency of botulinal toxin as influenced by body weight and mode of exposure. In: *Botulism 1966*. Ingram M, Roberts TA eds. Chapman and Hall, London p. 370.

41. MacDonald KL, Rutherford GW, Friedman SM *et al.* (1985) Botulism and botulism-like illness in chronic drug abusers. *Ann Intern Med* **102**, 616.

42. McMahon HT, Foran P, Dolly JO *et al.* (1992) Tetanus toxin and botulinum toxins type A and B inhibit glutamate, γ-aminobutyric acid, aspartate, and met-enkephalin release from synaptosomes. *J Biol Chem* **267**, 21338.

43. Merson MH, Dowell VR Jr (1973) Epidemiologic, clinical, and laboratory aspects of wound botulism. *N Engl J Med* **289**, 1105.

44. Mezaki T, Kaji R, Kohara N *et al.* (1995) Comparison of therapeutic efficacies of type A and F botulinum toxins for blepharospasm: A double-blind, controlled study. *Neurology* **45**, 506.

45. Montecucco C, Schiavo G (1993) Tetanus and botulism neurotoxins: A new group of zinc proteases. *Trends Biochem Sci* **18**, 324.

46. Niemann H (1991) Molecular biology of clostridial neurotoxins. In: *A Sourcebook of Bacterial Protein Toxins*. Alouf JE, Freer JH eds. Academic Press, New York/London p. 303.

47. Oguma K, Yamaguchi T, Sudou K *et al.* (1986) Biochemical classification of *Clostridium botulinum* type C and D strains and their nontoxigenic derivatives. *Appl Environ Microbiol* **51**, 256.

48. Oguma K, Yokota K, Hayashi S *et al.* (1990) Infant botulism due to *Clostridium botulinum* type C toxin. *Lancet* **336**, 1449.

49. Olney RK, Aminoff MJ, Gelb DJ *et al.* (1988) Neuromuscular effects distant from the site of botulinum neurotoxin injection. *Neurology* **38**, 1780.

50. Otto H, Hanson PI, Chapman ER *et al.* (1995) Poisoning by botulinum neurotoxin A does not inhibit formation or disassembly of the synaptosomal fusion complex. *Biochem Biophys Res Commun* **212**, 945.

51. Pickett J, Berg B, Chaplin E *et al.* (1976) Syndrome of botulism in infancy: Clinical and electrophysiologic study. *N Engl J Med* **295**, 770.

52. Poulet S, Hauser D, Quanz M *et al.* (1992) Sequences of the botulinal neurotoxin E derived from *Clostridium botulinum* type E (strain beluga) and *Clostridium butyricum* (strains ATCC43181 and ATCC43755). *Biochem Biophys Res Commun* **183**, 107.

53. Rosales RL, Arimura K, Takenaga S *et al.* (1996) Extrafusal and intrafusal muscle effects in experimental botulinum toxin-A injection. *Muscle Nerve* **19**, 488.

54. Schiavo G, Benfenati F, Poulain B *et al.* (1992) Tetanus and botulinum-B neurotoxins block neurotransmitter release by proteolytic cleavage of synaptobrevin. *Nature* **359**, 832.

55. Schiavo G, Rossetto O, Benfenati F *et al.* (1994) Tetanus and botulinum neurotoxins are zinc proteases specific for components of the neuroexocytosis apparatus. *Ann N Y Acad Sci* **710**, 65.

56. Schiavo G, Rossetto O, Catsicas S *et al.* (1993) Identification of the nerve terminal targets of botulinum neurotoxin serotypes A, D, and E. *J Biol Chem* **268**, 23784.

57. Schiavo G, Rossetto O, Santucci A *et al.* (1992) Botulinum neurotoxins are zinc proteins. *J Biol Chem* **267**, 23479.

58. Schiavo G, Shone CC, Bennett MK *et al.* (1995) Botulinum neurotoxin type C cleaves a single Lys-Ala bond within the carboxyl-terminal region of syntaxins. *J Biol Chem* **270**, 10566.

59. Schiavo G, Shone CC, Rossetto O *et al.* (1993) Botulinum neurotoxin serotype F is a zinc endopeptidase specific for VAMP/synaptobrevin. *J Biol Chem* **268**, 11516.

60. Schnider P, Brichta A, Schmied M (1993) Gallbladder dysfunction induced by botulinum A toxin. *Lancet* **342**, 811.

61. Sellin LC, Thesleff S, Dasgupta BR (1983) Different effects of types A and B botulinum toxin on transmitter release at the rat neuromuscular junction. *Acta Physiol Scand* **119**, 127.

62. Sheean GL, Lees AJ (1995) Botulinum toxin F in the treatment of torticollis clinically resistant to botulinum toxin A. *J Neurol Neurosurg Psychiat* **59**, 601.

63. Shone CC, Quinn CP, Wait R *et al.* (1993) Proteolytic cleavage of synthetic fragments of vesicle-associated membrane protein, isoform-2 by botulinum type B neurotoxin. *Eur J Biochem* **217**, 965.

64. Simpson LL (1989) *Botulinum Neurotoxin and Tetanus Toxin.* Academic Press, New York.

65. Simpson LL, Coffield JA, Bakry N (1993) Chelation of zinc antagonizes the neuromuscular blocking properties of the seven serotypes of botulinum neurotoxin as well as tetanus toxin. *J Pharmacol Exp Ther* **267**, 720.

66. Smith LDS (1977) *Botulism: The Organism, Its Toxins, the Diseases.* Charles C Thomas Bannerstone House, Springfield, Illinois.

67. Smith LDS (1979) *Clostridium botulinum*: Characteristics and occurrence. *Rev Infect Dis* **1**, 637.

68. Söllner T, Whiteheart SW, Brunner M *et al.* (1993) SNAP receptors implicated in vesicle targeting and fusion. *Nature* **362**, 318.

69. Sonnabend OA, Sonnabend WF, Heinzle R *et al.* (1981) Isolation of *Clostridium botulinum* type G and identification of type G botulinal toxin in humans: Report of five sudden unexpected deaths. *J Infect Dis* **143**, 22.

70. Sonnabend OA, Sonnabend WF, Krech U *et al.* (1985) Continuous microbiological study of 70 sudden and unexpected infant deaths: Toxigenic intestinal *Clostridium botulinum* infection in 9 cases of sudden infant death syndrome. *Lancet* **1**, 237.

71. Steinhardt RA, Bi G, Alderton JM (1994) Cell membrane resealing by a vesicular mechanism similar to neurotransmitter release. *Science* **263**, 390.

72. Suen JC, Hatheway CL, Steigerwalt AG *et al.* (1988) *Clostridium argentinense* sp. nov.: A genetically homogeneous group composed of all strains of *Clostridium botulinum* toxin type G and some non toxigenic strains previously identified as *Clostridium subterminale* or *Clostridium hastiforme*. *Int J Syst Bacteriol* **38**, 375.

73. Sugiyama H (1979) Animal models for the study of infant botulism. *Rev Infect Dis* **1**, 683.

74. Sugiyama H (1980) *Clostridium botulinum* neurotoxin. *Microbiol Rev* **9**, 419.

75. Terranova W, Breman JG, Locey RP *et al.* (1978) Botulism type B: Epidemiologic aspects of an extensive outbreak. *Amer J Epidemiol* **108**, 150.

76. Terranova W, Palumbo JN, Breman JG (1979) Ocular findings in botulism type B. *J Amer Med Assn* **241**, 475.

77. Thompson DE, Brehm JK, Oultram JD *et al.* (1990) The complete amino acid sequence of the *Clostridium botulinum* type A neurotoxin, deduced by nucleotide sequence analysis of the encoding gene. *Eur J Biochem* **189**, 73.

78. Thompson DE, Hutson RA, East AK *et al.* (1993) Nucleotide sequence of the gene coding for *Clostridium baratii* type F neurotoxin: Comparison with other clostridial neurotoxins. *FEMS Microbiol Lett* **108**, 175.

79. Trimble WS, Cowan DM, Scheller RH (1988) VAMP-1: A synaptic vesicle-associated integral membrane protein. *Proc Nat Acad Sci USA* **85**, 4538.

80. Tsujihata M, Kinoshita I, Mori M *et al.* (1987) Ultrastructural study of the motor end-plate in botulism and Lambert-Eaton myasthenic syndrome. *J Neurol Sci* **81**, 197.

81. van Ermengem E (1979) A new anaerobic bacillus and its relation to botulism. *Rev Infect Dis* **1**, 701.

82. Whelan SM, Elmore MJ, Bodsworth NJ *et al.* (1992) Molecular cloning of the *Clostridium botulinum* structural gene encoding the type B neurotoxin and determination of its entire nucleotide sequence. *Appl Environ Microbiol* **58**, 2345.

83. Woodruff BA, Griffin PM, McCroskey LM *et al.* (1992) Clinical and laboratory comparison of botulism from

toxin types A, B, and E in the United States, 1975–1988. *J Infect Dis* **166**, 1281.

84. Yamasaki S, Baumeister A, Binz T *et al.* (1994) Cleavage of members of the synaptobrevin/VAMP family by types D and F botulinal neurotoxins and tetanus toxin. *J Biol Chem* **269**, 12764.

85. Yamasaki S, Binz T, Hayashi T *et al.* (1994) Botulinum neurotoxin type G proteolyses the Ala^{81}-Ala^{82} bond of rat synaptobrevin 2. *Biochem Biophys Res Commun* **200**, 829.

86. Yee WC, Pestronk A (1987) Mechanisms of postsynaptic plasticity: Remodeling of the junctional acetylcholine receptor cluster induced by motor nerve terminal outgrowth. *J Neurosci* **7**, 2019.

87. Zhou L, de Paiva A, Liu D *et al.* (1995) Expression and purification of the light chain of botulinum neurotoxin A: A single mutation abolishes its cleavage of SNAP-25 and neurotoxicity after reconstitution with the heavy chain. *Biochem* **34**, 15175.

88. Zhou Y, Sugiyama H, Nakano H *et al.* (1995) The genes for the *Clostridium botulinum* type G toxin complex are on a plasmid. *Infect Immunity* **63**, 2087.

CASE REPORT

A 45-year-old woman was brought to the emergency room with new onset of diplopia, blurred vision, dry mouth, and difficulty talking. The patient was well until the day prior to admission when she ate home-canned chili peppers and developed nausea, vomiting, and abdominal bloating within a few hours of the ingestion. The patient's 17-year-old son ate only a small portion of the same canned chili peppers because they "tasted bad" and remained asymptomatic. The patient complained of a severely dry mouth and constipation since the previous day. There were no sensory symptoms.

On examination, the patient was alert and oriented to person, place, and time. Blood pressure was 90/60 mm Hg in the supine, sitting, and standing positions. Speech was hoarse and dysarthric, and the patient repeatedly rinsed her mouth with water. Tongue and throat were red and very dry. The neck was supple. Lung fields were clear, and the heart was normal. The abdomen was moderately distended; bowel sounds were present. There were no skin lesions or superficial wounds. Visual fields were full, and the optic fundi appeared normal. Pupils were 4 mm and unreactive. There was bilateral partial ptosis, such that the patient could elevate both lids approximately half their normal excursion. There was complete inability to deviate either eye laterally, and poor medial deviation bilaterally. Mild bilateral facial weakness was evidenced by poor eye and mouth closure, and impaired ability to raise the eyebrows. Palate elevation was sluggish, although a gag reflex was present. Tongue movement was very weak. Sensory testing to light touch, pin, and vibration was normal in the face as well as the trunk and extremities. Motor testing revealed 4/5 weakness in proximal arm muscles, including deltoid, biceps, and triceps. Deep tendon reflexes were ++ in the legs and + in the arms, and the plantar responses were flexor. Coordination was normal.

Nerve conduction studies revealed low-amplitude compound muscle responses in clinically weak muscles. Sensory nerve amplitudes and distal latencies were normal, as were motor nerve conduction velocities. Repetitive stimulation of clinically weak muscles at rates of 2 Hz produced a modest decremental response (9%). Fast stimulation rates (50 Hz) produced an incremental response of up to 20%. Postexercise facilitation was noted in several muscles, producing an increase in compound muscle amplitude ranging from 40% to 90%. Needle EMG revealed frequent fibrillation potentials and positive sharp waves, and an increased number of small, polyphasic motor unit potentials.

The following tests were within normal limits: hemoglobin, hematocrit and white-cell count, urinalysis, electrolytes and liver function tests, arterial blood gas, electrocardiogram, and chest x-ray. A film of the abdomen showed marked distention of the transverse colon, but no air-fluid levels were seen. A lumbar puncture yielded clear, colorless cerebrospinal fluid under an opening pressure of 210 mM; the fluid contained 2 lymphocytes/m², and the protein was 27 mg/dl.

The patient was admitted to the medical intensive care unit. Vital capacity was 1800 ml and deteriorated over the next 10 h to 1200 ml, when the patient was electively intubated. Extremity weakness progressed to involve the legs. The patient was treated with polyvalent (BoNT/A, BoNT/B, BoNT/E) botulinal antitoxin by intravenous and intramuscular routes. The patient's serum was positive for BoNT/A, and the contaminated jar of peppers also contained BoNT/A. Following administration of antitoxin, there was no further progression of neurological deficits. Recovery was slow but steady, beginning with return of extremity strength within 2 days; extraocular movements were improved on the third day after therapy. The vital capacity reached 1300 ml 1 week after intubation, permitting extubation. Colonic activity was sluggish but resumed on the eighth hospital day. Pupillary responsiveness gradually returned, as did saliva and tear production. The patient was discharged on the 25th hospital day. She was without detectable neurological deficit two months after the onset of illness.

Comment

This case illustrates many of the classic features of botulism noted by van Ermengem in his original description, including decreased oropharyngeal secretions, external ophthalmoplegia, mydriasis, ptosis, and constipation (81). Of note is the absence of CNS dysfunction. Fever is found only if due to secondarily complicating infection. Weakness typically involves muscles innervated by the facial, glossopharyngeal, vagus, and hypoglossal nerves, followed by a descending pattern of weakness to the arms, then legs. Respiratory insufficiency may occur prior to significant extremity weakness; close monitoring of vital capacities is indicated, with early elective intubation if vital capacities fall. Clinical recovery can be prolonged and correlates with formation of new synaptic end plates (20).

Bradykinin Analogs

Tom Piek

Arg-Pro-Pro-Gly-Phe-Ser-Pro-Phe-Arg
BRADYKININ (BK)
$C_{50}H_{73}N_{15}O_{11}$

Lys-Arg-Pro-Pro-Gly-Phe-Ser-Pro-Phe-Arg
LYS-BRADYKININ (Lys-BK)
$C_{56}H_{85}N_{17}O_{12}$

Arg-Pro-Pro-Gly-Phe-Thr-Pro-Phe-Arg
THREONINE⁶-BRADYKININ (THR⁶-BK)
$C_{51}H_{75}N_{15}O_{11}$

$\begin{bmatrix} \text{Pro-Phe-Arg-Arg} \\ \text{Ser-Phe-Gly-Pro} \end{bmatrix}$ Pro
CYCLO-BRADYKININ (c-BK)
$C_{50}H_{71}N_{15}O_{10}$

$\begin{bmatrix} \text{Pro-Phe-Arg-Lys-Arg} \\ \text{Ser-Phe-Gly-Pro-Pro} \end{bmatrix}$
CYCLO-LYS-BRADYKININ (c-N$^{\alpha}$-Lys-BK)
$C_{56}H_{83}N_{17}O_{11}$

$\begin{bmatrix} \text{Pro-Phe-Arg-Arg} \\ \text{Thr-Phe-Gly-Pro} \end{bmatrix}$ Pro
CYCLO-THREONINE⁶-BRADYKININ (c-Thr⁶-BK)
$C_{51}H_{73}N_{15}O_{10}$

NEUROTOXICITY RATING

Experimental

A   Smooth muscle agonist

A   Ion channel dysfunction (presynaptic nicotinic inhibition)

Kinins, like bradykinin, are small polypeptides (MW, 1–2.5 kDa). Some are released from mammalian tissues during pathogenic disorders such as anaphylactic and hemorrhagic shock, arthritis, burns, liver cancer and cirrhosis, inflammation, migraine, pancreatitis, etc. (3). Although in the mammalian CNS the function and mode of action of bradykinin, or related kinins, is still obscure, bradykinin is considered to be a brain peptide (11). Moreover, studies on the role of kinins in the mammalian brain have demonstrated that these peptides significantly affect various aspects of behavior (1,14).

Wasp kinin, a bradykinin-like substance, is the first of several similar agents to have been isolated from the venom of social wasps (12,17). Threonine⁶-bradykinin (Thr⁶-BK) is present in the venom of a solitary wasp (15). Intraganglionic perfusion of insect ganglia with kinins induces a delayed and irreversible block of synaptic transmission (9,10), an effective mechanism to render the wasp's prey immobile.

Cyclic bradykinins also possess specific kininergic (bradykinin-like) activity in mammalian tissues. N^{α}-cyclobradykinin and N^{ε}-cyclo-Lys-bradykinin (=N^{ε}-cyclokallidin) are less potent than bradykinin in the isolated rat uterus (2). Similarly, N^{α}-cyclo-kinins are 50–300 times less active than bradykinin and 30–5000 times less potent than straight-chain analogs, in mammalian intestinal muscle preparations (6–8). Cyclic kinins studied recently include cyclo-bradykinin (6), N^{α}-cyclo-Lys-bradykinin (6), N^{ε}-cyclo-Lys-bradykinin (7), cyclo-Thr⁶-bradykinin (7), N^{ε}-(1-8 VSK1)-cyclo-N^{α}-Lys-bradykinin, N^{ε}-[(Galβ)Thr³, (Galβ)Thr⁴, 1-8 Vespulakinin 1], cyclo-N^{α}-Lys-bradykinin (6), cyclo-Vespakinin A (8), and cyclo-Vespakinin T (8). Interest in the activity of these substances relates to the development of new pesticides and drugs (16).

The bradykinin-potentiating snake venom peptide BPP$_{5a}$ (4,5), which has no properties as a kininase inhibitor (18), potentiates the effect of cyclo-N^{α}-Lys-bradykinin as it does the straight-chain analog. Moreover, 10^{-5} M of the antagonist of bradykinin: N^{α}-adamantaneacetyl-D-Arg[Hyp³, Thi⁵,⁸, D-Phe⁷] bradykinin (13), completely blocks the effects of 10 pmol Lys-bradykinin and 500 pmol N^{α}-cyclo-Lys-bradykinin, when given topically to mammalian intestinal muscle preparations mounted in a cascade. A ten-times-higher dose of agonist partially restores the effects.

Preliminary results of experiments on the action of straight and cyclic (wasp) kinins at the level of synaptic (nicotinic) transmission in the insect CNS indicate that cyclic analogs of kinins are about equiactive with their straight-chain analogs.

REFERENCES

1. Capek R (1962) Some effects of bradykinin on the central nervous system. *Biochem Pharmacol* **10**, 61.

2. Chipens GJ, Mutuli EK, Myshlyakova NV *et al* (1985) Cyclic analogues of bradykinin. *Int J Peptide Protein Res* **26**, 460.

3. Erdös EG (1966) Hypotensive peptides, bradykinin, kallidin and eledosin. *Adv Pharmcol* **4**, 1.

4. Feirreira SH (1965) A bradykinin potentiating factor (BPF) present in the venom of *Bothrops jararaca*. *Brit J Pharmacol* **24**, 163.

5. Feirreira SH, Bartelt DC, Greene LJ (1970) Isolation of bradykinin-potentiating peptides on isolated smooth muscle. *Eur J Pharmacol* **44**, 89.

6. Gobbo M, Biondi L, Filira F *et al.* (1994) Synthesis and biological activity of some linear and cyclic kinin analogues. *Int J Peptide Protein Res* **44**, 1.

7. Gobbo M, Biondi L, Filira F *et al.* (1995) Cyclic analogues of Thr⁶-bradykinin, Nᵉ-Lys-bradykinin and endo-Lys⁸ᵃ-vespulakinin 1. *Int J Peptide Protein Res* **45**, 459.

8. Gobbo M, Biondi F, Filira F *et al.* (1995) Cyclic analogues of wasp kinins from *Vespa analis* and *Vespa tropica*. *Int J Peptide Protein Res* **45**, 282.

9. Hue B, Piek T (1988) Effects of kinins and related peptides on synaptic transmission in the insect CNS. In: *Neurotox '88: Molecular Basis of Drugs and Pesticide Action*. Lunt GG ed. Elsevier, Amsterdam p. 27.

10. Hue B, Piek T (1989) Irreversible presynaptic activation-induced block of transmission in the insect CNS by hemicholinium-3 and threonine-6-bradykinin. *Comp Biochem Physiol* **93**, 87.

11. Iversen L (1983) Nonopioid neuropeptides in mammalian CNS. *Amer Rev Pharmacol Toxicol* **23**, 1.

12. Jaques R, Schachter M (1954) The presence of histamine, 5-hydroxytryptamine and a potent slow contracting substance in wasp venom. *Brit J Pharmacol* **9**, 53

13. Lammek B, Wang Y, Gravas I, Gravas H (1990) A new highly potent antagonist of bradykinins. *Peptides* **11**, 1041.

14. Moniouska-Jakonick J, Buczo W, Wiśniewski K (1986) Kallikrein effect on the acquisition and extinction of conditioned reflexes in rats. *Acta Physiol Pol* **37**, 25.

15. Piek T (1991) Neurotoxic kinins from wasp and ant venoms. *Toxicon* **29**, 139.

16. Piek T (1993) Arthropod-derived neurotoxic insecticides. A lead in pesticide science? In: *Pest Control with Enhanced Environmental Safety*. Duke SO, Menn JJ, Plimmer JR eds. American Chemical Society, Washington, DC p. 233.

17. Schachter M, Thain EM (1954) Chemical and pharmacological properties of the potent, slow contracting substance (kinin) in wasp venom. *Brit J Pharmacol* **9**, 352.

18. Ufkes JGR, Aarsen PN, Van der Meer C (1977) The mechanism of action of two bradykinin-potentiating peptides on isolated smooth muscle. *Eur J Pharmacol* **44**, 89.

Brevetoxins

Albert C. Ludolph

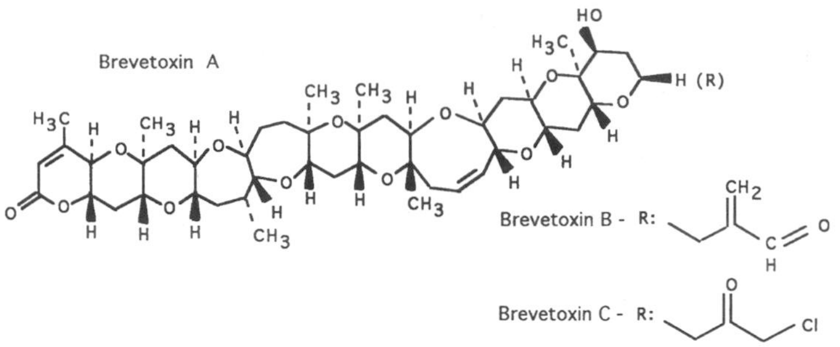

Brevetoxin A

BREVETOXIN-A
$C_{49}H_{70}O_{13}$

BREVETOXIN-B
$C_{50}H_{70}O_{14}$

BREVETOXIN-C
$C_{49}H_{69}ClO_{14}$

NEUROTOXICITY RATING

Clinical

A Ion channel syndrome (Na^+ channel)

A Ataxia

Experimental

A Ion channel dysfunction (Na^+ channel-inactivation blockade)

Brevetoxins are lipid-soluble marine poisons synthesized by the red tide dinoflagellate *Ptychodiscus brevis* (previously *Gymnodinium breve*). These cyclic polyethers and structural relatives of ciguatoxin may induce massive killings of fish and also cause neurotoxic shell fish poisoning (NSP). NSP is a nonlethal intoxication of humans and animals (3,4) prevalent around the Gulf of Mexico as an algal bloom-associated phenomenon caused by ingestion of oysters, clams and coquina. The disorder is milder than the saxitoxin-induced paralytic shellfish poisoning. Clinical signs and symptoms include the presence of gastrointestinal disturbances, a sensation of hot-cold reversal, ataxia, oral tingling, paresthesias, and numbness; the latter complaints may also involve the extremities. These phenomena usually disappear within 36 h. Methods to detect brevetoxins and other marine toxins relevant to human health have been summarized (6).

The brevetoxins have been characterized in experimental studies. The structures of ten compounds (PbTx-1–PbTx-10, previously GBTX) can be distinguished (4). They are derived from one of two structural types, PbTx-1 and PbTx-2; the latter is illustrated. Like ciguatoxin, each of these toxins specifically binds to site 5 (domain IV) of the α-subunit of the voltage-sensitive Na^+ channel; inactivation is inhibited and excitation results (10). Brevetoxins increase the amplitude of the peak Na^+ current (2) but do not change channel open time or conductance of the single channel (8).

Brevetoxins are ichthyotoxic; fish bioassays may be used to determine toxicity (5). In mice (3,5), they cause irritability, hindquarter paralysis and, finally, respiratory paralysis. In rats, PbTx-2 induces depression, ataxia, uncontrolled muscle movements, cardiac arrhythmias, respiratory depression, and reduced body temperature (9). Pharmacokinetic studies showed that after intravenous administration of PbTx-3 to the rat, 90% of the compound was cleared from the blood after 1 min (7). After 30 min, the radiolabeled compound was found in the skeletal muscle (69.5%), liver (18%), and intestine (8.0%). During the following 24 h, activity in muscle decreased but remained constant in liver and increased in intestine. PbTx-3 was eliminated *via* feces (75.1%) and urine (14.4%). Less than 1.5% of the compound was found in the brain. When PbTx-3 was applied to the guinea pig hippocampal slice, synaptic responses were depressed, likely due to reduced transmitter release after the presynaptic membrane is depolarized (1).

REFERENCES

1. Apland JP, Adler M, Sheridan RE (1993) Brevetoxin depresses synaptic transmission in guinea pig hippocampal slices. *Brain Res Bull* **31**, 201.
2. Atchison WD, Luke VS, Narahashi T, Vogel SM (1986) Nerve membrane sodium channels as the target sites of brevetoxins at neuromuscular junctions. *Brit J Pharmacol* **89**, 731.
3. Baden DG (1988) Public health problems of red tides. In: *Handbook of Natural Toxins. Vol 3. Marine Toxins and Venoms.* Tu AT ed. Marcel Dekker, New York p. 259.

4. Baden DG (1989) Brevetoxins: Unique polyether dinoflagellate toxins. *FASEB J* **3**, 1807.

5. Baden DG, Mende TJ (1982) Toxicity of two toxins from the Florida red tide dinoflagellate *Ptychodiscus brevis*. *Toxicon* **20**, 457.

6. Hokama Y (1993) Recent methods for detection of seafood toxins: Recent immunological methods for ciguatoxin and related polyethers. *Food Addit Contam* **10**, 71.

7. Poli MA, Templeton CB, Thompson WL, Hewetson JF (1990) Distribution and elimination of brevetoxin PbTx-3 in rats. *Toxicon* **28**, 903.

8. Sheridan RE, Adler M (1989) The actions of a red tide toxin from *Ptychodiscus brevis* on single sodium channels in mammalian neuroblastoma cells. *FEBS Lett* **247**, 448.

9. Templeton CB, Poli MA, LeClaire RD (1989) Cardiorespiratory effects of brevetoxin (PbTx-2) in conscious, tethered rats. *Toxicon* **27**, 1043.

10. Trainer VL, Moreau E, Guedin D *et al.* (1993) Neurotoxin binding and allosteric modulation at receptor sites 2 and 5 on purified and reconstituted rat brain sodium channels. *J Biol Chem* **268**, 17114.

Bromide

Peter C. Mabie

NEUROTOXICITY RATING

Clinical

A Acute encephalopathy (sedation, coma)

A Chronic encephalopathy (confusion, cognitive slowing)

Experimental

A GABA receptor binding

A CNS depression

Medical use of bromides began in the early nineteenth century when potassium bromide was administered as treatment for inflammation and splenomegaly (6). Since the mid-nineteenth century, the sodium, potassium, calcium, and ammonium salts of bromine have been used for a variety of neurological and mental disorders, including insomnia, chorea, *delirium tremens*, and especially epilepsy (13). Although bromide use declined following the introduction of phenobarbitol and phenytoin, there has been a resurgence of bromide use for epilepsy, primarily in children with intractible epilepsy. Bromide was a component of "patent medicines" used in treatment of insomnia and anxiety; currently, it appears in nonprescription medications such as dextromethorphan bromide plus acetaminophen, a cold remedy. The CNS is the primary site of action for bromide, and thus bromism is manifest predominantly by alterations in neurologic function, such as apathy, lethargy, confusion, weakness, ataxia and, in severe cases, coma (7). Cardiopulmonary insufficiency may occur in severe bromide toxicity.

Orally administered bromide is rapidly absorbed from the stomach and upper small intestine. Studies with rabbits suggest that at plasma concentrations of 0.5 mmol/l, the ratio of bromide in plasma to cerebrospinal fluid (CSF) is 1.30, but when the plasma bromide concentration reaches 20 mmol/l, brain, CSF, and plasma concentrations equilibrate (11). Bromide is rapidly cleared from the CSF by a saturable active transport process; oxidation to bromate may also occur (11). Bromide is primarily excreted unmetabolized in the urine. An organic bromine compound has been detected in human CSF (16,19).

The primary target of bromide is the CNS. The mechanism of action involves interaction with the anion channel of central inhibitory γ-aminobutyric acid receptors (2,4,12). Bromide also targets the kidney where it alters renal chloride excretion (18). Therapeutic doses may range up to 100 mg/kg in infants treated for severe myoclonic epilepsy, with corresponding therapeutic blood levels ranging up to 1590 mg/l (9). Toxicity has been reported with blood concentrations as low as 325 mg/l (15). Generally, toxicity occurs with blood concentrations of about 9–12 mmol/l (720–960 mg/l); however, the correlation between bromide blood levels and toxicity is unreliable (7,13). In addition to neurotoxicity, bromide causes an acneiform skin rash (bromoderma tuberosum) and gastrointestinal discomfort (7,10,13). Rarer untoward effects include necrotizing panniculitis and pancreatitis (5). There is no evidence of bromide toxicity on the peripheral nervous system.

Studies with rabbits demonstrate that a single injection of sodium bromide 3 g/kg resulted in an encephalopathy characterized by decreased responsiveness, weakness, and ataxia, progressing to coma, cardiopulmonary depression, and death (3). A case report of bromide toxicity in a dog treated with potassium bromide for refractory seizures describes progressive neurological signs, from depression to stupor, with anisocoria, apparent muscle pain, and hyporeflexia (20). Serum bromide concentration was elevated (2.7 mg/ml; therapeutic range, 1.0–2.0 mg/ml).

In humans, bromide toxicity occurs both in patients prescribed bromide as an anticonvulsant, and in individuals taking nonprescription bromide preparations (*see also* Sarin, this volume). The usual manifestations are skin rash, excessive lacrimation, gastrointestinal symptoms, and chronic encephalopathy with insidious onset of confusion and lethargy (7). The elderly appear more sensitive. In a study intended to determine the no-effect level of sodium bromide in healthy volunteers, administration of either 4 or 9 mg/kg of sodium bromide over 3 months caused α- and β-band abnormalities on electroencephalography (17). Loss of consciousness was reported in a patient who ingested cold syrup containing dextromethorphan bromide (0.4 mg/ml) plus acetaminophen daily for 4–5 years (8). Another case report describes fatigue, poor concentration, confusion, and altered speech in a patient who took a total of 60 g of bromide from nonprescription drug mixtures over a 6-week period (15).

The diagnosis of bromide toxicity should be considered in any patient with chronic or acute encephalopathy, a low anion gap, and hyperchloremia, even in the absence of known bromide exposure (1). Diagnosis is confirmed by blood bromide levels. Therapy consists of cessation of bromide intake and increasing sodium chloride intake in mild cases (14,15). Moderate cases may benefit from hydration and forced diuresis; however, severe cases should be treated with hemodialysis (8).

REFERENCES

1. Baumeister FA, Eife R (1993) Bromism or chronic bromide poisoning. *Klin Padiat* **205**, 432. [German]
2. Belhage B, Hansen GH, Schousboe A (1990) GABA agonist induced changes in ultrastructure and GABA receptor expression in cerebellar granule cells is linked to hyperpolarization of the neurons. *Int J Dev Neurosci* **8**, 473.
3. Bernoulli E (1913) Untersuchungen uber die Wirkung der Bromsalze. *Naunyn-Schmied Arch Exp Path Pharmakol* **73**, 355.
4. Catarzi D, Cecchi L, Filacchioni G *et al.* (1993) Synthesis and structure-activity relationships of 1-aminophthalazinium bromides as $GABA_A$ receptor ligands. *Drug Design Discov* **10**, 23.
5. Diener W, Kruse R, Berg P (1993) Halogen-induced panniculitis caused by potassium bromide. *Monatsschr Kinderheilk* **141**, 705. [German]
6. Garrod AB (1886) *The Essentials of Materia Medica and Therapeutics. 12th Ed* (revised and edited by N Tirard). Longmans, Green, London.
7. Goodman L, Gilman A (1941) *The Pharmacological Basis of Therapeutics. 1st Ed.* Macmillan, New York.
8. Ng YY, Lin WL, Chen TW *et al.* (1992) Spurious hyperchloremia and decreased anion gap in a patient with dextromethorphan bromide. *Amer J Nephrol* **12**, 268.
9. Oguni H, Hayashi K, Oguni M *et al.* (1994) Treatment of severe myoclonic epilepsy in infants with bromide and its borderline variant. *Epilepsia* **35**, 1140.
10. Pfeifle J, Grieben U, Bork K (1992) Bromoderma tuberosum caused by anticonvulsive treatment with potassium bromide. *Hautarzt* **43**, 792. [German]
11. Pollay M (1967) The processes affecting the distribution of bromide in blood, brain, and cerebrospinal fluid. *Exp Neurol* **17**, 74.
12. Sieghart W, Placheta P, Supavilai P, Karobath M (1981) GABA receptor associated drug receptors. In: *GABA and Benzodiazepine Receptors*. Costa E, Dichiora G, Gessa GL eds. Raven Press, New York p. 303.
13. Sourkes TL (1991) Early clinical neurochemistry of CNS-active drugs. Bromides. *Mol Chem Neuropathol* **14**, 131.
14. Steinhoff BJ, Kruse R (1992) Bromide treatment of pharmaco-resistant epilepsies with generalized tonic-clonic seizures: A clinical study. *Brain Develop* **14**, 144.
15. Steinhoff BJ, Paulus W (1992) Chronic bromide intoxication caused by bromide-containing combination drugs. *Deut Med Wochenschr* **117**, 106. [German]
16. Torri S, Mitsumori, K, Inubushi S, Yanagisawa I (1973) The REM-sleep-inducing action of a naturally occurring organic bromine compound in the encephale isolé cat. *Psychopharmacologia (Berlin)* **29**, 65.
17. van Gelderen CE, Savelkoul TJ, Blom JL *et al.* (1993) The no-effect level of sodium bromide in healthy volunteers. *Hum Exp Toxicol* **12**, 9.
18. Von Wyss H (1908) Uber das verhalten der bromsalze im menschlichen und tierischen organismus. *Naunyn-Schmied Arch Exp Path Pharmakol* **59**, 186.
19. Yanagisawa I, Yoshikawa H (1973) A bromine compound isolated from human cerebrospinal fluid. *Biochim Biophys Acta* **329**, 283.
20. Yohn SE, Morrison WB, Sharp PE (1992) Bromide toxicosis (bromism) in a dog treated with potassium bromide for refractory seizures. *J Amer Vet Med Assn* **201**, 468.

Bromocriptine

John D. Rogers

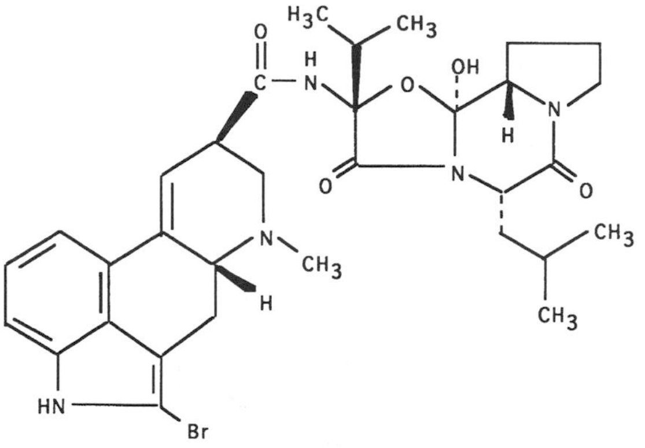

BROMOCRIPTINE
$C_{32}H_{40}BrN_5O_5$

(5'α)-2-Bromo-12'-hydroxy-2'-(1-methylethyl)-5'-
(2-methylpropyl)ergotaman-3',6',18-trione)

NEUROTOXICOLOGY RATING

Clinical

B   Acute encephalopathy (headache, confusion, hallucination)

Bromocriptine, a derivative of the ergotoxin group of ergot alkaloids, acts at the dopamine D_2 receptor and is a partial dopamine antagonist at the D_1 receptor, with weak antagonist properties at tryptaminergic and at α-adrenergic receptors (3). Bromocriptine is employed as an adjuvant to L-dopa for the treatment of parkinsonism (2,7) and may have neuroprotective effects (6,9,11). It inhibits prolactin secretion and is used in the treatment of prolactin-secreting pituitary tumors (4,5) and lactation suppression postpartum (the U.S. Food and Drug Administration has withdrawn its approval for this purpose due to reports of increased cardiovascular and cerebrovascular events) (8).

Bromocriptine toxicity usually appears when given in conjunction with L-dopa for the treatment of Parkinson's disease. Side effects, which can also occur when used independently, include orthostatic hypotension, confusion, hallucinations, headache, and nausea. As an ergot, it may also induce pleuropulmonary and retroperitoneal fibrosis, erythromyalgia, and peripheral vasospasm (1,3,7).

Chronic administration of bromocriptine has been reported to alter concentrations of essential metals in the guinea pig caudate, frontal cortex, and cerebellar hemisphere; specifically, there was a reduction of copper and increased manganese (10).

Bromocriptine is reported to suppress the action of free radicals and thereby protect against glutamate neurotoxicity in cultured rat mesencephalic neurons (9). Bromocriptine blocked behavioral dysfunction and depletion of glutathione and dopamine in mice treated with 1-methyl-4-phenyl-1,2,3,6-tetrahydropyridine (6).

REFERENCES

1. Boyd A (1995) Bromocriptine and psychosis: A literature review. *Psychiat Quart* 66, 87.
2. Duvoisin RC, Mendoza MM, Yahr MD (1980) A comparative study of bromocriptine and levodopa in Parkinson's disease. *Adv Biochem Psychopharmacol* 23, 271.
3. Giron-Forest DA, Schonleber WD (1979) Bromocriptine. In: *Analytical Profiles of Drug Substances. Vol 8.* Florey K ed. Academic Press, New York p. 47.
4. Klibanski A, Zervas NT (1991) Diagnosis and management of hormone secreting pituitary adenomas. *N Engl J Med* 324, 822.
5. Melmed S (1990) Acromegaly. *N Engl J Med* 322, 966.
6. Muralikrishnan D, Mohanakumar KP (1998) Neuroprotection by bromocriptine against 1-methyl-4-phenyl-1,2,3,6-tetrahydropyridine-induced neurotoxicity in mice. *FASEB J* 12, 905.
7. Pezzoli G, Martignoni E, Paschetti C *et al.* (1995) A crossover, controlled study comparing pergolide with bromocriptine as an adjunct to levodopa for the treatment of Parkinson's disease. *Neurology* 45, S22.
8. Rayburn WF (1996) Clinical commentary: Bromocriptine (Parlodel) controversy and recommendations for lactation suppression. *Amer J Perinatol* 13, 69.
9. Sawada H, Ibi M, Kihara T, Urushitani M *et al.* (1998) Dopamine D2-type agonists protect mesencephalic neurons from glutamate neurotoxicity: mechanisms of neuroprotective treatment against oxidative stress. *Ann Neurol* 44, 110.
10. Weiner WJ, Nausieda PA, Klawans HL (1978) The effects of levodopa, lergotrile, and bromocriptine on brain iron, manganese and copper. *Neurology* 28, 734.
11. Yamashita H, Kawakami H, Zhang YX (1995) Neuroprotective mechanism of bromocriptine. *Lancet* 346, 1305.

p-Bromophenylacetylurea

Richard M. LoPachin
Ellen J. Lehning

BROMOPHENYLACETYLUREA
$C_9H_9BrN_2O_2$

NEUROTOXICITY RATING

Experimental

A   Peripheral neuropathy

p-Bromophenylacetylurea (BPAU) is a brominated congener of the antiepileptic drug phenylacetylurea. Animal studies demonstrated the neurotoxic potential of BPAU (5,8) which, consequently, excluded potential clinical application of this compound. BPAU is of experimental neurotoxicological interest because of its ability to produce classic, delayed-onset central-peripheral distal axonopathy (2,6,16).

BPAU is a white crystalline powder (MW, 279.09; MP, 237°C) with limited solubility in aqueous and most organic solvents. Because of this insolubility, most animal studies have used dimethyl sulfoxide (DMSO) as a vehicle for BPAU administration. However, there is behavioral evidence suggesting that DMSO might produce neurotoxic effects that interact with the expression of BPAU toxicity (9).

The pharmacokinetic characteristics of BPAU have not been well characterized. Rats are the most sensitive to BPAU, whereas rabbits, guinea pigs, and chickens do not respond to the compound (6). Although gender does not affect the expression of functional deficits, young rats (3 weeks postpartum) appear to be less sensitive than adults (9–10 weeks postpartum) to the neurotoxic actions of BPAU (7). For induction of neuropathy in rats, BPAU has been administered by either gastric intubation (6) or intraperitoneal (i.p.) injection (10). Effective doses for both routes of administration range from 50–400 mg/kg in DMSO. Behavioral signs of neurotoxicity (*e.g.*, hindlimb weakness, gait abnormalities) and neuropathic structural correlates (*e.g.*, swollen axons) following a single oral or i.p. exposure develop after a dose-dependent "silent" period (6,10). Compromised liver function, either from partial hepatectomy or carbon tetrachloride intoxication, enhances the magnitude of BPAU neurotoxicity in rats (7). This suggests that BPAU is detoxified by the liver and the parent compound, rather than a liver metabolite, mediates induction of nerve injury. Studies of structure–activity relationships show that small changes in BPAU structure (*e.g.*, io-dine substitution) produce a significant loss of toxic potency (3,14).

Rats intoxicated with orally administered BPAU (50–400 mg/kg) develop delayed-onset body weight loss and hindlimb skeletal muscle weakness that, at higher doses, eventually involves the forelimbs (6–8). Morphological examination reveals distal axon degeneration in posterior tibial nerve and dorsal spinal cord columns. Dorsal root ganglion (DRG) and anterior horn cells exhibit only minimal neuropathic changes. The absence of a neuron perikaryal effect was also observed in a morphometric study which showed that BPAU intoxication (200–400 mg/kg, i.p.) did not alter the number or size distribution of DRG nerve cell bodies (16). However, distal sural nerve exhibited significant fiber loss and an increase in the frequency of axons undergoing wallerian degeneration, while proximal sural nerve showed comparable but less extensive effects. Similar distal changes were noted in the phrenic nerve of rats treated with BPAU (400 mg/kg, i.p.) (21). These findings clearly delineate the distal nature of BPAU-induced axonal lesions. Prior to axon degeneration, tubulovesicular profiles (presumably derived from smooth endoplasmic reticulum) accumulate in focal swellings (1,16,18,21). The behavioral and morpho-logical effects of BPAU are qualitatively similar when animals are treated on either an acute (400 mg/kg i.p., single injection) or chronic (10 mg/kg/day × 2–7 months, i.p.) dosing schedule (21). During recovery from either acute or chronic BPAU intoxication, regenerating axonal sprouts in phrenic nerve contained tubulomembranous structures that were interpreted as reflecting a persistent toxic effect (21). Although the foregoing indicates that nonterminal regions of distal fibers are affected in BPAU treatment, other evidence suggests that axonal terminals are impacted. In the early stages of BPAU intoxication, preterminal regions of distal axons were spared, whereas evoked muscle action potentials displayed a marked reduction in amplitude (11). Direct skeletal muscle toxicity did not appear to be involved and, therefore, it was concluded that nerve terminal function was compromised by BPAU treatment.

The mechanism underlying BPAU-induced distal axonopathy remains to be determined. An early study demonstrated reduced radiolabeled amino acid incorporation (^{14}C-glycine) into rat DRG proteins during the onset of BPAU neurotoxicity (5). However, the mechanistic significance of this finding is unclear. Moreover, although it has been suggested that defective neuronal energy metabolism might be responsible for distal axonopathies induced by certain chemical neurotoxicants (20), several lines of evidence suggest that such a mechanism is not involved in BPAU neuropathy (4,12). It has been consistently demonstrated that BPAU treatment impairs turnaround processing of fast-transported proteins in distal portions of sensory and motor neurons (10,13,14). Turnaround processing in nerve terminals initiates the return of axonally transported proteins to the cell body *via* retrograde movement. The effect of BPAU on turnaround is (a) specific, since it can be demonstrated before the onset of neurological dysfunction and (b) selective, since the effect is not a generalized impairment of axonal transport (*i.e.*, slow anterograde transport in rat motor neuron does not appear to be a significant event) (13,15). In addition to an effect on turnaround, BPAU is associated with an abnormality in the onset of fast anterograde axonal transport; in peripheral sensory nerves, the entry of proteins into the axon is delayed (13), whereas in motor neurons, a premature onset of fast anterograde transport is observed (17). The composition of retrogradely transported axonal proteins in peripheral nerve was altered during the later stages of BPAU intoxication; three proteins were missing (42, 41, and 25 kDa), while four other proteins were more prominent (63, 56, 50, and 26 kDa) relative those in controls (17). It was suggested that these compositional changes might reflect abnormal posttranslational modifications or proteolysis of transported proteins in terminal or preterminal regions of affected axons. Considered together, these data suggest that the mechanism of BPAU axonopathy involves defective axonal transport, which might be a product of dysfunctional cell body processing of material (17), perturbed posttranslational modification of transported proteins (19), and/or a deficient turnaround mechanism (14).

REFERENCES

1. Bacci B, Cochran E, Nunzi MG *et al.* (1994) Amyloid *β* precursor and ubiquitin epitopes in human and experimental dystrophic axons. *Amer J Pathol* **144**, 702.
2. Blakemore WF, Cavanagh JB (1969) "Neuroaxonal dystrophy" occurring in an experimental "dying back" process in the rat. *Brain* **92**, 789.
3. Brimijoin S, Carlson G, Nguyen NN, Jakobsen J (1982) Analogs of *p*-bromophenyl-acetylurea: A structure-activity study of their neurotoxicity in rats. *Muscle Nerve* **5**, S122.
4. Brimijoin S, Mintz KP (1984) Unimpaired energy metabolism in experimental neuropathy induced by *p*-bromophenylacetylurea. *Muscle Nerve* **7**, 725.
5. Cavanagh JB, Chen FCK (1971) Amino acid incorporation in protein during the "silent phase" before organomercury and *p*-bromophenylacetylurea neuropathy in the rat. *Acta Neuropathol* **19**, 216.
6. Cavanagh JB, Chen FCK, Kyu MH, Ridley A (1968) The experimental neuropathy in rats caused by *p*-bromophenylacetylurea. *J Neurol Neurosurg Psychiat* **31**, 471.
7. Chen FCK, Cavanagh JB (1971) Factors affecting neurotoxicity by *p*-bromophenylacetylurea in rats. *Brit J Exp Pathol* **52**, 315.
8. Diezel PB, Quadbeck G (1960) Nervenschädigung durch *p*-bromophenylacetyl-Harnstoff. *Naunyn-Schmied Arch Exp Pathol Pharmakol* **238**, 534.
9. Fossom LH, Messing RB, Sparber SB (1985) Long lasting behavioral effects of dimethyl sulfoxide and the peripheral toxicant *p*-bromophenylacetylurea. *Neurotoxicology* **6**, 17.
10. Jakobsen J, Brimijoin S (1981) Axonal transport of enzymes and labeled proteins in experimental axonopathy induced by *p*-bromophenylacetylurea. *Brain Res* **229**, 103.
11. Jakobsen J, Lambert G, Carlson G, Brimijoin S (1982) Clinical and electrophysiological characteristics of the experimental neuropathy caused by *p*-bromophenylacetylurea. *Exp Neurol* **75**, 158.
12. LoPachin RM, Moore RW, Menahan LA, Peterson RE (1984) Glucose-dependent lactate production by homogenates of neuronal tissues prepared from rats treated with 2,4-dithiobiuret, acrylamide, *p*-bromophenylacetylurea and 2,5-hexanedione. *Neurotoxicology* **5**, 25.
13. Nagata H, Brimijoin S (1986) Axonal transport in the motor neurons of rats with neuropathy induced by *p*-bromophenylacetylurea. *Ann Neurol* **19**, 458.
14. Nagata H, Brimijoin S (1986) Neurotoxicity of halogenated phenylacetylureas is linked to abnormal onset of rapid transport. *Brain Res* **385**, 136.
15. Nagata H, Brimijoin S, Schmelzer JD (1987) Slow axonal transport in experimental hypoxia and in neuropathy induced by *p*-bromophenylacetylurea. *Brain Res* **422**, 319.
16. Ohnishi A, Ikeda M (1980) Morphometric evaluation of primary sensory neurons in experimental *p*-bromophenylacetylurea. *Acta Neuropathol* **52**, 111.
17. Oka N, Brimijoin S (1990) Premature onset of fast axonal transport in bromophenylacetylurea neuropathy: An electrophoretic analysis of proteins exported into motor nerve. *Brain Res* **509**, 107.
18. Oka N, Brimijoin S (1992) Tubulomembranous lesions in *p*-bromophenylacetylurea neuropathy reflect local stasis of fast axonal transport: Evidence from electron microscopic autoradiography. *Mayo Clin Proc* **67**, 341.
19. Oka N, Brimijoin S (1993) Altered spectrum of retrogradely transported axonal proteins in *p*-bromophenylacetylurea neuropathy. *Neurochem Res* **18**, 675.
20. Spencer PS, Sabri MI, Schaumburg HH, Moore C (1979) Does a defect in energy metabolism in the nerve fiber cause axonal degeneration in polyneuropathies? *Ann Neurol* **5**, 501.
21. Troncoso JC, Griffin JW, Price DL, Hess-Kozlow KM (1982) Pathology of the peripheral neuropathy induced by *p*-bromophenylacetylurea. *Lab Invest* **46**, 215.

p-Bromophenylisothiocyanate

John L. O'Donoghue

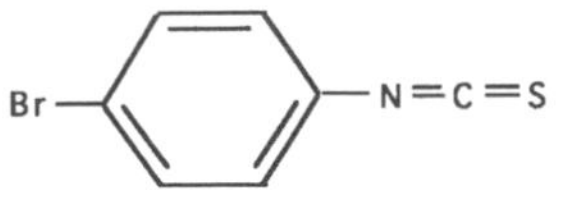

p-BROMOPHENYLISOTHIOCYANATE
C_7H_4BrNS

4-Bromophenylisothiocyanate; 1-Bromo-
4-*iso*thiocyanatobenzene; Bromobenzene-
4-*iso*thiocyanatobenzene

NEUROTOXICITY RATING

Experimental

A   Spinal cord degeneration

p-Bromophenyl*iso*thiocyanate has been used to treat dermatomycoses and studied for use as a veterinary anthelmintic. Experimental administration of single oral doses of 150 or 200 mg/kg to 8-week-old unweaned lambs resulted in ataxia and paraplegia after a 2-week delay (2). The lumbar spinal cord showed the most severe lesions, which included swollen, degenerating axons, degenerating myelin sheaths, and degeneration and lysis of neurons. Weaned lambs, rabbits, cats, and dogs given 200 mg/kg and rats and hens given 400 mg/kg did not develop neurotoxicity. The lack of neurotoxicity in weaned lambs may be due to dilution of the test material by the rumen contents or detoxication of the test substance by rumen microorganisms (1,2).

REFERENCES

1. Cavanagh JB (1969) Toxic substances and the nervous system. *Brit Med Bull* **25**, 268
2. Lessel B, Towlerton RG (1967) Neurotoxicity of *p*-bromophenyl isothiocyanate. *Food Cosmet Toxicol* **5**, 741.

Buspirone

Herbert H. Schaumburg

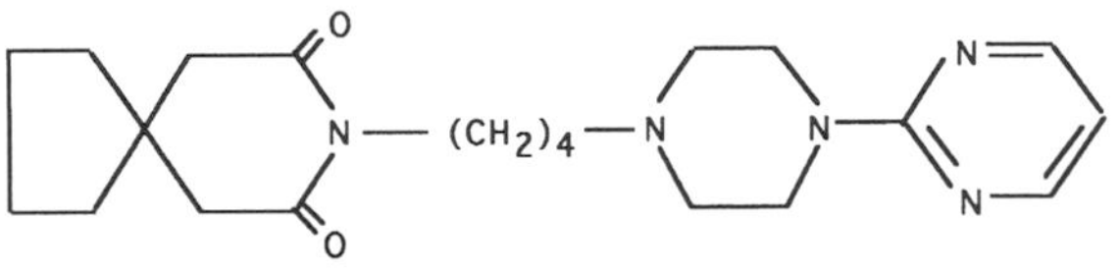

BUSPIRONE
$C_{21}H_{31}N_5O_2$

8-[4-[4-(2-Pyrimidinyl)-1-piperazinyl]butyl]-
8-azaspiro[4.5]decane-7,9-dione

NEUROTOXICITY RATING

Clinical

B   Extrapyramidal syndrome (dyskinesias, dystonia)

Experimental

A   Dopaminergic receptor blockade

Buspirone, an azaspirodecanedione compound, is the prototype of a class of anxiolytic agents, the azaspirones. The azaspirones display moderate anxiolytic potential with a lesser degree of two major undesired side effects associated with benzodiazepine therapy, sedation and fatigue, and are not susceptible to dependency or abuse (7). Because these side effects are mild and well tolerated, buspirone is primarily used for chronic anxiety states (generalized anxiety disorder) that require long-term maintenance therapy; it has no anticonvulsant or muscle relaxant activity. The anxiolytic effects of azaspirones are widely held to stem primarily from suppression of 5-hydroxytryptaminergic activity, especially in the raphe nuclei (8). They also both mildly enhance and antagonize dopaminergic activity, probably reflecting a moderate affinity for dopamine D_2 receptors (1). The azaspirones, in contrast to the benzodiazepines, have no effect on γ-aminobutyric acid (GABA)-ergic cells.

Buspirone therapy is associated with few systemic side effects. The coadministration of monoamine oxidase inhibitors is contraindicated because "hypertensive crisis" may occur, as is the coadministration of haloperidol because of the development of unstable serum levels of haloperidol.

Mild generalized neurological side effects are occasionally associated with buspirone; they include dizziness, dream disturbances, insomnia, and lightheadedness. Rare, isolated reports of extrapyramidal reactions probably reflect the dopaminergic action of this class of agents; there are case descriptions of transient, reversible akathisia (4), orofacial dyskinesia (6), and dystonia (7). There is one report of persistent dystonia (2) and one of acute myoclonus (5). Instances have occurred at variable intervals during treatment at conventional dosages of 5–10 mg *q.i.d.* Buspirone overdose resulted in generalized seizures in one case (3). Tardive dyskinesia is not a feature of buspirone therapy.

REFERENCES
1. Alford C, Bhatti JZ, Curran S *et al.* (1991) Pharmacodynamic effects of buspirone and clobazam. *Brit J Clin Pharmacol* **32**, 91.
2. Boylan K (1990) Persistent dystonia associated with buspirone. *Neurology* **49**, 1904.
3. Catalano G, Catalano MC, Hanley PF (1998) Seizures associated with buspirone overdose: case report and literature review. *Clin Neuropharmacol* **21**, 647.
4. Patterson JF (1988) Akathisia associated with buspirone. *J Clin Psychopharmacol* **8**, 296.
5. Ritchie EC, Bridenbaugh RH, Jabbari B (1988) Acute generalized myoclonus following buspirone administration. *J Clin Psychiat* **49**, 242.
6. Strauss A (1988) Oral dyskinesia associated with buspirone use in an elderly woman. *J Clin Psychiat* **49**, 322.
7. Taylor DP, Moon SL (1991) Buspirone and related compounds as alternative anxiolytics. *Neuropeptides* **19**, 15.
8. Tunnicliff G (1991) Molecular basis of buspirone's anxiolytic action. *Pharmacol Toxicol* **69**, 149.

2-Butenenitrile

Kevin M. Crofton
Mary Beth Genter

$$CH_2 = C(CH_3)C \equiv N$$

2-BUTENENITRILE
C_4H_5N

2-Methyl-2-propenenitrile; α-Methylacrylonitrile

NEUROTOXICITY RATING
Experimental

A   Ototoxicity (ataxia)
B   Ototoxicity (hearing loss)

2-Butenenitrile (2-BN) is an unsaturated short-chain aliphatic nitrile that has been used as a comonomer with unsaturated esters and as a plasticizer for synthetic resins (17). Production quantities and potential for human exposure are unknown. No workplace standards, drinking water standards, or reference concentrations have been established for 2-BN (1,19).

2-BN is excreted rapidly, with complete excretion of a single dose occurring within 24 h (20). Two major pathways are believed to be important in the metabolism of 2-BN. The predominant pathway, accounting for approximately 90% of the urinary metabolites of 2-BN, involves direct, nonenzymatic conjugation of 2-BN with glutathione (*i.e.*, Michael addition) producing a cyanomercapturic acid. The other major metabolic pathway is mediated by cytochrome P-450 oxidation, producing an epoxide intermediate. Subsequent conjugation results in the excretion of a hydroxymercapturic metabolite (20). *In-vitro* studies reveal that glutathione enhances cyanide release, perhaps by shunting more of the parent compound *via* the P-450 metabolism pathway (4). In the environment, 2-BN also serves as a substrate for aliphatic nitrilase from *Rhodococcus rhodochrous* K22; this enzyme catalyzes the cleavage of nitriles to the corresponding acid and ammonia (8).

Little neurotoxicity testing has been performed on 2-BN. The LD_{50} in rats is 50–80 mg/kg subcutaneously and, in mice, 200 mg/kg intraperitoneally (i.p.), with equivalent oral dosages in the 200 to 500 mg/kg range for both species (11–13).

Treatment of rats and mice with 2-BN induces circling, hyperactivity, head bobbing, and retropulsion (14–16), a syndrome comparable to that seen after exposure to β,β'-iminodipropionitrile (*see* 3,18). While changes in CNS catecholamines may occur (14,16), the syndrome probably results from damage to vestibular sensory epithelia (10). Both 2-BN and β,β'-iminodipropionitrile destroy vestibular hair cells in all areas of the vestibular apparatus, with a gradient of effects in the crista, utricle, and saccule (9,10). Destruction of the vestibular apparatus, *via* either physical or chemical trauma, results in a similar syndrome of toxicity in rats (*see* 7,10). Evidence that 2-BN is an ototoxicant comes from a study in which animals received three daily i.p. exposures of 75–125 mg/kg (6). This dose regimen caused a complete, persistent, broad-band loss of auditory function. The characteristics of this hearing loss—rapid onset, broad-band, persistent—are similar to that seen after β,β'-iminodipropionitrile exposure (2) and suggest that hair cells in the cochlea may be damaged in addition to destruction of vestibular hair cells.

Several other toxicological end points have been investigated with respect to 2-BN. Very high doses of 2-BN were associated with enlarged thyroid, loss of colloid, desquamation, and necrosis of follicular epithelium, as well as adrenal necrosis and duodenal ulcers (13). Olfactory mucosal damage was not noted following i.p. exposure to 2-BN, in contrast to the results of other aliphatic nitriles (*e.g.*, 2-pentenenitrile; *see* 5,6).

There is no information on human exposures to 2-BN.

REFERENCES

1. American Conference of Governmental Industrial Hygienists (1994) Threshold Limit Values, Cincinnati, Ohio.

2. Crofton KM, Janssen R, Prazma G *et al.* (1994) The ototoxicity of β,β'-iminodipropionitrile: Functional and morphological evidence of cochlear dysfunction. *Hear Res* **80**, 129.

3. Delay J, Pichot P, Thuillier J, Marquiset J-P (1952) Action de l'amino-dipropionitrile sur le comportement moteur de la souris blanche. *C R Soc Biol* **146**, 37.

4. Farooqui MYH, Massa E (1991) Effect of glutathione on *in vitro* metabolism of unsaturated aliphatic nitriles to cyanide. *Bull Environ Contam Toxicol* **46**, 431.

5. Genter MB, Llorens J, O'Callaghan JP *et al.* (1992) Olfactory toxicity of β,β'-iminodipropionitrile in the rat. *J Pharmacol Exp Ther* **263**, 1432.

6. Genter MB, Zhao X, Crofton KM (1995) Structure-activity studies on the audio-vestibular and olfactory toxicity of nitriles. *Toxicologist* **15**, 22.

7. Hunt MA, Miller SW, Neilson HC, Horn KM (1987) Intratympanic injection of sodium arsanilate (Atoxyl) solution results in postural changes consistent with changes described for labyrinthectomized rats. *Behav Neurosci* **101**, 427.

8. Kobayashi M, Yanaka N, Nagasawa T, Yamada H (1992) Primary structure of an aliphatic nitrile-degrading enzyme, aliphatic nitrilase, from *Rhodococcus rhodochrous* K22 and expression of its gene and identification of its active site residue. *Biochemistry* **31**, 9000.

9. Llorens J, Demênes D (1994) Hair cell degeneration resulting from β,β'-iminodipropionitrile toxicity in the rat vestibular epithelia. *Hear Res* **76**, 78.

10. Llorens J, Demênes D, Sans A (1993) The behavioral syndrome caused by β,β'-iminodipropionitrile and related nitriles in the rat is associated with degeneration of the vestibular sensory hair cells. *Toxicol Appl Pharmacol* **123**, 199.

11. Kodak (1992) Toxic Substances Control Act 8th Submission to the U.S. Environmental Protection Agency (8EHQ-0892-6532), August 11, 1992.

12. NIOSH (1995) Registry of Toxic Effects of Chemical Substances. U.S. National Institute for Occupational Safety and Health, Cincinnati, Ohio.

13. Szabo S, Larsen PR, Kovacs K *et al.* (1977) Thyroid necrosis produced by pyrazole and certain alkenes: Ultrastructural and functional studies. *Amer J Pathol* **86**, 83A.

14. Tanii H, Hayshi M, Hashimoto K (1989) Nitrile-induced behavioral abnormalities in mice. *Neurotoxicology* **10**, 157.

15. Tanii H, Hayshi M, Hashimoto K (1990) Effects of neurotropic agents with a selectivity for alpha-adrenoreceptors on nitrile-induced dyskinetic syndrome in mice. *Pharmacol Biochem Behav* **36**, 317.

16. Tanii H, Hayshi M, Hashimoto K (1991) Behavioral syndrome induced by allylnitrile, crotononitrile or 2-pentenenitrile in rats. *Neuropharmacology* **30**, 877.

17. Thompson AR (1972) Organic nitrogen compounds. In: *Chemical Technology: An Encyclopedic Treatment.* Codd LW, Dijkoff K, Fearon JH *et al.* eds. Barnes & Noble, New York p. 532.

18. Thuillier J, Burger A (1954) Contribution à l'étude du syndrome moteur provoque chez la souris par l'amino-dipropionitrile (souris tournantes). *Experientia* **10**, 223.

19. US EPA (1995) *Drinking Water Regulations and Health Advisories.* Office of Water, U.S. Environmental Protection Agency, Washington, DC.

20. van Bladeren PJ, Delbressome LPC, Hoogeterp JJ *et al.* (1981) Formation of mercapturic acids from acrylonitrile, crotononitrile, and cinnamonitrile by direct conjugation and via an intermediate oxidation process. *Drug Metab Disposition* **9**, 246.

3-Butenenitrile

Kevin M. Crofton
Mary Beth Genter

$$CH_2 = CH - CH_2 - CN$$

3-BUTENENITRILE
C_4H_5N

Allylnitrile; Allyl cyanide

NEUROTOXICITY RATING

Experimental

A Ototoxicity (ataxia, hearing loss)

B Pontine degeneration—mulitfocal

B Autonomic peripheral neuropathy

3-Butenenitrile (3-BN) is found naturally in some mustard oils and has been produced commercially (6). The substance is also released by enzymatic decomposition of sinigrin in soil (3). Production quantities and potential for human exposure are unknown. No American workplace standards, drinking water standards, or reference concentrations have been established for 3-BN (2,25). There is a Russian Occupational Exposure Limit of 0.3 mg/m^3 (15).

3-BN is extensively absorbed through the gastrointestinal tract and distributed to all tissues examined, including liver, kidney, brain, heart, and lungs (6). The major route of excretion of 3-BN is *via* the urine and exhaled CO_2; 81% of an administered dose was eliminated 10 days following treatment, with the peak for excretion *via* CO_2 occurring between 0 and 3 h, and the peak of urinary excretion occurring between 6 h and 24 h after dosing (6).

Lethality associated with 3-BN exposure appears to result from cyanide release. Pretreatment of mice with the hepatotoxic agent carbon tetrachloride improved the survival of mice subsequently treated with 3-BN (18), presumably because of the destruction of microsomal xenobiotic-metabolizing enzymes that cause the generation of cyanide. Microsomal metabolism of 3-BN requires NADPH and O_2, suggesting metabolism by cytochrome P-450 enzymes (7). Enzymatic release of cyanide in liver microsomal preparations is increased when microsomes are prepared from phenobarbital-pretreated rats (7), is decreased when microsomes are prepared from rats pretreated with carbon tetrachloxide (19), and is decreased in the presence of either cytochrome P-450 inhibitors (*i.e.*, cobaltous chloride or SKF525) or epoxide hydrolase inhibitors. These observations suggest that P-450–mediated cyanide release may proceed through an epoxide intermediate (7). Glutathione (GSH) and other sulfhydryl compounds enhance the rate of cyanide release from 3-BN, and tissue GSH levels decrease following 3-BN exposure (1).

There is a paucity of information on the toxic effects of short-term exposure to 3-BN. In mice, an LD$_{50}$ of 67 mg/kg was estimated for intraperitoneal administration of 3-BN (19). An LD$_{50}$ of 115 mg/kg was calculated for oral exposure in rats (15).

In both mice and rats, acute 3-BN exposure results in signs of neurotoxicity, including circling, hyperactivity, head bobbing, and retropulsion (20–23). This syndrome is similar to that seen with β,β'-iminodipropionitrile (5,24) and possibly results in part from changes in CNS catecholamines (20–23). However, recent work with β,β'-iminodipropionitrile and 2-butenenitrile indicates that the 3-BN–induced behavioral syndrome results from vestibular damage (*see* 12,13). Both 2-butenenitrile and β,β'-iminodipropionitrile caused a loss of vestibular hair cells in all areas of the vestibular apparatus, with a gradient of greater effects in the crista, utricle, and saccule (12,13). Destruction of the vestibular apparatus, *via* either physical or chemical trauma, produced a syndrome of toxicity very similar to that seen after exposure to β,β'-iminodipropionitrile, 2-pentenenitrile, and 2-BN and 3-BN (*see* 10,13). Evidence that 3-BN is ototoxic comes from a study in which animals received three daily intraperitoneal doses of 75–125 mg/kg (9). This regimen caused a complete, persistent, broad-band (frequency-independent) loss of auditory function. The characteristics of 3-BN neurotoxicity—vestibular dysfunction and a broad-band persistent hearing loss with rapid onset—are very similar to that seen after exposure to other aliphatic nitriles (4,13) and suggest that 3-BN may damage hair cells in the cochlea and vestibular apparatus. In contrast to the results of other aliphatic nitriles (*e.g.*, 2-pentenenitrile, β,β'-iminodipropionitrile), olfactory mucosal damage was not noted following intraperitoneal exposure to 3-BN (8). Acute 3-BN exposure in mice pretreated with carbon tetrachloride revealed histopathological changes (*i.e.*, neuronal degeneration and demyelination) in the pons and midbrain (22). No other reports of CNS neurotoxicity have involved 3-BN. It is also interesting to note a report of urine retention in 3-BN–treated rats (6). This suggests that 3-BN may cause peripheral nerve damage in the bladder similar to that seen after exposure to dimethylaminopropionitrile (11,14,16).

The only longer-term exposure study with 3-BN involved inhalation exposure of pregnant rats for 6 h/day from gestational day 6–20 (17). This study revealed that 3-BN is teratogenic, causing significant increases in gastroschisis and unossified and split sternebrae in rats. These effects occurred with 50 ppm 3-BN, a concentration that was not associated with maternal toxicity (17).

There is no information on human exposures to 3-BN.

REFERENCES

1. Amed AE, Farooqui MYH (1982) Comparative toxicities of aliphatic nitriles. *Toxicol Lett* **12**, 157.
2. American Conference of Governmental Industrial Hygienists (1994) Threshold Limit Values, Cincinnati, Ohio.
3. Borek V, Morra MJ, Brown PD, McCaffrey JP (1994) Allelochemicals produced during sinigrin decomposition in soil. *J Agr Food Chem* **42**, 1030.
4. Crofton KM, Janssen R, Prazma G *et al.* (1994) The ototoxicity of β,β′-iminodipropionitrile: Functional and morphological evidence of cochlear dysfunction. *Hear Res* **80**, 129.
5. Delay J, Pichot P, Thuillier J, Marquiset J-P (1952) Action de l'amino-dipropionitrile sur le comportement moteur de la souris blanche. *C R Soc Biol* **146**, 37.
6. Farooqui MYH, Ybarra B, Piper J (1993) Toxicokinetics of allylnitrile in rats. *Drug Metab Disposition* **21**, 460.
7. Farooqui MYH, Ybarra B, Piper J (1993) Metabolism of allylnitrile to cyanide: *In vitro* studies. *Res Commun Chem Pathol Pharmacol* **81**, 355.
8. Genter MB, Llorens J, O'Callaghan JP *et al.* (1992) Olfactory toxicity of β,β′-iminodipropionitrile in the rat. *J Pharmacol Exp Ther* **263**, 1432.
9. Genter MB, Zhao X, Crofton KM (1995) Structure-activity studies on the audio-vestibular and olfactory toxicity of nitriles. *Toxicologist* **15**, 22.
10. Hunt MA, Miller SW, Neilson HC, Horn KM (1987) Intratympanic injection of sodium arsanilate (Atoxyl) solution results in postural changes consistent with changes described for labyrinthectomized rats. *Behav Neurosci* **101**, 427.
11. Jaeger RJ, Plugge H, Szabo S (1980) Acute urinary bladder toxicity of a polyurethane foam catalyst mixture: A possible new target organ for a propionitrile derivative. *J Environ Pathol Toxicol* **4**, 559.
12. Llorens J, Demênes D (1994) Hair cell degeneration resulting from β,β′-iminodipropionitrile toxicity in the rat vestibular epithelia. *Hear Res* **76**, 78.
13. Llorens J, Demênes D, Sans A (1993) The behavioral syndrome caused by β,β′-iminodipropionitrile and related ni-triles in the rat is associated with degeneration of the vestibular sensory hair cells. *Toxicol Appl Pharmacol* **123**, 199.
14. Mumtaz MM, Farooqui MYH, Ghanayem BI *et al.* (1991) Studies on the mechanism of urotoxic effects of *N,N′*-dimethylaminopropionitrile in rats and mice I. Biochemical and morphological characterization of the injury and its relationship to metabolism. *J Toxicol Environ Health* **33**, 1.
15. NIOSH (1995) Registry of Toxic Effects of Chemical Substances, U.S. National Institute for Occupational Safety and Health, Cincinnati, Ohio.
16. Pestronk A, Koegh JP, Griffin JW (1980) Dimethylaminopropionitrile. In: *Experimental and Clinical Neurotoxicology.* Spencer PS, Schaumburg HH eds. Williams and Wilkins, Baltimore p. 430.
17. Saillenfait AM, Bonnet P, Guenier JP *et al.* (1993) Relative developmental toxicities of inhaled aliphatic mononitriles in rats. *Fund Appl Toxicol* **20**, 365.
18. Tanii H, Hashimoto K (1984) Structure-activity relationship of aliphatic nitriles. *Toxicol Lett* **22**, 267.
19. Tanii H, Hashimoto K (1984) Studies on the mechanism of acute toxicity of nitriles in mice. *Arch Toxicol* **55**, 47.
20. Tanii H, Hayshi M, Hashimoto K (1990) Effects of neurotropic agents with a selectivity for alpha-adrenoreceptors on nitrile-induced dyskinetic syndrome in mice. *Pharmacol Biochem Behav* **36**, 317.
21. Tanii H, Hayshi M, Hashimoto K (1991) Behavioral syndrome induced by allylnitrile, crotononitrile or 2-pentenenitrile in rats. *Neuropharmacology* **30**, 877.
22. Tanii H, Kurosaka Y, Hayshi M, Hashimoto K (1989) Allylnitrile: A compound which induces long-term dyskinesia in mice following a single administration. *Exp Neurol* **103**, 64.
23. Tanii H, Okayama A, Yamatodani A *et al.* (1991) Alterations in the metabolism of serotonin and dopamine in the mouse brain following a single administration of allylnitrile, which induces long-term dyskinesia. *Toxicol Lett* **58**, 323.
24. Thuillier J, Burger A (1954) Contribution à l'étude du syndrome moteur provoque chez la souris par l'amino-dipropionitrile (souris tournantes). *Experientia* **10**, 223.
25. US EPA (1995) *Drinking Water Regulations and Health Advisories.* Office of Water, U.S. Environmental Protection Agency (EPA), Washington, DC.

Buthotus hottentota

Albert C. Ludolph

NEUROTOXICITY RATING

Experimental

A   Calcium channel opener

The venom of the African scorpion *Buthotus hottentota* contains a semipurified peptide fraction that selectively stimulates binding of ^{3}H-ryanodine to receptors of skeletal and cardiac sarcoplasmic reticulum and brain microsomes, resulting in opening of the Ca^{2+} channel (4). Ryanodine is an alkaloid that mediates the release of Ca^{2+} from intracellular stores in muscle and possibly brain *via* a specific binding site. There are no descriptions of the specific human toxicity of *Buthotus hottentota*. Nonspecific neurological abnormalities such as muscle rigidity, convulsions, and mental changes are rare complications of scorpion stings (1–3,5); however, the clinical picture after scorpion stings is commonly dominated by cardiovascular effects, which may be responsible for human lethality.

REFERENCES

1. Gueron M, Ovsyshcher I (1984) Cardiovascular effects of scorpion toxins. In: *Handbook of Natural Toxins. Vol 2. Insect Poisons, Allergens, and Other Invertebrate Venoms.* Tu AT ed. Marcel Dekker, New York p. 639.
2. Mebs D (1992) *Gifttiere: ein Handbuch für Biologen, Toxikologen, Ärzte und Apotheker.* Wissenschaftliche Verlagsgesellschaft, Stuttgart.
3. Rodichok LD, Barron KD (1979) Neurologic complications of bee sting, tick bite, and scorpion sting. In: *Handbook of Clinical Neurology, Intoxications of the Nervous System. Part II.* Vinken PJ, Bruyn GW eds. Elsevier, North Holland p. 107.
4. Santhanakrishnan BR, Gajalakshmi BS (1986) Pathogenesis of cardiovascular complications in children following scorpion envenoming. *Ann Trop Paediat* 6, 117.
5. Valdivia HH, Fuentes O, El-Hayek R *et al.* (1991) Activation of the ryanodine receptor Ca^{2+} release channel of sarcoplasmic reticulum by a novel scorpion venom. *J Biol Chem* 266, 19135.

2-*t*-Butylazo-2-hydroxy-5-methylhexane

Thomas L. Kurt

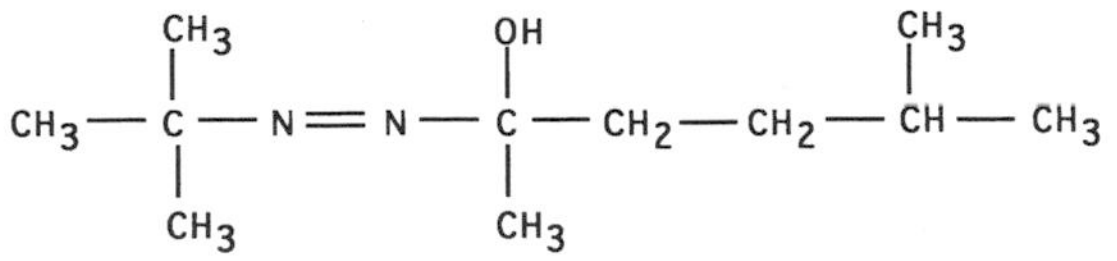

2-*t*-BUTYLAZO-2-HYDROXY-5-METHYLHEXANE
$C_{11}H_{24}N_2O$

NEUROTOXICITY RATING

Clinical

A   Peripheral neuropathy

A   Acute encephalopathy (memory impairment)

A   Visual dysfunction (color vision)

Experimental

A   Peripheral neuropathy

A   Optic neuropathy

2-*t*-Butylazo-2-hydroxy-5-methylhexane (BHMH) is an azo-substituted aliphatic hydrocarbon that was used in the manufacture of polyester-based plastics (6). It decomposes in the presence of polyester resin to form free radicals that cross-link the resin; it also releases bubbles of nitrogen, which cause the resin to foam (7).

In September, 1979, BHMH ("Lucel-7") was introduced in the manufacture of reinforced bathtubs in a newly designed plant in Lancaster, Texas, United States (3). BHMH took the place of the catalyst methyl ethyl ketone peroxide (MEKP) and was incorporated in a spray gun with layers of chopped fibrous glass, polyester resin, *t*-butylbenzoate, styrene, and ethyl acetate, and applied to bathtub molds. Ease of application and the formation of a better quality foam drove the decision to use BHMH. Within 2 weeks of its introduction, a microepidemic began when a spray gun operator developed distal weakness and dysesthesia. Six additional workers directly exposed to BHMH subsequently developed a syndrome consisting of weight loss, sensorimotor neuropathy, visual dysfunction, impaired memory or concentration, and emotional lability (2,3,10).

Limited premarket evaluation of BHMH in rats and rabbits demonstrated acute dermal, conjunctival, and pulmonary toxicity. In addition, tremors, subconvulsive jerking, and ataxia were noted in rats exposed by inhalation for 1 h at a concentration of 20 mg/l (1,4). Ataxia was noted in rats exposed for 1 h at 2.55 mg/l. Chronic toxicity tests were not performed. Information on BHMH distributed by its manufacturer did not warn of possible neurotoxicity (5).

The clinical picture began 2 weeks after the start of operations when the 27-year-old male worker assigned to spray-gun operation developed weakness in his extremities and dysesthesias with shooting pains in his back. He was replaced by the 33-year-old female supervisor, who had been brought initially to this new plant from another location for worker training. Within 10 weeks of BHMH introduction, 7 of 18 workers in the immediate work area developed neurological symptoms. The first three affected workers had not used protective clothing, and neuropathy developed in all 2–4 weeks after BHMH introduction. Protective clothing was used by the other affected workers, and neurological symptoms developed in these individuals after 4–10 weeks of exposure, including in one who had also used a respirator.

Common clinical features were weight loss; extremity weakness; and loss of peripheral, color, and/or night vision (Table 5). Severe extremity weakness, ataxia, paresthesias, decreased calculating ability, and memory deficits were experienced by workers with early onset. One individual developed posterior lenticular cataracts. Urinary incontinence, menstrual irregularity, loss of pain sensation, and muscle atrophy were also noted (Table 5).

Sensory examination revealed depressed deep tendon reflexes. One individual was initially totally areflexic at knees and ankles. Fasciculations were not noted, and Hoffmann's and Babinski's reflexes were uniformly absent. Electrodiagnostic studies revealed slowed or absent nerve conduction and/or increased nerve latencies in four of the affected workers. Results of laboratory tests, including complete blood counts, urinalysis, measurements of triiodothyronine, thyroxine, testosterone levels in men, and estradiol levels in women, were normal.

After these neurological findings were verified through an investigation requested by the U.S. National Institute for Occupational Safety and Health (NIOSH), BHMH was voluntarily withdrawn from the market by the manufacturer while an experimental animal study was performed on rats. NIOSH was called in because no OSHA (U.S. Occupational Safety and Health Administration) hazard guidelines had been established for this novel substance (2,3).

In the animal-modeling study, young adult male and female rats were percutaneously exposed to 250, 375, or 500 mg/kg of BHMH dissolved in ethanol; lethargy, hindlimb weakness, and tonic seizures developed after 2–3 weeks, with females exhibiting a lower threshold of susceptibility than males. Forelimb weakness, eye and nasal discharge, corneal opacity and urinary incontinence developed by 5 weeks (10). Neuropathological examination of the CNS and PNS of treated rats revealed axonal degeneration that first appeared in the spinal cord and optic tract, with similar changes in the sciatic-tibial-plantar nerve complex shortly thereafter. Optic nerves were among the most vulnerable distal to the chiasm and in the lateral geniculate nucleus. The spinal cord and medulla oblongata were also severely involved, with degenerative changes and loss of myelinated fibers in the dorsal columns (gracile tract). Isolated degenerated fibers were encountered in the corpus callosum and cerebellar vermis. While minimal axonal degeneration of myelinated fibers was found in hindlimb peripheral nerves, sensory neurons were generally intact. Control groups showed no abnormal clinical signs or neuropathological changes (10).

Both the human disorder and the experimental disease induced in rodents by BHMH were unusual for their rapidity of onset, severity of impairment, and extensive involvement of central and peripheral nervous systems. In both, neurological deficits occurred after 2–4 weeks of exposure. In the more seriously affected workers, while improved, there was still weakness and sensory loss in their extremities

TABLE 5. Clinical Findings in Workers Exposed to 2-*t*-Butylazo-2-Hydroxy-5-Methylhexane

| Case# | Age/Sex | Abnormalities (Physical Examination) | | | Dysfunction (Reported by Workers) | | | |
		Sensory	Motor	Nerve Conduction	Visual	Ataxia	Bladder/Bowel	Memory Loss
1	27 M	4+	4+	Abnormal	C/P/B	+	+	+
2	33 F	3+	4+	Abnormal	C/P/B	+	+	+
3	25 M	3+	4+	Abnormal	C/P/B	+	+	+
4	27 M	1+	1+	Abnormal	P	−	−	+
5	20 M	1+	1+	Normal	B	−	−	+
6	28 F	1+	—	Normal	D/B	−	−	+
7	21 M	1+	1+	Not done	D/B	−	−	+

Visual changes: B = blurring; C = loss of color vision; D = diplopia; P = loss of peripheral vision.

[Reproduced by permission from Horan JM *et al.* (2).]

after 2 years. With the pattern of axonal degeneration beginning distally, clinical manifestations tended first to appear distally and symmetrically; recovery followed a converse, proximal-to-distal progression. Urinary incontinence in the animals and in the first two more severely involved patients suggested some autonomic involvement. The optic tract involvement in the rats and the major visual symptoms in the patients were greater than in most other experimental toxic neuropathies (3,10).

Early in the investigation of this incident, styrene, a solvent with neurotoxic potential, was an etiological consideration (2,3). However, styrene was also used in a parallel production line in the plant, and three sister plants that were identical (save for their use of MEKP as the catalyst instead of BHMH) lacked workers with neurological disease. Additionally, styrene intoxication typically does not involve motor nerves (8), and the ventilation in the work area had been designed to keep styrene air levels below the OSHA Permitted Exposure Limit of 100 ppm. The primary reason for wanting to switch to BHMH was its ability to produce a finer and more uniform foam, as well as its relative ease of application (3).

Following this incident, NIOSH investigated 86 plants that the manufacturer indicated had received BHMH. Information was obtained from 68 (79%), most of which were small-volume customers, except for one plastic swimming pool plant that had received 370 gallons of BHMH (3). This plant had used the BHMH only 3 h/day, in contrast to 8 h/day at the Texas plant, and had provided organic vapor masks to all exposed workers. However, five workers, all members of spray teams, reported having subtle sensory or motor symptoms after starting work with BHMH. Three of the five consented to have examinations; one had decreased deep tendon reflexes. Four spray gun workers who did not have symptoms consented to be examined; all had decreased deep tendon reflexes. A survey of the workers at the plant where the BHMH was produced revealed no manifestations of neurotoxicity, probably because production took place in a completely enclosed system (3).

BHMH undergoes spontaneous decomposition to produce nitrogen and the hydrocarbons methyl isoamyl ketone and isobutylene. Methyl isoamyl ketone is an iso-branched heptacarbon with a keto at the 2-carbon position and a methyl branch at the iso-5-carbon; this is not metabolized to the neurotoxic hexacarbon 2,5-hexanedione and, thus, fails to produce peripheral neuropathy in experimental animals (9,11) (*see* Hexane, Metabolites, and Derivatives, this volume). Intact BHMH may therefore be required to induce axonal degeneration; the mechanism is unknown.

REFERENCES

1. Dean WP, Jessup DC (1977) Acute toxicity studies in rats and rabbits of Lucel-7 (2-*t*-butylazo-2-hydroxy-5-methylhexane). International Research & Development Corp. Study No. 164-070. IRDC, Mattawan, Missouri.

2. Horan JM, Kurt TL, Landrigan PJ *et al.* (1985) Neurologic dysfunction from exposure to 2-*t*-butylazo-2-hydroxy-5-methylhexane (BHMH): A new occupational neuropathy. *Amer J Public Health* **75**, 513.

3. Kurt TL, Webb CR Jr (1980) Toxic occupational neuropathy—Texas. *Morb Mort Weekly Rep* **29**, 529.

4. Leon BKJ, Jessup DC, Dean WP (1977) Acute one-hour LC50 inhalation study in rats of Lucel-7 (2-*t*-butylazo-2-hydroxy-5-methylhexane. International Research & Development Corp. Study No. 164-071. IRDC, Mattawan, Missouri.

5. Lucidol Division, Pennwalt Corp (1977) Product Bulletin for Luccl-7 (2-*t*-butylazo-2-hydroxy-5-methylhexane). Pennwalt, Buffalo, New York.

6. MacLeay RD, Sheppard CS (1977) Assignee: Pennwalt Corp: Asymmetrical tertiary-aliphatic azoalkanes. U.S. Patent #4,007,165. Feb 8, 1977.

7. Naitove MH (1980) With polyester foam, the payoff is productivity. *Plas Technol* March, p. 79.

8. Seppalaninen AM, Karkonen H (1976) Neuropsychologic findings among workers occupationally exposed to styrene. *Scand J Work Environ Health* **2**, 140.

9. Spencer PS (1982) Experimental evaluation of selected petrochemicals for subchronic neurotoxic properties. In: *Toxicology of Petroleum Hydrocarbons*. MacFarland HN, Holdsworth SE, MacGregor JA *et al.* eds. American Petroleum Institute, Washington, DC p. 249.

10. Spencer PS, Beaubernard CM, Bischoff-Fenton MC, Kurt TL (1985) Clinical and experimental neurotoxicity of 2-*t*-butylazo-2-hydroxy-5-methylhexane. *Ann Neurol* **17**, 28.

11. Spencer PS, Schaumburg HH (1975) Experimental neuropathy produced by 2,5-hexanedione, a major metabolite of the neurotoxic solvent methyl *n*-butyl ketone. *J Neurol Neurosurg Psychiat* **38**, 771.

N-Butylbenzenesulfonamide

Albert C. Ludolph

C₆H₅SO₂NHCH₂CH₂CH₂CH₃

$$C_6H_5SO_2NHCH_2CH_2CH_2CH_3$$

N-BUTYLBENZENESULFONAMIDE
$$C_{10}H_{15}NO_2S$$

NBBS

NEUROTOXICITY RATING

Experimental

A   Anterior horn cell degeneration

The plasticizing agent N-butylbenzenesulfonamide (NBBS) is a stable viscous, light-yellow liquid of pleasant odor with a BP of 372°–374°F (192°–195°C) at 4.5 mm Hg. The compound is soluble in alcohol and ether, but poorly soluble in water. In the United States, exposure limits are not established. NBBS and other amides of organic sulfonic acids (organic sulfonamides, such as N-ethyl-o,p-toluene sulfonamide and o,p-toluene sulfonamide) are commonly used in industry as plasticizers to increase the stability of polyamide materials. These compounds also play a role in the synthesis of sulfonyl carbamate herbicides (4).

NBBS has attracted attention because the compound apparently induces a spastic myelopathy in New Zealand white rabbits after single or repeated intracerebral or systemic injections (5,6). Twelve years before these publications appeared, a single study showed that NBBS is not only neurotoxic but may also suppress erythropoiesis in laboratory animals (1).

The neurotoxic effects of NBBS were discovered during the development of an experimental model for aluminum intoxication when rabbits injected intracisternally with saline (0.9%) developed a progressive spastic paraparesis comparable to the picture seen in aluminum-injected animals (5). Further analysis revealed that the NBBS content of the corresponding aluminum solution was fivefold higher (5), which may indicate that complexation with aluminum may facilitate leaching and solubilization of NBBS. Intraperitoneal injection of a 30-fold higher dosage reproduced the clinical syndrome and neuropathological findings indicating that the neurotoxic principle crosses the blood-brain barrier. On the motor-behavioral level, Strong and collaborators (5) observed dose-dependent neurological deficits, including limb splaying, hyperreflexia, hypertonia, gait impairment, and paralysis. Deficits were initially confined to the hindlimbs but, when animals were injected with larger amounts (50 or 100 µg), forelimbs were also affected (5).

Neuropathological examination (5,6) revealed the presence of abnormalities of dendritic processes of the nucleus motoris lateralis, with vacuoles and multilamellar bodies in the postsynaptic zones. Immunoreactivity to a monoclonal antibody against microtubule-associated protein-2 (MAP-2) was increased in the dendrites of spinal motor neurons. Fusiform thickening of the intraspinal portion of spinal motor neurons contrasted with normal neuropathology of the spinal roots and teased fiber preparations of more distal portions of the peripheral nerve. Axonal spheroids were detected in brainstem nuclei and spinal motor neurons. Although the pattern of damage induced by NBBS in the New Zealand white rabbit seems to be reproducible and well defined, it is unclear whether the progressive nature of the neurological deficits is simply due to repeated injections or an interesting example of a non–self-limited neurotoxic effect. Reportedly, neuropathological findings could be readily distinguished from aluminum toxicity (6). Coadministration of aluminum and NBBS potentiated the neurotoxicity of both compounds (6).

The neurotoxicity of NBBS was also assessed in glial and neuronal cell lines (3). In these systems, micromolar concentrations inhibit cell growth and DNA synthesis. In comparison to glial cells, neurons are ten times more vulnerable to NBBS. The neurotoxic effects of the compound were also studied in primary cultures of mouse hippocampus (7).

There is no evidence that NBBS has any impact on human health. However, previous authors pointed out (6) that, in the United States, NBBS was found as an industrial contaminant in the Delaware River in 1978. Italian investigators detected NBBS in drinking water (2). Organic plasticizers are among the most ubiquitous of all environmental contaminants (4); since they can easily migrate into any food, in particular, those foods with high fat content, the British government recently urged caution in the use of cling film.

REFERENCES

1. Bazarova LA, Migukina NV (1979) Evaluation of the toxicity and safety of benzenesulfonic acid butylamide. *Toksikol Nov Prom Khim Veshchestv* **15**, 110.
2. Brambilla AL, Broglia L, Nidasio G (1991) N-Butylbenzenesulfonamide in drinking water. *Boll Chim Igien* **42**, 779.
3. Nerurkar VR, Wakayama I, Rowe T *et al.* (1993) Preliminary observations on the *in vitro* toxicity of N-butylbenzenesulfonamide: A newly discovered neurotoxin. *Ann N Y Acad Sci* **679**, 280.
4. Sheldon LS, Hites RA (1979) Sources and movement of organic chemicals in the Delaware River. *Environ Sci Technol* **13**, 574.

5. Strong MJ, Garruto RM, Wolff AV *et al.* (1991) *N*-Butyl benzenesulfonamide: A neurotoxic plasticizer inducing a spastic myelopathy in rabbits. *Acta Neuropathol* 81, 235.

6. Strong MJ, Garruto RM (1991) Potentiation in the neurotoxic induction of experimental chronic neurodegenerative disorders: *N*-Butyl benzenesulfonamide and aluminum chloride. *Neurotoxicology* 12, 415.

7. Wakayama I, Nerurkar VR, Garruto RM (1992) *N*-Butylbenzenesulfonamide toxicity in primary neuronal cultures. *Soc Neurosci Abstr* 18, 1606.

6-*tert*-Butyl-3-methyl-2,4-dinitroanisole

Peter S. Spencer

6-*tert*-BUTYL-3-METHYL-2,4-DINITROANISOLE
$C_{12}H_{16}N_2O_5$

6-*tert*-Butyl-3-methyl-2,4-dinitroanisole; 5-*tert*-Butyl-1,3-dinitro-4-methoxy-2-methylbenzene; 4-*tert*-Butyl-3-methoxy-2,6-dinitrotoluene; 2,6-Dinitro-3-methoxy-4-*tert*-butyltoluene; Musk ambrette; Amber musk

NEUROTOXICITY RATING

Experimental

A   Distal axonopathy

A   Myelinopathy

First synthesized in 1892 (4), 6-*tert*-butyl-3-methyl-3,4-dinitroanisole [musk ambrette (MA)] was formerly widely used as an ingredient in fragrances (perfumes, soaps, detergents, and cosmetics) and foodstuffs (candy, chewing gum, beverages). The ability of high doses of dietary MA to paralyze rats and cause testicular atrophy was recognized in a brief scientific report from the U.S. Food and Drug Administration (FDA) in 1967 (5), and the murine oral and dermal neurotoxicity of this compound was defined in 1984 (8,18). An association between MA and human photoallergic contact dermatitis was first reported in 1979–1980 (18). Use of MA declined thereafter: In 1985 and 1986, over 40% of 125 finished fragrances surveyed by the FDA contained MA. It was present in 41% (29/41) of marketplace perfume and cosmetic products assayed by the FDA in 1989, 8% (3/36) in 1990, and 11% (2/18) in 1992; product levels of MA ranged from 0.045%–0.35% (1,12). The decline in product use of MA was driven by concerns primarily relating to human photoallergenicity; there are no reports of human neurotoxicity.

MA, together with musk xylene and musk ketone, form a group of compounds known as aromatic nitro musks; these are used in food and fragrances. U.S. consumption of MA in fragrance formulations, which began in the 1920s, exceeded 100,000 lb/year by the 1960s (2). Annual worldwide production of nitro musks was 7000 tonnes in 1987; this had declined in the early 1990s to 1000 tonnes, including 67% musk xylene, 21% musk ketone, and 12% musk ambrette, the latter mostly for internal markets in China and India (11,17,21).

In 1965, the Flavoring Extract Manufacturer's Association gave MA the status of a chemical that was Generally Regarded as Safe (GRAS). A 1979 report noted that the Council of Europe considered MA suitable for use in concentrations of 1 ppm as an artificial flavoring additive in foodstuffs (15). MA was removed from the GRAS list in the United States in 1984 (10). Reports of photosensitization in association with MA led the International Fragrance Association (IFRA) in 1981 to issue nonenforceable guidelines limiting use of MA to 4% in new fragrance compounds (10). In 1983, IFRA recommended that MA should not be used in fragrance products for cosmetics, toiletries, or other products (including rinse-off products) which, under normal conditions of use, come into contact with skin. For other applications, IFRA recommended that MA should not be used as a fragrance ingredient at a level over 4% in fragrance compounds (10). The low-level (<1%) use of fragrance compounds in products in which MA is allowed would result in final product concentrations of less than 0.04%. By 1992, MA reportedly was no longer used in the United States and its use in Europe was said to be very limited (21). Based on photosensitivity, neurotoxicity in animals, and accumulated evidence that MA can penetrate human skin and is only slowly excreted, IFRA, in July 1994, recommended that MA should not be used as a fragrance ingredient (Research Institute for Fragrance Materials, Englewood, NJ personal communication, 1998).

MA forms pale yellow granular crystals or powder with a sweet, heavy floral-musk odor. The taste is bitter, except at low concentrations (1 ppm). MA is virtually insoluble in water and soluble in 95% ethanol (3.3 g/100 g). The MP is 110°C and the BP > 200°C.

Typical concentrations of MA in fragranced commercial products reported in 1975 included soap, 0.03% (max. 0.2%); detergent, 0.003% (max. 0.02%); cream/lotion, 0.01% (max. 0.07%); and perfume, 0.2% (max. 2%) (15). Aftershave lotions contained *up to* 15% MA (22). A 1986 paper reported concentrations in 14 men's colognes ranging from 0.02%–0.39% w/v MA (9). A 1993 German report found 18 mg/kg MA in 1 of 13 shampoos tested for the presence of nitro musks; 5.3 mg/g in 1 of 13 detergents; and no MA in 23 perfumes, 24 lotions and creme samples, and 11 fabric softeners (19). Typical concentrations of MA in certain alcoholic beverages were 0.10 ppm (mg/kg) and 0.18 ppm (max. 0.42 ppm) in nonalcoholic beverages. Concentrations in certain foodstuffs included gelatin pudding, 0.45 ppm (max. 1.32 ppm); chewing gum, 36 ppm; and hard candy, 423 ppm (6). A 1986 paper reported that samples of Indian betel quid and tobacco contained 0.82–1.44 mg/g wet weight and 11.22–23.51 mg/g wet weight in perfumed tobacco (14). Maximum human exposure to MA in fragrances from all possible sources was estimated in 1981 to be 0.15–0.32 mg/kg/day (16). Analysis of human milk collected in 1991 and 1992 revealed MA in concentrations ranging from >0.01–0.29 mg/kg fat (mean, 0.04 mg/kg fat). The 1981–1983 U.S. National Occupational Exposure Survey estimated that 22,735 employees were potentially exposed to MA (10).

The rat oral LD_{50} for MA has been reported as 339 mg/kg body weight (13) and 4.8 g/kg body weight (10); the dermal LD_{50} is in excess of 2 g/kg (6). Photosensitivity is induced in guinea pigs and mice (10). No effects were observed in rats fed 0.67 mg/kg for 12 weeks (3). Subchronic feeding studies in rats receiving 500–4000 ppm (25–200 mg/kg body weight) found evidence of growth retardation and testicular atrophy (at 2500 ppm), with progressive paralysis of the hindlimbs (at 1500 ppm) beginning at 12–15 weeks (5). Complete hindlimb paralysis was seen after 16–40 weeks of treatment with higher MA dose levels. Female animals, which were more susceptible than males, also showed depressed erythrocyte counts, hemoglobin values, and icteric plasma when treated with doses >1500 ppm. Decreased clotting time was observed in all female groups and in males treated with 1500 or 2500 ppm. Postmortem and histological studies of paralyzed animals revealed brittle bones and enlarged adrenal glands in females, testicular atrophy in males, and muscle atrophy; the nervous system was not examined (5).

Repeated treatment of the shaven back of Sprague-Dawley rats with concentrations of MA in phenylethyl alcohol equivalent to 10, 40, 80, or 240 mg/kg was used to evaluate and define the neurotoxic effects of the nitromusk. Additional animals were given a diet containing 1500 ppm (75 mg/kg) (20). Depressed body weight gain was seen in these animals and in those receiving the two high dermal exposures of MA. Hematology, clinical chemistry and urinalysis parameters were comparable to control values at 6 and 12 weeks of treatment. At the latter timepoint, hindlimb weakness was observed in 1 of 30 animals receiving 40 mg/kg/day, 15 of 30 on 80 mg/kg/day, in all animals treated with 240 mg/kg/day, and in 20 of 40 animals receiving 1500 ppm MA in the diet. Diet-treated animals and rats treated percutaneously with 80 mg/kg/day showed testicular degeneration, and testicular weight was depressed in animals receiving 240 mg/kg/day (8). The testicular and neurotoxic properties of MA were not reproduced in animals treated with other nitromusks, including musk ketone, musk xylene, musk tibetene, and moskene (7).

Oral and topically MA-treated animals showed a common pattern of neuropathological changes in brain, spinal cord, lumbar spinal roots, and hindlimb peripheral nerves (20). Changes were most severe in animals treated topically with 240 mg/kg/day in 20% phenylethyl alcohol and somewhat less severe in those given MA in the diet; scattered early changes were found in animals exposed percutaneously to 80 mg/kg/day, some animals showed isolated abnormalities at 40 mg/kg/day, and no abnormalities were present at 10 mg/kg/day. Primary vacuolar demyelination was prominent in dorsal and ventral spinal roots; intramyelinic phagocytes participated in the removal of damaged myelin, leaving demyelinated and attenuated axon segments. Schwann cell proliferation and remyelination took place during the period of MA treatment. Myelin vacuolation was scattered in peripheral nerves, found throughout the white matter of the spinal cord, and occasionally present in the cerebellar vermis. Primary axonal degeneration of myelinated fibers first appeared with bilateral symmetry in the gracile tract at the level of the medulla oblongata, and in tibial nerve branches supplying the calf musculature. The most severely affected animals showed axonal degeneration to the lumbar level of the spinal cord, and of the sciatic nerve up to the sciatic notch. No clear pattern of differential sensitivity to MA with respect to gender was noted (20).

The mechanism of MA neurotoxicity is unknown. Musk xylene (5-*tert*-butyl-2,4,6-trinitro-*m*-xylene), a compound with some degree of structural relation to MA, reportedly did not show neurotoxicity in a study of topically treated albino rats in which MA was used as a positive control (7). The International Agency for Research on Cancer (IARC) states that MA is not classifiable as to its carcinogenicity in humans (IARC, group 3); there is inadequate evidence for carcinogenicity in humans and experimental animals (10).

REFERENCES

1. Anon (1987) Musk ambrette's persistence in fragrances. *FDC Reports Rose Sheet.* May 25, p. 4.
2. Arctander S (1969) *Perfume and Flavor Chemicals (Aroma Chemicals).* Arctander, Montclair, New Jersey.
3. Bär F, Griepentrog F (1967) State of safety evaluation of aromatics for food. *Med Ernahr* 8, 244. [German]
4. Bedoukian PZ (1986) *Perfumery and Flavoring Synthetics. 3rd Ed.* Allured Publ., Wheaton, Illinois p. 322.
5. Davis DA, Taylor JM, Jones WI, Brouwer JB (1967) Toxicity of musk ambrette. *Toxicol Appl Pharmacol* 10, 405.
6. Flavor and Extract Manufacturers' Association (1995) *Monograph: Musk Ambrette.* Washington, DC.
7. Ford RA, Api AM, Newberne PM (1990) 90-Day dermal toxicity study and neurotoxicity evaluation of nitromusks in the albino rat. *Food Chem Toxicol* 28, 55.
8. Giovinazzo VJ, Harber LC, Armstrong RB, Kochevar IE (1980) Photoallergic contact dermatitis to musk ambrette. Clinical report of two patients with persistent light reactor patterns. *J Amer Acad Dermatol* 3, 384.
9. Goh CL, Kwok SF (1986) A simple method of qualitative analysis of musk ambrette, musk ketone and musk xylene in cologne. *Contact Dermatitis* 14, 53.
10. International Agency for Research on Cancer (IARC) (1996) Musk Ambrette and Musk Xylene. *IARC Monographs on the Evaluation of Carcinogenic Risks to Humans. Vol 65. Printing Processes and Some Printing Inks, Carbon Black and Some Nitro Compounds.* World Health Organization, Geneva.
11. Ippen H (1994) Nitro musk. *Int Arch Occup Envir Health* 66, 283.
12. Jackson EM (1993) Substantiating the safety of fragrances and fragranced products. *Cosmet Toiletries* 108, 43.
13. Jenner PM, Hagan EC, Taylor JM *et al.* (1964) Food flavorings and compounds of related structure. *Food Cosmet Toxicol* 2, 327.
14. Nair J, Ohshima H, Malaveille C *et al.* (1986) Identification, occurrence and mutagenicity in *Salmonella typhimurium* of two synthetic nitroarenes, musk ambrette and musk xylene, in Indian chewing tobacco and betel quid. *Food Chem Toxicol* 24, 27.
15. Opdyke DL (1975) Fragrance raw material monographs: Musk ambrette; musk ketone; musk xylol. *Food Chem Toxicol* 13, p. 875.
16. Opdyke DL (1981) *Research Institute for Fragrance Materials.* NBB Information Bulletin 1, October 29.
17. Qinghua Z 1993) China's perfumery industry picks up. *Perfum Flavor* 18, 47.
18. Raugi GJ, Storrs FJ, Larsen WG (1979) Photoallergic contact dermatitis to men's perfumes. *Contact Dermatol* 5, 251.
19. Sommer C (1993) Gas chromatography determination of nitro musks in cosmetics and detergents. *Deut Lebensm-Rundsch* 89, 108. [German]
20. Spencer PS, Bischoff-Fenton MC, Moreno OM *et al.* (1984) Neurotoxic properties of musk ambrette. *Toxicol Appl Pharmacol* 75, 571.
21. Topfer K (1992) Chinese musk prices drop as polycyclic use grows. *Chem Mark Rep* 242, 26.
22. Wojnarowska F, Calnan CD (1986) Contact and photoallergy to musk ambrette. *Brit J Dermatol* 114, 667.

γ-Butyrolactone

Peter S. Spencer

BUTYROLACTONE
$C_4H_6O_2$

Dihydro-2(3*H*)-furanone; 1,2-Butanolide

NEUROTOXICITY RATING

Clinical

B   Seizure disorder

Experimental

A   Seizure disorder

γ-Butyrolactone is an oily liquid used as a polymer solvent in products such as paint and nail polish removers. Liquids and powders containing γ-butyrolactone were marketed as dietary supplements under product names such as Renewtrient, Revivarant, Blue Nitro, Gamma G; these generally claimed improved physical performance, muscle building, reduced stress, and enhanced sexual activity and sleep. In January 1999, after these products had been associated with at least 55 adverse health events and one death, the U.S. Food and Drug Administration urged a voluntary recall of all dietary supplements containing γ-butyrolactone.

The oral LD_{50} in rats is 17.2 ml/kg. Rats display absence-like seizures after systemic administration of γ-butyrolactone or microinfusion of its metabolite, γ-hydroxybutyric acid (GHB), into the ventrobasal nucleus of the thalamus. γ-Butyrolactone may possess limited γ-aminobutyric acid agonist (GABA) activity. GHB is used as a relatively specific inhibitor of central dopamine release (3). It is suggested that GHB modulates the basal and K^+-evoked release of GABA and glutamate in the thalamic ventrobasal relay nuclei (1). GHB-induced absence seizures may regulate GABA$_A$-receptor α-1 and α-4 gene expression in thalamic relay nuclei as a compensatory mechanism by which absence seizures are terminated (2).

Rapid onset of coma, respiratory depression, and bradycardia has been reported in adults and children intoxicated with products containing γ-butyrolactone (4,5). Seizures are also said to occur. A two-year-old was apneic, bradycardic, flaccid and unresponsive to deep painful stimuli after oral exposure to γ-butyrolactone; he responded well to oral intubation and atropine (4).

REFERENCES

1. Banerjee PK, Snead OC 3rd (1995) Presynaptic γ-hydroxybutyric acid (GHB) and γ-aminobutyric acid B (GABA$_B$) receptor-mediated release of GABA and glutamate (GLU) in rat thalamic ventrobasal nucleus (VB): a possible mechanism for the generation of absence-like seizures induced by GHB. *Pharmacol Exp Ther* **273**, 1534.
2. Banerjee PK, Tillakaratne NJ, Brailowsky S *et al.* (1998) Alterations in GABA$_A$ receptor α-1 and α-4 subunit mRNA levels in thalamic relay nuclei following absence-like seizures in rats. *Exp Neurol* **154**, 213.
3. Feigenbaum JJ, Howard SG (1996) Gamma hydroxybutyrate is not a GABA agonist. *Prog Neurobiol* **50**, 1.
4. Higgins TF Jr, Borron SW (1996) Coma and respiratory arrest after exposure to butyrolactone. *Emerg Med* **14**, 435.
5. Rambourg-Schepens MO, Buffet M, Durak C, Mathieu-Nolf M (1997) γ-Butyrolactone poisoning and its similarities to γ-hydroxybutyric acid: two case reports. *Vet Hum Toxicol* **39**, 234.

Butyrophenones

Matthias Riepe

Phenyl butylpiperidines

NEUROTOXICITY RATING
Clinical

A   Extrapyramidal syndrome (parkinsonism, tardive dyskinesia)

A   Neuroleptic malignant syndrome

A   Seizure disorder

Experimental

A   Dopamine D$_2$ receptor antagonist

B   Extrapyramidal dysfunction (dystonia—primates)

Since the discovery of butyrophenones in 1957 and their introduction into clinical practice in 1959, haloperidol and other butyrophenones have been widely used for the treatment of psychotic disorders. Treatment is effective for positive psychotic symptoms such as hallucinations and delusion. In general, antipsychotic potency correlates with antagonism at dopamine D$_2$ receptors. Butyrophenones are also used for nausea and vomiting, cough and cold treatments, and as supplementary agents for sedation for minor surgical or diagnostic procedures. The therapeutic index is high, with lethal doses ranging from 200–11,000 times the therapeutic levels (25). Clinically, the most common side effects are extrapyramidal and adrenolytic symptoms.

Butyrophenone-induced parkinsonism occurs in 20%–40% of patients (32), usually within 5–90 days of treatment initiation. With chronic neuroleptic therapy, 5%–40% of patients develop tardive dyskinesia (26).

Although a specific animal model of human psychosis does not exist, inhibition of amphetamine-induced stereotyped behavior correlates well with antipsychotic efficacy in humans. Alternatively, prolactin-increasing effects are used for predicting antipsychotic efficacy in humans (22). Apomorphine-induced antagonism of emesis in dogs serves as a useful predictor for duration of action. All butyrophenones are effective inhibitors of amphetamine- or apomorphine-induced stereotypies in rats and of apomorphine-induced emesis in dogs. At dose levels not significantly affecting gross behavior, they are specific inhibitors of conditioned operant behavior and of intracranial self-stimulation in most common laboratory species. Higher doses induce a state of catalepsy. At progressively higher doses they induce palpebral ptosis, inhibit epinephrine-induced motility and, finally, induce prostration. However, there are also some butyrophenone derivatives that lack antipsychotic activity (8). The ratio of norepinephrine antagonism over amphetamine antagonism can be used as an effective measure for the relative adrenolytic *vs.* antipsychotic activity, low ratios correlating with high potential for autonomic side effects. Sedative effects—oversedation, somnolence, and hypokinesia—can be effectively predicted with the ratio of palpebral ptosis over catalepsy, low ratios correlating with sedative side effects. Extrapyramidal side effects can be predicted less consistently. Apart from these side effects, adverse reactions from butyrophenones result from blockade of autonomic function; for example, the adrenolytic properties of butyrophenones induce orthostatic hypotension and tachycardia. Behavioral classification of neuroleptics into three different groups is comparable with the classification obtained by dopamine-receptor binding techniques *in vitro* (9).

Butyrophenones also have nonmedical usages. Those with a short half-life are employed in pig farming to reduce stress and thereby increase the quality of the meat (13). Butyrophenones are used in game capture because of their rapid onset of action, suppression of the alarm reaction, and facilitation of large-scale handling and translocation of captured animals. Extrapyramidal effects have been observed in some species (23).

Butyrophenones have a 4-fluorobenzoyl moiety linked by a straight unbranched propylene chain to the nitrogen atom of a 4-substituted piperidine ring or, less frequently, to a 4-substituted piperazine ring. The more potent butyrophenones are derived from 4-hydroxy-4-phenyl-piperidine or from 4-anilinopiperidine. All butyrophenones are characterized by a more or less fully extended side chain. The more potent compounds possess a planar aromatic ring, attached to the 4-position of the piperazidine (or piperidine) ring, which is capable of orienting itself perpendicular to the mean plane of this piperazine (piperidine) ring. The most potent compounds possess a hydrogen bond-donating moiety attached to the 4-position of the piperazine (or piperidine) ring and oriented with respect to the mean plane of the piperazine (piperidine) ring, toward the side opposite that of the lone pair of the basic nitrogen. All butyrophenones are very lipophilic.

Butyrophenones are largely metabolized before excretion (6,39). The principal biodegradation of haloperidol in the rat is oxidative dealkylation resulting in the formation of *p*-fluorobenzoylpropionic acid (39). Metabolism of butyrophenones, however, is species dependent. After intraperitoneal (i.p.) injection in guinea pigs, haloperidol is converted to reduced haloperidol with such rapidity that, 1 h after the injection, the concentration of haloperidol was only about one-fifth of that of reduced haloperidol. After a single dose of the butyrophenone neuroleptics, haloperidol and bromperidol (both at 1 mg/kg, i.p.), near-terminal elimination half-lives from brain were 6.6 and 5.8 days, respectively, and each was detectable for 21 days after dosing (10). A long-lasting formulation for intramuscular (i.m.)

application of haloperidol in humans is haldol decanoate. Most intramuscularly administered haloperidol decanoate is absorbed in blood after hydrolysis to haloperidol; absorption is rate limiting. Butyrophenone levels in regional lymph nodes suggest that the intramuscularly administered ester is absorbed *via* the lymphatic system where hydrolysis to haloperidol probably occurs (34). Haloperidol to a considerable extent passes through the milk in lactating animals, and up to 60% of maternal serum levels is reached in fetal serum (45). Recently, it has become possible to visualize binding of some butyrophenones directly by positron emission tomography, such as fluorinated melperone in the rat brain by *in vivo* [19]F nuclear magnetic resonance measurements (20).

Initial toxic symptoms in mice and rats consist of ptosis, sedation and catalepsy. The LD_{50} for mice and rats is similar; about 13–30 mg/kg intravenously, 60 mg/kg subcutaneously, and 100–800 mg/kg orally (p.o.). Death is preceded by clonic convulsions. Due to cumulative effects, the LD_{50} varies with observation time, particularly upon p.o. administration. In this case, increase of toxicity for up to 10 days has been reported. The LD_{50} for haloperidol was 285 mg/kg at 24 h, 129 mg/kg at 3 days, and 50 mg/kg at 7 days (25). Slight to moderate local irritation was reported after i.m. injection (36). No increased teratogenic risk was observed in several studies (16,21,24,36). Administration of haloperidol during and after gestation did not affect litter sizes, birth weights, or postnatal development in mouse, rat, or rabbit. However, one study reported a syndrome of malformations: exencephaly, craniorachischisis, kinking of the spinal cord, brachyury, and dilatation of the fourth brain ventricle (27).

Subacute and chronic side effects in monkeys manifest as dystonic reactions at 0.5 and 1.0 mg/kg of haloperidol for 2 months (19). No pathology was seen in rats given 33 mg/kg or dogs given 12 mg/kg of haloperidol for up to 1 year (36). Chronic treatment of animals with a daily i.p. dose of 5 µmol/kg resulted in markedly attenuated responses of plasma corticosterone to challenge of the same dose of the same drug. By contrast, acute treatment caused a large increase in the plasma corticosterone levels. This result indicates that the tolerance to the stimulatory action of the butyrophenones may occur in the hypothalamo-pituitary axis (1).

Suicidal overdosage with haloperidol can cause death (30), but fatalities are rare. Dose-independent fatalities result from neuroleptic malignant syndrome (38), dystonic airway obstruction (3), and *torsades de pointes* ventricular tachycardia (28).

Extrapyramidal side effects are most commonly observed during butyrophenone treatment. Up to 44% of patients show some tardive dyskinesia. The proportion of patients with tardive dyskinesia increases directly with age and number of years of neuroleptic treatment. Dose reduction may *exacerbate* the syndrome. Severity of dyskinesia correlates with anticholinergic drug use and with piperazine/butyrophenone neuroleptics (15,18). Dystonia is more common in males (41) and after prolonged drug treatment (2). When treated with depot formulation of haldol, the clinical condition of about two-thirds of the patients remains unchanged or improves, compared with the period of oral treatment. During the first 2 months of treatment, however, rigidity and tremor are increased. From the third month, the extrapyramidal signs are less pronounced than during the period of oral neuroleptics (11). Alcohol lowers the threshold of resistance to dystonic side effects (31).

Increased seizure activity has been observed experimentally and upon application of haloperidol in humans (35,40,42); however, the clinical incidence is lower than with other neuroleptic drugs. Neuroleptic malignant syndrome is rare and life threatening; phenothiazine and butyrophenones are most frequently implicated. Fever, muscle rigidity, and elevated creatine phosphokinase are the important criteria for diagnosis (17,29). (For more details, *see* Chlorpromazine and Other Neuroleptics, this volume.)

Toxic effects potentially can be mediated by a variety of mechanisms including *via* dopaminergic (side effects: extrapyramidal), muscarinic (accommodation, increased intraocular pressure, dry mouth), adrenergic (hypotension, reflex tachycardia), histaminergic (sedation), serotonergic, and opioid receptors.

Haloperidol suppresses action potentials by a nonspecific local anesthetic-like effect; specific inhibition of sodium conductance is mediated by means of an opiate drug receptor associated with the muscle fiber membrane. However, naloxone does not antagonize the effects on sodium conductance (12). Haloperidol also affects calcium channels (37).

It is generally accepted that the nigrostriatal degenerative properties of the parkinsonism-inducing agent 1-methyl-4-phenyl-1,2,3,6-tetrahydropyridine are mediated by the brain monoamine oxidase B-generated 1-methyl-4-phenylpyridinium ion metabolite (MPP^+), produced by the action of brain monoamine oxidase B. A similar haloperidol-derived pyridinium metabolite, a 1,4-disubstituted structural analog of the MPP^+ metabolite, HPP^+, has been found in haloperidol-treated rats and humans. Intrastriatal perfusion of HPP^+ has been shown to induce irreversible depletion of striatal dopamine and serotonin. Furthermore, HPP^+ is a potent inhibitor of NADH-supported mitochondrial respiration (5,14,43). It also has been shown that neuroleptics, in particular butyrophenones, inhibit both complex I of the electron transport chain (7) and the mitochondrial pyruvate dehydrogenase complex activity (33).

Supersensitivity as a cause of tardive dyskinesia is still under discussion (44). Drug holidays have been proposed as a strategy to prevent tardive dyskinesia. Three animal studies in which dopamine receptor hypersensitivity after chronic neuroleptic treatment was used as a model for tardive dyskinesia failed to find any reduction in dopamine-receptor hypersensitivity with intermittent, as opposed to continuous, treatment. Even drug-free periods fail to reduce the development of dopamine-receptor hypersensitivity (4).

REFERENCES

1. Aimoto T, Kaida M, Numazaki K *et al.* (1981) Development of tolerance to the stimulatory effect of neuroleptic butyrophenones on pituitary-adrenal activity in rats. *J Pharmacobiodyn* **4**, 827.
2. Altamura CA, Colacurcio F, Mauri MC *et al.* (1990) Haloperidol decanoate in chronic schizophrenia: A study of 12 months with plasma levels. *Prog Neuro-psych Biol Psych* **14**, 25.
3. Barach E, Dubin LM, Tomlanovich MC, Kottamasu S (1989) Dystonia presenting as upper airway obstruction. *J Emerg Med* **7**, 237.
4. Belmaker RH, Elami A, Bannet J (1985) Intermittent treatment with droperidol, a short-acting neuroleptic, increases behavioral dopamine receptor sensitivity. *Psychopharmacol Suppl* **2**, 194.
5. Bloomquist J, King E, Wright A *et al.* (1994) 1-Methyl-4-phenylpyridinium-like neurotoxicity of a pyridinium metabolite derived from haloperidol: Cell culture and neurotransmitter uptake studies. *J Pharmacol Exp Ther* **270**, 822.
6. Braun GA, Poos GI, Soudijn W (1967) Distribution, excretion and metabolism of neuroleptics of the butyrophenone type. II. Distribution, excretion and metabolism of haloperidol in Sprague-Dawley rats. *Eur J Pharmacol* **1**, 58.
7. Burkhardt C, Kelly JP, Lim YH *et al.* (1993) Neuroleptic medications inhibit complex I of the electron transport chain. *Ann Neurol* **33**, 512.
8. Cascio G, Erba R, Manghisi E *et al.* (1980) Omega-amino-2-hydroxy-*p*-fluorobutyro-phenones: Synthesis and preliminary pharmacological evaluation. *Farmaco Sci* **35**, 605.
9. Christensen AV, Arnt J, Hyttel J, Svendsen O (1984) Behavioural correlates to the dopamine D-1 and D-2 antagonists. *Pol J Pharmacol Pharm* **36**, 249.
10. Cohen BM, Tsuneizumi T, Baldessarini RJ *et al.* (1992) Differences between antipsychotic drugs in persistence of brain levels and behavioral effects. *Psychopharmacology* **108**, 338.

11. De Cuyper H, Bollen J, van Praag HM, Verstraeten D (1986) Pharmacokinetics and therapeutic efficacy of haloperidol decanoate after loading dose administration. *Brit J Psychiat* **148**, 560.

12. Durham HD, Frank GB, Marwaha J (1977) Effects of antipsychotic drugs on action potential production in skeletal muscle. II. Haloperidol: Nonspecific and opiate drug receptor-mediated effects. *Can J Physiol Pharmacol* **55**, 462.

13. Eikelenboom G (1975) [Use of neuroleptic agents in modern pig-farming]. *Tijdschr Diergeneeskd* **100**, 265. [Dutch]

14. Eyles DW, McLennan HR, Jones A *et al.* (1994) Quantitative analysis of two pyridinium metabolites of haloperidol in patients with schizophrenia. *Clin Pharmacol Ther* **56**, 512.

15. Ezrin WC, Seeman MV, Seeman P (1981) Tardive dyskinesia in schizophrenic outpatients: Prevalence and significant variables. *J Clin Psychiat* **42**, 16.

16. Godet PF, Marie CM (1991) Neuroleptics, schizophrenia and pregnancy. Epidemiological and teratologic study. *Encephale* **17**, 543.

17. Greenblatt DJ, Gross PL, Harris J *et al.* (1978) Fatal hyperthermia following haloperidol therapy of sedative-hypnotic withdrawal. *J Clin Psychiat* **39**, 673.

18. Grohmann R, Koch R, Schmidt LG (1990) Extrapyramidal symptoms in neuroleptic recipients. *Agents Actions Suppl* **29**, 71.

19. Gunne L-M, Barany S (1976) Haloperidol-induced tardive dyskinesia in monkeys. *Psychopharmacology* **50**, 237.

20. Gunther U, Albert K (1993) *In vivo* ^{19}F nuclear magnetic resonance of a monofluorinated neuroleptic in the rat. *NMR Biomed* **6**, 27.

21. Hara K (1990) [Psychiatric and nervous disorders]. *Nippon Sanka Fujinka Gakkai Zasshi* **42**, 847. [Japanese]

22. Hayashi T, Tadokoro S (1984) Parallelism between avoidance-suppressing and prolactin-increasing effects of antipsychotic drugs in rats. *Jpn J Pharmacol* **35**, 451.

23. Hofmeyr JM (1981) The use of haloperidol as a long-acting neuroleptic in game capture operations. *J S Afr Vet Assn* **52**, 273.

24. Imai S, Tauchi K, Huang KJ *et al.* (1984) Teratogenicity study on bromperidol in rats. *J Toxicol Sci* **1**, 109.

25. Janssen PAJ (1968) Toxicology and metabolism of butyrophenones. *Proc Eur Soc Study Drug Toxicol* **9**, 107.

26. Jenner P, Marsden CD (1985) Neuroleptic agents: Acute and chronic receptor actions. In: *Drugs in Central Nervous System Disorders.* Horwell ed. Marcel Dekker, New York p.149.

27. Jurand A, Martin LV (1990) Teratogenic potential of two neurotropic drugs, haloperidol and dextromoramide, tested on mouse embryos. *Teratology* **42**, 45.

28. Kriwisky M, Perry GY, Tarchitsky D *et al.* (1990) Haloperidol-induced torsades de pointes. *Chest* **98**, 482.

29. Kurien T, Rajeev KK, Abraham OC *et al.* (1993) Management of neuroleptic malignant syndrome—a series of eight cases. *J Assn Phys India* **41**, 91.

30. Levine BS, Wu SC, Goldberger BA, Caplan YH (1991) Two fatalities involving haloperidol. *J Anal Toxicol* **15**, 282.

31. Lutz EG (1976) Neuroleptic-induced akathisia and dystonia triggered by alcohol. *J Amer Med Assn* **236**, 2422.

32. Marsden CD, Jenner P (1980) The pathophysiology of extrapyramidal side-effects of neuroleptic drugs. *Psychol Med* **10**, 55.

33. Miernyk JA, Fang TK, Randall DD (1987) Calmodulin antagonists inhibit the mitochondrial pyruvate dehydrogenase complex. *J Biol Chem* **262**, 15338.

34. Oh EY, Miyazaki H, Matsunaga Y, Hashimoto M (1991) Pharmacokinetics of haloperidol decanoate in rats. *J Pharmacobiodyn* **14**, 615.

35. Satoh H, Nakanishi H, Shirakawa K *et al.* (1987) Comparative study of tiapride and neuroleptics with anti-dopamine activity on convulsive seizure in mice. *Jpn J Pharmacol* **43**, 27.

36. Seay PH, Field WE (1967) Toxicological studies on haloperidol. *Int J Neuropsychiat* **3**, 19.

37. Seth P, Maitra KK, Ganguly DK (1991) Haloperidol on rat phrenic hemidiaphragm. *Arch Int Pharmacodyn Ther* **310**, 87.

38. Shalev A, Hermesh H, Munitz H (1989) Mortality from neuroleptic malignant syndrome. *J Clin Psychiat* **50**, 18.

39. Soudijn W, Van Wijngaarden I, Allewijn F (1967) Distribution, excretion and metabolism of neuroleptics of the butyrophenone type. I. Excretion and metabolism of haloperidol and nine related butyrophenone-derivatives in the Wistar rat. *Eur J Pharmacol* **1**, 47.

40. Spatz R, Kugler J (1982) Abnormal EEG activities induced by psychotropic drugs. *Electroencephalogr Clin Neuro Suppl* **36**, 549.

41. Swett CJ (1975) Drug-induced dystonia. *Amer J Psychiat* **132**, 532.

42. Turski L, Cavalheiro EA, Bortolotto ZA *et al.* (1988) Dopamine-sensitive anticonvulsant site in the rat striatum. *J Neurosci* **8**, 4027.

43. Van der Schyf CJ, Castagnoli K, Usuki E *et al.* (1994) Metabolic studies on haloperidol and its tetrahydropyridine analog in C57BL/6 mice. *Chem Res Toxicol* **7**, 281.

44. Wolfarth S, Ossowska K (1989) Can the supersensitivity of rodents to dopamine be regarded as a model of tardive dyskinesia? *Prog Neuro-psych Biol Psych* **13**, 799.

45. Ziv G, Shani J, Givant Y *et al.* (1974) Distribution of tritiated haloperidol in lactating and pregnant cows and ewes. *Arch Int Pharmacodyn Ther* **212**, 154.

Cadmium

J. Michael Schröder

NEUROTOXICITY RATING

Clinical

B Acute encephalopathy (edema, endothelial damage)

B Olfactory syndrome

Experimental

A CNS/PNS vasculopathy (endothelial cells)

A Neuroteratogen (endothelial cells)

A Encephalomalacia (hemorrhage)

A Neuronopathy (dorsal root ganglion cell)

A Peripheral neuropathy

Cadmium (Cd) is almost exclusively found in nature in association with zinc; consequently, no distinction was made between the two metals until 1817. In the book, *On Marvels*, attributed to Aristotle (300 BC), first mention is made of a "peculiar earth." When utilized as an alloying constituent together with copper, it yielded an especially shiny type of bronze. This earth-like substance was named *Cadmia* by Dioscorides and Pliny in the first century AD. In 1817, the element cadmium was discovered by Strohmeyer.

Cd is extracted from zinc ores and zinciferous residues. It has an atomic weight of 112.40; specific gravity of 8.65; MP of 321.03°C; and BP of 765°C at a pressure of 760 mm Hg. It is rarely used as a metal, but it is a constituent of many alloys of low MP. It is softer than zinc (Zn) and harder than tin (Sn). It is insoluble in water but soluble in acids. The most important compounds are the oxide (CdO), sulfate ($CdSO_4 \cdot H_2O$), sulfide (CdS), chloride ($CdCl_2$), iodide (CdI_2), and bromide ($CdBr_2$). For simplicity, the symbol Cd^{2+} is used for any of these compounds, except when otherwise specified.

With the advent of industrialization, the demand for Cd^{2+} extracted from Zn^{2+} ores increased greatly; Cd^{2+} is used in the manufacture of alkaline accumulators, Cu^{2+}-Cd^{2+} alloys, paint pigments, silver polish, and plated metals, and as a pigment for coating photoelectric cells and cathode ray tubes (3).

Some 50 years ago, cadmiosis was essentially an occupational disease. Nowadays, the main source of intake of Cd^{2+} arises from the polluted environment, and it has become virtually impossible to avoid exposure to the metal. The atmosphere over industrialized cities may contain up to 0.062 μg Cd^{2+}/m³. Soft tap water remaining overnight in galvanized or black polyethylene pipes can take up considerable amounts of Cd^{2+}. Levels up to 220 ppb Cd^{2+} have been measured in polluted rivers of West Germany. Daily intakes of Cd^{2+} vary greatly according to the degree of environmental pollution, as well as sources and types of food.

Values of 4760 ppb Cd^{2+} have been measured in kidneys of freshwater fish. Oysters are especially rich in Cd^{2+}; 2–3 ppm Cd^{2+} wet weight have been recorded. The metal is highly concentrated in polished rice and wheat. Cigarette smoking is another nonoccupational source of Cd^{2+} contamination; the smoke of 20 cigarettes contains a median amount of 16 μg Cd^{2+}.

The upper limit set by the World Health Organization in 1992 (27) for the "provisional tolerable weekly cadmium intake" is 400–500 μg for an adult; the drinking water guideline value is 0.005 mg/l. The air quality guideline for rural area levels is <1–5 ng/m³; in urban and industrialized areas, 10–20 ng/m³; and for short-term occupational exposure, 250 μg/m³, provided the recommended time-weighted average (40 h/wk) of 10 μg/m³ is respected.

Cadmium is a highly toxic material. It has an extremely long biological half-life and may be considered a cumulative toxicant. It has sterilizing, teratogenic, and carcinogenic effects, and Cd accumulation might play an important role in senescence (2).

The human body contains a total of 30 mg Cd^{2+}, of which about 10 mg occur in the kidneys and 4.1 mg in the liver. Cd^{2+} is absent from the kidneys of the newborn. Concentrations of 30–40 ppm Cd^{2+} in the kidneys and 2–3 ppm in the liver of human adults are common. Renal levels of Cd^{2+} in Japanese individuals are twice those found in North Americans. The metabolism of Cd^{2+} is subject to considerable variation and is influenced by the relative intakes of Zn^{2+}, Cu^{2+}, and other metals. In turn, Cd^{2+} influences the metabolism of Zn^{2+}, Fe^{2+}, and Cu^{2+}. In contrast with Zn^{2+} and Mn^{2+}, the body has no means of homeostatic control of Cd^{2+}.

Cd^{2+} is a potent noncompetitive inhibitor of Ca^{2+} transport across the small intestine. Like Zn^{2+}, Cd^{2+} reduces the intestinal absorption of Cu^{2+}. A negative Ca^{2+} balance leading to osteomalacia is induced by Cd^{2+}. It is generally accepted that a mutual antagonism exists between Cd^{2+} and Zn^{2+}.

The relative binding constants for Cd^{2+} by sulfhydryl, acetate, imidazole, and amino groups are six to ten times those for Ca^{2+}, Zn^{2+}, Ni^{2+}, and Co^{2+}. Under physiological conditions, blood contains only minute amounts of Cd^{2+}. When poisoned with the metal, Cd^{2+} accumulates almost exclusively in erythrocytes (90%–95%) bound to hemoglobin. Rabbits fed Cd^{2+} develop hyperplastic bone marrow and hypochromic, microcystic anemia, reminiscent of that elicited by iron deficiency.

A protein containing up to 5.9% Cd^{2+} and 2.2% Zn^{2+}, termed *metallothionein*, was isolated from the kidney and liver of horses (14). It has a low molecular weight (6 kD), binds specifically to these two metals, and has the highest content of cysteine in known proteins. The amount of Cd^{2+} and Zn^{2+} in human metallothionein may vary, but the sum of the two elements remains constant, suggesting that Cd^{2+} and Zn^{2+} compete for the binding sites of metallothionein. Cd^{2+}-thionein, when given parenterally to rats and mice, is seven to eight times more toxic than the free cation. Since the injected protein is catabolized, it is reasoned that the liberated Cd^{2+} causes the acute damage of renal tubules.

Retention of Cd^{2+} is one of the characteristic features of the interaction of the metal with mammalian tissues. At a daily ingestion of 200 μg Cd^{2+} by human adults, and a urinary output totaling 40 μg, approximately 20% appears in the urine, 78.2%–79.1% is excreted by the feces, and the rest is retained for undefined periods of time. The extremely protracted elimination of the metal is documented in the case of an individual treated for syphilis with a total of 900 mg Cd^{2+}. During a 39-day period, only about 3% was eliminated from the body. The biological half-life is estimated to be >10 years in humans (23).

Cd^{2+} has complex effects on systemic biochemistry, especially that of the lung (6). Single exposure of Cd^{2+} aerosol to rats led to inflammation of the lung accompanied within hours by an alveolar exudation of polymorphonuclear leukocytes and alveolar macrophages. Acute emphysema could be provoked in rats by inhalation. Thirty minutes after a single exposure of mice to a Cd^{2+} aerosol, the element had passed the alveolar-blood barrier and, within days, accumulated in the liver and kidney. Degradation of liver polysomes and impairment of protein synthesis in these organelles was noticed in mice following injection of $CdCl_2$, 20 $\mu mol/kg$. Respiratory activity of liver mitochondria was inhibited by the metal only at low pH (11).

Cadmium is a reproductive toxin in rodents. In male rats, after intraperitoneal injection of $CdCl_2$, 10 ml/kg, edema and hemorrhage of the testes, as well as acute destruction of the germinal epithelium, are regular events. There is a selective response of testicular and epididymal blood vessels to Cd^{2+}; endothelial lesions invariably are the first to occur. These effects can be prevented by Zn^{2+}, which competes with Cd^{2+}, in testes and prostate. Se^{2+} is about 100 times as effective as Zn^{2+} in counteracting testicular injury; concurrent administration of Se^{2+} also prevented to some extent Cd^{2+}-induced hyperglycemia, and hypoinsulinemia in rats given $CdCl_2$ (2×1 mg/kg/day for 7 days).

Whereas most of the orally administered Cd^{2+} in rats is excreted in the feces, about 2% is taken up across the wall of the small intestine. In the blood, the metal is probably associated with plasma protein (23). It is rapidly removed from the vascular system and accumulates in the pancreas and kidneys of mice, rats, and rabbits. Destruction of renal convoluted tubules gives rise to proteinuria. With the help of ultrastructural cytochemistry for the localization of Cd^{2+}, it was found that administration of 50 ppm Cd^{2+} in the drinking water for up to 8 months led to the accumulation of the element in lysosomes of proximal tubule cells (17). An increase in pinocytotic activity of these cells was noted in rabbits subjected to a comparable procedure.

In whole isolated heart perfused for up to 30 min with $3CdSO_4 \cdot 8H_2O$ at concentrations between 3×10^{-2} and 3×10^{-5} mM, Cd^{2+}-induced bradycardia was followed by atrioventricular blocking. Histologically, these alterations were accompanied by a vacuolization of the conductile tissues.

Cd^{2+} can cross the placenta and cause somatic malformations in mice and rats. Cd and specified Cd compounds cause cancer in experimental animals (27). Cd^{2+} has been implicated in the genesis of testicular tumors. Proliferation of Leydig cells and neoplastic interstitial cells has been found in rats and mice.

Animal Studies

The neurotoxic effects of Cd^{2+} in animals were first documented in 1893. Reflexes and the sensation of pain were abolished following injection of Cd^{2+} glucosate in cats and dogs; the animals succumbed to pulmonary edema and respiratory paralysis. A comparable pattern of responses was described in frogs, birds, and mammals.

A more recent study reports changes of locomotor behavior of newborn rats subjected to intraperitoneal injection of 100 $\mu g/kg$ of Cd^{2+} for 30 days. These functional signs were linked to interference with monoamine metabolism. Activities of acetylcholinesterase and adenylate cyclase show a considerable decrease after Cd^{2+} exposure (5). Following a single intraperitoneal dose of 840 $\mu g/kg$ of Cd^{2+}, hexobarbital-induced sleeping time was significantly prolonged in adult rats. The effect of Cd^{2+} exposure in mice is similar to lead-induced hypothermia, depending on the level of metal absorbed by the brain and its rate of uptake (12). Cd^{2+} may accumulate to a modest extent in the rabbit brain. However, in a study on 6-day-old rats, no more than 6% of $^{115}Cd^{2+}$ was located in the brain and spinal cord.

Changes in the CNS caused by Cd^{2+} are most likely to occur during early stages of fetal development. A single dose of 2.0 mg Cd^{2+} administered to pregnant rats at day 20 of gestation led to endothelial damage in the vessels of the caudate nuclei of fetuses at day 21 (19).

Encephalopathy ensued after intraperitoneal injection of 10 mg/kg $CdCl_2$ to rats and rabbits during the immediate postnatal period (18). Lesions consisted of extensive hemorrhages in the deeper portions of the gray matter and in the white matter. The cerebellum was particularly damaged by hemorrhage, and there was widespread necrosis of granule cells. Ethanol rendered the brain more susceptible to cadmium neurotoxicity (16).

Subcutaneous administration of $CdCl_2$ to adult rats leads to massive hemorrhage inside spinal and trigeminal ganglia. Necrosis of spinal ganglion cells develops. A study on guinea pigs, golden hamsters, mice, and rats noted hemorrhagic suffusions and necrosis of nervous parenchyma (19). Bleeding into peripheral ganglia resulted from endothelial lesions that became apparent after an interval of 15–30 min (7). Arterioles (9), venules, and capillaries (21) were the primary target vessels.

A long-term study of young rats exposed to low doses (10–20 ppm Cd^{2+}) in drinking water revealed a Cd^{2+}-induced neuropathy unassociated with hemorrhagic alterations (20). Membrane-bound glycogen deposits were located inside axons. Spinal nerve roots and sciatic nerves displayed pronounced demyelination. An unspecified number of spinal ganglion cells disappeared, and a discrete numerical increase of satellite cells was noted.

In acute Cd^{2+} poisoning, the vasculature bears the brunt of pathological changes in the PNS and CNS. Cd^{2+} disrupts calcium-dependent cell–cell interactions and alters the distribution of E-cadherin in cultured cells (4). In addition, a direct interference with the nervous parenchyma is most likely to take place in subacute and subchronic Cd^{2+} intoxication. In organized cultures of rat peripheral ganglia, pharmacological concentrations of $CdCl^{2+}$ (4×10^{-4} mol) induce pathological changes in dorsal root ganglion cells (25). During a culture period up to 3 weeks, aggregates of glycogen, often intermingled with lipid droplets, gradually filled the neuronal perikarya. Glycogen particles were also abundant inside nerve fibers. Other conspicuous changes consisted of filamentous whorls in neurons, and the formation of exceptionally large mitochondrial matrix granules in neurons and in Schwann cells. Electron probe x-ray microanalysis revealed the presence of Cd^{2+} mainly inside glycogen deposits and nucleoli of spinal ganglion cells. The element was also traceable in Schwann cell cytoplasm (24).

Human Studies

In an experiment on himself, Burdach reported that vomiting was induced by ingestion of half a grain of $CdSO_4$. The health hazards of Cd^{2+} became apparent with the commencement of large-scale production of the metal for industrial purposes. Factory workers who sustained acute Cd^{2+} poisoning by inhalation of fumes presented with vehement coughing, nausea, and difficulty in breathing because of bronchopneumonia (6). Reduction of the lung capacity persisted. Dryness of throat, headache, rapid pulse, nausea, brown-colored urine, and a sensation of cold developed in three reported cases. One individual died and, at autopsy, findings included congestion of the respiratory system, stomach, and intestine; fatty degeneration of the heart; and acute inflammation of the kidneys. Additional manifestations of acute poisoning were registered when the metal was used for treatment of syphilis, tuberculosis, and malaria. Heavy dyspnea, edema of the face, and mucous diarrhea ranked first among the side effects.

The main systemic responses in chronic Cd^{2+} poisoning are pulmonary emphysema, anosmia, yellowing of dental necks, and marked proteinuria. Emphysema is suggested to be caused by the activation of proteases that overcome the proteinase inhibitor system, including α_1-antitrypsin. Incubation of human plasma with Cd^{2+} caused a marked decrease of α_1-antitrypsin (28), a factor that is deficient in inherited obstructive lung disease. Renal damage may be mild or severe and is predominantly localized to the convoluted tubules.

Cd^{2+}–specific proteinuria and emphysema usually become clinically manifest years after initial exposure. In Japan, from 1939 until 1945, some 200 persons fell ill because of chronic Cd^{2+} poisoning. Clinically apparent cases were limited to women over 40 years of age who had given birth to many children and who had lived in the area for more than 30 years. Drinking water and water for irrigation of rice fields were drawn from a polluted river. A syndrome called *itai-itai* disease developed in exposed subjects. The disorder comprised severe pains in the bones, waddling gait, aminoaciduria, glycosuria, decreased pancreatic function, pronounced osteomalacia, and multiple pathological fractures (15). Although the spinal ganglia were not studied, the experimental evidence quoted above suggests that the pain was caused by involvement of this part of the sensory system. Half of the patients died. This was the hitherto most alarming indication of the danger inherent in chronic exposure to Cd^{2+}.

Cadmium encephalopathy was noted in a boy of East Indian origin; energy dispersive x-ray microprobe analysis of his brain revealed the presence of cadmium and a marked increase of sulfur, predominantly intracellular, both within neuroglial and, to a lesser degree, endothelial cells; localization was predominantly in the nucleus (18). There was marked cerebral swelling with herniation and histological evidence of perivascular protein leakage indicative of disruption of the blood-brain barrier. Kidney analysis showed cadmium deposition in renal tubules and in the basal lamina of podocytes within glomeruli. The source of cadmium, however, remained unknown.

There is limited evidence that Cd and Cd^{2+} compounds are carcinogenic in humans. Cd is classified as a probable human carcinogen (group 2A) (27). A causal relationship of Cd^{2+} in prostatic cancer cannot be ruled out; in patients suffering from carcinoma of the prostate, elevated concentrations of Cd^{2+} are demonstrable by means of atomic absorption spectrophotometry. Testicular endocrine function is also disturbed (13).

There is no specific treatment for acute or chronic cadmiosis in humans. Efforts to increase the urinary output by edathamil calcium disodium, or dimercaprol (British antilewisite) were discontinued because of renal damage. In mice, Cd^{2+} mobilization was achieved by new monoaralkyl- and monoalkylesters of meso-2,3-dimercaptosuccinic acid and by a dithiocarbamate; however, these substances cannot be used for therapy in humans (10).

Toxic Mechanisms

Since wide gaps between adjacent endothelial cells are a consistent and early pathological finding in acute Cd^{2+} poisoning (7,21), Cd^{2+} might compete for Ca^{2+}-rich binding sites on the cell surface and in junctional complexes. This hypothesis is substantiated by the finding that cadmium inhibits endothelin-binding activity (26) and, as stated, alters the distribution of E-cadherin (4).

Binding of Cd^{2+} to membrane protein has been held responsible for the noted depolarization of ionic currents in squid giant axon following application of this cation (1). The effect of Cd^{2+} on mitochondrial respiratory activity (11) may be equally important for the accumulation of lipids within spinal ganglia (25). Functional impairment of phosphorylase could constitute the biochemical background for the accumulation of glycogen in neurons *in situ* and *in vitro*; this key enzyme in glycogen degradation is sensitive to metal ions and compounds reacting with sulfhydryl groups (24).

REFERENCES

1. Begenesich T, Lynch C (1974) Effects of internal divalent cations on voltage-clamped squid axons. *J Gen Physiol* 63, 675.

2. Bin OH, Garfinkel D (1994) The cadmium toxicity hypothesis of aging: A possible explanation for the zinc deficiency hypothesis of aging. *Med Hypotheses* 42, 380.

3. Cai SW, Yue L, Hu ZN et al. (1990) Cadmium exposure and health effects among residents in an irrigation area with ore dressing wastewater. *Sci Total Envir* 90, 67.

4. Chen B, Hales BF (1994) Cadmium-induced rat embryotoxicity *in vitro* is associated with an increased abundance of E-cadherin protein in the yolk sac. *Toxicol Appl Pharmacol* 128, 293.

5. Fasitsas CD, Theocharis SE, Zoulas D et al. (1991) Time-dependent cadmium neurotoxicity in rat brain synaptosomal plasma membranes. *Comp Biochem Physiol Pt C* 100, 271.

6. Fuortes L, Leo A, Ellerbeck PG, Friell LA (1991) Acute respiratory fatality associated with exposure to sheet metal and cadmium fumes. *Clin Toxicol* 29, 279.

7. Gabbiani G, Badonnel MC, Mathewson SM, Graeme BR (1974) Acute cadmium intoxication. Early selective lesions of endothelial clefts. *Lab Invest* 30, 686.

8. Gabbiani G, Baic D, Déziel C (1967) Toxicity of cadmium for the central nervous system. *Exp Neurol* 18, 154.

9. Gabbiani G, Gregory A, Baic D (1967) Cadmium-induced selective lesions of sensory ganglia. *J Neuropathol Exp Neurol* 26, 498.

10. Jones MM, Singh PK, Basinger MA et al. (1994) Cadmium mobilization by monoaralkyl- and monoalkyl esters of meso-2,3-dimercaptosuccinic acid and by a dithiocarbamate. *Pharmacol Toxicol* 72, 76.

11. Koizumi T, Yokota T, Shirakura H et al. (1994) Potential mechanism of cadmium-induced cytotoxicity in rat hepatocytes: Inhibitory action of cadmium on mitochondrial respiratory activity. *Toxicology* 92, 115.

12. Martinez F, Vicente I, Garcia F et al. (1993) Effects of different factors in lead- and cadmium induced hypothermia in mice. *Eur J Pharmacol* 248, 199.

13. Mason HJ (1990) Occupational cadmium exposure and testicular endocrine function. *Hum Exp Toxicol* 9, 91.

14. Munoz C, Vormann J, Dieter HH (1989) Characterization and development of metallothionein in fetal forelimbs, brain and liver from the mouse. *Toxicol Lett* 45, 83.

15. Murata J (1971) Chronic entero-osteo-nephropathy due to cadmium ("itai-itai" disease). *J Jpn Med Assn* 65, 15.

16. Pal R, Nath R, Gill KD (1993) Influence of ethanol on cadmium accumulation and its impact on lipid peroxidation and membrane bound functional enzymes (Na^+, K^+-ATPase and acetylcholinesterase) in various regions of adult rat brain. *Neurochem Int* 23, 451.

17. Popham JD, Webster WS (1976) The ultrastructural localization of cadmium. *Histochemistry* 46, 249.

18. Provias JP, Ackerley CA, Smith C, Becker LE (1994) Cadmium encephalopathy: A report with elemental analysis and pathological findings. *Acta Neuropathol* 88, 583.

19. Rohrer SR, Shaw SM, Lamar CH (1978) Cadmium-induced endothelial cell alterations in the fetal brain. *Acta Neuropathol* 44, 147.

20. Sato K, Iwamasa T, Tsuru T, Takeuchi T (1978) An ultrastructural study of chronic cadmium-induced neuropathy. *Acta Neuropathol* 41, 185.

21. Schlaepfer WW (1971) Sequential study of endothelial changes in acute cadmium intoxication. *Lab Invest* **25**, 556.

22. Schwartze EW, Alsberg CL (1923) Studies on the pharmacology of cadmium and zinc with particular reference to emesis. *J Pharmacol Exp Ther* **21**, 1.

23. Shaikh ZA, Tohyama C, Nolan CV (1987) Occupational exposure to cadmium: Effect on metallothionein and other biological indices of exposure and renal function. *Arch Toxicol* **59**, 360.

24. Tischner KH (1980) Cadmium. In: *Experimental and Clinical Neurotoxicology.* Spencer PS, Schaumburg HH eds. Williams & Wilkins, Baltimore p. 348.

25. Tischner KH, Schröder JM (1972) The effects of cadmium chloride on organotypic cultures of rat sensory ganglia. *J Neurol Sci* **16**, 383.

26. Wada K, Fujii Y, Watanabe H *et al.* (1991) Cadmium directly acts on endothelin receptor and inhibits endothelin binding activity. *FEBS Lett* **285**, 71.

27. WHO (1992) *Environmental Health Criteria 134, Cadmium.* International Programme on Chemical Safety, World Health Organization, Geneva.

Calycanthine

Albert C. Ludolph

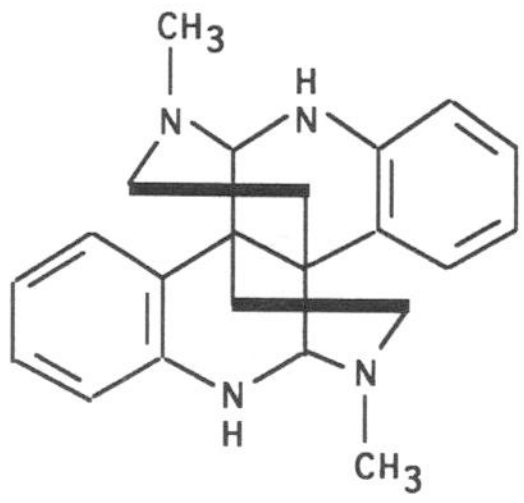

CALYCANTHINE
$C_{22}H_{26}N_4$

NEUROTOXICITY RATING

Experimental

A   Seizure disorder

Calycanthine is a powerful convulsant alkaloid of the order Calycanthaceae; it is also synthesized by *Chimonanthus praecox* and members of the genus *Psychotria* (Rubiaceae) (1,2). Little is known about the biological effects of this dimeric tetrahydroquinoline base (MW, 346.48). Reportedly, calycanthine alters behavioral parameters of mice (1) "similar to other neuropoisons such as strychnine." However, in the cockroach CNS, the effects of calycanthine are quite distinct from those of strychnine (1). In contrast to strychnine, calycanthine does not affect the axon membrane but, instead, interferes with synaptic transmission pre- and postsynaptically.

REFERENCES

1. Adjibade Y, Hue B, Pelhate M, Anton R (1991) Action of calycanthine on nervous transmission in cockroach central nervous system. *Planta Med* **57**, 99.

2. Budavari S (1996) *The Merck Index. 12th Ed.* Merck & Co, Rahway, New Jersey p. 280.

Canatoxin

Albert C. Ludolph

NEUROTOXICITY RATING

Experimental

B   Seizure disorder

Canatoxin is a powerful convulsant protein (MW, 115,000) present in seed of the Jack bean, *Canavalia ensiformis.* The compound is distinct from concanavalin A and canavanine, which are also present in this plant. Rats are reportedly 10- to 20-fold more sensitive to the toxic effects of canatoxin than mice. Parenteral administration to either species induces hypothermia, bradycardia, hypertension, and respiratory distress followed by tonic convulsions (3). Levels of the neurotransmitters γ-aminobutyric acid, dopamine, serotonin, and norepinephrine were unchanged in the CNS of treated animals (3), but rat brain synaptosomes revealed a concentration- and time-dependent increase of serotonin and dopamine release that could be blocked by lipoxygenase inhibitors (2). Subconvulsant doses of canatoxin produce hypoxemia, metabolic alkalosis, and long-lasting hypoglycemia *in vivo* (4). Hypoglycemia may reflect increased insulin secretion induced by canatoxin (4). The relationship between seizure activity and changes in carbohydrate metabolism is unclear (5,6). In rabbit skeletal muscle, canatoxin interacts dose-dependently with the Ca^{2+} pump; it uncouples Ca^{2+} uptake from Ca^{2+}-dependent ATP hydrolysis (1).

REFERENCES

1. Alves EW, Ferreira AT, Ferreira CT, Carlini CR (1992) Effects of canatoxin on the Ca^{2+}–ATPase of sarcoplasmic reticulum membranes. *Toxicon* 30, 1411.
2. Barja-Fidalgo TC, Carlini CR, Guimaraes JA (1988) The secretory effect of canatoxin on rat brain synaptosomes involves a lipoxygenase-mediated pathway. *Braz J Med Biol Res* 21, 249.
3. Carlini CR, Gomes CB, Guimaraes JA et al. (1984) Central nervous effects of the convulsant-protein canatoxin. *Acta Pharmacol Toxicol* 54, 161.
4. Carlini CR, Guimaraes JA (1991) Plant and microbial toxic proteins as hemilectins: Emphasis on canatoxin. *Toxicon* 29, 791.
5. Ribeiro-DaSilva G, Carlini CR, Pires-Barbosa R, Guimaraes JA (1986) Blood glucose alterations induced in rats by canatoxin, a protein isolated from Jack Bean (*Canavalia ensiformis*) seeds. *Toxicon* 24, 775.
6. Ribeiro-DaSilva G, Pires-Barbosa R, Prado JF, Carlini CR (1989) Convulsions induced by canatoxins in rats are probably a consequence of hypoxia. *Braz J Med Biol Res* 22, 877.

Cannabis

John C.M. Brust

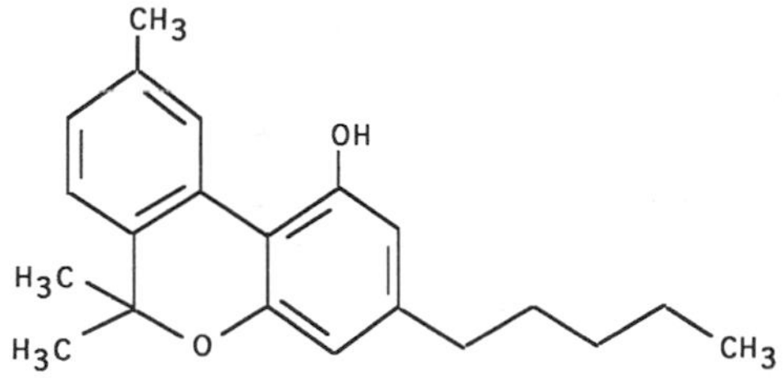

CANNABINOL
$C_{21}H_{26}O_2$

6,6,9-Trimethyl-3-pentyl-6*H*-dibenzo[b,d]pyran-1-ol

NEUROTOXICITY RATING

Clinical

A Acute encephalopathy (cognitive impairment, hallucinations)

A Physical dependence and withdrawal

C Chronic encephalopathy

Experimental

A Acute encephalopathy (sedation, memory impairment)

C Chronic encephalopathy

The hemp plant, *Cannabis sativa*, contain dozens of cannabinoid compounds (cannabinols) with different pharmacological properties. Isomers of tetrahydrocannabinol (THC), especially δ-9-THC, have psychoactive properties and are the basis of the plant's popularity as a recreational drug. Other cannabinols are sedating (cannabigerol), anticonvulsant (cannabinol, cannabidiol), analgesic (*9-β-*hydroxyhexahydrocannabinol), or antimicrobial (cannabidolic acid) (4,18).

A resin covering the flowers and leaves of the female plant contains the active substances. The resin protects the plant from dry heat and is more abundant in plants grown in tropical climates. "Marijuana" (also referred to as "ghanja," "bhang," "kif," or "dagga," as well as such street names as "grass," "pot," "tea," "reefer," and "weed") is made from cut tops and leaves of whole plants. "Hashish" ("charas") made from the resin itself, is much more potent (15).

Street marijuana may be contaminated with stramonium leaves, lysergic acid diethylamide, methamphetamine, or other drugs, and it is often deliberately taken with heroin, cocaine, or phencyclidine. Marijuana has additive or synergistic sedative effects with ethanol or barbiturates.

Although cannabinols are well absorbed from the gastrointestinal tract, marijuana and hashish are most often smoked. (The gummy, water-insolubility of the resin accounts for the rarity of parenteral abuse.) An average "good quality" marijuana cigarette delivers 2.5–5.0 mg δ-9-THC. Psychic effects begin within minutes of smoking, peak at 20–30 min, and last up to 2 or 3 h. After oral ingestion, effects begin after 30–60 min, peak after 2 or 3 h, and last up to 12 h. δ-9-THC is metabolized to 11-hydroxy-δ-9-THC, which is also psychoactive, and then to inactive metabolites that are excreted in urine and feces. Bile excretion leads to reabsorption, and both δ-9-THC and its metabolites are detected in blood for days or weeks after use (1).

Marijuana is classified by the U.S. Food and Drug Administration as a Schedule I controlled substance ("no accepted medical use; high potential for abuse"). Two commercial cannabinoid preparations are available (for appetite stimulation in patients with acquired immunodeficiency syndrome and for antiemesis in patients receiving cancer thermotherapy). Dronabinol is δ-9-THC. Nabilone is a synthetic compound. Both are taken orally (4).

Cannabinoids indirectly affect a number of CNS neurotransmitter systems, including the dopaminergic "reward circuit" from the midbrain ventral tegmental area to the nucleus accumbens and the medial prefrontal cortex (16). Directly, it acts at stereospecific receptors on neuronal membranes. Cannabinoid receptors are G-protein–coupled and inhibit adenyl cyclase dose-dependently (1). The cDNA for the cannabinoid receptor has been cloned; the gene resides on chromosome 6. An endogenous ligand (termed "anandamide," from the Sanskrit word for bliss) has also been identified; it is arachidonylethanol-amide, a C-20 fatty acid derivative (6).

The effects of psychoactive cannabinoids on animals often differ from those produced in humans. In mice, low doses of δ-9-THC induce simultaneous depression and stimulation, termed the "popcorn effect." The animals appear sedated until one mouse is stimulated, causing it to jump hyperreflexly; as it falls on another mouse, that animal jumps, and the ensuing chain-reaction resembles corn popping in a pan. Higher doses are more typically sedating but, in contrast to barbiturates or ethanol, they do not produce general anesthesia. δ-9-THC in animals also produces hypothermia and impairs memory and performance on complex tasks (7,17).

Animal studies on the reinforcing properties of psychoactive cannabinoids have been conflicting. Generally, animals are disinclined to self-administration. Tolerance develops to the psychoactive and hypothermic effects, but most studies have failed to identify a predictable abstinence syndrome (5). Also conflicting are animal studies of possible lasting CNS effects: rodents receiving δ-9-THC daily for months reportedly had impaired learning after several months of abstinence, but comparable studies in chimpanzees found no such effect. Abnormalities of hippocampal dendritic spines were described in rats after long-term δ-9-THC exposure; other studies in rodents and monkeys failed to demonstrate alterations in either cannabinoid or other neurotransmitter receptors.

Animal studies of cannabinoid exposure *in utero*, using pair-fed controls and surrogate fostering, have failed to identify behavioral or neurological abnormalities in the offspring.

Cannabidiol is anticonvulsant at all doses; δ-9-THC in animals is proconvulsant in low doses and anticonvulsant in high doses. Its effects on seizures, however, vary with species, seizure model, and route of administration (18).

Smoked marijuana may initially produce jitteriness or anxiety; there follows relaxed dreamy euphoria ("stoned"), often with jocularity or silliness (Table 6) (15). There is disinhibition or depersonalization, subjective slowing of time, and a sense of altered body proportion. Although many users report heightened awareness of events or stimuli, objective testing reveals decreased auditory and visual signal detection, reduced perception of the emotions of others, and impaired memory and problem-solving; decreased performance on cognitive tasks can last hours longer than subjective effects. Motor coordination is also compromised, as is driving (10).

Systemic effects include tachycardia, systolic hypertension, conjunctival injection, decreased salivation, urinary frequency, increased thirst and appetite, decreased intraocular pressure, bronchodilation, analgesia, and selective reduction of rapid-eye-movement sleep. In contrast to ethanol, marijuana-induced sleep is not followed by "hangover."

High doses cause auditory and visual illusions or hallucinations, unformed or formed. Still higher doses cause confusion, disorientation, psychotic depression or excitement, bradycardia, and hypotension, but fatal overdose has not been documented. Some users develop, in the absence of other signs of toxicity, acute adverse reactions consisting of intense anxiety, paranoia, delusions, depression, or panic ("freaking out"); such symptoms can last hours or days (12,19). "Flashbacks" consist of the spontaneous recurrence of cannabis effects, including hallucinations, weeks or months after last use. Their physiological basis is unknown (14).

TABLE 6. Acute Effects of Marijuana

Anxiety, jitteriness, paranoia
Euphoria, relaxation, jocularity
Depersonalization
Subjective time-slowing
Dizziness, sensation of floating
Impaired memory and problem-solving
Impaired balance and hand steadiness
Conjunctival injection
Decreased salivation
Urinary frequency
Tachycardia
Systolic hypertension and postural hypotension
Increased appetite and thirst
Decreased intraocular pressure
Analgesia
Auditory and visual illusions and hallucinations
Psychotic excitement or depression
Bradycardia, hypotension
Acute dysphoria, panic

Acute toxic reactions to cannabis can usually be managed with calm reassurance. Benzodiazepines or haloperidol can be used for severe symptoms.

Tolerance develops to marijuana's cardiovascular, motor, and psychic effects. Controversial is the possible occurrence in some users of "reverse tolerance" ("sensitization"), with repeated use more readily producing a "high." Withdrawal after several weeks of daily use in humans has produced anxiety, emotional lability, insomnia, anorexia, nausea, vomiting, tremor, sweating, and salivation, but such symptoms are unusual (11); most abrupt abstainers experience at most jitteriness, anorexia, headache, and mild gastrointestinal upset without objective signs. Craving for the drug is common (13).

Uncertain and highly controversial is whether cannabis use can cause lasting mental abnormalities (20). Early reports described on "antimotivational syndrome" in chronic users, consisting of diminished drive and ambition, apathy and flat affect, decreased attentiveness, and impaired recent memory. Most subsequent neuropsychological studies from different countries, comparing users to nonusers, found no significant differences; a frequent problem with studies claiming mental abnormalities in cannabis users is the absence of any measure of predrug cognitive functioning. A personality disorder could as well be the cause of marijuana use as its effect. Current evidence suggests that if cannabinoid exposure causes lasting behavioral or intellectual abnormalities, they are very subtle (11).

Cannabinoids easily cross the placenta, and newborns exposed in utero have had decreased birth weight and body length, and reduced nonfat mass. These findings are similar to those reported in the offspring of tobacco smokers; they implicate hypoxia or nonnutritional toxic effects (21). Whether such exposure also causes neurobehavioral abnormalities is less certain; studies claiming delays in motor development or impaired performance on verbal or memory tests have often been confounded by the presence of maternal malnutrition, exposure to other substances, and a pernicious home environment (8,9).

Cannabis users have reduced response of growth hormone and cortisol to hypoglycemia (2), as well as impaired secretion of follicle-stimulating hormone (FSH) and luteinizing hormone (3). There is impotence, decreased sperm count, and gynecomastia in men and menstrual irregularity with anovulatory cycles in women. Normal function returns with abstinence.

Anecdotal reports of stroke in cannabis users have been unconvincing as to cause and effect.

The acute effects of psychoactive cannabinoids presumably result from actions on specific neuronal receptors, with indirect actions on a multitude of other neurotransmitter systems. Claims that chronic or in utero cannabis exposure causes lasting neurobehavioral abnormalities are, to date, unsupported by convincing evidence.

REFERENCES

1. Abood ME, Martin BR (1992) Neurology of marijuana abuse. *Trends Pharmacol Sci* **13**, 201.
2. Benowitz NL, Jones RT, Lerner CB (1976) Depression of growth hormone and cortisol response to insulin-induced hypoglycemia after prolonged oral delta-9-tetrahydrocannabinol administration in man. *J Clin Endocrinol Metab* **42**, 938.
3. Block RI, Farinpour R, Schlechte JA (1991) Effects of chronic marijuana use on testosterone, luteinizing hormone, follicle stimulating hormone, prolactin, and cortisol in men and women. *Drug Alcohol Dependence* **28**, 121.
4. Brust JCM (1993) *Neurological Aspects of Substance Abuse*. Butterworth-Heinemann, Stoneham, MA p. 131.
5. Compton DR, Dewey WL, Martin BR (1990) Cannabis dependence and tolerance production. *Adv Alcohol Subst Abuse* **9**, 129.
6. Devane WA, Hanus L, Breuer A *et al.* (1992) Isolation and structure of a constituent that binds to the cannabinoid receptor. *Science* **258**, 1946.
7. Dewey WL (1986) Cannabinoid pharmacology. *Pharmacol Rev* **38**, 151.
8. Fried PA, Watkinson B (1988) 12- and 24-Month neurobehavioral follow-up of children prenatally exposed to marijuana, cigarettes, and alcohol. *Neurotoxicol Teratol* **10**, 305.
9. Fried PA, Watkinson B (1990) 36- and 48-Month neurobehavioral follow-up of children prenatally exposed to marijuana, cigarettes, and alcohol. *J Develop Behav Pediat* **11**, 49.
10. Heishman SJ, Huestis MA, Henningfield JE, Cone EJ (1990) Acute and residual effects of marijuana: Profiles of plasma THC levels, physiological, subjective, and performance measures. *Pharmacol Biochem Behav* **37**, 561.
11. Hollister LE (1986) Health aspects of cannabis. *Pharmacol Rev* **38**, 1.
12. Imade AG, Ebic JC (1991) A retrospective study of symptom patterns of cannabis-induced psychosis. *Acta Psychiat Scand* **83**, 134.
13. Jones RT, Benowitz N (1976) The 30-day trip—clinical studies of cannabis tolerance and dependence. In: *Pharmacology of Marijuana*. Braude MC, Szara S eds. Raven Press, New York p. 627.
14. Keller M, Reifler CB, Lipzin MB (1968) Spontaneous recurrence of marijuana effect. *Amer J Psychiat* **125**, 384.
15. Lieberman CM, Lieberman BW (1971) Marijuana—A medical review. *N Engl J Med* **284**, 88.
16. Martin BR (1986) Cellular effects of cannabinoids. *Pharmacol Rev* **38**, 45.

17. Pertwee RG (1988) The central neuropharmacology of psychotropic cannabinoids. *Pharmacol Ther* **36**, 189.
18. Seth R, Sinha S (1991) Chemistry and pharmacology of cannabis. *Prog Drug Res* **36**, 71.
19. Weil AT (1970) Adverse reactions to marijuana: Classification and suggested treatment. *N Engl J Med* **282**, 997.
20. Weinreib RM, O'Brien CP (1993) Persistent cognitive deficits attributed to substance abuse. *Neurol Clin* **11**, 663.
21. Zuckerman B, Frank DA, Hingson R *et al.* (1989) Effects of marijuana and cocaine use on fetal growth. *N Engl J Med* **320**, 762.

Cantharidin

Herbert H. Schaumburg

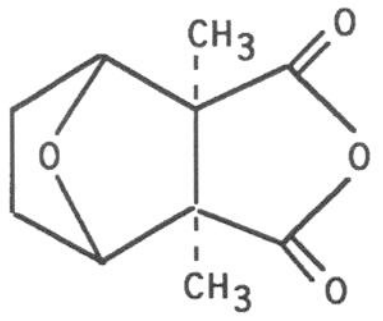

CANTHARIDIN
$C_{10}H_{12}O_4$

Hexahydro-3a,7a-dimethyl-4,7-epoxyisobenzofuran-1,3-dione

NEUROTOXICITY RATING

Clinical

B   Seizure disorder

Cantharidin, the anhydride of cantharidic acid, is derived from the dried and powdered blister beetle, *Cantharis ves-* *icatoria* (Spanish fly). It is used as an active ingredient of wart-removing compounds. Irritation of the membranes of the genitourinary tracts (priapism in men, pelvic congestion in women) account for its reputation as an aphrodisiac.

Cardiac arrhythmias, especially ventricular tachycardia and renal tubular necrosis, are the most serious systemic adverse effects.

Generalized seizures may accompany severe, sometimes fatal, cantharidin intoxication (1,2).

REFERENCES

1. Till J, Majmudar B (1981) Cantharidin poisoning. *Southern Med J* **74**, 444
2. Karras DJ, Farrell SE, Harrigan RA *et al.* (1996) Poisoning from "Spanish fly" (cantharidin). *Amer J Emerg Med* **14**, 478.

Capsaicin and Analogs

Rainer Amann
Peter Holzer

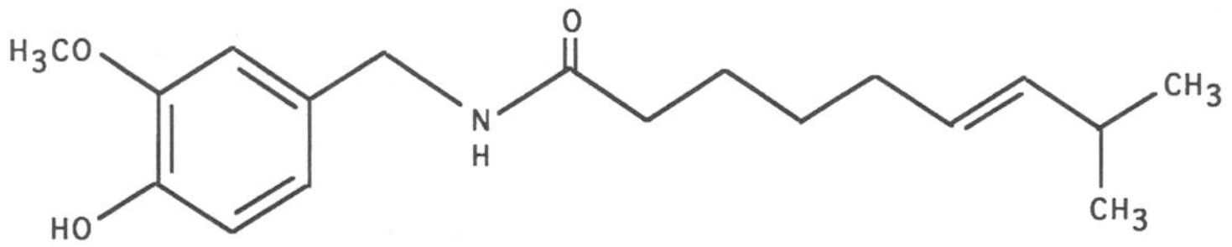

CAPSAICIN
$C_{18}H_{27}NO_3$

trans-8-Methyl-*N*-vanillyl-6-nonenamide

NEUROTOXICITY RATING

Clinical

A   Peripheral neuropathy (afferent terminal irritation)

Experimental

A   Neuronopathy (dorsal root ganglion cell)

A   Peripheral afferent terminal degeneration

Capsaicin, a derivative of vanillyl amide, is the pungent ingredient in a wide variety of red peppers of the genus *Capsicum*.

Capsaicin is a crystalline white-yellow powder soluble in organic solvents, such as ethanol or dimethyl sulfoxide (DMSO). It is found as an alimentary additive in a large variety of foods (15); consumption of a "hot spicy" meal can provide an oral intake of as much as 20 mg capsaicin (32).

Over-the-counter medications containing *Capsicum* extracts or capsaicin for topical application to the skin are available in several countries. Traditionally, these medications have been used to relieve various pain syndromes originating from the musculature. The subjective relief associated with this treatment may be due primarily to the acute effects of capsaicin: hyperemia, a feeling of warmth, and a mild burning sensation.

Because of the progress that has been made in understanding the mode of action of capsaicin on primary afferent neurons, the possible therapeutic effect of capsaicin has been studied in more detail. Repeated topical application of capsaicin causes a reversible loss of function of a population of primary afferent neurons that mediates perception of pain and promotes local inflammatory responses (22). Therefore, a possible effect of capsaicin-containing medications has been investigated for potential analgesic and anti-inflammatory actions (7). However, a major problem in conducting double-blind, placebo-controlled studies is the fact that the acute irritating effects of capsaicin cannot be concealed from patients or investigators.

General Toxicity

After oral intake in rats, capsaicin is readily absorbed from the gastrointestinal tract mainly *via* a nonactive process in the jejunum (30). After intestinal absorption, labeled dihydrocapsaicin is metabolized to a large extent in the liver before reaching the systemic circulation. When administered in low doses (50 mg), less than 5% unchanged compound is recovered in arterial blood (12). After intragastric application of 20 mg dihydrocapsaicin, 9% and 10% unchanged substance are detected in urine and feces, respectively (29). There are no data concerning cutaneous absorption after topical application of capsaicin.

After subcutaneous (s.c.) administration in rats, capsaicin is detectable in most tissues within 10 min and in adipose tissue 30 min after administration. It readily enters the CNS, where concentrations of capsaicin are similar to those in peripheral blood (38).

In the rat liver, capsaicin and dihydrocapsaicin undergo hydrolysis of the acid–amide linkage (29), oxidation of the vanillyl ring, or aliphatic hydroxylation (39). The metabolites (*e.g.*, vanillyl amine, vanillin, vanillyl alcohol, vanillic acid, and ω-hydroxycapsaicin), together with a small amount of the unchanged parent molecule, are excreted mainly in the urine (29,39).

With respect to target, potency, and mechanism of action, two effects of capsaicin can be differentiated (22): one action of capsaicin is grossly selective for thin primary afferent neurons of mammalian species. Initially, capsaicin causes excitation of C- and Aδ-afferent fibers, an effect that may soon subside and be followed by unresponsiveness of the neurons to further capsaicin exposure and to other stimuli. The initial excitation is accompanied by local release of proinflammatory neuropeptides from afferent nerve endings. Higher doses of capsaicin can cause prolonged defunctionalization and, when administered to newborn rats, irreversible damage of afferent neurons. The other action of capsaicin is cell-nonselective and consists usually of a transient depression of cell excitability. The concentrations of capsaicin required to produce these nonselective effects are commonly orders of magnitude higher than those sufficient to stimulate primary afferent neurons.

Animal Studies

Parenteral administration of high doses of capsaicin to rats causes hypotension, dyspnea and, finally, respiratory arrest (35). These effects are explained to some extent by capsaicin-induced excitation of afferent nerve endings and subsequent release of neuropeptides that cause vasodilation, edema, and bronchoconstriction (21). Topical application of capsaicin causes pain and local reddening of the skin (24) or, when inhaled, irritation of the airways and coughing (16). Exposure of the rat eye to capsaicin causes intense blepharospasm and a wiping response (42). Acute excitation of afferent neurons by capsaicin is followed by unresponsiveness to capsaicin and other irritant chemicals.

Higher doses of capsaicin cause age-dependent pathological changes in small sensory neurons of dorsal root ganglia. This neurotoxic action has been frequently used as an experimental tool to defunctionalize a subpopulation of primary afferent neurons in laboratory animals. For this purpose, capsaicin ($\geq$50 mg/kg) is administered s.c., the total dose being delivered often over several days to avoid acute adverse reactions, which arise from the irritant effect of capsaicin. Under these conditions, animals survive relatively high dosages of capsaicin (*i.e.*, several hundred mg/kg) and show deficits that are assumed to reflect a selective neurotoxic action of capsaicin on primary afferent neurons (22).

Capsaicin-induced degeneration of primary afferent neurons has been observed in the dog, cat, guinea pig, mouse, and rat (22).

Small primary afferent neurons in 1- to 12-day old rats are particularly sensitive to the neurotoxic action of capsaicin (25,26). The threshold dose for degeneration of unmyelinated axons in dorsal roots and axon terminals in the spinal cord lies between 5 and 15 mg/kg s.c. (25). A dose of 50 mg/kg s.c. is thought to cause maximal degeneration of afferent neurons that support unmyelinated axons. Functional deficits that arise from capsaicin administration to newborn rats persist during adult life (22).

In the adult rat, s.c. administration of 35–300 mg/kg capsaicin causes ultrastructural signs of damage in dorsal root ganglion cells and degeneration of peripheral afferent terminals (11,23,27,28). The functional deficits after treatment of adult rats with capsaicin usually reverse after several weeks to months.

Apart from its selective neurotoxic effects, prolonged capsaicin exposure may have carcinogenic effects in laboratory animals. In mice, capsaicin has been reported to induce duodenal adenocarcinomas (43) and to promote stomach and liver tumors (1).

In Vitro Studies

Intracellular recording from rat dorsal root ganglion (DRG) or nodose ganglion neurons has shown that capsaicin causes depolarization accompanied by increased membrane conductance. These responses become smaller upon repeated applications of capsaicin (20,34). Prolonged exposure of DRG cells to capsaicin (≥ 1 mM) causes rapid neuronal damage and eventually cell death of responsive cells (4,34). DRG cells that are cultured in the absence of nerve growth factor are largely unresponsive to capsaicin, and replacement of nerve growth factor restores the sensitivity to capsaicin (45).

Peripheral and central endings of primary afferent neurons respond to capsaicin in a manner similar to that of ganglion cell bodies. After initial stimulation of mediator release, application of capsaicin leads to unresponsiveness of afferent neurons to further capsaicin exposure (pharmacological desensitization) and, at higher concentrations, to general blockade (functional desensitization) of afferent neuron function (2,13,14).

A mutagenic activity of capsaicin was reported to occur in Chinese hamster lung cells (31) and in the Ames test (37,43). In transformed cells of human origin, but not in normal cells, capsaicin has been shown to inhibit reduced nicotinamide adenine dinucleotide oxidase and growth (36).

Human Studies

The acute effects of capsaicin in humans are caused by irritation of afferent nerve endings. On the skin, capsaicin produces local reddening and pain (24) and, in the airways, intense coughing (17). Asthmatic and nonasthmatic subjects seem to respond to capsaicin in a similar manner (6).

Various studies have addressed the possibility that capsaicin exposure may have carcinogenic/mutagenic effects,

but results have been negative (18,44). In view of the fact that capsaicin has been used as a food additive for centuries, the absence of firm epidemiological evidence for a carcinogenic action argues against such effects in humans. However, a recent study suggested, but did not prove, an association between chili pepper consumption and gastric cancer (33).

Toxic Mechanism

A capsaicin receptor has been proposed on the basis of structure–activity relationships of several synthetic capsaicin analogues (41). Studies using resiniferatoxin (RTX), an ultrapotent capsaicin analogue, and capsazepine, a competitive capsaicin antagonist, have provided convincing evidence for a specific vanilloid-binding site (40); this has been cloned and characterized as a nonselective cation channel (8).

Binding of capsaicin activates this cation channel, thus depolarizing the nerve cell. Subsequent challenges with capsaicin produce attenuated responses. At low concentrations, this phenomenon of desensitization probably reflects blockade of capsaicin-specific excitation mechanisms and has to be differentiated from cellular neurotoxicity (3).

Neuronal desensitization is probably caused by capsaicin-induced increase in intracellular calcium (3). Exposure of cells to capsaicin in calcium-free medium does not produce desensitization, even in the presence of carbonyl cyanide p-(tri-fluoromethoxy)phenyl hydrazone, which liberates calcium from internal stores (10). It seems, therefore, that desensitization depends on extracellular calcium that enters the cell *via* the capsaicin-operated channel and which acts locally, either near or within the activated channel.

The cellular neurotoxic effects of capsaicin can be explained by excess influx of calcium and sodium ions, and the concomitant influx of water, which produces osmotic swelling and cell damage (5). In addition, calcium-activated proteolytic enzymes, such as calpain, may play a part in the capsaicin-induced cell damage (9).

Capsaicin Analogues

Among the large number of capsaicin analogues that has been employed in experimental studies, the phorbol ester RTX has attracted most interest. RTX occurs naturally in the latex of *Euphorbia resinifera*, *E. poissonii*, and *E. unispina*. Isolated in 1975 (19), it is a diterpene esterified at C-20 with homovanillic acid. As a consequence, RTX lacks a free 20-hydroxyl group, which is essential for phorbol ester activity and thus fails to stimulate protein kinase C and to have tumor-promoting activity (40).

The vanillyl group relates RTX to capsaicin, and the structural similarity of the two compounds forms the basis for a common mechanism of action. The available evidence indicates that RTX and capsaicin share common binding site(s) on primary afferents and produce very similar effects, RTX being usually much more potent than capsaicin (40).

Administration of RTX, like capsaicin, induces ultrastructural changes in small dorsal root ganglion neurons of adult rats (41). Administration of RTX to newborn rats causes degeneration of about 50% of dorsal root ganglion cells and functional deficits that are similar to those produced by neonatal capsaicin, but RTX is at least two orders of magnitude more potent than capsaicin (22).

REFERENCES

1. Agrawal RC, Wiessler M, Hecker E (1986) Tumor-promoting effect of chili extract in Balb/c mice. *Int J Cancer* **38**, 689.

2. Amann R (1990) Desensitization of capsaicin-evoked neuropeptide release—Influence of Ca^{2+} and temperature. *Naunyn-Schmied Arch Pharmacol* **342**, 671.

3. Bevan SJ, Docherty RJ (1993) Cellular mechanisms of action of capsaicin. In: *Capsaicin in the Study of Pain*. Wood J ed. Academic Press, London p. 27.

4. Bevan SJ, James IF, Rang HP *et al.* (1987) The mechanism of action of capsaicin—a sensory neurotoxin. In: *Neurotoxins and Their Pharmacological Implications*. Jenner P ed. Raven Press, New York p. 261.

5. Bevan SJ, Szolcsanyi J (1990) Sensory neuron-specific actions of capsaicin: Mechanisms and applications. *Trends Pharmacol Sci* **11**, 330.

6. Blanc P, Liu D, Juares C, Boushey HA (1991) Cough in hot pepper workers. *Chest* **99**, 27.

7. Campbell E, Bevan S, Dray A (1987) Clinical applications of capsaicin and its analogues. In: *Capsaicin in the Study of Pain*. Wood J ed. Academic Press, London p. 255.

8. Caterina MJ, Schumacher MA, Tominaga M *et al.* (1997) The capsaicin receptor: Heat-activated ion channel in the pain pathway. *Nature* **389**, 816.

9. Chard PS, Savidge JR, Bleakman D, Miller RJ (1992) Calpain inhibitors prevent capsaicin-dependent neurotoxicity in dorsal root ganglion neurons. *Soc Neurosci (Abstr)* **18**, 465.9.

10. Cholewinsky A, Burgess G, Bevan S (1993) The role of calcium in capsaicin-induced desensitization in rat cultured dorsal root ganglion neurons. *Neuroscience* **55**, 1015.

11. Chung K, Klein CM, Coggeshall RE (1990) The receptive part of the primary afferent axon is most vulnerable to systemic capsaicin in the adult rat. *Brain Res* **511**, 222.

12. Donnerer J, Amann R, Schuligoi R, Lembeck F (1990) Absorption and metabolism of capsaicinoids following intragastric administration in rats. *Naunyn-Schmied Arch Pharmacol* **342**, 357.

13. Dray A, Bettany J, Forster P (1990) Actions of capsaicin on peripheral nociceptors of the neonatal rat spinal cord-tail *in vitro*: Dependence of extracellular and independence of second messengers. *Brit J Pharmacol* **101**, 727.

14. Dray A, Hankins MW, Yeats JC (1989) Desensitization and capsaicin-induced release of substance P-like immunoreactivity from guinea-pig ureter *in vitro*. *Neuroscience* **31**, 479.

15. Edwards SJ, Colquhoun EQ, Clark MG (1990) Levels of pungent principles in chili sauces and *Capsicum* fruit in Australia. *Food Aust* **42**, 432.

16. Forsberg K, Karlsson J-A, Theodorsson E *et al.* (1988) Cough and bronchoconstriction mediated by capsaicin-sensitive sensory neurons in the guinea-pig. *Pulm Pharmacol* **1**, 33.

17. Fuller RW, Dixon CM, Barnes PJ (1985) Bronchoconstrictor response to inhaled capsaicin in humans. *J Appl Physiol* **85**, 1080.

18. Godvindarajan VS, Sathyanarayana MN (1991) *Capsicum* production, technology, chemistry and quality. Part V: Impact on physiology, pharmacology, nutrition and metabolism; structure, pungency, pain and desensitization sequences. *Crit Rev Food Sci Nutr* **29**, 435.

19. Hergenhahn M, Adolph W, Hecker E (1975) Resiniferatoxin and other esters of novel polyfunctional diterpenes from *Euphorbia resinifera* and *unispina*. *Tetrahedron Lett* **19**, 1595.

20. Heyman I, Rang HP (1985) Depolarizing responses to capsaicin in subpopulation of rat dorsal root ganglion cells. *Neurosci Lett* **56**, 69.

21. Holzer P (1988) Local effector function of capsaicin-sensitive sensory nerve endings: Involvement of tachykinins, calcitonin gene-related peptide and other neuropeptides. *Neuroscience* **24**, 739.

22. Holzer P (1991) Capsaicin: Cellular targets, mechanism of action, and selectivity for thin sensory neurons. *Pharmacol Rev* **43**, 143.

23. Hoyes AD, Barber P (1981) Degeneration of axons in the ureteric and duodenal nerve plexuses of the adult rat following *in vivo* treatment with capsaicin. *Neurosci Lett* **25**, 19.

24. Jancsó G, Jancsó-Gábor A, Szolcsányi J (1968) The role of sensory nerve endings in neurogenic inflammation induced in human skin and in the eye and paw of the rat. *Brit J Pharmacol* **33**, 32.

25. Jancsó G, Király E (1981) Sensory neurotoxins: Chemically induced selective degeneration of primary sensory neurons. *Brain Res* **210**, 83.

26. Jancsó G, Király E, Jancsó-Gábor A (1977) Pharmacologically induced selective degeneration of chemosensitive primary sensory neurones. *Nature* **270**, 741.

27. Jancsó G, Király E, Joó F (1985) Selective degeneration by capsaicin of a subpopulation of primary sensory neurons in the adult rat. *Neurosci Lett* **59**, 209.

28. Joó F, Szolcsányi J, Jancsó-Gábor A (1969) Mitochondrial alterations in the spinal ganglion cells of the rat accompanying the long-lasting sensory disturbance induced by capsaicin. *Life Sci* **8**, 621.

29. Kawada T, Iwai K (1985) *In vivo* and *in vitro* metabolism of dihydrocapsaicin, a pungent principle of hot pepper, in rats. *Agr Biol Chem* **49**, 441.

30. Kawada T, Suzuki T, Takahashi M, Iwai K (1984) Gastrointestinal absorption and metabolism of capsaicin and dihydrocapsaicin in rats. *Toxicol Appl Pharmacol* **72**, 449.

31. Lawson T, Gannett P (1989) The mutagenicity of capsaicin and dihydrocapsaicin in V79 cells. *Cancer Lett* **48**, 109.

32. Limlomwongse L, Shaittauchawong C, Tongyai S (1979) Effect of capsaicin on gastric acid secretion and mucosal blood flow. *J Nutr* **109**, 773.

33. Lopez-Carrillo L, Avila MH, Dubrow R (1993) Chili pepper consumption and gastric cancer in Mexico: A case-control study. *Amer J Epidemiol* **139**, 263.

34. Marsh SJ, Stansfeld CE, Brown DA *et al.* (1987) The mechanism of action of capsaicin on sensory C-type neurons and their axons *in vitro*. *Neuroscience* **23**, 275.

35. Monsereenusorn Y, Kongsamut S, Pezalla PD (1982) Capsaicin—A literature survey. *Crit Rev Toxicol* **10**, 321.

36. Morre DJ, Chueh PJ, Morre DM (1995) Capsaicin inhibits preferentially NADH oxidase and growth of transformed cells in culture. *Proc Nat Acad Sci USA* **92**, 1831.

37. Nagabhushan M, Bhide SV (1985) Mutagenicity of chili extract and capsaicin in short-term tests. *Environ Mutagen* **7**, 881.

38. Saria A, Skofitsch G, Lembeck F (1982) Distribution of capsaicin in rat tissues after systemic administration. *J Pharm Pharmacol* **34**, 273.

39. Surh Y-J, Ahn HS, Kim K-C *et al.* (1995) Metabolism of capsaicinoids: Evidence for aliphatic hydroxylation and its pharmacological implications. *Life Sci* **56**, PL305.

40. Szallasi A, Blumberg PM (1990) Resiniferatoxin and its analogs provide novel insights into the pharmacology of the vanilloid (capsaicin) receptor. *Life Sci* **47**, 1399.

41. Szallasi A, Joó F, Blumberg PM (1989) Duration of desensitization and ultrastructural changes in dorsal root ganglia in rats treated with resiniferatoxin, an ultrapotent capsaicin analog. *Brain Res* **503**, 68.

42. Szolcsányi J, Jancsó-Gábor A (1975) Sensory effects of capsaicin congeners. I. Relationship between chemical structure and pain-producing potency of pungent agents. *Drug Res* **25**, 1877.

43. Toth B, Rogan E, Walker B (1984) Tumorigenicity and mutagenicity studies with capsaicin of hot peppers. *Anticancer Res* **4**, 117.

44. Winek CL, Markie DC, Shanor SP (1982) Pepper sauce toxicity. *Drug Chem Toxicol* **5**, 89.

45. Winter J, Forbes A, Sternberg J, Lindsay RM (1988) Nerve growth factor (NGF) regulates adult rat cultured dorsal root ganglion neuron responses to the excitotoxin capsaicin. *Neuron* **1**, 973.

Captopril

Herbert H. Schaumburg

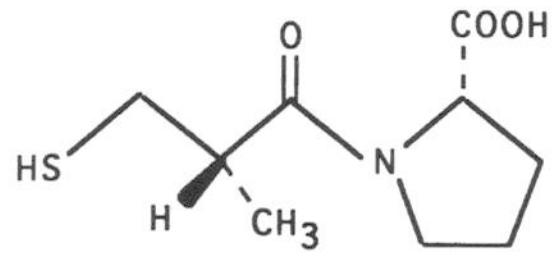

CAPTOPRIL
C₉H₁₅NO₃S

(S)-1-(3-Mercapto-2-methyl-1-oxopropyl)-L-proline

NEUROTOXICITY RATING

Clinical

B Headache

C Peripheral neuropathy

Captopril is an angiotensin-converting enzyme (ACE) inhibitor widely used in treatment of essential hypertension. It is considered safe and effective; principal systemic toxic reactions center around sudden decreases in blood pressure associated with commencement of therapy. In common with other ACE inhibitors, captopril may cause headache, fatigue, and lightheadedness. A 1980 report of two cases of peripheral nerve disease, Guillain-Barré syndrome and a peroneal palsy, suggested that captopril therapy may cause neuropathy (1). Since no similar cases have subsequently appeared, the association was likely fortuitous.

REFERENCE

1. Atkinson AB, Brown JJ, Lever AF *et al.* (1980) Neurological dysfunction in two patients receiving captopril and cimetidine. *Lancet* **2**, 36.

Carbamates

Donald J. Ecobichon

$$R_3 - O - \overset{\overset{\displaystyle O^{(S)}}{\|}}{C} - N \overset{\displaystyle R_1}{\underset{\displaystyle R_2}{<}}$$

(-S-)

CARBAMATES

Insecticides; Fungicides

NEUROTOXICITY RATING

Clinical

A Acute encephalopathy (cholinergic syndrome)

A Neuromuscular transmission syndrome

B Peripheral neuropathy

Experimental

A Neuromuscular transmission dysfunction (CNS-PNS anticholinesterase inhibition)

A Acute encephalopathy (cognitive dysfunction)

The basic structures of carbamates are either carbamic (the monoamide of carbon dioxide) or dithiocarbamic (the monoamide of carbon disulfide) acids, highly unstable molecules that decompose rapidly. However, with the introduction of one or more N-alkyl substituents (at R_1 and R_2 above), the synthesis of aliphatic or aryl esters (at R_3 above), or the incorporation of different cations (sodium, manganese, magnesium, zinc), these chemicals become stable, more lipophilic and less hydrophilic, and show varying biological potency and selectivity.

The salts and esters of carbamic and dithiocarbamic acids are widely used as insecticides, herbicides, and fungicides, with one chemical, disulfiram (tetraethylthiuram), having properties useful in treating alcoholism in aversion programs (*see* Disulfiram, this volume). Many of these chemicals are potential neurotoxicants, particularly following occupational, accidental, or suicidal exposure either to single, high concentrations or prolonged exposure to moderate levels. Here, the subject of carbamate toxicity is divided into: (a) agents possessing insecticidal properties and showing either direct or indirect actions on the nervous system; and (b) others used as fungicides that appear for the most part to act indirectly through their breakdown products.

INSECTICIDES

Most carbamate insecticides in use are N-monomethyl (N-methylcarbamates, methylcarbamates) carbamate esters with a broad array of substituents that influence the lipid solubility, species specificity (usually by way of selective bio-transformation and degradation), and potency of the agent as an anticholinesterase (Table 7). The newest group of methylcarbamate insecticides are derivatives of aliphatic oximes, resembling aldehydes or ketones in structure and being relatively water soluble (*e.g.*, aldicarb, methomyl) (Table 7). The general toxicology of carbamate insecticides has been reviewed extensively (1,12), while that associated specifically with neurotoxicity has been reviewed elsewhere (6).

General Toxicology

Carbamate insecticides (esters) decompose slowly in acidic, aqueous solutions but rapidly in alkaline medium. Stabilization of the ester bond occurs with mono- or dimethyl substitution of the carbamoyl nitrogen. N-Monomethylcarbamates degrade slowly, the half-life of carbaryl being approximately 10 days, whereas the N-dimethylcarbamates are exceedingly stable, the half-life of dimetilan being 100 days. Most of the carbamate insecticides are absorbed efficiently from the gastrointestinal tract and are distributed within body compartments according to their lipophilicity as measured by an oil/water coefficient (K_{ow}). It is stated that little storage of carbamates occurs, biotransformation being rapid. However, there are several cases reported in the literature mentioning episodic or prolonged biological effects following exposure, suggesting the possible cyclic release and storage of the biologically active agent.

Carbamate esters are susceptible to rapid hydrolysis by the ubiquitous carboxylesterases or aliesterases [E.C. 3.1.1.1] found in all mammalian tissues, the rate being governed by the molecular structure, the tissue level of enzyme activity, and the substrate specificity of the enzymes (5). In the rat, the percent hydrolysis for carbofuran, propoxur, carbaryl, aldicarb, zectran, and mobam is 23%, 31%, 39%–65%, 53%–62%, 76%, and 99%, respectively (18). Hydrolysis appears to be a minor pathway in most insect species (except the cockroach) and in the pig and the monkey.

The biotransformation of carbaryl has been studied extensively, but few other carbamates have received the same detailed attention. Phase I oxidative reactions, using the hemoprotein cytochrome P-450 (and P-448), occur, usually limited to the hydroxylation of the N-methyl group, oxidative cleavage of side chains, and the oxidation of methyl substituents on the aryl moiety to form hydroxymethyl groups (6). Thiocarbamate compounds, such as aldicarb, can undergo S-oxidation by the cytochromes, with the ini-

TABLE 7. Structures, Common and Trade Names, and Oral LD_{50} Values in Male Rats of Some Commercially Important Carbamate Ester Insecticides*

Structure	Common Name	Trade Name	Oral LD_{50} (mg/kg)
$CH_3-S-CH-NO-C-NH-CH_3$ (with CH_3, CH_3, and O substituents)	Aldicarb	Temik	0.93
$(CH_3)_2N-$ ring $-O-C-NH-CH_3$ with CH_3	Aminocarb	Matacil	30–40
CH_3- ring with Cl $-O-C-NH-CH_3$, CH_3	Carbanolate	Banol	293
naphthalene $-O-C-NH-CH_3$	Carbaryl	Sevin	550–850
benzofuran structure $-O-C-NH-CH$, CH_3, CH_3	Carbofuran	Furadan	8–14
CH_3, CH_3 cyclohexenone $-O-C-NH-N(CH_3)_2$	Dimetan		150
$(CH_3)_2N-C-N$ pyrazole $-O-C-N(CH_3)_2$, CH_3	Dimetilan	Snip	47–64
CH_3-S- ring with CH_3, CH_3 $-O-C-NH-CH_3$	Methiocarb	Mesurol	100
$CH_3-S-C-N-O-C-NH-CH_3$, CH_3	Methomyl	Lannate	17–24
$(CH_3)_2-N-$ ring with CH_3, CH_3 $-O-C-NH-CH_3$	Mexacarbate	Zectran	1500–2500
ring $-O-C-NH-CH_3$, $O-CH(CH_3)_2$	Propoxur	Baygon	83
benzothienyl $-O-C-NH-CH_3$	4-Benzothienyl-N-methylcarbamate	Mobam	150

*LD_{50} values were obtained from *The Pesticide Manual*, 6th and 8th editions, British Crop Protection Council, 1979 and 1987.

tial formation of a sulfoxide and a slower formation of a sulfone, both of which retain potent anticholinesterase properties.

Phase II conjugative reactions occur, the products formed being highly dependent on the species of animal being studied, the nature and specificity of the enzyme, and the insecticide being investigated (6). Once again, carbaryl tends to be the most extensively investigated agent. Following hydrolysis, glucuronide and sulfate derivatives of the released aryl groups have been detected. In some cases, reactions with glutathione result in products destined to become mercapturic acids detectable in the urine and feces.

Excretion of the biotransformation/degradation products is generally *via* the urine and/or the feces. However, the hydrolysis of different carbamate insecticides (mentioned above) was equated with the amount of carbon dioxide formed from the carbamoyl group and exhaled (18).

Animal Studies

The structural diversity found in carbamate insecticides has resulted in considerable variability in acute toxicity; this is reflected in the range of oral LD_{50} values for male rats shown in Table 7. The chemical structure influences not only hydrophilicity and/or lipophilicity, plus the rate of absorption and biotransformation/degradation, but also the affinity of the agent for acetylcholinesterase (AChE) and the severity and persistence of the toxic effects. Consider the low LD_{50} value for the highly water-soluble aldicarb (0.93 mg/kg) and the LD_{50} of 1500–2500 mg/kg for zectran.

The observed signs and symptoms should be comparable for the different agents, having administered adequate doses and given the fact that the inhibited product is a carbamoylated AChE. Animal studies with N-methylcarbamates show that agents that induce signs of short duration persist in the bloodstream for only 1–2 h, whereas those eliciting prolonged effects remain in the blood for more than 6 h. Considering carbaryl as a prototype insecticide of moderate toxicity, toxic signs will begin to appear within 15–30 min of treatment, reach an intensity/severity between 90 and 240 min, dissipate by 6 h with few visible, residual signs by 24 h following treatment (4). A similar spectrum of events, with different time courses, has been reported for other carbamates, the observed toxicity correlating well with their anticholinesterase potency over time, particularly with the inhibition of erythrocytic and brain AChE (1).

Administration of carbamate esters *via* the intravenous (i.v.) or intraperitoneal routes causes effects suggestive of another possible mechanism of action in addition to the inhibition of AChE. Within a few minutes of treatment, a marked anesthetic "narcotic" effect is produced; this is ac-

companied by severe respiratory depression (dyspnea) followed by respiratory failure. However, this effect is produced only by carbamates of low toxicity, and it is suggested that the administration of such high concentrations elicits a marked reduction in nerve conduction at motor end plates by way of a blockade of sodium ion transport across the membrane (6).

Short-term exposure of rats or dogs to repeated oral doses of carbamate insecticides or fungicides results in inhibition of plasma, erythrocytic, and brain cholinesterases accompanied by typical signs and symptoms of cholinergic toxicity but with little evidence of any persistent effects on the CNS or PNS (6).

Many carbamates and thiocarbamates have been tested in the domestic chicken, the short-term administration of several compounds eliciting a severe, delayed neurotoxicity in adult white leghorn hens distinct from the neuropathy associated with certain organophosphorus esters (10). Both aldicarb and carbaryl affected locomotor activity in 7- to 21-day-old chicks for some 6 weeks following a 7-day treatment period, the birds walking with an abnormal, high-stepping, short-stride, wide-based gait with some weakness up to the termination of the experiment at 40 days (6).

Carbamate esters have been assessed in rodents for neurobehavioral effects. Rats treated acutely with carbaryl (levels up to 6.76 mg/kg) developed mild tremors and decreased performance behavior in an activity-wheel cage (6). However, subchronic exposure (14 days) to carbaryl (2.24 mg/kg) was without significant effect in the same test system. The acute administration of carbaryl to rats (1.0, 3.0, 5.0, and 10.0 mg/kg) resulted in a dose-dependent decrease in variable interval response rates in a learned procedure for food reward (6). Both propoxur and carbaryl caused post-treatment reductions in motor activity (open-field and figure-eight mazes), but successful maze activity reappeared within 30 min (propoxur) and 60 min (carbaryl), even though the brain AChE activities remained depressed for 120 and 240 min for propoxur and carbaryl, respectively (17). These results suggest some threshold effect involving the spontaneous recovery of AChE activity. The chronic toxicity of carbaryl has received much more attention than that of other carbamate esters (4). Some studies suggest that long-term exposure to carbamates may result in neurotoxicity. Rats receiving carbaryl for 2 years, at doses not inhibiting erythrocytic AChE or eliciting clinical signs of toxicity, showed electroencephalographic (EEG) changes and decreased maze performance (4). In contrast, male rats receiving carbaryl at 200 mg/kg/day for 90 days showed no overt toxicity (4). Rats and dogs receiving oral aldicarb for up to 2 years showed no adverse effects (16). Tolerance to carbamates has been reported. The EEG patterns in monkeys receiving carbaryl at 10 mg/kg/day were not adversely affected (4,6).

In the other positive study, swine received oral carbaryl (150 mg/kg) for up to 83 days and showed a clinical syndrome characterized by a progressive myasthenia, incoordination, ataxia, intention tremor, and clonic muscular contractions terminating in paraplegia and prostration (4,6). CNS lesions involved moderate to severe edema, fragmentation of myelin sheaths, and swollen and ruptured axons in the cerebellum, brainstem, and upper spinal cord. Myodegeneration of a traumatic or ischemic type was evident in skeletal muscle. Effects were minimal when animals were at rest but became exaggerated when they were forced to move. Most characteristic were a reluctance to stand, a peculiar stance in which the hindlegs were carried well forward under the body, an exaggerated flexion of the rear legs, inability to sit down or back up, an overall muscle weakness following exercise, an inability to stand even when assisted, and prostration. While the high doses administered complicate interpretation of these results, it should be noted that, in an earlier study, single doses of carbaryl (20 mg/kg) administered to swine resulted in a 44% inhibition of cerebral cortex AChE and a 75% inhibition of brainstem AChE; the changes were accompanied by a hindlimb paralysis even though no obvious morphological damage was observed (4,6).

Carbaryl and propoxur have been tested in male rats to assess neurobehavioral changes. Animals received dietary carbaryl at an equivalent of 10 and 20 mg/kg body weight and dietary propoxur at an equivalent of 1.25 and 2.5 mg/kg body weight for up to 50 days (6). Having learned a task (finding food in a maze), shorter periods of time were required initially but, as the study progressed, the animals took longer to fulfill the task, even forgetting what they had learned. Minute changes in EEGs were found for both insecticides, wave components being decreased by propoxur but increased by carbaryl. Other experiments, in monkeys receiving carbaryl (0.01 and 1.0 mg/kg/day), demonstrated a reduction in the abundance of EEG waves of the 0.5- to 3.0-Hz frequency class (4,6). Squirrel monkeys receiving carbaryl (0.007 mg/kg/day for 26 months) showed an increase in abundance of intervals (interval histograms) longer than 1.5 sec along with an increased slow-wave amplitude (6). Other experiments of this type have been reviewed (6). Overall, it appears that carbamate esters can initiate some neurological and behavioral changes at dose levels that produce few obvious clinical signs of toxicity or significant reduction in nervous tissue AChE activity.

Human Studies

While carbamate insecticides are reported to be relatively "safe," producing only transient, short-term toxicity in an-

imals following acute exposure, toxicity does occur in humans, giving rise to both immediate, characteristic, mild to severe signs as well as some bizarre, unexplained, neurological sequelae of a delayed and/or prolonged nature (6).

Studies involving the volunteer-related ingestion or dermal application of carbamate insecticides have been summarized (6). In most cases, the doses were sufficiently low to produce only mild, transient, characteristic signs and symptoms of toxicity that dissipated with the rapid, spontaneous reactivation of the low to moderately inhibited erythrocytic AChE used frequently as a biomarker of intoxication. More germane to the concerns of neurotoxicity are the actual poisonings, even though exposure may be poorly defined.

Periodic incidents of aldicarb-induced poisonings first appeared in the late 1970s to the mid 1980s in both the United States and Canada following the illegal use of this agent on hydroponically grown cucumbers or on various melon crops (6,11). Aldicarb is not registered for use on fruits and vegetables that may contain a high water content. Not surprisingly, high concentrations of this systemic insecticide were found in both cucumbers and melons. The 1985 outbreak of watermelon-induced illness was the largest recorded incident, involving 1376 individuals of which 77% were considered to be aldicarb-poisoned on the basis of signs and symptoms (bradycardia, hypotension, vomiting, diarrhea, lacrimation, salivation, muscular twitching) within 30 min of ingesting the fruit. Estimations of the aldicarb ingested ranged from 0.002–0.057 mg/kg body weight (11). In another incident, groundwater contamination resulting from the legal usage of aldicarb raised concerns about toxicity associated with prolonged consumption of well water containing levels of 8.0–75 μg/l (20). A questionnaire-based survey showed a statistically significant but weak correlation between reported symptoms and increasing aldicarb levels in the drinking water. However, a Wisconsin study, where groundwater contained an aldicarb level of 1.0–61 μg/l, revealed no neurological symptoms.

In an incident in Jamaica, methomyl was inadvertently used as common salt in unleavened bread, in which it attained a concentration of 1000 ppm (6). Of the five individuals poisoned, three died, and it was estimated, from analysis of methomyl residues, that they had consumed 12–15 mg/kg body weight of toxicant. The two survivors showed characteristic muscarinic and nicotinic signs of toxicity. A successful suicide of a mother and of two of three children provided estimates of doses of methomyl of 55 mg/kg in the mother and 13 mg/kg in a 6-year-old child (1).

An unreported incident of the aerial application of carbofuran (substitution for carbaryl) to corn illustrates the rapid onset, the mild to moderate illness, and the quick recovery usually characteristic of carbamate insecticide poisonings (12). Within 12 h of application, 142 teenage boys and girls entered the sprayed corn field to remove tassels from the plants. Within 6 h, 74 complained of dizziness, nausea, and/or blurred vision, some 45 receiving medical aid. Twenty-nine were hospitalized but released within a few hours; only one person was detained overnight. Another incident in which a woman was intoxicated by 60 mg of carbofuran resulted in a 50%–80% inhibition of erythrocytic AChE; this recovered within 72 h and the symptoms disappeared in a similar timeframe.

Propoxur is frequently associated with occupational and suicidal intoxications, the severity of the poisonings being much greater in the latter cases with the use of agricultural formulations or tick and flea preparations. While moderate to severe signs and symptoms appear quickly, they disappear within 2–6 h depending on the dose and the rate of reactivation of the inhibited nervous tissue AChE. Several cases have been described in detail (1). In one case, complete inhibition of both erythrocytic AChE and plasma pseudocholinesterase occurred within 60 min of ingesting a flea/tick preparation but, by 6 h afterward, the plasma enzyme had been completely reactivated, leaving a 40% inhibited erythrocytic AChE and an improving condition of the patient.

Because of its widespread use and availability, several intoxications by carbaryl have been summarized in the literature (4). The severity of the poisonings were dose-related and included nausea, vomiting, lacrimation, blurred vision, salivation, and headache. While fatalities have occurred following high-level exposure (e.g., the ingestion of 500 ml of an 80% carbaryl concentrate), the usual pattern of intoxication at lower exposure levels begins with an early appearance of the characteristic muscarinic and nicotinic signs, attaining a peak in severity approximately 2–3 h after exposure, with few signs observed by 6–8 h.

The appearance of delayed and prolonged neurotoxicity following massive, single exposures to carbamate insecticides has been reported; two such incidents have involved carbaryl (6). While anecdotal and involving single cases, the sequelae of intoxication were similar, although the carbaryl exposure was by a drenching of clothes and dermal absorption in one and by ingestion in the second. Following treatment for the acute crisis, these patients returned to hospitals within 3–4 weeks showing weakness in the extremities, loss of deep tendon reflexes, peripheral paresthesia, incoordination, ataxia, lethargy, and fatigue. In the drenching case, interesting behavioral sequelae persisted: severe headache, mood changes, inability to control temper, frustrated rage, loss of recent memory, and short periods of blackout. While the individual never recovered totally, the other case required a 6- to 9-month recovery period, and some neurological incapacity remained.

Prolonged exposures of humans to carbamate insecticides at levels high enough to elicit neurotoxicity are infrequent, but one case involving a 6- to 8-month continuous exposure to carbaryl dust in a home is of interest, since the effects are contrary to everything written about carbamates and carbaryl in particular. The case has been described in detail and, while the typical signs and symptoms of acute toxicity appeared with frequent regularity, it is the chronic effects persisting after the individual was removed from the source that are of particular interest (2). Mild muscular weakness persisted for some 2 years afterward, as did CNS signs and symptoms, which included altered sleep patterns, headache, tinnitus, and mental confusion. A persistent neurological defect that became more severe was defined as a stocking-and-glove peripheral neuropathy. The inefficient biotransformation of carbaryl may have played a significant role in this case, since the patient was 75 years old and was also being treated with cimetidine, an H_2-receptor antagonist, that has been shown to inhibit carbaryl biotransformation in perfused rat liver and also to increase the systemic availability of carbaryl when ingested (2). However, this appears not to be an isolated case, since this author has had discussions with an individual showing similar signs and symptoms of chronic intoxication from carbaryl sprayed in a home.

The predominant symptoms of carbamate-induced toxicity are associated with accumulating unmetabolized neurotransmitter, acetylcholine being released at nerve endings of the parasympathetic and sympathetic ganglia, ganglia within the CNS (nicotinic actions), the postganglionic parasympathetic nerve endings (muscarinic actions), and at the neuromuscular junctions of somatic motor nerves (nicotinic actions), as a consequence of inhibiting nervous tissue AChE.

Atropine is the antidote of choice to counteract excessive acetylcholine activity at postganglionic, parasympathetic nerve terminals innervating exocrine glands, respiratory tract, gastrointestinal tract, eyes, bladder, and heart (6). Atropine also exerts a remarkable central effect, appearing to have some direct action on the respiratory system. Initially, small (0.5–1.0 mg) doses should be administered subcutaneously (s.c.), carefully titrating the patient by watching for the dilation (mydriasis) of a pinpoint pupil and/or flushing of the face. This is particularly important given the relatively rapid, spontaneous reactivation of carbamoylated AChE with destruction of the acetylcholine, and the possibility of atropine toxicity.

The myorelaxant diazepam (10 mg, s.c. or i.v.), should be considered in all but the mildest cases of carbamate intoxication, since this agent reduces muscular fasciculation, relieves the patient's anxiety, and appears to counteract some aspects of CNS-derived symptoms not affected by atropine.

The use of the oxime reactivators, such as pralidoxime (2-PAM), pralidoxime mesylate (P2S), and obidoxime, is *contraindicated* in carbamate-related intoxications, particularly for carbaryl (6). In both controlled animal experiments and in human carbaryl intoxication, the concomitant administration of 2-PAM enhances the agent's toxicity. While it is generally agreed that oximes are not effective antidotes in carbamate poisonings, this contraindication does not extend to all carbamate esters. In aldicarb-related intoxications in animals and one clinical case involving a child, 2-PAM and P2S reduced the toxicity and enhanced the therapeutic effects of administered atropine (6).

Toxic Mechanisms

The target site of all carbamate insecticides is the nervous tissue macromolecule, AChE, the enzyme that destroys neurotransmitter, acetylcholine (ACh), thereby terminating its biological activity at parasympathetic autonomic endings, at all ganglia, and at motor nerve endings. Carbamates also inhibit erythrocytic AChE, an enzyme identical in most respects to that found in the nervous tissue. Some carbamates inhibit plasma pseudocholinesterase and tissue nonspecific carboxylesterase, enzymes for which no clearly defined physiological roles exist.

With inhibition of nervous tissue AChE in an acute poisoning, characteristic muscarinic, nicotinic, and CNS signs and symptoms range from mild to intense severity depending on the carbamate involved. Clinical manifestations do not last beyond 3–6 h, since there is a rapid, spontaneous reactivation of the inhibited enzyme, with destruction of the accumulated ACh (6). In fact, carbamate esters are recognized as being rather poor substrates for AChE (5). An extensive study of structure–activity relationships with a series of phenyl N-methylcarbamates revealed the presence of a second molecular center in AChE functioning as a supplementary anionic site (15). The optimum distance between the carbonyl group site and this second site is 5.0 Å, a result in keeping with the known distance between the anionic and esteratic site of AChE.

The interaction of a carbamate insecticide with AChE occurs in three distinct steps (5,6). In the first, the enzyme (EOH) couples with the carbamate in a loosely attached manner (low-affinity constant, $K_A = k_{-1}/k_{+1}$) which is reversible; the complex can dissociate easily, releasing free enzyme and the insecticide, or it can proceed to the next stage. In step 2, there is decomposition of the complex into an N-methyl or N-dimethyl carbamoylated enzyme (E-O-CO-NR$_2$), with the loss of the aryl or aliphatic substituent forming the ester (carbamoylation constant, k_2). In step 3, the carbamoylated AChE is hydrolyzed in the presence of water to yield free enzyme (EOH) again and a mono- or dimethylated carbamic acid (HO-CO-NR$_2$), an unstable molecule degrading into carbon dioxide and a mono- or dimethylamine. Since all N-methylated insecticides produce the same carbamoylated enzyme, the rate constant (k_3) for step 3 is the same for all agents. A similar statement could be made for all N-dimethylated carbamoylated AChE. Thus, the variation in overall rates of inhibition and reactivation must be related to the properties contributed by the leaving group and associated with K_A and k_2. The half-life for the decarbamoylation of AChE has been calculated to be 30–40 min, depending upon the agent involved. In the absence of excess insecticide, the enzyme will begin to recover within a few minutes of inhibition and would be completely reactivated after a few hours.

FUNGICIDES

Fungicidal activity is associated with a broad range of chemical structures, carbamic acid esters being only one such class, including heterocyclic carbamates (benomyl, carbendazim, propham, thiophanate, and thiophanate-methyl) as well as a variety of dithiocarbamates. Only this last group of chemicals has been associated with neurotoxicity (7,8).

The dithiocarbamate esters, thio-derivatives of N-substituted carbamic acid, can be divided into four subclasses: methyldithiocarbamates; dimethyldithiocarbamates (DMDCs); diethyldithiocarbamates (DEDCs); and ethylene *bis*-dithiocarbamates (EBDCs) (Table 8). The common nomenclature of these agents arises from the metal cations (sodium, iron, manganese, zinc, selenium). Most of these fungicides are polymeric structures, providing environmental stability, yielding good foliar protection and having low acute as well as chronic toxicity except at high doses (Table 8).

General Toxicology

Because of the complex structures, these chemicals are not efficiently absorbed *via* the skin or gastrointestinal tract. However, the most likely route of occupational exposure is *via* the lungs, these agents being applied frequently as powders or dusts. The metal complexes do not appear to be absorbed well in the gastrointestinal tract; studies with ^{14}C-maneb revealed no elevated blood manganese levels, although 50% of the radiolabel appeared in urine and 1.0% in expired air (7).

The biotransformation of the absorbed fraction is relatively rapid, the metal moiety being lost during metabolism,

TABLE 8. Structures, Common and Trade Names, and Oral LD_{50} Values in Male Rats of Some Commercially Important Carbamate Ester Fungicides*

Structure	Common Name	Trade Name	Oral LD_{50} (mg/kg)
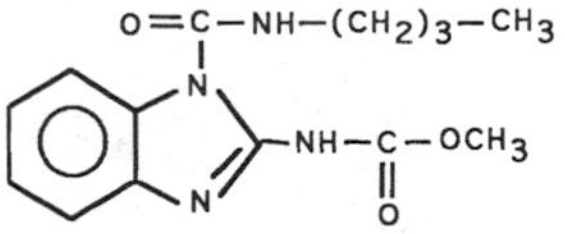 $O=C-NH-(CH_2)_3-CH_3$ on benzimidazole, $NH-C(=O)-OCH_3$	Benomyl	Benlate	10,000
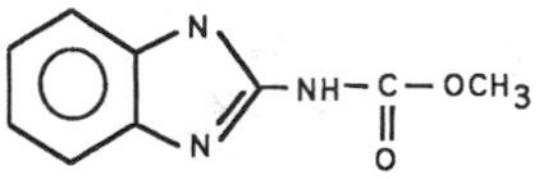 benzimidazole, $NH-C(=O)-OCH_3$	Carbendazim	Delsene	15,000
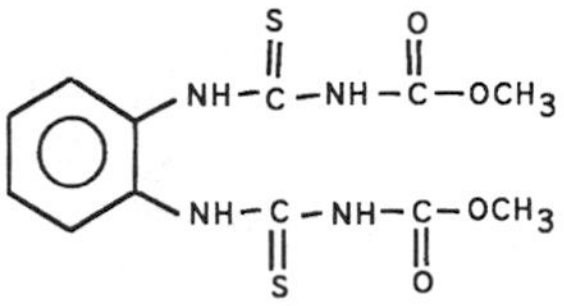 benzene ring with $NH-C(=S)-NH-C(=O)-OCH_3$ and $NH-C(=S)-NH-C(=O)-OCH_3$	Thiophanate-methyl	Mildothane	6000
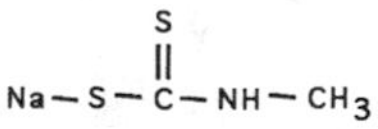 $Na-S-C(=S)-NH-CH_3$	Metam-sodium	Vapam	1800

Dimethyldithiocarbamates

Na^+, Fe^{3+}, Zn^{2+} $\left[-S-C(=S)-N(CH_3)_2 \right]_n$

	Common Name	Trade Name	Oral LD_{50} (mg/kg)
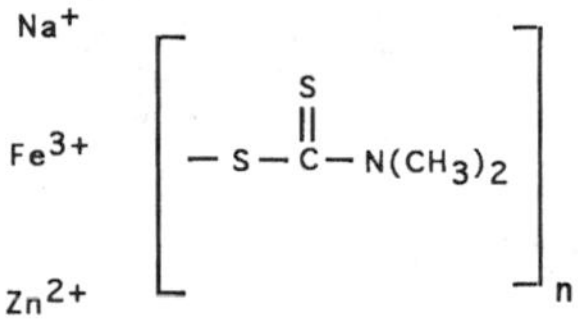	Sodium dimethyl dithiocarbamate	DDC	
	Ferric dimethyl dithiocarbamate	Ferbam	4000
	Zinc dimethyl dithiocarbamate	Ziram	1400

Diethyldithiocarbamates

Se^+, Te^{2+}, Zn^{2+} $\left[-S-C(=S)-N(C_2H_5)_2 \right]_n$

	Common Name	Trade Name	Oral LD_{50} (mg/kg)
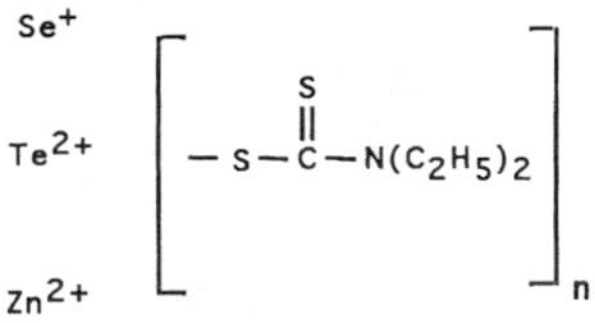	Selenium diethyl dithiocarbamate	Ethyl Selenac	
	Tellurium diethyl dithiocarbamate	Ethyl Tellurac	
	Zinc diethyl dithiocarbamate	Ethyl Zinate	
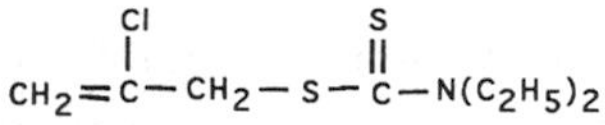 $CH_2=C(Cl)-CH_2-S-C(=S)-N(C_2H_5)_2$	2-Chloro-2-propenyl ester of diethyl dithiocarbamate	Sulfallate	850

Ethylene bis-dithiocarbamates

Structure	Common Name	Trade Name	Oral LD_{50} (mg/kg)
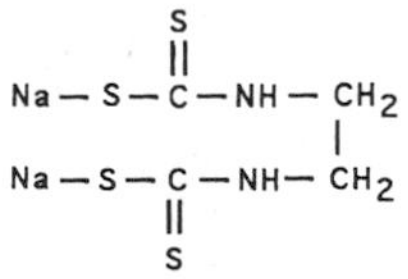 $Na-S-C(=S)-NH-CH_2$ / $Na-S-C(=S)-NH-CH_2$	Nabam	Parzate Dithane d	395
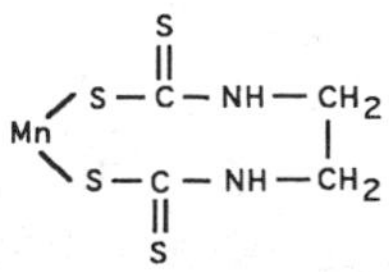 Mn with $S-C(=S)-NH-CH_2$ / $S-C(=S)-NH-CH_2$	Maneb	Manzate Dithane M-22	6750
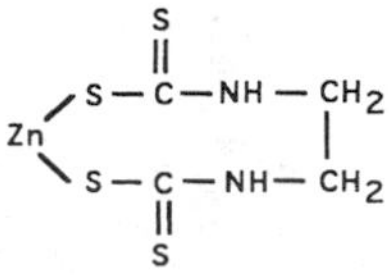 Zn with $S-C(=S)-NH-CH_2$ / $S-C(=S)-NH-CH_2$	Zineb	Dithane Z-78	5200

Table continued on following page

TABLE 8. Structures, Common and Trade Names, and Oral LD$_{50}$ Values in Male Rats of Some Commercially Important Carbamate Ester Insecticides (*Continued*)

Structure	Common Name	Trade Name	Oral LD$_{50}$ (mg/kg)
Zn^{++}_x $\begin{bmatrix} Mn-S-\overset{\overset{S}{\|}}{C}-NH-CH_2 \\ -S-\underset{\underset{S}{\|}}{C}-NH-CH_2 \end{bmatrix}_y$	Mancozeb Complex mixture of maneb & zineb	Dithane M-45 Manzidan	8000
$S-\overset{\overset{S}{\|}}{C}-NH(CH_3)_2$ $S-\underset{\underset{S}{\|}}{C}-NH(CH_3)_2$	Thiram	Arasan Tersan	780–865

*LD$_{50}$ values were obtained from *The Pesticide Manual*, 6th and 8th editions, British Crop Protection Council, 1979 and 1987.

with the formation of a number of identical metabolites from the remaining structure(s) (7,8). The DMDC and DEDC subclasses are metabolized to their respective dimethyl- or diethyl-amines, dithiocarbamic acids, and carbon disulfide (CS$_2$). For the EBDC subclass, the metabolites include ethylenethiourea (ETU), ethylenediamine, ethylenebis-isothiocyanate (EBIS, mustard oil), and CS$_2$. The single most common metabolite from all dithiocarbamates is CS$_2$; the fact that so little of this metabolite is exhaled is attributed to reactions with cellular constituents. A degradation product of CS$_2$, carbonyl sulfide, may also be involved in the neurotoxicity. Excretion is incomplete in all cases, the breakdown products being retained but, with many agents, upwards of 60% is excreted in the feces unchanged.

These chemicals are highly irritating to mucous membranes (eyes, nose, throat, upper respiratory tract) and the skin, causing severe contact dermatitis and allergic hypersensitivity in workers in the agricultural and greenhouse industries. While not particularly toxic to animals except at high doses, they are cytotoxic (their mechanism of action) and many give positive results in microbial mutagenicity assays. Several of these agents are mammalian teratogens, and a few have been shown to be potential carcinogens (8). The EBDC subclass are of particular concern in that one metabolite, ETU, is mutagenic, teratogenic, and carcinogenic in mammals. In addition, the dithiocarbamates interact with imbibed alcohol in the same manner as disulfiram, and workers should avoid the consumption of alcoholic beverages when working with these agents.

The similarity between the toxicity of dithiocarbamates and that of CS$_2$ has been reported, the latter being a potent neurotoxicant (7,8) (*see* Carbon Disulfide, this volume). These chemicals also possess specific antithyroid activity, originally thought to be due to the thiourea. However, other

studies, using ethylenethiourea, demonstrated the formation of ethyleneurea with the release of a highly reactive form of atomic sulfur that appeared to bind to macromolecules in the thyroid, causing a reduction in iodine uptake and in iodination of tyrosine, with resulting thyroid dysfunction (13). Single doses of dithiocarbamates can affect the thyroid gland, and goiters can occur with repeated exposures. This reactive sulfur might also be involved as a mechanism of target organ (liver, kidney, hematopoiesis, testis, spleen, *etc.*) toxicity reported in animal studies, possibly contributing to the disruption of enzymatic functions.

Animal Studies

Dithiocarbamate-related animal studies of short duration have reported some neurological sequelae (hyperactivity, ataxia, hindlimb weakness, loss of muscle tone, reduction in reflexes, incoordination, inactivity, stupor, convulsions), but extensive toxicity was also observed in other target organs due to the high doses administered (7,8). Agents studied have included maneb, thiram, zineb, and ziram.

Few long-term exposure studies with dithiocarbamates have focused on neurotoxicity (7,8). Thiram-induced poisoning in rats resulted in ataxia and hindlimb paralysis, later confirmed to be due to lower lumbar, ventral horn chromatolysis and pyknosis plus sciatic nerve axonal degeneration and myelin loss. Decreased nerve conduction velocities and abnormal electromyography were seen. Ziram administered to rats at 125 mg/kg/day (2500 ppm in diet) caused an abnormal reflex, the animals clasping or crossing their hindlimbs when picked up, rather than normally spreading and extending their legs. Maneb administered to rats caused hindlimb paralysis and ataxia as did EBIS, a metabolite of the EBDC subclass, although removal of EBIS from the diet resulted in a rapid reversal of the paralysis, suggesting reversible biochemical changes.

Dogs appeared to be particularly sensitive to ziram; hindlimb weakness, depression of reflexes and muscle tone, incoordination, tremors, and convulsions were observed in animals receiving 25 mg/kg/day.

Human Studies

The usual toxicity associated with single or repeated exposure to dithiocarbamate fungicides manifests mostly as contact dermatitis or thyroid dysfunction rather than as neurotoxicity. However, at least two interesting incidents have been reported. In the first, an agricultural worker twice applied a commercial mixture of maneb and zineb to cucumbers, walking afterward through the treated field each time without protective clothing (14). The initial exposure resulted in observed nervousness, dizziness, weakness, and fatigue. With a second exposure to a tenfold more concentrated preparation, there was a rapid appearance of muscle weakness, incoordination, disorientation, slurred speech, loss of consciousness, and tonic/clonic convulsions. With appropriate treatment and hospitalization, signs and symptoms began to abate by day 3 and disappeared within 4 days of exposure. No persistent effects were mentioned.

A second incident involved two Brazilian agricultural workers who showed Parkinson-like symptoms and were found to have a history of annual contact with maneb for over 4–5 years (9). The signs and symptoms observed in these patients included arm and leg rigidity, inability to walk, difficulty in talking, a short-stepped, shuffling gait, rigidity with cogwheeling, postural tremor, bradykinesia, brisk deep tendon reflexes, and emotional instability. A follow-up study of 50 rural workers, 84% of whom admitted to using maneb improperly or carelessly, revealed similar but less prominent signs and symptoms. Compared to control individuals, the exposed workers showed a significantly higher prevalence of plastic rigidity with cogwheeling, headache, fatigue, nervousness, memory loss, and sleepiness. An association between manganese and parkinsonism disease is reported (19) but, in these agricultural workers, blood manganese levels were not elevated. It is known that dithiocarbamates *in vivo* can bind various divalent cations, enhancing their penetration into the CNS (3). There is also the possibility that, if exposure to maneb was high enough, the observed toxicity might be attributed to CS_2, a common breakdown product of most dithiocarbamates that has been associated with parkinsonism (19).

The few reported intoxications by dithiocarbamates provide little definitive evidence concerning possible mechanisms of action and consist mostly of anecdotal, single cases. However, these poisonings do indicate that, given high-level exposure, sufficient active agent is absorbed to elicit a neurotoxic reaction.

REFERENCES

1. Baron RL (1991) Carbamate insecticides. In: *Handbook of Pesticide Toxicology*. Hayes WJ Jr, Laws ER eds. Academic Press, New York p. 1125.
2. Branch RA, Jacqz E (1986) Subacute neurotoxicity following long-term exposure to carbaryl. *Amer J Med* 80, 741.
3. Cantilena LR Jr, Klaassen CD (1981) Comparison of the effectiveness of several chelators after single administration on the toxicity, distribution and excretion of cadmium. *Toxicol Appl Pharmacol* 58, 452.
4. Cranmer MF (1986) Carbaryl. A toxicological review and risk analysis. *Neurotoxicology* 7, 247.
5. Ecobichon DJ (1979) Hydrolytic mechanisms of pesticide degradation. In: *Advances In Pesticide Science*. Geissbuhler H ed. Pergamon Press, New York p. 516.
6. Ecobichon DJ (1994) Carbamic acid ester insecticides. In: *Pesticides and Neurological Diseases. 2nd Ed*. Ecobichon DJ, Joy RM eds. CRC Press, Boca Raton, Florida p. 251.
7. Ecobichon DJ (1994) Fungicides. In: *Pesticides and Neurological Diseases. 2nd Ed*. Ecobichon DJ, Joy RM eds. CRC Press, Boca Raton, Florida p. 313.
8. Edwards R, Ferry DG, Temple WA (1991) Fungicides and related compounds. In: *Handbook of Pesticide Toxicology*. Hayes WJ Jr, Laws ER eds. Academic Press, New York p. 1409.
9. Ferraz HB, Bertolucci PHF, Pereira JS *et al.* (1988) Chronic exposure to the fungicide maneb may produce symptoms and signs of CNS manganese intoxication. *Neurology* 38, 550.
10. Fisher SW, Metcalf RL (1983) Production of delayed ataxia by carbamic esters. *Pestic Biochem Physiol* 19, 243.
11. Goldman LR, Smith DF, Neutra RR *et al.* (1990) Pesticide food poisoning from contaminated watermelons in California, 1985. *Arch Environ Health* 45, 229.
12. Hayes WJ Jr (1982) Carbamate pesticides. In: *Pesticides Studied In Man*. Williams & Wilkins, Baltimore p. 436.
13. Hunter A, Neal RA (1974) Response of the hepatic mixed function oxidase enzyme system to thionosulfur-containing compounds. *Pharmacologist* 16, 239.
14. Israeli R, Sculsky M, Tiberin P (1983) Acute intoxication due to exposure to maneb and zineb. A case with behavioral and central nervous system changes. *Scand J Work Environ Health* 9, 47.
15. Metcalf RL, Fukuto TR (1965) Effects of chemical structure on intoxication and detoxication of phenyl *N*-methylcarbamates in insects. *J Agr Food Chem* 13, 220.
16. Risher JF, Mink FL, Stara JF (1987) The toxicological effects of the carbamate insecticide aldicarb in mammals: A review. *Environ Health Perspect* 72, 267.

17. Ruppert PH, Cook LL, Dean KF, Reiter LW (1983) Acute behavioral toxicity of carbaryl and propoxur in adult rats. *Pharmacol Biochem Behav* **18**, 579.

18. Schlagbauer BGL, Schlagbauer AWJ (1972) The metabolism of carbamate pesticides—a literature analysis. Part I and Part II. *Residue Rev* **42**, 1.

19. Spencer PS, Butterfield P (1995) Environmental agents and Parkinson's disease. In: *Etiology of Parkinson's Disease*. Ellenberg HJ, Koller R eds. Marcek Dekker, New York p. 319.

20. Zaki MH, Moran D, Harris D (1982) Pesticides in groundwater: The aldicarb story in Suffolk County, NY. *Amer J Public Health* **72**, 1391.

Carbamazepine

Carol Eisenberg

Mark J. Sinnett

Shlomo Shinnar

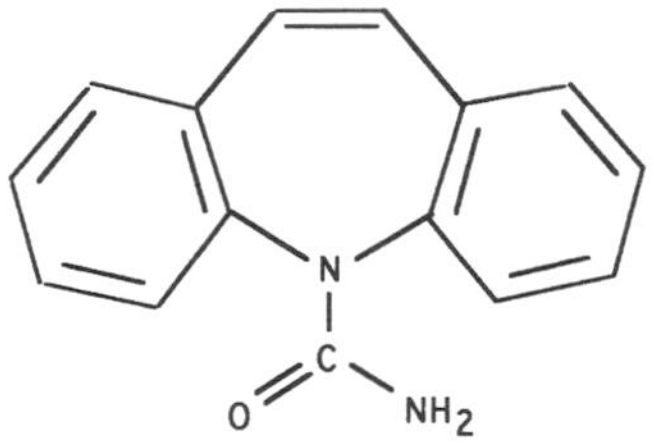

CARBAMAZEPINE
$C_{15}H_{12}N_2O$

5-Carbamoyl-5H-dibenz[b,f]azepine

NEUROTOXICITY RATING

Clinical

A Teratogenicity (spina bifida)

A Acute encephalopathy (sedation, diplopia, ataxia)

A Seizure disorder (children)

Experimental

A Acute encephalopathy (sedation, dysequilibrium)

Carbamazepine is an iminostilbene derivative developed in Switzerland in the late 1950s. The basic structure of carbamazepine is similar to other established antiepileptic drugs (AEDs) such as phenytoin. Its conformational structure, however, more closely resembles the tricyclic antidepressants imipramine and clomipramine. While a very effective drug, carbamazepine is associated with significant acute and chronic neurotoxicity. It is available only by prescription.

Carbamazepine is a white crystalline compound that is soluble in alcohol, acetone, and propylene glycol but is practically insoluble in water. The solubility in water at pH 7.4 is 288 mmol/l (72 mg/l) (40). It is a neutral lipophilic drug available both as a tablet and a suspension.

Carbamazepine is a primary treatment for generalized tonic-clonic, simple partial, and complex partial seizures (4). It is ineffective against generalized absence seizures. Its spectrum of efficacy against seizures appears to be similar to that of phenytoin. The typical maintenance dose is 10–20 mg/kg in adults. The usual therapeutic serum concentration for carbamazepine is 16–48 μg/l (4–12 mg/ml). It is also a first-line drug for symptomatic treatment of pain associated with true trigeminal neuralgia (56) and may be effective in the management of lithium-resistant bipolar disorders (75).

Carbamazepine is slowly and erratically absorbed from the gastrointestinal tract (59). Peak serum concentrations are usually obtained in 4–8 h. Carbamazepine is widely distributed throughout the body and has been detected in the cerebrospinal fluid (CSF), bile, saliva, duodenal fluids, and breast milk. Approximately 65%–80% of carbamazepine is protein-bound, particularly to albumin and α_1-acid-glycoprotein. The drug readily passes through the blood-brain barrier; the CSF/plasma concentration ratio ranges from 0.17–0.31 (43).

Carbamazepine undergoes almost complete hepatic biotransformation. An important product is the active carbamazepine-10,11-epoxide (CBZ-E) metabolite, which is rapidly and completely oxidized to trans-10,11-dihydroxy-10,11-dihydrocarbamazepine. The drug also undergoes N-glucuronidation and ring hydroxylation (Fig. 2). Seventy-two percent of the dose is excreted in the urine, 1%–3% as unchanged drug. Carbamazepine induces liver microsomal enzymes, particularly the cytochrome P-450 system. It also induces its own metabolism (autoinduction) (23). The half-life of carbamazepine ranges from 25–65 h on initial dosing and can decrease to 12–17 h after a few weeks of therapy. Autoinduction usually initially evolves over 1–3 weeks of carbamazepine administration but may continue over several months.

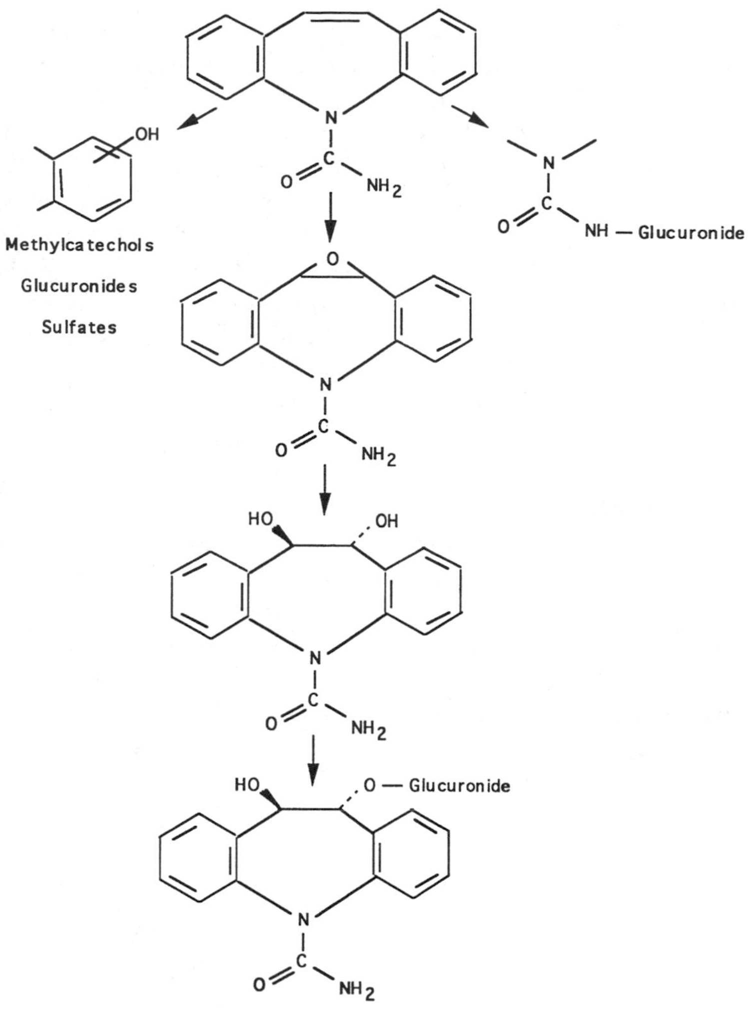

FIGURE 2. Metabolism of carbamazepine. Carbamazepine is primarily metabolized to an active 10,11 epoxide metabolite which is rapidly oxidized to trans-10,11-dihydroxy-10,11-dihydrocarbamazepine. The drug also undergoes minor *N*-glucuronidation and ring hydroxylation.

The mechanism of action of carbamazepine is similar to that of phenytoin. Carbamazepine and its active metabolite, CBZ-E, interact with neuronal sodium channels and appear to stabilize the inactive form of the channel in a voltage-dependent fashion (50). The overall effect is a reduction in the frequency of sustained, repetitive firing of action potentials.

Carbamazepine has major toxic effects on the CNS, and on gastrointestinal and hematological systems. To a lesser degree, it may also affect the hepatic, dermatological, musculoskeletal, and metabolic systems.

Carbamazepine neurotoxicity is evident in mice at oral doses of 24–220 mg/kg (5,28,29). Neurological deficits are demonstrated by the rotorod procedure [a test of the ability of the mouse to maintain its equilibrium for 1 min on a rotating rod (22)], positional sense, gait and stance tests, and the Irwin test (37). The median hypnotic dose, assessed by the loss of righting reflex, is reportedly 172 mg/kg in mice (28). A correlation between neurotoxic effects and plasma concentrations is demonstrable in both mice and rats (55). The protective index (median neurotoxic dose/median dose required to elicit an anticonvulsant effect) of carbamazepine in mice has varied between 4.8 and 14.6 (5,28,29). This was significantly lower than that reported in rats (28). The LD_{50} of carbamazepine in mice and rats is 628–3750 mg/kg (3,28) and 4025 mg/kg (3), respectively.

A major metabolite of carbamazepine, CBZ-E, is thought to contribute to the neurotoxic effects of the parent drug. Following short-term administration, carbamazepine and CBZ-E exhibited a similar degree of neurotoxicity in mice despite a one to two times higher brain/plasma concentration ratio for carbamazepine than for CBZ-E; in combination, the compounds' neurotoxic effects may be slightly synergistic (9).

There have been few studies examining the effect of carbamazepine on peripheral nerve function. A decline in sciatic nerve conduction developed in rats following 2 days of intraperitoneal carbamazepine administration (12 mg/kg) (34). A concentration-dependent depression of muscle spindle activity was shown in carbamazepine-treated cats at serum concentrations of $36-180$ μM/l ($9-45$ μg/ml). It is suggested that some neurotoxic effects (*i.e.*, ataxia, tremor, vertigo, and nystagmus) of the drug may be partly a consequence of the interruption of proprioceptive input caused by a decrease in muscle spindle activity (33).

Carbamazepine neurotoxicity was studied for 3 days in cultured cerebellar granule cells. Neuronal survival decreased in a concentration-dependent manner as evidenced by direct morphological examination and a loss of both ^{3}H-ouabain binding to Na$^+$, K$^+$-ATPase and ^{3}H-N-methyl scopolamine binding to muscarinic cholinergic receptors; N-methyl-D-aspartate administration reversed these effects (26). Carbamazepine slightly inhibited process formation and had no effect on the production of substrate-attached, neurite-promoting activity in embryonic chick dorsal root ganglia (19).

Common adverse neurological effects of carbamazepine therapy include diplopia, drowsiness, dizziness, ataxia, blurred vision, nausea, and headache. Less commonly, vertigo, depression, psychosis (6,42), and mania (20) are described (48,58), as well as restlessness, insomnia, agitation, anxiety, and asthenia (72). Note that neuropsychiatric/neurobehavioral problems are also seen in patients with epilepsy who are not taking carbamazepine (64).

Acute toxicity often occurs if the full maintenance dose is attained within 3 days or less (13). With rapid increases in drug dose, acute toxicity occurred even when carbamazepine levels were <10 mg/ml in patients who were asymptomatic a few days later at higher levels (9). Significantly higher serum levels were found in patients with neurotoxicity than in those without; no neurotoxic effects were seen at a serum level of <5.9 mg/ml (35,69). Ataxia occurred with low levels, diplopia with high levels, and sedation with low and high levels (11). Gradually increasing the dose over $7-14$ days minimizes these side effects.

The risk of carbamazepine-induced hyponatremia in adults increases with age and carbamazepine serum level (41). Although it is generally not severe enough to cause symptoms, carbamazepine-induced hyponatremia should be considered when headache, dizziness, nausea, and drowsiness occur with loss of seizure control. It is unclear whether carbamazepine-induced hyponatremia is due to a hypothalamic effect on osmoreceptors or to a direct effect on renal tubules.

Using the multiple sleep-latency test and visual reaction times, patients on carbamazepine monotherapy who reported daytime sleepiness had shorter daytime sleep latencies and longer reaction times (54); sleep latency did not correlate with carbamazepine plasma levels or seizure frequency.

Some studies have shown a connection between toxic side effects and the plasma concentration of the active metabolite carbamazepine-10,11-epoxide (63), but others have not (68). Although the incidence of neurotoxicity is generally 1%–5% (32,65), an incidence of 14% has been reported (16). The prevalence of neurotoxicity related to carbamazepine therapy seems to be higher in the elderly (27) and in patients with underlying brain damage and mental retardation (13).

Dyskinesias are reported in association with carbamazepine, but these are rare and tend to be associated with anticonvulsant polytherapy in brain-damaged patients or with toxic levels of carbamazepine (10,14,28,38).

In children, carbamazepine may exacerbate myoclonic, atonic, and absence seizures (71,74) and rarely may precipitate absence status epilepticus (12). It is also rarely associated with an increase in partial seizures of frontal and temporal lobe origin (18,36).

A correlation was found between carbamazepine-associated electroencephalogram (EEG) changes and seizure exacerbation (76). Seizure exacerbation occurred in 65% of children in whom, after starting carbamazepine, the EEG became markedly abnormal with new appearance of generalized spike/polyspike-and-wave discharges. Cryptogenic seizure disorders were more common in this group of children. None of the children in their study had childhood absence epilepsy or Lennox-Gastaut syndrome.

The occurrence of absence seizures is described in a woman with primary generalized tonic-clonic seizures and in a woman with juvenile myoclonic epilepsy, as well as exacerbation of absence seizures in two women with generalized tonic-clonic seizures and a remote past history of absence (47). Two of the women had 2.5- to 3-Hz generalized spike-and-wave activity with hyperventilation; one had a normal EEG and one had 4- to 5-Hz generalized spike-and-wave and polyspike-and-wave while awake or asleep and hyperventilation during carbamazepine therapy (47).

A "paradoxical intoxication" is described in association with an increase in serum carbamazepine level from 17.1 μg/ml to 22.6 μg/ml; this involved an increase in seizure frequency from none to six per month, with no other symptoms or clinical signs of toxicity. The phenomenon occurred in a patient with complex partial and generalized motor seizures; it resolved with decrease in dose (78).

EEG changes during the introduction of carbamazepine in 16 previously untreated patients are reported (7). Within 3 days of beginning treatment with 400 mg *b.i.d.*, the mean values of the total power and relative powers of the theta and delta bands increased, while those of the alpha band and central frequency decreased. There was no correlation between EEG parameters and serum levels of carbamazepine or carbamazepine-10,11-epoxide.

The alpha rhythm slowed during initiation of carbamazepine therapy in 16 previously untreated children, aged 5–14 years, with partial seizures (24). Decreased neuropsychological performance at 1 year, particularly in the Arithmetic and Picture Completion subtests of the Wechsler Intelligence Scale for Children, Revised, was seen in the children whose alpha frequency decreased the most (>0.5 Hz). Neither the degree of alpha slowing nor the neuropsychological status correlated with the carbamazepine blood level at that time (24). Others have found that most children on long-term carbamazepine monotherapy have little neuropsychological impairment (2,25). Although reports document no behavioral changes in children on carbamazepine (1,8), adverse behavioral changes associated with its use have been noted, more often in children with mental retardation and/or neurobehavioral problems (73).

In adults, most studies show little or no cognitive and behavioral impairment related to therapeutic levels of carbamazepine (21,53,57,66). Dose-related cognitive and behavioral problems are reported (52,66).

Acute toxicity due to overdosage of carbamazepine may result in nystagmus, ophthalmoplegia, cerebellar and extrapyramidal signs, impairment of consciousness evolving to a comatose state, respiratory compromise, and convulsions. The lethal dose of carbamazepine has ranged from 4–60 g (30), although there is a report of a patient surviving the ingestion of 80 g (61). It is suggested that the course of the intoxication may correlate more closely with the epoxide level than with that of carbamazepine itself (31,49). Gastric lavage (up to 12 h after overdosage) and hemoperfusion may be helpful (51,61).

Several studies address the neurodevelopmental effects of carbamazepine on the fetus. One study describes a pattern of minor anomalies including up-slanting palpebral fissures, epicanthal folds, short nose, long philtrum, hypoplastic nails, and microcephaly in 37 infants of mothers on carbamazepine monotherapy (39). Another described 34 Dutch cases of spinal defects associated with prenatal exposure to valproate only in 22, carbamazepine only in 6, and valproate plus carbamazepine in 3 (46; see also 62). Based on personal data and literature review, Rosa reported an association between carbamazepine and spina bifida (67), and on meta-analysis of published and unpublished prospective studies estimated the risk to be 0.5%–1.0%. It has been shown that either valproate or phenobarbital in combination with carbamazepine is associated with a higher teratogenic risk than carbamazepine alone, and produced levels of carbamazepine-10,11-epoxide three to five times higher than carbamazepine monotherapy (44).

A prospective study compared neurodevelopment (Bayley or McCarthy scale) from 18–36 months postnatally of children of mothers on phenytoin or carbamazepine monotherapy (70). Children exposed to carbamazepine in utero did not differ from the controls on any of the neurobehavioral tests, whereas those exposed to phenytoin had lower global IQ and Reynell language development scores than their controls.

The mechanism of carbamazepine and carbamazepine epoxide neurotoxicity is unknown. In regard to the 0.5% –1.0% risk of spina bifida in the fetuses of mothers receiving carbamazepine, some have recommended periconceptional folic acid supplementation. Studies in pregnant women who do not have epilepsy (and are not taking anticonvulsant medications) show that periconceptional folic acid supplementation decreases the incidence of neural tube defects (15,60). An association has been shown between maternal folic acid status and any adverse pregnancy outcome (17). However, carbamazepine and valproate affect folic acid status much less than phenytoin and barbiturates, both of which have a much lower risk than carbamazepine for fetal neural tube defects. In short, there is no proof that folic acid deficiency in and of itself is a pathogenetic mechanism of carbamazepine-induced teratogenesis. There is no proof that folic acid supplementation protects against carbamazepine-associated neural tube defects although, in animal experiments, folinic acid reduced the teratogenic action of valproate (77).

Carbamazepine alone and in combination with phenobarbital and valproate is associated with hyponatremia in 10%–15% of treated adults. It is unknown whether hyponatremia itself is teratogenic, but the teratogenic effects of patients' sera on rat embryos was correlated with the degree of hyponatremia (45).

REFERENCES

1. AldenKamp AP, Alpherts WC, Blennow G et al. (1993) Withdrawal of antiepileptic medication in children—effects on cognitive function: The multicenter Holmfrid study. Neurology 43, 41.
2. Aman MG, Werry JS, Paxton JW et al. (1990) Effects of carbamazepine on psychomotor performance in children as a function of drug concentration, seizure type and time of medication. Epilepsia 31, 51.
3. Anon (1984) Carbamazepine. In: Merck Index. 10th Ed. Windolz M, Buduvari S, Stroumtsis LY, Noether-Fertig M eds. Merck and Co, Rahway, New Jersey p. 226.
4. Anon (1994) Carbamazepine. In: American Hospital Formulary Service: Drug Information McEvoy GK ed. Amer-

ican Society of Hospital Pharmacists, Bethesda, MD p. 1366.

5. Ater SB, Swinyard EA, Tolman KG, Franklin MR (1984) Anticonvulsant activity and neurotoxicity of piperonyl butoxide in mice. *Epilepsia* 25, 551.

6. Berger, H (1971) An unusual manifestation of Tegretol (carbamazepine) toxicity. *Ann Intern Med* 74, 449.

7. Besser R, Hornung K, Theisohn M *et al.* (1992) EEG changes in patients during the introduction of carbamazepine. *Electroencephalogr Clin Neuro* 37, 329.

8. Bird CA, Griffin BP, Miklascewska JM, Galbraith AW (1966) Tegretol (carbamazepine): A controlled trial of a new anticonvulsant. *Brit J Psychiat* 112, 737.

9. Bourgeois BFD, Wad N (1984) Individual and combined antiepileptic and neurotoxic activity of carbamazepine and carbamazepine-10,11-epoxide in mice. *J Pharmacol Exp Ther* 231, 411.

10. Bradbury AJ, Bentick B, Todd PJ (1982) Dystonia associated with carbamazepine toxicity. *Postgrad Med J* 58, 525.

11. Callaghan N, O'Callaghan M, Duggan B, Feely M (1978) Carbamazepine as a single drug in the treatment of epilepsy. *J Neurol Neurosurg Psychiat* 41, 907.

12. Callahan DJ, Noetzel MJ (1992) Prolonged absence status epilepticus associated with carbamazepine therapy, increased intracranial pressure, and transient MRI abnormalities. *Neurology* 42, 2198.

13. Cereghino JJ, Brock JT, Van Meter JC *et al.* (1974) Carbamazepine for epileptic patients. A controlled prospective evaluation. *Neurology* 24, 401.

14. Crosley CJ, Swender PT (1979) Dystonia associated with carbamazepine administration: Experience in brain-damaged children. *Pediatrics* 63, 612.

15. Czeizel AE, Dudas I (1992) Prevention of the first occurrence of neural-tube defects by periconceptional vitamin supplementation. *N Engl J Med* 327, 1832.

16. Dallos V, Heathfield KW (1972) Tegretol in intractable epilepsy. In: *Tegretol in Epilepsy*. Wink CA ed. C. Nicholls, Manchester p. 89.

17. Dansky LV, Rosenblatt DS, Andermann E (1992) Mechanisms of teratogenesis: Folic acid and anticonvulsant therapy. *Neurology* 42, 32.

18. Dhuna A, Pascual-Leone A, Talwar D (1991) Exacerbation of partial seizures and onset of nonepileptic myoclonus with carbamazepine. *Epilepsia* 32, 275.

19. Dow KE, Riopelle RJ (1988) Differential effects of anticonvulsants on developing neurons *in vitro*. *Neurotoxicology* 9, 97.

20. Drake ME, Peruzzi WT (1986) Manic state with carbamazepine therapy of seizures. *J Nat Med Assn* 78, 1105.

21. Duncan JS, Shorvon SD, Trimble MR (1990) Effects of removal of phenytoin, carbamazepine, and valproate on cognitive function. *Epilepsia* 31, 584.

22. Dunham NW, Miya TS (1957) A note on a single apparatus for detecting neurological deficit in rats and mice. *J Amer Pharm Assn* 46, 208.

23. Eichelbaum M, Tomson T, Tybring G, Bertilsson L (1985) Carbamazepine metabolism in man: induction and pharmacogenetic aspects. *Clin Pharmacokinet* 10, 80.

24. Frost JD, Hrachovy RA, Glaze DG, Rettig GM (1995) Alpha rhythm slowing during initiation of carbamazepine therapy: Implications for future cognitive performance. *J Clin Neurophysiol* 12, 57.

25. Gallasi R, Morreale A, Lorusso S *et al.* (1988) Carbamazepine and phenytoin. Comparison of cognitive effects in epileptic patients during monotherapy and withdrawal. *Arch Neurol* 45, 892.

26. Gao X, Chuang D (1992) Carbamazepine-induced neurotoxicity and its prevention by NMDA in cultured cerebellar granule cells. *Neurosc Lett* 135, 159.

27. Gayford JJ, Redpath TH (1969) The side effects of carbamazepine. *Proc Roy Soc Med* 6, 615.

28. Goehring RR, Greenwood TD, Nwokogu GC *et al.* (1990) Synthesis and anticonvulsant activity of 2-benzylglutarimides. *J Med Chem* 33, 926.

29. Gower AL, Noyer M, Verloes R *et al.* (1992) ucb L059, a novel anti-convulsant drug: Pharmacological profile in animals. *Eur J Pharmacol* 222, 193.

30. Gram L, Jensen PK (1989) Carbamazepine toxicity. In: *Antiepileptic Drugs. 3rd Ed.* Levey R, Mattson R, Meldrum B *et al.* eds. Raven Press, New York p. 555.

31. Groot deG, Van Heijst ANP, Maes RAA (1984) Charcoal hemoperfusion in the treatment of two cases of acute carbamazepine poisoning. *Clin Toxicol* 22, 349.

32. Hanke NF (1972) Clinical tolerance of tegretol. In: *Tegretol in Epilepsy*. Wink CA ed. C. Nicholls, Manchester p. 113.

33. Hershkowitz N, Raines A (1978) Effects of carbamazepine on muscle spindle discharges. *J Pharmacol Exp Therap* 204, 581.

34. Honda H, Allen M (1973) The effect of an iminostilbene derivative (G32883) on peripheral nerves. *J Med Assn Ga* 62, 38.

35. Hoppener RJ, Kuyer A, Meijer JW, Hulsman J (1980) Correlation between daily fluctuations of carbamazepine serum levels and intermittent side effects. *Epilepsia* 21, 341.

36. Horn CS, Ater SB, Hurst DL (1986) Carbamazepine-exacerbated epilepsy in children and adolescents. *Pediat Neurol* 2, 340.

37. Irwin S (1968) Comprehensive observational assessment: 1a. A systematic quantitative procedure for assessing the behavioural and physiologic state of the mouse. *Psychopharmacologica (Berlin)* 13, 222.

38. Jacome D (1979) Carbamazepine induced dystonia. *J Amer Med Assn* 241, 2263.

39. Jones KL, Lacro RV, Johnson KA *et al.* (1989). Pattern of malformations in the children of women treated with carbamazepine during pregnancy. *N Engl J Med* 320, 1661.

40. Kutt H (1989) Carbamazepine: Chemistry and methods of determination. In: *Antiepileptic Drugs. 3rd Ed.* Levey R, Mattson R, Meldrum B *et al.* eds. Raven Press, New York p. 457.

41. Lahr MB (1985) Hyponatremia during carbamazepine therapy. *Clin Pharmacol Ther* 37, 693.

42. Leviatov VM, Vselowskaja TD, Marienko G, Chtchegoleva AP (1976) Psychoses au Tegretol chez des Epileptiques. *Ann Med Psychol* 1, 473.

43. Levy RH, Wilensky AJ, Anderson GD (1992) Carbamazepine, valproic acid, phenobarbital, and ethosuximide. In: *Applied Pharmacokinetics: Principles of Therapeutic Drug Monitoring. 3rd Ed.* Evans WE, Schentag JJ, Jusko WJ eds. Applied Therapeutics, Vancouver p. 26.

44. Lindhout D, Höppener RJEA, Meinardi H (1984) Teratogenicity of antiepileptic drug combinations with special emphasis on epoxidation (of carbamazepine). *Epilepsia* 25, 77.

45. Lindhout D, Meijer JWA, Verhoef A, Peters PWJ (1987) Metabolic interactions in clinical and experimental teratogenesis. In: *Pharmacokinetics in Teratogenesis. Vol. 1. Interspecies Comparison and Maternal/Embryonic-Fetal Drug Transfer.* Nau H, Scott WJ eds. CRC Press, Boca Raton, Florida p. 233.

46. Lindhout D, Omtzigt JGC, Cornel MC (1991) Spectrum of neural tube defects in 34 cases prenatally exposed to antiepileptic drugs. *Neurology* 42, 111.

47. Liporace JD, Sperling MR, Dichter MA (1994) Absence seizures and carbamazepine in adults. *Epilepsia* 35, 1026.

48. Livingston S, Pauli L, Berman W (1974) Carbamazepine (Tegretol) in epilepsy: Nine year follow-up study with special emphasis on untoward reactions. *Dis Nerv Sys* 35, 103.

49. Luke DR, Rocci ML, Schaible DH, Ferguson RK (1986) Acute hepatotoxicity after excessive high doses of carbamazepine on two occasions. *Pharmacotherapy* 6, 108.

50. Macdonald RL, Kelly KM (1994) Mechanisms of action of currently prescribed and newly developed antiepileptic drugs. *Epilepsia* 35, S41.

51. Mack RB (1985) Carbamazepine poisoning. *N C Med J* 46, 41.

52. MacPhee GJA, McPhail EM, Butler E, Brodie MJ (1986) Controlled evaluation of a supplementary dose of carbamazepine on psychomotor function in epileptic patients. *Eur J Clin Pharmacol* 31, 195.

53. Marchesi GF, Ladavas E, Provinciali L *et al.* (1980) Neuropsychological performances in patients treated with different antiepileptic drugs. *Monogr Neural Sci* 5, 258.

54. Massetani R, Galli R, Bonanni E *et al.* (1994) Daytime sleepiness in epileptic patients treated with carbamazepine monotherapy and receiving vigabatrin add-on treatment. *Epilepsia* 35, 65.

55. Masuda Y, Utsui Y, Shiraishi Y *et al.* (1979) Relationship between plasma concentrations of diphenylhydantoin,

56. Mauskop A (1993) Trigeminal neuralgia (tic douloureux). *J Pain Symptom Manage* 8, 148.

57. Meador KJ, Loring DW, Allen ME *et al.* (1991) Comparative cognitive effects of carbamazepine and phenytoin in healthy adults. *Neurology* 41, 1537.

58. Meinardi H, Stoel MK (1974) Side effects of antiepileptic drugs. In: *Handbook of Clinical Neurology. Vol 15.* Vinken PJ, Bruyn GW eds. North Holland, Amsterdam p. 705.

59. Morselli PL (1989) Carbamazepine: Absorption, distribution and excretion. In: *Antiepileptic Drugs. 3rd Ed.* Levy R, Mattson R, Meldrum R *et al.* eds. Raven Press, New York p. 473.

60. MRC Vitamin Study Research Group (1991) Prevention of neural-tube defects: Results of the Medical Research Council Vitamin Study. *Lancet* 338, 131.

61. Nilson C, Sterner G, Idvall J (1984) Charcoal hemoperfusion for treatment of serious carbamazepine poisoning. *Acta Med Scand* 216, 137.

62. Omtzigt JGC, Los FJ, Grobbee DE *et al.* (1992) The risk of spina bifida aperta after first trimester valproate exposure in a prenatal cohort. *Neurology* 42, 119.

63. Patzalos PW, Stephenson TJ, Korshna S *et al.* (1985) Side effects induced by carbamazepine-10,11-epoxide. *Lancet* 8, 496.

64. Perrine K, Congett S (1994) Neurobehavioral problems in epilepsy. In: *Neurologic Clinics. Epilepsy II: Special Issues. Vol. 12.* Devinsky O ed. WB Saunders, Philadelphia p. 129.

65. Reynolds EH (1975) Neurotoxicity of carbamazepine. In: *Advances in Neurology. Vol 11.* Penry JK, Daly DD eds. Raven Press, New York p. 345.

66. Ronnberg J, Samuelsson S, Soderfeldt B (1992) Memory effects following carbamazepine monotherapy in patients with complex partial seizures. *Seizure* 1, 247.

67. Rosa FW (1991) Spina bifida in infants of women treated with carbamazepine during pregnancy. *N Engl J Med* 324, 674.

68. Schmidt D, Corragia C, Fabian A (1984) Carbamazepine suspension for acute treatment of trigeminal neuralgia: Clinical effects in relation to plasma concentration. In: *Metabolism of Antiepileptic Drugs.* Levy R, Mattson R, Meldrum R eds. Raven Press, New York p. 35.

69. Schneider H (1975) Carbamazepine: An attempt to correlate serum levels with anticonvulsive and side effects. In: *Clinical Pharmacology of Anti-epileptic Drugs.* Schneider H, Janz D, Gardner-Thorpe C *et al.* eds. Springer-Verlag, Heidelberg p. 151.

70. Scolnik D, Nulman I, Rovet J *et al.* (1994) Neurodevelopment of children exposed in utero to phenytoin and carbamazepine monotherapy. *J Amer Med Assn* 271, 676.

phenobarbital, carbamazepine, and 3-sulfamoylmethyl-1-1,2-benzisoxazole (AD-810), a new anticonvulsant agent, and their anticonvulsant or neurotoxic effects in experimental animals. *Epilepsia* 20, 623.

71. Shields WD, Saslow E (1983) Myoclonic, atonic and absence siezures following institution of carbamazepine therapy in children. *Neurology* **33**, 1487.

72. Sillanpää M (1981) Carbamazepine pharmacology and clinical uses. *Acta Neurol Scand* **64** (Suppl 88).

73. Silverstein SS, Parrish MA, Johnston MV (1982) Adverse behavioral reactions in children treated with carbamazepine. *J Pediat* **101**, 785.

74. Snead O, Hosey LC (1985) Exacerbation of seizures in children by carbamazepine. *N Engl J Med* **313**, 916.

75. Stuppaeck C, Barnas C, Miller C *et al.* (1990) Carbamazepine in the prophylaxis of mood disorders. *J Clin Psychopharmacol* **10**, 39.

76. Talwar D, Arora MS, Sher PK (1994) EEG changes and seizure exacerbation in young children treated with carbamazepine. *Epilepsia* **35**, 1154.

77. Trotz M, Wegner C, Nau H (1987). Valproic acid-induced neural tube defects: reduction by folinic acid in the mouse. *Life Sci* **41**, 103.

78. Troupin AS, Ojemann LM (1975) Paradoxical intoxication—A complication of anticonvulsant administration. *Epilepsia* **16**, 753.

Carbolines and Isoquinolines

Michael A. Collins
Edward J. Neafsey

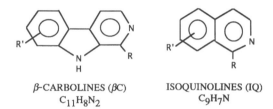

β-CARBOLINES (βC)
$C_{11}H_8N_2$

ISOQUINOLINES (IQ)
C_9H_7N

NEUROTOXICITY RATING

Experimental

A   Extrapyramidal dysfunction (dopaminergic neurotoxin; substantia nigra degeneration; parkinsonism—monkey)

β-Carbolines (βCs; 9H-pyrido[3,4-b]indoles), isoquinolines (IQs) and, in particular, their N-methylated derivatives are putative or potential neurotoxicants. Interest in N-methylated forms of βCs and IQs was kindled by the discovery of the meperidine contaminant, N-methyl-4-phenyl-1,2,3,6-tetrahydropyridine (MPTP), and its neurotoxic oxidation product, N-methyl-4-phenylpyridinium cation (MPP$^+$). MPTP induces a state of parkinsonism in humans that closely mirrors idiopathic Parkinson's disease (PD) (50). Its generally accepted neurotoxic mechanism involves inhibition (*via* MPP$^+$) of mitochondrial respiration that leads to death of dopaminergic neurons in the brain nigrostriatal system (95,103).

Interaction of potential environmental neurotoxins with genetic susceptibility is considered important in the etiology of idiopathic PD (43,64,101). N-Methylated βCs and IQs, which contain pyridinium moieties like MPP$^+$ and can inhibit mitochondrial respiration, are reasonable candidates for such environmentally derived agents (23). The βC and IQ structural classes encompass a large number of alkaloidal constituents of selected plants, especially angiosperms (46). However, because a number of simpler compounds in the βC class are generated by grilling or broiling protein-rich foodstuffs, by pyrolytic industrial processes, and presumably by fermentation, they are indisputably xenobiotic for most humans. Various IQs, including those related to 3,4-dihydroxyphenylethyl amine (dopamine), are normally present in certain plant-derived foods and alcoholic beverages, but their pyrolytic formation has not been widely documented. There is also convincing evidence that simple βC and IQ ring structures may form endogenously by condensation reactions within animal cells ("mammalian alkaloids"); this is reviewed in detail elsewhere (62,86).

The initial and, in the case of pyrolysis, no doubt transient products from "open chain" amine or amino acid precursors are believed to be 1,2,3,4-tetrahydro-β-carbolines (THβCs) and tetrahydroisoquinolines (TIQs), which, as shown in Figure 3, undergo 2-electron oxidation to 3,4-dihydro intermediates (DHβCs and DIQs), and then further dehydrogenation to the heteroaromatic βC and IQ forms. The premise of many investigations of βC and IQ neurotoxicity in humans is that bioactivation *via* N-methylation, hydroxylation, and/or oxidation is a requisite *in vivo* process. N-Methylation occurs with the tetrahydro forms in plants and with both hydrogenated and heteroaromatic forms in animals (shown in Fig. 4 with βCs). N-Methyltransferases were initially suggested to have a role in converting environmental pyridines into potential neurotoxins (7).

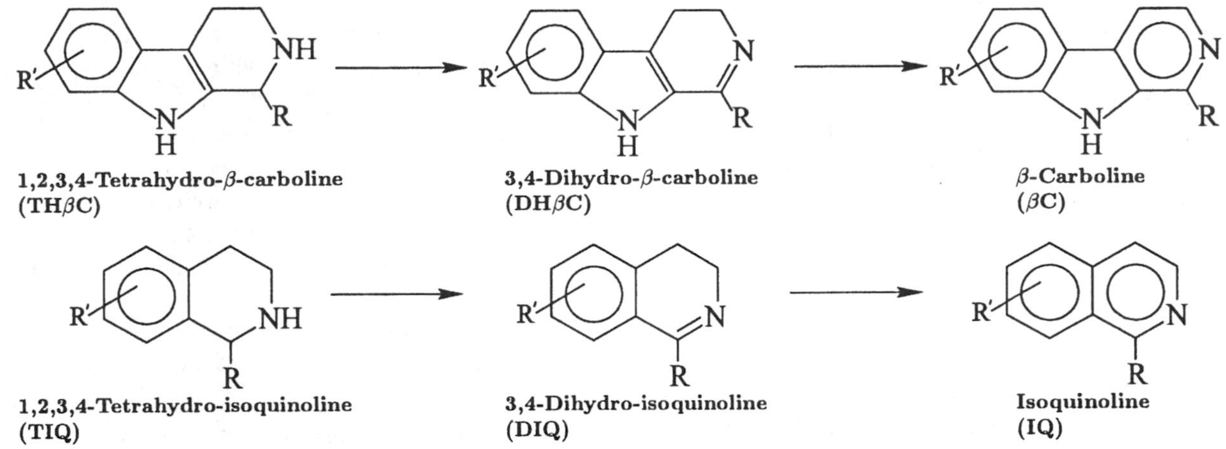

FIGURE 3. Dehydrogenation pathways for the β-carbolines and isoquinolines. R = hydrogen or methyl group; R′ = hydroxyl or methoxyl groups.

Brain bioactivation of environmental heterocyclic compounds in the βC and IQ classes by enzymatic processes such as N-methylation and perhaps methoxylation can produce potential neurotoxicants within the CNS. Such conversions might be important in idiopathic PD, since the cationic (quaternary) βC and IQ products are remarkably similar in structure to MPP⁺, the bioactive metabolite of the synthetic parkinsonian neurotoxin MPTP. The 2,9-di-N-methylated cationic derivatives of βCs, such as norharman, harman, and harmine display neurotoxic actions in animal models, as well as significant inhibition of monoamine oxidase (MAO). Furthermore, the 2,9-di-N-methylnorharmanium cation occurs along with its precursors in trace amounts in human brain, and may be selectively pres-

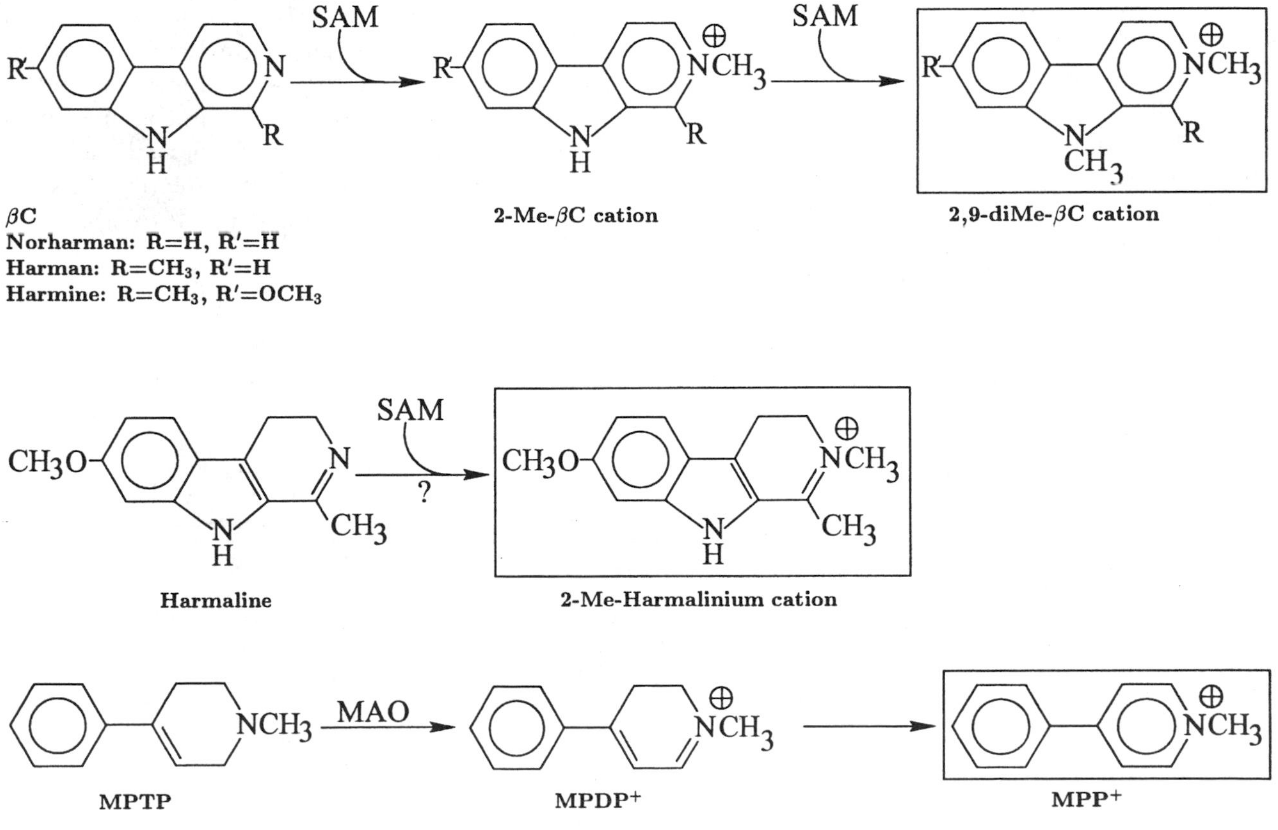

FIGURE 4. (Top) Sequential N-methylation of β-carbolines by S-adenosylmethionine (SAM)-dependent enzymes, to produce β-carbolinium cations. The most neurotoxic species are enclosed in boxes. (Bottom) MPTP and its neurotoxic oxidation product, MPP⁺. MAO = monoamine oxidase.

ent in cerebrospinal fluid (CSF) obtained from parkinsonian patients. Likewise, the N-methyl derivatives of IQ and 6,7-dihydroxy-1-methyl-IQ also induce neurotoxicity in animal models *in vitro* and *in vivo*. Their tetrahydro precursors have been detected in the human nervous system and can induce parkinsonian syndromes in primate models.

β-CARBOLINES

Avid interest in the potential oncogenic roles of carbolines arising from the diet or environment was initiated by the pioneering research of Sugimura and colleagues (97). For nearly two decades, simple βC heterocyclics have been examined as genotoxic agents that could augment the activities of otherwise relatively weakly mutagenic/carcinogenic compounds (thus the term, comutagens). The mechanisms appear to involve induction or inhibition of enzymes such as the cytochrome P-450 systems and DNA topoisomerases, and genomic DNA interactions (intercalation) (33). The specific βCs of interest in this regard have been norharman and harman (Fig. 4). Representative xenobiotic sources for these two carbolines are summarized in Table 9, with concentration ranges where available. With respect to mechanisms of formation during cooking, elevated temperatures induce reaction of tryptophan derived from (or in) proteins with aldehydic compounds and subsequent oxidations leading to carbolines. In addition to the β-forms, carbolines of the α- and γ-subclasses are produced in lesser amounts. It is these latter forms (referred to as AαC, Trp-P1, and Trp-P2) that are potent mutagens by virtue of a primary amino group on the β-carbon. Thorough discussions of the genomic activities of α-, β- and γ-carbolines are available in recent reviews (33,40,97).

When chronically infused into specific brain regions in rats, the βC harman promotes the consumption of high-alcohol solutions (3). Whether a permanent neurotoxic insult underlies this effect is not clear. A subclass of derivatives related to harman that has also been the focus of behavioral research are the 7-methoxylated derivatives, harmine and harmaline, the latter compound being the 3,4-dihydro reduction product of the former (Fig. 4). These and related βCs are best known in ethnopharmacology and ethnobiology as constituents of the hallucinogenic extracts of the Asian *Peganum harmala* and of the South American psychoactive "*ayuahasca*" or "*yahé*" beverage, made from *Banisteriopsis caapi* (6,46,90). Although these βCs may have direct psychotropic effects, harmine and particularly harmaline also may potentiate the intrinsic activities of open-chain tryptamines by virtue of their potent inhibition of the mitochondrial enzyme MAO (45). Neuropharmacologically, harmine and harmaline are somewhat equivalent in their tremorigenic potencies (believed to be due to activation of the olivocerebellar system) in rodent models (109). However, in terms of neural cell toxicity, the 2-mono-N-methylated cationic derivative of harmaline is considerably more potent than the analogous derivative of harmine (*vide infra*).

In addition, pharmacological research on βCs has focused on the remarkably high affinity of selected derivatives for the brain γ-aminobutyric acid (GABA)−benzodiazepine receptor complex. Studies revealed the high reversible binding affinity of 3-carboxylated methyl and ethyl esters of norharman to this complex (14), and important synthetic analogs have been successfully developed as anxiolytic and anxiogenic agents (2,88). A potent "natural" analog may be norharman-3-carboxylate *n*-butyl ester (Fig. 4), reported to be endogenous in mammalian brain (61).

Animal Studies

Table 10 summarizes analyses of norharman and harman in animal fluids and tissues. The extents to which they are

TABLE 9. Representative Xenobiotic Sources of β-Carbolines: Norharman and Harman

Source	Concentrations	References
Broiled/fried meats & fish	20−160 ng/g	(68)
Grilled bacon & drippings	0.1−30 ng/g	(44)
Tryptophan: pyrrolysates	ng/g amounts	(40,97)
Soy, corn, & rye flour	1−40 ng/g	(1)
Cigarette smoke	4−12 µg/g	(81,94)
Marijuana smoke	Qualitative i.d.	(48)
Airborne particulates	Qualitative i.d.	(51)
Beer	7.3−140 ng/ml	(12)
Wine, beer, liquor	0.2−8.5 ng/ml	(1)
Sake	67−600 ng/ml	(1,100)
Vinegar, soy sauce	15−700 ng/ml	(1)
Fungi & angiosperms	Descriptive review	(6)

TABLE 10. Norharman and Harman in Rat and Human Tissues

βC	Species	Tissue	References
Norharman	Rat	Plasma	(89)
	Rat	Brain, liver, kidney	(38)
	Human	Red cells	(86)
	Human	Plasma	(15,39,49,86)
	Human	Brain	(54)
	Human	Cerebrospinal fluid	(57)
Harman	Rat	Brain	(11,84,91)
	Rat	Urine	(84)
	Rat	Lung	(11)
	Human	Platelets	(10)
	Human	Urine	(84)
	Human	Red blood cells	(86)
	Human	Plasma	(15,49)
	Human	Brain	(54)
	Human	Cerebrospinal fluid	(57)

derived from external sources (*see* Table 9) *vs.* endogenous biosynthesis have not been precisely determined. In some circumstances, the environment probably constitutes a major source (1,104), but endogenous synthesis could be important, particularly in the case of norharman in smokers (15,85). When monomethylated on the β[2] nitrogen, norharman, harman, and related βCs are transformed into essentially superimposable structural analogs of MPP$^+$ (25,26,82) (Fig. 4). Whereas the N-methylated norharman and harman cations have yet to be found in the environment, they have been detected and estimated in human brain and CSF (54,57). They presumably arise *in vivo* and particularly within the nervous system, from S-adenosylmethionine–dependent N-methylation of the neutral lipophilic βCs (28). As shown in Figure 4, the initial 2-mono-N-methyl products can be subsequently methylated on the indole nitrogen to form 2,9-di-N-methylated β-carbolinium cations (58). Parenthetically, only 2-mono-N-methylation takes place with THβCs, possibly by a mammalian enzyme other than those acting on heteroaromatic βCs (55). The product, 2-Me-THβC, was the first N-methylated carboline to be quantified in animal tissues (9). Plants used by indigenous South American peoples to induce altered perception and hallucinations are also known to contain various 2-Me-THβCs (4).

Brain 9[indole]-N-methylation of a 2-Me-βC species generates a di-N-methylated carbolinium cation inside the blood-brain barrier that does not readily deprotonate (neutralize), and thus, with a possible exception, is a more potent "MPP$^+$-like" neurotoxicant than its precursor. For example, in isolated mitochondria, N-methylated βC cations are about as effective as MPP$^+$ with respect to respiratory inhibition at complex I (5,41,47), but the 2,9-di-N-methyl-ated species more closely resemble the inhibitory behavior of the pyridinium cation than do the 2-mono-N-methylated derivatives. Furthermore, inhibition of MAO-A from human brain by norharman and harmane is significantly increased by the addition of 2- and 9-N-methyl groups (45).

The *in vivo* neurotoxic effects of N-methylated βC cations on nigrostriatal brain neurons have been compared to MPP$^+$ in adult rats. Striatal microdialysis experiments revealed that the 2-Me-norharmanium cation exerted appreciable and apparently irreversible neurotoxicity (83), but that addition of a 9-[indole-N]methyl group to 2-methyl-ated cation resulted in a substantial increase in neurotoxic efficacy (28); nevertheless, the 2,9-dimethylated species was an order of magnitude less toxic to striatal dopaminergic terminals than MPP$^+$. After intranigral injection, comparisons of the extent of nigrostriatal toxicity indicated that 2-Me-norharmanium cation was several orders of magnitude less potent than MPP$^+$ (75,83). In a more detailed study, measurement of nigral lesion sizes and striatal dopamine and dopac levels following acute intranigral administration showed, in accord with *in vitro* results, that the 2,9-dimethylated norharman/harman derivatives and 2-Me-harmalinium cation were the most neurotoxic methylated βC cations (74). These neurotoxic cations caused nigral lesions that approached the size of the lesion induced by MPP$^+$, and significantly depleted the striatal levels of both dopamine and its acid metabolite. Neutral βCs and 2-mono-N-methylated βC cations other than 2-Me-harmalinium displayed little or no neurotoxic effect when histological and neurochemical end points were evaluated together.

Correlations between the toxic potencies of selected N-methylated βC cations *in vivo* and their potencies in a series of *in vitro* studies—namely, blockade of synaptosomal DA uptake, inhibition of mitochondrial respiration, toxicity in PC-12 cells, and inhibition of rat brain MAO-A (data from the laboratory of R. Ramsay)—revealed unexpected relationships (74). For example, the ability of βCs and *N*-methylated βC cations to inhibit dopamine uptake in isolated brain synaptosomes correlated well with the size of nigral lesions ($r = +0.78$; $p < 0.05$) or the percent depletions of striatal dopamine ($r = -0.70$) obtained in *in vivo* experiments; however, the opposite correlations should have been observed if the neurotoxicity of the cations depended on affinity for the dopamine-uptake system. Furthermore, in comparisons of just the *in vitro* studies, a surprisingly strong negative relationship ($r = -0.84$) emerged between the toxicities of *N*-methylated βC cations in PC-12 cells (cell protein) and their inhibition constants with MAO-A. Such a correlation might indicate that MAO-A further "bioactivates" the βC cations, in much the same fashion that MAO-B carries out the bioactivation of MPTP (103). Alternatively, the βC cation's primary toxic mechanism of mitochondrial respiratory inhibition could be potentiated by an amine that accumulates as a result of the MAO blockade.

Consistent with results obtained with primary mesencephalic culture studies, the most cytotoxic *N*-methylated βC cations, the 2,9-dimethylated forms and 2-Me-harmalinium cation, are not highly specific for nigral dopaminergic neurons *in vivo* (74). However, concerns about the lack of neuronal specificity in these experiments are somewhat lessened if the *N*-methylated products of xenobiotic carbolines tend to accumulate within a certain brain region or within specific brain cells. Measurements of the *N*-methylated species in human brain provide evidence for selective regional production or removal. In normal human brain, the levels of norharman, 2-Me-norharmanium cation, and 2,9-diMe-norharmanium cation were 7–15 times higher in substantia nigra, the principal site of neuronal degeneration in PD, than in frontal cortex (54). Although PD brain tissue has not yet been analyzed, approximately 50% of CSF from PD patients—but none of the samples from control individuals—contained detectable amounts of the neurotoxic 2,9-dimethylated norharmanium cation (57).

A somewhat different βC that has received consideration as a potential neurotoxicant underlying neurodegenerative conditions such as PD is 1-trichloromethyl-THβC or "TaClo" (16). The molecule could arise in the environment and in animal cells *via* tryptamine's condensation with the aldehydic form of the hypnotic, chloral hydrate. TaClo was detected by gas chromatography/mass spectrometry (GC/MS) in the blood and brain of 10%–30% of rats treated chronically with the above reactants. TaClo and its 2-*N*-

methyl derivative exert behavioral and neurochemical toxic effects in rats, but their potencies relative to MPTP and MPP⁺ have not been clearly delineated. Another environmental source of chloral hydrate would be from the metabolism of trichloroethylene, a widely used industrial and commercial solvent. If TaClo was a promoter of PD, occupations linked to trichloroethylene usage such as in the dry-cleaning industry might be expected to carry a higher risk for the disease.

An additional aspect of βC neurotoxicity concerns livestock: certain forage grasses contain intrinsic toxins that can result in chronic and long-lasting neurological damage in sheep, cattle, and other ruminants (17). Poisoning due to *Phalaris* grasses in sheep induces a nervous syndrome and a sudden death syndrome. The former syndrome is believed to be related to the indole alkaloid content of the grasses, of which key toxic constituents are THβCs and open-chain tryptamine derivatives. Furthermore, locomotor disturbances in sheep consuming Australian *Tribulus terrestis* are thought to be due to norharman and harman in the plant materials, since administration of the two βCs caused similar motor problems (limb paresis) in experimental studies (13). In these aforementioned cases, the specific mechanisms of neurological damage induced by the indoles remain obscure.

In Vitro Studies

The cytotoxicities of the *N*-methyl βC cations have been compared to MPP⁺ in rat PC-12 cells and fetal rat mesencephalic cultures. In PC-12 cells cultured in media with relatively low glucose concentrations, 2,9-diMe-βC cations and 2-Me-harmalinium cation (boxed structures in Fig. 4) are equivalent to MPP⁺ as cytotoxicants—other 2-mono-*N*-methylated βC cations are negligibly toxic or nontoxic (18). At relatively high glucose concentrations, however, the toxic potencies of MPP⁺ and the 2,9-diMe-βC cations (represented by 2,9-diMe-norharmanium cation) in PC-12 cells were greatly suppressed. This is inferred to mean that the principal cytotoxic mechanism of 2,9-diMe-βC cations, like MPP⁺, is interference with mitochondrial energy metabolism, which is readily overcome in these glycolytic cells by the additional glucose. However, the high glucose conditions did not reduce the potent cytotoxicity of 2-Me-harmalinium cation, indicating that this carbolinium species has a different mechanism of action (18).

In fetal rat primary mesencephalic cultures, the EC50s with respect to toxicity toward dopaminergic neurons (EC50$_{DA}$) for 2,9-diMe-norharmanium, 2,9-diMe-harmanium, and 2-Me-harmalinium cations were all approximately 10 μM under the conditions utilized (2-day exposures in 6-day-old cultures) (27,29). In comparison, MPP$^+$ was some 25-fold more effective as a dopaminergic neurotoxin in the primary cultures. Furthermore, the remarkably high toxic selectivity of exogenous MPP$^+$ for dopaminergic neurons (as manifested by the high value for EC50$_{GABA}$/EC50$_{DA}$) was not evident with any carbolinium toxicants. However, an aromatic methoxy group appeared significantly to potentiate the toxicity of the 2,9-dimethylated βC cations; the EC50$_{DA}$ for 2,9-diMe-harminium cation was <2 μM in mesencephalic cultures, nearly five times stronger than its nonmethoxylated analog (2,9-diMe-harmanium cation) and only six-fold less effective than MPP$^+$ (27).

ISOQUINOLINES

In plants and animals, IQs can be derived as shown in Figure 3 from TIQs that form *via* the bimolecular condensation reaction of a phenylethylamine and an aldehyde (62). Initial interest in TIQs as neurotoxicants in humans stemmed from alcoholism research (19,62) and the reactivity of dopamine with the acetaldehyde arising from ethanol oxidation (106). Salsolinol (the TIQ derived from the above two reactants; Fig. 5), apparently a human brain constituent (92), is increased in the brains of ethanol-intoxicated rats treated with an aldehyde dehydrogenase inhibitor (24). Some studies showed increased salsolinol in the urine of alcoholics early in detoxification, while others did not (22,37). Rats consuming ethanol *ad libitum* for many weeks were reported to have higher brain striatal levels of salso-

linol (93). However, this appears to depend upon coingestion of 3,4-dihydroxyphenylalanine (DOPA), the amino acid precursor to dopamine that is normally present in rat chow, since the brain levels of salsolinol were not significantly increased by ethanol in liquid diets lacking DOPA unless the amino acid was supplemented (30).

In reference to neurotoxicity in alcoholism, salsolinol and other dopamine-related TIQs, as readily oxidizable catechols, were suggested to generate quinoidimine forms of DIQs that might have the potential to be "6-hydroxydopamine–like" neurotoxicants (21). The catalytic oxidation by enzymes *in vitro* of salsolinol to form DIQs, IQs, and more complex adducts has been studied in some detail (36), but there is no definitive evidence that the quinoidimine products are neurotoxic factors in alcohol abuse. Another TIQ that has received attention *vis-à-vis* neurotoxicants is tetrahydropapaveroline (THP) (Fig. 5), a readily oxidizable Pictet-Spengler product of dopamine and dopaldehyde that is a morphinan alkaloid precursor (62). It was one of the initial "mammalian alkaloids" associated with alcohol metabolism (32); a GC/MS study has reported the presence of the (S)-enantiomer of THP in brain and heart of rats chronically ingesting ethanol (63).

Animal Studies

With the discovery of MPTP-induced parkinsonism, two structural types of TIQs and IQs (*see* Fig. 5) have been investigated as neurotoxic factors in PD: simple nonoxygenated IQs, mainly represented by TIQ itself (formally an adduct of formaldehyde with phenylethylamine) and its de-

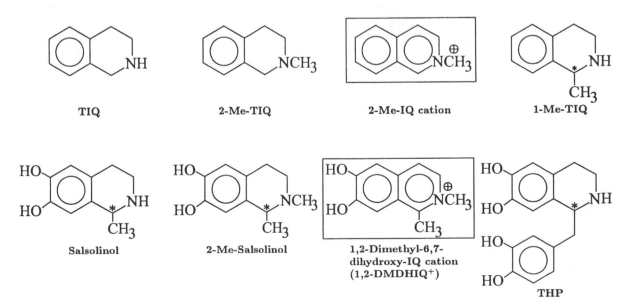

FIGURE 5. Tetrahydroisoquinoline (TIQ) structures and related IQ cations. * = chiral carbon. The most neurotoxic species are enclosed in boxes.

rivatives, and dopamine-derived salsolinol and its derivatives. The basic TIQ molecule and its N-methyl product (2-Me-TIQ) occur in similar amounts in brain samples from parkinsonian and control subjects (79). These nonoxygenated heterocyclics readily cross the blood-brain barrier and are most reasonably derived from environmental sources (23), but 2-Me-TIQ could result from N-methyl-transferase activity *in vivo* (78). By analogy with MPP^+, the formation of the aromatized isoquinoline cation (2-Me-IQ^+; Fig. 5) is of concern, and the cation can be produced from 2-Me-TIQ by the action of MAO (69). Interestingly, TIQ itself is a poor substrate for MAO oxidation. Most neurotoxicity investigations with the nonoxygenated IQ series have been carried out *in vivo*, but studies with primary cultures rich in dopaminergic neurons indicate that 2-Me-IQ^+ is more cytotoxic than TIQ or 2-Me-TIQ (76,77). TIQ, 2-Me-TIQ and 2-Me-IQ^+ have been examined as neurotoxicants *in vivo* in monkeys and in mice (42,107). Behavioral motor syndromes resembling parkinsonism were variably induced in monkeys by the three heterocyclics. Histological and neurochemical examination of the monkey substantia nigra indicated that reduced levels of tyrosine hydroxylase (TH) and dopamine neurotransmitter, rather than loss of dopaminergic neurons *per se*, might underlie the motor disturbances. In young adult mice, TIQ treatment also did not induce substantial cellular neurotoxicity (80), but suppression of immunoreactive TH has been observed (107). Comparatively, neurotoxic effects (reductions in TH-positive cell numbers in the substantia nigra and other brain regions) were evident in mice treated intraperitoneally with 2-Me-TIQ for several months (42).

Investigating the possibility that mitochondrial respiratory inhibition by the nonoxygenated IQ derivatives might subserve their varied neurotoxic effects, researchers showed that TIQ inhibits complex I–mediated respiration (98), but there was no direct comparison with MPP^+. More recent studies demonstrate that IQ and 2-Me-IQ cation are actually more potent than MPP^+ as inhibitors of complex I in mitochondrial fragments, but less effective with intact mitochondria (59,60). This has led to the postulate that respiratory inhibition by the IQ derivatives is controlled by transport into mitochondria rather than interaction with complex I enzymes.

Paradoxically, 1-Me-TIQ, a rat brain component that decreases with age (8), was reported to prevent the parkinsonian behavioral symptoms induced in mice by either TIQ or MPTP, but had little neurotoxic activity on its own (102). Its neuroprotection has been ascribed to inhibition of MAO, which would diminish the formation of hydrogen peroxide and derived free radicals (69). If this substance occurs in humans, age-dependent reductions in levels of neuroprotectant 1-Me-TIQ could lead to progressive vulnerability in environmentally determined neurodegenerative diseases (8).

A host of studies on the (R)- and (S)-enantiomers of the catecholic IQs, salsolinol, and its N-methylated/aromatized derivatives, has been spawned by the MPTP discovery. The (R)-enantiomers of salsolinol and N-methyl-salsolinol (Fig. 5) appear to be the principal forms existing endogenously in human brain (34), but (S)-salsolinol predominates in foods and beverages (96). Initial evidence has been presented for stereospecific brain biosynthesis of the (R)-enantiomer (72). The N-methyl (R)-derivative could be an *in vivo* N-methylation product, as evidenced by its formation after central microdialysis of racemic salsolinol in the rat (53). Furthermore, N-methyl-(R)-salsolinol forms the 1,2-dimethyl-6,7-dihydroxy-isoquinolinium cation ($1,2$-$DMDHIQ^+$ in Fig. 5) nonenzymatically in phosphate buffer, enzymatically in human brain mitochondria, and in various brain regions of rats following central injection (70,71,73). A related catecholisoquinoline, N-methyl-norsalsolinol, but not isomeric (racemic) salsolinol, was reported to be oxidized by MAO, presumably to the catecholic isoquinolinium cation (65).

Evidence for neurotoxic actions *in vivo* has been obtained with the N-methyl and oxidized derivatives of (R)-salsolinol, apparently the chief enantiomer in human brain. Acute central administration of N-methyl-(R)-salsolinol was reported to induce postural changes in rats that resembled parkinsonism (70). Neurochemical changes induced by chronic administration into rat brain of the aforementioned catecholic TIQ, or its aromatized isoquinolinium derivative, $1,2$-$DMDHIQ^+$, were indicative of marked toxicity to the nigrostriatal system (71); $1,2$-$DMDHIQ^+$ appeared to exert more selective cytotoxic effects than its TIQ precursor.

In Vitro Studies

The toxicity in SH-SY5Y neuroblastoma cell cultures of racemic salsolinol was reported to be equivalent to MPP^+ and MPTP (105). Unlike MPTP, salsolinol's cytotoxicity in these cultures remains to be clarified; it was neither dependent on catecholamine-uptake systems or MAO activity, nor was it prevented by free-radical trapping reagents. Nevertheless, oxidative stress may be a mechanism for degeneration of nigrostriatal neurons in PD (20,108). Catecholic isoquinolines such as salsolinol were less effective than dopamine in evoking generation of hydroxyl radicals *in vitro* and even suppressed generation by dopamine itself (35). As mentioned before, respiratory impairment in mitochondria is another possible reason for accelerated senescence of dopamine neurons in PD, but with mouse brain mitochondria, racemic salsolinol was a relatively weak inhibitor of complex I respiration (99).

Human Studies

N-Methyl-(R)-salsolinol was detectable in the CSF of all controls and PD patients who were not currently undergoing L-dopa therapy, whereas the (S)-enantiomer was below detection (52). Perhaps more significant were the two-fold higher levels of the (R)-enantiomer in the PD samples. Another study determined that the related TIQ, 2-me-norsalsolinol, was detectable in approximately 50% of CSF samples from PD patients (both with and without concurrent L-dopa therapy) but was absent from control samples (66). These latter findings are similar to results with 2,9-di-N-methylated norharmanium cation (*vide supra*). However, primarily because of its higher levels early in the disease process, 2-Me-norsalsolinol was proposed as a marker for compensatory initial increases in dopamine turnover rather than an etiological toxic factor. Of a related nature is a report that urinary levels of salsolinol (enantiomeric composition not specified) are three-fold higher in PD patients with visual hallucinations than in those without the disturbances (67); it was suggested that salsolinol *in vivo* may be a predictor or indicator of hallucinatory behavior. A recurring question concerns the therapeutic benefits of L-dopa for PD patients in the face of knowledge that formation of potentially neurotoxic catechol IQ precursors such as salsolinol, THP, and 1-carboxylated THP isomers, as well as endogenous morphine, may be promoted by the therapy itself (31,56,87). Clinical and animal studies are needed to assess the significance of these observations.

Editors' Note: A recent epidemiological study in Guadeloupe found a relationship between atypical parkinsonism and consumption of herbal tea and fruits of the Annonaceae family (*Annona muricata* and *A. squamosa*), which contain neurotoxic benzyltetrahydroisoquinoline compounds (Caparros-Lefebvre D, Elbaz A (1999) *Lancet* **354**, 281.

REFERENCES

1. Adachi J, Mizoi Y, Naito T *et al.* (1991) Determination of β-carbolines in foodstuffs by high-performance liquid chromatography and high-performance liquid chromatography-mass spectrometry. *J Chromatogr* **538**, 331.
2. Adamec R (1994) Modelling anxiety disorders following chemical exposures. *Toxicol Ind Health* **10**, 391.
3. Adell A, Myers RD (1994) Increased alcohol intake in low alcohol drinking rats after chronic infusion of the beta-carboline harman into the hippocampus. *Pharmacol Biochem Behav* **49**, 949.
4. Agurell S, Holmstedt B, Lindgren J-E *et al.* (1968) Identification of two new β-carboline alkaloids in South American hallucinogenic plants. *Biochem Pharmacol* **17**, 2487.
5. Albores R Jr, Neafsey EJ, Drucker G *et al.* (1990) Mitochondrial respiratory inhibition by N-methylated β-carboline derivatives structurally resembling N-methyl-4-phenylpyridine. *Proc Nat Acad Sci USA* **87**, 9368.
6. Allen MS, Holmstedt B (1980) The simple β-carboline alkaloids. *Phytochemistry* **19**, 1573.
7. Ansher SS, Cadet JL, Jacoby WB *et al.* (1986) Role of N-methyltransferases in the neurotoxicity associated with the metabolites of 1-methyl-4-phenyl-1,2,3,6-tetrahydropyridine (MPTP) and other 4-substituted pyridines in the environment. *Biochem Pharmacol* **35**, 3359.
8. Ayala A, Parrado J, Cano J *et al.* (1994) Reduction of 1-methyl 1,2,3,4-tetrahydroisoquinoline level in substantia nigra of the aged rat. *Brain Res* **638**, 334.
9. Barker S, Harrison R, Monti J *et al.* (1981) Identification and quantification of 1,2,3,4-tetrahydro-β-carboline, 2-methyl-1,2,3,4-tetrahydro-β-carboline, and 6-methoxy-1,2,3,4-tetrahydro-β-carboline as *in vivo* constituents of rat brain and adrenal gland. *Biochem Pharmacol* **30**, 9.
10. Bidder TG, Shoemaker DW, Boettger HG *et al.* (1979) Harman in human platelets. *Life Sci* **25**, 157.
11. Bosin T, Borg S, Faull KF (1989) Harman in rat brain, lung and human CSF: Effect of alcohol consumption. *Alcohol* **5**, 505.
12. Bosin T, Faull KF (1988) Harman in alcoholic beverages: Pharmacological and toxicological implications. *Alcohol Clin Exp Res* **12**, 679.
13. Bourke CA, Stevens GR, Carrigan MJ (1992) Locomotor effects in sheep of alkaloids identified in Australian *Tribulus terrestris*. *Aust Vet J* **69**, 163.
14. Braestrup C, Nielsen M, Olsen C (1980) Urinary and brain β-carboline-3-carboxylate as potent inhibitor of brain benzodiazepine receptors. *Proc Nat Acad Sci USA* **74**, 3805.
15. Breyer-Pfaff U, Wiatr G, Stevens I *et al.* (1996) Elevated norharman plasma levels in alcoholic patients and controls resulting from tobacco smoking. *Life Sci* **58**, 1425.
16. Bringmann G, Feineis D, God R *et al.* (1996) Neurotoxic effects on the dopaminergic system induced by TaClo (1-trichloromethyl-1,2,3,4-tetrahydro-β-carboline), a potential mammalian alkaloid: *in vivo* and *in vitro* studies. *Biog Amine* **12**, 83.
17. Cheeke PR (1995) Endogenous toxins and mycotoxins in forage grasses and their effects on livestock. *J Anim Sci* **73**, 909.
18. Cobuzzi R Jr, Neafsey EJ, Collins MA (1994) Differential cytotoxicities of N-methyl-β-carbolinium analogues of MPP$^+$ in PC12 cells: Insights into potential neurotoxicants in Parkinson's disease. *J Neurochem* **62**, 1503.

19. Cohen G (1976) Alkaloid products in the metabolism of alcohol and biogenic amines. *Biochem Pharmacol* **25**, **1123.**

20. Cohen G, Werner P (1994) Free radicals, oxidative stress, and neurodegeneration. In: *Neurodegenerative Disease.* Calne DB ed. WB Saunders Co, Philadelphia p. 138.

21. Collins MA (1982) A possible neurochemical mechanism for brain and nerve damage associated with chronic alcoholism. *Trends Pharmacol Sci* **3**, 373.

22. Collins MA (1988) Acetaldehyde and its amine condensation products as markers in alcoholism. *Recent Develop Alcohol* **6**, 387.

23. Collins MA (1994) Parkinsonian protoxicants within and without. *Neurobiol Aging* **15**, 277.

24. Collins MA, Bigdeli MG (1975) Tetrahydroisoquinolines *in vivo.* Rat brain formation of salsolinol, a condensation product of dopamine and acetaldehyde, under certain conditions during ethanol intoxication. *Life Sci* **16**, 585.

25. Collins MA, Neafsey EJ (1985) β-Carboline analogues of *N*-methyl-4-phenyl-1,2,5,6-tetrahydropyridine (MPTP): Endogenous factors underlying idiopathic parkinsonism? *Neurosci Lett* **55**, 179.

26. Collins MA, Neafsey EJ, Cheng BY *et al.* (1986) Endogenous analogs of *N*-methyl-4-phenyl-tetrahydropyridine: Indoleamine-derived tetrahydro-β-carbolines as potential causative factors in Parkinson's disease. *Ann Neurol* **45**, 179.

27. Collins MA, Neafsey EJ, Matsubara K (1996) β-Carbolines: Metabolism and neurotoxicity. *Biog Amine* **12**, 171.

28. Collins MA, Neafsey EJ, Matsubara K *et al.* (1992) Indole-*N*-methylated β-carbolinium ions as potential brain-bioactivated neurotoxins. *Brain Res* **570**, 154.

29. Collins MA, Slobodnik L, Neafsey EJ (1995) Inhibitors of NO synthase and poly (ADP-ribose) synthase (PARS) do not block toxic actions of β-carbolinium cations or MPP⁺ in mesencephalic cultures. *Soc Neurosci* **21**, 1259.

30. Collins MA, Ung-Chhun NS, Cheng B *et al.* (1990) Brain and plasma tetrahydroisoquinolines in rats: Effects of chronic ethanol intake and diet. *J Neurochem* **55**, 1507.

31. Coscia CJ, Burke W, Jamroz G *et al.* (1977) Occurrence of a new class of tetrahydroisoquinoline alkaloids in L-dopa-treated parkinsonian patients. *Nature* **269**, 617.

32. Davis VE, Walsh MJ (1970) Alcohol, amines and alkaloids: A possible biochemical basis for alcohol addiction. *Science* **167**, 1005.

33. de Meester C (1995) Genotoxic potential of beta-carbolines: A review. *Mutat Res* **339**, 139.

34. Deng Y, Maruyama W, Dostert P *et al.* (1995) Determination of the (*R*)- and (*S*)-enantiomers of salsolinol and *N*-methylsalsolinol by use of a chiral high-performance liquid chromatographic column. *J Chromatogr* **670**, 47.

35. Dostert P, La Croix R, Maruyama W *et al.* (1996) Effects of dopamine-derived isoquinolines on hydroxyl radical formation by dopamine autoxidation. *Biog Amine* **12**, 149.

36. Fa Z, Dryhurst G (1991) Interactions of salsolinol with oxidative enzymes. *Biochem Pharmacol* **42**, 2209.

37. Feest U, Kemper A, Nickel B *et al.* (1991) Comparison of salsolinol excretion in alcoholics and nonalcoholic controls. *Alcohol* **9**, 49.

38. Fekkes D, Bode WT (1993) Occurrence and partition of the beta-carboline norharman in rat organs. *Life Sci* **52**, 2045.

39. Fekkes D, Schouten MJ, Pepplinkhuizen L *et al.* (1992) Norharman, a normal body constituent. *Lancet* **339**, 506.

40. Felton JS, Knize MG (1990) Heterocyclic-amine mutagens/carcinogens in foods. In: *Chemical Carcinogenesis and Mutagenesis I.* Cooper CS, Grover PL eds. Springer-Verlag, Berlin p. 502.

41. Fields J, Albores R Jr, Neafsey EJ, Collins MA (1992) Inhibition of mitochondrial succinate oxidation: Similarities and differences between *N*-methylated β-carbolines and MPP⁺. *Arch Biochem Biophys* **294**, 539.

42. Fukuda T (1994) 2-Methyl-1,2,3,4-tetrahydroisoquinoline does dependently reduce the number of tyrosine hydroxylase-immunoreactive cells in the substantia nigra and locus ceruleus of C57BL/6J mice. *Brain Res* **639**, 325.

43. Gorrell JM, DiMonte D, Graham D (1996) The role of the environment in Parkinson's disease. *Environ Health Perspect* **104**, 652.

44. Gross GA, Turesky RJ, Fay LB *et al.* (1993) Heterocyclic aromatic amine formation in grilled bacon, beef and fish and in grill scrapings. *Carcinogen* **14**, 2313.

45. Hasegawa S, Matsubara K, Takahashi A *et al.* (1995) Inhibition of type A monoamine oxidase by *N*-methyl β-carbolinium ions. *Biog Amine* **11**, 295.

46. Holmstedt B (1982) Beta-carbolines and tetrahydroisoquinolines: Historical and ethnopharmacological background. In: *Beta-Carbolines and Tetrahydroisoquinolines.* Bloom FE, Barchas J, Sandler M, Usdin E eds. Alan R Liss, New York p. 3.

47. Hoppel CL, Greenblatt D, Kwok H *et al.* (1987) Inhibition of mitochondrial respiration by analogs of 4-phenylpyridine and 1-methyl-4-phenyl-pyridinium cation (MPP⁺), the neurotoxic metabolite of MPTP. *Biochem Biophys Res Commun* **148**, 684.

48. Kettenes-van den Bosch JJ, Salemink CA (1977) Cannabis XVI. Constituents of marijuana smoke condensate. *J Chromatogr* **131**, 422.

49. Kuhn W, Muller T, Grosse H *et al.* (1995) Plasma harman and norharman in Parkinson's disease. *J Neural Transm* **46**, 291.

50. Langston JW, Ballard P, Tetrud JW *et al.* (1983) Chronic parkinsonism in humans due to a product of meperidine-analog synthesis. *N Engl J Med* **219**, 979.

51. Lofroth G (1994) Airborne mutagens and carcinogens

from cooking and other food preparation processes. *Toxicol Lett* **72**, 83.

52. Maruyama W, Abe T, Tohgi H *et al.* (1996) A dopaminergic neurotoxin, (*R*)-*N*-methylsalsolinol, increases in parkinsonian cerebrospinal fluid. *Ann Neurol* **40**, 119.

53. Maruyama W, Nakahara D, Ota M *et al.* (1992) *N*-Methylation of dopamine-derived 6,7-dihydroxy-1,2,3,4-tetrahydroisoquinoline, (*R*)-salsolinol, in rat brains: *In vivo* microdialysis study. *J Neurochem* **59**, 395.

54. Matsubara K, Collins MA, Akane A *et al.* (1993) Potential bioactivated neurotoxicants, *N*-methylated β-carbolinium ions, are present in human brain. *Brain Res* **610**, 90.

55. Matsubara K, Collins MA, Neafsey EJ (1992) Mono-*N*-methylation of 1,2,3,4-tetrahydro-β-carbolines in brain cytosol: Absence of indole methylation. *J Neurochem* **59**, 505.

56. Matsubara K, Fukushima S, Akane E *et al.* (1992) Increased urinary morphine, codeine and tetrahydropapaveroline in parkinsonian patients undergoing L-DOPA therapy: A possible biosynthetic pathway of morphine from L-DOPA in humans. *J Pharmacol Exp Ther* **260**, 974.

57. Matsubara K, Kobayashi S, Kobayashi Y *et al.* (1995) β-Carbolinium cations, endogenous MPP$^+$ analogs, in the lumbar cerebrospinal fluid of patients with Parkinson's disease. *Neurology* **45**, 2240.

58. Matsubara K, Neafsey EJ, Collins MA (1992) Novel *S*-adenosylmethionine-dependent indole-*N*-methylation of β-carbolines in brain particulate fractions. *J Neurochem* **59**, 511.

59. McNaught KSt P, Thull U, Carrupt PA *et al.* (1995) Inhibition of complex I by isoquinoline derivatives structurally related to MPTP. *Biochem Pharmacol* **50**, 1903.

60. McNaught KSt P, Thull U, Carrupt PA *et al.* (1996) Effect of isoquinoline derivatives structurally related to MPTP on mitochondrial respiration. *Biochem Pharmacol* **51**, 1503.

61. Medina JH, de Stein ML, DeRobertis E (1989) *n*-[^{3}H]Butyl-β-carboline-3-carboxylate, a putative endogenous ligand, binds preferentially to subtype 1 of central benzodiazepine receptors. *J Neurochem* **52**, 665.

62. Melchior CM, Collins MA (1982) The routes and significance of endogenous synthesis of alkaloids in animals. *CRC Crit Rev Toxicol* **10**, 313.

63. Melzig MF, Haber H, Putscher I *et al.* (1996) Chronic alcohol intake induces formation of tetrahydropapaveroline in rat brain and heart. *Alcohol Clin Exp Res* **20**, 106A.

64. Mizuno Y, Mori H, Kondo T (1995) Parkinson's disease—from etiology to treatment. *Int Med* **34**, 1045.

65. Moser A, Kompf D (1992) Presence of methyl-6,7-dihydroxy-1,2,3,4-tetrahydroisoquinolines, derivatives of the neurotoxin isoquinoline, in parkinsonian lumbar CSF. *Life Sci* **50**, 1885.

66. Moser A, Scholz J, Nobbe F *et al.* (1995) Presence of *N*-methyl-salsolinol in the CSF: Correlations with dopamine metabolites of patients with Parkinson's disease. *J Neurol Sci* **131**, 183.

67. Moser A, Siebecker F, Vieregge P *et al.* (1996) Salsolinol, catecholamine metabolites, and visual hallucinations in L-dopa-treated patients with Parkinson's disease. *J Neural Transm* **103**, 421.

68. Nagao M, Honda M, Seino Y *et al.* (1977) Mutagenicities of smoke condensates and the charred surface of fish and meat. *Cancer Lett* **2**, 221.

69. Naoi M, Maruyama W (1993) Type B monoamine oxidase and neurotoxins. *Eur Neurol* **33**, 31.

70. Naoi M, Maruyama W, Dostert P *et al.* (1996) Animal model of Parkinson's disease induced by naturally-occurring 1(*R*), 2(*N*)-dimethyl-6,7-dihydroxy-1,2,3,4-tetrahydroisoquinoline. *Biog Amine* **12**, 135.

71. Naoi M, Maruyama W, Dostert P *et al.* (1996) Dopamine-derived endogenous 1(*R*),2(*N*)-dimethyl-6,7-dihydroxy-1,2,3,4-tetrahydroisoquinoline, *N*-methyl-(*R*)-salsolinol, induced parkinsonism in rat—biochemical, pathological and behavioral studies. *Brain Res* **709**, 285.

72. Naoi M, Maruyama W, Dostert P *et al.* (1996) A novel enzyme enantio-selectively synthesizes (*R*)salsolinol, a precursor of the dopaminergic neurotoxin, *N*-methyl (*R*)salsolinol. *Neurosci Lett* **212**, 183.

73. Naoi M, Maruyama W, Zhang JH *et al.* (1995) Enzymatic oxidation of the dopaminergic neurotoxin, 1(*R*),2(*N*)-dimethyl-6,7-dihydroxy-1,2,3,4-tetrahydro-isoquinoline, into 1,2(*N*)-dimethyl-6,7-dihydroxy-iso-quinolinium ion. *Life Sci* **57**, 1061.

74. Neafsey EJ, Drucker G, Raikoff K, Collins MA (1989) Striatal dopaminergic toxicity following intranigral injection in rats of 2-methyl-norharman, a β-carbolinium analog of *N*-methyl-4-phenylpyridinium ion. *Neurosci Lett* **105**, 344.

75. Neafsey EJ, Albores R Jr, Gearhart D *et al.* (1995) Methyl-β-carbolinium analogs of MPP$^+$ cause nigrostriatal toxicity after substantia nigra injections in rats. *Brain Res* **675**, 279.

76. Niijima K, Araki M, Ogawa M *et al.* (1991) *N*-Methyl-isoquinolinium ion destroys cultured mesencephalic dopamine neurons. *Biog Amine* **8**, 61.

77. Nishi K, Mochizuki H, Furukawa Y *et al.* (1994) Neurotoxic effects of MPP$^+$ and tetrahydroisoquinoline derivatives on dopaminergic neurons in ventral mesencephalic-striatal co-culture. *Neurodegeneration* **3**, 33.

78. Niwa T, Yshizumi H, Tatematsu A *et al.* (1990) Endogenous synthesis of *N*-methyl-1,2,3,4-tetrahydroisoquinoline, a precursor of *N*-methyl-isoquinolinium ion, in the brains of primates with parkinsonism after systemic ad-

ministration of 1,2,3,4-tetrahydroisoquinoline. *J Chromatog* 533, 145.

79. Ohta S, Kohno M, Makino Y *et al.* (1987) Tetrahydroisoquinoline and 1-methyl-tetrahydro-isoquinoline are present in human brain: Relation to Parkinson's disease. *Biomed Res* 8, 453.

80. Perry TL, Jones K, Hansen S (1988) Tetrahydroisoquinoline lacks dopaminergic nigrostriatal neurotoxicity in mice. *Neurosci Lett* 85, 101.

81. Poindexter EH, Carpenter RD (1962) The isolation of harmane and norharmane from tobacco and cigarette smoke. *Phytochemistry* 1, 215.

82. Ramsden D, Williams A (1985) Production in nature of a compound resembling methyl-phenyl-tetrahydropyridine, a possible cause of Parkinson's disease. *Lancet* i, 215.

83. Rollema H, Booth R, Castagnoli NJ (1988) *In vivo* dopaminergic neurotoxicity of the 2-β-methylcarbolinium ion, a potential endogenous MPP⁺ analog. *Eur J Pharmacol* 153, 151.

84. Rommelspacher H, Damm H, Schmidt L *et al.* (1985) Increased excretion of harman by alcoholics depends on events of their life history and the state of the liver. *Psychopharmacology* 87, 64.

85. Rommelspacher H, May T, Salewski B (1994) Harman (1-methyl-beta-carboline) is a natural inhibitor of monoamine oxidase A in rats. *Eur J Pharmacol* 252, 51.

86. Rommelspacher H, May T, Susilo R (1991) β-Carbolines and tetrahydroisoquinolines: Detection and function in mammals. *Planta Med* 57, s87.

87. Sandler M, Bonham-Carter S, Hunter KR *et al.* (1973) Tetrahydroisoquinoline alkaloids: *In vivo* metabolites of L-dopa in man. *Nature* 241, 439.

88. Schmiechen R, Seidelmann D, Huth A (1993) Beta-carboline-3-carboxylic acid ethyl ester: A lead for new psychotropic drugs. *Psychopharmacol Ser* 11, 7.

89. Schouten MJ, Bruinvels J (1986) Endogenously formed norharman (beta-carboline) in platelet-rich plasma obtained from porphyric rats. *Pharmacol Biochem Behav* 24, 1219.

90. Schultes RE (1982) The beta-carboline hallucinogens of South America. *J Psychoactive Drug* 14, 205.

91. Shoemaker DW, Cummins JT, Bidder TG *et al.* (1980) Identification of harman in the rat arcuate nucleus. *Arch Pharmacol* 310, 227.

92. Sjoquist B, Eriksson A, Winblad B (1982) Salsolinol and catecholamines in human brain and their relation to alcoholism. *Prog Clin Biol Res* 90, 57.

93. Sjoquist B, Liljequist S, Engel J (1982) Increased salsolinol levels in rat striatum and limbic forebrain following chronic ethanol treatment. *J Neurochem* 39, 259.

94. Snook ME, Chortyk OT (1982) Capillary gas chromatography of carbolines. Application to cigarette smoke. *J Chromatogr* 245, 331.

95. Snyder SH, D'Amato RJ (1986) MPTP: A neurotoxin relevant to the pathophysiology of Parkinson's disease. *Neurology* 36, 250.

96. Strolin Benedetti M, Bellotti V, Poanezola E *et al.* (1989) Ratio of the *R* and *S* enantiomers of salsolinol in food and human urine. *J Neural Transm* 77, 47.

97. Sugimura T, Sato S, Wakabayashi K (1988) Mutagens/carcinogens in pyrolysates of amino acids and proteins in cooked foods: heterocyclic aromatic amines. In: *Chemical Induction of Cancer: Structural Bases and Biological Mechanisms.* Woo TY, Lai DY, Arcose JC, Argus MF eds. Academic Press, New York p. 681.

98. Suzuki K, Muzuno Y, Yoshida M (1989) Selective inhibition of complex I of the brain electron transport system by tetrahydroisoquinoline. *Biochem Biophys Res Commun* 162, 1541.

99. Suzuki K, Mizuno Y, Yoshida M (1990) Inhibition of mitochondrial respiration by 1,2,3,4-tetrahydroisoquinoline-like endogenous alkaloids in mouse brain. *Neurochem Res* 15, 705.

100. Takase S, Murakami H (1966) Studies on fluorescence of sake. I. Fluorescence spectrum of sake and identification of harman. *Agr Biol Chem* 30, 869.

101. Tanner CM (1989) The role of environmental toxins in the etiology of Parkinson's disease. *Trends Neurosci* 12, 49.

102. Tasaki Y, Makino Y, Ohta S *et al.* (1991) 1-Methyl-1,2,3,4-tetrahydroisoquinoline, decreasing in 1-methyl-4-phenyl-1,2,3,6-tetrahydropyridine-treated mouse, prevents parkinsonism-like behavior abnormalities. *J Neurochem* 57, 1940.

103. Tipton KF, Singer TP (1993) Advances in our understanding of the mechanism of the neurotoxicity of MPTP and related compounds. *J Neurochem* 61, 1191.

104. Tsuchiya H, Yamada K, Todoriki H *et al.* (1996) Urinary excretion of tetrahydro-β-carbolines influenced by food and beverage ingestion implies their exogenous supply via dietary sources. *J Nutr Biochem* 7, 237.

105. Willets JM, Lambert DG, Lunec J *et al.* (1995) Studies on the neurotoxicity of 6,7-dihydroxy-1-methyl-1,2,3,4-tetrahydroisoquinoline (salsolinol) in SH-SY5Y cells. *Eur J Pharmacol* 293, 319.

106. Yamanaka, Davis VE, Walsh M (1970) Salsolinol, an alkaloid derivative of dopamine formed *in vitro* during alcohol metabolism. *Nature* 227, 1143.

107. Yoshida M, Ogawa M, Suzuki K *et al.* (1993) Parkinsonism produced by tetrahydroisoquinoline (TIQ) or the analogues. *Adv Neurol* 60, 207.

108. Youdim MBH, Riederer P (1993) The role of iron in senescence of dopaminergic neurons in Parkinson's disease. *J Neural Transm (Suppl)* 40, 57.

109. Zetler G, Singbartl G, Schlosser L (1972) Cerebral pharmacokinetics of tremor-producing harmala and iboga alkaloids. *Pharmacology* 7, 237.

Carbon Disulfide

Doyle G. Graham
William M. Valentine

CS₂

CARBON DISULFIDE

Dithiocarbonic anhydride

NEUROTOXICITY RATING

Clinical

A   Peripheral neuropathy (spasticity, distal axonopathy)

A   Psychobiological reaction (mania, suicide)

C   Chronic encephalopathy

Experimental

A   Distal axonopathy

A   Retinopathy (ganglion cell degeneration)

Carbon disulfide (CS_2) is employed in the synthesis of carbon tetrachloride and as an irreplaceable reactant in the manufacture of rayon fiber and cellophane. Other sources of CS_2 are dithiocarbamates used in cancer chemotherapy and in alcohol aversion therapy (disulfiram) (3), as well as those employed in agriculture (*see* Carbamates, this volume). Historically, CS_2 was widely used as a solvent for fats, rubber, phosphorus, and sulfur; as a grain fumigant; and as a treatment for parasitic infestations in animals (4). Recognition of the toxicity associated with occupational exposure to CS_2 occurred during the middle of the nineteenth century in Europe and was based on both clinical observations and animal studies. The high-dose effects of CS_2 were associated with the cold vulcanization of rubber; workers involved in this process developed an acute mania sometimes accompanied by suicidal tendencies. During the last century, as exposure levels in industry have been reduced, the effects of chronic exposure have been manifested in workers as peripheral neuropathies and accelerated atherosclerosis (4).

CS_2 is a clear liquid at room temperature, with a boiling point of 46.5°C and a vapor pressure of 352.6 mm Hg at 25°C. CS_2 is a volatile and highly flammable chemical that is miscible with organic solvents and soluble in water to 2.3 mg/ml at 22°C. Published conversion factor in air is 0.32 ppm = 1 mg/mm³.

World Health Organization occupational exposure limits are a Time-Weighted Average (TWA) in males of 3.2 ppm, in females, 0.96 ppm, with a Short-Term Exposure Limit (STEL) of 19.2 ppm. In the United States, OSHA final rule limits are a Permissible Exposure Limit TWA (8 h) of 20 ppm, STEL of 12 ppm, with a ceiling of 30 ppm. The American Conference of Governmental Industrial Hygienists

Threshold Limit Value TWA is 10 ppm, with a Biological Exposure Index for 2-thiothiazolodone-4-carboxylic acid (TTCA) in urine at the end of a shift of 5 mg/g creatinine. The U.S. National Institute for Occupational Safety and Health TWA (10 h) is 1 ppm, with STEL and 15-min ceiling both at 10 ppm. Acceptable ambient air concentrations vary from state to state within the United States.

In humans and animals, CS_2 is rapidly absorbed *via* inhalation, oral, or dermal routes and is distributed throughout the body. During continuous exposure, the fraction of an inhaled dose that is absorbed decreases from 80% to 40%; the majority of CS_2 absorbed is exhaled rather rapidly, with a terminal half-life of approximately 55 min, and less than 1% is excreted in urine as CS_2 (19). Because of the high fat solubility of CS_2, its distribution is greatest to brain and liver. CS_2 is metabolized by cytochrome P-450 to an unstable oxygen intermediate that either decomposes to atomic sulfur and carbonyl sulfide or hydrolyzes to atomic sulfur and monothiocarbonate. Monothiocarbonate degrades to carbonyl sulfide, carbon dioxide, and sulfide ion. In every tissue, including blood, CS_2 reacts with protein amino groups to form dithiocarbamates and with sulfhydryl groups to form trithiocarbonates; both of these reactions are reversible, particularly at low pH, and constitute an "acid-labile" pool. The trithiocarbonate derivatives of cysteine, either free or derived from glutathione, can cyclize to form TTCA, a urinary metabolite (4,15). As discussed later, the protein-bound dithiocarbamates can either serve as sources of CS_2 or can decompose to electrophilic isothiocyanate derivatives (2,5,21).

Although proteins of all tissues are derivatized and cross-linked after exposure to CS_2, the toxicologically relevant reactions are those that occur with long-lived proteins, such as the subunits of the neurofilament, the intermediate filament of the axon (9,16). It has been proposed that another significant target may be low-density lipoprotein (LDL) and that cross-linking of the protein moiety of LDL, apolipoprotein B (apoB), may alter the uptake by macrophages, leading to the formation of foam cells, the initial lesion in the pathogenesis of atherosclerosis (10). In addition, two other proteins with a lifetime of 2–4 months in rats and humans, respectively, are α and β spectrin within erythrocyte membranes; the cross-linking of these and related proteins appears to have excellent potential as a biomarker of absorbed dose (6,7,20,22,23).

Prolonged inhalation exposure of rats to CS_2 results in a toxic distal axonopathy that is identical to that which follows subchronic dosing with 2,5-hexanedione, the neurotoxic metabolite of *n*-hexane. Accumulations of neurofilaments grow to form large focal axonal swellings, often located just proximal to nodes of Ranvier. Myelin retraction from nodes of Ranvier can be followed by segmental demyelination. With continued exposure, swellings develop in more proximal locations, and the axon distal to the swellings undergoes degeneration, resulting in loss of muscle strength and of sensory modalities in the hindlimbs. The longest and largest myelinated axons appear to be the most sensitive, including peripheral nerves and both ascending and descending tracts of the spinal cord (8). The Lowest-Observed-Adverse-Effect level (for axonal swellings and loss of grip strength) are in the range of 300–500 ppm (8). Larger species, such as the rabbit, are vulnerable to the development of neuropathy; however, mice appear to be less vulnerable, perhaps a reflection of shorter axonal lengths. An additional neurotoxic effect has been documented in monkeys: the degeneration of retinal ganglion cells (4). Short-term effects on the nervous system (*e.g.*, mania) require higher doses and are apparently reversible (4).

In human workers, the most sensitive index of neurotoxicity is clinical and electrophysiological evidence of peripheral neuropathy. Symptoms of peripheral neuropathy follow exposure to higher concentrations of CS_2 than are generally experienced in the U.S. rayon industry today, but reports from central and eastern Europe continue to document this neurotoxic effect from exposures considerably higher than the U.S. TWA. Acute CNS effects require considerably higher exposure levels than are required for development of neuropathy (11,13). Exposure is documented by the presence of TTCA in the urine (15), and the diagnosis of an axonal neuropathy is supported by the characteristic electrophysiological changes seen in distal axonopathies, reductions in amplitude, and later in conduction velocity in the distal, but not proximal, regions of nerves. Diagnosis can be established by nerve biopsy, which discloses the characteristic neurofilament-filled axonal swellings, but this is seldom necessary (8). Treatment relies on early diagnosis and removal from conditions of exposure. Mild neuropathies are reversible, with residual effects seen in workers with more severe neuropathies (4,9). Reports of spasticity and tremor in individuals chronically exposed to CS_2 likely represent CNS manifestations of distal axonopathy (24).

Some historical studies attribute extrapyramidal dysfunction to chronic high-level industrial exposure to CS_2; these have been reviewed (8). Parkinsonism and dystonia are both described; some reports allege a frequency of Parkinson's-like disorders in 30%–55% of exposed individuals. It is difficult to evaluate these reports; most are

from the late nineteenth and early twentieth centuries, some persons were exposed to several agents (especially H_2S), or experienced loss of consciousness and anoxia. Likewise, anoxic episodes likely were an inadvertent feature of the degeneration of the globus pallidus and substantia nigra (17). It is curious that peripheral neuropathy, the salient feature of contemporary clinical studies of CS_2, is documented in few of the older human instances of parkinsonism. Two unconvincing contemporary clinical studies, one uncontrolled, the other self-selected, describe (respectively) cognitive dysfunction or an extrapyramidal syndrome in workers exposed to low levels of CS_2 (1,12).

Acute psychotic episodes appeared in workers with high-level, subacute exposure in poorly ventilated plants in the nineteenth century and during World War II. Following several months' exposure, affected individuals began to hallucinate, became manic, and occasionally attacked fellow workers or committed suicide.

An uncontrolled study describes a poorly defined chronic encephalopathy that appeared in some youthful workers who experienced high-level exposure in the viscose rayon industry during World War II; the relationship of CS_2 exposure to this syndrome is unclear (24).

The ability of CS_2 to react with amines to form dithiocarbamates has provided the basis for several proposed mechanisms of neurotoxicity (4). The copper- and zinc-chelating property of dithiocarbamates has been suggested to decrease the availability of these two cofactors resulting in enzyme inhibition. For example, it has been postulated that the chelation of copper leads to inhibition of dopamine-β-hydroxylase and abnormal catechol metabolism. Alternatively, dithiocarbamate formation on pyridoxamine has been proposed to result in vitamin B_6 deficiency (4). More recently, in attempts to establish a mechanistic relationship for the identical neuropathies produced by 2,5-hexanedione and CS_2, reactions subsequent to dithiocarbamate formation have been investigated (1,5,9,21). Because the ability to cross-link proteins covalently is required for the production of neurofilamentous swellings by γ-diketones (18), the potential for CS_2 to cross-link proteins has also been examined. It has been demonstrated that, under physiological conditions, a fraction of the dithiocarbamates decomposes to yield protein-bound isothiocyanate adducts, potent electrophiles that then react with protein nucleophiles to yield covalent cross-links within and between proteins. The reaction with sulfhydryl groups to form dialkyldithiocarbamate esters is reversible, while the reaction with amino groups to form thiourea cross-links is irreversible and, thus, probably the most biologically significant (2,5,21). Because of their stability and spatial proximity, the cross-linking of the neurofilament proteins renders the axon the most sensitive target, and suggests that covalent cross-linking may be the initiating event in the development of the axonal swellings. It has been postulated that targets in the axon other than the neurofilament may be involved in the genesis of axonal degeneration in both *n*-hexane and CS₂ neuropathies (9).

REFERENCES

1. Aaserud O, Gjerstad L, Mnakstad P *et al.* (1988) Neurological examination, computerized tomography, cerebral blood flow, and neuropsychological examination in workers with long-term exposure to carbon disulfide. *Toxicology* **49**, 277.
2. Amarnath V, Anthony DC, Valentine WM, Graham DG (1991) The molecular mechanism of the carbon disulfide mediated cross-linking of proteins. *Chem Res Toxicol* **4**, 148.
3. Ansbacher LE, Bosch EP, Cancilla, PA (1982) Disulfiram neuropathy: A neurofilamentous distal axonopathy. *Neurology* **32**, 424.
4. Beauchamp RO, Bus JS, Popp JA *et al.* (1983) A critical review of the literature on carbon disulfide toxicity. *CRC Crit Rev Toxicol* **11**, 169.
5. DeCaprio AP, Olajas ES, Chen X *et al.* (1992) Characterization of isothiocyanates, thioureas, and other lysine addition products in carbon disulfide-treated peptides and protein. *Chem Res Toxicol* **5**, 496.
6. Erve JCL, Amarnath V, Graham DG *et al.* (1998) Carbon disulfide and *N,N*-diethyldithiocarbamate generate thiourea cross-links on erythrocyte spectrin in vivo. *Chem Res Toxicol* **11**, 54.
7. Erve JCL, Amarnath V, Sills RC *et al.* (1998) Characterization of a valine-lysine thiourea cross-link on rat globin produced by carbon disulfide or *N,N*-diethyldithiocarbamate *in vivo*. *Chem Res Toxicol* **11**, 1128.
8. Gottfried MR, Graham DG, Morgan M *et al.* (1985) The morphology of carbon disulfide neurotoxicity. *Neurotoxicology* **6**, 89.
9. Graham DG, Amarnath V, Valentine WM *et al.* (1995) Pathogenetic studies of hexane and carbon disulfide neurotoxicity. *CRC Crit Rev Toxicol* **25**, 91.
10. Graham DG, Montine TJ, Amarnath V *et al.* (1995) Cross-linking of apolipoprotein B (apoB) in the acceleration of atherosclerosis by carbon disulfide. *Toxicologist* **5**, 126.
11. Johnson BL, Boyd J, Burg JR *et al.* (1983) Effects on the peripheral nervous system of workers' exposure to carbon disulfide. *Neurotoxicology* **4**, 53.
12. Peters H, Levine RL, Matthews CG, Chapman LJ (1988) Extrapyramidal and other neurologic manifestations associated with carbon disulfide fumigant exposure. *Arch Neurol* **45**, 537.
13. Putz-Anderson V, Albright DE, Lett ST *et al.* (1983) A behavioral examination of workers exposed to carbon disulfide. *Neurotoxicology* **4**, 67.
14. Richter R (1945) Degeneration of the basal ganglia in monkeys from chronic carbon disulfide poisoning. *Exp Neurol* **4**, 324.
15. Riihimaki V, Kivisto H, Peltonen K *et al.* (1992) Assessment of exposure to carbon disulfide in viscose production workers from urinary 2-thiothiazolidine-4-carboxylic acid determinations. *Amer J Indust Med* **22**, 85.
16. Schlaepher WW (1987) Neurofilaments: Structure, metabolism, and implications in disease. *J Neuropathol Exp Neurol* **46**, 117.
17. Spencer PS, Butterfield P (1995) Environmental agents and Parkinson's disease. In: *Etiology of Parkinson's Disease.* Ellenberg JH, Koller WC, Langston JW eds. Marcel Dekker, New York p. 319.
18. St. Clair MGB, Amarnath V, Moody MA *et al.* (1988) Pyrrole oxidation and protein cross-linking as necessary steps in the development of γ-diketone neuropathy. *Chem Res Toxicol* **1**, 179.
19. Teisinger J, Soucek B (1949) Absorption and elimination of carbon disulfide in man. *J Ind Hyg Toxicol* **31**, 67.
20. Valentine WM, Amarnath V, Amarnath K *et al.* (1998) Covalent modification of hemoglobin by carbon disulfide: III. A potential biomarker of effect. *Neurotoxicology* **19**, 99.
21. Valentine WM, Amarnath V, Graham DG, Anthony DC (1992) Covalent cross-linking of proteins by carbon disulfide. *Chem Res Toxicol* **5**, 254.
22. Valentine WM, Amarnath V, Graham DG *et al.* (1997) CS2-mediated cross-linking of erythrocyte spectrin and neurofilament protein: dose response and temporal relationship to the formation of axonal swellings. *Toxicol Appl Pharmacol* **142**, 95.
23. Valentine WM, Graham DG, Anthony DC (1993) Covalent cross-linking of erythrocyte spectrin by carbon disulfide *in vivo. *Toxicol Appl Pharmacol* **121**, 71.
24. Vigliani EC (1954) Carbon disulfide poisoning in viscose rayon factories. *Brit J Ind Med* **11**, 235.

Carbon Monoxide

Howard A. Crystal
Myron D. Ginsberg

CO

NEUROTOXICITY RATING

Clinical

A   Acute encephalopathy (sedation, coma)

A   Leukoencephalopathy

A   Headache

C   Peripheral neuropathy

Experimental

A   Neuronal degeneration (anoxia)

A   Leukoencephalopathy

Carbon monoxide intoxication (COI) is the most common fatal accidental poisoning in the United States (73). Mortality from acute CO exposure ranges from 2%–31% (73,75); 3%–30% of survivors are left with permanent neurological sequelae (12,30,55,81). CO has likely caused morbidity and mortality since fires were first used to heat caves. The history of research on COI began with Claude Bernard's discovery in 1857 that CO displaces oxygen from hemoglobin (41). Hyperbaric oxygen was first used to treat COI in 1868 (83). In 1895, Haldane used himself as a test subject to investigate the effects of CO on psychological function (34,41). In the past decade, advances in cellular biology have afforded new insights into the pathophysiology of COI and shown that endogenously produced CO acts as an intercellular messenger. The literature of COI is extensive; several reviews provide detailed discussions of specific topics including neuropsychological performance (77), epidemiology (73), physiology (16), pathology (44), and treatment (81).

CO, a neutral diatomic molecule, is an odorless, colorless, tasteless gas with a density of 0.97 relative to air. In size, molecular weight, and diffusion capacity, CO resembles oxygen.

Carbon monoxide is formed by the incomplete combustion of carbon-containing fuels; an inadequate supply of oxygen for combustion predisposes to its production (18). Sources of CO intoxication include smoke, the exhaust of motor vehicles and other gasoline-powered engines, furnaces, water heaters, wood stoves, and canned fuel (73). Although cigarette smoking is a widespread source of individual CO exposure, it makes an insignificant contribution to atmospheric CO. Another exogenous source of COI is methylene chloride (77,78), an agent used in industrial solvents and in household paint removers (16).

The concentration of CO in the lower atmosphere in the United States varies from 0.01–1.0 ppm in rural areas to 1–30 ppm in urban areas (44). During temperature inversions, CO concentrations near major highways may transiently exceed 100 ppm (77,88). CO levels in underground garages, tunnels, and near loading docks, may exceed 100 ppm for sustained periods. These levels are associated with decreased exercise tolerance in patients with coronary artery disease (1,3,28,29,88). In 1989, exhaust from motor vehicles accounted for 33,000 gigagrams of CO (50% of atmospheric CO in the United States) (62). Other important sources of atmospheric CO include aircraft, train, and ship engines (12.3%); stationary engines (12.4%); industrial processes (7.8%); solid waste combustion (2.8%); and forest fires (13.4%) (62). Proposed methods to remove excess CO from the lower atmosphere include oxidation of CO to CO_2 in the upper atmosphere, and metabolism by microorganisms. Despite an increased number of motor vehicles, the total CO emissions in the U.S. from motor vehicles declined by 50% from 1970–1989 (62). Most of this decline was attributed to the Clean Air Act of 1968; this mandated that, by 1975, all new cars were to be equipped with catalytic converters.

CO acts chiefly as a ligand, binding selectively to metals to form metal carbonyls (2,10). Most important among its interactions is its tenacious but reversible linkage with the ferrous iron complex of protoporphyrin IX in the hemoglobin molecule. In biological systems, CO binding is dependent on the availability of an appropriate site or upon its ability to displace other ligands. CO may act either as a σ-donor or a π-electron acceptor. The solubility of CO in body fluids is slight; arterial P_{CO} tension is therefore low even under conditions of elevated arterial carboxyhemoglobin (COHb) concentration. COHb levels in urban nonsmokers range from 1%–2%. Cigarette smokers usually have COHb levels from 2%–8%; occasionally they are as high as 18% (77). Patients with hemolytic anemias have increased red blood cell catabolism and may have COHb levels up to 5% (77).

Carbon monoxide shares several chemical properties with nitric oxide (88); both share free radicals of comparable size, both gases are toxic to man, and both are produced endogenously. Endogenous synthesis of CO or NO requires reduced nicotinamide adenine dinucleotide phosphate and cytochrome P-450. With the discovery that NO functions as an intracellular and intercellular messenger, several groups sought to determine whether CO might have a similar role (85). Endogenous CO is produced as a by-product of the conversion of heme to biliverdin, a reaction catalyzed by heme oxygenase (16,77). There are at least two forms of heme oxygenase in humans (85). Heme oxygenase-1 is located in reticuloendothelial cells in liver and spleen. Heme oxygenase-2 is more widely distributed throughout the body, and high levels are found in the brain in high levels. *In situ* hybridization studies in rat brain showed heme oxygenase-2 activity in granule cells of the cerebellum, hippocampus, and olfactory bulb, and within pyramidal cells of the hippocampus and Purkinje cells of the cerebellum. Endogenous production of CO in a normal human adult male accounts for 0.4 ml/h and is associated with a carboxyhemoglobin (COHb) level of less than 1% (77). Some endogenously produced CO acts as a second messenger in the CNS and as an intercellular messenger in other organ systems (19,33,77). Like NO, endogenous CO stimulates guanylate cyclase, leading to increased intracellular cyclic guanosine monophosphate (cGMP) levels, and causes relaxation of smooth muscle. Thus, like NO, CO can also cause vasodilatation.

The U.S. ambient outdoor air-quality primary standard for CO is 10 mg/m^3 (9 ppm) over an 8-h Time-Weighted Average (TWA), and 40 mg/m^3 (35 ppm) over a 1-h TWA (84). U.S. Occupational Safety and Health Administration industrial workplace standards are 55 mg/m^3 (50 ppm) TWA (cited in 84).

The U.S. Environmental Protection Agency does not provide recommendations for residential indoor CO levels. The World Health Organization working-group consensus of concern about indoor air pollutants as of 1984 indicated that CO levels of <0.19mg/m^3 or 2% COHb were of limited or no concern. Concentrations of concern were >0.32 mg/m^3 or COHb >3% (84).

General Toxicology

CO exerts its toxicity by binding tenaciously to the ferrous iron complex of hemoglobin and reducing the protein's ability to transport oxygen to tissues. Each hemoglobin molecule is a tetramer containing two α and two non-α (usually β) polypeptide chains (70); each α or non-α chain contains one heme group. Heme groups are coenzymes composed of a protoporphyrin ring coordinated with ferrous iron in its center (70). Ferrous iron has six electron pairs in its outer orbitals; one electron pair is bound to the nitrogen in each of the four pyrrole rings. One pair is bound to a histidyl group in each globin chain. The last pair is free to react with O_2. Thus, each hemoglobin molecule can bind from zero to four oxygen molecules.

The oxygen-hemoglobin dissociation curve normally has a sigmoid shape (Fig. 6) (16). The flat "upper tail" of the curve indicates that Hb is almost fully saturated at a P_{O_2} of 70. Normal alveolar P_{O_2} is around 95 mm Hg. Thus, this flat "upper tail" serves as a reserve, protecting against relative alveolar hypoxia. Only when alveolar P_{O_2} drops below 70 mm Hg will hemoglobin saturation drop significantly. The presence of a steep middle part of the curve between P_{O_2} levels of 10 and of 50 mm Hg means that even a small decrement between arteriolar and interstitial P_{O_2} will be associated with a significant release of O_2 from hemoglobin. The cytosolic P_{O_2} within cells and in the interstitial space in various body tissues is between 5 and 40 mm Hg (21). At these low P_{O_2} levels, oxygen dissociates from hemoglobin

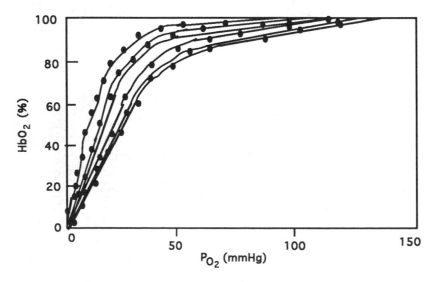

FIGURE 6. Observed and calculated effects of HbCO on the HbO$_2$ dissociation curve. Reproduced from Okada *et al.* (64).

and diffuses across capillary endothelial cells into the interstitial space, and then into cells. The presence of a flat tail to the curve implies that at P_{O_2} levels <20 mm Hg, the blood cannot carry enough oxygen to sustain life for more than a few minutes. The mass-action equation below describes the association and dissociation of O_2 and CO to Hb.

$$Hb + O_2 = O_2-Hb$$
$$O_2-Hb + CO = CO-Hb + O_2$$

The binding constant of CO to hemoglobin is comparable to its binding constant for O_2. However, the dissociation constant of CO from hemoglobin is 200–290 times less than that of oxygen from hemoglobin. The difference in dissociation constants means that, whereas hemoglobin is half-saturated with O_2 when P_{O_2} is 30 mm Hg, it is half-saturated with CO when the P_{CO} is 0.125 mm Hg (about 1600 ppm).

Figure 6 shows the influence of CO binding to hemoglobin on the oxyhemoglobin dissociation curve. At higher CO concentrations, the curve is shifted to the left, and the shape of the curve changes from sigmoid to hyperbolic (16). These changes are significant because at the same tissue P_{O_2}, less O_2 is released from hemoglobin into the surrounding tissue. Thus, a patient with a 50% COHb level and normal Hb level of 15 is more impaired than a subject with a Hb of 7.5 (assuming comparable maintenance of organ perfusion). The latter subject will have about 5 ml of oxygen per deciliter of blood available to the tissue, whereas the subject with CO intoxication will have only about 1.5 ml. The kinetics of COHb association are described by the Coburn-Forster-Kane equation (16). Factors influencing the rate of COHb association include the initial carboxyhemoglobin level, partial pressure of CO in the inspired gas, alveolar ventilatory rate, partial pressure of oxygen in alveolar capillaries, diffusion rate of CO, and altitude. Figure 7 shows the influence of CO concentration in ambient air on the kinetics of COHb association in human volunteers (16). The figure demonstrates that 30% COHb—usually sufficient to produce headache and lethargy—is reached in 5 min while breathing 1000 ppm CO, and in over 200 min while breathing 500 ppm CO.

CO is capable of transplacental diffusion and may affect fetal oxygenation. Factors affecting transplacental diffusion of CO have been thoroughly reviewed (45,46). Though oxygen and CO have traditionally been assumed to reach the fetus by passive diffusion, facilitated diffusion may also occur (45).

Fetal P_{O_2} is proportionate to maternal and fetal COHb levels (45). Since oxygen tension in the fetus is normally only 20%–30% of adult values, and because the fetus is unable to increase its cardiac output significantly above its already high resting levels, even mild reductions in fetal oxygen tension may lead to tissue hypoxia. This is of practical concern, since COHb levels of 5%–10% are commonly present in moderate to heavy cigarette smokers. Low birth weight, increased numbers of perinatal deaths, and possible long-term intellectual sequelae have been observed in the offspring of smoking mothers.

In addition to hemoglobin, CO binds to other extravascular proteins, including myoglobin, cytochrome-c oxidase, at least eight cytochrome P-450–associated enzymes, and dopamine β-hydroxylase. Other enzymes with heme or copper cofactors also probably bind CO. About 15% of CO in the body is bound to extravascular proteins (16,46).

Cardiac toxicity is a serious and common complication of CO exposure. ST-segment and T-wave abnormalities, atrial fibrillation, atrioventricular dissociation and heart block, and other arrhythmias occur in both experimental animals and humans (1,17,60). Electrocardiographic abnormalities may persist for several months in some instances. Pathological findings include multifocal myocardial necrosis, focal leukocyte infiltration and degeneration of myocardial fibers, punctate hemorrhages of the myocardium, and mural thrombi with coronary artery embolization (1,17). The clinical presentation may resemble an acute myocardial infarction. The mechanisms of cardiac injury in CO poisoning include both tissue anoxia, coronary ischemia secondary to hypotension, and possible direct toxic effects of CO on the myocardium (60).

CO inhalation normally leads to increased coronary blood flow to maintain myocardial oxygenation (4). CO may nonetheless decrease myocardial oxygen tension by (a) increasing ventricular work secondary to adrenergic stimulation, (b) decreasing oxygen extraction, and (c) decreasing capillary oxygen tension (3). Patients with coronary artery disease may be more vulnerable to myocardial hypoxia during CO exposure because of a limited capacity to increase coronary artery blood flow.

Animal Studies

The early literature on experimental CO intoxication was primarily neuropathological with little attention given to physiobiological abnormalities. Studies performed in the 1920s, in which mice, guinea pigs, rabbits, and dogs were exposed to CO, demonstrated cerebral hyperemia, particularly pronounced in the basal ganglia, following fatal exposures of 5–10 min. Symmetrical hemorrhagic softening of these nuclei occurred in animals surviving up to 2 days (66). Other early investigations described neuropathological alterations in cats and dogs receiving acute, fractionated CO exposure (54). Softening of the globus pallidus, affect-

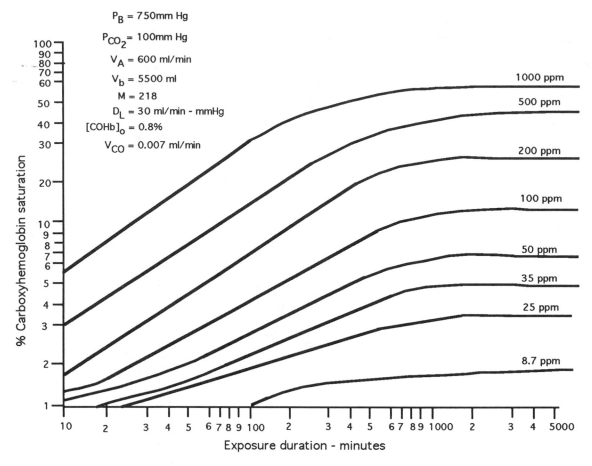

FIGURE 7. Carbon monoxide uptake in a normal human subject as a function of inspired [CO]. P_B, barametric pressure; P_{CO_2}, average partial pressure of O_2 in lung capillaries; V_A, alveolar ventilation rate; V_b, blood volume; M, equilibrium constant; D_L, diffusing capacity of the lungs; $[COHb]_o$, control value prior to CO exposure; V_{CO}, rate of endogenous CO production. Reproduced from Peterson & Stewart (65).

ing chiefly the anterior two-thirds but occasionally involving the contiguous internal capsule or putamen, occurred regularly, as did lesions of the deep cerebral white matter, which variably spared the subcortical U-fibers. Microscopically, white matter lesions displayed myelin loss, histiocyte accumulation and transformation into lipid-laden macrophages, perivascular cellular infiltrates, adventitial proliferation, and luminal dilatation of blood vessels. Investigations of animals subjected to multiple CO exposures showed neuronal loss in the hippocampus and the Purkinje cell layer of the cerebellum, alterations of vascular endothelium, and minimal diffuse glial reaction of the cerebral white matter (48).

Contemporary investigations have attempted to correlate physiological variables and neuropathology (69). Two-thirds of dogs exposed to 0.13%–1.7% CO for variable lengths of time survived the immediate intoxication and had changes in the cerebral white matter when sacrificed 3–7 days later. Severe lesions occurred in animals with 60 or more minutes of CO exposure and maximal COHb levels

of 40%–50%. Physiological alterations included an initial respiratory depression, elevated cerebrospinal fluid pressure and venous pressure, and later declines in arterial blood pressure with evidence of right-sided heart failure.

Studies of pentobarbital-anesthetized juvenile rhesus monkeys allowed to breathe 0.1%–0.3% CO for periods of 75–325 min showed that arterial COHb levels rose quickly, attaining plateau levels within 75 min (25). Animals breathing 0.2% CO achieved a mean COHb plateau of 76%. These levels remained constant during CO administration and declined smoothly following discontinuation. Arterial hypotension and metabolic acidosis evolved consistently during the insult, though variably from animal to animal. Central venous pressure remained normal. Premature ventricular contractions were observed in all animals receiving 0.2% and 0.3% CO within 75 min of the onset of CO exposure. Fourteen animals survived the intoxications; three displayed severe neurological deficits including limb paralysis, alteration of muscle tone, blindness, and deafness (26). Mild motor abnormalities were noted in three others. The remaining eight were unremarkable. The neuropathological lesion consistently created by this insult was a bilaterally symmetrical necrotizing leukoencephalopathy (26). In the least affected animals, there was only a hypercellularity in the parietal or inferior temporal white matter. More severely injured brains showed bilaterally symmetrical foci of central white matter softening, often with small peripheral areas of cavitation. These foci were most prominent in the parietal region where lesions often tended to parallel the contours of the overlying cortical gyri, separated by a zone of undamaged subcortical U-fibers. Microscopically, such lesions showed scattered regions of myelin pallor with a loosening of the neuropilar texture but with preservation of oligodendroglia. The most severely affected brains contained extensive necrotic lesions of the central white matter. A combination of hypoxia (associated with high COHb levels) and hypotension was necessary to induce the severe lesions.

Human Studies
Low-Level

Despite extensive investigations, it is uncertain whether low-dose CO exposure has an effect on human perceptual function and cognition. Ability to discriminate among small differences in light intensity was perturbed by COHb levels as low as 4.5% (51). COHb levels of 5% produced transient alterations of visual thresholds (51). There is a significant performance decrement in the ability to compare the duration of tones after exposure to 100 ppm CO for only 50 min, or 50 ppm CO for 90 min (6). Other studies, how-

ever, have failed to show an effect of comparably low doses of CO. Differences in experimental design, in particular the task duration, may in part account for the discrepant findings among studies (5,77). An excellent summary of these investigations concludes that, while visual perception may be subtly altered by COHb levels of 5%, complex tasks of judgment and motor coordination do not appear impaired unless COHb levels exceed 10% (77).

High-Level

Clinical symptoms and signs in the first minutes of high-level COI result, at least in part, from hypoxia of brain and heart (16,22,77). Cardiac dysfunction due to effects of CO binding to cardiac myoglobin may contribute to decreased perfusion of heart and brain (16). As COHb levels rise, there is a gradient of symptoms that reflects increasing brain and heart dysfunction (Table 11) (40,77). COHb levels of 10%–20% are associated with headache. A COHb level of 30% is associated with headache, nausea, lethargy, confusion, and fatigue. Levels above 50% usually cause coma, and levels over 60%–70% are usually fatal. Several factors modulate the clinical effects of CO exposure. Actively exercising patients have greater oxygen demand and are more susceptible to CO intoxication than sleeping patients (52). The degree and duration of hypotension, the presence of baseline cardiac or pulmonary disease or anemia, and any arrhythmias or other cardiac dysfunction induced by CO exposure also influence clinical outcome (22,77).

TABLE 11. Human Responses to Various Concentrations of Carboxyhemoglobin

Blood Saturation COHb (%)	Response of Healthy Adult	Response of Patient with Severe Heart Disease
0.3–0.7	Normal range due to endogenous CO production; no known detrimental effect	—
1–5	Selective increase in blood flow to certain vital organs to compensate for reduction in oxygen-carrying capacity of the blood	Patient with advanced cardiovascular disease may lack sufficient cardiac reserve to compensate
5–9	Visual light threshold increased	Less exertion required to induce chest pain in patients with angina pectoris
16–20	Headache; visual-evoked response abnormal	May be lethal for patients with severely compromised cardiac function
20–30	Throbbing headache; nausea; fine manual dexterity abnormal	—
30–40	Severe headache; nausea and vomiting; syncope	—
50–60	Coma; convulsions	—
67–70	Lethal if not treated	—

[From Stewart (77).]

Sequelae in patients who survive COI are attributable to variable combinations of (a) the direct result of brain hypoxia during the acute exposure, and medical complications that develop during recovery from the acute exposure, the "acute syndrome"; and (b) the findings that first appear weeks following exposure, the "delayed syndrome."

The Acute Syndrome

There is great variability in the clinical presentation of acute high-level CO intoxication. Evidence of mental abnormality is present in virtually all. Approximately two-thirds have some degree of altered consciousness ranging from mild somnolence to coma. Others may be merely apprehensive, disoriented, confused, or excitable. Fluctuation of signs is the rule. Striking evidence of focal cortical and subcortical dysfunction may cause a variable clinical profile; hyperreflexia, decerebrate rigidity, visual disturbances, apraxias and aphasia, and seizures are described in various reports. These patients can pose, if unaccompanied, formidable diagnostic problems in the emergency room. The "cherry red" skin discoloration, widely held as diagnostic of acute CO poisoning, is present in only 6% of living patients; it is more often seen postmortem (27).

Computed tomography (CT) and magnetic resonance imaging (MRI) are rarely helpful in the acute illness. As the patients emerge from initial alteration of consciousness, neurological sequelae appear that reflect neuropathological changes. The histopathological changes are identical to those of other hypoxic-ischemic insults. Individuals dying within days display only congestion of the vessels and scattered petechial hemorrhages. Patients dying after the first week show neuronal loss in the hippocampus and in a pattern of laminar necrosis in the cerebral neocortex. Necrosis of the inner globus pallidus is an especially consistent finding, as in other forms of hypoxic insult. A series of 22 cases of COI noted the most common lesion of gray matter was necrosis of the globus pallidus—found in 16 cases (44). Usually the necrosis was bilateral. In milder cases, necrosis was confined to the anterior superior region of the globus pallidus in contact with fibers of the internal capsule. The MRI and CT images of the pallidal lesions are considered hallmarks of the acute syndrome (9,13,31,74,89). The cortical lesions in the occipital pole correlate with the prolonged latency of the P100 on visual evoked potentials, considered a marker of poor prognosis. This report described two patterns of white matter pathology (44). In one, scattered necrotic foci, 1–3 mm in diameter, were frequently mixed with hemorrhagic areas. Axons were reduced in number. White matter pathology was found in the deep centrum semiovale, as well as the interhemispheric commissures. The second pattern also consisted of necrotic foci

involving both axons and myelin, but the softenings were more extensive, extending from frontal to temporal poles. The corpus callosum, fornix, and anterior commissure were affected, but the internal capsule, external capsule, extreme capsule, and optic tracts were usually spared. Studies utilizing single-photon-emission computed tomography and positron emission tomography imaging have neither correlated closely with the neuropathological findings nor been useful prognostic indicators (14,20).

Sequelae in comatose patients who survive COI severe enough to cause coma range from no deficits (*i.e.*, normal neurological and neuropsychological examinations) to a chronic vegetative state (23,30,75). Interposed between these extremes are consistent syndromes featuring varying degrees of memory impairment (24), gait disorders and parkinsonism (43), personality changes (47), and other cognitive dysfunction (57). There are anecdotal reports describing deafness (56), peripheral neuropathy (12,76), and Tourette's syndrome (68). It is unclear whether long-term sequelae occur in patients whose initial exposure was not severe enough to cause an altered level of consciousness.

Sequelae are described in 129 of 549 (23.6%) patients admitted to a Korean university hospital for treatment of acute COI from 1976–1981 (13,55). Data from the Korean study are consistent with a British survey from 1973 (75) reporting that 33% of survivors had personality changes and 43% had memory impairment. A more recent study showed that 32% of patients had neurological findings when evaluated 1 month after admission for COI (30).

Several studies have examined factors that might help predict prognosis in subjects with the acute syndrome. Although several reports have stated that there is "no relationship between COHb level and outcome," when taken out of context this phrase is misleading. A more precise statement would be that among patients with loss of consciousness from CO intoxication who do not die during the first weeks after exposure, there is no relation between COHb on admission and outcome. Certainly, during the period of acute exposure, there can be no question that death will occur within minutes with COHb levels of 60%–70%. Several reasons account for the poor correlation between COHb level and outcome. There can be considerable delay between the time when COHb was maximal, and the time a sample of blood to determine COHb level is obtained. Subjects who are exposed to CO during a fire are exposed to other substances (including cyanide) that can affect brain function.

The Delayed Syndrome

Following 4 days to 4 weeks of recovery from an acute COI-induced coma, about 3% of patients develop a severe, sometimes fatal, neurological condition (12,55). This delayed syndrome is widely held as a characteristic of COI; however, the identical illness can, less commonly, also appear following hypoglycemia, heroin overdose, strangling, and anesthetic accidents (67). It is best described as the delayed postanoxic encephalopathy syndrome. The reason for an increased incidence following COI may reflect, in part, an increase in free radical formation (see Toxic Mechanisms, below).

In most instances, the acute episode has been one of severe coma that lasted 1–3 days; the patient then awakened and was able to walk out of the hospital in a week in a lucid state. After 1–4 weeks, irritability, confusion, or mania suddenly appear soon followed by a spastic or parkinsonian gait. Rigidity and masked facies are common, and most become somnolent and no longer walk. A few become mute, comatose, and die. The illness may stop progressing at any stage, and some make a partial or complete recovery.

The initial report of the delayed COI-associated syndrome appeared in 1925; it affords a concise description of a 58-year-old woman with gastric carcinoma who had attempted suicide with illuminating gas (32). "She was initially comatose, but regained consciousness, and at first appeared neurologically unremarkable. Twenty-six days later she became poorly oriented and apathetic, had a masked facies, absence of limb movements, and a short-stepped gait. Her speech was slow and monotonous, and she had impaired remote memory." At postmortem there was bilateral necrosis of the globus pallidus and bilateral diffuse demyelination of the white matter of the centrum semiovale.

The most striking histopathological change is diffuse demyelination in the cerebral hemispheres with variable degree of axonal loss. Brainstem and cerebellar white matter are usually spared. The severity of lesions ranges from small isolated areas with indistinct borders to diffuse homogenous demyelination. Areas of maximal pathology are the deep centrum semiovale and the periventricular zones. Unlike the two patterns in the acute syndrome, the corpus callosum, fornix, and anterior commissure are usually spared. Axons are preserved, but myelin is severely affected. There is severe venostasis. Capillaries have swollen walls and hemosiderin, calcium, or pseudocalcium deposits (44). Cortical necrosis is not a feature of this condition, and the globus pallidus is affected to a variable extent. MRI assists in the diagnosis of this leukoencephalopathy. There are no accurate predictors of the advent of the delayed syndrome; most have been over 50 years of age and have experienced severe coma. It is suggested that exercise should be avoided following the acute illness to lessen the probability of the delayed illness. It is also suggested that hyperbaric oxygen (HBO) therapy may be especially helpful in the delayed illness on the rationale that oxidative phosphorylation will be restored sooner and free radical formation decreased.

Epidemiology

A review of all U.S. death certificates from 1979–1988 showed that CO intoxication was cited as contributing to 56,133 deaths (11,15). Forty-six percent were suicides, 28% were from severe burns or house fires, and 21% were unintentional. Fifty-seven percent of the unintentional deaths were associated with exhaust from motor vehicles; 83% of these occurred in stationary vehicles. The percentages of unintentional deaths declined by 58% over this 10-year interval (15). Possible factors accounting for this decline include decreased CO in motor vehicle emissions, improved ventilation in new buildings, and stricter occupational standards (15). Mortality data collected from death certificates likely underestimate the extent of CO-associated deaths. COHb levels are not routinely determined on patients presenting to emergency rooms with altered levels of consciousness. Thus, some cases of fatal or nonfatal CO intoxication are undiagnosed. Estimates of morbidity from acute, nonfatal intoxications are also difficult to determine. Mortality from acute carbon monoxide intoxication ranges from 1%–31% (73). If about 5000 deaths in the United States were associated with carbon monoxide intoxication, one could estimate that CO was a factor in 11,000–245,000 nonfatal hospital admissions per year. "Epidemics" of CO intoxication can result from widespread improper use of machinery. Such an outbreak occurred among Iowa farmers using a gasoline-powered pressure washer to clean livestock (82). When these devices were used indoors in the winter, five cases of CO poisoning—one fatal—ensued. Other causes of clusters of CO intoxication include indoor burning of charcoal briquettes (37), indoor use of forklifts (9), and riding in the back of pick-up trucks (38).

Since the symptoms of COI are nonspecific, physicians may overlook the diagnosis in settings where a source of CO is not obvious. A common source of carbon monoxide intoxication in the United States is faulty home-heating systems. One study found elevated COHb levels in 24% of emergency room patients from a Chicago hospital evaluated for headaches during the winter months (39). In considering a patient with symptoms such as headache, fatigue, nausea, and dizziness, physicians may fail to consider COI in the differential diagnosis and falsely attribute symptoms to a nonspecific viral infection. A history that several members of a household have all developed these same symptoms may be construed to mean that the family members are suffering from the same virus rather than the same exposure to CO. Tragedy occurs when such patients are told they have a self-limited illness, only to be found dead several days later from fatal exposure to CO. The key to the diagnosis of acute COI is awareness that its source—for example, a faulty home-heating system or faulty automobile exhaust system—can seem so trivial that it is not mentioned. "Routine" blood studies, such as a complete blood count, do not provide any indication of COI, and measurement of COHb levels must be specifically requested from the clinical laboratory. Arterial blood gases also do not provide direct evidence of COI (60) as the arterial P_{O_2} level is typically normal.

Treatment

HBO, first used therapeutically for COI in 1868, is widely used for the treatment of acute CO intoxication (59,60, 63,81). The rationale for treatment with HBO is provided by Henry's law, which states that the concentration of a gas in solution is proportional to its concentration in the surrounding gas (83,87). At normal atmospheric pressure, about 0.4 volume percent of O_2 is dissolved in every 100 ml blood (as compared to 15 vol% bound to hemoglobin). One hundred percent of O_2 at 3 atmospheres (atm) provides 6.4 vol% of oxygen in solution; this concentration of oxygen is sufficient to support life even if all the hemoglobin in blood is dysfunctional. Furthermore, HBO treatment markedly increases the rate of elimination of CO from hemoglobin. Despite its theoretical appeal, superior outcomes with HBO therapy have never been clearly demonstrated in studies free of design or statistical shortcomings. Even though all outcome studies have had limitations, some believe the efficacy of HBO is so clear-cut that further study would be unethical (83). Indeed, it is advocated that acutely ill patients should be transported, by helicopter if necessary, to facilities where HBO therapy is available.

Table 12 lists studies comparing outcome of treatment of COI with normobaric oxygen (NBO) or HBO (81). One study described 213 patients with COI treated with HBO or NBO (59). The 131 more severely affected patients (defined by abnormal mental status and/or COHb level >30%) received HBO treatment; 82 less-affected patients received NBO. Sequelae developed 1–21 days after exposure in ten of the patients treated with NBO, but in none of the HBO-treated subjects. All ten promptly recovered when treated with HBO. The study lacked a standardized follow-up protocol, and neuropsychological tests were not administered. A complementary study compared neuropsychological performance before and after treatment with HBO in patients with mild to moderate COI. Before treatment, patients scored within the "dysfunctional" range on the Trails B test and the Block-Design subtest of the Wechsler Adult Intelligence Scale, Revised, after treatment, all test scores fell within the normal range (53). Since many of these patients likely would have improved without treatment, these data are difficult to interpret. Furthermore, the patients were undoubtedly anxious when first tested. On repeat testing, they were calmer and had the benefit of practice on the test. A prospective randomized study found no difference in final clinical outcome between 15 patients with COI treated with NBO and 11 patients treated with HBO (21). Those treated with HBO seemed to improve faster than the NBO group. The study lacked neuropsychological testing; thus, differences in cognitive functioning between the groups may have been missed. Neuropsychological testing was performed 1 month after NBO or HBO treatment in a longitudinal study (30). Testers were blinded to treatment group. "Loss of higher functions" was found in three of six patients in the NBO group, 9 of 20 who received a single HBO treatment,

TABLE 12. Comparison of Normobaric Oxygen (NBO) and Hyperbaric Oxygen (HBO) Treatment for CO Intoxication with the Development of Neuropsychiatric Sequelae

Reference	No. of Patients (Characteristics)	Follow-up (Psychometric Testing)	Development of Neuropsychiatric Sequelae with NBO Treatment (%)	Development of Neuropsychiatric Sequelae with HBO Treatment (%)
72	40 (mostly severe)	Not stated (No)	6/20 (38)	0/20
59	213 (82, mild; 131, moderate to severe)	6 mo to 1 yr (Yes)	10/82 (12)	0/131
49	230 (27, mild; 203, moderate to severe)	At 1,3,6, & 12 months (No)	0/27	9/203 (4)
71	343 (mild to moderate)	1 mo (No)	50/148 (34)	51/159 (32)
21	26 (moderate to severe)	<12 h (Yes?)	5/13 (38)	0/13
		12–28 (Yes?)	0/13	0/13
30	32 (mild to severe)	At discharge and 1 mo (Yes)	5/8 (63)	11/24 (46)
			4/6 (67)	11/20 (55)

[From Tibbles and Perrotta (81)]

and 7 of 50 who received multiple HBO treatments. No neuropsychological data are presented, and neuropsychological scores used to assign patients to normal or abnormal (*i.e.*, loss of higher function) groups are not specified.

There are no other specific treatments indicated for CO intoxication. In 1976, a review of treatment for CO intoxication stated that "bedrest for 2–4 weeks seems necessary to avoid delayed onset of neuropsychiatric symptoms" (27). The efficacy of such therapy has never been demonstrated in controlled studies, and the risk of complications from prolonged bedrest may be high in older individuals. On the other hand, anecdotal evidence suggests the delayed syndrome commonly follows resumption of normal levels of physical activity.

Toxic Mechanisms

The initial COHb level-induced acute hypoxia likely accounts for the acute reaction. Factors that may precipitate the *delayed reaction* include the amount of free radical formation, the tissue availability of free-radical scavengers, the degree and duration of cytochrome-*c* oxidase dysfunction, and the extent of granulocyte-capillary adhesions.

If a tissue is deprived of all oxygen or circulation for 4–5 min, energy reserves are depleted, cells may be irreversibly damaged, and cell death occurs. If, instead of total anoxia/ischemia, the tissue is rendered partially ischemic, cells may not die but are able to survive utilizing energy reserves for the production of adenosine triphosphate (ATP). Partial ischemia creates an intracellular environment that predisposes to the formation of reactive oxygen metabolites when normal levels of oxygen are restored. These reactive metabolites such as O_2^- (superoxide), H_2O_2, and hydroxyl free radical, will attack and damage cellular macromolecules (90). Lipids are peroxidized; proteins, carbohydrates, and nucleic acids degraded; hemeproteins and cytochrome oxidases inactivated; and inflammatory mediators such as C5a and leukotriene B_4 formed (90). Of all cellular macromolecules, lipids may be most suspectible to free-radical reactions because free-radical attack can precipitate a self-perpetuating "chain reaction" in cell membranes. Peroxidized lipids are less flexible and cellular function is compromised because membrane fluidity is decreased (35,36). There are at least two reasons why COI is more likely than other causes of hypoxia to be associated with free radical formation. First, in addition to binding to the heme group in hemoglobin, CO also binds to the heme group in cytochrome-*c* oxidase (16). During (mitochondrial) oxidative phosphorylation, electrons are transferred by the electron carrier protein, cytochrome-*c*, from the cytochrome-*b*–c_1 complex to the cytochrome oxidase complex. Under conditions of hypoxia, both the copper and iron ions in cytochrome oxidase are in a reduced state. In that state, CO will bind with ferrous ion in cytochrome oxidase. The CO prevents oxygen from reacting with the ferrous iron; thus, oxygen is not available to accept electrons from the shuttle electron carrier cytochrome-*c*. This uncoupling of oxidative phosphorylation leads to both production of more free radicals, and decreased ATP synthesis. (CO remains bound to cytochrome-*c* oxidase even after oxygenation is restored. The cytochrome-*c* oxidase is dysfunctional: thus, electron transport is compromised, leading to increased release of free radicals. Furthermore, ATP synthesis is also inhibited.)

COI also predisposes to more severe free radical damage than other causes of hypoxia/ischemia because CO increases the activity of soluble guanylate cyclase (sGC) (50,58). CO binding to the heme cofactor is associated with a several-hundredfold increase in the activity of sGC, which, in turn, elevates concentrations of intracellular cGMP. cGMP activates various protein kinases and phosphodiesterases that act on smooth muscle proteins and ion channels. CO may also increase activity of membrane-bound Na^+, K^+-ATPase (58) and thereby promote free-radical production.

Excess vasodilation decreases blood pressure and impairs organ perfusion. Impaired cardiac perfusion can further decrease cardiac output. Vasodilation exposes tissues to polymorphonuclear leukocytes (PMNs) usually confined to the intravascular space. PMNs contain enzymes that, once activated, promote the production of superoxide anion and hypochlorous acid (90). A hypotensive episode during the CO exposure is a poor prognostic sign. Hypotension may reflect vasodilation with its associated emigration of PMNs. Free radical synthesis is exacerbated because of both relative tissue hypoxia and activated PMNs.

Other factors can exacerbate the free-radical chain reaction. The enzyme xanthine dehydrogenase (XDH) converts hypoxanthine to xanthine, and then xanthine to uric acid (80,90). XDH utilizes NAD^+ as an electron acceptor for this reaction. XDH can be converted to xanthine oxidase (XO) by proteolysis. XO utilizes oxygen as an electron acceptor with release of H_2O_2 and O_2^-. Conditions that favor the XO form promote free radical synthesis. Partial ischemia and a free-radical chain reaction help promote the proteolysis of XDH to XO.

Some experimental data support the role of free radicals in CO-induced brain injury. Focal increases in brain lipid peroxidation occurred in rats exposed to CO ischemia (86), and rats exposed to CO had a 75% increase in lipid peroxidation products over controls (79). The increase occurred after animals were returned to an environment with normal oxygenation. A brief period of hypotension was necessary to induce these changes. A later study showed that CO poisoning was associated with increased production of the irreversible form of XO (80).

In vivo cytochrome-*c* oxidase activity in rats exposed to 1% CO for 15 min (associated with a COHb level of 69%) was 35% of control (7). HBO prevented most of the decrease in cytochrome-*c* oxidase activity. This was an important observation because others had questioned whether the intracellular P_{CO} levels found in COI would be sufficient to affect cytochrome-*c* oxidase. HBO therapy may have an additional rationale for presenting the delayed deterioration than NBO therapy. HBO therapy accelerates release of CO from cytochrome-*c* oxidase; thus, oxidative phosphorylation should be restored sooner, and free radical formation should be decreased.

The same investigators (8) then compared the effects of CO-induced hypoxia and alveolar hypoxia on cellular energy metabolites in their rat model. Both types of hypoxia were associated with a marked decrease in phosphocreatine, and a concomitant increase in creatine. ATP levels from phosphocreatine were normal in both groups. Animals with alveolar hypoxia showed partial restoration of energy stores after 45 min treatment with 100% O_2 at 1 atm. In contrast, phosphocreatine levels 45 min after CO exposure continued to decrease when the mice were treated with 100% O_2 at 1 atm. Phosphocreatine levels were near normal in animals rescued from CO exposure with 100% O_2 at 2.5 atm for 45 min. Intracellular pH declined from 7 at baseline to 6.5 after 20 min of CO exposure. Hydrogen ion continued to decline for at least 25 min in animals rescued with 100% O_2 at 1 atm; 25 min after removal from CO, pH had increased in animals treated with HBO (86).

A more recent study showed that endogenous CO also up-regulated the activity of Na^+, K^+-ATPase in rat brain (61). The authors speculated that excess Na^+, K^+-ATPase activity might be excitotoxic.

REFERENCES

1. Anderson RF, Allensworth DC, DeGroot WJ (1967) Myocardial toxicity from carbon monoxide poisoning. *Ann Intern Med* **67**, 1172.
2. Antonini E (1967) Hemoglobin and its reactions with ligands. *Science* **158**, 1967.
3. Aronow WS, Harris CN, Isbell MW *et al.* (1972) Effect of freeway travel on angina pectoris. *Ann Intern Med* **77**, 66.
4. Ayres SM, Evans R, Licht D *et al.* (1973) Health effects of exposure to high concentrations of automotive emissions. *Arch Environ Health* **27**, 168.
5. Beard RR, Grandstaff N (1970) Carbon monoxide exposure and cerebral function. *Ann N Y Acad Sci* **174**, 385.
6. Beard RR, Wertheim GA (1967) Behavioral impairment associated with small doses of carbon monoxide. *Amer J Public Health* **57**, 2012.
7. Brown SD, Piantadosi A (1990) *In vivo* binding of carbon monoxide to cytochrome *c* oxidase in rat brain. *J Appl Physiol* **68**, 602.
8. Brown SD, Piantadosi A (1992) Recovery of energy metabolism in rat brain after carbon monoxide hypoxia. *J Clin Invest* **89**, 686.
9. Bruno A, Wagner W, Orrison WW (1993) Clinical outcome and brain MRI four years after carbon monoxide intoxication. *Acta Neurol Scand* **87**, 205.
10. Caughey WS (1970) Carbon monoxide binding in hemeproteins. *Ann N Y Acad Sci* **174**, 148.
11. Centers for Disease Control (1992) Unintentional deaths from carbon monoxide poisoning—Michigan. *J Amer Med Assn* **268**, 3419.
12. Choi IS (1982) A clinical study of peripheral neuropathy in carbon monoxide intoxication. *Yonsei Med J* **23**, 174.
13. Choi IS (1983) Delayed neurologic sequelae in carbon monoxide intoxication. *Arch Neurol* **40**, 433.
14. Choi IS, Lee KS (1993) Early hypoperfusion of technetium-99m hexamethylprophylene amine oxime brain single photon emission computed tomography in a patient with carbon monoxide poisoning. *Eur Neurol* **33**, 461.
15. Cobb N, Etzel RA (1991) Unintentional carbon monoxide-related deaths in the United States, 1979 through 1988. *J Amer Med Assn* **266**, 659.
16. Coburn RF, Forman HJ (1987) Carbon monoxide toxicity. In: *Handbook of Physiology. Vol 14.* Fahri LE, Tenney SM eds. Amer Physiol Soc, Bethesda, MD p. 439.
17. Cosby RS, Bergeron M (1963) Electrocardiographic changes in carbon monoxide poisoning. *Amer J Cardiol* **11**, 93.
18. Cotton FA, Wilkinson G (1988) *Advanced Inorganic Chemistry. 5th Ed.* John Wiley, New York p. 243.
19. Dawson TM, Snyder SH (1994) Gases as biological messengers: Nitric oxide and carbon monoxide in the brain. *J Neurosci* **14**, 5147.
20. DeReuck J, Decoo D, Lemahieu I *et al.* (1993) A positron emission tomography study of patients with acute carbon monoxide poisoning treated by hyperbaric oxygen. *J Neurol* **240**, 430.
21. Ducasse JL, Izard PH, Celsis P *et al.* (1990) Moderate carbon monoxide poisoning: Hyperbaric or normobaric oxygenation? Human randomized study with tomographic cerebral blood flow measurement. In: *Proceedings of the 2nd Swiss Symposium on Hyperbaric Medicine.* Schmutz J, Bakkers D eds. Foundation for Hyperbaric Medicine, Basel, p. 289.
22. Ehrich WE, Bellet S, Lewey FH (1944) Cardiac changes from CO poisoning. *Amer J Med Sci* **208**, 502.
23. Garland H, Pearce J (1967) Neurological complications of carbon monoxide poisoning. *Quart J Med* **36**, 445.

24. Garrel S, Perret J, Pellat J, Arnould P (1970) Neuropsychiatric syndrome following carbon monoxide poisoning. *Electroencephalogr Clin Neurol* **29**, 529.

25. Ginsberg MD, Myers RE (1974) Experimental CO encephalopathy in the primate. I. Physiological and metabolic aspects. *Arch Neurol* **30**, 282.

26. Ginsberg MD, Myers RE, McDonag BF (1974). Experimental carbon monoxide encephalopathy in the primate. II. Clinical aspects, neuropathology, and physiologic correlation. *Arch Neurol* **30**, 209.

27. Ginsburg R, Romano J (1976) Carbon monoxide encephalopathy: Need for appropriate treatment. *Amer J Psychiat* **133**, 317.

28. Goldsmith JR (1972) Carbon monoxide and coronary heart disease: Compelling evidence in angina pectoris. *Ann Intern Med* **77**, 808.

29. Goldsmith JR, Aronow WS (1975) Carbon monoxide and coronary heart disease: A review. *Environ Res* **10**, 236.

30. Gorman DF, Clayton D, Gilligan JE, Webb RK (1992) A longitudinal study of 100 consecutive admissions for carbon monoxide poisoning to the Royal Adelaide Hospital. *Anaesth Intensive Care* **20**, 311.

31. Gotoh M, Kuyama H, Asar S *et al.* (1993) Sequential changes in MR images of the brain in acute carbon monoxide poisoning. *Comput Med Imaging Graph* **17**, 55.

32. Grinker RR (1925) Über einen fall von leuchtgasvergiftung mit doppelseitiger pallidumerweichung und schwerer degeneration des tieferen grosshirnmarklagers. *Z Gesamte Neurol Psychiat* **98**, 433.

33. Gurchgott RF, Jothianandan D (1991) Endothelium-dependent and -independent vasodilation involving cyclic GMP: Relaxation induced by nitric oxide, carbon monoxide and light. *Blood Vessels* **28**, 52.

34. Haldane J (1895) The action of carbonic oxide on man. *J Physiol* **18**, 430.

35. Halliwell B, Gutteridge JMC (1989) The chemistry of oxygen radicals and other oxygen-derived species. In: *Free Radicals in Biology and Medicine*. Halliwell B, Gutteridge JMC eds. Oxford University Press, New York p. 22.

36. Halliwell B, Gutteridge JMC (1989) Lipid peroxidation: A radical chain reaction. In: *Free Radicals in Biology and Medicine*. Halliwell B, Gutteridge JMC eds. Oxford University Press, New York p. 188.

37. Hampson NB, Kramer CC, Dunford RG *et al.* (1994) Carbon monoxide poisoning from indoor burning of charcoal briquets. *J Amer Med Assn* **271**, 52.

38. Hampson NB, Norkool DM (1992) Carbon monoxide poisoning in children riding in the back of pick-up trucks. *J Amer Med Assn* **267**, 538.

39. Heckerling PS, Leikin JB, Maturen A *et al.* (1990) Screening hospital admissions from the emergency department for occult carbon monoxide poisoning. *J Emerg Med* **8**, 301.

40. Hillick EM (1940) Carbon monoxide anoxemia. *Physiol Rev* **20**, 313.

41. Jackson DL, Menges H (1980) Accidental carbon monoxide poisoning. *J Amer Med Assn* **243**, 772.

42. Jaffe LS (1970) Carbon monoxide in the environment, Part II. Sources, characteristics, and fate of atmospheric carbon monoxide. *Ann N Y Acad Sci* **174**, 76.

43. Klawans HL, Stein RW, Tanner CM, Goetz CG (1982) A pure parkinsonian syndrome following acute carbon monoxide intoxication. *Arch Neurol* **39**, 302.

44. LaPresle J, Fardeau M (1967) The central nervous system and carbon monoxide poisoning. II. Anatomical study of brain lesions following intoxication with carbon monoxide (22 cases). *Prog Brain Res* **24**, 31.

45. Longo LD (1976) Carbon monoxide: Effects of oxygenation of the fetus *in utero*. *Science* **194**, 523.

46. Longo LD (1977) The biological effects of carbon monoxide on the pregnant woman, fetus, and newborn infant. *Amer J Obstet Gynecol* **129**, 69.

47. Lugaresi A, Montagna P, Moreale A, Gallassi (1990) 'Psychic akinesia' following carbon monoxide poisoning. *Eur Neurol* **30**, 167.

48. Lund OE (1956) Histologische Befunde bei experimentellen akuten Kohlenoxydvergiftungen. *Arch Gewerbepathol Gewerbehug* **15**, 96.

49. Mathieu D, Nolf M, Durocher A *et al.* (1985) Acute carbon monoxide poisoning. Risk of late sequelae and treatment by hyperbaric oxygen. *J Toxicol-Clin Toxicol* **23**, 315.

50. Mayer B (1994) Regulation of nitric oxide synthase and soluble guanylyl cyclase. *Cell Biochem Funct* **12**, 167.

51. McFarland RA, Roughton FJW, Halperin MH, Niven JJ (1944) The effects of exposure to small quantities of carbon monoxide on vision. *J Aviat Med* **6**, 381.

52. Meredith T, Vale A (1988) Carbon monoxide poisoning. *Brit Med J* **296**, 77.

53. Messier LD, Myers RA (1991) A neuropsychological screening battery for emergency assessment of carbon monoxide intoxication. *J Clin Psychol* **47**, 676.

54. Meyer A (1928) Experimentelle Erfahrungen über die Kohlenoxydvergiftung des Zentralnervensystems. *Z Gesamte Neurol Psychiat* **112**, 187.

55. Min SK (1986) A brain syndrome associated with delayed neuropsychiatric sequelae following acute carbon monoxide poisoning. *Acta Psychiat Scand* **73**, 87.

56. Morris TMO (1969) Deafness following acute carbon monoxide poisoning. *J Laryngol Otol* **83**, 1219.

57. Motomura N, Yamadori A (1994) A case of ideational apraxia with impairment of object use and preservation of object pantomime. *Cortex* **30**, 167.

58. Murad F (1994) Regulation of cytosolic guanylyl cyclase by nitric oxide: The NO-cyclic GMP signal transduction system. *Adv Pharmacol* **26**, 19.

59. Myers RA, Linberg SE, Cowley RA (1979) Carbon monoxide poisoning: The injury and its treatment. *JACEP* **8**, 479.

60. Myers RA, Snyder SK, Emhof TA (1985) Subacute sequelae of carbon monoxide poisoning. *Ann Emerg Med* **14**, 1163.

61. Nathanson JA, Scavone C, Scanlon C, McKee M (1995) The cellular Na$^+$ pump as a site of action for carbon monoxide and glutamate: A mechanism for long-term modulation of cellular activity. *Neuron* **14**, 781.

62. National Air Pollution estimates 1940–1990. Washington, DC. US Environmental Protection Agency, 1991. US EPA publication EPA-450/4-91-004.

63. Neubauer RA (1979) Carbon monoxide and hyperbaric oxygen. *Arch Intern Med* **139**, 829.

64. Okada Y, Tyuma I, Ueda V, Sugimoto T (1976) Effect of carbon monoxide on equilibrium between oxygen and hemoglobin. *Amer J Physiol* **230**, 471.

65. Peterson JE, Stewart RD (1970) Absorption and elimination of carbon monoxide by inactive men. *Arch Environ Health* **21**, 165.

66. Photakis BA (1921) Anastomische Veranderungen des Zentralnervensystems bei Kohlenoxydvergiftungen. *Vierteljahrsh Gerlich Med* **62**, 42.

67. Plum F, Posner JB, Hain RF (1962) Delayed neurological deterioration after anoxia. *Arch Intern Med* **110**, 56.

68. Pulst SM, Walshe TM, Romero JA (1983) Carbon monoxide poisoning with features of Gilles de la Tourette's syndrome. *Arch Neurol* **40**, 443.

69. Preziosi TJ, Lindenberg R, Levy D, Christenson M (1970) An experimental investigation in animals of the functional and morphologic effects of single and repeated exposures to high and low concentrations of carbon monoxide. *Ann N Y Acad Sci* **174**, 369.

70. Ranney HM, Sharma V (1995) Structure and function of hemoglobin. In: *Williams Hematology. 5th Ed.* Bleutler E, Lichtman MA, Coller BS eds. McGraw-Hill, New York p. 417.

71. Raphael JC, Elkharrat D, Jars-Guincestre MC *et al.* (1989) Trial of normbaric and hyperbaric oxygen for acute carbon monoxide intoxication. *Lancet* **2**, 414.

72. Roche L, Bertoye A, Vincent P *et al.* (1968) [Comparison of 2 groups of 20 cases of carbon monoxide poisoning treated with normobaric and hyperbaric oxygen]. *Lyon Méd* **220**, 1483.

73. Sadovnikoff N, Varon J, Sternbach GL (1992) Carbon monoxide poisoning—An occult epidemic. *Postgrad Med* **92**, 86.

74. Silverman CS, Brenner J, Murtagh FR (1993) Hemorrhagic necrosis and vascular injury in carbon monoxide poisoning: MR demonstration. *Amer J Neurol Res* **14**, 168.

75. Smith JS, Brandon S (1973) Morbidity from acute carbon monoxide poisoning at three-year follow-up. *Brit Med J* **1**, 318.

76. Snyder RD (1970) Carbon monoxide intoxication with peripheral neuropathy. *Neurology* **20**, 1977.

77. Stewart RD (1976) The effect of carbon monoxide on humans. *J Occup Med* **18**, 304.

78. Stewart RD, Fisher TN, Hosko MJ *et al.* (1972) Experimental human exposure to methylene chloride. *Arch Environ Health* **25**, 342.

79. Thom SR (1990) Carbon monoxide mediated brain lipid peroxidation in the rat. *J Appl Physiol* **68**, 997.

80. Thom SR (1992) Dehydrogenase conversion to oxidase and lipid peroxidation in brain after carbon monoxide poisoning. *J Appl Physiol* **73**, 1584.

81. Tibbles PM, Perrotta PL (1994) Treatment of carbon monoxide poisoning: A critical review of human outcome studies comparing normobaric oxygen with hyperbaric oxygen. *Ann Emerg Med* **24**, 269.

82. Unintentional carbon monoxide poisoning from indoor use of pressure washers—Iowa, January 1992–January 1993. (1993) *J Amer Med Assn* **270**, 2034. [From the Centers for Disease Control and Prevention]

83. Van Meter KW, Harch PG, Andrews LC *et al.* (1994) Should the pressure be off or on in the use of oxygen in the treatment of carbon monoxide-poisoned patients. *Ann Emerg Med* **24**, 283.

84. Ventilation for acceptable indoor air quality. (1989) Amer Soc Heating, Refrigerating, and Air Conditioning Engineers, ANSI/ASHRAE standard 62-1989, Atlanta, GA.

85. Verma Λ, Hirsch DJ, Glatt CE *et al.* (1993) Carbon monoxide: A putative neural messenger. *Science* **259**, 381.

86. Watson BD, Busto R, Goldberg WJ *et al.* (1984) Lipid peroxidation *in vivo* induced by reversible global ischemia in rat brain. *J Neurochem* **42**, 268.

87. Weiss LD, van Meter KW (1992) The applications of hyperbaric oxygen therapy in emergency medicine. *Amer J Emerg Med* **10**, 558.

88. Winter PM, Miller JN (1976) Carbon monoxide poisoning. *J Amer Med Assn* **236**, 1502.

89. Zagami AS, Lethlean AK, Mellick R (1993) Delayed neurological deterioration following carbon monoxide poisoning: MRI findings. *J Neurol* **240**, 113.

90. Zimmerman BJ, Granger DN (1994) Mechanisms of reperfusion injury. *Amer J Med Sci* **307**, 284.

Carbon Tetrachloride

John L. O'Donoghue

CARBON TETRACHLORIDE
CCl_4

Tetrachloromethane; Carbon chloride; Perchloromethane

NEUROTOXICITY RATING

Clinical

A   Acute encephalopathy

B   Visual dysfunction

B   Optic neuropathy

C   Peripheral neuropathy

Experimental

A   Acute encephalopathy (sedation)

A   Optic neuropathy

Carbon tetrachloride (CCl_4), once commonly used in various solvent and degreasing applications, has been replaced because the compound induced hepatic and renal toxicity. It has also been used as refrigerant, fire-extinguisher fluid, and anthelmintic. The main use for CCl_4 today is for the production of fluorocarbon propellants; it is also used as a grain fumigant.

CCl_4 is rapidly absorbed following ingestion from the gastrointestinal tract; its vapors are also readily absorbed through the lungs. Percutaneous absorption of liquid CCl_4 is rapid, with CCl_4 appearing in the breath 10 min after immersion of a thumb in CCl_4; exposure of both hands in liquid CCl_4 for 30 min is equivalent to inhalation of 100–500 ppm vapor for 30 min (25). CCl_4 vapor can be absorbed through the skin, but not in toxicologically significant quantities. When inhaled repeatedly at 100 ppm, CCl_4 is primarily excreted as metabolites (60% of excreted dose) in the feces and urine (<8%) or exhaled unchanged (40% of excreted dose) in the breath with small amounts (<2%) exhaled as carbon dioxide (20). Following a single oral gavage dose of CCl_4, radiolabeled CCl_4 or its metabolites can be found extensively in the liver, but only low levels are found in the brain (28). After inhalation of radiolabeled CCl_4 vapor at 100 ppm (rats) or 46 ppm (rhesus monkeys), the ^{14}C label is present in highest concentration in body fat and liver, but significant levels can also be detected in the brain (17,21). Even though CCl_4 has a rapid elimination rate with repeated 8- or 11.5-h exposures to 100 ppm, low levels of residual ^{14}C radiolabel are present in the brain 2 weeks following exposure (21). Because humans eliminate CCl_4 more slowly than rats (26), residual CCl_4 or its metabolites may remain in the brain for longer periods of time. Metabolism of CCl_4 involves P-450 dehalogenation, formation of a trichloromethyl-free radical, binding to microsomal lipids and proteins; and formation of carbon dioxide, carbon monoxide, hexachloroethane, chloroform, phosgene, and other metabolic products (19). Metabolism of CCl_4 results in destruction of cytochrome P-450, consequently, metabolism of subsequent doses of CCl_4 is not as efficient following exposure to a toxic dose level.

At high vapor concentrations or following high-oral-dose exposure, CCl_4 has anesthetic properties producing unconsciousness and analgesia. These properties are the basis for its early use as a human anesthetic. If exposure is sufficiently severe, death may result from depression of the medullary respiratory centers. At lower concentrations, CCl_4 is a CNS depressant; however, hepatoxicity and, to a lesser extent in animals than humans, renal toxicity are the primary target organ effects.

At lethal oral or subcutaneous (s.c.) dose levels, neuronal changes and areas of necrosis have been reported in the pons of rabbits (13). Following administration of oral, s.c., or intravenous doses of CCl_4 to rabbits, necrosis of neurons in the spinal gray matter and lumbosacral dorsal root ganglia has been observed (13–15). Spongiosis of spinal myelin and hemorrhages into the leptomeninges and spinal gray matter are also reported (14). Cerebellar hemorrhage, loss of Purkinje cells, and astrocyte and oligodendroglial cell swelling have been reported in animals (dogs and rabbits) acutely intoxicated with CCl_4 (5,27).

Repeated exposures of laboratory animals to CCl_4 at levels that do not induce significant hepatotoxicity apparently do not result in neurotoxicity. Maximum CCl_4 vapor concentrations that do not result in adverse effects (hepatic or renal toxicity primarily) following 7 h/day exposures for 6 months have been reported for the rat (5 ppm), guinea pig (5 ppm), rabbit (10 ppm), and rhesus monkey (25 ppm) (1). Rhesus monkeys exposed to levels as high as 100 ppm CCl_4 for 7 h/day over a period of 232 days (163 exposures) developed mild histological changes in the liver, but no behavioral abnormalities or histological changes in the brain, optic nerve, sciatic nerve, or skeletal muscle (1). Female rats given up to 1.5 g/kg of CCl_4 for 14 days and then tested for neurotoxicity using a functional-observational battery and automated motor activity measurement showed decreased activity levels but no other effects (18). Male rats given 1 g/kg CCl_4 in corn oil by oral gavage for 3 days did not show changes in horizontal or vertical motor activity, acoustic startle reflex response, auditory threshold, or functional-observational end points (16).

Osmium black granules suggesting axonal degeneration have been reported in the optic nerves of guinea pigs and rats, and in the sciatic nerve and extraocular muscles of rats, guinea pigs, and rhesus monkeys exposed repeatedly to CCl₄ (typically 200–400 ppm); no clinical signs of neurotoxicity were associated with the histological changes (23). A small number of guinea pigs had optic nerve lesions at CCl₄ levels as low as 50 ppm (23). While the effects observed in these animals appeared to be related to dose and length of exposure, individual animal susceptibility seemed to play a role in whether or not effects were observed; the majority of animals exposed to CCl₄ did not show osmium black granules (23). Lesions were present in nerves 176 days after exposure to CCl₄ was discontinued (23). Reduction of Purkinje cells and alterations in astroglia have been observed in rats given repeated doses of CCl₄ sufficient to induce severe liver necrosis (0.25–0.40 ml two times a week for 8 weeks by oral gavage) (9,10).

Signs and symptoms of CCl₄ intoxication in humans include acute CNS depression at high exposure levels; dizziness, vertigo, headache, depression, mental confusion, and loss of consciousness at lower levels; and serious liver and kidney impairment with low-concentration long-term exposures. In contrast to the large body of data on liver and kidney effects, information on the neurotoxic effects of CCl₄ in humans exists primarily as individual case reports published prior to 1954 when exposures were typically higher than they are presently. While signs and symptoms of cerebellar damage are commonly observed in humans acutely intoxicated with CCl₄, and cerebellar hemorrhage and loss of Purkinje cells have been observed in fatal cases, cerebellar damage is not present in survivors (24). Persistent neuropsychiatric and electroencephalographic changes have been observed in survivors of acute intoxication (24).

The most significant effects observed in humans intoxicated with CCl₄ after either single or repeated exposures to CCl₄ have been liver and renal toxicity; many of these cases have been associated with previous or concurrent exposure to alcohol, but a number of the cases with signs or symptoms referable to the nervous system was not associated with alcohol consumption (19). Two different types of effects have been described; however, it is important to note that, in some of these cases, there was concurrent exposure to other substances. The first involves signs and symptoms suggesting a sensorimotor neuropathy with weakness, loss of position sense, hyporeflexia, and paresthesias (11,12,24, 29). The second includes abnormalities involving vision, including blurred vision, constriction of visual fields, pallor of the optic nerve, and optic nerve atrophy, which have occurred with or without hepatic or renal toxicity (11,12, 22–24,29). Epidemiological data supporting a clear link between repeated exposure to low concentrations of CCl₄ and neurotoxicity do not exist.

CCl₄ has been widely used as a model chemical for induction of hepatic toxicity and hepatic encephalopathy in laboratory animals. Much less effort has been directed to study of the direct effects of CCl₄ on the nervous system. CCl₄ exerts its toxic effects by the generation of free radicals. The activation of CCl₄ is dependent on the presence of cytochrome oxidases, which are present in highest amounts in the liver; however, the liver is not the only organ where free radicals can be formed, as the microsomal systems in the brain also appear capable of generating free radicals (2). The greater *in vitro* sensitivity of neurons as compared to astrocytes to CCl₄ appears to be due in part to higher levels of microsomal activation of CCl₄ in neurons. Exposure of neuron cultures to CCl₄ (1–4 mM) results in loss of membrane integrity leading to cell swelling and death; astrocytes are not affected (6). The sensitivity of neurons may be explained by their greater capacity to activate CCl₄ and the lower level of protection afforded by glutathione in neuronal cultures (6).

Lipid peroxidation following CCl₄ exposure *in vivo* follows a tissue distribution pattern that is similar to the distribution of cytochrome oxidases. The primary site for lipid peroxidation is the liver; no lipid peroxidation has been observed in the brain *in vivo* (4). Thiobarbituric acid levels, a measure of lipid peroxidation, were significantly increased in liver homogenates by CCl₄, but thiobarbituric acid levels in brain homogenates were not significantly increased, suggesting that CCl₄ may not have direct effects on the brain (2). CCl₄ may induce transient effects on cerebral calmodulin levels. Gerbils given a single intraperitoneal injection of 15 μl CCl₄ showed a decrease in Ca^{2+}-adenosine triphosphatase (ATPase) and calmodulin in the P2 and cytosol fractions isolated from the brain at 0.5 and 2 h following dosing; by 6 h following dosing, Ca^{2+}-ATPase was back to normal levels, and calmodulin levels had returned to 80% of the control value (7).

Irreversible liver cirrhosis can be induced in rats by repetitive dosing with CCl₄ (3,30). The cirrhosis induced by CCl₄ in rats is similar to that seen in humans and includes alterations in aromatic amino acid content, elevated ammonia levels, reduced zinc levels, and elevated insulin levels without changes in glucose levels in the blood or plasma. These changes occur without obvious changes in the brain morphology. In CCl₄-induced chronic liver failure, pyridoxal phosphate activity and γ-aminobutyric acid (GABA) synthesis are reduced, resulting in diminished efficiency of GABAergic neurotransmission (8).

Mechanistic data dealing with neurotoxicity following repeated exposures to CCl₄ at dose levels that do not induce hepatotoxicity are not available.

REFERENCES

1. Adams EM, Spencer HC, Rowe VK *et al.* (1952) Vapor toxicity of carbon tetrachloride determined by experiments on laboratory animals. *Arch Ind Hyg Occup Med* **6**, 50.

2. Ahmad FF, Cowan DL, Sun AY (1987) Detection of free radical formation in various tissues after acute carbon tetrachloride administration in the gerbil. *Life Sci* **41**, 2469.

3. Ariosto F, Riggio O, Cantafora A *et al.* (1989) Carbon tetrachloride-induced experimental cirrhosis in the rat: A reappraisal of the model. *Eur Surg Res* **21**, 280.

4. Benedetto C, Dianzani MU, Ahmed M *et al.* (1981) Activation of carbon tetrachloride and distribution of NADPH-cytochrome reductase, cytochrome P-450 and other microsomal enzyme activities in rat tissue. *Biochem Biophys Acta* **677**, 363.

5. Biancalani A (1934) Richerche sperimentali sulle alterazione del sistema nervosa centrale nella into sicazione da tetrachoruro di carbonio. *Riv Pat Erv Ment* **44**, 352.

6. Clemedson C, Romert L, Odland L *et al.* (1994) Biotransformation of carbon tetrachloride in cultured neurons and astrocytes. *Toxicol Vitro* **8**, 145.

7. Desaiah D, Pentyala SN, Trottman CH *et al.* (1991) Combined effects of carbon tetrachloride and chlordecone on calmodulin activity in gerbil brain. *J Environ Health* **34**, 219.

8. Diaz-Munoz M, Tapia R (1988) Glutamate decarboxylase inhibition and vitamin B6 metabolism in brain of cirrhotic rats chronically treated with carbon tetrachloride. *J Neurosci Res* **20**, 376.

9. Diemer NH (1976) Number of Purkinje cells and Bergmann astrocytes in rats with CCl₄-induced liver disease. *Acta Neurol Scand* **55**, 1.

10. Diemer NH (1976) Glial and neuronal alterations in the corpus striatum of rats with CCl₄-induced liver disease. *Acta Neurol Scand* **55**, 16.

11. Farrel C, Senseman L (1944) Carbon tetrachloride polyneuritis: A case report. *R I Med J* **27**, 334.

12. Lahl R (1973) Carbon tetrachloride poisoning and the CNS: Review of neurological and mental symptomatology in man. *Psychiat Neurol Med Psychol* **25**, 1.

13. Lahl R (1974) The pathomorphology of the CNS in carbon tetrachloride poisoning. IV. The histopathology of the rhombencephalon in experimental studies on random bred rabbits. *Zbl Allg Pathol Pathol Anat* **118**, 305.

14. Lahl R (1974) The pathomorphology of the CNS in carbon tetrachloride poisoning. V. The histopathology of the spinal cord in experimental studies on random bred rabbits. *Acta Morphol Acad Sci Hung* **22**, 47.

15. Lahl R (1975) The pathomorphology of the CNS in carbon tetrachloride poisoning. VII. The histopathology of lumbar spinal ganglia in experimental studies. *Zbl Allg Pathol Pathol Anat* **119**, 276.

16. Llorens J, Crofton KM (1991) Enhanced neurotoxicity of 3,3'-iminodipropionitrile following carbon tetrachloride pretreatment in the rat. *Neurotoxicology* **12**, 583.

17. McCollister DD, Beamer WH, Atchison WH, Spencer HC (1951) Absorption, distribution and elimination of radioactive carbon tetrachloride by monkeys upon exposure to low concentrations of vapor. *J Pharmacol Exp Ther* **102**, 112.

18. Moser VC, Cheek BM, MacPhail RC (1995) A multidisciplinary approach to toxicological screening: Neurobehavioral toxicity. *J Toxicol Environ Health* **45**, 173.

19. National Institute for Occupational Safety and Health (1975) *Criteria for a Recommended Standard: Occupational Exposure to Carbon Tetrachloride.* U.S. Department of Health, Education, and Welfare, Publ. No. 76-133, Washington, DC.

20. Paustenbach DJ, Carlson GP, Christian JE, Born GS (1986) A comparative study of the pharmacokinetics of carbon tetrachloride in the rat following repeated inhalation exposures of 8 and 11.5 h/day. *Fund Appl Toxicol* **6**, 484.

21. Paustenbach DJ, Christian JE, Carlson GP, Born GS (1986) The effect of an 11.5-h/day exposure schedule on the distribution and toxicity of inhaled carbon tetrachloride in the rat. *Fund Appl Toxicol* **6**, 472.

22. Smith AR (1950) Optic atrophy following inhalation of carbon tetrachloride. *Arch Ind Hyg Occup Med* **1**, 348.

23. Smyth HF, Smyth HF Jr, Carpenter CP (1936) The chronic toxicity of carbon tetrachloride; animal exposures and field studies. *J Ind Hyg Toxicol* **18**, 277.

24. Stevens H, Foster FM (1953) Effect of carbon tetrachloride on the nervous system. *Arch Neurol Psychiat* **70**, 635.

25. Stewart RD, Dodd HC (1964) Absorption of carbon tetrachloride, trichloroethylene, tetrachloroethylene, methylene chloride, and 1,1,1-trichloroethane through the human skin. *Amer Ind Hyg Assn J* **25**, 439.

26. Stewart RD, Gay HH, Erley DS *et al.* (1961) Human exposure to carbon tetrachloride vapor: Relationship of expired air concentration to exposure and toxicity. *J Occup Med* **3**, 586.

27. Tanohata K, Tagawa D (1932) Histopathologic study of the central nervous system in experimental carbon tetrachloride poisoning. *Nagasaki Igakkai Zasshi* **10**, 1505.

28. Watanabe A, Shiota T, Takei N *et al.* (1986) Blood to brain transfer of carbon tetrachloride and lipoperoxidation in rat brain. *Res Commun Chem Pathol Pharmacol* **51**, 137.

29. Wirtschafter ZT (1933) Toxic amblyopia and accompanying physiological disturbances in carbon tetrachloride intoxication. *Amer J Public Health* **23**, 1035.

30. Yamamoto H (1990) Brain phenylalanine and tyrosine levels and hepatic encephalopathy induced by CCl₄ in rats. *Toxicology* **61**, 241.

Carboxyatractyloside

Albert C. Ludolph

ATRACTYLOSIDE
$C_{30}H_{44}K_2O_{16}S_2$

$(2\beta,4\alpha,15\alpha)$-15-Hydroxy-2-[[2-O-(3-methyl-1-oxobutyl)-3,4-di-O-sulfo-β-D-glucopyranosyl]oxy]-19-norkaur-16-en-18-oic acid dipotassium salt; Atractyloside

NEUROTOXICITY RATING

Clinical

A   Acute encephalopathy (seizures, coma)

Experimental

A   Acute encephalopathy (seizures, coma)

Carboxyatractyloside is extracted from the plants *Atractylis gummifera* (birdlime thistle), *Xanthium strumarium* (cocklebur), and *Wedelia* spp. Carboxyatractyloside glycosides are highly specific inhibitors of adenine nucleotide translocases responsible for adenosine diphosphate/adenosine triphosphate transport across the inner mitochondrial membrane in the terminal stages of oxidative phosphorylation (1). In accidental and experimental poisonings, carboxyatractylosides cause hypoglycemia and primarily induce hepatic and renal lesions (2).

Swine fed *X. strumarium* experimentally develop hepatic necrosis, hypoglycemia, depression, "ataxia," "paddling of the limbs," convulsions, coma, and death (10). The same clinical picture is seen after oral or intravenous administration of the potassium salt of carboxyatractyloside (10), indicating that the glycoside is responsible for the clinical observations. Hepatic necrosis is the primary lesion; however, nephrotic changes and cerebral "ischemic" neuronal degeneration is also present (10). A comparable clinical picture has been observed in cattle (7,11). In laboratory rodents, hypoglycemia and centrilobular hepatic necrosis are described; lethargy, weakness, increased depth of respiration, seizures, and coma were observed, but the brain was not examined (6,9). Some workers describe the development of tolerance in animals accidentally poisoned by toxin-containing plants. Several cases of accidental human intoxication, in particular caused by the Mediterranean *A. gummifera*, are reported (3,4,8); clinical signs included hypoglycemia and hepatic and renal damage; convulsions, brain edema, and coma occurred in some.

Addition of a low concentration of carboxyatractyloside (0.075 μM) renders mitochondria *in vitro* susceptible to the opening of their non-specific pores by oleate, in a cyclosporin A-sensitive fashion. Mitochondrial permeability transition may result from an additive effect of carboxyatractyloside plus oleate on the ADP/ATP carrier (5).

REFERENCES

1. Brandolin G, Le Saux A, Trezeguet V *et al.* (1993) Chemical, immunological, enzymatic, and genetic approaches to studying the arrangement of the peptide chain of the ADP/ATP carrier in the mitochondrial membrane. *J Bioenerg Biomembrane* **25**, 459.
2. Bye SN, Dutton MF (1991) The inappropriate use of traditional medicines in South Africa. *J Ethnopharmacol* **34**, 253.
3. Capdevielle P, Darracq R (1980) L'intoxication par le chadon à glu (*Atractylis gummifera* L.). *Méd Trop* **40**, 137.
4. Catanzano G, Delons S, Benyahia TD (1969) A propos de 2 cas d'intoxication par le chadon à glu. *Maroc Med* **49**, 651.
5. Chavez E, Zazueta C, Garcia N (1999) Carboxyatractyloside increases the effect of oleate on mitochondrial permeability transition. *FEBS Lett* **445**, 189.
6. Hatch RC, Jain AV, Weiss R, Clark JD (1982) Toxicologic study of carboxyatractyloside (active principle in cocklebur—*Xanthium strumarium*) in rats treated with enzyme inducers and inhibitors and glutathione precursor and depletor. *Amer J Vet Res* **43**, 111.
7. Martin T, Stair EL, Dawson L (1986) Cocklebur poisoning in cattle. *J Amer Vet Med Assn* **189**, 562.
8. Santi R, Cascio G (1955) Richerche farmacologiche sul principie attivo dell'*Atractylis gummifera*. I. Azione generale. *Arch Ital Sci Farmacol* **5**, 534.
9. Seawright AA, Hrdlicka J, Lee JA, Ogunsan EA (1982) Toxic substances in the food of animals: Some recent findings of Australian poisonous plants investigations. *J Appl Toxicol* **2**, 75.
10. Stuart BP, Cole RJ, Gosser HS (1981) Cocklebur (*Xanthium strumarium*) intoxication in swine: Review and redefinition of the toxic principle. *Vet Pathol* **18**, 368.
11. Witte ST, Osweiler GD, Stahr HM, Mobley G (1990) Cocklebur toxicosis in cattle associated with the consumption of mature *Xanthium strumarium*. *J Vet Diagn Invest* **2**, 263.

Carmustine

William C. Welch
Paul L. Kornblith

CARMUSTINE
$C_5H_9Cl_2N_3O_2$

N,N'-Bis(2-chloroethyl)-N- nitrosourea;
N-(2-Chloroethyl)-N-nitrosourea;
1,3-Bis(β-chloroethyl)-1-nitrosourea;
1,3-Bis(2-chloroethyl)-1-nitrosourea;
1,3-Bis(chloroethyl)-1-nitrosourea;
Urea, N,N'-Bis(2-chloroethyl)-N-nitroso-;
Urea, 1,3-Bis(2-chloroethyl)-1-nitroso-;
Bis(2-chloroethyl) nitrosourea;
SRI 1720; SK 27702; FDA 0345;
CAS 154-93-8; HSC-409962;
NIOSH/RTECS YS 2625000;
NCI-c 04773; NCS 409962; WR 139021;
Nitrumon; Carmubris; Carmustin; BiCNC; BiCNU; BCNU

NEUROTOXICITY RATING
Clinical
B Retinopathy (vasculopathy)
B Leukoencephalopathy

Carmustine (BCNU) is a chloroethyl-nitrosourea (CNU) compound approved by the U.S. Food and Drug Administration (FDA) for the treatment of primary malignant brain tumors (glioma, medulloblastoma, ependymoma), multiple myeloma, Hodgkin's lymphoma, and other lymphoma (7,54). BCNU has also been used to treat malignant melanoma (11).

BCNU and related CNU compounds are soluble in water, lipids, or alcohols. BCNU is a highly lipid-soluble compound that is poorly ionized at physiological pH, properties that allow it readily to cross the blood-brain barrier (51). The agents can be synthesized with antimetabolites, amide groups, steroids, or other moieties (33,34).

Two mechanisms of action are responsible for the anticancer activities of BCNU. These actions include alkylative DNA cross-linking and carbamoylation (2,34). DNA cross-linking occurs through the generation of 2-chloroethyl diazohydroxides (CEDH) as a product of BCNU metabolism. The CEDH moieties alkylate O^6-guanine residues. This alkylation leads to complementary DNA strand cross-linking

through the formation of ethylene bridges attached to cytosine residues. Alkylated guanine residues may also lead to miscoding, damage, and interstrand cross-linking of the DNA chain (43). Cells can resist this cross-linking through the action of the suicide repair enzyme O^6-methylguanine-DNA-methyltransferase (41,53).

Carbamoylation activity occurs when organic isocyanates generated through the metabolic breakdown of BCNU react with intracellular proteins (16). This activity may inhibit cellular repair enzymes and enhance radiation effects (16,51). Alternatively, carbamoylation may potentiate bone marrow suppression (1).

BCNU is packaged as a powder that is reconstituted in absolute alcohol. The compound is administered to patients either in a hospital or outpatient clinic setting. It is now most commonly used for the treatment of malignant glial tumors. When combined with intracranial radiation therapy, it is effective in prolonging patient survival (12,15,21,36,46–48).

Carmustine is FDA-approved for intravenous administration, the most commonly employed method of drug delivery. Patients are administered 150–200 mg/m² as a single dose. Alternatively, BCNU can be given on 2 consecutive days at 75–100 mg/m². A course of therapy is given every 6–8 weeks. Treatment frequency is limited by bone marrow suppression with subsequent hematological recovery.

Following intravenous injection, BCNU is passively distributed throughout the body and is protein-bound (44). A generalized distribution of agent is noted with excellent CNS penetration (38). BCNU is inactivated by denitrosation reactions catalyzed by NADPH and glutathione in the liver (18,49); the biological half-life is 15 min (38). Sixty to 70% of the drug is excreted in the urine, and 10% is excreted as CO_2 from the lungs within 96 h.

BCNU has undergone an investigational study for intra-arterial use (26). Twenty patients received 50 courses of intra-arterial BCNU dissolved in 5% dextrose in water. Each patient received a dose of 150 mg/m². Nine patients had stabilization or reduction in tumor size. The extracorporeal removal of intra-arterially infused BCNU has been investigated as a means to reduce systemic toxicity (14,37).

BCNU has been impregnated into biodegradable polyanhydride polymer wafers for use in a clinical trial in patients with malignant primary glial tumors (5). The wafers were placed on the exposed cortical brain surface following tumor resection. BCNU leaches out of the wafers into the surrounding cortical tissue to kill malignant cells. Although the drug half-life is longer, the route of BCNU elimination is similar to that following intravenous administration (17). No systemic toxicity related to BCNU was noted in the phase I–II trial. A phase III trial has been completed (6).

Carmustine has also been administered topically for the treatment of mycosis fungoides (54). Solutions and ointments were prepared for topical and intralesional use. Patients generally received 10–60 mg daily for mean total body doses of 607 mg.

The most widely recognized serious toxicity following intravenous BCNU administration is delayed bone marrow suppression involving all marrow elements (9,11). Granulocytes and leukocytes are most sensitive to BCNU, and they may reach a nadir as late as 6 weeks after treatment. Hematological recovery typically occurs over the ensuing weeks. Bone marrow toxicity appears to be cumulative.

Another serious general toxicological reaction to BCNU is pulmonary fibrosis. This occurs with a high frequency in patients who receive a cumulative dosage of 1400 mg/m^2 or more (50). Other toxicological reactions are noted below.

Complications related to both short and prolonged animal exposures to BCNU are summarized in Table 13. These complications are similar to those noted in humans. Specifically, controlled exposures in animals have demonstrated CNS depression, bone marrow suppression, atrophy of organs associated with the immune system, hepatic and renal injury, and other pathological findings. The myelosuppressive effects of BCNU were reduced with the addition of interleukin-11 in a mouse model (32). Prolonged BCNU

exposure in rats caused pulmonary fibrosis (44). Carmustine is toxic to the reproductive system of animals; it affects fertility in male rats, it is toxic to developing embryos of rats and rabbits, and is a teratogen in rats (7).

The mechanisms of BCNU action, as discussed above, have been examined in cellular studies. Cellular resistance to BCNU through the generation of the DNA-repair enzyme O^6-methylguanine-DNA-methyltransferase has also been examined using in vitro models (41,53). Cells that generate this enzyme are phenotypically described as Mer^+ (29).

BCNU reduces glutathione disulfide reductase, which may increase the sensitivity of cells to oxidant stress. This has been demonstrated for human erythrocytes (19,20), human platelets (35), human granulocytes (13), human and bovine endothelial cells (22), and rat hepatocytes (3). Carbamoylating effects of BCNU have been noted in cell culture. Specifically, there is rapid, direct cell membrane and cytoplasmic effects following the addition of BCNU to glioma cell line growth medium (45).

Microcytotoxicity assays have been utilized to help predict in vivo responses. Seventy-two percent of treated cell cultures showed a statistically significant cytotoxic response to BCNU, which was predictive of the clinical response (30).

Most organ systems are affected by BCNU treatment. Hematological toxicities have included leukemia, bone marrow dysplasias, and hypoplasia (10,38,52). Gastrointestinal system toxicities include nausea and vomiting. Hepatic toxicity with reversibly elevated liver function tests, jaundice, and hepatic coma have been reported (18,23,40).

TABLE 13. Animal Studies with Carmustine

Species	Dose Range (mg/kg)	Courses of Chemotherapy	LD$_{50}$ (mg/kg)	Findings
Mouse	3.8–112.0	1–5	11.8–62.5	CNS depression, ptosis, ataxia, icterus, respiratory difficulties, weight loss, piloerection, others
Rat	4.6–50.1	1	20.0–25.0	CNS depression, respiratory difficulty, abnormal gait, weight loss, others
Rhesus monkey	1.2–20.0/day	7–17		Anorexia, malaise, emesis, shock, diarrhea, bone marrow depression, splenic atrophy, pneumonia, hemorrhagic and other lesions, elevated BUN, glucose, liver function tests, and alkaline phosphatase
Beagle	1–20/day 5–20/week	5–50 2–7		Anorexia, malaise, hyperthermia, respiratory depression, bone marrow suppression, spleen and lymph node atrophy, hemorrhages, pneumonia, pulmonary edema, gastric ulcers, liver swelling, other pathologic findings, elevated BUN, liver function tests, and alkaline phosphatase

BUN, blood urea nitrogen.

[Modified with permission from Carter and Newman (10)]

Nephrotoxicity including azotemia, decrease in renal size and renal failure was identified in patients receiving BCNU therapy (38). Also noted have been flushing of the skin at the intravenous injection site (4) and elsewhere (23), skin hyperpigmentation, burning, erythema, telangiectasia, dermatitis, superficial denudation, bullae formation, and transient hyperpigmentation at the application site when used topically (54). Some of these effects may have been due to the alcohol diluent (24). Cardiovascular effects have included hypotension, angina, and tachycardia (23,27). Gynecomastia has also been noted in patients whose treatment regimens included BCNU (42).

A number of neurological and optic toxicities has been reported with the intravenous and intra-arterial administration of BCNU. One study reported a subgroup of nonirradiated patients undergoing a phase I–II trial of BCNU therapy with autologous bone marrow transplant for Hodgkin's disease, embryonal cell carcinoma, and metastatic melanoma (8). Each of three patients received 1500–2850 mg/m^2 BCNU in divided doses over 3 days. A fourth received 1200 mg/m^2 BCNU in divided doses over 3 days and 2250 mg/m^2 BCNU in divided doses 6 weeks later. Each patient died within 3 months of BCNU treatment. Autopsy studies of the brains demonstrated discrete foci of swollen axons in all and larger areas of edema and fibrinoid necrosis in two.

Intra-arterial BCNU administration has been associated with hemiparesis and aphasia (31), ocular pain (26), ocular injuries (39), retinal hemorrhages (38), and vasculitis (26). Leukoencephalopathic changes have been found in isolated patients who received BCNU and other treatments (28).

There have been no reported uncontrolled exposures to BCNU. A single case of lomustine overdose is reported in the literature (25). Treatment for a suspected BCNU overdose is supportive (4).

REFERENCES

1. Ali-Osman F, Giblin J, Berger M et al. (1985) Chemical structure of carbamoylating groups and their relationship to bone marrow toxicity and antiglioma activity of bifunctionally alkylating and carbamoylating nitrosoureas. Cancer Res 45, 4185.
2. Ali-Osman F, Srivenugopal K, Berger MS, Stein DE (1990) DNA interstrand crosslinking and strand break repair in human glioma cell lines of varying [1,3-bis (2-chloroethyl)-1-nitrosourea] resistance. Anticancer Res 10, 677.
3. Babson JR, Abell NS, Reed DJ (1981) Protective role of the glutathione redox cycle against adriamycin-mediated toxicity in isolated hepatocytes. Biochem Pharmacol 30, 2299.
4. BCNU (1974–1995) Poisindex 85.
5. Brem H, Mahaley MS Jr, Vick NA et al. (1991) Interstitial chemotherapy with drug polymer implants for treatment of recurrent gliomas. J Neurosurg 74, 441.
6. Brem H, Piantadosi S, Burger PC et al. (1995) Placebo-controlled trial of safety and efficacy of intraoperative controlled delivery by biodegradable polymers of chemotherapy for recurrent gliomas. The Polymer-Brain Tumor Treatment Group. Lancet 345, 1008.
7. Bristol Myers Squibb Oncology Division (1995) BiCNU®. In: Physicians' Desk Reference: PDR, 1995. 49th Ed. Duffy MA, Dir. Production. Medical Economics Data Production Co, Oradell, NJ p. 659.
8. Burger PC, Kamenar E, Schold SC et al. (1981) Encephalomyelopathy following high-dose BCNU therapy. Cancer 48, 1318.
9. Calabresi P, Chabner BA (1990) Antineoplastic Agents. In: Goodman and Gilman's The Pharmacological Basis of Therapeutics. 8th Ed. Gilman AG, Rall TR, Nies AS, Taylor P eds. Pergamon Press, New York.
10. Carter SK, Newman JW (1968) Nitrosoureas: 1,3-Bis (2-chloroethyl)-1-nitrosourea (NSC-409962; BCNU) and 1-(2-chloroethyl)-3-cyclohexyl-1-nitrosourea (NSC-79037; CCNU)—Clinical Brochure. Cancer Chemother Rep 1, 115.
11. Cascino TL (1991) The nitrosoureas. In: Neurological Complications of Cancer Treatment. Rottenberg DA ed. Butterworth-Heinemann, Boston p. 131.
12. Chang CH, Horton J, Schoenfeld D et al. (1983) Comparison of postoperative radiotherapy and chemotherapy in the multidisciplinary management of malignant gliomas. Cancer 52, 997.
13. Cohen HJ, Tape EH, Novak J et al. (1987) The role of glutathione reductase in maintaining human granulocyte function and sensitivity to exogenous H_2O_2. Blood 69, 493.
14. Dedrick RL, Oldfield EH, Collins JM (1984) Arterial drug infusion with extracorporeal removal. I. Theoretic basis with particular reference to the brain. Cancer Treatment Rep 68, 373.
15. Deutsch M, Green SB, Strike TA et al. (1989) Results of a randomized trial comparing BCNU plus radiotherapy, streptozotocin plus radiotherapy, BCNU plus hyperfractionated radiotherapy, and BCNU following misonidazole plus radiotherapy in the postoperative treatment of malignant glioma. Int J Radiat Oncol Biol Phys 16, 1389.
16. Dive C, Workman P, Watson JV (1988) Inhibition of intracellular esterases by antitumor chloroethylnitrosoureas. Biochem Pharmacol 37, 3987.
17. Domb AJ, Rock M, Schwartz J et al. (1994) Metabolic disposition and elimination studies of a radiolabeled biodegradable polymeric implant in the rat brain. Biomaterials 15, 681.
18. Dorr RT, Fritz WL (1980) Cancer Chemotherapy Handbook. Elsevier North Holland Inc, New York p. 295.

19. Frischer H, Ahmad T (1977) Severe generalized glutathione reductase deficiency after antitumor therapy with BCNU [1,3-bis (chloroethyl)-1-nitrosourea]. *J Lab Clin Med* **89**, 1080.

20. Frischer H, Ahmad T (1987) Consequences of erythrocytic glutathione reductase deficiency. *J Lab Clin Med* **109**, 583.

21. Green SB, Byar DP, Walker MD et al. (1983) Comparisons of carmustine, procarbazine, and high-dose methylprednisolone as additions to surgery and radiotherapy for the treatment of malignant glioma. *Cancer Treatment Rep* **67**, 121.

22. Harlan JM, Levine JD, Callahan KS et al. (1984) Glutathione redox cycle protects cultured endothelial cells against lysis by extracellularly generated hydrogen peroxide. *J Clin Invest* **73**, 706.

23. Henner WD, Peters WP, Eder JP et al. (1986) Pharmacokinetics and immediate effects of high-dose carmustine in man. *Cancer Treatment Rep* **70**, 877.

24. Higby DJ (1987) Pharmacokinetics and immediate effects of high-dose carmustine in man. *Cancer Treatment Rep* **71**, 433.

25. Hornsten P, Sundman-Engberg B, Gahrton G, Johansson, B (1983) CCNU toxicity after an overdose in a patient with Hodgkin's disease. *Scand J Haematol* **31**, 9.

26. Johnson DW, Parkinson D, Wolpert SM et al. (1987) Intracarotid chemotherapy with 1,3-bis (2-chloroethyl)-1-nitrosourea (BCNU) in 5% dextrose in water in the treatment of malignant glioma. *Neurosurgery* **20**, 577.

27. Kanj SS, Sharara AI, Shpall EJ et al. (1991) Myocardial ischemia associated with high-dose carmustine infusion. *Cancer* **68**, 1910.

28. Kleinschmidt-DeMasters BK, Geier JM (1989) Pathology of high-dose intraarterial BCNU. *Surg Neurol* **31**, 435.

29. Kohn KW (1988) Prospects for improved chloroethylnitrosoureas and related haloethylating agents. In: *Advances in Neuro-Oncology*. Kornblith PL, Walker MD eds. Futura Publishing Co. Mount Kisco, New York p. 491.

30. Kornblith PL, Smith BH, Leonard LA (1981) Response of cultured human brain tumors to nitrosoureas: Correlation with clinical data. *Cancer* **47**, 255.

31. Mahaley MS Jr, Whaley RA, Blue M, Bertsch L (1986) Central neurotoxicity following intracarotid BCNU chemotherapy for malignant gliomas. *J Neuro-oncol* **3**, 297.

32. Maze R, Moritz T, Williams DA (1994) Increased survival and multilineage hematopoietic protection from delayed and severe myelosuppressive effects of a nitrosourea with recombinant interleukin-11. *Cancer Res* **54**, 4947.

33. McCormick JE, McElhinney RS (1986) Nucleoside analogues. 4. Molecular combinations of anti-tumour drugs: Synthesis of 5-fluorouracil seco-nucleosides with N-(2-chloroethyl)-N-nitrosourea residues by using aryl N-nitrosocarbamates. *Anti-Cancer Drug Des* **1**, 111.

34. McCormick JE, McElhinney RS (1990) Perspectives in cancer research. Nitrosoureas from chemist to physician: Classification and recent approaches to drug design. *Eur J Cancer* **26**, 207.

35. McKenna R, Ahmad T, Ts'ao CH, Frischer H (1983) Glutathione reductase deficiency and platelet dysfunction induced by 1,3-bis(2-chloroethyl)-1-nitrosourea. *J Lab Clin Med* **102**, 102.

36. Nelson DF, Diener-West M, Weinstein AS et al. (1986) A randomized comparison of misonidazole sensitized radiotherapy plus BCNU and radiotherapy plus BCNU for treatment of malignant glioma after surgery: Final report of an RTOG study. *Int J Radiat Oncol Biol Phys* **12**, 1793.

37. Oldfield EH, Dedrick RL, Chatterji DC et al. (1983) Reduced systemic drug exposure by combining intracarotid chemotherapy with hemoperfusion of jugular drainage. *Surg Forum* **34**, 535.

38. Olin BR ed. (1990) *Drug Facts and Comparisons*. JB Lippincott Co, Philadelphia.

39. Pickrell L, Purvin V (1987) Ischemic optic neuropathy secondary to intracarotid infusion of BCNU. *J Clin Neuroophthal* **7**, 87.

40. Reitemeier RJ, Moertel CG, Hahn RG (1966) 1,3-Bis (2-chloroethyl)-1-nitrosourea (BCNU) therapy in advanced gastrointestinal adenocarcinoma. *Proc Amer Assn Cancer Res* **7**, 59.

41. Sariban E, Kohn KW, Zlotogorski C et al. (1987) DNA cross-linking responses of human malignant glioma cell strains to chloroethylnitrosoureas, cisplatin, and diaziquone. *Cancer Res* **47**, 3988.

42. Schorer AE, Oken MM, Johnson GJ (1978) Gynecomastia with nitrosourea therapy. *Cancer Treatment Rep* **62**, 574.

43. Shapiro R (1968) Chemistry of guanine and its biologically significant derivatives. *Prog Nucleic Acid Res Mol Biol* **8**, 73.

44. Smith AC (1989) The pulmonary toxicity of nitrosoureas. *Pharmacol Ther* **41**, 443.

45. Smith BH, Vaughan M, Greenwood MA et al. (1983) Membrane and cytoplasmic changes in 1,3-bis(2-chloroethyl)-1-nitrosourea (BCNU)-sensitive and resistant human malignant glioma-derived cell lines. *J Neuro-oncol* **1**, 237.

46. Stewart DJ, Benoit B, Richard MT et al. (1984) Treatment of malignant gliomas in adults with BCNU plus metronidazole. *J Neuro-oncol* **2**, 53.

47. Walker MD, Alexander E Jr, Hunt WE et al. (1978) Evaluation of BCNU and/or radiotherapy in the treatment of anaplastic gliomas. *J Neurosurg* **49**, 333.

48. Walker MD, Green SB, Byar DP et al. (1980) Randomized comparisons of radiotherapy and nitrosoureas for the treatment of malignant glioma after surgery. *N Engl J Med* **303**, 1323.

49. Weber GF, Waxman DJ (1993) Denitrosation of the anticancer drug 1,3-bis(2-chloroethyl)-1-nitrosourea catalyzed by microsomal glutathione S-transferase and cyto-

chrome P450 monooxygenases. *Arch Biochem Biophys* **307**, 369.

50. Weinstein AS, Diener-West M, Nelson DF, Pakuris E (1986) Pulmonary toxicity of carmustine in patients treated for malignant glioma. *Cancer Treatment Rep* **70**, 943.
51. Welch WC, Kornblith PL (1994) Chemotherapy of brain tumors: Fundamental principles. In: *Brain Tumors, A Comprehensive Text*. Morantz RA, Walsh JW eds. Marcel Dekker, New York p. 717.
52. Wiemann MC, Calabresi P (1985) Pharmacology of anti-neoplastic agents. In: *Medical Oncology. Basic Principles and Clinical Management of Cancer*. Calabresi P, Schein PS, Rosenberg SA eds. Macmillan Publishing Co, New York p. 292.
53. Yarosh DB (1985) The role of O^6-methylguanine-DNA methyltransferase in cell survival, mutagenesis and carcinogenesis. *Mutat Res* **145**, 1.
54. Zackheim HS, Epstein EH Jr, McNutt NS *et al.* (1983) Topical carmustine (BCNU) for mycosis fungoides and related disorders: A 10-year experience. *J Amer Acad Dermatol* **9**, 363.

Cassava

Hans Rosling
Thorkild Tylleskär

$R_1 = CH_3$ LINAMARIN
$R_2 = C_2H_5$ LOTAUSTRALIN

NEUROTOXICITY RATING
Clinical
B Spastic paraparesis (*konzo*)
C Peripheral neuropathy (ataxic)

Cassava (*Manihot esculenta* Crantz) ranks fourth among the tropical food crops. The starchy roots of this 1- to 2-m-high perennial and drought-tolerant plant are the main supplier of dietary energy for about 400 million persons, half of whom live in Africa. Cassava is drought tolerant; the roots provide more carbohydrates per hectare than any other staple crop, and the edible leaves are also an important source of nutrients. In Africa, roots are mainly processed into flour to prepare the dumpling-like porridge that is eaten as a staple food. The low protein content of roots constitutes a nutritional disadvantage that should be balanced by protein-rich supplementary food (2,15).

The term *cassava cyanogenesis* refers to the process by which destruction of plant cells of cassava leads to release of cyanide from its natural content of cyanogenic glucosides. Roots and leaves of all cassava varieties contain varying amounts of the cyanogenic glucosides linamarin and lotaustralin in the proportions 93:7 (22). The levels of glucosides vary 25-fold between different genetic varieties (7),

and adverse environmental factors such as drought and poor soil increase the levels of glucosides (8). Bitterness of roots is associated with higher levels of glucosides (42), but many cassava farmers preferentially cultivate bitter varieties, since it protects plants from being eaten by wild animals (12,18).

Roots from nonbitter varieties are eaten fresh or directly boiled, whereas the high amount of glucosides in roots from bitter varieties is reduced through processing before consumption. Effective processing methods first achieve a cell disintegration that brings glucosides in contact with an endogenous glucosidase stored in a separate compartment of the intact cell. The enzymatic cleavage of linamarin leads to formation of acetone cyanohydrin that is relatively stable at low pH and low temperature. Cyanohydrin rapidly breaks down to hydrogen cyanide at higher temperatures and above pH 6. In a second processing step, drying or heating as well as an increased pH leads to formation of hydrogen cyanide that rapidly dissolves in water or disperses into the air. The glucosides, cyanohydrins, and hydrogen cyanide—jointly known as cyanogens—can all be reduced to negligible levels if the optimal length and sequence of each processing step are adhered to. However, if full cell disintegration is not achieved before drying or heating, the glucosides will remain in the consumed product. If the product is not well dried or sufficiently heated following cell disintegration, residual cyanohydrins will be consumed; this is especially common if cell disintegration has been achieved through lactic acid fermentation, which yields a low pH that stabilizes cyanohydrins (4,50).

Fermentation of roots by soaking for 3 days in water followed by sun-drying and pounding to make flour effectively reduces cyanogens in bitter and toxic roots, and it is a common processing method in Africa. Another effective method includes grating of fresh roots into a mash that is fermented in sacks under pressure and finally heat-dried in frying pans to obtain granules. This product, developed thousands of years ago in South America, is known as *gari* in West Africa (35). Boiling of fresh roots only results in leaching of glucosides and, depending on the size of root pieces, only 25%–75% of cyanogens are removed (33). Sun-drying roots removes about 80% of initial cyanogen levels or less if small chips are dried rapidly (29). The method by which cassava roots are processed is as important for the intake of cyanogens as are the initial glucoside levels and the amounts of cassava consumed (36).

General Toxicology

A high dietary intake of cyanogens from insufficiently processed cassava roots has been almost exclusively reported from poor populations which, during a period food shortage, are saved from hunger by availability of bitter cassava roots. These may either be populations that normally do not eat bitter cassava and have no knowledge of effective detoxication, or populations that normally eat well-processed roots from toxic varieties but take shortcuts in processing as a desperate measure to cope with famine (37). Varying degrees of low dietary intake of cyanogens are reported in many cassava-eating populations that use ineffective processing methods (direct sun-drying).

The three different cyanogens—glucosides, cyanohydrins, and hydrogen cyanide—have different fates in the human body. The majority of ingested linamarin is absorbed from the gut and rapidly excreted intact in the urine without causing any cyanide exposure (19); a small part of an oral linamarin dose releases cyanide. The cyanide release probably occurs in the gut through the action of microbial enzymes or dietary glucosidases that withstand the acidity of the stomach. Ingested cyanohydrins are stable in the low pH of the stomach but are presumably completely decomposed to cyanide in the alkali environment of the gut. Hydrogen cyanide (HCN) formed is rapidly absorbed throughout the gastrointestinal tract. Since HCN formed during processing is rapidly lost before consumption, the dietary cyanide exposure from cassava will almost entirely result from cyanide released in the gut. Daily cyanide exposure thus depends on the amount and type of cyanogens remaining in the food after processing and the degree of cyanide release from linamarin in the gut (36).

The body possesses two defense mechanisms against cyanide exposure. Once absorbed into the blood, up to 10 mg of cyanide can rapidly but reversibly be bound to the methemoglobin fraction of hemoglobin. Only when all methemoglobin has been converted to cyanomethemoglobin will an additional cyanide dose result in rapid increase in plasma cyanide levels and toxic effects (26). The second defense is the slow enzymatic conversion of cyanide to thiocyanate that occurs in several tissues. The rate-limiting factor is availability of sulfur substrate provided from sulfane sulfur compounds derived from different metabolic pathways originating from dietary sulfur amino acids. Even in severe protein malnutrition, available sulfur will preferentially be used for cyanide detoxification, and most of the cyanide dose will be converted into thiocyanate (43). Thiocyanate is therefore a reasonably good quantitative biomarker for cyanide intake (24). The rate of cyanide conversion will be decreased by protein malnutrition, and the same cyanide dose will exert a greater and possibly different biological effect in subjects with low intake of sulfur amino acids. It has been shown, in rats, that cyanide exposure leads to increased formation of two alternative metabolites if protein intake is low (43). These metabolites, 2-iminothiazolidine-4-carboxylic acid (25) and cyanate (23), are neurotoxic in animals (6,40) (*see also* Cyanides and Related Compounds, this volume). For several decades, cassava cyanogenesis has been implicated as a major or contributing factor in acute cassava poisonings, in the aggravation of cretinism and goiter, and in tropical ataxic neuropathy. In the last decade, an upper motoneuron disease, *konzo* (39), has been suggested to stem from cassava consumption. There is no satisfactory experimental animal model of cassava intoxication.

Human Studies
Acute Cassava Poisoning

The risk of acute poisoning following consumption of insufficiently processed bitter roots is known in many communities growing bitter and toxic varieties, but is sparsely reported in medical literature. Symptoms occur within a half hour to some hours following a meal of insufficiently processed bitter cassava roots; manifestations range from nausea, vomiting, diarrhea, and weakness to collapse and (occasionally) death. Such acute poisonings have been attributed to cyanide exposure from the cassava meal. The typical delay between the intake of cassava and the start of symptoms is compatible with the cyanide exposure resulting from release of cyanide in the gut from ingested cyanogens. Only one case report includes determination of blood cyanide levels that were made in eight fatal cases in Lagos, Nigeria (1). Blood cyanide ranged from 21 to 71 μmol/l, which is 100-fold the reference levels but slightly less than levels found in other cases of lethal cyanide intoxication. Severe acute poisoning of cyanide from other sources has resulted in permanent lesions in basal ganglia and parkinsonism (9). Parkinsonism has not been reported following acute cassava poisoning. This may reflect the fact that parkinsonism only has appeared following severe acute cyanide intoxication that required intensive care for survival; such facilities are unavailable to almost all subjects exposed to large amounts of cyanide from cassava.

Extensive outbreaks of acute cassava poisoning with thousands of symptomatic cases have occurred in rural areas with food shortages (13,31). Lethal cases are unusual in such outbreaks; it is possible that symptoms of acute cassava poisoning are not exclusively associated with cyanide but are due to several substances. Cyanide intoxication may be the cause of the few deaths through the general anoxia and direct effects on CNS neurons resulting from a single high dose of cyanide. However, most of the gastrointestinal symptoms reported in acute cassava poisoning may be caused by the intact cyanogenic glucoside linamarin or other substances that cause symptomatic but nonlethal intoxication.

Cretinism

Cretinism and milder forms of submental capacity stem from iodine-deficiency disorders and are among the most common forms of preventable CNS damage in the world. The thiocyanate load resulting from detoxification of dietary cyanide exposure from cassava has been implicated as an aggravating factor in iodine-deficiency disorders. It is suggested that the negative thiocyanate ion is a pseudohalide that can interfere with iodine uptake in the thyroid gland. This goitrogenic effect can be quenched by iodine supplementation, and populations with adequate iodine intake do not develop goiter and cretinism in spite of high thiocyanate levels originating from cassava cyanide (17).

Tropical Ataxic Neuropathy (TAN)

This neurological syndrome is dominated by loss of sensation in the lower limbs and optic atrophy; it has mainly been described among rural Nigerians. In extensive Nigerian studies, two of the following four components were required for diagnosis: myelopathy, bilateral optic atrophy, bilateral sensorineural deafness, and symmetrical peripheral neuropathy (34). In almost all cases, the syndrome developed slowly during several years and both sexes were equally affected. The peak incidence was in the fifth and sixth decades of life, and TAN only affected the poorest part of the population. Tendon reflexes were absent in the

lower limbs in about 50% and exaggerated in about 20% of the Nigerian cases. High prevalence, 1.8%–2.6%, was found in some rural populations with a monotonous cassava diet. The geographical distribution was associated with moderate chronic exposure to cyanide from cassava. Mean blood cyanide levels found in TAN cases were 1.0 μmol/l, and the serum level of the main metabolite (thiocyanate) was 114 μmol/l. These levels are higher than those found in subjects without known cyanide exposure and correspond to the levels emerging from the cyanide inhalation resulting from moderate tobacco smoking. The proportion of different symptoms and signs differs between case series of TAN reported from different countries. It appears unlikely that the same combination of etiological factors is responsible for this type of syndrome in different parts of the world. The Nigerian studies suggest that cyanide exposure from cassava in combination with protein deficiency were causative factors in TAN but that other dietary deficiencies also may have contributed to the etiology of the disorder (34).

Konzo

Konzo is an upper motoneuron disease that is held to be a distinct disease entity (21,39,55). It is named after the local designation among the initially affected population in Zaire (42). In the Yaka language, *konzo* means "tied legs," which describes the resulting spastic gait. Based on several epidemiological studies of outbreaks in rural parts of Africa, konzo has been attributed to the combination of high cyanide and low sulfur intake from the almost exclusive consumption of insufficiently processed bitter cassava roots. Konzo is clinically and epidemiologically distinct from TAN. The cyanide exposure found in konzo-affected populations is several times higher than the exposure linked to TAN (47).

Konzo is characterized by an abrupt onset of symmetrical permanent paraparesis within minutes to a few hours. Occasionally, progression occurs over 2–3 days. All eight published case series have similar clinical findings (39). Initial symptoms are heaviness or trembling of the legs and difficulty walking. The most severely affected are unable to stand immediately at onset. Severity of the impairment varies, and the legs are always affected first and to a greater extent than the arms. Deficits range from mild hyperreflexia in the legs to severe spastic paraparesis with associated weakness of the trunk and arms. Difficulty in speech and vision sometimes occurs at onset but usually disappears during the first month. Only the most severely affected patients retain spastic dysarthria and optic atrophy. About half can walk unaided with a spastic gait, whereas the remaining patients need one or two sticks to walk. About one in ten is unable to walk due to severe spastic paraparesis and associated weakness of the trunk and arms. Mental capacity is unaffected. Impairment is not progressive, but subjects disabled by konzo may experience further attacks of the disease in the following years. Such second or third attacks result in an abrupt and permanent deterioration of the paraparesis (10,21,52,53).

The only two autopsies of konzo patients were done in 1937 and were unremarkable (46). Recent magnetic resonance imaging examinations of two subjects severely disabled by konzo disclosed no abnormalities. Responses to transcranial magnetic stimulation were absent both in the paralyzed legs and in the apparently healthy arms (53).

The distribution of konzo is limited to geographical isolates in rural Africa; the majority of cases occurs in epidemic outbreaks during the dry season. More than 3700 cases have been confirmed from studies of eight different areas (47). Zaire has the largest number of cases reported, mainly from the Bandundu region. The first reported outbreak occurred in the southern part of Bandundu in 1936–37 (46); since 1974, cases occur annually during the dry season in the central part of the region (3,5,49). In Mozambique, an extensive outbreak occurred in Nampula province during a drought in 1981 (27,28), and further outbreaks have been reported from other parts of the same province during periods of drought (18) and civil war (16). Konzo has also been reported from two areas in Tanzania (21,22,30) and one in the Central African Republic (54). The sex and age distribution have been similar in all areas. No children below 2½ years of age have been found to contract konzo. In the affected areas, almost all children are breast-fed to this age. Incidence is highest among women of childbearing age and in children aged 3–13 years. Sharp geographical variations of occurrence are found in most affected areas. Prevalence typically varies from 2%–5% in most affected villages and decreases to zero over a distance of <20 km (3,14,16,27,32). The geographic, seasonal (11), and age variation in occurrence, as well as the abrupt onset, have facilitated epidemiological studies of possible etiological factors in konzo. However, as the disease is restricted to some of the poorest population groups in remote rural areas of Africa, only a handful of konzo patients have ever been admitted to a hospital and examined carefully.

The etiology of konzo has been proposed to be infectious based on the epidemic occurrence, familial clustering, and clinical similarities to human T-cell lymphotropic virus type I (HTLV-I)–associated myelopathy (10). However, konzo patients do not show any signs of infection, cerebrospinal fluid is normal, and extensive testing for infections have been negative. Konzo patients are seronegative for HTLV-I and other retroviruses (38,51). The current hypothesis is that the neurodegeneration in konzo results from a metabolic derangement resulting from the combination of a high continuous daily cyanide intake from insufficiently processed bitter cassava roots in concert with low dietary intake of sulfur amino acids that provide substrate for cyanide to thiocyanate conversion (39,47,53).

The chain of events leading to konzo outbreaks is as follows: intensive cultivation of bitter cassava in poor rural areas; a cassava-dominated diet; shortcuts in processing as indicated by high remaining levels of linamarin and acetone cyanohydrin in products consumed; high cyanide intake indicated by high urinary and serum thiocyanate levels; low intake of foods rich in sulfur amino acids indicated by low urinary inorganic sulfate levels and continuous high blood cyanide. The thiocyanate levels found in konzo cases and konzo-affected populations are severalfold higher than those in earlier reports from cyanide exposure from cassava linked to ataxic tropical neuropathy and aggravation of iodine-deficiency disorders, respectively. Likewise, levels of inorganic sulfate were lower than earlier reported from populations with low protein intake. The konzo-affected populations only constitute some few percent of the cassava-eating populations in Africa, and merely eating cassava is far from sufficient to cause konzo. Dietary interviews and chemical biomarkers of dietary exposure consistently show that the disease is associated with a very abnormal diet dominated by ill-processed toxic roots. Acute cassava poisoning following meals was frequently reported from the konzo-affected communities during the outbreaks, but symptoms of acute poisoning were not associated with the abrupt onset of limb weakness.

A strong association between high blood cyanide levels and onset of konzo has also been found on individual levels in case-referent studies in affected villages in Zaire. Cases had blood cyanide levels in the range of 20–80 μmol/l, 20-fold higher than the median of controls from the same village and 60-fold higher than the upper range of unexposed subjects (10). Likewise, an association was found between shortcuts in processing and occurrence of konzo at the household level with an odds ratio of 11 (95% confidence interval, 1.7–73) and a clear dose–response relationship (48). The absence of konzo in breast-fed children also supports the hypothesis, since they eat the least cassava and have the highest protein intake in the community.

The most valid argument against the cyanide hypothesis is that a similar disease has never been described following cyanide exposure from other sources. This apparent paradox may be explained by a different pattern of biologically effective exposure to cyanide resulting from regular and simultaneous high cyanide and low sulfur intake than from repeated high peaks of cyanide exposure in subjects with a better protein status. This paradox suggests that a metabolite other than cyanide *per se* is responsible for the neurological damage in konzo. One candidate is 2-iminothiazolidine-4-carboxylic acid; this is neurotoxic (6) and formed in higher proportions following cyanide exposure in protein-deficient animals (43). Another candidate is cyanate; it also is formed in higher proportion following cyanide exposure in protein malnutrition (43). Rats maintained on a diet free of sulfur amino acids and treated with cyanide in drinking water show increasing concentrations of plasma cyanate relative to comparably treated animals on a balanced diet (44,45). When used for treating sickle-cell anemia, cyanate was found to induce peripheral neuropathy in humans; when given in high doses to primates for several weeks, they abruptly developed a spastic paraparesis similar to konzo (40).

Editorial addition. Thiocyanate, the principal metabolite of cyanide, is a third etiologic candidate for konzo (41). Thiocyanate is a chaotropic agent that selectively promotes the neurotransmitter action of glutamate at the (RS)-α-amino-3-hydroxy-5-methyl-isoxazole-4-propionic acid (AMPA) subclass of neuronal glutamate receptors. AMPA receptors are the specific molecular targets of β-N-oxalylamino-L-alanine, the neurotoxin responsible for lathyrism, a konzo-like spastic paraparesis (*see β-N-Oxalylamino-L-alanine, this volume*).

REFERENCES

1. Akintowa A, Tunwashe OL (1992) Fatal cyanide poisoning from cassava based meal. *Hum Exp Toxicol* **11**, 47.
2. Akoroda MO (1995) Alleviating hunger in Africa with root and tuber crops. *Afr J Trop Root Crops* **1**, 41.
3. Banea M, Bikangi N, Nahimana G *et al.* (1992) Haute prévalence de konzo associée à une crise agro-alimentaire dans la région de Bandundu au Zaire. *Ann Soc Belg Med Trop* **72**, 295.
4. Banea M, Poulter N, Rosling H (1992) Shortcuts in cassava processing and risk of dietary cyanide exposure in Zaire. *Food Nutr Bull* **14**, 137.
5. Banea M, Tylleskär T, Rosling H (1997) Konzo and Ebola in Bandundu region in Zaire. *Lancet* **349**, 622.
6. Bitner RS, Kanthasamy A, Isom G *et al.* (1995) Seizures and selective CA-1 hippocampal lesions induced by an excitotoxic cyanide metabolite, 2-iminothiazolidine-4-carboxylic acid. *Neurotoxicology* **16**, 115.
7. Bokanga M (1994) Distribution of cyanogenic potential in the cassava germplasm. *Acta Hort* **375**, 11.
8. Bokanga M, Ekanayake IJ, Dixon AGO *et al.* (1994) Genotype-environment interactions for cyanogenic potential in cassava. *Acta Hort* **375**, 131.
9. Carella F, Grassi M, Savoiardo M *et al.* (1988) Dystonic-parkinsonian syndrome after cyanide poisoning: clinical and MRI findings. *J Neurol Neurosurg Psychiat* **51**, 1345.
10. Carton H, Kayembe K, Odio K *et al.* (1986) Epidemic spastic paraparesis in Bandundu (Zaire). *J Neurol Neurosurg Psychiat* **49**, 620.
11. Casadei E, Cliff J, Neves J (1990) Surveillance of urinary thiocyanate concentration after epidemic spastic paraparesis in Mozambique. *J Trop Med Hyg* **93**, 257.
12. Chiwona-Karltun L, Mkumbira J, Saka J *et al.* (1998) The importance of being bitter—A qualitative study on cassava cultivator preference in Malawi. *Ecol Food Nutr* (in press).
13. Cliff J, Coutinho J (1995) Acute intoxication from newly-introduced cassava during drought in Mozambique. *Trop Doct* **25**, 193.
14. Cliff J, Lundquist P, Mårtensson J *et al.* (1985) Association of high cyanide and low sulfur intake in cassava-induced spastic paraparesis. *Lancet* **ii**, 1211.
15. Cock JH (1985) Cassava: A basic energy source in the tropics. *Science* **218**, 755.
16. Davis A, Howarth J (1993) Konzo in Mogincual, Mozambique. Médicine Sans Frontières. *Med News* **2**, 16.
17. Delange F, Ekpechi L, Rosling H (1994) Cassava cyanogenesis and iodine deficiency disorders. *Acta Hort* **375**, 289.
18. Essers AJA, Alsén P, Rosling H (1992) Insufficient processing of cassava induced acute intoxications and the paralytic disease konzo in a rural area of Mozambique. *Ecol Food Nutr* **27**, 17.
19. Hernández T, Lundquist P, Oliveira L *et al.* (1995) The fate in humans of dietary intake of cyanogenic glycosides from roots of sweet cassava consumed in Cuba. *Nat Toxins* **3**, 114.
20. Howlett W, Brubaker G, Mlingi N *et al.* (1992) A geographical cluster of konzo in Tanzania. *J Trop Geogr Neurol* **2**, 102.
21. Howlett WP, Brubaker GR, Mlingi N *et al.* (1990) Konzo, an epidemic upper motor neuron disease studied in Tanzania. *Brain* **113**, 223.
22. Koch BM, Sibbesen O, Swain E *et al.* (1994) Possible use of a biotechnological approach to optimize and regulate the content and distribution of cyanogenic glucosides in cassava to increase food safety. *Acta Hort* **375**, 45.
23. Lundquist P, Backman-Gullers B, Kågedal B *et al.* (1993) Fluorometric determination of cyanate in plasma by conversion to 2,4(1*H*,3*H*)quinazolinedione and separation by high-performance liquid chromatography. *Anal Biochem* **211**, 23.
24. Lundquist P, Kågedal B, Nilsson L (1995) An improved method for determination of thiocyanate in plasma and urine. *Eur J Clin Chem Clin Biochem* **33**, 343.
25. Lundquist P, Kågedal B, Nilsson L *et al.* (1995) Analysis of the cyanide metabolite 2-aminothiazoline-4-carboxylic

acid in urine by high-performance liquid chromatography. *Anal Biochem* **228**, 27.

26. Lundquist P, Rosling H, Sörbo B (1985) Determination of cyanide in whole blood, erythrocytes and plasma. *Clin Chem* **31**, 591.

27. Ministry of Health Mozambique (1984) Mantakassa: An epidemic of spastic paraparesis associated with chronic cyanide intoxication in a cassava staple area in Mozambique. 1. Epidemiology and clinical and laboratory findings in patients. *Bull WHO* **62**, 477.

28. Ministry of Health Mozambique (1984) Mantakassa: An epidemic of spastic paraparesis associated with chronic cyanide intoxication in a cassava staple area in Mozambique. 2. Nutritional factors and hydrocyanic content of cassava products. *Bull WHO* **62**, 485.

29. Mlingi N, Bainbridge ZA, Poulter NH *et al.* (1995) Critical stages in cyanogen removal during cassava processing in southern Tanzania. *Food Chem* **53**, 29.

30. Mlingi N, Kimatta S, Rosling H (1991) Konzo, a paralytic disease observed in southern Tanzania. *Trop Doct* **21**, 24.

31. Mlingi N, Poulter N, Rosling H (1992) An outbreak of acute intoxications from consumption of insufficiently processed cassava in Tanzania. *Nutr Res* **12**, 677.

32. Mlingi NV, Assey V, Swai A *et al.* (1993) Determinants of cyanide exposure from cassava in a konzo-affected population in northern Tanzania. *Int J Food Sci Nutr* **44**, 137.

33. Nambisan B (1994) Evaluation of the effect of various processing techniques on cyanogen content reduction in cassava. *Acta Hort* **375**, 193.

34. Osuntokun BO (1981) Cassava diet, chronic cyanide intoxication and neuropathy in Nigerian Africans. *World Rev Nutr Diet* **36**, 141.

35. Padmaja G (1995) Cyanide intoxication in cassava for food and feed uses. *Crit Rev Food Sci Nutr* **35**, 299.

36. Rosling H (1994) Measuring effects in humans of dietary cyanide exposure from cassava. *Acta Hort* **375**, 271.

37. Rosling H (1996) Molecular anthropology of cassava cyanogenesis. In: *The Impact of Plant Molecular Genetics.* Sobral BWS ed. Birkenhäuser, Boston, p. 315.

38. Rosling H, Gessain A, de Thé G *et al.* (1988) Tropical and epidemic spastic paraparesis are different. *Lancet* i, 1222.

39. Rosling H, Tylleskär T (1995) Konzo, an epidemic upper motoneuron disease associated to cassava and agro-ecological collapse in Africa. In: *Tropical Neurology.* Shakir RA, Newman PK, Poser CM eds. WB Saunders Co, London p. 353.

40. Shaw CM, Papayannopoulou T *et al.* (1974) Neuropathology of cyanate toxicity in rhesus monkeys. *Pharmacology* **12**, 166.

41. Spencer PS (1999) Food toxins, AMPA receptors, and motor neuron diseases. *Drug Metab Rev* **31**, 561.

42. Sundaresan S, Nambisan B, Easwari-Amna CS (1987) Bitterness in cassava in relation to cyano-glucoside content. *Indian J Agr Sci* **57**, 37.

43. Swenne I, Eriksson UJ, Christofferssin R *et al.* (1996) Cyanide detoxification in rats exposed to acetonitrile and fed a low protein diet. *Fund Appl Toxicol* **32**, 66.

44. Tor-Agbidye J, Palmer VS, Lasarev MR *et al.* (1999) Bioactivation of cyanide to cyanate in sulfur amino acid deficiency: Relevance to neurological disease in humans subsisting on cassava. *Toxicol Sci* (in press).

45. Tor-Agbidye J, Palmer VS, Spencer PS (1999) Sodium cyanate alters glutathione homeostasis in rodent brain: relationship to neurodegenerative diseases in protein-deficient malnourished populations in Africa. *Brain Res* **820**, 12.

46. Trolli G (1938) Paraplégie spastique épidémique, Konzo des indigènes du Kwango. In: *Résumé des Observations Réunies, au Kwango, au Sujet de Deux Affections d'órigine Indéterminée.* Trolli G ed. Fonds Reine Elisabeth, Brussels p. 1.

47. Tylleskär T (1994) The causation of konzo. Studies on a paralytic disease in Africa. Thesis. Uppsala University, Sweden.

48. Tylleskär T, Banea M, Bikangi N *et al.* (1995) Dietary determinants of a non-progressive spastic paraparesis (konzo): A case-referent study in a high incidence area of Zaire. *Int J Epidemiol* **24**, 949.

49. Tylleskär T, Banea M, Bikangi N *et al.* (1991) Epidemiological evidence from Zaire for a dietary aetiology of konzo, an upper motor neuron disease. *Bull WHO* **69**, 581.

50. Tylleskär T, Banea M, Bikangi N *et al.* (1992) Cassava cyanogens and konzo, an upper motoneuron disease found in Africa. *Lancet* **339**, 208.

51. Tylleskär T, Banea M, Böttiger B *et al.* (1996) Konzo, an epidemic spastic paraparesis in Africa, is not associated with antibodies to HTLV-I, HIV, or HIV *gag*-encoded proteins. *J AIDS* **12**, 317.

52. Tylleskär T, Banea M, Rosling H (1995) Konzo, an upper motoneuron disease associated to cassava and agro-ecological collapse in Africa. In: *Recent Advances in Tropical Neurology.* Clifford Rose F ed. Elsevier Science, Amsterdam p. 355.

53. Tylleskär T, Howlett W, Rwiza H (1993) Konzo: A distinct disease entity with selective upper motoneuron damage. *J Neurol Neurosurg Psychiat* **56**, 638.

54. Tylleskär T, Légué F, Peterson S *et al.* (1994) Konzo in the Central African Republic. *Neurology* **44**, 959.

55. World Health Organization (1996) Konzo—A distinct type of upper motoneuron disease. *Weekly Epidemiol Rec* **71**, 225.

Catha edulis

Matthias Riepe

CATHINONE
$C_9H_{11}NO$

Cathinone; (S)-2-Amino-1-phenyl-1-propanone

NEUROTOXICITY RATING

Clinical

A   Psychobiological reaction (euphoria, paranoia, mania)

B   Optic neuropathy

Catha edulis Forsk. (Celastraceae) is an evergreen tree that grows at high altitudes in southern Africa, Afghanistan, Yemen, and Madagascar. The fresh tender parts are used as a chew (*khat*) in East Africa, the Arab Peninsula, and elsewhere (11,12). The syndrome caused by khat consumption is similar to that induced by amphetamine (11). Toxic effects include psychotic behavior and cardiovascular dysfunction. Only fresh leaves have a stimulating effect.

The alkaloid mainly responsible for the psychostimulant effect of khat is cathinone (11). Cathinone is structurally similar to amphetamine; the only difference is substitution of a carbonyl group for the methylene group in the α-position of the amphetamine side chain (11). In addition to cathinone, khat leaves contain two further alkaloids of the phenylpropylamine type, cathine and norephedrine (11). On average, 100 g fresh khat contain 36 mg cathinone, 120 mg cathine, and 8 mg norephedrine (5). Cathinone is an intermediate in the biosynthesis of cathine; this intermediate accumulates in young but not in old leaves. Cathinone is transformed into cathine during wilting of leaves (11).

Cathinone in khat is extracted by prolonged mastication. Chewing fresh khat leaves produced peak plasma levels after about 1.5–3.5 h. Maximum levels were 41–141 ng/ml (mean, 83 ng/ml) after chewing of 60 g khat with a cathinone content of about 0.9 mg/g fresh weight leaves (8). Since cathinone is metabolized rapidly, there is probably a limit to the cathinone plasma levels that can be reached by khat chewing. Cathinone is labile because of its α-aminoketone structure and is almost completely transformed to norephedrine by stereospecific keto reduction (11).

Cathinone has a potent adrenergic effect; it increases blood pressure and has a positive chronotropic and inotropic effect in isolated guinea pig atria (7). In sum, the cardiovascular effects are those of an indirectly acting sympathomimetic (11). Cathinone was found to have analgesic properties that in part are mediated by catecholamine pathways and in part by opioid mechanisms (11). Intravenous injection induces restlessness and tremor, as would be expected from an amphetamine-like compound (11). Mice fed a diet containing 200 mg/kg khat showed a higher death rate, an increase of tumors and a variety of inflammatory conditions, and abnormal behavior (waltzing movements) (1). Drug-conditioned animals do not distinguish between cathinone and amphetamine (10). The development of tolerance to cathinone is more rapid than to amphetamine (11). Like amphetamine, cathinone increases the metabolic rate and oxygen consumption of rats (11). A teratogenic effect in rats has been described (9).

Humans consuming khat leaves experience the same objective and subjective effects as low doses of amphetamine (11,14), in particular euphoria and reduction of hunger. In a double-blind random crossover study, increased blood pressure and heart rate were noted 30 min after 0.5 mg/kg body weight cathinone; this corresponds to 100 g of khat leaves. In a test battery 30 and 90 min after administration, the euphoria effect of khat was significantly higher than with placebo (3). Khat can induce psychotic behavior (10,12,15) and dependence (4). Two kinds of psychotic reaction have been observed: a paranoid psychosis with prominent persecutory delusions associated with intense fear and anxiety, or a hypomanic illness with grandiose illusions but without auditory hallucinations (12). Numerous chronic khat chewers experience persistent hypnagogic hallucinations (6). Abstinence may be associated with withdrawal, depression, homicide, and suicide; optic neuropathy and retinopathy are described in some khat users (2,13).

In summary, khat and amphetamines elicit neurotoxic effects that are mediated by release of neurotransmitters from presynaptic storage sites.

REFERENCES

1. Al-Meshal IA, Qureshi S, Ageel AM, Tariq M (1991) The toxicity of *Catha edulis* (khat) in mice. *J Subst Abuse* **3**, 107.
2. Baird DA (1952) A case of optic neuritis in a khat addict. *East Afr Med J* **29**, 325.
3. Brenneisen R, Fisch H-U, Koelbing U *et al.* (1990) Amphetamine-like effects in humans of the khat alkaloid cathinone. *Brit J Clin Pharmacol* **30**, 825.
4. Expert Committee on Addiction-Producing Drugs, World Health Organization (1964) Khat. *WHO Tech Rep Ser* **273**, 10.

5. Geisshhsler S, Brenneisen R (1987) The content of psychoactive phenylpropyl- and phenylpentenyl-khatamines in *Catha edulis* Forsk of different origin. *J Ethnopharmacol* **19**, 269.

6. Granek M, Shalev A, Weingarten AM (1988) Khat-induced hypnagogic hallucinations. *Acta Psychiat Scand* **78**, 458.

7. Gugelmann R, von Allmen M, Brenneisen R, Porzig H (1985) Quantitative differences in the pharmacological effects of (+) and (−) cathinone. *Experientia* **41**, 1568.

8. Halket JM, Karasu Z, Murray-Lyon IM (1995) Plasma cathinone levels following chewing khat leaves (*Catha edulis* Forsk). *J Ethnopharmacol* **49**, 111.

9. Islam MW, Al-Shabanah OA, Al-Harbi MM, Al-Gharably NMA (1994) Evaluation of the teratogenic potential of khat (*Catha edulis* Forsk.) in rats. *Drug Chem Toxicol* **17**, 51.

10. Kalix P (1984) Amphetamine psychosis due to khat leaves. *Lancet* **i**, 46.

11. Kalix P (1992) Cathinone, a natural amphetamine. *Pharmacol Toxicol* **70**, 77.

12. Pantelis CC, Hindler C, Taylor J (1989) Use and abuse of khat: Distribution, pharmacology, side effects and description of psychosis attributed to khat chewing. *Psychol Med* **19**, 657.

13. Roper JP (1986) The presumed neurotoxic effects of *Catha edulis*—an exotic plant now available in the United Kingdom. *Brit J Ophthalmol* **70**, 779.

14. Widler P, Mathys K, Brenneisen R *et al.* (1994) Pharmacodynamics and pharmacokinetics of khat: A controlled study. *Clin Pharmacol Ther* **55**, 556.

15. Yousef G, Huq Z, Lambert T (1995) Khat chewing as a cause of psychosis. *Brit J Hosp Med* **54**, 322.

Cephalosporins

Lebor Velísek

Solomon L. Moshé

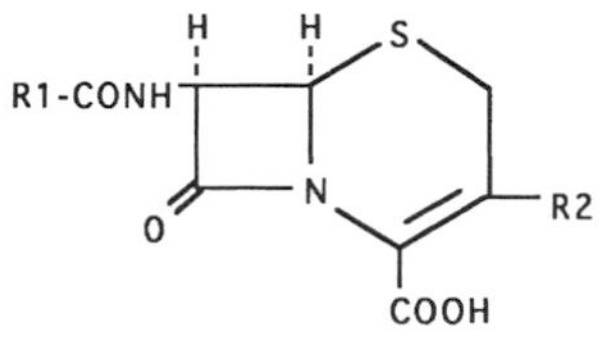

AMINOCEPHALOSPORANIC ACID
R1 = $C_5H_{10}O_5N$
R2 = $C_3H_5O_5$

7-Aminocephalosporanic acid derivatives

NEUROTOXICITY RATING

Clinical

A Seizure disorder

A Headache

B Acute encephalopathy (hallucinations, nystagmus)

Experimental

A Seizure disorder

Cephalosporins are products of the fungus *Cephalosporinum acremonium*. Nowadays, the term cephalosporins is used only for cephalosporin C and the derivatives of 7-aminocephalosporanic acid (Table 14). Cephalosporins are structurally related to penicillin and have a similar mechanism of action (*see* Penicillins, this volume); they inhibit the synthesis of the bacterial cellular wall. The spectrum of antimicrobial effects is similar to that of penicillins; however, cephalosporins impact bacteria that are penicillin resistant due to the production of penicillinase. Nevertheless, cephalosporins can be decomposed by some bacteria-produced β-lactamases. Currently, cephalosporin C serves as a significant source of 7-aminocephalosporanic acid. This acid is an essential component in the production of semisynthetic cephalosporins. Newly synthesized drugs from this group with the broadest antibacterial spectrum and with the least side effects are often referred to as third-generation cephalosporins (Table 15).

Cephalosporins differ in their stability in the acidic environment. Cefalexin, cephradine, cefaclor, and cefoxadril are well absorbed after oral administration and can be given by this route. Because cephalotin and cephapirin cause pain when given intramuscularly, they are usually administered intravenously. Most of the other agents can be given either intramuscularly or intravenously. Parenteral administration may provide sufficient therapeutic levels for up to 8 h. There are large differences among individual cephalosporins in binding with plasma albumins from ~20% (ceftazimide) to ~95% (ceftriaxone). Cephalosporins are readily distributed in all tissues except brain. However, several cephalosporins penetrate the blood-brain barrier in sufficient concentrations to be useful in the treatment of meningitis. There is almost no biotransformation of cephalosporins in the body; most of the administered drug (~90%) is excreted unchanged by the kidneys *via* glomerular filtration (9).

TABLE 14. 7-Aminocephaloranic Acid Derivatives

Drugs	R1 Position	R2 Position
Cefazolin		
Cefotiam		
Cephaloridine		
Ceftezole		
Cephapirin		$-CH_2OCOCH_3$
Cephalothin		$-CH_2OCOCH_3$
Ceftizoxime		$-H$
Cephalexin		$-CH_3$
Cephradin		$-CH_3$

Seizures are the most frequent and the most severe neurological effect that may occur as a consequence of cephalosporin therapy, especially following the administration of the first-generation cephalosporins. A pioneering study assessed in rats the epileptogenic property of ten different cephalosporins after a single intracerebroventricular administration and compared it to the epileptogenic potential of penicillin G (6). Of these cephalosporins, cefazolin had the most pronounced epileptogenic effects eliciting intense, repeated violent motor seizures and uninterrupted spike-and-wave electroencephalographic (EEG) complexes. The ED_{50} for both motor and EEG seizures was approximately 20 μg [compared to 45–90 μg (70–140 U) for penicillin G]. The epileptogenic reactions to cefotiam, ceftezole, and cephaloridine were less severe (ED_{50} for both EEG and motor seizures were 50–120 μg), compared to cefazolin and similar

TABLE 15. Cephalosporins

First Generation	Second Generation	Third Generation
Cefazolin	Cefamandole	Cefotaxime
Cephalotin	Cefuroxime	Ceftizoxime
Cephapirin	Ceforanid	Cefoperazone
Cephradine	Cefonicid	Ceftriaxone
Cephalexin	Cefoxitin	Ceftazidime
Cefadroxil	Cefmetazole	Moxalactam
	Cefotetan	Cefixime
	Cefaclor	
	Cefuroxime axetil	

[Adapted from Molavi (9)]

to those induced by penicillin. After the administration of cephapirin and cefmetazole (ED_{50} 200–1000 μg), there were only moderate epileptogenic phenomena consisting of clonic seizures of forelimbs. In contrast, intracerebroventricular cephalotin, ceftizoxime, cephalexin, and cephradine in doses up to 1000 μg did not produce any epileptic EEG changes or motor seizures (6). Not only intracerebroventricular administration but also a single systemic injection of cephalosporins may elicit seizures. Thus, after intravenous administration, ceftezol, cefotiam, and cefazolin (dosage <200 mg/kg) elicited epileptiform EEG as well as motor seizures in rats. After cephacetril and cephaloridine (dosage 200–1000 mg/kg), there was only EEG spiking in the frontal cortex without any behavioral seizures (14). Seizures also occurred after intravenous administration of cefazolin in rats (10) and cefotaxime in mice (2). The epileptogenic serum levels of cefotaxime in mice were 3.4 mmol/ml, which is rather low compared to that of penicillin (5.8 mmol/ml) (2). There are no chronic experiments to demonstrate possible long-term (kindling-like or potentiated) epileptiform effects of repeated administration of cephalosporins. There is probably a fair correlation between epileptogenic potential and the size of the substituent at position 7 (R1) and position 3 (R2) of 7-aminocephalosporanic acid (Table 14). The larger the substituent the more serious is the epileptogenic profile of the drug; cefazolin, with large substituents on both positions, has the most serious epileptogenic effects (6).

The *in vitro* brain-slice technique is a convenient system in which to demonstrate the epileptogenic effects of antibiotics. These employ hippocampal tissue, which has a low threshold for the development of epileptiform activity. There is no brain-blood barrier to prevent entry of the drug, and a specific drug concentration is easily maintained. Results obtained from these types of *in vitro* studies support *in vivo* experimental data. Cephalotin, at a concentration of 1 g/l, had significant epileptiform effects; it increased the number and amplitude of evoked population spikes in hippocampal area CA1. Cefuroxime and cefotaxime had no such epileptogenic effects (5).

Seizures are also known to be a complication of cephalosporin therapy in humans. This side effect may often occur after intracerebroventricular or intrathecal administration of the drug and especially of first- or second-generation compounds (8). The high risk of seizures makes cephalosporins less suited for intracerebroventricular therapy, although newly developed cephalosporins with reduced epileptogenic potential may be promising agents for local intracranial therapy (12). However, because cephalosporins penetrate the blood-brain barrier, seizures may also appear after systemic administration, especially if the drugs are used in patients with renal failure (1,13). This rare complication occurs mostly after the use of first- and second-generation cephalosporins with dosages exceeding 25 g/day and serum levels over 250 μmol/ml (4), although seizures were also reported after the administration of the third-generation ceftazidime (3). A large study on the effects of ampicillin in combination with a third-generation cephalosporin in the treatment of bacterial meningitis in children reported seizures as the most frequent short-term side effect (64.7% of 41 cases) (7). However, due to additional proconvulsant factors in this study (*i.e.*, median age 7 months, which represents a postnatal period with a high risk for seizures, add-on ampicillin, which may have proconvulsant effects similar to penicillin; and meningitis, which may induce seizures *per se*), cephalosporin therapy probably had only a small proconvulsant contribution. Rare side effects of cephalosporin therapy include headache, nystagmus, hallucinations, and paresthesias (3).

Cephalosporins appear to induce convulsions through the inhibiton of γ-aminobutyric acid (GABA) receptor binding (11). This mechanism is similar to penicillin, which is believed to inhibit the Cl^- conductance associated with the $GABA_A$ receptor.

REFERENCES

1. Craig WA, Welling PG, Jackson TC, Kunin CM (1967) Pharmacology of cefazolin and other cephalosporins in patients with renal insufficiency. *J Infect Dis* **128**, S347.

2. Eng RHK, Munsif AN, Yangco BG et al. (1989) Seizure propensity with imipenem. *Arch Intern Med* **149**, 1881.

3. Fekety FR (1990) Safety of parenteral third generation cephalosporins. *Amer J Med* **88**, 38.

4. Fishman RA (1966) Blood-brain and CSF barriers to penicillin and related organic acids. *Arch Neurol* **15**, 113.

5. Grøndahl TØ, Langmøen IA (1993) Epileptogenic effect of antibiotic drugs. *J Neurosurg* **78**, 938.

6. Kamei C, Sunami A, Tasaka K (1983) Epileptogenic activity of cephalosporins in rats and their structure activity relationship. *Epilepsia* **24**, 431.

7. Liu CC, Chen JS, Lin CH et al. (1993) Bacterial meningitis in infants and children in southern Taiwan: Emphasis on *Haemophilus influenzae* type B infection. *J Formosa Med Assoc* **92**, 884.

8. Manzella JP, Paul RL, Butler IL (1988) CNS toxicity associated with intraventricular injection of cefazolin. Report of three cases. *J Neurosurg* **68**, 970.

9. Molavi A (1991) Cephalosporins: Rationale for clinical use. *Amer Fam Physician* **43**, 937.

10. Nistico G, Musolino R, Naccari F, Di Perri R (1978) Experimental epilepsy in chicks and rats after intravenous benzylpenicillin and cefazolin. *Boll Soc Ital Biol Sper* **54**, 600.

11. Shimada J, Hori S, Kanemitsu K et al. (1992) A comparative study on the convulsant activity of carbapenems and beta-lactams. *Drug Exp Clin Res* **18**, 377.

12. Wen DY, Bottini AG, Hall WA, Haines SJ (1992) Infections in neurologic surgery. The intraventricular use of antibiotics. *Neurosurg Clin N Amer* **3**, 343.

13. Yost RL, Lee JD, O'Leary JP (1977) Convulsions associated with sodium cefazolin: A case report. *Amer Surg* **43**, 417.

14. Yu QH, Kitazumi K, Kamei C, Tasaka K (1984) Epileptogenic activity induced by intravenous injection of certain cephalalosporins in rats. *J Pharmacobio-Dynamics* **7**, 586.

CASE REPORT

A 63-year-old woman with no antecedent seizure history was severely injured in a car accident. The injuries consisted of a fractured pelvis, retroperitoneal pelvic hematoma, laceration of urinary bladder, fracture of the left humerus, and multiple fractures of the ribs; there was no obvious head injury. After surgery, she received morphine sulfate 3 mg every 4 h, 1 g of intravenous sodium cefazolin each 6 h (4 g/day), positive-pressure ventilation, and fluid replacement. Her renal function deteriorated progressively (fifth postoperative day: serum creatinine 8.5 mg/dl; blood urea nitrogen 118 mg/dl, total urine volume 377 ml). She was also hypoalbuminemic. On the fifth postoperative day, 3 h after the last cefazolin administration, she experienced two tonic-clonic seizures within a 2-h period. During the next 40 h, she experienced seven additional seizures. Cefazolin serum levels were determined following the second seizure. The level was 455 mg/ml. (In normal volunteer studies, the serum levels after 1 g of intravenous cefazolin do not exceed a peak of 190 mg/ml and decline to 40 mg/ml within 3 h.) The high serum level was probably due to the renal failure. The hypoalbuminemia further complicated the situation allowing for higher levels of unbound (free) cefazolin leading to the emergence of seizures.

[Modified from Yost et al. (13).]

Ceruleotoxin

Albert C. Ludolph

NEUROTOXICITY RATING

Clinical

A   Neuromuscular transmission syndrome

A   Myopathy (rhabdomyolysis)

Experimental

A   Neuromuscular transmission (presynaptic blockade of acetylcholine release)

Ceruleotoxin is a potent neurotoxin isolated from the venom of *Bungarus fasciatus*, a poisonous snake (krait) from central and southeast Asia (1). The slightly basic protein is composed of two identical polypeptides (MW, 13,000 each) that show amino acid sequence homology to toxic and nontoxic phospholipases; it possesses significant phospholipase A activity (1). The LD_{50} for mice is 0.03–0.07 mg/kg. Ceruleotoxin belongs to the group of β-bungarotoxins; at low concentrations (10^{-6} g/ml), it blocks neuromuscular transmission by inhibition of transmitter release in the chick biventer cervicis muscle preparation (3). The typical triphasic effect begins with a depression, is followed by an augmentation of transmitter release, and finally results in long-lasting inhibition (2,3). At higher concentrations (10^{-5} g/ml), ceruleotoxin also has a myotoxic effect but does not significantly interfere with peripheral nerve function (3). The effect of this toxin on vertebrate neuromuscular transmission is similar to the effects of notoxin (from *Notechis scutatus scutatus*) and a basic phospholipase A_2 trimucrotoxin isolated from the Formosan habu (*Trimeresurus mucrosquamatus*) venom (4,6).

Local pain is often minor. Life-threatening systemic symptoms of diffuse neuromuscular dysfunction usually appear after 1–12 h and may last up to 12 days (5). Initial manifestations of intoxication consist of paresthesias, abdominal pain, and fasciculations. In most patients, the edrophonium (Tensilon) test is negative, but reportedly may be variable in some cases. Rhabdomyolysis and myoglobinuria are infrequent complications of krait bites.

REFERENCES

1. Bon C, Saliou B (1983) Ceruleotoxin: Identification in the venom of *Bungarus fasciatus*, molecular properties and importance of phospholipase A2 activity for neurotoxicity. *Toxicon* 21, 681.
2. Harris JB (1985) Phospholipases in snake venoms and their effects on nerve and muscle. *Pharmacol Ther* 31, 33.
3. Ho CL, Lee CY (1983) Mode of neuromuscular blocking action of ceruleotoxin. *Toxicon* 21, 301.
4. Ho CL, Tang CM, Lee CY (1984) Presynaptic and musculotropic effects of a basic phospholipase A from the Formosan habu (*Trimeresurus mucrosquamatus*) venom. *Toxicon* 22, 813.
5. Sanmuganathan PS, Senanayake N (1991) Myasthenic syndrome of snake envenoming: A clinical and neurophysiological study. *Neurology* 41, 142.
6. Tsai IH, Wang YM (1998) Effect of site directed mutagenesis on the activity of recombinant trimucrotoxin, a neurotoxic phospholipase from *Trimeresurus mucrosquamatus* venom. *Toxicon* 36, 1591.

CGS 21595

Georg J. Krinke

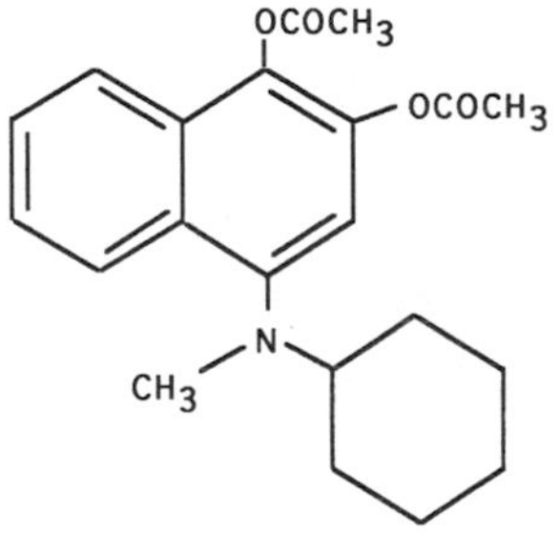

CGS 21595
$C_{21}H_{25}NO_4$

4-(Cyclohexylmethylamino)-1,2-naphthalenediol diacetate

NEUROTOXICITY RATING

Experimental

A   Peripheral neuropathy (segmental demyelination)

CGS 21595, a 5-lipoxygenase inhibitor, is an experimental anti-inflammatory agent that suppresses leukotriene formation from arachidonic acid. The 5-lipoxygenase inhibitors may be beneficial in conditions such as asthma, rheumatoid arthritis, and psoriasis. CGS 21595 is not used clinically because serious neurotoxicity emerged in experimental animal studies.

In vitro, CGS 21595 inhibits the formation of *S*-hydroxyeicosatetraenoic acid and leukotriene B_4 (LTB_4). When orally administered to dogs at 100 mg/kg, CGS 21595 caused a 32% inhibition of *ex vivo* LTB_4 formation. This inhibition persisted for up to 3 h, with significant inhibition still apparent at 6 h. CGS 21595 inhibited edema formation and the influx of mononuclear cells and polymorphonuclear leukocytes 48 h after administration (2). Autoradiographs using ^{14}C-labeled CGS 19213, the naphthoquinone metabolite of CGS 21595, showed that it was rapidly distributed to the liver, lung, brain, spinal cord, and myocardium.

Administration of CGS 21595 to rats produced demyelinating lesions in spinal nerve roots and sciatic nerves, and a reversible formation of cytoplasmic hyaline droplets in proximal renal tubules. No such lesions were observed in treated dogs (2).

Rats of either sex were given CGS 21595 at daily doses of 50, 150, 500, or 1000 mg/kg orally for 13 weeks. Animals in the higher dose groups had a reduced weight gain, but significant neurological signs were not routinely observed. A peripheral neuropathy consisting of myelin destruction in the spinal nerve roots and sciatic nerves was seen in male rats treated with 150 mg/kg or more and in females at all dose levels (2). Rats treated with 1000 mg/kg, 5 days a week, were examined at 2-week intervals until termination at 10 weeks. Neurotoxicity was first detected following 4 weeks of treatment. Functional examination showed a reduction of grip strength, reduced motor activity, and increased landing foot splay. Neuropathological examination revealed peripheral segmental demyelination predominantly affecting ventral spinal nerve roots. In a subsequent study, the dose–effect relationship was examined in rats treated with 50, 200, or 1000 mg/kg/day, 5 days a week. Neurotoxicity occurred only in animals treated with 1000 mg/kg. Presumably because the treatment schedule included two "drug holidays" per week, the no-effect level was much higher than in the previous study using continuous administration for 7 days a week (1,2).

CGS 21595 is a prodrug that is metabolized to the active form, CGS 19213, a naphthoquinone that is more soluble in lipid than water, and likely to enter myelin of Schwann cells. It may interact with Schwann cell membrane components in peripheral myelin and produce demyelination. Another naphthoquinone and potent 5-lipoxygenase inhibitor, CGS 8515, inhibits several nerve growth factor–mediated responses *in vitro* (4). By that means, some lipoxygenase inhibitors might disrupt myelination of axons affected by suppression of nerve growth factor effects. The demyelinating effect of CGS 21595, however, appears unrelated to the pharmacological suppression of leukotriene formation *via* 5-lipoxygenase inhibition, since no similar effects have been reported with other 5-lipoxygenase inhibitors (1,2). The microscopic features of segmental demyelination induced with CGS 21595 resemble the spontaneous radiculopathy seen in aged rats (3). The lesion induced by CGS 21595 showed a distinct perivascular location, suggesting that the demyelinating agent is blood borne (1).

REFERENCES
1. Classen W, Gunson DE, Iverson WO et al. (1994) Functional and morphological characterization of neuropathy induced with 5-lipoxygenase inhibitor CGS 21595. *Exp Toxicol Pathol* **46**, 119.
2. Gunson DE, Sahota PS, Iverson WO et al. (1992) Toxic peripheral neuropathy with demyelination in Sprague-Dawley rats given CGS 21595—a 5-lipoxygenase inhibitor. *Vet Pathol* **29**, 145.
3. Krinke GJ (1988) Spontaneous radiculopathy, aged rats. In: *Nervous System, Monographs on Pathology of Laboratory Animals.* Jones TC, Mohr U, Hunt RD eds. Springer Verlag, Berlin p. 203.
4. Steel DJ, Wasley JWF, Greene LA (1989) Suppression of NGF actions by the 5-lipoxygenase inhibitor CGS 8515. *Soc Neurosci Abst* **15**, 869.

Charatoxin

Albert C. Ludolph

CHARATOXIN
C₄H₈S₃

4-Methylthio-1,2-dithiolane

NEUROTOXICITY RATING

Experimental

A   Neuromuscular transmission dysfunction (postsynaptic blockade of acetylcholine receptor)

Charatoxin is an insecticidal product of the alga *Chara globularis* Thuillier (1). The compound resembles nereistoxin (2); a methionyl group (−S−CH₃) replaces the dimethyl group of nereistoxin. Charatoxin is less potent than nereistoxin. In high concentrations, it is a competitive antagonist at the nicotinic acetylcholine receptor of the frog sartorius muscle (4,5); in lower concentrations it potentiates acetylcholine binding (4). Charatoxin activity is similar to that of nereistoxin (3).

REFERENCES
1. Anthoni U, Christopherson C, Madsen JO et al. (1980) Biologically active sulfur compounds from the green alga, *Chara globularis. Phytochemistry* **19**, 1228.
2. Anthoni U, Christopherson C, Jacobsen N, Svendsen A (1982) Synthesis of 4-methylthio-1,2-dithiolane and 5-methylthio-1,2,3-trithiolane. Two naturally occurring bioactive compounds. *Tetrahedron* **38**, 2425.
3. Jacobsen N, Pedersen LE (1983) Synthesis and insecticidal properties of derivatives of propane-1,3-dithiol (analog of the insecticidal derivatives of dithiolane and trithiolane from the alga *Chara globularis* Thuillier). *Pestic Sci* **14**, 90.
4. Nielsen LE, Pedersen LE (1984) The effect of charatoxin, 4-methylthio-1,2-dithiolane, on the frog sartorius neuromuscular junction. *Experientia* **40**, 186.
5. Sherby SM, Eldefrawi AT, David JA et al. (1986) Interactions of charatoxins and nereistoxin with the nicotinic acetylcholine receptors of insect CNS and *Torpedo* electric organ. *Arch Insect Biochem Physiol* **3**, 431.

Charybdotoxin

Albert C. Ludolph

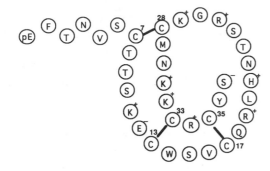

CHARYBDOTOXIN
$C_{176}H_{277}N_{57}O_{55}S_7$

NEUROTOXICITY RATING

Experimental

A   Ion channel dysfunction (certain potassium channels)

Charybdotoxin (ChTX) is a minor component of the venom of the scorpion *Leiurus quinquestriatus hebreus* (3). Venoms of the scorpions *Buthus occitanus, martensi* and *arenicola*, and *Centruroides sculpturatus* have similar activity (6,9). ChTX is a 37-amino-acid, highly basic peptide with six cysteine residues and a molecular weight of 4.3 kDa; it has been synthesized (10). ChTX is a reversible blocker of high- and lower-conductance Ca^{2+}–activated K^+ channels in mammalian skeletal muscle (2,5) and rat brain (2,8); it binds through an electrostatic mechanism to the outer face of the open or closed channel (2). Blockade is achieved by an interaction between positive charges on the ChTX molecule and negative charges within the external mouth of the channel. ChTX does not interact with Na^+ or Ca^{2+} channels. However, since ChTX also potently blocks slowly inactivating, voltage-gated Ca^{2+}–insensitive K^+ channels in rat brain and human T lymphocytes (2), the compound is nonselective. There is biochemical evidence that the C-terminal domain of ChTX is of major importance for its differential action on both channel types (4). The three-dimensional structure of the protein has been analyzed (1). Reliable information on human neurotoxicity is unavailable. Deaths in children who have been stung by *L. quinquestriatus* (7) cannot be ascribed to effects of this experimental neurotoxin, especially since clinical manifestations did not suggest neurotoxicity.

REFERENCES

1. Bontems F, Roumestand C, Gilquin B *et al.* (1991) Refined structure of charybdotoxin: Common motifs in scorpion toxins and insect defensins. *Science* **254**, 1521.
2. Garcia ML, Galvez A, Garcia-Calvo M *et al.* (1991) Use of toxins to study potassium channels. *J Bioenerg Biomembrane* **23**, 615.
3. Gimenez-Gallego G, Navia MA, Reuben JP *et al.* (1988) Purification, sequence, and model structure of charybdotoxin, a potent selective inhibitor of calcium-activated potassium channels. *Proc Nat Acad Sci USA* **85**, 3329.
4. Giangiacomo KM, Sugg EE, Garcia-Calvo *et al.* (1993) Synthetic charybdotoxin-iberiotoxin chimeric peptides define toxin binding sites on calcium-activated and voltage-dependent potassium channels. *Biochemistry* **32**, 2363.
5. Miller C, Moczydlowski E, Latorre R, Philips M (1985) Charybdotoxin, a protein inhibitor of single Ca^{2+}-activated K^+-channels from mammalian skeletal muscle. *Nature* **313**, 316.
6. Moczydlowski E, Lucchesi K, Ravindran A (1988) An emerging pharmacology of peptide toxins targeted against potassium channels. *J Membrane Biol* **105**, 95.
7. Osman El, Amin E (1992) Issues in management of scorpion sting in children. *Toxicon* **30**, 111.
8. Reinhart PH, Chung S, Levitan SB (1989) A family of calcium-dependent potassium channels from rat brain. *Neuron* **2**, 1031.
9. Romi-Lebrun R, Lebrun B, Martin-Eauclaire MF *et al.* (1997) Purification, characterization, and synthesis of three novel toxins from Chinese scorpion *Buthus martensi*, which act on K^+ channels. *Biochemistry* **36**, 13473.
10. Sugg EE, Garcia ML, Reuben JP *et al.* (1990) Synthesis and structural characterization of charybdotoxin, a potent peptidyl inhibitor of the high-conductance Ca^{2+}-activated K^+ channel. *J Biol Chem* **265**, 18745.

Cheilanthes sieberi

Albert C. Ludolph

NEUROTOXICITY RATING

Clinical

A   Chronic encephalopathy
    (polioencephalomalacia in sheep)

Experimental

A   Thiaminase toxicity

Cheilanthes sieberi (rock fern) is neurotoxic to grazing animals because it contains the enzyme thiaminase I (2). This enzyme destroys thiamine (vitamin B_1) by degradation; thus, consumption of rock fern, similar to the ingestion of bracken fern (*Pteridium aquilinum*), horse tail (*Equisetum arvense* and *palustre*), or nardoo (*Marsilea drummondii*), causes neurological symptoms in animals. Phosphorylated thiamine (vitamin B_1) is an important coenzyme for several metabolic steps in carbohydrate metabolism; in particular, the mitochondrial enzymes pyruvate and α-ketoglutarate dehydrogenase, and the branched-chain dehydrogenase complex. Transketolase, the cytoplasmic enzyme that rearranges sugars in the pentose phosphate pathway, is also thiamine-dependent. Therefore, insufficient intake or breakdown of this essential nutrient leads to severe neurological deficits, exemplified by the Wernicke-Korsakoff syndrome or by polyneuropathy (central-peripheral distal axonopathy) in humans. Thiaminases are found in several plants, and reportedly are produced by fish, shellfish, and bacteria (2).

Only monogastric animals and young ruminants are susceptible to the neurotoxic effects of dietary thiamine deficiency, since adult ruminants are able to synthesize vitamin B_1 by microbiota (2). Oral intake of significant amounts of *C. sieberi* leads to the syndrome of "staggers" in sheep. The disease, described in Australia (1,3), is characterized predominantly by hindlimb paresis that leads to a staggering gait. Diarrhea, increased respiratory rate, and depression also occur (1,3). Evidence for the causal role of plant intake are the presence of rock fern during disease outbreak, significant amounts of enzyme levels in the rumen of the animals, a latency to disease onset consistent with feeding trials, increased blood lactate and pyruvate, significantly decreased transketolase activity, and a therapeutic response to thiamine hydrochloride (1). Autopsies in 41 animals (out of 480) demonstrated the presence of a polioencephalomalacia (cerebrocortical necrosis), which is considered to be typical of thiaminase poisoning in animals (5). The results of feeding trials, however, were equivocal (3), and it is uncertain whether compounds other than thiaminase in *C. sieberi* contribute to the clinical picture. For treatment of thiaminase intoxication, intravenous or subcutaneous application of 100–200 mg thiamine hydrochloride to sheep and 1–2 g thiamine hydrochloride to cattle is recommended (1,2).

There are no convincing, well-documented examples of human poisoning with *Cheilanthes* spp. A possible exception is the tragic outcome of the Burke and Wills expedition through the interior of Australia in 1860–1861 (4). On their return journey, the explorers reportedly had to rely on staple foods such as the freshwater mussel *Velesunio ambiguus* and a flour prepared from *M. drummondii* (4). They developed symptoms consistent with beriberi (4). Three of the four men died, and the fourth reportedly developed a poorly reversible paresis of the legs, which was retrospectively ascribed to a polyneuropathic syndrome (4).

REFERENCES

1. Chick BF, Carroll SN, Kennedy SN, McCleary BV (1981) Some biochemical features of an outbreak of polioencephalomalacia in sheep. *Aust Vet J* 57, 251.
2. Chick BF, McCleary BV, Beckett RJ (1989) Thiaminases. In: *Toxicants of Plant Origin*. Cheeke PR ed. CRC Press, Boca Raton, Florida p. 73.
3. Clark IA, Dimmock CR (1971) The toxicity of *Cheilanthes sieberi* to sheep and cattle. *Aust Vet J* 47, 149.
4. Earl JW, McCleary BV (1994) Mystery of the poisoned expedition. *Nature* 368, 683.
5. Edwin EE, Lewis G, Allcroft R (1968) Cerebrocortical necrosis: A hypothesis for the role of thiaminases in its pathogenesis. *Vet Rec* 83, 176.

Chelidonium majus

Albert C. Ludolph

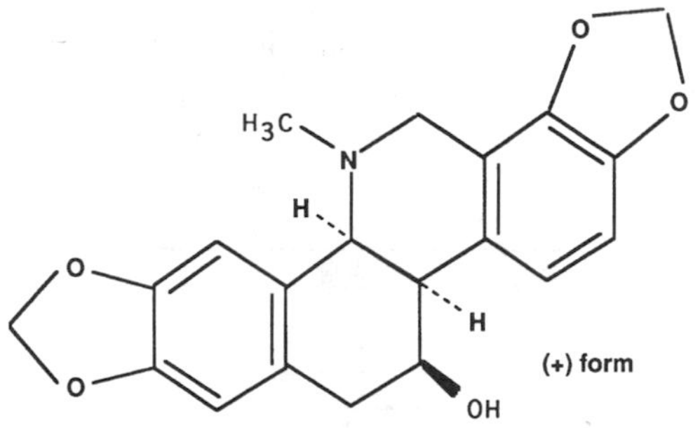

CHELIDONINE
$C_{20}H_{19}NO_5$

(+) form

Chelidonine; Stylophorin; (+)-Form: [5bR-(5bα,6β,12bα)]-
5b,6,7,12b,13,14-hexahydro-13-
methyl[1,3]benzodioxolo[5,6-c]-1,3-dioxolo[4,5-i]-
phenanthridin-6-ol

NEUROTOXICITY RATING

Experimental

A   Acute encephalopathy (sedation)

The plant *Chelidonium majus* (greater celandine) has been traditionally used in European folk medicine, in particular as a spasmolytic (2,3). Young blind swallows were reported to have been cured by the milk-like sap of the plant (3). Interest in this folk medicine continued through the Middle Ages; the plant was used during epidemics of plague and was considered a cure for warts. Human neurotoxicity is controversial and based on a single questionable case (2). However, *C. majus* contains several alkaloids (including chelidonine, chelerythine, and bereberine), one of which (sanguinarin) is used experimentally for the induction of glaucoma. Oral intake of the plant reportedly induces some sedation in experimental animals. Observations in horses and cattle showed that systemic toxicity developed after intake of 500 g of *C. majus*; neurotoxicity was not shown (1).

REFERENCES

1. Bentz H (1969) *Nutztiervergiftungen, Erkennung und Verhütung*. Gustav Fischer Verlag, Jena.
2. Frohne D, Pfänder HJ (1987) Giftpflanzen. In: *Handbuch für Apotheker, Ärzte, Toxikologen und Biologen*. Wissenschaftliche Verlagsgesellschaft mbH, Stuttgart.
3. Hahn G (1981) *Chelidonium majus*—eine alte Arzneipflanze. *Acta Med Emp* 6, 427.

Chloral Hydrate

Herbert H. Schaumburg

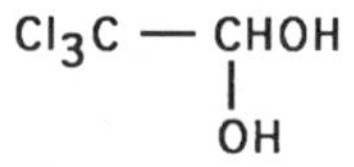

$$Cl_3C - CHOH$$
$$|$$
$$OH$$

CHLORAL HYDRATE
$C_2H_3Cl_3O_2$

2,2,2-Trichloro-1,1-ethanediol

NEUROTOXICITY RATING

Clinical

A   Acute encephalopathy (sedation, coma)
A   Physical dependence and withdrawal
C   Optic atrophy

Choral hydrate (CH), once widely used as a hypnotic, has been largely replaced by benzodiazepines. Orally administered CH is rapidly adsorbed and metabolized to trichloroethanol, which is responsible for most of its pharmacological and toxicological effects (1).

There is considerable variation in individual response to CH; an oral dose of 10 g is usually needed to produce acute intoxication in an adult, but death has occurred after administration of as little as 4 g. Initial acute toxic effects are nausea and vomiting, soon followed by stupor and signs of brainstem dysfunction that may include pupillary constriction. Aberrant eye movements and perturbed vision of unknown origin are common in the early stages (1). Acute intoxication closely resembles barbiturate overdose, and death is from respiratory depression.

Chronic abuse of CH, a persistent problem in India, is associated with hepatic dysfunction, proteinuria and emaciation. Hepatic dysfunction, in time, may produce even higher circulating levels of trichloroethanol because of impaired detoxification. Withdrawal from chronic high-level consumption has been accompanied by seizures and death. Anecdotal reports (pre-1930 literature) of transient and persistent visual impairment accompanying chronic consumption of CH are difficult to evaluate. There are no reports since 1931 (2).

REFERENCES
1. Adams WL (1940) The toxicity of chloral hydrate. *J Pharmacol Exp Ther* **69**, 273.
2. Grant WM, Shuman JS (1993) *Toxicology of the Eye. 4th Ed*. Charles C Thomas, Springfield, Illinois p. 349.

Chloramphenicol

Herbert H. Schaumburg

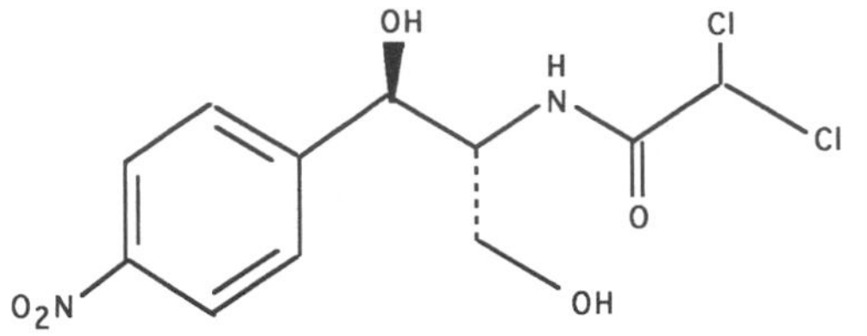

CHLORAMPHENICOL
$C_{11}H_{12}Cl_2N_2O_5$

[R-(R*,R*)]-2,2-Dichloro-N-[2-hydoxy-1-(hydoxymethyl)-2-(4-nitrophenyl)ethyl]acetamide

NEUROTOXICITY RATING

Clinical

A   Optic neuropathy

A   Peripheral neuropathy

B   Acute encephalopathy (delerium)

Chloramphenicol is a nitrobenzene antibiotic especially useful in treatment of salmonella infections, *Haemophilus influenzae* meningitis, amebiasis, and rickettsial diseases. The drug is now rarely used in North America because of the unpredictable appearance of severe blood dyscrasias (especially aplastic anemia) at customary doses. Therapy with this agent is currently restricted to circumstances where there is no effective alternate (8).

Chloramphenicol inhibits the synthesis of proteins of the inner mitochondrial membrane probably by inhibiting ribosomal peptidyltransferase. Both the toxicity and antibacterial effects of the drug are considered to be related to inhibition of protein synthesis. The inhibition is so predictable that it has been widely used as a tool in neuroscience (5).

Chloramphenicol is readily absorbed from the gastrointestinal tract; peak plasma concentrations appear in 2 h. It is widely distributed, readily enters the CNS, and may accumulate in the brain. The major route of excretion is hepatic conjugation to the glucuronide, which is then secreted into the urine.

There are no experimental animal studies that replicate the neurotoxic effects of chloramphenicol in humans. Humans experience optic neuropathy or peripheral neuropathy generally following prolonged high-level treatment (2–4,7,8). The mean duration of therapy is 229 days (range, 10–1513 days) and the mean dose is 225 g (range, 10–1600 g). Most instances of neurotoxicity have been children with cystic fibrosis receiving prolonged antibiotic treatment for pulmonary infections. Optic neuropathy is more common and usually is the sole manifestation of chloramphenicol neurotoxicity; peripheral neuropathy has appeared in about 10% of individuals who developed visual dysfunction.

Optic neuropathy is usually heralded by mild orbital pain; blurred vision follows with obvious visual compromise within a few days. The optic discs are usually hyperemic, visual acuity is diminished, and central or paracentral scotomata are demonstrable in all cases. Postmortem examination of eyes from five individuals disclosed severe loss of ganglion cells and axonal degeneration within the nerve fiber layer of the retina (1). The histopathological study did not indicate the primary site of the lesion. Most patients have commenced recovery within a week of drug withdrawal and most regained normal vision.

Chloramphenicol neuropathy commences as symmetrical mild foot numbness soon followed by calf pain. Burning sensations in the feet appear if the drug is not promptly stopped. The upper limbs are usually spared. Objective signs are few—diminished pain and touch sensation and loss of patellar and Achilles reflexes. Recovery begins within 2 weeks and is usually complete within 6 months, even in severe instances. Treatment with high doses of B vitamins is advocated, but the rationale and efficacy are questionable.

The mechanism of chloramphenicol neurotoxicity is unclear. Because there has been a large number of patients who received prolonged therapy without problems, host susceptibility factors may predispose to illness in some. It is suggested that color vision or visual acuity be carefully monitored during prolonged drug administration.

An acute toxic delirium has occasionally accompanied prolonged chloramphenicol treatment (6); this condition has promptly resolved following drug withdrawal. Most instances have occurred in patients under treatment for typhoid or pneumonia, or in hepatic-compromised patients with metastatic neoplasms; its pathophysiology is unclear.

REFERENCES

1. Cogan DG, Truman JT, Smith TR (1973) Optic neuropathy, chloramphenicol, and infantile genetic agranulocytosis. *Invest Ophthalmol* 12, 534.
2. Godel F, Nemet P, Lazar M (1980) Chloramphenicol optic neuropathy. *Arch Ophthalmol* 98, 1417.
3. Hill CFL, Armstrong JV, McDonald CK, Allott EN (1950) Treatment of typhoid fever with chloramphenicol. *Lancet* 259, 802.
4. Joy RJT, Scalettar R, Sodee DB (1960) Optic and peripheral neuritis. *J Amer Med Assn* 173, 1731.
5. Kang H, Schuman EM (1996) A requirement for local protein synthesis in neurotrophin-induced hippocampal synaptic plasticity. *Science* 273, 1402.
6. Levine PH, Regelson W, Holland JF (1970) Chloramphenicol-associated encephalopathy. *Clin Pharmacol Ther* 11, 194.
7. Ramilo O, Kinane BT, McCracken GH (1988) Chloramphenicol neurotoxicity. *Pediat Inf Dis J* 7, 358.
8. Snavely SR, Hodges GR (1984) The neurotoxicity of antibacterial agents. *Ann Intern Med* 101, 92.

Chlordecone

John R. Taylor
John B. Selhorst
Vincent P. Calabrese
Martha Neff-Smith

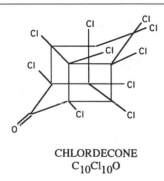

CHLORDECONE
$C_{10}Cl_{10}O$

1,1a,3,3a,4,5,5,5a,5b,6-Decachloro-octahydro-1,3,4-metheno-2*H*-cyclobuta[*cd*]pentalen-2-one

NEUROTOXICITY RATING

Clinical

A Cerebellar syndrome (tremor)

A Opsoclonus

B Benign intracranial hypertension

B Chronic encephalopathy (cognitive dysfunction)

Experimental

A Ataxia, tremor

Chlordecone was developed by the Allied Chemical Corporation (ACC) and registered as a pesticide in 1955. It is a chlorinated hydrocarbon insecticide that is among the general group of insecticides spawned by chlorophenothane (DDT). (*See also* Chlorinated Cyclodienes, this volume)

Chlordecone was manufactured by ACC until 1973 when production of the chemical was turned over to Life Science Products Company (LSPC) of Hopewell, Virginia, USA. From March 1974 through July 1975, LSPC was the only manufacturer of chlordecone in the world. Production achieved an annual rate of 400,000 kg. LSPC supplied 90% pure, powdered chlordecone to a chemical concern in West Germany, where it was utilized to make another pesticide known as Kelevan. This latter pesticide was exported to banana-producing areas of Central and South America for use against the banana borer weevil. Small amounts of chlordecone were retained in the United States to formulate poison traps for ants and roaches. During the production period, chlordecone was not registered with the U.S. Environmental Protection Agency (EPA) as a pesticide because it was considered a chemical product under shipment to another manufacturer. In July 1975, production of chlordecone was halted at LSPC by the Virginia State Health Department (VSHD) (8). A Hopewell internist, concerned about the illness manifest in one of his patients, had submitted serum containing a high concentration of chlordecone to the U.S. Centers for Disease Control in Atlanta, Georgia, and a nearby neurologist suspected widespread, industrial chlordecone intoxication because a confused and markedly tremulous patient told of a similar affliction in fellow workers. Both had duly informed the VSHD. Gross overexposure of the pesticide was found about the plant site and among symptomatic employees. Subsequent investigation by VSHD revealed chlordecone contamination of the local environment through the air and more extensively in the waterways draining the refuse from LSPC. Fish and shellfish were discovered to contain variable quantities of chlordecone (33). As a consequence, taking marine life from the James River was stopped by the Governor of Virginia on December 18, 1975 (39). In 1980, the sport-fishing ban was lifted, followed by lifting of most of the restrictions on commercial fishing. In 1988, all restrictions expired and there remains only a consumption advisory (62).

Chlordecone (Kepone) is a chlorinated polycyclic ketone with an empirical formula of $C_{10}C1_{10}O$ (MW, 491) (51). It has a rigid caged structure and is closely related to Mirex ($C_{10}C_{10}$) (47). It also has many structural similarities to the cyclodienes such as chlordane, aldrin, and dieldrin, but is quite different from other halogenated pesticides such as 1,1'-(2,2,2-trichloroethylidene)bis[4-chlorobenzene] (DDT).

Chlordecone is an odorless white to tan powder. It readily forms a hydrate resulting in a gem-diol (dialcohol). It is nonvolatile, sublimes, and decomposes at 350°C. Its water solubility is only 4 g/l at 100°C, but is soluble in acid or alkali solutions because of its hydration. It is soluble in organic solvents, but it is relatively less soluble in nonpolar solvents such as n-hexane and benzene than in oxygenated solvents such as acetone, diethylether, and the lower aliphatic alcohols. The molecule is not affected by acids or bases. Because of this relative increase in water solubility and a decrease in nonpolar solvent solubility, distribution in the body is somewhat different from that seen with the less polar organic pesticides.

The chlorides on the molecule are relatively unreactive; they cannot undergo elimination reactions, since the resultant double bonds would put too much stress on the bridgehead carbon atoms (Bredt's rule), and low-energy elimination reactions and displacement reactions are difficult because of the stereoscopy of the molecule (1). However, the carbonyl portion can undergo the usual reactions of this functional group, such as ketal and hemiketal formation (30), reduction to an alcohol (19,26), and the formation of oxazolidiones (55) with amino acids. The keto group can be removed by various procedures forming the compound Mirex (27). Other environmental reactions include degradation by photo-oxidation in the presence of air and water (46). These degradation reactions in the environment are very slow, however, as seen by the very small changes in chlordecone levels in the James River (Virginia) sediment. According to a report from the Virginia Institute of Marine

Science, there was no significant change in the sediment concentration of chlordecone from December, 1976 to July, 1977 (R.J. Huggett: Project Manager, The Virginia Institute of Marine Science, personal communication, 1978).

Chlordecone is a synthetic compound that was commercially produced by the dimerization of hexachlorocyclopentadiene in the presence of sulfur trioxide, with subsequent hydrolysis to the ketone (28). Chlordecone can also be produced from Mirex by a slow photolytic dechlorination; a significant concentration of chlordecone has been found in soil and water contaminated with Mirex (9). Therefore, despite the cessation of chlordecone production in 1975, the environment may still be undergoing contamination with this pesticide. Analysis of chlordecone has been difficult because of insufficient sensitivity of the methods or changes in the compound during analysis. The method used most commonly involves extraction using acid/organic solvent and analysis by gas-liquid chromatography with an electron-capture detector (2).

General Toxicology

Gastrointestinal absorption of chlordecone is nearly complete (>90%), as measured in animals (20,38,43). The pharmacokinetics and toxicology of chlordecone have been thoroughly reviewed (31). Absorption through the skin has been documented, though the relevance of this to human disease is unclear. Illness following absorption of the related chemical dieldrin has been documented in humans (59); however, this case report deals with a patient with chronic skin disease. Absorption via respiratory pathways is presumed to occur.

The distribution of chlordecone after ingestion has been elucidated extensively in animals and, to a lesser extent, in humans. Rats fed ^{14}C-chlordecone and sacrificed 2 weeks later (5) were found to have the highest concentration of radioactive chlordecone in liver, adrenal glands, and lung. The total radioactivity in these tissues, together with the feces and urine, accounted for 80% of the administered radioactivity. A group of patients was studied (14) following a period of industrial exposure to chlordecone. The distribution of unlabeled chlordecone in various body tissues was greatest in liver and muscle. The tissue-to-blood ratio is very low in both the animal and human studies compared to that seen with other organochlorines, where the ratio can be extremely high. The distribution of chlordecone, unlike other lipophilic pesticides, shows that it accumulates more in liver than in fat. Subcellular fractionation studies of liver show very little chlordecone in the cytosol; most of the pesticide is probably bound to the cell membrane (31).

The high blood concentration could indicate either a high free chlordecone fraction or significant protein binding. The latter is most likely since only a small fraction has been shown to be "free," and a significant amount is found bound to albumin or the lipoprotein fraction (65).

As with other organochlorines (44), chlordecone is an inducer of hepatic mixed oxidase systems (24). These systems are not important in the metabolism of the pesticide, unlike dieldrin, which can be removed from the body faster if a mixed-oxidase system is induced by phenobarbital or phenytoin (44), two well-known liver mixed oxidase inducers. The pattern of oxidases induced by chlordecone is different from that induced by Mirex (42), indicating that this is not a nonspecific induction even though the enzymes induced may affect many unrelated compounds. Irrespective of the reason, blood levels are a relatively good index of body stores of chlordecone.

The major metabolite of chlordecone is the reduced form, chlordecone alcohol (3), some of which is conjugated to glucuronic acid. Not all animals show the same metabolites, including the excretion pathways noted below, so care should be taken in extrapolating experimental results to humans.

Chlordecone has not been detected in sweat, and only small amounts have been found in urine, saliva, and gastric juice. Most of the excreted chlordecone is passed in the feces of humans and experimental animals (14,21). Chlordecone excretion follows a linear log curve and, in exposed workers, the half-life is 153 days for blood and 125 days for fat (13). Unlike most organochlorine pesticides, there is rapid equilibrium between blood and other tissues.

A substantial portion of body chlordecone is excreted into the gut *via* a classic biliary pathway linked to bile salt excretion. The majority of this bile chlordecone is reabsorbed and recirculated in the liver (14); because of this, cholestyramine, a nonabsorbable anion exchange resin that binds chlordecone, speeds up excretion of the chlorohydrocarbon (4). Cholestyramine treatment shortened the blood half-life to 80 days. Chlordecone is also excreted into the gut *via* a nonbiliary pathway, probably by transmucosal transport (5). This finding is not without precedence, since the other lipophilic hydrocarbons [*e.g.*, the closely related compounds, Mirex (53) and dieldrin] have an extrabiliary excretion into the intestine (35).

The major metabolite of chlordecone is the reduced molecule, chlordecone alcohol (3), some of which is conjugated to glucuronic acid. Not all animals show the same metabolic pathways as in humans (31).

Chlordecone has been shown to have a number of effects on subcellular systems; most have been related to membrane systems, particularly transport mechanisms. The adenosine triphosphatases (ATPases), in particular mitochondrial Mg^{2+}–ATPase, appear to be the most vulnerable to chlordecone (16,17). Chlordecone produces a reversible inhibition of this enzyme in brain, heart, and liver with an I_{50} of 5×10^{-8} M chlordecone. Brain and heart Na^+,K^+–ATPase is somewhat less sensitive with an I_{50} of 5×10^{-6} M chlordecone (16,18); however, inhibition may be irreversible. Of note is the observation that the degree of tremor induced in rats is very strongly correlated with the degree of inhibition of both Mg^{2+}–ATPase and Na^+,K^+–ATPase. Unequivocal cause and effect, however, has not been shown.

Chlordecone is a potent inhibitor of brain mitochondrial oxidative phosphorylation as well as an inhibitor of Ca^{2+} uptake by the cell (Ca^{2+}–ATPase) (22). The I_{50} was in the 10^{-7}M range, similar to that for Mg^{2+}–ATPase. Thus, mitochondrial Mg^{2+}–ATPase and Ca^{2+}–ATPase appear to be more sensitive to chlordecone than the membrane Na^+,K^+–ATPase. In keeping with these findings, active transport across liver membranes is inhibited by chlordecone (56).

Neurotransmitters are also affected (16,37). Little effect on serotonin and norepinephrine was noted in the mouse brain, but chlordecone did affect the steady-state level of dopamine (37). Chlordecone also affected synaptosomal catecholamine uptake (10) in a concentration-dependent manner (10); this effect is secondary to decreased binding of dopamine in the presence of chlordecone. No effect was found on rat brain levels of catecholamine or the precursor, tyrosine (22). At the electron microscopic level, however, morphological changes were seen in synaptosomes exposed to chlordecone.

Chlordecone has a concentration-dependent effect on K^+-dependent γ-aminobutyric acid (GABA) uptake by synaptosomes (11). The cholinergic system may also be affected, since the closely related compound dieldrin causes a marked increase in cholinergic activity, at least in insects (58). Thus, while changes in transmitter levels are not found universally, there is some evidence that the changes may be pathophysiologically significant. Other enzyme systems are also affected; lactic acid dehydrogenase is inhibited to a great extent by chlordecone (36).

Although the effect of chlordecone on the nervous system is the most obvious, other parts of the body are also affected. Hepatic changes include increased fat and proliferation of the endoplasmic reticulum, as well as the appearance of numerous dense bodies (13). Hepatomegaly was noted in exposed humans, but liver function did not decompensate (*vide infra*). However, hepatomas have been reported in rodents treated with chlordecone (54). Exposure to chlordecone has also caused significant reproductive problems in animals (23,38,52,64) and humans (63). Other effects of exposure include arthralgias and pleuritic pain of uncertain pathogenesis, as well as skin rash.

Animal Disease

The most consistent observation regarding behavior of laboratory animals is the presence of severe body tremors, ataxia, and emaciation (23,29,38,48). This syndrome is usually accompanied by weight loss and commonly culminates in death. Minnows develop scoliosis, darkening of the posterior body, cessation of feeding, fin rot, and uncoordinated swimming (22). A single juvenile rhesus monkey (weight, 2.5 kg) was fed 140 mg/kg of chlordecone over a 56-day period. When a blood level of 11,850 ng/ml was reached (after 24 days), jitteriness and tremor were noted, but no abnormal ocular movements were seen. Death occurred at 56 days (J.R. Taylor et al., unpublished data, 1977).

Although some investigators made brief statements regarding the nervous system [e.g., hemorrhaging near the brain in sheepshead minnows (32)], the literature contains little regarding neuromorphology. In the single monkey mentioned before, a grossly normal brain was evident at necropsy. Light microscopy disclosed nonspecific axonal swelling. Electron microscopy revealed a large collection of poorly preserved spheroidal organelles with triple membranes in the decussation pyramis; this was interpreted as degeneration. In studies of chlordecone-induced scoliosis in fish, precaudal trunk flexures due to abnormally contorted muscle bundles were observed (15); in severe cases, the vertebrae were fractured. Though no histological lesions in the CNS were found, it was proposed that the bone changes were caused by tetany from an undetermined neuromuscular dysfunction or molecular alteration in the CNS.

Dogs fed the related chemical DDT displayed the characteristic syndrome of tremor and ataxia leading to death (34). At necropsy, cerebellar damage consisting of swollen and hyperchromatic cytoplasm and pyknotic nuclei in the Purkinje cells was noted. Whether similar changes occur with chlordecone has not been established.

Distribution of chlordecone in primate brain was studied in a single monkey treated as previously discussed (J.R. Taylor et al., unpublished data, 1977). The chlordecone level in the liver was 828 ng/g, higher than in any other organ. Levels in brain ranged from 259 ng/g in the occipital lobe, to 286 ng/g in the frontal lobe, and 338 ng/g in the spinal cord. These levels were similar to that (294 ng/g) found in subcutaneous fat. The blood level 1 month prior to death was 16.9 ng/g, and 12.5 ng/g at the time of death. Thus, while organs high in fat content readily partition

chlordecone, the liver appears actively to concentrate the chemical.

Few neuroteratogenic data are available. One study of rats and mice fed chlordecone reported "enlarged ventricles" in offspring of dams fed 10 mg/kg/day (12). This finding might suggest the presence of a syndrome of psychomotor retardation in offspring of animals intoxicated with chlordecone; however, these investigators hastened to point out that the noted morphological effects might be nonspecific, since there was "a considerable degree of maternal toxicity."

Cataracts were observed in offspring of rats treated with Mirex (25); however, suckling of the dams was not prevented, and when other sucklings were placed with untreated dams after birth, the cataracts did not develop.

Human Disease

In the Hopewell epidemic (vide supra), the physical plant was a renovated gasoline service station that was connected by an open-paved area to several outbuildings. In the synthesis of chlordecone, a wet form of the pesticide was developed, and this liquid frequently leaked from collecting tanks onto the paved area. Workers walked through a slurry of the pesticide without boots or protective clothing. Following synthesis, chlordecone was dried for shipment. In the drying areas of the plant, exhaust ventilation was poor and a particulate haze of dust often filled the air. Consequently, a powdery residue of chlordecone soiled workers' clothing, caked their skin, accumulated on walls, and layered machinery. Protective masks were rarely used. Workers ate midday meals on plant premises, sometimes in the company of visiting family members, where they were exposed to the chlordecone dust that filled the air. Showers following work were taken infrequently at the plant; more often the workers wore their contaminated clothes home to be washed. No single portal of entry resulting in human chlordecone can be presumed to have caused chlordecone intoxication in these workers. Indeed, not only the food they ate and the air they breathed, but also their skin was heavily exposed to the insecticide dust.

The only known human intoxication with chlordecone resulted from the industrial overexposure at LSPC. This epidemic among the chemical workers was thoroughly summarized (8). Of 148 workers employed by LSPC over the 17 months of chlordecone production, 133 were contacted and subsequently cooperated with VSHD investigators. Among these workers, 76 (57%) reported a sensation of nervousness and/or visible tremulousness after beginning employment at LSPC.

The attack rate among employees correlated with the respective responsibilities of workers at the plant. Secretarial and office personnel, who were the only women employed at LSPC, reported no illness. Workers employed in the dryer and filter operation, an area where chlordecone dust was almost constantly in the air, had an attack rate of 70%. An attack rate of 51% was found among maintenance workers, and janitors had only a 30% incidence of illness. Among ACC workers involved in chlordecone production 18 or more months before, 77% (30 of 39) had detectable levels of the pesticide in their blood. Family members of affected workers had low blood chlordecone levels and few objective signs of intoxication.

The effect of the plant's operation upon the surrounding community was also studied (8). Nearby collection of air samples by the U.S. EPA showed that small amounts of chlordecone were discharged into the air apparently by the ACC production process. The amount of contaminated air greatly increased after production commenced at LSPC in March 1974. Other information disclosed that spilled chlordecone was washed from the plant into the sewage treatment plant. The effluent from this plant drained into Bailey's Creek, down the James River and into the Chesapeake Bay.

A community survey was undertaken from randomly selected households and businesses to study the effect of the air and water contamination. None of the 215 persons who were interviewed had ever worked in the manufacture of chlordecone. No one manifested an illness consistent with chlordecone intoxication at the time of evaluation, although some reported prior symptoms. Blood levels of chlordecone in 40 (19%) community residents ranged from 5.1–32.5 ppb. The majority of these persons lived within 0.4 km of the plant. Detectable blood chlordecone levels were also found in 75% (23 of 32) of neighborhood workers and in 60% (six of ten) of sewage treatment plant workers.

Symptomatic employees of LSPC were found to have a mean blood chlordecone of 2.53 ppm (2.0–333.0 ppm), whereas asymptomatic workers had a mean level of 0.6 ppm (0–10.0 ppm). Twenty-three employees with signs and symptoms persisting after 1 month cooperated in a serial study of their illness (63).

Pleuritic chest pains were variable in location and intensity, but troublesome in many of the chronically intoxicated men. Mild, constant pain in larger joints, such as the knees or hip, occurred in most. This discomfort migrated from joint to joint and was not sensitive to climatic changes. A small effusion occurred in two patients, and chlordecone was detected in the aspirated fluid of one. Weight loss, up to 130 kg, occurred in ten workers; its cause was not clear.

Mild enlargement of the liver was found in nine workers, and several also had a slightly palpable spleen.

A sense of trembling and tremor itself were the most pervasive effects of chlordecone intoxication. The workers referred to the trembling as the "Kepone shakes." The tremor was usually small in amplitude and irregular in direction. It was most manifest with voluntary acts or fixed postures, but in those most affected it was present at rest as well. The tremor stopped in sleep and increased with anxiety or fatigue. Tremorgrams showed a frequency of 6–8 Hz. Commonly, the upper extremities were involved, but visible trembling of the hand, the trunk, and lower limbs occurred in those with high tissue concentrations of chlordecone. Involvement of the trunk and lower limbs resulted in a mild instability that widened the station and slowed the gait. A distinct cerebellar type of incoordination that exceeded the tremor's range of motion during the purposeful movements was not evident.

Generally, tremor began after 6 weeks or more of exposure to the industrial conditions at LSPC. Eventually, the constant, progressive trembling impaired dexterity for handling small tools, fastening clothing, drinking from containers, or eating with utensils. Onset and intensity of the tremor from worker to worker correlated with degree and duration of exposure. Over the year following closure of LSPC, the tremor slowly diminished and stopped in all but several workers.

A series of quick eye movement (saccades), usually small in amplitude and multidirectional, was observed in 15 patients. These aberrant eye movements caused patients to complain of brief blurring of images. Visual acuity that involved reading or driving was somewhat hampered by this ocular trembling. The saccades were both conjugate and dysconjugate, and although spontaneous, they were often elicited by requesting the patient to make a refixation saccade from one stationary target to another. In one patient, touch of the eyelid or globe of the eye induced a conjugate burst of saccades. These chaotic eye movements had all the appearance of opsoclonus; this appears to be the first description of human opsoclonus in which a toxic agent has been identified as the cause.

Over 3–6 months, opsoclonus became smaller in amplitude and less frequent. Subsequent infrared recordings of ocular abnormality in six patients showed several additional perturbations of eye movements. Recordings of steady fixation showed interruptions by several small-amplitude, square-topped (indicating a latency for a controlled go, stop-and-go signal within the ocular motor mechanism) eye movements that are known as *Gegenrücken*. Hypometric saccades were frequent, and a very small postsaccadic tremor replaced the opsoclonus. Refixation opsoclonus was recorded in one patient. The recording shows a series of saccades without intervening latencies. Convergence also occurs in this tracing, much like voluntary nystagmus. However, previous clinical observations and AC oculography excluded concomitant convergence during many other saccadic bursts. Recordings and high-speed cinematographic analysis suggested that the form and velocity of these saccades were normal; this indicated that there was no aberration of neuronal units lying in the pontine pathway for saccade formation. Rather, the postsaccadic induction of opsoclonus implied that neuronal circuits suppressing the oculomotor neuron pool between saccades had been disinhibited. Neurons in the pontine reticular formation of monkeys appear to have an inhibiting relationship to neurons that have burst discharges during saccades (45). Momentary suppression of such "pause cells" would permit a brief discharge of saccadic eye movements and is proposed as a basis for opsoclonus (D.A. Robinson, personal communication, 1977).

Irritability and mild memory loss were present in 13 of 23 patients. These persisted for only several weeks after chlordecone exposure was halted. The first worker to be hospitalized and diagnosed presented in a confused and disoriented state; he had the highest blood chlordecone level (33.0 ppm). He exhibited auditory and visual hallucinations and a startle response to tactile or auditory stimulation that consisted of a series of brief but incapacitating whole-body myoclonic jerks. Nine workers complained of a mild, persistent headache. Three had low-grade papilledema. Each of the three workers had elevated cerebrospinal fluid (CSF) pressures (400, 310, 290 mm H$_2$O) and abnormal CSF infusion tests, implying impaired CSF absorption. Elevated blood, serum, and fat chlordecone levels were found in these three patients. Neuroradiological studies eliminated an intracranial mass, which in the absence of drug use or systemic illness established a clinical diagnosis of pseudotumor cerebri (57). Headache diminished, and papilledema resolved as tissue chlordecone levels declined over the subsequent year. Fluid obtained by lumbar puncture in four more of the nine patients was normal. In all nine workers, headaches abated as the months passed.

To assay for chlordecone (2), adipose tissue was biopsied by aspiration of abdominal subcutaneous tissue, and liver was obtained by needle aspiration. High levels of chlordecone were regularly found in whole blood, adipose tissue (50–90 ppm), and the liver (13–173 ppm). Modest amounts of chlordecone were found in muscle, gall bladder, bile, and stool. Trace amounts were present in CSF, urine, saliva, synovial fluid, and gastric juice.

Routine laboratory tests of blood, urine, electrolytes, and renal and liver function were normal. Roentgenograms and electrocardiograms were within normal limits. Radioisotope scans showed in nine workers mild enlargement of the liver that was occasionally associated with splenomegaly. Histological examination of liver biopsy specimens was generally unremarkable.

Oligospermia was observed in 13 men. The severity of this varied from no motile sperm in two workers to an immediate count of 38,350,000 (normal, 50,000,000 motile sperm/mm^3). After a follow-up period of 18 months, sperm counts in seven men had recovered to normal levels, and of the six that remained low, all had increased substantially. The two workers with the initial counts of zero had improved to 37,000,000 sperm/mm^3 and 49,750,000 sperm/mm^3.

Neurological tests included electromyography, nerve conduction velocities, electroencephalography, radioisotope brain scan, computed tomography of the head, and CSF analysis, all of which were normal. Results of the tremorgram, eye-movement recordings, CSF pressure at lumbar puncture, and CSF infusion tests are given above. Muscle biopsies in six patients contained increased lipofusion and lipid-like droplets, as well as a predominance of type 1 fibers (49). Sural nerve biopsies in five patients disclosed decreased numbers of unmyelinated fibers, general increase in endoneural collagen, various inclusions, and redundant cytoplasmic folds of Schwann cells.

Initially, over half of the active employees at LSPC were moderately ill. A few required hospitalization for several months. In the subsequent 18 months, most symptoms and signs gradually diminished. After 4 years, several workers continued to manifest a mildly incapacitating tremor.

Sixteen of 23 patients were evaluated between 1980 and 1982, five to 7 years following cessation of exposure (61). Nine were asymptomatic; of the remainder, five complained of persistent tremor or "nervousness." Of these, three stated their tremor was present only when they were emotionally upset, and the other two complained of constant tremor. Only one showed objective tremor at the time of evaluation. Other symptoms included three with psychiatric complaints and one with headache. The remaining patients were normal on neurological and general physical examination. Twelve of the former workers who were being re-evaluated agreed to some laboratory evaluations. In all twelve subjects, a chlordecone level could not be detected in the blood but was detected in the fat in ranges of 5–29 ppb. There was no correlation between fat levels or findings on examination. Eight patients submitted semen for analysis; the sperm count was normal in all but one. This patient who previously had a low sperm count showed a low count of 27,500,000. At that time, two had sired normal children.

A 1995 survey of the 23 well-studied former workers who were severely affected was performed using both telephone contact and a mailed questionnaire. The questionnaire was either completed by telephone or confirmed by telephone if one was received by mail. Twelve of the former workers were contacted and completed a questionnaire. Eleven were lost to follow-up; none appeared on the Commonwealth of Virginia Death Certificate Register. The present ages of those contacted ranged from 39–67 years. Six reported they were still working, and two were unemployed for undisclosed reasons. One was retired. Three were disabled, one each from systemic scleroderma, results of a fall, and from stroke and coronary artery disease. Specific cardinal symptoms of chlordecone intoxication were sought. Five reported that they still had a tremor; however, four of these reported that the tremor only occurred when they were anxious. Seven reported no tremor. Three reported occasional eye jerks, and one reported eye jerks specifically when looking quickly to one side or the other. Only one of these had any visual symptoms; however, this former worker had lost one eye due to trauma following his employment at LSPC. None reported cancer. Ten noted that the health of the family was good; one related that his wife had breast cancer, and one related that his wife had diabetes mellitus. Ten children (six males and four females) had been sired and born since the Hopewell epidemic. One of the males has congenital hearing loss, and another male is hyperactive and a "slow learner." One of the females is a "slow learner" and is sister to the boy with congenital hearing loss; they are the only two children fathered since 1975 by that worker. The remainder of the children are normal and healthy. An open question concerning general health was asked: six reported good health, one reportedly had acquired diabetes mellitus, and a seventh reported fair health. The five who reported otherwise gave as the main reason for their health impairment the effects of a fall, systemic scleroderma, pancreatic disease, stroke and coronary artery disease, and chronic breathing problems. This last patient also reported that he smoked cigarettes.

The numbers are sufficiently small that conclusions relating to various health problems relative to chlordecone cannot be drawn. It is clear that some of the symptoms persist, particularly tremor, although none related any disability due to the tremor other than difficulty with fine movement tasks reported by one.

As noted previously, the half-life of chlordecone in untreated workers averaged 165 days. Cholestyramine significantly increased fecal excretion of the pesticide (14). Following 16 g/day of this resin, the observed half-life of chlordecone in blood was reduced to a mean of 80 days. Chlordecone concentrations in fat were similarly reduced.

Other forms of therapy, such as activated charcoal (40 g/day) and plasmapheresis were not effective in lowering blood chlordecone levels (14). In some patients exposed to chlordecone, propanolol in dosages up to 200 mg/day was effective in ameliorating tremor.

Pathogenesis and/or Toxic Mechanisms

The most striking manifestations of chlordecone intoxication are tremor and opsoclonus. The central origin of chlordecone-induced tremor was demonstrated in mice by transecting the spinal cord and observing the tremor continue rostral but not caudal to the transection (40). Limb and ocular tremors were observed in dogs given tremorine (6). This is the only tremorogenic agent used in the laboratory that affects ocular movements. Destructive lesions of the mesencephalic reticular formation of rats were found to be the most effective in reducing tremorine-induced tremors (60). By analogy, chlordecone may alter neural stabilizing mechanisms for the motor system that are localized about the mesencephalic reticular formation but outside the direct cerebellar-thalamic-cortical-spinal pathway for the programming of motor movement.

The patients who had pseudotumor cerebri associated with chlordecone poisoning showed a CSF absorption block similar to that seen in the idiopathic form of pseudotumor cerebri (7,41,50). The underlying mechanism of this block is unknown.

REFERENCES

1. Benson WR (1969) The chemistry of pesticides. *Ann N Y Acad Sci* **160**, 7.
2. Blanke RV, Fariss MW, Griffith FD Jr, Guzelian PS (1977) Analysis of chlordecone (Kepone) in biological specimens. *J Anal Toxicol* **1**, 57.
3. Blanke RV, Fariss MW, Guzelian PS *et al.* (1978) Identification of a reduced form of chlordecone (Kepone^R) in human stool. *Environ Contam Toxicol* **20**, 782.
4. Boylan JJ, Cohn WJ, Egle JL Jr (1979) Excretion of chlordecone by the gastrointestinal tract: Evidence for a nonbiliary mechanism. *Clin Pharmacol Ther* **25**, 579.
5. Boylan JJ, Egle JL, Guzelian PS (1978) Cholestyramine: Use as a new therapeutic approach for chlordecone (Kepone) poisoning. *Science* **199**, 893.
6. Brumlik I, Means ED (1969) Tremorine-tremor, shivering and acute cerebellar ataxia in the adult and child—a comparative study. *Brain* **92**, 157.
7. Calabrese VP, Selhorst JB, Harbison JW (1979) Cerebrospinal fluid infusion test in pseudotumor cerebri. *Trans Amer Neurol Assn* **103**, 8.
8. Cannon SB, Veazey JM Jr, Jackson RS *et al.* (1978) Epidemic Kepone poisoning in chemical workers. *Amer J Epidemiol* **17**, 529.

9. Carlson DA, Konyha KD, Wheeler WB *et al.* (1976) Mirex in the environment: Its degradation to kepone and related compounds. *Science* **194**, 939.

10. Chang-Tsu Y-YH, Ho IK (1980) Effect of Kepone^R (Chlordecone) on synaptosomal catecholamine uptake in the mouse. *Neurotoxicology* **1**, 643.

11. Chang-Tsu Y-YH, Ho IK (1979) Effect of Kepone^R (chlordecone) on synaptosomal gamma aminobutyric acid uptake in the mouse. *Neurotoxicology* **1**, 357.

12. Chernoff N, Rogers EH (1976) Fetal toxicity of kepone in rats and mice. *Toxicol Appl Pharmacol* **38**, 1896.

13. Cohn WJ, Blanke RV, Griffith FD Jr, Guzelian PS (1976) Distribution and excretion of Kepone (KP) in humans. *Gastroenterology* **71**, 90.

14. Cohn WJ, Boylan JJ, Blanke RV *et al.* (1978) Treatment of chlordecone (Kepone) toxicity with with cholestyramine. *N Engl J Med* **298**, 243.

15. Couch JA, Winstead JT, Goodman LR (1977) Keponeinduced scoliosis and its histological consequences in fish. *Science* **197**, 585.

16. Desaiah D (1981) Interaction of chlordecone with biological membranes. *J Toxicol Environ Health* **8**, 707.

17. Desaiah D, Ho I, Menhendale H (1977) Effects of kepone and mirex on mitochondrial Mg-ATPase activity in rat liver. *Toxicol Appl Pharmacol* **39**, 219.

18. Desaiah D, Koch RB (1975) Inhibition of ATPase activity in channel catfish brain by kepone and its reduction product. *Bull Environ Contam Toxicol* **13**, 153.

19. Dilling W, Braendlin H, McBee EM (1967) Pentacyclodecane chemistry; II. Some reactions of dodecachloropentacyclo-(5.3.0.0.^{2,6}.0^{3,9}..0^{4,8}) decane and related compounds. *Tetrahedron* **23**, 1211.

20. Egle JL Jr, Fernandez SB, Guzelian PS, Borzelleca JF (1978) Distribution and excretion of chlordecone (kepone) in rats. *Pestic Biochem Physiol* **6**, 91.

21. Ellenberger C Jr, Keltner JL, Stroud MH (1972) Ocular dyskinesia in cerebellar disease. Evidence for the similarity of opsoclonus, ocular dysmetria and flutter-like oscillations. *Brain* **95**, 685.

22. End DW, Carchman RA, Dewey WL (1981) Neurochemical correlates of chlordecone neurotoxicity. *J Toxicol Environ Health* **86**, 707.

23. Eroschenko VP, Wilson WO (1974) Photoperiods and age as factors modifying the effects of kepone in Japanese quail. *Toxicol Appl Pharmacol* **29**, 329.

24. Fabacher DL, Hodgson E (1976) Induction of hepatic mixed function oxidase enzymes in adult and neonatal mice by Kepone and Mirex. *Toxicol Appl Pharmacol* **38**, 71.

25. Gaines TB, Kimbrough RD (1970) Oral toxicity of mirex in adult and suckling rats. *Arch Environ Health* **21**, 7.

26. Gilbert E, Lombardo P, Rumanowski EJ, Walker GL (1966) Preparation and insecticidal evaluation of alcoholic analogs of Kepone. *J Agr Food Chem* **14**, 111.

27. Gilbert EE, Giolito SL (1953) *Chem Abst* **47**, 2424 e.

28. Gilbert EE, Giolito SL (1952) U.S. Patent 2,616,928.

29. Good EE, Ware GW, Miller DF (1965) Effects of insecticides on reproduction in the laboratory mouse; I. Kepone. *J Econ Entomol* **53**, 751.

30. Griffin GW, Price AR (1964) *Chem Abst* **61**, 159, 566.

31. Guzelian PS (1982) Comparative toxicology of chlordecone (Kepone) in humans and experimental animals. *Ann Resp Pharmacol Toxicol* **22**, 89.

32. Hansen DJ, Goodman LR, Wilson AJ Jr (1977) Kepone: Chronic effects on embryo, fry, juvenile, and adult sheepshead minnors (*Cyprinodon variegatus*). *Chesapeake Sci* **18**, 227.

33. Hansen DJ, Wilson AJ, Nimmo DR *et al.* (1976) Kepone: Hazard to aquatic organisms. *Science* **193**, 5286.

34. Haymaker W, Gingler AM, Ferguson RL (1946) The toxic effects of prolonged ingestion of DDT on dogs with special reference to lesions in the brain. *Amer J Med Sci* **212**, 423.

35. Heath D, Vandekar M (1964) Toxicity and metabolism of dieldrin in rats. *Brit J Ind Med* **21**, 269.

36. Hendrickson CM, Bowden JA (1975) The *in vitro* inhibition of rabbit muscle lactate dehydrogenase by mirex and Kepone. *J Agr Food Chem* **23**, 407.

37. Ho IK, FujimorI K, Huang TP, Chang-Tusi H (1981) Neurochemical evaluation of chlordecone toxicity in the mouse. *J Toxicol Environ Health* **8**, 707.

38. Huber J (1965) Some physiologic effects of the insecticide Kepone in the laboratory mouse. *Toxicol Appl Pharmacol* **7**, 516.

39. Huff JE, Gerstner JB (1977) Kepone I. A literature summary. National Technical Information Service, U.S. Department of Commerce, Springfield, Va.

40. Hwang EC, Van Woert MH (1979) Serotonin-norepinephrine interaction in the tremorlytic actions of phenoxybenzamine and trazodone. *Pharmacol Biochem Behav* **10**, 27.

41. Johnston I, Gilday DL, Hendrick EB (1975) Experimental effects of steroids and steroid withdrawal on cerebrospinal fluid absorption. *J Neurosurg* **42**, 690.

42. Kaminsky LS, Piper LJ, McMartin DN, Fasco MJ (1978) Induction of hepatic microsomal cytochrome P-450 by mirex and Kepone. *Toxicol Appl Pharmacol* **43**, 327.

43. Kavloch RJ, Chernoff N, Rogers E, Whitehouse D (1980) Comparative tissue distribution of mirex and chlordecone in fetal and neonatal rats. *Pestic Biochem Physiol* **14**, 227.

44. Kay K (1973) Toxicology of pesticides: Recent advances. *Environ Res* **6**, 202.

45. Keller EL (1974) Participation of medial pontine reticular formation in eye movement generation in monkey. *J Neurophysiol* **37**, 316.

46. Knoevenagel K, Himmelreich R (1976) Degradation of compounds containing carbon atoms by photooxidation in the presence of water. *Arch Environ Contam Toxicol* **4**, 324.

47. McBee ET, Roberts CW, Idol JD Jr, Earle RH Jr (1956)

An investigation of the chlorocarbon $C_{10}Cl_{10}O$, M.P. 349°. *J Amer Chem Soc* **78**, 1511.

48. McFarland LZ, Lacy PB (1969) Physiologic and endocrinologic effects of the insecticide Kepone in the Japanese quail. *Toxicol Appl Pharmacol* **15**, 441.

49. Martinez AJ, Taylor JR, Dyck PJ *et al.* (1978) Chlordecone intoxication in man; II. Ultrasound of peripheral nerves and skeletal muscle. *Neurology* **28**, 631.

50. Martins AN (1973) Resistance to drainage of cerebrospinal fluid: Clinical measurement and significance. *J Neurol Neurosurg Psychiat* **36**, 313.

51. *Merck Index* (1976) Windholz M ed. Merck & Co, Rahway, New Jersey p. 263.

52. Naber E, Ware G (1965) Effect of Kepone and mirex on reproductive performance in the laying hen. *Poultry Sci* **44**, 875.

53. Pittman KA, Wiener M, Treble DH (1976) Mirex kinetics in the rhesus monkey. *Drug Metab Disposition* **4**, 288.

54. Reuber MD (1978) Carcinogenicity of Kepone. *J Toxicol Environ Health* **4**, 895.

55. Roberts CW, Travis GD, Heeschen JP (1967) The synthesis of a series of 1,1a,3,3a,4,5,5a,5b,6-decachloro-octahydro-4-substituted spiro (1,3,4-metheno-2*H*-cyclobuta(*c,d*)pentalene-2,2′-oxazolidine)-5′-ones. *J Org Chem* **32**, 3194.

56. Rochelle LG, Curtis LR (1994) Distribution of chlordecone to liver plasma membranes and recovery from hepatobiliary dysfunction. *Manage Toxicol* **86**, 123.

57. Sanborn GE, Selhorst JB, Calabrese VP, Taylor JR (1979) Pseudotumor cerebri and insecticide intoxication. *Neurology* **19**, 1222.

58. Shankland DL, Schroeder ME (1973) Pharmacological evidence for a discrete neurologic action of dieldrin (HEOD) in the American cockroach *Periplaneta americana*. *Pestic Biochem Physiol* **3**, 77.

59. Starr HG Jr, Clifford JN (1971) Absorption of pesticides in chronic skin disease. *Arch Environ Health* **22**, 369.

60. Tasker RR, Kertesz A (1965) The physiology of tremorine-induced tremor. *J Neurosurg* **22**, 449.

61. Taylor JR (1965) Neurological manifestations in humans exposed to chlordecone: Follow-up results. *Neurotoxicology* **6**, 231.

62. Taylor JR, Selhorst JB, Calabrese, VP (1980) Chlordecone. In: *Experimental and Clinical Neurotoxicology*. Spencer PS, Schaumburg HH eds. Williams & Wilkins, Baltimore p. 407.

63. Taylor JR, Selhorst JB, Houff S, Martinez J (1978) Chlordecone intoxication in man. *Neurology* **28**, 626.

64. Ware E, Good E (1977) Effects of insecticide on reproduction in the laboratory mouse; II. Mirex, Telodrine, DDT. *Toxicol Appl Pharmacol* **10**, 54.

65. Weikel JH Jr, Lau GE, Tomchick R (1958) Ion movement across the rabbit erythrocyte membrane as affected by chlorinated insecticides. *Arch Int Pharmacodyn Ther* **113**, 261.

Chlorhexidine Gluconate

Herbert H. Schaumburg

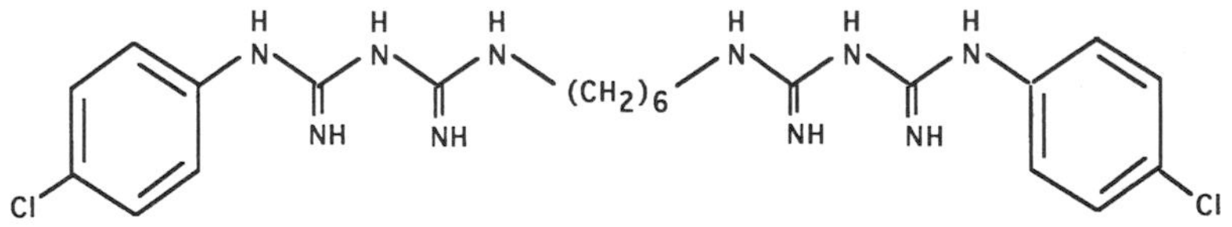

CHLORHEXIDINE
$C_{22}H_{30}Cl_2N_{10}$

N,N″-Bis(4-chlorophenyl)-3,12-diimino-2,4,11,13-tetraazatetradecanediimidamide

NEUROTOXICITY RATING

Clinical

A Ototoxicity (topical, hearing loss)

A Olfactory syndrome

Experimental

A Ototoxicity (necrosis of organ of Corti)

Chlorhexidine gluconate is a chlorophenyl biguanide with a broad spectrum of antimicrobial activity. It is widely used as a topical antiseptic, antiseptic mouthwash, and contact lens cleaner; these uses have been associated with systemic side effects. Topical application of chlorhexidine gluconate in the nasal cavity causes reversible anosmia from desquamation of the olfactory epithelium; oral use is associated with discoloration of the teeth.

Perfusion of the myringoplasty operative site with chlorhexidine gluconate was associated with sensorineural deafness in 15% of cases in a 1971 report (3). Subsequent experimental studies clearly demonstrate that topical, subtympanic application of chlorhexidine gluconate to the guinea pig ear causes damage to the organ of Corti and vestibular neuroepithelium (1,2).

REFERENCES

1. Aursnes J (1981) Vestibular damage from chlorhexidine in guinea pigs. *Acta Oto-Laryngol* **92**, 89.
2. Aursnes J (1981) Cochlear damage from chlorhexidine in guinea pigs. *Acta Oto-Laryngol* **92**, 259.
3. Bicknell PG (1971) Sensorineural deafness following myringoplasty operations. *J Laryngol Otol* **85**, 957.

Chlorinated Cyclodienes

Peter S. Spencer
Herbert H. Schaumburg

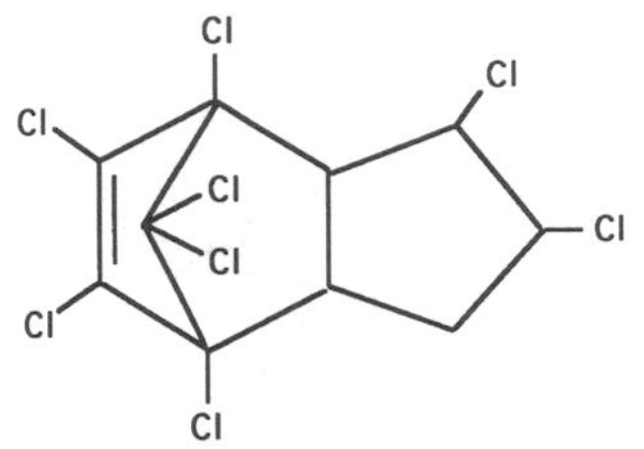

CHLORDANE
$C_{10}H_6Cl_8$

Chlordane; 1,2,4,5,6,7,8,8-Octachloro-2,3,3a,4,7,7a-hexahydro-4,7-methano-1*H*-indene (*cis* isomer > *trans* isomer)

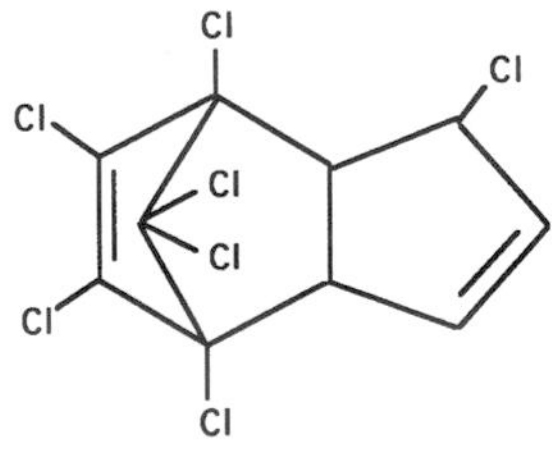

HEPTACHLOR
$C_{10}H_5Cl_7$

Heptachlor; 1*H*-1,4,5,6,7,8,8-Heptachloro-3a,4,7,7a-tetrahydro-4,7-methanoindene; E-3314

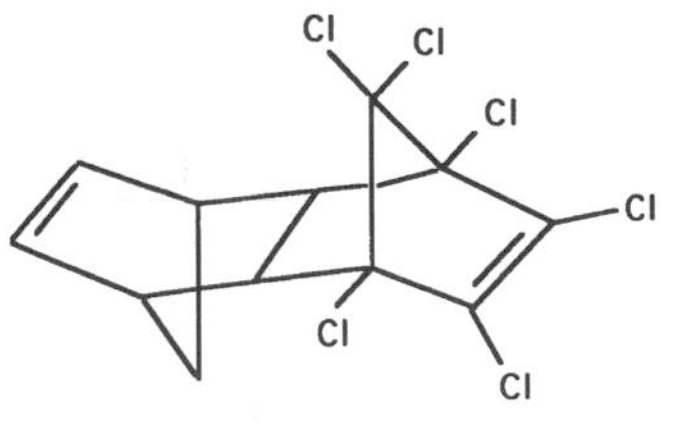

ALDRIN
$C_{12}H_8Cl_6$

Aldrin; 1,2,3,4,10,10-Hexachloro-1,4,4a,5,8,8a-hexahydro-1,4:5,8-dimethanonaphthalene; HHDN

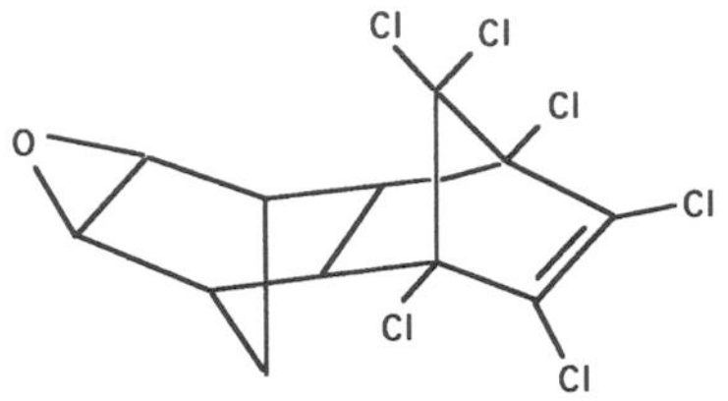

DIELDRIN
$C_{12}H_8Cl_6O$

Dieldrin; 1,2,3,4,10,10-Hexachloro-6,7-epoxy-1,4,4a,5,6,7,8,8a-octahydro-*endo*,*exo*-1,4:5,8-dimethanonaphthalene; HEOD

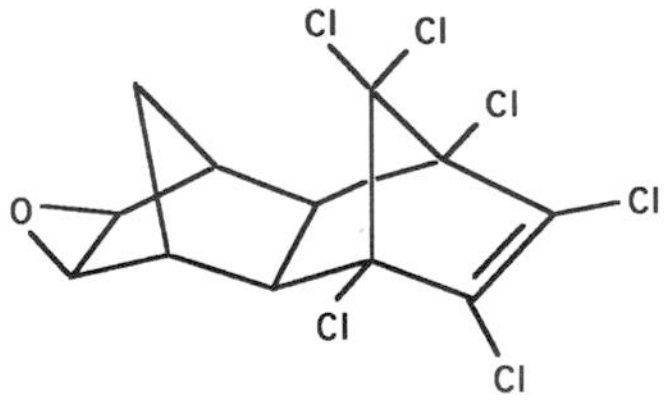

ENDRIN
$C_{12}H_8Cl_6O$

Endrin; 1,2,3,4,10,10-Hexachloro-6,7-epoxy-1,4,4a,5,6,7,8,8a-octahydro-*endo*,*endo*-1,4:5-8-dimethanonaphthalene; ENT-17251

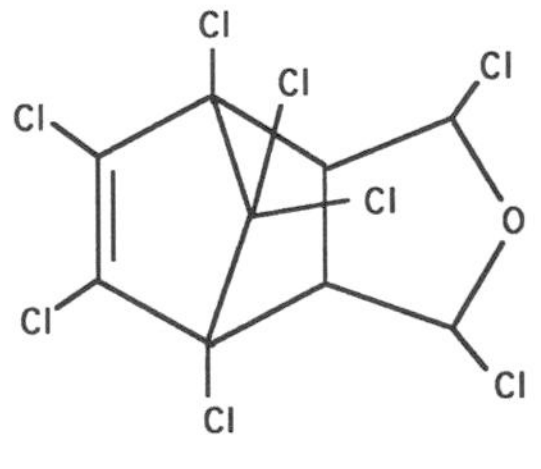

ISOBENZAN
$C_9H_4Cl_8O$

Isobenzan; 1,3,4,5,6,7,8,8-Octachloro-1,3,3a,4,7,7a-hexahydro-4,7-methanoisobenzofuran; SD-4402

ENDOSULFAN
$C_9H_6Cl_6O_3S$

Endosulfan; Stereoisomeric mixture of 6,7,8,9,10,10-Hexachloro-1,5,5a,6,9,9a-hexahydro-6,9-methano-2,4,3,-benzodioxathiepin 3-oxide; Endosulfan I and II, *exo* and *endo* configurations, respectively

NEUROTOXICITY RATING
Clinical
A   Seizure disorder
Experimental
A   Seizure disorder
A   GABA synapse inhibition

Chlorinated cyclodiene insecticides (CCIs) and related compounds (endosulfan) represent one of several classes of organochlorine insecticides (*see* Dichlorodiphenyltrichloroethane and Derivatives, and Toxaphene, this volume) (58). With the exception of mirex and chlordecone (*see* Chlordecone, this volume), which are nonconvulsant caged cyclodienes, CCIs produce a reversible seizure disorder in humans and animals by interfering with the function of γ-aminobutyric acid (GABA), the major inhibitory neurotransmitter in the vertebrate and insect CNS. Neurotoxic potency of the convulsant CCIs varies markedly among stereoisomers of individual compounds, and the metabolic conversion of some members to epoxides results in increased toxicity (78). A detailed description of the use and properties of CCIs and other organochlorine insecticides compounds is available (58).

Chlordane in impure form was introduced in 1945; the composition and insecticidal activities of aldrin and dieldrin were described in 1949 and those of endosulfan in 1956. From the 1940s to the 1960s, organochlorine insecticides were widely used in North America in vast quantities and with great effect to control a wide variety of insect pests in agriculture, forestry, and construction. Chlordane and heptachlor are also effective termiticides. However, the environmental persistence of many organochlorine insecticides, coupled with their potential for bioconcentration and biomagnification in various food chains, caused avian and other species to accumulate body burdens that were linked to disrupted reproductive success. From the early 1970s, usage of organochlorine insecticides was progressively restricted to specific applications and then phased out in many countries. While banned in North America and Europe, extensive use of organochlorine insecticides continues in less-developed parts of the world where the risk-benefit ratio for human health and food supply is considered to be heavily weighted in their favor (22).

Physical Properties and Formulations

The physical properties of CCIs depend on the purity of the formulation. The pure compounds are generally highly soluble in aromatic hydrocarbon solvents and almost insoluble in water. Technical chlordane is a viscous, amber-colored liquid containing as many as 45 constituents; the early product (1945–1951) contained variable concentrations of hexachlorocyclopentadiene, an unreacted intermediate (58). Refined chlordane, a mixture of less toxic *cis* and more toxic *trans* isomers with melting points (MP) of 104°–106°C, has a vapor pressure (VP) of 1×10^{-5} mm Hg at 25°C (58,78). Heptachlor forms white crystals with a MP of 95°–96°C and VP of 3×10^{-4} mm Hg at 25°C. Technical heptachlor is a wax that melts in the range of 45°–74°C. Pure forms of aldrin (HHDN) and dieldrin (HEOD) are white crystalline solids with MPs of 104°C and 176°–177°C, and VPs of 6×10^{-6} and 1.8×10^{-7} mm Hg at 25°C, respectively. The technical forms of aldrin and dieldrin are defined as containing not less than 85.5% HHDN or 80.75% HEOD, not less than 4.5% or 14.25% of insecticidally active related compounds, and not more than 10% or 5% of other compounds, respectively. They are brown-colored materials with "chemical" odors and MPs of 49°–60°C (technical aldrin) and not less than 95°C (technical dieldrin). Technical endrin, which contains 85% endrin, is a powder with a distinctive odor; the pure compound has a VP of 2×10^{-7} mm Hg at 25°C. Technical endosulfan contains 95% of a purified mixture of alpha (endosulfan I) and beta (endosulfan II) isomers in a 7:3 ratio; it forms impure brown crystals with a VP of 9×10^{-3} mm Hg. Isobenzan (Telodrin) contained approximately 95% of the pure material; manufacture of the insecticide was discontinued in 1965; it was never registered in the United States (58).

Formulations of cyclodiene insecticides include dusts, seed dressings, water-wettable powders, granules, emulsifiable concentrates, and oil solutions. They are effective as soil insecticides, in the control of insects on a wide range of agricultural products, and in the extermination of household insects, termites, and other pests (58).

Threshold limit values for workplace exposure to CCIs are given in mg/m³ (and in mg/kg/day): endrin and endosulfan, 0.1 (0.014); aldrin, 0.25 (0.036); heptachlor 0.5 (0.07) (58).

General Toxicology

Chlorinated hydrocarbon insecticides enter the body *via* respiratory, oral, and dermal routes. Absorption from skin is variable (low for DDT and high for dieldrin). Intestinal absorption varies with dietary composition and total food intake (dieldrin absorption increases in starvation) (58). In rats, peak levels of dieldrin in blood (where it is largely bound to hemoglobin) were reported 2.5 h after dosing (50,65). Whether dosages are subclinical (10 mg/kg body weight) or lethal (150 mg/kg), brain levels of dieldrin peak at 4 h and then decline; levels in fat increase over a 24-h period (34). A steady state of dieldrin storage in fat and blood (474:1) is reached in 16 days or longer (7,17,18,74). Loss of dieldrin from rats fed dieldrin (*ca.* 0.5 mg/kg/day for 8 weeks) was exponential from fat (half-life 10.3 days) and brain (3 days); loss from blood and liver was initially rapid (1.3 days) and then slower (10.2 days) (57). Biphasic loss of dieldrin from serum was apparent in a single, severely poisoned human subject: an initial rapid rate of loss (during which redistribution of dieldrin to fat was likely) was reduced from day 3 forward, when the half-life of dieldrin in serum was 34 days (9). In contrast, a mean half-life of 369 days was reported in volunteers given small daily doses of dieldrin (40). Others have reported a biological half-life for dieldrin in human blood of 267 days and, for isobenzan, 2.77 years (42,66).

Dieldrin and heptachlor epoxide accumulate in fatty tissue to a much greater extent than either endrin or chlordane. Dieldrin is stored avidly, and trace amounts are present throughout the general population. While environmental dieldrin levels reportedly dropped from the mid-1960s, levels in human adipose tissue and milk fat (0.16–0.22 ppm) were judged not to have declined up to 1976 (2). Levels of CCIs in humans, animals, and their food supplies continue to be monitored.

Metabolism by the microsomal cytochrome P-450 system converts the lipophilic chlorinated cyclodienes to hydroxyl derivatives. For example, in the rabbit, endrin is metabolized to *anti*-12-hydroxyendrin and *syn*-12-hydroxyendrin; these are excreted as sulfur and glucuronide conjugates (8). Aldrin and heptachlor are converted by oxidative reactions in humans and rodents to stable and more toxic epoxides, namely, dieldrin and heptachlor epoxide, respectively. Dieldrin is metabolized very slowly (especially in female animals) to a wide range of detoxication products found in feces and urine (58). Biotransformation of chlordane (LD_{50}, 283 mg/kg) produces a range of metabolites that includes oxychlordane (LD_{50}, 19 mg/kg) and *trans*-chlordane; the latter is metabolized to heptachlor (LD_{50}, 90 mg/kg) and then to heptachlor epoxide and its metabolites (20,48,78). *Trans*-nonachlor, a component of technical chlordane, is metabolized to a greater extent by rats than by humans (51). The human fat concentration of chlordane-related materials was nonachlor > oxychlordane > chlordane 3 years after use of chlordane had been discontinued in Japan (37).

Organochlorine compounds, including CCIs, can influence their own metabolism in species-specific manners. For example, dogs "store" less dieldrin and more DDT when the compounds are given together instead of individually (19). DDT suppresses storage of dieldrin or heptachlor in rats (54,61,62). Hexachlorobenzene reduces storage of aldrin but increases storage of DDT and mirex (12). Storage of DDT in guinea pigs is decreased by co-exposure to dieldrin (73).

Animal Studies

Controlled studies show that the acute toxicity of CCIs in rats is characterized by hypothermia, loss of appetite, convulsions, and death (78). Single lethal doses can be administered dermally or orally. Oral LD_{50} values illustrate the range of acute toxicity (in mg/kg body weight) and differential gender susceptibility: chlordane, 150–700; heptachlor, 100 (male), 163 (female); dieldrin, 25–170; oxychlordane, 20; endosulfan 43 (male), 18 (female); aldrin, 10–70; endrin, 6–43 (male), 5–16 (female); isobenzan, 6–11. Rats treated with a single, comparable dose of isobenzan display lethargy and piloerection, tremor, muscle twitching, labored breathing, opisthotonus, and convulsions. Animals die after about 20 h or rapidly recover. Repeated oral doses of 2.5 mg/kg/day isobenzan are lethal after 1 week. Animals given 0.86 mg/kg/day in the diet show irritability and occasional convulsions, but partial recovery occurs over a number of weeks and animals survive for 2 years; this suggests the possibility of adaptive or metabolic tolerance (43,79).

Adult rats are more vulnerable than young animals to the acute toxic effects of endrin (58); a low-protein diet increases susceptibility to this compound (11). Loss of appetite or refusal of food is a prominent feature of dieldrin intoxication (36,45). Nonconvulsive doses of organochlorine insecticides increase susceptibility of animals to convulsions by electroshock and other poisons (58).

The temporal evolution of acute neurotoxic phenomena in rodents is illustrated by the following graphic description (43):

> For example, mice given LD_{50} doses of dieldrin orally exhibit hyperexcitability, piloerection, salivation, and other signs of autonomic stimulation during the first hr. Tremoring, when it develops, is intermittent and more akin to myoclonus than to the continual tremor seen after DDT [*see* Dichlorodiphenylethane and derivatives, this volume.] In time, the my-

oclonus becomes so severe that the mice adopt very characteristic postures with all four feet widely spread and all limbs extended. Some prop themselves into corners of the cage and maintain a constant push against the cage through their extended limbs. Intermittent, severe clonus occurs abruptly without warning, and the mouse may rear and paw the air near his face, looking much like a shadowboxer. This process is eventually terminated by a seizure which often starts as an especially severe jerk or series of jerks accompanied by vocalization. The mouse begins to run rapidly around the cage only to eventually collapse onto his side. The seizure which follows develops rapidly and usually exhibits four components: (1) a short phase of clonic activity, (2) the development of a tonic flexion followed by a transition to (3) a tonic extension phase. The mouse may die at this point or progress to (4) a final clonic period followed by a postictal prostration. Those that survive the seizures may experience one of three fates. They may remain stuporous and inactive for a period, then recover without further incidence. They may die during the postictal period. They may recover and repeat the process up to and including additional seizures. Similar phenomena have been reported in various species for aldrin and dieldrin,[10,143] [(42,76)] endrin,[10,143] [(42,76)] Telodrin[R],[10,137] [(42,79)] toxaphene,[136] [(6)] endosulfan,[139,144] [(29,30)] and lindane.[138,145] [(38,59)] [From Joy (43).]

Development of apparently reversible blindness reportedly has been associated with some cyclodiene compounds, notably endosulfan (58). Sheep apparently became blind 1 week after their first exposure to a pasture sprayed with endosulfan, with recovery over a period of 1 month (21). Pigs and lambs reportedly developed ataxia and inability to stand after a comparable exposure (67).

Human Studies

Controlled studies have been carried out in adult male humans treated orally with pure dieldrin (*i.e.*, >99.9% HEOD). Subjects received a daily dose of 0.211 mg (*n* = 3), 0.050 mg (*n* = 3), 0.010 mg (*n* = 3), or vehicle (*n* = 3) for 18 months. The two highest dose groups continued at the same dosage level for a further 6 months, while the other two groups were both given 0.211 mg/day per person. All reportedly remained healthy, and there were no treatment-related electroencephalographic changes (*vide infra*) (39,40,55).

Single or repeated accidental exposures by ingestion or extensive skin contamination have been responsible for cases of human poisoning. Gastrointestinal exposure to chlordane has been associated with death (28–56 mg/kg body weight, adult with alcoholism), convulsions and re-

covery (10–28 mg/kg, infants; 32 mg/kg, adult), and relatively mild illness (0.53–2.9 mg/kg) (15,31,49).

Individuals with violent convulsions following chlordane intoxication showed serum levels of 2.7–3.4 ppm; these levels dropped rapidly over 3–4 days but remained detectable for 3 months during which recovery was complete. No changes in the electroencephalogram (EEG) were seen in three cases >24 h after chlordane exposure when neurological signs had subsided (5,13,15). Plasma levels in a fatal case were 4.87 ppm 2 h after death, with higher levels in liver (59.9 ppm), brain (23.3 ppm), and adipose tissue (22 ppm) (46).

Poisoning with aldrin, dieldrin, endrin, and other pesticides has been associated with ingestion of contaminated seed grain or flour. Homicidal and suicidal cases have also occurred. Mortality rates for consumption of endrin-contaminated bread have ranged between 0% (150 ppm contamination) and 1.4% (48 ppm) to as high as 9% (1339–1807 ppm) (14,16,77). Occupational exposure during manufacture or application of CCIs has also resulted in intoxication. Dieldrin manufacture has been associated with clinical poisoning of some factory workers (42). Some groups of dieldrin sprayers rapidly (2 days) or slowly (up to 2 years) experienced high rates of illness (2%–40%), and 47%–100% of ill subjects had convulsions (32,33,53). Neurological illness has followed workplace exposure to endosulfan powder (24).

Poisoning by aldrin or dieldrin has been seen in individuals with blood levels >200 μg/l of dieldrin. Aldrin (which is rapidly metabolized to dieldrin) was fatal in a baby girl who received an estimated amount of 120 mg; a dose of 25.6 mg/kg caused serious poisoning in a young man who survived and recovered completely (58,60). For endrin, the single convulsive threshold is estimated as 0.25 mg/kg; multiple, sublethal convulsions are expected to occur at 1 mg/kg (58). A fatal case of endrin intoxication showed blood levels of 0.45 ppm at 4 h, 0.086 ppm at 6 h, and 0.071 ppm 11 days after ingestion when the subject died (58). Mortality rates for consumption of endrin-contaminated bread have ranged between 0% (150 ppm contamination) and 1.4% (48 ppm) to as high as 9% (1339–1807 ppm) (14,16,77). Levels up to 0.030 ppm have been found in convulsive and nonconvulsive subjects exposed to isobenzan.

Signs and symptoms of CCI poisoning include headache, dizziness, nausea, vomiting, muscular weakness, ataxia, and eventually convulsions; these may appear early in the course of illness, there is no aura, those affected are unconscious during the seizure, and they wake in a dazed state. Both acute and chronic intoxication may trigger convulsions in the absence of premonitory signs and symptoms (66).

Circumoral numbness, anorexia, nausea, fatigue, and myoclonic jerks were reported in a woman exposed to chlordane for 1–4 weeks (27). Convulsions induced by chlordane are accompanied by confusion, incoordination, excitability and, in some cases, coma (52). Symptoms of isobenzan poisoning in the presence or absence of dieldrin have featured headache, dizziness, drowsiness, irritability, and paresthesias in the lower extremities; recovery was slow and complete but sometimes took months. On occasion, EEG changes remained abnormal for more than 1 year; no untoward effects were seen in follow-up studies performed on average 24 years later (42,56,72).

Hyperthermia and decerebrate rigidity have been reported in children poisoned with endrin (31,41).

Occupational exposure to endosulfan has been associated with violent convulsions preceded by malaise, headache, vomiting, dizziness, weakness, and confusion, and followed by unconsciousness and confusion for 24 h (24). One case had persistent amnesia for the 1.75-h period immediately preceding and following the convulsion, and EEG findings were consistent with epilepsy 7 and 21 days later when neurological examination was otherwise normal (35). Prolonged occupational exposure to low levels of CCIs may increase sensitivity to an additional acute exposure, or lead to slow accumulation of insecticide and progressive symptomatology (42).

Symptoms of intoxication, including myoclonic jerking, irritability, and memory loss, were reported for up to 1 year following 6–12 months of oral exposure to grain containing aldrin and lindane (28). Postconvulsion changes in brain function are probably associated with repeated episodes of seizure-related hypoxia.

Biological monitoring of exposure to chlorinated cyclodiene insecticides requires determination of the concentration of the specific compound in blood or serum. Dieldrin serves as a biological marker of exposure to both aldrin or dieldrin. Exposure to endrin is determined from urinary metabolites (12-hydroxyendrin), since this CCI has a very short biological half-life in blood (66). The EEG also serves as a biological monitor of patients suspected of CCI poisoning; characteristic findings consist of bilateral, synchronous theta wave activity, and occasional bilateral, synchronous spike-and-wave complexes are said to be typical (43).

Treatment of organochlorine insecticide intoxication is symptomatic. Contaminated skin is washed with soap and water; eyes are flushed with water for at least 10 min. Treatment for ingestion consists of gastric lavage, avoiding aspiration into the lungs, followed by intragastric administration of 3–4 tablespoonfuls of activated charcoal and 30 g of magnesium or sodium sulfate in 30% solution. Fats, oils, and milk should be avoided because these promote absorption of organochlorine insecticides from the intestinal tract. Convulsions are treated with single or, if required, repeated intravenous (i.v.) application of an anticonvulsant benzodiazepine (diazepam, 0.3 mg/kg i.v., maximum dose of 10 mg) (22,66).

Toxic Mechanisms

Chlorinated cyclodiene insecticides inhibit binding of [^{35}]t-butylbicyclophosphorothionate (TBPS) to the picrotoxinin-binding site of the GABA receptor in rat brain synaptic membranes (47). They interfere with chloride ion flux through GABA-gated chloride channels (GABA$_A$) responsible for maintaining excitable membranes in a hyperpolarized state, thereby decreasing neuronal excitability (1,10,23,25,26). The neurotoxic potency of CCIs generally matches their ability to displace TBPS binding to the GABA$_A$ receptor (i.e., endrin > endosulfan I > endosulfan II > heptachlor epoxide > dieldrin > lindane > heptachlor and aldrin) (78).

Repeated administration of dieldrin accelerates amygdaloid kindling, the process by which repeated, subconvulsive electrical stimulation of the brain eventuates in seizures (43,44). The limbic system seems to have an important role in the convulsant effects of dieldrin (63,64).

Peripheral nerves are largely unaffected by CCIs. Dieldrin has no appreciable effect on the neurophysiological properties of invertebrate (fish, squid) or vertebrate nerve fibers (3,4,68–70). A single report claimed that endrin produced selective alterations in unmyelinated fibers of mouse sciatic nerve (75). Skeletal muscle of rats treated with large doses of dieldrin or telodrin exhibit higher twitch tensions than controls, and tetanus develops at lower stimulus frequencies (71).

REFERENCES

1. Abalis IM, Eldefrawi ME, Eldefrawi AT (1986) Effects of insecticides on GABA-induced chloride influx into rat brain microsacs. *J Toxicol Environ Health* **18**, 13.

2. Ackerman LB (1980) Overview of human exposure to dieldrin residues in the environment and current trends of residue levels in tissue. *Pestic Monit J* **14**, 64.

3. Akkermans LMA, van der Bercken J, van der Zalm JM, van Straaten HWM (1974) Effects of dieldrin (HEOD) and some of its metabolites on synaptic transmission in the frog motor end-plate. *Pestic Biochem Physiol* **4**, 313.

4. Akkermans LMA, van der Bercken J, Verluijs-Helder M (1975) Comparative effects of DDT, allethrin, dieldrin and aldrin-transdiol on sense organs of *Xenopus laevis*. *Pestic Biochem Physiol* **5**, 451.

5. Aldrich FD, Holmes JH (1969) Acute chlordane intoxication in a child. *Arch Environ Health* **19**, 129.

6. AMA Committee on Pesticides (1952) Pharmacologic properties of toxaphene, a chlorinated hydrocarbon insecticide. *J Amer Med Assn* **149**, 1135.

7. Baron RL, Walton MS (1971) Dynamics of HEOD (dieldrin) in adipose tissue of the rat. *Toxicol Appl Pharmacol* **18**, 958.

8. Bedford CT, Harrod RK, Hoadley EG, Hutson DG (1975) The metabolic fate of endrin in the rabbit. *Xenobiotica* **5**, 485.

9. Black AMS (1974) Self poisoning with dieldrin: A case report and pharmacokinetic discussion. *Anaesthesiol Intensive Care* **2**, 369.

10. Bloomquist JR, Adams PM, Soderlund DM (1986) Inhibition of gamma-aminobutyric acid-stimulated chloride flux in mouse brain vesicles by polychlorocycloalkane and pyrethroid insecticides. *Neurotoxicology* **7**, 11.

11. Boyd EM, Stefec J (1969) Dietary protein and pesticide toxicity, with particular reference to endrin. *Can Med Assoc J* **101**, 335.

12. Clark DE, Ivie GW, Camp BJ (1981) Effects of dietary hexachlorobenzene or *in vivo* biotransformation, residue deposition, and elimination of certain xenobiotics by rats. *J Agric Food Chem* **29**, 600.

13. Curley A, Garrettson LK (1969) Acute chlordane poisoning. *Arch Environ Health* **18**, 211.

14. Curley A, Jennings RW, Mann HT, Sedlak V (1970) Measurement of endrin following epidemics of poisoning. *Bull Environ Contam Toxicol* **5**, 24.

15. Dadey JL, Kammer AG (1953) Chlordane intoxication: A report of a case. *J Amer Med Assn* **153**, 723.

16. Davies GM, Lewis I (1956) Outbreak of food poisoning from bread made from chemically contaminated flour. *Brit Med J* **2**, 393.

17. Davison KL (1973) Dieldrin ^{14}C balance in rats, sheep and chickens. *Bull Environ Contam Toxicol* **10**, 16.

18. Deichmann WB, Dressler I, Keplinger M, McDonald WE (1968) Retention of dieldrin in blood, liver and fat of rats fed dieldrin for six months. *Ind Med Surg* **37**, 837.

19. Deichmann WB, MacDonald WE, Cubit DA (1971) DDT tissue retention: Sudden rise induced by the addition of aldrin to a fixed DDT intake. *Science* **172**, 275.

20. Dequidt J, Erb F, Brice A, Van Aerde C (1973) Accumulation and transformation of heptachlor by the rat. *Bull Soc Pharm Lille* **4**, 153. [French]

21. Doman I (1971) Thiodan poisoning in sheep. *Magy Allatorv Lapja* **26**, 342. [Hungarian]

22. Ecobichon DJ (1996) Toxic effects of pesticides. In: *Casarett and Doull's Toxicology. The Basic Science of Poisons. 5th Ed.* Klaassen CD ed. McGraw-Hill, New York p. 187.

23. Eldefrawi AT, Eldefrawi ME (1987) Receptors for gamma-aminobutyric acid and voltage-dependent chloride channels as targets for drugs and toxicants. *FASEB J* **1**, 262.

24. Ely TD, MacFarlane JW, Galen WP, Hine CH (1967) Convulsions in Thiodan workers: A preliminary report. *J Occup Med* **9**, 35.

25. Fishman BE, Gianutsos G (1988) CNS biochemical and pharmacological effects of the isomers of hexachlorocyclohexane (lindane) in the mouse. *Toxicol Appl Pharmacol* **93**, 146.

26. Gant DB, Eldefrawi ME, Eldefrawi AT (1987) Cyclodiene insecticides inhibit GABA$_A$ receptor-regulated chloride transport. *Toxicol Appl Pharmacol* **88**, 313.

27. Garrettson LK, Guzlian PS, Blake RV (1985) Subacute chlordane poisoning. *J Toxicol Clin* **22**, 565.

28. Gupta PK (1975) Neurotoxicity of chronic chlorinated hydrocarbon insecticide poisoning—a clinical and electroencephalographic study in man. *Ind J Med Res* **63**, 601.

29. Gupta PK (1976) Endosulfan-induced neurotoxicity in rats and mice. *Bull Environ Contam Toxicol* **15**, 708.

30. Gupta PK, Chandra SV (1975) The toxicity of endosulfan in rabbits. *Bull Environ Contam Toxicol* **14**, 513.

31. Hayes WJ Jr (1963) *Clinical Handbook on Economic Poisons: Emergency Information for Treating Poisoning.* Publ Health Serv Publ No 476. U.S. Government Printing Office, Washington, DC.

32. Hayes WJ Jr (1957) Dieldrin poisoning in man. *Publ Health Rep* **72**, 1087.

33. Hayes WJ Jr (1959) The toxicity of dieldrin to man. *Bull WHO* **20**, 891.

34. Hayes WJ Jr (1974) Distribution of dieldrin following a single oral dose. *Toxicol Appl Pharmacol* **28**, 485.

35. Hayes WJ Jr (1982) *Pesticides Studied in Man.* Williams & Wilkins, Baltimore p. 172.

36. Hayes WJ Jr, Ferguson FF, Cass JS (1951) The toxicology of dieldrin and its bearing on field use of the compound. *J Trop Med* **31**, 519.

37. Hirai Y, Tomokuni K (1991) Levels of chlordane, oxychlordane and nonachlor in human adipose tissues. *Bull Environ Contam Toxicol* **47**, 173.

38. Hulth L, Larsson M, Carlsson R, Kihlstrom JE (1976) Convulsive action of small single oral doses of the insecticide lindane. *Bull Environ Contam Toxicol* **16**, 133.

39. Hunter CJ, Robinson J (1967) Pharmacodynamics of dieldrin (HEOD). I. Ingestion by human subjects for 18 months. *Arch Environ Health* **15**, 614.

40. Hunter CJ, Robinson J, Roberts M (1969) Pharmacodynamics of dieldrin (HEOD). Ingestion by human subjects for 18 to 24 months and postexposure for 8 months. *Arch Environ Health* **18**, 12.

41. Jacobziner H, Raybin HW (1959) Briefs on accidental chemical poisonings in New York City. *N Y State J Med* **59**, 2017.

42. Jager KW (1970) *Aldrin, Dieldrin, Endrin and Telodrin.* American Elsevier, New York.

43. Joy RM (1982) Chlorinated hydrocarbon insecticides. In: *Pesticides and Neurological Diseases.* Ecobichon DF, Joy RM eds. CRC Press, Boca Raton, Florida, p. 91.

44. Joy RM (1985) The effects of neurotoxicants on kindling and kindled seizures. *Fund Appl Toxicol* **5**, 41.

45. Keane WT, Zavon MR (1969) Dieldrin poisoning in dogs: Relationship to obesity and treatment. *Brit J Ind Med* **26**, 338.

46. Kutz FW, Strassman SC, Sperling JF *et al.* (1983) A fatal chlordane poisoning. *J Toxicol Clin Toxicol* **20**, 167.

47. Lawrence LJ, Casida JE (1984) Interactions of lindane, toxaphene and cyclodienes with brain specific *t*-butylcyclophosphorothionate receptor. *Life Sci* **35**, 171.

48. Matsumura F, Nelson JO (1970) Identification of the major metabolite product of heptachlor epoxide in rat feces. *Bull Environ Contam Toxicol* **5**, 489.

49. Menconi S, Clark JM, Langenberg P, Hryhorczyk D (1988) A preliminary study of potential human health effects in private residences following chlordane application for termite control. *Arch Environ Health* **43**, 349.

50. Moss JA, Hathway DE (1964) Transport of organic compounds in the mammal—partition of dieldrin and Telodrin between the cellular components and soluble proteins of blood. *Biochem J* **91**, 384.

51. Nomeir AA, Hajjar NP (1987) Metabolism of chlordane in mammals. *Rev Environ Contam Toxicol* **100**, 1.

52. Olanoff LS, Bristow WJ, Colcolough J, Reigart JR (1983) Acute chlordane intoxication. *J Toxicol-Clin Toxicol* **20** 291.

53. Patel TB, Rao VN (1958) Dieldrin poisoning in man. A report of 20 cases in Bombay State. *Brit Med J* **1**, 919.

54. Pearl W, Kupfer D (1972) Stimulation of dieldrin elimination by a thiouracil derivative and DDT in the rat: Enhancement of dieldrin oxidative metabolism? *Chem-Biol Interact* **4**, 91.

55. Prior PF, Deacon PA (1969) Spontaneous sleep in healthy subjects in long-term serial electroencephalographic recordings. *Electroencephalogr Clin Neurophysiol* **27**, 422.

56. Ribbens PH (1985) Mortality studies of industrial workers exposed to aldrin, dieldrin and endrin. *Int Arch Occup Environ Health* **56**, 75.

57. Robinson J, Roberts M, Baldwin M, Walker AIT (1969) The pharmacokinetics of HEOD (dieldrin) in the rat. *Food Cosmetic Toxicol* **7**, 317.

58. Smith AG (1991) Chlorinated hydrocarbon insecticides. In: *Handbook of Pesticide Toxicology. Vol 2. Classes of Pesticides.* Hayes WJ Jr, Laws ER Jr eds. Academic Press, San Diego p. 731.

59. Solomon LM (1977) Gamma benzene hydrochloride toxicity. A review. *Arch Dermatol* **113**, 353.

60. Spiotta EJ (1951) Aldrin poisoning in man. Report of a case. *Arch Ind Hyg Occup Med* **4**, 560.

61. Street JC, Chadwick RW, Wang M, Phillips RL (1966b) Insecticide interactions affecting residue storage in animal tissues. *J Agric Food Chem* **14**, 545.

62. Street JC, Wang M, Blau AD (1966a) Drug effects on dieldrin storage in rat tissue. *Bull Environ Contam Toxicol* **1**, 6.

63. Swanson KL, Woolley DE (1978) Neurotoxic effects of dieldrin. *Toxicol Appl Pharmacol* **45**, 339.

64. Swanson KL, Woolley DE (1980) Dieldrin induced changes in hippocampal evoked potentials in the rat. *Proc West Pharmacol Soc* **23**, 81.

65. Tanaka R, Fujisawa S, Nakai K (1981) Study on the absorption and protein binding of carbaryl, dieldrin and paraquat in rats fed on protein diet. *J Toxicol Sci* **6**, 1.

66. Tordoir WF, van Sittert NJ (1994) Organochlorines. *Toxicology* **91**, 51.

67. Utklev HE, Westbye C (1971) Endosulfan poisoning. *Nor Veterinaertidsskr* **83**, 31. [Swedish]

68. van der Bercken J (1972) The effect of DDT and dieldrin on myelinated nerve fibers. *Eur J Pharmacol* **20**, 205.

69. van der Bercken J, Akkermans LMA, van Langen RG (1973) The effect of DDT and dieldrin on skeletal muscle fibers. *Eur J Pharmacol* **21**, 89.

70. van der Bercken J, Narahashi T (1974) Effects of aldrintransdiol—a metabolite of the insecticide dieldrin—on nerve membrane. *Eur J Pharmacol* **27**, 255.

71. Van Genderen H, Ibrahim TM (1965) The action of dieldrin on striated muscle of the rat. *Acta Physiol Pharmacol Neerl* **13**, 193.

72. Versteeg JPJ, Jager KW (1973) Long-term exposure to the insecticides aldrin, dieldrin, endrin and Telodrin. *Brit J Ind Med* **30**, 201.

73. Wagstaff DJ, Street JC (1971) Antagonism of DDT storage in guinea pigs by dietary dieldrin. *Bull Environ Contam Toxicol* **6**, 273.

74. Walker AIT, Stevenson DE, Robinson J *et al.* (1969) The toxicology and pharmacodynamics of dieldrin (HEOD): Two-year oral exposure of rats and dogs. *Toxicol Appl Pharmacol* **15**, 345.

75. Walker JF, Philips DE (1987) An electron microscope study of endrin-induced alterations in unmyelinated fibers of mouse sciatic nerve. *Neurotoxicology* **8**, 55.

76. Walsh GM, Fink GB (1972) Comparative toxicity and distribution of endrin and dieldrin after intravenous administration in mice. *Toxicol Appl Pharmacol* **23**, 408.

77. Weeks DE (1967) Endrin food-poisoning. A report on four outbreaks caused by two separate shipments of endrin-contaminated flour. *Bull WHO* **37**, 499.

78. Woolley DE (1995) Organochlorine insecticides: Neurotoxicity and mechanisms of action. In: *Handbook of Neurotoxicology.* Chang LW, Dyer DS eds. Marcel Dekker, New York p. 475.

79. Worden AN (1969) Toxicity of Telodrin. *Toxicol Appl Pharmacol* **14**, 556.

6-Chloro-6-deoxyglucose

Peter S. Spencer

6-CHLORO-6-DEOXYGLUCOSE
$C_6H_{11}ClO_5$

NEUROTOXICITY RATING

Experimental

A   CNS toxin (astrocyte, oligodendrocyte, neuron)

6-Chloro-6-deoxyglucose (6-CDG), a chlorinated sugar developed as a male contraceptive (2), inhibits D-glucose transport into the brain and preferentially disrupts regions with high glucose consumption (7).

6-CDG is transported into the brain of adult, anesthetized rats; its affinity for the glucose carrier is greater than that for D-glucose (1). The chlorosugar inhibits D-glucose transport (K_i, 3.01 mM) in the same system (1). Glucose oxidation by brain, liver, kidney, and diaphragm was unchanged in rats given oral 6-CDG (40 mg/kg/day) for 14 days. By contrast, glucose oxidation in seminiferous tubules and activity of sperm glyceraldehyde-3-phosphate dehydrogenase [E.C. 1.2.1.12] were reduced in animals treated for the same period by oral gavage with 240 mg/kg/day and 24 mg/kg/day, respectively. Animals given single or repeated doses of 240 mg/day developed spermatoceles in ductili efferentes or caput epididymes (3). Whereas these rats were infertile, those treated with 24 mg/kg/day for periods >4 days showed reversible infertility, an effect likely mediated by inhibition of glucose utilization by spermatozoa (2). Reversible infertility was also found in marmosets treated with low doses of 6-CDG (25 mg/kg/day); however, tenfold higher doses produced hindlimb paralysis accompanied by striking CNS changes (6). Similar CNS lesions were found in male CD-1 mice treated with high doses of 6-CDG (480 mg/kg/day). Females impregnated by 6-CDG–treated males gave birth to live offspring that appeared normal.

Mice (13/24) treated with 480 mg/kg/day developed hindlimb paralysis by day 8; death occurred 2–4 days after onset of paralysis, which was associated with rapid weight loss, cervical kyphosis, and urinary retention. Withdrawal of 6-CDG treatment was followed by recovery of body weight and hindlimb function. CNS vacuolar lesions, first evident at 2 days, advanced with daily dosing. Regions most consistently affected were the spinal cord (Rexed's laminae V, VI, VII) and medullary nuclei (n. of spinal tract of trigeminal nerve, dorsal and ventral cochlear n., facial n., vestibular n., superior olivary n., paramedian reticular n.). Other lesions were variably found in the cerebellum, midbrain, and forebrain (7).

Ultrastructural study revealed early swelling of astrocyte processes (especially those in a perivascular location) and the mitochondria therein. Extracellular edema was marked. Oligodendrocytes showed vacuolar changes by day 6; thereafter, with continued dosing, neuronal and axonal degeneration were evident in affected regions of the brain and spinal cord. Peripheral axons in lumbar ventral roots and sciatic nerves were largely spared (7).

The basis for the selective neurotoxicity of 6-CDG is unknown. However, regions of the brain affected by 6-CDG correspond to areas with high glucose consumption, as demonstrated by their accumulation of 2-deoxy-D-(^{14}C)glucose from blood (10). Lesions resembling those produced by 6-CDG both in mice and marmosets are produced in rats by metronidazole and misonidazole (4,8), by the testicular toxin, 1-amino-3-chloro-2-propanol, in the rhesus monkey (5), and by 6-amino-nicotinamide (6-AN) in a number of species including rats (9). 6-AN causes accumulation of 6-phosphogluconate, which inhibits phosphoglucoisomerase with a resulting decrease in glucose consumption (7).

REFERENCES

1. Cremer JE, Cunningham VJ (1979) Effects of some chlorinated sugar derivatives on the hexose transport system of the blood/brain barrier. *Biochem J* **180**, 677.
2. Ford WCL, Waites GMH (1978) A reversible contraceptive action of some 6-chloro-6-deoxy sugars in the rat. *J Reprod Fertil* **52**, 153.
3. Ford WCL, Waites GMH (1981) The effect of high doses of 6-chloro-6-deoxyglucose on the rat. *Contraception* **24**, 577.
4. Griffin JW, Price DL, Kuethe DO, Goldberg AM (1979) Neurotoxicity of misonidazole in rats. I. Neuropathology. *Neurotoxicology* **1**, 299.
5. Heywood R, Sortwell RJ, Prentice DE (1978) The toxicity of 1-amino-3-chloro-2-propanol hydrochloride (CL88,236) in the rhesus monkey. *Toxicology* **9**, 219.
6. Jacobs JM, Duchen LW (1980) Effects of 6-chloro-6-deoxyglucose on the nervous system of the marmoset. *Neuropathol Appl Neurobiol* **6**, 236.
7. Jacobs JM, Ford WCL (1981) The neurotoxicity and antifertility properties of 6-chloro-6-deoxyglucose. *Neurotoxicology* **2**, 405.

8. Rogulja PV, Kovac W, Schmid H (1973) Metronidazole encephalopathie der Ratte. *Acta Neuropathol* 25, 36.

9. Schneider H, Cervos-Navarro J (1974) Acute gliopathy in spinal cord and brain stem induced by 6-amino-nicotinamide. *Acta Neuropathol* 27, 11.

10. Sokoloff L, Reivich M, Kennedy C et al. (1977) The (¹⁴C)deoxyglucose method for the measurement of local cerebral glucose utilization; theory, procedure and normal values in the conscious and anesthetized albino rat. *J Neurochem* 28, 897.

(2-Chloroethyl)-*N*-ethyl-2-bromo-benzylamine

Albert C. Ludolph

$$(C_6H_5CH_2)_2NCH_2CH_2Cl$$

(2-CHLOROETHYL)-*N*-ETHYL-2-BROMO-BENZYLAMINE
$C_{16}H_{19}Cl_2N$

N-(2-Chloroethyl)dibenzylamine; DSP-4

NEUROTOXICITY RATING

Experimental

A Locus ceruleus retrograde neuronal degeneration

(2-Chloroethyl)-N-ethyl-2-bromo-benzylamine (DSP-4) is a xylamine analogue and experimental neurotoxin used to deplete noradrenaline in rodent brain (2,6). The remarkable selective effect of DSP-4 is explained by its presynaptic uptake by noradrenergic neurons. Blockers of noradrenaline uptake, such as desipramine, significantly protect against DSP-4 toxicity, indicating that the high-affinity noradrenaline transporter is critical for the selectivity of the compound. Among noradrenergic cells, terminals of locus ceruleus neurons are particularly sensitive; the affinity of axon terminals of these neurons for DSP-4 and noradrenaline is two to three times higher than the affinity of noradrenergic nerve terminals originating in the tegmentum (7). After selective uptake, aziridinium ions are formed and alkylate nucleophilic cell components (8). This results in long-lasting irreversible damage to terminals of target axons of unknown specificity. Additionally, the cell bodies of the locus ceruleus degenerate, indicating that DSP-4 causes retrograde degeneration of vulnerable neurons (4).

The monoamine oxidase B (MAO B) inhibitor deprenyl, but not a monoamine oxidase A (MAO A) inhibitor such as clorgyline, protects neurons from DSP-4 toxicity. This effect apparently is unrelated to MAO B inhibition since MDL 72974—an equipotent selective inhibitor of the enzyme—does not protect against the toxic effect (3). It is possible that deprenyl blocks the uptake of DSP-4 into noradrenergic neurons by its metabolites amphetamine and methamphetamine (2).

The neurotoxic effect of DSP-4 is age-dependent. Old rats appear more vulnerable than young animals (5); this may reflect the decline of function in locus ceruleus neurons with aging. If DSP-4 is administered prenatally or in newborn rats, noradrenaline levels only decrease in the cortex, not in brain stem and cerebellum (2).

REFERENCES

1. Baumgarten HG, Zimmermann B (1992) Neurotoxic phenylalkylamines and indolalkylamines. In: *Handbook of Experimental Pharmacology. Vol. 102. Selective Neurotoxicity.* Herken H, Hucho H, eds. Springer-Verlag, Berlin, Heidelberg, New York p. 225.

2. Dudley MW, Howard BD, Cho AK (1990) The interaction of the beta-haloethyl benzylamines, xylamine, and DSP-4 with catecholaminergic neurons. *Ann Rev Pharmacol Toxicol* 30, 387.

3. Finnegan KT, Skratt JJ, Irwin I et al. (1990) Protection against DSP-4-induced neurotoxicity by deprenyl is not related to its inhibition of MAO B. *Eur J Pharmacol* 184, 119.

4. Fritschy J-M, Grzanna R (1991) Experimentally-induced neuron loss in the locus coeruleus of adult rats. *Exp Neurol* 111, 123.

5. Riekkinen P Jr, Riekkinen M, Valjakka A et al. (1992) DSP-4, a noradrenergic neurotoxin, produces more severe biochemical and functional deficits in aged than in young rats. *Brain Res* 570, 293.

6. Ross SB (1976) Long term effects of N-2-chloroethyl-N-ethyl-2-bromobenzylamine hydrochloride on noradrenergic neurons in the rat brain and heart. *Brit J Pharmacol* 58, 521.

7. Zaczek R, Fritschy J-M, Culp S et al. (1990) Differential effects of DSP-4 on noradrenaline axons in cerebral cortex and hypothalamus may reflect heterogeneity of noradrenaline uptake sites. *Brain Res* 522, 308.

8. Zieher LM, Jaim-Etcheverry G (1980) Neurotoxicity of N-(2-chloro-ethyl)-N-ethyl-2-bromobenzylamine hydrochloride (DSP-4) on noradrenergic neurons is mimicked by its cyclic aziridinium derivative. *Eur J Pharmacol* 65, 249.

2-Chloropropionic Acid

John L. O'Donoghue

$$CH_3 - \underset{\underset{Cl}{|}}{CH} - \underset{\underset{O}{\|}}{C} - OH$$

2-CHLOROPROPIONIC ACID
$C_3H_5ClO_2$

2-Chloropropanoic acid; α-Chloropropionic acid

NEUROTOXICITY RATING

Experimental

A   Cerebellar degeneration (granule cells)

2-Chloropropionic acid (CPA) is a highly irritating liquid with a pungent odor. It is used as an intermediate in the production of agrochemicals and pharmaceuticals. CPA exists as two stereoisomers; commercial samples may include either isomer or a mixture of the two. The L-isomer is used for the manufacture of some agrochemicals but is not present in the final product (3). The toxicity of the two isomers and the mixture appear to be toxicologically equivalent; the specific form of the CPA tested is indicated when it is known.

There are no significant data available on the systemic absorption, distribution, excretion, or metabolism of CPA. Observation of cerebellar damage and testicular atrophy following oral administration indicates that CPA is readily absorbed by the oral route of exposure. As it is highly irritating to the skin, it is likely to be absorbed percutaneously; lung absorption of vapors should also be expected. Propionic acid itself is metabolized through an interaction with coenzyme A and carboxylation to form methylmalonyl-coenzyme A, followed by conversion to succinic acid, which can enter the citric acid cycle. Because propionic acid may be incorporated into carbohydrates and lipids, metabolism of CPA may be expected to alter these pathways. 2-Chloropropionate has been shown to be an activator of pyruvate dehydrogenase in rats and dog (2,4,6,8,14). A consequence of activation of this pathway is stimulation of pyruvate metabolism that could result in hypoglycemia and, possibly, neurotoxicity (3). Intravenously administered 2-chloropropionate decreases blood glucose, lactate, and pyruvate in fasted rats (2) and stimulates leucine metabolism in the perfused rat heart (6). Oral 2-chloropropionate decreases plasma triglycerides but does not alter glucose levels in rats (14). In dogs given 2-chloropropionate, lactate and pyruvate were reduced, but glucose, β-hydroxybutyrate, and acetoacetate levels in the blood were unchanged (5). When a neurotoxic dose (750 mg/kg) of either the D- or L-isomer of CPA was given by oral gavage, blood glucose levels were not altered, but both isomers produced a rapid decrease in plasma pyruvate and, to a lesser degree, lactate concentration (3). Glucose, pyruvate, and lactate levels in the cerebellum were not altered by either isomer when examined at a time prior to the onset of cerebellar toxicity (3). Pyruvate and glucose oxidation in cerebellar slices taken from animals given neurotoxic doses of both isomers were not impaired 24 h after dosing (3). Cerebellar brain slices incubated with up to 10 mM of either isomer for 2 h did not show alterations in oxidation of glucose or pyruvate (3). While CPA can alter pyruvate metabolism, this change is not associated with a decrease in blood or cerebellar glucose levels; thus, the change in metabolism does not appear to be linked to the induction of cerebellar damage (3).

A single oral dose of either the L- or D-isomer of CPA (7) or a mixture of the isomers (4) can result in cerebellar damage. The oral LD_{50} of the mixture in rats was 800 mg/kg; rats surviving this dose exhibited tremors that were likely to be related to cerebellar damage (4). Single oral doses of either isomer at 750 mg/kg also resulted in cerebellar toxicity (7). A single dose of 500 mg/kg of the L-isomer was not sufficient to induce neurotoxicity, but administration of three daily doses of 250 mg/kg of the L-isomer produced effects comparable to a single dose of 750 mg/kg (7).

Rats develop neurotoxicity following exposure to CPA at significantly lower dose levels if exposure is repeated. Rats fed 0.04-mmol/kg diets of 2-chloropropionate consumed about 4–2.5 mmol/kg/day or about 434–271 mg/kg/day (1) of the salt for 12 weeks (14). Within 2–4 weeks on the diet, rats developed hindlimb weakness and abnormal gaits that were associated with a slight reduction in motor nerve conduction velocity. These effects were assumed to be due to PNS damage; the CNS was not examined. Testicular atrophy and growth retardation were also noted.

Among groups of rats fed 1.0%, 0.5%, 0.25%, or 0.1% diets containing mixed isomers of CPA (dose levels were 207–320, 220, 171, and 78 mg/kg, respectively), clinical abnormalities were seen in all dose groups but the lowest (4). The 1.0% group began to have difficulty walking and developed gross ataxia and tremors after 3–4 days on the diet. Animals that were taken off the diet after 8 days showed little or no improvement over a 36-day recovery period. The 0.5% diet group developed comparable signs of neurotoxicity in 6 days. Rats fed the 0.25% diet for 6 days began to show signs of increased sensitivity to stimulation, especially to sound, and ataxia; however, the clinical signs in these animals did not change even though the diet was fed for another 36 days. The 0.1% diet group did not show clinical evidence of toxicity, even after 38 days. When 1% sodium 2-chloropropionate diets were fed, the onset of ataxia was delayed from 3–4 days to 10 days, but neutralization of the acid had no effect on the eventual outcome. In feeding studies with L-CPA, male rats were slightly more sensitive to its neurotoxic effects than females (7).

Morphological studies with the L-isomer (7) and a mixed isomer preparation (4) produced essentially similar lesions. The gross appearance of the unfixed brains from intoxicated animals was either normal or displayed an edematous cerebellum (4,7). After a single dose of CPA, lesions were well developed by 3 days (7). In affected areas, individual granule cells showed condensation of the nuclear chromatin, pyknosis, karyorrhexis, and karyolysis. Lesions typically were focal in nature with confluency of foci into large areas of granule cell loss. Astrocyte hypertrophy and hyperplasia were limited to areas with degenerating granule cells (7). In affected areas, the region around degenerating granule cells showed edema or vacuolization (4,7). Small numbers of Purkinje cells in areas with extensive granule cell necrosis were condensed and eosinophilic (7). The first appearance of Purkinje cell degeneration was observed 36 h after a single neurotoxic dose of D- or L-CPA (7). In more chronic lesions, areas of gliosis became mineralized (4). Other regions of the brain and the PNS showed no pathologic changes (4,7).

The reason for the selectivity of this neurotoxin on the cerebellar granule cells is unknown. Rats given sufficient L-CPA to cause near-total loss of cerebellar granule cells in 5 days (250 mg/kg/day for 3 days) produced a marked reduction in cerebellar kainate and N-methyl-D-aspartate (NMDA) receptor concentrations, which are known to be associated with granule cell somata (9). Concentrations of the granule-cell neurotransmitters, aspartate and glutamate, were reduced. Density of adenosine A1 receptors in the cerebellar cortex was not altered, suggesting that granule cell axons were not affected during early stages of intoxication. Changes in the concentrations of γ-aminobutyric acid, glutamine, and taurine in the cerebellar cortex were considered secondary to granule cell loss (9). Increased ^{125}I-endothelin-1 binding in the molecular layer of the cerebellar cortex was observed following the period of acute granule cell necrosis; this change is regarded as a secondary effect associated with an increase in astrocyte processes in the molecular layer (10).

Two factors that appear to play significant roles in the appearance of neurotoxicity following exposure to CPA are hepatic and cerebellar glutathione levels, and activation of a subpopulation of NMDA receptors located on granule cells. There is a rapid, dose-, and time-dependent reduction in hepatic nonprotein sulfhydryl levels and a slower reduction in cerebellar nonprotein sulfhydryl level prior to the onset of neurotoxicity (12). A single dose of 750 mg/kg of L-CPA produced an 85% reduction in total glutathione levels in the cerebellum, but no increase in oxidized glutathione (12). Recovery of glutathione levels was relatively rapid in the liver, but slower in the cerebellum such that repeated doses of L-CPA caused increasingly sharper declines in total glutathione levels prior to the onset of granule cell necrosis. *In vitro* data suggest that the depletion in hepatic glutathione is due to the formation of a 2-S-glutathionyl propanoic acid adduct catalyzed by a theta-class glutathione S-transferase. Neither the transferase nor adduct formation was observed *in vitro* in cerebellar cytosol (12). Administration of buthionine sulfoximine, an inhibitor of glutathione synthesis, enhances the neurotoxicity and transmitter changes caused by L-CPA (13).

Supplementation of glutathione levels with the isopropyl ester of glutathione protected rats against the neurotoxic effect of L-CPA (13). The depletion of glutathione in the rat cerebellum may be due to a reduction in the delivery of glutathione precursors by the cysteine conjugate of L-CPA formed in the liver (13). While glutathione depletion may increase the susceptibility of the cerebellum to CPA, it is not clear that it causes the observed neurotoxicity. Administration of dizocilpine (MK-801)—an irreversible open-channel NMDA receptor antagonist—prior to administration of L-CPA, completely prevents CPA-induced neurotoxicity and the neurochemical changes that precede it (11). Current data suggest that CPA produces its effects through the activation of a discrete subpopulation of NMDA receptors located on cerebellar granule cells (11).

There are no reported cases of human or domestic animal neurotoxicity due to CPA. The American Conference of Governmental Industrial Hygienists has established a Threshold Limit Value (TLV) of 0.1 ppm for CPA (1). The TLV is based on the presence of testicular atrophy in rats at 78 mg/kg and provision of an adequate safety margin (1).

REFERENCES

1. American Conference of Governmental Industrial Hygienists (1991) 2-Chloropropionic acid. In: *Documentation of Threshold Limit Values. Vol 1. 6th Ed.* Cincinnati, Ohio p. 305.
2. Crabb DW, Harris RA (1979) Mechanism responsible for the hypoglycemic actions of dichloroacetate and 2-chloropropionate. *Arch Biochem Biophys* **198**, 145.
3. Lock EA, Gyte A, Widdowson P *et al.* (1995) Chloropropionic acid-induced alterations in glucose metabolic status: possible relevance to cerebellar granule cell necrosis. *Arch Toxicol* **69**, 640.

4. O'Donoghue JL (1985) Aliphatic halogenated hydrocarbons, alcohols, acids, and their thioacids. In: *Neurotoxicity of Industrial and Commercial Chemicals. Vol II.* O'Donoghue JL ed. CRC Press, Boca Raton, Florida p. 99.

5. Ribes G, Valette G, Valette JF, Loubatieres-Mariani MM (1981) Sodium 2-chloropropionate: Its effects on experimental hyperlactemia in the dog. *J Pharmacol Exp Ther* **216**, 172.

6. Sans RM, Jolly WW, Harris RA (1980) Studies on the regulation of leucine catabolism. III. Effects of dichloroacetate and 2-chloropropionate on leucine oxidation in the heart. *J Mol Cell Cardiol* **12**, 1.

7. Simpson MG, Wyatt I, Jones HB *et al.* (1996) Neuropathological changes in rat brain following oral administration of 2-chloropropionic acid. *Neurotoxicology* **17**, 471.

8. Whitehouse S, Cooper RH, Randle P (1974) Mechanisms of activation of pyruvate dehydrogenase by dichloroacetate and other halogenated carboxylic acids. *Biochem J* **141**, 761.

9. Widdowson PS, Gyte A, Simpson MG *et al.* (1996) Changes in cerebellar amino acid neurotransmitter concentrations and receptors following administration of the neurotoxin L-2-chloropropionic acid. *Toxicol Appl Pharmacol* **136**, 57.

10. Widdowson PS, Simpson MG, Wyatt I, Lock EA (1995) [^{125}I]endothelin binding in rat cerebellum is increased following L-2-chloropropionic acid-induced granule cell necrosis. *Peptides* **16**, 897.

11. Widdowson PS, Wyatt I, Gyte A *et al.* (1996) L-2-Chloropropionic acid-induced neurotoxicity is prevented by MK-801: Possible role of NMDA receptors in the neuropathology. *Toxicol Appl Pharmacol* **136**, 138.

12. Wyatt I, Gyte A, Mainwaring G *et al.* (1996) Glutathione depletion in the liver and brain produced by 2-chloropropionic acid: Relevance to cerebellar granule cell necrosis. *Arch Toxicol* **70**, 380.

13. Wyatt I, Gyte A, Simpson MG (1996) The role of glutathione in L-2-chloropropionic acid induced cerebellar granule cell necrosis in the rat. *Arch Toxicol* **70**, 724.

14. Yount EA, Felton SY, O'Connor BL *et al.* (1982) Comparison of the metabolic and toxic effects of 2-chloropropionate and dichloroacetate. *J Pharmacol Exp Ther* **222**, 501.

Chloroquine

William A. Meier-Ruge
Herbert H. Schaumburg

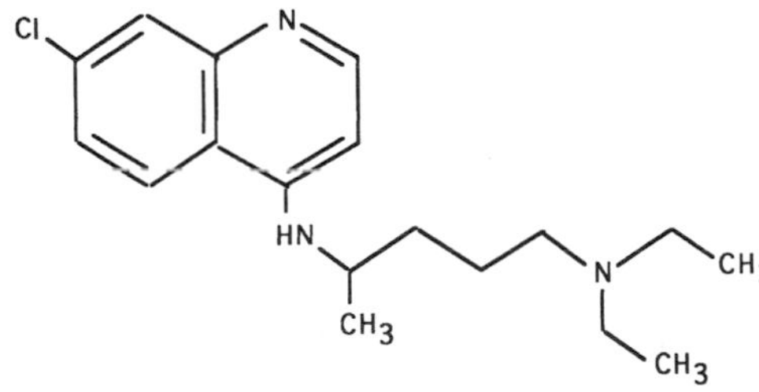

CHLOROQUINE
$C_{18}H_{26}ClN_3$

7-Chloro-4-(4-diethylamino-1-methylbutylamino)quinoline

NEUROTOXICITY RATING

Clinical

A Retinopathy (pigmentary degeneration)

A Ototoxicity

B Acute encephalopathy (psychosis, cognitive dysfunction)

B Neuromuscular transmission syndrome

B Peripheral neuropathy

B Myopathy

Experimental

A Retinopathy (pigment epithelium degeneration)

A Myopathy

Chloroquine an antimalarial and anti-inflammatory 4-aminoquinoline derivative, is dispensed as chloroquine phosphate ($C_{18}H_{26}ClN_2 \cdot 2H_3PO_4$; MW, 516; 500 mg equivalent to 300 mg chloroquine base) or chloroquine hydrochloride (MW 516; 500 mg are equivalent to 400 mg chloroquine base). Hydroxychloroquine (7-chloro-4-[4'-[ethyl-(2-hydroxyethyl) amino]-1'-methylbutylamino] quinoline; $C_{18}H_{26}ClN_3O$; MW, 335.87) is used mainly as hydroxychloroquine sulfate ($C_{18}H_{28}ClN_3O_5S$); 500 mg is equivalent to 387.5-mg hydroxychloroquine base).

Chloroquine phosphate forms water-soluble colorless crystals. The compound is stable in solution at pH 4.0–6.5. The solubility of chloroquine decreases at pH >7.0; it is insoluble in ethanol or diethylether. Chloroquine phosphate is sensitive to light and exhibits photodegradation.

Chloroquine is primarily used to treat malaria. It is effective against the asexual erythrocytic forms of *Plasmodium vivax* and *P. falciparum*. In much higher doses, chloroquine is used to treat rheumatoid arthritis and discoid lupus erythematosus (10). Similar doses are employed in treatment of porphyria cutanea tarda and solar urticaria.

Chloroquine is active on clonorchis and opisthorchis liver flukes. *Onchocerca volvulus* does not infect patients on antimalarial chloroquine prophylaxis.

General Toxicology

Inhibition of DNA replication is held as the primary chloroquine effect in malaria. Chloroquine inactivates DNA by combining with it 1:4 stoichiometrically (2). Incorporation of ^{32}P-labeled phosphate into RNA and DNA is inhibited by chloroquine (20,52); the RNA polymerase is only moderately inhibited (8). Interaction of chloroquine with DNA polymerase has been demonstrated. Chloroquine is completely absorbed after oral administration in humans. Plasma levels peak 1–3 h after a single oral dose; 55%–60% is bound to plasma proteins (mainly albumin and a glycoprotein), granulocytes, and thrombocytes. Only 15% of chloroquine remains free in the plasma.

Chloroquine is rapidly distributed throughout the body. Relative to the plasma concentration, 200–700 times higher levels occur in liver, kidney, spleen, and lung. Chloroquine is found at lower concentrations in erythrocytes, CNS, and the gut. Very high concentrations are observed in melanin-containing structures such as the iris, uvea, and pigment epithelium in the retina.

Fifty-five to 70% of chloroquine is slowly excreted unchanged in the urine, 25%–30% is metabolized in the liver (31,32). Principal metabolites are desethylchloroquine and bisdesethylchloroquine. Five to 10% appears in the feces.

Clearance occurs in three phases, with half-lives of 50 h, 6–7 days, and 17 days. After cessation of chloroquine therapy, small amounts of chloroquine are found in urine for as long as 5 years. The slow excretion explains the progression of toxic lesions following drug withdrawal.

Chloroquine, in doses used for antimalarial treatment and prophylaxis, has few side effects. Neuromyopathy and acute encephalopathy are rare; they occur at prolonged high doses used for lupus and rheumatoid disease. Chloroquine accumulates in melanin-bearing structures (choroid, iris, pigment epithelium) and, in the high levels used to treat rheumatoid arthritis, may cause a time- and dose-related irreversible retinopathy (33,34,46). The primary retinal lesion of chloroquine is damage to the pigment epithelium; the visual cells are affected secondarily (33,37,38).

Animal Studies

Chloroquine retinopathy was first reported in rabbits and cats in 1965 (27,33,39,46). Funduscopic examination showed a finely punctate pigmentation of the retina; retinal changes progressed even after withdrawal of chloroquine.

The morphological changes, a markedly thickened pigmentary epithelium, resemble postmortem human tissues (5,42). Increased acid phosphatase activity and an increased level of periodic acid–Schiff (PAS)-positive substances are also present in the pigmentary epithelium. The material stored in the pigmentary epithelium is an acidic phospholipid (25). Melanin is lost and, in later stages, degenerative changes of visual cells occur (33,34,37,38). Chloroquine retinopathy has also been produced in monkeys (49), rats (53), and pigs (18,26). Retinal lesions are directly related to the melanin-binding property of chloroquine (37–39).

Administration of 25 mg/kg of chloroquine to rats for periods up to 100 days produced a vacuolar myopathy (29) resembling the changes in humans. Vacuolation and splitting of muscle fibers were widespread. Ultrastructural analysis suggested that vacuole formation resulted from proliferation of tubular and sarcoplasmic membranes, with encirclement of small cytoplasmic spaces by the membranes.

In Vitro Studies

The effect of chloroquine on cellular differentiation and viability has been examined in primary cell cultures of embryonic chicken retina, pigmentary epithelium, and brain (6). Reduced viability was observed maximally in the pigmentary epithelium. Differentiation of neural cells was affected at much lower chloroquine concentrations in the following order: brain neurons > astroglia > retinal neurons.

Human Studies
Retinopathy

The safe daily dose of chloroquine is considered to be 100–120 mg (23,43). Retinopathy is extremely rare in conventional antimalarial dosages. High daily chloroquine doses of >250 mg (3.5–4.0 mg/kg), used for the long-term treatment of rheumatoid arthritis, can cause irreversible retinopathy (7,11,30,45). The threshold dose for chloroquine retinopathy is 5.1 mg/kg/day (hydroxychloroquine 7–8 mg/kg/day) (43). With a cumulative dose of 300 g chloroquine administered over a period of 3 years, the probability of a toxic retinopathy is in the range of 80% (43). The incidence of chloroquine retinopathy is three times greater in patients with lupus erythematosus than in rheumatoid arthritis (43,56). The risk of developing chloroquine retinopathy increases with age, in particular after age 60. Exposure to intense light amplifies the risk of retinopathy (14,34,44,49). The advanced retinal lesions have distinctive funduscopic findings. The characteristic chloroquine maculopathy, the "bull's-eye" (an intact fovea surrounded by a depigmented ring, in turn surrounded by a hyperpigmented area) is accompanied by optic atrophy. Central scotomata with decline of central visual acuity is common (21). There are no totally reliable easy means of detecting chloroquine retinopathy (1,3). The electroretinogram may show nonspecific decrements in b- and c-wave amplitudes (51). Color vision is disturbed and, sometimes, the c-wave disappears (7,19). Amsler grid testing is sometimes a simple, rapid, reproducible and sensitive diagnostic screening procedure for chloroquine retinopathy (4,12,13).

Morphological studies show the finely punctate chloroquine retinopathy to be characterized by a marked thickening and enlargement of the pigment epithelium (5,42). These cells contain PAS-positive substances and increased sulfhydryl groups. In supravitally stained cryostat sections, the pigment epithelium is swollen up to five times its original thickness. These lesions are initially scattered but eventually become diffuse (4,33,35,36). Retinotoxic side effects at dose levels used for malarial prophylaxis are rare (14,40,44,55). The chloroquine derivative hydroxychloroquine is less retinotoxic than chloroquine (31). A mild pigmentary maculopathy developed in 29% of patients treated with a cumulative dose of 900 g (15,41). Two cases of systemic lupus erythematosus developed atypical maculopathy after 10 years of treatment with hydroxychloroquine (cumulative doses of 1788 g and 2920 g) (17,57). Dosages under 6.5 mg/kg/day (<455 mg/day/70 kg) for more than 10 years have not caused retinopathy (4,24).

Neuromuscular Transmission Syndrome

Long-term administration of high dosages of chloroquine (250–750 mg/day) can cause a vacuolar myopathy in humans, similar to the condition it produces in experimental animals (16). Patients experience insidious onset of proximal weakness accompanied by elevated serum levels of serum glutamic oxaloacetic transaminase, serum glutamate pyruvate transaminase, and creatine phosphokinase. Muscle biopsy findings include acid phosphatase–positive vacuoles, myofiber necrosis, and curvilinear body inclusions. Discontinuing chloroquine is followed by recovery in most instances. Cardiomyopathy and axonal polyneuropathy sometimes accompany the vacuolar myopathy. Cardiomyopathy is manifested as biventricular heart failure with diminished ventricular ejection fractions. The axonal polyneuropathy is characterized by mild limb distal sensory loss and areflexia. Sural nerve biopsy in one instance disclosed myeloid and dense bodies in Schwann cell cytoplasm and curvilinear bodies in pericytes. Chloroquine also may impair neuromuscular dysfunction and should not be given to individuals with myasthenia gravis (47).

Acute Encephalopathy

Psychotic symptoms (paranoia, aggressiveness, depression, confusion) may occur within weeks of commencing therapy. Long-term therapy may be accompanied by impairment of memory and perception. Children may experience a reversible acute extrapyramidal syndrome that includes torticollis and dystonia.

Chloroquine can cause tinnitus and deafness. Deafness mainly appears after prolonged application of high drug dosages (54). The pathogenesis of chloroquine ototoxicity is unclear. In albino rats, no accumulation of chloroquine is observed in the inner ear. It is suggested that ototoxicity is associated with damage to the stria vascularis (9).

Toxic Mechanisms

Toxic retinopathy occurs when chloroquine has been given for a sufficiently long time and is associated with a high level of the drug in the choroidal capillaries (37–39). The concentration of the compound is always higher in the choroidal capillaries than in the systemic circulation; the difference is due to the steady adsorption of chloroquine by melanin. Since the melanin content of the choroid is similar in both eyes, the toxic levels attained and the subsequent deterioration in the metabolism of pigmented epithelium and/or visual cells is symmetrical (35–38). Conversely, the blood level of chloroquine in the vessels of the retina (inner retinal layers) is low, as in the brain.

Chloroquine interferes with the enzymatic activity of melanocytes by inhibiting protein metabolism (28,50), causing melanin depletion from melanin-bearing cells of the pigment epithelium.

The defect of color vision observed in chloroquine retinopathy is a consequence of disturbed protein metabolism (19,43) and inhibition of outer rod segment regeneration (22).

The irreversible blindness associated with chloroquine retinopathy stems from the inability of the pigmentary epithelium to isomerize all-*trans* retinene to 11-*cis* retinene. Vitamin A metabolism, which depends on an intact protein metabolism of the pigment epithelium, is severely disturbed (36–38).

Accumulation of chloroquine in the uvea, coupled with slow urinary excretion, explains the progression of a chloroquine retinopathy after drug discontinuation (50).

Myotoxicity may reflect lysosomal accumulation of chloroquine with subsequent enzyme inhibition. Chloroquine accumulates in lysosomes causing an elevation in intralysosomal pH and inhibition of acidic lysosomal hydrolases. Subsequent accumulation of phospholipids, glycogen, and curvilinear bodies occurs. The phospholipid-containing myeloid bodies in Schwann cells have also been experimentally demonstrated to be lysosomal in origin. Chloroquine-treated cells are unable to process lipids at a normal rate and myeloid bodies accumulate.

REFERENCES

1. Adlakha D, Crews SJ, Shearer ACI, Tonks EL (1968) Electrodiagnosis in drug-induced disorders of the eye. *Trans Ophthal Soc UK* **87**, 267.

2. Allison JL, O'Brien RL, Han FE (1965) DNA: reaction with chloroquine. *Science* **149**, 1111.

3. Bernstein HN (1983) Ophthalmologic considerations and testing in patients receiving longterm antimalarial therapy. *Amer J Med* **75**, 25.

4. Bernstein HN (1991) Ocular safety of hydroxychloroquine. *Ann Ophthalmol* **23**, 292.

5. Bernstein HN, Ginsberg J (1964) The pathology of chloroquine retinopathy. *Arch Ophthalmol* **71**, 238.

6. Bruinink A, Zimmermann G, Riesen F (1991) Neurotoxic effects of chloroquine *in vitro*. *Arch Toxicol* **65**, 480.

7. Crews SJ (1969) Some aspects of retinal drug toxicity. *Ophthalmologia* **158**, 232.

8. Cohen SN, Yielding KL (1965) Inhibition of DNA and RNA polymerase reactions by chloroquine. *Proc Nat Acad Sci USA* **54**, 521.

9. Dencker L, Lindquist NG (1975) Distribution of labelled chloroquine in the inner ear. *Arch Otolaryngol* **101**, 185.

10. Dubois EL (1978) Antimalarials in the management of discoid and systemic lupus erythematosus. *Semin Arthritis Rheum* **8**, 33.

11. Elman A, Gullberg R, Nilsson E *et al.* (1976) Chloroquine retinopathy in patients with rheumatoid arthritis. *J Rheumatol* **5**, 161.

12. Easterbrook M (1984) The use of Amsler grids in early chloroquine retinopathy. *Ophthalmology* **91**, 1368.

13. Easterbrook M (1988) Ocular effects and safety of antimalarial agents. *Amer J Med* **85**, 23.

14. Easterbrook M (1992) Long-term course of antimalarial maculopathy after cessation of treatment. *Can J Ophthalmol* **27**, 237.

15. Ehrenfeld M, Nesher R, Merin S (1986) Delayed-onset chloroquine retinopathy. *Brit J Ophthalmol* **70**, 281.

16. Estes ML, Ewing-Wilson D, Chou SM *et al.* (1987) Chloroquine neuromyotoxicity. *Amer J Med* **82**, 447.

17. Finbloom DS, Silver K, Newsome DA, Gunkel R (1985) Comparison of hydroxychloroquine and chloroquine use and the development of retinal toxicity. *J Rheumatol* **12**, 692.

18. Gleiser CA, Dukes TW, Lawwill T *et al.* (1969) Ocular changes in swine associated with chloroquine toxicity. *Amer J Ophthalmol* **67**, 399.

19. Grutzner P (1969) Acquired color vision defects secondary to retinal drug toxicity. *Ophthalmologica* **158**, 592.

20. Hahn FE (1968) Interaction of antimalarials with DNA. *Hoppe Seyler's Z Physiol Chem* **349**, 955.

21. Henkind P, Carr RE, Siegel IM (1964) Early chloroquine retinopathy. *Arch Ophthalmol* **71**, 157.

22. Ivanina TA, Sakina NL, Lebedva MN, Borovjagin VL (1988) A study of the mechanisms of chloroquine retinopathy. Chloroquine effect on protein synthesis of retina. *Ophthalmic Res* **21**, 272.

23. Jeremy R (1986) A critical appraisal of therapy in rheumatoid arthritis. *Med J Australia* **1**, 818.

24. Johnson MW, Vine AK (1987) Hydrochloroquine therapy in massive total doses without retinal toxicity. *Amer J Ophthalmol* **104**, 139.

25. Klinghardt GW (1981) Pathology of the neuron, preferences and differences in the participation of neuronal system in experimental storage dystrophy due to chloroquine. *Acta Histochem Suppl* **24**, 41.

26. Klinghardt GW, Fredman P, Svennerholm L (1981) Chloroquine intoxication induces ganglioside storage in nervous tissue: A chemical and histopathological study of brain, spinal cord, dorsal root ganglia, and retina in the miniature pig. *J Neurochem* **37**, 897.

27. Kuhn H, Steiger A (1981) Structural alterations of tapetal cells in the retina of cats induced by prolonged treatment with chloroquine. *Cell Tissue Res* **215**, 263.

28. Lefler CF, Filja HS, Holdbrook DJ (1973) Inhibition of aminoacylation and polypeptide synthesis by chloroquine and primaquine in rat liver *in vitro*. *Biochem Pharmacol* **22**, 715.

29. MacDonald RD, Engel AG (1973) Experimental chloroquine myopathy. *J Neuropathol Exp Neurol* **29**, 479.

30. Marks JS (1982) Chloroquine retinopathy: Is there a safe daily dose? *Ann Rheumatol Dis* **41**, 52.

31. McChesney EW (1983) Animal toxicity and pharmacokinetics of hydroxychloroquine sulfate. *Amer J Med* **75**, 11.

32. McChesney EW, Fasco MJ, Banks WF Jr (1967) The metabolism of chloroquine in man during and after repeated oral dosage. *J Pharmacol Exp Ther* **158**, 323.

33. Meier-Ruge W (1965) Experimental investigation of the morphogenesis of chloroquine retinopathy. *Arch Ophthalmol* **73**, 540.

34. Meier-Ruge W (1968) The pathophysiological morphology of the pigment epithelium and its importance for retinal structures and functions. *Mod Probl Ophthalmol* **8**, 32.

35. Meier-Ruge W (1972) Eye toxicity. *Excerpta Med Intern Cong Ser* **288**, 133.

36. Meier-Ruge W (1972) Drug induced retinopathy. *CRC Crit Rev Toxicol* **1**, 325.

37. Meier-Ruge W (1981) Drug induced retinopathy: Causal and clinical aspects. In: *Lecture in Toxicology. Vol. 6.* Zbinden G ed. Pergamon Press, London, New York.

38. Meier-Ruge W (1981) Drug induced retinopathy: Pathogenesis and experimental pathology. In: *Lecture in Toxi-*

cology. *Vol. 7*. Zbinden G ed. Pergamon Press, London, New York.

39. Meier-Ruge W, Cerletti A (1968) The significance of the melanin-bearing choroid in the retina. In: *Biochemistry of the Eye*. Dardenne U ed. Karger, Basel, New York p. 521.

40. Metge P, Rodor F (1980) Retinopathie à la chloroquine lors de la prophylaxie du paludisme à posologie correcte. *Therapie* **35**, 439.

41. Mills PV, Beck M, Power BJ (1981) Assessment of the retinal toxicity of hydrochloroquine. *Trans Ophthalmol Soc UK* **101**, 109.

42. Monahan RH, Horns RC (1964) The pathology of chloroquine in the eye. *Amer Acad Ophthalmol Otolaryngol* **68**, 40.

43. Nylander U (1967) Ocular damage in chloroquine therapy. *Acta Ophthalmol Copenh Suppl* **92**, 1.

44. Obikilia AG (1990) A type of macular degeneration in adult Nigerians; a possible role of chloroquine. *East Afr Med J* **67**, 614.

45. Potts AM (1968) Agents which cause pigmentary retinopathy. *Dis Nerv Syst* **29**, 16.

46. Ramsey MS, Bloodworth JMB, Engerman RL (1970) Chloroquine retinopathy in the rabbit. *J Ophthalmol* **5**, 264.

47. Robberecht W, Bednarik J, Bourgeois P *et al.* (1989) Myasthenic syndrome caused by direct effect of chloroquine on neuromuscular junction. *Arch Neurol* **46**, 464.

48. Rosenthal AR, Kolb H, Bergsma D *et al.* (1978) Chloro-quine retinopathy in the rhesus monkey. *Invest Ophthalmol Vis Sci* **17**, 1158.

49. Rubin M, Bernstein HN, Zvaifler NJ (1963) Studies on the pharmacology of chloroquine. Recommendation for the treatment of chloroquine retinopathy. *Arch Ophthalmol* **70**, 474.

50. Rubin M, Slonicki A (1966) A mechanism for the toxicity of chloroquine. *Arthritis Rheum* **9**, 537.

51. Sassaman FW, Cassidy JT, Alpern M, Maaseidvaag F (1970) Electroretinography in patients with connective tissue diseases treated with hydroxychloroquine. *Amer J Ophthalmol* **70**, 515.

52. Schellenberg KA, Coatney GR (1960) The influence of antimalarial drugs on nucleic acid synthesis in *Plasmodium gallinaceum* and *Plasmodium berghei*. *Biochem Pharmacol* **6**, 143.

53. Tobin DR, Krohel G, Rynes RI (1982) Hydrochloroquine. Seven-year experience. *Arch Ophthalmol* **100**, 81.

54. Toone EC, Hayden GD, Ellman HM (1965) Ototoxicity of chloroquine. *Arthritis Rheum* **8**, 475.

55. Vedy J, Graveline J, Carrica J *et al.* (1979) La retinopathie par les amino-4-quinolines dans la prophylaxie du paludisme. *Bull Soc Pathol Exot Filiales* **72**, 353.

56. Voipio H (1966) Incidence of chloroquine retinopathy. *Acta Ophthalmol* **44**, 349.

57. Weiner A, Sandberg MA, Gaudio AR *et al.* (1991) Hydroxychloroquine retinopathy. *Amer J Ophthalmol* **112**, 528.

Chlorpromazine and Other Neuroleptics

Arnold E. Merriam

CHLORPROMAZINE HYDROCHLORIDE
$C_{17}H_{19}ClN_2S \cdot HCl$

HALOPERIDOL
$C_{21}H_{23}ClFNO_2$

Chlorpromazine hydrochloride
2-Chloro-*N*,*N*-dimethyl-10*H*-phenothiazine-10-propanamine

Haloperidol
4-[4-(4-Chlorophenyl)-4-hydroxy-1-piperidenyl]-1-(4-fluorophenyl)-1-butanone

MOLINDONE HYDROCHLORIDE
$C_{16}H_{24}N_2O_2 \cdot HCl$

Molindone Hydrochloride
   3-Ethyl-1,5,6,7-tetrahydro-2-methyl-5-(4-morpho-
   linylmethyl)-4H-indol-4-one

PIMOZIDE
$C_{28}H_{29}F_2N_3O$

Pimozide
   1-[1-[4,4-Bis(4-fluorophenyl)butyl]-4-piperidinyl]-1,3-
   dihydro-2H-benzimidazol-2-one

THIOTHIXENE
$C_{23}H_{29}N_3O_2S_2$

Thiothixene
   N,N-Dimethyl-9-[3-(4-methyl-1-
   piperazinyl)propylidene]thioxanthene-2-sulfonamide

NEUROTOXICITY RATING
Clinical
A Extrapyramidal syndrome (parkinsonism, dystonia, akathesia,
   tardive dyskinesia)
A Neuroleptic malignant syndrome
A Seizure disorder
Experimental
A Dopamine receptor blockade

Generically referred to as "neuroleptics," these agents share common neurochemical properties, therapeutic indications, and neurotoxicological propensities, despite their heterogeneous structural forms. They form classes that are constituted of multiple agents in therapeutic use. Prototypical examples of agents within each family are shown: chlorpromazine is an example of a phenothiazine compound and represents the first neuroleptic agent to be used clinically; haloperidol is an example of a butyrophenone neuroleptic; molindone falls into the dihydroindolone category; pimozide is a diphenylbutylpiperidine agent; and thiothixene is a thioxanthene neuroleptic. Because of their clinical importance, butyrophenones are presented in a separate chapter (*see* Butyrophenones, this volume).

Neuroleptic compounds have been widely used since the mid-1950s for the treatment of psychosis, a common manifestation of schizophrenia and certain phases of the affective disorders. They have also been used with good effect in treating secondary psychotic manifestations of various neurological disorders (*e.g.*, certain of the psychiatric manifestations of dementing diseases). Finally, they have earned a place in the treatment of various hyperkinetic movement disorders (*e.g.*, chorea of diverse etiologies, hemiballismus, and tics, including those seen in Tourette's syndrome).

General Toxicology

All neuroleptic compounds are well absorbed *via* the gastrointestinal tract but exhibit a first-pass effect as they traverse the hepatic circulation, during which as much as two-thirds of the ingested dose is inactivated. Neuroleptic agents are for the most part highly lipophilic, membrane- and protein-bound; important exceptions to this statement are thioridazine and its metabolite mesoridazine, which are water-soluble. Neuroleptics accumulate not only in the brain, the site of their presumed target tissue, and the dopamine receptor components of the mesolimbic and mesocortical tracts, but also in lipid stores and in highly vascular tissues. Metabolism is primarily oxidative and is mediated by hepatic microsomal enzymes; conjugation with glucuronic acid is another important metabolic route. Multiple metabolites of neuroleptic compounds—not all of them well characterized—are known; in some cases, metabolites may exhibit biological activity. Plasma half-lives are markedly variable, both between agents and between patients, ranging from 10–40 h; the half-life of these agents' biological effect in the human brain is unknown but persists long after they clear from the plasma. This lingering effect is supported by animal studies showing behavioral drug effects that persist long after the administered drug is no longer biochemically detectable. In the human being, neuroleptic metabolites have been observed in the urine for months after cessation of drug treatment.

The principal biochemical action of these compounds is blockade of dopamine receptors, a property thought to underlie their therapeutic effect. While the limbic striatum is often mentioned as a likely key site of antipsychotic effect, this has not been conclusively demonstrated. Each of the agents discussed here displays widespread dopamine-blocking actions in other brain regions as well, including other portions of the basal ganglia, thus accounting for the agents' propensities for the induction of motor side effects. In addition to their blocking actions on dopamine receptors of diverse types, neuroleptics have blocking effects on α_1-noradrenergic receptors, muscarinic cholinergic receptors, H_1 histamine receptors, and diverse types of serotonin receptors. The various agents display widely differing affinities for these various receptor types; relevant aspects of the biochemical profile of commonly used agents are shown in Table 16 (4). It has been speculated that actions on other than the dopaminergic system may be relevant to antipsychotic efficacy; serotonin receptor blockade in particular may be an important feature. The diverse receptor blocking actions of these drugs are certainly an important aspect of their neurotoxicology, insofar as these agents trigger not only many types of motor abnormalities but also anticholinergic behavioral syndromes, autonomic symptoms, and neuroendocrine abnormalities.

Animal Studies

Neuroleptic agents demonstrate an extremely low risk of lethality even when administered in massive doses, both to the laboratory animal and to humans. The ratio of the lethal dose to the pharmacologically effective dose in laboratory animals is 25–200 for the phenothiazines and more than 1000 for the butyrophenones.

Animal studies have demonstrated a variety of chemical and ultrastructural nervous system alterations following neuroleptic exposure. The changes best documented are in the basal ganglia and affiliated structures, a localization compatible with the principal biochemical action of these dopamine-receptor blocking agents. Changes include an increase in the number of striatal dopamine receptors assessed behaviorally and *via* tritiated receptor-binding studies, in rodents exposed to haloperidol and other neuroleptics for periods of 1 week to 1 year (8,9,18,23,26). Increased size of some neurons and axon terminals in the corpus striatum, as well as collateral axonal sprouting in the substantia nigra, have been demonstrated in rats treated with 3 mg/kg/day of haloperidol for a period of 16 weeks (2,3). Selective striatal neuronal loss has been identified (13) in rats treated

with fluphenazine for a year, and an increase in the synaptic density on dendritic shafts in the medial prefrontal cortex has been seen in rats treated with chronic haloperidol (15). An increase in the number of synapses containing perforated postsynaptic densities, thought to represent the ultrastructural correlate of "strengthened" or more efficient synapses, has been identified in the caudate nuclei of rats treated with 0.5 mg/kg/day of haloperidol for 2 weeks (19). An accumulation of manganese and copper in the caudate nuclei of guinea pigs treated with 10 mg/kg/day of chlorpromazine for 10 days has also been documented (30).

In Vitro Studies

Haloperidol has been noted to be structurally similar to the neurotoxin 1-methyl-4-phenyl-1,2,3,6-tetrahydropyridine (MPTP), a poison that induces permanent parkinsonism, probably through inhibition of mitochondrial reduced nicotinamide adenine dinucleotide:ubiquinone oxidoreductase (complex I), thereby leading to cell death (*see* MPTP, this volume). Like MPTP, chlorpromazine, thiothixene, and haloperidol have been shown *in vitro* to inhibit complex I of rat brain mitochondria (6).

Neuroleptic agents are known to lower the human seizure threshold; *in vitro* techniques using perfused guinea pig hippocampal slices have been used to clarify the relative effects of different neuroleptics on penicillin-induced spike activity (24). In this model, chlorpromazine emerges as the most, and molindone the least, epileptogenic of the agents tested, parallel to the profiles of these agents in humans.

Human Studies

The neuroleptic agents have been documented to induce a variety of movement disorders, a lowering of the seizure threshold, and a potentially lethal syndrome of febrile catatonia, the neuroleptic malignant syndrome (NMS). Additionally, on the basis of blockade of adrenergic and cholinergic receptors, these agents may cause autonomic derangements, including postural hypotension, sexual dysfunction, impaired ocular accomodation, and delirium.

The movement disorders evoked by neuroleptics may be divided into those seen from the initiation of treatment and those whose appearance is delayed until exposure is persistent, typically for a matter of months or years; the latter group of movement disorders is characterized as *tardive*. Movement disorders seen early on in treatment include drug-induced parkinsonism, dystonia, and akathisia; those seen after chronic exposure include choreiform tardive dyskinesia, tardive dystonia, tardive Tourette's syndrome, tardive Meige's syndrome, tardive akathisia, tardive stereotypy, tardive myoclonus, and tardive tremor. The existence of a so-called tardive dysmentia has been claimed by some but has been difficult to disentangle from the behavioral consequences of the underlying psychiatric disorder.

Drug-induced parkinsonism is clinically similar to the idiopathic variety. Most parkinsonian manifestations disappear within a matter of weeks after cessation of neuroleptic treatment, but some individuals fully normalize only after many months. Evidence that neuroleptic agents are a cause of permanently persistent parkinsonism is lacking. In those in whom the parkinsonism is purely drug-induced and reversible, L-6-^{18}F-fluorodopa positron emission tomography demonstrated putamen ^{18}F-dopa uptake by the putamen to be normal (7), while abnormal findings were found in some patients with persistent and some with transient parkinsonism. Treatment of neuroleptic-induced parkinsonism consists of the administration of anticholinergic compounds or of amantadine; use of L-dopa (3,4-dihydroxyphenylalanine) or of other dopamine receptor agonists is not favored since such agents generally reverse the therapeutic effects of the neuroleptic agent.

Acute transient dystonia involving oral, lingual, mandibular, facial, ocular, pharyngeal, laryngeal, and/or limb musculature is common in the first several days of neuroleptic treatment, but is not likely to occur subsequently except in the wake of a substantial increase in drug dose. The diagnosis is usually clear if the physician is aware of the patient's exposure to neuroleptics.

A third acute extrapyramidal syndrome, akathisia, consists of aimless motor activity in the form of pacing, fidgeting, and postural readjustment, accompanied by a subjective sense of uncomfortable restlessness. It is encountered in the early weeks of treatment and typically lessens or spontaneously remits with time. The syndrome is sometimes mistaken for motor excitement secondary to the underlying psychiatric illness; the diagnosis is purely clinical. Treatment consists of the administration of β-adrenergic blocking agents, anticholinergic compounds, amantadine, or benzodiazepines.

The tardive syndromes are distinguished from those just described both by virtue of their delayed appearance after prolonged exposure and either their persistence, for months to years, or their actual permanence. It is estimated that about 15%–20% of patients chronically treated with neuroleptics will develop tardive dyskinesia; of these, the majority will resolve within 5 years of drug cessation. In some cases the movements are permanent and disfiguring, and may interfere with the patient's functional status. The most common form of tardive dyskinesia is a choreiform disorder involving the oral, buccal, and lingual structures; other facial muscles, the limbs, and respiratory muscles may be affected. The differential diagnosis of choreiform tardive dyskinesia includes all disorders causing chorea; Huntington's disease and neuroacanthocytosis bear particular mention, since these disorders are commonly associated with behavioral disturbance and may thus mimic the entire picture of coincident movement and psychiatric disorders. Other variants of tardive dyskinesia resemble Meige's syndrome, with blepharospasm and oromandibular movements (29); Tourette's syndrome, with vocal and/or motor tics (22); and tardive dystonia, with persistent posturing of the neck, torso, or limbs (31). These three conditions closely resemble their idiopathic counterparts and are distinguished chiefly by their appearance following prolonged neuroleptic

TABLE 16. Affinity* of Certain Antipsychotic Agents for Several Neurotransmitter Receptors[†]

Antipsychotic Agents Generic Name (Trade Name)	Receptor					
	Dopamine D-2	Histamine		Adrenergic		Muscarinic
		H$_1$	H$_2$	α$_1$	α$_2$	
Chlorpromazine (Thorazine)	5.3	11	0.03333	38	0.13	1.4
Chlorprothixene (Taractan)	13	—	—	—	—	—
Fluphenazine (Permil, Prolixin)	125	4.8	—	11	0.064	0.053
Haloperidol (Haldol)	25	0.053	0.0034	16	0.026	0.0042
Loxapine (Loxitane)	1.4	20	—	3.6	0.042	0.22
Mesoridazine (Serentil)	5.3	55	—	50	0.062	1.4
Molindone (Moban)	0.83	0.00081	0.00142	0.040	0.16	0.00026
Perphenazine (Trilafon)	71	12	—	10	0.20	0.067
Prochlorperazine (Compazine)	14	5.3	—	4.2	0.059	0.18
Thioridazine (Mellaril)	3.8	6.2	—	20	0.12	5.6
cis-Thiothixene (Navane)	222	17	0.0213	9.1	0.50	0.034
Trifluoperazine (Stelazine)	38	1.6	—	4.2	0.038	0.15

*$10^{-7} \times 1/K_d$ in which K_d is the equilibrium dislocation constant in molarity. All receptors were from human brain except the histamine H$_2$ receptor, which was from guinea pig brain.

[†]A high numerical value indicates greater binding and greater antagonism of a given receptor.

[From Black et al. (4).]

exposure. Tardive akathisia, another variant, is manifest, as is acute akathisia, by motor restlessness; in some cases the movements appear without the subjective discomfort accompanying acute akathisia, in which case the condition may be better described as tardive stereotypy (25,28). Other less common tardive variants include tardive myoclonus and tardive tremor (25).

Many treatments for choreiform tardive dyskinesia have been proposed; none is so effective to be endorsed with enthusiasm, with the possible exception of oral reserpine (11) and, in certain cases, intramuscular botulinum toxin injection (14).

Of all neurotoxic responses to neuroleptic administration, the most calamitous is NMS, a sometimes lethal syndrome characterized by the precipitous development of fever without infectious source, catatonic muscle rigidity, diminution in the level of consciousness, tachycardia, elevation and instability of the blood pressure, tachypnea, and diaphoresis. Abnormal laboratory measures include elevations in serum creatine phosphokinase, leukocytosis, and sometimes myoglobinuria. The syndrome carries the risk of death, usually due to unchecked hyperthermia or intercurrent infection. Management of a full-blown case consists of intensive care, stabilization of metabolic and hydrational parameters, and normalization of body temperature. The administration of dantrium sodium has been recommended for the purpose of relieving muscle rigidity, and the use of bromocriptine has been endorsed for the purpose of reversing CNS dopamine receptor blockade, the putative cause of the disorder (17). Cerebellar dysfunction and peripheral neuropathy have been described in survivors, compatible with nervous system damage from hyperthermia and other manifestations of critical illness. Cognitive compromise with prominent memory impairment has also been described (27), although most survivors exhibit no sequelae. Neuropathological studies of a patient who succumbed has shown indications of injuries to the hypothalamus and cerebellum (12,16).

Neuroleptics are known to lower the seizure threshold; however, the relative propensities of the various neuroleptics to evoke seizures has been difficult to ascertain. The overall risk of this complication is thought to be about 1%. Impressions based on multiple clinical series suggests that the risk of seizure is highest with chlorpromazine and lowest with molindone, haloperidol, and fluphenazine; these conclusions are compatible with rodent *in vitro* studies (24).

Neuroleptics also disinhibit the release of prolactin from the pituitary, a function under dopaminergic control; in most patients, the prolactin becomes elevated acutely but then drops toward normal (5); rarely, patients develop galactorrhea and amenorrhea. Some important neurotoxic complications of treatment result from effects on nondopaminergic neurohumoral systems involving adrenergic and cholinergic transmission. Toxic antiadrenergic effects include postural hypotension and sexual dysfunction; anticholinergic effects include impaired ocular accommodation and cognitive dysfunction, including memory and attentional impairment. Anticholinergic toxicity is more common in the context of treatment with tricyclic antidepressants, as discussed elsewhere (*see* Tricyclic Antidepressants, this volume).

Overdose is rarely fatal but may be complicated by respiratory depression, severe parkinsonism, anticholinergic delirium, and autonomic dysregulation.

Toxic Mechanisms

The elicitation of drug-induced parkinsonism by neuroleptic agents is compatible with the dopamine receptor-blocking actions of these compounds. Inhibition of complex I of the mitochondrial electron transport chain (*vide supra*) may also play a role in the production of drug-induced parkinsonism: neuroleptic-treated patients have been shown to exhibit depressed platelet mitochondrial complex I activity, similar to that reported in idiopathic Parkinson's disease (6).

The precise pathophysiology of acute dystonic reactions is unknown; it likely involves a drug-induced imbalance in the relationship between dopamine and acetylcholine in the striatum. Dystonic reactions are both relieved and prevented by the administration of anticholinergic agents.

The mechanism underlying the tardive movement disorders is likewise unknown, but the existence of these persistent or permanent sequelae implies that neuroleptics are capable of creating lasting neurochemical or structural alterations in humans, as they have been shown to do in laboratory animals. The loss of neurons in the striatum of neuroleptic-treated rats (13) has been interpreted as representing damage to cholinergic interneurons (20) and has been considered a candidate substrate of the tardive movement syndromes. The neuroradiologic identification of possible structural consequences of neuroleptic administration and of possible structural correlates of the tardive syndromes is made more difficult by the presence of morphologic abnormalities in the brains of schizophrenics and other psychiatric patients. Magnetic resonance imaging (MRI) has shown the caudate nuclei of schizophrenics with tardive dyskinesia to be smaller than those of their counterparts without tardive dyskinesia (21). In a study in which MRI was performed in schizophrenic patients prior to and then following treatment with neuroleptics, the volumes of the caudate nuclei were found to have significantly enlarged in the interim, a finding interpreted as demonstrating some intervening response to dopamine receptor blockade (10).

NMS is chiefly thought to represent the consequences of extensive dopamine receptor blockade in the basal ganglia and hypothalamus. Because of symptomatic commonalities between this syndrome and malignant hyperthermia, evidence of an abnormal interaction between neuroleptic agents and muscle cell membranes has also been sought, albeit with little success (1,17).

REFERENCES

1. Araki M, Takagi A, Higuchi I, Sugita H (1988) Neuroleptic malignant syndrome: Caffeine contracture of single muscle fibers and muscle pathology. *Neurology* **38**, 297.

2. Benes FM, Paskevich PA, Davidson J, Domesick VB (1985) The effects of haloperidol on synaptic patterns in the rat striatum. *Brain Res* **329**, 265.

3. Benes FM, Paskevich PA, Domesick VB (1983) Haloperidol-induced plasticity of axon terminals in rat substantia nigra. *Science* **221**, 969.

4. Black JL, Richelson E, Richarson JW (1985) Antipsychotic agents: A clinical update. *Mayo Clin Proc* **60**, 777.

5. Brown-Armin W, Laughren TP (1981) Tolerance to the prolactin-elevating effect of neuroleptics. *Psychiat Res* **5**, 317.

6. Burkhardt C, Kelly JP, Lim Y-H et al. (1993) Neuroleptic medications inhibit complex I of the electron transport chain. *Ann Neurol* **33**, 512.

7. Burn DJ, Brooks DJ (1993) Nigral dysfunction in drug-induced parkinsonism: An ^{18}F-dopa PET study. *Neurology* **43**, 556.

8. Burt DR, Creese I, Snyder SH (1977) Antischizophrenic drugs: Chronic treatment elevates dopamine receptor binding in brain. *Science* **196**, 326.

9. Chakos MH, Lieberman JA, Bilder RM et al. (1994) Increase in caudate nuclei volumes of first-episode schizophrenic patients taking antipsychotic drugs. *Amer J Psychiat* **151**, 1430.

10. Clow A, Jenner P, Marsden CD (1979) Changes in dopamine-mediated behavior during one year's neuroleptic administration. *Eur J Pharmacol* **57**, 365.

11. Fahn S (1985) A therapeutic approach to tardive dyskinesia. *J Clin Psychiat* **46**, 19.

12. Horn E, Bolesaw L, Lapierre Y, Hrdina P (1988) Hypothalamic pathology in the neuroleptic malignant syndrome. *Amer J Psychiat* **145**, 617.

13. Jeste DV, Lohr JB, Manley M (1992) Neuropathological changes following 4, 8 and 12 months of treatment with fluphenazine in rats. *Psychopharmacology* **106**, 154.

14. Kaufman DM (1994) Use of botulinum toxin injections for spasmodic torticollis of tardive dystonia. *J Neuropsychiat Clin Neurosci* **6**, 50.

15. Klintzova ZJ, Haselhorst NA, Ranova NA et al. (1989) The effects of the haloperidol on synaptic plasticity in rat's medial prefrontal cortex. *J Hirnforsch* **1**, 51.

16. Lee S, Merriam A, Kim T-S et al. (1989) Cerebellar degeneration in neuroleptic malignant syndrome: Neuropathologic findings and review of the literature concerning heat-related nervous system injury. *J Neurol Neurosurg Psychiat* **52**, 387.

17. Levenson JL (1985) Neuroleptic malignant syndrome. *Amer J Psychiat* **142**, 1137.

18. McKenzie RG, Zigmond MJ (1985) Chronic neuroleptic treatment increases D-2 but not D-1 receptors in rat striatum. *Eur J Pharmacol* **113**, 159.

19. Meshul CK, Casey DE (1989) Regional, reversible ultrastructural changes in rat brain with chronic neuroleptic treatment. *Brain Res* **489**, 338.

20. Miller R, Chouinard G (1993) Loss of striatal cholinergic neurons as a basis for tardive and L-dopa-induced dyskinesias, neuroleptic-induced supersensitivity psychosis and refractory schizophrenia. *Biol Psychiat* **34**, 713.

21. Mion CC, Andreasen NC, Arndt S et al. (1991) MRI abnormalities in tardive dyskinesia. *Psychiat Res-Neuroimag* **40**, 157.

22. Mueller J, Aminoff MJ (1982) Tourette-like syndrome after long-term neuroleptic drug treatment. *Brit J Psych* **141**, 191.

23. Muller P, Seeman P (1977) Brain neurotransmitter receptors after long-term haloperidol: Dopamine, acetylcholine, serotonin, alpha noradrenergic and naloxone receptors. *Life Sci* **21**, 1751.

24. Oliver AP, Luchins DJ, Wyatt RJ (1982) Neuroleptic-induced seizures. *Arch Gen Psychiat* **39**, 206.

25. Stacy M, Cardoso F, Jankovic J (1993) Tardive stereotypy and other movement disorders in tardive dyskinesias. *Neurology* **43**, 937.

26. Tarsy D, Baldessarini RJ (1974) Behavioral supersensitivity to apomorphine following chronic treatment with drugs which interfere with the synaptic function of catecholamines. *Neuropharmacology* **13**, 927.

27. van Harten PN, Kemperman JF (1991) Organic amnestic disorder: A long-term sequel after neuroleptic malignant syndrome. *Biol Psychiat* **29**, 407.

28. Weiner WJ, Luby ED (1983) Persistent akathisia following neuroleptic withdrawal. *Ann Neurol* **13**, 466.

29. Weiner WJ, Nausieda PA, Glantz RH (1981) Meige syndrome (blepharospasm-oromandibular dystonia) after long-term neuroleptic therapy. *Neurology* **31**, 1555.

30. Weiner WJ, Nausieda PA, Klawans HL (1977) Effects of chlorpromazine on central nervous system concentrations of manganese, iron, and copper. *Life Sci* **20**, 1181.

31. Wojcik JD, Falk WE, Fink JS et al. (1991) A review of 32 cases of tardive dystonia. *Amer J Psychiat* **148**, 105.

Cicutoxin

Albert C. Ludolph

CICUTOXIN
$C_{17}H_{22}O_2$

(E,E,E)-(—)-8,10,12-Heptadecatriene-4,6-diyne-1,14-diol

NEUROTOXICITY RATING

Clinical

A   Seizure disorder (status epilepticus)

B   Myopathy

Experimental

A   Seizure disorder (acute administration)

Cicutoxin is the active principle of the poisonous water hemlock, a member of the family Umbelliferae (2). Cicutoxin has a MW of 258.35; is soluble in alcohol, chloroform, ether, hot water, and alkali hydroxides; and has a MP of 67°C. The plant *Cicuta virosa* is common in Europe; in North America, the varieties *C. douglasii* and *C. maculata* are potential causes of intoxication. The roots of *Cicuta* spp. are particularly hazardous, and toxin levels peak during spring (10). Even the dry plant is known to be toxic (10), and leaves and stem of *Cicuta* spp. may contain significant quantities of cicutoxin. The plant typically occupies swampy or wet habitats along rivers or in marshes.

Cicutoxin is a highly unsaturated aliphatic alcohol that is isomeric with oenanthotoxin from the genus *Oenanthe* (1). The pharmacology and general toxicology of cicutoxin are only partly explored. Death in sheep occurs at *C. occidentalis* doses of 0.2%–0.5% body weight, in cattle at 0.1%, and in horses at 0.5% body weight (8). A study of pea chloroplasts showed that cicutoxin inhibited NADP⁺ photoreduction by 50% and the electron transport at the cytochrome *f* level by 25%–30% (13). Studies with oenanthotoxin revealed that this isomer of cicutoxin reversibly blocks K⁺ and Na⁺ channels (6), and that batrachotoxin can prevent the blocking effect on the latter (5).

Accidental livestock poisonings by *Cicuta* spp. (8,10) are most frequent in early spring. Animals develop excessive salivation, tremors, weakness, incoordination, and violent convulsions 15–60 min after oral intake; this may result in death after 60 min to 8 h (8,10). The syndrome was reproduced in a short-term feeding study of sheep (10) that recovered after nonlethal doses. CNS neuropathology was not reported, but "moderate myofiber degeneration" was observed in muscle (10). Greatly increased muscle enzyme levels were explained by the violent convulsions (10). The clinical picture in rabbits treated with oenanthotoxin is said to be indistinguishable from seizures induced by picrotoxin, a noncompetitive blocker of γ-aminobutyric acid A responses (7). In another small study in dogs (*n* = 4), injection of an alcoholic extract from *C. douglasii* produced a hypotensive effect and convulsions (15).

Water hemlock is a potent, often lethal, human poison (3,4,9–12,15). Eighty human intoxications are reported; about 30% were lethal. In some cases, death occurred 5–15 min after oral intake of water hemlock (12). The ingestion of even a small amount of roots, leaves, or stem causes a stereotyped dramatic clinical effect (3,4,9,12,15): after 15–60 min, the patient may initially complain of gastrointestinal disturbances, nausea, vertigo, and dizziness. Excessive salivation and bronchial secretion may follow. Coma soon develops, and a series of *grand mal* seizures appears. Extremely rigid generalized muscle spasms with features of opisthotonus then supervene. After recovery, patients consistently report complete amnesia, which may sometimes even be retrograde. Electroencephalographic changes persist as long as 7 days after acute poisoning (9). Laboratory investigations during the acute intoxication reveal a substantial increase of creatine kinase and other muscle enzymes. Serum creatine is also greatly increased, whereas liver enzymes are more or less unremarkable. A severe metabolic acidosis accompanies coma and seizures, and body temperature may be moderately increased during intoxication. In a single patient, electrophysiological studies of peripheral nerves were performed and yielded normal results (14). It remains unclear whether the increase of muscle enzymes is secondary to seizures and severe muscle rigidity or indicates the presence of a direct myotoxic effect.

Treatment recommendations for the acute intoxication include early gastric lavage, if possible, use of intravenous barbiturates and/or benzodiazepines to treat seizures and spasmodic movements, and intravenous administration of bicarbonate to correct metabolic acidosis. Administration of atropine is also suggested (14). Hemodialysis and hemoperfusion may be helpful, since the cicutoxin molecule was found to be dialyzable (9). Artificial ventilation may be necessary.

In summary, although the precise pharmacological background of cicutoxin poisoning is still unknown, experience from accidental poisonings in humans and domestic animals suggests that the CNS is a primary target. There is some evidence that primary muscle damage may occur.

REFERENCES

1. Anet EFLJ, Lythgoe B, Silk MH, Trippett S (1953) Oenanthotoxin and cicutoxin. Isolation and structures. *J Amer Chem Soc* 66, 309.
2. Bohlmann F (1971) Acetylenic compounds in the *Umbelliferae*. In: *The Biology and Chemistry of the Umbelliferae*. Heywood VH ed. Academic Press, London p. 279.
3. Carlton BE, Tufts E, Girard DE (1979) Water hemlock poisoning complicated by rhabdomyolysis and renal failure. *Clin Toxicol* 14, 87.
4. Costanza DJ, Hoversten VW (1973) Accidental ingestion of water hemlock. *Calif Med* 119, 78.
5. Dubois JM, Khodorov BI (1982) Batrachotoxin prevents sodium channels from the blocking action of oenanthotoxin. *Pflugers Arch* 395, 55.
6. Dubois JM, Schneider MF (1981) Block of Na-current and intramembrane charge movement in myelinated nerve fibers poisoned with a vegetable toxin. *Nature* 289, 685.
7. Grundy HF, Howarth F (1956) Pharmacological studies on hemlock water dropwort. *Brit J Pharmacol* 11, 225.
8. Kingsbury JM (1964) *Poisonous Plants of the United States and Canada*. Prentice-Hall Inc, Englewood Cliffs, NJ.
9. Knutsen OH, Patzkowski P (1984) New aspects in the treatment of water hemlock poisoning. *J Toxicol-Clin Toxicol* 22, 157.
10. Panter KE, Keeler RF, Baker DC (1988) Toxicoses in livestock from the hemlocks (*Conium* and *Cicuta* spp.). *J Anim Sci* 66, 2407.
11. Rizzi D, Basile C, Di Maggio A *et al.* (1991) Clinical spectrum of accidental hemlock poisoning: Neurotoxic manifestations, rhabdomyolysis and acute tubular necrosis. *Nephrol Dialysis Transplant* 6, 939.
12. Robson P (1965) Water hemlock poisoning. *Lancet* ii, 1274.
13. Roshchina VV, Solomatkin VP, Roshchina VD (1980) Cicutoxin as an inhibitor of electron transport in photosynthesis. *Fiziol Rast (Mosc)* 27, 704.
14. Starreveld E, Hope CE (1975) Cicutoxin poisoning. *Neurology* 25, 730.
15. Withers LM, Cole FR, Nelson RB (1969) Water-hemlock poisoning. *N Engl J Med* 281, 566.

Ciguatoxin

Jerry G. Kaplan

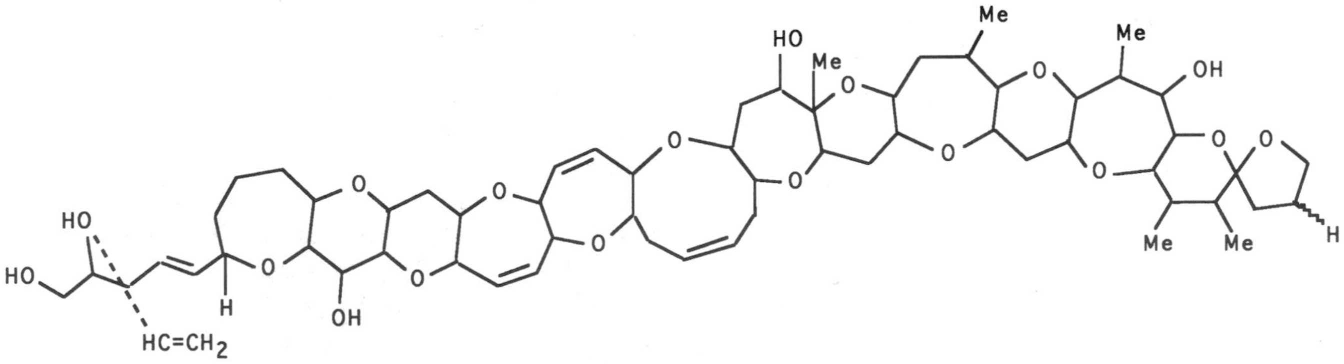

CIGUATOXIN

NEUROTOXICITY RATING

Clinical

A   Ion channel syndrome (sodium ion)

B   Autonomic neuropathy (postural hypotension)

C   Myopathy

Experimental

A   Ion channel dysfunction (sodium channel agent)

Ciguatoxin is a partially characterized, heat-stable, lipid-soluble compound elaborated by the photosynthetic dinoflagellate *Gambierdiscus toxicus* (40). The toxin is stored in the viscera of fish and passed along the food chain to progressively larger carnivorous fish. Ingestion of these fish leads to neurological, autonomic, gastrointestinal, and cardiac dysfunction (3), collectively known as *ciguatera*. Ciguatera is the most common food-borne illness caused by a chemical toxin in the United States (21) and is the most common illness related to fish consumption in the world (3).

The principal active component is a lipophilic compound named ciguatoxin (33). The isolation of ciguatoxin for structural elucidation has proven extremely difficult because of its high potency (LD_{50}, 0.45 μg/kg), (22,23), low concentration in toxic fish, sporadic distribution of cases, and toxin instability during purification (40). Studies suggest that ciguatoxin is a complex polyether of approximate MW 1100. Nuclear magnetic resonance study revealed the presence of four olefins, five hydroxyl, and five methyl groups with the oxygen atoms bound by ether linkages. Ciguatoxin is chemically similar to, and chromatographically indistinguishable from, okadaic acid. The precise structural characterization will likely depend on x-ray crystallography because of the microquantities and limited solubility of ciguatoxin (40).

Maitotoxin, a large nonpeptide (MW, 145,000), has also been implicated in cases of ciguatera. This substance is also produced by *G. toxicus* (40,41).

Other lipophilic chemicals, principally scaritoxin, have been identified in ciguatoxin-laden fish. Most are poorly characterized (41).

Ciguatoxin is widely distributed in fish. Assays suggest it is most concentrated in the viscera, particularly the liver. Fish liver is the source of most ciguatoxin used in basic research (39).

Attempts to produce ciguatoxin from *G. toxicus* in culture have failed, though wild specimens of *G. toxicus* collected from coral have yielded significant amounts of ciguatoxin. The observation that maitotoxin is readily produced from *G. toxicus* cultures has led some to postulate a biosynthetic association between ciguatoxin and okadaic acid. Okadaic acid produces similar symptoms in mice and is chromatographically similar to ciguatoxin. Others have postulated a metabolic contribution from host macroalgae or bacterial populations (40).

Ciguatera was formerly a tropical disease encountered only in those warm water reefs where *G. toxicus* is endemic (21); increasingly, outbreaks are encountered in temperate climes as improvements in refrigeration and transportation have increased the availability of tropical fish in these areas (11). A recent report suggests ciguatera can result from ingestion of farm-raised salmon (12). As ciguatera cannot be prevented by cooking, freezing, or drying fish (40), early recognition of this increasingly common problem is essential. A recent review calls for a permanent monitoring program for marine toxins on Mexican coasts (35).

General Toxicology

G. toxicus lives in association with algae that grow in channels in coral reefs. Herbivorous fish feed on the algae, accidentally consuming the dinoflagellates, and carnivorous fish, in turn, feed on the herbivorous fish. Thus, the toxin tends to accumulate in large predatory fish (*e.g.*, grouper, barracuda, red snapper). The illness is found wherever there are reefs; it is most prevalent in the waters of Florida, the Caribbean, Hawaii, and the South Pacific.

After ingestion of contaminated fish, ciguatoxin is widely distributed in the body and is probably stored in body fat (21). Clinical experience indicates that multiple exposures give rise to increasingly severe and permanent deficits, which suggests that ciguatoxin is incompletely metabolized or excreted (3,13,15). The inherently great neurotoxicity of ciguatoxin gives rise to clinical symptomatology after ingestion of minimal quantities of this tasteless, colorless, and odorless compound. Ciguatoxin is unmeasurable by current techniques, so little is known regarding its metabolism or excretion (40).

The primary action of ciguatoxin is to increase the permeability of excitable membranes to Na^+ by binding to Na^+ channel 5 and causing depolarization (2,5,10,24,26,28). Its target organs are, therefore, characterized by dependence on maintenance of the transmembrane resting potential (5,24,28). The PNS is most sensitive, especially autonomic and somatosensory components (8,27). Cardiac (14,27) and, less commonly, skeletal muscle may also be affected by ciguatoxin (27,35,37).

Animal Studies

Ciguatoxin is said to have no effect on the fish that harbors the compound. When injected intraperitoneally into mice, animals develop a stereotyped pattern of hypothermia, gait dysfunction, areflexic diarrhea, cyanosis, respiratory distress, convulsions, and death. Oral administration of toxin to chicks gives rise to internal hypersalivation, weight loss, and acute ataxia (40).

Human Studies

Ciguatera is usually characterized by neurological dysfunction following or coincident with a brief period of gastroenteritis lasting 1–2 days (20,40). Paresthesias, the hallmark of ciguatera, occur typically within 6–12 h of a meal and are prominent in the extremities and circumoral regions. Temperature reversal in which cold is misperceived as hot, referred to as the "dry-ice phenomenon," is highly characteristic of ciguatera. Generalized weakness, sensory loss, and ataxia may worsen within several days of poisoning and, following partial recovery, may persist for months or even years. Cardiovascular instability occurs less frequently, but may give rise to life-threatening hypotension and bradycardia. Retrospective studies suggest that short-term gastrointestinal symptoms are most common (90% diarrhea, 79% vomiting), but neurological dysfunction is the most common cause of morbidity; weakness and pain occur in three-fifths, and a similar number complain of sensory dysfunction. Rare cases of inflammatory myopathy (36,37), coma (11), retrobulbar pain (17), urinary frequency, and cerebellar dysfunction (19) have been ascribed to ciguatera.

Several factors, including physical exertion and sexual intercourse immediately following intoxication, have been alleged to enhance the toxic effects of ciguatera. Further ingestion of nontoxic fish, protein, or alcohol have been claimed to cause recurrence of symptoms months to years later. Repeated poisoning appears to result in a more severe disorder than the illness observed in patients experiencing ciguatera for the first time (3,15,16).

The clinical features of ciguatera have been intensely studied in the U.S. Virgin Islands (27). Clinical data obtained on 33 patients demonstrated that gastrointestinal symptoms occur in all, with 30 patients (91%) complaining of diarrhea and 23 (70%) vomiting; these events occurred early in the course and were short-lived. Twenty-three (70%) experienced malaise, 19 (58%) had leg weakness, and sensory symptoms occurred in an equal number of patients. The median duration of sensory symptoms was 2 weeks; in some, they persisted for more than 2 months. Hypotension and bradycardia, which occurred in the acute phase, were less common. It has been suggested that ingestion of herbivorous fish leads to preponderance of gastrointestinal symptoms because of a high concentration of maitotoxin in these fish (15). Several cases of polymyositis have been ascribed to severe ciguatera (36,37), attributed to myocyte toxicity. These reports are unconvincing.

Orthostatic hypotension may persist after ciguatera. Studies of autonomic function including measurement of plasma catecholamine levels in the standing and supine positions, and pressor responses to infusion of norepinephrine, atropine, and propanolol were performed and suggest that orthostatic hypotension in ciguatera is the result of parasympathetic excess and sympathetic failure. Volume depletion has been excluded as a cause of hypotension (14).

Many treatment regimens have been suggested to combat ciguatera. Since no specific antidote exists, treatment is symptomatic. Atropine may combat bradycardia and hypotension in the acute phase, but has no effect against neurological or musculoskeletal symptoms (40). Similarly, antidiarrheal, antiemetic and parenteral fluids are indicated against the gastrointestinal effects of ciguatera. Pralidoxime is ineffective (4). Amitriptyline can sometimes ameliorate pain and dysesthesias (20,21). Intravenous mannitol has been reported to blunt the effects of ciguatera. Several reports suggest that an early infusion (1 g/kg over 3–4 h) given within 48 h of ingestion dramatically decreases the acute morbidity of ciguatera (6,29), including neurological and gastrointestinal compromise (30). Reduction in intracellar edema and scavenger effects have been suggested as a mechanism for the mannitol effect (32).

Prevention of ciguatera is difficult given the inherent potency of these odorless, tasteless toxins. A good rule is to eat only small fish; many instances follow a shared meal of a large grouper or red snapper. Native tests such as discoloration of metallic coins or wire, and repulsion in insects are ineffective. Oral feeding of fish to cats or mongoose is complicated by regurgitation and latency of onset of symptoms (40).

Animal bioassays are often nonspecific for individual toxins. Alternative assays based on immunochemical technology show the greatest promise for use in seafood safety monitoring (31). Early enzyme-linked immunosorbent assay tests have been replaced by solid-phase immunofeed assays (S-PIA), which have great potential as a marketplace screening tool to remove toxic fish. This technique may also be used to monitor reefs for ciguatoxicity (31). An inexpensive ($20.00 U.S.), portable, simple, 25-minute, visual colorimetric screening test kit is now available for in-boat use by recreational fishers (Cigua-Check™ from *Oceanit Test Systems*, Honolulu, HI). Other screening S-PIA test kits are under evaluation (18,31).

Toxic Mechanisms

The primary action of ciguatoxin and its congeners is to increase the permeability of excitable membranes to Na^+, causing depolarization. Ciguatoxin acts at neurotoxin receptor site 5 of the sodium channel, which contains at least five receptor sites. Site 5 is located on the α-subunit of the sodium channel. Ciguatoxin-induced depolarization is blocked by tetrodotoxin, and both depolarization and subsequent changes in membrane excitability are antagonized by increased extracellular Ca^{2+} ion concentration (10).

Purified ciguatoxin at 0.1–10 mg/ml inhibits the net accumulation of neurotransmitters (γ-aminobutyric acid and dopamine) by brain synaptosomes through stimulation of neurotransmitter release. This effect, due to membrane depolarization, is blocked by tetrodotoxin. This correlates with influx of Na^+ *via* the action of ciguatoxin on the Na^+ channel. Under appropriate conditions, ciguatoxin causes spontaneous oscillations in membrane polarization levels and repeated action potentials, which are inhibited by tetrodotoxin in a noncompetitive manner; this suggests a unique site of action for ciguatoxin (5).

Studies of the action of ciguatoxin on acetylcholine (ACh) release from motor terminals or cholinergic synaptosomes indicate that ciguatoxin affects Ca^{2+}-dependent ACh release *via* distinct actions mediated by Na^+. These actions alter presynaptic excitability and Ca^{2+} influx through both voltage-sensitive channels and the reversed operations of the Na^+/Ca^{2+} exchange system. The external calcium-independent ACh release induced by ciguatoxin in motor terminals seems to be due to a Na^+-dependent and tetrodotoxin-sensitive mechanism that mobilizes Ca^{2+} from intraterminal stores (25,26).

Studies of the effects of ciguatoxin on frog neuromuscular junction (NMJ) showed fibrillations after a brief delay; these could be suppressed by tetrodotoxin, spontaneous firing of muscle action potentials, and repetitive firing of action potentials after a single stimulus, triggered by repetitive end-plate potentials (EPPs) (25,26).

Ciguatoxin produces a positive inotropic effect on cardiac muscle. At low levels, this is primarily due to indirect action *via* noradrenaline release, whereas high concentrations produce inotropic effects by direct action on voltage-dependent Na^+ channels of cardiac muscles as well (34). Repetitive administration of ciguatoxin to guinea pigs resulted in endothelial swelling, accumulation of platelets in capillaries causing necrosis of cardiac cells and, eventually diffuse myocardial fibrosis (38). Similar changes may occur in skeletal muscles, leading to the observed cases of myopathy (*vide supra*).

The effects of ciguatoxin on peripheral nerve have been well studied. Human pathological studies demonstrate striking edema of adaxonal Schwann cell cytoplasm, presumably as a result of increased membrane permeability to sodium ions (1). Electrophysiological studies in animals and humans show slowing of nerve conduction, with diminution of amplitudes and prolongation of absolute and supernormal periods. These data suggest a direct effect of ciguatoxin on sodium channel activation (8), which is modified by lidocaine (9). The paradoxical reversal of temperature perception ("dry-ice phenomenon"), in which cold stimuli are misperceived as burning, hot, tingling, or electric, has been postulated to result from exaggerated and intense nerve depolarization occurring in peripheral $A\delta$ myelinated and, in particular, c-polymodel nociceptor fibers (7).

Ciguatoxin induces a marked release of norepinephrine from presynaptic sites in the guinea pig vas deferens causing contraction. The agent also releases acetylcholine from nerves in the guinea pig ileum, resulting in sustained contraction and bursts of contractile activity (39). Use of a fractionated toxin preparation on ileal tissue showed a striking increase in transepithelial electrical potential difference and short circuit current seemingly mediated by calcium as a second messenger, directly stimulating intestinal fluid secretion without accompanying tissue damage. Maitotoxin probably acts as a novel activator of calcium channels and thereby stimulates intestinal mucosa (40).

REFERENCES

1. Allsop JL, Martini L, Lebris H *et al.* (1986) Neurologic manifestations of ciguatera. 3 cases with a neurophysiologic study and examination of one nerve biopsy. *Rev Neurol* 142, 590.
2. Baden DG (1989) Brevetoxins: Unique polyether dinoflagellate toxins. *FASEB J* 3, 1807.
3. Bagnis R, Kuberski T, Laugier S (1979) Clinical observations on 3,009 cases of ciguatera (fish poisoning) in the South Pacific. *Amer J Trop Med Hyg* 28, 1067.
4. Bagnis R, Spiegel A, Boutin JP *et al.* (1992) Evaluation of the efficiency of mannitol in the treatment of ciguatera in French Polynesia. *Med Trop* 52, 67.
5. Bidard JN, Vijverberg HP, Frelin C *et al.* (1984) Ciguatoxin is a novel type of Na^+ channel toxin. *J Biol Chem* 259, 8353.
6. Blythe DG, De Sylva DP, Fleming LE *et al.* (1992) Clinical experience with i.v. mannitol in the treatment of ciguatera. *Bull Soc Pathol Exot* 85, 425.
7. Cameron J, Capra MF (1993) The basis of the paradoxical disturbance of temperature perception in ciguatera poisoning. *J Toxicol-Clin Toxicol* 31, 571.
8. Cameron J, Flowers AE, Capra MF (1991) Effects of ciguatoxin on nerve excitability in rats (Part I). *J Neurol Sci* 101, 87.
9. Cameron J, Flowers AE, Capra MF (1993) Modification of the peripheral nerve disturbance in ciguatera poisoning in rats with lidocaine. *Muscle Nerve* 16, 782.
10. Catterall WA, Trainer V, Baden DG (1992) Molecular properties of the sodium channel: A receptor for multiple neurotoxins. *Bull Soc Pathol Exot* 85, 481.
11. DeFusco DJ, O'Dowd P, Hokamay, Ott BR (1993) Coma due to ciguatera poisoning in Rhode Island. *Amer J Med* 95, 240.
12. DiNubile MJ, Hokama Y (1995) The ciguatera poisoning syndrome from farm-raised salmon. *Ann Intern Med* 122, 113.
13. Eason RJ, Harding E (1987) Neurotoxic fish poisoning in the Solomon Islands. *Papua New Guinea Med J* 30, 49.
14. Geller RJ, Benowitz NL (1992) Orthostatic hypotension in ciguatera fish poisoning. *Arch Intern Med* 152, 2131.
15. Glaziou P, Martin PM (1992) Study of factors that influence the clinical response to ciguatera fish poisoning. *Bull Soc Pathol Exot* 85, 419.

16. Glaziou P, Martin PM (1993) Study of factors that influence the clinical response to ciguatera fish poisoning. *Toxicon* **31**, 1151.

17. Hamburger HA (1986) The neuro-ophthalmologic signs of ciguatera poisoning: A case report. *Ann Ophthalmol* **18**, 287.

18. Hokama Y, Takenaka WE, Nishimura KL, Ebesu JSM (1998) A simple membrane immunobead assay for detecting ciguatoxin and related polyethers from human ciguatera intoxication and natural reef fishes. *J AOAC Internat* **81**, 727.

19. Jones HR Jr (1980) Acute ataxia associated with ciguatera-type (grouper) tropical fish poisoning. *Ann Neurol* **7**, 491.

20. Lange WR (1994) Ciguatera fish poisoning. *Amer Fam Physician* **1**, 579.

21. Lang WR (1987) Ciguatera toxicity. *Amer Fam Physician* **36**, 51.

22. Lewis RJ, Hoy AW, Sellin M (1993) Ciguatera and mannitol: *In vivo* and *in vitro* assessment in mice. *Toxicon* **31**, 1039.

23. Lewis RJ, Sellin M (1993) Recovery of ciguatoxin from fish flesh. *Toxicon* **31**, 1333.

24. Lobet A, Bidard JN, Lazdunski M (1987) Ciguatoxin and brevetoxins share a common receptor site on the neuronal voltage-dependent Na$^+$ channel. *FEBS Lett* **27**, 355.

25. Molgo J, Comella JX, Legrand AM (1990) Ciguatoxin enhances quantal transmitter release from frog motor nerve terminals. *Brit J Pharmacol* **99**, 695.

26. Molgo J, Shimahara T, Gaudry-Talarmain YM *et al.* (1992) Ciguatoxin-induced changes in acetylcholine release and in cytosolic calcium levels. *Bull Soc Pathol Exot* **85**, 486.

27. Morris JG Jr, Lewin P, Hargrett NT *et al.* (1982) Clinical features of ciguatera fish poisoning: A study of the disease in the U.S. Virgin Islands. *Arch Intern Med* **142**, 1090.

28. Ohizumi Y, Ishida Y, Shibata S (1982) Mode of the ciguatoxin-induced supersensitivity in the guinea-pig vas deferns. *J Pharmacol Exp Ther* **221**, 748.

29. Palafox NA (1992) Review of the clinical use of intravenous mannitol with ciguatera fish poisoning from 1988 to 1992. *Bull Soc Pathol Exot* **85**, 423.

30. Palafox NA, Jain LG, Pinano AZ *et al.* (1988) Successful treatment of ciguatera fish poisoning with intravenous mannitol. *J Amer Med Assn* **13**, 2740.

31. Park DL (1994) Evolution of methods for assessing ciguatera toxins in fish. *Rev Environ Contam Toxicol* **136**, 1.

32. Pearn JH, Lewis RJ, Ruff T *et al.* (1989) Ciguatera and mannitol: Experience with a new treatment regimen [see comments]. *Med J Australia* **151**, 77.

33. Scheuer P (1982) Marine ecology—some chemical aspects. *Naturwissenschaften* **69**, 528.

34. Seino A, Kobayashi M, Momose K *et al.* (1988) The mode of inotropic action of ciguatoxin on guinea-pig cardiac muscle. *Brit J Pharmacol* **95**, 876.

35. Sierra-Beltran AP, Cruz A, Nunez E *et al.* (1998) An overview of the marine food poisoning in Mexico. *Toxicon* **36**, 1493.

36. Stommel EW, Jenkyn LR, Parsonnet J (1993) Another case of polymyositis after ciguatera toxin exposure. *Arch Neurol* **50**, 571.

37. Stommel EW, Parsonnet J, Jenkyn LR (1991) Polymyositis after ciguatera toxin exposure. *Arch Neurol* **48**, 874.

38. Terao K, Ito E, Yasumoto T (1992) Light and electron microscopic studies of the murine heart after repeated administrations of ciguatoxin or ciguatoxin-4c. *Nat Toxins* **1**, 19.

39. Vernoux JP, Lahlou N, Abbad el Andaloussi S *et al.* (1985) A study of the distribution of ciguatoxin in individual Caribbean fish. *Acta Trop* **42**, 225.

40. Withers NW (1988) Ciguatera fish toxins and poisoning. In: *Handbook of Natural Toxins. Vol 3. Marine Toxins and Venoms.* Tu A ed. Marcel Dekker, New York p. 31.

41. Yasumoto T, Kanno K (1976) Occurrence of toxins resembling ciguatoxin, scaritoxin and maitotoxin in a turban shell. *Bull Jpn Soc Sci Fish* **42**, 1399.

CASE REPORT

A 46-year-old woman developed nausea, vomiting, and diarrhea several hours after eating grouper while on vacation in the Caribbean. She noted acral paresthesias, limb weakness, and orthostatic dizziness 1 day later. Strength normalized within a week, but paresthesias and orthostasis persisted for 2 months. On examination, blood pressure was 120/80 lying and 90/70 standing; pulse was 105 without compensatory change on standing. Sensory examination revealed distal shading to all modalities and Romberg's sign was present. Ankle reflexes were absent. Strength was normal. Six months later, the only symptoms were burning paresthesias of the feet when immersed in cold water. The patient no longer drinks alcohol, since this results in flushing. She avoids seafood.

Cimetidine

Herbert H. Schaumburg

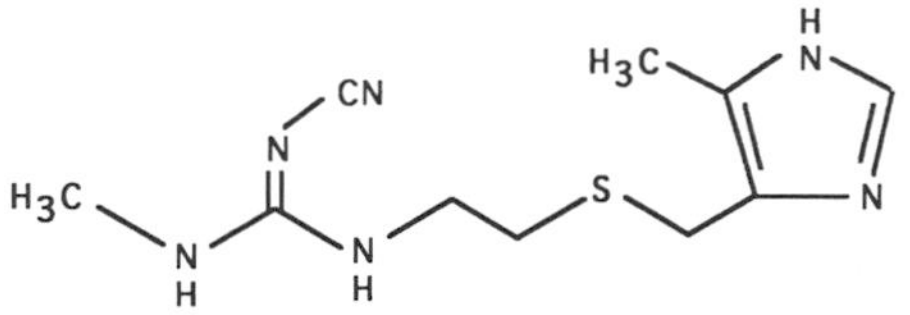

CIMETIDINE
$C_{10}H_{16}N_6S$

N-Cyano-N'-methyl-N''-[2-[[(5-methyl-1H-imidazol-4-yl) methyl]thio]ethyl]guanidine

NEUROTOXICITY RATING
Clinical

A Acute encephalopathy (confusion, psychosis)

A Extrapyramidal syndrome (dystonia, chorea)

Cimetidine is a histamine H_2 receptor antagonist used to treat uncomplicated cases of gastric or duodenal ulcers. Cimetidine is rapidly absorbed from the stomach and has a half-life for elimination (unchanged) by the kidneys of 3 h. Normally, little is metabolized by the liver. Cimetidine is widely disseminated in many organs and crosses the blood-brain barrier. The low incidence of side effects from this widely prescribed drug is attributed to the limited function of H_2 receptors in organs other than the stomach.

Two types of acute neurotoxic reaction are associated with cimetidine therapy: encephalopathy and dystonic movements. Acute encephalopathy is dose-related and usually occurs after weeks of therapy at conventional regimens of 660–900 mg daily in individuals with hepatic or renal dysfunction, or following high doses in the elderly. Elevated cerebrospinal fluid levels of the drug have been demonstrated in such cases, suggesting that blockade of CNS H_2 receptors may be a factor (2). The encephalopathic features generally are confusion and mild disorientation; occasionally, progressive cognitive impairment occurs, and rare cases present as toxic psychosis with hallucinations, myoclonic jerks, and abnormal electroencephalograms (3). The encephalopathy gradually abates following withdrawal.

Acute dystonic reactions are considered idiosyncratic and, in healthy individuals, generally appear after only a few doses at conventional levels. Occasionally, restless leg syndrome or chorea may be the initial movement disorder. These episodes usually respond promptly to intravenous administration of diphenylhydramine (1).

REFERENCES
1. Romischer S, Falter R, Dougherty (1987) Tagemet-induced acute dystonia. *Ann Emerg Med* **16**, 1162.
2. Schentag JJ, Cerra FB, Calleri G *et al.* (1979) Pharmacokinetic and clinical studies in patients with cimetidine-associated mental confusion. *Lancet* **1**, 177.
3. Van Sweden B (1985) Toxic "ictal" confusion in middle age: Treatment with benzodiazepines. *J Neurol Neurosurg Psychiat* **48**, 472.

Cinnarizine

John D. Rogers

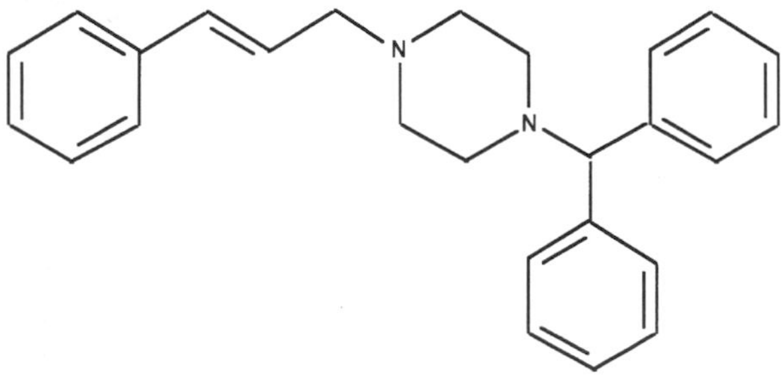

CINNARIZINE
$C_{26}H_{28}N_2$

1-(Diphenylmethyl)-4-(3-phenyl-2-propenyl)piperazine

NEUROTOXICITY RATING
Clinical

A Acute encephalopathy (sedation, depression)

A Extrapyramidal syndrome (parkinsonism, akathisia, dyskinesia)

Cinnarizine is an antiallergic and antivasoconstricting agent with slow calcium-channel blocking activity. Since the 1970s, and principally in Latin America and Europe, it has been used as an antihypertensive agent, for treatment of vertigo and for peripheral circulatory disorders (2). Cinnarizine has antihistaminic and serotonin-antagonist properties; because it is a piperazine derivative, it also has mild

D_2 receptor-blocking effects. Striatal single photon emission computed tomography D_2 receptor studies using ^{123}I-iodobenzamide as a ligand demonstrated lower values (14%–63%) compared with age-matched controls. Older subjects, those treated for >6 months, and those with parkinsonian signs, showed a greater reduction of D_2 receptor binding (1).

Side effects of cinnarizine include drowsiness and depression, asthenia, parkinsonism, akathisia, dyskinesias, and tremor (4,5). In long-term follow-up of patients developing parkinsonism while initially treated with cinnarizine or the calcium-entry blocker flunarizine, a majority had persistent parkinsonism as well as perioral and upper limb dyskinesias despite cessation of the drug for up to 7 years (6). Clinical symptoms appeared 7 months from initial exposure to cinnarizine or flunarizine; rigidity, bradykinesia, and postural instability were found in >75% of these patients, with 5 of 13 patients worsening in terms of gait and balance disturbance during the mean 5-year period of follow-up. In addition, pharmacological studies have suggested the potential neurotoxic significance of the cinnamyl moiety 1-(diphenylmethyl)-4-[3-(4'-hydroxyphenyl)-2-propenyl] piperazine.

There is an increased relative D_2 receptor affinity for this ring-hydroxylated metabolite of cinnarizine (3).

REFERENCES
1. Brucke T, Wober C, Podreka I et al. (1995) D_2 receptor blockade by flunarizine and cinnarizine explains extrapyramidal side effects. A SPECT Study. *J Cerebr Blood Flow Metabol* 15, 513.
2. Gotfraind T, Tows G, Van Gnathion JM (1982) Cinnarizine: A selective calcium entry blocker. *Drugs Today* 18, 27.
3. Kariya S, Isozaki S, Masubuchi Y et al. (1995) Possible pharmocokinetic and pharmacodynamic factors affecting parkinsonism inducement by cinnarizine and flunarizine. *Biochem Pharmacol* 50, 1645.
4. Micheli FE, Pardal MF, Gatt M et al. (1987) Flunarizine and cinnarizine-induced extrapyramidal reactions. *Neurology* 37, 881.
5. Micheli FE, Pardal MF, Gianaula R (1989) Movement disorders and depression due to flunarizine and cinnarizine. *Movement Disord* 4, 139.
6. Negrotti A, Calzetti S (1997) A long term follow-up study of cinnarizine and flunarizine-induced parkinsonism. *Movement Disord* 12, 107.

Cisplatin

Anthony J. Windebank

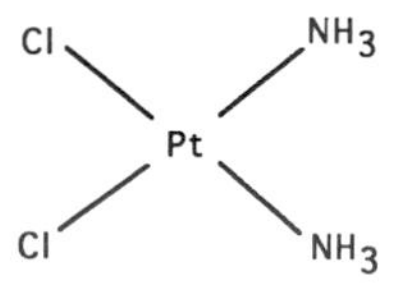

CISPLATIN
$Cl_2H_6N_2Pt$

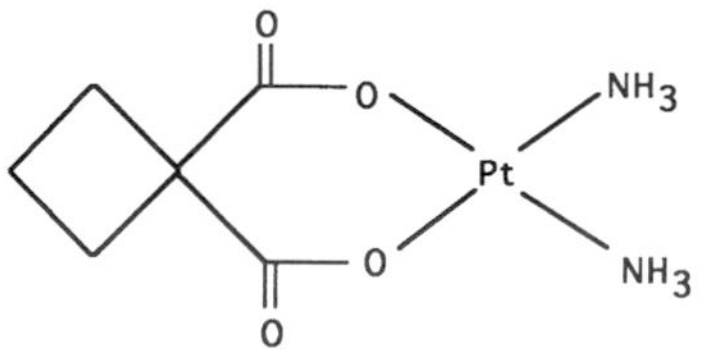

CARBOPLATIN
$C_6H_{12}N_2O_4Pt$

Cisplatin; *cis*-Diaminedichloroplatinum
Carboplatin; 1,1-Cyclobutanedicarboxylic acid platinum complex

NEUROTOXICITY RATING
Clinical
A   Peripheral neuropathy (sensory)
A   Ototoxicity
Experimental
A   Cochlear hair cell damage
A   Peripheral neuropathy (*in vitro*)

Over 1000 platinum compounds have been synthesized and tested for antitumor activity; two, cisplatin and carboplatin, are used in cancer chemotherapy. Cisplatin is a yellow solid moderately soluble in aqueous solution (0.25 g/100 g at 25°C). Cisplatin changes gradually in aqueous solution to the *trans* form, which has no antineoplastic activity. Stability of the *cis* form is enhanced by the presence of excess chloride ions. Since aluminum reacts with and inactivates cisplatin, aluminum-containing intravenous connectors or needles must not be used to deliver the drug.

Both cisplatin and carboplatin are used extensively as cancer chemotherapeutic agents. The typical intravenous regimen of cisplatin is 20 mg/m^2 for 5 days given every 4 weeks. It is used as the primary agent in the treatment of ovarian and testicular cancer and as adjunctive therapy for many other solid tumors.

Cisplatin dust may be absorbed through skin or mucous membranes and is potentially toxic. There are regulations governing appropriate handling by pharmacy staff who formulate intravenous solutions and for medical staff who administer solutions to patients. In the United States, these rules are set out in guidelines of the Occupational Safety and Health Administration (OSHA Medical Records Rule 47,30420,82).

General Toxicology

Cisplatin may be absorbed through skin or mucous membranes and, therefore, poses a theoretical risk for those working in the manufacture or administration of the drug. Practically, because of strict enforcement of regulations, toxicity from this route of absorption is never encountered in clinical practice. After therapeutic intravenous administration, the drug is eliminated from plasma in two phases. The first has a half-time of 30–60 min; the second, 24 h. Ninety percent of cisplatin in blood is covalently bound to plasma proteins (10). The drug distributes rapidly to kidneys, liver, intestine, and testes; it does not readily cross the blood-brain barrier. During the first 24 h, 25% of the drug is excreted by the kidneys and, after 5 days, 43% is excreted. There is little biliary excretion, and the drug is not metabolized.

Cisplatin has three major dose-limiting toxicities; nephrotoxicity, ototoxicity, and peripheral neurotoxicity. Nephrotoxicity is significantly reduced by aggressive hydration and diuresis. Typically, 1–2 liters of normal saline are given intravenously to the patient prior to cisplatin administration. Ototoxicity is manifest by tinnitus and high-tone hearing loss; it is not prevented by hydration. Ototoxicity occurs with both carboplatin and cisplatin, but is reported to be less common and less severe with carboplatin (15). For both agents, ototoxicity involves damage to the outer hair cells of the cochlea. Vestibular damage has been minimal or absent in humans (21) and animals (34). Although several agents have been reported to protect against ototoxicity (4,42,45), the most reliable approach appears to be prevention by monitoring with frequent audiometry (14,38).

Cisplatin is one of the most emetic drugs used in cancer chemotherapy. Nausea may be reduced by pretreatment with the 5-HT$_3$ antagonist ondansetron or high-dose corticosteroids (10). Marrow toxicity is relatively mild with cisplatin. Hypocalcemia, hypomagnesemia, hypokalemia, and hypophosphatemia are common. Careful electrolyte monitoring is important especially in interpreting unusual neurological side effects such as weakness, tetany, alterations in consciousness, or fluctuating paresthesias. Peripheral neurotoxicity is the major dose-limiting side effect.

Animal Studies

Development of animal models for the study of cisplatin neurotoxicity has been difficult. The major problem has been that animals, particularly rodents, develop severe nephrotoxicity before neurotoxicity appears. Renal failure usually causes death of animals. Careful attention to hydration and dose schedule has reduced these difficulties. Animal studies have involved intravenous (9) or intraperitoneal doses of cisplatin; in most cases, 1–2 mg/kg once or twice each week have been used with follow-up for an additional 3–10 weeks. None of the animal studies has demonstrated an obvious clinical deficit. Behavioral studies in mice that stress balance function have demonstrated a deficit in cisplatin-treated mice (1). This was associated with biochemical abnormalities in dorsal root ganglia and slowing of tail-nerve conduction. Several other groups have demonstrated similar slowing of nerve conduction in rats (7,9,18,22,30). Using comparable dosage schedules, changes in dorsal root ganglion neurons of rats have been identified; these include neuronal shrinkage, nucleolar abnormalities, and both decreased and increased neurotransmitter levels (1,2,8,9,40). Examination of distal nerve segments has not generally provided additional information.

In Vitro Studies

Most of the extensive *in vitro* studies of the effect of cisplatin on cancer cells have focused on the mechanism by which cisplatin kills tumor cells. These studies have also examined drug efficacy—alone or in combination—in killing specific types of tumor cells. Both neuronal cell lines (37) and primary sensory neurons (28,29,39,48) have been used to study the mechanism of cisplatin neurotoxicity; these methods have demonstrated that cisplatin causes sensory neuron injury *in vitro* at concentrations similar to those found in patients (20). *In vitro* models have also been used to study potential therapeutic approaches to separating the chemotherapeutic and neurotoxic effects of cisplatin.

Human Studies

All human cisplatin neurotoxicity results from controlled exposures during chemotherapeutic protocols. The neuropathy was reported soon after the drug was introduced (44,46), although neurotoxicity was not predicted from preclinical studies. CNS toxicity is relatively rare (3,33). The neuropathy is stereotyped, dose-limiting, and probably most closely related to total cumulative drug dose (16,20,26,32). Lhermitte's phenomenon may occur (25), but most patients present with complaints of symmetrical, distal paresthesias beginning in the feet during therapy. Rarely, symptoms commence 1 or 2 months following therapy. Positive symptoms are generally not painful but are described as a tingling or as vibration-like. Negative symptoms of gait ataxia, loss of feeling, or dropping of small objects are common. Burning dysesthesias and lightning pain may occur but are rare. Abnormalities on examination correspond to the symptoms; most commonly, there is distal loss of vibration and joint position sense. Sensory threshold to superficial pain and touch may be distally increased, but motor function is well preserved. Sensory ataxia may be present and reflexes are reduced. Cases with pronounced upper-limb involvement may display pseudoathetotic movements. Electrophysiological studies show reduction of sensory nerve action potentials with relative preservation of conduction velocity and motor responses.

Progression of neuropathy may produce severe limb ataxia if the drug is continued. Progression ceases when the drug is stopped, although coasting occasionally occurs. This phenomenon involves progression of neuropathy for several weeks, but not more than 2 months, after the drug has been discontinued. Neuropathy improves slowly thereafter. Extent of recovery, which is often incomplete, depends upon the severity of maximum involvement.

Cisplatin neurotoxicity is potentiated by and appears to potentiate the neurotoxicity produced by other agents. This has been demonstrated most clearly for the interaction between cisplatin and taxol (6,13,35) and occurs in patients treated simultaneously or sequentially with this drug combination. Human studies have not demonstrated whether this effect is additive or synergistic.

Diagnosis of cisplatin-induced neuropathy is straightforward when made in the context of a well-defined exposure. Because cisplatin is used to treat both ovarian and small-cell lung cancer, there may be some difficulty in distinguishing drug-induced from paraneoplastic or idiopathic sensory neuropathy. Each may produce predominantly sensory, large-fiber polyneuropathy (12,47). ANNA-1 or other antibody tests will not help distinguish these patients, since those with cancer or idiopathic neuropathy may have negative antibody studies (11), while those with cancer, in the absence of paraneoplastic neuropathy, may have positive antibodies. Clinical features do not reliably distinguish these types of sensory neuropathy. Helpful clues include the observation that paraneoplastic neuropathy may begin asymmetrically and in the upper limbs. It is likely to be painful and also affect small-fiber sensory modalities of pain and temperature (12). Ultimately, diagnosis may depend upon discontinuing the drug followed by at least 3–6 months of observation. Drug-induced coasting will cease within 2 months, while paraneoplastic neuropathy is usually relentlessly progressive.

Treatment of cisplatin neuropathy involves stopping the drug exposure. This requires experience on the part of the oncologist and neurologist to balance potential benefit against risk. Since the neurotoxic effects appear to be dose-cumulative, the balance usually weighs in favor of stopping the drug once significant symptoms or deficits appear.

Much attention has focused on the use of neuroprotective agents. Ideally, a protective agent administered with or before the drug will prevent neurotoxicity without interfering with chemotherapeutic efficacy. Various agents have been used *in vitro*, in animal models, and in humans with varying degrees of efficacy. These include glutathione (5,7,22,36,41); the radioprotectant WR2721 (27,42); the MSH (melanocyte stimulating hormone) analog $ACTH_{4-9}$ (adrenocorticotrophic hormone) (18,19,23,37,43); and polypeptide growth factors, including IGF-1 (insulin-derived growth factor), NGF (nerve growth factor), BDNF (brain-derived neurotrophic factor), NT3 (neurotrophin), and NT4/5 (17,32,49,50). A well-substantiated treatment effect has yet to be demonstrated.

Carboplatin appears to be equally effective in treating cancer, but less neurotoxic than cisplatin. This may relate to tissue access. Carboplatin is not appreciably bound to plasma proteins. The major dose-limiting toxicity of carboplatin is myelosuppression (10).

Toxic Mechanism

The mechanism of cisplatin neurotoxicity in unknown. Chemotherapeutic efficacy almost certainly depends upon cisplatin binding to DNA. This modifies the structure of DNA, which interferes with replication (24). Since sensory neurons do not mitose, this mechanism is not associated with neurotoxicity. Cisplatin binds to DNA, RNA, and protein in neurons, but the cellular mechanism of damage is unknown. The drug does interfere with axonal transport *in vitro* (37) or *in vivo* (31).

The reason for predominant sensory neuron toxicity probably relates to drug access rather than selective neuronal vulnerability. Cisplatin does not cross the blood-brain barrier and, therefore, motor neurons and other CNS neurons are not exposed to toxic levels of drug. By contrast, sensory neurons are exposed to serum levels of drug because dorsal root ganglia are supplied with fenestrated capillaries. This has been confirmed in one human autopsy study (20). The primary site of cisplatin neurotoxicity may therefore be in the nerve cell body, not the distal axon where degeneration takes place. Motor and sensory fibers are equally protected by the blood-nerve barrier along the course of the nerve.

REFERENCES
1. Apfel SC, Arezzo JC, Lipson L, Kessler JA (1992) Nerve growth factor prevents experimental cisplatin neuropathy. *Ann Neurol* **31**, 76.
2. Barajon I, Bersani M, Quartu M *et al.* (1996) Neuropeptides and morphological changes in cisplatin-induced dorsal root ganglion neuronopathy. *Exp Neurol* **138**, 93.
3. Berman IJ, Mann MP (1980) Seizures and transient cortical blindness associated with *cis*-platinum(II) diamminedichloride (PDD) therapy in a thirty-year-old man. *Cancer* **45**, 764.

4. Capizzi RL (1994) Protection of normal tissues from the cytotoxic effects of chemotherapy by amifostine (Ethyol): Clinical experiences. *Semin Oncol* **21**, 8.

5. Cascinu S, Cordella L, Del Ferro E *et al.* (1995) Neuroprotective effect of reduced glutathione on cisplatin-based chemotherapy in advanced gastric cancer: A randomized double-blind placebo-controlled trial. *J Clin Oncol* **13**, 26.

6. Cavaletti G, Bogliun G, Marzorati L *et al.* (1995) Peripheral neurotoxicity of taxol in patients previously treated with cisplatin. *Cancer* **75**, 1141.

7. Cavaletti G, Minoia C, Schieppati M, Tredici G (1994) Protective effects of glutathione on cisplatin neurotoxicity in rats. *Int J Radiat Oncol Biol Phys* **29**, 771.

8. Cavaletti G, Tredici G, Marmiroli P *et al.* (1994) Off-treatment course of cisplatin-induced dorsal root ganglia neuronopathy in rats. *In Vivo* **8**, 313.

9. Cece R, Petruccioli MG, Cavaletti G *et al.* (1995) An ultrastructural study of neuronal changes in dorsal root ganglia (DRG) of rats after chronic cisplatin administrations. *Histol Histopathol* **10**, 837.

10. Chabner BA, Allegra CJ, Curt GA, Calabresi P (1996) Antineoplastic agents. In: *Goodman and Gilman's The Pharmacological Basis of Therapeutics. 9th Ed.* Hardman JG, Limbird LE, Molinoff PB *et al.* eds. McGraw-Hill Inc, New York p. 1233.

11. Chalk CH, Lennon VA, Stevens JC, Windebank AJ (1993) Seronegativity for type 1 antineuronal nuclear antibodies ("anti-Hu") in subacute sensory neuronopathy patients without cancer. *Neurology* **43**, 2209.

12. Chalk CH, Windebank AJ, Kimmel DW, McManis PG (1992) The distinctive clinical features of paraneoplastic sensory neuronopathy. *Can J Neurol Sci* **19**, 346.

13. Chaudhry V, Rowinsky EK, Sartorius SE *et al.* (1994) Peripheral neuropathy from taxol and cisplatin combination chemotherapy: Clinical and electrophysiological studies. *Ann Neurol* **35**, 304.

14. Fausti SA, Henry JA, Schaffer HI *et al.* (1993) High-frequency monitoring for early detection of cisplatin ototoxicity. *Arch Otolaryngol Head Neck Surg* **119**, 661.

15. Freilich RJ, Kraus DH, Budnick AS *et al.* (1996) Hearing loss in children with brain tumors treated with cisplatin and carboplatin-based high-dose chemotherapy with autologous bone marrow rescue. *Med Pediat Oncol* **26**, 95.

16. Fu KK, Kai EF, Leung CK (1995) Cisplatin neuropathy: A prospective clinical and electrophysiological study in Chinese patients with ovarian carcinoma. *J Clin Pharm Ther* **20**, 167.

17. Gao WQ, Dybdal N, Shinsky N *et al.* (1995) Neurotrophin-3 reverses experimental cisplatin-induced peripheral sensory neuropathy. *Ann Neurol* **38**, 30.

18. Gerritsen van der Hoop R, Hamers FP, Neijt JP *et al.* (1994) Protection against cisplatin induced neurotoxicity by ORG 2766: Histological and electrophysiological evidence. *J Neurol Sci* **126**, 109.

19. Gispen WH, Hamers FP, Vecht CJ *et al.* (1992) ACTH/MSH like peptides in the treatment of cisplatin neuropathy. *J Steroid Biochem Mol Biol* **43**, 179.

20. Gregg RW, Molepo JM, Monpetit VJ *et al.* (1992) Cisplatin neurotoxicity: The relationship between dosage, time, and platinum concentration in neurologic tissues, and morphologic evidence of toxicity. *J Clin Oncol* **10**, 795.

21. Hallmark RJ, Snyder JM, Jusenius K, Tamimi HK (1992) Factors influencing ototoxicity in ovarian cancer patients treated with *cis*-platinum based chemotherapy. *Eur J Gynaecol Oncol* **13**, 35.

22. Hamers FPT, Brakkee JH, Cavalletti E *et al.* (1993) Reduced glutathione protects against cisplatin-induced neurotoxicity in rats. *Cancer Res* **53**, 544.

23. Hol EM, Mandys V, Sodaar P *et al.* (1994) Protection by an $ACTH_{4-9}$ analogue against the toxic effects of cisplatin and taxol on sensory neurons and glial cells in vitro. *J Neurosci Res* **39**, 178.

24. Huang H, Zhu L, Reid BR *et al.* (1995) Solution structure of a cisplatin-induced DNA interstrand cross-link. *Science* **270**, 1842.

25. Inbar M, Merimsky O, Wigler N, Chaitchik S (1992) Cisplatin-related Lhermitte's sign. *Anti-cancer Drug* **3**, 375.

26. Krarup-Hansen A, Fugleholm K, Helweg-Larsen S *et al.* (1993) Examination of distal involvement in cisplatin-induced neuropathy in man. An electrophysiological and histological study with particular reference to touch receptor function. *Brain* **116**, 1017.

27. Lewis C (1994) A review of the use of chemoprotectants in cancer chemotherapy. *Drug Safety* **11**, 153.

28. Lorenzo NY, Ames MM, Windebank AJ (1993) Dissociation of *cis*-platinum induced neurotoxicity and chemotherapeutic efficacy. *Soc Neurosci Abstr* **19**, 1482.

29. Lorenzo NY, Ames MM, Windebank AJ (1993) The role of *cis*-platinum-induced DNA damage in neurotoxicity. *Ann Neurol* **34**, 267.

30. Lorenzo NY, Brimijoin WS, Windebank AJ (1994) Cisplatin-induced *in vivo* neurophysiological changes and its prevention by $ACTH_{4-9}$. *Ann Neurol* **36**, 284.

31. Malgrange B, Delrée P, Rigo JM *et al.* (1994) Image analysis of neuritic regeneration by adult rat dorsal root ganglion neurons in culture: Quantification of the neurotoxicity of anticancer agents and of its prevention by nerve growth factor or basic fibroblast growth factor but not brain-derived neurotrophic factor or neurotrophin-3. *J Neurosci Meth* **53**, 111.

32. McKeage MJ (1995) Comparative adverse effect profiles of platinum drugs. *Drug Safety* **13**, 228.

33. Mead GM, Arnold AM, Green JA *et al.* (1982) Epileptic seizures associated with cisplatin administration. *Cancer Treatment Rep* **66**, 1719.

34. Mount RJ, Takeno S, Wake M, Harrison RV (1995) Carboplatin ototoxicity in the chinchilla: Lesions of the ves-

tibular sensory epithelium. *Acta Otolaryngol Suppl* **519**, 60.

35. Pirker R, Krajnik G, Zochbauer S *et al.* (1995) Paclitaxel/ cisplatin in advanced non-small-cell lung cancer (NSCLC). *Ann Oncol* **6**, 833.

36. Pirovano C, Balzarini A, Bohm S *et al.* (1992) Peripheral neurotoxicity following high-dose cisplatin with glutathione: Clinical and neurophysiological assessment. *Tumori* **78**, 253.

37. Russell JW, Windebank AJ, McNiven MA *et al.* (1995) Effect of cisplatin and ACTH$_{4-9}$ on neural transport in cisplatin induced neurotoxicity. *Brain Res* **676**, 258.

38. Simpson TH, Schwan SA, Rintelmann WF (1992) Audiometric test criteria in the detection of cisplatin ototoxicity. *J Amer Acad Audiol* **3**, 176.

39. Smith AG, Windebank AJ (1992) The effect of ACTH analogs on cisplatin neurotoxicity using embryonic rat dorsal root ganglia explant as an *in vitro* model. *Neurology* **42**, 144.

40. Tomiwa K, Nolan C, Cavanagh JB (1986) The effects of cisplatin on rat spinal ganglia: A study by light and electron microscopy and by morphometry. *Acta Neuropathol* **69**, 295.

41. Tredici G, Cavaletti G, Petruccioli MG *et al.* (1994) Low-dose glutathione administration in the prevention of cisplatin-induced peripheral neuropathy in rats. *Neurotoxicology* **15**, 701.

42. Treskes M, van der Vijgh WJ (1993) WR2721 as a modulator of cisplatin- and carboplatin-induced side effects in comparison with other chemoprotective agents: A molecular approach. *Cancer Chemother Pharmacol* **33**, 93.

43. van Gerven JMA, Hovestadt A, Moll JWB *et al.* (1994) The effects of an ACTH (4-9) analogue on development of cisplatin neuropathy in testicular cancer: A randomized trial. *J Neurol* **241**, 432.

44. Von Hoff DD, Schilsky R, Reichert CM *et al.* (1979) Toxic effects of *cis*-dichlorodiammineplatinum(II) in man. *Cancer Treatment Rep* **63**, 1527.

45. Walker EM Jr, Fazekas-May MA, Heard KW *et al.* (1994) Prevention of cisplatin-induced toxicity by selected dithiocarbamates. *Ann Clin Lab Sci* **24**, 121.

46. Walsh TJ, Clark AW, Parhad IM, Green WR (1982) Neurotoxic effects of cisplatin therapy. *Arch Neurol* **39**, 719.

47. Windebank AJ, Blexrud MD, Dyck PJ *et al.* (1990) The syndrome of acute sensory neuropathy: Clinical features and electrophysiologic and pathologic changes. *Neurology* **40**, 584.

48. Windebank AJ, Smith AG, Russell JW (1994) The effect of nerve growth factor, ciliary neurotrophic factor, and ACTH analogs on cisplatin neurotoxicity *in vitro*. *Neurology* **44**, 488.

49. Zheng JL, Stewart RR, Gao WQ (1995) Neurotrophin-4/5 enhances survival of cultured spiral ganglion neurons and protects them from cisplatin neurotoxicity. *J Neurosci* **15**, 5079.

50. Zheng JL, Stewart RR, Gao WQ (1995) Neurotrophin-4/5, brain-derived neurotrophic factor, and neurotrophin-3 promote survival of cultured vestibular ganglion neurons and protect them against neurotoxicity of ototoxins. *J Neurobiol* **28**, 330.

Clioquinol

Herbert H. Schaumburg

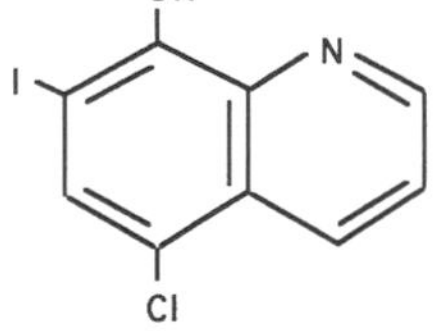

CLIOQUINOL
C$_9$H$_5$ClINO

5-Chloro-7-iodo-8-quinolinol; Iodochloroxyquin

NEUROTOXICITY RATING
Clinical
A   Myelopathy
A   Optic neuropathy

Experimental
A   Central axonopathy

Clioquinol, a dihalogenated derivative of 8-hydroxyquinoline, was initially developed in 1934 as a topical antiseptic. The drug was widely used for the treatment of intestinal amebiasis and as a self-administered remedy for traveler's diarrhea until 1970, when it was associated with an epidemic of a myelo-optic neuropathy syndrome in Japan (6,22).

Clioquinol is a crystalline, tasteless, brown powder with a MP between 177° and 180°C. It is poorly soluble in water (0.4 mg/dl), saline, and urine; slightly more soluble in serum and bile; and highly lipid soluble. There are few studies of the biochemical properties of clioquinol, and the mechanism of its amebicidal activity is unknown. The hydroxyquinolines bind metal ions avidly. Metal binding by clioquinol, especially exogenous iron, is responsible for the green fecal pigment and the "green hairy tongue" associated with high-level dosage (34). Zinc binding has been credited for its former therapeutic role in ameliorating acrodermatitis enteropathica.

Clioquinol is currently available in North America only as a cream or ointment for topical antisepsis. Another 8-hydroxyquinoline, diiodohydroxyquinolinol, is used as an amebicide (18) and has not been associated with myelo-optic neuropathy while the brominated derivative, 5,7-dibromohydroxyquinoline has; the latter is no longer available (27).

General Toxicology

There is considerable species variation in the gastrointestinal absorption of clioquinol (relatively high in rodents and low in dogs and monkeys) and the drug appears rapidly in blood (7,20). Increasing the dose produces a proportional increase in both the amount absorbed and the plasma level. Repeated administration over a 1-month period does not cause any appreciable change in the rate of absorption. Whereas gastrointestinal absorption is not affected by prefeeding in rodents, it is much greater in fed than fasting dogs.

Dogs fed radiolabeled clioquinol rapidly clear the compound; after 48 h, only 1.7% of the dose remains in the body and by 120 h, 99.5% of the dose has been excreted (15.3% in urine, 84.2% in the feces). Clioquinol and its metabolites do not accumulate in the blood, and its pharmacokinetics are not modified by repeated administration (21). Absorbed clioquinol is conjugated with glucuronic or sulfuric acid and not further metabolized; the conjugates are highly water soluble and rapidly excreted in the urine and bile.

Quantitative distribution studies show that only the liver, kidney, and thyroid contain higher levels than the plasma (20). A small amount of orally administered clioquinol appears in the brain and peripheral nerve and is rapidly cleared. Dogs receiving repeated oral doses of large amounts of clioquinol over a period of weeks develop detectable levels in the spinal fluid.

Humans absorb between 13% and 32% of an orally administered dose. Absorbed clioquinol is conjugated and excreted by the kidney as the glucuronide (9,20). Considerable amounts, presumably unabsorbed, appear in the feces. The brominated derivative is less well absorbed and the diiodinated derivative hardly at all; for this reason, the diiodinated form is considered unlikely to be neurotoxic and is still used for amebiasis therapy (4,18). Claims that up to 40% of clioquinol is absorbed through the intact skin have led to its disuse as a topical treatment for diaper rash. Studies with isotope-labeled clioquinol suggest that human elimination is as rapid and complete as in animals. Simultaneous feeding does not affect absorption (20).

Animal Studies

Oral administration to dogs or cats of single doses of clioquinol in excess of 400 mg/kg may provoke status epilepticus, hyperexcitability, and death. No specific changes have been noted in the viscera, and the nervous system displays findings consistent with anoxic encephalopathy (13).

Oral administration to dogs and baboons of repeated doses has elicited clinical signs, electrophysiological abnormalities and neuropathological changes indicative of a distal axonopathy confined to the CNS (16). This neuropathological pattern of changes mirrors the clinical and histopathological profile of humans with the myelo-optic neuropathy syndrome (17,26,28,29).

Oral administration of 250–400 mg/kg/day to beagles produced, after about 20 days, an unsteady, stiff-legged gait. Sensory dysfunction and visual dysfunction were not detected, even in animals dosed for 5 months (14,33). Lower-limb motor nerve conduction velocities were normal. Histopathological study, performed on animals examined at monthly intervals, revealed axonal degeneration of the rostral regions of long ascending tracts (gracile, spinocervical, dorsal spinocerebellar), caudal regions of long descending tracts, and the distal portion of the optic tracts.

Granular axonal swelling was the earliest detected change in these regions; more advanced stages were featured by fiber degeneration with myelin collapse and disappearance of the axon (14). Electrophysiological studies of sural nerve stimulation-evoked potentials in the gracile nucleus of subchronically dosed cats has confirmed the exquisite vulnerability of the dorsal column lower-limb afferent fibers and suggests that dysfunction of this system is responsible for the early paresthesias in humans (1,12). One report, based on experiments with peripheral receptor function in clioquinol-dosed dogs, proposed that peripheral receptor aberration may also contribute to early sensory symptoms (15).

Baboons, dosed with escalating amounts of clioquinol (600–1500 mg/kg/day) developed clinical signs at extremely variable doses and intervals; likewise, the severity of lesions correlated poorly with blood levels of clioquinol (30). All animals displayed histopathological evidence of distal axonal degeneration of ascending (gracile, cuneate, spinocerebellar) tracts; only one of ten developed degenerative changes in the distal optic tracts. Electrophysiological and histopathological examination of multiple levels of the PNS detected no significant abnormalities.

Most studies in murine species have failed to demonstrate clinical or convincing histopathological changes.

Human Studies

Massive consumption of clioquinol (4 g in one instance) may be followed in 12–36 h by a toxic encephalopathy with a prominent amnestic component (10). Some consider this a model of the naturally occurring transient global amnesia syndrome; they suggest it is the human equivalent of the hippocampal electrical dysrhythmia seen in canine clioquinol encephalopathy. This notion is supported by the subsequent appearance—12 years following toxic encephalopathy—of partial complex seizures in two individuals (5).

Isolated optic atrophy has been the predominant neurotoxic reaction in children and is associated with high doses (2 g/day) for 6 months—used for the treatment of acrodermatitis enteropathica (3). Recovery has been poor and some have been left with severely diminished visual acuity; central scotoma and selective impairment of color vision are not described. Children with optic atrophy, in contrast to adults, rarely develop evidence of coincident myelopathy.

The most common and infamous toxic effect of clioquinol is myelopathy, sometimes combined with optic nerve degeneration. Myelopathy is most consistently associated with oral intake of at least 2 g/day for 3 weeks or longer. Considerable variation in dose, duration, and intensity has been reported (11,25). Transient symptoms have appeared after 1500 mg/day for 10 days. A daily dosage of 3 g for 4 months, with continued intake after symptom onset, results in the apoplectic appearance of a devastating myelopathy and visual impairment. Diminished or absent Achilles reflexes of unclear cause initially suggested the presence of peripheral neuropathy, but subsequent human and experimental animal studies determined the disorder is essentially confined to the CNS (28,29).

Numbness and pain in the lower limbs were the initial complaints in almost all cases. Early objective signs were loss of pain and touch senses from sole to knees or up to mid-thigh; frequently, vibration sense was initially impaired to a level of the iliac crest. Stimulation of the hypesthetic areas caused unpleasant, painful sensations. About one-half developed weakness and stiffness in the lower limbs; this was accompanied by increased patellar reflexes and variably increased or diminished Achilles reflexes. One-quarter had some degree of visual dysfunction; 5% developed optic atrophy. Greenish discoloration of the tongue was an oc-

casional finding in Japanese cases and probably reflected the variable coconsumption of iron. Laboratory evaluation of cerebrospinal fluid and peripheral electrodiagnosis were unhelpful.

Most made a satisfactory recovery from the motor impairment; many were left with some sensory loss in the distal limbs. Mild visual dysfunction improved; if severe, there was almost always residual impairment. Recurrence is attributed to recommencement of dosage with clioquinol.

Postmortem studies of 132 Japanese cases described large-fiber degeneration in cervical gracile tracts and lumbar corticospinal tracts; one report found optic tract degeneration adjacent to the geniculate nucleus (24,26).

The Japanese Epidemic

Beginning in the mid-1950s, there appeared in Japan cases of an unusual, seriously disabling, gastrointestinal and neurological syndrome. Because of a steadily increasing incidence, the Japanese government launched an extensive epidemiological and scientific investigation of this condition, which they called the subacute myelo-optico neuropathy (SMON) syndrome (11,22–26). Because many cases appeared in clusters, the cause was felt to be infectious or due to local pollution. However, exhaustive environmental studies produced uncertain leads. The malady seemed of mysterious origin until 1970 when studies of the green tongue, urine, and feces, found in some cases of SMON, revealed the presence of an iron chelate of clioquinol. Such individuals had been taking iron dietary supplements as well as clioquinol. Initially, the linkage of SMON to clioquinol was strongly challenged, and the exact number of cases has been disputed. However, there is now no doubt that clioquinol produced instances of severe myelopathy and cases of optic nerve damage in Japan during this period. Several individuals became very debilitated and eventually died from various causes. The distribution of the postmortem findings in the CNS of these individuals closely resembles that found in dogs and baboons intoxicated with large amounts of clioquinol. Further evidence of the role of clioquinol was the disappearance of SMON from Japan only after the drug was withdrawn from the market.

Repeated epidemiological analyses of the alleged 10,000 cases in the 1956–1972 Japanese SMON outbreak, and a study of the only 220 reported cases of non-Japanese clioquinol neurotoxicity, have failed to explain fully the numerical and geographical discrepancies (2,11,23). Furthermore, at the time, it seemed incredible to many that this presumed harmless and minimally absorbed gastrointestinal agent, used worldwide for 35 years with few reported side effects, would suddenly prove to be neurotoxic. Claims of a "SMON virus" isolated in Japan, an ethnic predisposition, dietary idiosyncrasy, or impurity in the clioquinol, have not been confirmed.

In retrospect, several factors were probably critical:

1. Repeat studies of the pharmacokinetics revealed that considerable amounts of ingested clioquinol *are* absorbed and appear in the circulation.
2. Most of the Western consumption of clioquinol was for the prophylaxis and transient treatment of travelers' diarrhea; toxic levels were rarely approached. Retrospective analysis by experienced neurologists in the tropics disclosed that there had been occasional cases in the past; these were usually attributed to nutritional or demyelinating disease (32).
3. In Japan, it is likely that under public and governmental pressure the vaguely defined clinical SMON syndrome was enthusiastically overdiagnosed, especially since general physicians, not neurologists, examined the majority of the cases (11). This notion was strongly supported when a critical analysis by experienced neurologists of the 220 alleged clioquinol-caused SMON cases occurring outside of Japan was able to establish a relationship to the drug in only 42 (2).
4. Most important, Japanese consumption and domestic production of clioquinol increased dramatically after 1951. The drug became widely available both as an over-the-counter and as a prescription drug; it was also widely used as a prophylactic "gastrointestinal conditioner" by the Japanese (11). In North America, where only a handful of world travelers experienced the illness, it was a prescription-only drug; its use was so narrowly defined that most pharmacies did not even carry it.

Differential diagnosis is simple if a history of clioquinol ingestion is forthcoming, since improvement in all myelopathic symptoms and signs usually commences within 3 months following withdrawal. Diagnosis is extremely difficult without an ingestion history, since the symptoms and signs may be recapitulated *in toto* by several conditions, such as combined system disease, multiple sclerosis, celiac disease, human T-cell leukemia/lymphoma virus infection, nutritional disease, and cassava intoxication.

Toxic Mechanisms

The mechanisms remain unclear. Two unconvincing hypotheses have been advanced; one proposes that clioquinol increases the penetration of metals into the CNS by forming lipophilic metal chelates (19,31), the other suggests that it abolishes the nerve growth factor-induced stimulation of RNA synthesis in sensory ganglion cells (8). It is perhaps noteworthy that other zinc-chelating agents (ethambutol, pyridinethione) induce axonal degeneration with involvement of optic nerve, spinal tracts, and peripheral nerves.

REFERENCES

1. Arasaki K, Nakanishi T (1989) Selective neurotoxicity of clioquinol on the function of the posterior column nuclei. *Neurosci Lett* **107**, 85.
2. Baumgartner G, Gawel MJ, Kaeser HE *et al.* (1979) Neurotoxicity due to halogenated hydroxy quinolines: A clinical analysis of cases reported outside Japan. *J Neurol Neurosurg Psychiat* **42**, 1073.
3. Berggren L, Hansson O (1966) Treating acrodermatitis enteropathia. *Lancet* **1**, 52.
4. Berggren L, Hansson O (1967) Absorption of intestinal antiseptics derived from 8-hydroxyquinolines. *Clin Pharmacol Ther* **9**, 67.
5. Ferrier TM, Schwieger AC, Eadie MJ (1987) Delayed onset of partial epilepsy of temporal lobe origin following acute clioquinol encephalopathy. *J Neurol Neurosurg Psychiat* **50**, 93.
6. Gholz LM, Arons WL (1964) Prophylaxis and therapy of amebiasis and shigellosis with iodochlorohydroxyquin. *Amer J Trop Med Hyg* **13**, 296.
7. Heywood R, Chesterman H, Worden AM (1976) The oral toxicity of clioquinol (5-chloro-7-iodo-8-hydroxyquinoline) in beagle dogs. *Toxicology* **6**, 41.
8. Hori S, Kayanuma K, Ohtani S *et al.* (1988) Effects of 5-chloro-7-iodo-8-hydroxyquinoline (clioquinol) and nerve growth factor on DNA, RNA and protein syntheses in neonatal rat superior cervical ganglia. *Pharmacol Toxicol* **63**, 225.
9. Jack DB, Reiss W (1973) Pharmacokinetics of iodochlorohydroxyquinoline in man. *Amer J Pharm Sci* **62**, 1929.
10. Kaeser HE (1984) Transient global amnesia due to clioquinol. *Acta Neurol Scand Suppl* **100**, 175.
11. Kono R (1978) A review of the S.M.O.N. studies in Japan. In: *Epidemiological Issues in Reported Drug-Induced illnesses—S.M.O.N. and Other Examples.* Gent M, Shigematsu I eds. McMaster University Library Press, Hamilton, Ontario, Canada p. 121.
12. Koyama N, Terada M, Yokota T (1989) Electrophysiological changes in the fasciculus gracilis of the cat following chronic clioquinol administration. *J Neurol Sci* **94**, 271.
13. Krinke G, Pericin C, Thomann P, Hess R (1978) Toxic encephalopathy with hippocampal lesions. *Zbl Veterinaermed, Reihe A* **25**, 277.
14. Krinke G, Schaumburg H, Spencer PS *et al.* (1979) Clioquinol and 2,5-hexanedione induce different types of distal axonopathy in the dog. *Acta Neuropathol* **47**, 213.
15. Kumazawa T, Mizumura K (1984) Abnormal activity of polymodal receptors induced by clioquinol (5-chloro-7-iodo-8-hydroxyquinoline). *Brain Res* **310**, 185.
16. Lannek B, Jonsson L (1974) Toxicity of halogenated oxyquinolines in dogs. A clinical study. V. Pathological findings. *Acta Vet Scand* **15**, 461.

17. Meade TW (1975) Subacute myelo-optic neuropathy and clioquinol. *Brit J Prevent Soc Med* **29**, 157.

18. Oakley, GP (1973) The neurotoxicity of the halogenated hydroxyquinolines. *J Amer Med Assn* **225**, 395.

19. Okada H, Aoki K, Ohno Y *et al.* (1984) Effects of metal-containing drugs taken simultaneously with clioquinol upon clinical features of SMON. *J Toxicol Sci* **9**, 327.

20. Schmid K (1977) The pharmacokinetics of clioquinol in animals and man. *Lakartidningen* **74**, 3003.

21. Schmid K, Krinke G, Fruh F, Keberle H (1973) Studies of the distribution and excretion of clioquinol in the animal. *Arzneim-Forsch* **23**, 1560.

22. Shigematsu I, Yanagawa H (1978) Data on clioquinol and S.M.O.N. *Lancet* **11**, 945.

23. Shigematsu I, Yanagawa H, Yamamoto S, Nakae K (1975) Epidemiological approach to SMON (subacute myelo-optico neuropathy). *Jpn J Med Sci Biol* **28**, 23.

24. Shiraki H (1975) The neuropathology of subacute myelo-optico neuropathy, SMON, in the human. *Jpn J Med Sci Biol* **28**, 101.

25. Sobue I (1978) Clinical features of S.M.O.N. In: *Epidemiological Issues in Reported Drug-Induced Illnesses—S.M.O.N. and Other Examples.* Gent M, Shigematsu I eds. McMaster University Library Press, Hamilton, Ontario, Canada p. 137.

26. Sobue I, Mukoyama M, Takayanagi T *et al.* (1972) Myeloneuropathy with abdominal disorders in Japan. Neuropathologic findings in seven autopsied cases. *Neurology* **22**, 1034.

27. Strandvik B, Zetterstrom R (1968) Amaurosis after broxyquinoline. *Lancet* **2**, 922.

28. Tateishi J, Kuroda S, Saito A, Otsuki A (1971) Myelo-optic neuropathy induced by clioquinol in animals. *Lancet* **2**, 1263.

29. Tateishi J, Kuroda S, Saito A, Otsuki S (1972) Experimental myelo-optico neuropathy induced by clioquinol. *Acta Neuropathol* **24**, 304.

30. Thomas PK, Bradley DJ, Bradley WA *et al.* (1984) Correlated nerve conduction, somatosensory evoked potential and neuropathological studies in clioquinol and 2,5-hexanedione neurotoxicity in the baboon. *J Neurol Sci* **64**, 277.

31. Tjalve H (1984) The aetiology of SMON may involve an interaction between clioquinol and environmental metals. *Med Hypotheses* **15**, 293.

32. Wadia NH (1984) SMON as seen from Bombay. *Acta Neurol Scand Suppl* **100**, 159.

33. Worden AN, Heywood R, Prentice DE *et al.* (1978) Clioquinol toxicity in the dog. *Toxicology* **9**, 227.

34. Yoshioka M, Tamura Z (1970) On the nature of the green pigment found in SMON patients. *Igaku no Ayumi* **74**, 320.

CASE REPORT

A 65-year-old, recently retired, North American nurse enrolled in an art college in Mexico. She developed severe diarrhea 1 week later and began taking clioquinol at a dose of 500 mg/day with no effect. Diarrhea stopped on increasing the dose to 1500 mg/day, and she continued this regimen as prophylaxis against further attacks. Four months later, she noticed onset of tingling and numbness in the soles; within 4 days, the abnormal sensations were experienced over the entire lower limbs and buttocks. A local physician performed a lumbar puncture that yielded unremarkable CSF and obtained lumbar spine x-rays that were normal. He prescribed vitamins and a visit to a local thermal spa. Two weeks later, the abnormal sensations spread over the abdomen as well, her gait became unsteady, and she was unable to climb the stairs unaided because of lower limb weakness. There were no visual or upper-extremity symptoms. She returned to the United States, stopped the self-administration of clioquinol, and consulted a neurologist. Examination revealed neurological abnormalities confined to the lower extremities. There was profound loss of vibration and position sense in the toes, less severe at the ankles, and mild at the knees. There was mild impaired pin and touch senses over the entire lower limbs to a level of the umbilicus. Strength was normal throughout, save for slight weakness of toe and ankle dorsiflexon. Tone and resistance to rapid passive movements of the lower limbs was normal. The gait was unsteady and slightly broad based; she could stand on a narrow base with eyes open but toppled when the eyes closed. She was unable to walk on her heels but able to walk on the toes. Patellar reflexes were abnormally brisk with a few beats of clonus, Achilles reflexes could only be elicited with reinforcement maneuvers.

Extensive laboratory evaluation was unremarkable; it included: three serum B_{12} and vitamin E assays, Schilling test, D-xylose urinary excretion, ova and parasite stool analysis, and a repeat CSF analysis that included oligoclonal band determinations. Visual and brainstem auditory evoked potentials were unremarkable. Cervical to lumbar myelography disclosed minor osteoarthritic degenerative changes at the C5–C6 interspace, with no significant impingement of the spinal roots or spinal cord. Sensory symptoms gradually disappeared over the following 8 months, and strength and gait returned to normal. A repeat examination disclosed moderately diminished position and vibration senses as the sole residual. Achilles tendon reflexes were readily elicited.

Comment

This case displayed the cardinal features of the illness: subacute onset, predominance of sensory dysfunction, and paradoxically diminished Achilles reflexes. The incomplete recovery of pedal position and vibration senses likely reflects incomplete regeneration in the vulnerable rostral dorsal column axons originating from the bipolar lumbar dorsal root ganglion cells.

Clioxanide

Albert C. Ludolph

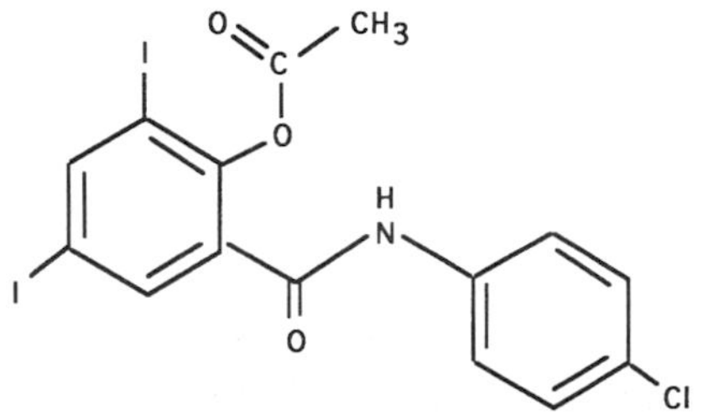

CLIOXANIDE
$C_{15}H_{10}CII_2NO_3$

2-(Acetyloxy)-N-(4-chlorophenyl)-3,5-diiodobenzamide; Halogenated salicylamide

NEUROTOXICITY RATING
Experimental
A Myelinopathy (CNS and PNS)

There are no reports of human neurotoxicity from the anthelmintic drug clioxanide. A single experimental study of rats fed about 350 mg/kg for 3 weeks reported no clinical findings (2). Histopathological study describes vacuolation of CNS white matter and peripheral nerves; these changes were reversible within 6–8 weeks following withdrawal. The related halogenated antimicrobial and fungistatic compound, 3,4′,5-tribromosalicylanilide, is not neurotoxic in the rat (1).

REFERENCES
1. Benitz K-F, Iatrapoulos MJ, Fabian RJ, Coulston F (1974) Morphologic effects of 3,4′,5-tribromosalicylanilide in male rats. *Toxicol Appl Pharmacol* **27**, 591.
2. Kurtz SM, Schardein JL, Fitzgerald JE, Kaump DH (1969) Toxicologic studies with a halogenated salicylamide. *Toxicol Appl Pharmacol* **14**, 652.

Clofibrate

Byron A. Kakulas

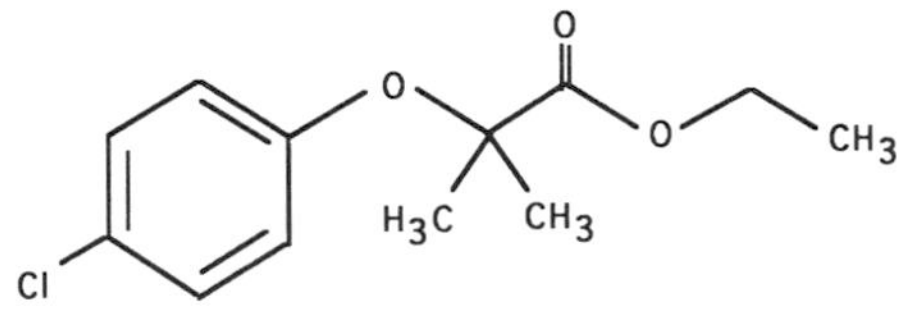

CLOFIBRATE
$C_{12}H_{15}ClO_3$

2-(4-Chlorophenoxy)-2-methylpropanoic acid ethyl ester

NEUROTOXICITY RATING
Clinical
A Myopathy (necrotizing)
A Myotonia
C Peripheral neuropathy

Clofibrate is an oil with a BP of 148°–150°C. It is practically insoluble in water but is miscible with ethanol, acetone, chloroform, and ether (12). Clofibrate and related drugs are branched-chain fatty acid esters. Clofibrate is used in the treatment of hyperlipidemia (types IIb, III, IV, and V) and central diabetes insipidus. The recommended dose for clofibrate is 1 g twice daily. Absorption of clofibrate occurs rapidly with peak serum levels in 3–6 h. Ninety-five percent is protein-bound. Clofibrate is converted in the liver to an inactive glucuronide ester, and the resultant metabolite (40%–70%) is eliminated by the kidneys within 48 h (4). The LD_{50} of clofibrate taken orally in mice is 1.28 g/kg. In rats, the LD_{50} is slightly higher at 1.65 g/kg (12).

Clofibrate and related drugs (see Lovastatin, this volume) may cause, in humans, a necrotizing myopathy, cholesterol-lowering agent myopathy (CLAM), and cardiomyopathy (7,9). Clofibrate reduces fatty acid and branched-chain amino acid oxidation and carnitine palmityl transferase activity. Which of these different actions or other unknown effects cause the myopathy is unclear (2). Patients with renal insufficiency are predisposed to clofibrate myopathy (3,9,15,17,18). The nephrotic syndrome also increases the risk of clofibrate myopathy (9). However, 20 patients with normal renal function also developed this complication (17). CLAM often presents as painful muscle weakness within 2–3 months of starting the drug. It is associated with an elevation in serum creatine kinase (CK) activity and occasionally myoglobinuria (18). Cautious monitoring of serum CK, muscle strength, and renal function is of critical importance to anticipate potential problems when this family of medicines is used therapeutically.

The myopathy appears to be dose-dependent and is uncommon when the drug is administered in conventional therapeutic doses. Five patients with clofibrate-induced myopathy continued to take the drug at lower doses and all recovered. Symptoms develop quite abruptly, usually within 3 weeks of the start of therapy, possibly when the concentration of the drug in the blood reaches a critical level (20). In almost all patients, muscle enzyme activity in the serum is increased.

The mechanism whereby clofibrate and related drugs causes muscle necrosis is uncertain, but the observation that the drug increases muscle lipoprotein lipase activity may be relevant (11). Disturbances in muscle energy metabolism were found in rats treated with clofibrate (14). Experimental clofibrate myopathy in rats is associated with mitochondrial swelling, dilatation of sarcoplasmic reticulum, and vesicular bodies (1,20). A single dose of clofibrate in rats produces myotonia accompanied by T-tubule dilatation and swelling of mitochondria (13).

In patients with renal or hepatic dysfunction, myopathy usually develops within 36 h to 2 years following initiation of therapy. Severe myalgia is the prominent clinical symptom. The degree of increased CK activity may be impressive. Levels as high as 22,700 IU/l (normal, 31–270 IU/l) have been reported. Recovery has averaged 35 days from discontinuation of the drug (18). One report describes a 70-year-old male with chronic renal failure who received the drug in doses of 2 g daily for 6 days. He developed severe and generalized muscle pain, weakness, and tenderness, with elevation of muscle enzyme activity. Myalgia subsided 5 days following withdrawal; strength returned 2 weeks later (17). In another report (15), clofibrate 500 mg administered two to four times daily over 2 weeks to 6 months

induced muscle damage in five patients. Clofibrate-induced enzyme changes correlated with the intensity of myalgia, muscle cramps, and weakness (5). Of 60 patients receiving clofibrate 2–4 g/day for hyperlipoproteinemia, five patients had elevated transaminases and CK. Onset of elevated enzyme activity varied from 7 days to over 6 months. Two patients experienced myalgia, stiffness, and malaise (unspecified onset). Withdrawal of the drug led to resolution of muscular symptoms and elevated enzyme levels within 5–7 days (10).

Another patient is instructive—a 36-year-old diabetic patient receiving clofibrate 500 mg ranging from twice daily to every 4 h for 1 year. The patient developed atrophy and weakness of the thigh muscles 6 months after treatment commenced (8). Laboratory analysis revealed increased serum glutamic oxaloacetic transaminase (SGOT), CK, and lactate dehydrogenase. Upon withdrawal of clofibrate, laboratory values returned to normal after 15 days, but symptoms did not improve. Also reported are two patients with histories of clofibrate intolerance (19); the patients were rechallenged with doses ranging from 500 mg twice daily to 4 times daily. In the first patient, onset of muscle pain, cramps, and tenderness in calves and thighs occurred in 9 days. CK activity rose as high as 258 IU (base normal, 5–50 IU) and SGOT was normal. The syndrome did not appear to be dose-related. Clinical symptoms improved and the CK level eventually dropped to normal 7–10 days after discontinuing clofibrate. The second patient was asymptomatic on a dose of clofibrate 500 mg twice daily for 34 days. When the dose was increased to 500 mg four times daily, the patient experienced muscle pain and elevated CK and SGOT, 13 days later. Symptoms subsided and enzyme levels returned to normal within 10 days of drug withdrawal.

Similar reactions to clofibrate are reported in a patient with diabetes insipidus. Within 9 days of treatment, the patient complained of muscular pain and tenderness in the shoulders and calf. Serum CK was elevated after 11–12 days. Upon discontinuing clofibrate, muscle symptoms resolved and CK levels returned to normal. When rechallenged, muscle pain returned with an elevated serum CK (1).

Clinical and electrophysiological evidence of peripheral nerve degeneration was found in two patients with clofibrate myopathy (6,16). The cause of the neuropathy in these cases is uncertain.

REFERENCES

1. Abourizk N, Khalil BA, Bahuth N, Afifi AK (1979) Clofibrate-induced muscular syndrome. Report of a case with clinical, electromyographic and pathologic observations. J Neurol Sci 42, 1.

2. Argov Z, Mastaglia FL (1994) Drug-induced neuromuscular disorders in man In: *Disorders of Voluntary Muscle. 6th Ed.* Walton JN, Kaparti G, Hilton-Jones D eds. Churchill Livingstone, Edinburgh p. 989.

3. Bridgman JF, Rosen SM, Thorp JM (1972) Complications during clofibrate treatment of nephrotic-syndrome hyperlipoproteinemia. *Lancet* **2**, 506.

4. DRUGDEX Editorial Staff (1995) *Clofibrate*. DRUGDEX Micromedex Inc, Denver, Colorado, USA.

5. Fabre J *et al.* (1973) Hypolipemic and myotoxic action of clofibrate in nephrotic syndrome. *Praxis* **62**, 732.

6. Gabriel R, Pearce JMS (1976) Clofibrate-induced myopathy and neuropathy. *Lancet* **2**, 906.

7. Kakulas BA (1982) Toxic and drug-induced myopathies In: *Skeletal Muscle Pathology* Mastaglia FL, Walton JN eds. Churchill Livingstone, Edinburgh, p. 409.

8. Katsilambros N *et al.* (1972) Muscular syndrome after clofibrate. *N Engl J Med* **286**, 1110.

9. Kuncl RW, Wiggins WW (1988) Toxic myopathies. *Neurol Clin* **6**, 593.

10. Langer T, Levy RI (1968) Acute muscular syndrome associated with the administration of clofibrate. *N Engl J Med* **279**, 856.

11. Lithell H, Boberg J, Hellsing K *et al.* (1978) Increase in the lipoprotein lipase activity in human skeletal muscle during clofibrate administration. *Eur J Clin Invest* **8**, 67.

12. *Merck Index* (1983) Merck & Co, Rahway, New Jersey p. 338.

13. Ontell M, Paul HS, Adibi SA, Martin JL (1979) Involvement of transverse tubules in induced myotonia. *J Neuropathol Exp Neurol* **38**, 596.

14. Paul HS, Abidi SA (1979) Paradoxical effects of clofibrate on liver and muscle metabolism in rats. *J Clin Invest* **64**, 405.

15. Pierides AM, Alvarez-Ude F, Kerr DNS *et al.* (1975) Clofibrate induced muscle damage in patients with renal failure. *Lancet* **2**, 1279.

16. Pokroy N, Ress S, Gregory MC (1977) Clofibrate induced complications in renal disease. *S Afr Med J* **52**, 806.

17. Rimon D, Ludatscher R, Cohen L (1984) Clofibrate induced muscular syndrome. Case report with ultrastructural findings and review of the literature. *J Med Sci* **20**, 1082.

18. Rush P, Baron M, Kapusta M (1986) Clofibrate myopathy: A case report and review of the literature. *Semin Arthritis Rheum* **15**, 226–229.

19. Sekowski I, Samuel P (1972) Clofibrate induced acute muscular syndrome. *Amer J Cardiol* **30**, 572.

20. Tervainen H, Larsen A, Hillborn M (1977) Clofibrate induced myopathy in the rat. *Acta Neuropathol* **39**, 135.

Clonidine

Herbert H. Schaumburg

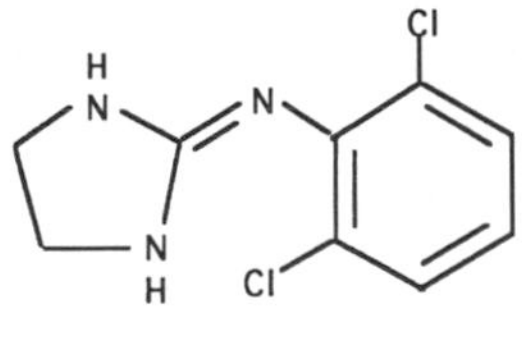

CLONIDINE
C$_9$H$_9$Cl$_2$N$_3$

2,6-Dichloro-*N*-2-imidazolidinylidenebenzenamine

NEUROTOXICITY RATING

Clinical

B Acute encephalopathy (hallucinations, depression)

Clonidine is an imidazoline α-adrenergic agonist. Although a powerful vasoconstrictor when given intravenously, oral administration of clonidine produces a sustained hypotensive response secondary to decreased central sympathetic outflow. Its primary use is in treatment of systemic hypertension; it is also employed to treat diarrhea in diabetic autonomic neuropathy, to ameliorate the symptoms that accompany narcotic withdrawal, and as a spinal analgesic (3).

Its major systemic adverse effects are mild (dry mouth, bradycardia) and dose related; they can usually be avoided by transdermal administration, which eliminates the high peaks associated with oral use.

Two neurological reactions are associated with clonidine therapy; one is an abrupt withdrawal syndrome of anxiety and hypertensive encephalopathy, the other an acute toxic encephalopathy associated with augmentation of dosage (1,2,4). The toxic encephalopathy is rare; both depression/sedation and acute psychosis with hallucinations are described—all disappear following withdrawal. One individual developed reversible cognitive changes without hallucinations (5).

REFERENCES

1. Brown MJ, Salmon D, Rendell M (1980) Clonidine hallucinations. *Ann Intern Med* **93**, 456.

2. Elizur A, Liberson Z (1980) An acute psychotic episode at the beginning of clonidine therapy. *Prog Neuro-psycho* **4**, 211.
3. Hodgson PS, Neal JM, Pollock JE, Liu SS (1999) The neurotoxicity of drugs given intrathecally (spinal). *Anesth Analg* **88**, 797.
4. Hoffmann WF, Ladogana L (1981) Delirium secondary to clonidine therapy. *N Y State J Med* **81**, 382.
5. Lavin P (1975) Dementia associated with clonidine therapy. *Brit Med J* **15**, 628.

Clozapine

Albert C. Ludolph

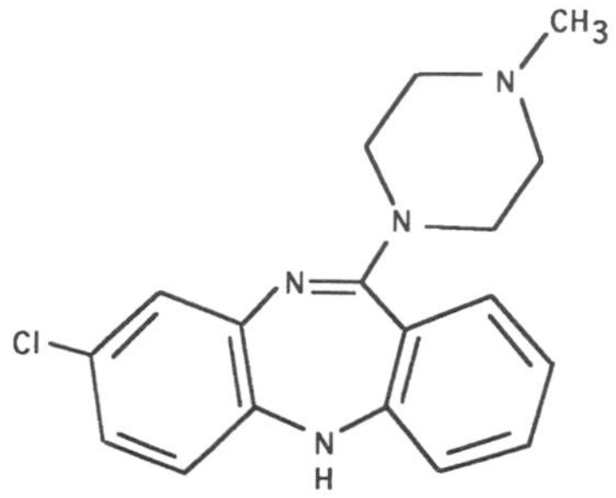

CLOZAPINE
$C_{18}H_{19}ClN_4$

8-Chloro-11-(4-methyl-1-piperazinyl)-5*H*-dibenzo[*b,e*][1,4]diazepine

NEUROTOXICITY RATING

Clinical

A   Seizure disorder
B   Extrapyramidal syndrome (tardive dystonia)
B   Acute encephalopathy (delirium)
B   Neuroleptic malignant syndrome

The dibenzazepine clozapine relieves psychotic symptoms with minimal extrapyramidal side effects (3). The compound has a MW of 326.83 and a MP of 183°–184°C.

Pharmacologically, clozapine shows the highest affinities for 5-HT$_{1C}$ and 5-HT$_2$ serotonin receptors, α_1- and α_2-adrenergic receptors, the muscarinic acetylcholine, and histamine H$_1$ receptors (6,14). Its affinity for dopamine D$_4$ receptors is comparably high (27), whereas affinity for dopamine D$_1$, D$_2$, D$_3$, and D$_5$ receptors is only moderate (6,14). It is of clinical importance that this atypical neuroleptic influences receptor density in the basal ganglia on repeated or chronic administration in a different way from classical neuroleptics. The number of dopamine D$_2$ receptors in the striatum does not increase after chronic clozapine treatment, an adaptive change characteristic for conventional neuroleptics (6,14). Positron emission tomography studies show that haloperidol has a higher affinity for D$_2$ receptors than clozapine (10). After chronic clozapine administration, D$_1$ receptor density increases and 5-HT$_2$ receptors are down-regulated, whereas haloperidol does not alter expression of these receptors (6,14).

Plasma levels of clozapine and its metabolites, clozapine-N-oxide and demethylclozapine, can be assayed by high-performance liquid chromatography (14). These metabolites are less pharmacologically active than the parent compound (14). There is significant inter-patient variability of plasma levels, in particular after higher doses (14).

Compared to conventional neuroleptics, clozapine strongly reduces the convulsive threshold. One to 5% of patients treated with clozapine develop seizures dose-dependently (17,18,20,21,25). In a series of 5629 patients, 1.3% developed generalized seizures in the first 6 months of treatment (21); the cumulative seizure rate was 1.9% at 6 months. Seizures induced by clozapine may commence with myoclonic movements (12,18,19,21). Dose-dependency does not imply that seizures are restricted to higher dosages; unexpectedly, a significant number of seizures also has occurred in those patients treated with a low dose of the drug (21). This may reflect uncautious titration (21,24); in addition, one-half of these patients had a positive history of seizures. Numerous studies (13,18–20,26) have shown that electroencephalographic changes often precede seizures and may indicate an increased seizure risk of the individual patient. Treatment with anticonvulsants is suggested in individuals whose recurrent seizures cannot be controlled by dose reduction. Administration of phenytoin may greatly reduce clozapine plasma levels (20). Use of the anticonvulsant carbamazepine should also be avoided, since it may increase the risk of agranulocytosis during clozapine treatment.

Toxic delirium has occurred in patients treated with clozapine (14,20); this is secondary to the anticholinergic properties of clozapine and can be readily diagnosed by the administration of physostigmine. One acute intoxication has occurred following 10 g of clozapine. The patient was unconscious, developed pulmonary edema, and required ventilatory support. The edema did not respond to furosemid but could be treated with 500 mg methylprednisolone (22). Coma induced by 150 mg clozapine was reported in a single patient (29); possibly, concomitant propranolol medication (120 mg/day) and pre-existing brain damage played a role in that case.

Extrapyramidal dysfunction is very rarely induced by clozapine. This may reflect previous medication with neuroleptics (4,5,16,20,25). Judgment on the importance of some of the observations is therefore difficult (see also 10). Although separation from effects of conventional neuroleptics is difficult in each case, some well-documented case reports exist on acute (9,15) and tardive dystonia (8) under clozapine treatment. The neuroleptic malignant syndrome is also rare during clozapine treatment (1,7,28). Finally, transient obsessive-compulsive symptoms were observed in seven patients (2,23) during clozapine treatment. However, the relation to the syndrome of schizophrenia remains unclear in these reports, and a causal relationship is unproven.

REFERENCES

1. Andersen ES, Powers PS (1991) Neuroleptic malignant syndrome associated with clozapine use. J Clin Psychiat 52, 102.
2. Baker RW, Roy Chengappa KN, Baird JW et al. (1992) Emergence of obsessive compulsive symptoms during treatment with clozapine. J Clin Psychiat 53, 439.
3. Baldessarini RJ, Frankenburg FR (1991) Drug therapy: Clozapine—a novel antipsychotic agent. N Engl J Med 324, 746.
4. Claghorn J, Honigfeld G, Abuzzahab FS et al. (1987) The risks and benefits of clozapine vs. chlorpromazine. J Clin Psychopharmacol 7, 377.
5. Cohen BM, Keck PE, Satlin A, Cole JO (1991) Prevalence and severity of akathisia in patients on clozapine. Biol Psychiat 29, 1215.
6. Coward DM (1992) General pharmacology of clozapine. Brit J Psychiat 160, 5.
7. DasGupta K, Young A (1991) Clozapine-induced neuroleptic malignant syndrome. J Clin Psychiat 52, 105.
8. De Leon J, Moral L, Camunas C (1991) Clozapine and jaw dyskinesias: A case report. J Clin Psychiat 52, 494.
9. Döpp S, Buddeberg C (1975) Extrapyramidale Symptome unter Clozapin. Nervenarzt 46, 589.
10. Farde L, Wiesel FA, Nordstrom AL, Sedvall G (1989) D-1 and D-2 dopamine receptor occupancy during treatment with conventional and atypical neuroleptics. Psychopharmacology 99, 28.
11. Gelenberg AJ, Hopkins HS (1996) Antipsychotics in bipolar disorder. J Clin Psychiat 57(Suppl. 9), 49.
12. Gouzoulis E, Grunze H, Bardeleben UV (1991) Myoclonic epileptic seizures during clozapine treatment: a report of three cases. Eur Arch Psychiat Clin Neurosci 240, 370.
13. Isermann H, Haupt R (1976) Auffällige EEG-Veränderungen unter Clozapin-Behandlung bei paranoid-halluzinatorischen Psychosen. Nervenarzt 47, 268.
14. Jann MW, Grimsley SR, Gray EC, Chang WH (1993) Pharmacokinetics and pharmacodynamics of clozapine. Clin Pharmacokinet 24, 161.
15. Kastrup O, Gastpar M, Schwarz M (1994) Acute dystonia due to clozapin. J Neurol Neurosurg Psychiat 57, 119.
16. Kuha S, Miettinen E (1986) Long-term effect of clozapine in schizophrenia. A retrospective study of 108 chronic schizophrenics treated with clozapine for up to 7 years. Nord Psykiat Tidsskr 40, 225.
17. Lindström LH (1988) The effect of long-term treatment with clozapine in schizophrenia. A retrospective study in 96 patients treated with clozapine for up to 13 years. Acta Psychiat Scand 77, 524.
18. Liukkonen J, Koponen HJ, Nousiainen U (1992) Clinical picture and long-term course of epileptic seizures that occur during clozapine treatment. Psychiat Res 44, 107.
19. Malow BA, Reese KB, Sato S et al. (1993) Clozapine, myoclonus, and EEG abnormalities. Epilepsia 34, 129.
20. Naber D, Holzbach R, Perro C, Hippius H (1992) Clinical management of clozapine patients in relation to efficacy and side effects. Brit J Psychiat 160, 54.
21. Pacia S, Devinsky O (1994) Clozapine-related seizures: Experience with 5629 patients. Neurology 44, 2247.
22. Pall H, Kleinberger G, Kotzaurek R et al. (1976) Severe intoxication with Leponex and its intensive treatment. Klin Wochenschr 88, 179.
23. Patil VJ (1992) Development of transient obsessive-compulsive symptoms during treatment with clozapine. Amer J Psychiat 149, 272.
24. Perry PJ, Miller DD, Arndt-Stephan V, Cadoret-Remi J (1991) Clozapine and norclozapine plasma concentrations and clinical response of treatment-refractory schizophrenic patients. Amer J Psychiat 148, 231.
25. Poulsen UJ, Noring U, Fog R, Gerlach J (1985) Tolerability and long-term effect of clozapine. A retrospective investigation of 216 patients treated with clozapine for up to 12 years. Acta Psychiat Scand 71, 176.
26. Tiihonen J, Nousiainen U, Hakola P et al. (1991) EEG abnormalities associated with clozapine treatment. Amer J Psychiat 148, 1406.
27. van Tol HHM, Bunzow JR, Guan H-C et al. (1991) Cloning of the gene for a human dopamine D_4 receptor with high affinity for the antipsychotic clozapine. Nature 350, 610.
28. Vetter P, Proppe D, Hoppe-Seyler S (1991) Neuroleptisches malignes Syndrom (NMS) unter Clozapinmonotherapie und benigne Hyperthermie bei abklingendem NMS unter Clozapin. Nervenarzt 62, 55.
29. Vetter PH, Proppe DG (1992) Clozapine-induced coma. J Nerv Ment Dis 180, 58.

Clupeotoxin

Albert C. Ludolph
Peter S. Spencer

NEUROTOXICITY RATING

Clinical

B   Seizure disorder

Clupeotoxin poisoning is an acute disorder most commonly caused by plankton-feeding fish such as herring and sardines (Clupeidae) or anchovies (Engraulidae) (3). Tarpon (Elopidae), bonefish (Albulidae), deep-sea bonefish (Pterothrissidae), and deep-sea slickhead (Alepocethalidae) may also cause poisoning (3). Intoxications are frequent during the warm months in the tropical islands of the Indian and Pacific Ocean, the tropical Caribbean Sea and along the African coastline. Rarely, intoxications are reported from the Mediterranean region.

Coastal Madagascar has been heavily impacted by seafood poisoning, and some cases have involved clupeotoxin. Mass intoxication was described in the nineteen sixties, including lethal cases following ingestion of sardines containing clupeotoxin. From July 1993 to May 1996, nine seafood poisoning outbreaks occurred in coastal villages among individuals who had eaten meals of turtle (chelonitoxin suspected), shark (two previously unknown biotoxins, *viz.* carchatoxins, identified) and sardine (clupeotoxin isolated). Sardine intoxication affected two subjects; both had gastrointestinal (vomiting) and neurological (paresthesias) symptoms, and one died. The Madagascan Ministry of Health has implemented a Seafood Poisoning National Control Programme: this includes an epidemiological surveillance network, disease prevention through education, and research on the marine eco-environment (4).

The culpable toxic agent has not been identified. The unidentified toxin may be taken up from planktonic blue-green algae and surface dinoflagellates (2). Viscera of contaminated fish are highly toxic. Clupeotoxin contamination of fish is sporadic and unpredictable; poisonous fish reportedly do not look or smell different from normal specimens. The poisoning may be more frequent after heavy rainfalls during summer months in the tropics (6). Therapy is nonspecific and includes early gastric emptying and attempts to stabilize the cardiovascular system.

Within 30–120 min of oral ingestion (2,5,6), initial signs and symptoms of gastrointestinal disturbances occur; they include a characteristic sharp metallic taste, nausea, vomiting, and diarrhea; hypotension and tachycardia soon follow. Severe metabolic acidosis develops (6). Later, severe headaches, dilated pupils, hypersalivation, numbness, tingling, paresthesia, muscle cramps and paralysis, and convulsions and coma appear. Lethal poisoning within 15 min of consuming contaminated fish is reported (1,6) and mortality is said to be as high as 45% (2,5).

After an acute fatal poisoning by *Sardinella marquesensis*, autopsy revealed the presence of enterocolitis and heart failure (6); a detailed neuropathological examination was not performed, although macroscopically "no abnormalities of the brain were seen" (6).

REFERENCES

1. Alcala AC (1983) Recent cases of crab, cone shell, and fish intoxication on Southern Nigros island, Phillipines. *Toxicon* 3, 1.
2. Auerbach PS (1988) Clinical therapy of marine envenomation and poisoning. In: *Handbook of Natural Toxins. Vol 3. Marine Toxins and Venoms.* Tu AT ed. Marcel Dekker, New York p. 542.
3. Bagnis R, Berglund F, Elias PS *et al.* (1970) Problems of toxicants in marine food products. 1. Marine biotoxins. *Bull WHO* **42**, 69.
4. Champetier de Ribes G, Rasolofonirina RN, Ranaivoson G *et al.* (1997) Intoxication by marine animal venoms in Madagascar (ichthyosarcotoxism and chelonitoxism): recent epidemiological data. *Bull Soc Pathol Exot* **90**, 286. [French]
5. Halstead BW (1988) *Poisonous and Venomous Marine Animals of the World. 2nd Revised Ed.* Darwin Press, Princeton.
6. Melton RJ, Randall JE, Fusetani N *et al.* (1984) Fatal sardine poisoning. A fatal case of fish poisoning in Hawaii associated with the Marquesan sardine. *Hawaii Med J* **43**, 114.

Cobra Venom

Albert C. Ludolph

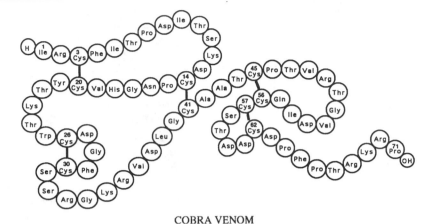

COBRA VENOM

NEUROTOXICITY RATING

Clinical

A Neuromuscular transmission syndrome

Experimental

A Nicotinic acetylcholine receptor binding

Cobra venom (*Naja* spp.) is a colorless, protein-rich liquid containing a complex mixture of toxic substances that are best divided into two groups. One major group has broad-spectrum lytic effects on a wide range of cells, such as blood cells, muscle, and the heart ("cardiotoxins," "lytic factor," "cytotoxin," "membrane toxins") (2). The others are α-neurotoxins that competitively bind to the α-subunit of the nicotinic acetylcholine receptor, produce a nondepolarizing block, and induce myasthenia-like symptoms (7,10). Neuromuscular blockade is induced after binding to one or both α-subunits of the receptor, since two acetylcholine molecules are required to activate current flow (8). Cobra venom contains long *and* short α-neurotoxins (10,12). For example, cobrotoxin from the venom of the Taiwan cobra *Naja naja atra* (12) is a short, basic α-neurotoxin of 62 amino acids with 4 internal disulfide bonds and a MW of 7 kDa. In contrast, the *N. nivea* toxin α is a long α-neurotoxin with 71–74 amino acids and 5 disulfide bonds (12).

After envenomation, cobra neurotoxins are rapidly distributed throughout the body; they do not cross the blood-brain barrier. α-Neurotoxins present in cobra venom bind to the acetylcholine receptor competitively; they produce a clinical profile similar to a postsynaptic myasthenic syndrome. After repetitive nerve stimulation, the amplitude of muscle responses decreases and postactivation exhaustion is present.

Toxic effects of snake bites are variable and depend on the composition of the toxin mixture (geographical varia-

tion), the amount of toxin injected, and characteristics of the victim (4,5,11). Children and the elderly are most susceptible. Reportedly, 20%–60% of all snake bites do not result in major envenomation (4,5,11); however, every venomous snake bite must be considered a potential life-threatening intoxication; an observation period of 12–24 h is customary (4). The clinical course and laboratory findings distinguish serious envenomations. Immediate identification of the snake species is critical. Manipulations at the wound, such as acute surgical intervention or "electrical treatment," are inadvisable (1,4,11). The affected extremity should be immobilized to reduce systemic distribution of toxin (4,11). In most cases, cobra bite induces major local reactions, such as edema, pain, or necrosis (4,5,7). Neurotoxic effects are infrequent with *N. nigricollis* and *N. mosambica* bites but, in many cases, bites induce severe local tissue necrosis that may culminate in loss of an extremity. Typically, 30–60 min after a cobra bite, ptosis and external ophthalmoplegia may develop; slurred speech, difficulty swallowing, facial diplegia, and neck muscle paralysis follow (4,5,7). Pupils may be dilated and, finally, respiratory paralysis and complete tetraplegia with fasciculation and areflexia may appear. CNS dysfunction does not reflect a direct neurotoxic effect; it is due to secondary hypoxia or hemorrhagic complications. Repetitive nerve stimulation shows a typical decremental response that is sensitive to inhibitors of acetylcholine esterase. Enzyme-linked immunosorbent assays may be used for detection of snake toxins in the blood (3,9); however, they are not generally available and are no substitute for clinical observation.

Diagnosis of a cobra bite relies on history, inspection of the wound (fang marks), and the presence of local pain and edema. A coagulation profile is part of the early evaluation of the consequences of a snake bite. If ptosis, blurred vision, diplopia, or bulbar symptoms develop after cobra bites, treatment with antivenin should commence (4,5,7). Antivenins are useful in the treatment of serious systemic effects of envenomation (4,5). Anaphylactic reactions to antivenin may occur, and serum sickness is common (4,5). If respiratory paralysis develops, ventilatory support is lifesaving. Paralysis is commonly reversible within a week. Anticholinesterase treatment is of limited benefit; it may be used to reduce the amount of antivenin required (6).

REFERENCES

1. Bucknall NC (1991) Electrical treatment of venomous bites and stings. *Toxicon* **29**, 397.
2. Harvey AL (1991) Cardiotoxins from cobra venoms. In *Handbook of Natural Neurotoxins. Vol. 5. Reptile Venoms and Toxins.* Tu AT ed. Marcel Dekker, New York p. 85.
3. Ho M, Warrell MJ, Warrell DA *et al.* (1986) A critical reappraisal of the use of enzyme-linked immunosorbent assays in the study of snake bite. *Toxicon* **24**, 211.
4. Mebs D (1992) *Gifttiere. Ein Handbuch für Biologen, Toxikologen, Ärzte, Apotheker.* Wissenschaftliche Verlagsgesellschaft mB, Stuttgart.
5. Minton SA (1990) Neurotoxic snake envenoming. *Semin Neurol* **10**, 52.
6. Mitrakul C, Dhamkrong-At A, Futrakul P *et al.* (1984) Clinical features of neurotoxic snake bite and response to antivenom in 47 children. *Amer J Trop Med Hyg* **33**, 1258.
7. Myint T, Mra R, Maung C *et al.* (1991) Bites by the king cobra (*Ophiophagus hannah*) in Myanmar: Successful treatment of severe neurotoxic envenoming. *Quart J Med* **80, 751.**
8. Sennayake N, Roman GC (1992) Disorders of neuromuscular transmisson due to natural environmental neurotoxins. *J Neurol Sci* **107**, 1.
9. Theakston RDG (1983) The application of immunoassay techniques, including enzyme-linked immunosorbent assay (ELISA) to snake venom research. *Toxicon* **21**, 341.
10. Tu AT (1994) Neurotoxins from snake venoms. In: *Handbook of Neurotoxicology.* Chang LW, Dyer RS eds. Marcel Dekker, New York p. 637.
11. Wingert WA (1991) Management of crotalid envenomations. In: *Handbook of Natural Neurotoxins. Vol. 5. Reptile Venoms and Toxins.* Tu AT ed. Marcel Dekker, New York p. 611.
12. Yang CC (1994) Structure and function of cobrotoxin. *J Toxicol-Toxin Rev* **13**, 275.

Cocaine

Randall Berliner

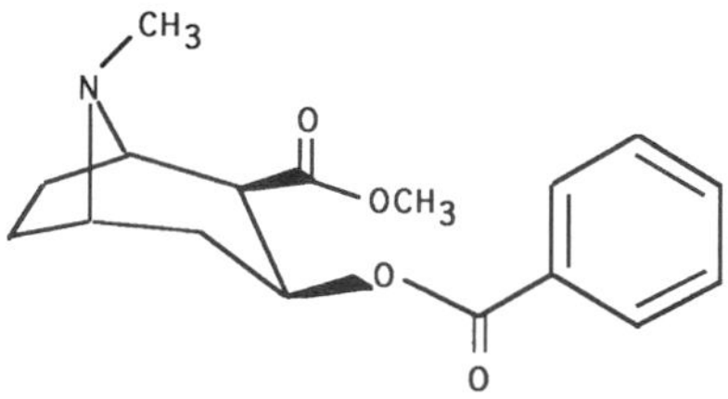

COCAINE
$C_{17}H_{21}NO_4$

[1*R*-(*exo*,*exo*)]-3-(Benzoyloxy)-8-methyl-8-azabicyclo[3.2.1]octane-2-carboxylic acid methyl ester

NEUROTOXICITY RATING
Clinical
A   Acute encephalopathy (psychosis, anxiety)
A   Encephalomalacia
A   Intracranial hemorrhage
A   Physical dependence and withdrawal
A   Seizure disorder
B   Teratogenicity
B   Extrapyramidal syndrome (dystonia, tics)
B   Headache
Experimental
A   Dopaminergic dysfunction

Cocaine is derived from the leaves of the coca tree, *Erythroxylon coca*, a species indigenous to South America. South American Indians have, for centuries, chewed its leaves for their stimulating effect. Despite their initial reservation, Spanish conquerors continued to allow their Inca slaves to chew coca leaves when they realized that the slaves worked harder under its influence (5). With the isolation of cocaine in the latter half of the nineteenth century, importation of cocaine into Europe and the United States became possible. Cocaine was then consumed in beverages such as Vin Mariani, a coca wine, and Coca Cola, an elixir containing both cocaine and caffeine, and originally marketed as a headache remedy and stimulant. Cocaine was used in various forms by President William McKinley, Thomas Edison, the Czar of Russia, Charles Gounod, Jules Verne, and

Sigmund Freud (5,24). In 1914, the first U.S. federal anti-cocaine law, the Harrison Act, required a physician's prescription to obtain cocaine (24). From then until the 1970s, cocaine use was primarily limited to entertainers, especially jazz musicians (5). In the 1960s and 1970s, cocaine use increased again. "Crack," the free base of cocaine, emerged in 1985 and, by 1989, the most common mode of cocaine abuse was by smoking (7). Injection and sniffing the drug are less common. A cocaine "epidemic" stimulated tougher legislation in an attempt control its use. Despite the Anti-Drug Abuse Acts of 1986 and 1988, cocaine abuse and its adverse effects on health continue to be a major problem in the United States. The number of people who report having used cocaine increased from 5.4 million in 1974 to 21.6 million in 1982 (9). More recent surveys indicate that cocaine abuse probably peaked in 1985 and then declined (14). The 1985 National Household Survey on Drug Abuse reported that almost 6 million people had used cocaine within the past 30 days but, by 1991, that number had declined to less than 2 million (14). With the falling cost of cocaine and, particularly, the wide availability of crack (which is relatively inexpensive), cocaine abuse has become more prevalent among lesser-educated and underprivileged people (14).

Although the bulk of cocaine used in the United States is for illegal "recreational" purposes, it is used therapeutically as a local ophthalmic anesthetic. The 1970 Comprehensive Drug Abuse Prevention and Control Act lists cocaine as a Schedule II controlled substance, indicating that while it has a high potential for abuse and psychic or physical dependence, cocaine also has legitimate medical indications. Cocaine hydrochloride is available commercially in 4% and 10% aqueous solution.

Cocaine is benzoylmethylecgonine, an ester of benzoic acid and methylecgonine. Ecgonine is an amino base, structurally related to tropine, the amino alcohol in atropine (6). Cocaine has a basic structure similar to other local anesthetics such as benzocaine and lidocaine, and was the first local anesthetic to be discovered.

General Toxicology

Cocaine may be insufflated ("snorted"), smoked, injected, or absorbed through other mucous membranes. Onset of action is rapid. Following any route of administration, the plasma half-life is about 40–60 min (5); however, a waning "high" results in more frequent use in both smoked and injected cocaine (11). The most rapid onset of action is achieved by smoking the alkaloidal (free base, "crack") form of the drug (cocaine hydrochloride is destroyed at the high temperatures associated with smoking).

One additional route of absorption that bears mentioning results from "body packing," a term that refers to the intracorporeal concealment of illicit drugs for the purpose of smuggling. Packets of cocaine may be swallowed prior to transport with the expectation that they will be "passed" at a later time. These packets may rupture in transit, resulting in massive overdose (34).

The route of administration affects the bioavailability of the drug (27). Total bioavailability is achieved by intravenous administration of cocaine. Cocaine that is smoked has a bioavailability of only 57%, and intranasal cocaine, 25% (27).

Cocaine is metabolized both in the liver and in the plasma. Plasma cholinesterases hydrolyze cocaine to ecgonine methyl ester; cocaine also undergoes nonenzymatic hydrolysis to benzoylecgonine. Variability in the elimination half-life of cocaine in the blood may in part be accounted for by variability in the concentrations and types of plasma cholinesterases (5,27). Minor metabolites detected in human urine include ecgonine, ecgonidine methyl ester, norcocaine, p-hydroxycocaine, m-hydroxycocaine, ecgonidine, norecgonine methyl ester, and m-hydroxybenzoylecgonine (27).

Concomitant use of alcohol and cocaine occurs in 60%–90% of cocaine abusers (14); this combination results in the additional metabolite cocaethylene. Cocaethylene has similar pharmacological properties to cocaine but a significantly longer half-life and a lower LD_{50} in mice (14). Concomitant alcohol use also increases the blood level of cocaine after nasal insufflation, perhaps by causing dilatation of the blood vessels lining the nasal mucosa (14). These factors may in part explain the frequency of mixed abuse but may also introduce additional toxicity.

The ability to detect cocaine use has become important for a number of medical, industrial, civil, legal, and scientific purposes. In one study, 24% of pregnant women who had denied using cocaine tested positive for cocaine metabolites in their urine (10). In hospitals and drug-treatment programs, urine is usually tested for cocaine metabolites. Cocaine can be detected in blood, sweat, saliva, and hair (31). Smoking cocaine produces anhydroecgonine methyl ester, which can be detected in the urine and serves as a marker for abuse *via* this route (14).

The level of cocaine metabolites in urine is dependent upon a number of factors. Time of last administration is important, with cocaine usually detectable 36–48 h after the last dose (27). Higher dosages and prolonged use allows detection up to 10 days later and sometimes longer (27). Because the pretest probability of cocaine use strongly influences the positive predictive value of a result, caution must be used and the application of the test must be borne in mind in selecting a threshold. For example, in employment testing, where the pretest likelihood of cocaine exposure is relatively low, a low threshold for identifying a test result as positive would result in an unacceptably large number of "false-positive results."

Cocaine blocks nerve-terminal reuptake of dopamine, norepinephrine, and serotonin at nerve terminals and causes the release of dopamine from storage vesicles; a mechanism of action similar to that of other psychostimulants (*e.g.*, amphetamines). Likewise, cocaine intoxication is similar to intoxication with other psychostimulants. Experienced users are often unable to discriminate the effects of cocaine from those of amphetamine, other than by the length of the intoxication (5). An immediate and intense euphoria ("rush") marks the onset of intoxication. The effects of this "rush" are probably heightened by intravenous use and particularly by smoking "crack." During acute intoxication, users report feelings of increased confidence, giddiness, and sometimes sexiness. The user may appear more garrulous, with racing thoughts, rapid, pressured speech, and even tangential thinking. Cocaine may also induce suspiciousness or even frank paranoid psychosis. These effects may last hours or may even, in severe cases, persist for weeks. This psychosis may occur in patients without predrug psychiatric history (5).

Animal Studies

Given an unlimited supply of cocaine, rats will administer themselves cocaine, forgoing food and water, enduring electric shocks, until they die (5,8,9,33). In one study, rats addicted to heroin eventually integrated feeding and grooming into their lives, whereas cocaine-addicted rats failed to groom and lost weight. After 30 days, cocaine-addicted rats had a mortality of 90%, whereas only 36% of heroin-addicted rats died (2). Rhesus monkeys given access to 0.2 mg/kg cocaine infusion died in less than 5 days. Monkeys given access to 0.05 mg/kg of methamphetamine or 0.025 mg of amphetamine also died but survived longer (9). Monkeys choose cocaine over both food and social access to another monkey (9).

Although cocaine blocks the reuptake of dopamine, norepinephrine, and serotonin in the CNS, dopamine excess appears to be most closely associated with the highly reinforcing and addictive nature of the drug (5,9,14,33,35). This hypothesis is supported by a number of lines of research. Mesolimbic and mesocortical dopamine systems are strongly involved in the pleasure and reward systems of the brain (35). Cocaine (and other abused drugs) increase the release of dopamine in the ventral tegmental-nucleus accumbens pathway, a major reward center (35). Cocaine-induced 6-hydroxydopamine—which specifically damages dopaminergic nerve terminals—is infused into the nucleus

accumbens, and motor activation and cocaine administration are diminished (35). The same phenomena are seen with dopamine-blocking medication such as antipsychotics. Recent data indicate that the cocaine "receptor" and the dopamine transporter are the same protein (14). Dopamine antagonists alter cocaine self-administration, whereas norepinephrine antagonists do not (35).

Studies have suggested a role for D_1, D_2, and D_3 receptors in the reinforcing properties of cocaine, but the differential effects of each of these receptors has yet to be elucidated (14,35). No analogs of ligands that bind to any of these receptors have completely substituted for cocaine in discrimination studies of reinforcing behavior (14).

Aside from being a strongly reinforcing agent, cocaine withdrawal also produces an abstinence syndrome (5,35). Stimulation of the medial forebrain bundle is highly reinforcing in animal models (35). Administration of cocaine reduces the threshold for self-stimulation of the medial forebrain bundle. However, when animals are allowed to administer unlimited amounts of cocaine over an extended period of time, withdrawal of cocaine results in an elevation of the threshold for stimulation of the medial forebrain bundle, compared to both pre-"addiction" levels and those in control animals (14,35). Similar effects have been shown in rats using *in vivo* microdialysis models, where extracellular dopamine levels in the nucleus accumbens dropped to 30%–40% of baseline levels (35).

Human Studies

Seizures are a major neurotoxic effect and occur immediately or shortly after administration of cocaine. Several series have examined the prevalence of seizures in cocaine-related admissions and have reported rates ranging from 1.4%–10% (5). Seizures may be focal or generalized, and may be brief or present as intractable status epilepticus.

Cocaine and antidepressants each accounted for 29% of 191 patients with seizures seen by the San Francisco Bay Area Regional Poison Control Center in 1988 and 1989 (26). Cocaine-associated seizures were generally brief, more likely to be multiple, but less likely to lead to medical complications than those with antidepressant use.

Cocaine has been implicated in 45%–57% of strokes associated with illicit drug use (17). Most cocaine-related strokes occur around the time of administration but, occasionally, the deficits are gradually progressive (17). Various routes of administration are implicated in producing stroke; presumably, no route is without risk (16). Both ischemic infarction and hemorrhages occur.

Both large-vessel ischemia (such as middle cerebral artery) and small-vessel (lacunar) strokes are associated with cocaine abuse. One study compared the computed tomography scans of 35 habitual cocaine users with a group of first-time users and a group of headache patients (28). The chronic cocaine users had a greater degree of cerebral atrophy, which reached statistical significance. Repeated episodes of microinfarction contribute to these changes.

Mechanisms of ischemic infarction are multiple, and more than one mechanism may play a role in any one case. Intravenous administration of cocaine places the user at risk for bacterial endocarditis and, thus, stroke. Another purported mechanism of infarction is catecholamine-mediated vasospasm. Although few angiograms performed after cocaine-related strokes have shown vasospasm, one study demonstrated increased cerebral blood velocity by transcranial Doppler ultrasound, suggesting vascular narrowing (5). One heavy cocaine user who experienced transient monocular blindness was observed to have diffuse narrowing of the retinal arterioles in the affected eye (21). Cocaine may also exacerbate pre-existing risk factors, such as atherosclerosis, hypertension, or antiphospholipid antibodies (5).

The role of toxic vasculitis in cocaine-associated stroke remains a point of controversy. Biopsy (or autopsy) proven cases of vasculitis in patients with stroke or hemorrhage following cocaine use are rare. Slightly more frequent are cases where angiography demonstrates vascular narrowing (15). Whether these cases are demonstrative of vasospasm or vasculitis is not certain. One patient who presented as angiographically demonstrated cerebral vasculitis following cocaine abuse (15) might, in actuality, have been a case of vasospasm associated with subarachnoid hemorrhage due to a ruptured aneurysm (20). There are two cases of biopsy-proven vasculitis; one had a normal angiogram (19). In one instance, angiography suggested vasculitis, but the biopsy failed to show signs of inflammation (22). Given the rarity of biopsy or autopsy-proven cases of cocaine-related vasculitis and the lack of an animal model, the existence of cocaine-induced vasculitis remains *sub judice*.

Intracranial hemorrhage associated with cocaine use may be either intracerebral or subarachnoid (23). Frequently, there is an underlying aneurysm or arteriovenous malformation (5). It is held that pre-existent vascular malformations or aneurysms may rupture during transient hypertensive episodes associated with cocaine use (12).

Benign headaches can also result from cocaine use; these may even have migrainous features. One survey reported that 12% of patients reporting to an emergency department for cocaine-related problems complained of headache (3). Cocaine may also abort vascular headaches, and there is a case report of a woman who developed a cocaine addiction while medicating her migraines (5).

Movement disorders have been associated with cocaine use: acute dystonia and chorea may be precipitated by co-caine, and cocaine appears to be an additional risk factor for the development of dystonic reactions to neuroleptic administration (13). Cocaine may precipitate exacerbations of previously well-controlled Tourette's syndrome (5). Opsoclonus and myoclonus had been reported in a young woman following cocaine use (29). Stereotypic behavior (tics) has been observed in cocaine-treated rats and also in humans who have abused cocaine (5).

Several reports depict a condition resembling neuroleptic malignant syndrome with delirium, extreme hyperpyrexia, and dystonic movements (5).

In one woman, cocaine unmasked and then caused the exacerbation of myasthenia gravis (1); the mechanism is unknown.

Prolonged exposure to cocaine through illicit recreational abuse can result in chronic behavioral changes. Perhaps the most importance of these is dependence. The large number of cocaine detoxification programs and rehabilitation programs is testament to the highly addictive nature of this substance.

A prolonged dysphoric state has been observed in abstinent cocaine users; conceivably, this may be related to persistent drops in dopamine availability in the nucleus accumbens or mesial forebrain bundle areas. Dysphoria may also be present in cocaine addiction as a result of inability to overcome the addiction. In other individuals, cocaine abuse may be an attempt to self-medicate an underlying depression.

Psychoses, which take a number of forms, have been observed both in acute and chronic cocaine abuse (5). A pure paranoid delusional disorder may be the primary manifestation in some cases while, in others, hallucinations (visual, auditory, or even tactile) may predominate. Thought disorder in cocaine abuse, without an underlying psychotic or mood disorder, is rare. Psychosis is usually short-lived, particularly in brief cocaine abuse. With chronic cocaine abuse, the psychotic disorder may be more prolonged. Psychosis, as well as some other toxic sequelae of cocaine abuse, may be subject to a phenomenon referred to as "sensitization," where repeated use results in increasing likelihood of the toxic effect. Using microdialysis methods, sensitization has been demonstrated on a cellular level (14,35). Synaptic dopamine levels are higher in the nucleus accumbens after repeated administration of cocaine than after single doses. Increased synaptic dopamine correlates with increased locomotor activity following repeated administration. This is further augmented by changes in presynaptic dopamine autoreceptor sensitivity with cocaine exposure. In addition, postsynaptic receptors may become supersensitive to cocaine effects. Serotonergic mechanisms have also been suggested to play a role in cocaine sensitization (14).

Cocaine use during pregnancy is a special problem, both for the woman and her fetus. Cocaine's low molecular weight and water and lipid solubility all contribute to its ability to cross the placental barrier, and also the fetal blood-brain barrier (32). It is suggested that cocaine may be a teratogen, but this is not proven (25,32). Cocaine probably causes constriction of the blood flow within the uterus, leading to a higher rate of birth defects (30,32). Actual human studies of maternal cocaine use are confounded by the fact that cocaine-abusing pregnant women often abuse other drugs as well. In addition, prenatal medical follow-up and nutrition are often poor. Findings of specific cranial abnormalities have been inconsistent (30,32). Maternal cocaine use is associated with low birth weight and decreased head circumference in the offspring (30,32). Various neonatal behavioral abnormalities have been described, including an "excitable" state and a "depressed" state, wherein the child is less alert and responsive to the environment (32). Studies of the long-term postnatal sequelae of prenatal cocaine exposure are confounded by the often deprived developmental conditions of the children (32).

Prevention efforts focus on abuse, both through educational materials and legal restrictions, and through the treatment of cocaine addiction. A number of short-term "detox" programs, longer term "rehabilitation" programs and ongoing "12-step" programs exists for the treatment of cocaine (and other drug) addiction. Several pharmacological approaches have been attempted, but these have had mixed results (5,14,18). The tricyclic antidepressant desipramine was found to be effective in preventing relapse in a double-blind trial, but more recent studies have reported inconsistent findings (5,14,18). Dopamine agonists, such as bromocriptine and amantadine, have also had mixed results (5,14). Despite the fact that they do tend to reduce craving in many users, no pharmacological agent has consistently been shown to prevent relapse in cocaine abuse and dependence (14). Rehabilitation programs have been shown to be effective in reducing relapse (14), and perhaps a combination of rehabilitation programs, ongoing 12-step or other behaviorally oriented "group therapy" programs with appropriate pharmacological intervention, and the attention to comorbid psychiatric conditions may ultimately produce the best results.

REFERENCES

1. Berciano J, Oterino A, Rebollo M, Pascual J (1991) Myasthenia gravis unmasked by cocaine abuse. *N Engl J Med* **325**, 892.

2. Bozarth MA, Wise RA (1985) Toxicity associated with long-term intravenous heroin and cocaine self-administration in the rat. *J Amer Med Assn* **254**, 81.

3. Brody SL, Slovis CM, Wrenn KD (1990) Cocaine-related medical problems: Consecutive series of 233 patients. *Amer J Med* **88**, 325.

4. Brown E, Prager J, Lee HY, Ramsey R (1992) CNS complications of cocaine abuse: Prevalence, pathophysiology, and neuroradiology. *Amer J Roentgenol* **159**, 137.

5. Brust JC (1993) *Neurologic Aspects of Drug Abuse*. Butterworth, Stoneham, MA.

6. Catterall WA, Mackie K (1996) Local anesthetics. In: *Goodman and Gilman's The Pharmacological Basis of Therapeutics. 9th Ed.* Hardman JG, Limbird LE, Molinoff PB *et al.* eds. McGraw-Hill Co, New York p. 338.

7. Colliver JD, Kopstein AN, Hughes AL (1992) Cocaine-related medical crises: Evidence from the drug abuse warning network. *Natl Inst on Drug Abuse Res Monog* **123**, p. 20.

8. Fibiger HC, Phillips AG, Brown EE (1992) The neurobiology of cocaine-induced reinforcement. In: *Cocaine: Scientific and Social Dimensions*. Bock GR, Whelan J eds. John Wiley & Sons Inc, West Sussex, England, *Ciba Fdn Symp* **166**, 7.

9. Fischman MW (1987) Cocaine and the amphetamines. In: *Psychopharmacology: The Third Generation of Progress*. Meltzer HY ed. Raven Press, New York p. 1543.

10. Frank D, Zuckerman BS, Amaro H *et al.* (1988) Cocaine use during pregnancy: Prevalence and correlates. *Pediatrics* **82**, 888.

11. Gold MS (1992) Cocaine (and crack): Clinical aspects. In *Substance Abuse: A Comprehensive Textbook*. Lowinson JH, Ruiz P, Millman RB, Langrod JG eds. Williams & Wilkins, Baltimore p. 205.

12. Goldfrank LR, Hoffman RS (1992) The cardiovascular effects of cocaine—update 1992. *Natl Inst on Drug Abuse Res Monog* **123**, 70.

13. Hegarty AM, Lipton RB, Merriam AE, Freeman K (1991) Cocaine as a risk factor for acute dystonic reactions. *Neurology* **41**, 1670.

14. Johanson CE, Schuster CR (1995) Cocaine. In: *Psychopharmacology: The Fourth Generation of Progress*. Bloom FE, Kupfer DJ eds. Raven Press, New York p. 1685.

15. Kaye BR, Fainstat M (1987) Cerebral vasculitis associated with cocaine abuse. *J Amer Med Assn* **258**, 2104.

16. Klonoff DC, Andrews BT, Obana WG (1989) Stroke associated with cocaine use. *Arch Neurol* **46**, 989.

17. Kokkinos J, Levine SR (1993) Stroke. *Neurol Clin* **11**, 577.

18. Kosten TR (1992) Clinical and research perspectives on cocaine abuse: The pharmacotherapy of cocaine abuse. *Natl Inst on Drug Abuse Res Monog* **135**, 48.

19. Krendel DA, Ditter SM, Frankel MR *et al.* (1990) Biopsy-proven cerebral vasculitis associated with cocaine abuse. *Neurology* **40**, 1092.

20. Levine SR, Welch KMA, Brust JCM (1988) Letter to the editor. *J Amer Med Assn* **259**, 1648.

21. Libman RB, Masters SR, de Paula A, Mohr JP (1993) Transient monocular blindness associated with cocaine abuse. *Neurology* **43**, 228.

22. Martin K, Rogers T, Kavanaugh A (1995) Central nervous system angiopathy associated with cocaine abuse. *J Rheumatol* **22**, 780.

23. Miller BL, Chiang F, McGill L *et al.* (1992) Cerebrovascular complications from cocaine: possible long-term sequellae. *Natl Inst on Drug Abuse Res Monog* **123**, 129.

24. Musto DF (1992) Cocaine's history, especially the American experience. In: *Cocaine: Scientific and Social Dimensions.* Bock GR, Whelan J eds. John Wiley & Sons, Inc, West Sussex, England *Ciba Fdn Symp* **166**, 7.

25. Olsen GD (1995) Potential mechanisms of cocaine-induced developmental neurotoxicity: A minireview. *Neurotoxicology* **16**, 159.

26. Olson KR, Kearney TE, Dyer JE *et al.* (1994) Seizures associated with poisoning and drug overdose. *Amer J Emerg Med* **11**, 392.

27. Osterloh J (1993) Testing for drugs of abuse: Pharmacokinetic considerations for cocaine in urine. *Clin Pharmacokinet* **24**, 355.

28. Pascual-Leone A, Dhuna A, Anderson DC (1991) Cerebral atrophy in habitual cocaine users: A planimetric CT study. *Neurology* **41**, 250.

29. Scharf D (1989) Opsoclonus-myoclonus following the intranasal use of cocaine. *J Neurol Neurosurg Psychiat* **52**, 1447.

30. Scherling D (1994) Prenatal cocaine exposure and childhood psychopathology: A developmental analysis. *Amer J Orthopsychiat* **64**, 9.

31. Selavka CM, Rieders F (1995) The determination of cocaine in hair: A review. *Forensic Sci Int* **70**, 155.

32. Singer L, Arendt R, Minnes S (1993) Neurodevelopmental effects of cocaine. *Clin Perinatol* **20**, 245.

33. Spealman RD, Bergman J, Madras BK *et al.* (1992) Role of D_1 and D_2 dopamine receptors in the behavioral effects of cocaine. *Neurochem Int* **20**, 147S.

34. Wetli CV (1992) The pathology of cocaine: Perspectives from the autopsy table. *Natl Inst on Drug Abuse Res Monog* **123**, 172.

35. Withers NW, Pulverenti L, Koob GF, Gillin JC (1995) Cocaine abuse and dependence. *J Clin Psychopharmacol* **15**, 63.

Colchicine

Herbert H. Schaumburg

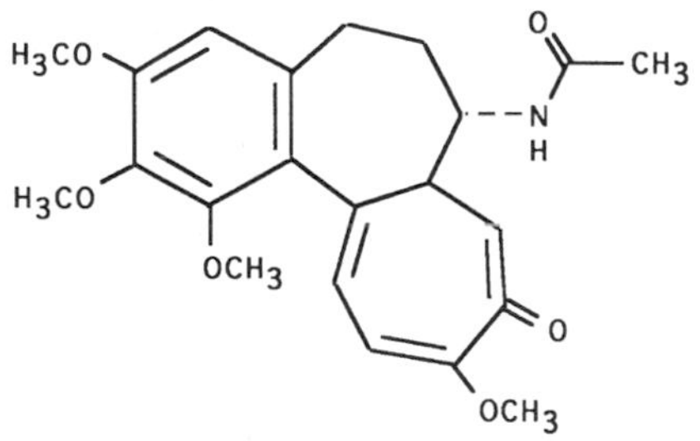

COLCHICINE
$C_{22}H_{25}NO_6$

(S)-N-(5,6,7,9-Tetrahydro-1,2,3,10-tetramethoxy-9-oxobenzo[a]heptalen-7-yl)acetamide

NEUROTOXICITY RATING

Clinical

A Myopathy

A Peripheral neuropathy

Experimental

A Myopathy (myofibril & myotubule degeneration)

Colchicine is a major alkaloid of *Colchicum autumnale* L. (autumn crocus, meadow saffron). The alkaloid was isolated from *Colchicum* in 1820. It forms pale yellow scales or powder with a MP of 142°–150°C. The material is freely soluble in alcohol and is also soluble in water, ether, and benzene. Synthetic colchicine is used as an anti-inflammatory agent in the treatment and prevention of acute attacks of gouty arthritis; it is also employed in therapy of amyloidosis, familial Mediterranean fever, primary biliary cirrhosis, and proliferative vitreoretinopathy. Colchicine's therapeutic effect in acute gout likely stems from inhibition of granulocyte migration into inflamed joints. Colchicine binds tubulin and causes depolymerization of microtubules; the binding site has been identified (4,17,19). Microtubule depolarization affects cell motility and is held responsible for inhibition of granulocyte migration. Colchicine's effect on microtubules causes metaphase arrest in mitosis and disrupts rapid axonal transport (1,13); its antimitotic property has led to the drug's use as an experimental agent in the study of cell division and function (2,6). Serious, dose-limiting neurotoxicity from colchicine therapy is rare in persons with normal renal function.

Colchicine is rapidly absorbed following oral dosage, and peak plasma levels are achieved within 2 h. It is excreted mostly in the feces; about 20% appears in the urine. Colchicine and its metabolites achieve high concentrations in the intestinal mucosa, liver, kidney, and spleen; there is poor penetration into muscle and CNS unless plasma concentrations are elevated.

Therapeutic dosages of 0.5–1.5 mg every 2 h are used to abort acute attacks of gouty arthritis; this usually meets with success within 2 days, and total amounts of 4–8 mg are generally not associated with serious side effects. Systemic toxicity may eventually accompany prophylactic daily doses of 0.6–1.2 mg, especially in persons with gout-associated renal dysfunction. Signs of upper gastrointestinal tract dysfunction (nausea, vomiting, diarrhea, abdominal pain) constitute the most common and disabling systemic toxic effect; these presumably represent a local effect of colchicine on the proliferating cells of the intestinal mucosa and can be circumvented by intravenous dosing (11). Leukopenia and eventual leukocytosis reflect a direct effect upon the bone marrow.

Disabling myopathy accompanies chronic colchicine therapy in individuals with renal dysfunction and has been produced in experimental animals; mild axonal polyneuropathy may accompany human myopathy. Cats develop weakness and atrophy of hindlimb muscles following doses of 0.2 mg/day for 4 weeks; conventional histological studies show atrophy and "slight edema" (18). Ultrastructural studies demonstrate degenerative changes in muscles of rats after a single intraperitoneal injection of 1.6 mg/kg (12) or following 22 days of daily injections of 0.8 mg/kg (16). Myofibrillar degeneration occurred in animals receiving a single dose, while myofilamentous disorientation developed in animals receiving 22 days of colchicine; complex spheromembranous inclusions were present in muscles from both groups. *In vitro* studies demonstrate that colchicine causes developing muscle fibers to lose their longitudinal geometry, myotubes fragment, and myoblasts are arrested at metaphase (5).

Colchicine myoneuropathy is alleged to be a common, unrecognized cause of weakness in gouty patients with renal dysfunction (9,10). It occurs at customary doses of 0.6 mg twice daily and almost always is associated with prolonged (2–3 years) treatment; myopathy has appeared in one instance following only 1–2 weeks of treatment (15). A serum colchicine level of 74 ng/dl (normal therapeutic level, 2–5 ng/dl) is reported in an individual with myoneuropathy (20). Colchicine myopathy may be disabling; the axonal neuropathy is mild (8,9,14).

Onset of disease is insidious (3 months) or subacute (2 weeks); proximal limb weakness that may render patients unable to walk or rise from a chair unaided and limits ability to lift objects over the head. Some experience paresthesias in distal limbs. Signs of proximal weakness without wasting may be pronounced, especially in iliopsoas and del-

toid muscles; tendon reflexes are absent in the legs, and there may be mild diminution in perception of pinprick and vibration stimuli in the feet. Clinical laboratory findings usually include mild elevation of serum creatinine (1.2–3.0) and marked (10 to 19-fold) elevations of creatine kinase. Electromyographic studies disclose myopathic motor unit potentials, early recruitment, and fibrillation potentials; nerve conduction abnormalities are consistent with mild sensory-motor axonopathy (9). Muscle biopsies feature accumulations of lysosomes and autophagic vacuoles, with perinuclear aggregates of densely packed filamentous material. These aggregates are similar to the caps of intermediate filaments characteristic of other eukaryotic cells treated with antimicrotubule agents (7). Nerve biopsy has failed to disclose significant abnormalities. Improvement in strength and reduction in creatine kinase levels commence within 2 weeks of discontinuing therapy, and most individuals recover strength within 3 months. Elevation of creatine kinase is an early indication of myopathy. This test may be a sensitive monitor for those at risk for colchicine myoneuropathy, except for individuals who have recently received renal transplants and have normal creatine kinase levels (3).

The pathogenesis of colchicine myopathy is unclear; vincristine, which also disaggregates microtubules, causes a similar vacuolar myopathy. It is suggested that colchicine may alter a microtubular network that "localizes, moves, allows normal extrusion of lysosomes and autophagosomes in skeletal muscles" (10). The pathogenesis of the mild axonal neuropathy is likely related to defective axonal transport caused by impaired microtubular assembly (13).

REFERENCES

1. Archer DR, Dahlin LB, McLean WG (1994) Changes in slow axonal transport of tubulin induced by local application of colchicine to rabbit vagus nerve. *Acta Physiol Scand* **150**, 57.
2. Bonfoco E, Ceccatelli S, Manzo L, Nicotera P (1995) Colchicine induces apoptosis in cerebellar granule cells. *Exp Cell Res* **218**, 189.
3. Cook M, Ramos E, Peterson J, Croker B (1994) Colchicine neuromyopathy in a renal transplant patient with normal muscle enzyme levels. *Clin Nephrol* **42**, 67.
4. Engelborghs Y, Dumortier C, D'Hoore A *et al.* (1993) Evidence for an alternative pathway for colchicine binding to tubulin, based on the binding kinetics of the constituent rings. *J Biol Chem* **268**, 107.
5. Godman GC, Murray MR (1953) Influence of colchicine on the form of skeletal muscle in tissue culture. *Proc Soc Exp Biol* **84**, 668.
6. Gold BG, Austin DR (1991) Regulation of aberrant neurofilament phosphorylation in neuronal perikarya. I. Production following colchicine application to the sciatic nerve. *J Neuropathol Exp Neurol* **50**, 615.

7. Holzer H, Forry-Schaudies S, Dlugosz A et al. (1985) Interactions between IFs, microtubules, and myofibrils in fibrogenic and myogenic cells. Ann N Y Acad Sci 455, 106.

8. Kontos HA (1962) Myopathy associated with chronic colchicine toxicity. N Engl J Med 266, 38.

9. Kuncl RW, Cornblath DR, Avila O, Duncan G (1989) Electrodiagnosis of human colchicine myoneuropathy. Muscle Nerve 12, 260.

10. Kuncl RW, Duncan G, Watson D et al. (1987) Colchicine myopathy and neuropathy. N Engl J Med 316, 1562.

11. Naidus RM, Rodvien R, Mielke H (1977) Colchicine toxicity. Arch Intern Med 137, 394.

12. Markand ON, D'Agostino AN (1971) Ultrastructural changes in skeletal muscle induced by colchicine. Arch Neurol 24, 72.

13. Paulson JC, McClure WO (1975) Inhibition of axoplasmic transport by colchicine, podophyllotoxin, and vinblastine: An effect on microtubules. Ann N Y Acad Sci 253, 517.

14. Riggs JE, Schochet SS, Gutmann L et al. (1986) Chronic human colchicine neuropathy and myopathy. Arch Neurol 43, 521.

15. Schiff D (1992) Rapid-onset colchicine myoneuropathy. Arthritis Rheum 35, 1535.

16. Seiden D (1973) Effects of colchicine on myofilament arrangement and the lysosomal system in skeletal muscle. Z Zellforsch 144, 467.

17. Skoufias DA, Wilson L (1992) Mechanism of inhibition of microtubule polymerization by colchicine: Inhibitory potencies of unliganded colchicine and tubulin-colchicine complexes. Biochemistry 31, 738.

18. Sternberg SS, Ferguson FC (1953) Colchicine III. Pathology and hematology in cats and rats. Cancer 7, 608.

19. Uppuluri S, Knipling L, Sackett DL, Wolff J (1993) Localization of the colchicine-binding site of tubulin. Proc Nat Acad Sci USA 90, 11598.

20. Younger DS, Mayer SA, Weimer LH et al. (1991) Colchicine-induced myopathy and neuropathy. Neurology 41, 943.

Conium maculatum

Albert C. Ludolph
Peter S. Spencer

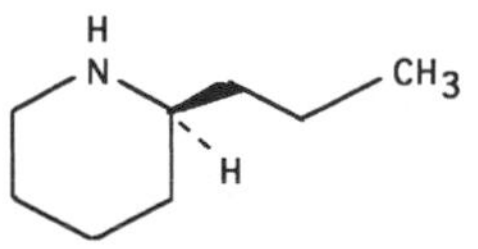

CONIINE
$C_8H_{17}N$

Coniine; (S)-2-Propylpiperidine; Cicutine; Conicine

NEUROTOXICITY RATING

Clinical

B   Neuromuscular transmission syndrome

B   Seizure disorder

Experimental

B   Neuromuscular transmission dysfunction

The neurotoxic plant *Conium maculatum* (hemlock, poison hemlock, spotted hemlock, poison fools parsley, California or Nebraska fern) is responsible for rare human and more frequent accidental poisonings of animals, although its distinct odor often prevents consumption. The herb is indigenous to Europe but, today, can also be found in large parts of Asia and North and South America. In parts of Europe in the nineteenth century, the dried leaf and juice of *C. ma-culatum* was used as an antispasmodic or sedative. It is likely that the execution of Socrates was performed by *Conium* poisoning (3,12); the clinical symptomatology is consistent with the known effects of coniine on neuromuscular transmission. Others (3) hypothesize that two of Moses' nephews were victims of a homicide committed by the use of vaporized coniine from charcoal glows. Individual lots of aniseed *Conium* fruit are currently available.

The toxic moiety of *C. maculatum* is coniine, a piperidine alkaloid with a MW of 127.22. Coniine is a colorless alkaline oil with mousy odor and an MP of −2°C and a BP of 166°C. The highest concentrations of coniine are found in the fruit (3.5%) (1).

Other potentially neurotoxic chemicals present in *C. ma-culatum* are pseudoconhydrine, conhydrine, *n*-methylconiine, γ-coniceine, and other low-molecular-weight piperidine alkaloids of less importance, such as conhydrinone, *N*-methyl pseudoconhydrine, and 2-methylpiperidine (7,14). Related compounds are produced by animals (anabaseine, *Aphaenogaster* ants) and fungi such as *Streptomyces* and *Actinomyces* (14).

Laboratory animals fed with plant material develop depression, muscular weakness, and flaccid paralysis; death is by respiratory failure. Signs are similar in cows, horses, pigs, sheep, and hamsters (14). In mice, fasciculation of skeletal muscles, clonic and tonic contraction, convulsions, and fetal repiratory depression occur after oral adminstration or injection of coniine, γ-coniceine, or N-methylconiine (2).

Accidental poisonings of farm animals are more likely to occur in spring when *C. maculatum* is one of the earliest plants to grow; also, the young plant contains the highest alkaloid concentrations. Poisonings during regrowth in autumn are uncommon. In accidental poisonings of cattle and other species exposed to *C. maculatum*, signs include initial stimulation followed by depression, muscular weakness, ataxia, and respiratory paralysis resulting in death (6,10,14). Convulsions are not seen. After recovery, goats, pigs and cows may show craving for the plant (1,14). Young animals are reportedly more sensitive to the neurotoxin (1), and piperidine alkaloids can be detected in the milk of cows grazing on *C. maculatum* (9). *C. maculatum* is also teratogenic: when fed during specific gestation days, the plant induces skeletal malformations in chicks, cattle, and pigs that resemble arthrogryposis (4,9,15,16).

Human poisoning ascribed to *C. maculatum* is rare. Following consumption, paralysis commences in the distal lower extremities and subsequently ascends to include the respiratory and bulbar muscles. Sensory loss is prominent; however, pain, seizures, and impairment of consciousness do not occur (3,8,11). One report describes a 13-year-old child who recovered from respiratory failure after 3 days in an intensive care unit without sequelae (3). Toxicity may also follow dermal absorption. Treatment includes gastric lavage with careful clinical observation.

The neurotoxic mechanisms underlying the effects of *C. maculatum* and its principal neurotoxin coniine are complex and incompletely elucidated (14). The effects of hemlock alkaloids on neuromuscular transmission have a curare-like component (14); a stimulative effect on parasympathetic ganglia is also likely (2). It is suggested that the curare-like effect is related to teratogenicity (4), since curare itself also induces an arthrogryposis-like picture in chicks (14). Differences in apparent affinity of coniine for nicotinic receptors, or differences in the "quantity" of nicotinic receptors between the rat and chick, have been advanced to explain the greater susceptibility of the chick relative to the rat to coniine-induced teratogenesis (5).

REFERENCES

1. Bentz H, Voigt O (1969) X. Giftpflanzen. In *Nutztiervergiftungen, Erkennung und Verhütung*. Bentz H ed. Gustav Fischer-Verlag, Jena p. 361.
2. Bowman WC, Snaghvi IS (1963) Pharmacological actions of hemlock (*Conium maculatum*) alkaloids. *J Pharm Pharmacol* 15, 1.
3. Davies ML, Davies TA (1994) Hemlock: Murder before the Lord. *Med Sci Law* 34, 331.
4. Forsyth CS, Frank AA, Watrous BJ, Bohn AA (1994) Effect of coniine on the developing chick embryo. *Teratology* 49, 306.
5. Forsyth CS, Speth RC, Wecker L *et al.* (1996) Comparison of nicotinic receptor binding and biotransformation of coniine in the rat and chick. *Toxicol Lett* 89, 175.
6. Galey FD, Holstege GM, Fisher EG (1992) Toxicosis in dairy cattle exposed to poison hemlock (*Conium maculatum*) in hay: Isolation of *Conium* alkaloids in plants, hay and urine. *J Vet Diagn Invest* 4, 60.
7. Habermehl G (1985) *Mitteleuropäische Giftpflanzen und ihre Wirkstoffe*. Springer-Verlag, Berlin, Heidelberg, New York.
8. Hardin JW, Arena JW (1974) *Human Poisoning from Native and Cultivated Plants*. Duke University Press, Durham, NC.
9. Keeler RF, Balls LD (1978) Teratogenic effects in cattle of *Conium maculatum* and conium alkaloids and analogues. *Clin Toxicol* 15, 417.
10. Kubik M, Refholec J, Zachoval Z (1980) Outbreak of hemlock poisoning in cattle. *Veterinarstvi* 30, 157.
11. Millspaugh CF (1974) *American Medicinal Plants*. Dover Publications, New York p. 265.
12. Ober WB (1977) Did Socrates die of hemlock poisoning? *N Y State J Med* 77, 254.
13. Panter KE, James LF, Gardner DR (1999) Lupines, poison-hemlock and *Nicotiana* spp.: toxicity and teratogenicity in livestock. *J Nat Toxins* 8, 117.
14. Panter KE, Keeler RF (1989) Piperidine alkaloids of poison hemlock (*Conium maculatum*). In: *Toxicants of Plant Origin. Vol I. Alkaloids*. Cheeke P ed. CRC Press, Boca Raton, Florida p. 109.
15. Panter KE, Keeler RF, Buck WB (1985) Congenital skeletal malformations induced by maternal ingestion of *Conium maculatum* (poison hemlock) in newborn pigs. *Amer J Vet Res* 46, 2064.
16. Panter KE, Keeler RF, Buck WB (1985) Induction of cleft palate in newborn pigs by maternal ingestion of poison hemlock (*Conium maculatum*). *Amer J Vet Res* 46, 1368.

Conotoxins

Lourdes J. Cruz
Baldomero M. Olivera

Conus peptides; *Conus* venoms

NEUROTOXICITY RATING

Clinical

B Neuromuscular transmission syndrome

B Ion channel syndrome

Experimental

A Muscle sodium channel agent

A Nicotinic acetylcholine blockade

Conotoxins are small, disulfide-rich peptides produced by venomous marine snails belonging to the genus *Conus* ("cone snails") (2,18,21). There are likely to be *ca.* 500 different species of cone snails; every one is venomous and produces a large number of conotoxins. The venoms of cone snails ("*Conus* venoms") typically contain a large complement of peptides (>50) of diverse pharmacological specificity. The purified components, *conotoxins* (6,7), are thought to play a direct role in immobilization of prey; the appellation is also used for *Conus* peptides more generally, including those that are not necessarily toxic. Here, *conotoxin* is used in its narrow sense, only for those peptides presumed to play a direct role in immobilizing prey; the term *Conus* peptide is applied to any peptide found in a *Conus* venom. The venom itself is of primary concern in relation to human intoxication, particularly in tropical areas. Purified conotoxins are presently being explored for potential therapeutic application.

The cone snails capture prey by injecting venom through a hollow harpoon-like tooth (11,19). Human envenomation occurs in the same manner. Animals that have been restrained (such as putting them in a pocket), or whose shells have been damaged (by spear-fishermen), seem most likely to sting.

Some cone snail species have venoms that are lethal to *Homo sapiens*. There are 26 human fatalities with reliable documentation; these have recently been surveyed by Cruz and White (4). Although the literature contains a number of reports indicting other large *Conus* species, in all cases where the details have been carefully verified, the species causing human fatality is a fish-hunting snail, *Conus geographus*. Over 60% of human stings reported for this species have been fatal (25). Based on clinical reports, the following species in addition to *C. geographus* should be regarded as having the potential for lethal stings: *C. textile* (4,10), *C. marmoreus* (4), and *C. omaria* (9), all of which are snail hunters. Some of these reports suggest severe allergic reactions, rather than an intrinsic neurotoxic property of the venom. However, the toxicity of a venom may depend on where it is injected.

The venom of *C. geographus* has been investigated in some detail, and the structures of some of the components likely to be dangerous to humans because of their mammalian toxicity are depicted (*i.e.*, α-conotoxin GI and μ-conotoxin GIII; *see* Fig. 8). The neurotoxic mechanism of many of these individual components is well understood. The α-conotoxins are small peptides, 13–15 amino acids in length, that block the nicotinic acetylcholine receptor at the neuromuscular junction (6,8); these act in much the same way as the α-neurotoxins in snakes (*i.e.*, cobratoxin, erabutoxin, and α-bungarotoxin) by preventing the neurotransmitter (acetylcholine) from signaling the muscle through the receptor. The μ-conotoxins are inhibitors of the muscle subtype of voltage-gated sodium channels (1); in this respect, their mechanism of action is similar to the guanidinium alkaloids tetrodotoxin and saxitoxin; indeed, μ-conotoxin competes for the same site on voltage-gated sodium channels found in muscle membranes. In effect, these toxins inhibit propagation of the muscle action potential. The two families of toxins found in *C. geographus* venom

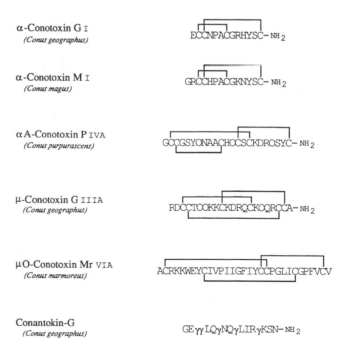

α-Conotoxin G I
(Conus geographus)
ECCNPACGRHYSC−NH₂

α-Conotoxin M I
(Conus magus)
GRCCHPACGKNYSC−NH₂

αA-Conotoxin P IVA
(Conus purpurascens)
GCCGSYONAACHOCSCKDROSYC−NH₂

μ-Conotoxin G IIIA
(Conus geographus)
RDCCTOOKKCKDRQCKOQRCCA−NH₂

μO-Conotoxin Mr VIA
(Conus marmoreus)
ACRKKWEYCIVPIIGFIYCCPGLICGPFVCV

Conantokin-G
(Conus geographus)
GEγγLQγNQγLIRγKSN−NH₂

FIGURE 8. Conotoxins: Sequences. One-letter amino acid code is used: O = 4-transhydroxyproline; γ = γ-carboxyglutamate; −NH₂ = amidated C-terminus.

TABLE 17. *Conus* Peptide and Conotoxin Families

Family	Mechanism, Target	Example(s)	References
α-Conotoxins	Inhibit nicotinic acetylcholine receptor	α-GI; α-MI	6, 14
αA-Conotoxins		αA-PIVA	8
μ-Conotoxins	Inhibit voltage-gated Na^+ channel	μ-GIIIA	1
μO-Conotoxins		μO-MrVIA	16
ω-Conotoxins	Inhibit voltage-gated Ca^{2+} channel	ω-GVIA	13
δ-Conotoxins	Delay or inhibit inactivation of voltage-gated Na^+ channel	σ-TxVIA	5
		δ-PVIA	24
Conantokins	Inhibit NMDA receptor	Conantokin-G	17
Conopressins	Vasopressin analog; agonist for vasopressin receptor	Conopressin-G	3
Conodipines	Phospholipase A_2	Conodipine-M	15

NMDA; *N*-Methyl-D-aspartate-preferring.

are probably responsible for the most severe effects in mammals. In combination, they would cause skeletal muscle paralysis; it is therefore likely that human fatality results from failure of the diaphragm muscle to contract, resulting in an inhibition of respiration and subsequent cardiac arrest (*see* later under Case History).

The α-conotoxins and μ-conotoxins are large families of peptides found in many different species of *Conus*; structures of some examples are shown above. Although the disulfide bonding pattern is conserved among peptides belonging to the same family (*i.e.*, α-conotoxins GI and MI), the primary sequences may diverge significantly (22). In some snails, peptides with entirely different structures have the same physiological mechanism. Thus, αA-conotoxin PIVA (8) has no obvious homology to α-conotoxin GI (*see* Fig. 8), but both block the binding of neurotransmitter to the ligand-binding site of the acetylcholine receptor.

It should be noted that although conotoxins from fish-hunting *Conus* are undoubtedly the major venom components with potential for serious toxicity to humans, other *Conus* peptides can be toxic if applied directly to the CNS. Thus, μO-conotoxin MrVIA (16) from a snail-hunting species (*C. marmoreus*) is extremely toxic to mice when injected directly into the CNS. Another example of a peptide that is toxic only when applied centrally is conantokin-G (20), also from *C. geographus* venom. This peptide does not show any obvious biological effects when injected peripherally into mice, but when injected centrally it induces a sleep-like state in young mice, and hyperactivity in older mice. At higher doses, it can cause fatality in young mice. This *Conus* peptide specifically targets and is an antagonist of the *N*-methyl-D-aspartate receptor, a pharmacological subtype of glutamate receptor (17).

A summary of the major conotoxin families is given in Table 17; in principle, all of these can cause toxicity in some animal systems, but there is considerable variation with respect to mammalian toxicity. For example, even among the α-conotoxins, some members of the family are lethal to

mammals, while other peptides in this group cause paralysis in fish but elicit only weak effects in mammalian systems (23, 26). There is little doubt that many more potent toxins will be isolated from *Conus* venoms.

REFERENCES

1. Cruz LJ, Gray WR, Olivera BM *et al.* (1985) *Conus geographus* toxins that discriminate between neuronal and muscle sodium channels. *J Biol Chem* **260**, 9280.

2. Cruz LJ, Gray W, Yoshikami D *et al.* (1985) *Conus* venoms: A rich source of neuroactive peptides. *J Toxicol-Toxin Rev* **4**, 107.

3. Cruz LJ, de Santos V, Zafaralla GC *et al.* (1987) Invertebrate vasopressin/oxytocin homologs. Characterization of peptides from *Conus geographus* and *Conus striatus* venoms. *J Biol Chem* **262**, 15821.

4. Cruz LJ, White J (1995) Clinical toxicology of *Conus* snail stings. In: *CRC Handbook on Clinical Toxicology of Animal Venoms and Poisons*. Meier J, White J eds. CRC Press, Boca Raton, Florida.

5. Fainzilber M, Kofman O, Zlotkin E *et al.* (1994) A new neurotoxin receptor site on sodium channels is identified by a conotoxin that affects sodium channel inactivation in molluscs and acts as an antagonist in rat brain. *J Biol Chem* **269**, 2574.

6. Gray WR, Luque A, Olivera BM *et al.* (1981) Peptide toxins from *Conus geographus* venom. *J Biol Chem* **256**, 4734.

7. Gray WR, Olivera BM, Cruz LJ (1988) Peptide toxins from venomous *Conus* snails. *Ann Rev Biochem* **57**, 665.

8. Hopkins C, Grilley M, Miller C *et al.* (1995) A new family of *Conus* peptides targeted to the nicotinic acetylcholine receptor. *J Biol Chem* **270**, 22361.

9. Kohn AJ (1958) Recent cases of human injury due to venomous marine snails of the genus *Conus*. *Hawaii Med J* **17**, 528.

10. Kohn AJ (1963) Venomous marine snails of the genus *Conus*. In: *Venomous and Poisonous Animals and Noxious Plants of the Pacific Region*. Keegan HC, McFarlane WV eds. Pergamon Press, Oxford p. 83.

11. Kohn AJ, Saunders PR, Wiener S (1960) Preliminary stud-

ies on the venom of the marine snail *Conus. Ann N Y Acad Sci* **90**, 706.

12. Makalinao IR, Castillo S, Dionisio AR, Dela Cruz J (1995) The clinical course and outcome of a nearly fatal conotoxin poisoning: A case report. *Proceedings of the Sea Western Pacific Regional Meeting of Pharmacologists: Towards Rational Drug Therapy at the Turn of the Century.* p. 521.

13. McCleskey EW, Fox AP, Feldman D *et al.* (1987) Calcium channel blockade by a peptide from *Conus*: Specificity and mechanism. *Proc Nat Acad Sci USA* **84**, 4327.

14. McIntosh M, Cruz LJ, Hunkapiller MW *et al.* (1982) Isolation and structure of a peptide toxin from the marine snail *Conus magus. Arch Biochem Biophys* **218**, 329.

15. McIntosh JM, Ghomashchi F, Gelb MH *et al.* (1995) Conodipine-M, a novel phospholipase A_2 isolated from the venom of the marine snail *Conus magus. J Biol Chem* **270**, 3518.

16. McIntosh JM, Hasson A, Spira ME *et al.* (1995) A new family of conotoxins which block sodium channels. *J Biol Chem* **270**, 16796.

17. Mena EE, Gullak MF, Pagnozzi MJ *et al.* (1990) Conantokin-G: A novel peptide antagonist to the N-methyl-D-aspartate acid (NMDA) receptor. *Neurosci Lett* **118**, 241.

18. Myers RA, Cruz LJ, Rivier J *et al.* (1993) *Conus* peptides as chemical probes for receptors and ion channels. *Chem Rev* **93**, 1923.

19. Olivera BM, Gray WR, Zeikus R *et al.* (1985) Peptide neurotoxins from fish-hunting cone snails. *Science* **230**, 1338.

20. Olivera BM, McIntosh JM, Clark C *et al.* (1985) A sleep-inducing peptide from *Conus geographus* venom. *Toxicon* **23**, 277.

21. Olivera BM, Rivier J, Clark C *et al.* (1990) Diversity of *Conus* neuropeptides. *Science* **249**, 257.

22. Olivera BM, Rivier J, Scott JK *et al.* (1991) Conotoxins. *J Biol Chem* **266**, 22067.

23. Ramilo CA, Zafaralla GC, Nadasdi L *et al.* (1992) Novel α- and ω-conotoxins from *Conus striatus* venom. *Biochemistry* **31**, 9919.

24. Shon K, Grilley MM, Marsh M *et al.* (1995) Purification, characterization, synthesis and cloning of the lockjaw peptide from *Conus purpurascens* venom. *Biochemistry* **34**, 4913.

25. Yoshiba S (1984) An estimation of the most dangerous species of cone shell *Conus geographus* venoms lethal dose in humans. *Jpn J Hyg* **39**, 565.

26. Zafaralla GC, Ramilo C, Gray WR *et al.* (1988) Phylogenetic specificity of cholinergic ligands: α-Conotoxin SI. *Biochemistry* **27**, 7102.

CASE REPORT 12

A case of *Conus* sting in Batangas, Luzon, Philippines (May 1995): *A 26-year-old male spear-fishing in a reef area at night with two companions picked up a crawling specimen of* Conus geographus *and placed it under the elastic band of his swimming trunks. Shortly thereafter, he complained of being stung by the cone on the right side of his abdomen. In about 10–20 min, he complained of dizziness and malaise. After ~30–45 min, he felt as if he were dying; his legs were paralyzed, he had difficulty speaking and breathing, and his vision was blurred. On the way to the hospital, he mentioned that he had a severe headache. On arrival at the town hospital after about 1.5 h, he was shaking heavily. He continued complaining of a very severe headache and looked pale. Salucortef and diazepam were administered intravenously and benadryl intramuscularly. At around the third hour, he lost consciousness after vomiting a blackish material. He stopped breathing, then went into cardiac arrest. The doctor administered cardiopulmonary resuscitation, and he was able to breathe again in a few minutes. He was intubated with oxygen, and atropine and epinephrine were administered intravenously. The following morning, he was able to talk but was still weak, partially paralyzed, and numb.*

He was transferred to the Philippine General Hospital (~12 h after the sting) with intubation, although he was already breathing spontaneously. He was also awake and communicative. A pinpoint erythematous area was observed at the site of the sting. Neurological examination indicated slight circumoral numbness and right-sided sensory loss particularly in the lower leg. The electrocardiogram revealed peaked T waves. The medications given were amoxicillin, hydrocortisone, famotidine, and antitetanus prophylaxis. He was extubated on the second day at the city hospital. Hydrocortisone was discontinued; oral feeding and medication were started. On the third day, intravenous fluid was discontinued; vital signs were still monitored. On the fourth day, he still had peaked T waves but was otherwise asymptomatic. At the patient's insistence, he was sent home but advised to take a daily dose of vitamin B complex and to have minimal activity and bed rest for possible ischemia.

On the sixth day after the sting, he was readmitted to the city hospital complaining of headache in the left frontal area, which became generalized as a feeling of tightness around the head. This was accompanied by blurring of vision, weakness, and numbness of upper extremities. His blurred vision was attributed to edema due to optic neuritis, which responded to prednisone. He still had peaked T waves. His pulse rate remained low for a few days. On the 13th day, he was asymptomatic with normal cardiac findings, and was released from the hospital.

Corticosteroids

Byron A. Kakulas

CORTICOSTERONE
$C_{21}H_{30}O_4$

Corticosterone; (11β)-11,21-Dihydroxypregn-4-ene-3,20-dione

NEUROTOXICITY RATING

Clinical

A   Myopathy (vacuolar)

A   Psychobiological reaction (euphoria, mania)

A   Cushing's syndrome

Experimental

A   Myopathy (necrotizing)

Corticosteroids represent a family of naturally occurring or synthetic adrenocortical hormones. The natural glucocorticoids are hydrocortisone and corticosterone. Hydrocortisone, prednisolone, and prednisone are the most commonly used therapeutically. Corticosteroids have wide medical applications mainly as anti-inflammatory agents or immunosuppressives and also as membrane stabilizers (*e.g.*, as antiepileptics or antimyotonics), and in the treatment of cerebral edema. The usual oral dose range for prednisolone is 5–60 mg/day for adults. Immunosuppressive and anti-inflammatory dosage for children ranges from 0.2–1.0 mg/kg/day. The acute treatment of asthma in children can require between 1.0 and 2.0 mg/kg/day (1).

Corticosteroids, given in prolonged or high dosage, are associated with many unwanted side effects. The more important of these are cushingoid features, risk of infection, peptic ulceration, hypertension, diabetes mellitus, and growth retardation in children. Changes in mental state, ranging from mood alterations to psychosis, also occur (3). Euphoria and mania are especially common. Withdrawal from corticosteroids is risky and must be done gradually because of secondary adrenal cortical hypofunction from inhibition of adrenocorticotropic hormone secretion.

Experimental animal studies clearly demonstrate that corticosteroids cause muscle fiber necrosis (10,14). The synthetic analogs fluorocortisone (19,28) and triamcinolone

(48) are even more toxic to muscle. In severe cases, there is polyfocal myonecrosis or vacuolar degeneration of muscle (33,35). Myofilament loss is apparent on ultrastructural study (19). Physiological changes of muscle fiber function also appear (9,17). Severe myonecrosis follows the administration of methylchlorocortisol and NaH_2PO_4 in rabbits (6); this can be prevented by chloride administration (41).

Most of the naturally occurring and synthetic corticosteroids are known to produce side effects similar to the clinical features of Cushing's disease, including muscle weakness (23,33). This myopathy is usually dose-dependent (4) and varies with the type of corticosteroid (13,18,49). Myopathy is unlikely when the daily dose of the steroid is kept below 10 mg of prednisone or its equivalent (7,49).

Severe human corticosteroid myopathies are uncommon. Accurate determination of the frequency of mild (subclinical) myopathies is difficult to ascertain because mild forms may be overlooked, particularly in patients with an underlying musculoskeletal disorder such as rheumatoid arthritis. Quantitative studies of muscle function show significant reductions in muscle performance in these patients (24,37). Electromyographic findings also indicate subclinical myopathy to be common (8,49).

Symmetrical involvement of proximal limb muscles, particularly in lower limbs, with atrophy and weakness of the quadriceps, is prominent. Muscle pain is not usually a feature and the tendon reflexes are preserved. Serum muscle enzyme levels are normal and, if found to be elevated, should suggest the possibility of another myopathy. Creatinuria occurs, and urinary creatine levels have been held to be useful in diagnosis and in monitoring progress (4). Electromyography shows changes typical of primary muscle disease, particularly in proximal groups; spontaneous discharges are rare.

In contrast to experimental corticosteroid myopathy, the histological changes in human steroid myopathy are slight. Muscle biopsy shows selective atrophy of type 2B fibers (26). Necrosis, regeneration, and vacuolar change are uncommon. Strength usually returns on stopping the drug or, to some extent, on substituting prednisone for the offending steroid (46,48). Anabolic steroids and B-group vitamins, which prevent the development of corticosteroid myopathy in the rat (39), are ineffective in patients with steroid myopathy (9). A regular program of physical activity may partially prevent or reverse muscle atrophy and weakness (21,22). Inhaled corticosteroids may cause local myopathy of the laryngeal muscles with dysphonia (47). Electron microscope study reveals thickening of the basement membrane (2,30), focal aggregations of mitochondria, vacuolation of the sarcoplasmic reticulum, and glycogen accumulation (15,32). Similar abnormalities characterize experimental steroid myopathy in the rat and rabbit (1,10,16,36). The increase in glycogen content is consistent with the elevated glycogen synthetase activity in experimental steroid myopathy (42). Lipid droplets are increased in muscle fibers in iatrogenic steroid myopathy, as well as in Cushing's disease (10,16,20). Fat accumulation does not occur in all cases (3). Necrosis and calcification of muscle fibers in acute, high-dose animal experiments (2,16) parallel the acute necrobiotic myopathy in patients with status asthmaticus treated with large intravenous doses of hydrocortisone (27,45). Myopathy may occur in Cushing's syndrome associated with acromegaly (31). Aldosterone or high doses of aldosterone-like substance ("licorice-abuse syndrome") hypokalemia may be associated with diffuse weakness and necrotizing myopathy (5,40).

Although usually subacute or chronic, steroid myopathy may also be acute. There have been reports of patients with status asthmaticus who were treated with high doses of intravenous hydrocortisone and developed a severe generalized myopathy with involvement of respiratory muscles and elevation of serum creatine kinase (CK) (27,29,45). Muscle biopsy showed vacuolar changes in both histochemical fiber types with evidence of regeneration. These features resembled experimental steroid myopathy in rabbits (1). Recovery was slow in these patients.

The combination of high-dose corticosteroids and prolonged administration of nondepolarizing muscle relaxants (pancuronium, vecuronium) may result in a unique myopathic condition commonly encountered by anesthesiologists. In this syndrome, severe diffuse muscle weakness, atrophy, and areflexia suddenly appear following termination of ventilatory support (11,12). Ophthalmoplegia may also occur (44). Serum creatine kinase activity can be elevated or normal. Most recover within weeks to months. Electron microscope study of muscle biopsy in one case showed selective loss of thick filaments (11); this is held to result from the combination of steroids and pharmacological denervation, similar to the effects of steroids on denervated rat muscle (38). Other cases have shown large areas of myofilament loss and resulting loss of staining in both fiber types (12).

The toxic mechanism involved in steroid myopathy is poorly understood; it is widely held to be related to its catabolic functions. Experimental studies show that specific corticosteroid receptors are present in muscle (42), and that corticosteroids interfere with oxidative metabolism (25) and enhance glycogen synthesis and degradation (43). Corticosteroids also inhibit the synthesis of messenger RNA, which may modify the translation and synthesis of muscle-specific proteins (34).

REFERENCES

1. Afifi AK, Bergman RA (1969) Steroid myopathy. A study of the evolution of the muscle lesion in rabbits. *Johns Hopkins Med J* **124**, 66.
2. Afifi AK, Bergman RA, Harvey JC (1968) Steroid myopathy. Clinical, histologic and cytologic observations. *Johns Hopkins Med J* **123**, 158.
3. Argov Z, Mastaglia FL (1994) Drug-induced neuromuscular disorders in man. In: *Disorders of Voluntary Muscle. 6th Ed.* Walton JN, Kaparti G, Hilton-Jones D eds. Churchill Livingstone, Edinburgh, p. 989.
4. Askari A, Vignos PJ, Moskowitz RW (1976) Steroid myopathy in connective tissue disease. *Amer J Med* **61**, 485.
5. Atsumi T, Isikawa S-E, Miyatake T, Yoshida M (1979) Myopathy and primary aldosteronism: Electronmicroscopic study. *Neurology* **29**, 1348.
6. Bajusz E (1965) Experimental myopathies: Influence of various factors as reflected by histochemical and morphological studies. In: *Myopathien*. Beckmann R ed. George Thieme, Stuttgart p. 121.
7. Bowyer SL, La Monthe MP, Hollister JR (1985) Steroid myopathy: Incidence and detection in a population with asthma. *J Allerg Clin Immunol* **76**, 234.
8. Coomes EN (1965) Corticosteroid myopathy. *Ann Rheum Dis* **24**, 465.
9. Coomes EN (1965) The rate of recovery of reversible myopathies and the effects of anabolic agents. *Neurology* **15**, 523.
10. D'Agostino AN, Chiga M (1966) Corticosteroid myopathy in the rabbit. A light and electron microscopic study. *Neurology* **16**, 257.
11. Dalakas MC (1992) Inflammatory and toxic myopathies. *Curr Opin Neurol Neurosurg* **5**, 645.
12. Danon MJ, Carpenter S (1991) Myopathy with thick filament (myosin) loss following prolonged paralysis with vecuronium during steroid treatment. *Muscle Nerve* **14**, 1131.
13. Dropcho EJ, Soong S (1991) Steroid induced weakness in patients with primary brain tumors. *Neurology* **41**, 1235.
14. Ellis JT (1956) Necrosis and regeneration of skeletal muscle in cortisone-treated rabbits. *Amer J Pathol* **32**, 993.
15. Engel AG (1966) Thyrotoxic and corticosteroid-induced myopathies. *Mayo Clin Proc* **41**, 785.
16. Freund-Molbert E, Ketelsen UP, Beckmann R (1973) Ultrastructural study of experimental steroid myopathy. In: *Basic Research in Myology*. Kakulas BA ed. Excerpta Medica, Amsterdam p. 593.
17. Gardiner PF, Edgerton VR (1979) Contractile responses of rat fast-twitch and slow-twitch muscles to glucocorticoid treatment. *Muscle Nerve* **2**, 274.

18. Golding DN, Begg TB (1960) Dexamethasone myopathy. *Brit Med J* **2**, 1129.

19. Golding DN, Murray SM, Pearce GW, Thompson M (1961) Corticosteroid myopathy. *Ann Phys Med* **6**, 171.

20. Harriman DGF, Reed L (1972) The incidence of lipid droplets in human muscle in neuromuscular disorders. *J Pathol* **106**, 1.

21. Hickson RC, Davis JR (1981) Partial prevention of glucocorticoid-induced muscle atrophy by endurance training. *Amer J Physiol* **241**, E226.

22. Horber FF, Scheidegger JR, Grunig BE, Frey FJ (1985) Thigh muscle mass and function in patients treated with glucocorticoids. *Eur J Clin Invest* **15**, 302.

23. Kakulas BA, Adams RD (1985) *Diseases of Muscle: Pathological Foundations of Clinical Myology. 4th Ed.* Harper & Row, Philadelphia p. 603.

24. Khaleeli AA, Edwards RHT, Gohil K *et al.* (1983) Corticosteroid myopathy: A clinical and pathological study. *Clin Endocrinol* **18**, 115.

25. Koski CL, Rifenberick DH, Max SR (1974) Oxidative metabolism of skeletal muscle in steroid atrophy. *Arch Neurol* **31**, 407.

26. Livingstone IR, Johnson MA, Mastaglia FL (1981) Effects of dexamethasone on fibre subtypes in rat muscle. *Neuropathol Appl Neurobiol* **7**, 381.

27. MacFarlane IA, Rosenthal FD (1977) Severe myopathy after status asthmaticus. *Lancet* **2**, 615.

28. Maclean K, Schurr PH (1959) Reversible amyotrophy complicating treatment with fludrocortisone. *Lancet* **1**, 701.

29. Mastaglia FL, Argov Z (1982) Immunologically-mediated drug-induced neuromuscular disorders. In: *Pseudo-allergic Reactions—Involvement of Drugs and Chemicals. Vol 3. Cell Mediated Reactions.* Dukor P, Kallos P, Schlumberger HD, West GB eds. Karger, Basel p. 1.

30. Mastaglia FL, McCollum JPK, Larson PF, Hudgson P (1970) Steroid myopathy complicating McArdle's disease. *J Neurol Neurosurg Psychiat* **33**, 111.

31. Muller R, Kugelberg E (1959) Myopathy in Cushing's syndrome. *J Neurol Neurosurg Psychiat* **22**, 314.

32. Pearce GW (1964) Tissue culture and electron microscopy in muscle disease. In: *Disorders of Voluntary Muscle.* Walton JN ed. Churchill, London.

33. Perkoff GT, Silber R, Tyler FH *et al.* (1959) Studies in disorders of muscle. XII. Myopathy due to the administration of therapeutic amounts of 17-hydroxycorticosteroids. *Amer J Med* **26**, 891.

34. Rannels SR, Rannels DE, Pegg AE, Jefferson LS (1978) Glucocorticoid effects on peptide-chain initiation in skeletal muscle and heart. *Amer J Physiol* **235**, E134.

35. Rewcastle NB, Humphrey JG (1965) Vacuolar myopathy, clinical histochemical and microscopic study. *Arch Neurol* **12**, 570.

36. Ritter RA (1967) The effect of cortisone on the structure and function of skeletal muscle. *Arch Neurol* **17**, 493.

37. Rothstein JM, Delitto A, Sinacore DR, Rose SJ (1983) Muscle function in rheumatic disease patients treated with corticosteroids. *Muscle Nerve* **6**, 128.

38. Rouleau G, Karpati G, Carpenter S (1987) Glucocorticoid excess induces preferential depletion of myosin in denervated skeletal muscle fibres. *Muscle Nerve* **10**, 428.

39. Sakai Y, Kobayashi K, Iwata N (1978) Effects of an anabolic steroid and vitamin B complex upon myopathy induced by corticosteroids. *Eur J Pharmacol* **52**, 353.

40. Sambrook MA, Heron JR, Aber GM (1972) Myopathy in association with primary hyperaldosteronism. *J Neurol Neurosurg Psychiat* **35**, 202.

41. Selye H, Bajusz E (1960) The prevention of experimental myopathies by various chlorides. *J Nutr* **72**, 37.

42. Shoji S, Pennington RJT (1977) Binding of dexamethasone and cortisol to cytosol receptors in rat extensor digitorum longus and soleus muscles. *Exp Neurol* **57**, 342.

43. Shoji S, Pennington RJT (1977) The effect of cortisone on protein breakdown and synthesis in rat skeletal muscle. *Mol Cell Endocrinol* **6**, 159.

44. Sitwell LD, Weinshenker BG, Monpetit V, Reid D (1991) Complete ophthalmoplegia as a complication of acute corticosteroid- and pancuronium-associated myopathy. *Neurology* **41**, 921.

45. Van Marle W, Woods KL (1980) Acute hydrocortisone myopathy. *Brit Med J* **3**, 271.

46. Walton JN (1977) *Brain's Diseases of the Nervous System. 8th Ed.* Oxford University Press, Oxford.

47. Williams AJ, Baghat MS, Stableforth DE *et al.* (1983) Dysphonia caused by inhaled steroids: recognition of a characteristic laryngeal abnormality. *Thorax* **38**, 813.

48. Williams RS (1959) Triamcinolone myopathy. *Lancet* **1**, 698.

49. Yates DAH (1970) Steroid myopathy. In: *Muscle Diseases.* Walton JN, Canal N, Scarlato G eds. Excerpta Medica, Amsterdam p. 482.

Cotyledon Spp.

Albert C. Ludolph

NEUROTOXICITY RATING

Clinical

A Extrapyramidal syndrome (in livestock, torticollis)

Plants of *Cotyledon, Kalanchoe* and *Tylecodon* spp. contain toxic glycosides, bufadienolides; these are named after the toad of the genus *Bufo* (1,2), which also harbors these compounds in venom. Toad venom may kill dogs and, occasionally, humans (5). The glycoside orbicuside A-C is present in *Cotyledon orbiculata*; lanceotoxin A and B and 3-O-acetylhelelbrigenin are the toxic principles of *Kalanchoe lanceolata*; and *Tylecodon wallichii grandiflorus* contains cotyledoside and tyledosides A-D, F, and G (2). Methods for extraction and identification of bufadienolides from each of the plants are available (2). Reportedly, consumption of these plants by goats leads to large livestock losses, in particular among young animals in southern Africa (2).

Acute poisoning of cattle, sheep, and goats is dominated by the cardiac effects of the glycoside (2,3); after chronic consumption of *Cotyledon* spp. or *Tylecodon* spp., sheep and goats show weight loss and develop a neuromuscular disorder ("cotyledonosis," "*krimpsiekte*," "nenta poisoning") characterized by muscle cramps and a torticollis-like picture (4). Labored breathing, a drooping lower jaw, a dangling head, and intolerance to exercise consitute the syndrome. After ingestion of bufadienolides, a torticollis-like picture appears in dogs and horses (4).

The popular house and garden plant *Kalanchoe blossfeldiana* also contains the same agents; minor intoxications in children may follow the ingestion of its leaves (1,6). Childhood intoxications should be treated by standard means (activated charcoal, increased fluid intake) (1,6). Experimental studies of chicks given *Kalanchoe* spp. have failed to identify the causative agent (7).

REFERENCES

1. Frohne D, Pfänder HJ (1987) *Giftpflanzen. Ein Handbuch für Apotheker, Ärzte, Toxikologen und Biologen*, 3. Auflage. Wissenschaftliche Verlagsgesellschaft mbH, Stuttgart.
2. Joubert JBJ (1989) Cardiac glycosides. In: *Toxicants of Plant Origin. Vol II. Glycosides.* Cheeke PR ed. CRC Press, Boca Raton, Florida p. 61.
3. Masvingwe C, Mavenyengwa M (1997) *Kalanchoe lanceolata* poisoning in Brahman cattle in Zimbabwe: the first field outbreak. *S Afr Vet Assn* **68**, 18.
4. Naude TW (1977) The occurence and significance of South African cardiac glycosides. *J S Afr Biol Soc* **18**, 7.
5. Otani A, Palumbo N, Read G (1969) Pharmacodynamics and treatment of mammals poisoned by *Bufo marinus* toxin. *Amer J Vet Res* **30**, 1865.
6. Ritter S, Krienke EG (1986) D. Vergiftungsunfälle mit Pflanzen. In: *Vergiftungen im Kindesalter.* Krienke EG, Mühlendahl KE, Oberdisse U eds. Ferdinad Enke Verlag, Stuttgart p. 222.
7. Williams MC, Smith MC (1984) Toxicity of *Kalanchoe* spp. to chicks. *Amer J Vet Res* **45**, 453.

Crotalaria Spp.

Albert C. Ludolph

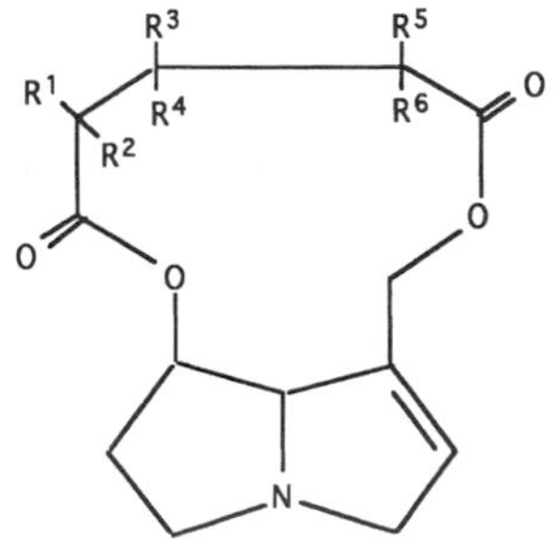

R¹–R⁶: *See* Table 18, page 424.

NEUROTOXICITY RATING

Clinical

B Hepatic encephalopathy (secondary)

B Acute encephalopathy (cattle)

Several species of the plant genus *Crotalaria* contain pyrrolizidine alkaloids (Table 18) with hepatotoxic, pneumotoxic, and carcinogenic properties (1,2,3). In humans, acute or chronic intoxication leads to severe liver necrosis from veno-occlusive disease and eventually causes hepatic encephalopathy; the genus is not primarily neurotoxic. En-

TABLE 18. Pyrrolizidine Alkaloids in *Crotalaria* Implicated in Human Intoxications

	R^1	R^2	R^3	R^4	R^5	R^6
Fulvine	CH$_3$	H	CH$_3$	OH	CH$_3$	H
Monocrotaline	CH$_3$	H	CH$_3$	OH	CH$_3$	OH
Cronaburmine	CH$_3$	H	CH$_3$	H	CHOHCH$_3$	H
Spectabiline	CH$_3$	H	CH$_3$	CH$_3$	CH$_3$	OH
Junceine	CH$_3$CH	H	CH$_3$	OH	CH$_2$OH	OH
Retusine	CH$_3$	H	CH$_3$	H	CH$_3$	OH

[Modified from Huxtable (3).]

demic hepatic disorders among children in Jamaica were traced to the practice of administering teas collected from the leaves of the scrub bush (3). A clinically similar picture is induced by the pyrrolizidine-containing genera *Cynoglossum*, *Heliotropum*, *Petasites*, *Senecio* and *Symphytum*. Pyrrolizidines are allegedly neurotoxic for horses, and the intoxication is associated with disease names such as "stomach staggers," "walking disease," "walkabout disease," and "dzhalangarsk encephalitis." Cows become manic.

REFERENCES

1. Cheeke PR (1988) Toxicity and metabolism of pyrrolizidine alkaloids. *J Anim Sci* **66**, 2343.
2. Huxtable RJ (1980) Problems with pyrrozilidines. *Trends Pharmacol Sci* **1**, 299.
3. Huxtable RJ (1989) Human health implications of pyrrolizidine alkaloids and herbs containing them. In: *Toxicants of Plant Origin. Vol I. Alkaloids.* Cheeke PR ed. CRC Press, Boca Raton, Florida p. 41.

Crotamine

Albert C. Ludolph

NEUROTOXICITY RATING

Clinical

A   Myopathy (contraction, vacuolar myopathy)

Experimental

A   Muscle sodium channel activation

Most venoms of *Crotalus* spp., in particular the venom of three *Crotalus durissus* subspecies, have myotoxic properties; these may cause myoglobin release and renal failure (9). Myotoxic effects are caused by the β-neurotoxin and phospholipase A$_2$ crotoxin; the 40 to 46-amino-acid peptide crotamine (MW, 5000) is also myotoxic (7). Crotamine is structurally similar to other myotoxic compounds in *Crotalus* spp. venom, such as myotoxin a [from *Crotalus v. viridis* (4)], CAM-toxin [from *C. adamanteus* venom (8)], peptide c [from *C. v. helleri* (5)], myotoxin I and II [from *C. v. concolor* (1,3)], and toxin III [from *C. horridus horridus*, (6)]. These myotoxic peptides and their effects are distinguished from the myotoxic property of phospholipase A$_2$.

After injection *in vivo*, crotamine causes muscle contracture that may last for several hours; it is associated with vacuolar changes on biopsy (2). Crotamine binds to the muscle membrane and activates sodium channels, reduces the membrane potential, and induces muscle contraction; these effects are antagonized by tetrodotoxin.

Crotamine is very similar to myotoxin a; differences exist only at three positions in the molecule. Myotoxin a inhibits Ca^{2+}–adenosine triphosphatase.

REFERENCES

1. Bieber AL, McParland RH, Becker RR (1987) Amino acid sequences of myotoxins from *Crotalus viridis concolor* venom. *Toxicon* **25**, 677.
2. Cameron DL, Tu AT (1978) Chemical and functional homology of myotoxin a from prairie rattlesnake venom and crotamine from South American rattlesnake venom. *Biochim Biophys Acta* **532**, 147.
3. Engle CM, Becker RR, Bailey T, Bieber AL (1983) Characterization of two myotoxic proteins from venom of *Crotalus viridis concolor*. *J Toxicol-Toxin Rev* **2**, 267.
4. Laure CJ (1975) Die Primärstruktur des Crotamins. *Hoppe-Seyler's Z Physiol Chemie* **356**, 213.
5. Maeda N, Tamiya N, Pattabhiraman TR, Russell FE (1978) Some chemical properties of the venom of the rattlesnake *Crotalus viridis helleri*. *Toxicon* **16**, 431.
6. Mebs D, Ehrenfeld M, Samejima Y (1983) Local necrotizing effects of snake venoms on skin and muscle: Relationship to serum creatine kinase. *Toxicon* **21**, 393.
7. Mebs D, Ownby CL (1990) Myotoxic components of snake venoms: Their biochemical and biological activities. *Pharmacol Ther* **48**, 223.
8. Samejima Y, Aoki Y, Mebs D (1988) Structural studies on a myotoxin from *Crotalus adamanteus* venom. In: *Progress in Venom and Toxin Research.* Gopalakrishnakone O, Tan CK eds. Academic Press, New York p. 186.
9. Santoro ML, Sousa-e-Silva MC, Goncalves LR *et al.* (1999) Comparison of the biological activities in venoms from three subspecies of the South American rattlesnake. *Comp Biochem Physiol Pt C* **122**, 61.

Crotoxin

Albert C. Ludolph

NEUROTOXICITY RATING

Clinical

A Neuromuscular transmission syndrome

A Myopathy (necrotizing)

Experimental

A Presynaptic nicotinic blockade

Crotoxin is a dimeric polypeptide (molecular mass, 23.5 kDa) from the venom of the southern Brazilian rattlesnake (*Crotalus durissus terrificus*) (8,11). The agent acts presynaptically at motor nerve terminals. In isolated nerve-muscle preparations, its effect on transmitter release occurs in three stages (2): An initial transient inhibition of acetylcholine release (first few minutes), resulting in a decrease of muscle contraction, is followed by facilitation of acetylcholine release over 30–60 min. Frequency of miniature end-plate potentials is increased during this time. Finally, the output of acetylcholine and frequency of miniature end-plate potentials decrease and block of neuromuscular transmission becomes complete. Neurotoxicity may reflect selective, site-directed hydrolysis of membrane phospholipids. Exocytotic release sites are also affected since, in common with other β-neurotoxins, crotoxin also has phospholipase A activity (2).

Crotoxin consists of two subunits; uncombined, each is comparatively nontoxic. The noncovalent link of the acidic subunit A (crotapotin) and the basic subunit B (crotactin) greatly enhances toxicity (10). Both the entire protein and the 140-amino-acid subunit B possess phospholipase A activity, whereas subunit A is enzymatically nonactive. Subunit B has hemolytic properties, interacts with fatty acids, and—in contrast to β-bungarotoxin—also binds to the receptor postsynaptically (1). Subunit A is relatively nontoxic but responsible for specific presynaptic binding of the protein at a receptor site (3,4) and increases the toxicity of crotoxin B at least 20-fold. *Crotalus* bites are frequently followed by elevation of serum creatine kinase levels and myoglobinuria; renal failure may result from myoglobin release. This myotoxic component is partly from an effect of crotoxin but is mostly caused by crotamine (*see* Crotamine, this volume). Crotamine is a major component of the venom of *C. durissus terrificus*.

The bite of the southern American rattlesnake (*C. durissus*) often induces severe minor local swelling, edema, and necrosis. Muscle paralysis (ophthalmoplegia, facial paralysis, danger of involvement of respiratory muscles), hypovolemia, and coagulopathy develop after the majority of bites (5,6). Rhabdomyolysis and renal failure are often prominent and life-threatening. Bites of North American rattlesnakes more often induce hypovolemic shock and coagulopathy; local reactions are more severe. Toxic effects on the muscle and the neuromuscular junction are less pronounced (5,6).

Therapeutically, general measures are similar to those described after cobra bites (*see* Cobra Venom, this volume). In particular, a coagulation profile, blood count and hematocrit, blood-gas tension and pH, creatine kinase serum levels, electrolytes, myoglobinuria, and renal function should be repeatedly monitored during the observation period (12). Surgical intervention is not part of the acute treatment of snakebites (7,9,12). Polyvalent antivenom (Wyeth antivenin) should be used if coagulopathy or paresis of external ocular and facial muscles develop (12). Local changes after snake bites often do not respond to antivenom treatment, and serum sickness is common after higher dosages of antivenom.

REFERENCES

1. Bon C, Changeux JP, Jeng TW, Fraenkel-Conrat H (1979) Post-synaptic effects of crotoxin and of its isolated subunits. *Eur J Biochem* **99**, 471.

2. Hawgood B, Bon C (1991) Snake venom pre-synaptic toxins. In: *Handbook of Natural Neurotoxins. Vol 5. Reptile Venoms and Toxins.* Tu AT ed. Marcel Dekker, New York p. 3.

3. Hendon RA, Tu AT (1979) The role of crotoxin subunits in tropical rattlesnake neurotoxic action. *Biochim Biophys Acta* **578**, 243.

4. Hseu M, Guillory RJ, Tzeng MC (1990) Identification of a crotoxin-binding protein in membranes from guinea pig brain by photoaffinity labelling. *J Bioenerg Biomembr* **22**, 39.

5. Mebs D (1992) *Gifttiere. Ein Handbuch für Biologen, Toxikologen, Ärzte, Apotheker.* Wissenschaftliche Verlagsgesellschaft mB, Stuttgart.

6. Minton SA (1990) Neurotoxic snake envenoming. *Semin Neurol* **10**, 52.

7. Russell FE (1980) *Snake Venom Poisoning.* JB Lippincott Co, Philadelphia.

8. Slotta K, Fraenkel-Conrat H (1938) Two active proteins from rattlesnake venom. *Nature* **142**, 213.

9. Stewart RM, Page CP, Schwesinger WH *et al.* (1989) Antivenin and fasciotomy/debridement in the treatment of severe rattlesnake bite. *Amer J Surg* **158**, 543.

10. Trivedi S, Kaiser II, Tanaka M, Simpson LL (1989) Pharmacological experiments on the interaction between crotoxin and the mammalian neuromuscular junction. *J Pharmacol Exp Ther* **251**, 490.

11. Tu AT (1994) Neurotoxins from snake venoms. In: *Handbook of Neurotoxicology*. Chang LW, Dyer RS eds. Marcel Dekker, New York p. 637.

12. Wingert WA (1991) Management of crotalid envenomations. In: *Handbook of Natural Neurotoxins. Vol 5. Reptile Venoms and Toxins*. Tu AT ed. Marcel Dekker, New York p. 611.

Cuprizone

Thomas W. Bouldin

CUPRIZONE
$C_{14}H_{22}N_4O_2$

Bis-cyclohexanone oxaldihydrazone

NEUROTOXICITY RATING

Experimental

A Leukoencephalopathy (intramyelinic edema)

A Hydrocephalus (aqueductal stenosis)

A Peripheral neuropathy

Cuprizone is a disubstituted hydrazine with a MP of 214°–216°C. It is a copper chelator and has been used in a quantitative spectrophotometric procedure for copper analysis (17). In a study of an animal model of swayback (a copper-deficiency disease of sheep and calves), cuprizone caused hydrocephalus, spongiform change, demyelination, and an Alzheimer's type II astrocytosis in the CNS of weanling mice (6). The spongiform change was due to intramyelinic edema, and giant mitochondria and proliferated smooth endoplasmic reticulum appeared in hepatocytes (19). Remyelination occurs quickly after cuprizone is withdrawn from the diet, making cuprizone a useful neurotoxicant for producing experimental models of demyelination and remyelination in the CNS (2–4,14). There are no reports of cuprizone toxicity in humans.

The absorption, distribution, metabolism, and excretion of cuprizone are unknown. The CNS, PNS and liver are target organs in experimental animal models.

Weanling mice fed a diet containing 0.1% cuprizone over a 7-week period have slightly reduced growth rates and develop spongiform edema of the brain (6). A diet with 0.5% cuprizone is much more toxic, causing marked growth retardation, hindlimb paresis, seizure activity, fetal wastage, and a high mortality rate (6,10,19). Within 5 days of treatment, vacuolation appears in myelin (spongiform change) in cerebellum, cerebrum, and brain stem (19). The myelin-associated vacuoles represent intramyelinic edema, with separation of myelin lamellae at the intraperiod line (2,14,19). Degenerative changes appear in oligodendrocytes at 1 week and peak after 2 weeks of treatment; oligodendrocytes are greatly reduced in number after 4 weeks (2,14,19). Degeneration of myelin becomes evident after 2–3 weeks of exposure, and completely demyelinated axons are present after 4–7 weeks (2,14). Myelin debris is removed by macrophages that appear during the third week of intoxication (2,14). Remyelination begins within 1 week after stopping cuprizone, and almost all axons are remyelinated within 4 weeks (3,14). Remyelinated axons have thin myelin sheaths and short internodal lengths (3,4,14). Astrocytes show cellular swelling, vacuolation, and proliferation (14,19). The blood-brain barrier remains intact during cuprizone-induced demyelination (1,12).

Cuprizone-induced hydrocephalus is secondary to aqueductal stenosis; it becomes evident after 3 weeks of treatment (7,9). The aqueductal stenosis is postulated to be secondary to compression of the aqueduct by edematous myelin sheaths in the midbrain (9).

Giant mitochondria appear in hepatocytes and oligodendrocytes during cuprizone intoxication and display a variety of degenerative changes (13,14,19). Giant hepatic mitochondria return to normal size by dividing within hours of stopping cuprizone treatment (20).

Cuprizone inhibits beef-liver mitochondrial monoamine oxidase, a copper protein, *in vitro* (18). Human plasma monoamine oxidase is also inhibited by cuprizone *in vitro* (15).

Cuprizone toxicity varies with strain and with species (14). Mice are most vulnerable to the myelinotoxic effects of cuprizone, with both weanling and old male mice showing demyelination and remyelination (3,4,14). Female mice do not show demyelination (14). Rats and guinea pigs develop myelin edema, but not hydrocephalus or demyelination (8,13).

Rats also develop peripheral neuropathy of the distal axonopathy type. Although neuropathy primarily affects myelinated fibers, peripheral nerve myelin is not edematous.

The pathogenesis of the peripheral neuropathy and its relationship to cuprizone-induced degeneration of oligodendrocytes and CNS demyelination are unclear (13).

It is generally accepted that cuprizone demyelination in the CNS is secondary to degeneration of oligodendrocytes (2). The pathogenesis of oligodendrocytic cell injury is unknown. The pathogenesis of the reversible cuprizone-induced intramyelinic edema is also unknown. Cuprizone decreases the copper content of the brain and alters the expression and distribution of the glial enzymes, carbonic anhydrase II and glutathione-S-transferase (5,11,21,22). It also depresses the activities of monoamine oxidase and cytochrome oxidase in brain and liver (22). Cuprizone depresses mRNA for myelin-associated glycoprotein, myelin basic protein, and ceramide galactosyltransferase before the morphological appearance of demyelination. However, mRNA levels recover in the face of massive demyelination. Upregulation of mRNA for these myelin genes does not correlate with initiation of remyelination (16). Copper-chelated cuprizone does not produce neurotoxic or hepatotoxic effects; it is suggested that the copper-chelating properties of cuprizone are important in the pathogenesis of cuprizone toxicity (20). Supplementation of the diet with copper does not ameliorate the neurotoxic effects of cuprizone (6).

REFERENCES

1. Bakker DA, Ludwin SK (1987) Blood-brain barrier permeability during cuprizone-induced demyelination. *J Neurol Sci* **78**, 125.
2. Blakemore WF (1972) Observations on oligodendrocyte degeneration, the resolution of status spongiosus and remyelination in cuprizone intoxication in mice. *J Neurocytol* **1**, 413.
3. Blakemore WF (1973) Remyelination of the superior cerebellar peduncle in the mouse following demyelination induced by feeding cuprizone. *J Neurol Sci* **20**, 73.
4. Blakemore WF (1974) Remyelination of the superior cerebellar peduncle in old mice following demyelination induced by cuprizone. *J Neurol Sci* **22**, 121.
5. Cammer W, Zhang H (1993) Atypical localization of the oligodendrocytic isoform (PI) of glutathione-S-transferase in astrocytes during cuprizone intoxication. *J Neurosci Res* **36**, 183.
6. Carlton WW (1966) Response of mice to the chelating agents sodium diethyldithiocarbamate, α-benzoinoxime, and biscyclohexanone oxaldihydrazone. *Toxicol Appl Pharmacol* **8**, 512.
7. Carlton WW (1967) Studies on the induction of hydrocephalus and spongy degeneration by cuprizone feeding and attempts to antidote the toxicity. *Life Sci* **6**, 11.
8. Carlton WW (1969) Spongiform encephalopathy induced in rats and guinea pigs by cuprizone. *Exp Mol Pathol* **10**, 274.
9. Kesterson JW, Carlton WW (1970) Aqueductal stenosis as the cause of hydrocephalus in mice fed the substituted hydrazine. *Exp Mol Pathol* **13**, 281.
10. Kesterson JW, Carlton WW (1971) Histopathologic and enzyme histochemical observations of the cuprizone-induced brain edema. *Exp Mol Pathol* **15**, 82.
11. Komoly S, Jeyasingham MD, Pratt OE, Lantos PL (1987) Decrease in oligodendrocyte carbonic anhydrase activity preceding myelin degeneration in cuprizone induced demyelination. *J Neurol Sci* **79**, 141.
12. Kondo A, Nakano T, Suzuki K (1987) Blood-brain barrier permeability to horseradish peroxidase in twitcher and cuprizone-intoxicated mice. *Brain Res* **425**, 186.
13. Love S (1988) Cuprizone neurotoxicity in the rat: Morphologic observations. *J Neurol Sci* **84**, 223.
14. Ludwin SK (1978) Central nervous system demyelination and remyelination in the mouse. *Lab Invest* **39**, 597.
15. McEwen CM (1965) Human plasma monoamine oxidase. *J Biol Chem* **240**, 2003.
16. Morell P, Barrett CV, Mason JL *et al.* (1998) Gene expression in brain during cuprizone-induced demyelination and demyelination. *Mol Cell Neurosci* **12**, 220.
17. Peterson RE, Bollier ME (1955) Spectrophotometric determination of serum copper with biscyclohexanone oxalyldihydrazone. *Anal Chem* **27**, 1195.
18. Sakari N, Yasunobu KT (1966) Some recent advances in the field of amine oxidases. In: *The Biochemistry of Copper.* Peisach J, Aisen P, Blumberg WE eds. Academic Press, New York p. 423.
19. Suzuki K, Kikkawa Y (1969) Status spongiosus of CNS and hepatic changes induced by cuprizone (biscyclohexanone oxalyldihydrazone). *Amer J Pathol* **54**, 307.
20. Tandler B, Hoppel CL (1973) Division of giant mitochondria during recovery from cuprizone intoxication. *J Cell Biol* **56**, 266.
21. Tansey FA, Zhang H, Cammer W (1997) Rapid upregulation of the Pi isoform of glutathione-S-transferase in mouse brains after withdrawal of the neurotoxicant, cuprizone. *Mol Chem Neuropathol* **31**, 161.
22. Venturini G (1973) Enzymic activities and sodium, potassium and copper concentrations in mouse brain and liver after cuprizone treatment *in vivo. J Neurochem* **21**, 1147.

Cyanides and Related Compounds

John Tor-Agbidye
Peter S. Spencer

CN

Hydrogen cyanide—HCN
Sodium cyanide—NaCN
Sodium cyanate—NaOCN
Sodium thiocyanate—NaSCN
Cyanogen, ethanedinitrile—C_2N_2
Cyanogen chloride—CNCl

NEUROTOXICITY RATING

Hydrogen cyanide

Clinical

A   Seizure disorder

Experimental

A   Convulsant

B   Encephalopathy

B   Striatal necrosis

Sodium cyanate

Clinical

A   Peripheral neuropathy

B   Spastic paraparesis

Experimental

A   Peripheral neuropathy

B   Spastic paraparesis

Cyanides (CN) and compounds releasing cyanide have well-established acute neurotoxic properties. Many flora and fauna are armed with cyanide-releasing compounds, presumably for the purposes of defense against predators. Humans have used hydrogen cyanide (HCN) for chemical warfare and as a tool for suicide, murder, and judicial execution. Cyanide and cyanate have different neurotoxic properties. Cyanocobalamin (vitamin B_{12}) is required for normal health, and endogenous cyanide might have a physiological role in modulating synaptic activity.

Cyanogens are present in certain bacteria (*e.g.*, *Chromobacterium violaceum*); algae (*Chorella vulgaris*); fungi (30 species in five families); higher plants (>1000 species), and certain centipedes (seven species), millipedes, and insects (ten species) (86). Higher plants contain a wide range of cyanogenic glucosides (60 known) that release cyanohydrin and HCN when hydrolyzed by β-glucosidases (85). Many cyanophoric plants are used for animal feed (sorghum) and human food, including cassava (tapioca), sorghum, soybeans, spinach, lima beans, sweet potato, sugarcane, and bamboo shoots. Sorghum leaves contain 192–1250 mg/g and apricot pits 89–2170 mg/g CN⁻

w/w (16,48). For cassava root, a staple for several hundred million people, the cyanide equivalent of total cyanogenic content (cyanogenic glucosides, cyanohydrins, and HCN) reportedly ranges from 86–1458 mg/g CN⁻ dry weight (63). A 1976 publication noted the presence of hydrocyanic acid in stone fruit juices (notably cherry) that were homemade (5–25 mg/l) or prepared commercially (<5 mg/l) (82). Many other edible plants (cabbage, kale, broccoli, brussels sprouts, cauliflower) contain thiocyanates or glucosinolates that are hydrolyzed to thiocyanate (26). Laetrile, a product containing the cyanogenic glucoside amygdalin, was formerly used in clinical trials for the treatment of cancer (41) and may still be encountered as a self-medicament. The antihypertensive drug sodium nitroprusside reacts with hemoglobin to form cyanomethemoglobin, with the concomitant release of excess free cyanide (78). Cyanide is a common product of combustion (18,36), notably of nitriles (45) and nitrogen-containing plastics, and is present in tobacco smoke (72) and automobile exhaust (1). It is found in certain rodenticides and pesticides, metal and silver polishes, photographic solutions, and fumigating products.

HCN is produced commercially by direct synthesis and as a by-product of acrylonitrile manufacture; annual demand in the United States approximates 1.5 billion pounds (1), principally for the production of adiponitrile, methyl methacrylate, and sodium cyanide. Potassium cyanide (KCN), sodium cyanide (NaCN), and calcium cyanide are used in the steel, electroplating, mining, and chemical industries: they serve as analytical reagents; as insecticides and fumigants; in the extraction of gold and silver from metal-bearing ores; in metal cleaning; and in the manufacture of fibers, plastics, dyes, pigments, and nylon. Cyanogen is used as a rocket propellant, and cyanogen chloride is deployed as a chemical-warfare agent (1). HCN was used as a chemical-warfare agent by France in World War I, to kill political prisoners in German concentration camps in World War II, and as a means to execute criminals (57).

NaCN and KCN are white solids. Alkaline cyanides are strongly dissociated in aqueous solution and may decompose upon exposure to air or light. HCN is a colorless gas or a colorless to yellow-brown liquid with a tendency to polymerize and explode (controlled by addition of phosphoric acid); the MP is −13.24°C and the BP is 25.7°C. HCN is highly volatile, has a low density, and forms a weakly acidic solution with a dissociation constant (pKa) of 9.2 (1). HCN, NaCN, KCN, and cyanogen (a colorless gas) exude an almond-like odor that is reportedly unde-tectable to 20% of the population. The lowest detectable concentration of HCN gas by nose is 1–10 ppm (50).

Detailed regulations, advisories, and guidelines relating to the presence of cyanide in air, water, food, and other sources are available (1). The intermediate oral Minimal Risk Level for cyanide is 0.05 mg/kg/day; this is based on a rat study that established a no-observed-adverse-effect level (NOAEL) of 4.5 mg/kg/day NaCN in drinking water (59). The U.S. Environmental Protection Agency sets 200 μg/l of water as the Maximum Contaminant Level of cya-nide. Tolerances for cyanides in food range from 5–250 ppm. The oral Minimal Risk Level for cyanide is 0.05 mg/kg/day based on a NOAEL of 4.5 mg/kg/day (59). The U.S. Occupational Safety and Health Administration posts a time-weighted Permissible Exposure Limit of 5 mg/m^3 cy-anide. The American Conference of Governmental Indus-trial Hygienists' Threshold Limit Values are similar to the recommended exposure limits for occupational exposure set by the U.S. National Institute for Occupational Safety and Health (in milligrams per cubic meter), namely, for cyano-gen, 21 and 20; HCN, KCN, and NaCN, 5 and 5; and cyanogen chloride, 0.75 and 0.6, respectively.

Cyanide gas and certain cyanide salts are quickly ab-sorbed into the systemic circulation following inhalation, oral, and dermal exposure. HCN is absorbed through the lungs within seconds and distributed throughout the body; however, more than half reportedly may be retained in the lungs (46). Occupational exposures of 135 to 200 ppm HCN for periods up to 30 min have proved fatal (20). The inhalation LC$_{50}$ for HCN for rats ranged from 3417 ppm for 10 min to 143 ppm for 60 min; those for rabbits ranged from 2200 ppm for 45 sec to 188 ppm for 30 min (5). The human, rat, and mouse oral LD$_{50}$s are 2.95 and 8.5 mg/kg, respectively (6). In rats, up to 53% of ingested cyanide was reported to have been absorbed after 24 h of administration (23). The rat and mouse LD$_{50}$s in milligrams per kilogram are, respectively, 9 and 6.5 for subcutaneous (s.c.) exposure, 4 and 6 for intraperitoneal (i.p.) administration, and 3.6 and 2.6 for the intravenous (i.v.) route (1).

Cyanide is readily distributed by the blood to different organs and tissues. A man who fatally inhaled HCN had tissue levels (in milligrams per kilogram) of 0.75 (lung), 0.42 (heart), 0.42 (blood), 0.33 (kidney), and 0.32 (brain) (1). Blood cyanide levels in smokers are approximately 100-fold lower (17). Cyanide levels (mg HCN/100 g tissue) ranged from 0.06–1.37 in brain and 0.22–0.91 in liver of humans who had ingested fatal doses of cyanide (29). Rab-bits treated by gavage with 11.9 to 20.3 mg CN$^-$ per kil-ogram as HCN had blood and serum cyanide levels of 480 and 252 μg/dl respectively, and tissue levels (μg/100 g wet

tissue) at the time of death were 512, 83, 95, 105, 107, and 72 for liver, kidney, brain, heart, lung, and spleen, respec-tively (5). Rats that had received 7 or 21 mg CN$^-$ per kil-ogram by gavage showed average tissue concentrations of cyanide (in micrograms per gram) of: liver, 8.9; lung, 5.8; blood, 4.9; spleen, 2.1; and brain 1.5 (93).

Cyanide is a normal metabolite in human blood where it occurs in concentrations of 0–14 μg/dl (25). Free cyanide in blood is removed by exhalation of HCN and by met-hemoglobin trapping (which can be modulated by environ-mental factors such as nitrate) and metabolism. The major metabolic pathway utilizes mitochondrial rhodanese (thio-sulfate:cyanide sulfurtransferase, E.C. 2.8.1.1) in the pres-ence of sulfane sulfur (from cysteine, methionine) to form thiocyanate (favored at high pH) (34,47). Tissue distribu-tion of rhodanese is variable among different species (3). In dogs, enzyme activity is highest in the adrenal gland and ~2.5 times greater than activity in the liver. Monkeys, rabbits, and rats have the highest rhodanese activity in the liver and kidney. In other species, low levels of rhodanese activity are reported in brain, testes, lungs, spleen, and mus-cles. Rhodanese may be regulated by protein phosphory-lation involving protein kinase C (51,54). Thiocyanate has been shown to account for 60%–80% of a given cyanide dose in sheep (8). Once formed, thiocyanate is excreted in the urine as the major metabolite. Minor cyanide detoxi-cation pathways include (a) nonenzymatic formation of 2-aminothiazoline-4-carboxylic acid (an experimental con-vulsant) and its tautomer 2-imino-4-thiazolidine-carboxylic acid in the presence of cysteine (accounts for 15% of CN given to experimental animals and is favored at low pH) (13); (b) reaction with mercaptopyruvate *via* mercaptopy-ruvate sulfurtransferase to form pyruvate (56); (c) reaction with pyruvate, mercaptopyruvate, α-ketoglutarate, glycer-aldehyde, or ascorbate to form cyanohydrin derivatives (58,81) (pyruvate can abolish cyanide-induced seizures) (92); (d) reaction with hydroxycobalamin to form vitamin B$_{12}$, which cannot be synthesized in the human body (4); and (e) metabolism to cyanate, especially in malnourished states. Blood cyanate levels increased in rats treated with a source of cyanide when maintained on a protein-deficient diet or a diet free of the sulfur amino acids methionine and cystine (83,87).

The mean lethal dose of sodium cyanide in the Sprague-Dawley rat was 4.6 mg/kg when the agent was infused *via* jugular cannula; blood glucose and lactate increased 45 min after initial cyanide treatment (75). Constant intravenous infusions of cyanide in rats cause rapid, progressive reduc-tion of oxidative-reduction responses of cerebrocortical cytochrome-*c* oxidase activity (Cox) concomitant with in-creases (up to 200% of normal) in cerebral blood flow.

Brain oxygen metabolism is maintained near normal limits until cerebral oxygen delivery begins to fall (49).

Mouse whole-brain calcium levels increased markedly and dose-dependently within 15 min of s.c. administration of 10–15 mg/kg KCN when centrally mediated tremors were evident; levels remained elevated for 3 h and returned to normal after 12 h. Pretreatment with diltiazem, a calcium channel blocker, blocked KCN-induced increases in whole-brain calcium and corresponding behavioral signs (35).

The mouse ED_{50} for KCN, as measured by induction of tonic and clonic seizures, was significantly increased by 1.5- or 1.8-fold by s.c. preinjection of melatonin (20, 100 or 345 mg/kg). The LD_{50} for KCN, based on 24-h mortality, was also significantly increased 1.3-fold by preinjection of melatonin. KCN (8 mg/kg, s.c.) increased lipid peroxidation in whole brain of mice, and the increased lipid peroxidation was completely abolished when cyanide-induced seizures were stopped by preadministration of melatonin. These results suggest that melatonin, a pineal hormone, may protect mice against cyanide-induced neurotoxicity via a free-radical scavenging effect (93).

Sodium cyanide (5–20 mg/kg) rapidly perturbed rat brain glutamatergic, dopaminergic, and γ-aminobutyric acid (GABA)–dependent pathways. Within 60 sec of i.p. administration: (a) striatal dopamine levels decreased rapidly and dose-dependently and (b) levels of the dopamine metabolite, 3-methoxy-4-hydroxyphenylacetic acid, decreased in striatum and olfactory tubercle, while (c) levels of the oxidatively deaminated metabolite 3,4-hydroxyphenylacetic acid remained unaltered. GABA concentrations diminished at high NaCN doses in all regions studied. Glutamic acid levels increased in the cerebellum, striatum, and frontal cortex up to 10 mg/kg NaCN; higher dosages decreased glutamate levels. A selective antagonist of the N-methyl-D-aspartate (NMDA) glutamate-receptor subtype blocked cyanide-induced changes in the transcriptional regulatory protein Fos (but not c-Jun) in rat cerebral cortex, cerebellum (increased levels), and hippocampus (decreased level) (69). Dopamine levels were significantly decreased in the striatum (41%), hippocampus (31%), and cerebral cortex (13%) of KCN-treated mice that displayed L-dopa–sensitive decreased locomotor activity, akinesia, and reduced numbers of tyrosine hydroxylase–positive cells in substantia nigra (38,39).

Cats given a continuous infusion of NaCN (0.2%) resulting in acidosis had tissue damage in the deep cerebral white matter, corpus callosum, pallidum, and substantia nigra, with less damage in the cerebral cortex and hippocampus. More severe damage in a similar distribution was seen in comparably treated animals given a ganglion-blocking

agent to promote hypotension (<100 mm Hg). The topographic selectivity of feline cyanide-induced leukoencephalopathy appeared to be related to the characteristic of the cerebral vascular system, and the severity of lesions to the intensity of both hypoxia and hypotension during cyanide infusion, but not to the cyanide dose or degree of acidosis (28).

Lightly anesthetized macaques (Macaca mulatta) given an i.v. infusion of sodium cyanide initially developed hyperventilation with tetany. Rapid infusion led to apnea. Bradycardia and hypotension precipitated an isoelectric or near-isoelectric electroencephalogram (EEG); there was no EEG or clinical evidence of seizures. Brain damage was evident in animals surviving up to 98 h; one animal displayed neuronal changes that were attributed to major circulatory alterations, while others showed involvement of white matter (11).

Relatively few long-term animal studies have been undertaken, and there are no animal models of the neurodegenerative disorders seen in humans dependent on a cyanogenic diet (vide infra). Male weanling rats fed a diet supplemented with 1500 mg/kg potassium cyanide or 2240 mg/kg for 11.5 months showed a consistent reduction in weight gain, both in well-nourished animals and in animals on a diet restricted in methionine, vitamin B_{12}, and iodine (71). However, rodents treated for prolonged periods with sodium cyanate develop a mixed axonal and demyelinating peripheral neuropathy (85). Prolonged treatment with cyanate induces neuronal damage in cerebral cortex, basal ganglia, spinal cord, and peripheral nerves of macaques (76) and sensorimotor neuropathy in humans (64). In rodents, treatment with low doses of cyanate causes weakness, spasticity of the hindlimbs, and seizures usually triggered by noise (14,85). Chronic administration of high doses of cyanate causes hindlimb paralysis in rats (2) and spastic quadriplegia in monkeys (76). The potential of chronic sodium cyanate therapy to induce sensory and motor neuropathy (64) led to its discontinuation as a therapy for sickle cell anemia.

Cyanide appears to equilibrate rapidly across the neuronal plasma membrane and then slowly accumulates in mitochondria (10). Treatment of rat pheochromocytoma cells or mouse brain slices with KCN increases membrane lipid peroxidation and cytosolic free calcium; prior or simultaneous administration of chlorpromazine decreases these effects (55). Administration of cyanide to differentiated PC-12 cell cultures induces neuronal degeneration that is blocked by MK-801, an antagonist of the glutamate-receptor NMDA subtype (31). Endogenous cyanide has been proposed to modulate the NMDA receptor response in PC-12 cells (9).

Most victims of acute HCN poisoning either die acutely or recover fully (22). Exposure to high concentrations of HCN is followed by increased depth of respiration (seconds), violent seizures (20–30 sec), shallow gasps (1 min), and asystole (a few minutes). Skin color may be pink. Moderate HCN concentrations induce vertigo, nausea, and headache followed by seizures and coma. Prolonged exposure to low concentrations of HCN leads to tissue hypoxia, coma, and seizures, with residual CNS effects (irrational behavior, altered reflexes, ataxia) that may persist for a few weeks (22).

Manifestations of acute cyanide intoxication include headache, vertigo, and agitation followed by combative behavior, coma, seizures, and death (91). Survival may occur after doses as high as 1–1.5 g KCN (73,88). Survivors rarely display personality changes, memory deficits, and extrapyramidal syndromes. The latter are characterized by progressive parkinsonism (akinesia, rigidity) and dystonia; bilaterally symmetrical lesions in the basal ganglia, cerebellum, and cerebral cortex are evident by computed tomography (CT) and magnetic resonance imaging (MRI) (12,24,73). MRI evidence of cyanide-induced brain damage may be delayed for up to 1 year following exposure (73). Follow-up of one 37-year-old subject 21 years after development of a cyanide-induced, L-dopa-responsive syndrome, showed mild dystonia, athetoid hand movements, and symmetrical putaminal hypodensities on CT scan (89). Autopsy of a 19-year-old, severely parkinsonian male who died 19 months after a KCN-mediated suicide attempt revealed major destructive changes of the globus pallidus and putamen, with preservation of the melanin-containing zone of the substantia nigra (89). Bilateral necrosis of the globus pallidus attributed to cyanide is also reported in an individual treated with sodium nitroprusside for malignant hypertension (42).

Acute intoxication with cyanogen chloride is associated with signs of cyanide poisoning and intense irritation of mucous membranes (nose, throat, eyes, bronchi). Dyspnea and dizziness may progress to unconsciousness, failing respiration, seizures, retching, involuntary urination and defecation, and death within minutes (22).

Ingestion of food plants probably constitutes the principal source of exposure to cyanide for a large proportion of *Homo sapiens*, especially those of low socioeconomic status in tropical and subtropical regions. Notable populations from a toxicological viewpoint are the Tuskanoan Indians of northwest Amazonia who reportedly remain healthy despite an estimated daily intake of >20 mg CN (predominantly from bitter cassava) (21) and certain protein-deficient African populations with epidemic cassava-associated neurological disorders (*see* Cassava, this volume).

Chronic cyanide exposure may be associated with headache, vertigo, tremor, weakness, fatigue, dizziness, confusion, optic neuropathy, myelopathy, peripheral neuropathy and, possibly, persistent mental impairment. Occupational exposure has been linked to headache, vertigo, fatigue, poor appetite, disturbed sleep (19,74), and seizures (27). Prolonged ingestion of cyanogenic plant materials appears to precipitate neurodegenerative disorders in protein-malnourished individuals. As described elsewhere in this text (*see* Cassava, this volume), cassava-associated neurological disease is a particular and pressing problem in parts of Africa where minimally nourished individuals subsist on incompletely detoxified cassava, which contains the cyanogenic glucosides linamarin and lotaustralin; by contrast, cassava-related neurological disease has not been reported in cassava-consuming communities in South and Central America. Affected African populations that use cassava as a staple contain a high prevalence of either (a) mostly young female children and women of childbearing age with spastic paraparesis of acute onset (Cameroon, Central African Republic, Zaire, Mozambique) (88), or (b) largely middle-aged subjects with an ataxic myeloneuropathy of insidious onset (Nigeria). Largely reversible visual and sensorineural deficits may accompany these disorders. Visual system deficits followed by peripheral neuropathy were the prime features of an epidemic of neurological disease (Strachan's syndrome) that reportedly affected tens of thousands of Cubans at a time of food shortages, dependence on locally grown materials including cassava, and high energy consumption associated with bicycle transportation during a period of gasoline shortage (33).

Generalized muscle weakness was reported in a middle-aged male who ingested 500 mg of amygdalin daily for 6 months; resolution occurred rapidly after dosing ceased (77). Peripheral neuromyopathy was reported in a 67-year-old woman with lymphoma following treatment with the cyanogenic glucoside amygdalin (Laetrile); blood and urinary thiocyanate and cyanide levels were elevated, and clinical improvement followed drug discontinuation. The patient had received prior treatment with vincristine (37), an established cause of human neuromyopathy.

The standard treatment for CN poisoning in the United States involves administration of amyl nitrite (immediate inhalation) and sodium nitrite (i.v.) to induce methemoglobin, which reversibly binds with CN; and administration of thiosulfate, which converts CN to SCN with the assistance of rhodanese (92). The appearance of slight cyanosis may indicate the desired methemoglobin is forming (22). A drawback of nitrites is that they are slow methemoglobin inducers (43) and, in addition, may cause hypotension (32). Intravenous 4-dimethylaminophenol, which also oxidizes hemoglobin to methemoglobin, is used in Germany (22). Cobalt compounds have high affinity for cyanide (92), and dicobalt edetate is used in Britain and France to treat cyanide poisoning (22). Likewise, hydroxocobalamin can be used to treat cyanide toxicity, because it combines with cyanide to form cyanocobalamin (vitamin B_{12}). ^{31}P-Nuclear magnetic resonance spectroscopic imaging of the awake rat brain showed that hydroxocobalamin suppresses cyanide-induced decreases in brain content of phosphocreatine and corresponding increases in inorganic phosphate; adenosine triphosphate levels remained constant at i.p. doses of <6 mg/kg KCN body weight (7).

Experimental antidotes for acute CN poisoning include the combination of sodium nitrite, sodium thiosulfate, and chlorpromazine pretreatment (53,70). Pretreatment of mice or pigs with 1-(5-isoquinoline-sulfonyl)-2-methylpiperazine (H-7), a potent protein kinase inhibitor, attenuates the CNS effects of cyanide toxicity (54). KCN intoxication in mice is effectively antagonized by dihydroxy acetone (DHA), particularly if administered in combination with sodium thiosulfate (61). Cyanide-induced seizures are also prevented by DHA treatment, either alone or in combination with thiosulfate. Injection (i.p.) of DHA (2 g/kg) 2 min after or 10 min before cyanide (s.c.) increased LD_{50} values of CN (8.7 mg/kg) by factors of 2.1 and 3.0, respectively. Pretreatment with a combination of DHA and thiosulfate increased the LD_{50} of cyanide to 83 mg/kg. Administration of α-ketoglutarate (2.0 g/kg), but not pyruvate, 2 min after CN increased the LD_{50} of CN by a factor of 1.6. DHA, glyceraldehyde, pyruvate, and α-ketoglutarate rapidly restored CN-inhibited mitochondrial respiration as a result of trapping CN to form cyanohydrin (60,62).

DHA combined with thiosulfate has been recommended for the treatment of CN poisoning, particularly in cases of smoke inhalation when carbon monoxide is present (60). In this situation, induction of methemoglobin formation may be dangerous because a large amount of hemoglobin may already have been bound to carbon monoxide (32,44).

Cyanide (as HCN) cytotoxicity is classically considered to result from histocytic anoxia caused by inhibition of oxygen uptake by cytochrome-c oxidase (Cox), the terminal enzyme of the mitochondrial respiratory chain (15,92). Mitochondrial respiration declines only after >50% depression of Cox activity (70). Heart Cox activity reportedly is inhibited to a greater degree than brain Cox activity in cyanide-treated mice. In addition to Cox, cyanide binds to catalase, peroxidase, xanthine oxidase, and succinic dehydrogenase (1).

Central suppression of breathing caused by cyanide has been proposed to result from changes in neuronal excitability in respiratory-modulating populations rather than to perturbation of cellular oxidative metabolism of neurons within rhythm-generating centers. Support for this hypothesis comes from observations *in vitro* in which concentrations of cyanide greatly exceeding those that would prove lethal *in vivo* failed to disrupt the function of rat neonatal brainstem neuronal networks that regulate respiratory function (30).

The cellular consequences of cyanide exposure appear to involve changes in calcium regulation and glutamate-mediated excitotoxic mechanisms (65). The cyanide-induced shift from aerobic to anaerobic metabolism results in increased levels of nicotinamide adenine dinucleotide, a powerful stimulant of calcium mobilization from inositol 1,4,5-triphosphate−sensitive stores (40). Cyanide-stimulated influx of extracellular calcium also occurs as a consequence of decreased energy charge and failure of plasmalemmal ion pumps (52,55). ATP-sensitive potassium channels (K_{ATP}) are activated by nonlethal concentrations of cyanide (67). Cyanide enhances NMDA-mediated Ca^{2+} influx and inward current by interacting with the Mg^{2+} block of the NMDA receptor (66), which mediates cyanide-induced excitotoxicity (68). NMDA receptor activation concurrently generates nitric oxide and reactive oxygen species, which are held responsible for cytotoxicity (31).

The syndrome of delayed striatal degeneration with parkinsonism and dystonia that occurs in some survivors of acute cyanide intoxication might also result from a glutamate-mediated neuronotoxic effect comparable to that seen with other agents (carbon monoxide, 3-nitropropionic acid) that interfere with mitochondrial respiration (79). Given that this devastating extrapyramidal disorder occurs in only a proportion of subjects who are intoxicated with any of these chemicals, activation of excitotoxic damage may require the combination of hypoxia (during seizures/coma) and ischemia (from hypoperfusion), as well as agent-induced inhibition of brain oxidative phosphorylation.

Chronic cyanide intake from cassava dependency causes self-limiting neurodegenerative disorders only in the setting of protein-calorie malnutrition. These are likely to be primary disorders of long central and peripheral axons or neuron cell bodies. It is plausible that ataxic myeloneuropathy results from prolonged, relatively low-level intoxication in minimally malnourished subjects, whereas subacute spastic paraparesis accompanies heavy cyanide exposure in the setting of severe nutritional privation. The apparent special susceptibility of young females and those of child-bearing age suggests a possible hormonal influence on neuronal survival in cassava intoxication. Degeneration of neurons or axons might be mediated by cyanate (87), an established cause of peripheral neuropathy in humans and rodents, and of spastic paraparesis in macaques (84,85). While cyanate carbamylates proteins (76), it is unknown whether this property mediates its neurotoxic properties.

Editorial Note. It has also been suggested that the greatly elevated levels of thiocyanate in cassava-dependent populations may have a role in the genesis of motor neuron degeneration in konzo (79). Thiocyanate selectively increases the binding of glutamate to the α-amino-2,3-dihydro-5-methyl-3-oxo-isoxazole-propionate (AMPA) subclass of glutamate receptors, which might mediate an excitotoxic response on AMPA-bearing neurons. This suggestion was advanced as a common mechanism to explain the clinical and neurophysiological similarities between konzo and lathyrism, an upper-motor-neuron disorder apparently triggered by the potent AMPA agonist β-N-oxalylamino-L-alanine (see β-N-oxalylamino-L-alanine, this volume).

REFERENCES

1. Agency for Toxic Substances and Disease Registry (1997) *Toxicological Profile for Cyanide (Update)*. U.S. Department of Health and Human Services, Washington, DC.
2. Alter BP, Kan YW, Nathan DG (1974) Toxic effects of high-dose cyanate administration in rodents. *Blood* 43, 69.
3. Aminlari M, Vaseghi T, Kargarr A (1994) The cyanide-metabolizing enzyme rhodanese in different parts of the respiratory systems of sheep and dog. *Toxicol Appl Pharmacol* 124, 67.
4. Ansell M, Lewis FAS (1970) A review of cyanide concentrations found in human organs: A survey of literature concerning cyanide metabolism, normal, non-fatal, and fatal body cyanide levels. *J Forensic Med* 17, 148.
5. Ballantyne B (1983) The influence of exposure route and species on the acute lethal toxicity and tissue concentrations of cyanide. In: *Developments in the Science and Practice of Toxicology*. Hayes AW, Schnell RC, Miya TS eds. Elsevier, New York p. 583.
6. Ballantyne B (1988) Toxicology and hazard evaluation of cyanide fumigation powders. *Clin Toxicol* 26, 325.
7. Benabid AL, Decorps M, Remy C et al. (1987) [31]P Nuclear magnetic resonance *in vivo* spectroscopy of the metabolic changes induced in the awake rat brain during KCN intoxication and its reversal by hydroxocobalamine. *J Neurochem* 48, 804.
8. Blakley RL, Coop IE (1949) The metabolism and toxicity of cyanides and cyanogenic glycosides in sheep. II. Detoxication of hydrocyanic acid. *N Z J Sci Technol* 31, 1.
9. Borowitz JL, Gunasekar PG, Isom GE (1997) Hydrogen cyanide generation by μ-opiate receptor activation: Possible neuromodulatory role of endogenous cyanide. *Brain Res* 768, 294.
10. Borowitz JL, Rathinavelu A, Kanthasamy A et al. (1994) Accumulation of labeled cyanide in neuronal tissue. *Toxicol Appl Pharmacol* 129, 80.
11. Brierley JB, Brown AW, Calverley J (1976) Cyanide intoxication in the rat: Physiological and neuropathological aspects. *J Neurol Neurosurg Psychiat* 39, 129.
12. Carella F, Grassi MP, Savoiardo M (1988) Dystonia-parkinsonism syndrome after cyanide poisoning: Clinical and MRI findings. *J Neurol Neurosurg Psychiat* 51, 1345.
13. Catsimpoolas N, Wood JL (1966) Specific cleavage of cystine peptide by cyanide. *J Biol Chem* 241, 1790.
14. Cerami A, Allen TA, Graziano JH et al. (1973) Pharmacology of cyanate. 1. General effects on experimental animals. *J Pharmacol Exp Ther* 185, 653.
15. Chance B, Erecinska M (1971) Flow flash kinetics of the cytochrome 3-oxygen reaction in coupled and uncoupled mitochondria using the liquid dye laser. *Arch Biochem Biophys* 143, 675.
16. Chand K, Dixit ML, Arora SK (1992) Yield and quantity of forage sorghum as affected by phosphorus fertilization. *J Indian Soc Soil Sci* 40, 302.
17. Chandra H, Gupta BN, Ghargava SK et al. (1980) Chronic cyanide exposure: A biochemical and industrial hygiene study. *J Anal Toxicol* 4, 161.
18. Clark CJ, Cambell D, Reid WH (1981) Blood carboxyhemoglobin and cyanide levels in fire survivors. *Lancet* 1, 1332.
19. Colle R (1972) L'Intoxication cyanohydrique chronique. *Maroc Médicale* 50, 750, 1972.
20. Dudley HC, Sweeney TR, Miller (1942) Toxicology of acrylonitrile (vinyl cyanide) II: Studies of effects of daily inhalation. *J Ind Hyg Toxicol* 24, 255.
21. Dufour DL (1988) Dietary cyanide intake and serum thiocyanate levels in Tukanoan Indians in northwest Amazonia. *Amer J Phys Anthropol* 75, 205.
22. Ellenhorn MJ (1997) *Medical Toxicology: Diagnosis and Treatment of Human Poisoning. 2nd Ed.* Williams & Wilkins, Baltimore p. 1267.
23. Farooqui MYH, Ahmed AE (1982) Molecular interaction of acrylonitrile and potassium cyanide with rat blood. *Chem Biol Interact* 38, 145.
24. Feldman JM, Feldman MD (1988) Sequelae of attempted suicide by cyanide ingestion: A case report. *Int J Psychiat Med* 20, 173.
25. Feldstein M, Klendshoj NC (1954) The determination of cyanide in biologic fluids by microdiffusion analysis. *J Lab Clin Med* 44, 166.
26. Fenwick GR, Heaney RK, Mawson R (1989) Glucosinolates. In *Toxicants of Plant Origin. Vol 2. Glycosides.* Cheeke PR ed, CRC Press, Boca Raton, Florida p. 1.
27. Finkel AJ (1983) *Hamilton and Hardy's Industrial Toxicology.* John Wright, PSG Inc. Boston.
28. Funata N, Song SY, Okeda R et al. (1984) A study of experimental cyanide encephalopathy in the acute phase—physiological and neuropathological correlation. *Acta Neuropathol* 64, 99.

29. Gettler AO, Baine JO (1938) The toxicology of cyanide. *Amer J Med Sci* **195**, 182.

30. Greer JJ, Carter JE (1995) Effects of cyanide on the neural mechanisms controlling breathing in the neonatal rat *in vitro*. *Neurotoxicology* **16**, 211.

31. Gunasekar PG, Sun PW, Kanthasamy AG *et al.* (1996) Cyanide-induced neurotoxicity involves nitric oxide and reactive oxygen species generation after N-methyl-D-aspartate receptor activation. *J Pharmacol Exp Ther* **277**, 150.

32. Hall AH, Kuling KW, Rumack BH (1989) Suspected cyanide poisoning in smoke inhalation: Complications of sodium nitrite therapy. *J Toxicol Clin Exp* **9**, 3.

33. Hernandez T, Lundquist P, Oliveira L *et al.* (1995) Fate in humans of dietary intake of cyanogenic glycosides from roots of sweet cassava consumed in Cuba. *Nat Tox* **3**, 114.

34. Himwich WA, Saunders JP (1948) Enzymatic conversion of cyanide to thiocyanate. *Amer J Physiol* **153**, 348.

35. Johnson JD, Mesienheimer TL, Isom GE (1986) Cyanide-induced neurotoxicity: Role of neuronal calcium. *Toxicol Appl Pharmacol* **84**, 464.

36. Jones M, McMullen MJ, Dougherty J (1987) Toxic smoke inhalation: Cyanide poisoning in fire victims. *Amer J Emerg Med* **5**, 318.

37. Kalyanaraman UP, Kalyanaraman K, Cullinan SA, McLean JM (1983) Neuromyopathy of cyanide intoxication due to "laetrile" (amygdalin). A clinicopathologic study. *Cancer* **51**, 2126.

38. Kanthasamy AG, Borowitz JL, Isom GE (1991) Cyanide-induced increases in plasma catecholamines: Relationship to acute toxicity. *Neurotoxicology* **12**, 777.

39. Kanthasamy AG, Borowitz JL, Pavlakovic G, Isom GE (1994) Dopaminergic neurotoxicity of cyanide: Neurochemical, histological, and behavioral characterization. *Toxicol Appl Pharmacol* **126**, 156.

40. Kaplin AI, Snyder SH, Linden DJ (1996) Reduced nicotinamide adenine dinucleotide-selective stimulation of inositol 1,4,5-trisphosphate receptors mediates hypoxic mobilization of calcium. *J Neurosci* **16**, 2002.

41. Khandekar JD, Edelman H (1979) Studies of amygdalin (laetrile) toxicity in rodents. *J Amer Med Assn* **242**, 169.

42. Kim YH, Foo M, Terry RD (1982) Cyanide encephalopathy following therapy with sodium nitroprusside: Report of a case. *Arch Pathol Lab Med* **106**, 392.

43. Kruszyna R, Kruszyna H, Smith RP (1982) Comparison of hydroxylamine, 4-dimethyaminophenol and nitrite protection against cyanide poisoning in mice. *Arch Toxicol* **49**, 191.

44. Kuling KW (1991) Cyanide antidote and fire toxicology. *N Engl J Med* **325**, 1801.

45. Kurt TL (1992) Chemical asphyxiants. In: *Environmental and Occupational Medicine*. Rom WN ed. Little Brown, Boston p. 539.

46. Landahl HD, Herrmann RG (1950) Retention of vapors and gases in the human nose and lung. *Arch Ind Hyg Occup Med* **1**, 36.

47. Lang K (1933) Die rhodanbildung in tierkorper. *Biochem Z* **259**, 243.

48. Lasch EE, El Shawa R (1981) Multiple cases of cyanide poisoning by apricot kernels in children from Gaza. *Pediatrics* **68**, 5.

49. Lee PA, Sylvia AL, Piantadosi CA (1988) Cyanide-related changes in cerebral O_2 delivery and metabolism in fluorocarbon-circulated rats. *Toxicol Appl Pharmacol* **94**, 34.

50. Lundquist P, Rosling H, Sorbo B (1988) The origin of hydrogen cyanide in breath. *Arch Toxicol* **61**, 270.

51. Maduh EU, Baskin SI (1994) Protein kinase C modulation of rhodanese-catalyzed conversion of cyanide to thiocyanate. *Res Commun Mol Pathol Pharmacol* **86**, 155.

52. Maduh EU, Borowitz JL, Isom GE (1991) Cyanide-induced alteration of the adenylate energy pool in a rat neurosecretory cell line. *J Appl Toxicol* **11**, 97.

53. Maduh EH, Johnson JD, Ardelt BK *et al.* (1988) Cyanide-induced neurotoxicity: Mechanisms of attenuation of chlorpromazine. *Toxicol Appl Pharmacol* **96**, 60.

54. Maduh EU, Nealley EW, Song H *et al.* (1995) A protein kinase C inhibitor attenuates cyanide toxicity *in vivo*. *Toxicology* **100**, 129.

55. Maduh EU, Turek JJ, Borowitz JL *et al.* (1990) Cyanide-induced neurotoxicity: Calcium mediation of morphological changes in neuronal cells. *Toxicol Appl Pharmacol* **103**, 214.

56. Martensson J, Sorbo B (1978) Human β-mercaptopyruvate sulfur-transferase: Distribution in the cellular compartments of blood and activity in erythrocytes from patients with hematological disorders. *Clin Chim Acta* **87**, 11.

57. Maynard RL (1993) Toxicology of chemical warfare agents. In: *General and Applied Toxicology*. *Vol 2*. Ballantyne B, Marrs T, Turner P eds. Stockton Press, New York p. 1253.

58. Moore SJ, Norris JC, Ho IK, Hume AS (1986) The efficacy of α-ketoglutaric acid in the antagonism of cyanide intoxication. *Toxicol Appl Pharmacol* **82**, 40.

59. National Toxicology Program (1993) Technical report on toxicity studies of sodium cyanide (CAS No 143-33-9) administered in drinking water to F344-N rats and B6C3F1 mice. *National Institutes of Health publication* 94-3386. U.S. Department of Health and Human Services.

60. Niknahad H, Khan S, Sood C, O'Brien PJ (1994) Prevention of cyanide-induced cytotoxicity by nutrients in isolated rat hepatocytes. *Toxicol Appl Pharmacol* **128**, 271.

61. Niknahad H, O'Brien PJ (1996) Antidotal effect of dihydroxyacetone against cyanide toxicity *in vivo*. *Toxicol Appl Pharmacol* **138**, 186.

62. Norris JC, Utley WA, Hume AS (1990) Mechanism of antagonizing cyanide-induced lethality by α-ketoglutaric acid. *Toxicology* **62**, 275.

63. O'Brien GM, Mbome L, Taylor AJ *et al.* (1992) Variations in cyanogen content of cassava during village processing in Cameroon. *Food Chem* 44, 131.

64. Ohnishi A, Peterson CM, Dyck PJ (1975) Axonal degeneration in sodium cyanate-induced neuropathy. *Arch Neurol* 32, 530.

65. Patel MN, Ardelt BK, Yim GK, Isom GE (1991) Cyanide induces Ca(2+)-dependent and -independent release of glutamate from mouse brain slices. *Neurosci Lett* 131, 42.

66. Patel MN, Peoples RW, Yim GK, Isom GE (1994) Enhancement of NMDA-mediated responses by cyanide. *Neurochem Res* 10, 1319.

67. Patel MN, Yim GK, Isom GE (1992) Potentiation of cyanide neurotoxicity by blockade of ATP-sensitive potassium channels. *Brain Res* 593, 114.

68. Patel MN, Yim GK, Isom GE (1993) N-Methyl-D-aspartate receptors mediate cyanide-induced cytotoxicity in hippocampal cultures. *Neurotoxicology* 14, 35.

69. Pavlakovic G, Rathinavelu A, Isom GE (1994) MK-801 prevents cyanide-induced changes of Fos levels in rat brain. *Neurochem Res* 19, 1289.

70. Pettersen JC, Cohen SD (1985) Antagonism of cyanide poisoning by chlorpromazine and sodium thiosulfate. *Toxicol Appl Pharmacol* 81, 265.

71. Philbrick DJ, Hopkins JB, Hill DC *et al.* (1979) Effects of prolonged cyanide and thiocyanate feeding in rats. *J Toxicol Environ Health* 5, 579.

72. Rickert WS, Robinson JC, Young IC (1980) Estimating the hazards of "less hazardous" cigarettes. I. Tar, nicotine, carbon monoxide, acrolein, hydrogen cyanide and total aldehyde deliveries of Canadian cigarettes. *J Toxicol Environ Health* 6, 351.

73. Rosenberg NL, Myers JA, Martin WRW (1989) Cyanide-induced parkinsonism: Clinical, MRI and 6-fluorodopa PET studies. *Neurology* 39, 142.

74. Saia B, DeRosa E, Galzigna L (1970) Considerations on chronic cyanide poisoning. *Med Lav* 62, 580.

75. Salkowski AA, Penney DG (1995) Metabolic, cardiovascular, and neurologic aspects of acute cyanide poisoning in the rat. *Toxicol Lett* 75, 19.

76. Shaw CM, Papayannopoulou T, Stamatoyannopuolos G (1974) Neuropathology of cyanate toxicity in rhesus monkeys. *Pharmacology* 12, 166.

77. Smith FP, Butler TP, Cohan S, Schein PS (1978) Laetrile toxicity: A report of two patients. *Cancer Treatment Rep* 62, 169.

78. Smith RP, Kruszyna H (1976) Toxicology of some inorganic antihypertensive anions. *Fed Proc* 35, 69.

79. Spencer PS (1999) Food toxins, AMPA receptors, and motor neuron diseases. *Drug Metab Rev* 31, 561.

80. Spencer PS, Butterfield PG (1995) Environmental agents and Parkinson's disease. In: *Etiology of Parkinson's Disease*. Ellenberg JH, Koller WC, Langston JW eds. Marcel Dekker, New York p. 319.

81. Sprince H, Smith GG, Parker CM, Rinehimer DA (1982) Protection against cyanide lethality in rats by L-ascorbic acid and dehydroascorbic acid. *Nutr Rep Int* 25, 463.

82. Stadelemann W (1976) Content of hydrocyanic acid in stone fruit juices. *Fluess Obst* 43, 45.

83. Swenne I, Eriksson U, Christoffersson R (1996) Cyanide detoxification in rats exposed to acetonitrile and fed a low-protein diet. *Fund Appl Toxicol* 31, 66.

84. Tellez-Nagel I, Johnson D, Nagel RL, Cerami A (1979) Neurotoxicity of sodium cyanate. New pathological and ultrastructural observations in *Macaca nemestrina*. *Acta Neuropathol* 36, 351.

85. Tellez-Nagel I, Korthals JK, Vlassara HV, Cerami A (1977) An ultrastructural study of chronic sodium cyanate-induced neuropathy. *J Neuropathol Exp Neurobiol* 36, 352.

86. Tewe OO, Iyayi EA (1989) Cyanogenic glycosides. In: *Toxicants of Plant Origin. Vol 2. Glycosides.* Cheeke PR ed. CRC Press, Boca Raton, Florida p. 43.

87. Tor-Agbidye J (1997) *Cyanide Metabolism in Sulfur Amino Acid Deficiency: Relevance to Cassava-Related Neurodegenerative Diseases.* PhD Thesis, Oregon State University.

88. Tylleskär T, Legue FD, Peterson S (1994) Konzo in the Central African Republic. *Neurology* 44, 959.

89. Uitti RJ, Rajput AH, Ashenhurst EM, Rozdilsky B (1985) Cyanide-induced parkinsonism: A clinicopathologic report. *Neurology* 35, 921.

90. Valenzuela R, Court J, Godoy J (1992) Delayed cyanide induced dystonia. *J Neurol Neurosurg Psychiat* 55, 198.

91. Vogel SN, Sultan B, Ten Eyck RP (1981) Cyanide poisoning. *Clin Toxicol* 18, 367.

92. Way JL (1984) Cyanide intoxication and its mechanism of antagonism. *Ann Rev Pharmacol Toxicol* 24, 451.

93. Yamamoto H, Tang HW (1996) Antagonistic effect of melatonin against cyanide-induced seizures and acute lethality in mice. *Toxicol Lett* 87, 19.

Cycasin, Methylazoxymethanol and Related Compounds

Peter S. Spencer
Glen E. Kisby
Valerie S. Palmer
Peter Obendorf

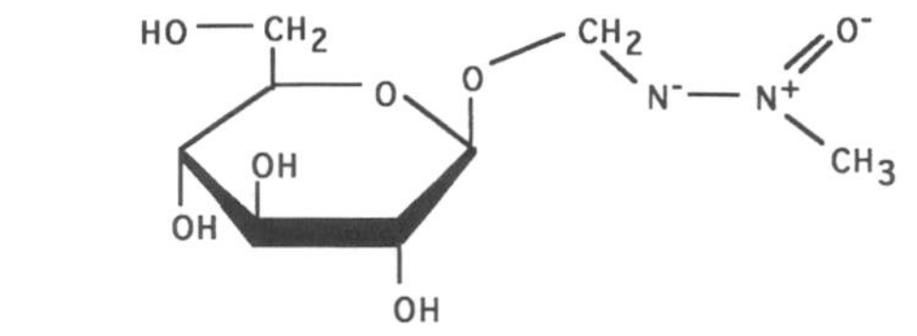

CYCASIN*
$C_8H_{16}N_2O_7$

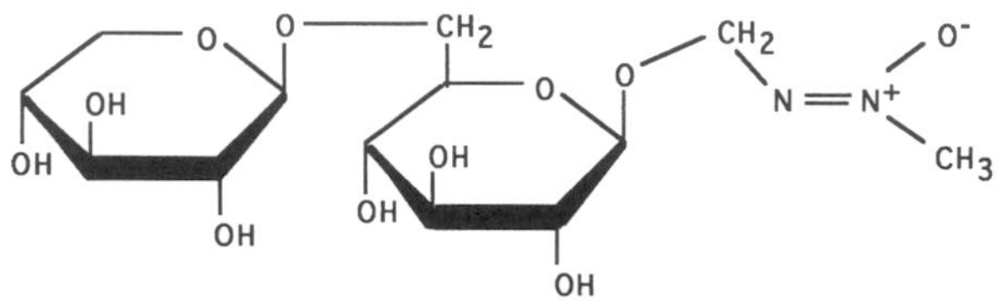

MACROZAMIN*
$C_{13}H_{23}N_2O_{11}$

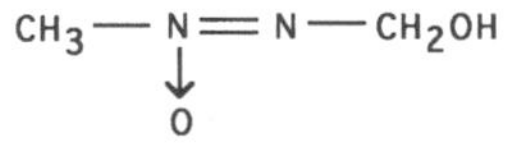

METHYLAZOXYMETHANOL, MAM
$C_2H_6N_2O_2$

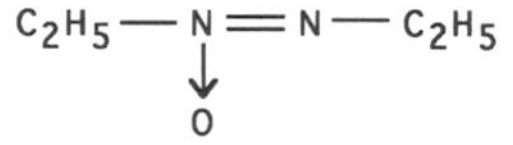

AZOXYETHANE
$C_4H_{10}N_2O$

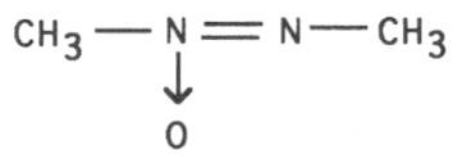

AZOXYMETHANE
$C_2H_6N_2O$

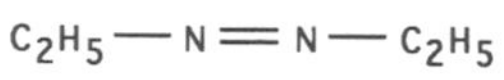

AZOETHANE
$C_4H_{10}N_2$

Methylazoxymethanol-β-D-glucoside; (Z)-β-O-D-glucopyranosyloxy-*NNO*-azoxymethane; cycasin
Methylazoxymethanol-β-D-primeveroside; (Z)-β-O-D-xylopyranosyl-(1-6)-β-D-glucopyranosyloxy-*NNO*-azoxymethane; macrozamin
Methylazoxymethanol, MAM

---

*The two canonical structures of these compounds are shown (122).

NEUROTOXICITY RATING

Experimental

A   Microcephaly (cycasin, MAM)

A   Gliomas (all)

Methylazoxymethanol (MAM) is the active component of azoxyglucosides, compounds found in primitive, nonflowering seed plants (gymnosperms) known as cycads (79). These are long-lived, perennial, unisexual, tropical and subtropical plants that develop pollen (microspore)-producing and seed-producing cones (56). Ruminants that consume plant material of various cycad genera (*Cycas, Macrozamia*) develop an incompletely described neuromuscular disorder (116). Epidemiological studies have implicated food and medicinal use of cycads in the etiology of a declining neurodegenerative disease—amyotrophic lateral sclerosis and parkinsonism-dementia complex (ALS/PDC)—that has been present in high incidence among three ethnically distinct populations in the western Pacific region (62,110,113,138). The neuropathology of ALS/PDC includes features suggestive of brain maldevelopment (102,136), an experimentally proven property of cycasin attributable to the genotoxic action of its aglycone. This property of MAM is exploited in the experimental setting as a tool to study perturbations of brain development (105–107). MAM and related azo, azoxy, and hydrazo compounds (*see* Hydrazine, this volume) also induce central (CNS) and peripheral nervous system (PNS) glial tumors in laboratory animals (137). In addition to the well-studied oncogenic actions of MAM on dividing cells (132), MAM induces long-lasting abnormalities in postmitotic neurons (31,51,63).

The 11 genera of the single surviving order of the Cycadales include: the Australian genera *Macrozamia* (east, central, and southwest), *Bowenia* (northeast Queensland), and *Lepidozamia* (northeast Queensland and New South Wales); *Zamia* of the Americas (southern Florida, USA, West Indies, southern Mexico to the Amazon and Peru); *Encephalartos* and *Stangeria* of central and southern Africa, respectively; and *Cycas*, which extends from northern Australia, through Oceania, across to the Indian subcontinent, and along the east African coast. Detailed examination of the distribution of cycad species is available elsewhere (56).

Because cycads have food and medicinal potential, and are resistant to drought, cyclone, and fire, they appear to have served throughout human history as a subsistence and famine food (129). Cycad seed and sago (extracted from the overground stem) have been used for food in certain cultures since ancient times. Australian Aboriginal groups used cycads for food for at least 4500 years (9); in 1996, certain aboriginal groups in the Northern Territory, Australia, continued their practice of careful seed detoxification for occasional food use (unpublished data). In the Florida Panhandle of North America, *Zamia floridana* was eaten by aboriginal people (sixteenth century), subsequently by Seminole Indians, and later by slaves and white settlers; the last cycad-processing plant closed in Miami, Florida, in 1926 (111). At their peak, mills along the Miami river processed tons of the tuberous underground stem of *Zamia floridana* and *Z. pumila*, most of which was marketed under the name Florida arrowroot for use in infant foods, biscuits, chocolate, and spaghetti. One of the first editions of the *Journal of the American Medical Association* noted the fine quality of starch and tapioca prepared from *Zamia* spp. (17). By 1950, nearly 6 million pounds of sago (prepared from *C. revoluta*) was imported into the United States for use in the preparation of food, syrup, beer, and adhesives, as well as sizing for paper and textiles (111). Cycasin-free material has been used as an emergency foodstuff and a delicacy by inhabitants of the Ryukyu Islands of southern Japan (64) and, in 1997, in the absence of other available food, by inhabitants of Moyo Island, Indonesia (unpublished data). Incompletely detoxified cycad flour (*Cycas* spp.) was an important source of food for the Chamorro people of Guam during and following the Second World War (130). In the 1980s, estimated daily ingestion of cycasin by Chamorros from consumption of cycad-derived *tortillas* was measured in milligrams (62,116); cycad flour is now used in this culture more as a delicacy for festive occasions. There is an extremely high and statistically significant correlation between the incidence of ALS (both of males and females) in districts of Guam during the period 1956–1985 and the cycasin content found in cycad flour prepared in those districts in the 1980s (138).

The poisonous properties of cycads have been exploited in former times as instruments of chemical warfare (Costa Rica), homicide (Celebes), and state-approved execution (Honduras) (130). In various parts of Oceania (*e.g.*, Guam, New Guinea), the highly toxic seed pulp of cycads has been used until the latter part of the twentieth century as a poultice to treat superficial and deep wounds (15,115, 130). Dried seed of *Cycas revoluta* was used until the 1960s to prepare a tonic for young children in Kii peninsula, Honshu Island, Japan (114). Cycad leaves are today found in the armamentarium of apothecaries in Beijing, China (unpublished data), and the underground caudex of *Stangeria er-iopus* is used by South African ethnic groups as an emetic and ingredient in magical potions (89).

General Toxicology

Macrozamia spp. and *Cycas* spp. contain the primeveroside macrozamin and/or the glucoside cycasin, and macrozamin undergoes conversion to cycasin (122). Cycasin, present in cycad seed in concentrations of 2%–4% (w/v) (135), forms colorless, monoclinic crystals with a MP of 144°–145°C (*Cycas revoluta* Thunb.) (88) or 154°C (*Cycas circinalis* L.) (94). Cycasin is soluble in water and insoluble in most organic solvents. The ultraviolet absorption spectrum has a maximum around 217 nm and an inflexion at 275 nm (132). Cycasin readily undergoes hydrolysis with 0.1 N hydrochloric acid at 100°C to yield methanol, formaldehyde, nitrogen, and glucose (132). Breakage of the β-D-glucopyranosyloxy linkage of cycasin by bacterial, plant, or mammalian β-glucosidase hydrolysis liberates MAM, a colorless liquid with an amine-like odor that is miscible with water and aqueous ethanol (67,79). Unlike MAM, azoxyethane, azoxymethane, and azoethane are not known to occur in nature (137). MAM is unstable at room temperature, especially in the presence of acid or alklai (132). The half-life in neutral aqueous solution is 11.5 h at 37°C, pH 7.8; it is less stable in alkaline solution (half-life 2.8 h, pH 10) (32). Most studies examining the biological actions of methylazoxymethanol employ MAM acetate because this compound is more stable than MAM; in particular, MAM acetate can withstand decomposition in aqueous solution when heated at 75°C for 30 min (132). Some investigators have used MAM benzoate (65). MAM spontaneously breaks down into reactive molecules, such as methyladiazonium ions and carbon-centered free radicals (potent alkylating agents) that methylate nucleic acids in the O^6-, N^7-, and C^8-positions of guanine (61,77,86,98). While MAM and its glucosides are the principal toxic moieties of cycads, these plants contain a number of other potentially neurotoxic materials, including the nonprotein amino acids β-N-methylamino-L-alanine (*Cycas* spp.) and β-N-oxalylamino-L-alanine (*Macrozamia* spp.) (90).

A synthesis of MAM is available (78). Cycasin is challenging to synthesize and yields are impractically small (D.N. Roy, unpublished data). Biological methods have employed insect larvae and plant material (119). Calluses produced from plant tissue of *Cycas revoluta* contain a glucosyltransferase that catalyzes the production of cycasin from uridine diphosphate-glucose and MAM (119,123).

Cycasin, MAM, and MAM acetate have teratogenic, mutagenic, hepatotoxic, and carcinogenic properties in rodents and primates (65,103). Hepatic and spinal lesions develop in ruminants fed cycasin (100). The glucoside is transported by the intestinal Na^+/glucose cotransporter, but has a lower affinity for the transporter than D-glucose (47). In contrast, cycasin is efficiently (100X lower concentrations) transported by the brain Na^+/glucose cotransporter (80), suggesting that a CNS capillary transport system accounts for the reported entry of cycasin into the brain of orally fed rats (19,80). Cycasin is hydrolyzed by gut bacteria and hepatic metabolism to form MAM, which is also able to enter the brain (60).

Animal Studies
Uncontrolled Observations

Acute effects of cycad poisoning in animals include hepatotoxicity, enterotoxicity, and death. Rapid twitching of the eyelids, nostrils, lips, jaw muscles, with periodic tremors of the body are reported in sheep, and muscle fasciculation has been seen in cycad-poisoned heifers (130). Delayed effects of cycad consumption are characterized by a progressive (?) and irreversible paralysis of the hindlimbs (neurocycadism). Initially, there is a staggering, weaving gait, with crossing of the legs, incoordination, and ataxia. More severe forms are characterized by posterior motor weakness, dragging of extended hindlimbs and, occasionally, a stringhalt-like action of the hocks. Function of the bladder, anus, and tail is unimpaired (52,130). Neuropathological examination reportedly shows degeneration of descending spinal tracts, readily observed in the lumbar region, with similar involvement of the fasciculus gracilis and dorsal spinocerebellar tracts, most prominent in the cervical region (59). Peripheral nerves and muscle have not been examined.

Neurocycadism, or cycadism (derriengue), occurs in cattle and sheep that graze on leaves and other components of cycad plants in Australia (*Bowenia, Cycas, Macrozamia*), New Guinea (*Cycas circinalis*), Dominican Republic and Puerto Rico (*Zamia*), and Mexico (*Dioon edule*) (52,130). Derriengue (literally, dancing feet) is associated with incomplete loss of power in the hindlimbs, coupled with an absence of muscle atrophy, loss of muscle tone and fasciculation, a clinical picture suggestive of an upper-motor-neuron disorder (76).

Controlled Studies

Mature Animals. The mouse oral LD_{50} for cycasin is 500–1000 mg/kg; the corresponding value for the rat is 270–562 mg/kg while that for the rabbit is only 30 mg/kg. The rat oral LD_{50} for macrozamin is 218 mg/kg. The lowest lethal dose for rats treated by the intraperitoneal route with MAM is 35 mg/kg, while the corresponding LD_{50} for MAM acetate is 90 mg/kg (132).

Reports of neuromuscular disease in ruminants grazing on cycads, and the possible relationship to the high incidence of motor neuron disease in the cycad-consuming Chamorro population of Guam, stimulated a flurry of experimental animal research on the toxicity of cycad between 1962 and 1972 (74,75,131). Discovery of the hepatotoxic and carcinogenic properties of cycasin and MAM in rodents was held responsible for reports of acute illness in humans ingesting cycad materials and for the allegedly high rate of hepatomas among Chamorros. Unfortunately, there was no detailed study of the incidence of liver disease or cancer on Guam, or of the relationships among these conditions and ALS/PDC. The suggestion that neurodegenerative disease resulted from exposure to cycad fell into disfavor when experimental feeding trials in laboratory rodents elicited malignant tumors rather than overt neurological disease. While cycasin is carcinogenic in rodents (107) and to some extent in nonhuman primates (19,103), there is no direct evidence that MAM, cycasin, or cycad seed are human carcinogens, nor is the prevalence of cancer known in regions endemic for cycad-associated ALS (49,66).

Few studies have examined the long-term consequences of newborn or adult exposure to materials derived from cycads. Newborn mice injected subcutaneously with MAM acetate (0.2–0.4 mg) and observed for 1 week to 1 year showed low body weight, required longer to develop, had difficulty walking, and dragged their hindlimbs. Adult mice fed for 4 days with 15% seed preparations from *Lepidozamia peroffskyana* developed cellular apoptosis of gut and brain tissue; cell types involved were not identified (41). Rats treated with intragastric cycasin (50 mg) showed weakness of legs on one side and general slowness of movement. Rats fed a 50-mg dose showed weakness of legs, tendency to fall on one side, and disinclination to move (19). Cycasin was detected in brain, liver, and kidneys of both rat groups (19). Feeding fresh leaves of *C. circinalis* produced a motor system disorder in a cow after 85 days (76). Spheroids were found in spinal white matter several months after a single intraruminal administration of cycad leaves to goats (101). Goats treated orally for 88–124 days with an oral solution of cycasin showed weakness in the hindquarters. Pathologic examination revealed hepatic lesions and, "In the whole length of spinal cord white matter of all treated cases axons were swollen or disappeared with [secondary] demyelination in the lateral and ventral funiculi," but with no obvious predilection for corticospinal and spinocerebellar tracts, as reported in some bovine cases of cycadism (101).

Neurological disease has also been reported in rhesus monkeys fed *chapatis* prepared from washed cycad flour containing (by paper chromatography) "almost no cycasin" (18, D.B. Dastur, personal communication). Weakness and wasting, especially of one upper limb, with neuropathological evidence of degeneration of anterior horn cells in spinal cord and of pyramidal cells in motor cortex, developed in a young animal fed for 4–9 months (18). A second, mature animal fed for 2 years showed "argyrophilic dystrophic plaques amongst the degenerating neurites of the cerebral white matter, without any amyloid or neurofibrillary tangles" (20). Additionally, one of two animals fed cycad seed boiled for 80 min (containing "clearly detectable amounts" of cycasin) showed "swelling and chromatolysis of anterior horn cells, as well as of axons of the anterior nerve roots, with accumulations of neurofilaments in both" (20). While the cycad flour was prepared according to the methods used by Chamorro people on Guam and was thought by the authors to be free of cycasin, the presence of liver changes in the treated primates suggests, retrospectively, that cycasin and/or its aglycone were present. Both groups of animals displayed hepatocellular changes characteristic of cycasin toxicity, and these were severe in animals fed the poorly detoxified boiled cycad (112). Another primate study assessed the carcinogenicity and hepatotoxicity of cycasin and MAM in rhesus, cynomolgus, and African green monkeys. Eight animals treated from birth up to 11 years of age with various combinations of cycad meal, cycasin, and MAM acetate displayed postmortem evidence of toxic hepatitis, centrilobular necrosis, hyperplastic nodules, and cirrhosis. The neurological status and CNS morphology were not described. One monkey showed a well-differentiated hepatocellular carcinoma, and a second had multiple malignant tumors. No histological evidence of liver damage was found in an additional animal fed cycad meal containing 3% cycasin for 8 months (103).

Developing Animals. A transplacental effect of cycasin was suggested by experiments showing that hamsters given intravenous MAM on gestation day (GD) 8 produced malformed fetuses (108). This was confirmed by the demonstration that cycad meal given to pregnant hamsters results in the appearance of cycasin and MAM in the fetus (109). MAM reacts with maternal and fetal nucleic acids by methylating guanine in the N^7-position in both DNA and RNA (85). Growth deficiencies occur if MAM (20 mg/kg) is administered to rats on day 13 of gestation when hypothalamic growth hormone-releasing factor cells are forming, while animals exposed later in gestation (when inhibitors of growth hormone release are forming) exhibit enlarged pituitaries and gigantism (95–97). Repeated subcutaneous

administration of MAM (5 mg/kg/day) twice daily on postnatal days 1–4 reduced body weight at day 28 by 24% relative to controls (118).

Brain development is reproducibly perturbed when MAM or its glucoside is administered to rodents. MAM kills or arrests neuroblasts undergoing mitosis. Cell death induced by MAM has been reported to be apoptotic in nature (35,41,69) and "independent both of the DNA fragmentation characteristic of apoptosis and of p53 expression" (133). An early study also reported extensive cellular necrosis in retinoblasts in hamsters and rats (42,99). Examination of the visual system shows that MAM reduces cell numbers both from a primary antimitotic action and also from increased loss of nerve cells that lack their normal cell targets (4). Despite a severe loss of cells in layers III and IV of the occipital cortex, the laminar distribution of vascular profiles, branch points, and cytochrome *c* oxidase activity, are similar to those in control animals (2,3). By contrast, there is severe disruption of the layered distribution of vascular trunks in rats treated with MAM acetate administered on embryonic day 14 (8). There is no delay in the formation of tight junctions, basal lamina, or loss of fenestrations (84).

Single intraperitoneal administration of MAM acetate (seven doses ranging from 0–25 mg/kg) to the pregnant rat on day 15 of gestation produces dose-dependent reductions in brain weight and DNA content at 60 days of postnatal age. With higher dosage, content of noradrenaline, dopamine, and 5-hydroxytryptamine increases dose-dependently (120). Neocortical somatostatin immunoreactivity also increases (87). Serotonergic neurons are reduced in number and irregularly distributed in dorsal and median raphe nuclei (38).

Effects of maternal administration of MAM acetate are illustrated by the persistent postnatal presence in the offspring of ectopic hippocampal neurons (CA1, CA2) (16,40,104,105). Exposure of developing rats at 15 days of gestation results in forebrain microencephaly; major losses are evident postnatally in cortical laminae II–IV, with deeper layers showing relative preservation and a higher density of calbindin interneurons (14,55). Glutamatergic and γ-aminobutyric acid (GABA)-ergic neuronal populations are severely reduced, while the shrunken cortex is relatively hyperinnervated by noradrenergic and cholinergic neurons (55,127). Basal forebrain cholinergic neurons are spared and, despite a massive loss of target cortical neurons, cholinergic innervation is preserved in offspring of MAM-treated dams up to 20 months of age (82,83). Acetylcholinesterase activity is markedly increased in the cerebral cortex of MAM-treated rats; by contrast, no significant changes occur in the striatum or hippocampus of these animals (6).

However, choline acetyltransferase activity is significantly decreased in the hippocampus and cerebral cortex of rats exposed to MAM on days 13–15 of gestation (50). Proliferation of neurons bearing excitatory amino acid receptors in animals treated on GD 15 is marked in the cortex and hippocampus, less so in the striatum (121). Susceptibility to kainate-induced seizures is increased in MAM-exposed rats with severe abnormalities of neuronal migration (40). There is marked loss of striatal aspiny interneurons in which somatostastin and neuropeptide Y coexist (125). The number of caudate-putamen neurons reactive to vasoactive intestinal polypeptide (VIP) or neuropeptide Y (NPY) is unchanged in rats treated with MAM acetate of gestational day 15, while cholecystokinin (CCK) and NPY-immunoreactive neurons in the neorcortex, and CCK- and VIP-immunoreactive neurons in the hippocampus, decrease (139). Cortical somatostatin immunoreactivity is increased (12).

Rodents treated with MAM acetate *in utero* or within days of birth show strikingly abnormal development of the cerebellum associated with partial destruction of the external germinal layer (45,49,53,57,73,99). The primary targets of MAM are the precursors of glutamatergic and GABA-receptive cells (5). Apoptotic cells in the external granule cell layer appear 24 h after MAM treatment, peak at 48 h, and decrease at 72 h (36,41). In adulthood, Purkinje and Golgi epithelial cells are found scattered ectopically within the internal granule cell layer and molecular layer, respectively; mature granule cells may form a separate ectopic layer (39). Alignment of Purkinje cells is disturbed, primary dendrites are reduced in length; they are less branched and have naked dendritic spines; basket cells are present (10,21,22,39,44,92,106). Multinucleated cells representing neuroblasts arrested during the process of cell division are reported in the cerebellum of rodents treated with cycasin or MAM (45,58). Heterologous synapses between mossy fibers and Purkinje cell dendrites develop early but are not seen after postnatal day 20 (22). Cerebellar ^{3}H-GABA$_B$ binding is unchanged in MAM-treated rodents (124). MAM lesions that reduce granule but not Golgi cells in the granule cell layer, and reduce basket and stellate cells in the molecular layer, markedly attenuate the ability of N-methyl-D-aspartate to increase cerebellar cyclic guanine mononucleotide (134).

Behavioral effects of early postnatal injection of MAM acetate include retarded development of the righting reflex, reduced locomotor activity, disrupted associative eyeblink conditioning, reduced acoustic startle amplitudes, and oral dyskinesia in the form of increased chewing movements (33,37,54,70). Rats with mild cortical hypoplasia exhibit hyperactivity (1,43,81) or are hyperreactive to environmental stimuli (31); this may be associated with augmented dopaminergic function (128). Rats allowed to survive for 26 months did not show any modification of spontaneous activity (43). MAM microcephalic rats display impaired learning of patterns but not brightness discrimination (91). Learning impairment is paralleled by a change in the phosphorylation of B-50/GAP-43 in hippocampus but not in cerebral cortex (23). Learning and memory capacity in rats treated prenatally with MAM reportedly improve after treatment with the phosphatidylcholine precursor, cytidine disphosphocholine (24). Performance of microcephalic rats aged 6, 15, or 24 months in a Morris water maze was impaired on acquisition and retention, and the acquisition deficit increased with age in a premature decline of cognitive function (71). This decline is ameliorated by surgical placement during infancy of normal fetal neocortical tissue (72).

Neurotropic Carcinogenesis. Pregnant rats fed crude meal containing 3% cycasin have produced litters free of malformations but with an increased propensity for glial malignancy in adult life. In one study of offspring surviving more than 6 months, 18.5% had tumors at various sites, five occurring in the brain (gliomas), four in the jejunum, and others being located, one each, in the uterus, kidney, colon, lung, chest wall, and muscles of the leg (68). Rats exposed *in utero* to MAM or MAM acetate (20 mg/kg) showed microencephaly and some developed endocrine adenomas, oligodendrogliomas and schwannomas, or tumors at peripheral sites (68).

Cycasin has limited potential to induce tumors relative to other azoxyalkanes (137). For example, CNS and PNS tumors develop in nearly all offspring of rats that inhaled azoethane during pregnancy (24), and 10% of adult animals developed brain tumors after subcutaneous administration of this compound (27). Application of 1,2-diethylhydrazine, as well as azo- and azoxyethane on the same day of gestation, resulted in development of nervous system tumors in the offspring (25,26,137). Predominantly brain tumors developed in 20% of animals after subcutaneous administration of 1,2-diethylhydrazine (28). Rats treated subcutaneously or periorally with 1-methyl-2-benzylhydrazine developed CNS and PNS tumors (137).

In Vitro Studies

Mouse cerebral cortex explants take up cycasin in a concentration- and time-dependent manner. Significant levels of MAM are detectable in cortical tissue but not in culture medium 24 h after treatment, suggesting that transported glycone is hydrolyzed to MAM by intracellular β-glucosidase (63). Cycasin (1 μM–1 mM) induces selective neuronal degeneration in mouse cortex that was blocked by pretreatment with a N-methyl-D-aspartate receptor antagonist (63). Astrocyte cultures treated with 1 mM cycasin exhibit no pathological changes (63). Similarly, concentrations of MAM that interfere with neuronal mitosis *in vitro* do not affect astrocyte proliferation (13). Treatment of early postmitotic hippocampal neurons at 0–1 days *in vitro* with micromolar concentrations of MAM persistently inhibits neurite outgrowth (51). Exposure to MAM depletes microtubule-associated protein 1B (MAP 1B) and MAP 2, which are required for axonal elongation (51). Brain slices from MAM-treated rats are less susceptible to excitotoxic injury induced by hypoxia or by glutamate agonists (126). Marked alteration of muscarinic and α_1-adrenergic receptor–stimulated phosphoinositide metabolism is found in cerebral cortical slices of brains removed from rats exposed to MAM on GD 15 (7).

Brains of Guam Chamorros ALS/PDC contain intraneuronal paired helical filaments composed of accumulated phosphorylated tau protein. Tau mRNA expression in rat neuronal cultures—normally modulated by glutamate—increases after MAM (10 μM) pretreatment. Elevated *tau* gene expression *in vitro* is coincident with MAM-related DNA adducts and reduced levels and activity of the DNA-repair enzyme, apurinic/apyridiminic endonuclease (31).

Human Studies

Twelve to 40 h after ingestion of poisonous cycad materials, there is sudden onset of nausea and vomiting, enlargement of the liver, convulsions, loss of consciousness, and death or recovery (48). In past times, Chamorro children were said to fall sick after eating cycad products; a few died if preparation was very poor, whereas the majority ingested the material without noticeable adverse health effects (111). Chamorro folklore links the practice of handling and consuming cycad materials to a disease known locally as *lytico*, many cases of which are diagnosed as ALS (129–131). Epidemiological study shows that preference for traditional Chamorro food is the only one of 23 tested variables significantly associated with an increased risk for parkinsonism-dementia (93). Other studies show a very highly significant positive association between ALS and the cycasin content of flour prepared by Chamorros (62,138). ALS was diagnosed in Japanese and Melanesian subjects within 10–15 years of repeated oral or subcutaneous exposure to cycad seed in the first or second decade of life (114,115), and ALS developed in a Caucasian woman with heavy exposure to *Macrozamia* seed prepared for ornamental purposes (*see* later under Case Report). Some Japanese and Guamanian patients with ALS/PDC revealed (in addition to the well-described cerebral neurofilamentous pathology of this disease) multinucleated and ectopic neurons in the cerebellum and vestibular nuclei, an observation that suggested exposure during the later phases of brain development (up to the age of 1 year) to an agent (such as MAM) that arrests the developmental mitotic and migratory responses of neurons (102,136). Taken together, these data are consonant with the proposal that western Pacific ALS/PDC is a long-latency disorder that may be acquired years or decades prior to clinical expression (112,113). The declining patterns of cycad utilization in all western Pacific communities at risk for ALS/PDC fulfill the requirement for a diminishing environmental factor required as an etiological link to this disappearing neurodegenerative disorder (111). On the island of Saipan, where cycads were totally cleared by the mid-1920s, ALS/PDC had declined to very low levels by the 1950s (117).

Toxic Mechanisms

Use of cycad seed for food and/or medicine is epidemiologically associated with western Pacific ALS/PDC among Chamorros of Guam, Japanese of the Kii peninsula of Honshu Island, and the Auyu and Jaqai linguistic groups of Irian Jaya (west New Guinea), Indonesia (113). While the culpable agent is unknown, there is a very strong geographical correlation between Guam ALS and cycasin concentration in cycad flour used for food (62,138). This association, coupled with the genotoxic properties of cycasin (rather than the cycad excitotoxic amino acid; *see* β-N-Methylamino-L-alanine, this volume), make it the leading candidate for the proposed environmental trigger ("slow toxin") of ALS/PDC (110,116). It is suggested that this trigger may also be responsible for the very high prevalence of glucose intolerance and diabetes mellitus among Chamorros with this neurodegenerative disease (19,30,110). Cycasin and MAM impair both rodent and human β-islet function and may cause death of these pancreatic cells *in vitro*. Cytotoxic mechanisms appear to include DNA alkylation, nitric oxide generation (29,30), and perturbed DNA repair (31, C.A. Delaney *et al.*, unpublished data).

The relationship between cycasin and western Pacific ALS/PDC is based largely on epidemiological evidence; there is no satisfactory animal model of Guam neurofibrillary degeneration (50), and the long-term CNS effects of early exposure to cycasin are unexplored other than one report of premature cognitive decline in aging microcephalic rats (71). Noteworthy, however, is the presence of ectopic and multinucleated cells in the cerebellum of rodents treated with cycasin or MAM (58) and in the cerebellum of Chamorros who died in middle age with ALS (102,136). MAM also appears to interfere with the normal development of differentiating postmitotic neurons *in vitro*, causing retraction and persistently shortened axons (51). MAM increases glutamate-stimulated neuronal tau mRNA expression and cell loss in neuronal cultures, raising the possibility that MAM produces long-term perturbation in neuronal responses to physiological levels of glutamate (31). Additionally, protein kinase C, activation of which stimulates release of secreted amyloid precursor protein (APPs) in several cell lines, is permanently hyperactivated in the cerebral cortex and hippocampus of MAM-treated rats. Synaptosomes derived from these brain areas show decreased membrane-bound APP concentration and a concomitant increase in soluble fractions (11).

REFERENCES

1. Archer T, Hiltunen AJ, Jarbe TU *et al.* (1988) Hyperactivity and instrumental learning deficits in methylazoxymethanol-treated rat offspring. *Neurotoxicol Teratol* **10**, 341.

2. Ashwell K (1987) Altered morphology of dorsal lateral geniculate nucleus neurons in methylazoxymethanol acetate induced microencephaly. *Exp Brain Res* **68**, 329.

3. Ashwell KW, Webster WS (1987) Vascularity and cytochrome oxidase distribution in the occipital cortex in MAM Ac-induced microencephaly. *Brain Res* **430**, 301.

4. Ashwell KW, Webster WS (1988) The contribution of primary and secondary neuronal degeneration to prenatally-induced microencephaly. *Neurotoxicol Teratol* **10**, 65.

5. Bacon E, Girard C, de Barry J, Gombos G (1992) [^{3}H]-Muscimol and [^{3}H]-flunitrazepam binding sites in the developing cerebellum of mice treated with methylazoxymethanol at different postnatal ages. *Neurochem Res* **17**, 707.

6. Balduine W, Lombardelli G, Peruzzi G, Cattabeni F (1992) Cholinergic hyperinnervation in the cerebral cortex of microencephalic rats does not result in muscarinic receptor down-regulation or in alteration of receptor-stimulated phosphoinositide metabolism. *Neurochem Res* **17**, 761.

7. Balduine W, Lombardelli G, Peruzzi G, Cattabeni F (1995) Effect of prenatal treatment with methylazoxymethanol on carbachol-, norepinephrine- and glutamate-stimulated phosphoinositide metabolism in the neonatal, young and adult offspring. *Neurochem Res* **20**, 1211.

8. Bardosi A, Ambach G, Hann P (1987) The angiogenesis of the microencephalic rat brains caused by methylazoxymethanol acetate. III. Internal angioarchitecture of cortex. *Acta Neuropathol* **75**, 85.

9. Beaton JM (1977) *Dangerous Harvest: Investigations in the Late Prehistoric Occupation of Southeast Central Queensland*. PhD Dissertation. Australian National University, Canberra.

10. Bradley P, Berry M (1978) Quantitative effects of methylazoxymethanol acetate on Purkinje cell dendritic growth. *Brain Res* **143**, 499.

11. Caputi A, Barindelli S, Pastorino L *et al.* (1997) Increased secretion of the amino-terminal fragment of amyloid precursor protein in brains of rats with a constitutive up-regulation of protein kinase C. *J Neurochem* **68**, 2523.

12. Cattabeni F, Abbracchio MP, Cimino M *et al.* (1989) Methylazoxymethanol-induced microcephaly: Persistent increase of cortical somatostatin-like immunoreactivity. *Dev Brain Res* **47**, 156.

13. Cattaneo E, Reinach B, Caputi A *et al.* (1995) Selective *in vitro* blockade of neuroepithelial cell proliferation by methylazoxymethanol, a molecule capable of inducing long lasting functional impairments. *J Neurosci Res* **41**, 640.

14. Ciani E, Contestabile A (1994) Immunohistochemical localization of calbindin-D28K in telencephalic regions of microencephalic rats. *Neurosci Lett* **171**, 41.

15. Close K, Close A, Gelegel N (1975) Medicinal plants of the Maprik Area. *Papua New Guinea Med J* **18**, 153.

16. Collier PA, Ashwell KW (1993) Distribution of neuronal heteropiae following prenatal exposure to methylazoxymethanol *Neurotoxicol Teratol* **15**, 439.

17. Cuzner AT (1898) Arrowroot, cassava, and koonti. *J Amer Med Assn* **1**, 366.

18. Dastur (1964) Cycad toxicity in monkeys: Clinical, pathological, and biochemical aspects. *Fed Proc* **23**, 1368.

19. Dastur DK, Palekar RS (1974) The experimental pathology of cycad toxicity, with special reference to oncogenic effects. *Ind J Cancer* **2**, 33.

20. Dastur DK, Palekar RS, Manhani DK (1993) Toxicity of various forms of *Cycas circinalis* in rhesus monkeys. Pathology of brain, spinal cord and liver. In: *ALS: New Advances in Toxicology and Epidemiology*. Rose C, Norris F eds. Smith-Gordon, London p. 129.

21. De Barry J, Gombos G (1989) Immunohistochemistry with anti-calbindin and anti-neurofilament antibodies in the cerebellum of methylazoxymethanol-treated mice. *J Neurosci Res* **23**, 330.

22. De Barry J, Gombos G, Klupp T, Hamori J (1987) Alteration of mouse cerebellar circuits following methylazoxymethanol treatment during development: Immunohistochemistry of GABAergic elements and electron microscopic study. *J Comp Neurol* **261**, 253.

23. Di Luca M, Merazzi F, DeGraan PN *et al.* (1993) Selective alteration in B-50/GAP-43 phosphorylation in brain areas of animals characterized by cognitive impairment. *Brain Res* **607**, 329.

24. Drago F, Mauceri F, Nardo L *et al.* (1993) Effects of cytidine-diphosphocholine on acetylcholine-mediated behaviors in the rat. *Brain Res Bull* **31**, 485.

25. Druckrey H (1973) Chemical structure and action in transplacental carcinogenesis and teratogenesis. In: *Transplacental Carcinogenesis*, #4. Tomatis L, Mohr I

eds. International Agency for Research on Cancer Press, Geneva p. 45.

26. Druckrey H, Ivankovic S, Preussmann R et al. (1968) Transplacental induction of neurogenic malignomas by 1,2-diethyl-hydrazine, azo-, and azoxy-ethane in rats. *Experientia* **24**, 561.

27. Druckrey H, Preussmann R, Ivakovic D et al. (1965) Carcinogene Wirkungon Azoëthan und Azoxyäthan an Ratten. *Z Krebforsch* **67**, 31.

28. Druckrey H, Preussmann R, Matzkies F, Ivankovic S (1966) Carcinogene Wirkung von 1,2-Diäthylhydrazin an Ratten. *Naturwissenschaften* **53**, 557.

29. Eizirik DL, Kisby GE (1995) Cycad toxin-induced damage of rodent and human pancreatic cells. *Biochem Pharmacol* **50**, 335.

30. Eizirik DL, Spencer PS, Kisby G (1996) Potential role of environmental genotoxic agents in diabetes mellitus and neurodegenerative diseases. *Biochem Pharmacol* **51**, 1585.

31. Esclaire F, Kisby G, Spencer PS et al. (1999) The Guam cycad toxin methylazoxymethanol damages neuronal DNA and modulates Tau mRNA expression and excitotoxicity. *Exp Neurol* **155**, 11.

32. Feinberg A, Zedeck MS (1980) Production of a highly reactive alkylating agent from the organospecific carcinogen methylazoxymethanol by alcohol dehydrogenase. *Cancer Res* **40**, 4446.

33. Ferguson SA, Paule MG, Holson RR (1996) Functional effects of methylazoxymethanol-induced cerebellar hypoplasia in rats. *Neurotoxicol Teratol* **18**, 529.

34. Ferguson SA, Racey FD, Paule MG, Holson RR (1993) Behavioral effects of methylazoxymethanol-induced microencephaly. *Behav Neurosci* **107**, 1067.

35. Ferrer I, Pozas E, Marti M et al. (1997) Methylazoxymethanol acetate-induced apoptosis in the external granule cell layer of the developing cerebellum of the rat is associated with strong c-Jun expression and formation of high molecular weight c-Jun complexes. *J Neuropathol Exp Neurol* **56**, 1.

36. Ferrer I, Pozas E, Planas AM (1997) Ubiquitination of apoptotic cells in the developing cerebellum of the rat following ionizing radiation or methylazoxymethanol injection. *Acta Neuropathol* **93**, 402.

37. Freeman JH Jr, Barone S Jr, Stanton ME (1995) Disruption of cerebellar maturation by an antimitotic agent impairs the ontogeny of eyeblink conditioning in rats. *J Neurosci* **15**, 7301.

38. Funahashi A, Inouye M, Yamamura H (1992) Developmental alteration of serotonin neurons in the raphe nucleus of rats with methylazoxymethanol-induced microencephaly. *Acta Neuropathol* **85**, 31.

39. Garcia-Ladona FJ, de Barry J, Girard C, Gombos G (1991) Ectopic granule cell layer in mouse cerebellum after methyl-azoxy-methanol (MAM) treatment. *Exp Brain Res* **86**, 90.

40. Germano IM, Sperber EF (1998) Transplacentally induced neuronal migration disorders—an animal model for the study of the epilepsies. *J Neurosci Res* **51**, 473.

41. Gobé GC (1994) Apoptosis in brain and gut tissue of mice fed a seed preparation of the cycad *Lepidozamia peroffskyana*. *Biochem Biophys Res Commun* **30**, 327.

42. Goerttler K, Arnold HP, Michael DV (1970) Uber Carcinogeninduzierte diaplacentare Wirkungen bei Ratten (Histologische Befunde und Kinetik des DNS-Stoffwechsels nach Gabe von Aflatoxin B1, Methylazoxymethanolacetat und Athylnitrosoharnstoff). *Z Krebsforsch* **74**, 396.

43. Greiner PO, Charles P, Bonnet M et al. (1992) Neuropharmacological study of aged MAM-treated rats. *Neurobiol Aging* **13**, 527.

44. Hartkop TH, Jones MZ (1977) Methylazoxymethanol-induced aberrant Purkinje cell dendritic development. *J Neuropathol Exp Neurol* **36**, 519.

45. Hillman DE, Chen S, Ackman J (1988) Perinatal methylazoxymethanol acetate uncouples coincidence of orientation of cerebellar folia and parallel fibers. *Neuroscience* **24**, 99.

46. Hirano A, Jones M (1972) Fine structure of cycasin-induced cerebellar alterations. *Fed Proc* **31**, 1517.

47. Hirayama B, Hazama A, Loo DF et al. (1994) Transport of cycasin by the intestinal Na$^+$/glucose cotransporter. *Biochim Biophys Acta* **1193**, 151.

48. Hirono I, Kachi H, Kato T (1970) A survey of acute toxicity of cycads and mortality rate from cancer in the Miyako Islands, Okinawa. *Acta Pathol Jpn* **20**, 327.

49. Hirono I, Shibuya C (1967) Induction of a neurological disorder by cycasin in mice. *Nature* **216**, 1311.

50. Hof PR, Perl DP, Loerzel AJ et al. (1994) Amyotrophic lateral sclerosis and parkinsonism-dementia from Guam: Differences in neurofibrillary tangle distribution and density in the hippocampal formation and neocortex. *Brain Res* **650**, 107.

51. Hoffman JR, Boyne LJ, Levitt P, Fischer I (1996) Short exposure to methylazoxymethanol causes a long-term inhibition of axonal outgrowth from cultured embryonic rat hippocampal neurons. *J Neurosci Res* **46**, 349.

52. Hooper PT (1983) Cycad poisoning. In: *Handbook of Natural Toxins. l. Plant and Fungal Toxins*. Keeler RF, Tu AT eds. Marcel Dekker, New York p. 463.

53. Ji Z, Hawkes R (1996) Partial ablation of the neonatal external granular layer disrupts mossy fiber topography in the adult rat cerebellum. *J Comp Neurol* **371**, 578.

54. Johansson P (1990) Methylazoxymethanol (MAM)-induced brain lesions and oral dyskinesia in rats. *Psychopharmacology* **100**, 72.

55. Johnston MV, Coyle JT (1979) Histological and neurochemical effects of fetal treatment with methylazoxymethanol on rat neorcortex in adulthood. *Brain Res* **170**, 135.

56. Jones DL (1993) *Cycads of the World. Ancient Plants in Today's Landscape.* Reed, Chatswood, New South Wales.

57. Jones MZ, Gardner E (1976) Pathogenesis of methylazoxymethanol-induced lesions in the postnatal mouse cerebellum. *J Neuropathol Exp Neurol* **35**, 413.

58. Jones MZ, Yang M, Mickelsen O (1972) Effects of methylazoxymethanol glucoside and methylazoxymethanol acetate on the cerebellum of the postnatal Swiss albino mouse. *Fed Proc* **31**, 1508.

59. Jubb KVF, Kennedy PC, Palmer N (1985) *Pathology of Domestic Animals. 3rd Ed.* Academic Press, Orlando, Florida p. 265.

60. Kabel JP, Kisby GE, Mako SC et al. (1992) Rodent brain metabolism of cycasin and DNA alkylation by methylazoxymethanol (MAM). *Soc Neurosci Abst* **18**, 1249.

61. Kisby GE, Eizirik D, Sweatt C, Spencer PS (1995) Reactive oxygen species produced by the cycad toxin methylazoxymethanol, a candidate etiological factor for western Pacific ALS/P-D. *J Cell Biochem* **21B**, 99.

62. Kisby GE, Ellison M, Spencer PS (1992) Content of the neurotoxins cycasins (methylazoxymethanol β-D-glucoside) and BMAA (β-N-methylamino-L-alanine) in cycad flour prepared by Guam Chamorros. *Neurology* **42**, 1336.

63. Kisby GE, Ross SM, Spencer PS et al. (1992) Cycasin and BMAA: Candidate neurotoxins for western Pacific amyotrophic lateral sclerosis/parkinsonism-dementia complex. *Neurodegeneration* **1**, 73.

64. Kobayashi A (1972) Cycasin in cycad materials used in Japan. *Fed Proc* **31**, 1476.

65. Kobayashi A, Matsumoto H (1965) Studies on methylazoxymethanol, the aglycone of cycasin: Isolation, biological and chemical properties. *Arch Biochem Biophys* **110**, 371.

66. Kurland LT (1972) An appraisal of the neurotoxicity of cycad and the etiology of amyotrophic lateral sclerosis on Guam. *Fed Proc* **31**, 1540.

67. Lacqueur GL, Matsumoto H (1966) Neoplasms in female Fischer rats following intraperitoneal injection of methylazoxymethanol. *J Natl Cancer Inst* **37**, 217.

68. Lacqueur GL, Spatz M (1973) Transplacental induction of tumors and malformations in rats with cycasin and methylazoxymethanol. In: *Transplacental Carcinogenesis, #4.* Tomatis L, Mohr I eds. International Agency for Research on Cancer Press, Geneva p. 59.

69. Lafarga M, Lerga A, Andres MA et al. (1997) Apoptosis induced by methylazoxymethanol in developing rat cerebellum—organization of the cell nucleus and its relationship to DNA and rRNA regulation. *Cell Tissue Res* **289**, 25.

70. Lai H, Quock RM, Makous W et al. (1978) Methylazoxymethanol acetate: Effect of postnatal injection on brain amines and behavior. *Pharmacol Biochem Behav* **8**, 251.

71. Lee MH, Rabe A (1992) Premature decline in Morris water maze performance of aging microencephalic rats. *Neurotoxicol Teratol* **14**, 383.

72. Lee MH, Rabe A (1998) Protective effects of fetal neocortical transplants on cognitive function and neuron size in rats with congenital microencephaly. *Behav Brain Res* **90**, 147.

73. Lovell KL, Jones MZ (1980) Partial external germinal layer regeneration in the cerebellum following methylazoxymethanol administration: Effects on Purkinje cell dendritic spines. *J Neuropathol Exp Neurol* **39**, 541.

74. Lyon Arboretum (1964) Proceedings of the Third Conference on the Toxicity of Cycads. *Fed Proc* **23**, 1337.

75. Lyon Arboretum (1972) Proceedings of the Sixth Conference on the Toxicity of Cycads. *Fed Proc* **31**, 1465.

76. Mason MM, Fredrickson TN (1965) Derriengue investigations. The Fourth Conference on the Toxicity of Cycads In: *Toxicity of Cycads: Implications for Neurodegenerative Diseases and Cancer. Transcripts of Four Cycad Conferences (1988).* Whiting MG ed. Third World Medical Research Foundation, New York p. 72.

77. Matsumoto H, Higa HH (1966) Studies on methylazoxymethanol, the aglycone of cycasin: Methylation of nucleic acids *in vitro. Biochem J* **98**, 20c.

78. Matsumoto H, Nagahama T, Larson HO (1965) Studies on methyl-azoxy-methanol, the aglycone of cycasin: A synthesis of methylazoxymethanol acetate. *Biochem J* **95**, 13c.

79. Matsumoto H, Strong FM (1963) The occurrence of methylazoxymethanol in *Cycas circinalis* L. *Arch Biochem* **101**, 299.

80. Matsuoka T, Nichizaki T, Kisby GE (1998) Na$^+$-dependent and phlorizin-inhibitable transport of glucose and cycasin in brain endothelial cells. *J Neurochem* **70**, 772.

81. Mercugliano M, Hyman SL, Batshaw ML (1990) Behavioral deficits in rats with minimal cortical hypoplasia induced by methylazoxymethanol acetate. *Pediatrics* **85**, 432.

82. Minger SL, Davies P (1992) Persistent innervation of rat neocortex by basal forebrain cholinergic neurons despite the massive reduction of cortical target neurons. I. Morphometric analysis. *Exp Neurol* **117**, 124.

83. Minger SL, Davies P (1992) Persistent innervation of rat neocortex by basal forebrain cholinergic neurons despite the massive reduction of cortical target neurons. II. Neurochemical analysis. *Exp Neurol* **117**, 139.

84. Misztal DR, Ahwell KW, Zhang LL (1994) Response of the fetal cerebral vasculature to prenatal cytotoxic brain damage. *Neurotoxicol Teratol* **16**, 593.

85. Nagata Y, Matsumoto H (1969) Studies on methylazoxymethanol: Methylation of nucleic acids in the fetal rat brain. *Proc Soc Exp Biol* **122**, 383.

86. Nagasawa HT, Shirota FN, Matsumoto H (1972) Decomposition of methylazoxymethanol, the aglycone of cycasin, in D$_2$O. *Nature* **236**, 234.

87. Naus CC, Cimino M, Wood GR *et al.* (1992) Cellular expression of somatostatin in MAM-induced microencephaly in the rat. *Devel Brain Res* **70**, 39.

88. Nishida K, Kobayashi A, Nagahama T (1955) Studies on cycasin, a new toxic glucoside, of *Cycas revoluta* Thunb. *Bull Agr Chem Soc* **19**, 77.

89. Osborne R, Grove A, Oh P *et al.* (1994) The magical and medicinal usage of *Stangeria eriopus* in South Africa. *J Ethnopharmacol* **43**, 67.

90. Pan M, Mabry TJ, Cao P, Moini M (1997) Identification of nonprotein amino acids from cycad seeds as *N*-ethoxy-carbonyl ethyl ester derivatives by positive chemical-ionization gas chromatography-mass spectrometry. *J Chromatogr* **787**, 288.

91. Rabe A, Lee MH (1990) Visual discrimination by rats with transplacentally induced microencephaly. *Neurotoxicol Teratol* **12**, 399.

92. Rabie A, Selme-Matrat M, Clavel MC *et al.* (1977) Effects of methylazoxymethanol given at different stages of postnatal life on development of the rat brain. Comparison with those of thyroid deficiency. *J Neurobiol* **8**, 337.

93. Reed D, Labarthe D, Chen K-M, Stallones R (1987) A cohort study of amyotrophic lateral sclerosis and parkinsonism-dementia on Guam and Rota. *Amer J Epidemiol* **125**, 92.

94. Riggs NV (1956) Glycosyloxyazoxymethane: A constituent of the seeds of *Cycas circinalis*. *Chem Ind* 926.

95. Rodier PM, Kates B, White AL (1991) A comparison of hypothalamic cell numbers in dwarf and normal weight rats exposed prenatally to methylazoxymethanol (MAM). *Neurotoxicol Teratol* **13**, 591.

96. Rodier PM, Kates B, White AL, Muhs A (1991) Effects of prenatal exposure to methylazoxymethanol (MAM) on brain weight, hypothalamic cell number, pituitary structure, and postnatal growth in the rat. *Teratology* **43**, 241.

97. Rodier PM, Kates B, White WA, White AL (1991) The relationship of rat brain weight and pituitary weight to postnatal growth after prenatal exposure to methylazoxymethanol. *Neurotoxicol Teratol* **13**, 583.

98. Shank RD, Magee PN (1967) Similarities between the biochemical actions of cycasin and dimethylnitrosamine. *Biochem J* **105**, 521.

99. Shimada M, Langman J (1970) Repair of the external granular layer of the hamster cerebellum after prenatal and postnatal administration of methylazoxymethanol. *Teratology* **3**, 119.

100. Shimizu J, Tamaru M, Katsukura T *et al.* (1991) Effects of fetal treatment with methylazoxymethanol acetate on radial maze performance in rats. *Neurosci Res* **11**, 209.

101. Shimizu T, Yasuda N, Kono I *et al.* (1986) Hepatic and spinal lesions in goats chronically intoxicated with cycasin. *Jpn J Vet Sci* **8**, 1291.

102. Shirake H, Yase (1975) ALS in Japan. In: *Handbook of Clinical Neurology. Vol 22. System Disorders and Atrophy Pt 2*. Vinken PJ, Bruyn GW eds. American Elsevier, New York p. 353.

103. Sieber SM, Correa P, Dalgard DW *et al.* (1980) Carcinogenicity and hepatotoxicity of cycasin and its aglycone methylazoxymethanol acetate in non-human primates. *J Natl Cancer Inst* **65**, 177.

104. Singh SC (1977) Ectopic neurons in the hippocampus of the postnatal rat exposed to methylazoxymethanol during foetal development. *Acta Neuropathol* **40**, 111.

105. Singh SC (1978) Redirected perforant and commissural connections of eutopic and ectopic neurons in the hippocampus of methylazoxymethanol-acetate treated rats. *Acta Neuropathol* **44**, 197.

106. Singh SC (1980) Deformed dendrites and reduced spine numbers on ectopic neurones in the hippocampus of rats exposed to methylazoxymethanol-acetate. A Golgi-Cox study. *Acta Neuropathol* **49**, 193.

107. Spatz M (1969) Toxic and carcinogenic alkylating agents from cycads. *Ann N Y Acad Sci* **163**, 848.

108. Spatz M, Dougherty WJ, Smith DWE (1967) Teratogenic effects of methylazoxymethanol. *Proc Soc Exp Biol* **124**, 476.

109. Spatz M, Lacqueur GL (1968) Evidence for transplacental passage of the natural carcinogen cycasin and its aglycone. *J Natl Cancer Inst* **38**, 233.

110. Spencer PS (1987) Guam ALS/Parkinsonism-dementia: A long-latency neurotoxic disorder caused by "slow toxin(s)" in food? *Can J Neurol Sci* **14**, 347.

111. Spencer PS (1990) Are neurotoxins driving us crazy? Planetary observations of neurodegenerative diseases of old age. In: *Behavioral Measures of Neurotoxicity*. Russell RW, Flattau PE, Pope AM eds. National Academy Press, Washington, DC p. 11.

112. Spencer PS, Kisby G (1992) Slow toxins and amyotrophic lateral sclerosis. In: *Handbook of Amyotrophic Lateral Sclerosis*. Smith RA ed. Marcel Dekker, New York p. 575.

113. Spencer PS, Kisby GE, Ludolph AC (1991) Slow toxins, biologic markers, and long-latency neurodegenerative disease in the western Pacific region. *Neurology* **41**, 62.

114. Spencer PS, Ohta M, Palmer VS (1987) Cycad use and motor neurone disease in Kii Peninsula of Japan. *Lancet* **ii**, 1462.

115. Spencer PS, Palmer VS, Herman A, Asmedi A (1987) Cycad use and motor neuron disease in Irian Jaya. *Lancet* **ii**, 1273.

116. Spencer PS, Ross SM, Kisby GE, Roy DN (1990) Western Pacific amyotrophic lateral sclerosis: Putative role of cycad toxins. In: *Amyotrophic Lateral Sclerosis: Concepts in Pathogenesis and Etiology*. Hudson AJ ed. University of Toronto Press, Toronto p. 263.

117. Steele JC, Guzman RQ, Driver MG *et al.* (1990) Nutritional factors in amyotrophic lateral sclerosis on Guam: Observations from Umatac. In: *Amyotrophic Lateral*

Sclerosis. Concepts in Pathogenesis and Etiology. Hudson AJ ed. University of Toronto Press, Toronto p. 193.

118. Sullivan-Jones P, Ali SF, Gough B, Holdon RR (1994) Postnatal methylazoxymethanol: sensitive periods and regional selectivity of effects. *Neurotoxicol Teratol* **16**, 631.

119. Tadera K, Ginya H, Sawada R *et al.* (1995) Cycasin formation in tissue cultures of Japanese cycad. *Phytochemistry* **38**, 1199.

120. Tamaru M, Hirata Y, Nagayoshi M, Matsutai T (1988) Brain changes in rats induced by prenatal injection of methylazoxymethanol. *Teratology* **37**, 149.

121. Tamaru M, Yoneda Y, Ogita K *et al.* (1992) Excitatory amino acid receptors in brains of rats with methylazoxymethanol-induced microencephaly. *Neurosci Res* **14**, 13.

122. Tate ME, Delaere IM, Jones GP, Tierkink ERT (1995) Crystal and molecular structure of (Z)-β-O-D-glucopyranosyloxy-NNO-azoxymethane. *Aust J Chem* **48**, 1059.

123. Teas HJ (1967) Cycasin synthesis in *Seirarctia echo* (Lepidoptera) larvae fed methylazoxymethanol. *Biochem Biophys Res Commun* **26**, 686.

124. Turgeon SM, Albin RL (1993) Pharmacology, distribution, cellular localization, and development of GABA$_B$ binding in rodent cerebellum. *Neuroscience* **55**, 311.

125. Vincent SR, Semba K, Radke JM *et al.* (1990) Loss of striatal somatostatin neurons following prenatal methylazoxymethanol. *Exp Neurol* **110**, 194.

126. Virgili M, Vandi M, Contestabile A (1997) Ischemic and excitotoxic damage to brain slices from normal and microencephalic rats. *Neurosci Lett* **233**, 53.

127. Watanabe M, Kinuya M, Ohtakeno S *et al.* (1992) Effects of treatment with methylazoxymethanol on noradrenergic synapses in rat cerebral cortex. *Pharmacol Toxicol* **71**, 314.

128. Watanabe M, Shimizu K, Kodama Y *et al.* (1995) Potentiating effects of methamphetamine on the hyperactivity of microencephalic rats treated prenatally with methylazoxymethanol: Possible implication of hyperdopaminergia. *Brain Res* **670**, 173.

129. Whiting MG (1964) Food practices in ALS foci in Japan, the Marianas and New Guinea. *Fed Proc* **23**, 1343.

130. Whiting MG (1963) Toxicity of cycads. *Econ Bot* **17**, 271.

131. Whiting MG (1988) *Toxicity of Cycads: Implications for Neurodegenerative Diseases and Cancer. Transcripts of Four Cycad Conferences.* Third World Medical Research Fdn, New York.

132. Woo YT, Lai DY, Arcos JC, Argus MF (1988) *Chemical Induction of Cancer. Structural Basis and Biological Mechanisms, Vol IIIc. Natural, Metal, Fiber and Macromolecular Carcinogens (Sect 5.3.2.2, Cycasin and Related Compounds).* Academic Press, San Diego p. 178.

133. Wood KA, Youle RJ (1995) The role of free radicals and p53 in neuron apoptosis *in vivo. J Neurosci* **15**, 5851.

134. Wood PL, Emmett MR, Wood JA (1994) Involvement of

granule, basket and stellate neurons but not Purkinje or Golgi cells in cerebellar cGMP increases in vivo. *Life Sci* **54**, 615.

135. Yagi F, Tadera K (1987) Azoxyglucoside contents in seed of several cycad species and various parts of Japanese cycad. *Agric Biol Chem* **51**, 1719.

136. Yase Y (1972) The pathogenesis of amyotrophic lateral sclerosis. *Lancet* **ii**, 292.

137. Zeller WJ (1992) Neurotropic carcinogenesis. In: *Selective Neurotoxicity.* Herken H, Harkin F eds. Springer-Verlag, Berlin p. 192.

138. Zhang ZX, Anderson DW, Mantel N, Roman GC (1996) Motor neuron disease on Guam: Geographic incidence and familial occurrence, 1956–85. *Acta Neurol Scand* **94**, 51.

139. Zoli M, Pich EM, Cimino K *et al.* (1990) Morphometrical and microdensitometrical studies on peptide- and tyrosine hydrolase-like immunoreactivities in the forebrain of rats prenatally exposed to methylazoxymethanol acetate. *Brain Res* **51**, 45.

CASE REPORTS

Kii Peninsula, Japan. From the age of 1 through 12, a Japanese female (who resided in a region with an unusually high historical incidence of ALS) received baskets of immature seed of Cycas revoluta (sotetsu) *collected from the garden by her grandmother. The young girl used the seed to fashion necklaces, marbles, and whistles. The girl was plagued by diarrhea during the first 6 years of life and had received oral infusions of a steep prepared from crushed mature seed. She grew into a strong teenager and a good long-distance runner. She developed muscle weakness at age 20, received a diagnosis of ALS from a distinguished neurologist, and died at age 25. [As recently as 1990, certain pharmacists in Mie prefecture, Kii peninsula, Honshu Island, rarely filled prescriptions written by practitioners (ki-toshi) of Japanese folk medicine. A textbook of Chinese Medicine and Folk Medicine states that daily oral doses of an aqueous steepe of 3–10 g/day are said to be useful for the treatment of diarrhea, tuberculosis, dysmenorrhea, neuralgia, and "to strengthen the body."]*

Irian Jaya, Indonesia. In 1987, a 29-year-old indigenous male of the Auyu linguistic group (who resided in a remote riverine village with an unusually high historical incidence of ALS) with a neurological picture typical of ALS denied oral contact with cycad seed (kurru). However, he reported that on a single occasion at the age of 15, he used the poisonous milky pulp of mature Cycas *seed to prepare a poultice that was applied to a 5- to 10-cm open sore on the ankle for a period up to 1 month. Typical practice in the area was to apply the material on a leaf that was strapped* in place and replaced with fresh material daily. The man's mother, who had instructed him, was "similarly" paralyzed prior to death at age 50. He refused examination on the grounds that bodily contact might prove fatal to him.

New South Wales, Australia. A husband and wife (both aged 64), both of European descent, collected thousands of bright red seed (nuts) of Macrozamia communis from their garden during a period of massive seed production (summer 1985 or 1986). Over the ensuing weeks and months, the husband drilled each seed and removed the (poisonous) wet starch, while his wife scraped off the fleshy seed cover, washed the seed in detergent water, dried the seed in a tray and strung them to form colorful necklaces. Both sustained heavy dermal exposure; neither knew the seed contents were hazardous. Hands were not washed, and food might have been contaminated. At about the same time, they also tried to make starch (sago) from the trunks of some old cycad plants. They cut up the overground stem, soaked the pieces in water, and forcibly extracted the starch by application of the material against a sieve. In addition, trays of seed were heated (by wife) in the kitchen oven in an attempt to stimulate germination. Both experienced mild illness (nausea, headache) during this time of heavy cycad exposure.

Beginning approximately 1 year later, the woman developed difficulty rising and walking, muscle fasciculation, and slowly progressive weakness; her condition was diagnosed by a neurologist as motor neuron disease (ALS). Examination in 1990 revealed predominantly weakness greater on the left side, ability to walk, and no bulbar signs. Eye movements and retina (abnormal in Guam ALS/PDC) were unremarkable. She died approximately 7 years after heavy contact with the cycad seed. Six other people within this community of approximately 10,000 reportedly had developed motor neuron disease over a preceding 10-year period.

In late November or early December 1992, the man collected a sack of male cones that had recently opened to reveal pollen. Inside his study, he shook the cones to release the pollen, which was then transferred to sample bottles. No precautions were taken to prevent inhalation of pollen (which contain azoxyglucoside). In January, 1993, loss of appetite and weight, and "bad taste in the mouth" led a visit to a physician and to the diagnosis of lymphoma; he died less than 1 year later.

Cyclobenzaprine

Herbert H. Schaumburg

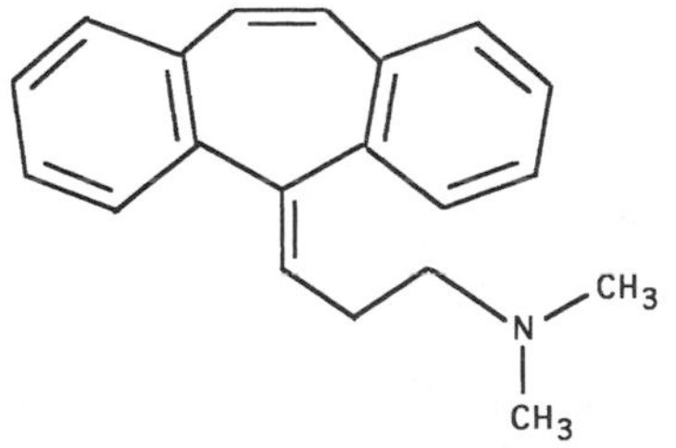

CYCLOBENZAPRINE
$C_{20}H_{21}N$

3-(5H-Dibenzo[a,d]cyclohepten-5-ylidene)-N,N-dimethyl-1-propanamine

NEUROTOXICITY RATING

Clinical

A Acute encephalopathy (sedation, mania)

Cyclobenzaprine is a centrally acting skeletal muscle relaxant that is structurally similar to the tricyclic antidepressants. Its use has been limited by nervous system side effects that frequently appear at therapeutic doses (1,2). Adverse effects of this drug constitute a mixture of muscarinic inhibition (dry mouth, somnolence) and adrenergic stimulation (tachycardia, mania). The neurotoxicity profile of cyclobenzaprine is identical to that of the tricyclic antidepressants (see Tricyclic Antidepressants, this volume).

REFERENCES

1. Azoury FJ (1979) Double-blind comparison of Parafon Forte and Flexeril in the treatment of acute musculoskeletal disorders. Curr Ther Res 26, 189.
2. Nibbelink DW, Strickland SC (1980) Cyclobenzaprine (Flexeril): Report of a post-marketing surveillance program. Curr Ther Res 28, 894.

Cycloleucine

Henry C. Powell

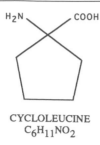

CYCLOLEUCINE
$C_6H_{11}NO_2$

1-Aminocyclopentanecarboxylic acid, ACPC; NSC-1026

NEUROTOXICITY RATING

Clinical

B   Leukoencephalopathy

B   Peripheral neuropathy

Experimental

A   Leukoencephalopathy (demyelination, intramyelinic edema)

A   Peripheral neuropathy

Originally developed as an anticancer drug, cycloleucine (CL) underwent clinical trials during which its neurotoxic properties came to light. It is now used as a biological testing material for immunosuppressive properties in mice, as an experimental agent in amino acid transport studies, and as a metabotropic agent in studies of amino acid excitotoxicity. It has found an important application in experimental neuropathology as an animal model for vitamin B_{12} deficiency. The following references are suggested for further reading (18,20,23).

CL is a synthetic amino acid thought to act as a valine antagonist. It is a white, odorless, crystalline powder at room temperature, and is soluble in water.

CL is an α-substituted nonmetabolizable amino acid that was first synthesized more than three decades ago in an effort to develop a new antineoplastic agent (19). Because of its structural differences from naturally occurring amino acids, it acts as an amino acid antagonist (2) and can inhibit protein synthesis (22). Its chemotherapeutic efficacy was limited, since it failed to control the growth of advanced solid tumors in human patients (19) despite the promise shown in the treatment of murine tumors. It was somewhat more effective in the treatment of hematological malignancies, including multiple myeloma and also leiomyosarcoma. Other uses of CL include treatment of malaria and immunosuppression (1,7,13).

At present, CL is used as an experimental drug only, although it has antineoplastic and antimalarial properties. Because of its neurotoxic effects, use of this agent is now largely confined to experimental studies of demyelination and amino acid antagonism. This latter property led to a surge of publications (20,23), notably in the fields of epilepsy and pain research. CL is a rigid glutamate analogue that activates phosphoinositide hydrolysis in brain slices at concentrations that do not affect ionotropic glutamate receptors (20). Its properties as an amino acid analogue have also led to many experiments on renal and intestinal transport. It is also used as an experimental immunosuppressant.

Because CL is poorly absorbed from the intestinal tract, the usual route of administration is by intraperitoneal (i.p.) injection (8,9). The dynamics of transmucosal absorption have been studied in equine cecal tissue (6) in which absorption from the lumen is weak, but transport from the serosal surface is much stronger, reflecting a mechanism for delivery of nutrients to cells in the crypts and other deeply placed mucosa.

The drug competes with certain naturally occurring amino acids for transport across the blood-brain barrier (BBB). Since BBB amino acid transport can be saturated, the reduced amino acid influx into the brain associated with cycloleucine toxicity is thought to contribute to impaired protein synthesis in this condition. It seems to function as an amino acid antagonist being itself an unnaturally constituted amino acid (2) that inhibits protein synthesis *in vivo* and *in vitro* (22). CL penetrates the nervous system by facilitated diffusion across the BBB and competes with certain other amino acids such as phenylalanine and valine. Because of these properties, it has even found use in experiments monitoring toxic damage to the BBB induced by mercury. With respect to impaired protein synthesis, other mechanisms are involved; specifically, CL interferes with the formation of adenosylmethionine, thus blocking a transmethylation reaction that converts homocysteine to methionine.

CL is a nonmetabolizable synthetic amino acid. Excretion is slow, the rate varying with the species (16).

The brain, spinal cord, and peripheral nerves appear to be the principal targets for CL toxicity. Multiple mechanisms of neurotoxicity are involved, including competition with other amino acids and inhibition of protein synthesis. CL shares a common transport system with DL-methionine and is an inhibitor of methionine adenosyltransferase (14). It can thus abrogate transmethylation by S-adenosylmethionine (SAM), resulting in severe depletion of an important component of myelin synthesis. Synthesis of myelin basic protein (MBP) is specifically inhibited through interference with its methylation. MBP is located at the intraperiod line of myelin lamellae and helps maintain the close apposition of these membranes that is necessary for compaction of the myelin sheath (4,19,23). Methylation of a single arginine residue at position 107, one of the posttranslational modifications essential for this process, is interfered with by CL. The sensitivity of nervous tissue to cycloleucine is due to interference with myelin synthesis, hence the greater vulnerability of developing brains to this neurotoxin (8).

When adult rats and mice are given a single dose of CL (1000–3000 mg/kg) by i.p. injection, the animals become weak, anorexic, and lose weight, dying within 5–7 days of treatment. Weanling mice receiving a single dose of 1000 mg/kg respond in the same way (9,12). Physical evidence of toxicity is present within 24 h of administration when the fur is ruffled and stiff. When mice are picked up by the tail, they fail to extend their limbs and spread their toes. If placed on a wire grid, they can hold the bars with their forepaws but not with their toes (12). Sensory functions remain undisturbed. Signs of paralysis extend to abdominal and respiratory muscles with apparent costal recession. When examined postmortem, 1 week after exposure, they have notably diminished muscle mass, loss of body fat, and empty gastrointestinal tracts.

Premortem injection of the supravital dye trypan blue stained extraneural organs but spared the brain parenchyma, thereby demonstrating the integrity of the BBB. Paraffin sections of brain tissue revealed status spongiosus of cerebral, cerebellar, and brainstem white matter, which was especially prominent in the optic tracts and forniccal columns (9). In brain tissue processed for electron microscopy, thin sections of white matter showed edema characterized by vacuolation of the myelin sheaths. Ultrastructural examination indicated that myelin vacuoles result from splitting of the myelin lamellae at the intraperiod line. There was no sign of extracellular edema, and the neuropil surrounding affected myelin sheaths did not itself appear edematous. Oligodendrocytes responded to cycloleucine treatment by increasing cytoplasmic volume and their Golgi apparatus. Within astrocytes, there was an increase in glycogen granules, a typical though nonspecific glial response to injury. Neurons and their processes appeared intact. Endothelial cells were uninjured (9).

Similar changes were detected in the spinal cord and the PNS (5,12) in plastic sections of tissue prepared for electron microscopy. The first PNS abnormalities to be detected involved motor end plates in which patches of electronlucent cytoplasm appeared. This was followed by involvement of other organelles and interposition of Schwann cell processes into the space between terminating axons and the underlying muscle. These changes were evident within 24 h, but more extensive axonal damage could be detected after 48 h. Collapse of axons and the appearance of myelin ovoids indicated the severity of these changes. It was noted that while motor nerve endings were severely affected, sensory nerves were spared (12). This selective toxic effect was most clearly appreciated in muscle where motor nerves innervating extrafusal fibers responded differently from those innervating muscle spindles. As in the CNS, valine administration after CL exposure greatly mitigated its toxic effects (11). In contrast to the CL-only treated experimental animals, regeneration of nerves was accelerated in valine-treated mice and innervation of injured end plates occurred. Other organs appeared unremarkable except for the liver in which occasional hepatocytes exhibited cytoplasmic vacuolation.

Similar abnormalities of the myelin sheath were detected in the brains of chickens (21). Concurrent biochemical studies determined that CL, an inhibitor of S-adenosyl methionine, decreased the incorporation of methyl groups into methyl arginine in MBP in vitro. The need for methylcobalamin for the conversion of homocysteine to methionine, and the requirement that myelin basic protein be methylated, help explain the mechanism of demyelination in affected experimental animals. It was noted that, while the overall brain weight in experimental chickens was not diminished, MBP concentration was halved relative to controls (21). The hydrophobic properties of MBP contribute to its critical role as a structural cement that binds myelin lamellae. Methylation of MBP is crucial with respect to its ability to augment hydrophobicity and enhance this binding property.

Administration of sublethal doses induced weakness, and wasting in adult mice receiving single i.p. doses of 250–900 mg/kg appeared to depend on the dose (8). Surviving animals recovered completely. The impression of dose dependence was supported by microscopic findings of barely detectable to mild status spongiosus in mice exposed to lower doses (250–500 mg/kg) vs. mild to moderate spongiosus in animals treated with 900 mg/kg. These histological abnormalities were present 4 weeks after CL administration (9).

Some additional changes were encountered in mice and rats that received repeated sublethal doses over a several-week period. Weekly doses of 100 mg/kg resulted in anorexia, weakness, and loss of weight. The severity of these symptoms appeared to be dose-related, since those animals that received a smaller dose lost less weight initially and showed only a small decrease in activity during the first 2 weeks, recovering after that time and resuming normal appearance and activity. Larger doses, on the other hand, eventually killed the animals. Neuropathological evaluation at the light microscopic level showed no difference from findings in acutely intoxicated animals. At the ultrastructural level, however, there were differences attributable to prolonged intoxication. While the myelinopathic abnormalities were indistinguishable from those seen with short-term intoxication, other changes of glia indicated toxic effects of a more widespread nature. Intracytoplasmic inclusions of two types were found in reactive astrocytes. Most of these were non–membrane–bound whorls of filaments measuring 9 nm in diameter. A smaller number of membrane-bound inclusions was found within cisternae of endoplasmic reticulum in astrocytic cytoplasm (9). These inclusions had a granular matrix; their appearance within the endoplasmic reticulum may reflect inhibition of protein synthesis, a well-established property of CL.

One report describes the neurotoxicity of CL for cultured cerebellar neurons (15), and also notes that these effects are antagonized by valine (15). More recently, astrocyte swelling has been induced in vitro by CL administration (10).

Cycloleucine was synthesized in the early 1960s as an anticancer agent (19) but showed disappointing results when used in patients with solid tumors that were far advanced. It was somewhat more effective against multiple myeloma and leiomyosarcoma and found further therapeutic application as an antimalarial drug (1). Clinical use of CL came to an end when the drug was found to have neurological side effects. Its neurotoxic properties came to light when symptoms of spinal cord degeneration and peripheral neuropathy were detected in patients who received doses of 220 mg/kg/day. Neurological complications also occurred in 41% of a series of 140 patients that were given 300 mg/kg daily for 8–10 days (3). Similar abnormalities were detected in mice exposed to the drug and were shown to be the consequence of CNS demyelination. Unfortunately, there is no neuropathological information on any of these patients.

CL gains access to the nervous system without disturbing the BBB (9). This synthetic amino acid competes with naturally occurring amino acids for transport across the BBB (17), and it has been suggested that saturation of amino acid transport mechanisms by this neurotoxin contributes to the reduction in protein synthesis that is associated with CL neurotoxicity. Increasing the dietary intake of valine for Cl-intoxicated rats mitigated the neuropathological effects of CL administration (11).

Both biochemical and pathological studies have helped to elucidate the mechanisms involved in CL neurotoxicity. The parenchymal effects of CL toxicity involve blockage of transmethylation reactions. By competitively inhibiting methionine adenosyltransferase, it reduces production of SAM. The latter is a substrate in the production of methylated MBP, an important component of compact myelin. Methylation increases the hydrophobicity of arginine, in turn increasing the hydrophobicity of MBP. This increases its capacity to act as a cementing agent, binding myelin lamellae more closely together. The posttranslational modification of MBP appears to be critical for membrane compaction, since interference with this mechanism by cycloleucine results in splitting of myelin lamellae giving the familiar fluid-filled appearance of spongiform myelinopathy (9,12). MBP can cross-link lipid vesicles, thus facilitating the approximation of adjacent myelin lamellae. The greater vulnerability of weanling mice and rats may reflect the impact of reducing methylation at a time of increased myelin formation.

The mechanism for peripheral nerve injury is not known, although inhibition of protein synthesis may be involved. MBP is less important in the PNS, in which it is a minor component; hence the absence of vacuolation from peripheral myelin (12). In common with other agents that cause intramyelinic vacuolation in the CNS, cuprizone, isoniazid, and triethyltin, CL leads to distal axonopathy without myelin vacuolation. Intramyelinic edema does occur in the PNS in hexachlorophene intoxication and is followed, after hexachlorophene withdrawal, by distal axonopathy. Since the distal neuropathic abnormalities are manifest in motor nerves, it is also conceivable that compression of central axons by intramyelinic edema may impair axonal transport of proteins and contribute to these rather nonspecific injuries. A more specific explanation for the injuries occurring in CL-treated mice has been put forward: It is suggested that abnormalities in phopholipid composition of the axolemma in motor nerve terminals might cause an increase in microviscosity of the axolemma and thus contribute to decreased efficiency of ion channels and pumps controlling electrochemical gradients essential for maintaining structural and functional integrity of the neuromuscular junction (5).

REFERENCES

1. Aviado DM, Reuter HA (1969) Pathologic physiology and chemotherapy of Plasmodium berghei, IX. Gastric secretion and interference of 1-amino cyclopentane carboxylic acid (WR14997 or Cycloleucine). Exp Parasitol 24, 314.
2. Berlinguet L, Begin N, Sarkar NK (1962) Mechanism of antitumor action of 1-amino cyclopentane carboxylic acid. Nature 194, 1082.
3. Carter SK (1970) 1-Aminocyclopentane carboxylic acid (NSC-1026) a review. Chemother Fact Sheet, NCI July, 1.
4. Crang AJ, Jacobson W (1980) The methylation in vitro of myelin basic protein by arginine methylase from mouse spinal cord. Biochem Soc Trans 8, 619.

5. Edwards JP, Lee C-C, Duchen LW (1994) The evolution of an experimental distal motor axonopathy. Physiological studies of changes in neuromuscular transmission caused by cycloleucine, an inhibitor of methionine adenosyltransferase. *Brain* **117**, 959.

6. Freeman DE, Donawick WJ (1991) *In vitro* transport of cycloleucine by equine cecal mucosa. *Amer J Vet Res* **52**, 540.

7. Frisch AW (1969) Inhibition of antibody synthesis by cycloleucine. *Biochem Pharmacol* **18**, 256.

8. Gandy G, Jacobson W, Sidman RL (1973) Inhibition of a transmethylation reaction in the CNS—an experimental model for subacute combined degeneration of the cord. *J Physiol-London* **233**, 1P-3P.

9. Greco CM, Powell HC, Garrett RS, Lampert PW (1980) Cycloleucine encephalopathy. *Neuropathol Appl Neurobiol* **6**, 349.

10. Hansson E (1994) Metabotropic glutamate receptor activation induces astroglial swelling. *J Biol Chem* **269**, 21955.

11. Lee C-C, Duchen L (1994) Reversal by valine of intramyelinic vacuolation and motor axonopathy produced by cycloleucine. *Brain Pathol* **4**, 572.

12. Lee C-C, Surtees R, Duchen LW (1992) Distal motor axonopathy and central nervous system myelin vacuolation by cycloleucine, an inhibitor of methionine adenosyltransferase. *Brain* **115**, 935.

13. Levine S, Sowinski R (1977) Effects of cycloleucine on macrophages and EAE. *Exp Mol Pathol* **26**, 103.

14. Lombardini JB, Coulter AW, Talalay P (1970) Analogues of methionine as substrate inhibitors of the methionine adenoxytransferase reaction. *Mol Pharmacol* **6**, 481.

15. Nixon RA, Suva M, Wolf MK (1976) Neurotoxicity of non-metabolizable amino acid 1-ACPC, antagonism by amino acids in cultures of the cerebellum. *J Neurochem* **27**, 245.

16. Owen G, Ruelis HW, Janssen F, Pollock JJ (1969) Species differences in the disposition of cycloleucine. *Toxicol Appl Pharmacol* **14**, 630.

17. Pardridge WM, Oldendorf WH (1975) Kinetic analysis of blood brain barrier transport of amino acids. *Biochim Biophys Acta* **401**, 128.

18. Powell HC (1989) Cycloleucine encephalopathy in rats and mice. In: *Monographs on Pathology of Laboratory Animals, Nervous System*. Jones TC, Mohr U, Hunt RD eds. Springer-Verlag, Berlin p. 77.

19. Ross RB, Noll CI, Ross WCJ *et al.* (1961) Cycloaliphatic amino acids in cancer therapy. *J Med Pharm Chem* **3**, 1.

20. Schoepp DD (1993) The biochemical pharmacology of metabotropic glutamate receptors. *Biochem Soc Trans* **21**, 97.

21. Small DH, Carnegie PR, Anderson R McD (1981) Cycloleucine-induced vacuolation of myelin is associated with inhibition of protein methylation. *Neurosci Lett* **21**, 287.

22. Sterling WR, Henderson JR (1963) Studies of the mechanism of action of 1-aminocyclopentane carboxylic acid. *Biochem Pharmacol* **12**, 303.

23. Verity MA (1993) Environmental neurotoxicity of chemicals and radiation. *Curr Opin Neurol Neurosurg* **6**, 437.

Cyclopentolate

Herbert H. Schaumburg

CYCLOPENTOLATE
$C_{17}H_{25}NO_3$

α-(1-Hydroxycyclopentyl)benzeneacetic acid 2-(dimethylamino)ethyl ether

NEUROTOXICITY RATING

Clinical

A   Acute encephalopathy (CNS muscarinic inhibition syndrome)

Cyclopentolate hydrochloride is a potent antimuscarinic drug widely used as a topical mydriatic. It shares a dimethylated side chain with certain hallucinogens (bodenine, bufotine) that might explain the drug's abuse. Following local application to the eye, cyclopentolate travels along the nasolacrimal duct and is rapidly absorbed from the nasal mucosa. The neurotoxic manifestations of cyclopentolate are those associated with overdose of atropine or other competitive inhibitors of cholinergic muscarinic receptors. Neurotoxicity is the rare, primary adverse effect of a single dose of cyclopentolate; little systemic dysfunction is associated with routine clinical use. Most instances are transient, develop within 1 h of application, and have been associated with use of a 2% solution (1,4). Ataxia, dysarthria, somnolence, generalized seizures, disorientation, auditory and visual hallucinations, and amnesia are all described.

Generalized urticaria has also been described after a single application of 1% cyclopentolate (2).

Abuse of cyclopentolate is described in two persons who instilled up to 200 ocular drops daily for 4 months to induce hallucinogenic effects; prominent findings were photophobia, punctate keratitis, and dilated pupils that were unresponsive to light (3). Withdrawal was followed by a period of nausea, vomiting, and intense tremors.

REFERENCES

1. Fitzgerald DA, Hanson RM, West C et al. (1990) Seizures associated with 1% cyclopentolate eyedrops. J Pediat Child Health 26, 106.
2. Novack GD (1997) Ocular toxicology. Curr Opin Ophthalmol 8, 88.
3. Sata EH, DeFreita D, Foster SC (1992) Abuse of cyclopentolate hydrochloride (cyclogyl) drops. N Engl J Med 326, 1363.
4. Shihab ZM (1980) Psychotic reaction in an adult after topical cyclopentolate. Ophthalmologica 181, 228.

Cycloserine

Herbert H. Schaumburg
Peter S. Spencer

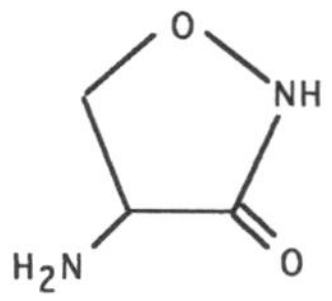

CYCLOSERINE
$C_3H_6N_2O_2$

D-4-Amino-3-isoxazolidinone

NEUROTOXICITY RATING

Clinical

A   Acute encephalopathy (confusion, anxiety, hallucinations)

A   Seizure disorder

D-Cycloserine, a structural analog of alanine, is a broad-spectrum antibiotic used in the treatment of tuberculosis. Its antibiotic action stems from competitive inhibition of the uptake of alanine into bacteria, disrupting cell wall synthesis. Orally administered, cycloserine is readily absorbed and reaches a peak plasma level within 2 h. The drug rapidly equilibrates throughout the body; plasma and cerebrospinal fluid concentrations are similar in individuals receiving daily dosage. Severe neurotoxicity has limited the use of cycloserine to individuals with drug-resistant tuberculosis; there are few systemic adverse effects of chronic therapy. Antituberculous treatment of female adults with cycloserine is considered compatible with infant breastfeeding (5).

Ten percent of individuals receiving a therapeutic daily dose of 1 g experience an acute encephalopathy. Generalized seizures and transient confusion are the most common adverse reactions, and the drug is contraindicated in patients with epilepsy or high alcohol consumption (1,2).

Paradoxically, recent experimental studies indicate that cycloserine has anticonvulsant and cognitive-enhancing properties; both are suggested to stem from its ability to act as a partial agonist of the strychnine-insensitive glycine site of the N-methyl-D-aspartate receptor complex (3,4). Other manifestations of cycloserine-induced neurotoxicity include tremor, anxiety, and visual hallucinations.

Partial Gly-B agonists have been studied as potential therapeutic agents for Alzheimer's disease. Administration of D-cycloserine (6 mg/kg, for 10 days) to rats had no effect on a spatial-working-memory deficit induced by entorhinal cortex lesions. The same dosage did reverse scopolamine-induced amnesia in a passive avoidance test; this was attributed to a cholinergic-glutamatergic interaction in the hippocampus (6).

REFERENCES

1. Addington WW (1979) The side effects and interactions of antituberculosis drugs. Chest 76S, 782S.
2. Moulding T, Davidson PT (1974) Tuberculosis II: Toxicity and intolerance to antituberculosis drugs. Drug Ther 4, 39.
3. Peterson SL, Schwade ND (1993) The anticonvulsant activity of D-cycloserine is specific for tonic convulsions. Epilepsy Res 15, 141.
4. Thompson LT, Moskal JR, Disterhoft JF (1992) Hippocampus-dependent learning facilitated by a monoclonal antibody or D-cycloserine. Nature 359, 638.
5. Tran JH, Montakantikul P (1998) The safety of antituberculosis medications during breastfeeding. J Hum Lact 14, 337.
6. Zajaczkowski W, Danysz W (1997) Effects of D-cycloserine and aniracetam on spatial learning in rats with entorhinal cortex lesions. Pharmacol Biochem Behav 56, 21.

Cyclosporine

Matthias Riepe
Herbert H. Schaumburg

CYCLOSPORIN A
$C_{62}H_{111}N_{11}O_{12}$

NEUROTOXICITY RATING

Clinical

A   Leukoencephalopathy (posterior)
C   Peripheral neuropathy

Cyclosporine is an immunosuppressive drug widely used in transplantation medicine and treatment of autoimmune diseases (7,10,15); it is derived from the fungus *Tolypocladium inflatum* Gams. The mechanism of immunosuppression is selective inhibition of adaptive immune responses of T cells and B cells (16). Serious systemic side effects, including nephrotoxicity, and dermal, hematological, and gastrointestinal dysfunction, are associated with prolonged administration (10,11,15,17,23). In addition, clinical and experimental data show a carcinogenic, nongenotoxic effect of cyclosporine (1,2,11,13,20–22). The principal neurotoxicity is acute, diffuse leukoencephalopathy (6,14).

Cyclosporine is a neutral, lipophilic, cyclic endecapeptide; the amino acids, in positions 11, 1, 2, and 3, form the hydrophilic active immunosuppression site (15). The relative bioequivalence of oral and intravenous doses is 1:3 (15). Cyclosporine is extensively metabolized in the liver by the cytochrome P-450 system and has a median half-life of 6.4–8.7 h (8,15). Less than 10% of cyclosporine is bound to either erythrocytes or lipoproteins. A cytosolic-binding protein, cyclophilin, influences the distribution of cyclosporine in the body. Despite its lipophilicity, cyclosporine does not cross the blood-brain barrier in healthy laboratory animals. The distribution of metabolites, which are less immunosuppressive than the parent drug, differs from that of cyclosporine. Elimination of metabolites (7,8) is mainly in the bile. Side effects correlate with blood levels of cyclosporine, not with the drug's cumulative dosage (3).

Cyclosporine has no genotoxic activity or DNA-binding property. In experimental studies, it does not cause cancer in the absence of an initiating event (*e.g.*, chemical mutagen) (14). However, by its immunosuppressive property, the drug may favor growth of initiated tumor cells or metas-

tases (22,23,28). Reversible hypertrichosis has occurred in nude mice along with dose-dependent weight loss and decreased survival (12,26).

Embryonic cultures exposed to microgram concentrations of cyclosporine developed a significant increase in the incidence of malformations, including defects in the neural tube, head folds, and facial arches. The mechanism of this *in vitro* embryopathy includes inhibition of the arachidonic acid pathway (24).

Signs and symptoms of CNS white-matter toxicity (leukoencephalopathy) from cyclosporine are clearly documented in patients at varying intervals following liver transplantation; these include headaches, confusion, disorientation, psychosis, anxiety, blurred vision, incontinence, cortical blindness, spasticity, quadriplegia, and seizures (5,6,9,14,17–20).

Seizures, focal or generalized, usually herald the illness and are usually soon followed by signs of visual dysfunction (hemianopsia, cortical blindness), hemiparesis, memory impairment and altered consciousness. Magnetic resonance (MR) and computed tomography imaging disclose edema of the white matter, often most prominent in the posterior cerebral hemispheres, with sparing of the calcarine and paramedian occipital lobe structures. Most patients recover with complete resolution of the MR-visualized abnormalities within weeks of discontinuing the drug. The imaging studies and the clinical syndrome featuring prominent cortical blindness indicate that cyclosporine neurotoxicity frequently exemplifies the reversible posterior leukoencephalopathy syndrome (14). This nebulous clinical entity has also been associated with transplant immunosuppression from other agents (tacrolimus-FK506), acute hypertensive encephalopathy, and eclampsia.

There are no postmortem studies on humans and no experimental animal model of cyclosporine leukoencephalopathy.

The mechanism of cyclosporine neurotoxicity is unclear. Drug levels are usually within the therapeutic range, and other suggested factors (hypercholesteremia, solvent vehicle toxicity, hypomagnesemia, aluminum intoxication) are absent in many isolated case reports (27).

It is suggested that its pathophysiology is analogous to eclampsia and acute hypertensive encephalopathy. These two conditions are attributed to an initial failure of autoregulation; regions of focal vasodilatation and constriction then appear in CNS white-matter vasculature causing a breakdown of blood-brain barrier with focal perivascular transudates of fluid and petechial hemorrhages. There is no explanation for the posterior distribution of brain involvement.

Although cyclosporine has not been shown to be directly neurotoxic to CNS tissue, it can cause vasculopathy and has toxic effects on endothelial cells that could disrupt the blood-brain barrier (4,16,25). The presence of cyclosporine and metabolites in the cerebrospinal fluid of liver transplant recipients with leukoencephalopathy support this notion (9). It is also proposed that toxicity occurs only in patients whose blood-brain barrier is already disrupted. Finally, many of the patients with leukoencephalopathy also are hypertensive and experience nephrotoxicity before CNS dysfunction; it is possible that these may be additive factors in the development of this condition. Two case reports suggest peripheral nerve dysfunction may accompany leukoencephalopathy (6,19).

REFERENCES

1. Arellano F, Krupp P (1993) Malignancies in rheumatoid arthritis patients treated with cyclosporin A. *Brit J Rheumatol* 1, 72.
2. Armitage JM, Kormos RL, Stuart RS *et al.* (1991) Post-transplant lymphoproliferative disease in thoracic organ transplant patients: Ten years of cyclosporine-based immunosuppression. *J Heart Lung Transplant* 10, 877.
3. Azoulay D, Lemoine A, Dennison A *et al.* (1993) Incidence of adverse reactions to cyclosporine after liver transplantation is predicted by the first blood level. *Hepatology* 17, 1123.
4. Benigni A, Morigi M, Perico N *et al.* (1992) The acute effect of FKC 506 and cyclosporine on endothelial cell function and renal vascular resistance. *Transplantation* 54, 775.
5. Belli LS, De CL, Romani F, Rondinara GF *et al.* (1993) Dysarthria and cerebellar ataxia: Late occurrence of severe neurotoxicity in a liver transplant recipient. *Transplant Int* 6, 176.
6. De Groen PC, Aksamit AJ, Rakela J *et al.* (1987) Central nervous system toxicity after liver transplantation. *N Engl J Med* 317, 861.
7. Doria A, Di LL, Vario S, Calligaro A (1992) Cyclosporin A in a pregnant patient affected with systemic lupus erythematosus. *Rheumatol Int* 12, 77.
8. Fahr A (1993) Cyclosporin clinical pharmacokinetics. *Clin Pharmacokinet* 24, 472.
9. Gottrand F, Largilliere C, Farriany JP *et al.* (1991) Cyclosporine neurotoxicity. *N Engl J Med* 324, 1744.
10. Grieve EM, Hawksworth GM, Simpson JG, Whiting PH (1993) The reversal of experimental cyclosporin A nephrotoxicity by thromboxane synthetase inhibition. *Biochem Pharmacol* 45, 1351.
11. Guerci AP, Burtin P, Mattei S, Lederlin P (1992) Lympho-proliferative syndromes after cardiac transplantation and treatment with cyclosporine. Report of 4 cases. *Ann Med Intern* 143, 155.
12. Henke W, Nickel E, Jung K (1992) Cyclosporine A inhibits ATP net uptake of rat kidney mitochondria. *Biochem Pharmacol* 43, 1021.
13. Hewit CW, Black KS, Gratwohl A *et al.* (1990) Lethal cyclosporine associated toxicity in the rabbit: Similar findings in two distant and independent transplant laboratories. *J Clin Lab Immunol* 31, 23.
14. Hinchey J, Chaves C, Appignani B *et al.* (1996) A reversible posterior leukoencephalopathy syndrome. *N Engl J Med* 334, 494.
15. Jiang T, Acosta D (1993) An in vitro model of cyclosporine-induced nephrotoxicity. *Fund Appl Toxicol* 20, 486.
16. Mehring N, Neumann KH, Rahn KH, Zidek W (1992) Mechanisms of cyclosporin A-induced vasoconstriction in the isolated perfused rat kidney. *Nephron* 60, 477.
17. Min DI, Monaco AP (1991) Complications associated with immunosuppressive therapy and their management. *Pharmacotherapy* 11, 119S.
18. Monteiro L, Almeida PJ, Rocha N *et al.* (1993) Case report: Cyclosporin A-induced neurotoxicity. *Brit J Radiol* 66, 271.
19. Porschke H, Strenge H, Stauch C (1991) Polyneuropathy and central nervous system diseases before and after heart transplantation. Is cyclosporin neurotoxic? *Deutsche Med Wochenschr* 116, 1577.
20. Reece DE, Frei LD, Sheherd JD *et al.* (1991) Neurologic complications in allogeneic bone marrow transplant patients receiving cyclosporin. *Bone Marrow Transplant* 8, 393.
21. Rosenkranz HS, Klopman G (1992) A structural analysis of the genotoxic and carcinogenic potentials of cyclosporin A. *Mutagenesis* 7, 115.
22. Ryffel B (1992) The carcinogenicity of ciclosporin. *Toxicology* 73, 1.
23. Tibell A, Larsson M, Alvestrand A (1993) Dissolving intravenous cyclosporin A in a fat emulsion carrier prevents acute renal side effects in the rat. *Transplant Int* 6, 69.
24. Uhing MR, Goldman AS, Goto MP (1993) Cyclosporin A-induced embryopathy in embryo culture is mediated through inhibition of the arachidonic acid pathway. *Proc Soc Exp Biol Med* 202, 307.
25. Verbeke M, Van de Voorde D, de Ridder L *et al.* (1994) Functional analysis of vascular dysfunction in cyclosporin treated rats. *Cardiovasc Res* 28, 1152.
26. Watanabe S, Mochizuki A, Wagatsuma K *et al.* (1991) Hair growth on nude mice due to cyclosporin A. *J Dermatol* 18, 714.
27. Windebank AJ, Blexrud MD, DeGroen PC (1994) Potential neurotoxicity of the solvent vehicle for cyclosporine. *J Pharmacol Exp Ther* 268, 1051.
28. Yamada T, Mogi M, Kage T *et al.* (1992) Enhancement by cyclosporin A of metastasis from hamster cheek pouch carcinoma. *Arch Oral Biol* 37, 593.

CASE REPORT

A 36-year-old woman with end-stage, chronic glomerulopathy underwent kidney transplantation in December 1987. The immunosuppressive regimen included prednisolone, antilymphocyte globulin, and azathioprine. Signs of kidney rejection developed in October 1988 and April 1990; on both occasions, bolus doses of corticosteroids and cyclosporine (2 mg/kg/day) were used to treat the condition. In June 1992, she had two right-sided focal seizures followed by generalized seizures. Neurological examination showed drowsiness and confusion. T_2-Weighted MRI showed severe diffuse hyperintensity of the hemispheric white matter. The electroencephalogram showed moderate generalized dysrhythmia. The cerebrospinal fluid contained 2 red cells/ml and 56 mg of protein per deciliter. Biochemical testing showed a blood urea nitrogen level of 67 mg/dl (23 mmol/l) and a serum creatinine level of 5.3 mg/dl (470 μmol/l). The serum cholesterol and magnesium concentrations were normal, and the cyclosporine level was maintained within therapeutic ranges. After cyclosporine was withdrawn, the patient made a full, gradual recovery within 2 weeks. Cyclosporine was not reintroduced. A follow-up MRI 1 month later showed almost complete resolution of the brain lesions.

[Reprinted with permission from Hinchey et al. (14)]

Comment

This patient had a cyclosporine-induced syndrome without the usual predilection for the posterior hemisphere white matter. The onset, heralded by seizures, the MRI profile, and recovery are typical of this syndrome.

Cyclotrimethylenetrinitramine

Steven A. Sparr

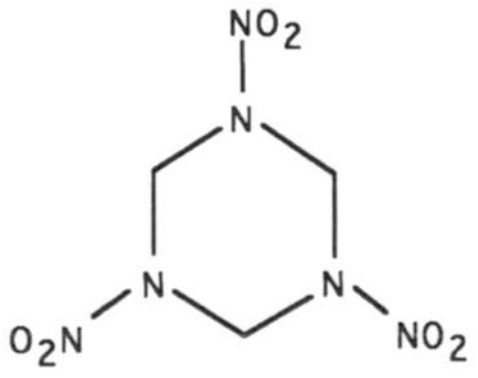

CYCLOTRIMETHYLENETRINITRAMINE
$C_3H_6N_6O_6$

RDX; Cyclonite; T_4; Hexogen; Hexahydro-1,3,5-trinitro-1,3,5-triazine

NEUROTOXICITY RATING

Clinical

A   Seizure disorder

A   Acute encephalopathy (confusion, anxiety, insomnia)

Cyclotrimethylenetrinitramine, also known as RDX, T_4, and cyclonite, is a high explosive in use since World War II as the major component of the plastic explosive C-4. It has demonstrated major neurotoxicity in humans, chiefly due to its powerful convulsant effects, in exposures of workers in munitions plants (1,9,10) and in military personnel (4,5,6,7,8). Animals develop similar neurotoxicity (2,3).

RDX, a white, crystalline powder at room temperature, is insoluble in water and ethyl alcohol, but soluble in acetone (6). When combined with polyisobutylene, motor oil, and an inert plasticizer, it has a putty-like consistency and is known as "C-4," a plastic explosive (7). C-4 is a malleable solid that is resistant to impact or friction (8); it burns readily but does not explode unless detonated with a blasting cap (7). It was used by American soldiers during the Vietnam War; many toxic ingestions were reported in soldiers who used C-4 to cook their food in the field, sometimes cutting the plastic explosive with the same knife they used to eat (7). During that period, it was also abused by ingestion to produce an intoxication similar to that of ethanol (4,5,7,8).

RDX may be absorbed into the body by inhalation of particulate matter, percutaneously, or by oral ingestion (5,6). Excretion of orally administered RDX is through the feces, with only 1%–2% eliminated in the urine (6). Measurable levels of RDX have been demonstrated in the feces and serum for up to 144 h following ingestion, suggesting a slow excretion of RDX into the gut (5). There is some metabolism of RDX in the liver; this may be enhanced by coadministration of phenobarbital, which induces hepatic microsomal enzymes (2). Plasma half-life is approximately 48 h with high-dose administration ($\geq$50 mg/kg) but may be shorter with lower doses (2).

The mechanism of RDX neurotoxicity is unknown. The hypothesis that, like other organic nitrate intoxications, RDX can induce methemoglobinemia with secondary cerebral anoxia, has not been corroborated by experience (7). It is generally considered that RDX itself, and not a metabolite, is the principal neurotoxic agent, as intravenous administration can provoke seizures in laboratory animals within seconds (2,6). Animals (mice, rats, cats, dogs) administered RDX by oral or intravenous routes develop behavioral changes that include irritability and viscousness, followed by seizures that are often fatal (2,3,6,7,9). The LD_{50} in rats is 200 mg/kg with acute ingestion, and 50 mg/kg/day with chronic ingestion (6). The LD_{50} is lower in cats (6).

A study of the effects of RDX on the development of spontaneous and audiogenic seizures in a rat model found that dosages as low as 12.5 mg/kg orally were associated with spontaneous seizures, usually occurring within 2 h of administration of RDX (2). At higher dosage, 60 mg/kg, seizures could be provoked by loud sounds (audiogenic seizures), but not until at least 4 h after ingestion, and peaking at 8 h after ingestion. Rats treated with 6 mg/kg RDX required fewer stimulations to achieve kindling in the amygdala.

The nervous system of animals treated with lethal doses of RDX is often morphologically intact. Nonspecific changes of uncertain significance include neuronal loss in cortex and spinal cord, and brainstem tract degeneration (6).

Reports of RDX neurotoxicity in humans in the late 1940s and early 1950s involved munitions workers with cutaneous exposure or by inhalation of dust particles (1,9). Subsequent reports from the Vietnam War involved intoxications of military personnel due to deliberate ingestion of C-4 or exposure to fumes when using C-4 for heating food (4–7). Accidental exposures have been reported through use of cooking bowls previously used to mix RDX, and in a child of a munitions worker who ingested bits of plastic explosive brought home on her clothing (4,10).

Nonneurological toxicity is primarily gastrointestinal, with nausea, vomiting, and abdominal pain; and renal, with hematuria, and rarely, oliguria and renal failure (5–7).

Neurological toxicity of acute intoxications is stereotypical (1,4–10). Following exposure by 8–12 h, patients develop confusion, irritability, and myoclonic jerks. These signs are followed by generalized convulsions, usually multiple. With more chronic exposures, in munitions plant workers, prodromal signs of anxiety, irritability, and insomnia may precede convulsions by hours (6) or several days (1). Patients may continue to have seizures for several hours and then have prolonged postictal periods. Recovery is usually complete. Routine laboratory tests, including serum electrolyes and complete blood counts, are normal in patients presenting with seizures. Cerebrospinal fluid is also within normal limits (7). Skeletal muscle biopsy is normal (8).

A study of 18 military personnel with acute RDX intoxication found that 82% had multiple seizures and 15% had status epilepticus (7). Seizures continued intermittently for up to 5 days, despite administration of diphenylhydantoin or phenobarbital. Postictal confusion and memory impairment, seen in most patients, typically lasted for a week, but lasted several weeks in some.

Electroencephalogram (EEG) performed prior to the onset of convulsions typically shows two to three per second spike-and-wave discharges or multiple spikes, usually maximal bifrontally (7). Postical EEG may be normal (5) but often shows generalized slowing, and it may take up to 3 months for EEG abnormalities to resolve (7).

Acute management of RDX intoxication includes airway control, treatment of seizures with anticonvulsants, and maintenance of urine output; RDX is not significantly removed by dialysis (5).

REFERENCES

1. Barsotti M, Crotti G (1949) Epileptic attacks as manifestations of industrial intoxication caused by trimethylenetrinitroamine (T4). *Med Lav* **40**, 107.
2. Burdette LJ, Cook LL, Dyer RS (1988) Convulsant properties of cyclotrimethylenetrinitramine (RDX): Spontaneous, audiogenic, and amygdaloid kindled seizure activity. *Toxicol Appl Pharmacol* **92**, 436.
3. Dilley DV, Tyson CA, Spaggord RJ (1982) Short-term oral toxicity of a 2,4,6-trinitrotoluene and hexahydro-1,3,5-trinitro-1,3,5-triazine mixture in mice, rats and dogs. *J Toxicol Environ Health* **9**, 587.
4. Goldberg DJ, Green ST, Nathwani D *et al.* (1992) RDX intoxication causing seizures and a widespread petechial rash mimicking meningococcaemia. *J Roy Soc Med* **85**, 181.
5. Harrell-Bruder B, Hutchins KL (1995) Seizures caused by ingestion of composition C-4. *Ann Emerg Med* **26**, 746.
6. Kaplan AS, Berghout CF, Peczenik A (1965) Human intoxication from RDX. *Arch Environ Health* **10**, 877.
7. Ketel WB, Hughes JR (1972) Toxic encephalopathy with seizures secondary to ingestion of composition C-4, a clinical and electroencephalographic study. *Neurology* **22**, 871.
8. Stone WJ, Paletta TL, Heiman EM *et al.* (1969) Toxic effects following ingestion of C-4 plastic explosive. *Arch Intern Med* **124**, 726.
9. Vogel W (1951) Hexogen poisoning in human beings. *Zbl Arbeitsmed* **1**, 51.
10. Woody RC, Kearns GL, Brewster MA *et al.* (1986) The neurotoxicity of cyclotrimethylenetrinitramine (RDX) in a child: A clinical and pharmacokinetics evaluation. *J Toxicol Clin Toxicol* **24**, 305.

L-Cysteine

John W. Olney

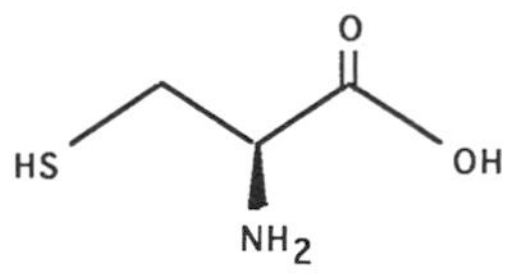

L-CYSTEINE
C₃H₇NO₂S

α-Amino-β-thiolpropionic acid

NEUROTOXICITY RATING

Experimental

A Excitant amino acid

L-Cysteine (Cys) is a common sulfur-containing amino acid which, like glutamate, is found ubiquitously in nature, is a normal constituent of foods, and is present in the human body and CNS. Cys administered orally or subcutaneously can damage many regions of the fetal or infant forebrain in pregnant rodents or their neonatal offspring (6). Cys neurotoxicity has been shown to be a form of excitotoxicity mediated by N-methyl-D-apartate (NMDA) receptors (and prevented by NMDA receptor antagonists) (2,8). Cys neurotoxicity is augmented by bicarbonate (*i.e.*, in the presence of physiological concentrations of bicarbonate, Cys is transformed from a relatively weak to a more potent excitotoxin). This may stem from the ability of bicarbonate to facilitate the conversion of Cys to an α-amino carbamate molecule that stereochemically resembles the potent excitotoxin, NMDA (5). Cys appears to be a unique excitotoxin that can penetrate both placental and blood-brain barriers and, after entering the brain, may undergo conversion to a molecule that potently interacts with NMDA receptors to destroy neurons in the immature forebrain. Cys has also been proposed to act synergistically with glutamate to produce neurotoxicity in immature rat arcuate nucleus *in vivo* (9). Cys-induced tonic seizures in mice are attenuated by N(G)-nitro-L-arginine, an inhibitor of nitric oxide synthase (10).

The potential significance of Cys neurotoxicity stems from the hypersensitivity of immature NMDA receptors. Immature NMDA receptors, during certain developmental periods, are hypersensitive to excitotoxic stimulation (relative to immature non-NMDA receptors or to mature NMDA receptors). Therefore, hypoxic/ischemic (H/I) brain damage in infant rodents may be mediated exclusively by interaction of endogenous Glu with NMDA receptors (1,4). Cys preferentially destroys neuronal populations that are also most sensitive to H/I injury (18) and the NMDA antagonist, MK-801, prevents either Cys-induced (2,8) or H/I (3,7) damage in infant rat brain. Moreover, it appears that within a several-week period, during which the postnatal rodent brain is hypersensitive to NMDA neurotoxicity, each of the vulnerable neuronal populations may be governed by its own timetable for reaching peak sensitivity (1).

REFERENCES

1. Ikonomidou C, Mosinger JL, Shahid Salles K *et al.* (1989) Sensitivity of the developing rat brain to hypobaric/ischemic damage parallels sensitivity to N-methyl-D-aspartate neurotoxicity. *J Neurosci* 9, 2809.
2. Lehmann A, Hagberg H, Orwar O (1993) Cysteine sulphinate and cysteate: Mediators of cysteine toxicity in the neonatal rat brain? *Eur J Neurosci* 5, 1398.
3. McDonald JW, Silverstein FS, Johnston MV (1987) MK-801 protects the neonatal brain from hypoxic-ischemic damage. *Eur J Pharmacol* 140, 359.
4. McDonald JW, Silverstein FS, Johnston MV (1988) Neurotoxicity of N-methyl-D-aspartate is markedly enhanced in developing rat central nervous system. *Brain Res* 459, 200.
5. Nunn PB, Davis AJ, O'Brien P (1991) Carbamate formation and the neurotoxicity of L-α amino acids. Technical comment. *Science* 251, 1619.
6. Olney JW, Ho OL, Rhee V (1972) Cysteine-induced brain damage in infant and fetal rodents. *Brain Res* 45, 309.
7. Olney JW, Ikonomidou C, Mosinger JL (1989) MK-801 prevents hypobaric-ischemic neuronal degeneration in infant rat brain. *J Neurosci* 9, 1701.
8. Olney JW, Zorumski C, Price MT (1990) L-Cysteine, a bicarbonate-sensitive endogenous excitotoxin. *Science* 248, 596.
9. Puka-Sundvall M, Eriksson P, Nilsson M *et al.* (1995) Neurotoxicity of cysteine: interaction with glutamate. *Brain Res* 705, 65.
10. Yamamoto H (1996) Preventive effect of N(G)-nitro-L-arginine against L-cysteine-induced seizures in mice. *Toxicol Lett* 84, 1.

Cytarabine

Mark F. Mehler

CYTARABINE
$C_9H_{13}N_3O_5$

4-Amino-1-β-D-arabinofuranosyl-2(1H)-pyrimidinone; 1-β-D-Arabinofuranosylcytosine

NEUROTOXICITY RATING

Clinical

A Acute encephalopathy (confusion, memory loss)

A Cerebellar syndrome (Purkinje cell degeneration)

B Peripheral neuropathy

B Seizure disorder

Experimental

A Neonatal granule cell degeneration (diminished DNA synthesis in progenitor cells)

Cytarabine is a synthetic nucleoside that differs from the normal nucleosides, cytidine and deoxycytidine, by the presence of the sugar moiety arabinose rather than ribose or deoxyribose. The antineoplastic agent is a white to off-white crystalline powder that is freely soluble in water and slightly soluble in chloroform and alcohol. The drug exhibits antitumor activity *in vivo*; deoxycytidine reverses the antitumor effects, both *in vitro* and *in vivo* (1). There is a lack of cross-resistance with other antineoplastic agents. Cytarabine inhibits growing mammalian cells and is cytotoxic *in vitro*. The drug exhibits a limited incorporation into DNA and RNA. Its primary action is inhibition of deoxycytidine synthesis; it can also inhibit cytidylic acid kinases. Cytarabine is therefore both cytostatic and cytocidal. It induces chromosomal breaks in human leukocytes *in vitro*, and inhibits DNA synthesis in mammalian cell culture. Cytarabine inhibits cell proliferation in lymphocytic leukemia, mast cell leukemia, granulocytic leukemia, reticulum cell sarcoma, lymphosarcoma, and solid tumors in mice (1).

The chemotherapeutic effect is useful for remissions in acute granulocytic leukemia of adults, and secondarily in acute leukemias of children and adults (2). Lesser responses have been seen with lymphomas and Hodgkin's disease; it is ineffective against solid tumors. Remissions can be extended with maintenance therapy (2). Intrathecal administration is used in prevention and treatment of meningeal leukemia. Cytarabine may cure acute myelogenous leukemia in a regimen of 7 days of continuous infusion (100–200 mg/m^2/day).

The antimetabolite is not active orally. Intravenous (i.v.) injection or infusion constitutes the favored route of systemic introduction of the drug; subcutaneous (s.c.) administration may be adequate for maintaining or inducing remissions (1). For continuing therapy, rapid injection (2 mg/kg/day for 10 days, with dose doubling for lack of initial efficacy) or continuous infusion (0.5–1.0 mg/kg/day, 1 to 24-h infusion) are used. Children often tolerate higher dosages. Cytarabine enters leukemic cells by the same mechanisms of facilitated diffusion utilized by naturally occurring nucleosides. Intracellularly, the drug is a substrate for deoxycytidine kinase, which converts it to the 5'-monophosphate (ara-CMP). The metabolite is then phosphorylated twice to the 5'-triphosphate (ara-CTP). Cytotoxicity stems from incorporation of ara-CTP into DNA. Cellular levels of ara-CTP rapidly decline with reductions in plasma or extracellular cytarabine concentrations (3).

In leukemic blast cells in acute leukemias, nucleoside transport capacity is less than in normal cultured cells; there are slower transport rates and wide interpatient variability (1). When the rate of transport is low in comparison with the rate of phosphorylation, cytarabine is converted to ara-CMP as rapidly as it enters the cell. Therefore, the transport limit slows the rate of ara-CTP accumulation by restricting the availability of substrate for deoxycytidine kinase (1). The rate of cytarabine transport exhibits first-order kinetics over the full range of clinically significant drug concentrations. Transport is rate-limiting at low concentrations. The impact of transport on cellular drug accumulations over a range of extracellular concentrations can be examined by calculation of the control strength (C_t), which is a measure of the kinetic constants for transport and intracellular phosphorylation. Uridine triphosphate, rather than adenosine triphosphate, appears to be the true phosphate donor.

The relative contribution of dephosphorylation *vs.* deamination in the elimination of ara-CMP varies among cell types. Deamination predominates in human leukemia cells in isolation (1). The low activity of nucleoside transport carriers in patient blast cells is a major factor in determining the mechanism of ara-CTP degradation. In patient blast cells, deamination to ara-UMP and dephosphorylation to ara-U (1β-D-arabinofuranosyl uracil) together form the predominant pathway for the net catabolism of ara-CTP. At high drug concentrations associated with high-dose therapeutic regimens, intracellular cytarabine is five- to tenfold higher than is necessary to saturate the phosphorylation capacity of the cell, and transport rates are no longer the determinants of either the rate of ara-CTP formation or its steady-state levels (1). The amount of ara-CMP incorporated into DNA correlates with cytotoxicity, and is related to concentration of cytarabine and duration of exposure. High-dose therapy may impair DNA synthesis and limit the amount of cytarabine residues at internucleotide positions. Ara-CMP is inserted opposite dGMP in the DNA template. With single insertions, chain elongation slows but does not stop.

Systemic pharmacokinetics are dose-dependent, and primarily affected by metabolism to ara-U by cytidine-deoxycytidine deaminase (1). Ara-U is a metabolically inert detoxification product. After bolus injection or following the standard dose regimen, plasma elimination profiles are a biexponential function ($t_{1/2}$ = 7–12 and 111–157 min). However, after high-dose administration (3 g/m^2), plasma elimination displays triphasic kinetics, with steady-state plasma concentrations of 60–166 μmol/l. At a drug concentration of 3 g/m^2, ara-U peak plasma concentration is 310 $\pm$ 106 μmol/l and the elimination half-life is 3.75 $\pm$ 1.8 h. Nine hours after high-dose treatment, plasma concentrations of ara-U are 83 $\pm$ 26 μmol/l. Increasing concentrations of ara-U interfere with deamination in competitive fashion (apparent K_i = 5.6 μmol/l). High concentrations of ara-U accumulate in leukemic cells during S phase, associated with an increase in the specific activity of deoxycytidine kinase, the rate-limiting enzyme in the accumulation of cytarabine, with enhanced incorporation of the antimetabolite into DNA.

Following i.v. administration, 5%–8% of the initial drug dose is excreted unaltered within 12–24 h. Cytarabine is rapidly metabolized in the liver and perhaps the kidney, and excretion is mainly as the deamination product (1). After a single high i.v. drug dose, blood levels are unmeasurable within 15 min of administration. With daily injections, the total tolerated dose of the antimetabolite decreases. The duration of continuous or repeated exposures to the antineoplastic agent is the primary determinant of efficacy and toxicity.

Intrathecal cytarabine is used in conjunction with methotrexate and hydrocortisone (30–100 mg/m^2, once or twice a week) (2). This therapeutic regimen results in a prolonged cerebrospinal fluid (CSF) half-life, due to lower concentrations of cytidine deaminase in the brain. Following a 30-mg intraventricular dose, there is a byphasic elimination profile ($t_{1/2}$ = 1, 3.4 h.). Peak CSF levels are 2 mmol/l, with significant drug retention (>1 μmol/l for at least 24 h). Divided doses (30 mg/dose $\times$ 3) result in the maintenance of cytotoxic drug levels for significantly longer temporal intervals (>72 h). Intravenous cytarabine penetrates the blood-brain barrier more readily than methotrexate (2). Persistent CSF cytotoxic concentrations are maintained with high-dose (3 g/m^2 every 12 h) systemic therapy. The elimination half-life of cytarabine in the CSF is eight times longer than in the plasma, and CSF levels eventually exceed plasma levels (2). Unlike methotrexate, the CSF:plasma ratio of cytarabine is dose-dependent. High-dose cytarabine therapy for meningeal leukemia is associated with significant systemic toxicity, and the lack of a rescue agent limits applicability (2). Serious systemic toxicity includes bone marrow suppression with anemia, leukopenia, and thrombocytopenia. Less severe toxic drug manifestations include nausea, vomiting, abdominal pain, oral ulcers, and hepatic dysfunction.

Cytarabine, administered s.c. to suckling mice 2–4 days after birth at a dose of 30 or 50 mg/kg, causes extensive necrosis of undifferentiated cells in the external granule layer of the cerebellum within 24 h (13). Partial regeneration of the external granule layer, most pronounced in the posterior lobes, appears 2 weeks later (13). Additional findings include generalized cerebellar hypoplasia, heterotopic granule cells in the molecular layer, poor cellularity in the internal granule layer, and irregularly arranged Purkinje cells, changes that correlate with cytarabine's role in interfering with DNA synthesis in actively dividing neural progenitor cells. Systemic administration of cytarabine to rabbits results in uptake of the drug into brain cells and phosphorylation of the molecule to ara-CTP, an active metabolite that may represent an injury signal. In primates, intraventricular administration of ara-U causes diffuse slowing in the electroencephalogram (EEG). There is a suggestion that definitive cerebellar toxicity may not be achieved after intrathecal administration of cytarabine; the duration of action is much shorter, although greater drug levels are achieved by this route. Continuous infusion of 1% cytarabine into the ventricles or cisternae magnae of adult, female Sprague-Dawley rats completely blocks the proliferation response of microglial cells that follows hypoglossal nerve transection (15).

Cytarabine's actions on the differential ontogeny of neural cell adhesion molecule (NCAM) expression was assayed in cerebellar neuronal lineage species following subcutaneous injections of 30 mg/kg to mice at days 2–4 postnatally (7). Neonatal administration causes destruction of the glial palisades and consequent stagnation of external granule layer cells in the mouse cerebellum, a histological profile resembling that of the cerebellar mutants, *Weaver*, *Reeler*, and *Staggerer*. NCAM normally mediates neuron-to-glia appositions and promotes granule cell migration. In normal mice, an embryonic, polysialyated form of NCAM (E-NCAM) is expressed in the cerebellum until postnatal day 7. However, in mice treated with cytarabine, E-NCAM expression persists until day 14 (7). The aberrant expression of E-NCAM in the external granule layer is attributed to abnormal cellular interactions between external granule layer cells and Bergmann glia. In cytarabine-treated preparations, the external granule layer displays an irregular, thin cell layer and superficial portion at postnatal day 7 that persists until postnatal day 14. This is associated with a delayed conversion of E-NCAM to NCAM, which is finally accomplished by postnatal day 21. This late reversion to the normal developmental program differs from the persistence of the embryonic NCAM isoform in the murine mutant, *Staggerer*.

In neonatal murine cerebellar organotypic cultures, cytarabine reduces the expression of granule neurons and eliminates oligodendrocytes, but has no demonstrable effect on astrocytes; in contrast, Purkinje cells exhibit increased survival, with sprouting of excessive recurrent axon collaterals that form heterotypical synapses with Purkinje cell dendritic spines (12). These functional alterations are associated with astrocytic ensheathment of Purkinje cells and apposition of unattached dendritic spines, encasement of heterotypical synapses in astrocytic processes, loss of Purkinje cell somatic spines, and an absence of somatic hyperinnervation of Purkinje cells by recurrent axon collateral terminals. These changes are held to be a response to the loss of granule cells and parallel fibers, and may be reversed only by transplantation of granule cells and astroglial cells. The pattern of astrocytic envelopment of heterotypical synapses is similar to the *in vivo* astrocyte ensheathment of parallel fiber–Purkinje cell dendritic spine synapses that occur. With a permanent loss of, or a significant reduction in, the number of parallel fibers, the astrocyte environment enhances heterotypical synapse formation (12). These findings contrast with the reductions in axo-spinous cortical synapses that are seen with cytarabine-treated cerebellar cultured cells, transplanted with postnatal day 7 optic nerve glial cells and examined after 13–14 days in culture. This suggests that immature astroglial cells may facilitate neurite

elaboration and cellular differentiation. The heterotypical recurrent axon collateral–Purkinje cell dendritic spine synapses are functionally significant and may mediate abnormal neuronal circuits (12). In a related study, murine neonatal cerebellar explant cultures were treated with cytarabine (10 µg/ml): Histological examination of treated tissue preparations revealed the graded loss of granule neurons and astrocytes, and the absence of myelinated fiber tracts. There was also evidence of unsheathed Purkinje cell somatas, hyperinnervated by sprouted inhibitory axonal terminals, with retained somatic spines.

Cerebral explants of sensorimotor cortex from embryonic day 20 rats, exposed to cytarabine (10^{-5} M) at days 7–10 and allowed to develop for 8 additional days in culture, exhibited an increase in the total volume of neurites from neuronal cellular forms with a corresponding reduction in the volume of nonneuronal cells in outgrowth zones (8). These experimental findings occurred without an alteration in total neuronal cell number, reflecting a decrease in nonneuronal cell division. Cytarabine inhibits cell division of neuroblastoma cells and increases neurite production through regulation of dividing cells. In postmitotic peripheral neurons, cytarabine application can induce cell death when applied at days 0–4 or 7–12 *in vitro*. Neurotoxicity is apparent by day 4 following antimetabolite application and is associated with a concentration of 5×10^{-5} M (EC_{50}). There is some experimental evidence that cytarabine may exert a primary cellular action on astrocytes; this effect involves the delayed secretion of neurotrophic factors to increase neurite production or to enhance the development of cells with cholinergic traits.

At standard doses (100–200 mg/m^2), cytarabine is generally not neurotoxic (1). At high doses (3.0 g/m^2 or more by infusion every 12 h for 4–16 doses), treatment with the antimetabolite is associated with an acute encephalopathy and cerebellar dysfunction; rarely, peripheral neuropathy, leukoencephalopathy, optic neuropathy, and additional neurological dysfunction appear (1,4,16). The incidence and severity of neurotoxic manifestations are related most directly to dose (>18 g/m^2/ course), course schedule, and age (incidence: 3%, ages 20–50; 19%, ages >50) (10).

Neurological dysfunction occasionally follows modest doses of cytarabine. One report describes paraplegia after intrathecal administration of cytarabine (100 mg/m^2/day every fifth day). Postmortem evaluation revealed multifocal demyelination and microvascular changes in the spinal cord and cerebral white matter, with minimal inflammatory reaction (9). Seizures may occur 1 day after intrathecal administration, especially when benzyl alcohol is the vehicle; they are difficult to control, remit after an additional 24 h, and are associated with elevated CSF protein. Necrotizing leukoencephalopathy may follow whole-brain radiation therapy and concomitant intrathecal administration of cytarabine, methotrexate, and hydrocortisone for treatment of meningeal Burkitt's lymphoma. The syndrome is characterized by somnolence and seizures, and pathological examination reveals the presence of multiple foci of necrosis, demyelination, and axonal damage within the cerebral white matter. Additional examples of iatrogenic leukoencephalography have been documented with combination radiation and high-dose intrathecal or systemic administration of cytarabine, methotrexate, and hydrocortisone.

Seizures from high-dose cytarabine treatment are usually generalized or partial complex (17). They appear during or after drug infusion or within 13 days of antimetabolic administration; they do not persist.

An acute encephalopathy, characterized by confusion, disorientation, somnolence, memory loss, additional cognitive dysfunction, psychosis, and frontal lobe release signs, may appear soon after drug infusion. The syndrome usually resolves spontaneously, is accompanied by diffuse slow-wave activity on EEG recordings, and occurs more frequently following rapid drug infusion.

A syndrome of prominent cerebellar dysfunction is the most common manifestation of high-dose therapy (1,6,14). The incidence is 10.5% and the majority of patients exhibits severe or life-threatening illness (grades 3–4). The neurological syndrome usually commences 3–8 days after initiation of treatment, and is associated with dysarthria, dysdiadochokinesia, dysmetria, and ataxia. Ataxia and nystagmus may precede other signs by as long as 24 h. In the majority of individuals, neurological dysfunction remits within 5 days of stopping treatment, although 30% of patients are left with permanent sequelae. Pathologically, there is selective loss of cerebellar Purkinje cells in the vermis and hemispheres; deep nuclei are unaffected. There is a high incidence of recurrence of the cerebellar signs with resumption of therapy. Significant risk factors include total therapeutic dose, initial subclinical damage with incipient treatment, meningeal leukemia, prior CNS disorders, age (>50 years), renal insufficiency (creatinine clearance ≥60 ml/dl), and hepatic dysfunction (bilirubin >3.0 mg/dl) (5).

Peripheral nerve dysfunction of various types develops in 0.6%; it is associated with high-dose therapy and increasing cumulative doses (600 mg to 36 g/m^2). Save for the convincing cases of sensory neuropathy (11), most reports of cytarabine neuropathy probably reflect effects of the underlying condition.

The mechanism of cytarabine neurotoxicity is unclear (1). Experimental studies suggest several possibilities. Cytarabine exhibits facilitated diffusion through the choroid plexus and rapidly gains entry into the CNS following systemic administration. Cytarabine interferes with DNA synthesis and cell cycle regulation, and shows differential cytotoxic actions on neural lineage species. Neuronal progenitors require that the timing of cell cycle exit be precisely linked to associated developmental events to prevent the induction of an active cell death program. In addition, the differential sensitivity of interrelated lineage species to the toxic effects of cytarabine could significantly alter their cooperative developmental interactions and profiles of maturation and effector molecule inductions. The action of cytarabine on DNA synthesis could also alter the temporal expression of surface proteins, such as NCAM, that are crucial for neuronal migration and the regulated elaboration of intercellular connections. Alterations in the developmental expression of these molecular and cellular signals could impair the viability of nascent lineage species, disrupt the expression of trophic signals necessary for their cellular differentiation, and short-circuit the neuronal signaling cascades essential for the propagation of regional instructional signals and the elaboration of a dynamic microenvironment. The pathological underpinnings of these postulated pathogenetic mechanisms have been demonstrated with the developmental persistence of E-NCAM expression, the formation of heterotypical synapses, and by the induction of neurotrophic factor secretion by targeted astroglial cells. Finally, metabolites of cytarabine, such as ara-CMP or ara-U, may represent "injury signals" with direct neurotoxic actions on specific neural lineage species or regional neuronal ensembles.

REFERENCES

1. Baker WJ, Royer GL Jr, Weiss RB (1991) Cytarabine and neurologic toxicity. *J Clin Oncol* **9**, 679.
2. Blaney SM, Balis FM, Poplack DG (1991) Current pharmacological treatment approaches to central nervous system leukaemia. *Drugs* **41**, 702.
3. Capizzi RL, White JC, Powell BL, Berrino F (1991) Effect of dose on the pharmacokinetic and pharmacodynamic effects of cytarabine. *Semin Hematol* **28**, 54.
4. Hoffman DL, Howard JR Jr, Sarma R, Riggs JE (1993) Encephalopathy, myelopathy, optic neuropathy and anosmia associated with intravenous cytosine arabinoside. *Clin Neuropharmacol* **16**, 258.
5. Jolson HM, Bosco L, Bufton MG *et al.* (1992) Clustering of adverse drug events: Analysis of risk factors for cerebellar toxicity with high-dose cytarabine. *J Nat Cancer Inst* **84**, 500.
6. Lundquist DM, Holmes W (1993) Documentation of neurotoxicity resulting from high-dose cytosine arabinoside. *Oncol Nurs Forum* **20**, 1409.

7. Ono K, Tokunaga A, Mizukawa K *et al.* (1992) Abnormal expression of embryonic neural cell adhesion molecule (N-CAM) in the developing mouse cerebellum after neonatal administration of cytosine arabinoside. *Brain Res* **65**, 119.

8. Oorschot DE, Jones DG (1991) Neuronal survival and neurite growth in cultured cerebral explants: Assessment of the effect of cytosine arabinoside using improved stereology. *Brain Res* **546**, 146.

9. Ozon A, Topalglu H, Cila A *et al.* (1994) Acute ascending myelitis and encphalopathy after intrathecal cytosine arabinoside and methotrexate in an adolescent boy with acute lymphoblastic leukemia. *Brain Develop* **16**, 246.

10. Rubin EH, Andersen JW, Berg DT *et al.* (1992) Risk factors for high-dose cytarabine neurotoxicity: An analysis of a cancer and leukemia group B trial in patients with acute myeloid leukemia. *J Clin Oncol* **10**, 948.

11. Russell JA, Poules PD (1974) Neuropathy due to cytosine arabinoside. *Brit Med J* **14**, 232.

12. Seil FJ, Drake-Baumann R, Herndon RM, Leiman AL (1992) Cytosine arabinoside effects in mouse cerebellar cultures in the presence of astrocytes. *Neuroscience* **51**, 149.

13. Shimada M, Wakaizumi S, Kasubuchi Y, Kusonoki T (1975) Cytarabine and its effect on cerebellum of suckling mouse. *Arch Neurol* **32**, 555.

14. Stentoft J (1990) The toxicity of cytarabine. *Drug Safety* **5**, 7.

15. Svensson M, Aldskogius H (1993) Infusion of cytosine-arabinoside into the cerebrospinal fluid of the rat brain inhibits the microglial cell proliferation after hypoglossal nerve injury. *Glia* **7**, 286.

16. Watterson J, Toogood I, Nieder M *et al.* (1994) Excessive spinal cord toxicity from intensive central nervous system-directed therapies. *Cancer* **74**, 3034.

17. Winick NJ, Bowman WP, Kamen BA *et al.* (1992) Unexpected acute neurologic toxicity in the treatment of children with acute lymphoblastic leukemia. *J Nat Cancer Inst* **84**, 252.

Dactinomycin (Actinomycin D)

Herbert H. Schaumburg

DACTINOMYCIN
$C_{62}H_{86}N_{12}O_{16}$

NEUROTOXICITY RATING

Experimental

A   Inhibition of RNA-dependent protein synthesis

A   CNS vacuolar myelinopathy (local administration)

A   CNS neuronopathy (local administration)

Dactinomycin is a naturally occurring chromopeptide antibiotic and antineoplastic agent; it is one of a group of actinomycins isolated from the culture broth of a species of *Streptomyces*. The most important use of dactinomycin is in the treatment of rhabdomyosarcoma and Wilms' tumor, where it is curative when employed in concert with radiotherapy and other chemotherapeutic agents. Dactinomycin has not been reported to cause human neurotoxic disease, presumably because it does not cross the blood-brain barrier; it is not administered intrathecally.

Serious systemic side effects are associated with dactinomycin therapy. Gastrointestinal dysfunction (nausea and vomiting) occurs within hours of commencing intravenous dosing. Hematological effects, including pancytopenia, may appear in the first week of therapy. Oral ulcers, glossitis, and alopecia are common. Standard, gradually increasing, week-long treatment regimens are usually well tolerated; high-dose pulse therapy in children has caused severe hepatotoxicity (1). Its antineoplastic and cytotoxic potencies stem from its firm, stable binding to DNA, blocking the transcription of DNA by RNA polymerase. In addition, dactinomycin causes single-strand breaks in DNA (2). It inhibits rapidly proliferating cells of normal and neoplastic origin and is one of the most potent antineoplastic agents known. Dactinomycin's ability to inhibit RNA and, secondarily, protein synthesis, has been widely used in experimental neurobiology. Since the neuronal perikaryon actively synthesizes and degrades RNA, the agent can function as a cytological probe for correlating biochemical

and structural events in the nucleus in intact animals following CNS injection. It has also been extensively used in *in vitro* studies, most recently employed to characterize cellular and molecular events in programmed cell death (4).

Dactinomycin injected into the parenchyma or cerebrospinal fluid of rats, cats, and monkeys causes behavioral and electroencephalographic changes (6). Two days after intrathecal administration to dogs, animals become listless and display myoclonic jerks. Status epilepticus develops on the third day. A similar pattern occurs in cats; this is heralded by spike discharges on the electroencephalogram.

Two distinctively different morphological patterns of CNS toxic reaction follow intracerebral and intrathecal administration to experimental animals: myelin vacuoles and neuronal chromatin condensation. Both reactions reflect the ability of dactinomycin to inhibit RNA-dependent protein synthesis, the former in the oligodendrocyte and the latter in the neuron.

Direct injection of dactinomycin into rat brain produces three distinct loci of vacuoles: between the inner tongue and the remainder of the myelin sheath, enlargement of the periaxonal space, and splitting of the myelin lamellae between the intraperiod lines (5).

Intrathecal and direct intracerebral injection of dactinomycin into cat and rat CNS both produce alterations in nuclear morphology in glial cells and small neurons (3). These changes become evident within 30 min and include formation of clumps of dense chromatin through compaction of loose chromatin, agglomeration and enlargement of nucleoplasmic granules, and rarefaction of intervening nucleoplasm. It is suggested that dactinomycin, upon binding to nuclear DNA or histones, cross-links the extended nucleohistone microfibrils. This converts the euchromatin and nucleolar chromatin into a contracted, impervious mass of dense (hetero)chromatin incapable of functioning as a template for RNA transcription. It is also suggested that the euchromatin of larger neurons may be less susceptible to cross-linkage because it is dispersed in a larger volume (3).

REFERENCES

1. D'Angio GJ (1987) Hepatotoxicity with actinomycin D. *Lancet* ii, 104.
2. Goldberg IH, Beerman TA, Poon R (1977) Antibiotics: Nucleic acids as targets in chemotherapy. In: *Cancer 5: A Comprehensive Treatise*. Becker FF ed. Plenum Press, New York p. 427.
3. Koenig H, Nayyar R, Sanghavi P *et al.* (1977) Neurotoxicity of actinomycin D and related inhibitors of RNA syn-

thesis: The role of nuclear heterochromatinization. In: *Neurotoxicology*. Roizin L, Shiraki RH eds. Raven Press, New York p. 391.

4. Pittman RN, Wang S, DiBenedetto AJ (1993) A system for characterizing cellular and molecular events in programmed neuronal cell death. *J Neurosci* **13**, 3669.

5. Rizzuto N, Gambetti PL (1976) Status spongiosus of rat central nervous system induced by actinomycin D. *Acta Neuropathol* **36**, 21.

6. Taira M, Kojima K, Takeuchi H (1972) A comparative study of the action of actinomycin D and actinomycinic acid on the central nervous system when injected into the cerebrospinal fluid of higher animals. *Epilepsia* **13**, 649.

Dapsone

Ludwig Guttmann

DAPSONE
$C_{12}H_{12}N_2O_2S$

4,4'-Diaminodiphenyl sulfone

NEUROTOXICITY RATING

Clinical

A   Peripheral neuropathy (motor)

Dapsone is a sulfone derivative that has both antibacterial and anti-inflammatory properties. It is effective in the treatment of a variety of infectious diseases including leprosy, malaria, and *Pneumocystis carinii* pneumonia in acquired immunodeficiency syndrome patients (1). It has also been effective in treating some patients with Crohn's disease associated with *Mycobacterium paratuberculosis* (8). Dapsone inhibits the bacterial synthesis of dihydrofolic acid through competition with *para*-aminobenzoate for the active site of dihydropteroate synthetase (1). Dapsone is reported to act as a neuroprotective agent against excitotoxicity induced by direct injection of glutamate receptor agonists into the brains of rats. Circling behavior and striatal γ-aminobutyric acid depletion induced by intrastriatal injection of either kainic acid or quinolinic acid (a *N*-methyl-D-aspartate agonist) were attenuated by systemic treatment with dapsone (10).

Dapsone's effectiveness is established for dermatitis herpetiformis; it is occasionally used in bullous pemphigus, leukocytoclastic vasculitis, rheumatoid arthritis, relapsing polychondritis, pyoderma gangrenosum, acne conglobata, acne vulgaris, and subcorneal pustular dermatosis (2,11). Its anti-inflammatory action is unclear. Neutrophils release myeloperoxidase which, when combined with hydrogen peroxide, forms a potent oxidant. Dapsone facilitates the conversion of myeloperoxidase to an inactive form, preventing tissue damage (1). Another anti-inflammatory effect is inhibition of neutrophil adherence to vascular endothelium. This prevents neutrophil release into tissues and the subsequent inflammatory response (1).

Dapsone is well absorbed from the gastrointestinal tract. Peak levels are obtained in 2–6 h. It is largely protein bound and widely distributed in body fluids (1,13).

Metabolism of dapsone by the liver occurs by (a) *N*-acetylation to monoacetyldapsone (MADDS) in hepatocyte cytosol, and (b) *N*-hydroxylation to *N*-hydroxydapsone (NOH-dapsone) in the smooth endoplasmic reticulum. MADDS is highly protein bound and does not undergo extensive glomerular filtration. Deacetylation of MADDS to dapsone and *N*-hydroxylation appear necessary for excretion. Dapsone is excreted 15% unchanged and 85% as metabolites in urine. Small amounts of dapsone are excreted in bile. In therapeutic doses, dapsone has an elimination half-life of 30 h. *N*-Hydroxylation is the major mechanism of elimination (1,13).

Dapsone has hematological and neurological toxicity. The dose-dependent hematological side effects are the most common; they include methemoglobinemia and hemolysis (1,3,7). Less commonly, sulfhemoglobinemia occurs (6). Long-term dapsone usage in conventional doses of 100 mg daily in normal individuals may result in methemoglobinemia. Levels under 20% are not usually associated with symptoms but may become significant in patients with methemoglobin reductase deficiency or in the face of compromised tissue oxygen delivery (1). Most reported cases with significant morbidity result from acute intoxication with dapsone (3,7). Hemolytic anemia, due to the action of dapsone or its metabolites on erythrocytes, is compensated by a bone marrow response. It becomes severe and life threatening in the presence of glucose-6-phosphate dehydrogenase deficiency (1,13). Agranulocytosis due to dapsone usually occurs in the initial 3 months of therapy and most often with treatment of dermatitis herpetiformis than with other disorders (1). Peripheral neuropathy, predominantly motor, results from its neurotoxic effect (2,11).

Attempts to produce dapsone-induced peripheral neuropathy in rats and guinea pigs have been unsuccessful (2,12).

Dapsone motor neuropathy is less common than the hematological side effects and is not clearly dose-dependent (2,4,5,9,11). Primarily a motor neuropathy, weakness and atrophy are the major clinical features. In contrast to most toxic neuropathies, initial weakness frequently appears in distal upper limbs (2,11). Most cases have few sensory symptoms (2), and sensory findings are unusual unless a meticulous sensory examination is performed (5). Optic neuropathy has been reported in one patient with motor neuropathy (4).

Onset of weakness occurs most often 6 weeks to 5 years after the initiation of dapsone therapy but, in four cases, it surfaced after 10–16 years. The earliest onset was at 13 days. The age of involved patients was 17–60 years, and 76% of patients were males (11). Dosages of dapsone ranged from 200–600 mg daily, higher than the more conventional dose of 100 mg daily (2,11). The patient with onset of symptoms at 13 days received 600 mg daily (4).

Nerve conduction studies reveal small or absent compound muscle action potentials. Motor conduction velocities are sometimes mildly reduced; this likely reflects loss of the fastest conducting axons. Sensory nerve action potentials and latencies are invariably normal. Needle electromyography shows fibrillations and loss of motor unit potentials in involved muscles (2,5).

The motor neuropathy improves or resolves within 1 year after discontinuation of dapsone. Improvement may also occur with a marked reduction in dosage (11). Electrophysiological measurements have documented progressive enlargement of evoked compound muscle action potentials over 5 years after dapsone discontinuation. Fibrillations disappear and motor unit potentials increase in size and number as recovery occurs (2).

In sum, the clinical profile consists of progressive weakness and atrophy involving mostly distal muscles in the arms, legs, or all four extremities with few sensory symptoms and findings. Recovery occurs when dapsone is discontinued. Electrophysiological studies document a motor axonopathy without sensory axon involvement. The motor axonopathy induced by dapsone likely reflects a "dying back" of motor axons. The reason for dapsone's predilection for motor axons is not known.

N-Acetylation of dapsone occurs in a polymorphic fashion as is the case with isoniazid, hydralazine, sulfamethazine, and procainamide. Some patients are slow acetylators and others rapid acetylators (1,2,13). However, the need for ultimate N-hydroxylation for drug excretion means the N-acetylated form of dapsone, MADDS, requires subsequent deacetylation and ultimate N-hydroxylation (1).

Slow acetylation, as opposed to rapid, appears to have no effect on dapsone's half-life and the hematological side effects. The toxic factor (*e.g.*, dapsone or a metabolite) that causes neuropathy is not known, but slow acetylation may well be a factor. Slow acetylation has been documented in several cases of dapsone motor neuropathy (5,9,11).

REFERENCES

1. Coleman MD (1993) Dapsone: Modes of action, toxicity and possible strategies for increasing patient tolerance. *Brit J Dermatol* **129**, 507.
2. Gutmann L, Martin JD, Welton W (1976) Dapsone motor neuropathy—An axonal disease. *Neurology* **26**, 514.
3. Hansen DG, Challoner KR, Smith DE (1994) Dapsone intoxication: Two case reports. *J Emerg Med* **12**, 347.
4. Homeida M, Babikr A, Daneshmend TK (1980) Dapsone-induced optic atrophy and motor neuropathy. *Brit Med J* **281**, 1180.
5. Koller WC, Gehlmann LK, Malkinson FD, Davis FA (1977) Dapsone-induced peripheral neuropathy. *Arch Neurol* **34**, 644.
6. Lambert M, Sonnet J, Mahieu P, Hassoun A (1982) Delayed sulfhemoglobinemia after acute dapsone intoxication. *J Toxicol-Clin Toxicol* **19**, 45.
7. Linakis JG, Shannon M, Woolf A, Sax C (1989) Recurrent methemoglobinemia after acute dapsone intoxication in a child. *J Emerg Med* **7**, 477.
8. Prantera C, Bothamley G, Levenstein S *et al.* (1989) Crohn's disease and mycobacteria; two cases of Crohn's disease with high anti-mycobacterial antibody levels cured by dapsone therapy. *Biomed Pharmacotherapy* **43**, 295.
9. Rosen I, Sorras R (1982) Peripheral motor neuropathy caused by excessive intake of dapsone (Avlosulfon). *Arch Psychiat Nervenkr* **232**, 63.
10. Santamaria A, Ordaz-Moreno J, Rubio-Osornio M (1997) Neuroprotective effect of dapsone against quinolinate- and kainate-induced striatal neurotoxicities in rates. *Pharmacol Toxicol* **81**, 271.
11. Waldinger TP, Siegle RJ, Weber W, Voorhees JJ (1984) Dapsone-induced peripheral neuropathy. *Arch Dermatol* **120**, 356.
12. Williams MH, Bradley WG (1972) An assessment of dapsone toxicity in the guinea pig. *Brit J Dermatol* **86**, 650.
13. Zuidema J, Hilbers-Modderman ESM, Merkus FWHM (1986) Clinical pharmacokinetics of dapsone. *Clin Pharmacokinet* **11**, 299.

Datura stramonium

Albert C. Ludolph

SCOPOLAMINE
$C_{17}H_{21}NO_4$

Scopolamine; [7(S)-(1α,2β,4β,5α,7β)]-α-
(Hydroxymethyl)benzeneacetic acid 9-methyl-3-oxa-
9-azatricyclo[3.3.1.0^{2,4}]non-7-yl ester

NEUROTOXICITY RATING

Clinical

A   Psychobiological reaction (hallucinations, agitation, euphoria)

Datura stramonium (jimsonweed, thorn-apple), a member of the family Solanaceae, contains a number of alkaloids that are competitive antagonists of acetylcholine and other muscarinic agonists. The major compounds atropine, hyoscyamine, and scopolamine are present in the seeds, flowers, leaves, and roots of the plant. Extracts of *Datura* spp. were used by the Egyptians and Greeks to induce hallucinations. In the Middle Ages, *Datura* spp. served as witch ointments and were used for medicinal purposes. In 1597, the use of ointments containing *Datura* spp. was recommended to induce hallucinations (6). Since ingestion of *D. stramonium* was the obvious cause of unusual behavior in the Jamestown colony, the plant is also known as Jamestown or Jimson weed. Accidental poisoning is rare because the plants are much less attractive than *Atropa belladonna* plants; the deliberate use of *Datura* to induce hallucinations and euphoria is frequently associated with poisonings (11). In some parts of the world, *Datura* spp. historically were and continue to be used for homicide and suicide; criminals have administered plant extracts to use the hallucinogenic and amnesic properties of the alkaloids (2,3).

The principal pharmacological syndrome is caused by a dose-dependent blockade of peripheral and central muscarinic receptors; atropine only affects the CNS if a higher dosage is used, whereas scopolamine, which crosses the blood-brain barrier more readily, affects the CNS at lower dosages (4). Early peripheral effects are bradycardia, dryness of mouth, mydriasis, photophobia and cycloplegia,

tachycardia, cardiac arrhythmias, and a rise of body temperature. CNS effects at low doses are variable; however, after higher doses, excitement, euphoria, restlessness, irritability, disorientation, hallucinations, and delirium appear (4). Convulsions are rare. Children and the elderly are more susceptible to anticholinergic effects.

In farm animals, the species *D. stramonium* and *D. ferox* are the most common causes of intoxications (9). Although acute poisoning is rare, chronic intoxications are seen in pigs (apparently the most sensitive species), cattle, horses, and chicken (9). The clinical picture is characterized by eating less, dry mouth, increase of respiration and heart rate, and reduced gastrointestinal motility. Sheep and rabbits are resistant to Datura toxicity, since they synthesize the enzyme atropine esterase.

Accidental Datura poisoning in humans is rare, although cases have been repeatedly reported, partly caused by rare events such as poisoning by self-made sandwiches contaminated with *Datura* seeds (1), the apparently accidental use of *Datura* spp. for teas (12), or the contamination of bread (7,10). More frequently, *Datura* spp. are deliberately employed to induce euphoria and hallucinations (5). *D. stramonium* is usually used for this purpose, but *D. sauveolens* (angel's trumpet) is also popular. Inhalation of smoke, eating Datura flowers, chewing roots, or drinking teas are all employed (5). Since Datura contains atropine and scopolamine, intoxication is characterized by peripheral and central anticholinergic effects. The symptomatology of human poisoning reflects the peripheral effects of antagonists to muscarinic receptors such as dryness of mouth, mydriasis, flushing, reduced gastrointestinal motility and secretion, tachycardia, and urinary retention. However, after a latency of 4–6 h, central effects of euphoria, agitation, and usually visual hallucinations are a part of the picture in most patients. At even higher dosages, CNS symptomatology predominates and includes disturbances of vision, hallucinations, later delirium, coma, possibly accompanied by seizures, and respiratory failure, circulatory collapse, and death (5). Electroencephalographic recordings are characterized by paroxysms and diffuse slowing (8). Adults may survive doses of 500 mg of scopalamine and 1000 mg of atropine; however, 10 mg of either drug may be fatal for children (5). Long-term use is associated with development of tolerance, withdrawal symptomatology may occur, and animal studies suggest that long-term hippocampal damage develops after experimental application of scopolamine and *Datura* spp. (5). The long-term human effects are unknown.

If an intoxication with anticholinergics is suspected, an intramuscular injection of 1 mg physostigmine is a diagnostic and therapeutic measure. If the syndrome can be reversed, slow parenteral administration of physostigmine (1–4 mg in adults, 0.5 mg in children) is used therapeutically (4). Treatment must often be repeated after 1–2 h. Other routine measures are gastric lavage, administration of activated charcoal, symptomatic treatment of fever by ice bags and alcohol sponges, and bladder catheterization (4).

REFERENCES

1. Anon. (1984) Datura poisoning from hamburger—Canada. *Morbid Mort Weekly Rep* 33, 282.

2. Ardila A, Moreno C (1991) Scopolamine intoxication as a model of transient global amnesia. *Brain Cognition* 15, 236.

3. Brizer DA, Manning DW (1982) Delirium induced by poisoning with anticholinergic agents. *Amer J Psychiat* 139, 1343.

4. Brown JH, Taylor P (1996) Muscarinic receptor agonists and antagonists. In: *Goodman & Gilman's The Pharmacological Basis of Therapeutics. 9th Ed.* Hardman JG, Limbird LE eds. McGraw-Hill, New York p. 141.

5. Brust JCM (1993) *Neurological Aspects of Substance Abuse.* Butterworth-Heinemann, Boston p. 185.

6. Gerard J (1964) *Gerard's Herbal Edition of 1636.* Spring Books, London p. 94.

7. Malorny G (1952) Stechapfelsamenvergiftungen nach Genuß von Buchweizenmehlzubereitungen. Sammlung von Vergiftungsfällen. *Arch Toxicol* 14, 181.

8. Mikolich JR, Paulson GW, Cross CJ, Calhoun R (1976) Neurologic and electroencephalographic effects of jimsonweed intoxication. *Clin Electroencephalogr* 7, 49.

9. Piva G, Piva A (1995) Antinutritional factors of *Datura* in feedstuffs. *Nat Toxins* 3/4, 238.

10. Pulewka P (1949) Die Aufklärung einer ungewöhnlichen, durch *Datura stramonium* in Brotmehl hervorgerufenen Massenvergiftung. *Klin Wochenschr* 27, 672.

11. Tiongson J, Salen P (1998) Mass ingestion of Jimson Weed by eleven teenagers. *Del Med J* 70, 471.

12. Vollmer H, Roberg M (1943) Vergiftung durch Stechapfelblätter. Sammlung von Vergiftungsfällen. *Arch Toxicol* 13, 189.

Delphinium Spp.

Albert C. Ludolph

Larkspur

NEUROTOXICITY RATING

Clinical

A Neuromuscular transmission syndrome (livestock)

Experimental

A Neuromuscular transmission dysfunction (postsynaptic)

Delphinium spp. (*Delphinium barbeyi*, tall larkspur; *D. andersonii*, low larkspur) are a significant cause of livestock loss in the western mountains and higher plains of North America (1). In contrast, the European *D. elatum* and *Consolida elatum* are far less toxic, and data on documented intoxications are not available. *Delphinum* spp. contain a mixture of neurotoxic diterpenoid alkaloids of which the most important is the neuromuscular blocking agent methyllycaconitine. The neurotoxicity of the plants depends on a number of factors: the potency, concentration and interaction of the various toxins present in the plant, species, their growth stages, specific plant parts, and external factors such as soil composition and climate. A precise chemotaxonomy for *Delphinium* spp. based on alkaloid contents in North America does not exist (6). Animal species, ingestion rate, ruminal metabolism, kinetics of absorption, and excretion influence larkspur neurotoxicity quantitatively and qualitatively.

The chemistry of the more than 100 diterpenoid alkaloids present in *Delphinium* spp. has been reviewed (6,9,10), as well as current methods of separation and synthesis (6). Several neurotoxins are identified (their relative potency in mice in relation to the major toxin methyllycaconitine is described in brackets) (6): methyllycaconitine [1], delphinine [2], elatine [1/8], delsemine [1/2], lappaconitine [1/3], anthranoyllycactonine [1/3], condelphine [1/10, rats], karakoline [1/17], delcosine [1/34], delsoline [1/55, rats], lycoctonine [1/110], and deltaline [<1/100]. Other larkspur alkaloids of low toxic potency are tricornine, browniine, browniine 14-acetate, denudatine and geyerline [N-(methylsuccinimido)anthranoyllycoctonine norditerpenoid alkaloid] (4,6). Studies of structure–activity relationships in a mouse bioassay revealed the importance of the tertiary nitrogen atom and of anthranilic acid esterification for the neurotoxic effect (3). Because of the comparatively large amount present in *Delphinium* spp., and its potent curare-like effect on skeletal muscle, methyllycaconitine is likely to be the compound of major practical importance in rangeland poisonings (*see* Methyllycaconitine, this volume).

Signs and symptoms in accidental field poisonings are primarily characterized by dose-dependent failure of neuromuscular transmission that may be exacerbated by exertion: Animals develop generalized weakness which, in severe poisoning, results in paralysis, sternal or lateral recumbency, asphyxiation and respiratory failure, and death (6,7). Sensory deficits seem to be absent. In comparative studies using plant extracts, *D. barbeyi* was the most toxic species in a rat assay (5). A numerical rating scale has been developed for the clinical signs of larkspur poisoning (8), and calculations of the effective toxic dosage ("total toxic alkaloid") reveal an LD_{50} for cattle of 25–40 mg/kg body weight (13). Daily consumption of non-acutely toxic amounts over a 4-day period results in toxic signs; these do not not persist longer than 4 days after intake ceases (8).

Controlled feeding of *D. barbeyi* extracts to mice, hamsters, rats, and sheep reveal that dose–response curves and primary clinical signs of poisoning are similar in each of the species examined (8), and are comparable to those observed in accidental poisoning. Mice are recommended for bioassay since they are highly susceptible, respond rapidly, and require low doses for intoxication. In controlled feeding trials of *D. barbeyi* (single oral dose of 1.5–3 g/kg body weight), the serial administration (intravenous, intraperitoneal, or subcutaneaous) of physostigmine reversed neurotoxicity, indicating that this treatment may reduce mortality from larkspur poisoning (12). An attempt to create taste aversions to prevent larkspur ingestion has been partly successful (14).

The major mechanism of intoxication is the impairment of neuromuscular transmisison by diterpenoid alkaloids, although effects on central cholinergic systems and the autonomic nervous system are also a likely part of the picture (11). The central effect may be related to the very-high-affinity binding of methyllycaconitine (nanomolar concentrations) to ^{125}I-α-bungarotoxin binding sites in rat brain (2,15).

REFERENCES

1. Cronin EH, Nielsen DB (1978) Tall larkspur and cattle on high mountain ranges. In: *Effects of Poisonous Plants on Livestock*. Keeler RF, van Kampen KR, James LF eds. Academic Press, New York p. 521.
2. Macallan DRE, Lunt GG, Wonnacott S *et al.* (1988) Methyllycaconitine and (+)-anatoxin-a differentiate between nicotinic receptors in vertebrate and invertebrate nervous systems. *FEBS Lett* 226, 357.
3. Manners GD, Panter KE, Pelletier SW (1995) Structure-activity relationships of nonditerpenoid alkaloids occuring in toxic larkspur (*Delphinium*) species. *J Nat Prod* 58, 863.
4. Manners GD, Panter KE, Pfister JA *et al.* (1998) The characterization and structure-activity evaluation of toxic norditerpenoid alkaloids from two *Delphinium* species. *Nat Prod* 61, 1086.
5. Olsen JD (1977) Rat bioassay for estimating toxicity of plant material from larkspur (*Delphinium* spp.). *Amer J Vet Res* 38, 277.
6. Olsen JD, Manners GD (1989) Toxicology of diterpenoid alkaloids in rangeland larkspur (*Delphinium* spp.). In: *Toxicants of Plant Origin. Vol 1. Alkaloids.* Cheeke PR ed. CRC Press, Boca Raton, FL p. 291.
7. Olsen JD (1978) Tall larkspur poisoning in cattle and sheep. *J Amer Vet Med Assn* 173, 762.
8. Olsen JD, Sisson DV (1991) Toxicity of extracts of tall larkspur (*Delphinium barbeyi*) in mice, hamsters, rats and sheep. *Toxicol Lett* 56, 33.
9. Pelletier SW, Page SW (1984) Diterpenoid alkaloids. *Nat Prod Rep* 1, 375.
10. Pelletier SW, Page SW (1986) Diterpenoid alkaloids. *Nat Prod Rep* 3, 451.
11. Pfister JA, Gardner DR, Panter KE *et al.* (1999) Larkspur (*Delphinium* SPP.) poisoning in livestock. *Nat Toxins* 8, 81.
12. Pfister JA, Panter KE, Manners GD, Cheney CD (1994) Reversal of tall larkspur (*Delphinium barbeyi*) poisoning in cattle with physostigmine. *Vet Human Toxicol* 36, 511.
13. Pfister JA, Panter KE, Manners GD (1994) Effective dose on cattle of toxic alkaloids from tall larkspur (*Delphinium arbeyi*). *Vet Human Toxicol* 36, 10.
14. Ralphs MH, Olsen JD (1992) Comparison of larkspur alkaloid extract and lithium chloride in maintaining cattle aversion to larkspur in the field. *J Anim Sci* 70, 1116.
15. Ward JM, Cockcroft VB, Lunt G *et al.* (1990) Methyllycaconitine: A selective probe for neuronal α-bungarotoxin binding sites. *FEBS Lett* 270, 45.

Dendroaspis angusticeps Toxins

Frank Bretschneider
Albert C. Ludolph

NEUROTOXICITY RATING

Clinical

A Neuromuscular transmission syndrome

Experimental

A Muscarinic receptor toxins

A Neuronal potassium channel blocker

Dendroaspis angusticeps, East African green mamba or eastern green mamba (family, Elapidae), is a long (6–8 ft) and very slender bright-green tree snake. It is often confused with the rear-fanged boomslang and harmless green bush snakes. It differs from the black mamba, the only other mamba in its range, by its color and the light color of the inside of its mouth. It is found in a narrow range in the forests and bushy country of East Africa from Kenya southward to South Africa (southern Natal, northeastern Cape Provence), and on the island of Zanzibar. Identified toxins in *D. angusticeps* are dendrotoxins (DTx), fasciculins, and muscarinic toxins (MTx).

Humans bitten by *Dendroaspis* (mamba) initially develop slight pain and local swelling. "Preparalytic symptoms" follow; they include headache, pain and tenderness of local lymph nodes, vomiting, abdominal pain, and sweating. Slight ptosis or impaired ocular movements herald the paralytic phase and are followed by bulbar symptoms and respiratory weakness. Apnea and unconsciousness develop within 30–60 min if the dose of the venom is large (6).

The main active fraction of the venom responsible for the effect on neuromuscular transmission is dendrotoxin (6, 14–16). The fraction of the venom responsible for the prolonged generalized muscle fasciculations in injected mice contains fasciculins (31,44). There is a third group of unique toxins, muscarinic toxins, that bind exclusively to muscarinic cholinergic receptors (1,2).

Dendrotoxins

The group of DTx includes more than seven polypeptides from *D. angusticeps* (α, β, γ, δ), *D. viridis*, and *D. polylepis*. They consist of 59- to 61-amino-acid residues in single polypeptide chains containing three to five intramolecular disulfide bonds. DTx have been shown to block K⁺ channels and have protease activity. They are active in the nanomolar range and have high-affinity binding sites in the brain. They have little effect with systemic administration, but toxicity increases 10,000-fold by injection into the brain. DTx induce repetitive firing of neurons and also en-

hance transmitter release by increasing the amplitude of end-plate potentials. DTx specifically block neuronal K⁺ channels in motor nerve terminals and in neurons (6,13,35,41). DTx have been employed as CNS probes to distinguish and localize several K⁺ channel subtypes (4,28,46) and to characterize neuronal K⁺ channel proteins (39,47), and have allowed the purification of K⁺ channels from mammalian brain (27,30).

Fasciculins

Fasciculins from *D. angusticeps* (two), *D. polylepis*, and *D. viridis* (one) are 61-amino-acid residue polypeptides cross-linked by four disulfide bridges (8,31). Fasciculins, in particular fasciculin-2 (former toxin F7 from *D. angusticeps*), act as competitive inhibitors of acetylcholinesterase (3,6,37,41,44). The two fasciculins of *D. angusticeps* differ only by a single amino acid (tyrosine-47 instead of asparagine) (7) (*see also* Fasciculins, this volume).

Muscarinic Toxins

Two toxins (MTx1, MTx2) bind to muscarinic cholinergic receptors; their MWs are about 7000 and they each contain 65 amino acids (1,20). The subtypes bind to different muscarinic receptors (21,40). The MTx1 and MTx2 toxins have an agonist-like action (18,20), whereas the m1 toxin from the same snake is an antagonist (25). Twelve MTx from venoms of green and black mambas have been isolated. They have 60%–90% sequence identity with each other, and are similar to many (about 180) other snake venom components, such as α-neurotoxins (which bind to nicotinic acetylcholine receptors), cardiotoxins (which increase permeability of membranes), and fasciculins (which inhibit acetylcholinesterases, *vide supra*). In contrast to α-neurotoxins, MTx do not bind to nicotinic acetylcholine receptors, nor do they inhibit acetylcholinesterase (2,10,21–23,25,42). Muscarinic acetylcholine receptors are found in the CNS and peripherally [regulation of smooth muscle tone, heart rate, several secretions, motor and sensory modulation, arousal (5,17,26)], which explains the large number of potential effects of MTx (32). The MTx are useful experimentally as selective muscarinic ligands (45).

Following subcutaneous administration, elapine venoms appear in the blood of monkeys within 15 min. Peak levels are reached within an hour (6).

DTx from *D. angusticeps* injected intraperitoneally into mice caused hypersensitivity to sound and touch (22), and complex stereotyped behavior including biting, head nodding, and rearing. DTx cross the blood-brain barrier and affect the limbic system (33,34). When DTx are injected intraventricularly into rat brain, they induce pronounced, fatal seizures. Seizures reflect an overall elevation of neuronal activity, including facilitated release of both excitatory and inhibitory transmitters, which can be explained, at least in part, by a selective block of different voltage-dependent K^+ channels (9,11,29,36,43). Intrastriatal injection of α-DTx produces an increased turnover of monoamines in rats (34).

A gel-filtration-purified (fasciculin) fraction of *D. angusticeps* venom produces hypersensitivity to touch and, later, long-lasting fasciculations in mice; that is, uncontrolled muscle twitches, salivation, lacrimation, and secretion from the nose (31). Studies of neuromuscular junctions of fasciculin-injected mice demonstrates the anticholinesterase activity of fasciculins with increasing amplitude and duration of end-plate potentials (3,24). Injection of MTx1 and MTx2 into dorsal hippocampus of rats immediately after training of an inhibitory avoidance task improves memory consolidation, as does oxitremorine. This improvement is antagonized by the muscarinic antagonist scopolamine (19).

It is suggested that these toxins have a synergistic action and cause the lethal effects of green mamba venom (38). DTx, MTx, and fasciculins have a common structural motif: a core, containing mostly four disulfide bridges, from which three loops ("three-fingered" toxin family) protrude like the central fingers of a hand (12,48). The structure of the central core is conserved, but the orientation of the fingers can vary considerably.

The principal effect of the venom of *D. angusticeps* is potentiation and prolongation of the action of acetylcholine. Fasciculins cause signs of neuromuscular block, as well as signs of central respiratory failure by inhibition of cholinesterase. DTx facilitate neuromuscular transmission by increase of acetylcholine quantal release after nerve stimulation because of their blocking effect on presynaptic K^+ channel subtypes, thereby depolarizing nerve terminals. It is unclear if the muscarinic toxins contribute to the toxicity of the venom.

REFERENCES

1. Adem A, Jolkkonen M, Bogdanovic N *et al.* (1997) Localization of M1 muscarinic receptors in rat brain using selective muscarinic toxin-1. *Brain Res Bull* **44**, 597.
2. Adem A, Karlsson E (1985) Mamba venom toxins that bind to muscarinic cholinergic receptors. *Toxicon* **23**, 551.
3. Anderson AJ, Harvey AL, Mbugua PM (1985) Effects of fasciculin 2, an anticholinesterase polypeptide from green mamba venom, on neuromuscular transmission in mouse diaphragm preparations. *Neurosci Lett* **54**, 123.
4. Bidard JN, Mourre C, Gandolfo G *et al.* (1989) Analogies and differences in the mode of action and properties of binding sites (localization and mutual interactions) of two K^+ channel toxins, MCD peptide and dendrotoxin I. *Brain Res* **495**, 45.
5. Brown HJ (1989) *The Muscarinic Receptors*. The Humana Press, Clifton, New Jersey.
6. Campbell CH (1995) Snake bite and snake venoms: Their effects on the nervous system. In: *Handbook of Clinical Neurology*. de Wolff FA ed. Elsevier Science BV, Amsterdam p. 177.
7. Cervenansky C, Engstrom A, Karlsson E (1995) Role of arginine residues for the activity of fasciculin. *Eur J Biochem* **229**, 270.
8. Cervenansky CF, Dajas F, Harvey AL, Karlsson E (1991) Fasciculins, anticholinesterase toxins from mamba venoms: Biochemistry and pharmacology. In: *Snake Toxins*. Harvey AL ed. Pergamon Press, New York p. 303.
9. Dolly J, Halliwell J, Black J *et al.* (1984) Botulinum neurotoxin and dendrotoxin as probes for studies on transmitter release. *J Physiol* **79**, 280.
10. Ducancel F, Rowan EG, Cassar E *et al.* (1991) Amino acid sequence of a muscarinic toxin deduced from the cDNA nucleotide sequence. *Toxicon* **29**, 516.
11. Halliwell JV, Othman IB, Pelchen-Matthews A, Dolly JO (1986) Central action of dendrotoxin: Selective reduction of a transient K^+ conductance in hippocampus and binding to localized acceptors. *Proc Nat Acad Sci USA* **83**, 493.
12. Harel M, Kleywegt GJ, Ravelli RB *et al.* (1995) Crystal structure of an acetylcholinesterase-fasciculin complex: Interaction of a three-fingered toxin from snake venom with its target. *Structure* **15**, 1355.
13. Harvey AL (1990) K^+ channel toxins. *Int Rev Neurobiol* **32**, 207.
14. Harvey AL, Andersson AJ, Mgubua PM, Karlsson E (1984) Toxins from mamba venoms that facilitate transmitter release. *J Toxicol-Toxin Rev* **3**, 91.
15. Harvey AL, Karlsson E (1979) Dendrotoxin from the green mamba, *Dendroaspis angusticeps*: A new type of snake venom neurotoxin. *Toxicon* **17**, 69.
16. Harvey AL, Karlsson E (1980) Dendrotoxin from the venom of the green mamba, *Dendroaspis angusticeps*. *Naunyn-Schmied Arch Pharmacol* **312**, 1.
17. Hulme EC, Birdsall NJM, Buckley NJ (1990) Muscarinic receptor subtypes. *Ann Rev Pharmacol Toxicol* **30**, 633.
18. Jerusalinsky D, Harvey AL (1994) Toxins from mamba venoms; small proteins with selectivities for different subtypes of muscarinic acetylcholine receptors. *Trends Pharmacol Sci* **15**, 424.
19. Jerusalinsky D, Kornisiuk E, Bernabeu R *et al.* (1995)

Muscarinic toxins from the venom of *Dendroaspis* snakes with agonist-like actions. *Toxicon* **33**, 389.

20. Jolkkonen M, Adem A, Hellman U *et al.* (1995) A snake toxin against muscarinic acetylcholine receptors: Amino acid sequence, subtype specificity and effect on guinea-pig ileum. *Toxicon* **33**, 399.

21. Jolkkonen M, Van-Giersbergen PL, Hellman U *et al.* (1995) Muscarinic toxins from the black mamba *Dendroaspis polylepis*. *Eur J Biochem* **234**, 579.

22. Karlsson E, Jolkkonen M, Sataypan M *et al.* (1994) Protein toxins that bind to muscarinic acetylcholine receptors. *Ann N Y Acad Sci* **710**, 153.

23. Karlsson E, Risinger C, Jolkkonen M *et al.* (1991) Amino acid sequence of a snake venom toxin that bind to muscarinic acetylcholine receptor. *Toxicon* **29**, 521.

24. Lee CY, Lee SY, Chen YM (1986) A study on the cause of death produced by angusticeps-type toxin F7 isolated from eastern green mamba venom. *Toxicon* **24**, 33.

25. Max SI, Liang JS, Potter LT (1993) Purification and properties of m1-toxin, a specific antagonist of m1 muscarinic receptors. *J Neurosci* **13**, 4293.

26. Nathanson NM (1987) Molecular properties of the muscarinic acetylcholine receptor. *Annu Rev Neurosci* **10**, 195.

27. Parcej DN, Dolly JO (1989) Dendrotoxin acceptor from bovine synaptic plasma membranes. *Biochem J* **257**, 899.

28. Pelchen-Matthews A, Dolly JO (1989) Distribution in the rat central nervous system of acceptor sub-types for dendrotoxin, a K$^+$ channel probe. *Neuroscience* **29**, 347.

29. Penner R, Peterson M, Pierau F-K, Dreyer F (1986) Dendrotoxin: A selective blocker of a non-inactivating potassium current in guinea-pig dorsal root ganglion neurones. *Pflugers Arch* **407**, 365.

30. Rehm H, Lazdunski M (1988) Purification and subunit structure of a putative K$^+$-channel protein identified by its binding properties for dendrotoxin I. *Proc Nat Acad Sci USA* **85**, 4919.

31. Rodriquez-Ithurralde D, Silveira R, Barbeito L, Dajas F (1983) Fasciculin, a powerful anticholinesterase polypeptide from *Dendroaspis angusticeps* venom. *Neurochem Int* **5**, 267.

32. Segelas I, Roumestand C, Zinn-Justin S *et al.* (1995) Solution structure of a green mamba toxin that activates muscarinic acetylcholine receptors, as studied by nuclear magnetic resonance and molecular modeling. *Biochemistry* **34**, 1248.

33. Silveira R, Barbeito L, Dajas F (1988) Behavioral and neurochemical effects of intraperitoneally injected dendrotoxin. *Toxicon* **26**, 287.

34. Silveira R, Siciliano J, Abo V *et al.* (1988) Intrastriatal

dendrotoxin injection: Behavioral and neurochemical effects. *Toxicon* **26**, 1009.

35. Smith LA, Olson MA, Lafaye PJ, Dolly JO (1995) Cloning and expression of mamba toxins. *Toxicon* **33**, 459.

36. Stansfeld CE, Marsh SJ, Parcej DN *et al.* (1987) Mast cell degranulation peptide and dendrotoxin selectivity inhibit a fast activating potassium current and bind to common neuronal proteins. *Neuroscience* **23**, 893.

37. Strydom DJ (1976) Snake venom toxins. Purification and properties of low-molecular weight polypeptides of *Dendroaspis polylepis* (black mamba) venom. *Eur J Biochem* **69**, 169.

38. Strydom DJ, Botes DP (1970) Snake venom toxins. I. Preliminary studies on the separation of toxins of Elapidae venoms. *Toxicon* **8**, 203.

39. Stuhmer W, Ruppersberg JP, Schroter KH *et al.* (1989) Molecular basis of functional diversity of voltage-gated potassium channels in mammalian brain. *EMBO J* **8**, 3235.

40. Toomela T, Jolkkonen M, Rinken A *et al.* (1994) Two-step binding of green mamba toxin to muscarinic acetylcholine receptor. *FEBS Lett* **352**, 95.

41. Tu AA (1995) Neurotoxins from snake venoms. In: *Handbook of Neurotoxicology*. Chang LW, Dyer LW II eds. Marcel Dekker, New York p. 637.

42. Vandermeers A, Vandermeers-Piret MC, Rathe J *et al.* (1995) Purification and sequence determination of a new muscarinic toxin (MT4) from the venom of the green mamba (*Dendroaspis angusticeps*). *Toxicon* **33**, 1171.

43. Velluti JC, Caputi A, Macadar O (1987) Limbic epilepsy induced in the rat by dendrotoxin, a polypeptide isolated from the green mamba (*Dendroaspis angusticeps*) venom. *Toxicon* **25**, 649.

44. Viljoen CC, Botes DP (1973) Snake venom toxins: The purification and amino acid sequence of toxin VII from *Dendroaspis angusticeps* venom. *J Biol Chem* **248**, 4915.

45. Waelbroeck M, De Neef P, Domenach V *et al.* (1996) Binding of the labelled muscarinic toxin ^{125}I-MT1 to rat brain muscarinic M1 receptors. *Eur J Biochem* **305**, 187.

46. Wang FC, Bell N, Reid P *et al.* (1999) Identification of residues in dendrotoxin K responsible for its discrimination between neuronal K$^+$ channels containing Kv1.1 and 1.2 alpha subunits. *Eur J Biochem* **263**, 222.

47. Wang FC, Parcej DN, Dolly JO (1999) Alpha subunit compositions of Kv1.1-containing K$^+$ channel subtypes fractionated from rat brain using dendrotoxins. *Eur J Biochem* **263**, 230.

48. Wonnacott SM, Dajas F (1994) Neurotoxins: Nature's untapped bounty. *Trends Pharmacol Sci* **15**, 1.

20,25-Diazacholesterol

Jorge N. Larocca

20,25-DIAZOCHOLESTEROL
$C_{25}H_{44}N_2O$

$(3\beta,17\beta)$-17-[[3-(Dimethylamino)propyl]-methylamino]androst-5-en-3-ol

NEUROTOXICITY RATING

Clinical

A Myopathy (myotonic)

Experimental

A Myopathy (myotonic)

20,25-Diazacholesterol (DAC), a cholesterol analog, was developed as an anticholesterolemic agent (6). The compound inhibits several steps of the cholesterol biosynthetic pathway (17). Early studies showed that DAC effectively reduced serum cholesterol in humans and laboratory animals (17,24,27). Prolonged treatment with this drug produced myotonia in patients and precluded its continued clinical use (1,24,27).

Studies performed in normal and hypercholesterolemic rats demonstrated that oral or parenteral administration of DAC, 0.2–2.0 mg/kg/day for 9 days, resulted in a marked reduction of the serum cholesterol level, caused by inhibition of hepatic cholesterol synthesis (17).

Daily subcutaneous injections of DAC (0.15 mg/kg, during 25 days) induced myotonia in developing and adult rats (16). Administration of single high doses of DAC (200 mg/kg, administrated orally) also produced myotonia (7). Morphological abnormalities, such as changes of fiber outlines, numerous "moth-eaten" fibers, and rare ring fibers were observed in both fast and slow muscles of rats treated with DAC (5). Evaluation of extensor digitorum longus of myotonic animals revealed moderate hypotrophy of type I and type II fibers, with an increase in the numbers of type I and type III and a parallel decrease of type II fibers (5).

Biochemical analysis of muscle from DAC-treated rats revealed a reduction in cholesterol level, an increase in the amount of desmosterol (16), and a reduction in the total

level of phospholipids (14,15). Studies performed with plasma membranes isolated from muscles of DAC-treated rats showed changes of enzymatic activities related to ion transport, including reduction of Na^+,K^+-adenosine triphosphatase (ATPase) activity (14). In addition, the Ca^{2+}-dependent ATPase and Ca^{2+}-transport activities were reduced in sarcoplasmic reticulum (21). DAC caused a large decrease in Cl^- conductance (19), which produced an increase in the total membrane resistance. The Na^+ permeability was also reduced (7).

DAC reduces the synthesis of cholesterol in the brain (25). Biochemical analysis of the brains of rats treated with DAC (30–60 mg/kg/day, for 15–32 days) revealed a massive accumulation of desmosterol (25), and the presence of a minor sterol component tentatively identified as 5,7,24-cholestatriene-3-ol. Histological studies of these animals showed osmiophilic inclusions in the cytoplasm of cortical neurons and, to a lesser extent, of oligodendrocytes (25). Treatment of rats with DAC also produced a delay in the formation of myelin (8), and myelin isolated from these animals showed a marked accumulation of desmosterol (8). In addition, it was shown that treatment of retinal explants with DAC inhibited neurite outgrowth (11). This effect was overcome by addition of mevalonolactone, but not cholesterol, to the culture medium (11).

Mice treated with DAC (30–60 mg/kg/day, for 6–9 weeks) developed a generalized scaling disorder. Total stratum corneum sterol content was markedly decreased, and topical or systemic repletion with cholesterol corrected the scaling abnormalities (26).

A single administration of DAC in high dosage (100 mg/kg) or treatment with SC-12397 at 10 or 30 mg/kg for 10 days caused spermatogenesis inhibition without affecting accessory organ function in rats (23).

Treatment of hypercholesterolemic patients with DAC (25–50 mg/day) produced a marked and sustained fall in serum cholesterol (1,24,27). After approximately 5 months, 80% of treated subjects showed muscle cramping and, in a smaller group, muscle weakness (27). Electromyography (EMG) disclosed myotonia in 96% of cases (1,27). Abnormal EMG was observed in asymptomatic patients (27). In addition, approximately 20% of the subjects developed a palmoplantar keratoderma (1). Associated with the myotonia and reduced levels of cholesterol in serum was the appearance of desmosterol in sera, erythrocyte membranes and muscles (24,27). Muscle biopsies from patients with muscle weakness revealed histological changes compatible with myopathy (27). Following cessation of DAC treatment, symptoms disappeared, usually within 2 months, and follow-up EMGs within 3–7 months were normal (1,24,27).

It is highly probable that DAC toxicity is associated with its ability to inhibit cholesterol synthesis. The molecular mechanisms that cause myotonia are not fully understood. However, it is known that DAC inhibits several steps of the cholesterol biosynthetic pathway, including formation of mevalonate and conversion of desmosterol to cholesterol (17). Since the DAC-dependent accumulation of desmosterol leads to an increase in membrane fluidity (4), it was proposed that DAC-induced myotonia is caused by an increase in the membrane fluidity (4). Indeed, evidence indicated that some of the biochemical alterations observed in the muscle of DAC-treated animals can be the result of changes in the membrane fluidity (3,4,22).

It is noteworthy that mevalonate is also used for the synthesis of isoprenoid metabolites (20). Posttranslational modification of protein by isoprenyl groups is necessary for their intracellular localization and biological activities (12,2). Interestingly, the monomeric and trimeric guanosine 5′-triphosphatase-binding proteins are isoprenylated (12,13). These proteins regulate important cellular processes including cell growth (10), cell differentiation (4), transduction of extracellular signals (9), membrane formation, and cytoskeletal organization (10). Since DAC inhibits the formation of mevalonate, it is possible that DAC toxicity is in part due to deficient protein isoprenylation. This hypothesis is supported by the fact that DAC inhibition of neurite outgrowth can be reversed by increasing the levels of mevalonate, but not by the addition of cholesterol (11). Furthermore, DAC disrupts processes that involve isoprenylated proteins, such as the coupling of the β-adrenergic receptor with the adenylate cyclase second-messenger system (18).

REFERENCES

1. Anderson PC, Mart JM (1965) Myotonia and keratoderma induced by 20,25 diazacholesterol. *Arch Dermatol* **92**, 181.
2. Bourne HR, Sanders DA, McCormick F (1991) The GTPase superfamily: Conserved structure and molecular mechanism. *Nature* **349**, 117.
3. Butterfield DA, Chesnut DB, Roses AD, Appel SH (1976) Electron spin label study of erythrocyte membrane fluidity in myotonic and Duchenne muscular dystrophy and congenital myotonia. *Nature* **263**, 159.
4. Butterfield DA, Watson WE (1976) Electron spin resonance studies of an animal model of human congenital myotonia. *J Membrane Biol* **32**, 165.
5. Caccia MR, Parvis VP, Brambillia M, Diffidenti D (1979) A histological and histochemical study of changes of fiber types in experimental myotonia. *J Neurol* **220**, 131.
6. Counsell RE, Klimstra PD, Ranney RE (1962) Hypocholesterolemic agents. III. *N*-Methyl-*N*-(dialkylamino)alkyl-17β-aminoandrost-5-en-3β-ol derivatives. *J Med Pharm Chem* **5**, 1224.
7. DeCoursey TE, Bryant SH, Owenburg KM (1981) Dependence of membrane potential on extracellular ionic concentrations in myotonic goats and rats. *Amer J Physiol* **240**, C56.
8. Fumagalli R, Smith ME, Urna G, Paoletti R (1969) The effect of hypocholesteremic agents on myelinogenesis. *J Neurochem* **16**, 1329.
9. Gilman AG (1987) G proteins: Transducers of receptor-generated signals. *Ann Rev Biochem* **56**, 615.
10. Hall A (1990) The cellular functions of small GTP-binding proteins. *Science* **249**, 653.
11. Heacock AM, Klinger PD, Seguin EB, Agranoff BW (1984) Cholesterol synthesis and nerve regeneration. *J Neurochem* **42**, 987.
12. Maltese WA (1990) Posttranslational modification of proteins by isoprenoids in mammalian cells. *FASEB J* **4**, 3319.
13. Maltese WA, Sheridan KM, Repko EM, Erdman RA (1990) Post- translational modification of low molecular mass GTP-binding proteins by isoprenoid. *J Biol Chem* **265**, 2148.
14. Niebroj-Dobosz I, Kwiecinski H, Mrozck K (1976) Plasma membranes of muscle in experimental myotonia in rats. *J Neurol* **213**, 353.
15. Niebroj-Dobosz I, Kwiecinski H, Mrozek K, Szymanowski S (1976) Sarcoplasmic reticulum in experimental myotonia in rats. *J Neurol* **213**, 361.
16. Ramsey RB, McGarry JD, Fischer VW, Sarnat HB (1978) Alteration of developing and adult rat muscle membranes by zuclomiphene and other hypochelsterolemic agents. *Acta Neuropathol* **44**, 15.
17. Ranney RE, Cook DL (1965) The hypocholesterolemic action of 20,25-diazacholesterol. *Arch Int Pharmacodyn* **1**, 154.
18. Reddy NB, Askanas V, Oliver KL et al. (1982) Biochemical and morphological effects of 20,25-diazacholesterol on cultured muscle cells. *Biochem Pharm* **31**, 91.
19. Rudel R, Senges J (1972) Mammalian skeletal muscle reduced chloride conductance in drug-induced myotonia and induction of myotonia by low-chloride solution. *Naunyn-Schmied Arch Pharmacol* **274**, 337.
20. Rudney H, Sexton RC (1986) Regulation of cholesterol biosynthesis. *Annu Rev Nutr* **6**, 245.
21. Salviati G, Biasia E, Betto R, Danieli Betto D (1986) Fast to slow transition induced by experimental myotonia in rat ED muscle. *Pflugers Arch* **406**, 266.
22. Singer SJ (1971) The molecular organization of biological membranes. In: *Structure and Function of Biological Membranes*. Rothfield LI ed. Academic Press, New York p. 145.

23. Sinha Hikim AP, Chakraborty J (1986) Effects of diazacholesterol dihydrochloride (SC-12937), an avian antifertility agent, on rat testis. *J Androl* 7, 277.

24. Somers JE, Winer N (1964) Reversible myopathy and myotonia following administration of a hypocholesterolemic agent. *Neurology* 16, 761.

25. Suzuki K, Zagoren JC, Chen SM, Suzuki K (1974) Effects of triparanol and 20,25-diazacholesterol in CNS of rat:

26. Williams ML, Feingold KR, Grubauer G, Elias PM (1987) Ichthyosis induced by cholesterol-lowering drugs. *Arch Dermatol* 123, 1535.

27. Winer N, Martt JM, Somers JE *et al.* (1964) Induced myotonia in man and goat. *J Lab Clin Med* 64, 1019.

Morphological and biochemical studies. *Acta Neuropathol* 29, 141.

Dichloroacetic Acid

Peter S. Spencer

DICHLOROACETIC ACID
$C_2H_2Cl_2O_2$

Bichloracetic acid; Dichlorethanoic acid

NEUROTOXICITY RATING

Clinical

A Peripheral neuropathy

Experimental

A CNS demyelination

Dichloroacetic acid (DCAA) was used in the experimental treatment of diabetes mellitus and hyperlipoproteinemia until chronic oral administration was shown to be neurotoxic to humans (16). More recent therapeutic interest has centered on DCAA's ability to reduce lactic acid levels in experimental stroke injury (7,8) and in human mitochondrial disease (18). Diisopopylamine DCAA was also a component of a product sold in the United States as "vitamin B_{15}" or "pangamic acid," materials with variable formulations that were offered as a method of improving physical activity by minimizing lactate buildup during exercise. The potential toxicity of pangamic acid has been highlighted (9); it was apparently withdrawn from U.S. health-food stores *ca.* 1980.

Dichloroacetic acid is a water-miscible liquid with a pungent odor; its BP is 193°–194°C (5). Diisopopylamine DCAA is a solid that dissociates in water into diisopropylamine and DCAA (9). Chloroacetic acids are produced in drinking water as a result of disinfection, and they are metabolites of widely used halogenated hydrocarbons (3).

DCAA prevents the phosphorylation of pyruvate dehydrogenase complex (PDHC) by blocking the action of pyruvate dehydrogenase kinase (PDHK); this increases PDHC activity, stimulates glucose oxidation and reduces lactate production. In mitochondrial fractions of rat brain, heart, or liver, DCAA inhibited phosphate incorporation into the α-subunit of PDHC and the autophosphorylation of succinyl coenzyme A (CoA) synthetase (1,19); it also inhibited PDHK and increased active PDHC in rat brain slices (1,2). DCAA did not affect succinate- or adenosine triphosphate (ATP)–supported mitochondrial accumulation of calcium (4). Intraperitoneal administration of DCAA to starved rats increased the percentage of the active form of the PDHC in brain, liver, and muscle, while significantly lowering lactate and glucose concentrations in brain and blood (10). DCAA activated cerebral PDHC and improved recovery following reperfusion in animal models of ischemia (8,12).

The oral LD_{50} for rats is 2.82 g/kg body weight. DCAA lowers blood lactate and glucose levels in suckling rats (20). Intravenous administration of DCAA to 20- to 25-day-old rats markedly increased rates of glucose utilization and decreased lactate levels in all brain regions tested; there were no significant changes in ATP, creatine phosphate, or glycogen (11). DCAA reduced postischemic neuronal damage in the gerbil (7) and promoted recovery of spinal cord function after aortic occlusion (13).

Intravenous administration of DCAA to rats (up to 250 mg/kg for 38 days) and dogs (up to 100 mg/kg for 30 days) produced no demonstrable adverse effects (17). Subchronic (90-day) oral administration of mono-, di- (DCAA), and trichloroacetic acids at less than or equivalent to 0.25 times the LD_{50} dose per day produced variable changes in the lung (perivenular inflammation) and liver (enlarged portal triads and veins; bile duct proliferation; fibrosis) in all three groups. Testicular atrophy was noted in animals treated with DCAA (3) or 2-chloropropionate (20). Focal vacuolation and gliosis were present in the forebrain and brainstem of animals treated with DCAA but not in animals given mono- or trichloroacetic acid (3). "Oral administration for 90 consecutive days to rats in doses of 125, 500 and 2000 mg/kg body weight produced hind-limb paralysis, germinal epithelium degeneration of the testes, and vacuolation of the myelinated white tracts of the cerebrum" (17). Drug withdrawal was associated with functional recovery over a 4-week period. "In dogs receiving oral doses of 50, 75 and 100 mg/kg of dichloracetate for 13 consecutive weeks, hind-limb muscular weakness, testicular epithelial degeneration and vacuolation of Leydig cells and of both cerebral and cerebellar myelinated white tracts were among the changes observed" (17). Some animals developed ocular lesions consisting of bilateral lenticular opacities (irreversible), bulbar conjunctivitis, superficial corneal vascularization, and a tendency to keratoconjunctivitis sicca. Oral treatment of rats with 2 g/kg/day DCAA resulted in development (one animal) of transverse myelopathy in the upper thoracic region. Cross-sections of the myelopathic region revealed primary demyelination of the entire white matter, save the dorsal columns. Remyelination of denuded lengths of spinal axons had occurred during the period of treatment; this was accomplished both by oligodendrocytes and by Schwann cells that had invaded the cord lesion. Gray matter vacuolation was also evident. Spinal roots were normal (14).

Early DCAA treatment of patients with cerebrovascular disease has been considered. DCAA has been used with some therapeutic success in Leigh's syndrome and other mitochondrial disorders (6,18). In diabetes mellitus, DCAA stimulates peripheral glucose utilization and inhibits gluconeogenesis (16). In hyperlipidemic states, DCAA decreases circulating lipid and lipoprotein levels by decreasing lipogenesis and cholesterolgenesis (16). Mild sedation may be noted during DCAA therapy (16). Prolonged treatment with DCAA has been associated with a reversible peripheral neuropathy that reportedly may be related to thiamine deficiency and ameliorated or prevented by thiamine supplementation (15). Peripheral neuropathy developed in a 21-year-old patient with severe homozygous familial hypercholesterolemia who received an oral (daily?) dose of 50 mg/kg DCAA for 16 weeks; it resolved after discontinuation of drug therapy. The neurological picture was characterized by weakness of facial, finger, and lower-extremity muscles; diminished deep-tendon reflexes; and reduced nerve conduction velocity. Visual-field and slit-lamp examination yielded normal results (17).

REFERENCES

1. Abemayor E, Kovachich GB, Haugaard N (1984) Effects of dichloracetate on brain pyruvate dehydrogenase. *J Neurochem* 42, 38.

2. Baudry M, Kessler M, Smith EK, Lynch G (1982) The regulation of pyruvate dehydrogenase activity in rat hippocampal slices: Effect of dichloracetate. *Neurosci Lett* 31, 41.

3. Bhat HL, Kanz MF, Campbell GA, Ansari GA (1991) Ninety day toxicity study of chloroacetic acids in rats. *Fund Appl Toxicol* 17, 240.

4. Browning M, Baudry M, Bennett WF, Lynch G (1981) Phosphorylation-mediated changes in pyruvate dehydrogenase activity influence pyruvate-supported calcium accumulation by brain mitochondria. *J Neurochem* 36, 1932.

5. Budavari S (1996) *The Merck Index. 12th Ed.* Merck & Co. Whitehouse Stn, New Jersey p. 6167.

6. DeStefano N, Matthews PM, Ford B (1995) Short-term dichloroacetate treatment improves indices of cerebral metabolism in patients with mitochondrial disorders. *Neurology* 45, 1193.

7. Dimlich RV, Marangos RJ (1994) Dichloracetate attenuates neuronal damages in a gerbil model of brain ischemia. *J Mol Neurosci* 5, 69.

8. Dimlich RV, Nielsen MM (1992) Facilitating postischemic reduction of cerebral lactate in rats. *Stroke* 23, 1145.

9. Herbert V (1982) Pangamic acid ("Vitamin B_{15}"). In: *Nutrition Cultism, Facts and Fictions*. Herbert V ed. George F. Stickley, Philadelphia p. 107.

10. Kuroda Y, Toshima K, Watanabe T *et al.* (1984) Effects of dichloroacetate on pyruvate metabolism in rat brain *in vivo*. *Pediat Res* 18, 936.

11. Miller AL, Hatch JP, Prihoda TJ (1990) Dichloroacetate increases glucose use and decreases lactate in developing rat brain. *Metab Brain Dis* 5, 195.

12. Peeling J, Sutherland G, Brown RA, Curry S (1996) Protective effect of dichloroacetate in a rat model of forebrain ischemia. *Neurosci Lett* 208, 21.

13. Robertson CS, Goodman JC, Grossman RG, Priessman A (1990) Reduction in spinal cord postischemic lactic acidosis and functional improvement with dichloroacetate. *J Neurotrauma* 7, 1.

14. Spencer PS, Schaumburg HH (1985) Organic solvent neurotoxicity. *Scand J Work Environ Health* 11 (Suppl 1), 53.

15. Stacpoole PW (1989) The pharmacology of dichloroacetate. *Metab Clin Exp* 38, 1124.

16. Stacpoole PW, Moore GW, Kornhauser DM (1978) Metabolic effects of dichloroacetate in patients with diabetes mellitus and hyperlipoproteinemia. *N Engl J Med* 298, 526.

17. Stacpoole PW, Moore GW, Kornhauser DM (1979) Toxicity of chronic dichloroacetate. *N Engl J Med* 300, 372

18. Takanishi J, Sugita K, Tanabe Y *et al.* (1996) Dichloroacetate treatment in Leigh syndrome caused by mitochondrial DNA mutation. *J Neurol Sci* 145, 83.

19. Yang J, Smith RA (1983) The effect of dichloracetate on the phosphorylation of mitochondrial proteins. *Biochem Biophys Res Commun* **111**, 1054.

20. Yount EA, Fekten SY, O'Connor *et al.* (1982) Comparison of the metabolic and toxic effects of 2-chloropropionate and dichloracetate. *J Pharmacol Exp Ther* **222**, 501.

Dichloroacetylene

Herbert H. Schaumburg

$$Cl - C \equiv C - Cl$$

DICHLOROACETYLENE

$$C_2Cl_2$$

NEUROTOXICITY RATING

Clinical

A Cranial neuropathy

B Acute encephalopathy

C Peripheral neuropathy

Experimental

B Cranial neuropathy

Dichloroacetylene (DCA) is a noncommercial, undesired product of the dehydrochlorination of trichloroethylene (TCE). DCA is generated from exposure of TCE vapor to soda lime in closed, rebreathing general anesthesia machines and to alkali in closed submarines. It can be formed from exposure of TCE liquid to caustics in degreasing tanks. DCA is also an unwanted by-product in the synthesis of vinylidine chloride. Acute exposure to DCA can cause cranial nerve dysfunction; it appears likely that the trigeminal neuropathy widely attributed to TCE is secondary to DCA exposure.

Experimental animal studies in rats indicate two metabolic pathways are operative in DCA metabolism (8). Cytochrome P-450–dependent oxidation represents a minor pathway, accounting for the formation of 1,1-dichloro compounds after chlorine migration. The major pathway is the biosynthesis of toxic glutathione conjugates. Organ-specific toxicity and carcinogenicity may be due to the topographical distribution of γ-glutamyl transpeptidase (9).

The major systemic toxic effect in experimental animals (rabbits) is renal tubular necrosis, following a single 6-h inhalation exposure of 17 ppm (10). Renal tumors, cystadenomas and cystadenocarcinomas, appeared after 18-month exposures of rats and mice to levels of 9 ppm (12).

Two unconvincing experimental animal studies also claim trigeminal neuropathy from exposure to DCA. A recent experimental study exposed rats to DCA or to TCE and measured the trigeminal nerve somatosensory evoked potential (TNSEP) as a measure of dysfunction (1). The group of six rats exposed one time to 300 ppm of DCA displayed reduction in TNSEP amplitude and slowing of conduction velocity. Rats exposed to TCE experienced no alteration in TNSEP, nor did control animals. None of the animals displayed histopathological changes in the trigeminal ganglia. Rabbits received inhalation exposure for 1 h at levels up to 307 ppm and subsequently displayed impaired corneal and facial sensation. Postmortem examination of immersion formaldehyde-fixed brain and cranial nerve tissue revealed pyknotic change in trigeminal neurons and axonal fragmentation (11). Rats given 17 mg/kg orally for 10 weeks were perfused with glutaraldehyde, and teased fiber analysis of the trigeminal nerve showed reduction in internodal length and mean fiber diameter. Fiber degeneration was not observed, and neither the trigeminal nucleus nor axonal morphology were examined in this study (2).

There have been many reports of variably reversible trigeminal neuropathy following short-term high-level anesthetic or industrial inhalation exposure to TCE; sometimes there has been an association with orofacial herpes. In every instance, the exposure has occurred in association with heat and caustic or soda-lime chemicals, and it is widely held that these so-called instances of TCE neurotoxicity actually reflect the effects of DCA.

Severe industrial exposures to TCE have been followed by dysfunction in the facial, oculomotor, and optic nerves with limited recovery (3,5). An especially well-documented case of multiple cranial neuropathy after massive 5-min industrial exposure to TCE has been followed for 12 years (5,6). The patient was giddy following exposure but did not lose consciousness. Ten hours later, he developed nausea, vomiting, and numbness of the face, mouth, and oropharynx accompanied by facial and jaw muscle weakness (5). On examination, he appeared passive and easily confused and had the following findings: pupillary inequality, constricted visual fields, bifacial paralysis, and anesthesia to all modalities in the entire trigeminal distribution. There followed gradual recovery of vision and facial strength and robust improvement in facial sensation over the following 18 months. Eighteen years later, there remained slight abnormalities of sensation over the snout and malar areas;

neuropsychological testing indicated mild cognitive dysfunction (6).

There is one meticulous postmortem study of a male who died 51 days following industrial exposure to TCE. He was one of four individuals cleaning a tank, all of whom were affected to a degree proportionate to their duration of TCE exposure; three displayed cranial neuropathy (3). The subject spent 4 h in the tank and became giddy and ataxic. Within 2 days, he developed diplopia, facial numbness, and weakness; by day 8, he could barely speak. He eventually displayed facial diplegia and inability to speak or swallow; death was from pneumonia. At postmortem, there was severe axonal loss in the trigeminal nerves and nerve cell loss in the spinal and main sensory nuclei (the trigeminal ganglion was unavailable). Lesser degrees of neuronal degeneration were present in facial, abducens, and vestibular nuclei, and in the nucleus of the tractus solitarius.

There are two reports of facial numbness following documented (by analysis) environmental exposure to DCA. The first describes two individuals, meticulously documented by neurologists, exposed to a mixture of mono- and dichloroacetylene; both experienced nausea and vomiting 6 h following exposure and were admitted to the hospital. One subject displayed trigeminal and abducens dysfunction; the other, trigeminal and glossopharyngeal deficits (7). Both individuals experienced the onset of paresthesias and loss of sensation in the trigeminal nerve distribution within 12 h of inhalation exposure, and displayed abnormalities on blink reflex studies. Neither showed significant improvement in facial hypesthesia 4 months following exposure. The other report describes military personnel who developed facial numbness after accidental exposure to DCA in the ambient atmosphere in a mock-up of a space capsule and others in a submarine (13).

The pathophysiology of DCA cranial neuropathy is obscure. It is suggested that the human clinical data are compatible with a demyelinating neuropathy, but the autopsy study suggests a neuronal effect. The frequent association of orofacial herpes has suggested that some findings may stem from reactivation of the virus (4).

REFERENCES

1. Albee RR, Nitschke KD, Mattsson JL, Stebbins KE (1997) Dichloroacetylene: Effect on the rat trigeminal nerve somatosensory evoked potential. *Neurotoxicol Teratol* **19**, 27.
2. Barret L, Torch S, Leray CL *et al.* (1992) Morphometric and biochemical studies in trigeminal nerve of rat after trichloroethylene or dichloroacetylene oral administration. *Neurotoxicology* **13**, 601.
3. Buxton PH, Hayward M (1967) Polyneuritis cranialis associated with industrial trichloroethylene poisoning. *J Neurol Neurosurg Psychiat* **30**, 511.
4. Cavanagh JB, Buxton PH (1989) Trichloroethylene cranial neuropathy: Is it really a toxic neuropathy or does it activate latent herpes virus? *J Neurol Neurosurg Psychiat* **52**, 297.
5. Feldman RG, Mayer RM, Taub A (1970) Evidence for peripheral neurotoxic effect of trichloroethylene. *Neurology* **20**, 599.
6. Feldman RG, White RF, Currie JN *et al.* (1985) Long-term follow-up after single toxic exposure to trichloroethylene. *Amer J Ind Med* **8**, 119.
7. Henschler D, Broser F, Hopf HC (1970) 'Polyneuritis cranialis' following poisoning with chlorinated acetylenes while handling vinylidene chloride copolymers. *Arch Toxicol* **26**, 62.
8. Kanhai W, Dekant W, Henschler D (1989) Metabolism of the nephrotoxin dichloracetylene by glutathione conjugation. *Chem Res Toxicol* **2**, 51.
9. Kanhai W, Koob M, Dekant W, Henschler D (1991) Metabolism of ^{14}C-dichloroethylene in rats. *Xenobiotica* **21**, 905.
10. Reichert D, Henschler D, Bannasch P (1978) Nephrotoxic and hepatotoxic effects of dichloroacetylene. *Food Cosmet Toxicol* **16**, 227.
11. Reichert D, Liebaldt G, Henschler D (1976) Neurotoxic effects of dichloroacetylene. *Arch Toxicol* **37**, 23.
12. Reichert D, Spengler U, Romen W, Henschler D (1984) Carcinogenicity of dichloroacetylene: An inhalation study. *Carcinogenesis* **5**, 1411.
13. Saunders RA (1967) A new hazard in closed environmental atmospheres. *Arch Environ Health* **14**, 380.

Dichlorodiphenyltrichloroethane and Derivatives

Peter Spencer
Herbert H. Schaumburg

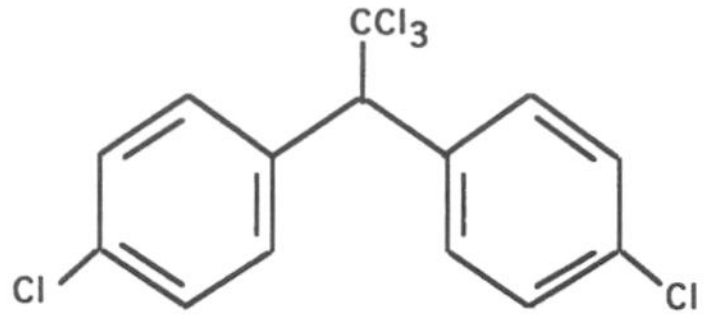

$$CCl_3$$

p,p'-DDT
$C_{14}H_9Cl_5$

1,1,1-Trichloro-2,2-bis(p-chlorophenyl)ethane; 1,1-Bis(4-chlorophenyl)-2,2,2-trichloroethane; 1,1'-(2,2,2-Trichloroethylidene)bis[4-chlorobenzene]; Chlorophenothane; Dicophane; Dichlorophenyltrichloroethane; p,p'-DDT; DDT

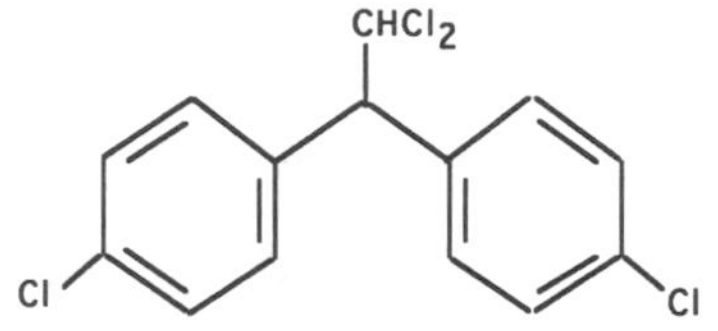

$$CHCl_2$$

p,p'-DDD
$C_{14}H_{10}Cl_4$

1,1-Dichloro-2,2-bis(p-chlorophenyl)ethane; TDE, p,p'-DDD

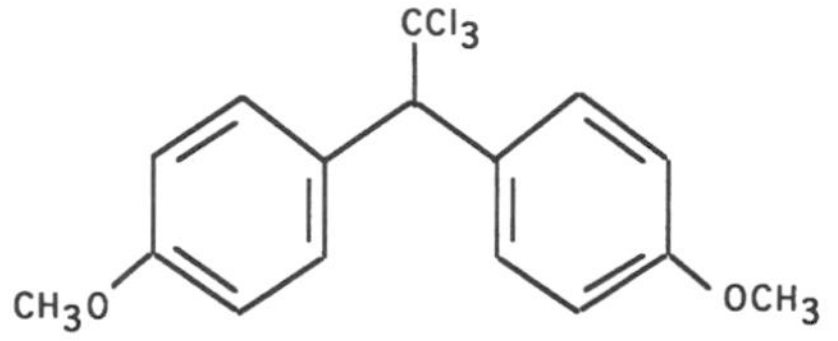

$$CCl_3$$

DMDT
$C_{16}H_{15}Cl_3O_2$

1,1,1-Trichloro-2,2-bis(p-methoxyphenyl)ethane; Dianisyltrichloroethane; DMDT; Methoxychlor

NEUROTOXICITY RATING (technical DDT)

Clinical

A Ion channel syndrome (paresthesias)

A Seizure disorder (myoclonus, generalized rarely)

A Tremor

C Peripheral neuropathy

Experimental

A Ion channel dysfunction (sodium ion)

A Seizure disorder

A Tremor

The insecticidal properties of 1,1,1-trichloro-2,2-bis(p-chlorophenyl) ethane (p,p'-DDT), which were discovered in 1939 and heavily exploited in medicine and agriculture since that time, have played an important role in worldwide human health promotion and disease prevention (41). The public health importance of DDT became apparent in 1944 when DDT dusting of 1.3 million civilians successfully arrested a major outbreak of typhus for the first time in history (5,6). DDT and chlorinated cyclodiene insecticides were massively deployed during World War II to kill mosquitoes that serve as vectors of diseases such as malaria, dengue fever, and filariasis. Public health programs in tropical regions of the world continue to use DDT for the control of malaria and in human de-lousing programs for the control of typhus (15,36). o,p-DDD (mitotane), which reduces adrenocorticotrophic hormone–stimulated glucocorticoid secretion, is used in human and veterinary medicine to treat Cushing's syndrome and inoperable adrenal carcinoma (73).

DDT and other organochlorine insecticides have also been used in vast quantities and with great effect to control a wide variety of insect pests in agriculture, forestry, and construction. Use of DDT in the United States increased rapidly until 1959 and then declined in association with growing evidence of the environmental persistence, bioconcentration, and biomagnification of the chemical and its metabolites in various food chains (20,73). Avian and other wildlife species were found to have body burdens of dichlorodiphenylethanes that were linked to changes in their reproductive success, the subject of a recent critical review (60). From the early 1970s, usage of organochlorine insecticides was progressively restricted to specific applications and then phased out in many countries. Use of DDT was banned in Sweden in 1969 and in the United States in 1972; it continues to be used in agriculture in less-developed parts of the world (73).

DDT and DDD, the primary environmental degradation product of DDT, are tasteless, crystalline solids with MPs of 109°C; that of methoxychlor is 69°C. Both DDD and DDT are stable compounds that break down slowly under ambient conditions. Methoxychlor undergoes environmental dechlorination more rapidly. The vapor pressure of DDT is 1.5×10^{-7} mm Hg at 20°C. DDT is soluble in most organic solvents; water solubility is extremely low (2 ppb). Technical DDT, a waxy solid, contains both the p,p' isomer (ca. 70%) and the o,p-isomer of DDT (34).

Methoxychlor is rapidly metabolized by O-dealkylation and P-450–mediated hydroxylation; consequently, there is little deposition of the parent compound in fat. Metabolism of p,p'-DDT is slow and complex, and there is heavy deposition in adipose and other fatty tissues (51). The major metabolic routes of p,p'-DDT are (a) oxidation to form water-soluble isomers of 2,2-bis(p-chlorophenyl)acetic acid (DDA), which are readily excreted in conjugated form in urine; (b) dehydrochlorination to 1,1-dichloro-2,2-bis(4-chlorophenyl) ethane (p,p'-DDE), and (c) reductive dechlorination to DDD, which is excreted or metabolized to DDA (73). DDA occurs in urine in concentrations of 1–2 ppm in workers exposed to 15–35 mg/day DDT (37,48).

DDT and DDE are highly lipophilic compounds that accumulate in adipose tissue where they reside for prolonged periods. DDT is found in other tissues, including the brain (52). The biological half-life DDT in human fat is reported as 3.4 years (59). DDE which, relative to DDT, increases in concentration with time, may persist for decades (25,51). Hundreds of parts per million of total DDT have been found in adipose tissue of workers engaged in the manufacture, formulation, or use of DDT; one healthy worker reportedly had a level of 1131 ppm (DDT, 648 ppm; DDE, 437 ppm) (27). Much lower concentrations are found in the general population. Levels of total DDT-related compounds in body fat of U.S. citizens increased from ca. 5 ppm in 1950 to ca. 16 ppm in 1955–56; levels decreased to about 8 ppm in 1970 and 3 ppm in 1980. Less than 2 ppm of total DDT-derived material was detectable in human adipose tissue in 1990 (50,51,54). The amount of DDT stored in tissues is gradually reduced if exposure to the compound is discontinued or diminished. DDT and metabolites are excreted in urine, bile, and milk (up to 10 ppm) (51). Reports in 1997–98 continued to document DDT and/or DDE contamination of human or bovine milk in various parts of the world (3,11,17,30,67,68). A 1989 report noted serum concentrations of p,p-DDE (1–379 ppb) in 99.5% of 5994 residents of the United States (53).

Organochlorine insecticides influence their own metabolism in species-specific manners. In rodents, DDT induces microsomal enzymes and associated morphological changes in liver cells. DDT promotes its own metabolism in the hamster but not in the mouse or squirrel monkey (10,23). Dogs store more DDT and less dieldrin when the compounds are given together instead of individually (16). DDT suppresses storage of dieldrin or heptachlor in rats (9,49,55,56). Hexachlorobenzene reduces storage of aldrin but increases storage of DDT and mirex (13). Storage of DDT in guinea pigs is decreased by co-exposure to dieldrin (66).

Acute Toxic Effects

The rat dermal LD_{50} for DDT is 2500 mg/kg; the oral LD_{50}s are 113 mg/kg for DDT and DDD and 5000 mg/kg for methoxychlor. Susceptibility to acute toxicity of DDT is greater in young than old animals, and in fasted relative to well-fed animals. Starvation results in mobilization of fat residues, deposition in brain, and neurotoxic signs (14,58). Insects and fish are very sensitive to DDT. Among mammals, susceptibility increases roughly in the following order: goat, sheep, pig, monkey, dog, cat, rat, mouse. Birds and humans are comparatively resistant to the acute neurotoxic effects of DDT (34).

Acute toxic effects result from the direct action of DDT or methoxychlor on the nervous system of animals. Insects display incoordination, ataxia, tremulous movements of the legs, and death or recovery (34). Rats and rabbits initially display increased respiration, hyperexcitability, increased spontaneous activity, and increased responses to stimuli; as intoxication advances, blepharospasm, hyperreflexia, and twitching of ears and vibrissae occur, with massive myoclonic jerks that can be antagonized by agents that increase brain serotonin levels (12,34,73). Intention tremor is prominent during voluntary movement; in rats it may persist for up to several days and result in hyperthermia. Convulsive seizures appear at later stages. However, both acute and long-term exposure of rats results in anticonvulsant effects, as demonstrated by changes in the duration of phases of maximal electroshock seizures, notably decreased during tonic hindlimb extensions (70,71).

Cats develop a condition akin to status epilepticus. Death occurs by ventricular fibrillation or respiratory failure (34). Cats, dogs, and monkeys develop tremors that spread from the neck to the body, myoclonic jerks follow sensory stimulation of attempts to move, convulsions occur abruptly, status epilepticus prevails, a coma-like status ensues, and death supervenes. The acute toxic effects of DDT in several species are attenuated by intravenous injection of calcium, as is the action of DDT on isolated preparations of rat nerve and muscle (21). Glucose given to animals before or after an LD_{33} dosage of DDT reduced convulsions and mortality (35).

Chronic intoxication may be associated with loss of weight, anorexia, mild anemia, muscular weakness, and tremors; high exposure levels trigger convulsive episodes followed by muscular weakness, paralysis, coma, and death (22,38). Accompanying changes include hepatic centrolobular necrosis, fatty degeneration of renal tubular epithelium, and focal necrosis of cardiac and skeletal muscle (34). Specific CNS pathology has not been reported save in one study of heavily dosed dogs (180–150 mg/kg/day in peanut oil) who displayed severe tremor and ataxia, but no observed convulsive seizures, and cerebellar degeneration perhaps consistent with hypoxia.

Human Studies

Human dermal and respiratory absorption of DDT is low. Oral doses are well absorbed. Controlled studies show that a single oral dose of <250 mg has little or no clinical effect. Variable hyperesthesia of the mouth is reported after an oral dose of 250–1000 ppm in oil solution. At 750 ppm, gait becomes unsteady and, at the peak time of reaction (6 h after dosing), subjects report malaise and have cold moist skin, normal reflexes, and hypersensitivity to contact. Doubling this dose causes paresthesias of the tongue and around the mouth and nose within 2.5 h of dosing. Subjects report dizziness, are confused, and develop tremor of the extremities; the peak reaction occurs at 10 h after ingestion and is characterized by malaise, headache, fatigue, and vomiting. Neurological examination at the height of symptoms reveals slight nystagmus, variable abnormalities in perception of touch and heat in the distribution of the trigeminal nerve, tremor in all extremities, and inability to stand on one leg for any length of time. Complete recovery occurs within 24 h of ingestion (64,65).

These experimental observations are consistent with estimates of the relation between dose and effect gleaned from accidental and other exposures. Available data suggest that a single dose of 10 mg/kg produces nonconvulsive illness in some subjects; dosages up to 20 mg/kg may be tolerated with little effect or result in convulsions; and dosages up to 285 mg/kg may not prove fatal (51). The lowest reported dose introduced by any route over any given period of time that resulted in death is 50 mg/kg for DDT, 500 mg/kg for DDD, and 6430 mg/kg for methoxychlor (24). Small, repeated doses (0.36–0.61 mg/kg/day) of technical DDT in food for up to 18 or 21 months produced no symptoms and no neurological signs either during treatment or up to 27 months thereafter (26,27).

Clinical manifestations of DDT poisoning begin 0.5–6.0 h after exposure and are heralded by hyperesthesia followed by paresthesias of the mouth, lower part of the face, and tongue. This is followed by objective disturbance of equilibrium, paresthesias and tremor of the extremities, confusion, malaise, headache, fatigue, and delayed vomiting. Recovery occurs within 24 h. Recovery takes place over several days in severe poisoning when convulsions have occurred. Residual weakness and ataxia of the hands has been reported 5 weeks after ingestion (51).

Chronic exposure to DDT is reportedly characterized by loss of weight, anorexia, mild anemia, muscular weakness, and tremors. Anxiety, nervous tension, hyperexcitability, and fear are common symptoms. Myoclonic jerks and generalized seizures may occur. Electroencephalography may reveal sharp waves, excessive theta waves, spike-and-wave complexes, and low-voltage, rhythmic spikes; these are reported to occur in the absence of clinically evident abnormality (40).

Extensive dermal and respiratory exposure to DDT in occupational settings has generally not resulted in neurological illness (51). Dermatitis, irritability, and fatigue noted on occasion have been attributed to dermal and inhalation exposure to the DDT vehicle kerosene. Factory workers exposed to air concentrations of 500–4200 mg/m^3 or higher have developed illness characterized by extremity paresthesias, headache, dizziness, and tremor of tongue and hands (2,8). Visuomotor functions were found to be significantly depressed in Indian DDT sprayers with 8.5 times higher DDT levels than controls (42). Other studies of workers have reported various clinical manifestations that are difficult to relate to the known effects of DDT (51). DDT has been linked unconvincingly to sensorimotor and predominantly motor neuropathies in subjects exposed to a variety of substances (34).

Serious neurological and neuropsychological side effects have been claimed following prolonged therapeutic use of mitotane (o,p'-DDD) for the treatment of adrenocortical carcinoma and Cushing's syndrome (4,19). Twelve patients treated for 9 years developed neurological manifestations (19) that were listed as depression, memory impairment, peripheral neuropathy VIIIth nerve symptoms, dysarthria, ataxia, Parkinson's disease, and confusion (18).

There is no specific treatment for DDT poisoning. Animal studies indicate that sedatives, ionic calcium, and glucose (or other energy source) might be useful. Diazepam has been suggested (51).

Toxic Mechanisms

DDT interferes with the movement of sodium ions across excitable membranes, which is required for the formation of an action potential (29). Voltage-clamp studies suggest that voltage-sensitive sodium channels are retained in the open state for prolonged periods, thereby disrupting normal propagation of the action potential (26,44–46). Single-channel studies reveal a prolonged open time of sodium channels (44). Whereas p,p'-DDT acts as a Na$^+$ channel opener, p,p'-hydroxy-DDT rapidly blocks the sodium channel. DDT appears to bind to a pyrethroid-binding site on the sodium channel. Phenytoin, which reduces repetitive firing by acting on Na$^+$ channels, reduces the tremor and hyperexcitability induced by p,p'-DDT and permethrin (28,57). DDT stimulates brain protein kinase C (PKC) activity, and both DDT and pyrethroids promote PKC-induced phosphorylation of the α-subunit of the sodium channel (32,43). DDT reportedly may induce hyperexcitability by inhibition of Ca^{2+}-dependent and Na$^+$,K$^+$-

adenosine triphosphatase (39). It is unclear whether various changes in CNS neurotransmitters and receptors are primary or secondary effects of DDT (31,51,73). Unlike the convulsant organochlorine insecticides (lindane, cyclodienes, toxaphene), p,p'-DDT does not appear to enhance synaptic activity by antagonism of the action of γ-aminobutyric acid (GABA) at the GABA$_A$ receptor (73).

Increased axonal excitability appears to be the primary mechanism by which DDT perturbs the functional integrity of the nervous system. By interfering with ionic conductance in excitable membranes, DDT prolongs the duration of the recovery phase of the action potential, increases the excitability of the nerve to stimulation, and thereby induces repetitive axonal discharges to stimuli that normally elicit a single response. While all levels of the neuraxis are potentially impacted by DDT, certain regions may be more exposed to the agent or more sensitive to its action. Function of peripheral sensory nerve fibers of rats and other species appears to be perturbed to a greater extent than motor fibers (1,61–63). Hyperreflexia and tremor seem to arise segmentally in the spinal cord, and to be modified by enhanced suprasegmental input. Seizures are associated with a widespread increase in CNS excitability, but the cerebral cortex appears to have a dominant role in the initiation and maintenance of convulsive activity (34). DDT has a direct effect on the rat cerebellum by potentiating responses evoked by auditory and visual stimuli (33,69,72).

DDT isomers bind to the estrogen receptor and are weakly estrogenic. The hierarchy of receptor binding is o,p'-DDT > o,p'-DDD > o,p'-DDE > methoxychlor > p,p'-DDT > p,p'-DDD and p,p'-DDE are inactive at this site (47). o,p'-DDT induces synthesis of functional progesterone receptors in the rat hypothalamus and pituitary gland (7).

REFERENCES

1. Akkermans LMA, van der Bercken J, Verluijs-Helder M (1975) Comparative effects of DDT, allethrin, dieldrin and aldrin-transdiol on sense organs of *Xenopus laevis*. *Pestic Biochem Physiol* **5**, 451.

2. Aleksieva T, Vasilev G, Spasovski M (1959) Study of the toxic effects of DDT. *J Hyg Epidemiol Microbiol Immunol* **5**, 8. [Russian]

3. Al-Saleh I, Echeverria-Quevedo A, Al-Dgaither S, Faris R (1998) Residue levels of organochlorinated insecticides in breast milk: A preliminary report from Al-Kharj, Saudi Arabia. *J Environ Pathol Toxicol Oncol* **17**, 37.

4. Bollen E, Lanser JB (1992) Reversible mental deterioration and neurological disturbances with o,p'-DDD therapy. *Clin Neurol Neurosurg* **94** (Suppl), S49.

5. Brooks GT (1974) *Chlorinated Insecticides. Vol 1.* CRC Press, Boca Raton, Florida.

6. Brooks GT (1974) *Chlorinated Insecticides Vol 2. Biological and Environmental Aspects.* CRC Press, Boca Raton, Florida.

7. Brown TJ, Blaustein JD (1984) 1-(o-Chlorophenyl)-1-(p-chlorophenyl)-2,2,2-trichlorethane induces functional progestin receptors in the rat hypothalamus and pituitary gland. *Endocrinology* **115**, 2052.

8. Burkatzkaya EN, Voitenko GA, Krasniuk EP (1961) Working conditions and health status of workers at DDT production plants. *Gig Sanit* **26**, 17. [Russian]

9. Chadwick RW, Cranmer MF, Peoples AJ (1971) Comparative stimulation of gamma-HCH metabolism by treatment of rats with gamma-HCH, DDT, and DDT + gamma-HCH. *Toxicol Appl Pharmacol* **18**, 685.

10. Chadwick RW, Cranmer MF, Peoples AJ (1971) Metabolic alterations in the squirrel monkey induced by DDT administration and ascorbic acid deficiency. *Toxicol Appl Pharmacol* **20**, 308.

11. Chikuni O, Nhachi CF, Nyazema NZ *et al.* (1997) Assessment of environmental pollution by PCBs, DDT and its metabolites using human milk of mothers in Zimbabwe. *Sci Total Environ* **199**, 183.

12. Chung Hwang E, Van Woert M (1978) p,p'-DDT-induced neurotoxic syndrome: Experimental myoclonus. *Neurology* **18**, 1020.

13. Clark DE, Ivie GW, Camp BJ (1981) Effects of dietary hexachlorobenzene or *in vivo* biotransformation, residue deposition, and elimination of certain xenobiotics by rats. *J Agric Food Chem* **29**, 600.

14. Clark DR Jr, Prouty RM (1977) Experimental feeding of DDE and PCB to female big brown bats (*Eptesicus fuscus*). *J Toxicol Environ Health* **2**, 917.

15. Coulston F (1985) Reconsideration of the dilemma of DDT for the establishment of an acceptable daily intake. *Regul Toxicol Pharmacol* **5**, 332.

16. Deichmann WB, MacDonald WE, Cubit DA (1971) DDT tissue retention: Sudden rise induced by the addition of aldrin to a fixed DDT intake. *Science* **172**, 275.

17. Dua VK, Pant CS, Sharma VP (1997) HCH and DDT residues in human and bovine milk at Hardwar, India. *Indian J Malariol* **34**, 126.

18. Dukes MNG (1992) *Meyler's Side Effects of Drugs. An Encyclopedia of Adverse Reactions and Interactions. 12th Ed.* Elsevier, Amsterdam p. 1112.

19. Du Rostu H, Krempf M, Mussini JM *et al.* (1987) Neurotoxicity of mitotane therapy of adrenocortical carcinoma (5 cases) and Cushing's syndrome (7 cases). *Presse Med* **16**, 951.

20. Ecobichon DJ (1996) Toxic effects of pesticides. In: *Casarett & Doull's Toxicology. The Basic Science of Poisons. 5th Ed.* Klaassen CD ed. McGraw Hill, New York p. 641.

21. Eyzaguirre C, Lilienthal JL Jr (1981) Veratrinic effects of pentamethylenetetrazol (Metrazol) and 2,2-bis(p-chlorophenyl)-1,1,1-trichloroethane (DDT) on mamma-

lian neuromuscular function. *Proc Soc Exp Biol Med* **70**, 272.

22. Fitzhugh OG, Nelson AA (1947) The chronic oral toxicity of DDT (2,2-bis(*p*-chlorophenyl)1,1,1-trichloroethane). *J Pharmacol Exp Ther* **89**, 18.

23. Gingell R, Wallcave L (1974) Species differences in the acute toxicity and tissue distribution of DDT in mice and hamsters. *Toxicol Appl Pharmacol* **28**, 385.

24. Hayes WJ Jr (1963) *Clinical Handbook on Economic Poisons*. Public Health Services Publ. No 476. U.S. Government Printing Office, Washington, DC p. 144.

25. Hayes WJ Jr (1982) *Pesticides Studied in Man*. Williams & Wilkins, Baltimore p. 172.

26. Hayes WJ Jr, Dale WE, Pirkle C (1971) Evidence of safety of long-term, high, oral doses of DDT for man. *Arch Environ Health* **22**, 119.

27. Hayes WJ Jr, Durham WF, Cueto C Jr (1956) The effect of known repeated oral doses of chlorophenothane (DDT) in man. *J Amer Med Assn* **162**, 890.

28. Herr DW, Hong JS, Tilson HA (1985) DDT-induced tremor in rats: Effects of pharmacological agents. *Psychopharmacology* **86**, 426.

29. Hille B (1968) Pharmacological modifications of the sodium channels of frog nerve. *J Gen Physiol* **51**, 199.

30. Hooper K, Hopper K, Petreas MX *et al.* (1997) Analysis of breast milk to assess exposure to chlorinated contaminants in Kazakstan: PCBs and organochlorine pesticides in southern Kazakstan. *Environ Health Perspect* **105**, 1250.

31. Hrdina PD, Singhal RL, Peters DAV, Ling GM (1973) Some neurochemical alterations during acute DDT poisoning. *Toxicol Appl Pharmacol* **25**, 276.

32. Ishikawa Y, Charalambous P, Matsumura F (1989) Modification by pyrethroids and DDT of phosphorylation activities of rat brain sodium channel. *Biochem Pharmacol* **38**, 2449.

33. Joy RM (1973) Electrical correlates of preconvulsive and convulsive doses of chlorinated hydrocarbon insecticides in the CNS. *Neuropharmacology* **12**, 63.

34. Joy RM (1982) Chlorinated hydrocarbon insecticides. In: *Pesticides and Neurological Diseases*. Ecobichon DF, Joy RM eds. CRC Press, Boca Raton, Florida p. 91.

35. Koster R (1947) Differentiation of gluconate, glucose, calcium, and insulin effect on DDT poisoning in cats. *Fed Proc Fed Amer Soc Exp Biol* **6**, 346.

36. Kutz FW, Wood PH, Bottimore DP (1991) Organochlorine pesticides and polychlorinated biphenyls in human adipose tissue. *Rev Environ Contam Toxicol* **120**, 1.

37. Laws ER Jr, Maddrey WD, Curley A, Burse VW (1973) Long-term occupational exposure to DDT. *Arch Environ Health* **27**, 318.

38. Lillie RD, Smith MI, Stohlman EF (1947) Pathologic action of DDT and certain analogs and derivatives. *Arch Pathol* **43**, 127.

39. Matsumura F, Ghiasuddin SM (1979) Characteristics of DDT-sensitive Ca-ATPase in the axonic membrane. In: *Neurotoxicology of Insecticides and Pheromones*. Narashashi T ed. Plenum Press, New York p. 245.

40. Mayersdorf A, Israeli R (1974) Toxic effects of chlorinated hydrocarbon insecticides on the human electroencephalogram. *Arch Environ Health* **28**, 159.

41. Metcalfe RL (1973) A century of DDT. *J Agric Chem* **21**, 511.

42. Misra UK, Nag D, Murti CR (1984) A study of cognitive functions in DDT sprayers. *Indian Health* **22**, 199.

43. Moser GL, Smart RC (1989) Hepatic tumor-promoting chlorinated hydrocarbons stimulate protein kinase C activity. *Carcinogenesis* **10**, 851.

44. Narahashi T (1992) Nerve membrane Na^+ channels as targets of insecticides. *Trends Pharmaceut Sci* **13**, 236.

45. Narahashi T (1994) Role of ion channels in neurotoxicity. In: *Principles of Neurotoxicology*. Chang L ed. Marcel Dekker, New York p. 609.

46. Narahashi T, Haas HG (1968) Interaction of DDT with the components of lobster nerve membrane conductance. *J Gen Physiol* **51**, 178.

47. Nelson JA (1974) Effects of DDT analogues and PCB mixtures on 17β-3H-estradiol binding to rat uterine receptor. *Biochem Pharmacol* **23**, 447.

48. Ortelee MF (1958) Study of men with prolonged intensive occupational exposure to DDT. *Arch Ind Health* **18**, 433.

49. Pearl W, Kupfer D (1972) Stimulation of dieldrin elimination by a thiouracil derivative and DDT in the rat: Enhancement of dieldrin oxidative metabolism? *Chem-Biol Interact* **4**, 91.

50. Redetzke KA, Applegate HG (1993) Organochlorine pesticides in adipose tissue of persons from El Paso, Texas. *J Environ Health* **56**, 25.

51. Smith AG (1991) Chlorinated hydrocarbon insecticides. In: *Handbook of Pesticide Toxicology. Vol 2. Classes of Pesticides*. Hayes WJ Jr, Laws ER Jr eds. Academic Press, San Diego p. 731.

52. Smith MI, Stohlman EF (1944) The pharmacologic action of 2,2-bis(*p*-chlorophenyl)-1,1,1-trichloroethane and its estimation in the tissues and body fluids. *Public Health Rep* **59**, 984.

53. Stehr-Green PA (1989) Demographic and seasonal influences on human pesticide residue levels. *J Toxicol Environ Health* **27**, 405.

54. Stevens MF, Ebell GF, Psaila-Savona P (1993) Organochlorine pesticides in Western Australia nursing mothers. *Med J Aust* **158**, 238.

55. Street JC, Chadwick RW, Wang M, Phillips RL (1966) Insecticide interactions affecting residue storage in animal tissues. *J Agric Food Chem* **14**, 545.

56. Street JC, Wang M, Blau AD (1966) Drug effects on dieldrin storage in rat tissue. *Bull Environ Contam Toxicol* **1**, 6.

57. Tilson HA, Hong JS, Mactutus CF (1985) Effects of 5,5-

diphenylhydantoin (phenytoin) on neurobehavioral toxicity of organochlorine insecticides and permethrin. *J Pharmacol Exp Ther* **233**, 285.

58. To-Figueras J, Gomez-Catalan J, Rodamilans M, Corbella J (1988) Mobilization of stored hexachlorobenzene and *p,p*-dichlorodiphenyldichloroethylene during partial starvation in rats. *Toxicol Lett* **42**, 79.

59. Tordoir WF, van Sittert NJ (1994) Organochlorines. *Toxicology* **91**, 51.

60. Tyler CR, Jobling S, Sumpter JP (1998) Endocrine disruption in wildlife: A critical review of the evidence. *Crit Rev Toxicol* **28**, 319.

61. van der Bercken J (1972) The effect of DDT and dieldrin on myelinated nerve fibers. *Eur J Pharmacol* **20**, 205.

62. van der Bercken J, Akkermans LMA (1971) Negative temperature coefficient of the action of DDT in a sense organ. *Eur J Pharmacol* **16**, 241.

63. van der Bercken J, Akkermans LMA, van Langen RG (1973) The effect of DDT and dieldrin on skeletal muscle fibers. *Eur J Pharmacol* **21**, 89.

64. Velbinger HH (1947) Contribution on the toxicology of "DDT"—active substances of dichlorodiphenyltrichloromethylmethane. *Pharmazie* **2**, 268. [German]

65. Velbinger HH (1947) Question of "DDT"—toxicity for humans. *Deut Gesundheitswes* **2**, 355. [German].

66. Wagstaff DJ, Street JC (1971) Antagonism of DDT storage in guinea pigs by dietary dieldrin. *Bull Environ Contam Toxicol* **6**, 273.

67. Waliszewski SM, Pardio VT, Waliszewski KN *et al.* (1997) Organochlorine residues in cow's milk and butter in Mexico. *Sci Total Environ* **208**, 127.

68. Wong SK, Lee Wo (1997) Survey of organochlorine pesticide residues on milk in Hong Kong (1993–1995). *J AOAC Int* **80**, 1332.

69. Woolley DE (1968) Toxicological and pharmacological studies of visual and auditory potential evoked in the cerebellum of the rat. *Proc West Pharmacol Soc* **11**, 69.

70. Woolley DE (1970) Effects of acute and chronic exposure to DDT and DDT-drug interactions on experimental seizure responses. *Ind Med* **39**, 50.

71. Woolley DE (1970) Effects of DDT and drug-DDT interactions on electroshock seizures in the rat. *Toxicol Appl Pharmacol* **16**, 521.

72. Woolley DE (1976) Some aspects the neurophysiological basis of insecticide action. *Fed Proc* **35**, 2610.

73. Woolley DE (1995) Organochlorine insecticides: Neurotoxicity and mechanisms of action. In: *Handbook of Neurotoxicology*. Chang LW, Dyer DS eds. Marcel Dekker, New York p. 475.

2,4-Dichlorophenoxyacetic Acid

Herbert H. Schaumburg

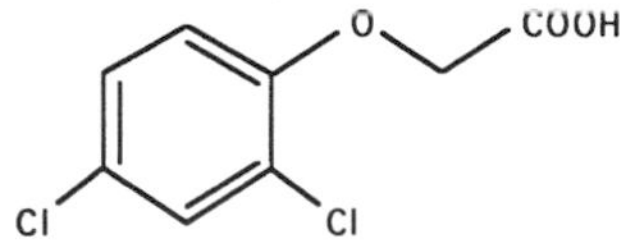

2,4-DICHLOROPHENOXYACETIC ACID
$C_8H_6Cl_2O_3$

2,4-D; Trinoxol

NEUROTOXICITY RATING

Clinical

B   Myopathy

C   Peripheral neuropathy

Experimental

A   Myopathy (myotonic)

2,4-Dichlorophenoxyacetic acid (2,4-D) is one of a group of chlorophenoxy compounds widely used as herbicides. The chlorophenoxy herbicides act as synthetic auxins (plant hormones) that alter the metabolism and enhance the growth of plants. The abnormal growth interferes with the transport of nutrients and destroys the plant. 2,4-D is a component of Agent Orange, a jungle defoliant contaminated with 2,3,7,8-tetrachlorodibenzo-*p*-dioxin (TCDD); its use in South Vietnam attracted considerable attention to this group of substances and blame for a variety of subsequent health problems. Although the chlorophenoxy herbicides act as plant growth hormones, they have no hormonal action in mammals. 2,4-D has long been known to cause myotonia and myonecrosis in experimental animals; isolated case reports of human 2,4-D–related myopathy are convincing; reports of peripheral neuropathy and myotonia are not.

Studies with rats indicate that orally administered 2,4-D is rapidly absorbed and widely distributed; absorption following topical application is much slower, it may take 10 h to reach peak plasma levels (13). Regardless of route of administration, small doses (4 mg/kg) are rapidly excreted; large doses (100 mg/kg) only reach peak concentration 17 h after termination of administration (7). 2,4-D is excreted in the urine unchanged. Several studies indicate a saturable accumulation of 2,4-D by isolated choroid plexus: one suggests that facilitated transport of 2,4-D operates at the cerebrospinal fluid/plasma interface, critically affecting the efficiency of its removal from the CNS (14).

Repeated administration of 2,4-D to rats and rabbits lowers serum cholesterol. Clofibrate, an analog of 2,4-D, is used in human medicine to reduce cholesterol levels. One study suggests that the chlorophenoxy herbicides cause hypolipidemia by enhancing lipid utilization in the liver (25).

Humans receiving intravenous 2,4-D excrete the compound in the urine; almost 100% is eliminated within 2 days. Orally administered 2,4-D is rapidly absorbed, and 76% is excreted in the urine within 4 days (20). Absorption following dermal application is very limited; only 5.8% appears in the urine within 5 days (11). Distribution in humans is widespread following massive doses (suicidal administration). A postmortem report provides the following organ distribution of 2,4-D: muscle (118 ppm), brain (93 ppm), blood (58 ppm), kidney (193 ppm), and liver (408 ppm) (9). This report also describes multifocal perivascular demyelination in the CNS, attributed to 2,4-D; it is more likely secondary to anoxia.

2,4-D intoxication is associated with little systemic toxicity in experimental animals or in humans. Acute occupational inhalation exposure is accompanied by headache, vertigo, and partial loss of the senses of taste and smell. Massive suicidal self-administration causes hypotension, tachycardia, muscle twitching, coma, and sometimes fatal diffuse hepatic necrosis.

Experimental animal studies clearly indicate that 2,4-D produces myotonia following a single dose and myopathy after subacute (3–14 days) administration. It readily evokes myotonia in many mammalian species (10). A singe oral dose of 100 mg/kg causes, in the dog, a clinical and electrophysiological episode of hindlimb myotonic spasm and opisthotonos lasting an hour (22). Three intraperitoneal injections of 200 mg/kg, repeated every 4 h, will maintain a guinea pig in a steady hindlimb myotonic state for 12 h (8). Electrophysiological studies indicate that 2,4-D–induced myotonia is identical to the naturally occurring idiopathic condition in humans and goats.

Repeated administration of 200 mg/kg/day of 2,4-D to rats for intervals up to 14 days causes diffuse weakness, weight loss, and muscle necrosis in one-third of the animals. One study describes myopathy mainly involving myosin of fast muscles, with elevated calcium-activated adenosine triphosphatases and alterations in heavy chains; another reports proliferation of myofilaments in the periphery of myocytes in concert with fiber necrosis (8,18). Myopathic changes are not secondary to myotonia.

Two experimental animal studies, one in the dog and another in rats, have failed to produce peripheral neuropathy following 12 weeks of daily intraperitoneal dosing at levels of 80 mg/kg body weight (22,24).

Four publications describe recent industry-sponsored studies that have assessed the toxic properties of different forms of 2,4-D acid (4–6,16). Male and female Fischer 344 rats treated by gavage with 75 or 250 mg/kg 2,4-D displayed transient (day 1) changes in gait and coordination, and decreased motor activity (16). Dietary treatment for 52 weeks with 150 mg/kg/day produced retinal degeneration in female rats (16). A slight increase in astrocytomas observed (in males only) at 45 mg/kg/day in a previously conducted chronic rat study was not confirmed in animals treated with 150 mg/kg/day (4). Subchronic studies in rats treated with 1–300 mg/kg/day 2,4-D acid, 2,4-D dimethylamine salt, or 2,4-D 2-ethylhexyl ester revealed similar treatment-related decreases in red cell mass, decreases in T3 and T4 levels, decreases in ovary and testes weights, increases in liver, kidney, and thyroid weights, and cataracts and retinal degeneration (high-dose females) (5). Subchronic toxicity studies in dogs treated with 1–7.5 mg/kg/day the diet showed comparable effects with the three compounds, namely reduction in body weight gain and food consumption, and increases in blood urea nitrogen, creatinine and alanine aminotransferase activity (6).

It is claimed that hypomyelination occurs in chicks after fertilized eggs are externally treated with a single dose of 2,4-D (17); this is proposed to reflect damage to oligodendrocytes or their precursors. No morphological data support this assertion.

Human myopathy from 2,4-D is described in one convincing case report (2) of a farmer who accidentally ingested 110 mg/kg of the commercial compound. Immediate nausea, headache, and vomiting was followed, 24 h later, by profound weakness of intercostal muscles, diffuse muscle "fibrillary twitching and irritability," elevated serum enzymes (lactic dehydrogenase, aldolase, creatine kinase, transaminase) reflecting myonecrosis, and myoglobinuria. The farmer gradually recovered but had limb weakness and painful limb muscles for 2 weeks. No signs or symptoms of peripheral neuropathy appeared, and electrodiagnostic studies were not reported.

While myotonia is the most consistent nervous system sign of intoxication in experimental animals, there is only one human report; a 39-year-old man experienced 2 months of weakness and muscle spasms following ingestion of a mixture of 2,4-D and 2-methyl-4-chloro-phenoxyacetic acid (19). The spasms were not characterized as myotonic by electrodiagnosis. Another report of incapacitating myotonia lasting 2 years following topical occupational 2,4-D exposure is implausible (26).

There are four case reports of distal symmetrical predominately motor polyneuropathy following (1 week) isolated dermal contact with 2,4-D (1,12,23,24). It is improbable that these few instances of diffuse neuropathy, following so soon after trivial exposure, represent toxic neuropathy; most likely they are coincidental instances of acute inflammatory demyelinating polyradiculoneuropathy (Guillain Barré syndrome). An epidemiological study of workers exposed to 2,4-D describes minor abnormalities in nerve conduction attributed to a peripheral neuropathy (21); this study is poorly controlled, lacks any environmental analysis, and utilizes unacceptable neurophysiological techniques.

The toxic mechanism underlying 2,4-D myopathy is unclear; it clearly occurs independently of myotonia. It is of interest that clofibrate, a lipid-lowering agent structurally related to 2,4-D, causes a toxic myopathy in humans. Possibly, the myopathy stems from effects on lipid metabolism (25). A myopathic condition, cholesterol-lowering agent myopathy, is caused by several antilipid agents (15).

The proposed biochemical mechanism of 2,4-D–induced myotonia is that 2,4-D enhances the activity of p-nitrophenylphosphatase (p-NPPase) in muscle microsomes; increased activity of p-NPPase increases the passive flux of potassium ions, leading to a compensatory decrease in chloride ions and myotonia (3).

REFERENCES

1. Berkley MC, Magee KR (1963) Neuropathy following exposure to a dimethylamine salt of 2,4-D. *Arch Intern Med* **111**, 351.
2. Berwick P (1970) 2,4-Dichlorophenoxyacetic acid poisoning in man: Some interesting clinical and laboratory findings. *J Amer Med Assn* **214**, 1114.
3. Brody IA (1973) Myotonia induced by monocarboxylic aromatic acids. A possible mechanism. *Arch Neurol* **28**, 243.
4. Charles JM, Bond DM, Jeffries TK *et al.* (1966) Chronic dietary toxicity/oncogenicity studies on 2,4-dichlorophenoxyacetic acid in rodents. *Fundam Appl Toxicol* **33**, 166.
5. Charles JM, Cunny HC, Wilson RD, Bus JS (1996) Comparative subchronic studies on 2,4-dichlorophenoxyacetic acid, amine, and ester in rats. *Fundam Appl Toxicol* **33**, 161.
6. Charles JM, Dalgard DW, Cunny HC *et al.* (1996) Comparative subchronic and chronic dietary toxicity studies on 2,4-dichlorophenoxyacetic acid, amine, and ester in the dog. *Fundam Appl Toxicol* **29**, 78.
7. Clark DE, Young JE, Younger RL *et al.* (1964) The fate of 2,4-dichlorophenoxyacetic acid in sheep. *J Agr Food Chem* **12**, 43.
8. Danon JM, Karpati G, Carpenter S, Wolfe LS (1976) Experimental myotonic myopathy. *Neurology* **26**, 384.
9. Dudley AW Jr, Thapar NT (1972) Fatal human ingestion of 2,4-D, a common herbicide. *Arch Pathol* **94**, 270.
10. Eyzaguirre C, Folk BP, Zierler KL, Lilienthal JL Jr (1948) Experimental myotonia and repetitive phenomena: The veratrinic effects of 2,4-dichlorophenoxyacetate (2,4-D) in the rat. *Amer J Physiol* **55**, 69.
11. Feldmann RJ, Maibach HI (1974) Percutaneous penetration of some pesticides and herbicides in man. *Toxicol Appl Pharmacol* **28**, 126.
12. Goldstein NP, Jones PH, Brown JR (1959) Peripheral neuropathology after exposure to an ester of dichlorophenoxyacetic acid. *J Amer Med Assn* **171**, 1306.
13. Khanna S, Fang SC (1966) Metabolism of C_{14}-labeled 2,4-dichlorophenoxyacetic acid in rats. *J Agr Food Chem* **14**, 500.
14. Kim CS, O'Tuama LA (1981) Choroid plexus transport of 2,4-dichlorophenoxyacetic acid: Interaction with the organic acid carrier. *Brain Res* **224**, 209.
15. London SF, Gross KF, Ringel SP (1991) Cholesterol-lowering agent myopathy (CLAM). *Neurology* **41**, 1159.
16. Mattsson JL, Charles JM, Yano BL *et al.* (1997) Single-dose and chronic dietary neurotoxicity screening studies on 2,4-dichlorophenoxyacetic acid in rats. *Fundam Appl Toxicol* **40**, 111.
17. Mori de Moro G, Duffard R, Evangelista de Duffard AM (1993) Neurotoxicity of 2,4-dichlorophenoxyacetic butyl ester in chick embryos. *Neurochem Res* **18**, 353.
18. Muhlrad A, Friedman M (1978) Myosin changes in experimental 2,4-dichlorophenoxyacetate myopathy. *Muscle Nerve* **1**, 471.
19. Prescott LF, Park J, Darrien L (1979) Treatment of severe 2,4-D and mecrorop intoxication with alkaline diuresis. *Brit J Clin Pharmacol* **7**, 111.
20. Sauerhoff MW, Braun WH, Blau GE, Gehring PJ (1977) The fate of 2,4-dichlorophenoxyacetic acid (2,4-D) following oral administration to man. *Toxicol Appl Pharmacol* **37**, 136.
21. Singer R, Moses M, Valciukas J *et al.* (1982) Nerve conduction velocity studies of workers employed in the manufacture of phenoxy herbicides. *Environ Res* **29**, 297.
22. Steiss JE, Braund KG, Clark EG (1987) Neuromuscular effects of acute 2,4-dichlorophenoxyacetic acid (2,4-D) exposure to dogs. *J Neurol Sci* **78**, 295.
23. Todd RL (1962) A case of 2,4-D intoxication. *J Iowa Med Soc* **52**, 663.
24. Toyoshima E, Mayer RF, Max SR, Eccles C (1985) 2,4-Dichlorophenoxyacetic acid (2,4-D) does not cause polyneuropathy in the rat. *J Neurol Sci* **70**, 225.
25. Vainio H, Linnairmas K, Kahonen M *et al.* (1983) Hyperlipidemia and peroxisome proliferation induced by phenoxyacetic acid herbicides in rats. *Biochem Pharmacol* **32**, 277.
26. Wallis WE, Van Poznak A, Plum F (1970) Generalized muscular stiffness, fasciculations, and myokymia of peripheral nerve origin. *Arch Neurol* **22**, 430.

Dideoxycytidine and Other Nucleoside Analogs

Joseph C. Arezzo

DIDEOXYCYTIDINE
$C_9H_{13}N_3O_3$

DIDEOXYINOSINE
$C_{10}H_{12}N_4O_3$

Zalcitabine (2',3'-dideoxycytidine—ddC)
Didanosine (2',3'-dideoxyinosine—ddI)
Stavudine (2',3'-didehydro-2',3'-dideoxythymidine—d4T)

NEUROTOXICITY RATING

Clinical

A   Peripheral neuropathy

C   Retinopathy

Experimental

A   Inhibition of mitochondrial DNA polymerase

A   Peripheral neuropathy (demyelinating—rabbit; axonal—monkey, rodent)

Antiviral nucleoside analogues (ANAs) are a class of compounds that resemble natural nucleotide bases. When phosphorylated, they compete with endogenous nucleotides for binding to reverse transcriptase and cause termination of viral DNA chain elongation. Thus, they are potent inhibitors of the early phase of both HIV-1 and HIV-2 replication. Their use in patients with acquired immunodeficiency syndrome (AIDS) and AIDS-related complex (ARC) has been associated with rapid suppression of serum p24 antigen levels, reduced infectious human immunodeficiency virus (HIV) titers in mononuclear cells, increases in CD4 cell counts, and in some studies, improvement in the patient's reported quality of life (27,30,33,44). In the past decade, multiple ANAs have been developed and tested *in vivo* and *in vitro*. Three ANAs, zalcitabine (ddC), didanosine (ddI), and stavudine (d4T), are considered here. Each of these compounds has been approved by the U.S. Food and Drug Administration, and each has received widespread clinical use against HIV infection. These ANAs are similar in structure, have a common mechanism of action, and are associated with a remarkably similar neurotoxic profile. Data are presented for zalcitabine, with differences among compounds emphasized when relevant. Zidovudine (AZT) is discussed in a separate section.

General Toxicology

Peak plasma concentrations of ANAs occur 1–2 h following oral administration, with bioavailability in adults ranging from 40%–88% (6,43). Concentration in the cerebrospinal fluid is approximately 20% of that in the plasma in adults, but is variable in children, with levels of stavudine reported as high as 55%. ANAs enter cells by facilitated diffusion *via* nucleoside carriers. In the case of zalcitabine, the compound is first phosphorylated by cellular deoxycytidine kinase to the 5'-monophosphate, and then to the active triphosphate compound (2',3'-dideoxycytidine 5'-triphosphate) (43). The major route of excretion is renal, with approximately 70% of the compounds found unchanged in urine following intravenous dosing. In a limited study in patients with AIDS, clearance of zalcitabine at doses of 0.03–0.3 mg/kg was similar to that reported in normal volunteers. The half-life of zalcitabine is approximately 2 h, but this can be significantly prolonged in patients with impaired renal function.

Recent therapeutic regimens for the treatment of HIV have stressed polypharmacy, combining various ANAs, including AZT and protease inhibitors. Preliminary studies suggest that the pharmacokinetic properties of zalcitabine are not significantly altered by combination with other ANAs, as judged by peak serum concentrations, area under the plasma concentration-time curve, and serum half-life (26). However, a recent study reports that concentrations of didanosine are increased by 50% or more when coadministered with another ANA, ganciclovir (38).

Although the principal toxic insult associated with ANAs, other than AZT, has been peripheral neuropathy (*vide infra*), muscle, pancreas, liver, and heart may also be affected (for review, *see* 23). Pancreatitis has been especially associated with didanosine (18). In clinical trials, largely with HIV-infected subjects, ANA therapy has been associated with peripheral neuropathy, skin rash, anemia, fever, headaches, and insomnia.

Animal Studies

The principal animal model of ANA neurotoxicity is the rabbit. Marked morphological and electrophysiological changes were seen in New Zealand white rabbits treated with zalcitabine for periods up to 18 weeks (2,14). Myelin pathology consisted of severe myelin splitting, intramyelinic edema, myelin folding, and demyelination. Myelin changes were seen in the majority of large-diameter fibers and remyelination was prominent. Axonal changes were less evident and characterized by axonal loss and rare shrunken axons or intraluminal phagocytes replacing axons within myelin sheaths. Changes were present in both sensory and motor fibers, including cells in both the dorsal and ventral spinal roots. The changes were associated with profound reductions in both sensory and motor electrophysiological measures (>30% in velocity, >70% in amplitude). No abnormalities of myelin, axons, or neurons were observed in sections of the cervical, thoracic, or lumbar spinal cord, brainstem at the level of the gracilis nucleus, retina, or brain (2).

In a subsequent study, mitochondrial changes were associated with 35 mg/kg of zalcitabine in the rabbit (13). Pathology consisted of the presence of cup-shaped mitochondria that were arrayed in unusual patterns and complex aggregations. The earliest changes in mitochondria were seen at 16 weeks and were positively correlated with myelin pathology in individual animals. Neither didanosine nor stavudine was found to induce myelin, axonal, or mitochondrial changes in rabbits, even when administered at near lethal doses (e.g., 1500 mg/kg) for up to 24 weeks (40).

The behavioral, electrophysiological and pathological features of the zalcitabine-induced neuropathy in the rabbit appear to differ substantially from the clinical features of zalcitabine neuropathy in humans. The rabbit data suggest a myelinopathy of large-diameter fibers, with only secondary axonal involvement. They also indicate a significant involvement of motor fibers. In contrast, human exposure to zalcitabine is more consistent with a sensory, distal axonopathy (vide infra). These differences may be related to the relatively high doses used in the rabbit study, to a possible unusual susceptibility of Schwann cell mitochondria in the rabbit, or to the interaction of HIV infection and zalcitabine toxicity in the human population studied.

Zalcitabine at doses of 3–10 mg/kg has produced electrophysiological and axonal changes in cynomolgus monkeys, with no evidence of demyelination (3). Initial changes consisted of a subtle slowing of maximal sensory nerve conduction velocity (~10%) and an associated reduction in compound sensory amplitudes. No neuropathological alteration was evident at the time of these early electrophysiological changes. Following 38 weeks of treatment, axonal changes consisted of a statistically significant reduction in mean cross-sectional diameter of myelinated axons in the sural nerve and a reduction in the density of unmyelinated fibers.

Didanosine has been reported to cause axonal neuropathy, electrophysiological changes, and ultrastructural changes in axonal mitochondria in rats (34). However, these results have been published only in abstract form and have not been confirmed by subsequent investigations.

In Vitro Studies

Each of the ANAs evaluated has clear effects on mitochondrial DNA (mtDNA) in tissue culture. Exposure of the neuronal cell line PC-12 to zalcitabine and didanosine results in a decrease in mtDNA, destruction of mitochondria, and an increase in lactate production (20). These effects can be prevented in part by the administration of uridine and pyruvate (19).

Chronic treatment of dorsal root ganglion cultures with zalcitabine resulted in a reduction in mtDNA associated with a decrease in the buffering of Ca^{2+} transient currents, which are partially mediated by mitochondria (41). Separate studies using a human lymphoblastoid cell line, CEM, have confirmed that zalcitabine is more potent than stavudine, which, in turn, is more potent than didanosine in ability to alter mtDNA (11,25). Mitochondrial ultrastructure was changed by each drug, with distortions in and reductions of cristae and the presence of numerous vesicles. Unique features were seen for each compound evaluated (25). These differences may partly explain why various ANAs affect different targets (i.e., Schwann cell, axon, muscle, pancreas), although each appears principally to alter mitochondrial function.

Human Studies

Zalcitabine is associated with a painful, sensory, distal polyneuropathy that is sometimes a dose-limiting side effect (7,8,16,27,28,44). The neuropathy was evident in all HIV-1–positive patients evaluated at the highest dose tested (i.e., 0.06 mg/kg every 4 h for up to 12 weeks) (7). The predominant, and often presenting symptom was bilateral burning or shooting pain in the feet. This was soon followed by complaints of paresthesias, numbness, and weakness. Hyporeflexia of the Achilles reflex was the most consistent sign of neuropathy, followed by clinically evident sensory loss, gait disturbances, and weakness. Elevation of vibration threshold in the great toe was the initial laboratory abnormality. This deficit had a mean onset time of 7.3 weeks of treatment and often preceded onset of pain. At the time of maximal symptoms, mild to moderate nerve conduction abnormalities, suggestive of axonal dysfunction, were evident in 80% of the patients (7). Lower doses (0.03–0.005 mg/kg every 4 h) were associated with a similar but less intense sensory neuropathy. The incidence of neuropathy was reduced to approximately 33% in subjects receiving 0.005 mg/kg every 4 h (7) and 34% of subjects receiving 2.25 mg/day (8). Progressive zalcitabine-induced neuropathy was confirmed in one patient by nerve-fiber degenerative changes in a series of skin punch biopsies (24). There were no autonomic symptoms or evidence of cranial nerve dysfunction at any dose. Significant recovery occurred in 67%–83% of subjects with clinically evident zalcitabine-induced neuropathy; however, there was often a period of "coasting" in which the neuropathy intensified immediately following cessation of treatment (7). The presence of diabetes mellitus (8), previous exposure to ANA compounds (22), and a history of heavy ethanol consumption (15), were identified as significant risk factors for the development of zalcitabine-induced neuropathy. Sensory neuropathy characterized by pain and paresthesias has also been associated with didanosine (1,12,30,32,35) and stavudine (5,9,31,36).

There has been limited exposure of children to ANA; however, studies to date indicate little evidence of induced peripheral neuropathy (21). One study of a 6-year-old girl with AIDS-associated didanosine treatment with the development of multiple, well-circumscribed retinal lesions characterized by hypertrophy or hypopigmentation of the retinal pigment epithelium (42).

The differentiation of true ANA-induced peripheral neuropathy is often difficult because signs and symptoms are similar to those seen in patients infected with HIV. At least four distinct (nontoxic) peripheral neuropathy syndromes have been identified in AIDS patients, the most common being a distal painful sensory neuropathy (29). ANA-induced neuropathy is principally distinguished from the painful sensory neuropathy of AIDS by the speed of onset (of ANA neuropathy) and by its recovery following cessation of treatment.

As polypharmacy is increasingly used for the treatment of AIDS, interactions among compounds and the use of alternating *vs.* intermittent dosing regimens will take on added significance. For instance, a much lower incidence of neuropathy was seen when the same total dose of zalcitabine was given in a monthly-alternating rather than weekly-alternating regimen (37). Neuropathy was evident in only 2 of 56 patients receiving combinations of AZT and zalcitabine at clinically effective doses (26), and no serious neuropathy was evident in a second study that included didansine (17).

Toxic Mechanisms

The common mechanism of ANA toxicity appears to be interference with mtDNA and defective mitochondrial gene expression (4,10,23). These deficits lead to alterations in mitochondrial function and ultrastructure and ultimately to failure of cellular processes that depend heavily on energy consumption. The specific subcellular target may be mitochondrial DNA polymerase, which is essential for DNA homeostasis (39). Mitochondria in select elements of the peripheral nervous system, such as axons and Schwann cells, are especially sensitive to zalcitabine, didanosine, and stavudine, while mitochondria in skeletal muscle are more readily affected by AZT. The reason for the differential susceptibility remains unclear.

REFERENCES

1. Allan JD, Connolly KJ, Fitch H *et al.* (1993) Long-term follow-up of didanosine administered orally twice daily to patients with advanced human immunodeficiency virus infection and hematologic intolerance of zidovudine. *Clin Infect Dis* **16**, S46.
2. Anderson TD, Davidovich A, Arceo R *et al.* (1991) Peripheral neuropathy induced by 2',3'-dideoxycytidine: A rabbit model of 2',3'-dideoxycytidine neurotoxicity. *Lab Invest* **66**, 63.
3. Anderson T, Davidovich A, Arezzo J, Brosnan C (1992) Comparative neurotoxicity of dideoxycytidine in monkeys and rabbits. *Toxicol Lett* Suppl 191.
4. Anderson TD, Davidovich A, Feldman D *et al.* (1994) Mitochondrial schwannopathy and peripheral myelinopathy in a rabbit model of dideoxycytidine neurotoxicity. *Lab Invest* **70**, 724.
5. Bacellar H, Munoz A, Miller EN *et al.* (1994) Temporal trends in the incidence of HIV-1-related neurologic diseases: Multicenter AIDS cohort study, 1985–1992. *Neurology* **44**, 1892.
6. Balis FM, Pizzo PA, Butler KM *et al.* (1992) Clinical pharmacology of 2',3'-dideoxyinosine in human immunodeficiency virus-infected children. *J Infect Dis* **165**, 99.
7. Berger AR, Arezzo JC, Schaumburg HH *et al.* (1993) 2',3'-Dideoxycytidine (ddC) toxic neuropathy: A study of 52 patients. *Neurology* **43**, 358.
8. Blum CS, Dal Pan GJ, Feinberg J *et al.* (1996) Low-dose zalcitabine-related toxic neuropathy: Frequency, natural history, and risk factors. *Amer Acad Neurol* **48**, 989.
9. Browne MJ, Mayer KH, Chafee SB *et al.* (1993) 2',3'-Didehydro-3'-deoxythymidine (d4T) in patients with AIDS or AIDS-related complex: A phase I trial. *J Infect Dis* **167**, 21.
10. Chen CH, Cheng YC (1989) Delayed cytotoxicity and selective loss of mitochondrial DNA in cells treated with the anti-human immunodeficiency virus compound 2',3'-deoxythymidine. *J Biol Chem* **264**, 119.
11. Chen CH, Vazquez-Padua M, Cheng YC (1991) Effect of anti-human immunodeficiency virus nucleoside analogs on mitochondrial DNA and its implication for delayed toxicity. *Mol Pharmacol* **39**, 625.
12. Connolly KJ, Allan JD, Fitch H *et al.* (1991) Phase I study of 2',3'-dideoxyinosine administered orally twice daily to

patients with AIDS or AIDS-related complex and hematologic intolerance to zidovudine. *Amer J Med* **91**, 471.

13. Feldman D, Anderson TD (1994) Schwann cell mitochondrial alterations in peripheral nerves of rabbits treated with 2′,3′-dideoxycytidine. *Acta Neuropathol* **87**, 71.

14. Feldman D, Brosnan C, Anderson T (1992) Ultrastructure of peripheral neuropathy induced in rabbits by 2′,3′-dideoxycytidine. *Lab Invest* **66**, 75.

15. Fichtenbaum CJ, Clifford DB, Powderly WG (1995) Risk factors for dideoxynucleoside-induced toxic neuropathy in patients with the human immunodeficiency virus infection. *J Acq Immun Defic Synd Hum R* **10**, 169.

16. Fischl MA, Olson RM, Follansbee SE *et al.* (1993) Zalcitabine compared with zidovudine in patients with advanced HIV-1 infection who received previous zidovudine therapy. *Ann Intern Med* **118**, 762.

17. Jablonowski H (1995) Studies of zidovudine in combination with didanosine zalcitabine. *J Acq Immun Defic Synd Hum R* **10** (Suppl 1), S52.

18. Kahn J (1993) New developments in the clinical use of didanosine. *J Acq Immun Defic Synd* **6**, S47.

19. Keilbaugh SA, Habbos GA, Simpson MV (1993) Anti-human immunodeficiency virus type 1 therapy and peripheral neuropathy: Prevention of 2′,3′-dideoxycytidine toxicity in PC 12 cells, a neuronal model, by uridine and pyruvate. *Mol Pharmacol* **44**, 702.

20. Keilbaugh SA, Prusoff WH, Simpson MV (1991) The PC-12 cell as a model for studies of mechanism of induction of peripheral neuropathy by anti-HIV 1 dideoxynucleoside analogs. *Biochem Pharmacol* **42**, R5.

21. Kline MW, Fletcher CV, Federici ME *et al.* (1996) Combination therapy with stavudine and didanosine in children with advanced human immunodeficiency virus infection: Pharmacokinetic properties, safety, and immunologic and virologic effects. *Pediatrics* **97**, 886.

22. LeLacheur SF, Simon GL (1991) Exacerbation of dideoxycytidine-induced neuropathy with dideoxyinosine. *J Acq Immun Defic Synd* **4**, 538.

23. Lewis W, Dalakas MC (1995) Mitochondrial toxicity of antiviral drugs. *Nature Med* **1**, 417.

24. McCarthy BG, Hsieh ST, Stocks A *et al.* (1995) Cutaneous innervation in sensory neuropathies: Evaluation by skin biopsy. *Neurology* **45**, 1848.

25. Medina DJ, Tsai CH, Hsiung GD, Cheng YC (1994) Comparison of mitochondrial morphology, mitochondrial DNA content, and cell viability in cultured cells treated with 3 anti-human immunodeficiency virus dideoxynucleosides. *Antimicrob Agents Chemother* **38**, 1824.

26. Meng TC, Fischl MA, Boota AM *et al.* (1992) Combination therapy with zidovudine and dideoxycytidine in patients with advanced human immunodeficiency virus infection. A phase I/II study. *Ann Intern Med* **116**, 13.

27. Merigan TC, Skowron G (1990) Safety and tolerance of dideoxycytidine as a single agent. Results of early-phase studies in patients with acquired immunodeficiency syndrome (AIDS) or advanced AIDS-related complex. *Amer J Med* **88**, 11S.

28. Merigan TC, Skowron G, Bozzette SA *et al.* (1989) Circulating p24 antigen levels and responses to dideoxycytidine in human immunodeficiency virus (HIV) infections: A phase I and II study. *Ann Intern Med* **110**, 189.

29. Miller RG (1994) Neuromuscular complications of human immunodeficiency virus infection and antiretroviral therapy. *West J Med* **160**, 447.

30. Moyle GJ, Nelson MR, Hawkins D, Gazzard BG (1993) The use and toxicity of didanosine (ddI) in HIV antibody-positive individuals intolerant to zidovudine (AZT). *Quart J Med* **86**, 278.

31. Peterson EA, Ramirez-Ronda CH, Hardy WD *et al.* (1995) Dose-related activity of stavudine in patients infected with human immunodeficiency virus. *J Infect Dis* **171**, S131.

32. Rathbun RC, Martin ES (1992) Didanosine therapy in patients intolerant of or failing zidovudine therapy. *Ann Pharmacol* **26**, 1347.

33. Riddler SA, Anderson RE (1995) Antiviral activity of stavudine. *Antivir Res* **27**, 189.

34. Russel JW, Cupler EJ, Dalakas MC (1995) Electrophysiological and pathological changes in 2′,3′-dideoxycytidine (ddC)-induced neuropathy in an animal model. *Ann Neurol* **38**, 306.

35. Shelton MJ, O'Donnell AM, Morse GD (1992) Didanosine. *Ann Pharmacother* **26**, 660.

36. Skowron G (1995) Biologic effects and safety of stavudine: An overview of phase I and II clinical trials. *J Infect Dis* **171**, S113.

37. Skowron G, Bozzette SA, Lim L *et al.* (1993) Alternating and intermittent regimens of zidovudine and dideoxycytidine in patients with AIDS or AIDS-related complex. *Ann Intern Med* **118**, 321.

38. Taburet AM, Singlas E (1996) Drug interactions with antiviral drugs. *Clin Pharmacokinet* **30**, 385.

39. Wallace DC (1992) Diseases of the mitochondrial DNA. *Ann Rev Biochem* **61**, 1175.

40. Warner WA, Bregman CL, Comereski CR *et al.* (1995) Didanosine (ddI) and stavudine (d4T): Absence of peripheral neurotoxicity in rabbits. *Food Chem Toxicol* **33**, 1047.

41. Werth JL, Zhou B, Nutter LM, Thayer SA (1994) 2′,3′-Dideoxycytidine alters calcium buffering in cultured dorsal root ganglion neurons. *Mol Pharmacol* **45**, 1119.

42. Whitcup SM, Dastgheib K, Nussenblatt RB *et al.* (1994) A clinicopathologic report of the retinal lesions associated with didanosine. *Arch Ophthalmol* **112**, 1594.

43. Whittington R, Brogden RN (1992) Zalcitabine: a review of its pharmacology and clinical potential in acquired immunodeficiency syndrome (AIDS). *Drugs* **44**, 656.

44. Yarchoan R, Perno CR, Thomas RV *et al.* (1988) Phase I studies of 2′,3′-dideoxycytidine in severe human immunodeficiency virus infection as a single agent and alternating with zidovudine (AZT). *Lancet* **1**, 76.

Diethylbenzene

Peter S. Spencer

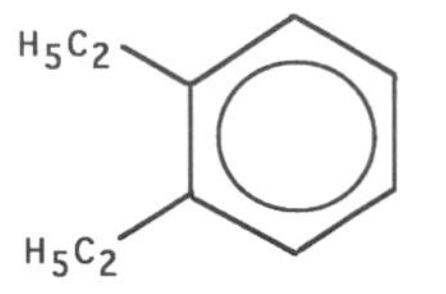

o-DIETHYLBENZENE
$C_{10}H_{14}$

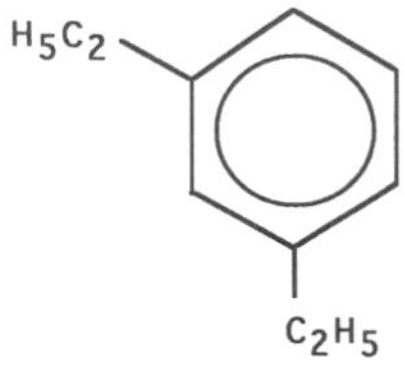

m-DIETHYLBENZENE
$C_{10}H_{14}$

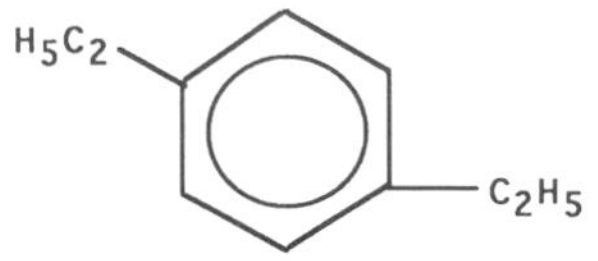

p-DIETHYLBENZENE
$C_{10}H_{14}$

1,2-Diethylbenzene
1,3-Diethylbenzene
1,4-Diethylbenzene

NEUROTOXICITY RATING

Experimental

A   Sensorimotor neuropathy

A   Cranial nerve (VIII) dysfunction

Diethylbenzene (DEB) is a component of aromatic organic solvents that are widely used in industry (3). It is a colorless, flammable liquid that exists as three isomers: 1,2- (*ortho*), 1,3- (*meta*), and 1,4- or *p*-diethylbenzene; proportions of 25%, 40%, and 35%, respectively, are reported in some commercial preparations (2), while others may contain a smaller (*e.g.*, 6%) percentage of 1,2-diethylbenzene (1,2-DEB) (5). o-Diethyl and *m*-diethylbenzene, plus a number of related aromatic hydrocarbons, produce a blue discoloration of tissues and/or excretion of green-colored urine (Table 19). There appears to be a direct relationship between the neurotoxic and chromogenic properties of these compounds; this was discovered in studies with acetyl ethyl tetramethyl tetralin (AETT) (13–15) (*see* Acetyl Ethyl Tetramethyl Tetralin, this volume) and subsequently reported for 1,2-DEB (8). This principle and the possible human health implications of exposures to a wide range of chomogenic aromatic hydrocarbons were noted in 1980 (14).

The physical properties and toxicity data of each of the three isomers have been summarized (2). The American Conference of Governmental Industrial Hygienists (ACGIH) has not established a Threshold Limit Value (TLV) for occupational exposure to commercial DEB, but the ACGIH TLV for ethylbenzene (100 ppm) may apply (2).

Much information is available on the biotransformation of ethylbenzene (12). In humans, metabolism of ethylbenzene proceeds principally through oxidation of the ethyl side chain to form 1-phenylethanol and then acetophenone. This metabolite undergoes hydroxylation to form ω-acetophenone and, to a minor extent, *p*- and *m*-hydroxyacetophenones. Over 90% of ethylbenzene metabolites in humans are mandelic and phenylglyoxylic acids, the end products of further side-chain modification. In rabbits and rats, hippuric acid (*N*-benzoyl glycine) is a principal metabolite, and oxidation of the ω-methyl group of the side chain leads to formation of phenylacetic acid. Limited ring oxidation occurs with the formation and excretion of 4-ethylphenol. Metabolites are largely excreted as glucuronides (4).

In the case of 1,2-DEB, oxidation of the ω-1 carbons of the ethyl side chains results in formation of 1,2-diacetylbenzene (1,2-DAB), a neurotoxic compound in rats that forms a blue pigment on contact with tissue (6,7,14). Similarly, 1,2-diacetyl derivatization of the benzene ring of the neurotoxin AETT confers a chomogenic property when this tetralin-based compound is reacted with amino acids, peptides, some proteins, and tissue. Substitition of the 2-ethyl group for a 2-methyl group on the benzene ring of the AETT derivative abolished both chromogenic and neurodegenerative properties (14).

TABLE 19. List of Aromatic Hydrocarbons Reportedly Associated with Production of Colored Urine (14)

Monocyclic	Dicyclic
Benzene*	Indane*
o-Xylene*	Indene*
o-Ethyltoluene*	Tetralin*,†
o-Diethylbenzene* (1,2-DEB)	Diphenyl*
m-Diethylbenzene* (1,3-DEB)	Diphenylmethane*
o-Diisopropylbenzene*	1-Methylnaphthalene*,‡
Triethylbenzene* (mixture)	2-Methylnaphthalene*,‡
Diethyldiisopropylbenzene*	1-Ethylnaphthalene*,‡
	2-Ethylnaphthalene*,‡

*Rats, single subcutaneous dose ~5 ml/kg body weight.

†,‡Humans may also excrete colored (green) urine following exposure to tetralin (1) or naphthalene (16).

Tetralin: *see* Acetyl Ethyl Tetramethyl Tetralin, this volume.

Diphenyl: *see* Diphenyl, this volume.

[From Gerarde (9).]

Consonant with the effects of orally or percutaneously administered AETT—which produces a remarkable blue discoloration of brain, spinal cord, and peripheral nerves (among other tissues) of treated rats (15) (*see* Acetyl Ethyl Tetramethyl Tetralin, this volume)—oral administration of 1,2-DEB to rats causes a bluish discoloration of skin, internal organs, and urine in combination with neurotoxic disease (7). Administration of the *o*- or *m*-isomer of diethylbenzene reportedly results in the excretion of a blue pigment in the urine of males and female rats and hamsters (1). The sclera, blood, and tissues are stained deep blue after a single subcutaneous injection of approximately 5 ml/kg (Table 19); this effect persists for many days. Rabbits receiving subcutaneous *o*- or *m*-diethylbenzene fail to excrete blue urine, although large doses of these chromogenic isomers will stain the sclera. The *p*-isomer of diethylbenzene is not chromogenic in the rat, hamster or rabbit (1).

Rats treated with 120 mg/kg DEB reportedly developed "slight hemorrhages and dystrophic changes in the liver, gastric mucosa, duodenum, spleen, and kidneys, and also decreases in hepatic protein and glycogen" (2). Oral administration of 1,2-DEB (75 or 100 mg/kg/day) or 1,2-DAB (10–15 mg/kg/day), 4 days per week for 8 weeks, produced time- and dose-dependent increases both in the peak latencies of all components of the brainstem auditory evoked responses (BAER) and in interpeak (I–V) differences, and a decrease in amplitude of all the components (5). Whereas there was a long-lasting decrease in peak amplitudes of the BAER, absolute and interpeak latencies recovered partially over an 8-week (1,2-DEB) or 10-week (1,2-DAB) period (5). Daily oral administration 4 or 5 days per week of 500 or 750 mg/kg of a commercial DEB (containing 6% 1,2-DEB) or of 100 mg/kg 1,2-DEB, produced blue discoloration of tissues and urine and a time-dependent decrease both of tail-nerve motor and sensory conduction times and of the amplitude of the sensory action potential (7). Comparable electrophysiological changes were reported in the PNS and CNS of rats treated with 500–800 ppm of commercial DEB. No changes developed in rats treated orally with 1,3-DEB and 1,4-DEB (500 mg/kg daily, 5 days per week for 8 weeks) (7). A preliminary neuropathological study of rats treated for one week via the intraperitoneal route with 20 mg/kg/d 1,2-DAB reported proximal giant axonal swellings and secondary demyelination in lumbar spinal cord, spinal nerve roots, and dorsal root ganglia (10).

In humans, 1,2-DEB is said to be mildly toxic by ingestion, and an eye, skin, and respiratory-tract irritant; 1,3-DEB is moderately toxic by ingestion (11). Reports of other adverse human health effects have not been encountered; however, acute neurotoxic effects (headache, stupor) have been noted in painters exposed to tetralin-containing var-

nishes in a poorly ventilated area; these painters also excreted green-colored urine (*see* Acetyl Ethyl Tetramethyl Tetralin, this volume).

Available data indicate that the chromogenic and neurotoxic properties of 1,2-DAB are directly related. Chromogenicity is proposed to result from the formation of a ninhydrin-like compound that reacts with proteinaceous material to generate a colored pigment (Ruhemann's purple) (14). For this to occur, the 1,2-diacetyl moiety of 1,2-DAB would have to undergo internal aldol condensation, followed by oxidation, loss of water, and further oxidation to yield a triketo structure representing an oxidized form of ninhydrin (14). How this putative chromogenic mechanism relates to the induction of neuronal and glial pathology is unknown.

REFERENCES

1. Browning E (1953) *Toxic Solvents*. Edward Arnold, London p. 44.
2. Cavender F (1994) Aromatic hydrocarbons. In: *Patty's Industrial Hygiene and Toxicology. 4th Ed. Vol IIB*. Clayton DE, Clayton FE eds. Wiley, New York p. 1301.
3. Czerski B, Kostrzewski P (1995) Alkyl derivatives of benzene, indene, naphthalene, diphenyl and fluorene as a potential source of occupational and environmental exposure. *Med Pr* **46**, 359.
4. Engström K, Rihimäki V, Hänninen O (1987) Ethylbenzene. In: *Ethel Browning's Toxicity and Metabolism of Industrial Solvents. 2nd Ed.* Snyder R ed. Elsevier, Amsterdam p. 85.
5. Gagnaire F, Becker MN, De Ceaurriz J (1992) Alteration of brainstem auditory evoked potentials in diethylbenzene and diacetylbenzene-treated rats. *J Appl Toxicol* **12**, 343.
6. Gagnaire F, Becker MN, Marignac B *et al.* (1992) Diethylbenzene inhalation-induced electrophysiological deficits in peripheral nerves and changes in brainstem auditory potentials in rats. *J Appl Toxicol* **12**, 335.
7. Gagnaire F, Ensminger A, Marignac B, De Ceaurriz J (1991) Possible involvement of 1,2-diacetylbenzene in diethylbenzene-induced neuropathy in rats. *J Appl Toxicol* **11**, 262.
8. Gagnaire F, Marignac B, De Ceaurriz J (1990) Diethylbenzene-induced sensorimotor neuropathy in rats. *J Appl Toxicol* **10**, 105.
9. Gerarde HW (1960) Toxicology and biochemistry of aromatic hydrocarbons. In: *Elsevier Monographs on Toxic Agents*. Browning E ed. Elsevier, Amsterdam p. 73.
10. Kim MS, Kayton R, Muñiz J *et al.* (1999) 1,2-Diacetylbenzene neurotoxicity: A model to study the role of Schwann cells in maintenance of axonal integrity in toxic states. *Microsc Microanal Proc* **5**(**Suppl 2**), 128.
11. Lewis RJ Sr (1992) *Sax's Dangerous Properties of Industrial Materials. 8th Ed. Vol 11*. Van Nostrand Reinhold, New York p. 1210.

12. Longacre SL (1987) Tetralin. In: *Ethel Browning's Toxicity and Metabolism of Industrial Solvents. 2nd Ed.* Snyder R ed. Elsevier, Amsterdam p. 143.

13. Spencer PS (1982) Experimental evaluation of selected petrochemicals for subchronic neurotoxic properties. In: *The Toxicology of Petroleum Hydrocarbons.* MacFarland HN *et al.* eds. American Petroleum Institute, Washington, DC p. 249.

14. Spencer PS, Foster V, Sterman AB, Horoupian D (1980) Acetyl ethyl tetramethyl tetralin. In: *Experimental and Clinical Neurotoxicology.* Spencer PS, Schaumburg HH eds. Williams & Wilkins, Baltimore p. 296.

15. Spencer PS, Sterman AB, Horoupian D *et al.* (1979) Neurotoxic changes in rats exposed to the fragrance compound acetyl ethyl tetramethyl tetralin. *Neurotoxicology* **1**, 221.

16. Zuelzer WW, Apt L (1949) Acute hemolytic anemia due to naphthalene poisoning. *J Amer Med Assn* **141**, 185.

N,N-Diethyl-*m*-Toluamide and Other Dialkylamides

Peter S. Spencer

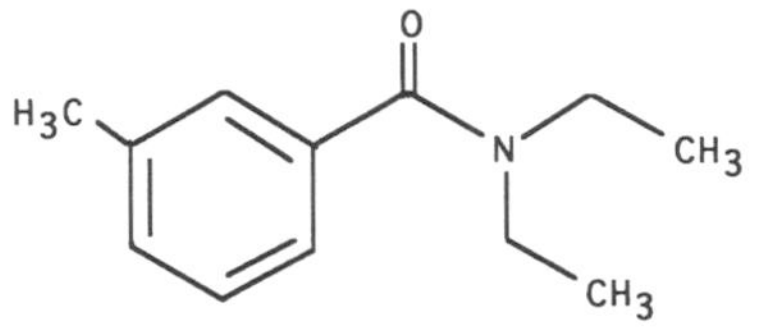

DEET
$C_{12}H_{17}NO$

N,N-Diethyl-3-methylbenzamide; DEET; *m*-DETA

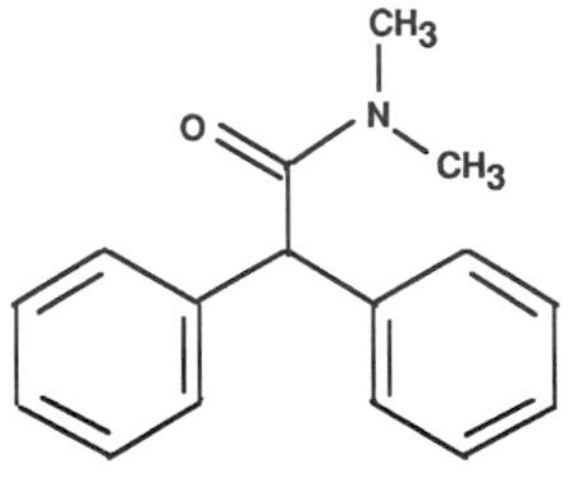

DIPHENAMID
$C_{16}H_{17}NO$

N,N-Dimethyl-2,2-diphenylacetamide; Diphenamid

NEUROTOXICITY RATING (DEET)

Clinical

C   Chronic encephalopathy

Experimental (large doses)

A   Ataxia

A   CNS myelinopathy

N,N-Diethyl-*m*-toluamide (DEET) is used worldwide as an effective insect and arachnid (tick) repellant. Several case reports, especially among young female children, show a temporal association between oral or dermal exposure to DEET and the appearance of acute encephalopathy that is either fatal or reversible; this rare condition has been modeled in rats (32). Controlled studies with rodents and hens administered single or repeated doses of DEET plus or mi-

nus the anticholinesterase agent pyridostigmine bromide (PB) and an organophosphorus or pyrethroid insecticide, suggest that the toxic potency of these substances may differ when they are administered in various binary and ternary combinations (1,2,16).

Since DEET formulations must contain a minimum of >95% of the *m*-isomer of N,N-diethyltoluamide, small percentages of the more toxic *ortho*- and less toxic *para*-isomers are likely to be present (20). Consumer products usually contain 10%–25% DEET in an ethanol or isopropanol base. Products are formulated as solutions, lotions, gels, aerosol sprays, sticks, and impregnated towlettes. Consumer products with higher DEET concentrations are available, including some listed as "pure" technical-grade DEET (33). Soldiers have been issued insect repellants containing 75% DEET (8,9), a formulation that may cause skin changes including contact dermatitis and urticaria (3,8,19). Cardiovascular (bradycardia and hypotension) effects have also been reported in animals and in a 61-year-old woman exposed dermally to a DEET-containing insect repellant (5,14).

Individuals living or employed in mosquito-infested areas may have high seasonal exposures to DEET (33). A 1986 study by the U.S. National Institute for Occupational Safety and Health reportedly estimated the upper 1% of the application dose of DEET by employees of the Everglades National Park, Florida, to be 1122 mg/kg/day or 392.6 g/week (1). A percentage of DEET applied topically to humans and animals accumulates in skin layers and exists in this site for weeks or months (19,28). Penetration of a topically applied dose is variable (9%–56%); percutaneous absorption predictably would be greater across immature skin (2–3 weeks postnatal) and with local skin maceration (29). Adult males dosed topically for 8 h on the volar surface of the forearm with radiolabeled DEET (either 100% or 15% DEET/ethanol solution) absorbed an average of 5%–10% transdermally. DEET was detectable in plasma within 2 h of application, and quantifiable radioactivity was present for 4 h after exposure termination (26). Peak blood radioactivity was found 1 h after application of 100 mg ^{14}C-DEET to mouse skin; elimination was complete by 2–3 days (27).

Two hours after dermal application of 15 mg/kg DEET to mice, the highest levels of activity were found in bile, intestine, and urine; high levels were also present in skin, liver, kidney, and nasal mucosa (4). High levels of DEET were detectable in the brain, lungs, and adrenal glands of mice given doses ≥2000 mg/kg body weight (20). Urinary metabolites in rats and rabbits exposed to DEET aerosol include benzoic acid and toluric acid (20). Humans oxidize the benzylic moiety of DEET to form *m*-carboxyl-*N,N*-diethylbenzoylamide and hydroxylate the side chain to produce the glucuronide of *N*-hydroxyethyl-*N*-ethyl-*m*-toluamide (34). Six major urinary metabolites were reported in a study of adult male volunteers (26). Excretion is initially rapid, but only one-half of absorbed DEET may be excreted in a 5-day period (20). Male and female rats excrete orally or transdermally administered radiolabeled DEET primarily in urine (75%–90%), with little (3%–7%) in feces (22).

The rat oral LD$_{50}$ for DEET is higher in male than female Lac:P Wistar-derived rats aged 11–56 days; the dose increases with the advance of age in animals of both genders, and it is lower in 31- to 57-day-old female rats pretreated with piperonyl butoxide (32). Predosing 48- to 58-day-old rats with piperonyl butoxide or 2,4-dichloro(6-phenylphenoxy)ethylamide did not alter the oral LD$_{50}$ for diphenamid (*N,N*-dimethyl-2,2-diphenylacetamide), a related compound used as a herbicide. Sublethal intraperitoneal injection of DEET (56–225 mg/kg) in anesthetized rats decreased mean blood pressure and heart rate in a dose-related manner (14). Dogs treated with 225 mg/kg DEET exhibited a similar hypotension and bradycardia (14). Excitation, stiffness of movement, and lack of coordination were observed in mice 15–120 min after topical treatment with large and lethal doses (20). Shaking, prostration, or loss of balance was noted in female rats (shaking only in male animals) exposed to DEET aerosols 4 h after exposure to 4100 mg/m^3 DEET (20). Pregnant rats and rabbits treated with 750 or 1000 mg/kg/day developed hypoactivity and ataxia (24). Tremor and hyperactivity were reported after each oral treatment with 0.1 and 0.3 ml/kg/day of 85% DEET and 10% other isomers for 13 weeks (20,31).

A single dose of either 1–3 g/kg (but not <1.5 g/kg) DEET induced CNS depression (accompanied by hypotension) interrupted by occasional head shakes and followed by myoclonic twitching; these were triggered by auditory or tactile stimuli. Loss of muscle tone was accompanied by marked slowing of the electroencephalogram (recorded from implanted electrodes) interrupted by spike discharges that were first detected in the auditory cortex; these evolved to spike trains that were accompanied by head and body twitches that persisted for up to 24 h (32). Some animals died, many recovered fully; others failed to recover muscle tone or righting reflex over 24 h, and a few remained ataxic. Respiration and arterial PO$_2$ were maintained until death supervened. Other animals were allowed to survive for 2 h to 8 days prior to controlled termination under anesthesia by intracardiac perfusion with fixatives suitable to provide optimal preservation of histological and ultrastructural tissue detail. Intramyelinic edema, evident from the earliest timepoint, evolved into a patchy and reversible spongiform myelinopathy largely restricted to the cerebellar roof nuclei, where it was bilaterally symmetrical. This was accompanied by withdrawal of astrocytic foot processes that normally surround synaptic boutons. Animals showing long-lasting prostration and partially controlled motor seizures displayed scattered neurons with edematous clefts of uncertain origin and significance (32). Taken in concert, these findings provide a valuable model of acute DEET-associated encephalopathy, with a predilection for young female animals that compares with the large percentage of reports in young female children.

A recent report describes the results of a large-scale, chronic oral toxicity study with CD-1 mice (2 years), CD rats (2 years), and dogs (1 year). Relative to control animals, dogs treated with 30–400 mg/kg/day DEET showed an increased incidence of "emesis and ptyalism, and levels of transient reduction in hemoglobin and hematocrit, increased alkaline phosphatase (males only), decreased cholesterol, and increased potassium. One male dog in the high-dose group also exhibited ataxia, tremors, abnormal head movements, and/or convulsions on several occasions during the course of the study." The highest no-observed-adverse-effect level was 100 mg/kg/day for dogs and rats, and 500 mg/kg/day for mice (25).

The toxicity and neurotoxicity of DEET coadministered with an organophosphate, carbamate, other anticholinesterase, and/or pyrethrin have been investigated for at least three reasons: (a) to identify repellent and pesticidal combinations with maximum efficacy against insect vectors of malarial and leishmanial parasites (13,17), (b) to understand unexpected toxicosis in domestic cats treated for fleas and ticks (6,7), and (c) to explore hypotheses relating to unexplained illness among U.S. and U.S.-led Coalition forces who were deployed to Southwest Asia during the 1991 Persian Gulf War, many of whom used the anticholinesterase drug pyridostigmine bromide prophylactically as a nerve-agent-antidote enhancer. Factor analysis of associations between exposures and symptoms reported by one battalion of 249 U.S. Gulf War veterans showed a significant association between the frequency and amount of skin application of a repellant containing 75% DEET in ethanol and risk for a nebulous set of postwar symptoms described as "arthro-myo-neuropathy" (9).

There was a significant increase in lethality relative to additive values when adult male rats were given by gavage DEET + PB, permethrin + PB, or DEET + PB + permethrin, and observed for up to 14 days (16). Hypersalivation, ataxia, depression, seizures, and death occurred in cats within 4–6 h of dermal application of DEET/fenvalerate; evidence was obtained for the presence of both compounds in the skin, kidney, liver, and brain (6). Measures of neurotoxicity were reportedly altered in hens treated 5 days a week for 2 months with binary (increased) and ternary (further increased) combinations of DEET [500 mg/kg/day subcutaneously (s.c.)], pyridostigmine bromide (PB, 5 mg/kg/day, in water), chlorpyrifos (10 mg/kg/day s.c., in corn oil), or permethrin (500 mg/kg/day s.c., in corn oil) relative to the effects of comparable treatment with any of the individual compounds (1,2). Locomotor dysfunction was absent in animals treated with DEET or PB alone, and present after 16–18 days in animals treated with DEET + PB or DEET + PB + chlorpyrifos (1).

Neuropathological examination of these animals employed methods that gave a quality of tissue preservation that does not permit accurate measurement of axonal diameter; nevertheless, there was a reported increase in the frequency of enlarged axons in spinal cord and peripheral nerves of animals treated with various chemical combinations, including DEET + PB (1). With the possible exception of one figure illustrating a longitudinal section of the lateral column of an animal treated with PB + DEET + chlorpyrifos (1), none of the illustrations shows convincing neuropathological findings.

Only reduced body weights were seen in the fetuses of Charles River CD rats treated by gavage on gestation days 56–15 with 750 mg/day DEET. No fetotoxic effects were seen in New Zealand white rabbits treated with a dose of DEET (325 mg/kg/day) that depressed body weight and food consumption in the dam (24). No evidence of reproductive or developmental toxicity was found in a rat study (33). The second generation of rats administered 5000 ppm DEET (maximal tolerated dose) continuously over two generations and then chronically for 9 months showed increased treatment-related exploratory locomotor activity in the absence of microscopic changes in central and peripheral nervous tissue (23).

Convincing evidence of human teratogenicity is lacking. There are two reports of three individuals with developmental abnormalities attributed to a teratogenic effect of DEET (10,21). Coarctation of the aorta was reported in male cousins with similar environmental exposure to DEET and insecticides (10). The mother of a 4-year-old boy with mental retardation, impaired sensorimotor coordination, and craniofacial dysmorphology applied DEET throughout her entire pregnancy, in addition to the prophylactic use of chloroquine (21).

Thirteen of 14 individuals with neurotoxic effects (convulsions, ataxia, weakness) presumptively attributed to DEET were between 1.5 and 8 years of age; the large majority was female (18,20). A 5-year-old boy with a history of mild developmental delay experienced a major motor seizure after relatively brief topical applications of DEET-containing insect repellents; DEET levels in urine were 0.003 mg/ml (15). Five subjects developed coma, seizures, and hypotension within 1 h of oral ingestion of DEET-containing insect repellant; two who died had serum DEET levels of 0.88 mmol/l and 1.25 mmol/l; the three others recovered without sequelae (30). Fatal encephalopathy developed in a 6-year-old heterozygote for ornithine carbomoyl transferase deficiency (12), an observation that led to the hypothesis that individuals with genetic or acquired defects in ammonia metabolism may be at special risk for DEET neurotoxicity (11).

A 30-year-old man who daily applied DEET-containing insect repellant, followed by a 1- to 2-h session in a light-bulb-heated box, exhibited sedation and incoherence after each application. Three days after discontinuing treatment, he developed an acute psychosis that lasted 2 weeks. He displayed aggression, psychomotor hyperactivity, rapid and pressured speech, tangentiality, flights of ideas, and grandiose delusions. Clinical improvement was complete within 6 days (28).

Possible neurotoxic effects (episodic confusion; abnormal sensation of decreased sweating) have been reported anecdotally in workers dermally exposed to estimated weekly amounts of DEET exceeding 4.25 g (20). A neurobehavioral survey of 143 U.S. National Park Service workers in the Florida Everglades found a significant increase of muscle cramping, insomnia, affective symptoms, and difficulty starting or stopping the urinary stream (19). A follow-up comparison of workers before (March) and after (August) DEET exposure revealed confounding factors that did not support the initial findings (18).

A detailed analysis of all reported cases of DEET toxicity has been presented and, for adult and pediatric cases, alternative etiologies suggested (18). An earlier review of the possible effects of dermal or oral exposure to DEET led

TABLE 20. Effects of Various Dialkylamides* Admininstered to Rats at the Maximum Tolerated Dose

Compound	Behavioral Phenomena	Cerebellar Roof Nuclei
N,N-Diethyl-m-toluamide (DEET)	Prostration, ataxia, protracted seizures	Myelinopathy, astrocytic foot retraction, neuronal clefts
N,N-Diethylacetamide	Prostration, tremor	No myelinopathy
N,N-Diethylformamide	Prostration	No myelinopathy
N,N-Diethylnicotinamide	Prostration, tremor, seizures	No myelinopathy
N,N-Diethylvanillamide	Prostration, tremor, seizures	No myelinopathy
N,N-Dimethyl-2,2-diphenylacetamide (diphenamid)	Hyperexcitability, ataxia	Myelinopathy, astrocytic foot retraction
N,N-Dimethylacetamide	Prostration	No myelinopathy, other
N,N-Dimethylformamide	Prostration	No myelinopathy
N,N-Dimethylpropionamide	Prostration	No myelinopathy

*Verschoyle et al. (32) refer to nine compounds in the Methods and eight compounds in the Results.

[From Verschoyle et al. (32).]

another group to conclude that human toxicosis is characterized by a highly variable and unpredictable clinical course (5). This group stated that highly concentrated DEET-containing insect repellents should be avoided to reduce the likelihood of toxicity in both children and adults. An industry-sponsored DEET Registry of Adverse Effects was established in 1995 (18).

The structure–activity neurotoxicity relationships for DEET and other dialkylamides are not clear. Like DEET, diphenamid produced a reversible ataxia associated with a spongiform myelinopathy largely confined to cerebellar roof nuclei (32). A similar distribution of myelin vacuolation is produced by long-term administration to rats of either ethanolamine-O-sulfate or 4-aminohex-5-enoate (γ-vinyl-γ-aminobuytric acid) (32). Other dialkylamides produced marked prostration at the maximally tolerated dose (Table 20): two caused hyperexcitability; none produced detectable intramyelinic edema.

The increased oral toxicity of DEET in rats pretreated with piperonyl butoxide supports a metabolic factor, since DEET is detoxified by a cytochrome P-450–linked microsomal system (32,35). Comparable pretreatment did not increase the susceptibilty of animals to the neurotoxic effect of diphenamid. Carbamylation of peripheral esterases (by pyridostigmine bromide) is proposed to reduce the hydrolysis of DEET and increase its availability to the nervous system (1).

Female carriers of ornithine carbamoyl transferase deficiency are hypothesized to be at risk for DEET neurotoxicity. DEET is proposed to inhibit urea cycle citrilline production leading to transient hyperammonemia and associated neurotoxicity. Ammonia levels rise in normal mice after intraperitoneal administration of 0.5 mg/kg DEET in corn oil (11).

The appearance in DEET/fenvalerate-treated cats and dogs of hypersalivation, bradycardia, mydriasis, ataxia, tremors, depression, and seizures is reminiscent of the effects of cholinesterase inhibition, but cholinesterase activity is uniformly unaltered. Female kittens are said to be especially vulnerable. Competition for excretory pathways is suggested as the cause of intoxication (see Chapter 3). DEET synergizes the insecticidal activity of some organophosphate and carbamate cholinesterase inhibitors by a mechanism other than acetylcholinesterase inhibition (17).

REFERENCES

1. Abou Donia MB, Wilmarth KR, Abdel Rahman AA et al. (1996) Increased neurotoxicity following concurrent exposure to pyridostigmine bromide, DEET, and chlorpyrifos. Fund Appl Toxicol 34, 201.

2. Abou Donia MB, Wilmarth KR, Jensen KG et al. (1996) Neurotoxicity resulting from coexposure to pyridostigmine bromide, DEET, and permethrin—Implications of Gulf War chemical exposures. J Toxicol Environ Health 48, 35.

3. Amichai B, Lazarov A, Halevey S (1994) Contact dermatitis from diethyltoluamide. Contact Dermatitis 30, 188.

4. Blomquist L, Thorsell W (1977) Distribution and fate of the insect repellent ^{14}C-N,N-diethyl-m-toluamide in the animal body. II. Distribution and excretion after cutaneous application. Acta Pharmacol Toxicol 37, 121.

5. Clem JR, Havemann DF, Raebel MA (1993) Insect repellant (N,N-diethyl-m-toluamide) cardiovascular toxicity in an adult. Ann Pharmacother 27, 289.

6. Dorman DC, Buck WB, Trammel RD (1990) Diethyltoluamide (DEET) insect repellant toxicosis. Vet Clin N Amer-Small Anim 20, 387.

7. Dorman DC, Buck WB, Trammel RD et al. (1990) Fenvalerate/N,N-diethyl-m-toluamide (Deet) toxicosis in two cats. J Amer Vet Med Assn 196, 100.

8. Fai FY, Lee L (1996) Perception and use of insect repellant among soldiers in the Singapore armed services. Milit Med 161, 113.

9. Haley RW, Kurt TL (1997) Self-reported exposure to neurotoxic chemical combinations in the Gulf War—A cross-sectional epidemiologic study. *J Amer Med Assn* **277**, 231.

10. Hall JG, McLaughlin JF, Stamm S (1975) Coarctation of the aorta in male cousins with similar maternal environmental exposure to insect repellant and insecticides. *Pediatrics* **55**, 425.

11. Heick HMC, Peterson RG, Dalpe-Scott M, Qureshi IA (1988) Insect repellant, N,N-diethyl-m-toluamide, effect on ammonia metabolism. *Pediatrics* **82**, 373.

12. Heick HMC, Shipman RT, Norman MG et al. (1986) Reye-like syndrome associated with use of insect repellent in a presumed heterozygote for ornithine carbamoyl transferase deficiency. *J Pediat* **97**, 471.

13. Kroeger A, Gerhardus A, Kruger G et al. (1997) The contribution of repellent soap to malaria control. *Amer J Trop Med Hyg* **56**, 580.

14. Leach GJ, Russell RD, Houpt JT (1988) Some cardiovascular effects of the insect repellent N,N-diethyl-m-toluamide (DEET). *J Toxicol Environ Health* **25**, 217.

15. Lipscombe JW, Kramer JE, Leikin JB (1992) Seizure following brief exposure to the insect repellent N,N-diethyl-m-toluamide. *Ann Emerg Med* **21**, 315.

16. McCain WC, Lee R, Johnson MS et al. (1997) Acute oral toxicity study of pyridostigmine bromide, permethrin, and DEET in the laboratory rat. *J Toxicol Environ Health* **50**, 113.

17. Moss JI (1996) Synergism of toxicity of N,N-diethyl-m-toluamide to German cockroaches (Orthoptera, Blattellidae) by hydrolytic enzyme inhibitors. *J Econ Entomol* **89**, 1151.

18. Osimitz TG, Murphy JV (1997) Neurological effects associated with use of the insect repellent N,N-diethyl-m-toluamide (DEET). *Clin Toxicol* **35**, 435.

19. Reuveni H, Yagupsky P (1982) Diethyltoluamide-containing insect repellent: Adverse effects in worldwide use. *Arch Dermatol* **118**, 582.

20. Robbins PJ, Cherniack MG (1986) Review of the biodistribution and toxicity of the insect repellent N,N-diethyl-m-toluamide (DEET). *J Toxicol Environ Health* **18**, 503.

21. Schaefer C, Peters PW (1992) Intrauterine diethyltoluamide exposure and fetal outcome. *Reprod Toxicol* **6**, 175.

22. Schoenig GP, Hartnagel RE, Osimitz TG, Llanso S (1996) Absorption, distribution, metabolism, and excretion of N,N-diethyl-m-toluamide in the rat. *Drug Metab Disposition* **24**, 156.

23. Schoenig GP, Hartnagel RE Jr, Schardein JL, Vorhees CV (1993) Neurotoxicity evaluation of N,N-diethyl-m-toluamide (DEET) in rats. *Fund Appl Toxicol* **21**, 355.

24. Schoenig GP, Neeper-Bradley TL, Fisher LC, Hartnagel RE Jr (1994) Teratologic evaluations of N,N-diethyl-m-toluamide (DEET) in rats and rabbits. *Fund Appl Toxicol* **23**, 63.

25. Schoenig GP, Osimitz TG, Gabriel KL et al. (1999) Evaluation of the chronic toxicity and oncogenicity of N,N-diethyl-m-toluamide (DEET). *Toxicol Sci* **47**, 99.

26. Selim S, Hartnagel RE, Osimitz TG et al. (1995) Absorption, metabolism, and excretion of N,N-diethyl-m-toluamide following dermal application to human volunteers. *Fund Appl Toxicol* **25**, 95.

27. Snodgrass HL, Nelson DC, Weeks MH (1982) Dermal penetration and potential for placental transfer of the insect repellent, N,N-diethyl-m-toluamide. *Amer J Ind Hyg Assn* **43**, 747.

28. Snyder JW, Poe RO, Stubbins JF, Garrettson LK (1986) Acute manic psychosis following the dermal application of N,N-diethyl-m-toluamide (DEET) in an adult. *J Toxicol-Clin Toxicol* **24**, 429.

29. Spencer TS, Hill JA, Feldman RJ, Maibach HI (1979) Evaporation of diethyltoluamide from human skin *in vivo* and *in vitro*. *J Invest Dermatol* **72**, 317.

30. Tenenbein M (1987) Severe toxic reactions and death following the ingestion of diethyltoluamide-containing insect repellents. *J Amer Med Assoc* **258**, 1509.

31. U.S. Environmental Protection Agency (1980) N,N-Diethyl-m-toluamide (DEET): Pesticide registration standard. U.S. Environmental Protection Agency, Office of Pesticide and Toxic Substances, Washington, DC.

32. Vershoyle RD, Brown AW, Nolan C et al. (1992) A comparison of the acute toxicity, neuropathology, and electrophysiology of N,N-diethyl-m-toluamide and N,N-dimethyl-2,2-diphenyl diacetamide in rats. *Fund Appl Toxicol* **18**, 79.

33. Wright DM, Hardin BD, Goad PW, Chrislip DW (1992) Reproductive and developmental toxicity of N,N-diethyl-m-toluamide in rats. *Fund Appl Toxicol* **19**, 33.

34. Wu A, Pearson ML, Shekoski D et al. (1979) High resolution gas chromatography/mass spectrometric characterization of urinary metabolites of N,N-diethyl-m-toluamide (DEET) in man. *J High Resolut Chromatogr Commun* **2**, 558.

35. Yeung JM, Taylor WG (1988) Metabolism of N,N-diethyl-m-toluamide (DEET) by liver microsomes from male and female rats. *Drug Metab Disposition* **16**, 600.

Digitalis and Other Cardiac Glycosides

Daniel M. Rosenbaum

Digoxin; (3β,5β,12β)-3-[(O-2,6-Dideoxy-β-D-ribo-hexopyranosyl-(1→4)-O-2,6-dideoxy-β-D-ribo-hexopyranosyl-(1→4)-2,6-dideoxy-β-D-ribo-hexopyranosyl)oxy]-12,14-dihydroxycard-20(22)-enolide — $C_{41}H_{64}O_{14}$

NEUROTOXICITY RATING

Clinical

A Visual dysfunction (color vision, photophobia)

A Acute encephalopathy (delirium, cognitive dysfunction, hallucinations)

B Seizure disorder

B Cranial neuropathy (trigeminal)

Experimental

A Seizure disorder

A Acute encephalopathy (agitation, coma)

Digitalis and other cardiac glycosides have in common a powerful action on the myocardium that traditionally has been relied upon for the treatment of congestive heart failure. Compounds containing the molecular motif common to these agents—a steroid nucleus with an unsaturated lactone at the C17 position and one or more glycosidic residues at 3C—are found in a number of plants as well as in the venom of certain toads. In the 1990s, digoxin became the most widely used of the cardiac glycosides because of its convenient pharmacokinetics and route of administration, and the widespread availability of techniques for its measurement in serum. The focus of this chapter is on digoxin.

The main pharmacodynamic property of digitalis is its ability to increase the degree of myocardial contraction. The beneficial effects of the drug in patients with heart failure—increased cardiac output; decreased heart size, venous pressure, and blood volume; diuresis and relief of edema—result mainly from the increased contractile force, a positive inotropic action. A second important action of digitalis is to slow the ventricular rate in atrial fibrillation or flutter (10). All cardiac glycosides are potent and highly selective inhibitors of the active transport of Na^+ and K^+ across cell membranes by binding to a specific site on the extracytoplasmic face of the α-subunit of Na^+, K^+-ATPase (10).

Absorption of digoxin after oral administration is somewhat variable. The fraction of the administered dose that is absorbed is related to the rate and extent of dissolution of various dosage forms and therefore depends strongly on the preparation used. Absorption of the encapsulated preparation in a hydroalcoholic vehicle is close to complete. However, absorption of other preparations may be as low as 4%; with others the fraction reaches 75%. After oral administration, the concentration of digoxin in plasma typically reaches a peak in 2–3 h; the maximal effect is apparent in 4–6 h. In the absence of a loading dose, near–steady-state blood levels are achieved in about 1 week (10).

Glycosides are distributed slowly in the body, in part due to their relatively large volume of distribution. The presence of congestive heart failure can slow the rate at which steady-state distribution is attained. About 25% of digoxin in the plasma is bound to proteins. Digitalis glycosides are distributed to most body tissues. At equilibrium, the concentrations in cardiac tissue are 15–30 times those in the plasma; the concentration in skeletal muscle is about half that in the heart (10).

Digoxin is eliminated primarily in the kidney. The drug is both filtered at the glomerulus and secreted by the tubules. A rare patient seems to form antibodies to digoxin, and this prevents its therapeutic effect. The half-time for elimination of digoxin, which averages 1.6 days, is strongly dependent on renal function; in most instances, there is a close correlation between the decrease in creatinine clearance and the concentration of digoxin in plasma that is attained with any given maintenance dose (10).

The number of drugs that exhibit potentially important pharmacokinetic drug interactions with digoxin is large and increasing. Many of these drugs, such as verapamil, guanidine, and amiodarone, are commonly administered with digoxin, and dosing of the cardiac glycoside must be adjusted appropriately.

Adverse reactions to cardiac glycosides may be cardiac or noncardiac, and are dose-related. Frequent cardiac reactions include ectopic dysrhythmias and heart block. Gastrointestinal effects (anorexia, vomiting, and diarrhea) are also common. Other less frequent reactions include thrombocytopenia and skin rashes (1).

In cats, intracerebroventricular administration of peruvoside, a cardiac glycoside obtained from the plant *Theretia neriifolia*, as well as ouabain, produce marked dose-dependent neurotoxic effects. Prior administration of reserpine or tetrabenazine suppressed the neurotoxicity. Perfusion with peruvoside or ouabain into the lateral ventricle of cats produced a massive release of 5-hydroxytryptamine, also in a dose-related manner (9).

Toxic effects of digoxin occur frequently in the nervous system. The incidence has been reported to be as high as 65% in patients with severe toxicity. Most series, however, report incidences in the range of 25% (13). Dizziness, drowsiness, restlessness, nervousness, agitation, and amnesia have been noted (1), as have chorea and cognitive impairment (17,19). Neuropsychiatric disturbances include acute pychoses and delirium, especially in the elderly (6). Serum digoxin levels were in the toxic range in patients with psychosis and withdrawal of the drug resulted in remission of psychosis. Psychiatric patients may be more susceptible to this effect. The overall occurrence is rare. Nightmares have been reported in patients on digoxin. Digoxin levels were in the toxic range, and the nightmares stopped upon withdrawal of the drug (5). There are reports of visual and auditory hallucination and digitalis delirium (1,18). Three case reports note seizures associated with digoxin toxicity (7,8,11). Accompanying electroencephalographic changes disappeared only when the plasma concentration of digoxin returned to the therapeutic range.

Trigeminal neuralgia involving all three branches of the trigeminal nerve has followed administration of digoxin in one case (4). Serum digoxin level measured 3.28 ng/ml. With discontinuation of digoxin, the facial pain ceased and serum digoxin levels measured 1.45 ng/ml. Rechallenge with the drug produced mild facial attacks a second time. Other reports describe involvement of the mandibular branch only (3,6).

Cardiac glycosides perturb vision; photophobia, blurred vision, scotomata, flickering sensations, and flashes of light are all described (1). Color vision may be altered, the most common form of abnormality being yellow vision ("xanthopsia"). Altered perception of green, red, brown, blue, or even white, can also occur (6). Clinical measurement of color vision has proven to be disappointing in diagnosing digoxin toxicity (2,12).

Measurement of plasma digitalis concentrations has become commonplace and has been useful in diagnosing toxicity. Plasma concentrations above 3 ng/ml toxicity are highly likely to be toxic (1). Toxicity can occur at lower concentrations but is unlikely below 1.5 ng/ml. Patients with hypokalemia are at particular risk for toxicity.

The most important complication of overdose in all age groups is a disturbance of cardiac conduction; CNS and visual disturbances can also occur. The pharmacokinetics of digoxin seem to be altered after overdosage, the half-time being reduced, but there is too little information to define the kinetics precisely (15). Treatment of overdosage includes withdrawal of digitalis (including ipecacuanha-induced emesis); correction of hypokalemia (if present), treatment of life-threatening dysthythmias and, most recently, antidigoxin antibody (Fab fragment). The latter should be reserved for the presence of life-threatening dysrhythmias, or heart block, and when the plasma K^+ concentration is above 5 mmol/l or rising (14). The role of hemoperfusion is still controversial (1).

There is considerable circumstantial evidence that digitalis toxicity results from direct or indirect inhibition of Na^+, K^+-adenosine triphosphatase (16).

REFERENCES

1. Aronson JK (1988) Positive inotropic drugs and drugs used in dysrhythmias. In: *Meyler's Side Effects of Drugs*. Dukes MNG ed. Elsevier, Amsterdam p. 333.
2. Aronson JK, Ford AR (1980) The use of colour vision measurement in the diagnosis of digoxin toxicity. *Quart J Med* 49, 273.
3. Baterman TL, Gutser LB (1948) Hitherto undescribed neurological manifestations of digitalis toxicity. *Amer Heart J* 36, 582.
4. Bernat JL, Sullivan JK (1979) Trigeminal neuralgia from digitalis intoxication. *J Amer Med Assn* 241, 164.
5. Brezis M, Michaele J, Hamburger R (1980) Nightmares from digoxin. *Ann Intern Med* 93, 639.
6. Chung EK (1969) *Digitalis Intoxication*. Williams & Wilkins, Baltimore.
7. Douglas EF, White PT, Nelson JW (1971) Three per second spike-wave in digitalis toxicity. *Arch Neurol* 25, 373.
8. Feurstein J, Mantz JM, Kurtz D *et al.* (1973) EEG and massive digitalis intoxication. A case of epilepsy with respiratory manifestations and prolonged apnoea. *Electroencephalogr Clin Neuro* 34, 313.
9. Gaitonde BB, Joglekar SN (1977) Mechanism of neurotoxicity of cardiotonic glycosides. *Brit J Pharmacol* 59, 223.
10. Kelly RA, Smith TW (1995) Pharmacological treatment of heart failure. In: *The Pharmacological Basis of Therapeutics. 9th Ed*. Hardman JG, Limbird LE eds. McGraw-Hill, New York p. 809.
11. Kerr DT, Elliott HL, Hillis WS (1982) Epileptic form seizures and electroencephalographic abnormalities as manifestations of digoxin toxicity. *Brit Med J* 284, 162.
12. Le Sage J (1984) Color vision testing to assist in diagnoses of digitalis toxicity. *Nurs Res* 33, 346.
13. Lely AH, Van Enter CHJ (1970) Large-scale digitoxin intoxication. *Brit Med J* 3, 737.
14. Lovejoy FH, Linden CH (1991) Acute poisoning and drug overdose. In: *Harrison's Principles of Internal Medicine*. Wilson JD, Braunwald E, Isselbacher KJ *et al.* eds. McGraw-Hill, New York p. 2171.
15. Rosenberg J, Benowitz NL, Pond S (1981) Pharmacokinetics of drug overdose. *Clin Pharmacokinet* 6, 161.
16. Schwartz A, Lindenmayer GE, Allen JC (1975) The sodium-potassium adenosine triphosphate: Pharmacological, physiological and biochemical aspects. *Pharmacol Res* 27, 3.
17. Tuck AR, Ng KT (1983) Digoxin-related impairment of learning and memory in cardiac patients. *Psychopharmacology* 81, 86.
18. Volpe BT, Soave R (1979) Formed visual hallucinations as digitalis toxicity. *Ann Intern Med* 91, 865.
19. Wedzicha J, Gibb WR, Lees AJ, Hoffbrand B (1984) Chorea in digoxin toxicity. *J Neurol Neurosurg Psychiat* 47, 419.

Dihydro-β-erythroidine

Albert C. Ludolph

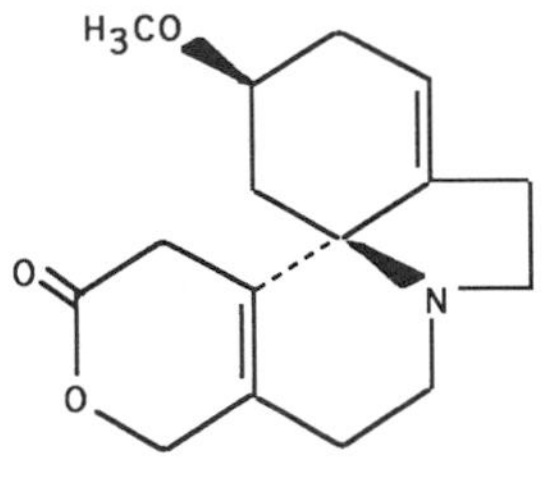

DIHYDRO-β-ERYTHROIDINE
$C_{16}H_{21}NO_3$

(3β)-1,6-Didehydro-14,17-dihydro-3-methoxy-
16(15H)-oxaerythrinan-15-one

NEUROTOXICITY RATING

Experimental

A   Neuromuscular transmission dysfunction (postsynaptic)

Dihydro-β-erythroidine is a hydrogenated derivative of erythroidine, an alkaloid isolated from seeds of trees and shrubs of the genus *Erythrina*. Crystals are soluble in ethanol and decompose at 85°–86°C. Like curare, this small molecule (MW, 275.34) is a competitive antagonist at muscle and neuronal nicotinic receptors (4). The effects of dihydro-β-erythroidine on the neuromuscular junction are partly reversed by neostigmine through a direct effect on the receptor (5). Dihydro-β-erythroidine binds with CNS high-affinity nicotinic agonist sites (3) and has an anticonvulsive effect (5). The agent is used experimentally to study differential nicotinic responses in the CNS (1,2).

REFERENCES

1. Alkondon M, Albuquerque EX (1993) Diversity of nicotinic acetylcholine receptors in rat hippocampal neurons. I. Pharmacological and functional evidence for distinct structural subtypes. *J Pharmacol Exp Ther* **265**, 1455.
2. Pereira EF, Reinhardt-Maelicke S, Schrattenholz A *et al.* (1993) Identification and functional characterization of a new agonist site on nicotinic acetylcholine receptors of cultured hippocampal neurons. *J Pharmacol Exp Ther* **265**, 1474.
3. Schneider M, Adee C, Betz H, Schmidt J (1985) Biochemical characterization of two nicotinic receptors from the optic lobe of the chick. *J Biol Chem* **260**, 14505.
4. Taylor P (1990) Agents acting at the neuromuscular junction and autonomic ganglia. In *The Pharmacological Basis of Therapeutics. 8th Ed.* Gilman AG, Rall TW, Nies AS, Taylor P eds. Pergamon Press, New York p. 166.
5. Unna K, Kniazuk M, Greslin JG (1944) Pharmacologic action of Erythrina alkaloids. I. β-Erythroidine and substances derived from it. *J Pharmacol* **80**, 39.

N,N'-Dimethylaminopropionitrile

Alan Pestronk

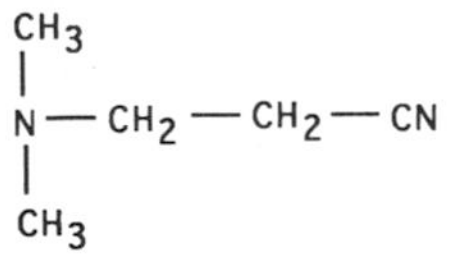

N,N'-DIMETHYLAMINOPROPIONITRILE
$C_5H_{10}N_2$

NEUROTOXICITY RATING

Clinical

A   Peripheral neuropathy
A   Autonomic neuropathy

Experimental

A   Motor nerve terminal degeneration

The propionitriles, a family of compounds containing the basic structures, $X—CH_2—CH_2—CN$, have a wide variety of toxic effects that depend on the identity of the X moiety (14). Two compounds, β,β'-iminodipropionitrile (5) and N,N'-dimethylaminopropionitrile (DMAPN) (14), have neurotoxic properties. The neurotoxic effects of DMAPN were first identified during an epidemic of urinary dysfunction and polyneuropathy that occurred when workers in plants manufacturing polyurethane foam were exposed to the compound in 1976 and 1977 (1,7–10,14).

DMAPN (Table 21) is a water-soluble liquid with an amine-type odor (14). It is colorless but becomes yellow on exposure to air. DMAPN is synthesized from acrylonitrile and dimethylamine. Before its toxicity was identified, DMAPN was a component in a catalyst used for the manufacture of polyurethane foam.

DMAPN may be absorbed through the skin, respiratory system, or gastrointestinal tract (14). Its metabolism varies among species. Rats excrete about 44% of administered DMAPN unchanged in the urine, while in mice the figure is only 6% (12,13). β-Aminopropionitrile, cyanoacetic acid,

TABLE 21. Physical Properties of DMAPN

Molecular weight	98.15
Boiling point	174.5°C
Freezing point	−44.3°C
Vapor pressure	1 mm Hg
Specific gravity	0.8715
Heat of vaporization at 1 atm	394 BTU/kg

and thiocyanate are urinary metabolites. Cyanide is also a metabolic by-product (2). Metabolism of DMAPN probably occurs *via* a cytochrome P-450–dependent mixed-function oxidase system. DMAPN, unlike other propionitriles, does not inhibit lysyl oxidase (19). DMAPN may inhibit the action of several glycolytic enzymes (3) but does not inhibit monoamine oxidase activity (18).

The LD_{50} in rats is 2.6 ml/kg given orally and 0.5–1.0 ml/kg after intraperitoneal administration (14). The dermal LD_{50} in rabbits is 1.4 ml/kg. After a single large dose, DMAPN produces irritability and then generalized, stimulus-sensitive, clonic movements. Death occurs after 5–10 min during tonic status epilepticus. If status epilepticus is prevented by sedation, then the LD_{50} is doubled.

Direct contact with DMAPN results in erythema and induration of the skin, and surface injury to the cornea (14,15). Doses of 175–700 mg/kg are followed by weight loss, reduced water consumption, urinary retention, and bladder wall injury (6,13). The bladder wall pathology includes edema, petechial hemorrhage, and inflammation. Bladder function normalizes 2 days after DMAPN is eliminated. DMAPN also produces systemic autonomic dysfunction (4). Heart rate and blood pressure cease to respond to stress for 2 h after treatment of rats with DMAPN. This effect may be due to central actions of DMAPN, since heart rate responded normally to systemically administered atropine and propranalol.

Prolonged exposure of rats to DMAPN produces swelling of nerve terminals (14). Animals that received 0.5% DMAPN in drinking water for 2–9 months developed abnormally enlarged motor nerve terminals containing disordered neurofilaments. Systemic effects of chronic DMAPN exposure include brown pigmentation of the skin, tail, and teeth similar to that in aged rats. Lifespan is halved. DMAPN does not produce the changes in bone associated with exposure to certain other propionitriles (11).

Several months after DMAPN was introduced into the manufacturing process of polyurethane foams, many exposed workers developed a characteristic syndrome (1,7–10,14). The initial symptoms were usually urinary hesitancy and abdominal discomfort. Many workers then noted a decreased urinary stream, reduced frequency of urination, and

urinary incontinence. In severely affected patients, a Credé or Valsalva maneuver was necessary to initiate urination.

Other systems became involved over time. Sexual function was impaired, with difficulty initiating or maintaining an erection. Paresthesias and numbness appeared, first in the feet, and then in the hands and more proximally in the legs. Other symptoms related to DMAPN included insomnia and feelings of tiredness and weakness.

Neurological examination showed a characteristic pattern of sensory loss in the more severely affected workers (14). Symptoms of pricking pain, temperature, and light touch were diminished in a symmetrical distribution confined to the lower sacral dermatomes, and the distal legs and hands. Vibratory sensation was diminished only in the feet. Muscle strength was decreased distally in the arms and legs. Tendon reflexes were generally preserved, but ankle jerks were often sluggish. Cranial nerve and cerebellar function was intact. Autonomic functions, such as pupillary reflexes and response of pulse and blood pressure to changes in position, were normal.

Routine hematological and blood chemistry tests on affected workers showed no consistent abnormalities. Cerebrospinal fluid from one severely affected worker was normal. Intravenous pyelograms, performed several weeks after DMAPN exposure was eliminated—a time when symptoms were abating—revealed significant postvoid residual urine in 28% of symptomatic workers. Cystometrograms in some patients showed flaccid neurogenic bladders with residual urine volumes up to 1 liter.

Nerve conduction studies showed mild abnormalities in severely affected patients. Sacral nerve latencies were prolonged in three subjects. Motor nerve conduction studies were normal, except for mild slowing and reduced amplitudes of compound muscle action potentials in several severely affected patients. Sensory potentials had small amplitudes and slightly prolonged terminal latencies. All measurements returned to normal 5 months after exposure to DMAPN was eliminated.

Pathological data on the effects of DMAPN in humans is available from one severely affected 38-year-old male, who was otherwise in good health (14). The gastrocnemius muscle showed mild denervation, including small angular muscle fibers and fiber-type grouping. An increased number of muscle fibers with internal nuclei, a nonspecific finding, was also noted. Axonal degeneration and collagen pockets surrounded by Schwann cell cytoplasm were evident in biopsied sural nerve. There was a mild reduction in the number of myelinated ($5400/mm^2$) and unmyelinated ($21,000/mm^2$) axons, and no evidence of demyelination or axonal regeneration. Occasional axons showed swellings with central cores of axoplasm containing disordered neurofilaments surrounded by an accumulation of densely packed particulate organelles, including mitochondria, membrane-bound vesicles of smooth endoplasmic reticulum, and dense bodies. These swellings resembled reactive swellings in interrupted axons, the terminal swellings in DMAPN-treated rats, and in axons regenerating after acrylamide intoxication. Myelin sheaths were not seen around these swellings, suggesting that they had either displaced the myelin sheath, or arisen in unmyelinated fibers.

The prognosis for recovery was generally good (14). Three months after exposure to DMAPN was eliminated, only 13% of workers in one plant still had symptoms. All patients with residual symptoms had urinary dysfunction. Half also had sexual dysfunction. After 10 years, at least one worker had persistent urinary and sexual complaints (A. Pestronk, unpublished observations). People with persistence of symptoms tended to be older and have more seniority at work. It is not clear whether persistence of symptoms was due to age or length and severity of exposure.

DMAPN was the major component of a catalyst (15) that was introduced into several workplaces several months before the onset of symptoms of urinary and sexual dysfunction in many exposed people. A second compound, dimethylaminoethylether (DMAEE), was also used in the catalyst (16). However, DMAEE was used without associated neurological symptoms, in the absence of DMAPN, in similar industrial processes and concentrations, before and after the epidemic.

During the months of exposure to DMAPN, its concentration in the manufacturing process was progressively increased (0.5%–2.0%). The prevalence of urological symptoms increased during this period, being highest in early 1978, just before the utilization of DMAPN was terminated. The latency between first exposure to DMAPN and the onset of symptoms varied inversely with the concentrations or amounts used. When DMAPN was first introduced and used in the lowest amounts (in mid-1977), workers were exposed for several months before noting urinary symptoms. Later, when use of DMAPN was at its peak (early 1978), several workers became symptomatic within 1–4 days of employment. No workers with new symptoms were identified after the use of DMAPN was discontinued. Most affected workers reported that their symptoms began to abate shortly (days to weeks) after DMAPN was removed from the workplace.

Airborne spread of DMAPN probably played a major role in the epidemic (14). In one factory, the highest incidence of symptoms occurred among workers in a room where hot, freshly produced foam was processed. Within that room, there was no difference in the incidence of the clinical syndrome between workers who had skin contact with the foam of high DMAPN content and those who handled foam with little or no DMAPN. Further, some workers with the most severe symptoms had no skin contact with the foam. The highest levels of organic vapors in factory air samples were in the areas with a high incidence of affected workers. No data are available on the air levels of DMAPN during its industrial use. High concentrations (11 mg/m^3) were found in the air of a warehouse where foam, produced 2 months previously, was stored. DMAPN was detectable, at much lower concentrations (0.11 mg/m^3), in a manufacturing plant 1 week after all use was discontinued (17). In a laboratory test simulating manufacturing conditions, DMAPN was detected as a reaction off-gas, and was also extractable from the cured foam. Although it seems likely that DMAPN intoxication resulted from inhalation, absorption through the skin from contaminated clothes cannot be ruled out.

The most common syndrome associated with DMAPN intoxication is urological and results from a flaccid urinary bladder. DMAPN and its metabolites may have a direct toxic effect on the bladder wall. Peripheral neuropathy probably also plays a role in the bladder dysfunction, and produces sensory loss, involving the sacral dermatomes and distal extremities, and some distal weakness. In humans and animals exposed to DMAPN, distal axons are enlarged with accumulations of neurofilaments similar to those found in proximal axons of animals given β,β'-iminodipropionitrile.

REFERENCES

1. Baker EL, Christiani DC, Wegman DH *et al.* (1981) Follow-up studies of workers with bladder neuropathy caused by exposure to dimethylaminopropionitrile. *Scand J Work Environ Health* 4, 54.

2. Froines JR, Postlethwait EM, LaFuente EJ, Liu WC (1985) *In vivo* and *in vitro* release of cyanide from neurotoxic aminonitriles. *J Toxicol Environ Health* 16, 449.

3. Froines JR, Watson AJ (1985) Evaluation of the inhibition of glycolytic enzymes by the neurotoxicant dimethylaminopropionitrile. *J Toxicol Environ Health* 16, 469.

4. Gad SC, McKelvey JA, Turney RA (1979) NIAX catalyst ESN: Subchronic neuropharmacology and neurotoxicology. *Drug Chem Toxicol* 2, 223.

5. Griffin JW, Price DL (1980) Proximal axonopathies induced by toxic chemicals. In: *Experimental and Clinical Neurotoxicology*. Spencer PS, Schaumburg HH eds. Williams & Wilkins, Baltimore p. 161.

6. Jaeger RJ, Plugge H, Szabo S (1980) Acute urinary bladder toxicity of a polyurethane foam catalyst mixture: A possible new target organ for propionitrile derivative. *J Environ Pathol Toxicol* 4, 555.

7. Keogh JP (1983) Classical syndromes in occupational medicine: Dimethylaminopropionitrile. *Amer J Ind Med* **4**, 479.

8. Keogh JP, Pestronk A, Wertheimer D, Moreland R (1980) An epidemic of urinary retention caused by dimethylaminopropionitrile. *J Amer Med Assn* **243**, 746.

9. Kreiss K, Wegman DH, Niles CA *et al.* (1980) Neurological dysfunction of the bladder in workers exposed to dimethylaminopropionitrile. *J Amer Med Assn* **243**, 741.

10. Landrigan PJ, Kreiss K, Xintaras C *et al.* (1980) Clinical epidemiology of occupational neurotoxic disease. *Neurobehav Toxicol* **2**, 43.

11. Levine CI (1961) Structural requirements for lathyrogenic agents. *J Exp Med* **114**, 295.

12. Mumtaz MM, Farooqui MY, Ghanayem BI, Ahmed AE (1991) The urotoxic effects of N,N'-dimethylaminopropionitrile. 2. *In vivo* and *in vitro* metabolism. *Toxicol Appl Pharmacol* **110**, 61.

13. Mumtaz MM, Farooqui MY, Ghanayem BI *et al.* (1991) Studies on the mechanism of urotoxic effects of N,N'-dimethylaminopropionitrile in rats and mice. 1. Biochemical and morphologic characterization of the injury and its relationship to metabolism. *J Toxicol Environ Health* **33**, 1.

14. Pestronk A, Keogh JP, Griffin JW (1980) Dimethylaminopropionitrile. In: *Experimental and Clinical Neurotoxicology.* Spencer PS, Schaumburg HH eds. Williams & Wilkins, Baltimore p. 422.

15. Union Carbide Corporation (1978) Toxicology Information Sheet: Dimethylaminopropionitrile.

16. Union Carbide Corporation (1978) Toxicology Information Sheet: Dimethylaminoethylether.

17. White G, Keogh JP (1978) Health Hazard Determination Report. TA 78-33 NIOSH, Cincinnati, OH.

18. Wilmarth KR, Froines JR (1991) Role of monoamine oxidase in aminopropionitrile-induced neurotoxicity. *J Toxicol Environ Health* **32**, 415.

19. Wilmarth KR, Froines JR (1992) *In vitro* and *in vivo* inhibition of lysyl oxidase by aminopropionitriles. *J Toxicol Environ Health* **37**, 411.

Dimethyl Sulfate

Peter S. Spencer

$$(CH_3)_2SO_4$$

$$C_2H_6O_4S$$

Sulfuric acid dimethylester

NEUROTOXICOLOGY RATING

Clinical

A Acute encephalopathy (secondary to hypoxia?)

Experimental

A Developmental CNS tumors

Dimethyl sulfate, a colorless, oily liquid with a faint onion odor, is a methylating agent used in chemical syntheses; it is also a potent alkylating agent for cellular macromolecules. Dimethyl sulfate is a corrosive, mutagenic, and carcinogenic compound for which there may be no safe level of exposure. A time-weighted Threshold Limit Value of 0.1 ppm has been set by the American Conference of Governmental Occupational Hygienists. The U.S. National Institute for Occupational Safety and Health has a Recommended Exposure Limit of 0.1 ppm averaged over a 10-h workshift. The Permissible Exposure Limit is 1 ppm averaged over an 8-h workshift.

The International Agency for Research on Cancer (IARC) considers there is sufficient evidence for carcinogenicity in animals. Rats treated with 3 ppm or 10 ppm dimethyl sulfate vapor for 1 h/day, 5 days a week for 130 days, with tissue examination at 643 days, developed three nervous system tumors, including a cerebellar tumor in the high-dose group (4). Malignant tumors of the nervous system (4/59) and liver (2/59) were also reported in the offspring of pregnant dams given a single intravenous dose of 20 mg/kg dimethyl sulfate on day 15 of gestation (3, *see also* 7).

Dimethyl sulfate induced differentiation and promoted neurite formation in mouse neuroblastomas N-18 cells (9).

Dimethyl sulfate can be absorbed in liquid or vapor form through the skin and respiratory tract. Overexposure may result in mucous membrane irritation, headache, giddiness, nausea, vomiting, diarrhea, photophobia, periorbital edema, aphonia, dysphonia, dysphagia, chest pain, pulmonary edema, cyanosis, dysuria, and hematuria (1,5). Headache and agitation are reported to be early signs of overexposure, but these effects may be delayed in onset for up to 10 h (5,6,8). Prostration, convulsions, delirium, paralysis, and coma are also reported. There my be delayed damage to the liver and heart, jaundice, albuminuria, and hematuria, and death (2,6). IARC considers that dimethyl sulfate may reasonably be anticipated to be a human carcinogen (1).

REFERENCES

1. Budavari S (1996) *The Merck Index. An Encyclopedia of Chemicals, Drugs, and Biologicals. 12th Ed.* Merck & Co. Whitehouse Station, New Jersey p. 3309.

2. Clayton GD, Clayton FE (1982) *Patty's Industrial Hygiene and Toxicology. Vol 2.* John Wiley-Interscience, New York p. 2094.

3. Druckrey H (1973) Chemical structure and action in transplacental carcinogenesis and teratogenesis. *IARC Sci Publ No.4*, p. 45.

4. Druckrey H, Kruse H, Preussmann S *et al.* (1970) Cancerogenic alkylating substances. Alkylhalogenides, -sulfates, -sulfonates and strained heterocyclic compounds. *Z Krebsforsch* **74**, 241.

5. Hathaway GJ, Proctor NH, Hughes JP *et al.* (1996) *Chem-ical Hazards of the Workplace. 4th Ed.* Van Nostrand Reinhold, New York p. 246.

6. Mohlau FD (1920) Report of two cases of dimethyl sulfate poisoning. *J Ind Hyg* **2**, 238.

7. Robbiano L, Brambilla M (1987) DNA damage in the central nervous system of rats after *in vivo* exposure to chemical carcinogens: correlation with the induction of brain tumors. *Terato Carcin Mut* **7**, 175.

8. Roux H, Gallet M, Vincent V, Frantz P (1977) Poisoning by dimethyl sulfate. Clinical and bibliographic study. *Acta Pharmacol Toxicol Suppl* **41**, 438.

9. Yoda K, Shimizu M, Fujimura S (1982) Induction of morphological differentiation in cultured mouse neuroblastoma cells by alkylating agents. *Carcinogenesis* **3**, 1369.

Diphenyl

Peter S. Spencer

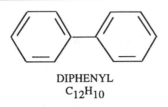

DIPHENYL
$C_{12}H_{10}$

Biphenyl; 1,1′-Biphenyl; Phenylbenzene

NEUROTOXICITY RATING

Clinical

B   Chronic encephalopathy

C   Peripheral neuropathy

Experimental

B   Suspect chromogenic neurotoxin

Diphenyl is used (a) as a citrus fungistat for fruit wrappings and shipping containers, (b) with diphenyl oxide as a heat-transfer fluid, (c) in methylated form as a freezing protectant, (d) in the compound diphenyl methane as an artificial flavoring substance and as a fragrance component in perfumes and soaps, and (e) in the synthesis of herbicides and chlorinated and brominated diphenyl oxides. Diphenyl has poorly defined neurotoxic properties. 2,2′-Dihydroxy-3,5,6,3′,5′,6′-hexachloro*diphenyl* methane has bactericidal and myelinotoxic effects (*see* Hexachlorophene, this volume) (2).

Diphenyl forms white to light-yellow leaflets that are soluble in alchohol and ether. The MP is 70°C and BP is 255°C; the odor is said to be pleasant and peculiar. For workroom air, a time-weighted Threshold Limit Value of 0.2 ppm has been adopted by the American Conference of Governmental Industrial Hygienists (2).

Diphenyl is one of several dicyclic aromatic hydrocarbons that appear to generate a metabolite that reacts with biological tissue to form a blue pigment (7) (*see* Diethylbenzene, Table 19). For those aromatic hydrocarbons (of which diphenyl is not one) that have been carefully studied for neurotoxic potential, the chromogenic property appears to predict neurotoxicity in rats (14) (*see* Acetyl Ethyl Tetramethyl Tetralin, this volume).

Biphenyl metabolism principally involves hydroxylation; the primary biphenyl metabolite is 4-hydroxybiphenyl in fish, amphibia, birds, and mammals, including humans (3,9,11). 2-Hydroxybiphenyl has been reported in young but not adult rats and rabbits (9). 4-Hydroxybiphenyl and 4,4′-hydroxybiphenyl were isolated as principal urinary metabolites in male albino rats given an oral dose of 100 mg/kg of carbon-labeled biphenyl (5); other metabolites include 3,4′-dihydroxy-, 3,4,4′-trihydroxy-, 3,4′-dihydroxy-4-methoxy-, and 4,4′-dihydroxy-3-methoxybiphenyl (5). Approximately 99% of the dose was eliminated within 96 h; fecal elimination was minor (5). 4-Hydroxybiphenyl was the principal urinary metabolite in male and female pigs given 100 mg/kg biphenyl in soya oil or propylene glycol; other metabolites included 2-hydroxy-, 3-hydroxy-, 4-hydroxy-, 3-hydroxy-4-methoxy or 4-hydroxy-3-methoxy, 3,4-dihydroxy-, 3,4′-dihydroxy-, 4,4′-dihydroxy-, 3,4′-dihydroxy-4-methoxy- or 4,4′-dihydroxy-3-methoxy-, and 3,4,4′-trihydroxybiphenyl. Unchanged biphenyl was detected in the feces of these animals (11). Mice and rats also generate intermediate epoxides that are reportedly rapidly converted to biphenylphenols (dihydrodiols, catechols, O-methylcatechol (2,9).

The acute oral LD_{50} in rats is 3280 mg/kg (6). Rats given a single, subcutaneous dose of ~5 ml/kg excrete green-colored urine (7). The identity of the chromogenic diphenyl metabolite is unknown; other chromogenic aromatic hydrocarbons form 1,2-diacetyl derivatives which are proposed to react directly with amino acids and peptides to form a blue pigment (see Diethylbenzene, this volume). Rats metabolize diphenyl oxide to a reactive metabolite that irreversibly binds to tissue proteins (2).

Diphenyl is not a teratogen in Wistar rats, but fetal toxicity can be produced when dams are treated with a dose (1000 mg/kg) sufficient to cause maternal toxicity (10). Hepatotoxic, nephrotoxic, and neurotoxic effects are reported in animals (2). Diphenyl-treated animals have also reportedly shown CNS depression, paralysis, and convulsions (2).

Like hexachlorophene (4), both diphenyl and diphenyl oxide inhibit respiration and uncouple oxidative phosphorylation of liver mitochondria in vitro (2).

Workplace exposures to diphenyl (0.7–20 ppm) have resulted in electroencephalographic and electromyographic abnormalities (13). Prolonged occupational exposures up to 19 ppm have been linked with headache, fatigue, giddiness, and aching limbs (8,12). Mood changes, memory loss, sexual "asthenia," nystagmus, facial paralysis, vertigo, insomnia, tremor, "sensory impairment," and extremity numbness have also been reported (1).

REFERENCES

1. Anger WK, Johnson BI (1985) Chemicals affecting behavior. In: Neurotoxicity of Industrial and Commercial Chemicals. Vol 1. O'Donoghue JL ed. CRC Press, Baton Rouge, Florida p. 51.
2. Benya TJ, Leber P (1994) Halogenated cyclic hydrocarbons. In: Patty's Industrial Hygiene and Toxicology. Vol II, Pt. D, 4th Ed. Clayton GD, Clayton FE eds. Wiley, New York p. 2430.
3. Block WD, Cornish HH (1959) Metabolism of biphenyl and 4-chlorobiphenyl in the rabbit. J Biol Chem 234, 3301.
4. Cammer W, Moore CL (1972) The effect of hexachlorophene on the respiration of liver and brain mitochondria. Biochem Biophys Res Commun 46, 1887.
5. Deichmann WB (1981) Halogenated cyclic hydrocarbons. In: Patty's Industrial Hygiene and Toxicology. 3rd Ed. Vol. IIB. Clayton GD, Clayton FE eds. Wiley, New York p. 3603.
6. Deichmann WB et al. (1947) Observations on the effects of biphenyl, o- and p-aminobiphenyl, o- and p-nitrophenyl, and dihydroxyoctachlorobiphenyl on experimental animals. J Ind Hyg Toxicol 29, 1.
7. Gerarde HW (1960) Toxicology and biochemistry of aromatic hydrocarbons. In: Elsevier Monographs on Toxic Agents. Browning E ed. Elsevier, Amsterdam p. 73.
8. Häkkinen I, Siltanen E, Hernberg S et al. (1973) Diphenyl poisoning in fruit paper production. Arch Environ Health 26, 70.
9. Halpaap K, Horning MG, Horning EC (1978) Metabolism of biphenyl in the rat. J Chromatogr 166, 479.
10. Khera KS et al. (1979) Assessment of the teratogenic potential of piperonyl butoxide, biphenyl, and phosalone in the rat. Toxicol Appl Pharmacol 47, 353.
11. Meyer T, Larsen JC, Hansen EV, Scheline RR (1976) The metabolism of biphenyl. III. Phenolic metabolites in the pig. Acta Pharmacol Toxicol 39, 433.
12. Proctor NH, Hughes JP (1978) Chemical Hazards of the Workplace. JB Lippincott Co, Philadelphia p. 236.
13. Seppäläinen AM, Häkkinen I (1975) Electrophysiological findings in diphenyl poisoning. J Neurol Neurosurg Psychiat 38, 248.
14. Spencer PS, Foster V, Sterman AB, Horoupian D (1980) Acetyl ethyl tetramethyl tetralin. In Experimental and Clinical Neurotoxicology, Spencer PS, Schaumburg HH eds. Williams & Wilkins, Baltimore p. 296.

Diphtheria Toxin

Herbert H. Schaumburg
Dennis A. Aquino
Kenneth R. Einberg

NEUROTOXICITY RATING

Clinical

A Peripheral neuropathy (demyelinating)

Experimental

A Peripheral myelinopathy (inhibition of myelin protein synthesis)

A CNS demyelination (local application)

Diphtheria toxin (DTX) is a polypeptide of approximately 60 kDa secreted by the bacterium *Corynebacterium diphtheriae*, a gram-positive nonsporulating rod. Infection with the bacterium in the nasopharynx and subsequent release of toxin into the circulation accounts for the local and systemic manifestations of diphtheria, a serious and potentially fatal disease. The malady was first described in the second century, the organism cultured in 1884, and the toxin isolated in 1888 (26). Tests for susceptibility and development of toxoid immunization were accomplished by 1920.

Epidemiological studies clearly indicate that humans are the only reservoir (21). Human-to-human transmission is typically mediated by airborne respiratory droplets and/or direct contact with the exudative secretions of infected skin lesions. The respiratory tract form of diphtheria is most common during the cooler months in temperate climates when indoor crowding is more prevalent. The identification of individuals in the incubation and convalescent stages of this illness, as well as asymptomatic carriers (respiratory and skin), is critical to the containment and prevention of *C. diphtheriae*. In endemic regions (Brazil, Nigeria, the Eastern Mediterranean, the Indian subcontinent, Indonesia, and the Philippines), up to 5% of healthy individuals may harbor *C. diphtheriae* (10). The prevalence of asymptomatic carriage is extremely low in North America; there have been only four reported cases between 1980 and 1995 (17). Worldwide total cases dropped from 69,475 to 5109 between 1980 and 1991 as a result of global childhood immunization (17). Russian cases have been reported recently (16,29).

DTX was once widely used as an experimental tool in neuropathology and neurophysiology laboratories to induce demyelination and remyelination. Current research focuses on the molecular biology of the sequence of events of toxin-mediated cell death; DTX is probably better characterized than any other bacterial membrane-translocating toxin, and it is a prototypical model for toxigenic disease.

DTX has been used to eliminate pathological or cancerous cells by combining the catalytic domain of DTX ($DAB_{486}IL-2$) with various cell-targeting agents. This toxin is cytotoxic *in vitro* for cells that express the high-affinity interleukin-2 (IL-2) receptor (*e.g.*, activated T lymphocytes, B lymphocytes, and monocytes). As a result of the limited distribution of the high-affinity IL-2 receptor, $DAB_{486}IL-2$ is viewed as a potential therapy for diseases in which activated lymphocytes play a pathogenic role (7,23,30).

General Toxicology

After arrival of *C. diphtheriae* at the site of infection (pharynx or skin), organisms proliferate and elaborate toxin. The rapidity of onset, severity of disease, and outcome are influenced by the rate of production, absorption, and dissemination of toxin and the immune status of the host. Infection of the pharynx is more threatening than that of skin because the former absorbs the toxin better; persons with immunity from prior immunization are rarely affected by localized carriage of organisms. DTX is graded as extremely potent; a dose as small as 0.1 μg/kg kills laboratory animals, and a single molecule is said to inhibit protein synthesis in a cell within several hours of toxin binding (36). Although receptors for DTX seem to be universal to all human cells, the most common target organs (presumably, harboring the most receptors) are heart (myocarditis), kidney (tubular necrosis), and peripheral nerve (segmental demyelination).

Mechanisms of Cellular Toxicity

DTX is inactive upon its release into the circulation of an infected host. Activation occurs within the host cell when DTX, a Y-shaped molecule of three domains, is proteolytically cleaved and reduced into two fragments—A and B. (6). Fragment A (~21 kDa) contains the catalytic domain, and fragment B (~37 kDa) both the receptor-binding and transmembrane domains. Fragments A and B are linked by a single, intramolecular disulfide bond. The target of DTX is diphthamide, a posttranslationally modified histidine residue that is present in the ribosomal binding site of, and unique to, the eukaryotic elongation factor-2 (eEF-2). eEF-2 is a G protein that binds guanosine triphosphate (GTP), which is then dephosphorylated to the diphosphate when eEF-2 binds to ribosomes. Fragment A of DTX catalyzes the adenosine diphosphate (ADP)–ribosylation of eEF-2 *via* transfer of the ADP-ribosyl moiety of nicotine adenine dinucleotide to diphthamide. The ADP-ribosylation of diphthamide inactivates eEF-2 by modifying eEF-2 so that it cannot productively interact with the ribosome. The functional consequence of this modification of eEF-2 leads to inhibition of the translocation step of protein chain elongation, and subsequently to cell death.

It has been proposed that cell death may also arise from intranucleosomal breakdown of chromosomal DNA, similar to apoptosis (programmed cell death), due to a DTX nuclease activity (14). The morphological changes that occur include condensation of chromatin, fragmentation of nuclei, a gradual loss of plasma membrane integrity, and cytolysis. It has been shown that ADP-ribosylation of eEF-2 is required for DTX-mediated apoptosis, but that inhibition of protein synthesis by DTX is not sufficient to mediate cell lysis (22).

The internalization and membrane translocation of DTX has been reviewed (15,24). DTX enters the target cell *via* receptor-mediated endocytosis and then translocates across the endosomal membrane into cell cytoplasm. The membrane-anchored precursor of heparin-binding epidermal growth factor (HB-EGF) has been shown to serve as the receptor for DTX. The number of HB-EGF/DTX receptor molecules on the cell surface determines a cell's susceptibility to DTX. DTX binds its receptor *via* fragment B, and toxin–receptor complexes are internalized by entrapment in clathrin-coated pits as part of a normal process for turnover of cell surface proteins (20). Increased hydrophobicity is envisioned as being partly responsible for insertion of DTX into the plasmalemma and translocation of fragment A into the cytosol.

The proteolytic or "nicking" site between fragments A and B is an arginine-rich region that has been shown to be easily cleaved by proteases (22). Proteolytic cleavage leaves only one disulfide bond connecting fragments A and B. Nicked DTX separates into free fragments A and B when this disulfide bond is exposed to the reducing environment of the cytoplasm during membrane translocation of the toxin. Reduction of this interchain disulfide bond is the rate-limiting step of the entire intoxication process (25). It has been proposed that a large number of fragment A molecules are released into the cytosol at the same time, rapidly inactivating eEF-2 molecules and inhibiting protein synthesis (23).

(10), clinical manifestations of disease appear in an infected host. Initial signs and symptoms of local infection appear at both sites (respiratory tract and skin). Subsequent symptoms originate from distant sites, secondary to hematogenous and lymphatic dissemination of DTX; symptoms are commonly categorized as either local or general. Local inflammation develops at the sites of infection. Within a few days following the appearance of a respiratory tract illness, a patchy gray-white pseudomembranous necrotic coagulum appears at the site of infection (*i.e.*, anterior nasal, proximal pharynx, laryngeal, or tracheobronchial); it is composed of fibrin, leukocytes, erythrocytes, dead respiratory tract epithelium, and organisms. The diphtheritic pseudomembrane can remain localized (*i.e.*, tonsils or nasal mucosa) or progress completely to line the pharynx and tracheobronchial tree. Severe cases can be accompanied by a profound cervical lymphadenitis resulting in the characteristic "bull neck" appearance. This combination of soft tissue edema, lymphadenopathy, and pseudomembranous material may cause fatal airway obstruction (17).

The local manifestation of skin infection is wound inflammation. Typically coexistent with *Staphylococcus aureus* and group A *Streptococcus* (17), the wound is a chronic nonhealing ulcer covered by a dirty-gray membrane. Skin infection rarely progresses to a state of general intoxication.

Generalized symptoms (headache, malaise, anorexia, diffuse myalgias, and irritability) follow dissemination of DTX from the primary site (10). There is usually a low-grade fever (rarely exceeding 103°F) associated with a rapid pulse, hypotension, serosanguinous nasal discharge, and nonproductive cough (17). These signs and symptoms gradually improve in mild cases. However, in moderate to severe forms, these initial manifestations may soon be followed by peripheral circulatory failure, cardiac arrhythmias, and congestive heart failure. Early or sudden death of patients with diphtheria is often due to inflammation of the myocardium and cardiac conduction system (4,12). In persons who eventually develop polyneuropathy, late-onset, resting tachycardia and fatal cardiac arrhythmias likely reflect involvement of the nodose ganglion of the vagus nerve. The majority of deaths occurs within the first 3–4 days as a result of either suffocation or cardiac involvement. The populations at greatest risk appear to be the very old and very young.

Human Systemic (Nonneurological) Toxicity

The two usual routes of entry into the host are the upper respiratory tract, following exposure to aerosolized respiratory droplets containing *C. diphtheriae*, or *via* an infected skin abrasion. Following an incubation period of 2–4 days

Animal Studies

Whereas *C. diphtheriae* does not infect animals, cats, rabbits, and guinea pigs subjected to subcutaneous injection of a mixture of diphtheria toxin-antitoxin mixtures readily and reliably develop diphtheritic neuropathy.

An exceptionally thorough study of diphtheritic neuropathy in cats defines a characteristic clinical syndrome and correlates the signs with histopathological and electrophysiological observations (18). There is a latent period of 2–19 days before the appearance of hindlimb splay and ataxia; strength is preserved at this stage. The neuropathy then evolves rapidly; unsteady forelimbs and swaying gait appear after a week. Depressed tendon reflexes and weakness develop in the most ataxic animals. Animals allowed to recover begin to improve within 10 days of achieving the peak neurological deficit; all display rapid improvement over 7 days, and no neurological abnormalities are detectable after 4 weeks.

Neuropathological findings in peripheral nerve and spinal roots of all species are virtually identical to those seen in human postmortem studies. Segmental demyelination with preservation of axons occurs at specific foci in the PNS (1,5,11,32–34). In somatic nerves, segments of dorsal root immediately proximal to the ganglion, the ganglion itself, and the immediate adjacent ventral root display the most severe demyelination. Nerve endings in tissue show variable amounts of change. The nodose ganglion of the vagus is the predominant site of autonomic nervous system involvement. These sites represent regions of high permeability of the blood-nerve interface. Studies utilizing ^{131}I-labeled toxin demonstrate the concentration of absorbed toxin coincides with the degree of damage in all species tested. Thus, in the rabbit, an animal with a well-formed blood-nerve barrier, the injected toxin and the lesions appear in the ganglia and roots with little in peripheral nerve. In the guinea pig, the lesions occur diffusely in the PNS, and there is entry of the labeled toxin throughout the nerve trunks (32). Lesions do not appear in the CNS of experimental animals following systemic administration of DTX; if toxin is locally injected into the CNS white matter, foci of demyelination appear at the sites of administration (35). One study suggests that DTX may reach spinal motor neurons *via* retrograde transport from the periphery and produce cytoskeletal disorganization (31).

Experimental histopathological studies with DTX have also yielded critical information on the evolution of toxin-induced nerve injury (1,11,33,34) and serve as classic models of the spatiotemporal cascade of events in segmental demyelination. In these studies, diphtheria toxin has been administered to a variety of experimental animals both parenterally and topically, and the evolution of the peripheral nerve lesions determined. There is a latent period of several days between administration of the toxin, by either route, and the onset of clinical findings. During this latent period, there is increased prominence of Schwann cell cytoplasm and early signs of myelin breakdown at paranodal regions.

In rats, the initial changes occurred in the outer terminal myelin loops and, in time, these loops became detached, resulting in nodal widening (1). Nodal widening and loss of Schwann cell processes develop after 1 week. Later, demyelination affects the entire internode, and substantial lengths of axon are denuded (11). Lesions are often hypercellular, due to proliferation of Schwann cells and macrophages. The extent of damage is dose-related. DTX has also had widespread use as a prototype in experimental neurophysiological studies of the slowing and blockade of peripheral nerve conduction associated with segmental demyelination. The results of these studies have usually correlated closely with histopathological abnormalities in nerves from the same animals (18,28). Indeed, DTX-induced peripheral nerve conduction block is so readily and reliably achieved that it has also been widely used to study the neurobiology of electrical excitability and conduction potential of the denuded internodal axon (3,28). Nerve conduction abnormalities encountered in human diphtheria appear identical to those in experimental animals (13). Studies of experimental CNS demyelination-associated conduction block have successfully utilized DTX focally injected into the dorsal columns of the spinal cord (19).

In Vitro Studies

The mechanism of peripheral nerve demyelination has been reported in an *in vitro* study (27). This investigation revealed that a 4-h *in vitro* incubation with diphtheria toxin produced no measurable degradation of myelin in the sciatic nerves of chick embryos. In contrast, a similar *in vitro* diphtheria toxin incubation succeeded in inhibiting the incorporation of L-U-^{14}C-leucine into myelin proteins by the nerve preparations after 1 h. The authors concluded that diphtheria toxin did not increase the degradation of preformed myelin lipids or proteins but that the toxin inhibited the synthesis of myelin proteolipid and basic proteins. This suggests that demyelination results from failure of myelin synthesis during normal turnover (27).

Human Studies

The estimated incidence of peripheral neuropathy in diphtheria is approximately 20% (18). Polyneuropathy may be extremely mild and escape detection; the reported figures for the incidence of diphtheritic paralysis have ranged from 8%–66%. The incidence and severity of the polyneuropathy increase in proportion to the magnitude of the primary infection. Two forms of neuropathy are recognized following faucial infection; a localized pharyngeal-extraocular type from local spread of toxin, and a later-onset generalized polyneuropathy reflecting systemic dissemination of toxin (10,17,18).

In the first 2 weeks, the initial neurological manifestation in patients with severe throat infection is the development of soft palate paralysis, which typically presents with the characteristic "nasal twang" speech followed by the nasal regurgitation of swallowed fluids. Examination at this time reveals diminished sensation over the palate and pharynx. By the fourth or fifth week, the patient may begin to experience dysfunction of ocular accommodation and near vision. Weeks 5–7 of the illness may be characterized by progressive dysphagia, dysphonia (or aphonia), and ventilatory compromise as a result of paralysis of the pharynx, larynx, and diaphragm. In addition, during this phase there may be the signs and associated symptoms of oculomotor, masticatory, facial, and sternocleidomastoid muscle weakness.

The generalized neuropathy, with rapid onset of sensory loss and paralysis, is similar to acute inflammatory demyelinating polyneuropathy (AIDP; Guillain-Barré syndrome); neuropathy appears in some by the eighth or twelfth week of illness. It is a generalized, sensorimotor neuropathy with pronounced distal-extremity involvement (18). Tenderness of the distal muscles, loss of tendon reflexes, and eventual muscle wasting are typical. Some individuals become quadriplegic and experience respiratory compromise. Less common is the appearance of bowel and/or bladder dysfunction. Paresthesias are an early manifestation of neurological dysfunction. Sensory examination typically reveals the involvement of all sensory modalities with an early and sometimes profound disturbance of vibratory and joint position sense. Referred to as "diphtheritic pseudotabes" (9), such patients can experience a marked sensory ataxia.

If the patient survives, recovery of neurological function typically begins within days to weeks from the time of presentation. Latency to the onset of recovery is highly dependent upon severity of illness. Complete recovery of motor and sensory function is the rule; typically it takes 3 months.

A series of meticulous clinicopathological studies has demonstrated concentration of pathological changes in the dorsal root ganglia and dorsal, ventral, and mixed spinal nerve roots (8). In some cases, less dramatic changes are present in more distal regions of the peripheral mixed nerve. Of note is the striking involvement of the nodose ganglion of the vagus nerve. The predominant feature of this polyneuropathy is patchy segmental and paranodal demyelination. While preserved axonal continuity is the rule, reportedly there is occasional axonal degeneration in demyelinated regions. Marked proliferation of Schwann cells is accompanied by macrophages, without evidence of polymorphonuclear leukocytes, plasma cells, or lymphocytes. The absence of the latter components argues against the likelihood of an allergic or inflammatory reaction.

A comprehensive analysis of the clinical neurophysiological effects of this disease upon human peripheral nerve appeared in 1979 (13). In this study, 11 patients (ages 4–16 years) had acute diphtheritic neuropathy. Most cases displayed increased distal motor latency and diminished motor nerve conduction velocity within the first 2 weeks of neurological illness. Electrophysiological dysfunction appeared to peak at approximately 5–7 weeks. Normalization of conduction velocity and/or distal motor latency did not occur prior to 17 weeks. There was marked dissociation of clinical and electrophysiological findings during the acute and convalescent stages of neurological illness (i.e., when patients initially demonstrated severe limb weakness, conduction velocities and distal motor latencies remained normal). Conversely, in some, the most abnormal electrophysiological values were recorded when the patient had returned to a state of clinical well-being. These observations are in precise agreement with experimental animal models in which the delayed nerve conduction and latency abnormalities are supported by the observation that demyelination in distally located peripheral nerves appears later than in the roots and ganglia (11,32). Late responses (F and H waves), which can lead to the early detection of proximal–nerve or nerve–root conduction abnormalities, may be important in the initial electrophysiological evaluation of patients with suspected diphtheritic neuropathy. Nine of the 11 patients demonstrated normal motor nerve conduction parameters at 33 weeks after the onset of neurological illness.

There are sporadic reports of CNS involvement in this disease (2). Most are careful to distinguish cases of diphtheritic delirium, similar to the reversible delirium seen in other toxic states, from a putative (probably nonexistent) diphtheritic encephalitis. In the rare instance of cases with proven cerebral lesions, the mechanism in a majority of cases is likely cerebral embolism originating from a cardiac thrombus developing in the setting of myocardial damage.

The diagnosis of diphtheritic neuropathy in an endemic area is a facile clinical exercise if the patient has a coexistent pseudomembranous pharyngeal inflammation and signs of cardiac dysfunction. North American cases presenting with subacute onset of craniofacial and subsequent diffuse polyneuropathy following pharyngitis will inevitably be suspected of having AIDP. It is extremely difficult to distinguish AIDP from diphtheritic polyneuropathy for the following reasons: the neuropathological distribution of demyelinative lesions is similar as are the neurophysiological changes; both have a subacute onset with severe limb and cranial nerve paralysis (accommodation paralysis is more common in diphtheria), and both may display moderate pleocytosis and elevated protein levels in the cerebrospinal fluid (CSF) (generally there are more cells in diphtheria and a higher protein level in AIDP). Serological tests to determine the presence of DTX, when positive, are helpful (*see* Case Report).

Diphtheria was the first disease in which specific antibody therapy was developed for the treatment of human disease. A hyperimmune antiserum produced from horses, diphtheria antitoxin (DAT), has been employed since the publication of its use in a controlled trial in 1898 (17). As its action is to neutralize toxin prior to its entry into cells, the prompt recognition of disease and early administration of antitoxin is crucial. Ten percent of patients may develop a hypersensitivity reaction to the antitoxin; all should be questioned about known allergies and then tested with a dilute solution of DAT. In addition to antitoxin, antibiotics should be administered in almost every case. The concomitant administration of appropriate antimicrobial therapy serves three major purposes: (a) the elimination of *C. diphtheriae* bacilli as a source of toxin production, (b) treatment of coexisting infections such as *Staphylococcus aureus*, and (c) elimination of the carrier state, which is a critical step in the containment of diphtheria.

Toxic Mechanism

Diphtheria toxin specifically inhibits the synthesis of myelin proteolipid and basic protein by the Schwann cell. Myelin degradation is unaffected. These findings suggest that demyelination in diphtheritic neuropathy results from failure of myelin synthesis during normal turnover (27). The major physiological effect of PNS demyelination is marked slowing of conduction in large, heavily myelinated axons. Complete conduction block occurs in severely involved fibers (18,28). These profound alterations in peripheral nerve conduction account for the diffuse weakness and sensory loss in diphtheria.

REFERENCES

1. Allt G, Cavanagh JB (1969) Ultrastructural changes in region of the node of Ranvier in the rat caused by diphtheria toxin. *Brain* 92, 459.
2. Baker AB, Noran HH (1944) The central nervous system in diphtheria. *J Nerv Ment Dis* 100, 24.
3. Bostock H, Sears TA (1978) The internodal axon membrane: Electrical excitability and continuous conduction in segmental demyelination. *J Physiol* 280, 273.
4. Burkhardt EA, Eggleston C, Smith LW (1938) Electrocardiographic changes and peripheral nerve palsies in toxic diphtheria. *Amer J Med Sci* 195, 301.
5. Cavanagh JB, Jacobs JM (1964) Some quantitative aspects of diphtheritic neuropathy. *Brit J Exp Pathol* 45, 309.
6. Choe S, Bennett MJ, Fujii G *et al.* (1992) The crystal structure of diphtheria toxin. *Nature* 357, 216.
7. Finberg RW, Wahl SM, Allen JB *et al.* (1991) Selective elimination of HIV-1-infected cells with an interleukin-2 receptor-specific cytotoxin. *Science* 252, 1703.
8. Fisher CM, Adams RD (1956) Diphtheritic polyneuritis—A pathological study. *J Neuropathol Exp Neurol* 15, 243.
9. Hall JAS (1963) Diphtheritic pseudotabes. *West Indian Med J* 12, 47.
10. Hoeprich PD (1994) Diphtheria. In: *Infectious Disease.* 5th Ed. Hoeprich PD, Jordan MC, Ronald AR eds. JB Lippincott Co, Philadelphia p. 373.
11. Jacobs JM (1967) Experimental diphtheritic neuropathy in the rat. *Brit J Exp Pathol* 48, 204.
12. James TN, Reynolds EW (1963) Pathology of the cardiac conducting system in a case of diphtheria associated with atrial arrhythmias and heart block. *Circulation* 28, 263.
13. Kurdi A, Abdul-Kader M (1979) Clinical and electrophysiologic studies of diphtheritic neuritis in Jordan. *J Neurol Sci* 42, 243.
14. Lessnick SL, Lyczak JB, Bruce C *et al.* (1992) Localization of diphtheria toxin nuclease activity to fragment A. *J Bacteriol* 174, 2032.
15. London E (1992) Diphtheria toxin: Membrane interaction and membrane translocation. *Biochem Biophys Acta* 1113, 25.
16. Lozhnikova SM, Pirogov VN, Piradov MA *et al.* (1997) Diphtheritic polyneuropathy: clinico-morphologic study. *Arkh Patol* 59, 11. [Article in Russian]
17. MacGregor RR (1995) *Corynebacterium diphtheriae.* In: *Principles and Practice of Infectious Disease.* 5th Ed. Mandell GL, Bennett JE, Dolin R eds. Churchill Livingstone, New York p. 1865.
18. McDonald WI, Kocen RS (1993) Diphtheritic neuropathy. In: *Peripheral Neuropathy.* 3rd Ed. Dyck PJ, Thomas PK, Griffin JW *et al.* eds. WB Saunders Co, Philadelphia p. 1412.
19. McDonald WI, Sears TA (1970) The effects of experimental demyelination on conduction in the central nervous system. *Brain* 93, 583.
20. Mitamura T, Iwamoto R, Umata T *et al.* (1992) The 27-kD diphtheria toxin receptor-associated protein (DRAP27) from Vero cells is the monkey homologue of human CD9 antigen: Expression of DRAP27 elevates the number of diphtheria toxin receptors on toxin-sensitive cells. *J Cell Biol* 118, 1389.
21. Morgan-Hughes JA (1968) Experimental diphtheritic neuropathy. A pathological and electrophysiological study. *J Neurol Sci* 7, 157.
22. Morimoto H, Bonavida B (1992) Diphtheria toxin- and Pseudomonas A toxin-mediated apoptosis. ADP ribosyla-

tion of elongation factor-2 is required for DNA fragmentation and cell lysis and synergy with tumor necrosis factor-alpha. *J Immunol* **149**, 2089.

23. Morimoto H, Safrit JT, Bonavida B (1991) Synergistic effect of tumor necrosis factor-alpha- and diphtheria toxin-mediated cytotoxicity in sensitive and resistant human ovarian tumor cell lines. *J Immunol* **147**, 2609.

24. Moskaug J, Sletten K, Sandvig K, Olsnes S (1989) Translocation of diphtheria toxin A-fragment to the cytosol. Role of the site of interfragment cleavage. *J Biol Chem* **264**, 15709.

25. Papini E, Rappuoli R, Murgia M, Montecucco C (1993) Cell penetration of diphtheria toxin. Reduction of the interchain disulfide bridge is the rate-limiting step of translocation in the cytosol. *J Biol Chem* **268**, 1567.

26. Pappenheimer AJ Jr (1993) The story of a toxin protein, 1888–1992. *Protein Sci* **2**, 292.

27. Pleasure DE, Feldmann B, Prockop DJ (1973) Diphtheria toxin inhibits the synthesis of myelin proteolipid and basic proteins by peripheral nerve *in vitro*. *J Neurochem* **20**, 81.

28. Rasminsky M, Sears TA (1972) Internodal conduction in undissected demyelinated nerve fibres. *J Physiol* **227**, 323.

29. Sakharova AV, Lozhnikova SM, Pirogov VN, Piradov MA (1999) Expression of NADPH-diaphorase in the peripheral nerve and its changes at different stages of diphtheritic polyneuropathy. *Arkh Patol* **61**, 39. [Article in Russian]

30. Strom TB, Kelley VR, Murphy JR *et al.* (1993) Interleukin-2 receptor-directed therapies: Antibody- or cytokine-based targeting molecules. *Annu Rev Med* **44**, 343.

31. Sunner K, Pullen AH (1995) Phosphorylated neurofilament antigen redistribution in intercostal nerve subsequent to retrograde axonal transport of diphtheria toxin. *Acta Neuropathol* **89**, 331.

32. Waksman BH (1961) Experimental study of diphtheritic polyneuritis in the rabbit and guinea pig. III. The blood-nerve barrier in the rabbit. *J Neuropathol Exp Neurol* **20**, 35.

33. Waksman BH, Adams RD, Mansmann HC (1957) Experimental study of diphtheritic polyneuritis in the rabbit and guinea pig. I. Immunologic and histopathologic observations. *J Exp Med* **105**, 591.

34. Webster HF, Spiro D, Waksman B, Adams R (1961) Phase and electron microscopic studies of experimental demyelination. II. Schwann cell changes in guinea pig sciatic nerves during experimental diphtheritic neuritis. *J Neuropathol Exp Neurol* **20**, 5.

35. Wiśniewski H, Raine CS (1971) An ultrastructural study of experimental demyelination and remyelination. V. Central and peripheral nervous system lesions caused by diphtheria toxin. *Lab Invest* **25**, 73.

36. Yamaizumi M, Mekada E, Uchida T, Okada Y (1978) One molecule of diphtheria toxin fragment A introduced into a cell can kill the cell. *Cell* **15**, 245.

CASE REPORT

A 29-year-old Haitian man was living in France for 10 years when he was admitted with a 2-day history of tingling in lower limbs. Recently, while on holiday in his native country, he had a sore throat with marked tonsillar exudate. He did not receive antibiotic therapy for the sore throat. At the time of his return in France, he noticed increasingly blurred vision preventing him from reading, accompanied by swallowing difficulties; these symptoms progressed from week 4 to week 6 after the sore throat.

From week 5 to week 7 after the sore throat, tingling developed in legs and hands, followed by increasing lower limb weakness. On admission (week 5), examination revealed nasal speech, difficulties in breathing, absent gag reflex, a left facial nerve palsy, areflexia, diffuse hypoesthesia to light touch, and decreased vibratory sensation in all four limbs (patient able to walk >10 m). Subsequently, weakness increased in the lower limbs, confining the patient to bed (patient able to raise the leg from the bed 20 cm up). There was a persistent tachycardia (between 100 and 120 pulses/min) with increased blood pressure (160/100 mm Hg). Temperature was normal. From week 8 to week 12, blurred vision and dysarthria improved, while motor deficit extended to all four limbs (tetraplegia with assisted ventilation). Motor improvement began at week 14, and was complete at week 18: the patient could walk, and there was return to normal of muscle stretch reflexes, sensation, strength, heart rate, and blood pressure. During his hospitalization, several courses of antibiotics, including amoxicillin, were administered for urinary and pulmonary infections.

Nerve conduction studies were carried out on four occasions from week 6 to week 18 after the onset of the sore throat. The initial study showed normal compound muscle action potential amplitudes, increased motor distal latencies, delayed F-wave latencies in left ulnar, right median, and both peroneal nerves; and conduction block in right median and both ulnar nerves. Sensory nerve action potential amplitudes were normal in the lower limbs and reduced in upper limbs. These features were inconsistent with an acute demyelinating polyneuropathy. Electrophysiological follow-up showed decrease of motor nerve conduction velocities in median and peroneal nerves. Sensory nerve action potential amplitudes continued to diminish over time.

On admission, CSF examination was normal. At week 8 after onset of the sore throat, CSF contained 27 cells/mm³ and protein 74 mg/dl. The following laboratory tests were negative or normal: antinuclear antibodies, latex and Rose-Waaler test, complement fractions, cryoglobulin, angiotensin-converting enzyme, porphobilinogen and coproporphyrin, thyroid tests, and vitamin B12. Serological testing yielded negative results for Herpes simplex virus; cytomegalovirus; human immunodeficiency virus types 1 and 2; human T-cell leukemia/lymphoma virus; paramyxovirus; Toxoplasma gondii; chlamydiae; measles virus; hepatitis virus A, B, and C; Lyme disease; brucellosis; syphilis; mycoplasma; and arboviruses. Neutralization of diphtheria toxin in vivo by the serum of the patient twice revealed antidiphtheritic toxin antibodies, titer higher than 10 IU/ml (Institut Pasteur, Paris). Serological tests for immunization against poliovirus and tetanus were negative. Diphtheria bacilli were absent in throat smears 3 months after the sore throat. Muscle and nerve biopsies were performed 8 weeks after onset of weakness. Muscle biopsy showed a slight atrophy of type I fibers, without inflammation or necrosis. Superficial peroneal nerve biopsy showed a mild loss of myelinated fibers and minute mononuclear infiltrates around epineural veins, without vasculitis.

(Reprinted with permission from Creange A *et al.* (1995) *Muscle Nerve* **18**, 1460.)

Comment

The peripheral neuropathy in this patient developed 1 month after a sore throat and met the clinical and electrophysiological criteria for an acute demyelinating polyneuropathy; rapid recovery is also characteristic of demyelinating neuropathy. Diphtheritic neuropathy was recognized by the combination of sore throat, a craniofacial stage of paralysis preceding the onset of a diffuse acute demyelinating polyneuropathy, and a high titer of serum antibodies for *C. diphtheriae* toxin (>10 IU/ml) indicating a recent specific infection in an unvaccinated patient.

Dipiperidinoethane

Albert C. Ludolph

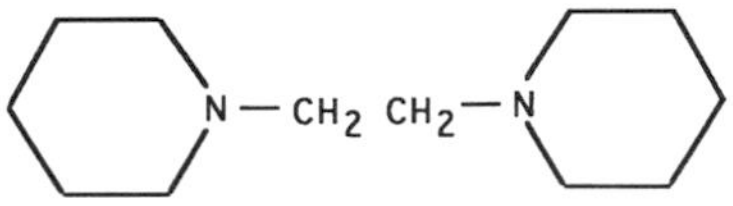

DIPIPERIDINOETHANE
$C_{12}H_{24}N_2$

NEUROTOXICITY RATING

Experimental

A   Seizure disorder

Dipiperidinoethane (DPE), an experimental convulsant, induces seizures following oxidation to DPE-di-N-oxide (2). Subcutaneous application of DPE induces seizures and associated brain damage. These characteristic clinical and morphological sequelae do not occur following direct injection of DPE into the amygdala. Direct injection of DPE-di-N-oxide in dosages exceeding 200 nM causes sustained limbic seizures similar to those seen after local kainate injection (2,3). Morphological lesions observed after local application of DPE-di-N-oxide also resemble kainate-induced lesions (2). Since DPE-N-oxide both inhibits acetylcholinesterase and is a muscarinic agonist, neurotoxicity is likely to arise from a cholinergic action (1,3,4).

REFERENCES

1. Baron BM, Kashman Y, Sokolovsky M (1985) Neurotoxicity of dipiperidinoethane due to *in vivo* conversion to a selective cholinesterase inhibitor. *Brain Res* **331**, 164.
2. Olney JW, Collins JF, De Gubareff T (1982) Dipiperidinoethane toxicity clarified. *Brain Res* **249**, 195.
3. Olney JW, Collins RC, Sloviter RS (1986) Excitotoxic mechanisms of epileptic brain damage. *Adv Neurol* **44**, 857.
4. Olney JW, de Gubareff T, Labuyere J (1983) Seizure-related brain damage induced by cholinergic agents. *Nature* **301**, 520.

Disulfiram

John C.M. Brust

DISULFIRAM
$C_{10}H_{20}N_2S_4$

Bis(Diethylthiocarbamoyl) disulfide;
Tetraethylthiuram disulfide

NEUROTOXICITY RATING

Clinical

B   Acute encephalopathy

A   Peripheral neuropathy

Disulfiram, an inhibitor of the enzyme aldehyde dehydrogenase (ALDH), is used to treat alcoholism (6). It is available as oral tablets of 250 or 500 mg (13).

About 80% of oral disulfiram is absorbed from the gastrointestinal tract; most is reduced to diethyldithiocarbamate and diethylamine by erythrocyte glutathione reductase. Interaction of disulfiram with sulfhydryl groups of albumin may also limit or delay its action. Metabolites are conjugated with glucuronic acid and excreted in the urine (5). Peak effects—signifying a symptomatic disulfiram-ethanol reaction—occur 8–12 h after taking disulfiram and within 30 min of ingesting ethanol. Ethanol may trigger an adverse reaction for up to 2 weeks after the last dose of disulfiram; diethyldithiocarbamate, which is itself pharmacologically active and probably contributes to symptoms, is slowly excreted; the enzyme ALDH is irreversibly inactivated, requiring generation of new enzyme in the liver before acetaldehyde metabolism can resume.

Ethanol is oxidized in the liver by alcohol dehydrogenase to acetaldehyde which, in turn, is oxidized by ALDH to acetate and ultimately to carbon dioxide and water. When ethanol is ingested by someone who has taken disulfiram, the blood concentration of acetaldehyde rises five to ten times higher than in untreated subjects, and this elevation accounts for most of the ensuing symptoms (5,8,16). Facial flushing quickly spreads to vasodilatation throughout the body. A throbbing headache develops. Anxiety, abdominal pain, nausea, vomiting, sweating, thirst, chest pain, tachycardia, shortness of breath, hypotension, and postural syncope follow. There may be weakness, vertigo, blurred vision, and confusion; pallor replaces flushing as blood pressure falls. Severe reactions, including seizures and coma, and shock or cardiac arrhythmia, can be fatal (12). Symptoms usually last 30 min to several hours and are followed by profound fatigue (5,13).

Most symptoms of the disulfiram-ethanol reaction are reproduced in normal humans by the infusion of acetaldehyde. The contribution of diethyldithiocarbamate to the syndrome is less certain. The metabolite chelates copper and other metals and thereby interferes with metalloenzymes including dopamine-β-hydroxylase; its inhibition might contribute to hypotension (14).

There is no antidote for the disulfiram-ethanol reaction; treatment is supportive. Vomiting makes gastric lavage superfluous; refractory vomiting can be treated with prochlorperazine or metoclopramide. Intravenous fluids generally relieve hypotension; if pressors are required, norepinephrine has theoretical advantages over dopamine; its action would be compromised by dopamine-β-hydroxylase inhibition. In life-threatening cases, hemodialysis has been employed to remove ethanol, disulfiram, and acetaldehyde (7).

Disulfiram inhibits enzymes with sulfhydryl groups; resulting delays in the metabolism of barbiturates, phenytoin, benzodiazepines, and other drugs can cause neurological symptoms (5). Patients taking disulfiram must avoid alcohol in other medications, in foods, and in household products.

Several other chemicals interfere with ALDH and produce disulfiram-like reactions with ethanol. Such agents include antimicrobials (*e.g.*, some cephalosporins, chloramphenicol, griseofulvin, metronidazole, quinacrine, and nitrofurantoin), sulfonylurea hypoglycemics, procarbazine, certain industrial compounds (*e.g.*, carbon disulfide, hydrogen sulfide, tetraethyl lead, and tetramethylthiuram disulfide), the mushroom *Coprinus atramentarius*, and animal charcoal (5,7). A drug with actions like disulfiram, calcium carbamide, is available in Canada for the treatment of alcoholism.

Disulfiram has neurotoxicity independent of its ethanol-acetaldehyde interactions. Some users report fatigue, restlessness, tremor, headache, dizziness, and reduced sexual potency. Psychosis and parkinsonism are also described, and there is evidence of teratogenicity. Inhibition of brain dopamine-β-hydroxylase and decreased brain levels of norepinephrine have been proposed as a mechanism for neurobehavioral abnormalities. Ethanol withdrawal could contribute (5,9,10).

The principal neurotoxic syndrome associated with disulfiram is peripheral neuropathy of the distal axonopathy type (3). Most cases occur at standard therapeutic doses

(250–500 mg daily) and commence within several months of starting treatment; one report describes an onset after 30 years' treatment with 250 mg daily (2). Tingling paresthesias in the feet, followed by unsteady gait, are initial complaints. Signs of diminished pain, temperature, and position sense in the feet; absent reflexes; and weakness of foot dorsiflexion are present in most cases. Eventually, distal upper extremities are involved. Cranial nerve palsies are not a feature of disulfiram neuropathy. Optic neuropathy may occur independently of peripheral neuropathy. Drug withdrawal is followed by remission of signs within months in most cases (11,15).

Mild slowing of motor nerve conduction, diminished amplitude of sensory action potentials, and electromyographic evidence of denervation in distal muscles are characteristic of disulfiram neuropathy. Sural nerve histological changes include loss of myelinated fibers and axonal degeneration. Biopsies have disclosed axonal swellings filled with intermediate filaments (4). The few experimental animal studies are unconvincing; one describes local axonal degeneration related to local injection of the drug (1,19). It is suggested that carbon disulfide, a metabolite of disulfiram, may have a role in the pathogenesis of the axonal swellings (*see* Carbon Disulfide, this volume).

Editorial addition: Disulfiram overdose reportedly may elicit extrapyramidal symptoms associated with bilateral lesions of lentiform nuclei. Experimental studies show that disulfiram antagonizes *in vitro* striatal binding of [^{3}H]tyramine, a putative marker of the vesicular transporter for dopamine, and the uptake of [^{3}H]dopamine into striatal synaptic vesicles, with inhibitory constants in the range of reported blood dithiocarbamate levels in treated alcoholics. In addition, when disulfiram is added directly to the incubation mixture, radioactivity is lost from [^{3}H]dopamine-preloaded striatal vesicles (18). Rats treated with diethyldithiocarbamate, the principal metabolite of disulfiram, exhibit an increase in extracellular glutamate that is blocked by 7-nitroindazole, a specific inhibitor of neuronal nitric oxide synthetase (17).

REFERENCES

1. Anzil AP, Duzic S (1978) Disulfiram neuropathy: An experimental study in the rat. *J Neuropathol Exp Neurol* 37, 585.
2. Borrett D, Ashby P, Bilbao J, Carlen P (1989) Reversible, late-onset disulfiram-induced neuropathy and encephalopathy. *Ann Neurol* 17, 396.
3. Bradley WG, Hewer RL (1966) Peripheral neuropathy due to disulfiram. *Brit Med J* 2, 449.
4. Dibao JM, Briggs SJ, Gray TA (1984) Filamentous axonopathy in disulfiram neuropathy. *Ultrastruct Pathol* 7, 295.
5. Eneanya DI, Bianchine JR, Duran DO et al. (1981) The actions and metabolic fate of disulfiram. *Annu Rev Pharmacol Toxicol* 21, 575.
6. Fuller RK, Branchey L, Brightwell DR et al. (1986) Disulfiram treatment of alcoholism: A Veterans Administration Cooperative Study. *J Amer Med Assn* 256, 1449.
7. Goldfrank LR, Bresnitz EA, Melinek M, Weisman RS (1990) Disulfiram. In: *Toxicologic Emergencies. 4th Ed.* Goldfrank LR, Flomenbaum NE, Lewin NA et al. eds. Appleton & Lange, Norwalk Connecticut p. 475.
8. Kitson TM (1977) The disulfiram-ethanol reaction. *J Stud Alcohol* 38, 96.
9. Knee ST, Razani J (1974) Acute organic brain syndrome: A complication of disulfiram therapy. *Amer J Psychiat* 131, 1281.
10. Liddon SC, Satran R (1967) Disulfiram (Antabuse) psychosis. *Amer J Psychiat* 123, 1284.
11. Morki B, Ohnishi A, Dyck PJ (1981) Disulfiram neuropathy. *Neurology* 31, 730.
12. Motte S, Vincent JL, Gillet JB (1986) Refractory hyperdynamic shock associated with alcohol and disulfiram. *Amer J Emerg Med* 4, 323.
13. Rall TW (1990) Disulfiram. In: *The Pharmacological Basis of Therapeutics. 8th Ed.* Gilman AG, Rall TW, Nies AS, Palmer T eds. Pergamon Press, New York p. 378.
14. Rogers WK, Benowitz NL, Wilson KM, Abbott JA (1979) Effect of disulfiram on adrenergic function. *Clin Pharmacol Ther* 24, 469.
15. Rothrock JF, Johnson PC, Rothrock SM, Merkley R (1984) Fulminant polyneuritis after overdose of disulfiram and ethanol. *Neurology* 34, 357.
16. Sanny CG, Weiner H (1987) Inactivation of horse liver mitochondrial aldehyde dehydrogenase by disulfiram: Evidence that disulfiram is not an active-site-directed reagent. *Biochem J* 242, 499.
17. Vaccari A, Ferraro L, Saba P et al. (1998) Differential mechanisms in the effects of disulfiram and diethyldithiocarbamate intoxication on striatal release and vesicular transport of glutamate. *J Pharmacol Exp Ther* 285, 961.
18. Vaccari A, Saba PL, Ruiu S et al. (1996) Disulfiram and diethyldithiocarbamate intoxication affects the storage and release of striatal dopamine. *Toxicol Appl Pharmacol* 139, 102.
19. Zuccarello M, Anzil AP (1979) Localized model of experimental neuropathy of topical application of disulfiram. *Exp Neurol* 64, 699.

2,4-Dithiobiuret

John L. O'Donoghue

$$H_2-N-\overset{\overset{\textstyle S}{\|}}{C}-NH-\overset{\overset{\textstyle S}{\|}}{C}-NH_2$$

2,4-DITHIOBIURET
$C_2H_5N_3S_2$

Thioimidodicarbonic diamide; Imidodicarbon-
imidothioic diamide; Imidodicarbonodithioic diamide

NEUROTOXICITY RATING

Experimental

A   Peripheral neuropathy

B   Ion channel dysfunction (muscle)

2,4-Dithiobiuret (DTB), a colorless, crystalline solid, is active as a strong, reversible reducing agent. It is a rubber accelerator and plasticizer and is used in the manufacture of resins, insecticides, and rodenticides. It has been proposed for use in horticulture to delay flower wilting and promote plant root growth (2), though it may not have been used commercially for these purposes.

Metabolism data for DTB are limited; those that have been collected are related to the intraperitoneal (i.p.) route of exposure because neurotoxicity studies with DTB have typically been conducted by this route. Twenty-four hours following an i.p. dose of 0.25–1 mg/kg DTB given to rats, 65%–70% of the dose is excreted in the urine while 3%–5% is present in the feces and <1% is present in the expired air (8). Repetitive daily doses do not alter this excretory pattern. Accumulation of DTB or it metabolites was highest in the thyroid glands, followed by the liver, skin, stomach, and kidneys. Brain concentrations of DTB radiolabel were lower than plasma levels, indicating that the brain is unlikely to concentrate DTB or its metabolites. The cumulative body burden of DTB at the point of induction of neurotoxicity (measured as rotarod failure) was similar (0.7–1.0 mg DTB equivalents/kg) at dose levels of 0.25–1.0 mg/kg/day (8). When rats are given 1 mg/kg DTB by i.p. injection, the parent compound and six metabolites (monothiobiuret, thiuret, sulfate, and three uncharacterized metabolites) were found in the urine (21). Thiuret can be formed by the reversible oxidation of the parent compound; therefore, redox cycling of DTB and thiuret may result in oxidative stress *in vivo*. Desulfurization of the parent compound to monothiobiuret appears to occur in the liver (21). About 60% of a 1-mg/kg dose of the parent compound was excreted in 24 h (21). The available data are not sufficient to indicate whether the parent compound or a metabolite(s) is responsible for induction of neurotoxicity. However, it

has been shown that increasing the dose level of DTB to 12 mg/kg (i.p.) can actually increase the latency to the appearance of neurotoxicity (20). Rats given 1–5 mg/kg doses of DTB (i.p.) developed neurotoxicity within 5–3 days (respectively), but rats treated with 12 mg/kg (i.p.) could be given DTB for 5–6 days before developing signs of neurotoxicity. These data suggest that DTB may be inhibiting its own metabolism to a toxic metabolite at high dose levels. Of the identified metabolites of DTB, thiuret but not monothiobiuret has been reported to produce a delayed-onset flaccid muscle weakness similar to that induced by DTB (18); however, since DTB-thiuret can redox cycle, thiuret neurotoxicity may reflect an *in vivo* equilibrium between the two materials that favors the formation of DTB.

Various substances that may alter the metabolism of DTB have been given concurrently with the diamide. Phenobarbital delays the appearance of DTB-induced neurotoxicity as do diethyldithiocarbamate, *d*-penicillamine, and disulfiram (6,16). In rats given 1 mg/kg (i.p.) DTB, neurotoxicity was seen in 5–6 days, but when the sulfur-containing antagonists were given, neurotoxicity was not seen until 21–26 days (6). Disulfiram given for 5 days reversed the muscle weakness caused by DTB (6). These results suggest that induction of hepatic P-450 enzymes and the presence of other sulfur-containing chemicals can ameliorate DTB-induced neurotoxicity.

DTB is acutely toxic to rats and mice. The 48–h LD_{50} for DTB is 29 mg/kg for male rats and 218 mg/kg for mice dosed by i.p. injection; phenobarbital pretreatment does not alter the LD_{50} for mice (7,14). With repeated i.p. dosing, the cumulative dose LD_{50} is 5.5–9.0 mg/kg for rats (8). Single doses of 5–20 mg/kg DTB do not result in neurotoxicity in rats (7) or mice (14); however, rabbits given 100 mg/kg by subcutaneous (s.c.) injection exhibit flaccid paralysis within several hours of dosing and remain paralyzed for up to 72 h prior to death (16).

Astwood and colleagues (3) first described the cumulative nature of DTB-induced neurotoxicity in rats. While large single s.c. or i.p. doses failed to produce neurotoxicity in rats, repeated doses of <0.5 mg given by s.c. injection or in drinking water resulted in profound neurotoxicity in 5 days. Drinking water DTB concentrations of 0.002% were capable of producing neurotoxicity on repeated exposure in rats, while 0.001% DTB was without effect (3). Whether given orally or by injection, there is a delay period before neurotoxicity appears following dosing (3). Using rotarod performance as an indicator for neurotoxicity, there is a latency threshold of 3–4 days and a cumulative dose threshold of 4–5 mg/kg for the onset of neurotoxicity in the rat (8). Female rats are in general more susceptible to DTB than male rats (4). Weanling rats are less sensitive than adult rats, and young adults are less sensitive than old adults (4). A no-observed-effect dose level of 0.125 mg/kg/day has been reported for rats exposed to DTB by i.p. injection for 52 days (8).

The neurotoxicity observed in rats begins as hindlimb weakness that can ascend until only the head, neck, and respiratory muscles are not obviously affected (3,7). If the dose level is increased above the level that causes limb weakness, the animals may die of respiratory paralysis. In affected animals, skeletal muscle tone is flaccid, but segmental spinal cord and cranial nerve reflexes remain intact (7). Rats can be kept in a state of severe skeletal muscle weakness by careful titration of the dose level (3). Even when animals are immobilized for weeks and muscle atrophy has occurred, the animals recover promptly if dosing is discontinued (3).

Rats are not the only species sensitive to DTB following repeated exposures; rabbits injected with 7–100 mg/kg DTB developed a flaccid paralysis in 1–12 days (16). The clinical signs observed in rabbits were similar to those seen in rats, except that the rabbits showed difficulty in voiding urine and enlarged bladders suggesting early autonomic system involvement. The rabbits also showed a significant increase in blood glucose that was not observed in rats (16). No cases of neurotoxicity have been reported in humans or domestic animals.

Various factors that might contribute to the weakness observed in rats treated with DTB have been investigated. Whole-blood cholinesterase was not affected by DTB exposure (7). Brain acetylcholine and acetylcholinesterase levels were not altered in affected rats, and administration of pilocarpine, prostigmine, atropine, epinephrine, ephedrin, vitamin A, vitamin B complexes, and biotin had no effect on DTB-intoxicated rats (3). Skeletal muscle Cl, Na, K, P, and creatinine, and plasma CO_2, Na, Ca, and K levels were also not altered in weak animals (3). Similar results were observed in rats or rabbits given DTB; skeletal muscle water, Cl, Na, K, P, and creatine, and plasma CO_2, Ca, Na, and K were unaffected (14). Total blood oxygen levels, and serum glucose, Na, K, Ca, Cl, and K were not altered in DTB-treated rats, indicating that hypoxia, hypoglycemia, and serum electrolyte imbalance did not play a role in DTB-induced neurotoxicity (18). Other investigations have shown that glucose-dependent lactate production in homogenates of neural tissue from DTB-intoxicated rats was not mechanistically linked to its neurotoxicity (13).

Observation of the clinical signs present in animals intoxicated with DTB led to the conclusion that DTB-induced neurotoxicity was primarily a motor deficit. Studies confirmed this conclusion by showing that all motor end points (motor activity, grip strength, and auditory startle amplitude) were decreased in a dose- and time-dependent manner, but all sensory functions (thermal sensitivity, auditory thresholds, pattern vision) with the exception of flash-elicited visual evoked potential were unaffected in DTB-intoxicated rats (9). The change in flash evoked potentials is interpreted to indicate that DTB alters cerebrocortical function affecting vision (9) and is therefore not a pure motor system toxicant. Electroencephalographic recordings of animals given DTB have not shown abnormalities, but at high dose levels, DTB did raise the threshold for electroconvulsive shock, which was suggested to be due to a spinal phenomenon (1).

Because many of the studies with DTB concluded that morphological changes in the nervous system (3,13,14,18) and changes in muscle electrophysiology (5,8) were not associated with DTB-induced neurotoxicity, except possibly during recovery from neurotoxicity, a primary defect in nerve terminal release of acetylcholine in response to nerve stimulation was considered a possible cause for the neurotoxicity (5). Contractile responses evoked by stimulation of peripheral nerves in DTB-intoxicated rats show a reduction in the quantal summation of motor units at higher stimulus intensities, a reduction in the magnitude of tetanic contractions, and an increase in susceptibility to junctional fatigue, indicating a prejunctional site of action for DTB (5). These effects in severely affected rats were also present in earlier stages of intoxication with DTB and closely followed decrements in treadmill performance and onset of flacidity in limb musculature (19). Voltage-clamp studies using *in vitro* mouse myotubes exposed to DTB and intact hemidiaphragms from DTB-intoxicated rats indicated that DTB decreased the open time of murine skeletal muscle acetylcholine receptor channels (17). Neurochemical studies using rat pheochromocytoma cells suggested that DTB can alter the release of acetylcholine by interrupting either the mobilization and/or release of the vesicular pool of acetylcholine (10). Decreased free calcium in the presynaptic terminal and alterations in the postjunctional acetylcholine nicotinic receptor-activated ion channel have also been implicated in DTB-induced toxicity in the rat (11).

Morphological lesions including axonal swelling and degeneration, and nerve terminal swelling and degeneration, have been observed in DTB-intoxicated rats but these findings were interpreted as indicating that axonal lesions were only present in late stages of intoxication (12,14,19). However, electron microscopy studies of peripheral nerves in DTB-intoxicated rats demonstrated morphological changes that correlate with electrophysiological changes and may be responsible for the physiological changes observed. Two reports describe branched tubulovesicular profiles that slowly accumulate in the motor nerve terminals of DTB-intoxicated rats (12,15). With progression of the lesion, motor nerve terminals were observed to swell and degenerate. Similar changes were also observed in the long descending spinal cord tracts and in the cerebellar vermis (15). Overall, the changes observed indicate that DTB induces a central-peripheral distal axonopathy that primarily results in motor nerve deficits.

REFERENCES

1. Altschul S (1947) Effects of dithiobiuret on the central nervous system. *Proc Soc Exp Biol Med* **66**, 448.

2. Anonymous (1952) Dithiobiuret. In: *Cyanamid New Products Bulletin Collective Vol. 1.* American Cyanamid Company, Princeton, New Jersey.

3. Astwood EB, Hughes AM, Lubin M *et al.* (1945) Reversible paralysis of motor function in rats from the chronic administration of dithiobiuret. *Science* **102**, 196.

4. Atchison WD, Dickens J, Peterson RE (1982) Age dependence of dithiobiuret neurotoxicity in male and female rats. *Neurotoxicology* **3**, 233.

5. Atchison WD, Lalley MP, Cassens RG, Peterson RE (1981) Depression of neuromuscular function in the rat by chronic 2,4-dithiobiuret treatment. *Neurotoxicology* **2**, 329.

6. Atchison WD, Peterson RE (1977) Alteration of dithiobiuret-induced rotarod failure by sulfur containing compounds. *Fed Proc* **36**, 405.

7. Atchison WD, Peterson RE (1981) Potential neuromuscular toxicity of 2,4-dithiobiuret in the rat. *Toxicol Appl Pharmacol* **57**, 63.

8. Atchison WD, Yang KH, Peterson RE (1981) Dithiobiuret toxicity in the rat: Evidence of latency and cumulative dose thresholds. *Toxicol Appl Pharmacol* **61**, 166.

9. Crofton KM, Dean KF, Hamrick RC, Boyes WK (1991) The effects of 2,4-dithiobiuret on sensory and motor function. *Fund Appl Toxicol* **16**, 469.

10. Ireland LM, Yan CH, Nelson LM, Atchison WD (1995) Differential effects of 2,4-dithiobiuret on the synthesis and release of acetylcholine and dopamine from rat pheochromocytoma cells. *J Pharmacol Exp Ther* **275**, 1453.

11. Jones HB (1989) Dithiobiuret neurotoxicity: An ultrastructural investigation of the lesion in pre-terminal axons and motor endplates in rat lumbrical muscles. *Acta Neuropathol* **78**, 72.

12. Kemplay S (1984) Effects of dithiobiuret intoxication on motor end plates in sternocostalis and hindlimb muscles of female rats. *Acta Neuropathol* **65**, 77.

13. LoPachin RM, Moore RW, Menahan LA, Peterson RE (1984) Glucose-dependent lactate production by homogenates of neuronal tissues prepared from rats treated with 2,4-dithiobiuret, acrylamide, *p*-bromophenylacetylurea and 2,5-hexanedione. *Neurotoxicology* **5**, 25.

14. Peterson RE, Sheth NK (1975) Acute toxicity and effect of dithiobiuret and acrylamide on rotarod performance in rats and mice. *Toxicol Appl Pharmacol* **33**, 142.

15. Sahenk Z (1990) Distal terminal axonopathy produced by 2,4-dithiobiuret: Effects of longterm intoxication in rats. *Acta Neuropathol* **81**, 141.

16. Seiffer S, Harkness DM, Muntwyler E, Seifter J (1948) The effect of dithiobiuret (DTB) on the electrolyte and water content of skeletal muscle and on carbohydrate metabolism. *J Pharmacol Exp Ther* **93**, 93.

17. Spitsbergen JM, Atchison WD (1995) The paralytic agent 2,4-dithiobiuret decreases open time of murine skeletal muscle acetylcholine receptor channels. *J Pharmacol Exp Ther* **272**, 645.

18. Williams KD, LoPachin RM, Atchison WD, Peterson RE (1987) Antagonism of dithiobiuret toxicity in rats. *Neurotoxicology* **7**, 33.

19. Williams KD, Miller MS, Boysen BG, Peterson RE (1987) Temporal analysis of dithiobiuret neurotoxicity in rats and assessment of potential non-neural causes. *Toxicol Appl Pharmacol* **91**, 212.

20. Williams KD, Peterson RE, Atchison WD (1992) High dose refractoriness to the neuromuscular toxicity of dithiobiuret in rats. *Neurotoxicology* **13**, 331.

21. Williams KD, Porter WR, Peterson RE (1982) Dithiobiuret metabolism in the rat. *Neurotoxicology* **3**, 221.

Dizocilpine

Albert C. Ludolph

DIZOCILPINE
$C_{16}H_{15}N$

(+)-5-Methyl-10,11-dihydro-5H-dibenzo[a,d]
cyclohepten-5,10-imine; MK-801 (as maleate)

NEUROTOXICITY RATING

Experimental

A   Glutamate receptor antagonist

A   Acute encephalopathy (hyperactivity)

Dizocilpine maleate (MK-801) is an open-channel, non-competitive antagonist of the N-methyl-D-aspartate (NMDA) glutamate receptor subtype. The compound was once held to have therapeutic potential for acute (stroke and epilepsy) and chronic (Huntington's chorea) neurological conditions that reflect disturbed glutamatergic neurotransmission ("excitotoxicity"). However, behavioral side effects have prevented widespread human use. MK-801 is a crystalline solid that readily crosses the blood-brain barrier; the MP is 208.5°–210°C.

Like competitive NMDA antagonists and other blockers of NMDA-associated ion channels (ketamine, phencyclidine), MK-801 (1 mg/kg body weight) produces vacuolar damage in pyramidal neurons of the posterior cingulate and retrosplenial cortices of the rat 2 h after administration of a single dose (7). This effect is reversible at low doses but irreversible at higher doses (1,4). Reversible changes induced by a dosage of 1 mg/kg body weight are accompanied by induction of hsp70 mRNA and HSP70 heat-shock protein in these vulnerable neurons (9); this may therefore serve as a marker for MK-801–induced injury. The pathogenetic relationship between induction of heat-shock protein and the morphological changes is unknown. The susceptibility of animals to morphological injury and functional changes may increase with age. The neurotoxic effect of MK-801 is prevented by haloperidol (9).

MK-801 produces phencyclidine (PCP)-like neurotoxicity in rodents (10,12). At a dosage of 0.05 mg/kg body weight, behavioral changes include hyperactivity and hyperreactivity (5). If dosages are increased, animals develop difficulties climbing, balancing, and orientation to tactile stimuli (0.3 mg/kg) (5). At 1.0 mg/kg body weight, animals cannot perform tongue extrusion, swimming behavior is impaired, and abnormal posture and gait develop (5). Similar to PCP, MK-801 produces stereotypic behavior in rats; catalepsy in pigeons; and calming, ataxia, and nystagmus in nonhuman primates (6). MK-801 substitutes for PCP in drug-discrimination studies (11) and has reinforcing properties; monkeys that have previously self-administered PCP or ketamine, but not cocaine, will self-administer MK-801 (2). Intracranial self-stimulation is facilitated by MK-801 (3). Nonspecific ultrastructural changes appear in lumbar spinal cord neurons of the rat after local administration of MK-801 (8).

REFERENCES

1. Allen HL, Iversen LL (1990) Phencyclidine, dizocilpine, and cerebrocortical neurons. *Science* **247**, 221.
2. Beardsley PM, Hayes BA, Balster RL (1990) The self-administration of MK801 can depend on drug reinforcement history, and its discriminative stimulus properties are phencyclidine-like in rhesus monkeys. *J Pharmacol Exp Ther* **252**, 953.
3. Corbett D (1989) Possible abuse potential of the NMDA antagonist MK801. *Behav Brain Res* **34**, 239.
4. Fix AS, Horn JW, Wightman KA *et al.* (1993) Light and electron microscopic evaluation of neuronal vacuolization and necrosis induced by the non-competitive N-methyl-D-aspartate antagonist MK(+)801 (dizocilpine maleate) in the rat retrosplenial cortex. *Exp Neurol* **123**, 204.
5. Hargreaves EL, Cain DP (1992) Hyperactivity, hyperreactivity, and sensorimotor deficits induced by low doses of the N-methyl-D-aspartate non-competitive channel blocker MK801. *Behav Brain Res* **15**, 23.
6. Koek W, Woods HJ, Winger GD (1988) MK801, a proposed noncompetitive antagonist of excitatory amino acid neurotransmission, produces phencyclidine-like behavioral effects in pigeons, rats, and rhesus monkeys. *J Pharmacol Exp Ther* **245**, 969.
7. Olney JW, Labruyere J, Price MT (1989) Pathological changes induced in cerebrocortical neurons by phencyclidine and related drugs. *Science* **244**, 1360.
8. Orendacova J, Marsala M, Marsala J (1995) Formation of filamentous and multivesicular bodies after intrathecal MK801 injection. *J Hirnforsch* **36**, 51.
9. Sharp FR, Butman M, Wang S *et al.* (1993) Haloperidol prevents induction of the hsp70 heat shock gene in neurons injured by phencyclidine, MK801, and ketamine. *J Neurosci Res* **33**, 605.
10. Sonders MS, Keana JFW, Weber E (1988) Phencyclidine and psychomimetic sigma opiates: Recent insights into their biochemical and physiological sites of action. *Trends Neurosci* **11**, 37.

11. Tricklebank MD, Singh L, Oles RJ *et al.* (1989) The behavioral effects of MK801: A comparison with antagonists acting non-competitively and competitively at the NMDA receptor. *Eur J Pharmacol* **167**, 127.

12. Willetts J, Balster RL, Leander JD (1990) The behavioral pharmacology of NMDA receptor antagonists. *Trends Pharmacol Sci* **11**, 423.

Domoic Acid

Neil R. Cashman
F. Cendes

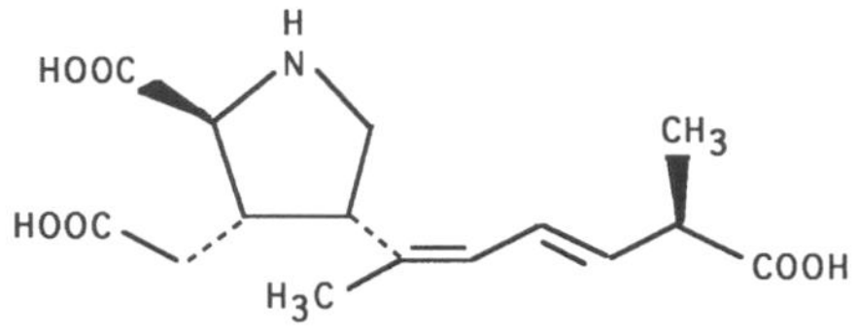

DOMOIC ACID
$C_{15}H_{21}NO_6$

[2S-[2α,3β,4β(1Z,3E,5S*)]]-2-Carboxy-4-(5-carboxy-1-methyl-1,3-hexadienyl)-3-pyrrolidineacetic acid

NEUROTOXICITY RATING

Clinical

A   Chronic encephalopathy (memory loss)

A   Acute encephalopathy (confusion, delirium, coma, seizures)

Experimental

A   Excitotoxic hippocampal necrosis

A   Acute encephalopathy (seizures)

Domoic acid (DA), a congener of the excitotoxin kainic acid (KA), is structurally related to the neurotransmitter glutamate (20,67,92). DA is found in the environment as a product of some sea organisms. This compound was first chemically identified following its isolation in 1957 from the seaweed *Chondria armata* found off the coast of Japan. In Japan, DA contained in seaweed extracts has been used as a home remedy to treat intestinal parasites, and as an insecticide (17,45). DA, purified from the seaweed, has been given orally to children in Japan at low doses (not exceeding 0.5 mg/kg; no ill effects have been reported (17).

In late November 1987, reports of individuals who acutely developed gastrointestinal symptoms, confusion, memory loss, and motor symptoms were received by the Canadian Department of National Health and Welfare (56,77). The four index cases had eaten mussels cultured in eastern Prince Edward Island within 24 h of symptom onset. Additional patients were rapidly identified throughout Canada by an active search. Leftover mussels were analyzed

for paralytic shellfish toxin by a mouse bioassay: test mice manifested involuntary scratching of their shoulders with their hindlegs, a reaction not typical of paralytic shellfish poisoning. The distribution of mussels was suspended, and a public warning against eating mussels from eastern Canada was issued (56,77).

DA was identified as the causative agent of toxicity in cultured mussels by a number of different bioassay-directed separation techniques including high-performance liquid chromatography, high-voltage paper electrophoresis, and ion-exchange chromatography; the toxin was characterized by a number of analytical techniques including mass spectrometry, and ultraviolet and infrared nuclear magnetic resonance spectroscopy (93). After DA had been identified as the toxin, its concentration was measured in samples of mussels from meals eaten by affected individuals. The DA levels in these samples ranged from 31–128 mg/100 g of mussel tissue. Estimates of total DA ingested by the patients ranged from 60–290 mg (56). The amount of DA consumed by victims of mussel poisoning in Canada was calculated to be as much as 5–6 mg/kg (20,56,77), ten times higher than the amounts administered as an anthelmintic in Japan (17).

The mussel's feeding response is controlled by algal density (2). During the search for the source of DA, investigators in the field found that over 90% of the algae available to these mussels was *Nitzschia pungens*, the major constituent of a plankton bloom at the time of the outbreak (1,37). Subsequently, DA was identified in the diatom *Pseudonitzschia australis* in the North Pacific coastline of the United States (88), and phytoplankton in the Gulf of Mexico (21). DA contamination of shellfish and crabs in these areas was also reported, and DA was linked to seabird fatalities in Monterey Bay, California, in 1991 (88,89,91).

In the 1987 Canadian epidemic, more than 250 reports of illness were received, and 145 were established as confirmed or probable affected patients (56). Eighty percent of affected individuals were over 40 years old, and 60% were between 40 and 60 years of age. The time from ingestion to onset of first symptoms varied from 15 min to 36 h. Onset of neurological symptoms ranged from 2-58 h after consumption of mussels. Both gastrointestinal and neurological symptoms ranged from mild to severe enough to require admission to an intensive care unit. Four deaths occurred within 24 h of hospitalization (56,77).

GENERAL TOXICOLOGY

DA is slowly and incompletely absorbed by the gastrointestinal tract when given orally to mice, rats, and cynomolgus monkeys (81–83). In rats, DA is cleared from plasma primarily by renal glomerular filtration and is not affected by probenecid (58,74). The acute illness that occurred in Canada in 1987, due to consumption of contaminated mussels, is evidence that DA is also absorbed by the gastrointestinal tract in humans (13,56,77,92). Decreased glomerular filtration with aging may be an explanation for the disproportionate severity of the DA intoxication syndrome in the elderly when compared to young individuals who received equivalent doses (77), although other mechanisms may apply (90) (*vide infra*).

Gastrointestinal symptoms were the predominant non-neurological manifestations in the Canadian DA intoxication. Victims of the mussel-poisoning epidemic had nausea within 5 h of mussel ingestion, with severity ranging from mild abdominal discomfort to severe vomiting requiring intravenous rehydration. Some also developed gastrointestinal bleeding (77). The gastrointestinal tracts of mice treated with extracts of DA-contaminated mussels displayed gastric and duodenal lesions, scarring and hyperemia, and proteinaceous peritoneal ascites, which correlated with the dose administered (26,27). Kynurenic acid, a nonspecific excitatory amino acid receptor antagonist, provided significant protection against gastrointestinal DA-induced lesions (26,27,57) at intraperitoneal (i.p.) doses of 300 and 600 mg/kg. Although many of the gastrointestinal effects of DA could be potentially attributed to CNS-mediated reflexes (*e.g.*, activation of the chemoreceptor trigger zone in the medulla), lesions of the mucosa, such as ulceration, suggest a direct effect of DA upon this system.

Neurotoxicity

Acute and chronic neurological dysfunction was the major manifestation of the 1987 Canadian DA intoxication (77). Neurological abnormalities developed in one-third of intoxicated persons. One study reported neurological manifestations in 14 of the more severely affected patients and presented neuropathological analysis of four other patients who died after their acute illness (77). Acute neurological manifestations of DA intoxication included headache, disequilibrium, confusion, an altered state of arousal ranging from agitation to mutism and coma, convulsions, and motor dysfunction. Chronic sequelae included memory impairment and a motor neuronopathy-axonopathy. Some survivors of the intoxication presented with psychomotor seizures after a "latent period" of a year or longer.

Acute Encephalopathy and Postintoxication Memory Loss
Animal Studies

Many similarities exist between the neuropathological lesions observed in human DA intoxication, and those in rats and mice following systemic injections of KA or DA (4,7,12,49,73,82). In rodents, DA-induced damage is most extensive in the hippocampal formation, specifically the subiculum, CA3 and CA1, but is also present in other structures including: the amygdala; basal ganglia; thalamus; and olfactory, insular, perirhinal, piriform, and entorhinal cortices (18,72,80). After 4 mg/kg of i.p. DA in mice, damage in the CA3 region of the hippocampus is evident as early as 4 h following injection (72). Early changes include edema in the vicinity of the CA3 cells resulting in a spongy vacuolated appearance, and pyknotic cells throughout the hippocampus, predominantly in the CA3 region. Some differences are apparent between humans and rodents with regard to kainate-domoate toxicity; for example, the involvement of the olfactory tubercle and dentate gyrus was common in the human syndrome, but is not observed in rodents (10,72,82).

As defined by classical pharmacological approaches, there are two main classes of receptor subtypes activated by glutamate: ionotropic (gating the flux of cations across the cell membrane) and metabotropic (G-protein–coupled receptors). Ionotropic receptors are generally divided into N-methyl-D-aspartate (NMDA) receptors and α-amino-3-hydroxy-5-methyl-isoxazolepropionic acid (AMPA)/KA receptors, each named for the exogenous ligands that most selectively activates that receptor. These receptors are differentially distributed in the CNS and activated under differing physiological conditions (reviewed in 15,51). KA receptors are concentrated in the hippocampus, particularly the CA3 region in rats (HA3 in humans). Experimental studies show that DA binds to kainate receptors: it is three times more potent than KA in producing cell depolarization and neuronal damage in the hippocampus (18,20). In addition, DA is eight times more potent than KA when administered systemically to mice (72,76). Studies have shown that DA and KA produce 20 times more depolarization and neuronal damage in the CA3 than in the CA1 region of the hippocampus in rats (19,20), whereas no such regional difference could be detected with all other glutamate analogues tested (19,72). Interestingly, when equally toxic doses of DA and KA are used, the general pattern of damage is quite similar (72), an exception being that the CA3 pyramidal cells are particularly vulnerable to the actions of DA (18,20,71,82). Recent data have suggested that DA may bind to some receptor subtypes that are poorly recognized by KA (75,78,94).

Human Studies

All 14 patients in the initial study (77) became confused and disoriented 1.5–48 h after eating DA-contaminated mussels. All but one displayed altered states of arousal, which ranged from agitation or somnolence to coma. Deficits were maximal within 4 h in the least severely affected individual, and up to 72 h in the most severely affected. Maximal improvement occurred 24 h to 12 weeks after intoxication. Patients who had been comatose took the longest time to recover.

Although the acute DA encephalopathy would be difficult to localize in the human brain, upon recovery from the acute syndrome a striking memory disorder was observed that was characteristic of a specific neuroanatomical substrate. All 14 patients underwent formal psychological testing 4–12 months after the acute phase (77,95). The patients had a predominantly anterograde memory disorder with relative preservation of other cognitive functions. Patients with moderate memory disturbances generally encoded information adequately, as demonstrated by normal immediate-recall scores, but had difficulty with delayed recall, particularly of visuospatial material. Patients with severe deficits initially had some difficulty in learning both verbal and visuospatial material, and their delayed recall was also extremely poor. Some severely affected patients also had retrograde amnesia, extending to several years before the intoxication (77,95).

The memory loss could not be explained by a nonselective general cortical injury in subjects surviving the intoxication. The average postintoxication full-scale IQ of the 14 patients was 104.8, which reflected the normal intellectual status of most patients. Scores ranged from 81–130 and were correlated with each patient's estimated abilities before the intoxication, according to age, education, and social status. Language tests did not reveal abnormalities in any of the patients, and the overall results suggested that the ability to form concepts was generally adequate (77,95). The neuropsychological features of the memory loss were similar to those of patients known to have sustained bilateral hippocampal damage (48).

Positron emission tomography (PET) studies with ^{18}F-fluorodeoxyglucose were performed in four subjects of the inital group (77) 2–3 months following the DA intoxication. Compared to a group of age-matched normal controls, two patients with severe memory disturbances displayed statistically significant glucose hypometabolism in the amygdala and hippocampus bilaterally; the less affected patients did not display a statistically significant difference. Notably, cranial computed tomography and magnetic resonance imaging (MRI) performed at this acute phase did not reveal abnormalities of the affected structures, although MRI follow-up studies performed more than 1 year after DA intoxication demonstrated late hippocampal atrophy (F. Cendes, F. Andermann, N.C. Cashman, unpublished data).

Neuropathological studies were performed in four patients not included in the clinical series who died 7 days to 3 months after eating contaminated mussels, and in one of the 14 patients described above, who died 3 years after the intoxication (10,13,77). The neuropathological lesions attributable to the intoxication were similarly distributed in the brains of the five subjects, although the character of the lesions varied with the stage of evolution at the time of death. There was severe involvement of the hippocampi and subicula, with moderate sparing in the H2 field of the hippocampus. The dentate gyrus was involved in four of the five subjects. All had involvement of the amygdala and pyriform cortex, with general sparing of the lateral nucleus of the amygdala. All patients showed some involvement of the following structures: the polymorphic layer of olfactory tubercle; the nucleus accumbens septi; the septal area; the claustrum; and the thalami, with nucleus submedialis being the area most involved. In addition, three brains showed involvement of the insular cortex and subfrontal cortex, limited to the sixth layer in one, and also involving the fifth layer in two others. The only patient without cortical lesions was the one surviving longest. The cerebellum was not involved in any subject.

Cellular pathology differed depending upon time of death following intoxication, showing longitudinal evolution of neuronal cell death following DA excitotoxicity. In a patient who died after 7 days, affected areas showed shrunken eosinophilic neurons often with a prominent perineuronal space. There was some tendency for fine vacuolation of the neuropil in severely affected areas of the hippocampus and subiculum. Astrocytic nuclei in affected areas tended to be enlarged and increased in number. In a patient who died 12 days after acute intoxication, the damaged areas of the brain also showed eosinophilic shrunken neurons. Some phagocytosis of neurons had begun in the most anterior part of the hippocampus. In a third patient who died after 24 days, most of the damaged neurons had disappeared. The main exception to that was the presence of eosinophilic neurons in the thalamus. In the field H1 of hippocampus, there was not only neuronal loss but also collapse of the tissue in the pyramidal layer. In a patient who died 98 days after intoxication, the pathological findings were quite similar to that of the third patient, except that no eosinophilic neurons remained. Neuropathological examination of a patient who died 3 years after the intoxication revealed complete neuronal loss in H1 and H3, almost total loss in H4, and moderate loss in H2 fields. Dentate cells were focally diminished in numbers. The amygdala showed patchy neuronal loss in medial and basal portions, with neuronal loss and gliosis in the overlying cortex (10,13,77).

DA INTOXICATION AND EPILEPSY

Acute Convulsive Activity
Animal Studies

KA causes seizures and seizure-related brain damage in animals (4,12,22,38,49,52,73,80). In rats, the behavioral signs of acute KA and DA intoxication include chewing, "wet dog shakes," rearing, forelimb clonus, and generalized tonic-clonic seizures. These behavioral manifestations are accompanied by electrophysiological hippocampal seizures (4,12,38,49,52,73). A selective lesion of the mossy fibers drastically reduces the excitatory effect of KA and DA in the CA3 region without affecting the response to the other substances tested (19,72). These data suggest that a major part of the neurotoxicity of DA is mediated by presynaptic input, probably from glutamate release by the mossy fiber terminals. Supporting this notion, KA or DA can potentiate the potassium-evoked release of glutamate from guinea pig hippocampal synaptosomes (78). However, a recent report has convincingly demonstrated that KA actually inhibits calcium-dependent glutamate release from rat synaptosomes (14).

Chemoanatomical studies have provided additional information regarding the selective vulnerability of hippocampal regions. The vulnerable sectors of the hippocampus are rich in kainate (endfolium and sector CA3) and NMDA receptors (sector CA1) (24). Activation of NMDA receptors (16,42) and of a subclass of AMPA/KA receptors (47) leads to Ca^{2+} influx into postsynaptic neurons. In the human hippocampus, the principal cells of the vulnerable sectors (i.e., the endfolium, and sectors CA3 and CA1) contain virtually no Ca^{2+}-binding proteins (calbindin or parvalbumin), while the relatively resistant structures such as the dentate granule cells and sector CA2 are rich in calbindin (68,69). A similar profile of hippocampal vulnerability to seizures presumably caused by the same pathogenetic mechanism is also seen in some experimental models of epilepsy (4,63,84).

Parenteral administration of DA in monkeys produced pathological changes comparable to those in mice and rats (81). In monkeys receiving 0.025–0.2 mg/kg DA intravenously (i.v.), the clinical signs of toxicity were preceded by a short presymptomatic period of 2–3 min. Animals developed chewing with frothing, varying degrees of gagging, and vomiting. At higher doses (0.5 mg/kg i.v. or 4 mg/kg i.p.), they exhibited additional signs that included abnormal head and body positions, rigidity of movements, loss of balance, and tremor (81). In another study, monkeys receiving 0.5–1.0 mg/kg of DA i.v. displayed no reliable behavioral signs of seizure activity comparable to those seen in rats (62). However, induction of c-fos immunoreactivity in most cells of the dentate gyrus was observed at 3 h, and in the CA1 pyramidal cells at 7 h after dosing, suggesting that subclinical seizures may have occurred (55,62).

The clinical and pathological effects of single oral doses of extracts of DA in cynomolgus monkeys (0.5–10 mg/kg) and rats (60–80 mg/kg) have been studied. While i.p. administration of DA in rats produced seizures and death at 4 mg/kg, oral administration produced toxicity only after 70 mg/kg. After oral administration of 5.0 mg/kg of DA, monkeys displayed gagging or vomiting. There was a wide variation of clinical and pathological responses to oral administration of DA in monkeys, which was attributed to a protective effect of vomiting and incomplete or slow gastrointestinal absorption (34,83).

In Vitro Studies

There is little in vitro work with DA. Neuroexcitatory and neurotoxic activities of DA in cultured hippocampal and retinal neurons have been evaluated (71). The neuroexcitatory properties of DA in rat hippocampal neurons were compared with those of KA, NMDA, and quisqualate. Currents induced in hippocampal neurons by DA and KA were identical and displayed a linear current/voltage relationship (in contrast to NMDA currents) and were nondesensitizing (in contrast to quisqualate currents). DA currents were not blocked by NMDA antagonists but were blocked by CNQX, an antagonist of non-NMDA receptors. Similar results were obtained with chick embryonic retina in vitro (71). Two studies have provided evidence that hippocampal neurons express a calcium-permeable AMPA/KA channel, and that DA may be a potent agonist of this channel (8,90).

Human Studies

A major CNS manifestation of the 1987 DA intoxication was epilepsy, both acute and chronic. Experimental data indicate that DA produces neuronal activation both by direct excitation of KA receptors, and by inducing acute recurrent seizures throughout limbic circuits (18–20,27,34,77,80,92). Moreover, neuronal death induced by DA excitotoxicity in the hippocampus and related structures resulted in the delayed onset of partial complex epilepsy (13), consistent with the latency of other hippocampal injuries.

Seizures were observed in 5 of the 14 patients in the initial study (77). Three subjects had generalized seizures, two had complex partial seizures, and one had partial motor attacks. It is likely that limbic ictal manifestations were unrecognized in some subjects; indeed, the acute intoxication was characterized by unusual motor activity reminiscent of grimacing or chewing. Recognized seizure activity was relatively resistant to intravenous infusion of phenytoin, and required high doses of i.v. diazepam and phenobarbital for control during the acute illness. Seven patients had electroencephalograms (EEGs) during the acute phase. Moderate to severe generalized disturbance of background activity was seen in all of the seven. Only one patient had clear epileptiform activity from EEG scalp recordings. Eight weeks after mussel ingestion seizures became progressively less frequent and ceased within 4 months in all subjects. Thus, the acute DA intoxication syndrome behaved as an excitatory insult to limbic structures, producing clinical seizure activity mimicking naturally occurring epilepsy of the hippocampus and related structures (77).

Treatment

Extensive *in vivo* and *in vitro* animal studies indicate that limbic damage induced by DA and KA occurs as a consequence of, or in association with, seizure-mediated mechanisms. Therefore, the treatment of accidental DA intoxication should be focused on achieving the best possible seizure control and, ideally, blocking any seizure activity until DA is fully excreted, thereby preventing limbic injury. According to previous experience of the epidemic mussel poisoning in Canada (53,77), seizures due to DA intoxication require intravenous infusion of large doses of diazepam, or of related agents such as midazolam and lorazepam (44,54). Benzodiazepines act as acute γ-aminobutyric acid (GABA) agonists, providing an inhibitory restraint on the excitatory activation induced by DA. Similarly, phenobarbital acts by enhancing GABA-mediated inhibition and, in addition, appears to reduce glutamate-mediated excitation, probably by acting on voltage-dependent potassium and calcium chan-

nels (for a review of pharmacological mechanisms of these drugs, *see* 60). If clinical or EEG evidence of seizure activity persists, a continuous infusion of barbiturate or benzodiazepine in anesthetic doses should be considered (44, 54). Theoretically, as animal studies would suggest (26,27,64,94), glutamate-receptor blocking agents (such as kynurenate), calcium-channel antagonists, or manipulation of other neurotransmitter systems, such as serotonin, may also limit excitotoxicity of a time-limited glutamatergic agonist, but further studies are necessary before clinical use could be recommended.

Chronic Convulsive Activity
Animal Studies

The development of limbic seizures long after acute hippocampal injury has many precedents in humans and animals (reviewed in 4,68). Limbic pathways in rats and a variety of other species are particularly vulnerable to activation with high-frequency trains of stimulation, or excitotoxins, that evoke brief electrographic and behavioral seizures with many features of complex partial seizures. Repeated activation results in progressive seizure activity that eventually evolves into spontaneous seizures and a permanent epileptic state, referred to as a kindling (12,63,73,84). The morphological alterations induced by kindling include progressive neuronal loss in the hilus of the dentate gyrus and reorganization of the mossy fiber pathway from granule cells. The axons of the granule cells, designated mossy fibers, normally establish synaptic contacts with a diverse population of polymorphic neurons in the hilus of the dentate gyrus, and with pyramidal neurons in the CA3 region of the hippocampus. Mossy fiber synaptic reorganization is observed both in animal models of epilepsy and in human epilepsy (12,63,68). There is a period of time between the cessation of the stimulus (or acute seizures) and the appearance of spontaneous seizures; this period differs among species. Experimental studies demonstrate that KA induces intense acute seizure activity in hippocampal pathways, followed by degeneration of hilar, CA3, and CA1 pyramidal neurons. The neuronal loss in the chronic KA-induced hippocampal lesion resembles the lesions of hippocampal sclerosis, is accompanied by abnormal excitability and seizures, and has been considered as a model of temporal lobe epilepsy (TLE) (4,12,63,68,73,84).

Hippocampal sclerosis is frequent in "naturally occurring" TLE, as seen at autopsy and in tissue resected during surgical treatment (28,46,96). The etiology and pathogenesis of hippocampal sclerosis and its relationship to TLE have been a source of controversy over the last century. It probably has several causes, but a major association with a history of prolonged early childhood convulsions, usually febrile, is a common finding (28,46,95). Classical hippocampal sclerosis has all the earmarks of an inert lesion acquired in the remote past. Fresh lesions with a distribution characteristic of hippocampal sclerosis have been reported in the hippocampi of children between 3 months and 7 years of age who died of status epilepticus, often but not necessarily associated with a febrile illness (28,95). It is therefore possible that hippocampal sclerosis is the consequence of a prolonged seizure or status that occurred within a period of childhood when the hippocampus is particularly vulnerable to convulsion-induced excitotoxic damage. The development of TLE and hippocampal sclerosis in a patient surviving acute DA intoxication strongly supports a role for excitotoxicity in "naturally occurring" hippocampal sclerosis in epilepsy.

Human Studies

Long after complete cessation of convulsive activity of the acute phase of the DA intoxication, two patients developed temporal lobe epilepsy. One of these, an 84-year-old man who, following consumption of contaminated mussels, had nausea, vomiting, and confusion, with subsequent coma, generalized convulsions, and complex partial status epilepticus (13). After 3 weeks, he improved and was seizure free with severe residual memory deficit. EEGs initially showed periodic epileptiform discharges, later evolving to epileptic abnormalities over frontotemporal regions with diffuse slow waves. Eight months after the intoxication, the EEG was normal. One year after the acute episode, he developed complex partial seizures. EEGs at that time showed epileptic discharges independently over both temporal lobes with left-sided predominance. MRI revealed hyperintense T2-weighted signal and severe atrophy of both hippocampi; a PET scan showed bitemporal decreased glucose metabolism. He developed pneumonia and died 3¼ years after the intoxication. Autopsy disclosed severe bilateral hippocampal sclerosis. Microscopically, the hippocampi showed complete neuronal loss in CA1 and CA3, almost total loss in CA4, and moderate loss in CA2. Numbers of dentate cells were focally diminished. The amygdala showed patchy neuronal loss in medial and basal portions, with neuronal loss and gliosis in the overlying cortex (13).

Motor Neuron Disease as an Acute Manifestation of DA Toxicity

Animal Studies

Despite the longstanding appreciation that excitatory amino acids can depolarize spinal motor neurons (5,32,33),

excitotoxicity has only been recently studied in these cells, particularly with regard to DA. In rats, intrathecal KA induced early and delayed degenerative changes most marked in spinal motor neurons (31,50). One *in vitro* study used the chick embryo spinal cord to evaluate the sensitivity of spinal neurons to the excitotoxic effects of DA and other excitatory amino acids agonists of NMDA and non-NMDA receptors. In this study, all agonists induced concentration-dependent acute degeneration of neurons distributed throughout the spinal cord, which was blocked by receptor-specific cognate antagonists (70). In spinal-cord slice cultures, chronic inhibition of glutamate uptake resulted in the slow degeneration of motor neurons over the course of weeks ("slow neurotoxicity"); interestingly, cell death was inhibited with non-NMDA antagonists, but not by NMDA antagonists (61). Motor neurons in dissociated mouse spinal cord cultures (identified by antibody staining for a hypophosphorylated neurofilament epitope) were differentially damaged by KA in a calcium-dependent manner (11), although acute glutamate-induced degeneration of most spinal cord neurons seems to be predominantly mediated by NMDA receptors (59). Considered in aggregate, these studies appear to demonstrate that: (a) spinal motor neurons bear receptors for glutamate, of both NMDA and AMPA/KA subtypes; (b) spinal motor neurons are differentially vulnerable to glutamatergic excitotoxicity when compared to other cells in the spinal cord; and (c) spinal motor neurons are particularly vulnerable to AMPA/KA excitotoxicity, through a calcium-dependent mechanism.

More recently, receptor-binding studies and *in situ*-hybridization studies have demonstrated the glutamate receptor subunits used by motor neurons. The predominant subtype ligand bound by rodent and human motor neurons is NMDA (41,65,66), which corresponds to mRNA studies showing high expression of NR1 NMDA receptor subunit (23,79). The minimal expression of an NR2 subunit (NR2D) has raised questions about NR1 homomeric complexes, an unknown NMDA receptor subunit, or some other feature of spinal cord neurons that would account for the atypical stoichiometry of subunits (79). KA binds at a low level to rodent and human motor neurons (41,65), and may be binding to AMPA sites through a low-affinity interaction. As might be expected from these data, *in situ* hybridization studies reveal KA-receptor subunits KA1 and GluR5 are expressed inconstantly in a small number of motor neurons in the rat, with no detectable expression of KA receptor subunits GluR6, GluR7, and KA2 (79). The non-NMDA ligand CNQX binds to motor neurons in mouse spinal cord sections (65), and AMPA receptor subunits GluR2, GluR3, and GluR4 are abundantly expressed in rat motor neurons, with a lesser but detectable expression of

GluR1 (23,35,36,79). Motor neurons do not express metabotropic glutamate receptors, which function as presynaptic regulators for axons synapsing on motor neurons (9,39).

How do these data relate to the neurotoxicity of DA? Recent data have suggested that a subset of AMPA/KA receptors can gate calcium influx in certain neurons (8,11,86,87,94), a property originally thought to be confined to NMDA receptors (51). AMPA/KA receptors with this property are not ubiquitous in the nervous system, but they have been observed on hippocampal neurons and motor neurons (11,94). Moreover, DA, originally thought to be a classical KA receptor agonist, has been recently found to interact with a subclass of AMPA receptors (94). Thus, it is likely that the differential vulnerability of hippocampal and motor neurons in DA toxicity is due to AMPA receptor-mediated calcium-induced neurotoxicity.

Human Studies

In DA intoxication, the prominent clinical involvement of neurons in the hippocampus and related structures was accompanied by injury to spinal motor neurons (77). The resultant acute denervating syndrome was clinically subtle (*i.e.*, it did not manifest as a diffuse flaccid paralysis), but caused weakness and was readily detected by electromyography (EMG) after the acute intoxication. During the acute phase of the illness, all 14 patients had nonspecific unsteadiness and generalized weakness. Two had symmetrical transient hyperreflexia and Babinski's signs, two developed alternating hemiparesis and hyperreflexia, and three had generalized fasciculations. Four experienced extraocular muscle weakness ranging from bilateral abducens palsies to complete external ophthalmoplegia. Four to 6 months after the intoxication, 11 of the 14 had distal atrophy and mild weakness of the extremities, and 8 had hyporeflexia.

Eleven of the 14 patients had at least one EMG evaluation (77). Two were studied within 1 month of the acute phase. Both had marked spontaneous activity (fibrillations and positive waves) and neurogenic recruitment shown by concentric needle examination with no evidence of slowed conduction velocity. These findings suggested acute denervation due to neuronopathy or axonopathy (*i.e.*, dysfunction of motor neurons or their axonal processes to muscle). Ten of the 14 patients underwent concentric needle EMGs at 6 months after the acute phase (77). Nine had findings suggesting varying degrees of acute denervation, such as spontaneous activity and unstable motor unit potentials. Seven who had well-preserved motor nerve conduction velocities had markedly diminished compound motor unit potentials (30%–50% of normal), suggesting that neurons or motor axons supplying muscle were reduced in number. Seven had a follow-up EMG 11–14 months after the acute phase; signs of acute denervation had partially resolved at this timepoint.

These electrophysiological results suggest that the DA intoxication induced either an acute, nonprogressive neuronopathy involving anterior horn cells, or a diffuse axonopathy predominantly affecting motor axons (77). Brainstem nuclei or axons supplying the extraocular muscles were also clinically involved acutely. However, no unequivocal motor neuron degeneration or cytopathology was observed in the brainstems of five autopsied individuals, or in the upper cervical spinal cord of a single individual from whom material was available (77). Thus, the injury occurring on DA intoxication engendered marked motor dysfunction, but not death of motor neurons detectable with conventional histopathological stains. Possibly, injury was subtle, such as neurofilament reorganization and phosphorylation that are seen in motor neurons exposed to kainate *in vitro* (30).

SIGNIFICANCE AND CONCLUSIONS

The Canadian epidemic confirms that selected human neurons *in vivo* display similar vulnerability to glutamatergic excitotoxins as neurons of rodents and other experimental animals. The clinical syndromes evoked by DA included acute intractable epilepsy and chronic anterograde memory deficits, both manifestations of the selective vulnerability of hippocampal neurons and related structures. A chronic deficit related to this selective vulnerability was complex partial epilepsy secondary to hippocampal injury and subsequent sclerosis, thus implicating the role of glutamate and other excitatory neurotransmitters in "naturally occurring" hippocampal sclerosis and complex partial seizures arising in childhood. Another acute manifestation of DA intoxication was injury of motor neurons, followed by nonprogressive and improving signs of chronic denervation. The naturally occurring disorders Alzheimer's disease and amyotrophic lateral sclerosis have been hypothesized to be due to glutamatergic excitotoxicity (*e.g.*, 15,43,65,85); perhaps information about them may be gleaned by comparison with human DA excitotoxicity.

It may be worthwhile to consider what the DA intoxication did not cause in humans. Despite theory and laboratory evidence linking excitotoxins with many neurological and psychiatric diseases, human DA intoxication was not associated with parkinsonian signs, chorea characteristic of Huntington's disease, visual loss consistent with retinal degeneration, or persistent schizophreniform psychosis.

Also, aside from the late development of psychomotor seizures due to ongoing plastic changes in hippocampal structures, DA did not produce gradually progressive syndromes, militating against a role for glutamate in "critical threshold" or "positive-feedback" models of human neurodegeneration.

In DA intoxication, the restricted involvement of certain structures with the sparing of others recapitulates the important question of selective vulnerability in neurodegenerative disease. At the ligand-binding level, selective vulnerability to DA cannot be fully explained; many neurons express binding sites for DA that are not killed by DA. Thus, DA excitotoxicity is not merely a distribution map of KA receptors in the human brain, but reflects some differential vulnerability of the neurons that are injured by the clinical intoxication. At least four potential mechanisms could be invoked to explain selective vulnerability of neuronal systems affected by DA.

1. Selective cell death is determined by activation of endogenous excitotoxic input. In the hippocampus, this mechanism explains a large part of the selective vulnerability of hippocampal pyramidal cells. In animals, sections of the mossy fiber input to hippocampal neurons ablates KA- and DA-induced toxicity (19). Thus, a structure may be differentially vulnerable to excitotoxins because of its "system circuitry." This mechanism cannot be applied to motor neurons, which lack a similar feed-forward-system anatomy.

2. Selective vulnerability is due to specific constellations of glutamatergic receptors. At the receptor level, differential vulnerability could be due to expression of receptor subtypes, as defined by agonist-antagonist studies of classical pharmacology, gene expression (glutamate receptor subunits and their stoichiometry), alternate splicing, and RNA editing modifying the function and ionic permeability of the receptor. Importantly, both hippocampal neurons and motor neurons appear to be somewhat unique in the nervous system for expressing calcium-permeable AMPA/KA receptors (8,11,94), a function that is classically thought to be restricted to the NMDA-type glutamate receptor (51). Lack of the RNA-editing capability that prevents calcium influx results in a progressive injury of hippocampal neurons (9). The role of calcium in triggering of cell death may predispose hippocampal and motor neurons to selective vulnerability in the DA intoxication.

3. Selective vulnerability is secondary to marginal cellular energy supply. Membrane depolarization frees the magnesium-dependent blockade of the NMDA receptor, allowing ready influx of calcium. Notably, spinal motor neurons and hippocampal neurons are both large cells, supporting large dendritic trees and long axons, necessitating that they be among the most metabolically active neurons in the neuroaxis. The maintenance of membrane potential may be more problematic in such cells than in smaller, metabolically less active cells. Moreover, in DA intoxication, a more severe syndrome was observed with advancing age. Perhaps mitochondrial dysfunction accumulating with aging (3) increases neuronal susceptibility to excitotoxicity.

4. Selective vulnerability devolves from differing cellular mechanisms for coping with excitotoxic stress. In addition to expressing appropriate glutamatergic receptors, vulnerable neurons must possess the proper complement of postreceptor transduction mechanisms to kill cells. Increased cytosolic calcium is a likely candidate for a major component of this second signal, originating from a specialized subset of AMPA/KA receptors, or secondary calcium influx from depolarization-activated NMDA receptors. In addition to calcium concentration, the cytosolic distribution of calcium is critical for how this increase will be interpreted by the cell—as a metabolic trigger for synaptic plasticity and gene expression, or the engagement of a cell death program (25). Moreover, the effects of calcium can be militated by intracellular binding proteins, such as calbindin and parvalbumin. Notably, both hippocampal neurons and spinal motor neurons are distinct from most neurons because they lack these calcium-buffering proteins (29,40,69). Downstream effects of calcium include activation of lipases, proteases, and nucleases, and activation of enzymes generating reactive oxygen species (6). Calcium-regulated kinases may participate in abnormal function and death of these neurons in disease (11,30). It is at least a formal possibility that selective vulnerability to excitotoxins is due to cells being "poised" to enter the apoptosis cascade.

In summary, the pattern of nerve cell damage associated with acute DA intoxication provides valuable information on the selective vulnerability of neuronal populations. Information garnered from the 1987 Canadian outbreak of human DA intoxication has impacted understanding of potential mechanisms of cell death in epilepsy, ischemia, and aging.

REFERENCES

1. Bates SS, Bird CJ, de Freitas ASW *et al.* (1989) Pennate diaton *Nitzschia pungens* as the primary source of domoic acid, a toxin in shellfish from eastern Prince Edward Island, Canada. *Can J Fisheries Aquat Sci* **46**, 1203.

2. Bayne BL, Widdows J, Thompson RJ (1976) Physiology of marine mussels. In: *Marine Mussels: Their Ecology and Physiology.* Bayne BL ed. Cambridge University Press, London p. 207.

3. Beal MF (1995) *Mitochondrial Dysfunction and Oxidative Damage in Neurodegenerative Diseases.* RG Landes Company, Texas.

4. Ben-Ari Y (1985) Limbic seizures and brain damage produced by kainic acid: Mechanisms and relevance to human temporal epilepsy. *Neuroscience* **14**, 375.

5. Biscoe TJ, Evans RH, Headley PM *et al.* (1976) Structure-activity relations of excitatory amino acids on frog and rat spinal neurones. *Brit J Pharmacol* **58**, 373.

6. Bondy SC, Lee DK (1993) Oxidative stress induced by glutamate receptor agonists. *Brain Res* **610**, 229.

7. Brusa R, Zimmerman F, Koh D-S *et al.* (1995) Early-onset epilepsy and postnatal lethality associated with an editing-deficient GluR-B allele in mice. *Science* **270**, 1677.

8. Burke SJ, Yin H-Z, Weiss JH (1995) Ca^{2+} and *in vitro* kainate damage to cortical and hippocampal SME-32(+) neurons. *NeuroReport* **6**, 629.

9. Cao CQ, Evans RH, Headley PM, Udvarhelyi PM (1995) A comparison of the effects of selective metabotropic glutamate receptor agonists on synaptically evoked whole cell currents of rat spinal ventral horn neurones in vitro. *Brit J Pharmacol* **115**, 1469.

10. Carpenter S (1990) The human pathology of encephalopathic mussel toxin poisoning. *Can Dis Wkly Rep* **16**, 73.

11. Carriedo SG, Yin H-Z, Lamberta R, Weiss JH (1995) *In vitro* kainate injury to large, SMI-32(+) spinal neurons is Ca^{2+} dependent. *NeuroReport* **6**, 945.

12. Cavazos JE, Golarai G, Sutula TP (1991) Mossy fiber reorganization induced by kindling: Time course of development, progression and permanence. *J Neurosci* **11**, 2795.

13. Cendes F, Andermann F, Carpenter S *et al.* (1995) Temporal lobe epilepsy caused by domoic acid intoxication: Evidence for glutamate receptor-mediated excitotoxicity in humans. *Ann Neurol* **37**, 123.

14. Chittajallu R, Vignes M, Dev KK *et al.* (1996) Regulation of glutamate release by presynaptic kainate receptors in the hippocampus. *Nature* **379**, 78.

15. Choi DW (1988) Glutamate neurotoxicity and disease of the nervous system. *Neuron* **1**, 623.

16. Collingridge GL, Bliss TVP (1987) NMDA-receptors—their role in long-term potentiation. *Trends Neurosci* **10**, 288.

17. Daigo K (1959) Studies on the constituents of *Chondria armata*. II. Isolation of an antihelmintical constituent. *J Jpn Pharm Assn* **79**, 353.

18. Debonnel G, Beauchesne L, de Montigny C (1989) Domoic acid, the alleged "mussel toxin," might produce its neurotoxic effect through kainate receptor activation: An electrophysiological study in the dorsal hippocampus. *Can J Physiol Pharmacol* **67**, 29.

19. Debonnel G, Weiss M, de Montigny C (1989) Reduced neuroexcitatory effect of domoic acid following mossy fiber denervation of the rat dorsal hippocampus: Further evidence that toxicity of domoic acid involves kainate receptor activation. *Can J Physiol Pharmacol* **67**, 904.

20. Debonnel G, Weiss M, de Montigny C (1990) Neurotoxic effect of domoic acid: Mediation by kainate receptor electrophysiological studies in the rat. *Can Dis Wkly Rep* **16**, 59.

21. Dickey RW, Fryxell GA, Granade HR, Roelke D (1992) Detection of the marine toxins okadaic acid and domoic acid in shellfish and phytoplankton in the Gulf of Mexico. *Toxicon* **30**, 355.

22. Fujita T, Tanaka T, Yonemasu Y *et al.* (1996) Electroclinical and pathological studies after parenteral administration of domoic acid in freely moving nonanesthetized rats—an animal model of excitotoxicity. *J Epilepsy* **9**, 87.

23. Furuyama T, Kiyama H, Sato K *et al.* (1993) Region-specific expression of subunits of ionotropic glutamate receptors (AMPA-type, KA-type and NMDA receptors) in the rat spinal cord with special reference to nociception. *Mol Brain Res* **18**, 141.

24. Geddes JW, Cotman CW (1986) Plasticity in hippocampal excitatory amino acid receptors in Alzheimer disease. *Neurosci Res* **3**, 672.

25. Ghosh A, Greenberg ME (1995) Calcium signaling in neurons: Molecular mechanisms and cellular consequences. *Science* **268**, 239.

26. Glavin GB, Pinsky C (1989) Kynurenic acid attenuates experimental ulcer formation and basal gastric acid secretion in rats. *Res Commun Chem Pathol Pharmacol* **64**, 111.

27. Glavin GB, Pinsky C, Bose R (1990) Domoic acid-induced neurovisceral toxic syndrome: Characterization of an animal model and putative antidotes. *Brain Res Bull* **24**, 701.

28. Gloor P (1991) Mesial temporal sclerosis: Historical background and an overview from a modern perspective. In: *Epilepsy Surgery*. Luders H ed. Raven Press, New York p. 689.

29. Heizmann CW, Braun K (1995) *Calcium Regulation by Calcium-Binding Proteins in Neurodegenerative Disorders*. RG Landes Company, Texas.

30. Hugon J, Vallat JM (1990) Abnormal distribution of phosphorylated neurofilaments in neuronal degeneration induced by kainic acid. *Neurosci Lett* **119**, 45.

31. Hugon J, Vallat JM, Spencer PS *et al.* (1989) Kainic acid induces early and delayed degenerative neuronal changes in rat spinal cord. *Neurosci Lett* **104**, 258.

32. Ishida M, Shinozaki H (1988) Acromelic acid is a much more potent excitant than kainic acid or domoic acid in the isolated rat spinal cord. *Brain Res* **474**, 386.

33. Ishida M, Shinozaki H (1991) Novel kainate derivatives: Potent depolarizing actions on spinal motoneurones and dorsal root fibres in newborn rats. *Brit J Pharmacol* **104**, 873.

34. Iverson F, Truelove J, Tryphonas L, Nera EA (1990) The toxicology of domoic acid administered systemically to rodents and primates. *Can Dis Wkly Rep* **16**, 15.

35. Jakowec MW, Fox AJ, Martin LJ, Kalb RG (1995) Quantitative and qualitative changes in AMPA receptor expression during spinal cord development. *Neuroscience* **67**, 893.

36. Jakowec MW, Yen L, Kalb RG (1995) *In situ* hybridiza-

tion analysis of AMPA receptor subunit gene expression in the developing rat spinal cord. *Neuroscience* **67**, 909.

37. Johnson GR, Hanic L, Judson I *et al.* (1990) Mussel culture and the accumulation of domoic acid. *Can Dis Wkly Rep* **16**, 33.

38. Knowles WD (1992) Normal anatomy and neurophysiology of the hippocampal formation. *J Clin Neurophysiol* **9**, 252.

39. Konnerth A, Keller BU, Lev-Tov A (1990) Patch clamp analysis of excitatory synapses in mammalian spinal cord slices. *Pflugers Arch—Eur J Physiol* **417**, 285.

40. Krieger C, Jones K, Kim SU, Eisen AA (1994) The role of intracellular free calcium in motor neuron disease. *J Neurol Sci* **124**, 27.

41. Krieger C, Lai R, Mitsumoto H, Shaw C (1993) The Wobbler mouse: Quantitative autoradiography of glutamatergic ligand binding sites in spinal cord. *Neurodegeneration* **2**, 9.

42. Kudo Y, Ogura A (1986) Glutamate-induced increase in intracellular Ca^{++} concentration in isolated hippocampal neurones. *Brit J Pharmacol* **89**, 191.

43. Lipton SA, Rosenberg PA (1994) Excitatory amino acids as a final common pathway for neurologic disorders. *N Engl J Med* **330**, 613.

44. Lowenstein DH, Simon RP (1992) Antiepileptic drugs useful in status epilepticus. In: *Drugs for Control in Epilepsy: Actions on Neuronal Networks Involved in Seizure Disorders*. Faingold CL, Fromm GH eds. CRC Press, Boca Raton, Florida p. 513.

45. Maeda M, Kodama T, Tanaka T *et al.* (1984) Insecticidal and neuromuscular activities of domoic acid and its related compounds. *J Pestic Sci* **9**, 27.

46. Meencke HJ, Veith G (1991) Hippocampal sclerosis in epilepsy. In: *Epilepsy Surgery*. Luders H cd. Raven Press, New York p. 689.

47. Miller RJ (1991) The revenge of the kainate receptor. *Trends Neurosci* **14**, 477.

48. Milner B (1958) Psychological effects produced by temporal lobe excision. *Res Publ Assn Res Nerv Ment Dis* **36**, 244.

49. Nadler JV, Cuthberston GJ (1980) Kainic acid neurotoxicity toward hippocampal formation: Dependence on specific excitatory pathways. *Brain Res* **195**, 47.

50. Nag S, Riopelle RJ (1990) Spinal neuronal pathology associated with continuous intrathecal infusion of N-methyl-D-aspartate in the rat. *Acta Neuropathol* **81**, 7.

51. Nakanishi S (1992) Molecular diversity of glutamate receptors and implications for brain function. *Science* **258**, 597.

52. Olney JW, Rhee VA, Ho OL (1974) Kainic acid: A powerful neurotoxic analogue of glutamate. *Brain Res* **77**, 507.

53. Olney JW, Teitelbaum J, Pinsky C, Debonnel G (1990) Domoic acid toxicity. Panel discussion: Treatment. *Can Dis Wkly Rep* **16**, 117.

54. Parent JM, Lowenstein DH (1994) Treatment of refractory generalized status epilepticus with continuous infusion of midazolam. *Neurology* **44**, 1837.

55. Peng YG, Ramsdell JS (1996) Brain *fos* induction is a sensitive biomarker for the lowest observed neuroexcitatory effects of domoic acid. *Fund Appl Toxicol* **31**, 162.

56. Perl TM, Bedard L, Kosatsky T *et al.* (1990) An outbreak of toxic encephalopathy caused by eating mussels contaminated with domoic acid. *N Engl J Med* **322**, 1775.

57. Pinsky C, Glavin GB, Bose R (1989) Kynurenic acid protects against neurotoxicity and lethality of toxic extracts from contaminated Atlantic coast mussels. *Prog Neuropsychopharmacol Biol Psychiat* **13**, 595.

58. Preston E, Hynie I (1991) Transfer constants for bloodbrain barrier permeation of the neuroexcitatory shellfish toxin, domoic acid. *Can J Neurol Sci* **18**, 39.

59. Regan RF, Choi DW (1991) Glutamate neurotoxicity in spinal cord cell culture. *Neuroscience* **43**, 585.

60. Rogawski MA, Porter RJ (1990) Antiepileptic drugs: Pharmacological mechanisms and clinical efficacy with consideration of promising developmental stage compounds. *Pharmacol Rev* **42**, 223.

61. Rothstein JD, Jin L, Dykes-Hoberg M, Kuncl RW (1993) Chronic inhibition of glutamate uptake produces a model of slow neurotoxicity. *Proc Nat Acad Sci USA* **90**, 6591.

62. Scallet AC, Binienda Z, Caputo FA *et al.* (1993) Domoic acid-treated cynomolgus monkeys (*M. fascicularis*): Effects of dose on hippocampal neuronal and terminal degeneration. *Brain Res* **627**, 307.

63. Schwartzkroin PA (1993) *Epilepsy: Models, Mechanisms, and Concepts*. University Press, Cambridge.

64. Sharma SK, Dakshinamurti K (1993) Suppression of domoic acid induced seizures by 8-(OH)-DPAT. *J Neural Transm—Gen Sect* **93**, 87.

65. Shaw PJ (1991) Excitotoxicity and motor neurone disease: A review of the evidence. *J Neurol Sci* **124**, 6.

66. Shaw PJ, Ince PG, Johnson M, Candy JM (1994) N-Methyl-D-aspartate (NMDA) receptors in the spinal cord and motor cortex in motor neuron disease: A quantitative autoradiographic study using [^{3}H] MK-801. *Brain Res* **637**, 297.

67. Shinozaki H (1978) Discovery of novel actions of kainic acid and related compounds. In: *Kainic Acid as a Tool in Neurobiology*. McGeer EG, Olney JW, McGeer PL eds. Raven Press, New York p. 17.

68. Sloviter RS (1994) The functional organization of the hippocampal dentate gyrus and its relevance to the pathogenesis of temporal lobe epilepsy. *Ann Neurol* **35**, 640.

69. Sloviter RS, Sollas AL, Barbaro NM, Laxer KD (1991) Calcium-binding protein (calbindin-D-28K) and parvalbumin immunocytochemistry in the normal and epileptic human hippocampus. *J Comp Neurol* **308**, 381.

70. Stewart GR, Olney JW, Pathikonda M, Snider WD (1991)

Excitotoxicity in the embryonic chick spinal cord. *Ann Neurol* 30, 758.

71. Stewart GR, Zorumski CF, Price MT, Olney JW (1990) Domoic acid: A dementia-inducing excitotoxic food poison with kainic acid receptor specificity. *Exp Neurol* 110, 127.

72. Strain SM, Tasker RA (1991) Hippocampal damage produced by systemic injections of domoic acid in mice. *Neuroscience* 44, 343.

73. Sutula TP (1990) Experimental models of temporal lobe epilepsy: New insights from the study of kindling and synaptic reorganization. *Epilepsia* 31, S45.

74. Suzuki CA, Hierlihy SL (1993) Renal clearance of domoic acid in the rat. *Food Chem Toxicol* 31, 701.

75. Takeuchi H, Watanabe K, Nomoto K *et al.* (1984) Effects of alpha-kainic acid, domoic acid and their derivatives on a molluscan giant neuron sensitive to beta-hydroxy-L-glutamic acid. *Eur J Pharmacol* 102, 325.

76. Tasker RA, Connell BJ, Strain SM (1991) Pharmacology of systemically administered domoic acid in mice. *Can J Physiol Pharmacol* 69, 378.

77. Teitelbaum JS, Zatorre RJ, Carpenter S *et al.* (1990) Neurologic sequelae of domoic acid intoxication due to the ingestion of contaminated mussels. *N Engl J Med* 322, 1781.

78. Terrian DM, Conner-Kerr TA, Privette TH, Gannon RL (1991) Domoic acid enhances the K(+)-evoked release of endogenous glutamate from guinea pig hippocampal mossy fiber synaptosomes. *Brain Res* 551, 303.

79. Tölle TR, Berthele A, Zieglgansberger W *et al.* (1993) The differential expression of 16 NMDA and non-NMDA receptor subunits in the rat spinal cord and in periaqueductal gray. *J Neurosci* 13, 5009.

80. Tryphonas L, Iverson F (1990) Neuropathology of excitatory neurotoxins: The domoic acid model [Review]. *Toxicol Pathol* 18, 165.

81. Tryphonas L, Truelove J, Iverson F (1990) Acute parenteral neurotoxicity of domoic acid in cynomolgus monkeys (*M. fascicularis*) [Erratum appears in *Toxicol Pathol* (1990) 18, 431]. *Toxicol Pathol* 18, 297.

82. Tryphonas L, Truelove J, Nera E, Iverson F (1990) Acute neurotoxicity of domoic acid in the rat. *Toxicol Pathol* 18, 1.

83. Tryphonas L, Truelove J, Todd E *et al.* (1990) Experimental oral toxicity of domoic acid in cynomolgus monkeys (*Macaca fascicularis*) and rats. Preliminary investigations. *Food Chem Toxicol* 28, 707.

84. Wada JA (1986) *Kindling 3*. Raven Press, New York.

85. Weiss JH, Choi DW (1991) Differential vulnerability to excitatory amino acid-induced toxicity and selective neuronal loss in neurodgenerative diseases. *Can J Neurol Sci* 18, 394.

86. Weiss JH, Turetsky D, Wilke G, Choi DW (1994) AMPA/kainate receptor-mediated damage to NADPH-diaphorase-containing neurons is Ca^{2+} dependent. *Neurosci Lett* 167, 93.

87. Weiss JH, Yin HZ, Choi DW (1994) Basal forebrain cholinergic neurons are selectively vulnerable to AMPA/kainate receptor-mediated neurotoxicity. *Neuroscience* 60, 659.

88. Walz PM, Garrison DL, Graham WM *et al.* (1994) Domoic acid-producing diatom blooms in Monterey Bay, California: 1991–1993. *Nat Toxins* 2, 271.

89. Wekell JC, Gauglitz EJ Jr, Barnett HJ *et al.* (1994) Occurrence of domoic acid in Washington State razor clams (*Siliqua patula*) during 1991–1993. *Nat Toxins* 2, 197.

90. Wozniak DF, Stewart GR, Miller JP, Olney JW (1991) Age-related sensitivity to kainate neurotoxicity. *Exp Neurol* 114, 250.

91. Wright JL (1998) Domoic acid—ten years after. *Nat Toxins* 6, 91.

92. Wright JL, Bird CJ, de Freitas AS *et al.* (1990) Chemistry, biology, and toxicology of domoic acid and its isomers. *Can Dis Wkly Rep* 16, 21.

93. Wright JLC, Boyd RK, de Freitas AS *et al.* (1989) Identification of domoic acid, a neuroexcitatory amino acid, in toxic mussels from eastern Prince Edward Island. *Can J Chem* 67, 481.

94. Xi D, Ramsdell JS (1996) Glutamate receptors and calcium entry mechanisms for domoic acid in hippocampal neurons. *Neuroreport* 7, 1115.

95. Zatorre RJ (1990) Memory loss following domoic acid intoxication from ingestion of toxic mussels. *Can Dis Wkly Rep* 16, 101.

96. Zimmerman HM (1940) The histopathology of convulsive disorders in children. *J Pediat* 13, 859.

Doxorubicin and Related Anthracyclines

Peter S. Spencer

DOXORUBICIN
$C_{27}H_{29}NO_{11}$

	Doxorubicin $C_{27}H_{29}NO_{11}$	Daunorubicin $C_{27}H_{29}NO_{10}$	Epirubicin $C_{27}H_{29}NO_{11}$	Idarubicin $C_{26}H_{27}O_9$
R_1	OCH₃	OCH₃	OCH₃	H
R_2	H	H	OH	H
R_3	OH	OH	H	OH
R_4	OH	H	OH	H

(8S-cis)-10-[(3-Amino-2,3,6-trideoxy-α-L-lyxo-hexopyranosyl)oxy]-7,8,9,10-tetrahydro-6,8,11-trihydroxy-8-(hydroxyacetyl)-1-methoxy-5,12-naphthacenedione; 14-Hydroxydaunomycin

NEUROTOXICITY RATING

Experimental

A Ganglioneuropathy

Doxorubicin and related anthracycline compounds are produced by the fungus *Streptomyces peucetius* var. *caesius*; they are used in combination with other cytotoxic drugs in the treatment of neoplasia. Doxorubicin is effective in acute leukemia, malignant lymphomas, and solid tumors—particularly breast cancer (12). Treatment is associated with a cumulative, dose-related, delayed cardiac toxicity (26,35); rats develop sensory and autonomic ganglioneuropathy. Opening the blood-brain barrier in animals allows doxorubicin to enter and damage the brain (24,32,41,42). The drug serves as an experimental neuronal lesioning agent (14).

General Pharmacology

Anthracycline antibiotics have tetracycline ring structures attached by a glucosidic linkage to the sugar daunosomine (12). Doxorubicin is the 14-hydroxy derivative of daunomycin. Doxorubicin hydrochloride (Adriamycin) forms orange-red colored needles with a MP of 204°–205°C; the compound is soluble in water and alcohol. Many anthra-cycline derivatives, such as idarubicin, have been prepared in a search for compounds with high antitumor activity and low cardiotoxicity (12).

The tetracycline moiety of doxorubicin imparts a unique orange-red fluorescence when tissue-bound drug is excited by ultraviolet light. The fluorescence spectrum has an optimum activation wavelength of 470 nm and an optimum emission wavelength of 595 nm. These properties are useful in studies of drug localization in tissue.

The pharmacokinetics, distribution, metabolism, and excretion of doxorubicin and metabolites have been reviewed (15). A clinically achievable drug concentration in patient serum is said to be 20 µg/ml (40). In humans and experimental animals, there is a rapid fall in the plasma concentration of the drug after intravenous (i.v.) injection. This is followed by a very low plasma concentration for a number of hours. A triphasic plasma disappearance curve in man includes a short half-life of 11.3 min, an intermediate half-life of 3.5 h, and a prolonged half-life of 28.1 h (2). The initial rapid plasma clearance corresponds to a marked accumulation of the drug in tissues such as the liver, kidney, lung, and heart. Doxorubicin is not detectable in human cerebrospinal fluid 1–18 h after i.v. administration (3). Average terminal half-life in humans is approximately 20 h (43).

Doxorubicin enters cells rapidly, imparting its characteristic fluorescence as early as 30 sec after intravenous injection of the drug in Syrian hamsters (20). The most intense fluorescence is localized to the nuclei of various tissues, including the heart, lung, kidney, and choroid plexus.

Metabolism of doxorubicin seems to occur principally in the liver. Six metabolites are found in plasma of patients treated with doxorubicin; these include doxorubicinol, aglycones, and other metabolites (1,2,12). The principal excretion route of doxorubicin and its metabolites is the biliary system.

Animal Studies

Systemic doxorubicin enters regions of the nervous system unprotected by blood-neural barriers. Orange-red fluorescence is detectable in cell nuclei of peripheral somatic and autonomic ganglia within minutes of i.v. injection in rats (14,28). Fluorescence is also found in the mouse choroid plexus and circumventricular organs (*i.e.*, median eminence, postremal area, subfornical organ, organum vasculosum of the lamina terminalis, pineal gland, neurohypophysis) (4,7,17). Doxorubicin autofluorescence is visible throughout the brains of rats with open blood-brain barriers, with patchy distribution in the caudate-putamen (33).

Rats treated with doxorubicin 20 mg/kg body weight die within 9 days; 10 mg/kg produces a mortality of 31% in 4 weeks, and 100% within 5 weeks (45). Rats given a single i.v. injection of doxorubicin (10 mg/kg body weight) develop severe posterior limb ataxia (11–12 days) and mild forelimb ataxia without apparent weakness (13,14). Drug-induced behavioral changes are associated with neuronal necrosis in spinal, paravertebral, and trigeminal ganglia. Comparable effects develop more slowly in animals treated with 5 mg/kg i.v. (28). Over 90% of primary sensory neurons in rats given a single i.v. injection (10 mg/kg) show initial pathological changes; by day 34, approximately half of the neuronal population undergoes necrosis and replacement of the vacated sites by satellite cells (nodes of Nageotte) (14). [Quelamycin is less neurotoxic than doxorubicin to rats; an i.v. dose of 10 mg/kg caused only 1% of dorsal root ganglion neurons to undergo necrosis (29).] This is accompanied by wallerian-like axonal degeneration of peripheral nerves (especially the sural nerve) and dorsal columns, notably the gracile tract (14). Cervical sympathetic and cardiac ganglia also display necrotic neurons at this time. Neuronal nuclei initially develop focal regions of clearing (within 3 h of injection), altered staining of chromatin, fibrillar changes, and nucleolar segregation and fragmentation (11,14,28). Cervical dorsal root ganglia of 11-week-old rats undergo neuronal degeneration after subcutaneous drug administration (10 mg/kg body weight) (19). Rabbits given cumulative doses of 2–24 mg/kg over a period of 5–28 weeks developed a dose-dependent ganglioneuropathy that was clinically evident as hindlimb paresis in 1 of 11 treated animals. Severe ganglioneuropathy was also produced in a single rhesus monkey (one of one tested) given 20 mg/kg over a 10-month period (9).

Intraperitoneal administration of doxorubicin (2 mg/kg) to rats twice weekly reduces body weight gain and has neurotoxic, cardiotoxic, and nephrotoxic effects (51). Vacuolar degeneration of myocardial cells develops progressively over 8 weeks in rats given 2 mg/kg once weekly; this is associated with decline of a ventricular wall marker (radiolabeled metaiodobenzylguanidine) of adrenergic neuronal function and integrity (54). Doxorubicin treatment induces a significant reduction of α- and β-adrenergic reactivity, and of baroreceptor activity (23).

Pathological changes are evident in restricted regions of the brain of mice given a single dose of doxorubicin systemically. Nucleolar segregation, rarefaction of nuclear chromatin, and cytoplasmic changes are found in the area postrema, with neuronal degeneration most evident by 30 days (6,7). Neurosecretory terminals in the neurohypophysis and median eminence undergo degeneration, and nuclear and cytoplasmic changes are seen in the pituicytes and glial cells of the median eminence (7).

Intravenous administration of doxorubicin immediately after opening the blood-brain barrier of rats with the hyperosmotic agent mannitol (1.4 M) results in hindlimb paresis. Cytotoxic effects are found in cerebral cortex and caudate-putamen; these include the aforementioned series of neuronal alterations plus hydropic degeneration of astrocytic end-feet (32). Dogs given unilateral intracarotid 25% mannitol plus Evans blue (which marks areas of blood-brain barrier permeability), followed 5 min later by 0.1–1 mg/kg doxorubicin, variably developed the following: petechial hemorrhages and ipsilateral necrosis of the hippocampus; median dorsal thalamus; and occipital, parietal, and temporal lobes, with additional changes in the brainstem, cerebellum, and basal ganglia (41).

Administration of doxorubicin into the subarachnoid space or the ventricular system of rats elicits dose-dependent toxicity characterized by head tremor, ataxic-dystonic posturing, and circling behavior; this is accompanied by histopathological changes in superficial cortical layers (mice) and the basal surface of the brainstem (rats) (47). Subpial necrotizing angiopathy was found in monkeys given intrathecal doxorubicin (38).

Intravitreal injection in rats elicits nuclear changes in retinal ganglion cells, transient axonal swellings filled with 10-nm neurofilaments, and neuronal degeneration (44).

Intraneural injection of doxorubicin into mouse sciatic nerve causes focal Schwann cell degeneration, demyelination, and remyelination (22). Lysosomal enzyme activities in sciatic nerve peak 30 days after epineurial injection of doxorubicin; pretreatment with cysteamine (sulfhydryl donor) or diethyl maleate (sulfhydryl depletor) neither prevents nor potentiates the doxorubicin-induced increase in enzyme activities (8).

Doxorubicin undergoes retrograde axonal transport in PNS neurons (5,21) and CNS neurons (31). For example, injection of doxorubicin into the rat caudate-putamen is followed, within 4 h, by the appearance of drug-related fluorescence in substantia nigra zona compacta and the ventral tegmental area; ipsilateral neuronal degeneration subsequently occurs in these nuclei (31). Injection of doxorubicin into the tongue of mice is followed 6 h later by the appearance of drug-related orange-red fluorescence in hypoglossal neurons (5,7). Early neuronal changes, such as rarefaction of nuclear chromatin and segregation and fragmentation of nucleolar components, are followed by cytoplasmic vacuolation, disappearance of ribosomes, and other changes indicative of neuronal degeneration (apparent at 14 days) (5). Similarly, microinjection of doxorubicin into rat tibial nerve precipitated progressive subacute anterior horn cell degeneration over a period of 35–39 days; dorsal root ganglion cells were relatively unaffected (21). By contrast, motor neurons were reportedly less sensitive than primary sensory neurons (especially small neurons) to doxorubicin transported retrogradely from the cut end of the proximal stump of a transected sciatic nerve (33).

Cyanomorpholinyl adriamycin (CMA) lacks the ionizable side group of doxorubicin, is 81 times more lipophilic, exhibits several hundred-fold greater in-vitro antineoplastic activity against a number of tumor cell lines, and is able to traverse blood-neural interfaces. CMA also binds to cellular nuclei in vitro but, unlike doxorubicin, autofluorescence cannot be detected in the brain or other organs of CMA-treated animals. Within 6–12 h of i.v. administration of CMA (equal to or greater than only 0.1 mg/kg), animals develop hypothermia, cyanosis, severe ataxia, hypoactivity, and tremor at rest (17).

Doxorubicin, like some other antitumor agents, is itself oncogenic and has induced neoplasms, such as mammary tumors in rats. It also has a teratogenic effect in rats, reflected in various gastrointestinal, urinary tract, and cardiovascular abnormalities (50).

In Vitro Studies

The spatial-temporal evolution of neuronal damage has been studied in structurally and functionally coupled mouse fetal spinal cord–ganglion cocultures treated with doxorubicin dissolved in nutrient fluid (55). Degree and type of pathological change were related to drug dosage, duration of treatment, age of the culture, and susceptibility of individual cells. Neuronal changes were seen over the range of 10^{-9}–10^{-5} M doxorubicin. Cultures treated for 20 min with 10^{-5} M doxorubicin showed strong orange fluorescence associated with the chromatin of satellite cells and discrete zones (nucleoli?) within the nuclei of primary sensory neurons (55). Weak orange fluorescence was seen in the cytoplasm of neurons and satellite cells. After 2 days of treatment, granular inclusions were evident in the majority of living neurons, and many displayed eccentrically displaced nuclei. Nucleoli were invariably altered in size and shape, with dissociation of the pars fibrosa and the pars granulosa. Beginning wallerian-like degeneration of proximal segments of some myelinated axons was seen at this time. Scattered blebbing of myelin sheaths was also apparent. Neurons eventually underwent complete breakdown: the nucleus and then the cytoplasm were transformed into a shrunken collection of dense granules. Satellite cells sometimes underwent necrosis, and occasional Schwann cells of unmyelinated fibers displayed nuclei with clumps of dense chromatin.

Neuroblastoma cell lines (SH-SY5Y and SMS-KCNR) underwent doxorubicin-induced apoptosis; cell differentiation triggered by retinoic acid induced bcl-2 expression and abolished sensitivity to doxorubicin (34). Doxorubicin increased tau expression and induced cell death in differentiated SH-SY5Y cells; pretreatment with sabeluzole, which protects cultured hippocampal neurons from N-methyl-D-aspartate neurotoxicity, inhibited neurotoxin-induced tau expression and cell death (52).

Doxorubicin reportedly depresses antioxidant enzymes (superoxide dismutase, catalase, glutathione peroxidase) and stimulates lipid peroxidation in rat CNS tissue in vitro and in vivo. Addition of glutathione or vitamin E to brain homogenates protects against doxorubicin-induced lipid peroxidation (30).

Doxorubicin increases the fluidity of dog brain synaptosomal plasma membranes (18).

Human Studies

The general toxic effects of doxorubicin are attributable to the drug's antimitotic activity; they involve rapidly proliferating tissues such as the hematopoietic system and the epithelium of the alimentary tract (45). This is reflected in doxorubicin-treated patients by leukopenia, stomatitis, nausea, vomiting, and alopecia.

The dose-limiting effect of doxorubicin is cardiomyopathy (10,16). Minor and transient changes in the electrocardiogram are seen shortly after doxorubicin administration. More importantly, a cumulative, dose-related cardiomyopathy appears months following the initial use of doxorubicin. This can lead to progressive congestive heart failure and cardiorespiratory decompensation. Evidence of cardiac sympathetic denervation may be present prior to deterioration of heart function and the appearance of clinical signs of cardiomyopathy (36,49,53). Neuronal changes in cardiac neurons have been reported postmortem in patients treated with daunomycin (48). Pathological studies of heart muscle reveal nonspecific changes such as myofibrillar lysis, vacuolar degeneration of myocytes, and interstitial edema with no inflammatory infiltrates.

Peripheral neurotoxicity may occur in subjects treated with drug combinations that include doxorubicin and other potentially neurotoxic drugs such as paclitaxel (25). Various clinical manifestations of neurotoxicity are common complications of cancer chemotherapy using high-dose combinations of cytotoxic drugs (37).

Pathological Mechanisms

The antiproliferative action of doxorubicin is attributed to DNA damage, including single- and double-strand breaks, and inhibition of DNA repair and synthesis (46). The four planar rings of the doxorubicin molecule intercalate with DNA, and the hydroxyl group on the side chain interacts with topoisomerase II; this enzyme enhances the action of DNA helicase, which unwinds DNA during DNA replication. Topoisomerase II is also an integral part of the DNA scaffold in mammalian cells (16). Scission of DNA by doxorubicin is mediated either by the action of topoisomerase II or the generation of hydroxyl free radicals (12). Depletion of DNA templates disrupts both DNA-dependent DNA and RNA polymerases, with consequent perturbation and cessation of protein synthesis (27,39).

Doxorubicin produces delayed degeneration in postmitotic cells, notably cardiac muscle cells and neurons (which have inefficient DNA repair). Blood-borne doxorubicin enters regions of the nervous system supplied with fenestrated blood vessels, including the circumventricular organs, and cranial, spinal, and autonomic ganglia. Drug binding to the nuclei of neurons, satellite cells, and Schwann cells is rapid. Pathological changes develop first in the neuronal nucleus, specifically the nucleolus, and later involve the entire perikaryon; subsequently, axonal and nerve fiber degeneration spreads in an anterograde wave as the neuron "dies forward" from its perikaryon distally. Nonpostmitotic neural cells, such as satellite cells in dorsal root ganglia, may die or survive concentrations of doxorubicin that kill neurons (14,15).

REFERENCES

1. Benjamin RS (1975) Clinical pharmacology of Adriamycin (NSC-123127). *Cancer Chemother Rep* 6, 183.
2. Benjamin RS, Riggs CE Jr, Bachur NR (1977) Plasma pharmacokinetics of Adriamycin and its metabolism in humans with normal hepatic and renal function. *Cancer Res* 37, 1416.
3. Benjamin RS, Wiernik PH, Bachur NR (1974) Adriamycin chemotherapy—efficacy, safety, and pharmacologic basis of intermittent single high-dose schedule. *Cancer* 33, 19.
4. Bigotte L, Arvidson B, Olsson Y (1982) Cytofluorescence localization of Adriamycin in the nervous system. I: Distribution of the drug in the central nervous system of normal adult mice after intravenous injection. *Acta Neuropathol* 57, 121.
5. Bigotte L, Olsson Y (1983) Cytotoxic effects of Adriamycin on mouse hypoglossal neurons following retrograde axonal transport from the tongue. *Acta Neuropathol* 61, 161.
6. Bigotte L, Olsson Y (1983) Toxic effects of Adriamycin on the central nervous system. Ultrastructural changes in some circumventricular organs of the mouse after intravenous administration of the drug. *Acta Neuropathol* 61, 291.
7. Bigotte L, Olsson Y (1984) Cytotoxic effects of Adriamycin on the central nervous system of the mouse—cytofluorescence and electron-microscopic observations after various modes of administration. *Acta Neurol Scand* 100, 55.
8. Boegman RJ, Scarth B, Dragovic L, Robertson DM (1985) Neurotoxicity of Adriamycin and misonidazole in the mouse. *Exp Neurol* 87, 1.
9. Bronson RT, Henderson TC, Fixlet H (1982) Ganglioneuropathy in rabbits and a rhesus monkey due to high cumulative doses of doxorubicin. *Cancer Treatment Rep* 66, 1349.
10. Carter JM, Bergin PS (1986) Doxorubicin cardiotoxicity. *N Engl J Med* 314, 1118.
11. Cavanagh JB, Tomiwa K, Munro PM (1987) Nuclear and nucleolar damage in Adriamycin-induced toxicity to rat sensory ganglion cells. *Neuropathol Appl Neurobiol* 13, 23.
12. Chabner BA, Allegra CJ, Curt GA, Calabresi P (1996) Antineoplastic agents. In: *Goodman & Gilman's The Pharmacological Basis of Therapeutics. 9th Ed.* Hardman JG, Limbird LE, eds. McGraw-Hill, New York p. 1233.
13. Cho ES (1977) Toxic effects of Adriamycin on the ganglia of the peripheral nervous system: A neuropathological study. *J Neuropathol Exp Neurol* 36, 907.
14. Cho ES, Spencer PS, Jortner BS (1980) Doxorubicin. In: *Experimental and Clinical Neurotoxicology.* Spencer PS, Schaumburg HH eds. Williams & Wilkins, Baltimore p. 430.
15. Cho ES, Spencer PS, Jortner BS, Schaumburg HH (1980) A single intravenous injection of doxorubicin (Adriamycin[R]) induces sensory neuronopathy in rats. *Neurotoxicology* 1, 583.
16. Coulson CJ (1994) *Molecular Mechanisms of Drug Action. 2nd Ed.* Taylor & Francis, London.
17. Cramer SC, Rhodes RH, Acton EM, Tökes ZA (1989) Neurotoxicity and dermatotoxicity of cyanorpholinyl Adriamycin. *Cancer Chemother Pharmacol* 23, 71.
18. Deliconstantinos G, Kopeikina-Tsiboukidou L, Villiotou V (1987) Evaluation of membrane fluidity effects and enzyme alterations in Adriamycin neurotoxicity. *Biochem Pharmacol* 36, 1153.
19. Eddy EL (1983) Neuronal loss from cervical dorsal root ganglia in Adriamycin-induced peripheral neuropathy—a quantitative study. *Anatomisch Anzeig* 153, 83.
20. Egorin MJ, Hildebrand RC, Cimino EF, Bachur NR (1974) Cytofluorescence localization of Adriamycin and daunorubicin. *Cancer Res* 34, 2243.
21. England JD, Asbury AK, Rhee EK, Sumner AJ (1988) Lethal retrograde axoplasmic transport of doxorubicin (Adriamycin) to motor neurons. A toxic motor neuronopathy. *Brain* 111, 915.
22. England JD, Rhee EK, Said G, Sumner AJ (1988) Schwann cell degeneration induced by doxorubicin (Adriamycin). *Brain* 111, 901.

23. Fillippelli W, Russo S, Marrazzo R (1994) Vasomotor responses in rats "intoxicated" with doxorubicin. *Res Commun Chem Pathol Pharmacol* **84**, 73.

24. Folb PI (1996) Cytostatics and immunosuppressive drugs. In: *Meyler's Side Effects of Drugs. 13th Ed.* Dukes MNG ed. Elsevier, Amsterdam p. 1336.

25. Frassineti GL, Zoli W, Silvestro L *et al.* (1997) Paclitaxel plus doxorubicin in breast cancer: An Italian experience. *Semin Oncol* **24**, S17.

26. Freter CR, Lee TC, Billingham ME *et al.* (1986) Doxorubicin cardiac toxicity mainifesting seven years after treatment. *Amer J Med* **80**, 483.

27. Goodman MF, Lee GM, Bachur NR (1977) Adriamycin interactions within T4 DNA polymerase. *J Biol Chem* **252**, 2670.

28. Jortner BS, Cho ES (1980) Neurotoxicity of Adriamycin in rats: A low-dose effect. *Cancer Treatment Rep* **64**, 257.

29. Jortner BS, Cho ES (1981) Neurotoxicity of quelamycin in the rat. *Neurotoxicology* **2**, 789.

30. Julka D, Sandhir R, Gill KD (1993) Adriamycin-induced oxidative stress in rat central nervous tissue. *Biochem Mol Biol Int* **29**, 807.

31. Koda LY, Van der Kooy D (1983) Doxorubicin: A fluorescent neurotoxin retrogradely transported in the central nervous system. *Neurosci Lett* **36**, 1.

32. Kondo A, Inoue T, Nagara H *et al.* (1987) Neurotoxicity of Adriamycin passed through the transiently disrupted blood-brain barrier by mannitol in the rat brain. *Brain Res* **412**, 73.

33. Kondo A, Ohnishi AM, Nagara H, Tateishi J (1987) Neurotoxicity in primary sensory neurons of Adriamycin administered through retrograde axoplasmic transport in rats. *Neuropathol Appl Neurobiol* **13**, 177.

34. Lasorella A, Iavarone F, Israel MA (1995) Differentiation of neuroblastoma enhances bcl-2 expression and induces alterations of apoptosis and drug resistance. *Cancer Res* **55**, 4711.

35. Lefrak EA, Pitha J, Rosenheim S, Gottlieb JA (1973) A clinicopathologic analysis of Adriamycin cardiotoxicity. *Cancer* **32**, 302.

36. Lekakis J, Prassopoulos V, Athanassiadis P *et al.* (1996) Doxorubicin-induced cardiac neurotoxicity: Study with iodine 123-labeled metaiodobenzylguanidine scintigraphy. *J Nuclear Cardiology* **3**, 37.

37. MacDonald DR (1991) Neurologic complications of chemotherapy. *Neurol Clin* **9**, 955.

38. Merker PC, Lewis MR, Walker MD, Richardson EP (1978) Neurotoxicity of Adriamycin (doxorubicin) perfused through the cerebrospinal fluid spaces of the rhesus monkey. *Toxicol Appl Pharmacol* **44**, 191.

39. Minow RA, Benjamin RS, Gottlieb JA (1975) Adriamycin cardiomyopathy—an overview with determination of risk factors. *Cancer Chemother Rep* **6**, 195.

40. Moriuchi S, Shimizu K, Mayao Y *et al.* (1996) *In vitro* assessment for neurotoxicity of antitumor agents before local administration into central nervous system. *Anticancer Res* **16**, 135.

41. Neuwelt EA, Glasberg M, Frenkel E, Barnett P (1983) Neurotoxicity of chemotherapeutic agents after blood-brain barrier modification: Neuropathological studies. *Ann Neurol* **14**, 316.

42. Neuwelt EWA, Pagel M, Barnett P *et al.* (1981) Pharmacology and toxicity of intracarotid Adriamycin administration following osmotic blood-brain barrier modification. *Cancer Res* **41**, 4466.

43. Ostrow S, Egorin MJ, Hahn D *et al.* (1980) Cis-Dichlorodiammine platinum and Adriamycin therapy for advanced gynecological and genitourinary neoplasms. *Cancer* **46**, 1715.

44. Parhad IM, Griffin JW, Clark AW, Koves JF (1984) Doxorubicin intoxication: Neurofilamentous axonal changes with subacute neuronal death. *J Neuropathol Exp Neurol* **43**, 188.

45. Philips FS, Gilladoga A, Marquardt H *et al.* (1975) Some observations on the toxicity of Adriamycin. *Cancer Chemother Rep* **6**, 177.

46. Schwartz HS (1976) Mechanisms and selectivity of anthracycline aminoglycosides and other intercalating agents. *Biomedicine* **24**, 317.

47. Siegal T, Melamed E, Sandbank U, Catane R (1988) Early and delayed neurotoxicity of mitoxantrone and doxorubicin following subarachnoid injection. *J Neuro-oncol* **6**, 135.

48. Smith B (1969) Damage to the intrinsic cardiac neurones by rubidomycin (daunorubicin). *Brit Heart J* **31**, 607.

49. Takano H, Ozawa H, Kobayashi I *et al.* (1995) Atrophic nerve fibers in regions of reduced MIBG uptake in doxorubicin cardiomyopathy. *J Nucl Med* **36**, 2060.

50. Thompson DJ, Molello JA, Strebling RJ, Dyke IL (1978) Teratogenicity of Adriamycin and daunomycin in the rat and rabbit. *Teratology* **17**, 151.

51. Tian Hu S, Brandle E, Zbinden G (1983) Inhibition of cardiotoxic, nephrotoxic and neurotoxic effects of doxorubicin by ICRF-159. *Pharmacology* **26**, 210.

52. Uberti D, Rizzini C, Galli P *et al.* (1997) Priming of cultured neurons with sabeluzole results in long-lasting inhibition of neurotoxin-induced tau expression and cell death. *Synapse* **26**, 95.

53. Valdes Olmos RA, ten Bokkel Huinink WW, ten Hoeve RF *et al.* (1995) Assessment of anthracycline-related myocardial adrenergic derangement by [^{123}I]metaiodobenzylguanidine scintigraphy. *Eur J Cancer* **31A**, 26.

54. Wakasugi S, Wada A, Hasegawa Y (1992) Detection of abnormal cardiac adrenergic neuron activity in Adriamycin-induced cardiomyopathy with iodine-125-metaiodobenzylguanidine. *J Nucl Med* **33**, 215.

55. Zagoren JC, Seelig M, Bornstein MB, Spencer PS (1984) The evolution of cellular degeneration in dorsal root ganglia exposed to doxorubicin in tissue culture. *J Neuropathol Exp Neurol* **43**, 384.

Enflurane

Herbert H. Schaumburg

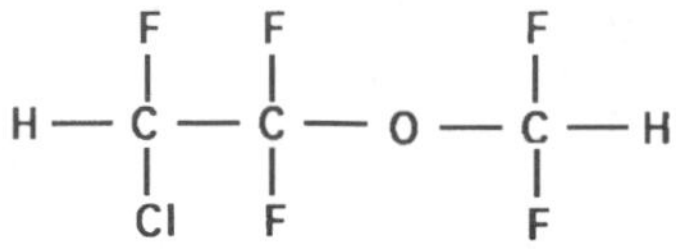

ENFLURANE
$C_3H_2ClF_5O$

2-Chloro-1-(difluoromethoxy)-1,1,2-trifluoroethane;
2-Chloro-1,1,2-trifluoroethyl difluoromethyl ether

NEUROTOXICITY RATING

Clinical

A Seizure disorder

B Acute encephalopathy (cognitive dysfunction)

Enflurane is a widely used volatile inhalant anesthetic agent. It is considered safe, is easily administered, and has fewer cardiac side effects than halothane, its chemically related predecessor.

Generalized and focal seizures have followed administration of high concentrations of enflurane, especially in the presence of hypocarbia. A characteristic electroencephalographic profile is associated with enflurane-induced seizures; a high-voltage, fast-frequency (14–18 Hz) pattern that progresses to spike-and-wave complexes. Seizures are of short duration, self-limited, and may occur at intervals from the immediate postoperative period up to 8 days later (2). Although there is no report of the drug aggravating a pre-existing seizure disorder, this agent is used with caution in epileptic individuals. Mild cognitive impairment develops during exposure to subanesthetic levels of enflurane; it is unclear if this is a potential hazard for operating room personnel (1,3).

REFERENCES

1. Bentin S, Collins GI, Adam N (1978) Decision-making behavior during inhalation of subanesthetic concentrations of enflurane. *Brit J Anesth* **50**, 1173.
2. Fahy LT (1987) Delayed convulsions after day case anesthesia with enflurane. *Anesthesia* **42**, 1327.
3. Lucchini R, Placidi D, Toffoletto F, Alessio L (1996) Neurotoxicity in operating room personnel working with gaseous and nongaseous anesthesia. *Int Arch Occup Environ Health* **68**, 188.

Erabutoxins

Albert C. Ludolph

NEUROTOXICITY RATING

Clinical

A Neuromuscular transmission syndrome

Experimental

A Neuromuscular transmission dysfunction (postsynaptic)

The erabutoxins a, b, and c (Ea, Eb, Ec) are basic, single, short-chain α-neurotoxins with four disulfide bonds isolated from the venom of the sea snake *Laticauda semifasciata*. Individual snakes carry different mixtures of these toxins. Erabutoxins a and c differ from erabutoxin b by a single amino acid residue at position 26 and 51, respectively. The molecules have a three-dimensional structure and fold into three loops (8,10). cDNA sequences for erabutoxins a, b, and c have been determined (3). Erabutoxins bind to the α-subunit of the nicotinic acetylcholine receptor of the neuromuscular junction; the precise site of binding is currently under investigation (5). The LD$_{50}$ of erabutoxin a and b in mice is 0.15 mg/kg body weight after intramuscular administration (9). Animals die of respiratory paralysis. Erabutoxins do not have an effect on the axon (4) but experimentally depress glutamatergic and nicotinic activity in the cerebral cortex (1,2). Clinical manifestations of sea snake bites, such as diplopia, and facial, bulbar, and generalized weakness, which may progress to respiratory failure, are ascribed to the action of erabutoxins at the neuromuscular junction (6,7,11,12). For more general information on sea snake neurotoxicity, *see* Hydrophiidae toxins.

REFERENCES

1. Burne JA (1978) The action of erabutoxin "b" in the cerebral cortex: Evidence for short latency potentially nicotinic neurons. *Life Sci* **23**, 775.
2. Burne JA, Webster MED (1977) The action of erabutoxins "b" on spontaneous and glutamate-induced cortical activity. *Life Sci* **20**, 2023.
3. Fuse N, Tsuchiya T, Nonomura Y *et al.* (1990) Structure

of the snake short-chain neurotoxin, erabutoxin c, precursor gene. *Eur J Biochem* **193**, 629.

4. Kato E, Kuba K, Koketsu K (1978) Effects of erabutoxins on neuromuscular transmission in frog skeletal muscles. *J Pharmacol Exp Ther* **204**, 446.

5. Pillet L, Tremeau O, Ducancel F *et al.* (1993) Genetic engineering of snake toxins. Role of invariant residues in the structural and functional properties of a curaremimetic toxin, as probed by site-directed mutagenesis. *J Biol Chem* **268**, 909.

6. Reid HA (1956) Sea-snake bite research. *Trans Roy Soc Trop Med Hyg* **50**, 417.

7. Reid HA (1975) Epidemiology of sea snake bites. *J Trop Med Hyg* **78**, 106.

8. Ruoppolo M, Moutiez M, Mazzeo MF *et al.* (1998) The length of a single turn controls the overall folding rate of "three-fingered" snake toxins. *Biochemistry* **37**, 16060.

9. Tamiya N, Arai H (1966) Studies on sea-snake venoms. *Biochem J* **99**, 624.

10. Tsernoglou D, Petsko GA (1976) The crystal structure of a postsynaptic neurotoxin from sea snake at 2.2 Å resolution. *FEBS Lett* **68**, 1.

11. Tu AT (1988) Sea snakes and their venoms. In: *Handbook of Natural Toxins. Vol 3. Marine Toxins and Venoms.* Tu AT ed. Marcel Dekker, New York p. 424.

12. Tu AT, Fulde G (1987) Sea snake bite. *Clin Dermatol* **5**, 118.

Ergot Alkaloids

Lawrence C. Newman
Richard B. Lipton

ERGOTAMINE
C$_{33}$H$_{35}$N$_5$O$_5$

12′-Hydroxy-2′-methyl-5′α-(phenylmethyl) ergotaman-3′,6′,18-trione; Ergotamine

NEUROTOXICITY RATING
Clinical

A Acute encephalopathy (confusion, polydipsia, coma)

A Chronic encephalopathy (confusion, encephalomalacia, seizures)

The ergot alkaloids can be divided into three groups: amino acid alkaloids, dihydrogenated amino acid alkaloids, and amine alkaloids. Ergotamine tartrate, a member of the amino acid group, is an ergopeptide consisting of a natural D-lysergic acid linked to a tricyclic moiety by a peptide bond.

Ergotamine tartrate was originally derived from the rye fungus *Claviceps purpurea*, a parasite of the head of rye stalks. Ergot poisoning, first described during the Middle Ages, was caused by eating grain contaminated by fungus. Epidemics of ergot poisoning were characterized by gangrene and intense burning of the extremities, giving rise to the terms "the holy fire" or "St. Anthony's fire" (10). Bizarre behavior, convulsions, and miscarriages were also reported during these outbreaks.

Efforts to isolate the active compound from the rye fungus led to the isolation and identification of ergotamine tartrate in 1918. The potent vasoconstricting effects of this isolate, combined with the theory that migraine pain was due to vasodilatation, led to its therapeutic use for migraine in 1925 (11). Today, ergotamine tartrate is widely used in migraine therapy, most often in combination with caffeine in oral tablets and rectal suppositories. Sublingual and inhalant preparations are no longer commercially available; parenteral formulations were never widely used.

The effects of the ergot alkaloids appear to result from their actions as both partial agonists and antagonists at adrenergic, dopaminergic, and tryptaminergic receptors (10). Ergotamine is poorly and erratically absorbed. Bioavailability depends not only on the route of administration, but can vary widely when given repeatedly to the same patient during different attacks (1,5–7). Bioavailability is <5% with oral formulations but considerably higher and more consistent with rectal administration (3,9). In normal volunteers, ergotamine given rectally produced blood levels 20- to 30-fold higher than oral doses (12). Peak plasma concentrations are attained approximately 1–3 h following oral dosing of ergotamine and within 1 h of rectal dosing (6,7,12).

When taken orally, ergotamine tartrate is absorbed from

the upper gastrointestinal tract, traverses the portal circulation to the liver, and then enters the systemic circulation (3). Ergotamine is metabolized by the liver, and 90% of the metabolites are excreted in the bile (4). Metabolism is believed to occur in two phases, the α phase having a plasma half-life of 1.5–2.5 h and the β phase, lasting 20–30 h (3). Orally administered ergotamine undergoes substantial degradation in the liver; rectal dosing limits first-pass hepatic metabolism yielding higher plasma levels.

In canine studies, ergotamine demonstrates potent vasoconstrictor activity, especially in the carotid arterial system (13). In experimental animal models, at therapeutic doses, ergotamine causes decreased shunting of blood from the carotid artery to the jugular vein (10). Intravenous injections of ergotamine prevented neurogenic inflamation of the rat dura mater (8). Although neurogenic inflammation is postulated to be a putative cause of migrainous pain, the dose required in these studies exceeded clinically relevant dosages.

When ergotamine tartrate is correctly used as an acute treatment of migraine, side effects are usually mild, self-limited, and do not require discontinuation of the drug. Doses should be limited to 6 mg/day and 10 mg/week. It should be avoided by patients with hypertension, claudication, angina, and other vascular diseases. At appropriate doses, in the selected patients, nausea is the most common side effect, occurring in 10%–75% of treated subjects (3,11). Less common are abdominal cramps, diarrhea, vertigo, distal paresthesias, and muscle cramps involving the lower extremities. Rare side effects include syncope, dyspnea, angina, drowsiness, and tremor.

At extreme doses, ergot alkaloids are highly toxic and may produce either acute or chronic poisoning. Acute poisoning is relatively uncommon and usually results from the ingestion of a large amount of ergot during an attempted abortion (10). Symptoms of acute ergotamine poisoning include vomiting, diarrhea, intense thirst, itching, tingling and cold skin, rapid and weak pulse, confusion, and coma. Fatal poisoning has occurred after oral administration of 26 mg ergotamine over several days, but has also been reported following single injections of 0.5–1.5 mg (10).

There have been 64 published reports relating to the adverse effects of chronic high-dose ergotamine tartrate (14). The most common serious adverse effect reported is ischemia of the extremities. Ergotamine tartrate use has rarely been linked to myocardial ischemia or infarction, cardiac arrest, and even sudden death (3,14). Renal artery spasm, cerebrovascular ischemia, bowel ischemia, retroperitoneal or intrathoracic fibrosis, and hepatic necrosis are also reported (14). Peroneal nerve palsies most likely caused by constriction of the vasa nevorum are described (3,11).

The most common potential serious consequence of long-term ergotamine overuse is ergotism. Ergotism usually occurs when ergotamine is taken in excessively large or frequently repeated doses. However, a few patients with an idiosyncratic sensitivity to ergotamine have developed ergotism after only brief exposure to the drug. Similarly, some patients are able to tolerate enormous doses of ergotamine on a long-term basis without identifiable sequelae. Ergotamine tartrate can induce profound peripheral vasospasm especially affecting the lower extremities. Superimposed secondary occlusions and thromboses of medium and small arteries may coexist and may lead to intermittent paresthesias of the distal extremities, cold digits, and claudication of the arms and legs followed by loss of arterial pulses with subsequent gangrene. The characteristic angiographic appearance of ergot-induced arterial insufficiency demonstrates distal segmental vessel spasm with increased collateral flow (2).

Ergotamine overuse has also been linked to encephalopathy, focal motor or sensory symptoms, seizures, and coma (3). Chronic ergotamine use may induce cerebral atrophy (3). There have been several reports of anal and rectal ulcers associated with ergotamine suppository use (14). The coadministration of erythromycin, methysergide, and β-blockers with ergotamine tartrate may increase a patient's risk of arteriospasm (14).

REFERENCES

1. Ala-Hurula V, Myllylä V, Arvela P et al. (1979) Systemic availability of ergotamine tartrate after three successive doses and during continuous medication. Eur J Clin Pharmacol 16, 355.
2. Bagby RJ, Cooper RD (1972) Angiography in ergotism: Report of two cases and review of the literature. Amer J Roentgenol 116, 179.
3. Davidoff RA (1995) Migraine: Manifestations, Pathogenesis and Management. FA Davis Co, Philadelphia.
4. Ekhart H, Kiechel JR, Rosenthaler J et al. (1978) Biopharmaceutical aspects: Ergot alkaloids and related compounds. In: Handbook of Experimental Pharmacology. Vol 49. Berde B, Schild HO eds. Springer-Verlag, New York p. 719.
5. Hakkarainen H, Vapaatalo H, Gothoni G et al. (1979) Tolfenamic acid is as effective as ergotamine during migraine attacks. Lancet 2, 326.
6. Ibraheem JJ, Paalzow L, Tfelt-Hansen P (1983) Low bioavailability of ergotamine tartrate after oral and rectal administration in migraine sufferers. Brit J Clin Pharmacol 16, 695.
7. Kanto J (1983) Clinical pharmacokinetics of ergotamine, dihydroergotamine, ergotoxine, bromocriptine, methysergide and lergotrile. Int J Clin Pharmacol 21, 135.
8. Markowitz S, Saito K, Moskowitz MA (1988) Neurogenically mediated extravasation in dura mater: Effect of ergot

alkaloids. A possible mechanism of action in vascular headache. *Cephalalgia* **8**, 83.

9. Perrin VL (1985) Clinical pharmacokinetics of ergotamine in migraine and cluster headaches. *Clin Pharmacokinet* **10**, 334.
10. Rall TW, Schleifer LS (1990) Oxytocin, prostaglandins, ergot alkaloids and other agents. In: *The Pharmacological Basis of Therapeutics. 7th Ed.* Gilman AG, Rall TW, Nies AS, Taylor P eds. Macmillan Publishing Company, New York p. 939.
11. Raskin NH (1988) Migraine: Treatment. In: *Headache.* Hurley RA, Terry D eds. Churchill Livingstone, New York p. 140.
12. Sanders SW, Haering N, Mosberg H, Jaeger H (1986) Pharmacokinetics of ergotamine in healthy volunteers following oral and rectal dosing. *Eur J Clin Pharmacol* **30**, 331.
13. Saxena PR, de Vlaam-Schluter GM (1974) Role of some biogenic substance in migraine and relevant mechanism in anti-migraine action of ergotamine—studies in an experimental model for migraine. *Headache* **13**, 142.
14. Silberstein SD, Young WB (1995) Safety and efficacy of ergotamine tartrate and dihydroergotamine in the treatment of migraine and status migrainosus. *Neurology* **45**, 577.

Erythromycin

Herbert H. Schaumburg

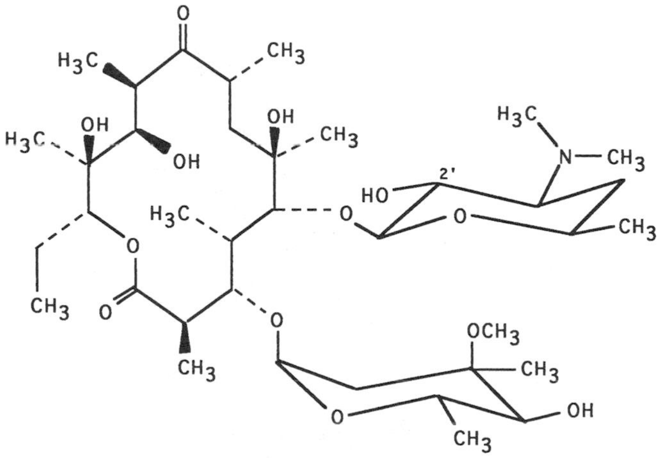

ERYTHROMYCIN A
$C_{37}H_{67}NO_{13}$

Erythromycin A

NEUROTOXICITY RATING

Clinical

A Ototoxicity (hearing loss)

B Psychobiological reaction

Experimental

A Ototoxicity (cochlear neuropathy)

Erythromycin is a widely used macrolide antibiotic effective in treatment of infections caused by gram-positive cocci. The mechanism of action involves inhibition of bacterial protein synthesis by binding reversibly to 50 S ribosomal subunits of the sensitive microorganism. Erythromycin is often administered orally but absorption is slow and incomplete; intravenous administration is advocated when high plasma levels are required. The drug has a plasma half-life of 1.6 h, is concentrated by the liver, and is excreted in the bile. Erythromycin diffuses rapidly into extracellular fluid compartments but has poor penetration into cerebrospinal fluid.

Serious systemic toxicity is unusual. Cholestatic hepatitis and epigastric distress are the most common untoward effects. Transient ototoxicity with auditory impairment may accompany high-level (4 g daily) intravenous administration and is the most serious, consistent effect upon the nervous system. Acute psychosis is rare.

The pathophysiology of erythromycin ototoxicity is unknown. Different anatomical sites of dysfunction are described in experimental animal studies. One report (2) delineates sensory cell loss in the cochlea following topical application in the middle ear of the guinea pig. Another notes an increased latency in the fourth wave of the brainstem auditory evoked response of systemically treated guinea pigs (1).

There are more than 25 clinical reports of reversible hearing loss in humans; most instances suggest end-organ dysfunction, since tinnitus, vertigo, and 50- to 75-db decrements on audiograms are common features (1). None of the studies features pretreatment audiograms or brainstem auditory response examinations. Hearing loss is dose-related, since higher doses or impaired elimination have been factors in almost every instance. Since hearing loss occurs at frequencies used for voice communication, as well as for higher frequencies, patients are immediately aware of auditory dysfunction. This is in striking contrast to the auditory dysfunction associated with aminoglycoside ototoxicity, which commences at high frequencies and often is unnoticed until serious damage ensues. In two instances, hearing loss only partially recovered.

There are several case reports of transient psychosis or nightmares in individuals receiving conventional doses of erythromycin (3,4).

REFERENCES

1. Brummett RE (1993) Ototoxic liability of erythromycin and analogues. In: *The Otolaryngologic Clinics of North America. Vol 26. Ototoxicity.* Rybak LP ed. WB Saunders Co, Philadelphia p. 811.

2. Stupp H, Kupper K, Lagler F *et al.* (1973) Inner ear concentrations and ototoxicity of different antibiotics in local and systemic application. *Audiology* **12**, 350.

3. Umstead GS, Neumann KH (1986) Erythromycin ototoxicity and acute psychotic reaction in cancer patients with hepatic dysfunction. *Arch Intern Med* **146**, 897.

4. Williams NR (1988) Erythromycin: A case of nightmares. *Brit Med J* **296**, 214.

Ethacrynic Acid

Herbert H. Schaumburg

ETHACRYNIC ACID
C13H12Cl2O4

[2,3-Dichloro-4-(2-methylene-1-oxobutyl)phenoxy]acetic acid

NEUROTOXICITY RATING

Clinical

A Ototoxicity (hearing loss)

Experimental

A Ototoxicity (stria vascularis degeneration)

Ethacrynic acid is a potent, short-acting, renal-loop diuretic; it is now infrequently used, since other loop diuretics, such as furosemide, have a less precipitous dose–response curve. Loop diuretics inhibit electrolyte reabsorption in the thick ascending limb of the loop of Henle; they act at the luminal face of the epithelial cells to inhibit the sodium, potassium, and chloride ion cotransport mechanism. Ethacrynic acid has little systemic toxicity aside from therapy-associated abnormalities of fluid and electrolyte imbalance. Hearing loss is the only serious adverse effect on the nervous system.

Guinea pigs dosed with ototoxic levels of ethacrynic acid display reduced endocochlear potentials, cochlear microphonics, and eighth-nerve compound action potentials; there is slow recovery following drug withdrawal (2). Ultrastructural examination discloses cellular atrophy and accumulation of intercellular fluid in the intermediate cell region of the stria vascularis (3). Freeze-fracture studies reveal alterations of gap junction morphology in the stria vascularis, suggesting that strial cells may uncouple in response to ethacrynic acid (5). The pathophysiology of these changes is unknown. While it is clear that ethacrynic acid decreases the potassium gradient between endolymph and perilymph, it is debated whether these changes in the stria vascularis stem from inhibition of potassium pumps or from inhibition of adenylate cyclase through an effect on the G-protein complex (6).

Acute-onset hearing impairment is well established as a human complication of high-dose ethacrynic acid therapy; one study estimates the incidence as 0.7% (4). Most reports describe reversible hearing loss, but permanent impairment and even deafness can develop; permanent hearing dysfunction is especially common in patients with renal disease (7). Postmortem light and electron microscopic examination demonstrates edematous changes in the marginal zone of the stria vascularis similar to the findings in laboratory animals (1).

REFERENCES

1. Arnold W, Nado JB Jr, Geidauer H (1981) Ultrastructural histopathology in a case of human ototoxicity due to loop diuretics. *Acta Otolaryngol* **91**, 414.

2. Bosher SK (1980) The nature of the ototoxic actions of ethacrynic acid upon the mammalian endolymph system. I. Functional aspects. *Acta Otolaryngol* **89**, 407.

3. Bosher SK (1980) The nature of the ototoxic action of ethacrynic acid upon the mammalian endolymph system. II. Structural-functional correlates in the stria vascularis. *Acta Otolaryngol* **90**, 40.

4. Boston Collaborative Drug Surveillance Program (1973) Drug-induced deafness: A cooperative study. *J Amer Med Assn* **224**, 515.

5. Forge A (1984) Gap junctions in the stria vascularis and effects of ethacrynic acid. *Hear Res* **13**, 189.

6. Koch T, Gloddek B (1991) Inhibition of adenylate-cyclase-coupled G protein complex by ototoxic diuretics and cis-platinum in the inner ear of the guinea pig. *Eur Arch Oto-Rhino-Laryngol* **248**, 459.

7. Rybak LP (1988) Ototoxicity of ethacrynic acid (a persistent clinical problem). *J Laryngol Otol* **102**, 518.

Ethambutol

Peter S. Spencer

ETHAMBUTOL
$C_{10}H_{24}N_2O_2$

2,2'-(1,2-Ethanediyldiimino)bis-1-butanol

NEUROTOXICITY RATING

Clinical

A Optic neuropathy

A Peripheral neuropathy

Experimental

A Optic neuropathy (axonal degeneration)

Ethambutol is a derivative of ethylenediamine, which chelates zinc and other metal ions. The D-isomer of ethambutol suppresses the growth of most isoniazid- and streptomycin-resistant tubercle bacilli; the L-isomer has little antituberculous effect and has greater neurotoxic potential (18).

D-Ethambutol hydrochloride was introduced in 1961 for use as a tuberculostatic drug active against *Mycobacterium tuberculosis*, *M. kansasii*, and a number of strains of *M. avium* complex. Prior to the use of rifampin for the treatment of tuberculosis, ethambutol was combined with isoniazid to provide a permissive environment for isoniazid to perform as a bactericide. Recent evidence suggests that ethambutol itself (at higher doses) possesses bactericidal properties, the agent apparently disrupting bacterial metabolism by interfering with essential metal-dependent enzymes, causing arrest in multiplication and cell death. These properties of ethambutol make the drug a key component of combination antimycobacterial therapy for the treatment of isoniazid- and multidrug-resistant tuberculosis that increasingly has affected patients with the acquired immunodeficiency syndrome (2). The most serious toxic effect of ethambutol is retrobulbar neuropathy and (rarely) peripheral neuropathy, especially in the elderly, in those with alcoholism or diabetes mellitus, and in subjects with renal impairment.

Ethambutol is well absorbed (80%) from the human gastrointestinal tract; peak plasma levels are reached in 2–4 h, and the half-life is 3–4 h (14). In mice treated with ^{14}C-ethambutol, radioactivity at 2 h following treatment is found principally in the liver, kidney, and lungs, and tissue-to-plasma concentration ratios greater than twofold are found in heart, spleen, and muscle, but not brain (11). Ethambutol reportedly "accumulates" in the brain, spinal cord, peripheral nerves, and retina of treated rats (16). Zinc concentration drops in rat plasma, liver, and kidney, and increases in the spleen of these animals (3). A ^{99m}Tc–ethambutol complex showed no significant renal retention in rodents (4), and two-thirds of an oral dose is excreted in human urine as the parent compound, with up to 15% as aldehyde and dicarboxylic acid metabolites (14). Uric acid excretion decreases and blood urate increases, an effect of ethambutol treatment possibly enhanced by isoniazid and pyridoxine (9).

While experimental animal studies of peripheral nerves are lacking, the effect of the drug on the optic pathway and other central pathways has been assessed. As in humans, rhesus monkeys, rabbits, and rats develop lesions in the optic pathway; dogs and cats (which possess a zinc-rich tapetum lucidum) display reversible changes in tapetal cells, decoloration of the tapetum lucidum, and (cats) retinal detachment. Rats treated with 105–2500 mg ethambutol for 18–102 days developed alopecia, epistaxis, lethargy, ataxia, and tremulousness; histological examination of epoxy sections of the retina, optic nerves, and chiasm revealed bilateral axonal swellings restricted to the optic chiasm and adjacent parts of the optic nerves (tracts not examined) (12). Rhesus monkeys receiving 800–1600 mg/kg/day ethambutol for up to 26 weeks developed blindness, impaired coordination, lower-limb weakness, respiratory distress, and dysphonia (18). Pathological changes culminating in nerve fiber degeneration (formalin-perfused tissues) first appeared in the central part of the optic chiasm, with or without extension into the proximal third of the optic tracts. Prolonged treatment with large doses sequentially involved additional areas, namely the reticular formation of the medulla oblongata, neurons in the nucleus ruber and anterior horn cells (especially the lumbar region) which displayed chromatolysis and, finally, the pyramidal decussation and lateral pyramidal tracts (18). "Mild demyelination and axonal fragmentation" were found in the optic nerves of two of seven rabbits fed ethambutol for 8–232 days (13).

Humans treated with large doses of ethambutol (usually >25 mg/kg/day) may develop catastrophic ocular toxicity resulting in optic atrophy and permanent blindness (2). Commonly, the drug is given in daily dosages of 25 mg/kg for 2 months and continued at a level of 15 mg/kg/day. Rare cases of irreversible optic neuropathy occur at the lower dosage, and the incidence is 6% and 15% at dosages of 25 and >35 mg/kg/day, respectively (1,5). Subjects with pretreatment zinc blood levels lower than 0.7 mg/l (normal, 0.9–1.0 mg/l) are at risk for visual changes (6). These may develop suddenly or slowly, and in one or both eyes. With early detection and prompt drug withdrawal, many ocular manifestations of ethambutol toxicity slowly reverse. Bilateral reduction in visual acuity associated with the development of cecocentral scotomata is the characteristic presentation. Changes in color vision may precede changes in visual acuity and provide an early-warning sign of toxicity. Peripheral visual field defects without loss of visual acuity may also occur. Rare cases, studied postmortem, show pathology in the optic chiasm or nerves comparable to that seen in intoxicated primates (10). Pretreatment assessment of renal function and visual acuity is recommended, children too young for objective visual assessment should not be treated with ethambutol, and adults must be instructed to stop the drug immediately if visual disturbances manifest during treatment (2).

A predominantly distal, sensory ethambutol neuropathy is much less common than optic neuropathy. Rarely, symptoms of neuropathy (distal-extremity numbness and tingling) are said to precede the onset of visual disturbances. Peripheral neuropathy is characterized by diminished response to pain, touch, and vibration in a stocking-and-glove distribution, with weak or absent ankle jerks. Increased distal latencies with modest changes in conduction velocity are found electrodiagnostically. Distal muscle weakness may occur in subjects treated with large doses of ethambutol. Improvement occurs after withdrawal of treatment (15).

Other side effects of drug treatment may include disorientation, mental confusion, dizziness, headache, abdominal and joint pain, pruritis and, in combined treatment with other tuberculostatics, various hypersensitivity reactions (7,9).

Mechanisms underlying the neurotoxicity of ethambutol are likely related principally to its property of chelating zinc and perhaps other metal ions; another zinc-chelating drug (pyridinethione, the zinc salt of which is used as an antiseborrheic agent in an over-the-counter shampoo) shows comparable experimental neurotoxicity (20). Zinc is found in high concentrations in the choroid, retina, and ganglion cells, and a zinc-containing enzyme (retinol dehydrogenase) is essential for color vision (7). Zinc in presynaptic mossy fiber terminals has an important role in hippocampal function, and the cuprozinc-dependent enzyme superoxide dismutase may protect neurons against damage by superoxide radicals. Zinc deficiency during development has been associated with brain malformations in humans and neurobehavioral changes in animals (8).

Ethambutol-induced inhibition of glucose metabolism in mycobacteria has been suggested (19), and it is perhaps noteworthy that several agents thought to perturb energy transformation are associated with optic and peripheral neuropathy. While the underlying pathology of ethambutol neuropathy has not been characterized, primary axonal degeneration (distal axonopathy) as in experimental zinc pyridinethione neuropathy seems a likely initial lesion. The following possibilities have been offered to explain the extraordinary predilection for axonal lesions to develop initially in the optic chiasm: (a) vascular or other peculiar local features promoting selective drug deposition; and (b) glial properties, enzyme activities, metal concentrations, or regional contact with cerebrospinal fluid (12).

REFERENCES

1. Addington WW (1979) The side effects and interactions of anti-tuberculosis drugs. *Chest* **76**, 782.
2. Alvarez KL, Krop LC (1993) Ethambutol-induced ocular toxicity revisited. *Ann Pharmacother* **27**, 102.
3. Bogden JD, Zadsielski E, Al-Rabiai D, Aviv A (1983) Effect of ethambutol on metabolism of copper, iron, manganese and zinc. *Trace Subst Environ Health* **17**, 327.
4. Causse JE, Pasqualini R, Cypriani B *et al.* (1990) Labeling of ethambutol with technetium-99m using a new reduction procedure. Pharmacokinetic study in the mouse and rat. *Appl Radiat Isotopes* **41**, 493.
5. Citron KM (1986) Ocular toxicity from ethambutol. *Thorax* **41**, 737.
6. Delacoux E, Moreau Y, Godefroy A *et al.* (1978) Prevention de la toxicité oculaire de l'ethambutol: interet de la zinemie et de l'analyse du sens chromatique. *J Fr Ophtalmol* **1**, 191.
7. Dukes MNG (1992) *Meyler's Side Effects of Drugs. 12th Ed.* Elsevier, Amsterdam.
8. Frederickson CJ, Howell GA, Kasarskis EJ (1984) *The Neurobiology of Zinc. Part A. Physiochemistry, Anatomy, and Techniques.* Alan R. Liss, New York.
9. Goodman Gilman AGG, Rall TR, Nies AS, Taylor P (1990) *The Pharmacological Basis of Therapeutics. 8th Ed.* Pergamon Press, New York.
10. Grant MW (1986) *Toxicology of the Eye. 3rd Ed.* Charles C Thomas, Springfield, Ilinois.
11. Kelly RG, Kaleita E, Eisner HJ (1991) Tissue distribution of (^{14}C)-ethambutol in mice. *Amer Rev Resp Dis* **123**, 689.
12. Lessell S (1976) Histopathology of experimental ethambutol intoxication. *Invest Ophthalmol* **15**, 765.
13. Matsuoka Y, Mukoyama M, Sobue I (1972) Histopathological study of experimental ethambutol neuropathy. *Clin Neurol* **12**, 453.
14. Peets EA, Sweeney WM, Place VA, Buyske DA (1965) The absorption, excretion and metabolic fate of ethambutol in man. *Amer Rev Respir Dis* **91**, 51.
15. Sahenk Z (1987) Toxic neuropathies. *Semin Neurol* **7**, 9.

16. Satoyoshi E, Mukoyama M (1984) Ethambutol neuropathy and neurotoxicity of chloramphenicol. *Excerpta Med* **662**, 209.

17. Schild HS, Fox BC (1991) Rapid-onset reversible ocular toxicity from ethambutol therapy. *Amer J Med* **90**, 404.

18. Schmidt IG, Schmidt LH (1966) Studies of the neurotoxicity of ethambutol and its racemate for the rhesus monkey. *J Neuropathol Exp Neurol* **25**, 40.

19. Silve G, Valeroguillen P, Quemard A *et al.* (1993) Ethambutol inhibition of glucose metabolism in mycobacteria —a possible target of the drug. *Antimicrob Agents Chemother* **37**, 1536.

20. Spencer PS, Schaumburg HH (1980) *Experimental and Clinical Neurotoxicology*. Williams & Wilkins, Baltimore.

CASE REPORT

A 49-year-old woman with a history of hypertension, hyperlipidemia, mild chronic renal failure, chronic hyperbilirubinemia secondary to hepatic congestion, and ischemic cardiomyopathy with orthotopic heart transplantation developed multiple nodular skin lesions positive for Mycobacterium kansasii *after 2 years of postoperative immunosuppression with cyclosporine, azathioprene, and prednisone. The 70-kg patient received 1700 mg ethambutol, 300 mg rifampin, and 300 mg isoniazid daily, with reduction in immunosuppression medication. Dim vision was reported after 2 days of treatment, progressed over the next week and, shortly thereafter, visual acuity was found to have changed in both eyes from 20/20 (baseline) to 20/40. Mild red-green and blue-yellow color vision defects were found. Optic discs and maculae appeared normal. Ethambutol medication was immediately discontinued; 4 days later, visual acuity and color vision showed improvement, a trend that continued over subsequent months until the retrobulbar optic "neuritis" resolved completely.*

[Abstracted from Schild and Fox (17)].

Ethanol

John C.M. Brust

$$CH_3CH_2OH$$

ETHANOL

$$C_2H_6O$$

NEUROTOXICITY RATING

Clinical

A Teratogenicity (fetal alcohol syndrome)

A Physical dependence and withdrawal

A Acute encephalopathy (agitation, sedation, ataxia, coma)

B Chronic encephalopathy (cognitive impairment, dementia)

B Myopathy

B Leukoencephalopathy

B Encephalomalacia

C Peripheral neuropathy

Experimental

A Acute encephalopathy (sedation, coma)

A Cerebral neuronal degeneration (hippocampus, cerebellum)

A CNS (frontal cortex) neuronal degeneration (thiamine-depleted animals)

A Tolerance and withdrawal syndrome

Beverages containing ethanol have been popular for tens of thousands of years, originally in the form of fermented beers and wines. The Arab invention of distillation and its introduction to Europe during the Middle Ages led to more concentrated products. Today, ethanol abuse is a worldwide public health problem, in the United States alone accounting for 100,000 premature deaths annually—nearly 5% of total mortality, and attributable to such diverse causes as cirrhosis of the liver, pancreatitis, cancer of the esophagus, cardiomyopathy, stroke, motor vehicle accidents, suicide, and homicide (4,15).

"Alcoholism" is difficult to define. The term usually refers to a pattern of drinking, whether continuous or episodic, that interferes with health or occupational and social functioning. The broader term "problem drinker" encompasses those either psychically dependent (*i.e.*, addicted) or physically dependent (*i.e.*, displaying withdrawal symptoms and signs), as well as those who, although they drink infrequently, get into trouble when they do. It is estimated that 19 million Americans—7% of adults and 19% of adolescents—are problem drinkers.

The ethanol content of most alcoholic beer ranges from 3.0%–6.5% and for nonfortified wine from 7%–15%. Distilled spirits vary markedly: 16%–18% for most vermouths and 40%–45% for most whiskeys. Medicinal "alcohol" contains 95%–96% ethanol; "rubbing alcohol" contains about 60%.

General Toxicology

Ethanol is rapidly absorbed from the gastrointestinal tract and distributed throughout body water. Ninety percent of ingested ethanol is metabolized in the liver by cytosolic alcohol dehydrogenase (ADH), producing acetaldehyde, which is further metabolized to acetate and then acetyl coenzyme A by mitochondrial aldehyde dehydrogenase (Fig. 9). The cofactor for both enzymes is nicotinamide adenine dinucleotide (NAD$^+$), which is thereby reduced to NADH. Ethanol is also metabolized by an inducible microsomal ethanol-oxidizing system (MEOS). Small amounts of ethanol are excreted unchanged by the lungs and the kidney.

Alcoholic liver disease—steatosis, alcoholic hepatitis, and cirrhosis—is more a result of direct toxicity than of nutritional deficiency. Complex mechanisms include replacement by ethanol of fatty acids as mitochondrial fuel, thereby decreasing lipid oxidation and resulting in lipid accumulation. In addition, MEOS oxidation of ethanol generates heat and induces hypermetabolism, increasing oxygen demand and leading to tissue hypoxia, and acetaldehyde produced by ethanol metabolism forms tissue-damaging adducts with a number of compounds and contributes to free radical formation.

Ethanol causes hypoglycemia by diverse mechanisms, including lack of eating and reduced hepatic glycogen secondary to liver damage. Of chief importance, however, is dependence of alcohol dehydrogenase and aldehyde dehydrogenase on NAD$^+$, converting it to NADH and thereby rendering it unavailable for gluconeogenesis. As a consequence, symptomatic hypoglycemia often occurs during periods of heavy drinking, and the symptoms—abnormal behavior, seizures, or coma—are mistakenly attributed to intoxication or withdrawal. Immediate treatment is required to prevent permanent brain damage: intravenous infusion of 50% glucose (plus thiamine and multivitamins).

Nonalcoholics can develop hypoglycemia by another mechanism. Ethanol stimulates intestinal secretion, which increases the insulin response to glucose. Such reactive hypoglycemia can follow a few drinks and a small meal. Small children may be especially vulnerable to this effect.

Alcoholic ketoacidosis consists of ketosis and an increased anion gap secondary to accumulation of acetoacetate and hydroxybutyrate (45). The precise mechanism is uncertain; starvation, increased lipolysis, and impaired fatty acid oxidation probably contribute. Typically affected are binge drinkers who become anorectic or nauseated and stop drinking; blood ethanol concentrations (BECs) are usually zero. Blood glucose may be elevated or decreased. Symptoms—depressed alertness and Kussmaul's respirations—usually respond promptly to correction of fluid and electrolyte imbalance. Glucose may be required. Insulin and bicarbonate are seldom necessary.

Ethanol has a number of endocrinological effects. In men, decreased testosterone production and increased estrogen levels (secondary to liver failure) cause impotence and gynecomastia. Alcoholic women develop hyperpolactinemia and amenorrhea. Ethanol-induced inhibition of antidiuretic hormone causes diuresis as the BEC is rising. Ethanol stimulates pituitary adrenocorticotropic hormone secretion, resulting in "pseudo-Cushing's syndrome," with characteristic symptoms and signs. By more than one mechanism, alcoholics are prone to hypocalcemia and osteoporosis. Through actions on the hypothalamus, ethanol increases skin blood flow and sweating, contributing to hypothermia.

Patients with alcoholism are immunosuppressed and at risk for infection, including bacterial and tuberculous meningitis. Ethanol-related trauma can cause subdural or epidural hematoma or spinal cord compression. Infectious or traumatic complications of ethanol are easily missed in the setting of intoxication or withdrawal. Deep sleep following ethanol ingestion can lead to pressure palsies of peripheral nerves or the brachial plexus.

In central pontine myelinolysis, demyelinating lesions in the basis pontis cause quadriplegia; if lesions extend into the tegmentum, there may be coma. The cause is overvigorous correction of hyponatremia. The condition is not restricted to those with alcoholism, but they are at special risk.

Animal Studies

Most animals do not like ethanol, and ingenious strategies, such as vapor-filled cages, have been adopted to study its effects. An exception is the Syrian hamster, which prefers ethanol to water. Other rodents have been inbred to produce strains that respond to ethanol in particular ways.

Some inbred strains differ in their initial sensitivity to ethanol; for example, long-sleep (LS) *vs.* short-sleep (SS) mice and high-sensitivity *vs.* low-sensitivity rats. Inbreeding has produced strains that are more or less sensitive to eth-

$$CH_3CH_2OH + NAD^+ \xrightarrow{\text{alcohol dehydrogenase}} CH_3CHO + NADH + H^+$$
ethanol   acetaldehyde

$$CH_3CHO + NAD^+ + H_2O \xrightarrow{\text{aldehyde dehydrogenase}} CH_3COO^- + NADH + H^+$$
acetaldehyde   acetate

FIGURE 9. Ethanol metabolism.

anol's hypothermic or ataxic effects. Differences are independent of blood ethanol concentrations. Some strains display altered responses to γ-aminobutyric acid (GABA)-ergic drugs such as barbiturates; in fact, in *Xenopus* oocytes injected with RNA from LS mice, ethanol facilitated GABA transmission, whereas in oocytes receiving SS RNA, GABA transmission was inhibited, implying different biophysical properties of GABA receptors in the two strains. In other mouse strains, mutation in the gene for the GABA$_A$ receptor—specific to cerebellar granule cells—produced animals hypersensitive to both ethanol and benzodiazepines. Other investigators have implicated differences in neurotensin, catecholamine synthesis, tryptophan hydroxylase, nicotine sensitivity, and synaptosomal gangliosides in such strains. Neuronal and erythrocyte membranes from LS mice are more easily "fluidized" by ethanol (31).

Inbreeding has also produced rodent strains that prefer ethanol; these include SS mice. Such rodents consume ethanol to intoxication, including direct intragastric administration and injection into the ventral tegmental area of the midbrain; as a result, they display both tolerance (less sedation and an increased locomotor response) and withdrawal signs. One strain of ethanol-preferring rats—the P strain—has decreased levels of serotonin in certain brain areas, including the cortex, hippocampus, thalamus, hypothalamus, and nucleus accumbens, as well as reduced levels of dopamine in the accumbens. Serotonin-reuptake blockers reduce ethanol drinking in these P rats. By contrast, another strain of ethanol-preferring rats—the AA strain—has elevated brain serotonin levels (82). The herb kudzu, thought to contain inhibitors of acetaldehyde dehydrogenase, reduces ethanol consumption in non-inbred Syrian hamsters (72).

The RAPP SS/Jr. strain of rats has low activity of the renin-angiotensin system and high ethanol preference; intraventricular transplants of fetal hypothalamic cells containing angiotensin produced a 40% decrease in voluntary ethanol intake (79). In another rat strain, voluntary ethanol intake was reduced following transplantation into the ventral striatum of fetal dopaminergic cells from the ventral mesencephalon (78).

Animals are also bred for severity of withdrawal signs. Withdrawal severity-prone (WSP) mice are more likely than withdrawal severity-resistant (WSR) mice to have tremor and seizures after even brief periods of ethanol intake, whether or not tolerance is demonstrated. WSR mice voluntarily drink more ethanol. With ethanol dependence, WSP mice display up-regulation of nitrendipine calcium channels and decreased hippocampal mossy fiber zinc, and during withdrawal they have reduced expression of GABA$_A$ receptor mRNA (29).

Experimental Studies

Animal models, which can be controlled for nutritional and other variables, offer the most persuasive evidence to date that ethanol is a CNS neurotoxin. Nutritionally maintained rodents—in experiments involving pair-fed controls and a sufficient period of abstinence to discount the effects of acute intoxication and withdrawal—have shown both behavioral and morphological abnormalities. Impaired learning—often subtle—is selective for some tasks but not others (38,40). Pathological changes in mature rats and mice include loss of dendritic spines and decreased dendritic branching is hippocampal neurons (37,43,69,73,89). Cerebellar Purkinje and granule cells are also affected (118). The cerebral cortex has not been studied in laboratory animals with chronic alcohol intoxication (75). Duration of exposure is critical; altered dendrites have been associated with only moderately elevated BECs (*e.g.*, 100–150 mg/dl) but are usually apparent only after at least several months of daily ingestion (or inhalation). Indeed, neurons appear resistant to brief ethanol exposure sufficient to cause apnea (122). Physiological counterparts to these morphological changes include decreased dentate granule cell response to perforant path input, depressed inhibitory postsynaptic potentials in dentate granule cells and CA1 cells, and reduced long-term potentiation (1,36).

Rats receiving daily ethanol to maintain a BEC of 80–120 mg/dl for 12 months had loss of hippocampal granule and pyramidal cells with preserved numbers of mossy fiber–CA3 synapses, suggesting new synapse formation; at 18 months, decreased numbers of synapses suggested collapse of this plastic response (16). In the cerebellum of 8-week-old ethanol-exposed rats, loss of granule cells and elongation of Purkinje cell dendritic spines suggested "searching" for new parallel fibers (119), and in rats exposed at 3 days of age for up to 8 weeks, synapses in the parietal cortex had a "perforated appearance," suggesting compensatory "splitting" to form additional synapses (70). Thirty-five-day-old rats consuming ethanol had decreased numbers of hippocampal CA1 cell basilar dendrites and reduced thickness of the strata oriens and radiatum of the CA1 field but no change in neuronal density; after 2 months of abstinence, there was recovery of dendritic branching. In these young animals, ethanol appeared to delay normal dendritic development, which, however, resumed upon alcohol withdrawal (85). The relevance of such improvement to the reversible radiographic brain abnormalities of adult humans with alcoholism is uncertain but intriguing. Consistent with human radiographic studies, young dogs receiving 36% of their calories as ethanol for a year had lateral ventricular enlargement but cortical thinning only in the temporal lobes; astrocytes and oligodendroglia were reduced in the temporal and frontal cortex, but there were no significant differences between the alcoholic and control groups in brain weight or neocortical neuronal populations. The findings indicated a selective shrinkage of white matter, but whether at the expense of axons, myelin, or both, could not be determined (56). In young rats, ethanol exposure led to *increased* number of dendritic spines on parietal lobe neurons, perhaps indicating abnormal persistence of redundant synapses during postnatal development (38).

Chronic ethanol administration to rats caused loss of presumably cholinergic neurons in the nucleus basalis (6), and exposure for up to 28 weeks caused "profound reductions" of brain acetylcholine (ACh) content, ACh synthesis and release, choline uptake, and activity of choline acetyltransferase and acetylcholinesterase (AChE), with impaired learning. There was also disruption of adrenergic and serotonergic pathways. Reduction of cholinergic markers and memory loss were partially reversible with abstinence in animals exposed for up to 18 weeks, but permanent in animals with longer exposure. Transplantation of cholinergic neurons into hippocampus or cerebral cortex corrected both the abnormal memory and the cholinergic deficit (5). In this study, control animals received plain water instead of water laced with ethanol; nutritional supplementation or pair-feeding was not commented on, and animals receiving ethanol did have "slightly lower" body weight than controls. Thus, although the authors found no changes in the mammillary bodies or thalamus to suggest Wernicke-Korsakoff disease (*vide infra*), the contribution of nutritional deficiency to the behavioral and biochemical abnormalities is uncertain.

In another study, diet and nutrition were carefully matched between ethanol-exposed and control rats. Animals were 3 months old, exposure was for 42 days, and BECs averaged 142–149 mg/dl. Although there was no change in the cytoarchitectonic organization of the cerebral cortex in ethanol-treated rats, the AChE-positive plexus was reduced in all cortical layers, and the density of AChE-positive neurons in the nucleus basalis was decreased without actual neuronal loss (87).

Human Studies
Addiction

In contrast to other drugs such as opioids, cocaine, or tobacco, psychic dependence develops in only a small proportion of those who drink ethanol. To varying degrees among different populations, genetic factors play a role in who becomes an alcoholic subject.

ADH and aldehyde dehydrogenase (ALDH) each consist of multiple isoenzymes. Differences in ADH produce differences in peak blood ethanol concentration after equivalent amounts of ethanol are ingested, providing a check on continued drinking in subjects who are more readily intoxicated. Differences in ALDH produce, in susceptible subjects, aversive symptoms when ethanol is ingested—flushing, tachycardia, and dysphoria—a consequence of elevated tissue levels of acetaldehyde. Such a response is common among Chinese, Japanese, and South American Indians, and ethanol dependence is much less common in these populations (50).

As shown by twin and adoption studies, heredity contributes to ethanol dependence in other ways as well, but the mechanisms are controversial and undoubtedly polygenetic. Among alcoholics, two major subtypes have been postulated: type I alcoholic subjects tend to be passive-dependent or anxious. Beginning as social drinkers, they start abusing ethanol in late adulthood, and, while able to remain abstinent for long periods, lose control when they drink. Type II alcoholic subjects tend to have antisocial personalities; they become alcoholic during adolescence or young adulthood and are unable to abstain from drinking. Men and women are equally susceptible to type I alcoholism; type II alcoholic subjects are predominantly male (24).

Not all investigators accept this classification, and some believe alcoholism is often simply one manifestation of a more fundamental psychiatric disturbance, such as antisocial personality disorder. Some workers believe that ethanol dependence is frequently secondary to depression; others maintain that when alcoholism and depression coexist, depression is most often a consequence of the alcoholism. Among primary alcoholics—those without other underlying psychiatric illness—a number of possible genetic markers has been studied. For example, compared with sons of nonalcoholic subjects, sons of alcoholic individuals had less ataxia and subjective intoxication at equivalent blood ethanol concentrations, and in a follow-up study 10 years later, the less responsive subjects, whether or not they were sons of alcohol-dependent fathers, were significantly more likely to have become alcoholic themselves (105). Other workers have identified differences between sons of nonalcoholic and of alcoholic subjects in electroencephalographic (EEG) alpha activity, in the P300 event-related potential, in platelet adenyl cyclase content, and in serum thyrotropin levels following administration of thyrotropin-releasing hormone (15).

In 1990, a report described linkage disequilibrium on chromosome 11 of an allele called "A1" and the gene for the dopamine receptor; the A1 allele was present in 64% of "alcoholics" compared with 17% of controls (11). A number of subsequent studies failed to demonstrate such an association (113). Others found the A1 allele over-represented among alcoholic individuals with serious medical problems, cocaine abusers; severely dependent polydrug abusers; or subjects with attention deficit disorder, autism, or Tourette's syndrome (25,64). Meta-analysis of nine published studies revealed association of the A1 allele with certain ethnic groups but not with alcoholic subjects (48). A sequence analysis of the dopamine D_2 receptor's seven coding exons (which do not include A1) showed no differences between alcoholic and nonalcoholic people (47). The prominence of dopamine in the mammalian "reward circuit" makes it plausible that dopamine receptors might play a role in alcohol dependence (and in other substance abuse). It is unlikely, however, that the dopamine D_2 receptor gene, (or any single gene) is responsible for something as heterogeneous (indeed, as difficult to define) as "alcoholism." Recently developed quantitative trait loci strategies offer the promise of better elucidating the biological basis of the polygenetic component of this disorder (28).

Acute Intoxication

Ethanol is a CNS depressant; the euphoria and hyperactivity of early intoxication are the result of disinhibition, not stimulation. Symptoms of intoxication correlate only roughly with BEC (Table 22) (15). At any BEC, intoxication is greater when the level is rising than when it is falling, when the level is reached rapidly, and when it has been recently achieved. Tolerance plays a major role. In most nontolerant 70-kg men, about 60 g (2 oz) of 100% ethanol (contained in approximately 4 oz of 90-proof spirits, 14 oz of wine, or 48 oz of beer) produces a mildly intoxicating BEC of 100 mg/dl. Ethanol metabolism reduces the BEC by 10–20 mg/dl/h (average, 16 mg/dl/h), therefore requiring 6 h to metabolize a 60-g dose. Induction of the MEOS system by ethanol contributes to tolerance, which, however, is more cellular (i.e., reduced CNS response) than pharmacokinetic. A tolerant individual may be entirely asymptomatic at BECs above 150 mg/dl, and although a BEC of 500 mg/dl causes fatal coma and respiratory depression in 50% of subjects, death has occurred at levels of <400 mg/dl, and alertness has accompanied documented levels >800 mg/dl.

Low to moderate BECs produce slow saccadic eye movements and jerky smooth pursuit, sometimes impairing visual acuity. Higher levels cause nystagmus and diplopia. Ethanol suppresses the rapid-eye-movement phase of sleep, with "rebound" vivid dreaming. Chronic drinkers often have marked disruption of sleep organization, with frequent awakenings. Even low BECs cause hypothermia, which can be profound and dangerous in drinkers subjected to cold environments. Acutely, ethanol can precipitate cardiac arrhythmia—including ventricular tachycardia—in the absence of evident underlying cardiomyopathy ("holiday heart syndrome").

Food in the stomach delays ethanol absorption, and aspirin and histamine H_2 receptor blockers, by reducing gastric ADH, enhance it. In addition, when taken with other agents—including general anesthetics, sedatives, antihistamines, tricyclic antidepressants, neuroleptics, and opioids—ethanol can produce additive or superadditive sedation. Cross-tolerance of ethanol with sedatives such as barbiturates, benzodiazepines, and chloral hydrate can cause initial resistance to sedation followed by life-threatening synergism.

When ethanol is taken with sulfonylurea hypoglycemics, procarbazine, sulfonamides, chloramphenicol, griseofulvin, quinacrine, or metronidazole, a disulfiram-like reaction occurs (see Disulfiram, this volume). When ethanol is taken with disulfiram itself, the reaction can be fatal.

Ethanol intoxication can mask or intensify depressed consciousness from coexisting disease, including meningitis, subdural hematoma, hypoglycemia, hepatic encephalopathy, and metabolic acidosis. A thorough assessment is essential in even the most obviously intoxicated subjects.

The treatment of severe ethanol poisoning is similar to that of other depressant drugs (Table 23).

Respiratory support is the mainstay. Neither sedation for obstreperousness nor stimulants for stupor are indicated. No drugs effectively accelerate ethanol metabolism; hemodialysis or peritoneal dialysis can be considered for extremely high BECs, severe acidosis, or additional drug ingestion and in severely intoxicated children. Anecdotal reports describe reversal of ethanol stupor with naloxone; the mechanism is unclear, and the effect is too unpredictable and transient to be practical. In animals, the imidazobenzodiazepine drug RO15-4513 reverses signs of mild ethanol intoxication but not stupor or apnea.

TABLE 22. Correlation of Signs and Symptoms with Blood Ethanol Concentration (BEC)

BEC (mg/dl)	Symptoms
50–150	Euphoria or dysphoria, shy or expansive, friendly or argumentative. Impaired concentration, judgment, and sexual inhibitions
150–250	Slurred speech and ataxic gait, diplopia, nausea, tachycardia, drowsiness, or labile mood with sudden bursts of anger or antisocial acts
300	Stupor alternating with combativeness or incoherent speech, heavy breathing, vomiting
400	Coma
500	Respiratory paralysis, death

TABLE 23. Treatment of Acute Ethanol Intoxication

For obstreporous or violent patients:
Isolation, calming environment, reassurance—avoid sedatives
Close observation

For stuporous or comatose patients:
If hypoventilation is present, artificial respiration in an intensive care unit
If serum glucose in doubt, i.v. 50% glucose
Thiamine 100 mg and multivitamins, i.m. or i.v.
Careful monitoring of blood pressure; correction of hypovolemia and of acid-base imbalance
Consider hemodialysis if patient is severely acidotic, deeply comatose, or apneic
Avoid emetics or gastric lavage
Avoid analeptics
Do not forget other possible causes of coma in an alcoholic subject, as well as concomitant drug use

i.m., intramuscularly; i.v., intravenously.

Two types of ethanol intoxication are poorly understood. "Pathological intoxication." also called "acute alcoholic paranoid state," consists of sudden extreme excitement, sometimes with delusions, hallucinations, and violence. Following sleep, there is amnesia for the episode. Some cases may represent psychological dissociative states; others may be the result of paradoxical excitation as encountered with barbiturates. Alcoholic "blackouts" consist of periods of drinking for which the subject has no recall, even though appearing awake and attentive at the time. It is disputed whether such a state affects only chronic drinkers. BECs as low as 40 mg/dl do impair memory encoding.

Ethanol Withdrawal

A single bout of heavy drinking is followed by "hangover"—headache, malaise, nausea, sweating, and tremulousness. Except for impaired coordination, symptoms are not harmful and do not signify dependence. By contrast, chronic heavy drinkers develop a variety of potentially dangerous abstinence syndromes.

Early withdrawal symptoms—usually within 48 h of abstinence—include tremor, hallucinations, and seizures, alone or in combination. Tremor, which is promptly relieved by ethanol, can be so coarse as to interfere with eating or even standing. It is often accompanied by anxiety, easy startling, insomnia, nystagmus, flushing, sweating, anorexia, nausea, vomiting, tachycardia, tachypnea, and systolic hypertension. Except for agitation and inattentiveness, however, the sensorium remains clear.

Hallucinations are visual, auditory, tactile, olfactory, or a combination ("alcoholic hallucinosis"). Most common are auditory and visual, with paranoid auditory accusation or imagery of insects, animals, or people. They tend to last minutes at a time over several days and can occur during active drinking or after more than a week of abstinence. Insight as to their unreality varies, but delirium is not present (this is *not* "delirium tremens," *vide infra*). Anecdotal reports suggest that even in the absence of previous schizophrenic symptoms, some subjects progress to a chronic hallucinatory state with flat affect, ideas of reference, and loose associations (122).

"Alcohol-related seizures"—occurring in the absence of pre-existing epilepsy or an underlying precipitant such as head injury or meningitis—are usually nonfocal major motor and occur singly or in brief clusters; <10% develop status epilepticus (124). Upon recovery, the EEG does not show epileptiform activity. [Early reports that ethanol withdrawal was associated with a high prevalence of EEG photomyoclonic or photoconvulsive response were not borne out by subsequent studies (41)]. Chronic drinkers consuming more than 50 g of ethanol daily are at risk for such seizures, and the risk increases with further intake, but whether a critical duration of drinking exists is uncertain (91). It is suggested that repeated bouts of ethanol withdrawal lower the threshold for alcohol-related seizures, a situation analogous to electrical "kindling." Others have reported less than clear temporal association between seizures and drinking cessation, with seizures frequently occurring during active drinking or more than a week after the last drink, suggesting that factors other than simply withdrawal are contributory in some cases (91). Ethanol can precipitate seizures in known epileptics, but the amount required is disputed.

Occasionally encountered during abstinence is either parkinsonism or chorea. Parkinsonism tends to appear within a few days of withdrawal and to clear over days or weeks. Chorea, especially oral-lingual, typically begins during the second week of abstinence and is similarly self-limited. Parkinsonism and chorea are likely related to ethanol suppression of striatal dopamine release (89).

Alcoholics are also prone to panic attacks, especially when they have had previous bouts of symptomatic withdrawal.

In contrast to tremor, hallucinosis, and seizures, "delirium tremens" typically begins 48–72 h after the last drink. It consists of tremor, delirium (defined as inattentiveness so severe that contact with the environment is impossible, and often is accompanied by agitation, hallucinations, or depressed alertness), and autonomic overactivity, with fever, tachycardia, hypertension, and profuse sweating. Because of the misconception that any alcoholic with tremor and hallucinations has delirium tremens, the condition is overdiagnosed. Seizures during delirium tremens are unusual and mandate a search for another possible cause. Fluid loss can be severe, and electrolyte imbalance is common. Mortality from delirium tremens is reportedly as high as 15%, usually, however, from associated illness. Patients with delirium tremens have often been hospitalized earlier for another reason.

Therapy for ethanol withdrawal depends on symptoms and severity. Treatment of withdrawal tremor is aimed at both symptomatic relief and preventing progression to delirium tremens (Table 24). Titrated doses of benzodiazepines, orally or parenterally, suffice. Hallucinosis does not usually require specific therapy; neuroleptics lower seizure threshold, cause hypotension, and have hepatic and other side effects, but they can be given to patients whose only symptoms are hallucinations or whose hallucinations have outlasted other symptoms.

Seizures have usually passed by the time treatment is considered. Repeated seizures or status epilepticus are treated in the usual fashion with parenteral agents. If no other cause is found, a patient with alcohol-related seizures does not need maintenance anticonvulsants.

Although it is the agent of choice when alcoholic subjects treat their own withdrawal symptoms, ethanol is inappropriate in the clinical setting. Parenterally, it has a small margin of safety, and by any route it causes direct organ damage.

The treatment of delirium tremens requires intensive care, with vigorous sedation and close monitoring of vital signs, fluids, and electrolytes. In contrast to withdrawal from other drugs such as opioids, delirium tremens is not immediately reversed by giving cross-tolerant drugs. Benzodiazepines are nonetheless the drug of choice, in parenteral dosage sufficient to produce sustained sedation. The equivalent of hundreds of milligrams of diazepam daily may be required initially, and a hazard of such treatment is that it can precipitate hepatic coma.

Other Neurological Complications of Ethanol

Ethanol is associated with a plethora of neurological complications besides acute intoxication and withdrawal. Some are indirect, the result of nutritional deficiency or damage to other tissues such as the liver or the cardiovascular system. Some complications may be the result of direct actions on the nervous system.

Indirect Effects of Ethanol—Nutritional
Wernicke's Disease

The result of thiamine deficiency, Wernicke's disease occurs in two phases (125). The syndrome consists of acutely or subacutely progressive altered mentation, abnormal eye movements, and ataxic gait. Mental abnormalities include inattentiveness, abulia, impaired memory, and lethargy progressing to coma. Abnormal eye movements include nystagmus, abducens paresis, and horizontal gaze paresis progressing to complete horizontal and vertical ophthalmoplegia. Gait ataxia appears to be both cerebellar and vestibular in origin. The distribution of the multifocal lesions of Wernicke's disease are often readily recognized on gross postmortem examination. Affected brain regions include medial thalamus and hypothalamus (especially the mammillary bodies) and the periaqueductal gray matter of the midbrain. Microscopic findings include atypical necrosis with relative preservation of neuronal cell bodies, endothelial hyperplasia, macrophages, reactive astrocytes, and sometimes petechiae.

Korsakoff's syndrome is a mental abnormality; it is not a histopathological entity and is not specific to Wernicke's disease. It has occurred following other lesions of the limbic system characterized by amnesia, both anterograde and retrograde. It most commonly emerges following recovery from Wernicke's syndrome; while improvement may continue during recovery, lasting impairment is common. Cognitive skills other than memory are affected to varying degrees.

Treatment of acute Wernicke's syndrome is an emergency; untreated, the disease is fatal, and prompt replacement therapy reduces the chance of lasting cognitive im-

---

TABLE 24. Treatment of Ethanol Withdrawal

Prevention or reduction of early symptoms

Diazepam 10–40 mg p.o. or i.v., repeated hourly until sedation or mild intoxication. If successive daily doses are required, taper by about one-fourth of preceding day's dose with resumption of higher doses if withdrawal symptoms recur. (Consider short-acting benzodiazepines in patients with abnormal liver function.)

Alternatively, pentobarbital 200 mg, p.o., i.m. or i.v., and then 100 mg hourly as needed. Maintenance dose and duration determined by symptoms.

Alternatively, paraldehyde 5–15 mg, p.o. or p.r., repeated hourly as needed. Maintenance and tapering titrated with symptoms.

Thiamine 100 mg and multivitamins, i.m. or i.v.

Magnesium, potassium, and calcium replacement as needed.

Delerium tremens

Diazepam 10 mg i.v., then 5 mg or more (up to 40 mg) i.v. or i.m. every 5 min until calming. Maintenance diazepam 5 mg or more i.v. or i.m. every 1–4 h as needed.

Careful attention to fluid and electrolyte balance; several liters of saline per day, or even pressors, may be needed.

Cooling blanket or alcohol sponges for high fever.

Prevent or correct hypoglycemia.

Thiamine and multivitamins.

Consider coexisting illness, *e.g.*, liver failure, pancreatitis, sepsis, meningitis, or subdural hematoma.

p.o., orally; i.v., intravenously; i.m., intramuscularly; p.r., rectally.

pairment. Thiamine (with other multivitamins) is given intravenously; it is not well-absorbed orally or intramuscularly. Mentation, ophthalmoplegia, and ataxia usually improve over hours, days, or weeks. Thiamine is a cofactor for enzymes required in glucose metabolism, and so administering glucose without thiamine to an alcoholic can precipitate Wernicke's syndrome.

Alcoholic Cerebellar Degeneration

Ataxic patients with Wernicke's syndrome have additional lesions of the anterior cerebellar vermis, consisting of neuronal loss of all three cortical layers, especially Purkinje cells. Such vermal degeneration can also occur without other clinical or pathological evidence of Wernicke-Korsakoff disease. The cause is probably nutritional deficiency, but the specific role of thiamine or some other vitamin is less clear. Truncal ataxia can progress over a few weeks to inability to stand; leg movements may also be ataxic, but the arms are usually spared. With abstinence and nutritional replacement, symptoms tend to improve, although incompletely.

Alcoholic Polyneuropathy

Peripheral neuropathy in alcoholics is also probably nutritional in origin. Thiamine deficiency may have a dominant role, but other vitamins and nutrients may also be lacking. A direct toxic component is suggested by some studies (75). Initial symptoms are sensory—paresthesias in the feet and later the hands, with early impairment of vibratory and pain sensation. With progression, paresthesias become painful, proprioceptive loss leads to ataxia, and weakness ascends proximally. Autonomic involvement, less common than with diabetic polyneuropathy, can cause hypotension, hypothermia, urinary incontinence, abnormal sweating, altered peristalsis, and cardiac arrhythmia. Nutritional replacement results in either stabilization or improvement in neuropathic symptoms.

Amblyopia

Although toxic roles for ethanol and tobacco cannot be excluded, alcoholic amblyopia was shown half a century ago to be chiefly nutritional in origin; as with cerebellar degeneration and polyneuropathy, the specific contribution of thiamine and other vitamins is unclear. Bilateral visual loss consists of achromatopsia progressing to central or centrocecal scotomata. Pathologically there is demyelination affecting the optic nerves with predilection for the maculopapular bundle; as a consequence, optic atrophy is most prominent at the temporal disc margins. Rarely is there progression to complete blindness, and improvement follows treatment.

Pellagra

Nicotinic acid deficiency in alcoholics produces the syndrome of pellagra, with dermatological, gastrointestinal, and neurological symptoms. Altered mentation can progress over hours, days, or weeks to amnesia, delusions, hallucinations, dementia, or delirium. Nicotinic acid or nicotinamide therapy (plus other vitamins) usually results in prompt improvement.

Hepatic Encephalopathy

Alcoholic liver failure causes encephalopathy, which can be symptomatically chronic, progressive, or abrupt. Altered behavior can progress to psychosis, inattentiveness to delirium, or lethargy to coma. Accompanying signs include asterixis, tremor, extensor posturing, abnormal eye movements, and sometimes focal signs such as hemiparesis. Seizures and myoclonus are rarely if ever attributable to hepatic encephalopathy. The most prominent neuropathological change is astrocytic swelling in the cerebral cortex and gray structures of the diencephalon, brainstem, and cerebellum.

If the nature of ethanol's hepatotoxicity has become at least partially understood, the encephalopathic toxins resulting from the damage are less readily defined. Candidates include ammonia, glutamine, α-ketoglutarate, short-chain fatty acids, mercaptans, tryptophan, quinolinic acid, and false neurotransmitters such as octopamine. Currently popular contenders are GABAergic compounds; if not GABA itself, then possibly an exogenous or endogenous benzodiazepine agonist acting at GABA receptors. Consistent with such a mechanism, the benzodiazepine antagonist flumazanil reverses—albeit only briefly—symptoms of hepatic encephalopathy (10).

Patients with repeated bouts of acute hepatic encephalopathy sometimes develop a more chronic condition—acquired chronic hepatocerebral degeneration—characterized by dementia, ataxia, tremor, choreoathetosis, and asterixis. Pathologically, CNS lesions progress to necrosis and microcavitation, and symptoms become irreversible.

Neurological Effects of Ethanol of Uncertain Cause
Marchiafava-Bignami Disease

Marchiafava-Bignami disease nearly always affects heavy drinkers; its cause is otherwise obscure. Defined pathologically, Marchiafava-Bignami disease consists of demyelinating lesions in the medial corpus callosum, spreading rostrally and caudally, and sparing the dorsal and ventral rims. There may be extension into the cerebral white matter with involvement of the anterior and posterior commissures and the middle cerebellar peduncle, but not the basis pontis. Marchiafava-Bignami disease and central pontine myelinolysis have rarely occurred together.

The symptoms of Marchiafava-Bignami disease are more severe than the pathological lesions would predict. Altered mentation—depression, mania, paranoia, or dementia—is soon accompanied by seizures, hemiparesis, aphasia, ataxia, dysarthria, or abnormal movements, often progressing to death within weeks or months. Autopsy reports have shown that the lesions can exist subclinically, and magnetic resonance imaging (MRI) has revealed callosal lesions which, along with symptoms, regressed with abstinence (8).

Alcoholic Dementia

The concept of "alcoholic dementia" has been controversial for decades. The term refers to cognitive impairment in heavy drinkers unexplained by nutritional deficiency, head injury, liver failure, anoxia, or other apparent cause. In other words, ethanol—in addition to causing acute intoxication and physical dependence—might directly and permanently damage the brain. Evidence for such neurotoxicity is based on clinical, radiological, and pathological studies in humans and on behavioral and pathological studies in animals. A recent controlled study of well-nourished alcoholic subjects strongly suggests that persistent cognitive impairment and cortical atrophy is caused by chronic alcohol consumption alone (90).

It has long been recognized that alcoholics often have cognitive impairment that does not fit the pattern of typical Korsakoff's syndrome. The onset is gradual rather than abrupt, prior features of Wernicke's syndrome are lacking, and the mental changes are not limited to amnesia. Moreover, it has been claimed that lasting cognitive impairment is unusual in nonalcoholics with Wernicke's syndrome. Such arguments are countered by psychological studies demonstrating not only that patients with pathologically verified Korsakoff's syndrome frequently display nonamnestic intellectual deficiencies (including abstract reasoning, visuospatial problem solving, and ability to shift sets) but also that such abnormalities can be more prominent than memory loss itself (14,123). The absence of prior Wernicke's syndrome in such patients may be more apparent than real; as noted above, the disease is underdiagnosed, and subtle residual signs (e.g., nystagmus or difficulty with tandem gait) may be overlooked on casual neurological examination.

Reports of "cerebral atrophy" have been based on pneumoencephalography, computed tomography (CT), and MRI (62,69). Ventricular enlargement and sulcal widening in some studies correlated with intellectual impairment and in other studies did not, and some demented patients did not show cerebral shrinkage at all (127). Moreover, some radiographic and cognitive abnormalities have reportedly improved with abstinence, especially in young subjects, indicating that whatever the radiographic changes signify, it is not neuronal loss and therefore should not be referred to as "atrophy" (123). [MRI studies have revealed increased rather than decreased water content in such brains, and so dehydration is not the basis of the shrinkage (60).]

Human pathological studies have been problematic. The neuropathology of alcohol-specific brain damage has been recently reviewed (57). Early descriptions of frontal lobe atrophy and neuronal loss probably involved nonspecific changes or artifacts (123). More convincing recent observations include increased pericerebral space, with or without reduced brain weight (59,60), reduced number or size of cortical neurons, and decreased cerebral blood flow [by single photon emission tomography and glucose metabolism [by positron emission tomography] in medial frontal areas (49,65,71,123,126). Volume loss in brains of those with alcoholism [greatest in subjects with clear-cut nutritional deficiency or liver disease (9,71)] disproportionately affects the subcortical white matter, and in the absence of obvious histopathological change, this shrinkage is presumed by its describers to be axonal (32,68). Loss of cerebral white matter was found in brains of nondemented alcoholic subjects with liver disease, but not in those of patients with nonalcoholic liver disease (21). It occurs in young as well as older subjects and is of sufficient magnitude to account for ventricular enlargement.

Brains of subjects with alcoholism contained reduced numbers of neurons in the superior frontal cortex (61). In the motor, anterior cingulate, or middle temporal gyri, there was no neuronal loss, but neuronal size was reduced in the superior frontal, cingulate, and motor areas, probably reflecting loss of dendritic arborization (58,76).

Alcoholic subjects also reportedly have loss of cholinergic neurons in the nucleus basalis and reduced brain levels of choline acetyltransferase (21,43). Others have been unable to confirm loss of cholinergic markers (108) and, in any event, pathological or biochemical changes in brains of alcoholic subjects could be the consequence of nutritional deficiency, ethanol neurotoxicity, or both.

Brains of "not-grossly-demented" alcoholic individuals demonstrated loss of synaptic receptors in the absence of morphological lesions. Compared to nonalcoholic control brains, there was 30%–40% reduction of muscarinic cholinergic receptors in frontal and temporal cortex and hippocampus and 25%–30% reduction in benzodiazepine receptors in hippocampus and temporal cortex. The brains were histologically normal, and there was no clinical evidence of Wernicke-Korsakoff disease or cirrhosis (44).

Myopathy

The spectrum of alcohol myopathy ranges from subclinical to fulminant. The subclinical variety consists of elevated serum creatine phosphokinase levels, electromyographic abnormalities, and mild myopathic changes histologically. Sometimes punctuated by bouts of cramps, weakness, or dark urine, subclinical myopathy is common among heavy drinkers. Failure of blood lactate to rise after ischemic exercise suggests disturbance of muscle phosphorylase in such patients.

Chronic alcoholic myopathy causes progressive proximal weakness with more pronounced pathological change. Acute rhabdomyolysis causes sudden marked weakness, painful muscle swelling, myoglobinuria, and renal shutdown. Potassium release can precipitate cardiac arrhythmia. Rhabdomyolysis most often occurs during heavy drinking, and abstinence leads to rapid improvement. Studies have shown better correlation with amount and duration of ethanol consumption than with nutritional status, and nonalcoholic volunteers consuming ethanol with adequate diets developed myopathic changes by electron microscopy. Acutely, ethanol reversibly inhibits muscle Na^+,K^+–adenosine triphosphate, mitochondrial fatty acid oxidation, protein synthesis, and calcium binding to troponin. Magnetic resonance spectroscopy of the brain of alcoholic patients suggests impaired glycolysis (12).

Ethanol also inducs cardiomyopathy. Congestive heart failure, conduction defects, arrhythmias, and embolism are common among alcoholic subjects; heart disease accounts for up to 15% of alcohol-related deaths. The three forms of myopathy (acute, chronic, cardiac) are held to be toxic disorders, not nutritional (121). All improve with abstinence.

Stroke

Most though not all epidemiological studies suggest that ethanol in low to moderate doses protects against coronary artery disease, whereas heavy doses increase the risk. The level at which protection changes to hazard has not been defined. Similar studies have addressed the role of ethanol in stroke. Not surprisingly, results have been less than uniform. A Finnish study reports an association between recent heavy drinking and both occlusive and hemorrhagic stroke,

but in a Chicago study the association disappeared when corrected for cigarette smoking (51).

Case-control and cohort studies of ethanol and stroke include the Framingham Study, the Honolulu Heart Study, the Yugoslavia Cardiovascular Disease Study, the Nurses' Health Study, the Lausanne Stroke Registry, and the Japanese Hisayama Study. End points have varied (total stroke, fatal stroke, occlusive or hemorrhagic stroke), as have sex, ethnicity, socioeconomic background, amount of ethanol consumed, and other risk factors such as hypertension and tobacco use (15).

Amid such confusion, a review of 63 epidemiological studies culled a number of useful conclusions. Among whites, moderate doses of ethanol (<1 oz, daily) appeared to protect against occlusive stroke, but higher doses increased risk. Among Japanese, there was little association between any dose of ethanol and ischemic stroke. In both populations, all doses of ethanol increased the risk of both intracerebral and subarachnoid hemorrhage. Data were insufficient to assess the risk in blacks (18).

Several mechanisms—some acting at cross-purposes—could underlie ethanol's influence on cerebrovascular disease. Acutely and chronically, ethanol causes hypertension (usually returning to normal with abstinence). Cerebral vasodilation occurs with both acute intoxication and withdrawal, although dehydration and hemoconcentration after heavy drinking could reduce cerebral perfusion. Chronic drinking leads to decreased cerebral blood flow secondary to reduced cerebral metabolism; and *in vitro*, ethanol causes constriction of both large and small cerebral vessels. Ethanol lowers blood levels of low-density lipoproteins (LDLs) and raises levels of high-density lipoproteins (HDLs), especially the HDL_2 and HDL_3 subfractions (46). Acutely, it raises levels of factor VIII, increases platelet reactivity, and shortens bleeding time; and independently of high-density lipoproteins, it increases plasma concentrations of endogenous tissue-type plasminogen activator (100). Others have reported inhibition of platelet function and increased levels of prostacyclin. Liver disease impairs coagulation, and alcoholic cardiomyopathy predisposes to embolic stroke (15).

Fetal Alcohol Syndrome

Children of alcoholic mothers frequently have low birth weight, congenital anomalies, and delayed psychomotor development (15,22). Full-blown, the condition is referred to as "fetal alcohol syndrome" (FAS) (Table 25); incomplete or subtle forms are called "fetal alcohol effects." The major clinical features are pre- and postnatal growth deficiency, distinctive facies, and mental retardation. Abnormalities can affect the skeleton, heart, urogenital organs, skin, and

TABLE 25. Clinical Features of the Fetal Alcohol Syndrome

Feature	Majority	Minority
CNS	Mental retardation Microencephaly Hypotonia Poor coordination Hyperactivity	
Impaired growth	Prenatal and postnatal for length and weight Diminished adipose tissue	
Abnormal face:		
Eyes	Short palpebral fissures	Ptosis Strabismus Epicanthal folds Myopia Microphthalmia Blepharophimosis Cataracts Retinal pigmentary abnormalities
Nose	Short, upturned Hypoplastic philtrum	
Mouth	Thin vermillion lip borders Retrognathia in infancy Micrognathia or prognathia in adolescence	Prominent lateral palatine ridges Cleft lip or palate Small teeth with faulty enamel
Maxilla	Hypoplastic	
Ears		Posteriorly rotated Poorly formed concha
Skeletal		Pectus excavatum or carinatum Syndactyly, clinodactyly, or camptodactyly Limited joint movements Nail hypoplasia Radioulnar synostosis Bifid xiphoid Scoliosis Klippel-Feil anomaly
Cardiac		Septal defects Great-vessel anomalies
Cutaneous		Abnormal palmar creases Hemangiomas Infantile hirsutism
Muscular		Diaphragmatic, inguinal, or umbilical hernias Diastasis recti
Urogenital		Labial hypoplasia Hypospadias Small rotated kidneys Hydronephrosis

muscles. Common are microphthalmia, malformed retinal vessels, optic atrophy, and blindness (63). Nearly 90% of those with full-blown FAS have microcephaly; other gross neuropathological abnormalities include agenesis of the corpus callosum, hydrocephalus, and cerebellar dysgenesis. Holoprosencephaly and septo-optic dysplasia have been reported (27). Microscopically there are abnormal neuronal migration and heteroptic cell clusters. The condition occurs independently of maternal malnutrition, age, tobacco use, and other drugs, and it may be associated more with binge drinking and high BECs at a critical period than with chronic exposure to ethanol.

Some children exposed to ethanol *in utero* are mentally deficient in the absence of other FAS signs. Exposed monozygotic twins are more likely than dizygotic twins to have identical syndromes (including low IQ), consistent with genetic influence on the expression of ethanol teratogenicity (112). Newborns with FAS are irritable and tremulous for weeks to months; seizures suggest withdrawal. Older children are hyperactive and clumsy, often deaf, and have impaired immune responses to infection. Follow-up studies show persistence of symptoms and signs. For example, a 30-year follow-up of 105 French victims of FAS revealed persistent facial dysmorphism, growth retardation, microcephaly, mental retardation, and abnormal behavior; several siblings without evident dysmorphism at birth also demonstrated psychological impairment (81). Another study of adolescents and adults with FAS found not only intellectual impairment (inattention, poor memory, impaired judgment, and extreme difficulty with abstraction) but also severe behavioral problems (hyperactivity, impulsivity, lying, stealing, lack of response to appropriate social cues, social withdrawal, and periodic high anxiety) (111). Some follow-up studies found catch-up growth in height and weight, especially in girls, but microcephaly is permanent in the majority, and mental retardation tends to persist even in those with relatively mild FAS (110).

Animal studies confirm that ethanol toxicity is the cause of FAS. In a variety of species, *in utero* ethanol exposure produces different combinations of bony anomalies in the face and limbs, microcephaly, reduced birth weight, impaired learning, microphthalmia, optic nerve hypoplasia, cardiac abnormalities, execephaly, and hydrocephalus (7,55,97). Endocrine abnormalities and immunosuppression are also present (54). Late gestational exposure of male rats to ethanol interferes with neurobehavioral sexual differentiation, perhaps a consequence of decreased postnatal testosterone surge (84). In pregnant mice, adrenalectomy (but not adrenal demedullation) prevented the growth-retarding effects of fetal ethanol exposure (120). Diminished mitogen-induced T-cell proliferation in rats exposed

in utero to ethanol was due to decreased responsiveness to interleukin-2 (20). Other exposed rats had markedly reduced lipopolysaccharide-induced fever (131). In male but not female rats, *in utero* ethanol exposure produced abnormalities of the anterior pituitary and of T lymphocytes that were prevented by maternal adrenalectomy (99). Midline structures of mouse brain exposed prenatally to ethanol had reduced numbers of neurons containing luteinizing hormone-releasing hormone (106). Rat fetal astrocyte cultures had reduced incorporation of tritiated thymidine, uridine, and valine, reflecting impaired synthesis of DNA, RNA, and protein (109). Failure of neuronal and glial migration is consistent with effects early in pregnancy (53,86), but subtle alterations in sleep patterns suggest later effects (2).

The basis of ethanol-induced damage is unknown (74). Candidate mechanisms include tissue hypoxia secondary to umbilical vasospasm; consistent with such an effect are neuronal changes in the CA-1 region of the hippocampus and in cerebellar Purkinje cells. Sheep and monkey fetuses exposed to ethanol develop metabolic acidosis and electroencephalographic slowing (3,88,129). In human placenta, ethanol inhibits progesterone synthesis and transport of pyridoxal (2,104). Other possible mechanisms are membrane damage secondary to lipid peroxidation, acetaldehyde toxicity, inhibition of nerve growth factors, and chromosomal damage (33). Offspring of ethanol-fed rats had decreased serum concentrations of insulin-like growth factors (IGF-I and IGF-II) and decreased amounts of hepatic IGF-II mRNA (107). Studies with mice suggest that ethanol inhibition of retinoic oxidation to retinoid acid (catalyzed by embryonal alcohol dehydrogenase) could contribute to neural tube defects (35). In fetal rat brain, ethanol (but not acetaldehyde) inhibited muscarinic receptor-stimulated phosphoinositide metabolism (117). Ethanol also inhibits development of serotonergic systems in rat brain, and this effect is partially blocked by the 5-HT$_{1A}$ agonist buspirone (116). Somatostatin concentration is increased in the retina of ethanol-exposed rat fetuses (39). Controversial is a possible role of paternal ethanol ingestion at the time of conception (23). The role of nutrition is also uncertain (34).

Also unknown is what represents a safe dose of ethanol during pregnancy. The incidence of FAS may be as high as 1–2 live births per 1000, with FEA affecting 3–5 per 1000 (26). FAS may affect 1% of children whose mothers drink 1 oz of ethanol per day early in pregnancy and over 30% of the offspring of heavy drinkers (93). One study, which corrected for nutrition and tobacco use, correlated reduced infant size with only 100 g of ethanol per week at the time of conception (130). Decreased head circumference, dysmorphism, behavioral effects, and EEG abnormalities have been associated with moderate "social drinking" during human pregnancy and with low levels of ingestion in pregnant animals (30,42,52,66,83). In fact, in mice, a single exposure to ethanol early in pregnancy produced craniofacial anomalies (114).

These observations suggest there may be no safe dose of ethanol during pregnancy. Moreover, by the time a woman becomes aware she is pregnant, fetal damage may already have occurred. Although some studies have been criticized on methodological grounds, the thousands of published reports on this subject are remarkably consistent in demonstrating ethanol teratogenicity over a wide range of doses (67,80). The burden of proof is therefore on those who would like to believe there is such a thing as a safe dose of ethanol during pregnancy. The American Academy of Pediatrics currently recommends "abstinence from alcohol for women who are pregnant or who are planning a pregnancy" (26).

Treatment of Chronic Alcoholism

Treatment of chronic alcoholism is controversial and often discouraging. There is no substitute medication comparable to methadone for heroin addiction. Therapeutic approaches include benzodiazepines, disulfiram, lithium, serotonin-uptake inhibitors, dopaminergic agents, opioid agonists and antagonists, acupuncture, and self-help groups such as Alcoholics Anonymous (15).

Toxic Mechanisms

Ethanol acts at many levels of the neuraxis, especially complex polysynaptic systems such as the reticular formation (decreased alertness) and the parietal association cortex (impaired eye-hand coordination). It affects a number of neurotransmitter systems, including GABA, norepinephrine, dopamine, serotonin, acetylcholine, adenosine, and glutamate, but such actions are probably indirect (77,101). More directly, ethanol disrupts the phospholipid bilayer of cell membranes, "fluidizing" them and producing secondary alterations in protein conformation and ion channels. (Such action is shared by general anesthetics, which, to varying degrees, are cross-tolerant with ethanol.) In animals, ethanol tolerance is associated with decreased membrane "fluidizability"—or increased membrane "stiffness"—and physical dependence is associated with persistence of "stiffness" following ethanol withdrawal. Increased "stiffness" with chronic ethanol intake is probably secondary to increased fatty acid and cholesterol content, which in turn reduces ethanol entry into the membrane.

Whether ethanol's CNS effects are entirely explained by membrane fluidization is controversial. Investigators have reported apparently direct actions on G proteins as well as lack of correlation between membrane fluidization and ethanol sensitivity. Such observations have led to the suggestion that ethanol, while acting on membranes rather than at particular receptors, does so semispecifically, interacting with particular membrane domains—patches of lipids that differ in chemical composition and fluidity. In any event, the overall effect is CNS depression, with inhibition of most excitatory receptors [including N-methyl-D-aspartate (NMDA) and kainate subtypes of glutamate receptors] and facilitation of most inhibitory receptors (including GABA receptors). Exceptions are the enhancement of excitatory nicotinic acetylcholine receptors and serotonergic 5-HT$_3$ receptors.

In animals, as in humans, thiamine deficiency and ethanol neurotoxicity could be additive or even superadditive in producing neuronal dysfunction and loss of these cells (75). Mice treated with ethanol and simultaneously fed a thiamine-deficient diet developed axon terminal degeneration in the olfactory bulbs and deep cerebellar nuclei; no cerebellar change and minimal olfactory bulb degeneration were seen in mice given the two treatments at different times (95,96). Rats chronically treated with ethanol and made thiamine deficient at varying intervals displayed frontal cortical neuronal degeneration if thiamine deficiency occurred early and alcohol administration was continued (75).

Ethanol metabolism increases tissue levels of lipid peroxides, both by enhancing free radical formation and by impairing antioxidant defences such as α-tocopherol, glutathione, and superoxide dismutase. The brain, with its high oxygen consumption and high content of easily oxidizable substrates (especially polysaturated fatty acids and catecholamines) would be particularly vulnerable (98). Upregulation of NMDA receptor-coupled ion channels occurred in brains of ethanol-dependent mice and in cultures of cerebellar neurons chronically exposed to ethanol (19,115).

Some of these effects might occur indirectly through the action of acetaldehyde which, in the liver, forms adducts with amino groups of many compounds, including enzymes and nucleic acids; it is also oxidized there to tissue-damaging free radicals. The escape of acetaldehyde from the liver allows it access to the brain, which locally metabolizes very little ethanol and where similar adduct and free radical formation could damage neurons (92). Disruption of neuronal tubulin might be especially important in this regard, and effects on thiamine-dependent enzymes, such as transketolase, could underlie possible synergism between ethanol neurotoxicity and nutritional deficiency.

Whatever the mechanism, studies such as these confirm that ethanol has neurotoxic potential. Two important clinical questions, however, remain. First, does ethanol neurotoxicity cause lasting cognitive impairment in humans? Second, if so, is there a safe dose? Mild cognitive impairment and brain shrinkage have been reported in "moderate" drinkers (usually defined as 30–80 g ethanol daily) (17,94,103); others have found no evidence of brain damage in such subjects (13,128). Until the matter is resolved, one must consider the possibility that there is no such thing as a truly safe repeated dose of ethanol.

REFERENCES

1. Abraham WC, Rogers CJ, Hunter BE (1984) Chronic ethanol-induced decreases in the response of dentate granule cells to perforant path input in the rat. *Exp Brain Res* 54, 406.

2. Ahluwalia B, Smith D, Adeyiga O *et al.* (1992) Ethanol decreases progesterone synthesis in human placental cells: Mechanism of ethanol effect. *Alcohol* 9, 395.

3. Altura BM, Altura BT, Corella A *et al.* (1982) Alcohol produces spasms of human umbilical vessels: Relationship to FAS. *Eur J Pharmacol* 86, 311.

4. Anonymous (1990) Alcohol-related mortality and years of potential life lost—United States, 1987. *Morbid Mort Wkly Rep* 39, 173.

5. Arendt J, Allen Y, Marchbanks RM *et al.* (1989) Cholinergic system and memory in the rat: Effects of chronic ethanol, embryonic basal forebrain transplants and excitotoxic lesions of cholinergic basal forebrain projection system. *Neuroscience* 33,435.

6. Arendt T, Henning D, Gray JA, Marchbanks R (1988) Loss of neurons in the rat basal forebrain cholinergic projection system after prolonged intake of ethanol. *Brain Res Bull* 21, 563.

7. Ashwell KW, Zhang LL (1994) Optic nerve hypoplasia in an acute exposure model of the fetal alcohol syndrome. *Neurotoxicol Teratol* 16, 161.

8. Baron R, Heuser K, Marioth G (1989) Marchiafava-Bignami disease with recovery diagnosed by CT and MRI: Demyelination affects several CNS structures. *J Neurol* 236, 364.

9. Barthauer L, Tarter R, Hirsch W, Van Thiel D (1992) Brain morphologic characteristics of cirrhotic alcoholics and cirrhotic nonalcoholics: An MRI study. *Alcohol Clin Exp Res* 16, 982.

10. Basile AS, Jones EA, Skolnick P (1991) The pathogenesis and treatment of hepatic encephalopathy: Evidence for the involvement of benzodiazepine ligands. *Pharmacol Rev* 43, 28.

11. Blum K, Noble EP, Sheridan PJ *et al.* (1990) Allelic association of human dopamine D-2 receptor gene in alcoholism. *J Amer Med Assn* 263, 2055.

12. Bollaert PE, Rodin-Lherbier B, Escayne JM *et al.* (1989) Phosphorus nuclear magnetic resonance evidence of abnormal skeletal muscle metabolism in chronic alcoholics. *Neurology* 39, 821.

13. Bowden SC (1987) Brain impairment in social drinkers? No cause for concern. *Alcohol Clin Exp Res* 11, 407.

14. Bowden SC (1990) Separating cognitive impairment in neurologically asymptomatic alcoholism from Wernicke-Korsakoff syndrome: Is the neuropsychological distinction justified? *Psychol Bull* 107, 355.

15. Brust JCM (1993) *Neurological Aspects of Substance Abuse.* Butterworth-Heinemann, Boston p. 190.

16. Cadete-Leite A, Tavares MA, Pacheco MM *et al.* (1989) Hippocampal mossy fibre-CA3 synapses after chronic alcohol consumption and withdrawal. *Alcohol* 6, 303.

17. Cala LA, Jones B, Burns P *et al.* (1983) Results of computerized tomography, psychometric testing, and dietary studies in social drinkers, with emphasis on reversibility after abstinence. *Med J Australia* 2, 264.

18. Camargo CA (1989) Moderate alcohol consumption and stroke: The epidemiologic evidence. *Stroke* 20, 1611.

19. Chandler IJ, Newsom H, Sumners C, Crews F (1993) Chronic ethanol exposure potentiates NMDA excitotoxicity in cerebral cortical neurons. *J Neurochem* 60, 1578.

20. Chang MP, Yamaguchi DT, Yeh M *et al.* (1994) Mechanism of the impaired T-cell proliferation in adult rats exposed to alcohol *in utero. Int J Immunopharmacol* 16, 345.

21. Charness ME (1993) Brain lesions in alcoholics. *Alcohol Clin Exp Res* 17, 2.

22. Chiriboga CA (1993) Fetal effects. *Neurol Clin* 11, 707.

23. Cicero TJ, Nock B, O'Connor L *et al.* (1994) Acute alcohol exposure markedly influences male fertility and fetal outcome in the male rat. *Life Sci* 55, 901.

24. Cloninger CR (1987) Neurogenetic adaptive mechanisms in alcoholism. *Science* 236, 410.

25. Comings DE, Muhleman D, Ahn C *et al.* (1994) The dopamine D_2 receptor gene: A genetic risk factor in substance abuse. *Drug Alcohol Dependence* 34, 175.

26. Committee on Substance Abuse and Committee on Children with Disabilities (1993) Fetal alcohol syndrome and fetal alcohol effects. *Pediatrics* 91, 1004.

27. Coulter CL, Leech RW, Schaefer B *et al.* (1993) Midline cerebral dysgenesis, dysfunction of the hypothalamic-pituitary axis, and fetal alcohol effects. *Arch Neurol* 50, 771.

28. Crabbe JC, Belknap JK, Buck KJ (1994) Genetic animal models of alcohol and drug abuse. *Science* 264, 1715.

29. Crabbe JC, Phillips TJ (1993) Selective breeding for alcohol withdrawal severity. *Behav Genet* 23, 171.

30. Day NL, Jasperse D, Richardson G *et al.* (1989) Prenatal exposure to alcohol: Effect on infant growth and morphologic characteristics. *Pediatrics* 84, 536.

31. Deitrich RA (1993) Selective breeding for initial sensitivity to ethanol. *Behav Genet* 23, 153.

32. de la Monte SM (1988) Disproportionate atrophy of ce-

rebral white matter in chronic alcoholics. *Arch Neurol* **45**, 990.

33. Devi BG, Henderson GI, Frosto TA, Schenker S (1993) Effect of ethanol on rat fetal hepatocytes: Studies on cell replication, lipid peroxidation and glutathione. *Hepatology* **18**, 648.

34. Dreosti IE (1993) Nutritional factors underlying the expression of the fetal alcohol syndrome. *Ann N Y Acad Sci* **678**, 193.

35. Duester G (1994) Retinoids and the alcohol dehydrogenase gene family. *Experientia* **71**, 279.

36. Durand D, Carlen PL (1984) Impairment of long-term potentiation in rat hippocampus following chronic ethanol treatment. *Brain Res* **308**, 325.

37. Durand D, St Cyr JA, Curevitch N, Carlen P (1989) Ethanol-induced dendritic alterations in hippocampal granule cells. *Brain Res* **477**, 373.

38. Ferrer I, Galofre E, Fabriques I, Lopez-Tejero D (1989) Effects of chronic ethanol consumption beginning at adolescence: Increased numbers of dendritic spines on cortical pyramidal cells in adulthood. *Acta Neuropathol* **78**, 528.

39. Ferriero DM, Sheldon RA, Domingo J (1992) Somatostatin is altered in developing retina from ethanol-exposed rats. *Neurosci Lett* **147**, 29.

40. File SE, Mabbutt PS (1990) Long-lasting effects on habituation and passive avoidance performance of a period of chronic ethanol administration in the rat. *Behav Brain Res* **36**, 171.

41. Fisch BJ, Hauser WA, Brust JCM *et al.* (1989) The EEG response to diffuse and patterned photic stimulation during acute untreated alcohol withdrawal. *Neurology* **39**, 434.

42. Forrest F, Du C, Florey V, Taylor D (1992) Maternal alcohol consumption and child development. *Int J Epidemiol* **21**, S17.

43. Freund G, Ballinger WE (1989) Loss of muscarinic cholinergic receptors from the temporal cortex of alcohol abusers. *Metab Brain Dis* **4**, 121.

44. Freund G, Ballinger WE (1991) Loss of synaptic receptors can precede morphologic changes induced by alcohol. *Alcohol Alcoholism* Suppl **1**, 395.

45. Fulop M (1989) Alcoholism, ketoacidosis, and lactic acidosis. *Diabetes Metab Rev* **5**, 365.

46. Gaziano JM, Buring JE, Breslow JL *et al.* (1993) Moderate alcohol intake increased levels of high density lipoprotein and its subfractions, and decreased risk of myocardial infarction. *N Engl J Med* **329**, 1829.

47. Gejman PV, Ram A, Gelernter J *et al.* (1994) No structural mutation in the dopamine D_2 receptor gene in alcoholism or schizophrenia. Analysis using denaturing gradient gel electrophoresis. *J Amer Med Assn* **271**, 204.

48. Gelernter J, Goldman D, Risch N (1993) The A1 allele at the D_2 dopamine receptor gene and alcoholism. A reappraisal. *J Amer Med Assn* **269**, 1673.

49. Gilman S, Adams K, Koeppe R *et al.* (1990) Cerebellar and frontal hypometabolism in alcoholic cerebellar degeneration studied with positron emission tomography. *Ann Neurol* **28**, 775.

50. Goedde HW, Agarwal DP (1990) Pharmacogenetics of aldehyde dehydrogenase (ALDH). *Pharmacol Ther* **45**, 345.

51. Gorelick PB, Rodin MB, Longenberg P *et al.* (1989) Weekly alcohol consumption, cigarette smoking, and the risk of ischemic stroke: Results of a case-control study at urban medical centers in Chicago, Illinois. *Neurology* **39**, 339.

52. Graham JM, Hansen JW, Darby BL *et al.* (1988) Independent dysmorphology evaluations at birth and four years of age for children exposed to varying amounts of alcohol *in utero*. *Pediatrics* **81**, 772.

53. Gressens P, Lammens M, Picard JJ, Evrard P (1992) Ethanol-induced disturbances of gliogenesis and neuronogenesis in the developing murine brain: An *in vitro* and *in vivo* immunohistochemical and ultrastructural study. *Alcohol Alcoholism* **27**, 219.

54. Grossman A, Astley SJ, Liggitt HD *et al.* (1993) Immune function in offspring of nonhuman primates (*Macaca nemestrina*) exposed weekly to 1.8 g/kg ethanol during pregnancy: Preliminary observations. *Alcohol Clin Exp Res* **17**, 822.

55. Hannigan JH, Abel EL, Kruger ML (1993) "Population" characteristics of birthweight in an animal model of alcohol-related developmental effects. *Neurotoxicol Teratol* **15**, 97.

56. Hansen LA, Natelson BH, Lemere C *et al.* (1991) Alcohol-induced brain changes in dogs. *Arch Neurol* **48**, 939.

57. Harper C (1998) The neuropathology of alcohol-specific brain damage, or does alcohol damage the brain? *J Neuropathol Exp Neurol* **57**, 101.

58. Harper C, Corbett D (1990) Changes in the basal dendrites of cortical pyramidal cells from alcoholic patients —a quantitative Golgi study. *J Neurol Neurosurg Psychiat* **53**, 856.

59. Harper CG, Kril JJ (1985) Brain atrophy in chronic alcoholic patients: A quantitative pathological study. *J Neurol Neurosurg Psychiat* **48**, 211.

60. Harper CG, Kril JJ (1990) Neuropathology of alcoholism. *Alcohol Alcoholism* **25**, 207.

61. Harper C, Kril J, Daly J (1987) Are we drinking our neurones away? *Brit Med J* **294**, 534.

62. Hayakawa K, Kumagai H, Suzuki Y *et al.* (1992) MR imaging in chronic alcoholism. *Acta Radiologica* **33**, 201.

63. Hinzpeter EN, Renz S, Loser H (1992). Eye manifestations of fetal alcohol syndrome. *Klin Monatsbl Augenheilk* **200**, 33.

64. Holden C (1994) A cautionary genetic tale: The sobering story of D_2. *Science* **264**, 1696.

65. Hunter R, McLuskie R, Wyoer D *et al.* (1989) The pat-

tern of function-related regional cerebral blood flow investigated by single photon emission tomography with 99mTc-HMPAO in patients with presenile Alzheimer's disease and Korsakoff's psychosis. *Psychol Med* **19**, 847.

66. Ioffe S, Chernick V (1988) Development of the EEG between 30 and 40 weeks gestation in normal and alcohol-exposed infants. *Develop Med Child Neurol* **30**, 797.

67. Jacobson JL, Jacobson SW, Sokol RJ (1993) Teratogenic effects of alcohol on infant development. *Alcohol Clin Exp Res* **17**, 174.

68. Jernigan TL, Butters N, DiTraglia G *et al.* (1991) Reduced cerebral grey matter observed in alcoholics using magnetic resonance imaging. *Alcohol Clin Exp Res* **15**, 418.

69. Jones DG, Colangelo W (1985) Ultrastructural investigation into influence of ethanol on synaptic maturation in rat neocortex. I. Qualitative assessment. *Develop Neurosci* **7**, 94.

70. Joyce EM (1994) Aetiology of alcoholic brain damage: Alcoholic neurotoxicity or thiamine malnutrition? *Brit Med Bull* **50**, 99.

71. Keung W-M, Vallee BL (1993) Daidzin and daidzein suppress free-choice ethanol intake by Syrian golden hamsters. *Proc Nat Acad Sci USA* **90**, 10008.

72. King MA, Hunter BE, Walker DW (1988) Alterations and recovery of dendrite spine density in rat hippocampus following long-term ethanol ingestion. *Brain Res* **439**, 381.

73. Kotch LE, Sulik KK (1992) Experimental fetal alcohol syndrome: Proposed pathogenic basis for a variety of associated facial and brain anomalies. *Amer J Med Genet* **44**, 168.

74. Kril JJ, Harper CG (1989) Neuronal counts from four cortical regions in alcoholic brains. *Acta Neuropathol* **79**, 200.

75. Kril JJ, Homewood J (1993) Neuronal changes in the cerebral cortex of the rat following alcohol treatment and thiamin deficiency. *J Neurol Exp Neuropathol* **52**, 586.

76. Kuriyama K, Ohkuma S (1990) Alteration in the function of cerebral neurotransmitter receptors during the establishment of alcohol dependence: Neurochemical aspects. *Alcohol Alcoholism* **25**, 239.

77. Lanca AJ (1994) Reduction of voluntary alcohol intake in the rat by modulation of the dopaminergic mesolimbic system: Transplantation of ventral mesencephalic cell suspensions. *Neuroscience* **58**, 359.

78. Lanca AJ, Grupp LA, Israel Y (1993) Reduction of voluntary alcohol consumption in the rat by transplantation of hypothalamic grafts. *Brain Res* **632**, 287.

79. Larroque B (1992) Alcohol and the fetus. *Int J Epidemiol* **21**, S8.

80. Lemoine P, Lemoine P (1992) Avenir des enfants de mères alcooliques (étude de 105 cas retrouvés à l'âge adult)

et quelques constatation d'intérêt prophylactique. *Ann Pediat* **29**, 226.

81. Li T-K, Lumeng L, Doolittle DP (1993) Selective breeding for alcohol preference and associated responses. *Behav Genet* **23**, 163.

82. Little RE, Asker RL, Sampson PD *et al.* (1986) Fetal growth and moderate drinking during pregnancy. *Amer J Epidemiol* **123**, 270.

83. McGivern RF, Handa RJ, Redei E (1993) Decreased postnatal testosterone surge in male rats exposed to ethanol during the last week of gestation. *Alcohol Clin Exp Res* **17**, 1215.

84. McMullen PA, St Cyr JA, Carlen PL (1984) Morphological alterations in rat CA1 hippocampal pyramidal cell dendrites resulting from chronic ethanol consumption and withdrawal. *J Comp Neurol* **225**, 111.

85. Miller MW (1993) Migration of cortical neurons is altered by gestational exposure to ethanol. *Alcoholism* **17**, 304.

86. Miller MW, Rieck RW (1993) Effects of chronic ethanol administration on acetylcholinesterase activity in the somatosensory cortex and basal forebrain of the rat. *Brain Res* **627**, 104.

87. Mukherjee AB, Hodgen GD (1982) Maternal ethanol exposure induces transient impairment of umbilical circulation and fetal hypoxia in monkeys. *Science* **218**, 700.

88. Neiman J, Lang AE, Fornazarri L, Carlen PL (1990) Movement disorders in alcoholism. A review. *Neurology* **40**, 741.

89. Ng SKC, Hauser WA, Brust JCM, Susser M (1988) Alcohol consumption and withdrawal in new-onset seizures. *N Engl J Med* **319**, 666.

90. Nicolas JM, Estruch R, Salamero M *et al.* (1997) Brain impairment in well-nourished chronic alcoholics is related to ethanol intake. *Ann Neurol* **41**, 590.

91. Nordmann R, Ribiere C, Rouach H (1990) Ethanol-induced lipid peroxidation and oxidative stress in extrahepatic tissues. *Alcohol Alcoholism* **25**, 231.

92. Oulette EM, Rosett HL, Rosman HP *et al.* (1977) Adverse effects on offspring of maternal alcohol abuse during pregnancy. *N Engl J Med* **297**, 528.

93. Parker ES, Noble EP (1977) Alcohol consumption and cognitive function in social drinkers. *J Stud Alcohol* **38**, 1224.

94. Phillips SC (1987) Neuro-toxic interaction in alcohol-treated, thiamine-deficient mice. *Acta Neuropathol* **73**, 171.

95. Phillips SC (1989) The threshhold concentration of dietary ethanol necessary to produce toxic effects on hippocampal cells and synapses in the mouse. *Exp Neurol* **104**, 68.

96. Pizano-Duran MD, Renau-Piqueras J, Guerri C (1993) Developmental changes in the optic nerve related to ethanol consumption in pregnant rats: Analysis of the ethanol-exposed optic nerve. *Teratology* **48**, 305.

97. Pratt OE, Rooprai HK, Shaw GK, Thomson AD (1990) The genesis of alcoholic brain tissue injury. *Alcohol Alcoholism* **25**, 217.

98. Redei E, Halasz I, Li LF *et al.* (1993) Maternal adrenalectomy alters the immune and endocrine functions of fetal alcohol-exposed male offspring. *Endocrinology* **133**, 452.

99. Ridker PM, Vaughan DE, Stampfer MJ *et al.* (1994) Association of moderate alcohol consumption and plasma concentration of endogenous tissue-type plasminogen activator. *J Amer Med Assn* **272**, 929.

100. Samson HH, Harris RA (1992) Neurobiology of alcohol abuse. *Trends Pharmacol Sci* **13**, 206.

101. Samson Y, Baron JC, Feline A *et al.* (1986) Local cerebral glucose utilisation in chronic alcoholics: A positron tomographic study. *J Neurol Neurosurg Psychiat* **49**, 1165.

102. Schaeffer KW, Parsons OA (1986) Drinking practices and the neuropsychological test performance in sober male alcoholics and social drinkers. *Alcohol* **3**, 175.

103. Schenker S, Johnson RF, Mahuren JD *et al.* (1992) Human placental vitamin B6 (pyridoxal) transport: Normal characteristics and effects of ethanol. *Amer J Physiol* **262**, R966.

104. Schuckit MA (1994) Low level of response to alcohol as a predictor of future alcoholism. *Amer J Psychiat* **151**, 184.

105. Scott HC, Paull WK, Rudeen PK (1992) Effects of *in utero* ethanol exposure on the development of LHRH neurons in the mouse. *Develop Brain Res* **66**, 119.

106. Singh SP, Srivenugopal KS, Ehmann S *et al.* (1994) Insulin-like growth factors (IGF-I and IGF-II), IGF-binding proteins, and IGF gene expression in the offspring of ethanol-fed rats. *J Lab Clin Med* **124**, 183.

107. Smith CJ, Perry EK, Perry RH *et al.* (1988) Muscarinic cholinergic receptor subtypes in hippocampus in human cognitive disorders. *J Neurochem* **50**, 847.

108. Snyder AK, Singh SP, Ehmann S (1992) Effects of ethanol on DNA, RNA, and protein synthesis in rat astrocyte cultures. *Alcohol Clin Exp Res* **16**, 295.

109. Spohr HL, Willms J, Steinhausen HC (1993) Prenatal alcohol exposure and long-term developmental consequences. *Lancet* **341**, 1993.

110. Streissguth AP, Aase JM, Clarren SK *et al.* (1991) Fetal alcohol syndrome in adolescents and adults. *J Amer Med Assn* **265**, 1961.

111. Streissguth AP, Dehaene P (1993) Fetal alcohol syndrome in twins of alcoholic mothers: Concordance of diagnosis and IQ. *Amer J Med Genet* **47**, 857.

112. Suarez BK, Parsian A, Hampe CL *et al.* (1994) Linkage disequilibria at the D_2 dopamine receptor locus (DRD2) in alcoholics and controls. *Genomics* **19**, 12.

113. Sulik K, Johnston MS, Webb MA (1981) Fetal alcohol syndrome: Embryogenesis in a mouse model. *Science* **214**, 936.

114. Tabakoff B, Hoffman PL (1993) Ethanol, sedative hypnotics, and glutamate receptor function in brain and cultured cells. *Behav Genet* **23**, 231.

115. Tajuddin NF, Druse MJ (1993) Treatment of alcohol-consuming rats with buspirone: Effects on serotonin and 5-hydroxyindoleacetic acid content in offspring. *Alcohol Clin Exp Res* **17**, 110.

116. Tan XX, Castoldi AF, Manzo L, Costa LG (1993) Interaction of ethanol with muscarinic receptor-stimulated phosphoinositide metabolism during the brain growth spurt in the rat: Role of acetaldehyde. *Neurosci Lett* **156**, 13.

117. Tavares MA, Paula-Barbosa MM (1982) Alcohol-induced granule-cell loss in the cerebellar cortex of the adult rat. *Exp Neurol* **78**, 574.

118. Tavares MA, Paula-Barbosa MM, Gray EG (1983) Dendritic spine plasticity and chronic alcoholism in rats. *Neurosci Lett* **42**, 235.

119. Tritt SH, Tio DL, Brammer GL, Taylor AN (1993) Adrenalectomy but not adrenal demedullation during pregnancy prevents the growth-retarding effects of fetal alcohol exposure. *Alcohol Clin Exp Res* **17**, 1281.

120. Urbano-Marquez A, Estruch R, Navarro-Lopez F *et al.* (1989) The effects of alcoholism on skeletal and cardiac muscle. *N Engl J Med* **329**, 409.

121. Victor M (1993) Persistent altered mentation due to ethanol. *Neurol Clin* **11**, 639.

122. Victor M, Adams RD, Collins GH (1989) *The Wernicke-Korsakoff Syndrome. 2nd Ed.* FA Davis Co, Philadelphia.

123. Victor M, Brausch CC (1967) The role of abstinence in the genesis of alcoholic epilepsy. *Epilepsia* **8**, 1.

124. Victor M, Hope JM (1958) The phenomenon of auditory hallucinations in chronic alcoholism. *J Nerv Ment Dis* **126**, 451.

125. Volkow ND, Wang G-J, Hitzemann R (1994) Recovery of brain glucose metabolism in detoxified alcoholics. *Amer J Psychiat* **151**, 178.

126. Wang GJ, Volkow ND, Roque CT *et al.* (1993) Functional importance of ventricular enlargement and cortical atrophy in healthy subjects and alcoholics as assessed with PET, MR imaging, and neuropsychologic testing. *Radiology* **186**, 59.

127. Waugh M, Jackson M, Fox GA *et al.* (1989) Effect of social drinking on neuropsychological performance. *Brit J Addict* **84**, 659.

128. Wiśniewski K (1983) A clinical neuropathological study of the fetal alcohol syndrome. *Neuropediatrics* **14**, 197.

129. Wright JT, Barrison IG, Richardson G *et al.* (1983) Alcohol consumption, pregnancy, and low birthweight. *Lancet* **1**, 663.

130. Yirmiya R, Pilati ML, Chiappelli F, Taylor AN (1993) Fetal alcohol exposure attenuates lipopolysaccharide-induced fever in rats. *Alcohol Clin Exp Res* **17**, 906.

131. Zajac CS, Abel EL (1992) Animal models of prenatal alcohol exposure. *Int J Epidemiol* **21**, S24.

Ethchlorvynol

Herbert H. Schaumburg

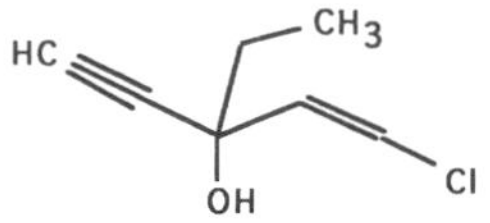

ETHCHLORVYNOL
C_7H_9ClO

1-Chloro-3-ethyl-1-penten-4-yl-3-ol

NEUROTOXICITY RATING

Clinical

A   Acute encephalopathy (sedation, coma)

A   Physical dependence and withdrawal

C   Peripheral neuropathy

Ethchlorvynol, a sedative-hypnotic drug with a rapid onset and short duration of action, has CNS effects similar to those of barbiturates. Oral ethchlorvynol has an effect within 15–30, min and maximum plasma concentration is attained within 1 h. The drug is largely metabolized by the liver. Ethchlorvynol is no longer widely prescribed in North America because of interactions with other agents, severe respiratory depression following overdose, and abuse potential. Save for hypersensitivity reactions and hypotension, there is little serious systemic toxicity. Neurotoxic reactions are similar to those of barbiturates; both dose-related CNS depression and withdrawal occur.

Most instances of CNS depression have followed suicide attempts and feature severe coma and prolonged respiratory depression, occasionally with pulmonary edema (1–3). Respiratory depression is far more profound with ethchlorvynol than with barbiturate overdose and is strongly enhanced by ingestion of ethanol. Lethal doses range from 10–25 g (therapeutic dose is 700 mg), but as little as 2.5 g has been fatal with coconsumption of ethanol. Chronic abuse is characterized by tolerance and intense withdrawal symptoms with terrifying hallucinations that resemble those associated with delirium tremens. It is likely that isolated descriptions of facial numbness or multifocal peripheral neuropathy reflect, respectively, hyperventilation and pressure-induced compromise of peripheral nerves (2).

REFERENCES

1. Oglivie R, Douglas DE, Lochead JR *et al*. (1966) Ethchlorvynol (Placidyl®) intoxication and its treatment by hemodialysis. *Can Med Assn J* 95, 954.
2. Teehan BP, Maher JF, Carey JJH *et al*. (1970) Acute ethchlorvynol (Placidyl®) intoxication. *Ann Intern Med* 72, 875.
3. Westervelt FB (1966) Ethchlorvynol (Placidyl®) intoxication experience with five patients, including treatment with hemodialysis. *Ann Intern Med* 64, 1229.

Ethidium Bromide

Peter S. Spencer

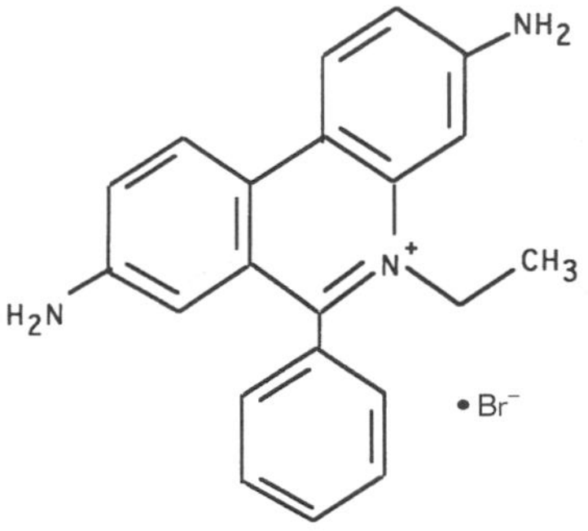

ETHIDIUM BROMIDE
$C_{21}H_{20}BrN_3$

3,8-Diamino-5-ethyl-6-phenylphenan-thridinium bromide; Homidium bromide

NEUROTOXICITY RATING

Experimental

A   DNA toxin

Ethidium bromide (EB), a phenanthridinium dye, is used as an antitrypanosomal drug in veterinary medicine and, in the research setting, as a membrane-permeant cell marker (11), a DNA stain, and an experimental arthropod and mammalian neurotoxin and cytotoxin.

EB forms bitter-tasting, dark-red crystals with a MP of 238°–240°C. Ethidium binds reversibly to DNA by intercalation with the minor groove of the nucleic acid, thereby causing the double helix partly to unwind; this property is exploited in separating plasmid DNA from genomic DNA in buoyant-density centrifugation. Presence of DNA-bound EB in living or formalin-fixed tissue is evident by the emission of a red fluorescence when illuminated with ultraviolet light (2,8). While the intercalation of EB with DNA does not stimulate topoisomerase II–mediated cleavage of DNA strands, covalent attachment of a photoreactive EB potently enhances activity of this enzyme (7).

EB suppresses DNA, RNA, and protein synthesis in mammalian cells; this appears to be the basis for its cytotoxic actions on directly exposed neuronal and glial cells. Treatment of DNA isolated from brain and liver cells of the chick embryo resulted in a concentration-dependent diminution of activity of the DNA-repair enzyme O^6-alkylguanine-DNA alkyltransferase (6). Neuroblastoma cell lines selectively deficient in enzyme complexes I and IV of the electron transport chain can be created by selective depletion of mitochondrial DNA through prolonged incubation with EB (9). At low concentrations, EB blocked the open ion channel of the nicotinic acetylcholine receptor and reduced its open time (13).

In animals, intravenously administered EB does not escape from blood vessels in neural tissue other than those regions lacking the capillary specializations that constitute blood-brain and blood-nerve barriers. Systemically circulating EB is therefore extravasated from capillaries supplying only spinal, cranial and autonomic ganglia, choroid plexus, area postrema and the circumventricular organs (neurohypophysis, organum vasculosum lamina terminalis, and median eminence). Red fluorescent material in the nucleus and cytoplasm of these areas appeared within minutes of intravenous injection of EB in mice; material was no longer apparent 24 h later. Unexpectedly, fluorescent material was also seen in the parenchyma of the olfactory lobes of some animals (2).

EB is transported retrogradely along nerve pathways; application to a transected mouse sciatic nerve or to neuromas formed 2 months post nerve transection resulted in labeling of both dorsal root ganglion neurons and associated satellite cells; there was only moderate sensory neuronal degeneration relative to that induced by retrogradely transported ricin, the lectin from *Ricinus communis*. (10).

Application of EB to cockroach CNS connectives caused extensive changes in neuroglia and disruption of axonal conduction within 24 h (12). In mice, intranasal irrigation with 2 mM EB resulted after 8 days in an inability to find food pellets; this was associated with a loss of thymidine incorporation into olfactory tissue and a dramatic decrease in activity of carnosine synthetase (a chemoreceptor marker) in the olfactory bulb (4,12). Intracisternal injection of EB in the rat induced status spongiosus with prominent degenerative changes in subpial oligodendrocytes; areas of axon demyelination with a total absence of oligodendrocytes were evident by the sixth day following injection, and remyelination by oligodendrocytes and Schwann cells had begun by the twelfth day (14). A comparable sequence of events followed injection of EB into the spinal cord of small mammals (1); repair of the demyelinated lesion by spontaneous remyelination was blocked by prior x-irradiation (3). EB-induced localized demyelination and remyelination in the dorsal funiculus of the rat cervical spinal cord correlated with a decrease in security of foot placement that recovered approximately 5 weeks after drug administration (5).

REFERENCES

1. Blakemore WF (1982) Ethidium bromide induced demyelination in the spinal cord of the cat. *Neuropathol Appl Neurobiol* 8, 365.

2. Cesarini K, Atillo A, Bigotte L *et al.* (1985) Cytofluorescence localization of ethidium bromide in the nervous system of the mouse. I. Ethidium bromide: Its distribution in regions within and without the blood-brain barrier after intravenous injection. *Acta Neuropathol* 68, 273.

3. Crang AJ, Franklin RJ, Blakemore WF *et al.* (1992) The differentiation of glial cell progenitor populations following transplantation into non-repairing central nervous system glial lesions in adult animals. *J Neuroimmunol* 40, 243.

4. Harding JW, Wright JW (1979) Effects of intranasal irrigation with mitotic inhibitors on olfactory behavior and biochemistry in mice. *Brain Res* 168, 31.

5. Jeffery ND, Blakemore WF (1997) Locomotor deficits induced by experimental spinal cord demyelination are abolished by spontaneous remyelination. *Brain* 120, 27.

6. Link A, Tempel K (1991) Inhibition of O^6-alkylguanine-DNA-alkyltransferase and DNase I activities by some alkylating substances and antineoplastic agents. *J Cancer Res Clin Oncol* 117, 549.

7. Marx G, Zhou H, Graves DE, Osheroff N (1997) Covalent attachment of ethidium bromide to DNA results in enhanced topoisomerase II-mediated DNA cleavage. *Biochemistry* 36, 15884.

8. McCarthy PW, Lawson SN (1988) Differential intracellular labelling of identified neurones with two fluorescent dyes. *Brain Res Bull* 20, 261.

9. Miller SW, Trimmer PA, Parker WD Jr, Davis RE (1996) Creation and characterization of mitochondrial DNA-depleted cell lines with "neuronal-like" properties. *J Neurochem* 67, 1897.

10. Nennesmo I, Kristensson K (1986) Effects of retrograde transport of *Ricinus communis* agglutinin I on neuroma formation. *Acta Neuropathol* 70, 279.

11. Pulliam L, Stubblebine M, Hyun W (1998) Quantification of neurotoxicity and identification of cellular subsets in a three-dimensional brain model. *Cytometry* 32, 66.

12. Smith PJ, Leech CA, Treherne JE (1984) Glial repair in an insect central nervous system: Effects of selective glial disruption. *J Neurosci* **4**, 2698.

13. Sterz R, Hermes M, Peper K, Bradley RJ (1982) Effects of ethidium bromide on the nicotinic acetylcholine receptor. *Eur J Pharmacol* **80**, 393.

14. Yajima K, Suzuki K (1979) Demyelination and remyelination in the rat central nervous system following ethidium bromide injection. *Lab Invest* **41**, 385.

Ethionamide

Herbert H. Schaumburg

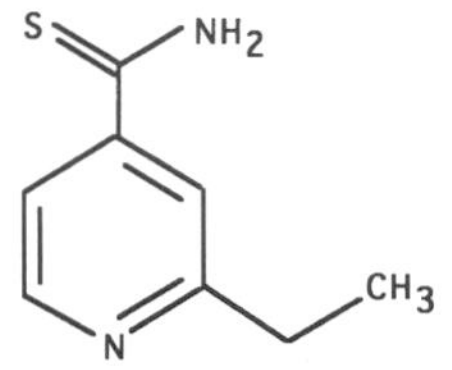

ETHIONAMIDE
$C_8H_{10}N_2S$

2-Ethyl-4-pyridinecarbothioamide

NEUROTOXICITY RATING

Clinical

B   Peripheral neuropathy

B   Acute encephalopathy

Ethionamide, a congener of isoniazid, is an effective antituberculosis agent; it is not used as primary therapy because systemic toxic reactions are common at conventional doses. It is used as a secondary agent concurrently with other drugs when therapy with primary agents has proven ineffective; as with isoniazid, the concomitant administration of pyridoxine is recommended. Orally administered ethionamide is rapidly absorbed and peak plasma levels appear within 3 h; the half-life is 2 h. The drug is widely distributed in the body, and significant concentrations appear in the cerebrospinal fluid. The principal, dose-limiting, systemic adverse effect of ethionamide is upper gastrointestinal distress; hepatitis develops in 5% of patients receiving conventional doses (6).

Neurotoxicity is uncommon (5). Tremor, generalized seizures, and confusional states are described in anecdotal case reports; these phenomena cease following drug withdrawal and persistent CNS dysfunction is not described (1,3). There are two case descriptions of distal-extremity paresthesias developing with therapeutic doses; only one experienced acral sensory loss and hyperreflexia (2,4). The symptoms and signs in both disappeared 2 weeks following drug withdrawal; neither of these individuals had peripheral electrophysiological studies, and both were receiving concurrent antituberculosis therapy with other agents (not isoniazid).

While most antituberculosis drugs appear to be safe for use with breastfeeding, there are no clear data on the safety of ethionamide (7).

REFERENCES

1. Addington WW (1979) The side effects and interactions of antituberculosis drugs. *Chest* **76S**, 782.

2. Leggat PO (1962) Ethionamide neuropathy. *Tubercle (Lond)* **43**, 95.

3. Moulding T, Davidson PT (1974) Tuberculosis II: Toxicity and intolerance to antituberculosis drugs. *Drug Therapy* **4**, 39.

4. Poole GW, Schneeweiss J (1961) Peripheral neuropathy due to ethionamide. *Annu Rev Resp Dis* **84**, 890.

5. Snavely SR, Hodges GR (1984) The neurotoxicity of antibacterial agents. *Ann Intern Med* **101**, 92.

6. Tala E, Tevola K (1969) Side effects and toxicity of ethionamide and prothionamide. *Ann Clin Res* **1**, 32.

7. Tran JH, Montakantikul P (1998) The safety of antituberculosis medications during breastfeeding. *J Hum Lact* **14**, 337.

Ethylcholine Aziridinium

Peter S. Spencer

$$HO - CH_2 - CH_2 - \overset{+}{\underset{\underset{CH_3}{\overset{|}{CH_2}}}{N}} \overset{\overset{CH_2}{\diagup}}{\underset{\diagdown}{}} \overset{|}{CH_2}$$

ETHYLCHOLINE AZIRIDINIUM
$C_6H_{14}NO$

AF64A

NEUROTOXICITY RATING
Experimental
A   Cholinotoxin

Ethylcholine aziridinium (AF64A), a neurotoxic choline analogue, is used as an experimental cholinotoxic tool. Within a certain concentration range, AF64A inhibits presynaptic high-affinity transport of choline and selectively induces cholinergic neuronal degeneration. Choline mustard aziridinium has a comparable action and potency. Related compounds, acetylcholine mustard aziridinium and ethoxycholine aziridinium, are much less potent inhibitors of choline transport (6). Propyl-, butyl-, and cyclopropyl AF64A analogues have higher IC_{50} values than that of AF64A (*vide infra*) (15).

Intracerebroventricular application of AF64A to the rat brain produces dose-dependent deficits in the cortex and hippocampus ranging from a reversible cholinergic hypofunction to a cholinotoxic effect that persists for at least 1 year (12). The CA3 region and ventral portion of the hippocampus are heavily affected (5,11), and several unidentified guanine/cytidine-rich transcripts are persistently induced (13). Secondary changes occur in other hippocampal neurotransmitter systems (6). Behavioral alterations associated with physostigmine-sensitive cognitive deficits are demonstrable in rats and mice with AF64A-induced hippocampal lesions (17).

AF64A damages cholinergic and, especially at higher concentrations, noncholinergic neurons in other regions of the brain, including the nucleus basalis of Meynert (10). Adult female rats, notably those in proestrus, are more susceptible than age-matched male rates to the cholinotoxic action of submaximal doses (7).

Intracarotid injection of AF64A in cats produces a selective, dose-dependent, and long-lasting inhibition of cholinergic transmission in the superior cervical ganglion (14). In guinea pigs, intraperitoneal injection of the drug selectively perturbs cholinergic neuromuscular transmission in the ileum and bladder, and cholinergic neuromodulation in the enteric nervous system of the distal colon (8). Single intravitreal administration of AF64A to rats induced delayed-onset retinal muscarinic supersensitivity (16).

In neuronal cell cultures, AF64A irreversibly inhibited choline acetyl transferase, choline kinase, choline dehydrogenase, and acetylcholinesterase, and it selectively reduces choline acetyl transferase activity (6). AF64A accumulates in axons in concentrations that induce neuronal DNA damage and cytotoxicity (2). Chick-embyro neuron-enriched CNS cultures responded to 10^{-3} M AF64A with widespread cell death by 24 h; by contrast, 10^{-5} M AF64A produced no morphological, DNA- or protein-content changes. At 10^{-4} M, astrocytes appeared intact, and some neurons survived with attenuated arbors (3). In agreement, rat brain primary neuronal cultures treated with AF64A appear to undergo retrograde axonal degeneration (1).

AF64A inhibits the high-affinity choline transport system in synaptic terminals and, in competition with choline, is transported into cholinergic neurons. Choline transport is reversibly inhibited at low concentrations (IC_{50}, 1.35–2.25 μM) and irreversibly inhibited (probably by alkylation of the transporter) at high concentrations (IC_{50}, 20–30 μM) (6). AF64A accumulates in the nerve terminal where it blocks enzyme activity, interferes with axonal transport, and triggers retrograde axonal degeneration (9). Oxidative stress appears to contribute to the cholinotoxic effects of AF64A (4).

REFERENCES

1. Amir A, Pittel Z, Shahar A *et al.* (1988) Cholinotoxicity of the ethylcholine aziridinium ion in primary cultures from rat central nervous system. *Brain Res* **454**, 298.
2. Barnes DM, Hanin I, Erickson LC (1988) Cytotoxic and DNA-damaging effects of AF64A in cholinergic and noncholinergic human cell lines. *Fed Proc* **47**, 1749.
3. Davies DL, Sakellaridis N, Valcana T, Vernadakis A (1986) Cholinergic neurotoxicity induced by ethylcholine aziridinium (AF64A) in neuron-enriched cultures. *Brain Res* **378**, 251.
4. Gulyaeva NV, Lazareva NA, Libe ML *et al.* (1996) Oxidative stress in the brain following intraventricular administration of ethylcholine aziridinium (AF64A). *Brain Res* **726**, 174.
5. Hörtnagl H, Berger ML (1989) Subregional differences of cholinergic deficit in rat hippocampus induced by ethylcholine aziridinium ion (AF64A). *J Neurochem* **52**, S94.
6. Hörtnagl H, Hanin I (1992) Toxins affecting the cholinergic system. In: *Selective Neurotoxicity*. Herken H, Harkin F eds. Springer-Verlag, Berlin p. 293.

7. Hörtnagl H, Hansen L, Kindel G *et al.* (1993) Sex differences and estrous cycle variations in the AF64A-induced cholinergic deficit in the rat hippocampus. *Brain Res Bull* **31**, 129.

8. Hoyle CHV, Moss HE, Burnstock G (1986) Ethylcholine mustard aziridinium (AF64A) impairs cholinergic neuromuscular transmission in the guinea-pig ileum and urinary bladder, and cholinergic neuromodulation in the enteric nervous system of the guinea-pig distal colon. *Gen Pharmacol* **17**, 543.

9. Kasa P, Hanin I (1985) Ethylcholine mustard aziridinium blocks the axoplasmic transport of acetylcholinesterase in cholinergic nerve fibres of the rat. *Histochemistry* **83**, 343.

10. Kozlowski MR, Arbogast RE (1986) Specific toxic effects of ethylcholine nitrogen mustard on cholinergic neurons of the nucleus basalis of Meynert. *Brain Res* **372**, 45.

11. Laganiere S, Marinko M, Corey J *et al.* (1990) Sector-dependent neurotoxicity of ethylcholine aziridinium (AF64A) in the rat hippocampus. *Neuropharmacology* **29**, 961.

12. Leventer SM, Wülfert E, Hanin I (1987) Time course of ethylcholine aziridinium ion (AF64A)-induced cholinotoxicity *in vivo*. *Neuropharmacology* **26**, 361.

13. Lev-Lehman E, el-Tamer A, Yaron A *et al.* (1994) Cholinotoxic effects on acetylcholinesterase gene expression are associated with brain-region specific alterations in G,C-rich transcripts. *Brain Res* **661**, 75.

14. Mantione CR, DeGroat WC, Fisher A, Hanin I (1983) Selective inhibition of peripheral cholinergic transmission in the cat produced by AF64A. *J Pharmacol Exp Ther* **255**, 616.

15. Mistry JS, Abraham DJ, Hanin I (1986) Neurochemistry of aging: I. Toxins for an animal model of Alzheimer's disease. *J Med Chem* **29**, 376.

16. Moroi-Fetters SE, Neff NH, Hadjiconstantinou M (1990) Ethylcholine aziridinium ion depletes acetylcholine and causes muscarinic receptor supersensitivity in rat retina. *Neurosci Lett* **109**, 304.

17. Nakahara N, Iga Y, Saito Y *et al.* (1989) Beneficial effects of FKS-508 (AF102B), a selective M$_1$ agonist on the impaired working memory in AF64A-treated rats. *Jpn J Pharmacol* **51**, 539.

Ethylene Glycol

Herbert H. Schaumburg

$$HOCH_2CH_2OH$$

ETHYLENE GLYCOL

$$C_2H_6O_2$$

1,2-Ethanediol

NEUROTOXICITY RATING

Clinical

A   Acute encephalopathy (sedation, cerebellar syndrome, papilledema)

A   Cranial neuropathy

Ethylene glycol, 1,2-ethanediol, is widely used as an antifreeze agent in automobiles and aircraft; its primary adverse effect is upon the kidney. Almost all human nephrotoxicity has occurred following deliberate ingestion of ethylene glycol as an ethanol substitute; there is little risk from industrial or common-use exposure.

Ethylene glycol is rapidly absorbed from the gastrointestinal tract and is widely distributed throughout body water. For the initial 2 h, about 20% is excreted in the urine unchanged, and there is a slow metabolism of the remainder by alcohol dehydrogenase (ADH) to form glycolaldehyde. This substance is rapidly metabolized to glycolic acid, which is then converted glyoxylic acid. Once glyoxylic acid is formed, a number of metabolic steps may occur; oxalic acid is among the most deleterious breakdown products (4). Deposition of oxalate crystals and severe metabolic acidosis are responsible for much of the systemic toxicity of ethylene glycol (6).

When taken orally, ethylene glycol is five to ten times more toxic to humans than to experimental animals; the single lethal dose for man is 1.4 ml/kg, or about 100 ml for a 70-kg person. The ethylene glycol toxic syndrome evolves in three stages: first is an acute encephalopathy that appears within 1–2 h (*vide infra*); second is a stage of cardiopulmonary failure that commences at 24–72 h and is usually attributed to acidosis and hypocalcemia; if the patient survives the first two stages, renal failure then gradually develops. Renal dysfunction can range from mild uremia to complete anuria and severe tubular necrosis. Although renal failure is usually attributed to oxalate crystal deposition, it is likely that other metabolites of glyoxylic acid (formate, malate, glycine) have a role. Treatment of ethylene glycol intoxication has its rationale in attempts to inhibit the action of ADH by dosing with 4-methylpyrazole (2,3) or to compete with ethylene glycol by administering ethanol (as in the treatment of methanol intoxication); other measures include reversal of acidosis, hemodialysis, and forced diuresis (5,6).

Encephalopathic symptoms usually appear within 2 h of a large dose; the characteristic early manifestation is an individual who appears inebriated but has no alcohol on the breath. Dysarthria, nausea, and ataxia are followed by hallucinations, progressive stupor, generalized and myoclonic seizures, ophthalmoparesis, and hypothermia. Postmortem reports describe cerebral edema, petechial hemorrhages, and a meningeal lymphocytic reaction. The pathogenesis of the CNS reaction is uncertain and is likely the result of multiple factors; ethylene glycol has a CNS depressant effect and profound acidosis and hypocalcemia (secondary to chelation of calcium by ethylene glycol) account for the signs of CNS irritability and edema. Deposition of calcium oxalate crystals in the CNS is occasionally beginning at this early stage but, in contrast to nephrotoxicity, is not considered to have a prominent role.

There are several clinical descriptions of facial diparesis as a delayed (weeks) complication, with onset after the commencement of renal failure (7); a postmortem report describes dense oxalate crystal deposits along the subarachnoid segments of the seventh and eighth cranial nerves (1).

REFERENCES

1. Anderson B (1990) Facial-auditory nerve oxalosis (Letter). *Amer J Med* **88**, 87.
2. Baud FJ, Galliot M, Astier A *et al.* (1988) Treatment of ethylene glycol poisoning with intravenous 4-methylpyrazole. *N Engl J Med* **319**, 97.
3. Brent J, McMartin K, Phillips S *et al.* (1999) Fomepizole for the treatment of ethylene glycol poisoning. Methylpyrazole for Toxic Alcohols Study Group. *N Engl J Med* **340**, 832.
4. Gabow PA, Clay K, Sullivan JB, Lepoff R (1986) Organic acids in ethylene glycol intoxication. *Ann Intern Med* **105**, 16.
5. Goldfrank LR, Flomenbaum NE, Lewin NA, Howland MA (1990) Methanol, ethylene glycol, and isopropanol. In: *Toxicologic Emergencies. 4th Ed.* Goldfrank LR, Flomenbaum NE, Lewin NA *et al.* eds. Appleton & Lange, Norwalk, Connecticut p. 481.
6. Jacobsen D, McMartin KE (1986) Methanol and ethylene glycol poisonings: mechanism of toxicity, clinical course, diagnosis, and treatment. *Med Toxicol* **1**, 309.
7. Spillane L, Roberts JR, Meyer AE (1990) Multiple cranial nerve deficits after ethylene glycol poisoning. *Ann Emerg Med* **208**, 138.

Ethylene Oxide

Akio Ohnishi

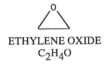

ETHYLENE OXIDE
C_2H_4O

1,2-Epoxyethane; Oxirane; Dimethylene oxide

NEUROTOXICITY RATING

Clinical

A Peripheral neuropathy
B Chronic encephalopathy (cognitive impairment)

Experimental

A Peripheral neuropathy

Ethylene oxide (EtO) (4,7) is produced by the direct oxidation of ethylene with air or oxygen over a catalyst. Its principal idustrial use is in the synthesis of ethylene glycol. EtO is also used to produce nonionic surfactants and to make polyethylene glycols, mixed polyglycols, glycol ethers, and other compounds. It is also used as a sterilant for medical and hospital supplies, and as a fumigant for furs and certain foods. The hazards associated with EtO stem from inhalation of vapor and contact of the eyes and skin with the liquid or solutions. When used as a sterilant or a fumigant, EtO is reported to cause peripheral neuropathy, seizures, and cognitive impairment.

EtO is a colorless gas or liquid with a MW of 44.05. Specific gravity is 0.8711 at 20°C. It is miscible with water, acetone, methanol, ether, benzene, and carbon tetrachloride. Its Threshold Exposure Limit, established by the American Conference of Governmental Industrial Hygienists, is 1 ppm (2 mg/m³); the principal hazard is mutagenicity and carcinogenicity (17).

General Toxicology

Hazards to health from EtO result from inhalation of the gas phase and contact of the eyes and skin with the liquid or solutions as dilute as 1%. EtO is a CNS depressant, an irritant, and a cytotoxin. The odor threshold is 700 ppm (9). EtO is highly reactive and alters many enzymatic reactions. After being absorbed into the cell, EtO undergoes hydrolysis to ethylene glycol, a compound that may cause cellular dysfunction. The metabolism and excretion of EtO are poorly understood (7,20). EtO is a potent respiratory irritant, and pulmonary edema may accompany high-level inhalation. Leukemia is reported in laboratory animals and humans exposed chronically to EtO. There is also evidence of adverse reproductive effects in humans and experimental animals exposed to EtO.

Animal Studies

High concentrations of EtO gas depress brain function. Concentrations exceeding 1000 ppm cause hindlimb weakness and death in various experimental animals (19). No detailed histopathological information is available on the effects of high-level EtO in the CNS, PNS, and skeletal muscles. Repeated (30–157 times) 7-h exposures to EtO gas at concentrations ranging from 204–400 ppm cause hindquarter weakness and decreased reflexes in dogs, rats, and monkeys (8,9). Histopathological examination of the CNS, PNS, and skeletal muscles was not performed in these studies. Rats exposed to moderately high concentrations of EtO gas (500 ppm) for 6 h three times a week for 13 weeks develop ataxia of the hindlimbs; histopathological study demonstrates distal axonal degeneration of myelinated fibers in hindleg nerves and in the fasciculus gracilis (13). Rats exposed by inhalation to 250 ppm EtO gas 6 h/day, five times a week for 9 months exhibit mild distal axonal degeneration of myelinated fibers in both hindleg nerves and the fasciculis gracilis; gait abnormality is not apparent (14). In addition, retardation of growth and maturation in the distal sural nerve is reported.

Rats exposed to EtO gas five times a week for 104 weeks developed skeletal muscle atrophy at an agent concentration of 100 ppm, but not 50 ppm, with no light microscopic changes in the sciatic nerve (11).

In Vitro Studies

Exposure of dorsal root ganglia cultures to an atmosphere containing 1 ppm EtO was followed by a 24-h period of normal axonal extension; varicosities and degeneration appeared after 48 h (20). This *in vitro* study is said to support the notion that small amounts of residual EtO in dialysis tubing have neurotoxic potential.

Human Studies

Short-term exposure to relatively high concentrations of EtO—mainly through accidents—seems to cause headache, vertigo, irritation with insomnia, convulsions, and loss of consciousness. Symptoms are reversible after termination of EtO exposure (15,18). Individuals exposed for long periods to EtO at variable, undetermined concentrations (months to years) experience mainly sensorimotor polyneuropathy (2,3,6,10,16). All cases have been engaged in sterilization work with EtO in a factory or hospital. An analysis of 12 cases from the literature reveals the following characteristics. In two, polyneuropathy developed within 3–5 months of exposure; they had been repeatedly exposed to EtO at concentrations of up to several hundred ppm. Other patients with a more insidious onset of polyneuropathy seem to have been exposed to approximately 10 ppm EtO. Initial symptoms included weakness, hypesthesia, and tingling sensations in the distal lower limbs, although the distal upper limbs were also involved in some. On neurological examination, 10 of 12 patients were weak and had decreased cutaneous sensations in the distal lower limbs. Ankle jerks were absent in nine and decreased in one of ten individuals. In two others—subjects who lacked weakness or decreased cutaneous sensations and who had normal ankle jerks—subclinical EtO polyneuropathy was determined from abnormalities of nerve conduction. Vibration sense was usually the most severely impaired sensory modality. Needle electromyography revealed neurogenic changes in 8 of 11 patients studied. Results of nerve conduction studies of limb nerves were abnormal in eight of ten patients. Relatively mild decreases in motor and sensory conduction velocities, with decreases in amplitude of nerve and muscle action potentials, suggesting axonal degeneration of both motor and sensory nerve fibers. Histopathological studies of the sural nerve in three individuals revealed mild abnormalities including decreased number of large myelinated fibers, presence of myelin ovoids and bands of Büngner (denervated columns of Schwann cells), and reduction of axonal circularity. Studies of cerebrospinal fluid in six individuals showed elevated protein levels in two (150 and 53 mg/dl). Both had histories of exposure to EtO at concentrations up to several hundred ppm. Most subjects with neuropathy improve after exposure to EtO ceases. In one report of three individuals, motor and sensory nerve conduction returned to normal and neurological function improved over a 4-year period (5).

One case report describes a woman who developed cognitive impairment and sensory loss following chronic low-level exposure to EtO (an 8-h time-weighted EtO average concentration of 2.4 ppm for 10 years) (1). In a cohort with long-term exposure to EtO (an 8-h time-weighted EtO average concentration of 3 to <1 ppm for 5–20 years), there was a dose-dependent decline in psychomotor performance and sural nerve conduction velocities (2). Therefore, impairments of cognitive function and hand-eye coordination may result from chronic exposure to EtO at levels encountered in hospital sterilization procedures. Prolonged exposure to EtO at an 8-h time-weighted EtO average concentration <10 ppm is documented in hospitals and companies that sterilize medical supplies (9). Short-term exposure to EtO at concentrations exceeding several hundred ppm may occasionally occur in accidents in factories where EtO is produced or in hospitals and companies that sterilize medical supplies.

The diagnosis of EtO neuropathy is established by a history of EtO exposure of concentration and duration sufficient to produce sensorimotor polyneuropathy with or without cognitive impairment, and improvement in symptoms after termination of EtO exposure. Analysis of EtO metabolites is not available for diagnostic purposes. There is no specific therapy. Most make a satifactory recovery within a year of termination of EtO exposure.

Toxic Mechanisms

The pathogenesis and biochemical basis of EtO neurotoxicity are unknown. EtO is completely soluble in water, and inhaled EtO is distributed to all organs via the circulation. Through alkylation, EtO reacts with virtually all cellular components, including proteins, vitamins, cofactors, DNA, and RNA (7). Distal axonal degeneration occurs in humans and rats both during and weeks after exposure to relatively low concentrations of EtO in the absence of apparent damage to other tissues. Fast axoplasmic transport is impaired in rats with neuropathy, which suggests the existence of a neuron-specific target for EtO (12). Results of tissue culture studies suggest involvement of a protein or other molecule synthesized in the cell body and transported to the growing axon for insertion into new membranes (20).

REFERENCES

1. Crystal HA, Schaumburg HH, Grober E *et al.* (1988) Cognitive impairment and sensory loss associated with chronic low-level ethylene oxide exposure. *Neurology* 38, 567.

2. Estrin WJ, Cavalieri SA, Wald P *et al.* (1987) Evidence of neurologic dysfunction related to long-term ethylene oxide exposure. *Arch Neurol* 44, 1283.

3. Finelli PF, Morgan TF, Yaar I, Granger CV (1983) Ethylene oxide-induced polyneuropathy. A clinical and electrophysiologic study. *Arch Neurol* 40, 419.

4. Glaser ZR (1979) Ethylene oxide: Toxicology review and field study results of hospital use. *J Environ Pathol Toxicol* 2, 173.

5. Greenberg MK, Swift TR (1982) Ethylene oxide peripheral neuropathy. Four-year following-up. *Muscle Nerve* 5, 557.

6. Gross JA, Haas ML, Swift TR (1979) Ethylene oxide neurotoxicity: Report of four cases and review of the literature. *Neurology* 29, 978.

7. Hine C, Rowe VK, White ER *et al.* (1981) Epoxy compounds. In: *Patty's Industrial Hygiene and Toxicology. 3rd Ed.* Clayton GD, Clayton FE eds. John Wiley & Sons, New York p. 2141.

8. Hollingworth RL, Rowe VK, Oyen F *et al.* (1956) Toxicity of ethylene oxide determined on experimental animals. *Arch Ind Health* 13, 217.

9. Jacobsen KH, Hackley EB, Feinsilver L (1956) The toxicity of inhaled ethylene oxide and propylene oxide vapors. *Arch Ind Health* 13, 237.

10. Kuzuhara S, Kanazawa I, Nakanishi T, Egashira T (1983) Ethylene oxide polyneuropathy. *Neurology* 33, 377.

11. Lynch DW, Lewis TR, Moorman WJ *et al.* (1984) Carcinogenic and toxicologic effects of inhaled ethylene oxide and propylene oxide in F344 rats. *Toxicol Appl Pharmacol* 76, 69.

12. Nagata H, Ohkoshi N, Kanazawa I *et al.* (1992) Rapid axonal transport velocity is reduced in experimental ethylene oxide neuropathy. *Mol Chem Neuropathol* 17, 209.

13. Ohnishi A, Inoue N, Yamamoto T *et al.* (1985) Ethylene oxide induces central-peripheral distal axonal degeneration of the lumbar primary sensory neurones in rats. *Brit J Ind Med* 42, 373.

14. Ohnishi A, Inoue N, Yamamoto T *et al.* (1986) Ethylene oxide neuropathy in rats. Exposure to 250 ppm. *J Neurol Sci* 74, 215.

15. Salinas E, Sasich L, Hall DH *et al.* (1981) Acute ethylene oxide intoxication. *Drug Intell Clin Pharm* 15, 384.

16. Schröder JM, Hoheneck M, Weis J, Deist H (1985) Ethylene oxide polyneuropathy: Clinical follow-up study with morphometric and electron microscopic findings in a sural nerve biopsy. *J Neurol* 232, 83.

17. Sheikh K (1984) Adverse health effects of ethylene oxide and occupational exposure limits. *Amer J Ind Med* 6, 117.

18. Thiess AM (1963) Beobachtungen über Gesundheits schädigungen durch Einwirkung von Äthylenoxyd. *Arch Toxicol* 20, 127.

19. Walker WJG, Greeson CE (1932) The toxicity of ethylene oxide. *J Hyg* 32, 409.

20. Windebank AJ, Blexrud MD (1989) Residual ethylene oxide in hollow fiber hemodialysis units is neurotoxic *in vitro. Ann Neurol* 26, 63.

CASE REPORT

A 21-year-old man first noticed paresthesias in his feet in March 1977, 6 months after he had started loading and unloading medical sterilizers (10). Subsequently, tingling and weakness of the hands developed, along with a staggering gait. Examination was performed in April 1977. There was moderate weakness of distal limb muscles without wasting; tendon reflexes were normal and plantar responses were flexor. Touch, pain, temperature, and vibration sense were mildly decreased symmetrically in the distal limbs, but position sense was normal.

Cerebrospinal fluid examination was normal. Results of an electromyographic examination of the limb muscles were normal except that long-duration and high-amplitude motor unit potentials were recorded in the triceps. Motor nerve conduction velocities were 48.2 m/sec in the right median nerve and 35.2 m/sec in the right superficial peroneal nerve. Sensory nerve conduction velocities were 44.7 m/sec in the distal sural nerve and 56.2 m/sec in the distal median nerve. Biopsies of left sural nerve and gastrocnemius muscle were performed on May 6. Teased fiber preparations of the sural nerve showed linear rows of myelin ovoids. A mild decrease of large myelinated fibers was observed in epoxy sections. Myelin figures and bands of Büngner were apparent. Histochemical studies of the gastrocnemius muscle showed atrophic fibers of both types 1 and 2, scattered or grouped, and target fibers. No necrotic fibers or inflammatory changes were found. Symptoms resolved 1 month later.

The work environment in the factory was as follows. The workers smelled gas for several minutes when the door of the sterilizer was open, indicating a concentration of >700 ppm. An EtO gas monitor automatically started a ventilator when the level exceeded 50 ppm, the Japanese 8-h time-weighted average standard. The ventilator operated twice a day for 40 min during each loading and unloading period. No information on concentrations of EtO in the work room were available.

Comment

This is a typical example of a patient with mild reversible sensorimotor axonal neuropathy caused by long-term exposure to EtO. Ventilation of the room was improved after intoxication was diagnosed.

Euphorbia Spp.

Thomas Meyer
Albert C. Ludolph

NEUROTOXICITY RATING

Clinical

B   Peripheral neuropathy

B   Afferent terminal irritation

Experimental

A   Ion channel dysfunction

A   Afferent terminal irritation

Euphorbia comprises a large number of species that all contain an irritant latex; the effects of the latex are only partly destroyed by drying. The white, milky sap causes severe blistering and intense pain when in contact with open cuts, mouth, and the eyes. The therapeutic potential of *Euphorbia* spp. was known and used at the time of the reign of the Roman Emperor Augustus (1); this included applications as a nose (to provoke sneezing) and skin irritant, and later as a purgative. The first medical use of *Euphorbia* was direct application on dental cavities to suppress chronic tooth pain (1). The active principle of *Euphorbia resinifera*, resiniferatoxin, was isolated in 1975 (3). This compound proved to be a capsaicin analogue (*see* Capsaicin and Analogues, this volume).

If horses, cattle, sheep, cats, dogs, or humans ingest *Euphorbia* spp., severe irritation of the mouth and gastrointestinal tract with vomiting, abdominal pain, and diarrhea results (1,2). Some reports of lethal poisonings in animals exist. Following topical application, resiniferatoxin interacts with a subset of primary sensory neurons and causes desensitization of vanilloid receptors. This is linked with the opening of an associated ion channel, which may explain the local irritation (4). Specific desensitization of receptor-associated pain pathways may be an approach to mitigate neurogenic pain. Although they contain pharmacologically potent compounds, systemic neurotoxicity of *Euphorbia* spp. is not reported. Major differences between species exist, and most of the widely cultivated plants [such as *Euphorbia pulcherrima* (Poinsettie, Poinsettia), Weihnachtsstern, or *Codiaeum variegatum*] seem to be considerably less harmful than *Euphorbium resinifera* (2).

REFERENCES

1. Appendino G, Szallasi A (1997) *Euphorbium*: Modern research on its active principle, resiniferatoxin, revives an ancient medicine. *Life Sci* **60**, 681.
2. Frohne D, Pfaender HJ (1986) Giftpflanzen. In: *Handbuch für Apotheker, Ärzte, Toxikologen und Biologen. 3. Auflage.* Wissenschaftliche Verlagsgesellscahft mbH, Stuttgart.
3. Hergenhahn M, Adolph W, Hecker E (1975) Diterpene esters from *Euphorbium* and their irritant and co-carcinogenic activity. *Tetrahedron Lett* **19**, 1595.
4. Szallasi A, Blumberg PM (1990) Specific binding of resiniferatoxin, an ultrapotent capsaicin analog, by dorsal root ganglia membranes. *Brain Res* **524**, 106.

Fasciculins

Albert C. Ludolph

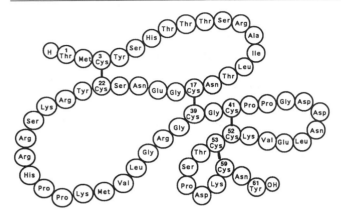

FASCICULIN

NEUROTOXICITY RATING

Clinical

A Neuromuscular transmission syndrome

Experimental

A Neuromuscular transmission dysfunction (acetylcholinesterase inhibition)

Fasciculins 1 (FAS1) and 2 (FAS2, synonym, toxin F_7) occur in green mamba (*Dendroaspis angusticeps*) snake venom; they bind to acetylcholinesterases and cause lethal impairment of neuromuscular transmission (3,9,10). Toxin C from *D. polylepis* (black mamba) venom is a homologous protein identical with another fasciculin (FAS3) isolated from *D. polylepis* venom (7). A fourth toxin has been isolated from *D. viridis* (1). The 57–61 polypeptide chains are cross-linked by four disulfide bonds (5).

Fasciculins bind irreversibly to acetylcholinesterase. Enzyme inhibition persists for days after injection of fasciculin into rat amygdala (8). Fasciculins bind to a peripheral regulatory anionic site of the enzyme by multipoint attachment; they do not interact with the catalytic site of the enzyme. Organophosphorus compounds, which phosphorylate the catalytic site, do not affect fasciculin binding (2,7). Amplitudes of end-plate potentials and miniature end-plate potentials are increased after application of fasciculins (10).

Rats and mice display generalized severe fasciculations and paralysis of skeletal muscles (6,9). Mamba venom also contains dendrotoxin, which increases presynaptic transmitter release from peripheral and central synapses by blocking voltage-sensitive potassium channels. The combi-nation of acetylcholinesterase inhibition, increased presynaptic release of acetylcholine, and the high acetylcholine content of mamba toxin (6–24 mg/g) (4) increases the lethal neurotoxic effect of the venom in humans. The human clinical profile includes ophthalmoplegia, ptosis, bulbar symptoms and, finally, flaccid tetraplegia and respiratory paralysis (*see also Dendroaspis angusticeps* Toxins, this volume).

REFERENCES

1. Cervenansky C, Dajas F, Harvey AL, Karlsson E (1991) Fasciculins, anticholinesterase toxins from mamba venoms: Biochemistry and pharmacology. In: *Snake Toxins.* Harvey AL ed. Pergamon Press, New York p. 303.

2. Duran R, Cervenansky C, Dajas F, Tipton KF (1994) Fasciculin inhibition of acetylcholinesterase is prevented by chemical modification of the enzyme at a peripheral site. *Biochim Biophys Acta* **1201**, 381.

3. Hawgood B, Bon C (1991) Snake venom presynaptic toxins. In: *Handbook of Natural Toxins. Vol 5. Reptile Venoms and Toxins.* Tu AT ed. Marcel Dekker, New York p. 3.

4. Karlsson E, Cervenansky, Jolkkonen M (1990) Chemistry of mamba toxins. *Toxicon* **28**, 154.

5. Le Du MH, Marchot P, Bougis PE, Fontecilla-Camps JC (1992) 1.9-Å resolution structure of fasciculin 1, an anticholinesterase toxin from green mamba snake venom. *J Biol Chem* **267**, 12122.

6. Lee CY, Lee SY, Chen YM (1986) A study on the cause of death produced by *angusticeps*-type toxin F7 isolated from eastern green mamba venom. *Toxicon* **24**, 33.

7. Marchot B, Khelif A, Ji YH *et al.* (1993) Binding of ^{125}I-fasciculin to rat brain acetylcholinesterase. The complex still binds diisopropyl fluorophosphate. *J Biol Chem* **268**, 12458.

8. Quillfeldt J, Raskovsky S, Dalmaz C *et al.* (1990) Bilateral injection of fasciculin into the amygdala of rats: Effects on two avoidance tasks, acetylcholinesterase activity, and cholinergic muscarinic receptors. *Pharmacol Biochem Behav* **37**, 439.

9. Rodriguez-Ithurralde D, Silveira R, Barbeito L, Dajas F (1983) Fasciculin, a powerful anticholinesterase polypeptide from *Dendroaspis angusticeps* venom. *Neurochem Int* **5**, 267.

10. Tu AT (1994) Neurotoxins from snake venoms. In: *Handbook of Neurotoxicology*, Chang LW, Dyer RS eds. Marcel Dekker, New York p. 637.

Fentanyl

John C.M. Brust

FENTANYL
$C_{22}H_{28}N_2O$

N-Phenyl-N-[1-(2-phenylethyl)-4-piperidinyl]propanamide

NEUROTOXICITY RATING

Clinical

A   Acute encephalopathy (sedation, coma, apnea)

A   Physical dependence and withdrawal

C   Chronic encephalopathy (persistent behavioral and cognitive disturbance)

Experimental

A   Opioid agonist

A   CNS depression

Fentanyl is a synthetic opioid agonist structurally similar to but more potent than meperidine; 100 μg of fentanyl are roughly equivalent to 10 mg morphine or 75 mg meperidine (6). As an anesthetic, it is available for parenteral use, sometimes combined with the neuroleptic droperidol. Commercially available related agents include sufentanil and alfentanyl. Fentanyl is classified by the U.S. Food and Drug Administration as a Schedule II drug ("high potential for abuse, currently accepted medical use").

Fentanyl undergoes considerable first-pass clearance by the liver; metabolites and small amounts of unchanged drug are excreted in the urine. The elimination half-life is 3–4 h. When given intravenously, fentanyl's onset of action is almost immediate, peaking after several minutes and lasting 30–60 min after a single 100-μg dose. Onset of action commences minutes after intramuscular injection and lasts 1–2 h.

Fentanyl's clinical effects are similar to those of morphine: analgesia, euphoria, narcosis, miosis, and respiratory depression (*see* Morphine and Related Opiates, this volume). It is less emetic, and respiratory depression often outlasts analgesia (with reduced respiratory response to CO_2 outlasting decreased respiratory rate). Maximal respiratory depression occurs 5–15 min after an intravenous dose.

High doses cause muscle rigidity that can interfere with surgery; the mechanism is unclear. Rigidity responds to naloxone; neuromuscular-blocking agents can be used without reversing desired opioid effects.

When combined with droperidol, fentanyl may provoke postoperative shivering and restlessness, hallucinations, akathesia, dystonia, tremor, and oculogyric crisis; these manifestations last up to 24 h and symptoms usually respond to anticholinergic agents.

Signs of fentanyl overdose include coma, pinpoint (but reactive) pupils, and apnea. Treatment, as with other opioid agonists, includes respiratory support and naloxone (which, however, has a much shorter duration of action than that of fentanyl, often necessitating repeated doses). Overdose with fentanyl plus droperidol is especially likely to cause bradycardia and hypotension.

Use of fentanyl as a spinal analgesic seems to have a low potential for neurotoxicity (6).

Fentanyl is abused recreationally by health care professionals (10). In the late 1970s, deaths occurred among southern California drug users who thought they were injecting high-grade "China White" heroin but had actually been sold a fentanyl analog, α-methyl-fentanyl (1). Abuse of this and other fentanyl derivatives spread throughout the southwest United States. By the 1980s, fentanyl "designer drugs" (at least ten varieties made street appearances) were being taken by an estimated 20% of California's 100,000 "heroin" addicts; usually injected intravenously, they were sometimes snorted (3,4,8). Use then declined in the western United States but, during the late 1980s and early 1990s, miniepidemics of sometimes fatal fentanyl analog overdose (called "Tango and Cash" in New York City) occurred in the eastern United States (2,5,9).

REFERENCES

1. Ayres WA, Starsiak MJ, Sokolay P (1981) The bogus drug: 3-Ethyl and alpha-methyl fentanyl sold as "China White." *J Psychoactive Drug* **13**, 91.

2. Brust JCM (1993) *Neurological Aspects of Substance Abuse.* Butterworth-Heinemann, Stoneham, Massachusetts p. 37.

3. Carroll FL, Boldt KG, Huang PT *et al.* (1990) Synthesis of fentanyl analogs. In: *Problems of Drug Dependence 1989.* Harris LS ed. Natl Inst Drug Abuse Research Monograph 95. U.S. Department of Human Health Services, Rockville, Maryland p. 497.

4. Henderson GL (1988) Designer Drugs: Past history and future prospects. *J Forensic Sci* **33**, 569.

5. Hibbs J, Perper J, Winek CL (1991) An outbreak of de-

signer drug-related deaths in Pennsylvania. *J Amer Med Assn* **265**, 1011.

6. Hodgson PS, Neal JM, Pollock JE, Liu SS (1999) The neurotoxicity of drugs given intrathecally (spinal). *Anesth Analg* **88**, 797.

7. Jaffe JH, Martin WR (1990) Opioid analgesics and antagonists. In: *The Pharmacological Basis of Therapeutics. 8th Ed.* Gilman AG, Rall TW, Nies AS, Taylor P eds. Pergamon Press, New York p. 485.

8. LaBarbera M, Wolfe T (1983) Characteristics, attitudes, and implications of fentanyl use based on reports from self-identified fentanyl users. *J Psychoactive Drug* **15**, 293.

9. Martin M, Hecker J, Clark R *et al.* (1991) China White epidemic: An eastern United States emergency department experience. *Ann Emerg Med* **20**, 158.

10. Silsby HD, Kruzich DJ, Hawkins MR (1984) Fentanyl citrate abuse among health care professionals. *Milit Med* **149**, 227.

Flecainide and Other Class Ic Antiarrhythmic Agents

Steven A. Sparr

FLECAINIDE
$C_{17}H_{20}F_6N_2O_3$

N-(2-Piperidinylmethyl)-2,5-bis(2,2,2-trifluoroethoxy)benzamide

NEUROTOXICITY RATING

Clinical

A Acute encephalopathy (dizziness, sedation, blurred vision)

A Headache

B Acute encephalopathy (encainide)

Flecainide is a benzamide derivative with local anesthetic properties and class Ic cardiac antiarrhythmic effects. Flecainide and other drugs in this class (including encainide, lorcainide, and propafenone) slow conduction in atrial, nodal, and ventricular conductive tissues, while minimally affecting refractoriness (19). All are highly effective in treating ventricular and supraventricular arrhythmias (15). The use of class Ic antiarrhythmics, however, has been severely curtailed since 1989 after the demonstration of excess mortality in post–myocardial infarction patients treated with these agents in the Cardiac Arrhythmia Suppression Trial (CAST) described below (2). These drugs are recommended only for treatment of patients with life-threatening arrhythmias and in patients with supraventricular arrhythmias without underlying organic heart disease (12).

Flecainide may be administered intravenously and is well absorbed after oral administration. Plasma concentration peaks 2–3 h after oral ingestion. Elimination half-life is 10–18 h, allowing for twice-daily dosing (9). The drug is eliminated by the kidneys unchanged and is metabolized by the liver to inactive or less active metabolites that are excreted primarily by the kidneys. Thus, elimination half-life increases markedly in patients with severe renal disease. Flecainide is widely distributed throughout the body, including the heart, but has poor penetration into the CNS (9).

Toxicity of class Ic agents is primarily cardiac and neurological. Pooled data from 80 published reports of patients treated with flecainide showed side effects in 7% of 695 subjects, including worsening of ventricular arrhythmias, conduction disturbances and, infrequently, congestive heart failure (1). A similar profile of cardiac toxicity was noted in a review of the literature on encainide (19) and with propafenone (3). CAST, conducted by the U.S. National Heart, Lung and Blood Institute was a randomized, double-blind study of the efficacy of class 1c agents (flecainide and encainide) in patients 2 days to 2 years after myocardial infarction with asymptomatic ventricular ectopy (2). Although these agents were effective in suppressing ventricular ectopy, those treated with class 1c agents showed a significant increase in mortality (7.7% *vs.* 3% at 10 months) principally due to an increase in sudden cardiac death (2,12). Risk of death was highest in those with multiple previous myocardial infarctions. This study has been interpreted to imply that class 1c antiarrhythmics can have significant proarrhythmic toxicity in the setting of cardiac ischemia or pump failure (12). As a result, these agents are now recommended only for patients with life-threatening arrhythmias or for supraventicular arrhythmias or symptomatic premature ventricular contractions in patients without underlying organic heart disease (12). Consequently, encainide was voluntarily withdrawn from the market by its manufacturer, and the use of flecainide has greatly diminished (12).

The major extracardiac side effects of class 1c agents are neurological. They include dizziness, visual disturbances, headache, fatigue, tremor, and paresthesias. These effects are usually mild and often respond to dose reduction but may lead to discontinuation of therapy (15). There are no animal models for neurological toxicity, although animals given large doses of flecainide develop ataxia, vomiting, and seizures (9). Flecainide has been shown to accumulate in pigmented ocular tissues, but the relationship of this finding to ocular toxicity is speculative (9).

The most common side effect of class 1c agents is dizziness. Loosely defined, dizziness includes symptoms of lightheadedness, faintness, near syncope, and visual blurring (4–6). In a multicenter trial of flecainide vs. quinidine, dizziness was reported in 30% of 141 patients treated with flecainide short-term (2 weeks) and 32% of 280 patients treated long-term (up to 6 months); medication was discontinued in 2%–4% of patients (5). Dizziness tends to be intermittent and dose-related, and has been attributed to a poorly defined effect on the CNS (9). Similar symptoms are described in patients treated with encainide (7,16,17,19), lorcainide (20), or propafenone (11).

Visual disturbances frequently complicate treatment with class 1c agents and often occur concurrently with symptoms of dizziness. Visual symptoms include blurred vision, and flashing lights and spots before the eyes; they occur in 28% of patients treated with flecainide short-term and 30% of those treated long-term, causing discontinuation of therapy in 3% (5). Similar symptoms are reported by patients treated with encainide (4,8).

Headache is experienced by about 10% of patients treated with flecainide (5,6) or encainide (19). Symptoms are usually mild and often respond to reduction of dosage. Rarely is headache cause for discontinuation of therapy (5).

Other less common neurological side effects of flecainide include fatigue (5%–6%), tremor (4%), and tinnitus (3%)—all usually mild (5). Paresthesias or hypesthesia affecting the distal extremities or perioral region are reported by 1%–3% of patients receiving flecainide (1,9). Vivid dreams, insomnia, and other forms of sleep disturbance are reported with various class Ic agents (9,20).

A single instance of dysarthria associated with formed visual hallucinations was reported in a patient with supratherapeutic serum levels of flecainide (14); symptoms promptly resolved with discontinuation of the drug. Another patient experienced hallucinations while on flecainide therapy, but these may have been related to alcohol withdrawal (13).

A single case of tardive dystonia commenced 3 days after initiation of flecainide therapy (10). Manifestations included chewing movements, facial grimacing, and masseter muscle spasm requiring botulinum toxin injections.

A patient with renal failure treated with standard doses of encainide developed an encephalopathy with memory disturbance, agitation, and confusion associated with asterixis (18). Symptoms improved with discontinuation of the medication and recurred with rechallenge. The author recommended decreased dosages for patients in renal failure to avoid toxicity.

Class 1c antiarrhythmics act by blocking fast sodium channels in cardiac conducting tissues, reducing the rate of rise of the phase 0 action potential and slowing conduction through the atrioventricular node and Purkinje fibers (6). These drugs do not significantly affect repolarization time. Thus, they prolong PR and QRS intervals on the electrocardiogram (depolarization) but have minimal effect on JT interval (repolarization) (15). Class Ic agents have little effect on refractoriness in normal conducting tissues but markedly increase refractoriness in retrograde anomolous pathways, making these drugs useful in the treatment of Wolf-Parkinson-White syndrome (15). These agents have been used to suppress premature ventricular contractions and other ventricular arrhythmias, as well as supraventricular arrhythmias such as paroxysmal supraventricular tachycardia and atrial fibrillation/flutter (9).

REFERENCES

1. Anderson JL, Jolivette DM, Fredell PA (1988) Summary of efficacy and safety of flecainide for supraventricular arrhythmias. *Amer J Cardiol* **62**, 62D.

2. CAST Investigators (1989) Preliminary report: Effect of encainide and flecainide on mortality in a randomized trial of arrhythmia suppression after myocardial infarction. *N Engl J Med* **321**, 406.

3. Chimienti M, Cullen MT, Casadel G (1996) Safety of long-term flecainide and propafenone in the management of patients with symptomatic paroxysmal atrial fibrillation: Report from the Flecainide and Propafenone Italian Study Investigators. *Amer J Cardiol* **77**, 60A.

4. DiBianco R, Fletcher RD, Cohen AI *et al.* (1982) Treatment of frequent arrhythmia with encainide: Assessment using serial ambulatory electrocardiograms, intracardiac electrophysiologic studies, treadmill exercise tests, and radionuclide cineangiographic studies. *Circulation* **65**, 1134.

5. Gentzkow GD, Sullivan JY (1984) Extracardiac adverse effects of flecainide. *Amer J Cardiol* **53**, 101B.

6. Hodges M, Salerno DM, Granrud G *et al.* (1984) Flecainide versus quinidine: Results of a multicenter trial. *Amer J Cardiol* **53**, 66B.

7. Kesteloot H, Stroobandt R (1979) Clinical experience of encainide (MJ 9067): A new antiarrhythmic drug. *Eur J Clin Pharmacol* **16**, 323.

8. Kunze KP, Kuck KH, Schlutter M *et al.* (1982) Electrophysiologic and clinical effects of intravenous and oral encainide in accessory arterioventricular pathway. *Amer J Cardiol* **54**, 323.

9. McEvoy GK (1995) *American Hospital Formulary Service Drug Information.* Amer Soc Hlth System Pharmacists p. 1094.

10. Miller LG, Jankovic J (1992) Persistent dystonia possibly induced by flecainide. *Movement Disord* 7, 62.

11. Morike K, Magadum S, Mettang T *et al.* (1995) Propafenone in the usual dose produces severe side-effects: The impact of genetically determined metabolic status on drug therapy. *J Intern Med* 238, 4692.

12. Naccarelli GV, Doughtery AH, Jalal S *et al.* (1992) Cardiac Arrhythmia Suppression Trial (CAST): Interpretation of the findings and effect on drug development and prescribing practices. *Hosp Formul* 27, 792.

13. Neuss H, Schlepper M (1988) Long-term efficacy and safety of flecainide for supraventricular tachycardia. *Amer J Cardiol* 62, 56D.

14. Ramhamadany E, Mackenzie S, Ramsdale DR (1986) Dysarthria and visual hallucinations due to flecainide toxicity. *Postgrad Med J* 62, 61.

15. Roden DM (1996) Antiarrhythmic drugs. In: *The Pharmacologic Basis of Therapeutics. 9th Ed.* Hardman JG, Goodman AG, Limbird LE eds. McGraw-Hill, New York p. 839.

16. Sami M, Harrison DC, Kraemer H *et al.* (1981) Antiarrhythmic efficacy of encainide and quinidine: Validation of a model of drug assessment. *Amer J Cardiol* 48, 147.

17. Soyka LF (1988) Safety considerations and dosing guidelines for encainide in supraventricular arrhythmias. *Amer J Cardiol* 62, 63L.

18. Tartini A, Keselbrenner M (1990) Encainide-induced encephalopathy in a patient with chronic renal failure. *Amer J Kidney Dis* 15, 178.

19. Tordjman T, Estes NA (1987) Encainide: Its electrophysiologic and antiarrhythmic effects, pharmacokinetics, and safety. *Pharmacotherapy* 7, 149.

20. Vlay SC, Mallis GI (1986) Intravenous and oral lorcainide: Assessment of central nervous system toxicity and antiarrhythmic efficacy. *Amer Heart J* 111, 452.

Fludarabine

Mark F. Mehler

FLUDARABINE
$C_{10}H_{12}FN_5O_4$

9-β-D-Arabinofuranosyl-2-fluoro-9H-purin-6-amine

NEUROTOXICITY RATING
Clinical
A   Leukoencephalopathy (diffuse)
A   Cerebellar syndrome
A   Acute encephalopathy (confusion, sedation)

Fludarabine is a fluorinated purine analog of the antiviral agent vidarabine. The antimetabolite is used in the treatment of lymphoproliferative malignancies, including chronic lymphocytic leukemia, prolymphocytic leukemia, and advanced low-grade non-Hodgkin's lymphoma associated with follicular pathology (8,16). The drug is also useful as a salvage agent (with cytarabine) for acute leukemias, and in the treatment of Waldenström's macroglobulinemia and mycosis fungoides (15). In culture or tumor models, fludarabine has been shown to be active against non-Hodgkin's lymphoma, leukemia, non–small cell carcinoma of the lung, and ovarian cancer. The antineoplastic agent is virtually inactive against solid tumors (8). The main cellular action of fludarabine is to terminate DNA or RNA synthesis by incorporation into elongating nucleotide chains (15). In addition, the compound can inhibit the enzyme activities of DNA and RNA polymerase, DNA primase, DNA ligase, and ribonucleotide reductase (16).

Fludarabine monophosphate is dephosphorylated and converted *via* deoxycytidine kinase to the metabolite 9β arabinofuranosyl-2-fluoroadenine (F-Ara-A) within 5 min of intravenous infusion (15). The drug is transported to the cell and exists in its active form, F-Ara-A-triphosphate (15). After a rapid intravenous drug bolus, there is a brief deposition phase ($t_{1/2}$ = 5 min), an intermediate phase ($t_{1/2}$ = 1–2 h), and a prolonged terminal elimination phase ($t_{1/2}$ = 10–30 h). Continuous infusion results in two elimination phases. Following bolus injection, 60% of the drug is excreted in the urine in 24 h. After a 30-min continuous infusion, $37 \pm 5\%$ of the drug is excreted in the urine within 24 h, and $57 \pm 7\%$ within 72 h. Dosage schedules include

30 mg/m^2/day for 3 days with 4-week cycles, or once per week for 4 weeks at the same dose levels. Lower response rates have been recorded with the weekly regimen. It is thought that clinical efficacy is correlated with the presence of minimal critical values of plasma F-ara-A concentration maintained for 3 consecutive days. The median peak F-ara-adenosine triphosphate (ATP) concentrations are proportional to the infusion dose in a fludarabine concentration range of 20–125 mg/m^2. F-ara-ATP, the long-lived active metabolite, has a monophasic elimination profile, with a half-life of several hours to several days (median, 15 h).

Fludarabine demonstrates a bioavailability of 70% following oral administration (9). After oral administration, the mean peak plasma concentration is 0.9 μmol/l at 1.5 h (t$_{max}$). However, the mean peak plasma concentration 30 min after intravenous infusion exceeds the oral value by threefold (3.4 μmol/l). Both routes of administration result in triexponential elimination kinetics, with equivalent terminal half-lives (31–32 h). Intracellular pharmacokinetics (F-ara-ATP), including peak concentrations and mean elimination half-lives, are also similar following oral or intravenous administration (14). The volumes of distribution are 44.2–96.2 vs. 10.8 l/m^2, and the plasma rates of clearance are 4.1 and 9.1 vs. 0.7 l/h/m^2 (15).

F-ara-ATP competes with deoxyATP for DNA incorporation, and this correlates with the degree of cytotoxicity. The anti-metabolite is more effective at DNA chain termination than cytarabine (15). The drug also exhibits a resistance to DNA proofreading activities (DNA polymerases) and is capable of inhibiting DNA primase (necessary for RNA primer-dependent inhibition of DNA synthesis) (15). With DNA ligase, the antineoplastic agent inhibits processing at two distinct steps: inhibition of the ligase–adenosine monophosphate complex, and inhibition of reactions at the 3′-terminus (13). The inhibition of RNA synthesis is dependent on the cellular concentrations of F-ara-ATP (88% efficacy on RNA polymerase II). Apoptosis of lymphocytes occurs after 24–72 h incubations in vitro. DNA cleavage is time- and dose-dependent, and these pathological effects are independent of the actions of the drug on DNA and RNA synthesis.

The principal toxic effects of the drug are severe myelosuppression, tumor lysis syndrome, pneumonitis, nausea and vomiting, and reversible neurotoxicity (15,17). Sustained adverse reactions necessitate a reduction in drug dose, a delay in administration, or frank withdrawal. Initial dose reductions are required for patients with creatinine clearance values <3 l/h, or in elderly patients with reduced bone marrow reserves (11,15). Lymphocytopenia usually develops rapidly (mean to nadir, 6 days), often is reversible

in 3 weeks, and T lymphocytes are more dramatically affected than B lymphocytes (90% vs. 50%).

Fludarabine enhances the antitumor activity of gallium nitrate, cytarabine, cisplatin, and mitoxantrone, and also demonstrates dose- and schedule-dependent radiosensitization (15). The synergistic interactions with radiotherapy are maximized by pretreatment with fludarabine (24 h), and the enhanced efficacy appears to be related to S-phase cell loss and tumor synchronization. When coadministered with cytarabine, fludarabine increases the therapeutic response profile in acute myelogenous leukemia (15). Sequential administration of fludarabine, cytarabine, and mitoxantrone results in a significant increase in the rate of complete remissions in acute lymphocytic leukemia, acute myelogenous leukemia, and chronic myelogenous leukemia. The combination of fludarabine, cytarabine, and cisplatin is the most effective therapeutic regimen for refractory cases of chronic lymphocytic leukemia (15). Fludarabine, when used with doxorubicin and prednisone, enhances the therapeutic responses in chronic lymphocytic leukemia and indolent lymphomas. Fludarabine with mitoxantrone and dexamethasone potentiate the response rate for follicular lymphoma (15). Finally, when combined with cytarabine and granulocyte colony-stimulating factor, fludarabine enhances the cytarabine-induced cytotoxic effects on myelodysplastic syndromes and in acute myelogenous leukemia.

High-dose fludarabine administered to mice implanted with leukemia L1210 resulted in neurotoxicity initially associated with hindlimb paralysis. This clinical syndrome eventually proved to be fatal. Coadministration of the 5′-phosphate of nitrobenzylthioinosine (NBMPR-P), a potent inhibitor of the equilibrative nucleoside transport system, reduced the incidence of the neurotoxicity (1). Coapplication also increased the fractional yield of mice that qualified as having been "cured" of leukemic involvement.

At standard doses, fludarabine causes neurotoxicity in approximately 15% of patients (7,12). The clinical manifestations may include confusion, agitation, coma, visual disturbances, headache, hearing loss, depression, incoordination, and peripheral nerve dysfunction with objective motor and sensory signs (2,15). These neurological signs and symptoms are often mild and ususally reversible (2). At high drug doses, severe and life-threatening neurotoxic syndromes are encountered. These clinical syndromes are occasionally delayed and often partially reversible. Severe progressive CNS demyelination is seen in one-third of patients treated with high-dose fludarabine (15). The clinical syndrome is encountered from 21–60 days after initiation of the last course of therapy and is associated with visual field deficits and mental status changes, progressing to coma and death (15). Pathological examination reveals diffuse demyelination of the brain and spinal cord with preferential involvement of the optic tracts. This clinical syndrome has occurred in acute leukemia, with a treatment regimen consisting of fludarabine doses in excess of 90 mg/m^2/day for 5 days. CNS demyelination with life-threatening consequences is also seen using low-dose fludarabine administration for treatment of acute leukemia and mycosis fungoides. In addition, there is the report of a case of uncertain significance in which a patient with chronic lymphocytic leukemia treated with standard-dose fludarabine developed severe neurological symptoms 6 months after termination of a six-cycle course of monotherapy (6,18). This patient, in clinical remission at the time, developed rapidly progressive cerebral dysfunction associated with mental status changes, including apraxia, agraphia, acalculia, and a slowly evolving hemiparesis with hemisensory involvement. Neuroimaging revealed subcortical white matter lesions and biopsy revealed the presence of progressive multifocal leukoencephalopathy. The patient progressed to irreversible coma in 2 weeks, and pathological examination confirmed the absence of CNS lymphoma.

In 6 of 62 patients treated for non-Hodgkin's lymphoma with standard-dose fludarabine (18 mg/m^2/day for 5 days), grade 3 neurotoxicity developed that was reversible with cessation of therapy (15). A similar clinical spectrum was seen in patients treated for chronic lymphocytic leukemia and mycosis fungoides. The occurrence of a listeria abcess has also been recorded for a patient treated with fludarabine for chronic lymphocytic leukemia (5). In patients treated with both cytarabine and fludarabine, the risk of developing a neurotoxic syndrome may be increased. In addition, the clinical syndrome may be more severe and involve additional neuroanatomical sites. In two of eight patients treated with both antineoplastic agents, a syndrome characterized by severe, progressive cerebellar dysfunction developed, and eventually proved to be fatal (10). Combination therapy is also associated with the occurrence of a myelopathy and a peripheral neuropathy (13). Therefore, the current recommendations for monotherapy with fludarabine consist of a regimen of 25 mg/m^2, administered over 30 min for 5 days. Lower doses or longer treatment intervals are associated with excess hematological and nonhematological toxicity. Three additional courses of treatment after attainment of the maximal response are recommended. In addition, oral drug administration may decrease morbidity in elderly patients.

The mechanisms of neurotoxicity with fludarabine are not known (3). Because fludarabine is capable of exerting its cytotoxicity by a spectrum of cellular actions on DNA and RNA synthesis, it may cause direct toxic effects on vulnerable neural progenitor cell species (4,15). The profile of clinical involvement in humans suggests that fludarabine may preferentially target regional oligodendroglial species and developing neuronal progenitor and maturing cellular lineage species. In addition, the ability of the antimetabolite to kill lymphocytes by an active cellular mechanism independent of its actions on nucleic acid synthesis suggests that fludarabine may activate an apoptotic signaling cascade in selectively vulnerable cellular subpopulations.

REFERENCES

1. Adjei AA, Dagnino L, Wong MM, Paterson AR (1992) Protection against fludarabine neurotoxicity in leukemic mice by the nucleoside transport inhibitor nitrobenzylthioinosine. Cancer Chemother Pharmacol 31, 71.

2. Cheson BD, Vena DA, Foss FM, Sorensen JM (1994) Neurotoxicity of purine analogs: A review. J Clin Oncol 12, 2216.

3. Chun HG, Leyland-Jones BR, Caryk SM, Hoth DF (1986) Central nervous system toxicity of fludarabine phosphate. Cancer Treatment Rev 70, 1225.

4. Chun HG, Leyland-Jones B, Cheson BD (1991) Fludarabine phosphate: A synthetic purine antimetabolite with significant activity against lymphoid malignancies. J Clin Oncol 9, 175.

5. Cleveland KO, Gelfand MS (1993) Listerial brain abscess in a patient with chronic lymphocytic leukemia treated with fludarabine. Clin Infect Dis 17, 816.

6. Cohen RB, Abdallah JM, Gray JR, Foss F (1993) Reversible neurologic toxicity in patients treated with standard-dose fludarabine phosphate for mycosis fungiodes and chronic lymphocytic leukemia. Ann Intern Med 118, 114.

7. Johnson PW, Fearnley J, Domizio P et al. (1994) Neurological illness following treatment with fludarabine. Brit J Cancer 70, 966.

8. Keating MJ, O'Brien S, Robertson LE et al. (1993) New initiatives with fludarabine monophosphate in hematologic malignancies. Semin Oncol 20, 13.

9. Kemena A, Keating M, Plukett W (1991) Oral bioavailability of plasma fludarabine and fludarabine triphosphate (F-ara-ATP) in peripheral CLL cells. Onkologie 14, 83.

10. Kornblau SM, Cortes-Franco J, Estey E (1993) Neurotoxicity associated with fludarabine and cytosine arabinoside chemotherapy for acute leukemia and myelodysplasia. Leukemia 7, 378.

11. Malspeis L, Grever MR, Staubus AE, Young D (1990) Pharmacokinetics of 2-F-ara-A (9-β-D-arabinofuranosyl-2-fluoroadenine) in cancer patients during the phase I clinical investigation of fludarabine phosphate. Semin Oncol 17, 18.

12. Merkel DE, Griffin NL, Kagan-Hallet K, Von Hoff DD (1986) Central nervous system toxicity with fludarabine. Cancer Treatment Rev 70, 1449.

13. Plunkett W, Gandhi V, Huang P *et al.* (1993) Fludarabine: Pharmacokinetics, mechanisms of action and rationales for combination therapies. *Semin Oncol* **20**, 2.

14. Plunkett W, Huang P, Gandhi V (1990) Metabolism and action of fludarabine phosphate. *Semin Oncol* **17**, 3.

15. Ross SR, McTavish D, Faulds D (1993) Fludarabine: A review of its pharmacological properties and therapeutic potential in malignancy. *Drugs* **45**, 737.

16. Saven A, Piro LD (1993) The newer purine analogs. *Cancer* **72**, 3470.

17. Vasova I, Penka M, Hajek R *et al.* (1997) A new purine analog in the treatment of hematologic malignancy. I. Fludarabine. *Vnitr Lek* **43**, 45. [Czech]

18. Zabernigg A, Maier H, Thaler J, Gattringer C (1994) Late-onset fatal neurological toxicity of fludarabine. *Lancet* **344**, 1780.

Flumazenil

Herbert H. Schaumburg

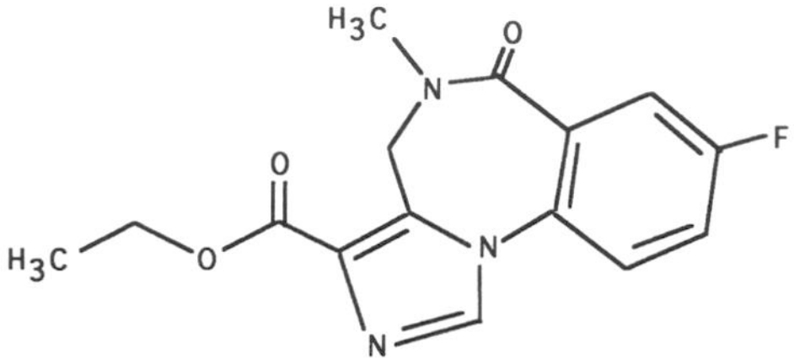

FLUMAZENIL
$C_{15}H_{14}FN_3O_3$

8-Fluoro-5,6-dihydro-5-methyl-6-oxo-4*H*-imidazo[1,5-a][1,4]benzodiazepine-3-carboxylic acid ethyl ester

NEUROTOXICITY RATING
Clinical
B   Seizure disorder

Flumazenil, an imidazobenzodiazepine, is a rapid-acting benzodiazepine antagonist that binds with high affinity to specific sites. It is widely used in the treatment of benzodiazepine overdose and occasionally employed to arouse patients with hepatic encephalopathy. The major limitation in the therapeutic use of flumazenil is its brief duration; it must be repeatedly administered intravenously every 2 h. There are no reports of serious systemic side effects.

Generalized seizures have occurred in some individuals with mixed drug (tricyclics/alcohol and benzodiazepine) overdoses (1).

REFERENCE
1. Curran HV, Birch B (1991) Differentiating the sedative, psychomotor and amnestic effects of benzodiazepines: A study with midazolam and the benzodiazepine antagonist, flumazenil. *Psychopharmacology* **103**, 519.

Flunarizine

John D. Rogers

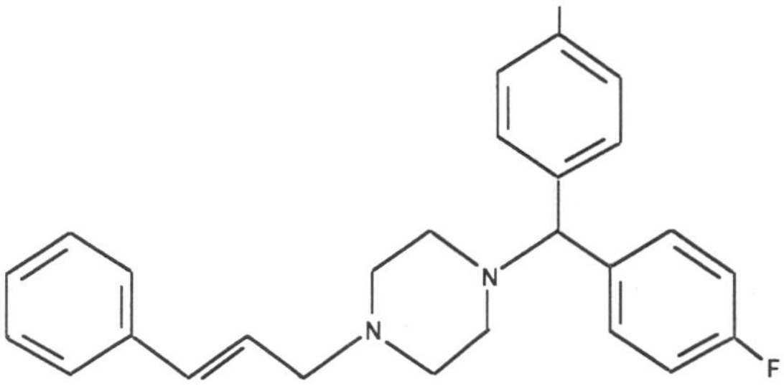

FLUNARIZINE
$C_{26}H_{26}F_2N_2$

(E)-1-[Bis(4-fluorophenyl)methyl]-4-(3-phenyl-2-propenyl)piperazine

NEUROTOXICOLOGY RATING
Clinical
B   Extrapyramidal syndrome (dyskinesias)

Flunarizine, a difluorinated derivative of cinnarizine, is a calcium antagonist with a greater potency and longer half-life than cinnarizine. As an antihypertensive agent, it has been used principally in Latin America and Europe since the 1970s for treatment of vertigo and peripheral circulatory disorders (11), and it has been advocated as prophylaxis for migraine headache (2).

Flunarizine has antihistaminic and serotonin-antagonist properties, and because it is a piperazine derivative it also has D_2 receptor–blocking effects (5). The drug depresses tyrosine hydroxylase immunoreactivity in nigrostriatal neurons (10) and inhibits the binding of ^{3}H-spiperone (1). Dopamine release may also be inhibited through calcium channel blockade. Striatal D_2 single photon emission computed tomography receptor studies using ^{123}I-iodobenzamide as a ligand demonstrated lower values (14%–63%) compared with age-matched controls. Greater reduction of D_2 receptor binding was seen in older subjects, those treated for >6 months, and those with parkinsonian signs (3).

Movement disorders have been more commonly reported with flunarizine than with cinnarizine. The most common side effects include drowsiness and depression, asthenia, parkinsonism, akathisia, dyskinesias, and tremor (4,7,8). A long-term follow-up of patients developing parkinsonism, initially treated with flunarizine or the calcium-entry blocker cinnarizine, demonstrated that most had persistent parkinsonism as well as perioral and upper limb dyskinesias despite cessation of the drug for up to a 7-year period (9). Symptoms appeared 7 months from initial exposure to cinnarizine or flunarizine; rigidity, bradykinesia, and postural instability were found in >75% of these patients with 5 of 13 patients worsening in terms of gait and balance disturbance during the mean 5-year period of follow-up. In addition, pharmacological studies have suggested the potential neurotoxic significance of the cinnamyl moiety 1-[bis(4-fluorophenyl)methyl]-4-[3-(4′-hydroxyphenyl)propenyl]piperazine. There is an increased relative D_2 receptor affinity for this ring-hydroxylated metabolite of flunarizine, which was found to be in higher concentration in the striatum than in plasma (6).

REFERENCES

1. Ambrosio C, Stefanini E (1991) Interaction of flunarizine with dopamine D2 and D1 receptors. *Eur J Pharmacol* **197**, 221.
2. Amery WK (1983) Flunarizine: A calcium channel blocker: New prophylactic drug in migraine. *Headache* **23**, 70.
3. Brucke T, Wober C, Podreka I *et al.* (1995) D$_2$ receptor blockade by flunarizine and cinnarizine explains extrapyramidal side effects. A SPECT Study. *J Cerebr Blood Flow Metabol* **15**, 513.
4. Chouza C, Scaramelli A, Caamano JL (1986) Parkinsonism, tardive dyskinesia, akathisia and depression induced by flunarizine. *Lancet* **1**, 1303.
5. Holmes B, Brogden RN, Heel RC *et al.* (1984) Flunarizine: A review of its pharmacodynamic and pharmacokinetic properties and therapeutic use. *Drugs* **27**, 6.
6. Kariya S, Isozaki S, Masubuchi Y *et al.* (1995) Possible pharmocokinetic and pharmacodynamic factors affecting parkinsonism inducement by cinnarizine and flunarizine. *Biochem Pharmacol* **50**, 1645.
7. Micheli FE, Pardal MF, Gatt M *et al.* (1987) Flunarizine and cinnarizine-induced extrapyramidal reactions. *Neurology* **37**, 881.
8. Micheli FE, Pardal MM, Gianaula R (1989) Movement disorders and depression due to flunarizine and cinnarizine. *Movement Disord* **4**, 139.
9. Negrotti A, Calzetti S (1997) A long term follow-up study of cinnarizine and flunarizine-induced parkinsonism. *Movement Disord* **12**, 107.
10. Takada M, Kono T, Kitai ST (1992) Flunarizine induces a transient loss of tyrosine hydroxylase immunoreactivity in nigrostriatal neurons. *Brain Res* **590**, 311.
11. Todd PA, Benfield P (1989) Flunarizine. A reappraisal of its pharmacological properties and therapeutic use in neurological disorders. *Drugs* **38**, 481.

Fluoroacetic Acid

Hans Kolbe

FLUOROACETIC ACID
$C_2H_3FO_2$

Sodium monofluoroacetate

NEUROTOXICITY RATING

Clinical

A Acute encephalopathy (sedation, seizures, tetany, coma)

Experimental

A Acute encephalopathy (sedation, seizures)

Fluoroacetic acid (FA), available as sodium monofluoroacetate (SMFA), is one of the most potent rodenticides; its use is restricted to experienced pest-control operators because of its high toxicity for all mammals. More than 17 fatalities have been reported with SMFA (17). It is the only organic fluorine-containing compound of toxicological significance to be found naturally. Leaves and fruits of South African "*Gifblaar*" (*Dichapetalum cymosum*) contain fluoroacetate and may fatally intoxicate cattle (15). FA-containing seed of the African plant *Dichapetalum toxicarium* causes human intoxication characterized by gastrointestinal symptoms, weakness, tremor, incoordination, and flaccid paraparesis. FA is also present in some *Acacia* (Australia) and *Palicourea* (South America) plants.

After its introduction as a rodenticide (12), it was used extensively worldwide, but rather soon, because of its hazards, its use was restricted to specially trained pest controllers. It has been an important research tool, leading the way to a new concept of toxicity mechanisms. In 1952, it was shown that physiological enzyme action within mammalian cells changes the nontoxic fluoroacetate into highly toxic fluorocitrate (18). The action of FA cannot be explained by fluorine toxicity because of the stability of the C-F bond in this molecule. The small size of the fluorine atom in FA enables this molecule to masquerade as acetic acid leading to the false synthesis of fluorocitrate (FC) *via* normal but erroneous enzyme action. FC inhibits the enzyme *cis*-aconitase [E.C. 4.2.1.3.] thereby blocking the Krebs cycle. This was termed "lethal synthesis" because of the subsequent energy breakdown of these cells. Targets are all mammalian cells that depend on energy production *via* the Krebs cycle, with a marked preference for cells and organs with high energy demands such as myocardial cells and CNS neurons.

FA, commercially available as SMFA (Compound 1080), is a white, tasteless powder, with a faint odor of vinegar. It burns with a green flame, is nonvolatile, highly water-soluble, and less soluble in solvents.

SMFA is readily absorbed after ingestion; however, even 17 h after intake, a considerable amount was found in the stomach contents of a subject who died (10). SMFA is less well absorbed through the intact skin, but easily taken up through cuts and abrasions. It may be absorbed through the lung by inhaling dust containing the poison (23).

Toxicological analysis of a man who died of FA intoxication showed a uniform content of the toxin in brain, liver, and kidney, and a very large amount of FA in urine indicating rapid renal excretion. An even distribution of the compound was also found in rats, with the exception of liver tissue, which contained only a relative small amount of the toxin (9).

The oral LD_{50} for rats is 0.2 mg/kg and 0.1 mg/kg for dogs and cats (11). The estimated fatal dose for humans is 3–7 mg/kg SMFA (17). The metabolism of fluoroacetate (FA) is well described (3). FA is activated by thiokinase to fluoro-acetyl-CoA which, by the action of citrate synthase [E.C. 4.1.3.7; Ochoa's "condensing enzyme"], condenses with oxaloacetate to form (2-R, 3-S)-fluorocitrate (FC). Fluoroacetyl-CoA is a competitive inhibitor of acetyl-CoA. The relative unspecific citrate synthase does not recognize the small fluorine atom and thus allows the "lethal synthesis" of FC. Low concentrations of FC inhibit *cis*-aconitase [E.C. 4.2.1.3] which, in turn, impairs the Krebs cycle at the

step where citrate is eventually converted to *cis*-aconitate and isocitrate. Citrate then accumulates in all tissues and in serum (2).

Toxic effects of FA are delayed up to several hours depending on the rate of conversion of nontoxic fluoroacetate to fluorocitrate. In addition to nonspecific signs of nausea and vomiting, toxic effects include cardiac irregularities, apprehension, clouded consciousness, cyanosis, tetanic phenomena, seizures, and coma. Death is caused by ventricular fibrillation or cardiorespiratory failure (4). There are apparent species differences premonitory to death: rabbits, horses, goats, and spider monkeys present mainly with cardiac manifestations; dogs, guinea pigs, and frogs exhibit only convulsions; and cats, pigs, chickens, and rhesus monkeys show cardiac and CNS effects (8). There is only one report of renal changes resembling nephrosis after repeated sublethal doses given to rats (6).

The toxic effects are also reflected by the accumulation of citrate in the affected organ (5). The most common explanation is that citrate accumulation mirrors the degree of enzyme inhibition in the Krebs cycle, leading eventually to a corresponding decrease in energy production and to functional impairment (19). There are, however, marked differences in adenosine triphosphate (ATP) depletion in metabolically active tissues not necessarily mirroring functional decline. Heart tissue shows a marked ATP loss in rats: eight hours after 3 mg/kg FA, ATP concentration dropped to 46% with a 15-fold increase of tissue citrate and a fivefold elevation of serum citrate. In dogs, the same experiment caused similar disturbances of myocardial function but only a twofold tissue citrate elevation and a threefold rise of the serum citrate concentration. ATP concentration remained in the physiological range (2). A close correlation was noted between serum citrate levels and the degree of clinical compromise. An inverse correlation was found between serum calcium and citrate levels in dogs; hypocalcemia has been advanced to explain tremors, tetany, and convulsions in fluoroacetate-intoxicated dogs. In cats, there was a 27.7% drop in ionized calcium in serum 45 min after 3 mg/kg FA, and a corresponding prolongation of electrocardiogram QT intervals was observed. A correction of serum calcium levels doubles the survival time but does not influence the fatal outcome (21). Only some of the toxic effects are due to calcium chelation by citrate. Many investigators failed to suppress seizures by giving calcium; some were unable to find any decrease in calcium levels (14). There are reports of animals with seizures and death without a significant increase of citrate. Thus, neither blockade of Krebs cycle nor hypocalcemia by chelation are generally accepted mechanisms of FA toxicity. There are, however, some other observations that can probably help solve the controversy: an increase of ammonia precedes that of citrate in brains of animals given FA (13). In cortex slices, no effect is observed after 1 mM FA. However, there is an increase of ammonia, caused by suppression of glutamine formation, the main mechanism of NH_4^+ removal in the brain.

Acetate and fluoroacetate are taken up in glial cells by an active transport system coupled to sodium transport (16). This transport system and a very active intracellular Krebs cycle lead to a fast conversion of fluoroacetate to fluorocitrate in glial cells, with marked blockade of energy production selectively in this cell population (20,22). Functional consequences are diminished glutamine synthesis and ammonia fixation, and decreased glutamate uptake due to diminished ATP, which is required for this transport mechanism (1). Synaptically released glutamate is elevated and acts in a proconvulsive manner.

No specific antidote is available for sodium fluoroacetate. Prompt gastric lavage with water is essential, followed by repeated application of activated charcoal and a cathartic. Glycerol monoacetate (Monactin, 0.1–0.5 ml/kg every half hour intramuscularly) inhibits the conversion of fluoroacetate to fluorocitrate in monkeys. Alternatively, a solution of ethyl alcohol can be used. Another possibility is the infusion of 500 ml of a 10% solution of acetamide in 5% dextrose over a period of 30 min every 4 h. Supportive treatment in an intensive care unit should be established at once with artificial respiration, antiarrhythmic drugs (procainamide), anticonvulsive measures (barbiturates), and calcium gluconate treatment against tetany. Hyperglycemia, drop of temperature, and a drop of blood pressure should be expected.

REFERENCES

1. Balcar VJ, Borg J, Mandel P (1977) High affinity uptake of L-glutamate and L-aspartate by glial cells. *J Neurochem* **28**, 87.
2. Bosakowski T, Levin AA (1986) Serum citrate as a peripheral indicator of fluoroacetate and fluorocitrate toxicity in rats and dogs. *Toxicol Appl Pharmacol* **85**, 428.
3. Brady RO (1955) Fluoroacetyl coenzyme A. *J Biol Chem* **217**, 213.
4. Brockmann JL, McDowell AV, Leeds WG (1955) Fatal poisoning with sodium fluoroacetate. *J Amer Med Assn* **159**, 1529.
5. Buffa P, Peters RA (1950) The *in vivo* formation of citrate induced by fluoroacetate poisoning and its significance. *J Physiol-London* **110**, 488.
6. Cater DB, Peters RA (1961) The occurrence of renal changes resembling nephrosis in rats poisoned with fluorocitrate. *Brit J Exp Pathol* **42**, 278.
7. Chenoweth MB (1949) Monofluoroacetic acid and related compounds. *Pharmacol Rev* **1**, 383.
8. Chenoweth MB, Kandel A, Johnson LB, Bennett DR (1950) Factors influencing fluoroacetate poisoning. Prac-

tical treatment with glycerol monoacetate. *J Pharmacol Exp Ther* **102**, 31.
9. Hagan EC, Ramsey LL, Woodard C (1950) Absorption, distribution, and excretion of sodium fluoroacetate (1080) in rats. *J Pharmacol Exp Ther* **99**, 432.
10. Harrisson JWE, Ambrus JL, Ambrus CM *et al.* (1952) Acute poisoning with sodium fluoroacetate (compound 1080) *J Amer Med Assn* **149**, 1520.
11. Hayes WJ (1975) *Toxicology of Pesticides*. Williams & Wilkins, Baltimore, MD.
12. Kalmbach ER (1945) Ten-eighty. War-produced rodenticide. *Science* **102**, 232.
13. Lahiri S, Quastel JH (1963) Fluoroacetate and the metabolism of ammonia in brain. *Biochem J* **89**, 157.
14. Liang CS (1977) Metabolic control of circulation: Effects of iodoacetate and fluoroacetate. *J Clin Invest* **60**, 61.
15. Marais ISC (1944) Monofluoroacetic acid, the toxic principle of "Gifblaar" *Dichapetalum cymosum*? (Hook) England onderstepoort. *J Vet Sci Anim Ind* **20**, 67.
16. Muir D, Berl S, Clarke DD (1986) Acetate and fluoroacetate as possible markers for glial metabolism *in vivo*. *Brain Res* **380**, 336.
17. Pattison FLM (1959) *Toxic Aliphatic Fluorine Compounds*. Elsevier Press Inc, New York.
18. Peters RA (1952) Lethal synthesis (Croonian lecture). *Proc Roy Soc Ser B* **139**, 143.
19. Peters RA (1972) Some metabolic aspects to fluoroacetate especially related to fluorocitrate. In: *Carbo-fluorine Compounds*. (Ciba Foundation Symposium, New Series, Vol. 2) Elsevier, Amsterdam p. 55.
20. Quastel JH (1974) Metabolic compartmentation in the brain and effects in metabolic inhibitors. In: *Metabolic Compartmentation and Neurotransmission*. Berl S, Clarke DD, Schneider D eds. Plenum Press, New York p. 337.
21. Shapira AR, Taitelman U, Bursztein S (1980) Evaluation of the role of ionized calcium in sodium fluoroacetate ("1080") poisoning. *Toxicol Appl Pharmacol* **56**, 216.
22. Szerb JC, Issekutz B (1987) Increase in the stimulation-induced overflow of glutamate by fluoroacetate, a selective inhibitor of the glial tricarboxylic cycle. *Brain Res* **410**, 116.
23. Williams AT (1948) Sodium fluoroacetate poisoning. *Hosp Corps* **Q21**, 16.

CASE REPORT

An alert and responsive 17-year-old boy, son of a professional rat exterminator, came to the hospital about 45–60 min after drinking a solution containing ~4 oz SMFA (4). Immediately after ingestion, he had vomited and since then had had severe epigastric pain. Gastric lavage was carried out but he became gradually unresponsive. He was comatose 2½ h after taking the poison, and 30 min later he had grand mal seizures. At this time, 3 h after SMFA ingestion, he was in deep coma, with a Babinski sign bilaterally. He was cyanotic, the skin was warm and dry, and pupils were constricted but reactive. The heart showed premature beats, and the QT interval was prolonged. He became irritable and showed carpopedal spasms. He started vomiting blood-containing material. Heart dilatation occurred. He became very "spastic." The next day, in even deeper coma, his pupils became fixed. Supraventricular tachycardia and pulmonary edema occurred; he became hypotensive. On day 3, his temperature had risen to 40.3°C. There was tremendous bronchial secretion. After starting therapy with ethyl alcohol, blood pressure stabilized, carpopedal spasms decreased remarkably, but he remained in deep coma. On the fifth hospital day, his temperature reached 42.3°C, respiration became rapid and labored, and tachycardia increased. He died in cardiorespiratory failure. Postmortem examination of the brain revealed marked edema (1600 g) with upward herniation of the cerebellum and small perivascular hemorrhages.

Fluoroquinolones

Herbert H. Schaumburg

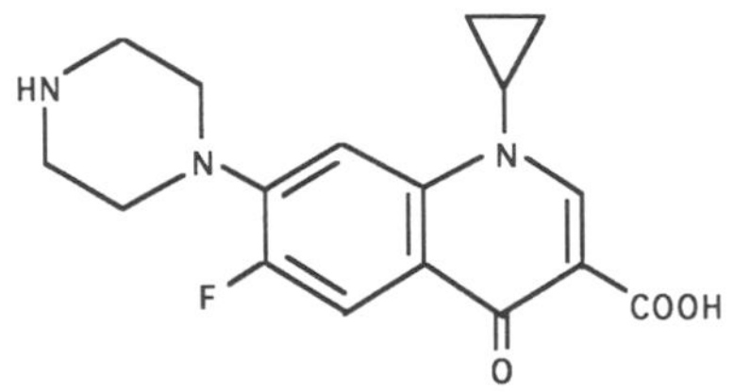

CIPROFLOXACIN
$C_{17}H_{18}FN_3O_3$

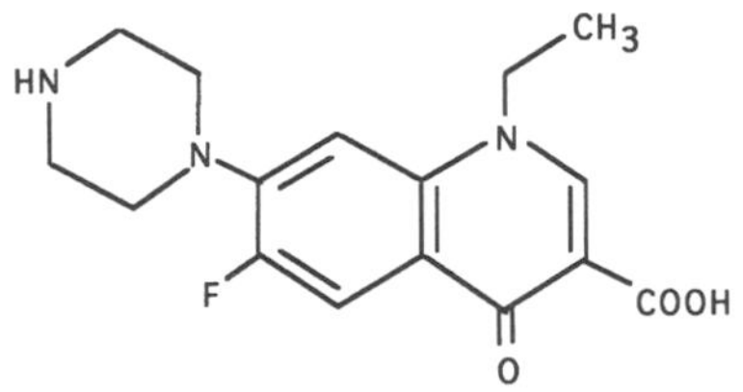

NORFLOXACIN
$C_{16}H_{18}FN_3O_3$

Ciprofloxacin; 1-Cyclopropyl-6-fluoro-1,4-dihydro-4-oxy-(1-piperazinyl)-3-quinolinecarboxylic acid
Norfloxacin; 1-Ethyl-6-fluoro-1,4-dihydro-4-oxo-7-(1-piperzinyl)-3-quinolinecarboxylic acid

NEUROTOXICITY RATING

Clinical

B   Acute encephalopathy

C   Seizure disorder

The fluoroquinolone antibiotics, norfloxacin and ciprofloxacin, are broad-spectrum, fluorine-substituted, 4-quinolone antibiotics primarily used in the treatment of urinary tract infections. Their antibiotic action stems from inhibition of gyrase-mediated bacterial DNA supercoiling. These drugs are well absorbed after oral administration and are widely distributed, although only 40% appears in the plasma. They are primarily excreted in urine; about 30% appears as the parent drug. There is little systemic toxicity aside from abdominal discomfort; arthropathy may occur in immature animals (1).

One percent of patients receiving conventional doses for more than 2 weeks experience headache, insomnia, restlessness, and tremor (1,5). These symptoms dissipate within a week of drug withdrawal. Generalized seizures are described in a few individuals with debilitating systemic illness; it is unclear if these are a genuine consequence of therapy or reflect facets of the underlying conditions. Two features of quinolone pharmacology support the convulsant potential of these drugs: one is their structural resemblance to amfenolic acid, a CNS stimulant (2); the other is that quinolones may inhibit the specific binding of the inhibitory neurotransmitter, γ-aminobutyric acid, to synaptic membranes (3,4).

REFERENCES

1. Ball P (1986) Ciprofloxacin: Overview of adverse experiences. *J Antimicrob Chemother* **18**, 187.
2. Juorio AV (1982) The effects of amfenolic acid and some other central stimulants on mouse striatal tyramine, dopamine, and homovanillic acid. *Brit J Pharmacol* **77**, 511.
3. Tsuji A, Sato H, Kume Y *et al.* (1988) Inhibitory effects of quinolone antibacterial agents on gamma-aminobutyric acid binding to receptor sites in rat brain membranes. *Antimicrob Agents Chemother* **32**, 190.
4. Unseld E, Ziegler G, Gemeinhardt A (1990) Possible interaction of fluoroquinolones with the benzodiazepine–GABA(A)-receptor complex. *Brit J Clin Pharmacol* **30**, 63.
5. Wang C, Sabbai J, Corrado M *et al.* (1986) World-wide clinical experience with norfloxacin: Efficacy and safety. *Scand J Infect Dis* **48**, 91.

5-Fluorouracil

Mark F. Mehler

5-FLUOROURACIL
$C_4H_3FN_2O_2$

5-Fluoro-2,4(1*H*,3*H*)-pyrimidinedione

NEUROTOXICITY RATING

Clinical

A Cerebellar syndrome

A Leukoencephalopathy (multifocal)

A Acute encephalopathy (confusion, sedation, seizures)

Experimental

A Leukoencephalopathy (local administration)

A Multifocal cerebellar and brainstem necrosis (local administration)

5-Fluorouracil (FU) is a fluorinated pyrimidine; it is a white crystalline powder, sparingly soluble in water, with a MW of 130.08. This antimetabolite and antineoplastic agent was initially introduced more than 30 years ago; it is used for palliative treatment of colorectal, metastatic breast, ovarian, and skin cancers, and as curative therapy for basal cell carcinoma (3). An analogue of the pyrimidine uracil, FU is metabolized *via* the same pathway (15); its mechanism of action is incompletely understood. Assays exist for the antimetabolite in plasma, serum, body fluids, and recipient tissues (5). Parenteral administration represents the major dosage form, either by intravenous bolus or by continuous infusion. Alternate routes of administration include hepatic arterial or intraperitoneal infusion, or topical application for remediation of skin cancer. FU was originally synthesized from acyclic precursors, with an alternate method of synthesis using direct fluorination of uracil by trifluoromethyl hypofluorite. It is stable in solution at physiological pH for weeks, and the unmetabolized compound is harmless to all cells.

Certain tumors can utilize uracil more avidly, and FU can interfere with nucleic acid synthesis and, thus, slow tumor growth (15). The 5' hydrogen is attractive for substitution. Mammalian cells may obtain thymidine 5-triphosphate needed for DNA synthesis from 2'-deoxyuridine-5' monophosphate by replacing the hydrogen on the 5' carbon with a methyl group. The antimetabolite is incorporated into ribosomal, messenger, and transfer RNA, and is thereby thought to cause functional damage. Antitumor effectiveness is increased with coadministration of folinic acid. Tumor resistance is thought to develop through a number of cellular mechanisms: increased catabolic rate with detoxification; deficiency of anabolic enzymes resulting in decreased production of active metabolites; alteration of intracellular target enzymes; cellular tolerance; and alteration in the turnover of enzymes, nucleic acids, and natural nucleotide precursors (17). Drug and metabolic assays are performed using gas chromatographic–mass spectrometric assays and reverse-phase high-pressure liquid chromatography. The latter technique is utilized for clinical pharmacokinetic analysis (3). Pharmacodynamic assays can be performed using serial needle biopsies.

Significant variations in bioavailability occur following oral administration (3). The most common intravenous dosage schedule is 10–15 mg/kg every week or daily for 5 days every month. The elimination half-life is 8–20 min; the volume of distribution, 14–54 l; and the plasma clearance, 48–114 l/h. The elimination half-life of catabolites is much longer than that of the parent compound (1–33 h). FU is rapidly cleared and degraded in the liver, but also in the intestines, lungs, pancreas, mucosa, and lymphatic system. This results in low systemic drug concentrations with consequent protection of the bone marrow and gastrointestinal tract. Hepatotoxicity is predominantly cholestatic rather than hepatocellular (3). The antimetabolite is eliminated primarily (80%) by reductive catabolism, with urinary excretion and trace biliary excretion. Reductions in dosage are advised for hepatic but not for renal dysfunction.

Continuous infusions reduce the type and severity of side effects and allow larger drug concentrations to be tolerated (3). Steady-state concentrations range from 0.8–71.0 μmol/l, with clearance values of 54–420 l/h. Continuous pump infusions result in circadian variations of 3- to 25-fold in plasma concentrations. Hepatic arterial infusions are performed using the hepatic artery or the portal vein. Intraperitoneal administration is used for drug-sensitive tumors, including those of the gastrointestinal tract and ovaries. With this therapeutic regimen, the remaining unmetabolized drug drains into the portal vein and is catabolized in the liver. Topical administration (1%–5% cream) is recommended for premalignant actinic keratosis, and is curative for basal cell carcinoma. Following systemic administration, the drug is distributed to all tissues, most notably the small intestines, bone marrow, liver, kidney, and spleen, and clinical studies have shown that 5-fluorouracil penetrates the extracellular spaces, ascites, cerebrospinal fluid, and ascites fluid.

The cytotoxicity of FU is related to the anabolism of nucleotides in actively proliferating cells (15). The antimetabolite and uracil enter cells by carrier-mediated transport with saturable entry at pharmacological or physiological concentrations that exhibit first-order kinetics (19). The availability of the drug for anabolism is regulated by catabolism (3). Dihydropyrimidine dehydrogenase (DPD) reduces the double bond of the pyrimidine ring and is the rate-limiting catabolic step. The product of this reaction, dihydrouracil, is unstable and is degraded to 5-fluoroureido propionic acid by dihydropyrimidinase. This transient catabolite is broken down to α-fluoro-β-alanine, the major urinary catabolite, by β-ureidoproprionase (20). Three separate biochemical pathways are utilized to convert the parent compound to cytotoxic ribophosphate metabolites: (a) uridine phosphorylase and uridine kinase convert the antimetabolite to 5-fluorouridine-5'-monophosphate (FUMP), (b) orotidine 5'-monophosphate phosphoribosyltransferase causes the direct conversion to FUMP, and (c) thymidine phosphorylase and thymidine kinase convert the drug to the deoxyribosyl nucleotide 5'-fluoro-2'-deoxyuridine-5'-monophosphate (FdUMP) (3). The exact nucleotides responsible for differential tumor cytotoxicity are not clear. FdUMP is known to disrupt thymidylate synthase with the resultant inhibition of DNA synthesis, but with continued RNA and protein synthesis (15). This progressive cellular and molecular metabolic imbalance results in cytotoxicity. To produce this effect, FdUMP forms ternary complexes with 5,10-methylene tetrahydrofolate and thymidylate synthase.

Methotrexate coapplication increases cytotoxicity by allowing the incorporation of FU into newly synthesized RNA (17). The drug also alters the transmembrane potential and surface charge to increase the susceptibility to cellular lysis. The concurrent use of other pyrimidines modulates drug activity and metabolism and increases toxicity (6). Simultaneous interference with pyrimidine synthesis has not been shown to have an additional therapeutic effect, although interest in this approach continues. The use of purine analogs with FU to modulate metabolism and toxicity has been demonstrated to have potential efficacy, and this is most evident with allopurinol. Finally, coapplication of misonidazole, which increases the radiosensitivity of hypoxic cells, reduces the therapeutic index of FU and increases toxicity.

General adverse reactions include diarrhea, anorexia, nausea and vomiting, stomatitis, and esophagopharyngitis. Additional organ system dysfunction includes anemia, pancytopenia, thrombocytopenia and agranulocytosis, gastrointestinal ulceration, myocardial ischemia, generalized allergic reactions, photosensitivity, palmar-plantar erythrodysesthesia syndrome, lacrimal duct stenosis, and thrombophlebitis.

Metabolites of FU have been implicated in the neurotoxicity of the antimetabolite. In one study, two metabolites, monofluoracetic acid (FA) and α-fluoro-β-alanine (FBAL) were administered by continuous osmotic pump (0.07 ml/day; concentration: FA, 0.75–2.25 mg/ml; FBAL, 0.1–2.4 mg/ml) to the lateral ventricles of the brains of cats for up to 1 month (14). The cumulative doses were: FU, 1.5–45 mg; FBAL, 0.2–4.8 mg. The FBAL metabolite exhibited greater neurotoxic potential than the parent compound when assessed by neuropathological examination. Pathological changes consisted of vacuolation and necrotic parenchymal softening (14). Vacuolation was seen with use of all drug preparations. The vacuoles were generally 20–50 μm in diameter and distributed within the cerebellar nuclei, white matter and tectum, and tegmentum of the brainstem. Electron microscopic examination revealed the presence of splitting between the myelin intraperiod lines or separation between axons and the innermost myelin layer. Parenchymal necrosis was preferentially seen in the FBAL-treatment group (14). The lesions were symmetrical and localized to the superior and inferior colliculus, oculomotor nucleus, and the thalamus. The characteristics of the drug-induced lesions were similar to those seen after oral administration of FU or its metabolites. Cumulative doses did not correlate with the severity of the neuropathological changes.

Attempts have been made to influence the neurotoxic profile of FU. 5-Ethynyluracil, which inactivates dihydropyrimidine dehydrogenase that normally catalyzes the rapid catabolism of FU, was coadministrated to dogs (subcutaneously, 1 mg/kg, 30 min before infusion and every 6 h thereafter) during continuous infusion of FU (40 mg/kg/24 h). In the absence of 5-ethynyluracil, the steady-state plasma concentration of the antimetabolite was 1.3 μM and a severe, often fatal neurotoxic syndrome ensued characterized initially by seizures, motor tremors, and ataxia (2). Coapplication of 5-ethynyluracil and a much reduced dose of FU (1.6 mg/kg/24 h) resulted in a lowering of the total clearance from 9.9 to 0.2 l/h/kg, with an associated steady-state concentration of 2.4 mM, and an absence of neurotoxicity (2). Coapplication of cyclophosphamide, dactomycin, and FU resulted in significant neurotoxicity in 40% of dogs tested (7).

To examine the pharmacodynamics of a potential neurotoxic derivative of FU, radiolabeled FBAL was administered to rats by intravenous bolus (10). Plasma disappearance rates reflected the sum of three exponential functions:

0.26, 12.1, 8426 min. Bile excretion commenced within 30 min of bolus and continued throughout the experimental protocol at concentrations in great excess of corresponding plasma levels. Urinary excretion consisted of mainly free FBAL, and was the major pathway of elimination with 40% excreted by 24 h, and 70% by 192 h. There was retention of radiolabel for extended periods in the brain, heart, and skeletal muscle at concentrations up to tenfold higher than plasma levels. High-pressure liquid chromatographic analysis failed to detect the presence of metabolites of FBAL other than biliary acid conjugates. These findings contradict the previous suggestion that at least three additional FBAL metabolites (fluorocitrate, fluoroacetic acid, and fluoroguanido propionic acid) could be found at significant systemic concentrations (3).

FU penetrates well into cerebrospinal fluid. The most common form of neurotoxicity is a pancerebellar syndrome associated with the rapid onset of gait ataxia, limb incoordination, hypotonia, nystagmus, and diplopia (11). Occasionally, therapeutic use of FU is associated with a subacute encephalopathy with confusion, headache, disorientation, lethargy, and seizures (18). With high-dose treatment, as many as 40% of patients exhibit an encephalopathy that may progress to coma. Peripheral neuropathy is not clearly associated with use of the antimetabolite. The spectrum of neurotoxic reactions is generally dose- and schedule-related. Reactions are usually reversible with cessation of treatment or dosage reduction. Concomitant use of interferon-α, cisplatin, folinic acid, N-phosphonacetyl-L-aspartate, or thymidine may potentiate the neurotoxicity.

Multifocal leukoencephalopathy has been seen following coapplication of FU and levamisole (8). This condition is characterized by ataxia, acute confusion, agitation, dysarthria, and diplopia, with diagnostic findings from magnetic resonance imaging and tissue pathology (4). Acute demyelinating lesions can improve following cessation of therapy and steroid treatment (9). High-dose continuous FU infusion is associated with transient hyperammonemia after 1.4–4 days, with restoration of normal biochemical indices after 2 days (10). Radiation myelitis has been observed after radiation therapy and concurrent FU and cisplatin application for metastatic uterine adenocarcinoma (1). Neurotoxicity has also been observed following a single therapeutic cycle with coapplication of levamisole and folinic acid (13).

Editors' Note. Recent data suggest that FU neurotoxicity is more common and more severe in DPD deficiency, a condition with an autosomal pattern of inheritance and a 3% estimated North American prevalence (12,16).

REFERENCES

1. Bloss JD, DiSaia PJ, Mannel RS *et al.* (1991) Radiation myelitis: A complication of concurrent cisplatin and 5-fluorouracil chemotherapy with extended field radiotherapy for carcinoma of the uterine cervix. *Gynecol Oncol* 43, 305.

2. Davis ST, Joyner SS, Badccanari DP, Spector T (1994) 5-Ethynyluracil (776C85): Protection from 5-fluorouracil-induced neurotoxicity in dogs. *Biochem Pharmacol* 48, 233.

3. Diasio RB, Harris BE (1989) Clinical pharmacology of 5-fluorouracil. *Clin Pharmacokinet* 16, 215.

4. Fassas AB, Gattani AM, Morgello S (1994) Cerebral demyelination with 5-fluorouracil and levamisole. *Cancer Invest* 12, 379.

5. Findlay MP, Leach MO (1994) *In vivo* monitoring of fluoropyrimidine metabolites: Magnetic resonance spectroscopy in the evaluation of 5-fluorouracil. *Anti-Cancer Drugs* 5, 260.

6. Gebbia V, Testa A, Borsellino N *et al.* (1993) Pharmacological modulation of 5-fluorouracil and its clinical implications: An overview. *In Vivo* 7, 639.

7. Hammer AS, Carothers MA, Harris CL *et al.* (1994) Unexpected neurotoxicity in dogs receiving a cyclophosphamide, dactinomycin, and 5-fluorouracil chemotherapy protocol. *J Vet Intern Med* 8, 240.

8. Hook CC, Kimmel DW, Kvols LK *et al.* (1992) Multifocal inflammatory leukoencephalopathy with 5-fluorouracil and levamisole. *Ann Neurol* 31, 262.

9. Kimmel DW, Schutt AJ (1993) Multifocal leukoencephalopathy: Occurrence during 5-fluorouracil and levamisole therapy and resolution after discontinuation of chemotherapy. *Mayo Clin Proc* 68, 363.

10. Liaw CC, Liaw SJ, Wang CH *et al.* (1993) Transient hyperammonemia related to chemotherapy with continuous infusion of high-dose 5-fluorouracil. *Anti-Cancer Drugs* 4, 311.

11. Macdonald DR (1991) Neurologic complications of chemotherapy. *Neurol Clin* 9, 955.

12. Milano G, Etienne MC, Pierrefite V *et al.* (1999) Dihydropyrimidine dehydrogenase deficiency and fluorouracil-related toxicity. *Brit J Cancer* 79, 627.

13. Neu IS (1993) Multifocal inflammatory leukencephalopathy caused by adjuvant therapy with 5-fluorouracil and levamisole after resection for an adenocarcinoma of the colon. *Acta Neurol Scand* 87, 70.

14. Okeda R, Shibutani M, Matsuo T *et al.* (1990) Experimental neurotoxicity of 5-fluorouracil and its derivatives is due to poisoning by the monofluorinated organic metabolites, monofluoroacetic acid and α-fluoro-β-alanine. *Acta Neuropathol* 81, 66.

15. Parker WB, Cheng YC (1990) Metabolism and mechanism of action of 5-fluorouracil. *Pharmacol Ther* 48, 381.

16. Shehata N, Pater A, Tang SC (1999) Prolonged severe 5-

fluorouracil-associated neurotoxicity in a patient with dihydropyrimidine dehydrogenase deficiency. *Cancer Invest* **17**, 201.

17. Sotos GA, Grogan L, Allegra CJ (1994) Preclinical and clinical aspects of biomodulation of 5-fluorouracil. *Cancer Treatment Rev* **20**, 11.
18. Tuxen MK, Hansen SW (1994) Neurotoxicity secondary to antineoplastic drugs. *Cancer Treatment Rev* **20**, 191.
19. van Groeningen CJ, Peters GJ, Pinedo HM (1992) Modulation of fluorouracil toxicity with uridine. *Semin Oncol* **20**, 148.
20. Zhang R, Soong S-J, Liu T *et al.* (1992) Pharmacokinetics and tissue distribution of 2-fluoro-β-alanine in rats: Potential relevance to toxicity pattern of 5-fluorouracil. *Drug Metab Disposition* **20**, 113.

Fluoxetine and Other Serotonin-Reuptake Blockers

Arnold E. Merriam

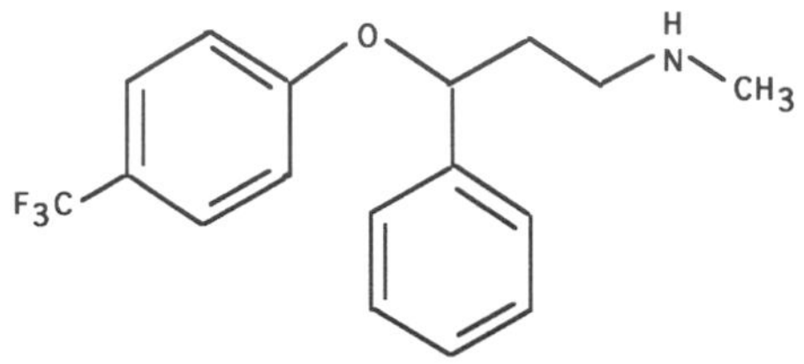

FLUOXETINE
$C_{17}H_{18}F_3NO$

($\pm$)-*N*-Methyl-3-phenyl-3-[(α,α,α-trifluoro-*p*-tolyl)oxy]propylamine (as hydrochloride)

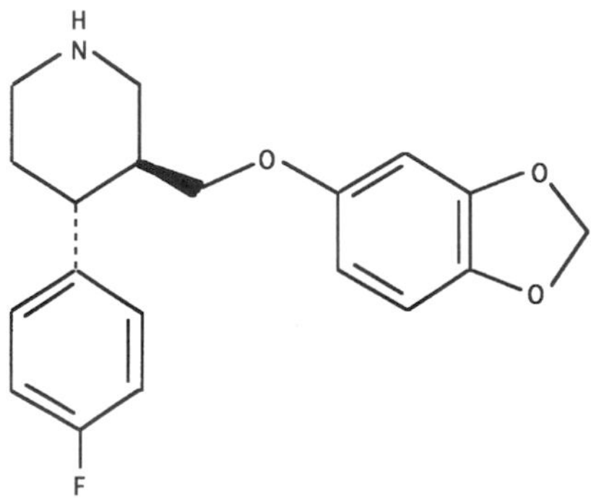

PAROXETINE
$C_{19}H_{20}FNO_3$

(3*S*-trans)-3-[(1,3-Benzodioxol-5-yl-oxy)methyl]-4-(4-fluorophenyl)piperidine

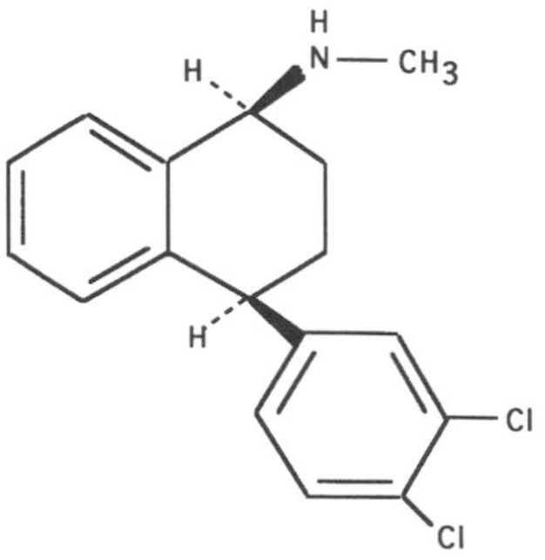

SERTRALINE
$C_{17}H_{17}Cl_2N$

(IS-*cis*)-4-(3,4-Dichlorophenyl)-1,2,3,4-tetrahydro-*N*-methyl-1-napthalenamine (as hydrochloride)

NEUROTOXICITY RATING

Clinical

A   Tremor

A   Extrapyramidal syndrome (parkinsonism)

A   Serotonin syndrome

Fluoxetine, paroxetine, and sertraline are structurally dissimilar agents that fall into the class of selective serotonin-reuptake inhibitors (SSRIs) by virtue of their potent inhibition of the neuronal reuptake pump for the neurotransmitter serotonin [5-hydroxytryptamine (5-HT)] and their relative paucity of direct effects on other neurotransmitter systems. They are discussed as a class because their therapeutic and neurotoxic profiles are similar. As a result of both their effectiveness and their comparative freedom from serious or dangerous side effects, the SSRIs are often used as first-line treatments for depression, anxiety disorders, and obsessive-compulsive disorder (OCD). Toxic effects on the nervous system include the precipitation of headache, tremor, extrapyramidal effects, and, in conjunction with other serotonin-active agents, the potentially lethal "serotonin syndrome," a constellation of symptoms and findings described in greater detail elsewhere (*see* Monoamine Oxidase Inhibitors, this volume).

Available data indicate that fluoxetine, paroxetine, and sertraline are well absorbed from the gastrointestinal tract following oral administration and undergo extensive first-pass metabolism in the liver, an effect that becomes partially saturated after repeated administration (15). There is wide interindividual variation in maximum plasma concentration in multiple-dose studies; steady-state concentrations are reached in 4–14 days; dose increases result in approximately linear inceases in plasma concentrations (12). Radiolabeling studies demonstrate that each of these agents distributes readily into tissues, with volumes of distribution ranging from 3.1–42 l/kg; plasma protein binding is estimated to be about 95%. Fluoxetine's *N*-demethylated metabolite norfluoxetine is as active a serotonin-reuptake inhibitor as is the parent compound. In distinction, sertraline's demethylated metabolite is much less potent than sertraline itself (13). Paroxetine is metabolized to glucuronide- and sulfate-conjugated metabolites that are pharmacologically inactive. Elimination half-life of both paroxetine and sertraline approximates 24 h (12,15), but is substantially longer for fluoxetine, the half-life of which has been measured at 8 days for the parent drug and 19.3 days for its active metabolite norfluoxetine. These prolonged plasma half-lives are responsible for the serious drug–drug interactions that may occur long after fluoxetine discontinuation: it is recommended to allow 5 weeks to pass before other agents likely to be incompatible with serotonin-enhancing drugs are introduced (17).

Animal studies document the relative selectivity of these agents' direct inhibitory effects upon serotonin uptake; at higher concentrations, some inhibition of reuptake of norepinephrine and, to a lesser extent, dopamine, is also encountered (16).

In contrast to the absence of significant direct actions of these agents on other than the serotonergic system, there is contradictory evidence, gleaned from animal studies, that they may indirectly influence the dopaminergic system. In a study of the effects of acute and chronic fluoxetine administration on the dopamine content of various rat brain regions, a significant inhibition of dopamine synthesis was noted acutely in the striatum, nucleus accumbens, hippocampus, and frontal cortex; this inhibition increased in the striatum and hippocampus after chronic drug treatment (1). In an attempt to replicate this work, the same investigators were unable to identify this effect (2), leaving the mechanism by which SSRIs induce extrapyramidal effects unresolved. Some sort of interaction between these two neurohumoral systems is supported by neuroanatomical evidence of serotonergic input to ventral tegmental dopaminergic neurons (8), and the fact that administration of 5-HT$_2$ antagonists reduce neuroleptic-associated extrapyramidal side effects (3).

The most commonly reported nervous system effects, noted in 25% or more of patients treated with these agents, are activation, insomnia, sedation, headache, and tremor (7). These symptoms rarely cause drug discontinuation.

SSRI administration has been reported, on a much less frequent basis, to engender the same gamut of extrapyramidal manifestations that is seen regularly in the context of neuroleptic drug treatment. Reports of extrapyramidal reactions with solo SSRI administration indicate these agents are capable of inducing such reactions in the absence of complicating pharmacological factors. Many patients reported to have sustained SSRI-induced extrapyramidal reactions, however, had also received neuroleptic treatment, either concurrently or in the immediately preceding period; it is possible in these cases that the SSRIs induce these symptoms by perturbing the dopaminergic system in the context of already partially blocked dopamine receptors.

SSRI-induced extrapyramidal symptoms include akathisia (14), a state of uncomfortable motor restlessness; acute dystonia (5), manifested by involuntary contraction of a muscle group, typically oral, nuchal, facial, or limb; dyskinesia (6), resembling choreiform tardive dyskinesia; and parkinsonism (4). In at least one report, the parkinsonian state was accompanied by delirium (19). SSRI-induced akathisia may be severe, may be extremely distressing to an already anxiety-ridden and depressed patient, and has been suggested as a factor contributing to the suicide of some patients early in antidepressant treatment. As is the case when this symptom occurs in the context of neuroleptic treatment, SSRI-induced akathisia may respond to the institution of β-adrenergic blocking agents. Acute dystonic reaction in the setting of SSRI use remains at the frequency level of occasional case reports, although there is little doubt that the complication is genuine.

In isolated cases, the SSRIs are reported to exacerbate the manifestations of pre-existent Parkinson's disease (10,11), an effect consonant with the observation that they exert an antidopaminergic action. All reports to date suggest that any SSRI-induced extrapyramidal side effects are transient and respond to removal of the offending agent.

Because SSRIs and monoamine oxidase inhibitors (MAOIs), when used in conjunction, have in some instances led to the potentially fatal "serotonin syndrome," this combination should be used with the utmost caution (*see* Monoamine Oxidase Inhibitors, this volume, for a discussion). A report indicates that SSRIs in combination with L-deprenyl, a type-B MAOI used in the treatment of Parkinson's disease, may precipitate hypomania in parkinsonian patients treated for depression (20).

Isolated reports suggest that the SSRIs may also be implicated in the appearance of a state resembling a frontal lobe dementia, with apathy, indifference, and sometimes disinhibition, which normalizes when the agent is withdrawn (9). The SSRIs have little seizure-provocative effect, except in overdose, and only a small number of case reports of seizures likely provoked by SSRIs has been published (18).

REFERENCES

1. Baldessarini RJ, Marsh ER (1990) Fluoxetine and side effects. *Arch Gen Psychiat* **47**, 191.
2. Baldessarini RJ, Marsh ER, Kula NS (1992) Interaction of fluoxetine with the metabolism of dopamine and serotonin in rat brain regions. *Brain Res* **579**, 152.
3. Bersani G, Grispini A, Marini S *et al.* (1986) Neuroleptic-induced extrapyramidal side effects: Clinical perspectives with ritanserin (R-5667), a new selective 5-HT2 receptor blocking agent. *Curr Ther Res* **40**, 205.

4. Bouchard RH, Pourcher E, Vincent P (1989) Fluoxetine and extrapyramidal side effects. *Amer J Psychiat* **146**, 1352.

5. Brod TM (1989) Fluoxetine and extrapyramidal side effects. *Amer J Psychiat* **146**, 1353.

6. Budman CL, Bruun RD (1991) Persistent dyskinesia in a patient receiving fluoxetine. *Amer J Psychiat* **148**, 1403.

7. Cooper GL (1988) The safety of fluoxetine—an update. *Brit J Psychiat* **153**, 77.

8. Herve D, Pickel VM, Joh TH, Beaudet A (1987) Serotonin axon terminals in the ventral tegmental area of the rat: Fine structure and synaptic input to dopaminergic neurons. *Brain Res* **435**, 71.

9. Hoehn-Saric R, Harris GJ, Pearlson GD *et al.* (1991) A fluoxetine-induced frontal lobe syndrome in an obsessive compulsive patient. *J Clin Psychiat* **52**, 131.

10. Jansen Steur ENH (1993) Increase of Parkinson disability after fluoxetine medication. *Neurology* **143**, 211.

11. Jimenez-Jimenez FJ, Tejeiro J, Martinez-Junqueera G *et al.* (1994) Parkinsonism exacerbated by paroxetine. *Neurology* **44**, 2406.

12. Kaye CM, Haddock RE, Langley PF *et al.* (1989) A review of the metabolism and pharmacokinetics of paroxetine in man. *Acta Psychiat Scand* **80**, 60.

13. Koe BK, Weissman A, Welch WM *et al.* (1983) Sertraline, 1S,4S - N - methyl - 4 - (3,4 - dichlorophenyl) - 1,2,3,4 -

tetrahydro-1-naphthylamine, a new uptake inhibitor with selectivity for serotonin. *J Pharmacol Exp Ther* **226**, 686.

14. Lipinski JF, Mallya G, Zimmerman RN *et al.* (1989) Fluoxetine-induced akathisia: Clinical and theoretical implications. *J Clin Psychiat* **50**, 339.

15. Lund J, Thayssen P, Mengel H *et al.* (1982) Paroxetine: Pharmacokinetics and cardiovascular effects after oral and intravenous single doses in man. *Acta Pharmacol Toxicol* **51**, 351.

16. Maitre L, Baumann PA, Jaekel J *et al.* (1982) 5-HT uptake inhibitors, psychopharmacological and neurochemical criteria of selectivity. In: *Serotonin in Biological Psychiatry.* Ho BT, Schoolar JC, Usdin E *et al.* eds. Raven Press, New York p. 229.

17. Pato MT, De Vane CL, Murphy DL (1991) Sustained plasma concentrations of fluoxetine and/or norfluoxetine 4 and 8 weeks after fluoxetine discontinuation. *J Clin Psychopharmacol* **12**, 224.

18. Prasher VP (1993) Seizures associated with fluoxetine therapy. *Seizure* **2**, 315.

19. Singh RK, Gupta AK, Singh B (1995) Acute organic brain syndrome after fluoxetine treatment. *Amer J Psychiat* **152**, 295.

20. Sucherowersky O, deVries JD (1990) Interaction of fluoxetine and selegiline. *Can J Psychiat* **35**, 571.

Fumitremorgen

Albert C. Ludolph

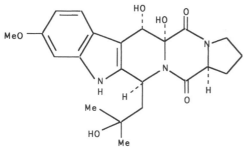

FUMITREMORGEN

NEUROTOXICITY RATING

Experimental

A　Seizure disorder

A　Tremor

The fumitremorgins A, B (synonym, lanosulin), and C, a group of indolic neurotropic mycotoxins, were first isolated from *Aspergillus fumigatus* from rice in 1971 and later detected in *Aspergillus caespitosus* and *Penicillium lanosum*

(1,12). The MWs of fumitremorgin A ($C_{32}H_{41}N_3O_7$) and fumitremorgin B ($C_{27}H_{33}N_3O_5$) are 579 and 479, respectively (8); the MPs are 206°–209°C and 211°–212°C (8). The corresponding data for fumitremorgin C ($C_{32}H_{25}N_3O_3$) are MW 499 and MP 125°–130°C. Elaboration of fumitremorgens is dependent on the presence of L-tryptophan in the culture; they can be detected by thin-layer chromatography (1) and cause tremors and convulsions in mice, rats, and rabbits (4,10,11). Their structure and clinical effects are similar to the mycotoxin verruculogen, isolated from *Penicillium verruculosum* (2) ("fumitremorgen-verruculogen group"). Fumitremorgin A is the most potent compound of this group (4); fumitremorgins B and C are less intensively studied (3,11,13).

In mice, fumitremorgin A induces tremor and generalized tonic-clonic convulsions (9,11) after parenteral and oral administration. Seizures (dosage, 10–200 μg/kg body weight) are not accompanied by electroencephalographic evidence of hypersynchronized cortical activity and were still present in the decorticated or decerebrated animal (4). Convulsions can be interrupted by transection of the spinal cord at an upper level and are associated with an increased excitability of midbrain reticular neurons, suggesting that abnormal excitation of the reticulospinal pathway may cause the seizures induced by fumitremorgin A (5,6). Convulsions can be antagonized by D,L-2-aminophosphonovalerate (AP5), an antagonist at the N-methyl-D-aspartate glutamate receptor subtype, indicating that excitatory amino acid transmitters may play a role. The structurally related compound verruculogen increases cerebral glutamate and aspartate release in rat and sheep synaptosomal preparations (7). Sporadic human and animal diseases from fumitremorgens are not reported (see also Penitrems and other Tremorgens, this volume).

REFERENCES

1. Betina V (1984) Indole-derived tremorgenic toxins. In: *Mycotoxins—Production, Isolation, Separation and Purification*. Betina V ed. Elsevier Science Publishers BV, Amsterdam p. 417.

2. Cole RJ, Kirksey JW, Moore JH et al. (1972) Tremorgenic toxin from *Penicillium verruculosum*. *Appl Microbiol* **24**, 248.

3. Nielsen PV, Beuchat LR, Frisvad JC (1988) Growth of and fumitremorgen production by *Neosartorya fischeri* as affected by temperature, light and water activity. *Appl Environ Microbiol* **54**, 1504.

4. Nishiyama M, Kuga T (1986) Pharmacological effects of the tremorgenic mycotoxin fumitremorgin A. *Jpn J Pharmacol* **40**, 481.

5. Nishiyama M, Kuga T (1989) Central effects of the neurotropic mycotoxin fumitremorgin A in the rabbit. (I). Effects on the spinal cord. *Jpn J Pharmacol* **50**, 167.

6. Nishiyama M, Kuga T (1990) Central effects of the neurotropic mycotoxin fumitremorgin A in the rabbit. (II). Effects on the brain stem. *Jpn J Pharmacol* **52**, 201.

7. Norris PJ, Smith CCT, De Belleroche J et al. (1980) Actions of tremorgenic fungal toxins on neurotransmitter release. *J Neurochem* **34**, 33.

8. Steyn PS, Vleggaar R (1985) Tremorgenic mycotoxins. *Fortschr Chem Org Naturst* **48**, 1.

9. Suzuki S, Kikkawa K, Yamazaki M (1984) Abnormal behavioral effects elicited by a neurotropic mycotoxin, fumitremorgen A, in mice. *J Pharmacobiodyn* **7**, 935.

10. Yamazaki M, Suzuki S (1986) Toxicology of tremorgenic mycotoxins, fumitremorgin A and B. *Develop Toxicol Environ Sci* **12**, 273.

11. Yamazaki M, Suzuki S, Kukita K (1979) Neurotoxicological studies on fumitremorgin A, a tremorgenic mycotocin, on mice. *J Pharmacobiodyn* **2**, 119.

12. Yamazaki M, Suzuki S, Miyaki K (1971) Tremorgenic toxins from *Aspergillus fumigatus*. *Fres Chem Pharm Bull (Tokyo)* **19**, 1739.

13. Weiser M, Fink-Gremmels J (1991) Effects of verruculogen and fumitremorgin B on neurotransmitter release *in vivo*. *Acta Vet Scand Suppl* **87**, 193.

Fumonisin

Albert C. Ludolph

FUMONISIN B$_1$
C$_{34}$H$_{59}$O$_{15}$

1,2,3-Propanetricarboxylic acid 1,1'-[1-(12-amino-4,9,11-trihydroxy-2-methyltridecyl)-2-(1-methylpentyl)-1,2-ethanediyl]ester; Fumonisin B$_1$

NEUROTOXICITY RATING

Clinical

A Leukoencephalopathy (livestock)

Experimental

A Leukoencephalopathy

Fumonisins A$_1$, A$_2$, B$_1$, B$_2$, B$_3$, and B$_4$ (FA$_1$, FA$_2$, FB$_1$, FB$_2$, FB$_3$, FB$_4$) are mycotoxins produced by strains of *Fusarium moniliforme*, *proliferatum*, *anthophilum*, *dlamini*, *napiforme*, and *nygamai* (1,7,8). They are hydroxylated long-chain alkylamines esterified with propanetricarboxylic acid moieties, which are *N*-acetylated (FA) or contain free amino groups (FB). Fumonisins are pulmotoxic for swine (3).

Fumonisin-producing *F. moniliforme* is detected in maize products in all parts of the world, but most reports are from South Africa and the United States (7). It is unknown whether milling and baking affect fumonisin levels, or if the food chain plays a role in the distribution of these neurotoxins in human and animal food (3,9). Thin-layer chromatography, high-performance liquid chromatography, and gas chromatography/mass spectroscopy can detect FB$_1$ and FB$_2$ fumonisins (12,14,19).

FB$_1$ in corn-based feeds causes equine leukoencephalomalacia (ELEM) (6,10,19), a disease observed worldwide in horses, donkeys, and mules. ELEM has been recognized for more than a century in corn-growing regions of North America. Outbreaks occur during late fall through early spring, and wet-harvest seasons after dry summers increase the prevalence of the disease (6). Initial clinical signs include sudden decrease of food intake, depression, and lethargy (6). Incoordination, walking in circles, agitation and hyperexcitability, blindness, severe ataxia, and paralysis follow. The majority dies within 2–3 days but, if exposure ceases, some may recover. There is no treatment; proper drying of corn is an effective preventive measure. FB$_1$ concentrations

>8 ppm in suspect feed are associated with disease (10). Massive necrotic lesions of white matter are the morphological hallmark, but hemorrhagic lesions of the brainstem also occur (19).

Experimental feeding studies with *F. moniliforme* have failed to cause disease in goats, monkeys, hamsters, and rabbits (18). A significant elevation of homovanillic acid (HVA) was observed in most brain regions of BALB/c mice treated with high doses (up to 6.75 mg) of fumonisin B$_1$ for 5 days (16). Decreased levels of 5-hydroxytryptamine (5-HT) were found in striatum. Ratios of neurotransmitters to metabolites, such as HVA/dopamine and 5-hydroxyindoleacetic acid/5-HT, were elevated in several brain regions. The accumulation of neurotransmitter metabolites suggested either increased neuronal activity or interference with metabolite efflux (16).

In a study using intravenous administration of fumonisin B$_1$ to horses for 7–12 days, neurological dysfunction appeared and was neuropathologically characterized by leukoencephalomalacia (5). Oral administration of fumonisin B$_1$ to horses (4) also induced a disease with clinical and neuropathological similarities to ELEM. Feeding fumonisin B$_1$ to ponies caused dose-dependent induction of ELEM (11).

The toxic mechanism is unknown. These compounds exhibit remarkable structural similarity to sphingosine, the long-chain (sphingoid) structural backbone of sphingomyelin, cerebrosides, sulfatides, gangliosides, and other sphingolipids present in the human and animal brain. These similarities prompted studies on the interaction of fumonisins with enzymes that play a role in sphingosin metabolism. Studies in rat hepatocytes show that fumonisins inhibit sphingolipid biosynthesis, more specifically, the enzyme sphingosine *N*-acyltransferase (ceramide synthase) (17). In cultured hippocampal neurons, the inhibition of sphingolipid synthesis by fumonisin leads to reduced synthesis of complex sphingolipids and decreased cellular levels (2). In hippocampal cells, fumonisins cause a disruption of axonal growth reversed by the administration of ceramide (2), consistent with inhibition of ceramide synthesis. Fumonisins also block Ca^{2+} currents in frog cardiac muscle (13). There are no human neurological diseases or neuroteratogenic effects induced by fumonisins (15).

REFERENCES

1. Gelderblom WC, Marasas WF, Vleggaar R et al. (1992) Fumonisins: Isolation, chemical characterization, and biological effects. *Mycopathologia* **117**, 11.

2. Harel R, Futerman AH (1993) Inhibition of sphingolipid synthesis affects axonal outgrowth in cultured hippocampal neurons. *J Biol Chem* **268**, 14476.

3. International Agency for Research on Cancer (IARC) (1993) Toxins derived from *Fusarium moniliforme*: Fumonisins B1 and B2 and fusarin C. *IARC Monogr Eval Carcinog Risks Hum* **56**, 445.

4. Kellermann TS, Marasas WF, Thiel PG et al. (1990) Leukoencephalomalacia in two horses induced by oral dosing of fumonisin B1. *Onderstepoort J Vet Res* **57**, 269.

5. Marasas WFO, Kellerman TS, Gelderblom WCA et al. (1988) Leucoencephalomalacia in a horse induced by fumonisin B_1 isolated from *Fusarium moniliforme*. *Onderstepoort J Vet Res* **55**, 197.

6. McCue PM (1989) Equine leucoencephalomalacia. *Compend Con Educ Pract Vet* **11**, 646.

7. Nelson PE, Plattner RD, Shackelford DD, Desjardins AE (1992) Fumonisin B1 production by *Fusarium* species other than *F. moniliforme* in section *Liseola* and by some related species. *Appl Environ Microbiol* **58**, 984.

8. Ross PF, Nelson PE, Richard JL et al. (1990) Production of fumonisins by *Fusarium moniliforme* and *Fusarium proliferatum* isolates associated with equine leukoencephalomalacia and a pulmonary edema syndrome in swine. *Appl Environ Microbiol* **56**, 3225.

9. Ross PF, Ledet AE, Owens DL et al. (1993) Experimental equine leukoencephalomalacia, toxic hepatosis, and en-

cephalopathy caused by corn contaminated with fumonisins. *J Vet Diagn Invest* **5**, 69.

10. Ross PF, Rice LG, Osweiler GD et al. (1992) A review and update of animal toxicoses associated with fumonisin-associated feeds and production of fumonisins by *Fusarium* isolates. *Mycopathologia* **117**, 109.

11. Ross PF, Rice LG, Reagor JC et al. (1991) Fumonisin B1 concentrations in feeds from 45 confirmed equine leukoencephalomalcia cases. *J Vet Diagn Invest* **3**, 238.

12. Rottinghaus GE, Coatney CE, Minor HC (1992) A rapid, sensitive thin layer chromatography procedure for the detection of fumonisin B1 and B2. *J Vet Diagn Invest* **4**, 326.

13. Sauviat M-P, Laurent D, Kohler F, Pellgrin F (1991) Fumonisin, a toxin from the fungus *Fusarium moniliforme* sheld, blocks both the calcium current and the mechanical activity in frog atrial muscle. *Toxicon* **29**, 1025.

14. Shephard GS, Thiel PG, Sydenham EW (1992) Determination of fumonisin B1 in plasma and urine by high-performance liquid chromatography. *J Chromatogr* **574**, 299.

15. Thiel PG, Marasas WF, Sydenham EW et al. (1992) The implications of naturally occurring levels of fumonisins in corn for human and animal health. *Mycopathologia* **117**, 3.

16. Tsunoda M, Dugyala RR, Sharma RP (1998) Fumonisin B1-induced increases in neurotransmitter metabolite levels in different brain regions of BALB/c mice. *Comp Biochem Physiol C Pharmacol Toxicol Endocrinol* **120**, 457.

17. Wang E, Norred WP, Bacon CW et al. (1991) Inhibition of sphingolipid biosynthesis by fumonisins. Implications for diseases associated with *Fusarium moniliforme*. *J Biol Chem* **266**, 14486.

18. Wilson BJ, Maronpot RR, Hildebrandt PK (1973) Equine leucoencephalomalacia. *J Amer Vet Med Assn* **163**, 1293.

19. Wilson TM, Ross FP, Rice LG et al. (1990) Fumonsin B1 levels associated with an epizootic of equine leukoencephalomalacia. *J Vet Diagn Invest* **2**, 213.

Funnel-Web Spider Toxins

Albert C. Ludolph
Peter S. Spencer

NEUROTOXICITY RATING

Experimental

A   Ion channel dysfunction (P-type calcium channel)—FTX

A   Ion channel dysfunction (sodium channel)—Atrachotoxins

Funnel-web spider toxin (FTX) is a polyamine neurotoxin from the venom of the spider *Agelenopsis aperta* (5). Intraperitoneal administration to mice results in lethal central respiratory failure (5). The effects of FTX differ from those of agatoxins, also isolated from the venom of this spider.

FTX has a polyamine-like structure (4) and, at submicromolar concentrations, selectively blocks P-type Ca^{2+} channels in the dendrites of mammalian Purkinje cells and in presynaptic terminals of squid giant synapses (5). These channels are also blocked by Cd^{2+} and Co^{2+}, but are insensitive to drugs acting at L-type Ca^{2+} channels (2,4). Studies with polyclonal antibodies demonstrate a wide distribution of the protein in the brain (2,4). P-type Ca^{2+} channels may initiate acetylcholine release at the mouse neuromuscular junction (11).

Additional insect and mammalian neurotoxins have been isolated from the venom of other species of funnel-web spider. Venom of *Hololena curta* contains a 38-amino-acid insecticidal peptide and ten acylpolyamine toxins (curtatoxins); the latter instantly paralyze lepidopteran larvae following injection (10). Australian funnel-web spider venom contain neurotoxins (δ-atracotoxins) that produce fatal neurotoxic illness in primates (1). Δ-Atracotoxin Arl (formerly, robustoxin), isolated from the Sydney funnel-web spider. *Atrax robustus*, is a 42-residue polypeptide cross-linked by four disulfide bonds (9). Another neurotoxic polypeptide, δ-atracotoxin-Hv1 (formerly versutoxin), is present in venom of the Australian Blue Mountains funnel-web spider, *Hadronyche versuta*. The actions of δ-atracotoxins on insect and rat brain sodium-channel gating and kinetics are similar to those of α-scorpion and sea anemone toxins; these bind to receptor site 3 on the voltage-gated sodium channel and markedly slow channel inactivation (1,3,6–8). While δ-atracotoxin-Hv1 shows no structural homology with either sea anemone or α-scorpion toxins, it contains charged residues that are topologically related to those implicated in the binding of sea anemone and α-scorpion toxins to mammalian voltage-gated sodium channels, suggesting similarities in their mode of interaction with these channels (1).

REFERENCES

1. Fletcher JI, Chapman BE, Mackay JP *et al.* (1997) The structure of versutoxin (delta-atracotoxin-Hv1) provides insights into the binding of site 3 neurotoxins to the voltage-gated sodium channel. *Structure* 15, 1525.
2. Hillman D, Chen S, Aung TT *et al.* (1991) Localization of P-type calcium channels in the central nervous system. *Proc Nat Acad Sci USA* 88, 7076.
3. Little MJ, Wilson H, Zappia C (1998) Delta-atracotoxins from Australian funnel-web spiders compete with scorpion alpha-toxin binding on both rat brain and insect sodium channels. *FEBS Lett* 439, 246.
4. Llinas RR, Sugimori M, Hillman DE, Cherksey B (1992) Distribution and functional significance of the P-type, voltage-dependent Ca^{2+} channels in the mammalian central nervous system. *Trends Neurosci* 15, 351.
5. Llinas R, Sugimori M, Lin JW, Cherksey B (1989) Blocking and isolation of a calcium channel from neurons in mammals and cephalopods using a toxin fraction (FTX) from funnel-web spider poison. *Proc Nat Acad Sci USA* 86, 1689.
6. Nicholson GM, Little MJ, Tyler M, Narahashi T (1996) Selective alteration of sodium channel gating by Australian funnel-web spider toxins. *Toxicon* 34, 1443.
7. Nicholson GM, Walsh R, Little MJ, Tyler MI (1998) Characterisation of the effects of robustoxin, the lethal neurotoxin from the Sydney funnel-web spider *Atrax robustus*, on sodium channel activation and inactivation. *Pflugers Arch* 436, 117.
8. Nicholson GM, Willow M, Howden ME, Narahashi T (1994) Modification of sodium channel gating and kinetics by versutoxin from the Australian funnel-web spider *Hadronyche versuta*. *Pflugers Arch* 428, 400.
9. Pallagy PK, Alewood D, Alewood PF, Norton RS (1997) Solution structure of robustoxin, the lethal neurotoxin from the funnel-web spider *Atrax robustus*. *FEBS Lett* 419, 191.
10. Quistad GB, Reuter CC, Skinner WS *et al.* (1991) Paralytic and insecticidal toxins from the funnel web spider, *Hololena curta*. *Toxicon* 29, 329.
11. Uchitel OD, Protti DA, Sanchez V *et al.* (1992) P-type voltage-dependent calcium channel mediates presynaptic calcium influx and transmitter release in mammalian synapses. *Proc Nat Acad Sci USA* 89, 3330.

Furaltadone

Herbert H. Schaumburg

FURALTADONE
$C_{13}H_{16}N_4O_6$

5-(4-Morpholinylmethyl)-3-[[(5-nitro-2-furanyl)methylene]amino]-2-oxazolidinone

NEUROTOXICITY RATING
Clinical

B Myopathy

Furaltadone, a synthetic nitrofuran derivative, is a broad-spectrum antibiotic introduced in 1959. It was withdrawn in 1961 following reports of diplopia accompanying dosage at conventional levels. Little systemic toxicity has been associated with furaltadone treatment aside from mild gastrointestinal distress and an occasional "disulfiram reaction" (flushed skin and dyspnea) when this drug is consumed with alcohol (4).

Extraocular muscle palsy is clearly associated with conventional doses of furaltadone for periods exceeding 6 weeks (1–3). Intermittent lateral rectus muscle weakness and horizontal diplopia herald this condition; the diplopia and paresis become persistent after 1 week if therapy continues. Clinical improvement commences within 2 weeks following drug withdrawal and is usually complete after another 3 weeks. There are no reports of permanent neurological impairment. Mild difficulty in swallowing and speaking occurred in two instances (1,2). The site and mechanism of action of furaltadone are unclear; the brief reports do not permit localization of an effect on the neuromuscular junction, cranial nerves, or brainstem.

REFERENCES

1. Hussain KK, Koilpillal H (1960) Toxic effects of furaltadone. *Lancet* **2**, 490.
2. Lee MLH (1960) Toxic effects of prolonged treatment with furaltadone. *Lancet* **2**, 374.
3. Loftus LR, Wagner AW (1960) New allergic reaction to furaltadone. *J Amer Med Assn* **173**, 362.
4. Kautz HD (1960) New and nonofficial drugs. *J Amer Med Assn* **128**, 1932.

Furosemide

Herbert H. Schaumburg

FUROSEMIDE
$C_{12}H_{11}ClN_2O_5S$

5-(Aminosulfonyl)-4-chloro-2-[(2-furanylmethyl)amino]benzoic acid

NEUROTOXICITY RATING

Clinical

A   Ototoxicity

Furosemide is a widely used, potent, renal-loop diuretic. The loop diuretics inhibit electrolyte reabsorption in the thick ascending limb of the loop of Henle; they act at the luminal face of the epithelial cells to inhibit the sodium, potassium, and chloride cotransport mechanism. Furosemide has little systemic toxicity aside from therapy-associated abnormalities of fluid and electrolyte imbalance. Hearing loss is the only serious adverse effect on the nervous system.

Cats, dogs, and guinea pigs dosed with ototoxic levels of furosemide display reduced endocochlear potentials and eighth-nerve compound action potentials; there is slow recovery following withdrawal (2). Ultrastructural examination reveals edema in the stria vascularis and degeneration of intermediate cells (6). Freeze-fracture studies of the tight junctions of the marginal cell of the stria vascularis disclose reduction in the number of apical ridges (7). The pathophysiology of these changes is unknown. While it is clear that furosemide decreases the potassium gradient between endolymph and perilymph, it is debated whether these changes in the stria vascularis stem from inhibition of K^+ pumps or from inhibition of adenylate cyclase through an effect on the G-protein complex (5).

Acute-onset hearing impairment is well established as a human complication of high-dose furosemide therapy; one study describes audiometric changes in 6.4% (8). Most reports describe reversible hearing loss, but permanent impairment can develop; permanent hearing dysfunction is especially common in patients with renal disease (4). Postmortem examination of one individual with renal failure who received large doses of furosemide disclosed marked cystic change in the stria vascularis with sparing of the inner and outer hair cells (1).

The risk of toxicity for pediatric patients treated with high doses of furosemide has been reviewed recently (3).

REFERENCES

1. Arnold W, Nadol JB Jr, Geidauer H (1981) Ultrastructural histopathology in a case of human ototoxicity due to loop diuretics. *Acta Oto-laryngol* **91**, 391.
2. Brusilow SW (1976) Propranolol antagonism to the effect of furosemide on the composition of endolymph in guinea pig. *Can J Physiol Pharmacol* **54**, 42.
3. Eades SK, Christensen ML (1998) The clinical pharmacology of loop diuretics in the pediatric patient. *Pediatr Nephrol* **12**, 603.
4. Gallagher KL, Jones JK (1979) Furosemide-induced ototoxicity. *Ann Intern Med* **91**, 744.
5. Koch T, Gloddek B (1991) Inhibition of adenylate cyclase-coupled G protein complex by ototoxic diuretics and cis-platinum in the inner ear of the guinea pig. *Eur Arch Oto-Rhino-Laryngol* **248**, 459.
6. Pike D, Bosher SK (1980) The time course of the strial changes produced by intravenous furosemide. *Hear Res* **3**, 79.
7. Rarey KE, Ross MD (1982) A survey of the effects of loop diuretics on the zonulae occludentes of the perilymph-endolymph barrier by freeze fracture. *Acta Oto-laryngol* **94**, 307.
8. Tuzel IH (1981) Comparison of adverse reactions to bumetanide and furosemide. *J Clin Pharmacol* **21**, 615.

Galactose

Andew P. Mizisin
Henry C. Powell

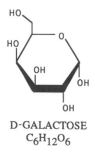

D-GALACTOSE
$C_6H_{12}O_6$

α-D-Galactose

NEUROTOXICITY RATING

Clinical

A   Chronic encephalopathy (cognitive retardation and seizures in
    hereditary galactosemia)

Experimental

A   Acute encephalopathy (seizures, ataxia)

A   Peripheral neuropathy (demyelination, endoneurial edema)

Galactose is a naturally occurring monosaccharide with α-
and β-stereoisomeric forms that have a MW of 180.16.
This hexose, which differs from glucose by the configuration of the hydroxyl group on the fourth carbon, is a white
crystalline powder at room temperature and soluble in water. Galactose is a constituent of many oligo- and polysac-
charides occurring in pectins, gums, and mucilages; it is also
present as a free sugar in fruits and vegetables (11). However, the principal dietary source of this sugar is the disaccharide lactose, the predominant carbohydrate of mammalian milk. Endogenous production of galactose can occur
as the result of synthesis from glucose or breakdown of
galactose-containing glycoproteins and glycolipids (8).
Aside from its nutritional importance, exogenously administered galactose is useful as a diagnostic aid in liver-
function tests; the rate of clearance of plasma galactose is
an index of hepatic blood flow (41).

Toxicity occurs as the result of deficiencies in enzymes of
galactose metabolism or when the capacity of galactose-
specific metabolic pathways is overwhelmed by dietary excess. Three inherited disorders of galactose metabolism
have been identified in humans; these result from different
enzyme deficiencies in the metabolic pathways that convert
galactose to glucose (Fig. 10). Toxicity resulting from high-
galactose diets has been studied in chickens and rodents in
which the enzymes of galactose metabolism are normal.
Galactose toxicity has also been noted in orphaned kan-
garoos bottle-fed with cow's milk and predicted in other
marsupials because many of these species have reduced levels of galactose-metabolizing enzymes, and females produce
milk with a low-lactose content (38). The impact of galactose toxicity depends on the particular pathway of galactose
metabolism present in various cells and the structure of the
tissues and organs containing these cells. Experimental
studies using high-galactose diets have demonstrated toxic
complications in tissues of the eye, liver, kidney, gonads,
and cardiovascular and nervous systems.

Absorption of free galactose or galactose derived from
the breakdown of lactose by lactase takes place in the intestine. Influx into intestinal epithelium occurs *via* a
sodium-dependent, carrier-mediated cotransporter with an
affinity for both D-glucose and D-galactose (5). Galactose
given orally or intravenously is rapidly cleared from the
blood, with the liver playing a major role in its subsequent
metabolism. A significant amount of the ^{14}C of radioactive
galactose given intravenously appears in the glucose stores
of the body, and the profile of $^{14}CO_2$ in expired air matches
that seen after administration of radioactive glucose (35),
suggesting the rapid conversion of galactose to glucose.

Galactose metabolism occurs *via* the uridine nucleotide
pathway and two alternative pathways (Fig. 10). The uridine nucleotide pathway contains three key enzymes: galactokinase, galactose 1-phosphate uridyltransferase, and
uridine diphosphate galactose 4-epimerase (*see* 34 and references therein). Under normal conditions, galactokinase
phosphorylates galactose with adenosine triphosphate
(ATP) to form galactose 1-phosphate. Galactokinase is
found in several human tissues, including erythrocytes, leukocytes, and in rat and pig liver. Galactose 1-phosphate and
uridine diphosphate glucose (UDP-glucose) are subsequently converted to UDP-galactose and glucose 1-
phosphate by galactose 1-phosphate uridyltransferase,
which is present in a variety of human and rat tissues including liver, intestinal mucosa, ovary, and cerebellum. The
UDP-galactose formed by galactose 1-phosphate uridyltransferase is converted to UDP-glucose by uridine diphosphate galactose 4-epimerase, which has been studied in
liver, intestinal mucosa, and erythrocytes. Subsequent
metabolism of UDP-glucose to glucose 1-phosphate occurs
in the presence of UDP-glucose pyrophosphorylase and
UTP. In humans, deficiencies of galactokinase, galactose
1-phosphate uridyltransferase, and uridine diphosphate
galactose 4-epimerase result in galactosemia of the
galactokinase-deficient, transferase-deficient, and epimerase-
deficient types, respectively.

Alternative pathways of galactose metabolism include re-

MAJOR PATHWAYS OF GALACTOSE METABOLISM

Galactose + ATP $\xrightarrow{1}$ Galactose 1-phosphate + ADP

Galactose 1-phosphate + UDP Glucose $\xleftrightarrow{2}$ Glucose 1-phosphate + UDP Galactose

UDP Galactose + NAD$^+$ $\xleftrightarrow{3}$ UDP Glucose + NADH

ALTERNATIVE PATHWAYS OF GALACTOSE METABOLISM

Galactose + NADPH $\xrightarrow{4}$ Galactitol + NADP$^+$

Galactose $\xrightarrow{5}$ Galactonate

FIGURE 10. Major and alternative pathways of galactose metabolism. Enzymes involved include galactosekinase (1); galactose 1-phosphate uridyltransferase (2); uridine diphosphate galactose 4-epimerase (3); aldose reductase (4); and an incompletely characterized oxidase or dehydrogenase (5). Deficiencies in enzymes 1, 2, and 3 result in galactokinase-, transferase-, and epimerase-deficient galactosemia, respectively. UDP Glucose and UDP Galactose, uridine diphosphoglucose glucose and galactose, respectively; ATP, adenosine triphosphate; ADP, adenosine diphosphate; UDP, uridine diphosphate; NAD$^+$, nicotinamide adenine dinucleotide; NADP$^+$, nicotine adenine dinucleotide phosphate; NADH and NADPH, reduced forms of NAD$^+$ and NADP$^+$.

duction to galactitol and oxidation to galactonate (*see* 34 and references therein). The reduction to galactitol is catalyzed by aldose reductase in the presence of reduced nicotinamide adenine dinucleotide phosphate. Aldose reductase is localized to a variety of insulin-independent tissues including lens, retina, peripheral nerve, artery, testis, and kidney (22,23). Galactitol appears in these tissues after feeding a high-galactose diet or as a consequence of both galactokinase- and transferase-deficient galactosemia and is associated with a decrease in myoinositol. The formation of galactonate from galactose by a metabolic pathway using an oxidase or dehydrogenase results in the accumulation of galactonate in the urine of galactosemic humans and in the urine, liver, intestine, heart, and kidney of rats fed a high-galactose diet.

Normally, galactose is metabolized to CO_2, which is excreted by the lungs. With galactose dysmetabolism, less galactose is excreted as expired CO_2, and plasma and tissue levels of galactose and its metabolites, galactose 1-phosphate, galactitol, and galactonate, increase (*see* 34 and references therein). These metabolites accumulate in the kidney and have been detected in the urine of galactosemic patients and galactose-fed rats.

Certain marsupials, including the kangaroo, have relatively low levels of galactokinase and/or uridyltransferase, such that orphaned pouch joeys fed cow's milk are predisposed to cataract formation (*see* 38 and references therein); no neurotoxic complications have been reported.

Galactose neurotoxicity in the chick can be observed within 36–48 h of feeding a diet containing 40% galactose by weight. The neurological disorder is characterized by ataxia, tremors, and epileptiform seizures that result in death after several days (*see* 32 and references therein). The tremor and convulsions represent an early neurotoxic effect

of galactose and are reversible upon withdrawal of the diet. The effects of galactose administration on chick brain metabolism include a decrease in ATP, glucose, glycolytic intermediates, and amino acid pools but no change in polyribosomal profiles and protein synthesis (3,9). Galactose and galactitol accumulations in chick retina and brain occur after 50–55 h of galactose feeding and are associated with delays in fast axoplasmic transport that are normalized 24 h after withdrawal from the diet (17). Degenerative changes of neurons within the basal ganglia accompanied by perineuronal edema have been described in galactose-fed chicks and may represent irreversible anoxic damage that culminates in death (32).

Early reports of short-term galactose feeding in rodents describe rapid declines in body weight and death, and the presence of "beriberi" convulsions accompanied by loss of muscular coordination in galactose-fed mice that received ample vitamin B in their diet (12). Subsequent studies investigating the effect of galactose feeding on fetal brain have shown galactose 1-phosphate and galactitol accumulations and reductions in brain weight and cell number in preterm and term fetuses, suggesting that galactose toxicity interferes with the rate of cell division in the fetal brain (15,45). In contrast, despite clinical and biochemical evidence of galactosemia, cerebral growth was not affected by feeding galactose to suckling rats (14). In adult rats, short-term effects of galactose feeding in peripheral nerve include accumulation of galactose and galactitol, and myoinositol and amino acid depletion, that are associated with increased water content (16,30). Increased endoneurial water content, manifest morphologically as edema, is associated with an increased permeability of the blood-nerve barrier to low-molecular-weight tracers (16).

The neurotoxic effects of prolonged exposure to high-galactose diets has been investigated primarily in rodents. As polyol accumulation has been implicated in long-term complications of diabetes mellitus (for review, see 40), localization of aldose reductase to nerve and spinal cord (6) prompted studies examining the consequences of sorbitol pathway activity in experimental models of diabetes. Since galactose-fed rats accumulate galactitol without the attendant complications associated with insulin deficiency, many studies have used galactose feeding to model the consequences of polyol accumulation in diabetic neuropathy.

A variety of galactose-induced functional defects of peripheral nerve have been reported, many of which are reversible by inhibiting aldose reductase. Defects include conduction velocity deficits (7), dose-dependent increases in Na^+,K^+-ATPase (25), impaired slow anterograde and retrograde axonal transport (37), decreased blood flow (28) and oxygen tension (21), and increased permeability of the blood-nerve barrier to low-molecular-weight tracers (42). These functional abnormalities have been documented in the context of an osmotic imbalance of the endoneurium characterized by dose-dependent increases in edema, interstitial fluid pressure, and electrolytes (26).

Galactose-induced structural injury occurs most frequently in Schwann cells of myelinated fibers, the major cellular repository of aldose reductase in peripheral nerve and, therefore, the site of galactitol synthesis and accumulation. Severe injury includes degenerative changes of Schwann cells that culminate in demyelination; these changes are ameliorated when galactitol accumulation is attenuated by inhibiting aldose reductase (27). Less severe Schwann cell injury is characterized by reactive changes that include cytoplasmic swelling associated with accumulation of lipid droplets, lysosomes and glycogen granules. Decreased levels of the Schwann cell–derived ciliary neuronotrophic factor (CNTF) have been documented after 1 month of galactose feeding (4) and may reflect direct or indirect consequences of polyol accumulation.

Decreased myoinositol levels in the tissues of galactosemic patients and galactose-fed rats (31,39,46) suggest that myoinositol metabolism may be adversely affected by galactitol accumulation. In vitro studies of brain slices from newborn rats exposed to galactose in utero demonstrate impaired conversion of glucose to myoinositol (45). In contrast, no impairment of myoinositol metabolism was observed in isolated synaptosomes prepared from similarly treated rats (44). These observations suggest that nonneuronal glial elements may be responsible for impaired myoinositol metabolism in brain slices (44). Further support for the involvement of the glial component of nervous tissue is derived from a study demonstrating that uptake of myo-inositol is inhibited by galactose in Schwann cells isolated from rat sciatic nerve (36). In vitro incubation of sciatic nerve in a high-galactose medium attenuates uptake of radiolabeled myoinositol and taurine and increases galactitol accumulation; these changes are prevented when aldose reductase is inhibited (30).

In humans, galactose-induced neurotoxicity results from inherited deficiencies of three enzymes of galactose metabolism that produce galactokinase-deficient, transferase-deficit, and epimerase-deficient galactosemia. Clinical descriptions of neurotoxic complications are most complete for transferase-deficient galactosemia. Retarded mental development noted after several months of life translates into delays in acquisition of language skills (43). While delayed speech and verbal dyspraxia are the most recognizable symptom of CNS dysfunction, specific learning disabilities are apparent and involve spatial relationships and mathematics. Behavioral and psychological problems include short attention spans and inadequate drive, shyness, and withdrawal (19). In older children and adolescents, cerebellar ataxia and tremor have been noted (see 18 and references therein). Magnetic resonance imaging scans have detected mild cerebral and cerebellar atrophy as well as multiple small white matter lesions; however, widespread neuropathological abnormalities are absent in cerebellar cortex (see 13 and references therein). Increased intracranial pressure and cerebral edema have been documented as has pseudotumor cerebri (see 1 and references therein).

In contrast to transferase-deficient galactosemia, clinical studies of galactokinase-deficient and epimerase-deficient galactosemia are based on fewer individuals and consequently the knowledge gathered about the transferase-deficiency condition has not been duplicated in these two disorders. Neurotoxic complications include seizures that developed in a 17-year-old youth with galactokinase deficiency and a report of pseudotumor cerebri (20). In severe forms of epimerase deficiency with systemic loss of enzymatic activity in liver and other tissues, nerve deafness has been reported in two children, with mental retardation in one (33).

All three forms of galactosemia are inherited as autosomal recessive disorders, with parents of severely affected individuals having one-half of normal enzyme activity. Estimates of incidence have been complicated by the presence of alleles that lower enzyme activity but do not have the capacity to cause galactosemia in the homozygous state (2). While the incidence varies with population, screening programs have detected an average frequency of the transferase-deficient disorder of 1 per 62,000. Estimates of the incidence of the galactokinase-deficient disorder range between 0 per 582,000 and 1 per 168,022. There are few reliable data on the incidence of epimerase-deficient galactosemia.

Key to the diagnosis of transferase-deficiency galactosemia within days of birth are the vomiting and diarrhea resulting from lactose intolerance precipitated by milk feedings that are associated with weight loss and jaundice (see 34 and references therein). Consistent laboratory findings are galactose in the blood and urine and increased levels of galactose metabolites, galactose 1-phosphate and galactitol, in tissue blood and urine. Galactonate has also been detected in urine following galactose ingestion. Galactokinase-deficiency galactosemia is distinguished from the transferase-deficient form by the absence of gastrointestinal dysfunction in the newborn period. Diagnosis in infancy depends on screening blood and urine for galactose and the demonstration of normal levels of uridyltransferase and no galactokinase in erythrocytes. Diagnosis of epimerase-deficient galactosemia depends on screening tissue and erythrocytes for uridine diphosphate galactose 4-epimerase. Individuals with the benign form of the epimerase-deficient disorder may have a normal galactose tolerance associated with a rise in erythrocyte galactose 1-phosphate. The severe form of epimerase-deficient galactosemia has been reported in one case to resemble the transferase-deficient form with respect to vomiting, weight loss, jaundice, and galactosuria in early infancy.

Treatment of galactosemia is dependent on the particular disorder; the main therapy for transferase- and galactokinase-deficiency galactosemia is *avoidance* of dietary lactose. Dietary restriction eliminates or reverses poor growth in infants, gastrointestinal dysfunction, jaundice, liver disease, kidney dysfunction, and cataracts. However, dietary therapy has no effect on the development and prevalence of CNS disease, and most patients placed on a lactose-restricted diet will exhibit some signs of nervous dysfunction (43). Treatment of the epimerase-deficient disorder requires a different strategy, as the complete lack of dietary galactose would compromise the ability to form galactose-containing glycoproteins and glycolipids. Therapy involves providing a diet containing enough galactose to promote the synthesis of galactoproteins and galactolipids but not enough to induce toxicity.

As noted earlier, investigations into the nature of the disruption of cellular processes induced by galactose dysmetabolism have been carried out mainly in animals, particularly chicks and rodents fed high-galactose diets. However, in these species, the enzymes of the major pathways of galactose metabolism (Fig. 10) are present, a situation not entirely analogous to human galactosemia. Therefore, toxic mechanisms of galactose-induced injury inferred from animal studies should be applied to the human disorders with caution.

Irreversible damage to neural tissue characterized by retarded mental development in human galactosemia is associated with the accumulation of end products of galactose metabolism including galactitol, galactose 1-phosphate, and galactose 6-phosphate. End-product accumulation in neural tissue is also common to animal fed high-galactose diets. Galactitol accumulations have been noted in rat and chick neural tissue, and galactose 1-phosphate and galactose 6-phosphate accumulations have been reported in chick brains. While no apparent galactose-induced brain abnormality develops in rats, neurotoxicity in chicks is characterized by tremor, ataxia, and convulsions. These abnormalities are reversible when galactose is removed from the diet, suggesting that neurotoxicity may be secondary to end-product accumulation. While it is unclear whether the neural symptoms observed in chicks are comparable to the mental retardation seen in human galactosemia, their acute onset and reversibility argue against this possibility.

One consequence of end-product accumulation is changes in the osmolality of neural tissue and other biological fluids. Perineuronal edema has been described in the basal ganglia of chicks fed high-galactose diets (32), and there is a report that chick neurotoxicity correlates with hyperosmolar dehydration resulting from galactose feeding (24). While no apparent brain abnormality is apparent in galactose-fed rats, as described above, a peripheral neuropathy does develop in the context of an osmotic-imbalance-characterized edema and dose-dependent increases in endoneurial electrolytes and interstitial fluid pressure. These changes are prevented when galactitol accumulation is attenuated by inhibiting aldose reductase. Interestingly, increased intracranial pressure and cerebral edema have been documented in a child with galactosemia (1), but whether these abnormalities are responsive to aldose reductase inhibition and thus due to galactitol accumulation is unknown. However, this observation and the finding of pseudotumor cerebri in both galactokinase- and transferase-deficient galactosemia (1,20) implicate changes in tissue osmolality as a toxic mechanism in humans.

Metabolite depletion is another consequence of the accumulation of end products of galactose metabolism. Myoinositol depletion has been linked to galactitol accumulation in galactose-fed rats, as aldose reductase inhibition not only prevents galactitol accumulation but also restores nerve myoinositol levels. In addition, impaired conversion of glucose to myoinositol has been reported in brains of newborn rats exposed to galactose *in utero* (45). Depletion of myoinositol has been suggested to disrupt phosphoinositide metabolism with consequent effects on intracellular signaling (for review, *see* 10). While there is evidence of myoinositol depletion associated with galactitol accumulation in galactokinase- and transferase-deficient galactose-mia, whether disrupted phosphoinositide metabolism contributes to neurotoxic complications in human galactosemia is unclear. Depletion of the sugar nucleotides, UDP-galactose and UDP-glucose, due to defective transferase activity, has been suggested to impair glycoprotein and glycolipid synthesis (29). However, whether depletion of sugar nucleotides compromises glycoconjugate synthesis, and what role this might have on neurotoxic complications in galactosemia, are unresolved questions.

Aside from the possible consequences described above, toxic effects of end-product accumulation on the cells that contain the enzymes of galactose metabolism need to be considered. In the peripheral nerve of galactose-fed rats, galactitol is produced by aldose reductase in Schwann cells, the major cellular repository of this enzyme. Structural injury, characterized by reactive and degenerative changes, occurs in Schwann cells in association with marked galactitol accumulation. Both galactitol accumulation and Schwann cell injury are attenuated when aldose reductase is inhibited (27), suggesting that either galactitol accumulation or indirect consequences of galactitol accumulation are responsible for the cellular injury. Disintegrating Schwann cells with hydropic cytoplasm are consistent with osmotic injury, and reports of reductions in CNTF (4) suggest that galactitol accumulation may compromise other aspects of metabolism prior to overt structural injury. While galactitol accumulation and white matter lesions have been reported in galactosemia (*see* 13 and references therein), there is no clear evidence that the cellular injury results from the accumulation of galactitol or another metabolite.

REFERENCES

1. Belman AL, Moshe SL, Zimmerman RD (1986) Computered tomographic demonstration of cerebral edema in a child with galactosemia. *Pediatrics* **78**, 606.
2. Beutler E (1991) Galactosemia: Screening and diagnosis. *Clin Biochem* **24**, 293.
3. Blosser JC, Wells WW (1972) Studies on amino acid levels and protein metabolism in the brains of galactose-intoxicated chicks. *J Neurochem* **19**, 69.
4. Calcutt NA, Muir D, Powell HC, Mizisin AP (1991) Reduced ciliary neuronotrophic factor-like activity in nerves from diabetic or galactose-fed rats. *Brain Res* **575**, 320.
5. Frizzel RA, Nellans HN, Schulz SG (1973) Effects of sugars and amino acids on sodium and potassium influx in the rabbit ileum. *J Clin Invest* **5**, 215.
6. Gabbay KH, Merola LO, Field RA (1966) Sorbitol pathway: Presence in nerve and cord with substrate accumulation in diabetes. *Science* **151**, 209.
7. Gabbay KH, Snider JJ (1972) Nerve conduction defect in galactose-fed rats. *Diabetes* **21**,295.
8. Gitzelmann R, Hansen RG, Steinman B (1975) Biogenesis of galactose, a possible mechanism of self-intoxication. In: *Normal and Pathological Development of Energy Metabolism.* Hommes F, Van den Berg G eds. Academic Press, London p. 25.
9. Grannett SE, Kozak LP, McIntyre JP, Wells WW (1972) Studies on cerebral energy metabolism during the course of galactose neurotoxicity in chicks. *J Neurochem* **19**, 1659.
10. Greene DA, Lattimer-Greene S, Sima AAF (1989) Pathogenesis of diabetic neuropathy: Role of altered phosphoinositide metabolism. *Crit Rev Neurobiol* **5**, 143.
11. Gross KC, Acosta PB (1991) Fruits and vegetables are a source of galactose: implications in planning diets of patients with galactosemia. *J Inherit Metab Dis* **14**, 253.
12. Guha BC (1931) On galactose as a dietary carbohydrate. *Biochem J* **25**, 1385.
13. Haberland C, Perou M, Brunngraber EG *et al.* (1971) The neuropathology of galactosemia: A histopathological and biochemical study. *J Neuropathol Exp Neurol* **30**, 431.
14. Haworth JC, Ford JD, Ho HK (1970) The effect of galactose toxicity on growth of the developing rat brain. *Brain Res* **21**, 385.
15. Haworth JC, Ford JD, Younoszai MK (1969) Effect of galactose toxicity on growth of the rat fetus and brain. *Pediat Res* **3**, 441.
16. Kalichman MW, Powell HC, Calcutt NA, Mizisin AP (1995) Mast cell degranulation and blood-nerve barrier permeability in rat sciatic nerve after seven days of hyperglycemia. *Amer J Physiol—Heart Circ Phy* **268**, H740.
17. Knull HR, Lobert PF, Wells WW (1974) Galactose neurotoxicity in chicks: Effects on fast axonal transport. *Brain Res* **79**, 524.
18. Koch TK, Schmidt KA, Wagstaff JE *et al.* (1992) Neurologic complications in galactosemia. *Pediat Neurol* **8**, 217.
19. Komrower GM, Lee DH (1970) Long-term followup of galactosemia. *Arch Dis Child* **45**, 367.
20. Litman N, Kanter A, Finberg L (1975) Galactokinase deficiency presenting as pseudotumor cerebri. *J Pediat* **86**, 410.
21. Low PA, Nukada H, Schmelzer JD *et al.* (1985) Endoneurial oxygen tension and radial topography in nerve edema. *Brain Res* **341**, 147.
22. Ludvigson MA, Sorenson RL (1980) Immunohistochemical localization of aldose reductase. I. Enzyme purification and antibody preparation—localization in peripheral nerve, artery and testis. *Diabetes* **29**, 438.
23. Ludvigson MA, Sorenson RL (1980) Immunohistochemical localization of aldose reductase. II. Rat eye and kidney. *Diabetes* **29**, 450.
24. Malone J, Wells H, Segal S (1972) Decreased uptake of glucose by brain of the galactose toxic chick. *Brain Res* **43**, 700.
25. Mizisin AP, Calcutt NA (1991) Dose-dependent altera-

tions in nerve polyols and (Na^+,K^+)-ATPase activity in galactose intoxication. *Metabolism* **40**, 1207.

26. Mizisin AP, Myers RR, Heckman HM, Powell HC (1988) Dose-dependence of endoneurial fluid sodium and chloride accumulation in galactose intoxication. *J Neurol Sci* **86**, 113.

27. Mizisin AP, Powell HC (1993) Schwann cell injury is attenuated by aldose reductase inhibition in galactose intoxication. *J Neuropathol Exp Neurol* **52**, 78.

28. Myers RR, Powell HC (1984) Galactose neuropathy: Impact of chronic endoneurial edema on nerve blood flow. *Ann Neurol* **16**, 587.

29. Ng WG, Xu YK, Kaufman FR, Donnell GN (1989) Deficit of uridine diphosphate galactose in galactosemia. *J Inherit Metab Dis* **12**, 257.

30. Nishimura C, Lou MF, Kinoshita JH (1987) Depletion of myo-inositol and amino acids in galactosemic neuropathy. *J Neurochem* **49**, 290.

31. Quan-Ma R, Wells W (1965) The distribution of galactitol in tissues of rats fed galactose. *Biochem Biophys Res Commun* **20**, 486.

32. Rigdon RH, Couch JR, Creger CR, Ferguson TM (1963) Galactose intoxication. Pathologic study in the chick. *Experientia* **19**, 349.

33. Sardharwalla IB, Wraith JE, Bridge C *et al.* (1988) A patient with severe type epimerase deficiency galactosemia. *J Inherit Metab Dis* **11**, 249.

34. Segal S, Berry GT (1995) Disorders of galactose metabolism. In: *The Metabolic and Molecular Basis of Inherited Disease. 7th Ed.* Scriver CR, Beaudet AL, Sly WS, Valle D eds. McGraw-Hill, New York p. 967.

35. Segal S, Blair A (1961) Some observations on the metabolism of D-galactose in normal man. *J Clin Invest* **40**, 2016.

36. Segal S, Hwang SM, Stern J, Pleasure D (1984) Inositol uptake by cultured isolated rat Schwann cells. *Biochem Biophys Res Commun* **120**, 486.

37. Sidenius P, Jakobsen J (1980) Axonal transport in rats after galactose feeding. *Diabetologia* **19**, 229.

38. Stephens T, Crollini C, Mutton P *et al.* (1975) Galactose metabolism in relation to cataract formation in marsupials. *Aust J Exp Biol Med Sci* **53**, 233.

39. Stewart MA, Sherman WR, Harris JT (1969) Effects of galactose on levels of free myoinositol in rat tissues. *Ann N Y Acad Sci* **165**, 609.

40. Tomlinson DR, Willars GB, Carrington AL (1992) Aldose reductase inhibitors and diabetic complications. *Pharmacol Ther* **54**, 151.

41. Tygstrup N, Winkler K (1958) Galactose clearance as a measure of hepatic blood flow. *Clin Sci* **17**, 1.

42. Wadhwani KC, Caspers-Velu LE, Murphy VA *et al.* (1989) Prevention of nerve edema and increased blood-nerve barrier permeability-surface area product in galactosemic rats by aldose reductase or thromboxane synthetase inhibitors. *Diabetes* **38**, 1469.

43. Waisbren SE, Norman TR, Schnell RR, Levy HL (1983) Speech and language deficits in early treated children with galactosemia. *J Pediat* **102**, 75.

44. Warfield AS, Segal S (1978) Myoinositol and phosphatidylinositol metabolism in synaptosomes from galactose-fed rats. *Proc Nat Acad Sci USA* **75**, 4568.

45. Wells HJ, Wells WW (1967) Galactose toxicity and myoinositol metabolism in the developing rat brain. *Biochemistry* **6**, 1168.

46. Wells W, Pittman T, Wells H, Egan T (1965) The isolation and identification of galactitol from brains of galactosemia patients. *J Biol Chem* **240**, 1002.

Ganciclovir

Steven A. Sparr

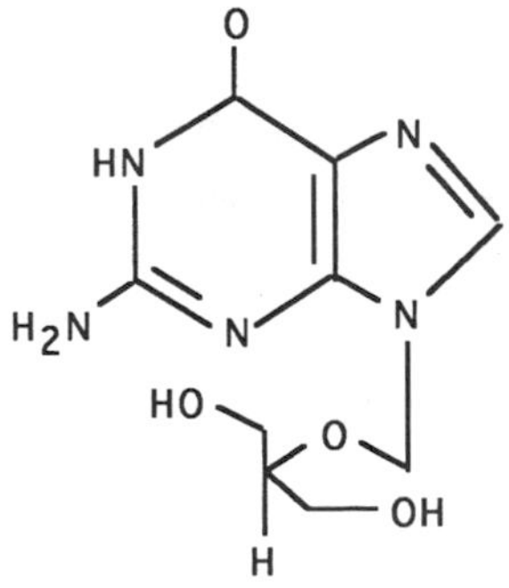

GANCICLOVIR
$C_9H_{13}N_5O_4$

9-[(1,3-Dihydroxy-2-propoxy)methyl]guanine

NEUROTOXICITY RATING

Clinical

B Retinopathy

B Seizure disorder

B Acute encephalopathy (confusion, psychosis, sedation)

Experimental

A Retinopathy (photoreceptor degeneration)

Ganciclovir, a nucleoside analog of guanine, has a similar structure to acyclovir and is used in treatment of herpes viruses, particularly cytomegalovirus (CMV) infections in immunocompromised hosts (7). The drug requires intracellular activation to ganciclovir triphosphate, which is accomplished by the action of viral thymidine kinase or by other enzymes induced by the host-cell virus (7). As triphosphorylation of ganciclovir is minimal in most noninfected host cells, the drug has selective activity in infected cells (10). Once activated, the drug competitively inhibits the incorporation of deoxyguanosine triphosphate into replicating DNA and is itself incorporated into DNA where it serves as a false nucleotide, inhibiting viral replication (7,10). Given its potential for severe toxicity, especially bone marrow suppression, the drug is recommended only for life-threatening CMV infections in immunocompromised hosts, or for averting potential blindness due to CMV retinitis (7). CNS and retinal toxicity have been reported, but it is unclear whether these effects are due to the drug or to the underlying disease processes (7).

Ganciclovir has been demonstrated *in vitro* to have activity against a wide variety of viruses in the herpes family: CMV, Epstein-Barr virus, varicella zoster, and *Herpes simplex* types I and II, although it is inactive against the latent phases of these viruses (7,10). Human studies have focused almost exclusively on patients with CMV infections and immune dysfunction due to acquired immunodeficiency syndrome (AIDS) or immunosuppressive drugs. Acyclovir, which has a better safety profile, is preferred for other herpes viridae infections (7). CMV infections of lungs, bowel, liver, and brain, and disseminated infections have been treated under compassionate-plea protocols (7,12); intravitreous infections have been used for sight-threatening CMV retinitis (7).

Ganciclovir may be administered intravenously or by vitreous injection. The drug has poor bioavailability by the oral route, with less than 7% absorption from the gastrointestinal tract (7,10). Following intravenous administration, peak plasma levels vary linearly with dose; the elimination half-life is 2–4 h (7,10), but may be as high as 30 h in patients with renal failure (1,7,10). The drug is minimally bound to plasma proteins and has wide distribution to body tissues, with spinal fluid concentrations 31%–67% of plasma concentrations, and intravitreous concentrations similar to those in serum (7,10). With normal renal function, virtually all of an intravenous dose of ganciclovir is excreted unchanged in the urine (7).

Activation of ganciclovir by mono- and then triphosphorylation is minimal in most noninfected cells (7), although rapidly dividing cells such as hematopoietic cells can achieve significant activation (10). In cells infected with *Herpes simplex*, varicella zoster and, to a lesser extent, Ebstein-Barr virus, viral thymidine kinase is responsible for most triphosphorylation. As CMV does not encode for thymidine kinase, mono- and triphosphorylation of the drug is accomplished by guanylate kinase and other enzymes induced in CMV-infected cells (7,10). Once incorporated into the genome, ganciclovir triphosphate interferes with DNA-chain elongation and with RNA transcription (7), ultimately decreasing viral replication. The drug is virustatic, not virucidal, and DNA synthesis resumes once the drug is withdrawn (10).

Adverse effects are frequent with ganciclovir therapy, causing cessation of therapy in about a third of treated patients (7). Bone marrow suppression is the most frequent and devastating side effect of ganciclovir, with neutropenia occurring in 40% of patients, thrombocytopenia in 20%, and anemia in only 2% (7). The hematological side effects are usually reversible with cessation of therapy (8). Fever, rash, and liver-function abnormalities occur in approximately 2% of patients (7,10). About 5% of patients monitored by the manufacturer were reported to have adverse neurological side effects after systemic therapy (7), and the incidence of adverse effects on the nervous system has been reported to be as high as 17% (10).

In animal toxicological studies, ganciclovir was well tolerated in dogs who were treated systemically with the drug after total body irradiation and autologous marrow transplantation (7). Intravitreal administration of ganciclovir did not produce electroretinographic or histological retinal toxicity in rabbits with doses that achieved vitreous concentrations of up to 30 μg/ml (9). However, multiple weekly injections of 100–1000 μg injected into the vitreous humor of rabbits led to vacuolization of retinal photoreceptor cells (13).

In human studies, ganciclovir has been reported to produce a variety of CNS side effects, including confusion, psychosis, nightmares, anxiety, ataxia, dysesthesias, seizures, and coma (7,8,10). In a European study of 120 non-AIDS patients with immune suppression treated with ganciclovir, 6% experienced CNS dysfunction during therapy, including seizures, confusion, and tremor (12). In another study of 26 patients (twenty-two with AIDS) treated with ganciclovir for CMV infection, one developed headache and myalgia, one developed disorientation, and one had hallucinations (4). It has been difficult to implicate ganciclovir causally with these side effects, as many patients have had concurrent CNS infections or other overwhelming infections, or were treated with other potentially neurotoxic drugs (2). For example, several patients reported to have generalized seizures were concurrently treated with imipenim-cilstatin, which may itself be epileptogenic (2,10). Headache was reported in 17% of renal transplantation patients receiving ganciclovir, but also in 11% of controls (10).

Several single case reports are suggestive of ganciclovir-induced CNS toxicity, especially in the setting of renal dysfunction (5). One described a patient with AIDS and CMV retinitis who developed nightmares and visual hallucinations while on ganciclovir therapy. Symptoms resolved with discontinuation of therapy but recurred with rechallenge (3). This individual had mild renal failure, perhaps with toxic accumulation of the drug. A renal transplant recipient with CMV hepatitis and duodenitis developed agitation and confusion while on ganciclovir therapy. Serum peak levels of ganciclovir were in the usual therapeutic range, and trough level was only borderline elevated; symptoms improved with dose reduction (6). Seizures appeared in a 32-year-old man with AIDS and disseminated CMV while on ganciclovir therapy (2). Seizures abated with cessation of the drug and recurred with resumption of therapy. Magnetic resonance imaging, however, showed focal pathology in the right temporal lobe.

Intravitreal injection is reserved for patients with CMV retinitis who cannot tolerate systemic administration of the drug. Ocular injection is usually well tolerated, although this has been associated with rhegmatogenous retinal detachment (10), a complication seen with the underlying disease. A single case was reported in which an inadvertent massive intravitreal injection of ganciclovir of 40 mg (usual dose, 0.2–0.4 mg) led to visual loss and permanent retinal damage (11). The authors could not be certain that the retinal toxicity was due to direct effects of the drug, osmolarity of the injection, or alkaline pH.

REFERENCES

1. Bastien O, Boulieu R, Bleyzac N, Estanove S (1994) Clinical use of ganciclovir during renal failure and continuous hemodialysis. *Intens Care Med* 20, 47.

2. Barton TL, Roush MK, Dever LL (1992) Seizures associated with ganciclovir therapy. *Pharmacotherapy* 12, 413.

3. Chen JL, Brocavich JM, Lin AY (1992) Psychiatric disturbances associated with gancyclovir therapy. *Ann Pharmacother* 26, 193.

4. Collaborative DHPG Treatment Study Group (1986) Treatment of serious cytomegalovirus infections with 9-(1,3-dihydroxy-2-propoxymethyl) guanine in patients with AIDS and other immunodeficiencies. *N Engl J Med* 314, 801.

5. Ernst ME, Franey R (1998) Acyclovir- and ganciclovir-induced neurotoxicity. *Ann Pharmacother* 32, 111.

6. Davis CL, Springmeyer S, Gmereo BJ (1990) Central nervous system side effects of ganciclovir. *N Engl J Med* 322, 933.

7. Faulds D, Heel RC (1990) Ganciclovir. A review of its antiviral activity, pharmacokinetic properties and therapeutic efficacy in cytomegalovirus infections. *Drugs* 39, 597.

8. Germann D, Schopfer K (1992) Antiviral drugs. In: *Myeler's Side Effects of Drugs. 12th Ed.* Dukes MNG ed. Elsevier Science Publishers, Amsterdam, p. 742.

9. Kao GW, Peyman GA, Fiscella R, House B (1987) Retinal toxicity of ganciclovir in vitrectomy infusion solution. *Retina* 7, 80.

10. McEvoy GK (1995) *American Hospital Formulary Service Drug Information.* American Society of Health System Pharmacists, p. 431.

11. Saran BR, Maguire AM (1994) Retinal toxicity of high dose intravitreal ganciclovir. *Retina* 14, 248.

12. Thomson MH, Jeffries DJ (1989) Ganciclovir therapy in iatrogenically immunosuppressed patients with cytomegalovirus disease. *J Antimicrob Chemother* 23, 61.

13. Yoshizumi MO, Lee D, Vinci V, Fajardo S (1990) Ocular toxicity of multiple intravitreal DHPG injections. *Graef Arch Clin Exp Ophthal* 228, 350.

Gangliosides

Horst Wiethölter

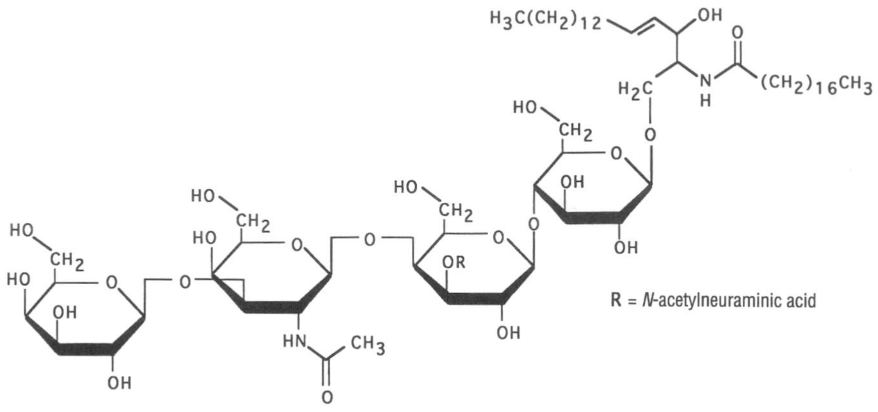

GANGLIOSIDE G$_{M1}$
$C_{73}H_{131}N_3O_{31}$

Sialic acid–containing glycosides; *e.g.*, monosialoganglioside GM$_1$

NEUROTOXICITY RATING

Clinical

B   Peripheral neuropathy

Gangliosides are sialic acid–containing glycosphingolipids primarily found in the plasma membrane of virtually all vertebrate tissues, with particular abundance in the nervous system. A mixture of purified bovine brain gangliosides (GM$_1$ = 2.1 mg, GD$_{1a}$ = 4.0 mg, GD$_{1b}$ = 1.6 mg, GT$_{1b}$ = 1.9 mg/ml solution) has been used for the treatment of alcoholic, diabetic, and uremic polyneuropathy; after peripheral nerve damage; and lumbar disc surgery. GM$_1$ alone has been used to treat spinal cord trauma and stroke (1,4,9,14).

Between 1985 and 1989, about 2 million doses of the ganglioside mixture Cronassial were distributed in Germany. After a report of six cases of a Guillain-Barré (GBS)–like syndrome, the drug was withdrawn in Germany, but it is still available in other European countries.

Gangliosides are administered parenterally by intramuscular injection. A peak blood level of GM$_1$ is reached after 12 h. Gangliosides injected into the circulation first bind to serum albumin and then find their way into many tissues. Small but significant quantities of GM$_1$ are taken up in the brain. Metabolites are excreted slowly after liver and renal degradation and synthetic conversions.

Exogenously administered gangliosides have been shown to promote neuronal regeneration and axonal sprouting in CNS and PNS tissues and have also been suggested to act as a neuronotrophic factor in noradrenergic, serotonergic, cholinergic, and dopaminergic systems.

Gangliosides have been considered nontoxic because, in several animal species, toxic effects could not be demonstrated after short-term or prolonged administration of excessive doses.

Problems may arise only with regard to the immunological effects of gangliosides; sialic acid–containing gangliosides are weakly immunogenic. In particular, GM$_1$ may modulate lymphocyte responses to antigenic or mitogenic stimuli. It may suppress early activation, and block accessory cell function and sequestration of interleukin-2 *in vitro* (2). *In vivo*, no evidence for a suppressive effect on humoral or cellular immunity has been observed (13).

In 1976, it was reported that brain gangliosides, GD$_{1a}$ and GM$_1$, were capable of inducing peripheral neuropathy by immunization [mixed with Freund's complete adjuvant (FCA)] in rabbits and, in a few cases, in Hartley guinea pigs (11). This experimentally induced disease [a form of experimental autoimmune neuritis (EAN)] was called "ganglioside syndrome." The lesions differed from most cases of classic EAN, which is induced by a mixture of peripheral nerve myelin with FCA, because of the presence of extensive axonal degeneration. Later, it was found that ganglioside syndrome can only be induced in a susceptible strain of rabbits (Japanese white—NIBS). Mild inflammation and demyelination in the PNS (EAN) was also reported after ganglioside administration (10). When gangliosides were mixed with the immunization compound (myelin with FCA), the development of myelin-induced EAN in rats was depressed and delayed (12,15).

Between September 1985 and June 1989, six patients in Germany developed a "GBS-like syndrome" within 16 days of commencing ganglioside therapy. This incidence rate was significantly higher than that expected from epidemiological data. The term "GBS-like syndrome" was chosen because of some special abnormalities seen only in variants of GBS.

1. Distal weakness appeared 7–16 days after commencing ganglioside treatment; sensory signs were absent or minor during the course of the disease.
2. Neurophysiological data documented mainly axonal degeneration with little or no conduction block and demyelination. Latencies of distally evoked compound muscle action potentials were prolonged.
3. Treatment of a few cases with plasma exchange had no beneficial effect.

There are further reports on patients with GBS-like syndrome after administration of GM_1 and mixtures of gangliosides (5–9). A report of a case of GBS with high titers of antibodies to monoganglioside suggested that gangliosides may induce an immune response under specific conditions (8). In seven patients with acute axonal GBS after ganglioside administration, immunoglobulin G antibodies against various gangliosides were detected; these recognized epitopes at nodes of Ranvier and motor end plates. Only 28% of a control group of 25 patients with ganglioside-unrelated GBS had high titers of antiganglioside antibodies (6). One report described 17 cases of mainly motor polyneuropathy after ganglioside administration (3); another reported 24 cases of GBS after ganglioside treatment (7).

Although most reports have limited neurological documentation, there seems to be little doubt that patients treated with gangliosides are at a statistically higher risk for a GBS-like syndrome.

REFERENCES

1. Bradley WG, Badger GJ, Tandan R et al. (1988) Double-blind controlled trials of Cronassail in chronic neuromuscular diseases and ataxia. Neurology 38, 1731.
2. Chieco-Bianchi L, Calabrò ML, Panozzo M et al. (1989) CD4 modulation and inhibition of HIV-1 infectivity induced by monosialoganglioside GM1 in vitro. AIDS 3, 501.
3. Figueras A, Morales-Olivas FJ, Capellà D et al. (1992) Bovine gangliosides and acute motor polyneuropathy. Brit Med J 305, 1330.
4. Geisler FH, Dorsey FC, Coleman WP (1991) Recovery of motor function after spinal-cord injury—a randomized, placebo-controlled trial with GM1-ganglioside. N Engl J Med 324, 1829.
5. Granieri E, Casetta I, Govoni V et al. (1991) Ganglioside therapy and the Guillain-Barré syndrome. A historical cohort study in Ferrera, Italy, fails to demonstrate an association. Neuroepidemiology 10, 161.
6. Illa I, Ortiz N, Gallardo E et al. (1995) Acute axonal Guillain-Barré syndrome (GBS) with IgG antibodies against motor axons following parenteral injection of gangliosides. J Neurol 242, S144.
7. Landi G, D'Alessandro R, Dossi BD et al. (1993) Guillain-Barré syndrome after exogenous gangliosides in Italy. Brit Med J 307, 1463.
8. Latov N, Koski CL, Walicke PA (1991) Guillian-Barré syndrome and parenteral gangliosides. Lancet 338, 757.
9. Lenzi GL, Grigoletto F, Gent M et al. (1994) Early treatment of stroke with monosialoganglioside GM-1. Efficacy and safety results of the Early Stroke Trial. Stroke 25, 1552.
10. Mizisin AP, Wiley CA, Hughes RAC, Powell HC (1987) Peripheral nerve demyelination in rabbits after inoculation with Fruend's complete adjuvant alone or in combination with lipid hapten. J Neuroimmunol 16, 381.
11. Nagai Y, Sakakibara K, Uchilda T (1980) Immunomodulatory roles of gangliosides in EAE and EAN. In: Search for Cause of Multiple Sclerosis and Other Chronic Diseases of the Central Nervous System. Boese A ed. Verlag Chemie, Weinheim p. 127.
12. Ponzin D, Menegus AM, Kirschner G et al. (1991) Effects of gangliosides on the expression of autoimmune demyelination in the peripheral nervous system. Ann Neurol 30, 678.
13. Presti D, Callegaro L, Toffano G, Marcus DM (1989) Lack of suppression by gangliosides of humoral or cellular immunity in vivo. J Neuroimmunol 22, 233.
14. Schneider JS, Yuwiler A (1989) GM1 ganglioside treatment promotes recovery of striatal dopamine concentrations in the mouse model of MPTP-induced parkinsonism. Exp Neurol 105, 177.
15. Weithölter H, Schabet M, Stevens A et al. (1992) Influence of gangliosides on experimental allergic neuritis. J Neuroimmunol 38, 221.

Gasoline

Herbert H. Schaumburg

NEUROTOXICITY RATING

Clinical

A Acute encephalopathy (sedation, coma)

B Chronic encephalopathy (cognitive dysfunction)

Gasoline is produced from light distillates during fractionation of petroleum; its main components are paraffins, olefins, naphthalenes, and aromatic hydrocarbons, including toluene. Ethyl alcohol is added in some instances. The threshold limit value set by the American Conference of Governmental Industrial Hygienists is 330 ppm (800 mg/m³). There is little toxicity from inhalation in the manufacture or industrial deployment of unleaded gasoline. Ingestion of as little as 10 g may be fatal. Gasoline is a severe irritant to pharyngeal and gastrointestinal muscosa and causes prolonged vomiting, hypotension, and vascular collapse. Confusion, vertigo, and convulsions have followed suicidal ingestion of large amounts.

Rodent inhalation studies have failed to disclose evidence of nervous system dysfunction (5).

Humans who repeatedly inhale gasoline for its euphoric effect, "gasoline sniffing," may acutely display ataxia, delirium, agitation, and psychotic behavior. If high levels are inhaled for a prolonged interval, signs of CNS depression and coma appear, and death may follow (1–4,6). Most reports depict adolescents who inhaled leaded gasoline, and many of the clinical features appear to represent a combination of organolead and aromatic hydrocarbon neurotoxicity. Repeated inhalant abuse over a period of years has resulted in an irreversible syndrome that includes both cognitive and cerebellar dysfunction (2,6).

REFERENCES

1. Boeckx RL, Postl B, Coodin FJ (1977) Gasoline sniffing and tetraethyl lead poisoning in children. *Pediatrics* **60**, 140.
2. Fortenberry JD (1985) Gasoline sniffing. *Amer J Med* **79**, 740.
3. Kaelan C, Harper C, Vieira BI (1986) Acute encephalopathy and death due to petrol sniffing: Neuropathological findings. *Aust N Z J Med* **16**, 804.
4. Valpey R, Sumi SM, Copass MK, Goble GJ (1978) Acute and chronic progressive encephalopathy due to gasoline sniffing. *Neurology* **28**, 507.
5. Vyskocil A, Tusl M, Obrsal J, Zaydlar K (1988) A subchronic inhalation study with unleaded petrol in rats. *J Appl Toxicol* **8**, 239.
6. Young RSK, Grzyb SE, Crismon L (1977) Recurrent cerebellar dysfunction as related to chronic gasoline sniffing in an adolescent girl. *Clin Pediat* **16**, 706.

Germanium Dioxide

Herbert H. Schaumburg

$$GeO_2$$

Germanic acid

NEUROTOXICITY RATING

Clinical

A Myopathy (vacuolar)

B Peripheral neuropathy

Experimental

A Myopathy (vacuolar)

B Peripheral neuropathy

Germanium, in elemental form, is widely distributed in the earth's crust and occurs as a natural component of many root plants, legumes, and some fish. There is no physiological requirement for germanium. Average daily intake is 1.5 mg; it is rapidly absorbed, appears promptly in many organs, and is 90% excreted by the kidney. The biological half-life is estimated as 1.5 days systemically and 4 days in the kidney; prolonged passage through the kidney is believed to account for the nephrotoxicity of most inorganic and organic germanium compounds.

Germanium dioxide is not a naturally occurring substance and has no accepted medicinal use. Germanium dioxide (GeO_2), inorganic germanium salts, and some novel organogermanium compounds (carboxyethyl germanium sesquioxide, germanium lactate citrate) are sold worldwide as nutritional supplements and for purported immunomodulatory effects in cancer patients. In Asia, germanium dioxide is especially widely consumed as treatment for endocrine conditions, hepatic failure, fatigue, and as a general health-enhancing elixir.

Early pharmacokinetic studies of germanium dioxide, which demonstrated rapid gastrointestinal absorption, diffusion throughout the body and prompt renal excretion, supported the belief that it has low toxicity and little risk associated with unregulated self-administration (7). Subsequent investigations with experimental animals utilizing radiolabeled $^{71}GeO_2$ disclosed that trace amounts remain in the kidneys long after clearance from other organs; this may account, in part, for recent reports of renal dysfunction in long-term users (8,9).

Nephrotoxicity is the most serious systemic undesired effect. Prolonged use (4–36 months; cumulative doses of 16–32 g) has been associated with 18 reports from Japan of acute or subacute renal failure, including two deaths (7,9). Biopsies of five of these cases show vacuolar degeneration of renal tubular epithelium with sparing of the glomeruli. Renal function improves after consumption is stopped, but recovery is incomplete (8). Identical morphological changes appear in rats following chronic treatment (6).

Diffuse weakness with elevated serum creatine kinase has accompanied about one-third of cases displaying renal dysfunction. Weakness appears following prolonged high-level consumption (22–26 months; cumulative doses of 36–70 g). This was initially attributed to nonspecific neuromuscular failure in debilitated patients with renal insufficiency, although vacuolar change in muscle is described in one instance.

A meticulous clinical-pathological report of a muscle biopsy from another (eventually autopsied) patient, accompanied by a murine experimental study, clearly establishes myotoxicity as a complication of extremely prolonged consumption of germanium dioxide (2). In this instance, diffuse muscle weakness accompanied renal failure in a 5-year-old diabetic subject after 20 months of parent-administered germanium dioxide. High levels were detected in hair, and muscle biopsy disclosed lipid accumulation and diffuse vacuolar fiber degeneration; rats chronically dosed (12 weeks with 150 mg/kg/day) with germanium dioxide showed similar vacuolar change but no lipid accumulation. Ultrastructural study of both human and rat muscle disclosed identical electron-dense mitochondrial inclusions, leading the authors to suggest that GeO_2 affects muscle by causing mitochondrial dysfunction; there have been no appropriate clinical biochemical/enzymatic studies in these patients to support this notion (2). It is likely these histopathological changes are truly related to GeO_2 and not to renal dysfunction, uremic neuropathy, or a toxic distal axonopathy; vacuolar myopathy is associated with none of these entities.

An experimental animal study, which employed contemporary histopathological techniques, has failed to produce evidence of axonal degeneration in sural nerve biopsies from rats intoxicated with up to 400 mg/kg/day for 8 weeks or monkeys dosed with 35 mg/kg/day for 8 months (5).

Evidence of renal dysfunction, proteinuria and elevated blood urea nitrogen, was present. Another experimental study treated rats with 100 mg/kg/day for 8 months and employed sophisticated histopathological techniques. Examination at 2-month intervals disclosed progressive hindlimb weakness; interval morphological analysis of sciatic nerves showed progressively intense, widespread segmental demyelination without significant axonal degeneration (4). This study did not include analysis of renal function.

In human studies, distal acral numbness accompanies about 40% of reported cases with renal dysfunction (1). There appears to be a relationship between dose level and time of onset of sensory symptoms, although this is not carefully documented in most reports; one case had onset after 24 months of daily 100-mg dosing and another had onset after 6 years at 35 mg daily. Several cases have displayed signs of stocking-and-glove distribution of large-fiber-type sensory loss and hyporeflexia; two subjects additionally displayed sensory ataxia in the lower limbs. Sensory nerve conductions are minimally abnormal but have been mostly studied in the upper limbs. Sural nerve biopsies are alleged to display axonal loss, but none has employed modern histological analytic techniques. Postmortem analysis of two especially advanced cases has revealed unequivocal loss of spinal dorsal root ganglion cells, and fiber loss with replacement gliosis in the dorsal columns of the spinal cord (1,3). Taken in concert, these clinical reports support the notion that a sensory distal axonopathy or neuronopathy accompanies some instances of chronic GeO_2 self-administration. Stronger support would stem from (a) an analysis of the consumed product, (b) a corresponding animal model, (c) documented recovery following withdrawal, and (d) occurence in a patient or experimental animal with only minor renal dysfunction.

REFERENCES

1. Asaka T, Nitta E, Makifuchi et al. (1995) Germanium intoxication with sensory ataxia. J Neurol Sci 130, 220.

2. Higuchi I, Izumo S, Suchara M et al. (1989) Germanium myopathy: Clinical and experimental pathological studies. Acta Neuropathol 79, 300.

3. Kamijo M, Yagihashi S, Kida S et al. (1991) An autopsy case of chronic germanium intoxication presenting peripheral neuropathy, spinal ataxia, and chronic renal failure. Clin Neurol 31, 191.

4. Matsumuro K, Izumo S, Higuchi I et al. (1993) Experimental germanium dioxide-induced neuropathy in rats. Acta Neuropathol 86, 547.

5. Ohnishi A, Yamamoto T, Murai Y et al. (1989) Evaluation of germanium dioxide neurotoxicity in rats and monkeys. Sangyo Ika Daigaku Zasshi 11, 323.

6. Sanai T, Okuda S, Onoyama K et al. (1990) Germanium

dioxide-induced nephropathy: A new type of renal disease. *Nephron* **54**, 53.

7. Schauss AG (1991) Nephrotoxicity and neurotoxicity in humans from organogermanium and germanium dioxide. *Biol Trace Elem Res* **29**, 267.

8. Tao SH, Bolger PM (1997) Hazard assessment of germanium supplements. *Regul Toxicol Pharmacol* **25**, 211.

9. Van der Spoel JI, Stricker BHCh, Esseveld MR, Schipper MEI (1990) Dangers of dietary germanium supplements. *Lancet* **ii**, 117.

Germine

Albert C. Ludolph

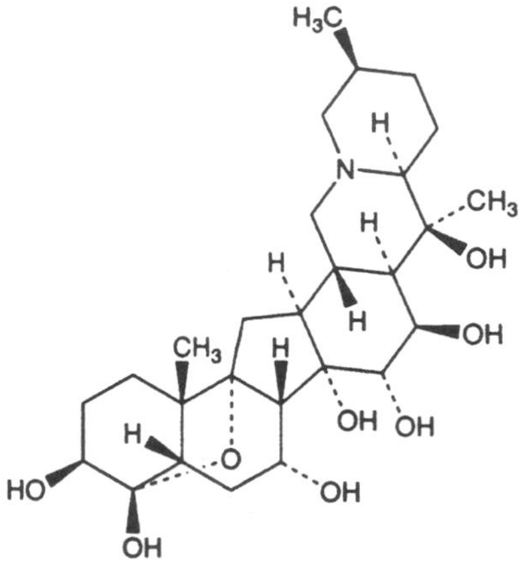

GERMINE
$C_{27}H_{43}NO_8$

$(3\beta,4\alpha,7\alpha,15\alpha,16\beta)$-4,9-Epoxycevane-3,4,7,14,15,16,20-heptol

NEUROTOXICITY RATING

Clinical

A   Ion channel syndrome

Experimental

A   Ion channel dysfunction (sodium channel)

Germine is a naturally occuring alkamine present in a number of polyester alkaloids obtained from *Veratrum* and *Zigadenus* spp. Germine crystals dissolve in chloroform, methanol, ethanol, acetone, and water; the MP is 221.5°–223°C. Germine-3-acetate ($C_{29}H_{45}NO_9$), an ester of germine, increases contractile strength of skeletal muscle, antagonizes *d*-tubacurarine– and succinylcholine–induced neuromuscular blockade (7) and, in large doses, blocks neuromuscular transmission (1). Germine-3-acetate was once used to treat myasthenia gravis (1,2). Germine is structurally similar to veratridine, which increases permeability of Na$^+$ channels in nerve and muscles. Germine and germine esters likely affect Na$^+$ channel inactivation.

Clinical manifestations associated with intravenous administration of germine diacetate in the treatment of myasthenia gravis included increased blood pressure; muscle fasciculation; tingling of hands, feet, and the perioral region; a bitter, metallic taste; a sensation of coolness in the mouth; and hot-cold reversal (2). These symptoms were less pronounced after oral administration and quickly disappeared after cessation of intravenous treatment.

Human intoxication with plants containing mixtures of veratrum alkaloids (*Veratrum album*, white hellebore) are rare. Shortly after consumption, oropharyngeal burning sensations and paresthesias appear, which then generalize and are accompanied by nausea, vomiting, and diarrhea. Arrhythmias and decreased blood pressure can be life-threatening. In several reports, ingestion of an alcoholic extract of veratrum roots caused gastrointestinal disturbances, cardiovascular symptoms, hallucinations, paresthesias, tingling, and muscle cramps (3,4,5). Veratrum poisoning is treated symptomatically, since no specific antidote exists. *Zigadenus* spp. poisoning has also occurred (6).

REFERENCES

1. Detwiler PB (1972) The effects of germine-3-acetate on neuromuscular transmission. *J Pharmacol Exp Ther* **180**, 244.

2. Flacke W, Caviness VS, Samaha FG (1966) Treatment of myasthenia gravis with germine diacetate. *N Engl J Med* **275**, 1207.

3. Hruby K, Lenz K, Krausler J (1981) Vergiftung mit *Veratrum album* (weißer Germer). *Wien Klin Wochenschr* **93**, 517.

4. Jaspersen-Schib R (1976) Pflanzenvergiftungen während 10 Jahren. *Schweiz Apoth Ztg* **114**, 265.

5. Seeliger J (1957) Über eine seltene Vergiftung mit weißer Nieswurz. *Arch Toxicol* **16**, 16.

6. Spoerke DG, Spoerke SE (1979) Three cases of *Zigadenus* (death cama) poisoning. *Vet Human Toxicol* **21**, 346.

7. Standaert FG, Detwiler PB (1970) The neuromuscular pharmacology of germine-3-acetate and germine-3,16-diacetate. *J Pharmacol Exp Ther* **171**, 223.

Gila Monster Venom

Albert C. Ludolph

NEUROTOXICITY RATING

Clinical

C Neuromuscular transmission syndrome

Gila monsters (Mexican beaded lizard, *Heloderma horridum horridum*) are nocturnal reptiles living in the deserts of the southern part of the North American continent (2,4). Bites are rare and only happen after provocation or careless handling of the animal (2). The venom of the gila monster contains a mixture of protein toxins but, in contrast to most reptilian venoms, does not contain primary neurotoxins (1,4). The major lethal factor, gilatoxin, lacks proteolytic, hemorrhagic, or hemolytic activity (3,4). The LD_{50} of the venom in mice reportedly is 0.45–1.0 mg/kg body weight after intravenous administration (2). In contrast to snake envenomation, the painful bite of the animal is always associated with injection of toxins (1). Reports of neurological complications of the bite of gila monsters, such as generalized weakness, tinnitus, or muscle fasciculation, are likely secondary to hypotension (1,2). Antivenin is not available, and treatment for envenomation is symptomatic (1,2,4).

REFERENCES

1. Mebs D (1992) Gifttiere. *Ein Handbuch für Biologen, Toxikologen, Ärzte, Apotheker.* Wissenschaftliche Verlagsgesellschaft mbH, Stuttgart.
2. Russell FE, Bogert CM (1981) Gila monster: Its biology venom and bite—a review. *Toxicon* 19, 341.
3. Tinkham ER (1971) The venom of the gila monster. In: *Venomous Animals and Their Venoms. Vol 2.* Bucherl W, Buckley EE eds. Academic Press, Orlando, Florida p. 415.
4. Tu AT (1991) A lizard venom: Gila monster (genus: *Heloderma*). In: *Handbook of Natural Toxins. Vol 5. Reptile Venoms and Toxins.* Tu AT ed. Marcel Dekker, New York p. 755.
5. Utaisincharoen P, Mackessy SP, Miller RA, Tu AT (1993) Complete primary structure and biochemical properties of gilatoxin, a serine protease with kallikrein-like and angiotensin-degrading activities. *J Biol Chem* 268, 21975.

Ginseng

Herbert H. Schaumburg

Panax spp.

NEUROTOXICITY RATING

Clinical

C Acute encephalopathy

"Ginseng" can refer to any of 22 related plant species, usually of the genus *Panax*, used in herbal medicine. Four species are most commonly employed: *P. ginseng* (Asian ginseng), *P. quinquefolium* (American ginseng), *Rumex hymenosepalus* (desert ginseng), and *Eleuthococcus senticosus* (Siberian ginseng) (3).

The root, which may resemble an extracted tooth or a vaguely human shape (the Chinese word ginseng—"man root"), grows worldwide. It is available in three forms in Asia: as the entire root (which must be steamed and pulverized), as an elixir, and as a powder; it is generally consumed in a tea, but may be used as a component in cooking. The pulverized root of *P. ginseng* has a sweet and aromatic taste. Ginseng preparations are available in the West, where there are an estimated 5–6 million users (8). It appears primarily in health-food stores; an illustrative label reads "500 mg tablets—Siberian ginseng." There is also a wide variety of North American commercial preparations, including capsules, extracts, gums, candies, and cigarettes.

Ginseng is a mainstay of Chinese traditional medicine; it is given as a stimulant to increase metabolism and as an antihypertensive. It is claimed that ginseng has increased the stamina of Chinese athletes, especially long-distance runners. The only recognized use in North America is as a demulcent in skin ointment (8). Ginseng also enjoys a phenomenal popularity in China as an inexpensive self-administered tonic, stimulant, aging retardant, and aphrodisiac (2,3). The recommended daily dose for dry ginseng root is generally 0.5–2.0 g (6).

Saponins, triterpenes, sesquiterpenes, and acetylenic compounds are the principal bioactive components of *P. ginseng*; the major sapogenin of ginseng is 20 (S)-protopanaxadiol (5,9). There are abundant analytical, biochemical, and pharmacological data that characterize and classify ginseng saponins ("the ginsenoids") in the Asian scientific literature. It is suggested that ginseng is best classified as a pharmacological "adaptogen," because some studies allege it helps experimental animals adapt to stress and corrects human adrenal and thyroid dysfunction (2). The Chinese claim opposite pharmacological effects with the two main groups of ginsenoids: Rg1 is said to stimulate the CNS and combat fatigue, while Rb1 is a CNS depressant. Experimental studies with specific ginsenoids describe stimulation of learning and memory, and enhancement of the effect of nerve growth factor on neurite outgrowth in tissue culture (6). An American experimental study of *P. quinquefolium* describes facilitation of release of acetylcholine in hippocampal slices (1).

Systemic toxicity is uncommon with ginseng use. Prolonged consumption may be associated with diarrhea and labile blood pressure; an instance of androgenization of a newborn is described following maternal ginseng consumption (4).

Nervous system adverse effects of short-term use are minor; they include headache, fatigue, and vertigo. One report describes severe headache and an angiographic appearance of cerebral arteritis in a woman who consumed an extract containing 22 g of ginseng (6).

Signs and symptoms attributed to CNS dysfunction, "ginseng-abuse syndrome," are claimed to accompany prolonged use in a neuropsychiatric study of 133 subjects (8). The most prominent effect was CNS stimulation with euphoria, nervousness, agitation, and insomnia. Hypertension, reversible after withdrawal, was documented in 22 subjects. The author concludes that most of the neurotoxicity reflects a corticosteroid effect of ginseng and urges avoidance of long-term ingestion. This provocative study lacks credibility; it suffers from lack of subject controls, absence of botanical or analytic chemical data on the nature or level of the substance consumed, and possible coconsumption of other agents by the subjects.

REFERENCES

1. Benishin CG, Lee R, Wang LCH, Liu HJ (1991) Effects of ginsenoid Rb1 on central cholinergic metabolism. *Pharmacology* **42**, 223.
2. Brekham II, Dardymov IV (1969) New substances of plant origins which increase nonspecific resistance. *Annu Rev Pharmacol* **9**, 419.
3. Keys JD (1976) *Chinese Herbs: Their Botany, Chemistry and Pharmacodynamics*. Charles Tuttle Co, Rutland, Vermont.
4. Koren G, Randor S, Martin S, Danneman D (1990) Maternal ginseng use associated with neonatal androgenization. *J Amer Med Assn* **264**, 2866.
5. Oakenfull D, Sidhu GS (1989) Saponins. In: *Toxicants of Plant Origin, Vol II*. Cheeke PR ed. CRC Press, Boca Raton, Florida p. 97.
6. Ryu SJ, Chein YY (1995) Ginseng-associated cerebral arteritis. *Neurology* **45**, 829.
7. Saito H, Suda K, Schwab M, Thoenen H (1976) Potentiation of the NGF-mediated nerve fiber outgrowth by ginsenoid Rb1 in organ cultures of chicken dorsal root ganglia. *Jpn J Pharmacol* **27**, 445.
8. Siegel RK (1979) Ginseng abuse syndrome. *J Amer Med Assn* **241**,1614.
9. Tang W, Eisenbrand G (1992) *Panax ginseng*. In: *Chinese Drugs of Plant Origin*. Springer-Verlag, Berlin p. 721.

Glutamic Acid

John W. Olney
Albert C. Ludoph

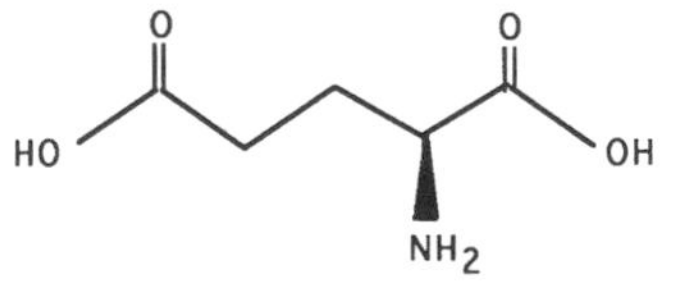

GLUTAMIC ACID
$C_5H_9NO_4$

L-Glutamic acid ← *configuration* → D-Glutamic acid

d-Glutamic acid ← *rotation* → *l*-Glutamic acid

(*S*)-2-Aminopentanedioic acid; Glutaminic acid; α-Aminoglutaric acid; 1-Aminopropane-1,3-dicarboxylic acid

NEUROTOXICITY RATING

Clinical

A   Chinese restaurant syndrome (transient sensory dysfunction)

Experimental

A   Excitotoxic CNS degeneration

L-Glutamic acid is an acidic nonessential amino acid, a major building block of protein, and a natural constituent of foods; it is present in the body tissues of all animal species; and is found in high concentrations throughout the mammalian CNS.

L-Glutamic acid (GLU) has a MW of 147.19; the orthorhombic bisphenoidal crystals decompose at 247°–249°C. The amino acid is soluble in water, but insoluble in acetone, ethanol, ether, and methanol. The monosodium salt [$C_5H_8NNaO_4 \cdot H_2O$; monosodium glutamate; MSG; glutamic acid monosodium salt monohydrate; monosodium L-glutamate monohydrate; sodium glutamate monohydrate; Chinese seasoning] is used widely as a flavor additive to foods. Its MW is 187.13; the white, odorless crystals are soluble in water, but much less so in alcohol. It is estimated that several million tons of monosodium glutamate are added to processed foods sold in the United States every year.

Hydrolyzed protein (HP) is also used widely and heavily as a flavor additive. Since a major purpose of using HP is to increase the GLU flavor level of food, HP is manufactured from protein sources that have a high content of GLU. In addition, GLU is sometimes added liberally to the hydrolysate so that the final product may contain up to 40% GLU (plus aspartate and various excitotoxic sulphur amino acids). Often, both HP and GLU are added to various food products. The primary reason for this practice is that GLU is a weak depolarizer of taste buds and must be incorporated into foods in very high concentration to confer the desired flavor impact.

Glutamate has received an increasing amount of attention in recent years because of its pivotal role in both physiological and pathological processes in the mammalian CNS. Glutamate is a key participant in intermediary metabolism, a major contributor to the synthesis of complex peptides and proteins and, of paramount importance, GLU is the predominant excitatory neurotransmitter in the CNS. In addition, GLU is the sole precursor molecule responsible for producing γ-aminobutyric acid (GABA), the predominant inhibitory neurotransmitter in the brain. Both GLU and GABA are synthesized in the CNS and their concentrations are homeostatically regulated.

In addition to its role in CNS physiology and pharmacology, GLU has neurotoxic (excitotoxic) potential to destroy CNS neurons directly or indirectly. In pathological conditions, such as cerebral ischemia, CNS trauma, status epilepticus, and profound hypoglycemia, excitotoxic activation of receptors by endogenous glutamate is the triggering event that leads to neuronal degeneration. Antagonist drugs that block glutamate receptors protect against this excitotoxic effect. Paradoxically, blockade of GLU receptors by these drugs can also have neurotoxic consequences that stem from a complex form of excitotoxicity. Thus, either hyper- or hypoactivation of GLU receptors can result in CNS neuronal death.

Although there has been considerable speculation on an adverse role for human health of exposure to *exogenous* glutamate-like compounds, the potential role of *endoge-nous* glutamate in CNS cell death has become a pillar of the concept of excitotoxicity. Based on the endogenous glutamate concept of CNS degenerative disease, a number of pharmacological approaches have been evaluated. Furthermore, the concept of indirect ("slow") excitotoxicity has stimulated investigations of mechanisms of cell death under conditions of reduced energy supply (1,3,20,21).

The excitotoxic concept holds that GLU is a major excitatory neurotransmitter and potential neurotoxin in the vertebrate CNS (9,19,25). These properties appeared unrelated until it was shown (34) that a select group of GLU structural analogs mimic both the neuroexcitatory and neurotoxic properties of GLU and display a parallel order of potencies for these two activities. Furthermore, the neurotoxicity of these agents appeared to be mediated by a predominant action on dendrosomal, not axonal, membranes (26,34,40). From these and related observations, the excitotoxic concept evolved that an excitatory mechanism and excitatory amino acid (EAA) synaptic receptors on dendrosomal membranes mediate GLU neurotoxicity.

The identification of EAA receptor subtypes has defined properties of EAA transmitter systems (53). The subtypes are differentially sensitive to specific agonists [N-methyl-D-aspartate (NMDA), amino-3-hydroxy-5-methyl-isoxazole-4-propionic acid (AMPA), and kainic acid (KA)]; there are also specific antagonists that block the excitatory (54) and toxic (32,35,37) actions of EAA agonists at such receptors. There has been successful cloning and sequencing of multiple numerous receptor subunits [six are differentially sensitive to NMDA, four to AMPA, five to KA, and eight additional subtypes of the metabotropic receptor (13)]. NMDA, AMPA, and KA receptor subunits form heteromeric receptor ionophore complexes, achieving signal transduction through activation of an ion channel. The metabotropic receptor subfamily achieves signal transduction by activation of G-protein–linked enzymatic processes. To date, all of the ionotropic receptor subtypes (NMDA, AMPA, KA) have been shown to mediate excitotoxic neurodegeneration, but excitotoxicity has not been linked to GLU metabotropic receptors.

General Toxicology

GLU is rapidly absorbed into the blood following oral intake; absorption is especially rapid following ingestion of GLU dissolved in liquids. Although GLU is metabolized to a variable extent by the liver, the rate of gastrointestinal absorption is the primary determinant of the blood concentration. Circulating GLU freely enters circumventricular regions of the brain that lack a blood-brain barrier; these are known collectively as the circumventricular organs

(CVO). Selective entry and accumulation of GLU and aspartate in CVO brain regions has been demonstrated in rodents by both microhistochemical and autoradiographic methods (15,41,44,45). Acute destruction of CVO neurons has been shown in all animal species appropriately tested to date (mice, rats, guinea pigs, hamsters, chicks, rabbits, cats, and monkeys). CVO neurons in immature animal brains are especially vulnerable to excitotoxic destruction. The basis for heightened vulnerability of immature CVO neurons is not only anatomically determined; a likely important factor is the hypersensitivity of the NMDA receptor (that mediates CVO damage in the immature brain) to excitotoxic stimulation during postnatal development (14,22,52). It is believed that NMDA receptors are programmed to undergo changes in heteromeric subunit composition at various stages in development; it has been shown in rodent brain that during the stage in postnatal life when NMDA receptors are most sensitive to excitotoxic stimulation, there is an overexpression of an NMDA receptor subunit (NR2D) that confers hyperexcitable properties to the NMDA receptor complex (24).

Animal Studies

Experimental animal studies showing the extreme sensitivity of the immature CNS to exogenous GLU generated the concept of GLU neurotoxicity and the general theory of excitotoxicity. Attempts to extrapolate neurotoxicity demonstrated in experimental animal studies to the risk of exposure to exogenous glutamate for the developing CNS of humans are controversial (27,28,30). The principal aspects of animal studies suggested as relevant to humans include the following:

1. The oral dose of GLU required to destroy neurons in the hypothalamus of an immature mouse is 250–500 mg/kg body weight. Extrapolated to humans, this appears to provide a two- to threefold margin of safety: A cup of soup containing 1300 mg GLU provides a 10-kg infant human with 130 mg GLU per kilogram of body weight. This safety margin is uncertain because much more of the ingested load of GLU ends up in the blood of humans (compared to the mouse).

2. A single feeding of GLU in an immature animal causes CVO neuronal degeneration. Animals display no signs of discomfort or neurological injury while neurons are being destroyed. This suggests that safety thresholds cannot be based on behavioral events associated with acute neurotoxicity. It is likely that the GLU lesion is a silent event because injured brain regions are concerned with endocrine regulation, not with sensory, motor, or cognitive functions. The eventual effects in GLU-treated laboratory animals include obesity, infertility, and delayed onset of puberty.

3. Ingestion of GLU causes blood GLU concentrations to rise in the adult human 20 times higher than in adult monkeys and five times higher than in adult mice (50). These findings suggest that humans may be five times more vulnerable than mice (the most sensitive animal species) and at least 20 times more vulnerable than monkeys; this difference challenges the suggested two- to threefold margin of safety. It also suggests that the mouse is a more appropriate species than the monkey for oral GLU safety testing.

4. Three pharmacokinetic points warrant emphasis (50): (a) Humans have by far the highest peak blood GLU values after oral loading, compared with mice and monkeys (vide supra); (b) in contrast to other primates, humans sustain GLU elevations of much longer duration with a much greater area under the plasma level curve; and (c) human blood GLU values show a remarkable individual variation, suggesting a pharmacokinetic basis for individual susceptibility.

5. Orally administered GLU causes substantially higher blood levels in infants than in adults of either animal species. It is unknown if the same infant-to-adult relationship is true for humans. Comparable data are not available for immature humans because it is unsafe to administer liquid preparations of GLU in high doses (e.g., 100–150 mg/kg) to immature humans.

6. Destruction of brain neurons is not the only possible mechanism of GLU neurotoxicity. GLU readily enters the endocrine hypothalamus (a CVO region that has no blood-brain barrier) and interacts with EAA receptors on the surfaces of hypothalamic neurons. These neurons, when stimulated by GLU or related EAA, secrete hypophysiotropic-releasing factors into the portal blood; the factors then move to the pituitary where they trigger release of pituitary hormones into the general circulation. This phenomenon, first demonstrated in the mid 1970s (31,43), indicated that repetitive exposure of immature humans to GLU throughout critical stages of development entails potential risk. Even if hypothalamic neuronal degeneration does not occur, hormonal biorhythms are likely to be disturbed with adverse effects on growth and development.

7. Recent studies indicate a significant role for endogenous GLU as an important excitatory transmitter involved in hypothalamic neuroendocrine regulatory physiology (33). Intravenous administration of GLU (23), or related analogs (11,42,55), to prepubertal monkeys induces an abrupt release of luteinizing hormone, growth hormone, and prolactin into the blood. Repetitive administration of NMDA to prepubescent monkeys induces premature onset of puberty (11,42); similar effects on sexual maturation and reproductive cycling have been reported in other species (2,18,51). This suggests that the NMDA subtype of GLU receptor is a factor in sexual maturation, and implies that erratic exposure of developing humans to exogenous GLU could result in erratic perturbations in hormonal mechanisms that

govern sexual maturation and reproductive function. While most studies have focused on the gonadotrophic axis, other neuroendocrine systems may be involved. For example, all of the neurons that regulate the growth hormone axis lie in the specific portion of the hypothalamus (arcuate nucleus) that is freely penetrated by GLU; furthermore, GLU administration to primates causes an abrupt increase in plasma levels of growth hormone (23,42).

8. Weanling mice (22 days old) are well beyond the newborn stage (at 45 days they reach puberty). They will drink enough GLU-enriched solution to destroy many neurons in the sensitive arcuate region of the hypothalamus (36). This indicates that these immature animals can develop CNS damage by voluntary oral ingestion of GLU.

9. It has been shown that infant monkeys are susceptible to GLU-induced brain damage (40).

In Vitro Studies

The detailed mechanism of toxicity of glutamate and its analogues ("excitotoxicity") has been largely defined in *in vitro* studies (6,7,37–39,55). *In vitro* studies of excitotoxic mechanisms during reduced neuronal energy supply have also been performed (12,56,57).

Human Studies

While GLU is added in high concentrations to the general food supply from which babies and children are fed indiscriminately, there is no convincing clinical evidence for acute or chronic CNS effects.

The Chinese restaurant syndrome is observed in some adults after ingestion of foods containing large amounts of glutamate on an empty stomach (48). After oral intake or parenteral adminstration of GLU, individuals develop sensations of subzygomatic pressure and burning, tingling, and numbness in the face, neck, and upper torso. Substantial discomfort may accompany the cutaneous sensory disturbances. A pressure-cuff experiment suggested the phenomenon is caused by a toxic interaction with the PNS, not the CNS (48).

As endogenous excitatory amino acids, GLU and aspartate (ASP) have long been suspected to be pathogenetic in neurodegenerative disorders because they are present in high concentrations in the CNS and because of their excitotoxic potential. A major impetus in understanding how the excitotoxic potential of endogenous GLU may be unleashed to cause neuronal degeneration came with the discovery that conditions such as hypoxia/ischemia (4,46), seizures (8), and head trauma (10) cause a marked outpouring of endogenous excitotoxins (GLU and ASP) from the intracellular to extracellular compartment of brain. Here, they interact with EAA receptors to trigger an excitotoxic cascade (increased excitation begets increased endogenous excitotoxin release which begets more excitation, *etc.*). The cascade concept extends beyond the cyclical process of excited GLU neurons releasing more GLU to excite more neurons. Other cascading chain reactions are triggered by this process within each hyperexcited neuron, each reaction involving other factors including calcium, arachidonic acid, nitric oxide, free radicals, and proteolytic or lipolytic enzymes; all may contribute to cell death. Compelling evidence has now linked endogenous excitotoxins, primarily GLU and aspartate, to acute brain injury syndromes; these include hypoxic/ischemic neurodegeneration in both the immature and adult CNS, neurodegeneration associated with trauma in both the immature and adult CNS, and neurodegeneration associated with status epilepticus and hypoglycemia.

It is also suggested that endogenous excitotoxins participate in chronic neurodegenerative disorders including sulfite oxidase deficiency, olivopontocerebellar degeneration, amyotrophic lateral sclerosis, dementia pugilistica, Huntington's disease, parkinsonism, Alzheimer's disease, and acquired immunodeficiency syndrome–associated dementia (6,17,29). In some of these human neurodegenerative disorders, the notion that an excitotoxic effect is pathogenetic may have impact on future therapies. In diseases of childhood, this is true for sulfite oxidase deficiency and nonketotic hyperglycinemia. Indirect excitotoxicity may be a factor in other diseases primarily affecting energy metabolism, such as glutaric aciduria and methylmalonic aciduria (20). Therapeutic attempts with NMDA antagonists were reportedly successful in control of seizures in children with nonketotic hyperglycinemia, although a protective effect on the process of degeneration has not been shown yet (49). There is evidence, based on studies of high-affinity glutamate transport (47), partially successful therapeutic attempts with antiglutamate compounds (16), and morphological features of transgenic animal models, that excitotoxicity may play a role in the pathogenesis of amyotrophic lateral sclerosis (21). The pathogenesis of Huntington's disease has been suggested to be linked to disruption of cellular energy metabolism and indirect excitotoxic mechanisms (3,5).

Toxic Mechanisms
Fast (Direct) Excitotoxicity

The basic mechanisms associated with fast (direct) excitotoxicity have been most clearly delineated in *in vitro* experiments. Physiological studies have demonstrated that excessive postsynaptic excitation of the neuron by glutamate and analogues lead to depolarization of postsynaptic membranes; this increases membrane permeability, and induces receptor-mediated ion (Na^+ and Cl^-) and water influx into postsynaptic structures. Water influx underlies the morphological hallmark of the lesion: postsynaptic dendrosomal swelling and vacuolation. Calcium influx initiates a cascade of intracellular metabolic alterations causing mitochondrial dysfunction and cellular energy depletion, disruption of the cytoskeleton, and excessive production of free radicals.

Slow (Indirect) Excitotoxicity

If the activity of neuronal ion pumps or the energy supplies of the cell are reduced, the effects of glutamate and its analogues are enhanced (1,3,5,56,57). In a first step, mildly reduced energy supplies lead to a decrease of the cell membrane potential; this causes an opening of the voltage-dependent Mg^{2+} block of the ion channel associated with the NMDA receptor that results in water and Ca^{2+} influx into the cell (56,57). If cellular energy metabolism becomes more compromised, the extracellular glutamate concentration will increase by failure of high-affinity transport mechanisms; the resulting pattern of vulnerability will include non−NMDA-mediated tissue injury. There is speculation that this mechanism contributes to chronic neuronal death in a wide spectrum of neurodegenerative diseases.

REFERENCES

1. Albin RL, Greenamyre JT (1992) Alternative excitotoxic hypotheses. *Neurology* **42**, 733.
2. Arslan M, Pohl CR, Plant TM (1988) DL-2-Amino-5-phosphonopentanoic acid, a specific N-methyl-D-aspartic acid receptor antagonist, suppresses pulsatile LH release in the rat. *Neuroendocrinology* **47**, 465.
3. Beal MF, Hyman BT, Koroshetz W (1993) Do defects in mitochondrial energy metabolism underlie the pathology of neurodegenerative disease? *Trends Neurosci* **16**, 125.
4. Benveniste H, Drejer J, Schousboe A (1984) Elevation of the extracellular concentrations of glutamate and aspartate in rat hippocampus during transient cerebral ischemia monitored by intracerebral microdialysis. *J Neurochem* **43**, 1369.
5. Brouillet E, Jenkins B, Hyman BT *et al.* (1993) Age-dependent neurotoxicity of the mitochondrial toxin 3-nitropropionic acid. *J Neurochem* **60**, 356.
6. Choi DW (1988) Glutamate neurotoxicity and diseases of the nervous system. *Neuron* **1**, 623.
7. Choi DW, Koh J, Peters S (1988) Pharmacology of glutamate neurotoxicity in cortical cell culture: Attenuation by NMDA antagonists. *J Neurosci* **8**, 185.
8. Clifford DB, Olney JW, Benz AM *et al.* (1990) Ketamine, phencyclidine and MK-801 protect against kainic acid induced seizure-related brain damage. *Epilepsia* **31**, 382.
9. Curtis DR, Watkins JC (1960) The excitation and depression of spinal neurons by structurally related amino acids. *J Neurochem* **6**, 117.
10. Faden AI, Demediuk S, Panter S (1989) The role of excitatory amino acids and NMDA receptors in traumatic brain injury. *Science* **244**, 798.
11. Gay VL, Plant TM (1988) Sustained intermittent release of gonadotropin-releasing hormone in the prepubertal male rhesus monkey induced by N-methyl-DL-aspartic acid. *Neuroendocrinology* **48**, 147.
12. Henneberry RL, Novelli A, Cox JA, Lysko PG (1989) Neurotoxicity at the N-methyl-D-aspartate receptor in energy-compromised neurons. An hypothesis for cell death in aging and disease. *Ann N Y Acad Sci* **568**, 225.
13. Hollmann M, Heinemann S (1994) Cloned glutamate receptors. *Ann Rev Neurosci* **17**, 31.
14. Ikonomidou C, Mosinger JL, Shahid Salles K *et al.* (1989) Sensitivity of the developing rat brain to hypobaric/ischemic damage parallels sensitivity to N-methyl-aspartate neurotoxicity. *J Neurosci* **9**, 2809.
15. Inouye M (1976) Selective distribution of radioactivity in the neonatal mouse brain following subcutaneous administration of ^{14}C-labeled monosodium glutamate. *Cong Anomalies* **16**, 79.
16. Lacomblez L, Bensimon G, Leigh PN *et al.* for the Amyotrophic Lateral Sclerosis/Riluzole Study Group-II (1996) Dose-ranging study of riluzole in amyotrophic lateral sclerosis. *Lancet* **347**, 1425.
17. Lipton SA, Rosenberg PA (1994) Excitatory amino acids as a final common pathway for neurologic disorders. *N Engl J Med* **330**, 613.
18. López FJ, Donoso AO, Negro-Vilar A (1990) Endogenous excitatory amino acid neurotransmission regulates the estradiol-induced LH surge in ovariectomized rats. *Endocrinology* **126**, 1771.
19. Lucas DR, Newhouse JP (1957) The toxic effect of sodium L-glutamate on the inner layers of the retina. *AMA Arch Ophthalmol* **58**, 193.
20. Ludolph AC, Riepe M, Ullrich K (1993) Excitotoxicity, energy metabolism and neuronal degeneration. *J Inherit Metab Dis* **16**, 716.
21. Ludolph AC, Spencer PS (1996) Neurotoxic models of upper motor neuron disease. *J Neurol Sci* **139**, 53.
22. McDonald JW, Silverstein FS, Johnston MV (1988) Neurotoxicity of N-methyl-D-aspartate is markedly enhanced in developing rat central nervous system. *Brain Res* **459**, 200.
23. Medhamurthy R, Dichek HL, Plant TM *et al.* (1990) Stimulation of gonadotropin secretion in prepubertal monkeys after hypothalamic excitation with aspartate and glutamate. *J Clin Endocrinol Metab* **71**, 1390.
24. Monyer H, Burnashev N, Laurie DJ *et al.* (1994) Developmental and regional expression in the rat brain and functional properties of four NMDA receptors. *Neuron* **12**, 529.

25. Olney JW (1969) Brain lesions, obesity and other disturbances in mice treated with monosodium glutamate. *Science* **164**, 719.

26. Olney JW (1971) Glutamate-induced neuronal necrosis in the infant mouse hypothalamus: An electron microscopic study. *J Neuropathol Exp Neurol* **30**, 75.

27. Olney JW (1980) Excitatory neurotoxins as food additives: An evaluation of risk. *Neurotoxicology* **2**, 163.

28. Olney JW (1984) Excitotoxic food additives—relevance of animal studies to human safety. *Neurobehav Toxicol Teratol* **6**, 455.

29. Olney JW (1990) Excitotoxic amino acids and neuropsychiatric disorders. *Annu Rev Pharmacol Toxicol* **30**, 47.

30. Olney JW (1994) Excitotoxins in foods. *Neurotoxicology* **15**, 535.

31. Olney JW, Cicero TJ, Meyer ER (1976) Acute glutamate-induced elevations in serum testosterone and luteinizing hormone. *Brain Res* **112**, 420.

32. Olney JW, Farber NB (1995) NMDA antagonists as neurotherapeutic drugs, psychotogens, neurotoxins, and research tools for studying schizophrenia. *Neuropsychopharmacology* **13**, 335.

33. Olney JW, Ho OL (1970) Brain damage in infant mice following oral intake of glutamate, aspartate or cysteine. *Nature* **227**, 609.

34. Olney JW, Ho OL, Rhee V (1971) Cytotoxic effects of acidic and sulphur-containing amino acids on the infant mouse central nervous system. *Exp Brain Res* **14**, 61.

35. Olney JW, Labruyere J, Collins JF (1981) D-Aminophosphonovalerate is 100-fold more powerful than D-alpha-aminoadipate in blocking N-methylaspartate neurotoxicity. *Brain Res* **221**, 207.

36. Olney JW, Labruyere J, deGubareff T (1980) Brain damage in mice from voluntary ingestion of glutamate and aspartate. *Neurobehav Toxicol* **2**, 125.

37. Olney JW, Price MT, Fuller TA *et al.* (1986) The antiexcitotoxic effects of certain anesthetics, analgesics and sedative-hypnotics. *Neurosci Lett* **68**, 29.

38. Olney J, Price MT, Labruyere J *et al.* (1987) Anti-parkinsonian agents are phencyclidine agonists and N-methyl-D-aspartate antagonists. *Eur J Pharmacol* **142**, 319.

39. Olney J, Price M, Shalid Salles K *et al.* (1987) MK-801 powerfully protects against N-methyl-D-aspartate neurotoxicity. *Eur J Pharmacol* **141**, 357.

40. Olney JW, Sharpe LG, Feigin RD (1972) Glutamate-induced brain damage in infant primates. *J Neuropathol Exp Neurol* **3l**, 464.

41. Perez JV, Olney JW (1972) Accumulation of glutamic acid in arcuate nucleus of infant mouse hypothalamus following subcutaneous administration of the amino acid. *J Neurochem* **19**, 1777.

42. Plant TM, Gray VL, Marshall GR (1989) Puberty in monkeys is triggered by chemical stimulation of the hypothalamus. *Proc Nat Acad Sci USA* **86**, 2506.

43. Price MT, Olney JW, Cicero TJ (1978) Acute elevations of serum luteinizing hormone induced by kainic acid, N-methylaspartic acid or homocysteic acid. *Neuroendocrinology* **26**, 352.

44. Price MT, Olney JW, Lowry OH (1981) Uptake of exogenous glutamate and aspartate by circumventricular organs but not other regions of brain. *J Neurochem* **36**, 1774.

45. Reynolds WA, Butler V, Lemkey-Johnston N (1976) Hypothalamic morphology following ingestion of aspartame or MSG in the neonatal rodent and primate: A preliminary report. *J Toxicol Environ Health* **2**, 471.

46. Rothman SM (1984) Synaptic release of excitatory amino acid neurotransmitter mediates anoxic neuronal death. *J Neurosci* **4**, 1884.

47. Rothstein JD, Martin LJ, Kuncl RW (1992) Decreased glutamate transport by the brain and spinal cord in amyotrophic lateral sclerosis. *N Engl J Med* **326**, 1464.

48. Schaumburg HH, Byck R, Gerstl R, Mashman JH (1969) Monsodium L-glutamate: Its pharmacology and role in the Chinese restaurant syndrome. *Science* **163**, 829.

49. Schmitt B, Steinmann B, Gitzelmann R *et al.* (1993) Nonketotic hyperglycinemia. Clinical and electrophysiological effects of dextromorphan: An antagonist of the NMDA receptor. *Neurology* **43**, 421.

50. Stegink LD, Reynolds WA, Filer LJ *et al.* (1979) Comparative metabolism of glutamate in the mouse, monkey and man. In: *Glutamic Acid: Advances in Biochemistry and Physiology.* Filer LJ, Garattini S, Kare MR *et al.* eds. Raven Press, New York p. 85.

51. Urbanski HF, Ojeda SR (1990) A role for N-methyl-D-aspartate (NMDA) receptors in the control of LH secretion and initiation of female puberty. *Endocrinology* **126**, 1774.

52. Wang GJ, Labruyere J, Price MT (1990) Extreme sensitivity of infant animals to glutamate toxicity: Role of NMDA receptors. *Soc Neurosci Abst* **16**, 198.

53. Watkins JC (1978) Excitatory amino acids. In: *Kainic Acid as a Tool in Neurobiology.* McGeer E, Olney JW, McGeer P eds. Raven Press, New York p. 37.

54. Watkins JC, Evans RH (1981) Excitatory amino acid transmitters. *Annu Rev Pharmacol Toxicol* **21**, 165.

55. Whetsell WO (1996) Current concepts of excitotoxicity. *J Neuropathol Exp Neurol* **55**, 1.

56. Zeevalk GD, Nicklas WJ (1990) Chemically-induced hypoglycemia and anoxia: Relationship to glutamate receptor-mediated toxicity in retina. *J Pharmacol Exp Ther* **253**, 1285.

57. Zeevalk GD, Nicklas WJ (1991) Mechanisms underlying initiation of excitotoxicity associated with metabolic inhibition. *J Pharmacol Exp Ther* **257**, 870.

Glutethimide

Albert C. Ludolph

GLUTETHIMIDE
$C_{13}H_{15}NO_2$

3-Ethyl-3-phenyl-2,6-piperidinedione

NEUROTOXICITY RATING

Clinical

A   Physical dependence and withdrawal

A   Acute encephalopathy (sedation, coma)

B   Peripheral neuropathy

The nonbarbiturate hypnotic glutethimide is no longer used today in most parts of the world because of its side effects and addiction potential. Although the practical importance of glutethimide has declined, it may have some clinical use as a tremor therapeutic (1). Its apparent beneficial effects in certain forms of tremor must be weighed against qualitatively and quantitatively significant undesirable effects. In combination with codeine, glutethimide abuse may be on the rise ("load") in some regions (3).

Since glutethimide is highly lipid soluble, it is rapidly taken up by the brain after absorption from the gastrointestinal tract. Fifty percent of the compound is bound to plasma proteins. The hypnotic effect lasts 4–8 h after an appropriate dose (250–500 mg). The drug is redistributed into kidneys, adipose tissues, and liver, where hydroxylation takes place. Elimination half-life is 5–22 h, and <2% of the oral drug is excreted unchanged in urine. Glutethimide induces microsomal enzymes in the liver. Although its precise mechanism of action is unknown, it is generally assumed that the compound exerts its pharmacological effect mainly by interacting with the benzodiazepine–γ-aminobutyric acid receptor chloride channel complex, possibly by prolongation of the opening time of the chloride channel.

The metabolite 4-hydroxy-2-ethyl-2-phenylglutarimide may accumulate after repeated administration or overdose and is suspected to contribute to the clinical picture of acute glutethimide intoxication (5).

The hallmark of acute glutethimide overdose, namely, prolonged coma, is complicated by the pronounced anticholinergic effect of the drug. The latter include mydriasis, hyperpyrexia, paralytic ileus, and an atonic bladder. Effects on motor control include tonic muscular spasm, and flaccid paralysis; rarely, seizures are described. Respiratory depression is usually less severe than after barbiturates, but hypotension may be intense. Treatment may include hemodialysis or hemoperfusion. Forced diuresis reportedly is without significant effect. The major undesired effects of glutethimide are development of tolerance and physical and psychic dependence. The withdrawal syndrome is characterized by seizures, myoclonic jerks, toxic psychosis, anxiety, delirium, hallucinations, abdominal cramps, and tachycardia.

Polyneuropathy may develop during glutethimide treatment. Two patients developed a sensory neuropathy after a daily oral intake of 2.5–3.0 g over 18 months and 1.5 g over 2 months (2). Partial recovery was observed after 4 months. Another patient had comparatively mild complaints after daily intake of 125 mg over a period of 3 years (4); muscle cramps and nail abnormalities were reported. A 39-year-old woman developed a typical distal polyneuropathy, cerebellar signs, and acute organic brain impairment after taking up to 3 g/day of glutethimide over 5 years (7). Electrophysiological recordings indicated that sensory fibers were predominantly affected. Recovery was poor. One reported case is questionable, since alcoholism also played a role (6).

The toxic mechanism of glutethimide-associated neuropathy is unknown—as is the neuropathy induced by the chemically related compound, thalidomide.

REFERENCES

1. Aisen ML, Holzer M, Rosen M *et al.* (1991) Glutethimide treatment of disabling action tremor in patients with multiple sclerosis and traumatic brain injury. *Arch Neurol* **48**, 513.
2. Bartholomew AA (1961) Neuropathy after thalidomide (Distaval). *Brit Med J* **11**, 1570.
3. Bender FH, Cooper JV, Dreyfus R (1988) Fatalities associated with an acute overdose of glutethimide (Doriden) and codeine. *Vet Human Toxicol* **30**, 332.
4. Chevers LCF (1961) Neuropathy after thalidomide. *Brit Med J* **11**, 1025.
5. Hobbs WR, Rall TW, Verdoorn TA (1996) Hypnotics and sedatives; ethanol. In: *Goodman and Gilman's The Pharmacological Basis of Therapeutics. 9th Ed.* Hardman JG, Limbird LE, Molinoff PB, Ruddon RW eds. McGraw-Hill, New York p. 361.
6. Lingle FA (1966) Irreversible effects of glutethimide addiction. *Amer J Psychiat* **123**, 349.
7. Nover R (1967) Persistent neuropathy following chronic use of glutethimide. *Clin Pharmacol Ther* **8**, 283.

α-Glycerotoxins

Frank Bretschneider
Albert C. Ludolph

NEUROTOXICITY RATING

Experimental

A   Neuromuscular transmission dysfunction (depolarizing)

α-Glycerotoxins (GTx) are components of venom produced by the jaw glands of the polychaete annelid worms *Glycera dibranchiata* and *G. convoluta*. Worms of the family Glyceridae, found along the Atlantic Coast and in the Caribbean Sea (7), possess four fangs on their proboscis that can be everted with great rapidity. This sting may result in an itchy inflammation in a diver or an angler; it can be lethal to a crustacean (1,4). A 300,000-Da partially purified venom protein is responsible for the toxic effect (8). GTx are used as tools in neurobiological studies.

The α-latrotoxin–like (black widow spider) venom increases the frequency of miniature end-plate potentials (MEPP) at crustacean and frog neuromuscular junctions (8,2,6). GTx also stimulate acetylcholine release from *Torpedo* electric organ synaptosomes but have no effect on PC-12 cells (a neurosecretory cell line) (5). GTx act upon synaptosomes from rat brain by depolarization of the synaptosomal plasma membrane with massive calcium influx; a marked increase in cytosolic calcium concentration follows with stimulation in catecholamine release independent of free cytosolic divalents (5). The supposed receptor for GTx action is different from that for α-latrotoxin binding (5), and is unidentified.

The toxic effect in man is solely a sting-induced painful local inflammatory reaction that may persist for days (3,7). The center of the wound usually has a small red macule surrounded by a blanched area. Since the venom does not contain proteolytic activity, there is no penetration into blood vessels or nervous system. The possible lethal effects of GTx in crustaceans may be due to a block of neurotransmitter release because of increased MEPP frequencies and loss of presynaptic transmitter vesicles (6).

REFERENCES

1. Halstead BW (1965) *Poisonous and Venomous Marine Animals of the World. Vol 1*. U.S. Government Printing Office, Washington, DC.
2. Howard BD, Gundersen CB (1980) Effects and mechanisms of polypeptide neurotoxins that act presynaptically. *Annu Rev Pharmacol Toxicol* 20, 307.
3. Kagan BL, Pollard HB, Hanna RB (1982) Induction of ion-permeable channels by the venom of the fanged bloodworm *Glycera dibranchiata*. *Toxicon* 20, 887.
4. Klawe WL, Dickie LH (1957) Biology of the bloodworm *Glycera dibranchiata* Ehlers and its relation to the bloodworm fishery of the marine provinces. *Bull Fish Res Bd Can* **115**, 1.
5. Madeddu L, Meldolesi J, Pozzan T *et al.* (1984) α-Latrotoxin and glycerotoxin differ in target specifity and in the mechanism of their neurotransmitter releasing action. *Neuroscience* 12, 939.
6. Manaranche R, Thieffry M, Israel M (1980) Effect of the venom of *Glycera convoluta* on the spontaneous quantal release of transmitter. *J Cell Biol* **85**, 446.
7. Mebs D (1992) Borstenwürmer. In: *Gifttiere: Ein Handbuch für Biologen, Ärzte und Apotheker*. Wiss Verl-Ges, Stuttgart p. 52.
8. Thieffry M, Bon C, Manaranche R *et al.* (1982) Partial purification of the *Glycera convoluta* components responsible for its presynaptic effects. *J Physiol* 78, 343.

Glycine

Thomas L. Slamovits

GLYCINE
$C_2H_5NO_2$

Aminoacetic Acid

NEUROTOXICITY RATING

Clinical

A   Retinal syndrome (transient)

Experimental

A   Retinal dysfunction (inhibition of neurotransmission)

Glycine is a natural, nonessential amino acid present in collagen and gelatin; the pure aminoacetic acid is a white, crystalline, water-soluble compound. As a nonelectrolyte, aqueous solutions are nonconductive, a property that has found wide use in a variety of electrosurgical procedures. Since its introduction as an irrigating solution for transurethral prostatectomy, aqueous glycine has been used in a variety of concentrations (1.1%, 1.3%, 1.5%), all hypotonic relative to extracellular fluid (280 mOsm/l). The commonly used solution of 1.5% (200 mOsm/l) offers a great advantage over plain water irrigation, since the latter is associated with a significant risk of intravascular hemolysis. Glycine irrigating solution is now used widely in urological procedures, primarily prostatic resection, and in gynecological (hysteroscopic) and orthopedic (arthroscopic) surgery.

Since aqueous glycine irrigation was first and is still most extensively used for transurethral prostate resection (TURP), to date most of the observed complications have been reported in the urological literature as TURP syndrome. This syndrome includes a wide range of symptoms, all attributable to excessive absorption of irrigating fluid through the prostatic venous sinuses. Dilutional hyponatremia can lead to orthostatic and electrocardiographic alteration. Neurological changes include nausea, irritability, confusion, blindness, encephalopathy, and cerebral edema. In severe cases, cardiogenic shock and renal failure may ensue. Metabolic disturbances, in addition to dilutional hyponatremia, include hyperglycemia and hyperammonemia (ammonia is a glycine metabolite), which can also contribute to the nausea and encephalopathy.

The TURP syndrome cannot be attributed entirely to the toxic effects of glycine, since many of the sequelae of glycine irrigation result from metabolic and fluid/electrolyte changes. The specific effect of hyperglycinemia in the TURP syndrome is held to be transient visual loss. Although the

TURP syndrome was initially described in 1947 (5), visual loss was not noted as a component until 1956, when glycine irrigation was first used (7).

There are at least two theoretical sites where glycine can have neurotoxic visual effects. Occipital cortical visual loss has been postulated in cases where pupillary light reactions were (presumably) normal during the episodes of transient loss of vision (1,6). The presence of elevated cerebrospinal fluid levels of glycine and its metabolites could lead to direct CNS toxicity (13). However, in most instances of presumed cortical visual loss, there is concurrent cerebral edema (1,6) which, independent of glycine, could affect visual function. Visual loss can also be attributed to direct glycine toxicity on the anterior visual pathway, as supported by clinical case reports of visual loss accompanied by subnormal or absent pupillary light responses (2,3,4,9,14).

The bulk of experimental and clinical studies implicate the retina as the site of glycine toxicity. Glycine is an inhibitory retinal neurotransmitter. In *Xenopus* and goldfish, the interplexiform cells of the retina are glycinergic (10,18, 19,23). In the cat, A II amacrine cells have been shown to release glycine (15,16). Cat and monkey studies have demonstrated the presence of glycine in retinal bipolar cells (8,11). Studies in rabbits after intravitreal glycine injection (12) and in mudpuppies (20) show reversible depression or loss of the oscillatory potential of the electroretinogram (ERG) b-wave, implying an effect on amacrine cells. Intravenous glycine infusion in dogs caused transient depression or extinction of visual evoked responses; recovery of waveforms paralleled glycine level normalization (22). Inhibition of the pupillary light response inhibition was noted in sheep after intravenous glycine administration (17). All of the above animal studies suggest a local (most likely retinotoxic) effect of glycine as an explanation for the transient visual loss.

Clinical studies (4,21) also support the proposed retinotoxicity of glycine. One study evaluated 20 patients undergoing TURP under spinal anesthesia (4). All had pre- and postoperative ERGs performed monocularly through a dilated pupil (the contralateral pupil remained undilated for assessment of pupillary response). Sixteen patients had no visual symptoms and no change from pre- to postoperative ERG; these visually asymptomatic patients had serum glycine levels in the range of 600–2000 μmol/l (5–15 mg/dl). Four patients had transient visual loss (ranging from light perception only to "count fingers" vision). All patients had postoperative ERG changes with reduction of the photopic b-wave and loss of the oscillatory potential b-wave, which normally appears on the ascending limb of the b-wave. All had serum glycine levels exceeding 4000 μmol/l (>30 mg/dl). The most profoundly affected patient (light perception only) had minimal pupillary responses. The remaining three had present (but unquantitated) pupillary responses. The authors also mention two additional patients—not part of their study—who had post-TURP visual loss to light perception only; both had minimal pupillary light responses. This study (4) offers convincing evidence that those patients with TURP syndrome who have transient visual loss also have simultaneous electrophysiological changes at the level of the retina. These changes can probably be attributed to glycine toxicity. Whether glycine breakdown products play a role remains unclear.

REFERENCES

1. Appelt GL, Benson GS, Corriere JN (1979) Transient blindness: Unusual initial symptoms of transurethral prostatic resection reaction. *Urology* 13, 402.

2. Barletta JP, Fanous MM, Hamed LM (1994) Temporary blindness in the TURP syndrome. *J Neuro-ophthalmol* 14, 6.

3. Burkhart SS, Barnett CR, Snyder SJ (1990) Transient postoperative blindness as a possible effect of glycine toxicity. *Arthroscopy* 6, 112.

4. Creel DJ, Wang JM, Wong KC (1987) Transient blindness associated with transurethral resection of the prostate. *Arch Ophthalmol* 105, 1537.

5. Creevy CD, Webb EA (1947) Fatal hemolytic reaction following transurethral resection: A discussion of its prevention and treatment. *Surgery* 21, 56.

6. Defalque RJ, Miller DW (1975) Visual disturbances during transurethral resection of the prostate. *Can Anaesth Soc J* 22, 620.

7. Harrison RH, Boren JS, Robison JR (1956) Dilutional hyponatremic shock: Another concept of the transurethral prostatic resection reaction. *J Urol* 75, 85.

8. Hendrickson AE, Koontz MA, Pourcho RG *et al.* (1988) Localization of glycine-containing neurons in the Macaca monkey retina. *J Comp Neurol* 273, 473.

9. Kaiser R, Adragna MG, Weiss FR Jr *et al.* (1985) Transient blindness following transurethral resection of the prostate in an achondroplastic dwarf. *J Urol* 133, 685.

10. Kalloniatis M, Marc RE (1990) Interplexiform cells of the goldfish retina. *J Comp Neurol* 297, 340.

11. Koontz MA, Hendrickson A, Pourcho R (1987) Glycine labelling of amacrine and bipolar cells by light and EM immunocytochemistry in macaque monkey retina. *Invest Ophthalmol Vis Sci* 28, 349.

12. Korol S, Leuenberger PM, Englert U *et al.* (1975) *In vivo* effect of glycine on retinal ultrastructure and averaged electroretinogram. *Brain Res* 97, 235.

13. Mahul P, Molliex S, Auboyer C *et al.* (1993) Neurotoxic role of glycocolle and derivatives in transurethral resection of the prostate. *Ann Fr Anesth Reanim* 12, 512. [French]

14. Ovasappian A, Joshi CW, Brunner EA (1982) Visual disturbances: An unusual symptom of transurethral prostatic resection reaction. *Anesthesiology* 57, 332.

15. Pourcho RG, Goebel DJ (1985) A combined Golgi and autoradiographic study of (^{3}H)glycine-accumulating amacrine cells in the cat retina. *J Comp Neurol* 233, 473.

16. Pourcho RG, Goebel DJ (1987) A combined Golgi and autoradiographic study of ^{3}H-glycine accumulating cone bipolar cells in the cat retina. *J Neurosci* 7, 1178.

17. Seggie J, Wright N (1989) Glycine inhibition of pupillary responses to pulses of light in conscious sheep. *J Ocul Pharmacol* 5, 343.

18. Smiley JF, Basinger SF (1988) Somatostatin-like immunoreactivity and glycine high-affinity uptake colocalize to an interplexiform cell of the *Xenopus laevis* retina. *J Comp Neurol* 274, 608.

19. Stone S, Witkovsky P (1984) The actions of γ-aminobutyric acid, glycine and their antagonists upon horizontal cells of the *Xenopus* retina. *J Physiol-London* 353, 249.

20. Wachtmeister L, Dowling JE (1979) The oscillatory potentials of the mudpuppy retina. *Invest Ophthalmol Vis Sci* 17, 1176.

21. Wang JM, Creel DJ, Wong KC (1989) Transurethral resection of the prostate, serum glycine levels, and ocular evoked potentials. *Anesthesiology* 70, 36.

22. Wang JM, Wong KC, Creel DJ (1985) Effects of glycine on hemodynamic responses and visual evoked potentials in the dog. *Anesth Analg* 64, 1071.

23. Yazzulla S, Studholme K (1990) Multiple subtypes of glycine-immunoreactive neurons in the goldfish retina. Single- and double-label studies. *Vis Neurosci* 4, 299.

Gold Salts

Steven Herskovitz

AUROTHIOGLUCOSE
$C_6H_{11}AuO_5S$

Aurothioglucose; (1-Thio-D-glucopyranosato-O2,-S1)gold

NEUROTOXICITY RATING
Clinical

A   Peripheral neuropathy

A   Acute encephalopathy (delirium, seizures)

A   Cranial neuropathy

B   Myopathy (myokymia)

Gold salt therapy (chrysotherapy) has been used in the treatment of rheumatoid arthritis for many years. The most common preparations are aurothioglucose and sodium aurothiomalate; these contain 50% gold by weight, are water soluble, and are administered intramuscularly. Auranofin is the only available gold compound for oral use. Chrysotherapy is reported to decrease synovial inflammation and retard cartilage and bone destruction. Neurotoxicity is uncommon; it may be characterized by encephalopathy, cranial neuropathy, myokymia, and peripheral neuropathy, including occasionally a clinical picture reminiscent of the Guillain-Barré syndrome.

Aurothioglucose and sodium aurothiomalate are rapidly absorbed after intramuscular injection (7). Peak serum concentration is reached in 2–6 h; 95% is bound to albumin. The plasma half-life is about 7 h for a 50-mg dose, but this lengthens substantially with successive doses. Tissue distribution is widespread but variable. Gold salts cross the blood-brain barrier into cerebrospinal fluid (CSF) (10). Residual gold can be found in the liver and skin many years after treatment cessation. Excretion is 60%–90% renal and 10%–40% fecal; it is increased by sulfhydryl agents such as dimercaprol, penicillamine, and N-acetylcysteine. Auranofin is more lipid soluble and absorbed orally, has plasma steady-state concentrations reached after 8–12 weeks, accumulates less in tissues, and has an elimination half-life of about 80 days.

Experimental animal studies of gold neurotoxicity are few. A dose-related neuropathy, similar to that observed in human studies, was demonstrated after prolonged exposure in hens; both axonal degeneration and segmental demyelination were evident (10). Mice develop paralysis, ataxia, and disorientation after repeated injections of aurothiosulphate (17).

The more common toxicities of gold therapy include mucocutaneous lesions, nephropathy, and blood dyscrasias (7). Auranofin is generally better tolerated but has a high incidence of gastrointestinal disturbances (3,9). There is a relationship between gold dosage and toxicity, but no clear correlation with plasma concentration of gold. Neurotoxicity is uncommon, and may appear with or without other systemic signs of gold toxicity. Reports of neurological syndromes in rheumatoid arthritis patients treated with gold are confounded by those of the underlying disease, but convincing cases of gold neurotoxicity are described.

Duration of treatment and total dose of gold vary widely in cases of gold neuropathy. The clinical course in most instances is a progressive, symmetrical, distal polyneuropathy, with predominant sensory, motor, or sensorimotor features evolving over days to weeks (5,6,10,11,19,21). Weakness may be severe and all sensory modalities involved. Clinical and electrophysiological evidence of myokymia may be prominent (1,2,13,15,20). Autonomic involvement can occur (12). CSF protein varies from normal to mildly to moderately elevated (more typical), occasionally even up to several grams per deciliter. Instances of rapid progression, areflexia, and albuminocytological dissociation have mimicked the Guillain-Barré syndrome (4,19). One case of Fisher's syndrome is reported (18). Electrophysiological data are few, with most reports describing signs of axonal degeneration, occasionally slowing of motor conduction, and sometimes myokymia. Morphological studies of sural nerve biopsies, including teased fibers, show both axonal degeneration and segmental demyelination (10), or almost exclusively axonal degeneration (21). Recovery over weeks to months is almost invariable after withdrawal of gold treatment, but neurological residua can occur in severe cases. It is unclear whether chelation therapy influences the course.

Cranial neuropathies may rarely occur either in association with polyneuropathy or in isolation (5). One case of gold-induced aseptic meningitis is purported (14). A few reports of gold-induced encephalopathy are described with delirium, psychiatric features, or focal abnormalities including hemiparesis, aphasia, or seizures (5,6,8,16). In one, reversible, contrast-enhancing white-matter lesions were demonstrated by computed tomography (5).

The mechanism of gold neurotoxicity, whether a hypersensitivity reaction or a direct toxic effect, or both, is uncertain. Experimental studies in hens showing dose-related neuropathy suggest a direct toxic effect in this species (10).

REFERENCES

1. Caldron PH, Wilbourn AJ (1988) Gold neurotoxicity and myokymia. *J Rheumatol* **15**, 528. [Letter]
2. Cavany JA, Chaignot A (1934) Accidents nerveux de la chrysothérapie. *Presse Med* **42**, 478.
3. Delafuente JC, Osborn TG (1984) Review of auranofin, an oral chrysotherapeutic agent. *Clin Pharmacy* **3**, 121.
4. Dick DJ, Raman D (1982) The Guillain-Barré syndrome following gold therapy. *Scand J Rheumatol* **11**, 119.
5. Fam AG, Gordon DA, Sarkozi J *et al.* (1984) Neurologic complications associated with gold therapy for rheumatoid arthritis. *J Rheumatol* **11**, 700.
6. Gambari P, Ostuni P, Lazzarin P *et al.* (1984) Neurotoxicity following a very high dose of oral gold (auranofin). *Arthritis Rheum* **27**, 1316. [Letter]
7. Gilman AG, Rall TR, Nies AS, Taylor P (1990) In: *Goodman & Gilman's The Pharmacological Basis of Therapeutics. 8th Ed.* Hardman JG, Gilman AG, Limbird LE eds. Pergamon Press, New York p. 670.
8. Gulliford MC, Archard NP, Vant Hoff W (1985) Gold encephalopathy. *Brit Med J* **290**, 1744.
9. Heuer MA, Pietrusko RG, Morris RW (1985) An analysis of the worldwide safety experience with auranofin. *J Rheumatol* **12**, 695.
10. Katrak SM, Pollock M, O'Brien CP *et al.* (1980) Clinical and morphological features of gold neuropathy. *Brain* **103**, 671.
11. Leiper EJR (1946) A case of polyneuritis due to gold. *Brit Med J* **2**, 119.
12. Meyer M, Haecki M, Ziegler W *et al.* (1978) Autonomic dysfunction and myokymia in gold neuropathy. In: *Peripheral Neuropathies. Proceedings of the International Symposium on Peripheral Neuropathies, Milan.* Canal N, Pozza G eds. Elsevier, Amsterdam p. 475.
13. Mitsumoto H, Wilbourn AJ, Subramony SH (1982) Generalized myokymia and gold therapy. *Arch Neurol* **39**, 449.
14. Myerson RM (1950) Meningitis during gold therapy. *J Amer Med Assn* **143**, 1336.
15. Nicholson D, Scalettar R, Jacobs RP (1986) Rheumatoid rigor: Gold induced myokymia. A report and review of the literature. *J Rheumatol* **13**, 195.
16. Perry RP, Jacobsen ES (1984) Gold induced encephalopathy: Case report. *J Rheumatol* **11**, 233.
17. Querido A (1947) Gold intoxication of nervous elements on the permeability of the blood-brain barrier. *Acta Psychiat Neurol Scand* **22**, 97.
18. Roquer J, Herraiz J, Maymo J *et al.* (1985) Miller-Fisher syndrome (Guillain-Barré syndrome with ophthalmoplegia) during treatment with gold salts in a patient with rheumatoid arthritis. *Arthritis Rheum* **28**, 838. [Letter]
19. Schlumpf U, Meyer M, Ulrich J, Friede RL (1983) Neurologic complications induced by gold treatment. *Arthritis Rheum* **26**, 825.
20. Vernay D, Dubost JJ, Thevenet JP *et al.* (1986) "Chorée fibrillaire de Morvan" followed by Guillain-Barré syndrome in a patient receiving gold therapy. *Arthritis Rheum* **29**, 1413. [Letter]
21. Walsh JC (1970) Gold neuropathy. *Neurology* **20**, 455.

Gossypol

Fengsheng He

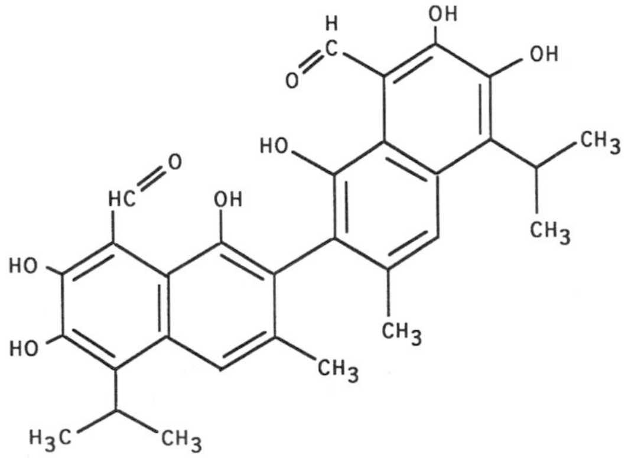

GOSSYPOL
$C_{30}H_{30}O_8$

1,1',6,6',7,7'-Hexahydroxy-5,5'-diisopropyl-3,3'-dimethyl-[2,2'-binaphthalene]-8,8'-dicarboxaldehyde

NEUROTOXICITY RATING
Clinical

A   Myopathy (hypokalemia)

Gossypol is a yellow pigment from the cotton plant flower of *Thespesia populnea* Soland., and the seed and root of *Gossypium herbaceum* L. In the 1960s, gossypol was found to be a cause of male infertility in many rural areas of China (9), where ingestion of raw cotton seed oil was common. Gossypol acetate was then developed as a contraceptive drug for men; it is now also used in China to treat female patients with essential uterine hemorrhage (5,7). The main side effect of gossypol treatment is hypokalemia (3–8).

The LD_{50} values of gossypol for rats ranges from 2.60–3.34 g/kg when administered in water; it is 10% more toxic when given in oil. Similarly, the oral LD_{50} values of gossypol administered in water to mice, rabbits, and guinea pigs are 500–950, 350–600, and 280–300 mg/kg, respectively (1,2). Rats retain gossypol in the liver after oral administration, and 70% of the intake is excreted in the feces after 72 h (7).

In most animals tested, feeding or treatment with gossypol results in weight reduction, loss of appetite, and consequently, growth retardation. Rabbits, dogs, and pigs develop diarrhea. Spastic paralysis has been observed in rabbits and cats. Poisoning can be fatal (1,2). Repeated oral dosing of gossypol to rats, 12–24 mg/day for 5 weeks, inhibits the motility of sperm and causes complete loss of sperm in the spermatic duct and epididymis (7).

The mechanism of gossypol toxicity is not clear. Gossypol uncouples the respiratory chain phosphorylation in rat liver mitochondria. Studies with mice show inhibition of DNA synthesis in primary spermatocytes (1,2,7).

Human studies on male contraception with oral administration of gossypol acetate 20 mg/day for 60 days in the loading phase and a maintenance dosage of 40 mg/week demonstrate an efficacy rate (in terms of sperm count <4 × 10^6) of 92% at the end of the loading phase and 98% after 12 months of the maintenance phase. Loss of spermatocyte and irreversible damage to the spermatogenic epithelium have been confirmed by testis biopsy (7).

Chronic gossypol poisoning usually occurs in cotton-growing areas of China where cottonseed oil is consumed without being processed by heating and alkalization, and more often in winter and spring when vegetable supplies are insufficient. Clusters of patients may appear in families or villages. The adverse effect of gossypol contraception manifesting as hypokalemia is found often after 0.5–1.5 years of treatment, at a prevalence of 0.88%–1.98% (5). Hypokalemia is linked to changes in potassium transport resulting from binding of gossypol to membrane phospholipids.

Patients may have prodromal symptoms such as nausea, loss of appetite, tingling in hands, and cramping and weakness of the legs. Symptoms may progress over 1 or 2 weeks. Patients then develop polydipsia, polyuria, nausea, vomiting, anorexia, palpitations, and flaccid paresis of extremities. Decreased muscle power (U.K. Medical Research Council Scale I-III) is more prominent proximally; however, wrist drop may appear. Muscle tone is reduced and tendon flexes are diminished or lost. Cranial nerves and sensation are not involved. No pathological reflexes are present. Serum potassium is <3 mEq/l in mild cases; in patients with severe weakness, values may be <2.5 mEq/l (3–5). Elevation of urinary potassium and distal renal tubular acidosis indicate a renal loss of potassium (4). Increased urinary protein and β_2-microglobulin are also found. Serum calcium may decrease; serum glutamate pyruvic transaminase activity is increased in some patients. Electrocardiogram shows hypokalemic changes including QT prolongation, flat T wave or inversion of the T wave, as well as ventricular premature beat and atrioventricular (AV) block (3–5).

After cessation of intake of gossypol and treatment with intravenous infusion or oral administration of potassium chloride for 1–3 weeks, serum potassium levels often recover first; this is followed by restoration of a normal electrocardiogram and strength in the extremities (3–5). A few patients with chronic gossypol poisoning died from Adams-Stokes syndrome or paralysis of respiratory muscles.

The differential diagnosis of chronic gossypol poisoning and periodic paralysis should be taken into consideration. Patients with chronic gossypol poisoning do not have history of hereditary disease, usually show an insidious onset and progression of symptoms within the first 2 weeks, and recover only after serum potassium has normalized.

The flaccid paresis in patients with chronic gossypol poisoning is due to hypokalemia induced by renal loss of potassium (4,6,8).

REFERENCES

1. Berardi LC, Goldblatt LA (1980) Gossypol. In: *Toxic Constituents of Plant Foods*. Liener IE ed. Academic Press, New York p. 183.
2. Concon JM (1988) *Food Toxicology. Part A: Principles and Concepts*. Marcel Dekker, New York p. 309.
3. Guo JC, Xu MX, Yuan TE (1989) Gossypol poisoning in 41 children. *Clin Pediat J* 7, 19.
4. Gao H, Yang ZX, Jin SX *et al.* (1985) Primary observations on distal renal tubule acidosis in 177 cases caused by gossypol intoxication. *Chin J Intern Med* 24, 419. [In Chinese.]
5. Han ML, Wang YF, Ma XH (1985) Gossypol induced hypokalemic paralysis. Three case reports. *Chin J Gynecol* 20, 379.
6. Kumar M, Sharma S, Lohiya NK (1997) Gossypol-induced hypokalemia and role of exogenous potassium salt supplementation when used as an antispermatogenic agent in male langur monkey. *Contraception* 56, 251.
7. Lei HP (1982) Review and prospect of gossypol research. *Acta Pharmacol Sin* 17, 1.
8. Liu GZ, Lyle KC (1987) Clinical trial of gossypol as a male contraceptive drug. Part II. Hypokalemia study. *Fert Steril* 48, 462.
9. Waites GM, Wang C, Griffin PD (1998) Gossypol: reasons for its failure to be accepted as a safe reversible male antifertility drug. *Int J Androl* 21, 8.

Grammostola spatulata

Albert C. Ludolph

NEUROTOXICITY RATING

Experimental

A Ion channel dysfunction (calcium channels, types N and P)

The venom of the South American chili rose tarantula spider, *Grammostola spatulata*, contains a 36-amino-acid peptide [ω-grammotoxin SIA (ω-GsTx SIA)] which blocks N- and P-type high-threshold voltage-sensitive neuronal Ca²⁺ channels (1–5). ³H-D-Aspartate release is inhibited in the hippocampal slice, and microdialysis studies of the hippocampus of freely moving rats show that K⁺-stimulated glutamate release is inhibited by the compound (3). The venom displays cardiac toxicity and causes arrhythmias. It is uncertain whether there is a direct systemic neurotoxic effect in humans.

REFERENCES

1. Chen Y, Simasko SM, Niggel J *et al*. (1996) Ca²⁺ uptake in GH₃ cells during hypotonic swelling: The sensory role of stretch-activated ion channels. *Amer J Physiol-Cell Physiol* 270, 39.
2. Keith RA, Defeo PA, Lampe RA *et al*. (1992) Inhibition of neuronal calcium channels by a fraction from *Grammostola spatulata* venom. *Pharmacol Commun* 1, 19.
3. Keith RA, Mangano TJ, Lampe RA *et al*. (1995) Comparative actions of synthetic omega-grammotoxin SIA and synthetic omega-Aga-IVA on neuronal calcium entry and evoked release of neurotransmitters *in vitro* and *in vivo*. *Neuropharmacology* 34, 1515.
4. Lampe RA, Defeo PA, Davison MD *et al*. (1993) Isolation and pharmacological characterization of omega-grammotoxin SIA, a novel peptide inhibitor of neuronal voltage-sensitive calcium channel responses. *Mol Pharmacol* 44, 451.
5. McDonough SI, Lampe RA, Keith RA, Bean BP (1997) Voltage-dependent inhibition of N- and P-type calcium channels by the peptide toxin omega-grammotoxin-SIA. *Mol Pharmacol* 52, 1095.

Grayanotoxins

Albert C. Ludolph

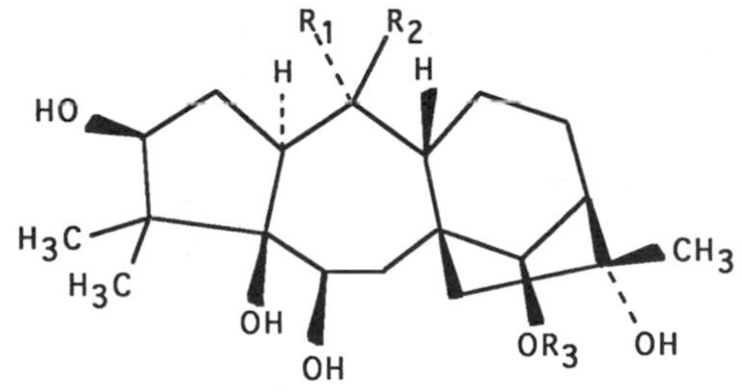

	R₁	R₂	R₃
GRAYANOTOXIN I	OH	CH₃	COCH₃
GRAYANOTOXIN III	OH	CH₃	H
GRAYANOTOXIN II	R₁R₂ = CH₂		R₃ = H

GTX I; (3β,6β,14R)- Grayanotoxane-3,5,6,10,14,16-hexol 14-acetate — C₂₂H₃₆O₇

GTX II; (3β,6β,14R)- Grayanotox-10(20)-ene-3,5,6,14,16-pentol — C₂₀H₃₂O₅

GTX III; (3β,6β,14R)- Grayanotoxane-3,5,6,10,14,16-hexol — C₂₀H₃₄O₆

Andromedotoxin; Asebotoxin; Acetylandromedol; Rhodotoxin

NEUROTOXICITY RATING

Clinical

A Acute encephalopathy (agitation, seizures)

Experimental

A Ion channel dysfunction (sodium channels)

More than 20 neurotoxic grayanotoxins are recognized; three are most important: grayanotoxin I (GTX I), GTX II, and GTX III. These diterpenoid toxins are found in the leaves of the genera *Rhododendron*, *Kalmia*, *Leucothoe*, *Pieris*, and other members of the family Ericaceae. The toxicity of the individual plant may vary considerably (5).

The MPs of GTX I and II are 258°–260°C and 199°–200°C, respectively. A single molecule of the lipid-soluble toxin induces membrane depolarization in skeletal and heart muscle, since it binds to site 2 on the Na⁺ channel and increases membrane permeability to sodium (2,14). GTX II (α-dihydrograyanotoxin II) modifies Na⁺ channels in depolarized squid giant axons to generate sustained inward current (15). Analytical methods for the detection of grayanotoxins have been described (4).

The oral LD_{50} for GTX I is 2–5 mg/kg body weight for rats (5). The intraperitoneal LD_{50}s in mice are 1.31 mg/kg (GTX I), 26.1 mg/kg (GTX II), and 0.84 mg/kg body weight (GTX III) (9). Mice develop postural abnormalities, torsion, retrocollis, spasm, and "locomotive ataxia" (9). Accidental poisoning has been observed in sheep, goats, and cattle (1,7,10,12). An experimental study of a goat fed a *Pieris* spp. (13) revealed a clinical picture dominated by nonspecific symptoms; there was no clear-cut evidence of neurological dysfunction and neuropathological examination was not performed. Prolonged feeding with grayanotoxins did not produce neurotoxicity (8).

In humans, the classical intoxication is induced by honey contaminated with grayanotoxins (3,5,6,11). The clinical picture has been inconsistent. A translated report of intoxication states: "*All soldiers who ate honey combs lost consciousness, suffered from vomiting and diarrhea and were unable to stand upright. Those who consumed only a small amount looked as if they were drunk; those who ate a lot of honey seemed to become mad, and some even died. Nobody died the day after the intoxication*" (6). Symptoms have appeared after the oral intake of only 20–75 ml Turkish honey (6); gastrointestinal disturbances such as diarrhea and nausea were followed by vertigo, abnormal sensations, and seizures (5,6). Agitation, euphoria, and aggressive behavior may appear along with arrhythmia and bradycardia (6). Treatment is gastric lavage and administration of charcoal (5,6) if andromedotoxin (grayanotoxin) intoxication is suspected or leaves of toxic plants have been ingested. Because of cardiac effects, electrocardiographic monitoring is mandatory (6).

REFERENCES
1. Bentz H (1969) *Nutztiervergiftungen, Erkennung und Verhütung*. Gustav Fischer Verlag, Jena.
2. Catterall WA (1980) Neurotoxins that act on voltage-sensitive sodium channels in excitable membranes. *Annu Rev Pharmacol Toxicol* **20**, 15.
3. Chambers AM (1984) Warning—rhododendrons may damage your health! *Scot Med J* **29**, 107.
4. Clarke EGC, Humphreys DJ, King T (1973) Nachweis von Andromedotoxin. In: *Tier- und Pflanzengifte*. Kaiser E ed. Wilhelm Goldmann Verlag, München.
5. Frohne-Pfändler (1987) *Giftpflanzen. Ein Handbuch für Apotheker, Ärzte, Toxikologen und Biologen*. Wissenschaftliche Verlagsgesellschaft mbH, Stuttgart.
6. Gössinger H, Hruby K, Pohl S et al. (1983) Vergiftungen mit andromedotoxinhaltigem Honig. *Deut Med Wochenschr* **108**, 1555.
7. Higgins RJ, Hannam DAR, Humphreys DJ, Stodulski JBJ (1985) Rhododendron poisoning in sheep. *Vet Rec* **116**, 294.
8. Hikino H, Ohizumi Y, Konno C et al. (1979) Subchronic toxicity of Ericaceous toxins and rhododendron leaves. *Chem Pharm Bull Tokyo* **27**, 874.
9. Hikino H, Ohta T, Ogura M et al. (1976) Structure-activity relationships of *Ericaceous* toxins on acute toxicity in mice. *Toxicol Appl Pharmacol* **35**, 303.
10. Humphreys DJ, Stodulski JBJ, Stocker JD (1983) *Rhododendron* poisoning in goats. *Vet Rec* **113**, 503.
11. Kerkvliet JD (1981) Analysis of a toxic *Rhododendron* honey. *J Apicult Res* **20**, 249.
12. Shannon D (1985) *Rhododendron* poisoning in sheep. *Vet Rec* **116**, 451.
13. Smith MC (1978) Japanese *Pieris* poisoning in the goat. *J Amer Vet Med Assn* **173**, 78.
14. Strichartz G, Rando T, Wang GK (1987) An integrated view of the molecular toxinology of sodium channel gating in excitable cells. *Annu Rev Neurosci* **10**, 237.
15. Yakehiro M, Seyama I, Narahashi T (1997) Kinetics of grayanotoxin evoked modification of sodium channels in squid giant axons. *Pflugers Arch* **433**, 403.

Griseofulvin

Herbert H. Schaumburg

GRISEOFULVIN
$C_{17}H_{17}ClO_6$

(1'S-trans)-7-Chloro-2',4,6-trimethoxy-6'-methylspiro[benzofuran-2(3H),1'-[2]cyclohexene]-3,4'-dione

NEUROTOXICITY RATING
Clinical
B   Acute encephalopathy (lethargy, coma)
B   Peripheral neuropathy

Griseofulvin is an orally administered, fungistatic agent used for serious infections with dermatophytes. Griseofulvin causes disruption of the mitotic spindle by interacting with polymerized microtubules (4). Absorption of orally administered drug is variable, since it is nearly insoluble in water; once absorbed, it is rapidly and widely distributed, and about 50% of the absorbed dose is excreted in the urine within 5 days. The drug binds tightly and persistently to newly formed keratin and makes the skin, hair, and nails resistant to fungal infection.

The incidence of systemic adverse effects is low (2). Nausea and vomiting occasionally occur, and there are well-documented instances of a severe "disulfiram-like reaction" in some individuals who coconsume alcoholic beverages (1). Since high doses may be carcinogenic and neuroteratogenic in experimental animals, griseofulvin is not advocated for trivial dermatophytoses.

Experimental studies indicate that griseofulvin interacts with microtubules (both *in vivo* and *in vitro*) and can reduce the rate and amount of fast axonal transport (3). There are no reports of peripheral neuropathy in experimental animals. Multiple congenital malformations in CNS and skeleton appear in kittens following chronic dosing of the pregnant mother (7).

Headache is common; it occurs in 15% and may be severe at onset but usually lessens with continued therapy. Other reversible encephalopathic effects include lethargy, psychosis, syncope, fatigue, and blurred vision (5). There are 11 case reports of peripheral paresthesias or peripheral neuropathy following chronic griseofulvin therapy at conventional doses; only one is well documented (6).

REFERENCES

1. Fett LD, Vukov LF (1994) An unusual case of severe griseofulvin-alcohol interaction. *Ann Emerg Med* **24**, 95.
2. Goldman L (1970) Griseofulvin. *Med Clin N Amer* **54**, 1339.
3. Hanson M, Edstrom A (1977) Fast axonal transport: Effect of antimitotic drugs and inhibitors of energy metabolism on the rate and amount of transported protein in frog sciatic nerves. *J Neurobiol* **8**, 97.
4. Knasmuller S, Parzefall W, Helma C et al. (1998) Toxic effects of griseofulvin: disease models, mechanisms, and risk assessment. *Crit Rev Toxicol* **27**, 495.
5. Lastnick G (1974) Psychotic symptoms with griseofulvin. *J Amer Med Assn* **229**, 1420.
6. Lecky BRF (1990) Griseofulvin-induced neuropathy. *Lancet* **335**, 230.
7. Scott FW, Lahunta A, Schultz RD et al. (1975) Teratogenesis in cats associated with griseofulvin therapy. *Teratology* **11**, 79.

Gyromitrin

Albert C. Ludolph

$$H_3C - CH = N - N < \begin{matrix} CH_3 \\ CHO \end{matrix}$$

GYROMITRIN
$C_4H_8N_2O$

Acetaldehyde *N*-methyl-*N*-formylhydrazone

NEUROTOXICITY RATING

Clinical

B   Acute encephalopathy (fatigue, headache, somnolence)

B   Hepatic encephalopathy (seizures, coma)

Gyromitrin is the toxin of the species *Gyromitra esculenta* (false morrel) (2,9), a mushroom found widely in Europe, in particular in central parts such as Poland and Germany, but also in North America (2,9). The mushroom also contains homologous hydrazones of minor importance (9). Other species, *G. gigas*, *G. fastigiata*, *G. infula*, *Helvella crispa*, and *H. lacunosa,* also contain gyromitrin (2,9). Consumption of *G. esculenta* causes severe poisoning; the mortality ratio is about 10% (4,9). Selling or trading the false morel is illegal in Germany and Switzerland (2).

Gyromitrin is a colorless, oily liquid with a BP of 143°C; its sensitivity to heat and its volatile character may partly explain the variation of the clinical effect of the poison (6–8). Gyromitrin is hydrolyzed under acidic conditions (such as in the stomach) to *N*-methyl-*N*-formylhydrazine (MFH) and, in a second slower step, to monomethylhydrazine (MH). *In vivo*, this hydrolysis is incomplete (9). Gyromitrin and its toxic metabolites are best detected by gas and thin-layer chromatography (2,9,12,13). Gyromitrin is hepatotoxic and renotoxic, induces hemolysis, and may be neurotoxic, presumably because it reduces pyridoxine (vitamin B_6) levels. A carcinogenic effect has been shown in rodents.

The $LD_{50}s$ for gyromitrin, MFH, and MH for mice are 344, 118, and 33 mg/kg body weight, respectively (10,14). The corresponding human estimated values are 20–50 mg/kg body weight for gyromitrin and 4.8–8 mg/kg body weight for MH (1,11). Fatal dosages for children may be lower (11).

Risk factors for an intoxication are the consumption of raw or poorly cooked mushrooms, and the intake of cooking juice or preservation liquid (2,4,9). It is unresolved whether repeated consumption increases toxicity (3). The clinical picture of the acute intoxication in humans (*Gyromitra* syndrome, *Helvella* syndrome) is characterized by two phases: fatigue, headache, nausea, vomiting, abdominal pain, and diarrhea appearing within 6–12 h of exposure. The patient recovers within 2-6 days. In the second phase, a late toxic response is dominated by a hepatorenal disorder accompanied by hepatosplenomegaly and icterus; finally, signs and symptoms develop in association with hepatic encephalopathy: drowsiness, restlessness, nystagmus, dysarthria, ataxia, delirium, coma, and tonic-clonic seizures. A comprehensive overview has noted that 14.5% of 513 patients died (4).

Gyromitra intoxications are mostly seen during spring. Subjects with *Gyromitra*-related gastrointestinal disturbances should be transferred to a hospital with an intensive care unit together with anyone who shared the culpable meal (2,5). Initial treatment includes gastric lavage with activated charcoal, and the replacement of fluids and electrolytes. Hemodialysis supports elimination of the toxin. Administration of vitamin B_6 during *Gyromitra* poisoning is suggested to prevent seizures (9). In practice, the *Gyromitra* syndrome must be distinguished from *Amanita* intoxication, which has a different clinical picture and typically occurs in the fall.

The neurotoxicity of hydrazine derivatives is related to their ability to bind to vitamin B_6; this leads to decreased activity of B_6-dependent decarboxylase reactions. As in isoniazid poisoning, inhibition of glutamate decarboxylase may lead to decreased brain levels of the inhibitory neurotransmitter γ-aminobutyric acid in the brain and possibly accounts for seizures. Since MFH is detoxified by acetylation, some of the differences in individual susceptibility to gyromitrin intoxication may be explained by genetic differences in the acetylation status of the individual.

Editors' Note: Information on the differential diagnosis and treatment of mushroom (including *Gyromitra* spp.) intoxication is available (i–iv).

i. Ellenhorn MJ (1997) *Ellenhorn's Medical Toxicology. Diagnosis and Treatment of Human Poisoning, 2nd Ed* Williams & Wilkins, Baltimore p 1880.

ii. Kohn R, Mot'ovska Z (1997) Mushroom poisoning—classification, symptoms and therapy. *Vnitr Lek* **43**, 230. [Slovak]

iii. Koppel C (1993) Clinical symptomatology and management of mushroom poisoning. *Toxicon* **31**, 1513.

iv. Michelot D, Toth B (1991) Poisoning by *Gyromitra esculenta*—a review. *J Appl Toxicol* **11**, 235.

REFERENCES

1. Andary C, Bourrier MJ, Privat G (1984) Teneur en toxine et inconstance de l'intoxication gyromitrienne. *Bull Soc Mycol Fr* **100**, 273.
2. Bresinsky A, Besl H (1985) *Giftpilze*. Wissenschaftliche Verlagsgesellschaft mbH, Stuttgart, p. 62.
3. Coulet M, Guillot J (1982) Poisoning by *Gyromitra*: A possible mechanism. *Med Hypotheses* **8**, 325.
4. Franke S, Freimuth U, List PH (1967) Über die Giftigkeit der Frühjahrslorchel, *Gyromitra* (*Helvella*) *esculenta*. *Arch Toxicol* **22**, 293.
5. Hanrahan J, Gordon M (1984) Mushromm poisoning: Case reports and review of therapy. *J Amer Med Assn* **251**, 1057.
6. List PH, Luft P (1967) Gyromitrin, das Gift der Frühjahrslorchel *Gyromitra* (*Helvella*) *esculenta* Fr. *Tetrahedron Lett* **20**, 1893.
7. List PH, Luft P (1968) Gyromitrin, das Gift der Frühjahrslorchel. *Arch Pharm* **301**, 294.
8. List PH, Luft P (1969) Nachweis und Gehaltsbestimmung von Gyromitrin in frischen Lorcheln. *Arch Pharm* **302**, 143.
9. Michelot D, Toth B (1991) Poisoning by *Gyromitra esculenta*—a review. *J Appl Toxicol* **11**, 235.
10. Niskanen A, Pyysalo H, Rimaila-Pänänen E, Hartikka P (1976) Short-term peroral toxicity of ethylidene gyromitrin in rabbits and chickens. *Food Cosmet Toxicol* **14**, 409.
11. Schmidlin-Meszaros J (1974) Gyromitrin in Trockenlorcheln (*Gyromitra esculenta* sicc.). *Mitt Geb Lebensm Hyg* **65**, 453.
12. Stijve T (1978) Ethylidene gyromitrin and *N*-methyl-*N*-formylhydrazine in commerciably available dried false morels, *Gyromitra esculenta* Fr. ex Pers. *Mitt Geb Lebensm Hyg* **69**, 492.
13. Stijve T (1981) High-performance thin-layer chromatographic determination of the toxic principles of some poisonous mushrooms. *Mitt Geb Lebensm Hyg* **72**, 44.
14. Wright A, Niskanen A, Pyysalo H, Korpela H (1978) The toxicity of some *N*-methyl-*N*-formylhydrazones from *Gyromitra esculenta* and related compounds in mouse and microbial tests. *Toxicol Appl Pharmacol* **45**, 429.

Halothane

Herbert H. Schaumburg

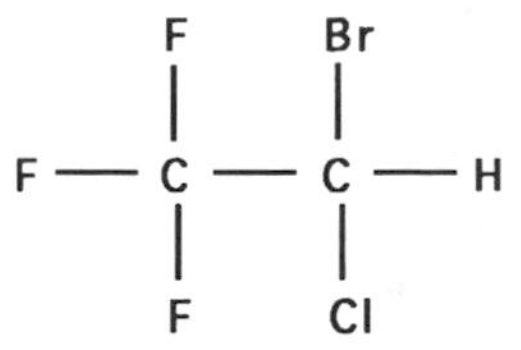

HALOTHANE
C₂HBrClF₃

2-Bromo-2-chloro-1,1,1-trifluoroethane

NEUROTOXICITY RATING

Clinical

A   Malignant hyperthermia syndrome

B   Seizure disorder

Halothane, a widely used, potent volatile anesthetic, is generally administered as a maintenance agent following thiopental-induced anesthesia. It is well tolerated, and there are few systemic toxic effects. Cardiovascular dysfunction may accompany high-level administration, and hepatitis has rarely occurred; it is uncertain whether hepatitis represents direct toxicity or a hypersensitivity reaction.

Cerebrospinal fluid pressure initially increases during halothane anesthesia as a result of elevated cerebral blood flow; this may aggravate pre-existing elevated intracranial pressure associated with many neurosurgical conditions (4). Cerebral blood flow gradually returns to normal when halothane anesthesia lasts for more than 2 h.

Prolonged psychological impairment has been reported following halothane anesthesia. Some reports of halothane administration in normal volunteers describe global cognitive dysfunction for as long as 1 week (3); other studies have only found mild postanesthetic psychological distress for 2 days, without definite cognitive impairment (1,2). Whether this is a genuine phenomenon specific to halothane is uncertain.

Generalized seizures have been described in three individuals immediately after halothane anesthesia (3). Electroencephalograms usually display generalized slowing with some posterior delta activity for 7 days after surgery; paroxysmal sharp-wave activity has also been observed in three instances (1). Susceptible individuals are at risk for malignant hyperthermia syndrome during halothane anesthesia.

REFERENCES

1. Burchiel KJ, Stockard JJ, Calverley RK et al. (1978) Electroencephalographic abnormalities following halothane anesthesia. *Anesth Analg* 57, 244.
2. Davison LA, Steinhelber JC, Eger EI et al. (1975) Psychological effects of halothane and isoflurane anesthesia. *Anesthesiology* 43, 313.
3. Smith PA, MacDonald TR, Jones CS (1966) Convulsions associated with halothane anaesthesia. *Anaesthesia* 21, 229.
4. Warner DS, Boarini DJ, Kassell NF (1985) Cerebrovascular adaptation to prolonged halothane anesthesia is not related to cerebrospinal fluid pH. *Anesthesiology* 63, 243.

Helichrysum Spp.

Helge Völkel
Albert C. Ludolph

NEUROTOXICITY RATING

Clinical

A   Leukoencephalopathy (cattle)

Experimental

A   CNS myelin edema

All 16 species of plants of the genus *Helichrysum* (Asteraceae) have neurotoxic potential. Definite evidence exists for the neurotoxicity of the South African *H. argyrosphaerum*, a plant used in traditional Zulu medicine that has caused lesions of the nervous system in cattle, sheep, and goats (1). Some members of the genus show antimicrobial effects against gram-positive bacteria (6,7); *H. aureonitens* has antiviral activity against *Herpes simplex* virus type 1 in human lung fibroblasts (6) and extracts of *H. nudifolium* inhibit cyclooxygenase (4).

The neurotoxicity of *H. argyrosphaerum* was first described in 1975 in sheep and cattle (1) in Namibia. Animals developed blindness, paresis, and cataracts. A second outbreak was described in 1988 among young sheep and goats in northwestern Cape Province, South Africa. Approximately 4–5 months after a heavy rainfall ended a 9-year drought, lambs and a few goat kids developed blindness, unresponsive pupils, nystagmus, and weakness (8). Light microscope studies revealed bilateral symmetrical status spongiosus of the white matter of the brain, in particular of the subendymal area adjacent to the lateral ventricles, cerebellar peduncles, and brainstem. Similar changes were found in the spinal cord and, less impressively, in the spinal nerve roots. Ultrastructurally, there was evidence of myelin edema; significant changes were absent in neurons, glial cells, and axons. Gliosis or inflammation was not detected. Myelin edema produced secondary axonal damage (wallerian degeneration by compression) of the optic nerve. Retinopathy was characterized by loss of photoreceptor outer segments predominantly in the nontapetal retina. These findings are largely consistent with the results of controlled feeding experiments in sheep done after the 1975 outbreak. Myelinic vacuolation was also seen, and the lesions were described in the periventricular white matter, middle cerebellar peduncles, and pyramidal and optic tracts (1). Degeneration of the photoreceptor layer was also part of the picture. *H. blandoskianum* also causes liver damage, hepatic encephalopathy, and spongiform changes in the CNS of sheep and cattle in Australia (5).

It is unknown which chemicals from the aerial parts of *Helichrysum* are responsible for its neurotoxicity. *Helichrysum* spp. of Greek origin (*H. stoechas*, *H. barrelieri*, *H. taenari*, *H. amorginum*, and *H. italicum*) have been analyzed (2,3). The chemical composition of *Helichrysum* spp. is heterogenous. In the first two species, β-elemene, β-caryophyllene, geraniol, and camphene were detected; in the latter, geraniol, geranyl acetate, and neryl acetate were the major constituents of the oil. Other compounds present in *Helichrysum* spp. are hydroxy-iso-pentenyl-acetophenones, triterpenoids, glycosylated and free steroids, phloroglucinol derivatives, and flavonoids (2,3).

REFERENCES

1. Basson PA, Kellerman TS, Albl P *et al.* (1975) Blindness and encephalopathy caused by *Helichrysum argyrosphaerum DC.* (Compositae) in sheep and cattle. *Onderstepoort J Vet Res* **42**, 135.
2. Chinou IB, Roussis V, Perdetzoglou D *et al.* (1997) Chemical and antibacterial studies of two *Helichrysum* species of Greek origin. *Planta Med* **63**, 181.
3. Chinou IB, Roussis V, Perdetzoglou D, Loukis A (1996) Chemical and biological studies of two *Helichrysum* species of Greek origin. *Planta Med* **62**, 377.
4. Jager AK, Hutchings A, van Staden J (1996) Screening of Zulu medical plants for prostaglandin-synthesis inhibitors. *J Ethnopharmacol* **52**, 95.
5. McAuliffe PR, White WE (1976) "Woolly everlasting daisy" (*Helichrysum blandoskianum*) toxicity in cattle and sheep. *Aust Vet J* **52**, 366.
6. Meyer JJ, Afolayan AJ, Taylor MB, Engelbrecht L (1996) Inhibition of herpes simplex virus type 1 by aqueous extracts from shoots of *Helichrysum aureonitens* (Asteraceae). *J Ethnopharmacol* **52**, 41.
7. Salie F, Eagles PF, Leng HM (1996) Preliminary antimicrobial screening of four South African Asteraceae species. *J Ethnopharmacol* **52**, 27.
8. van der Lugt JJ, Olivier J, Jordaan P (1996) Status spongiosis, optic neuropathy, and retinal degeneration in *Helichrysum argyrosphaerum* poisoning in sheep and a goat. *Vet Pathol* **33**, 495.

n-Heptane

Herbert H. Schaumburg

$$CH_3(CH_2)_5CH_3$$

n-HEPTANE
C_7H_{16}

NEUROTOXICITY RATING

Clinical

A Acute encephalopathy (sedation, stupor)

C Peripheral neuropathy

Experimental

A Acute encephalopathy (sedation, coma)

n-Heptane is a hydrocarbon solvent isolated from natural gas or crude oil. Following ingestion or inhalation, it is rapidly absorbed; the principal metabolites are 2-heptanol and 3-hepatanol. Minute amounts of 2,5-heptanedione are detectible in urine of humans and experimental animals following prolonged exposures (1,4).

n-Heptane is remarkably nontoxic. Acute or chronic exposure of experimental animals or humans to high levels of *n*-heptane causes little mucosal or upper airway irritation, bone marrow change, or hepatorenal dysfunction.

Mice exposed to 8000 ppm for 10 min become anesthetized; exposure to 32,000 ppm causes coma and irregular respiration within 3 min, and death after 5 min. One study of rats exposed to mixtures of heptane, methyl hexane, and other aliphatic hydrocarbons at levels of 1500 ppm for 5 months claimed that *n*-heptane caused peripheral neuropathy (6). A subsequent meticulous study of rats exposed to 3000 ppm of pure *n*-heptane failed to detect evidence of peripheral nerve dysfunction (5).

High-level human exposure (5000 ppm for 5 min) causes incoordination and unsteady gait; more prolonged exposure (5000 ppm for 15 min) produces stupor. The appearance of peripheral neuropathy in workers exposed to mixtures of *n*-hexane and *n*-heptane initially suggested that each was responsible (2). Subsequent studies of individuals exposed to one or the other disclosed that only *n*-hexane causes neuropathy in humans (3) (*see n*-Hexane, Metabolites, and Derivatives, this volume).

REFERENCES

1. Filser JG, Csanady GA, Dietz W *et al.* (1996) Comparative estimation of the neurotoxic risks of *n*-hexane and *n*-heptane in rats and humans based on the formation of the metabolites 2,5-hexanedione and 2,5-heptanedione. *Adv Exp Med Biol* **387**, 411.
2. Gaultier M, Rancurel G, Piva C, Efthymiou ML (1973) Polyneuritis and aliphatic hydrocarbons. *J Eur Toxicol* **6**, 294.
3. Herskowitz A, Ishii N, Schaumburg HH (1971) *n*-Hexane neuropathy—a syndrome occurring as a result of industrial exposure. *N Engl J Med* **285**, 82.
4. Perbellini L, Brugnone F, Cocheo V *et al.* (1986) Identification of the *n*-heptane metabolites in rat and human urine. *Arch Toxicol* **58**, 229.
5. Takeuchi Y, Ono Y, Hisanaga N *et al.* (1980) A comparative study on the neurotoxicity of *n*-pentane, *n*-hexane, and *n*-heptane in the rat. *Brit J Ind Med* **37**, 241.
6. Truhaut R, Laget P, Piat G *et al.* (1973) Preliminary electrophysiological results following experimental poisoning with technical hexane and heptane in white rats. *Arch Mal Prof* **34**, 417.

Heroin

John C.M. Brust

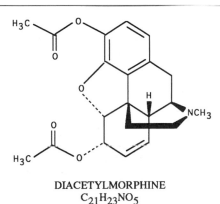

DIACETYLMORPHINE
$C_{21}H_{23}NO_5$

Diacetylmorphine; Diamorphine

NEUROTOXICITY RATING

Clinical

A Acute encephalopathy (sedation, coma)

A Physical dependence and withdrawal

B Encephalomalacia (occlusive stroke)

B Brachial plexus neuropathy

B Leukoencephalopathy

C Chronic encephalopathy

Experimental

A Acute encephalopathy (sedation, coma)

A Physical dependence (withdrawal)

Heroin is synthesized from morphine, a natural alkaloid contained in seed capsules of the poppy, *Paper somniferum*, indigenous to Southeast Asia, the Middle East and, more recently, Latin America (1).

Classified by the U.S. Food and Drug Administration as a Schedule I drug ("high potential for abuse, no accepted medical use"), heroin is illegal in most countries yet enjoys immense worldwide popularity as a recreational drug. In the United States, it is usually sold as a brown or white powder with heroin concentrations ranging from zero to over 90%. East Coast preparations often contain quinine, originally added in the 1930s for malaria prophylaxis and retained today because some users believe it enhances the "high" and also, from the dealer's standpoint, because its bitter taste disguises the true content of heroin present. Other impurities in the mixture include pharmacologically inactive substances such as lactose, mannitol, baking soda, talc, or starch, as well as, on occasion, pharmacologically active agents such as procaine, lidocaine, or strychnine. Heroin mixed with cocaine or amphetamine is called a "speedball."

In the United States, heroin ("horse," "smack," "junk," "dope") is most often taken parenterally either intravenously ("mainlining") or subcutaneously ("skin-popping"). Dissolved in unsterile water in a bottle cap or spoon and heated with a match, it is drawn into an eye dropper or syringe through cotton (purportedly to filter out impurities) and then injected. In parts of the world where heroin is plentiful and cheap, the drug is more often sniffed, snorted, or smoked; in the United States, fear of the acquired immunodeficiency syndrome (AIDS) has resulted in increased popularity of nonparenteral administration. A form of smoking, "chasing the dragon," consists of heating the drug on tinfoil and inhaling the vapor through a straw; this practice seems to have emerged in areas where most available heroin is a less pure "brown" variety, which is difficult to dissolve for injection (16).

Heroin's Schedule I classification has been opposed by those who advocate its use as an analgesic to treat cancer pain. There is little evidence, however, that heroin is more effective than morphine in such patients (12).

Heroin crosses the blood-brain barrier faster than morphine and is then metabolized to 6-acetylmorphine (which has opiate activity) and morphine. Three milligrams of heroin are equivalent to 10 mg of morphine (9). Experienced users cannot tell heroin from morphine when they are given the drugs subcutaneously but are able to do so when the drugs are given intravenously (13). Like that of morphine, heroin's duration of action is about 3–4 hours, and metabolites are detectable in urine for several days after a last dose (9).

Most if not all of heroin's CNS and PNS effects are mediated through its metabolites 6-acetylmorphine and morphine, acting at stereospecific neuronal receptors (*see* Morphine and Related Opiates, this volume) (10).

Studies addressing mechanisms of action of endogenous and exogenous opiate agonists are as relevant to heroin as to other morphine-related agents. Opiate reinforcement, demonstrated in animals using place preference, self-administration, and brain stimulation models, is dependent on the limbic "reward circuit" [ventral tegmental area (VTA), nucleus accumbens (NA), and medial prefrontal cortex]. Opiate agonists injected directly into either the VTA or the NA are rewarding, and rodents self-administer opiates at regular intervals with steady dosage escalation and preserved eating, drinking, and body weight. The extent to which drug-seeking behavior depends on positive or negative reinforcement (*i.e.*, euphoria *vs.* withdrawal avoidance) is controversial (18).

Some investigators claim that, in rodents, heroin and 6-acetylmorphine are more rewarding than morphine, and that heroin has direct CNS receptor specificities not shared by morphine. The relevance of such observations to heroin's greater popularity as a recreational drug is uncertain (8).

Animal studies of *in utero* exposure to heroin or other opiate agonists have been sparse. Variably described are low birth weight, behavioral abnormalities, and chromosomal aberrations (1,15).

Heroin has the same acute effects as morphine, including rapid development of tolerance, withdrawal symptoms and signs, and psychic dependence. Overdose, less likely when heroin is snorted or smoked, is managed in the same manner as overdose with other opiate agonists; ventilatory support and the specific antagonist naloxone are the mainstays of treatment (6). In adults, withdrawal is prevented or treated with titrated doses of methadone and in neonates with methadone or paregoric (4).

Heroin abuse is associated with a number of medical and neurological complications that are a consequence of its illegality. Trauma affects brain, spinal cord, and peripheral nerves. Infections include hepatitis (with subsequent hepatic encephalopathy), endocarditis [with cerebral infarction, brain abscess, meningitis, and ruptured septic ("mycotic") aneurysm], osteomyelitis (including vertebral), tetanus, botulism, malaria, AIDS, and human T-cell lymphotropic virus type I myelopathy. Heroin users are at increased risk for occlusive and hemorrhagic stroke, independent of endocarditis and sometimes affecting the spinal cord; possible mechanisms are hypertension secondary to heroin nephropathy, overdose with hypotension, particle embolism, and allergic vasculitis; a direct toxic effect of heroin or its impurities on blood vessels has not been demonstrated (2). Heroin-induced polyneuropathy (resembling Guillain-Barré syndrome) and brachial or lumbosacral plexopathy are probably immune-mediated. Rhabdomyolysis and myoglobinuria can follow prolonged coma but also occur without evidence of overdose, suggesting an allergic reaction to either the drug or impurities. Blindness occurred in a parenteral heroin user whose mixture contained large doses of quinine (3). Reports from Europe describe cerebral spongiform leukoencephalopathy in practitioners of "chasing the dragon." Abnormal behavior, ataxia, quadriparesis, chorea, and myoclonus often progress to death; the responsible toxin has not been identified (19). A report from North America illustrates the characteristic magnetic resonance image of this toxic leukoencephalopathy (11).

As with morphine and methadone, heroin use *per se* does not appear to cause any permanent neurobehavioral abnormalities (17).

In addition to the induction of a potentially lethal withdrawal syndrome, *in utero* exposure to heroin has been associated with developmental abnormalities. Infants are often of low birth weight and small for gestational age. The Moro reflex is hyperactive and persists beyond the usual 20 weeks. Respiratory distress and sudden infant death are common; later in life, there is disturbed sleep, hyperactivity, and impaired hearing. A problem with such reports is that, like those relating to other agents of abuse, they are confounded by poor prenatal care, additional drugs, ethanol or tobacco, and inadequate parenting. There is currently little evidence that *in utero* heroin exposure *per se* causes lasting neurobehavioral abnormalities in humans (4).

The treatment of heroin addiction is controversial. Those who view the condition as a chronic metabolic disturbance—an acquired opiate deficiency state—favor agonist-replacement therapy. The short duration of action of heroin and morphine render them impractical for such a purpose, and so the longer acting agonist methadone is now used in most countries. Doses sufficient not only to prevent withdrawal symptoms but to block CNS opiate receptors (thereby nullifying the effect of any administered heroin) are used, and most patients require methadone maintenance therapy indefinitely, relapsing to heroin when they discontinue methadone, even after years (5).

Those who view heroin addiction as a more psychologically determined, self-limited condition favor treatment with the opiate antagonist naltrexone, which, unlike naloxone, can be taken orally (7). The combined agonist-antagonist buprenorphine has also been recommended, especially for abusers of both heroin and cocaine (14).

The physiological mechanisms of intoxication, withdrawal, and dependence are the same for heroin as for morphine and other opiate agonists.

REFERENCES

1. Brust JCM (1993) *Neurological Aspects of Substance Abuse.* Butterworth-Heinemann, Stoneham, Massachusetts p. 16.
2. Brust JCM (1992) Stroke and substance abuse. In: *Stroke: Pathophysiology, Diagnosis, and Management.* Barnett HJM, Mohr JP, Stein BM, Yatsu FM eds. Churchill Livingstone, New York p. 875.
3. Brust JCM, Richter RW (1971) Quinine amblyopia related to heroin addiction. *Ann Intern Med* **74**, 84.
4. Chiriboga C (1993) Fetal effects. *Neurol Clin* **11**, 707.
5. Dole VP (1988) Implications of methadone maintenance for theories of narcotic addiction. *J Amer Med Assn* **260**, 3025.
6. Goldfrank LR, Bresnitz EA (1990) Opioids. In: *Toxicologic Emergencies. 4th Ed.* Goldfrank LR, Flomennbaum NE, Lewin NA *et al.* eds. Appleton & Lange, Norwalk, Connecticut p. 433.
7. Gonzalez JP, Brogden RN (1988) Naltrexone: A review of its pharmacodynamic and pharmacokinetic properties and therapeutic efficacy in the management of opioid dependence. *Drugs* **35**, 192.
8. Hubner CB, Kornetsky C (1992) Heroin, 6-acetylmorphine and morphine effects on threshold for rewarding and aversive brain stimulation. *J Pharmacol Exp Ther* **260**, 562.
9. Jaffe JH, Martin WR (1990) Opioid analgesics and antagonists. In: *The Pharmacological Basis of Therapeutics, 8th Ed.* Gilman AG, Rall TW, Nies AS, Taylor P eds. Pergamon Press, New York p. 491.
10. Koob GF, Bloom FE (1988) Cellular and molecular mechanisms of drug dependence. *Science* **242**, 715.
11. Krigstein AR, Armitage BA, Kim PY (1997) Heroin inhalation and progressive spongiform encephalopathy. *N Engl J Med* **336**, 589.
12. Levine MN, Sackett DL, Bush H (1986) Heroin vs morphine for cancer pain? *Arch Intern Med* **146**, 353.
13. Martin WR, Fraser HF (1961) A comparative study of physiological and subjective effects of heroin and morphine administered intravenously in postaddicts. *J Pharmacol Exp Ther* **133**, 388.
14. Resnick RB, Galanter M, Pycha C *et al.* (1992) Buprenorphine: An alternative to methadone for heroin dependence treatment. *Psychopharmacol Bull* **28**, 109.
15. Shafer DA, Falek A, Donahoe RM, Madden JJ (1990–91) Biogenetic effects of opiates. *Int J Addict* **25**, 1.
16. Strang J, Gossop M, Griffiths P, Farrel M (1989) The technology of dragon-chasing. *Brit J Addict* **84**, 699.
17. Weinreib RM, O'Brien CP (1993) Persistent cognitive deficits attributed to substance abuse. *Neurol Clin* **11**, 663.
18. Wise RA (1989) Opiate reward: Sites and substrates. *Neurosci Biobehav Rev* **13**, 129.
19. Wolters ECH, Van Winjungaarden GK, Stam FC *et al.* (1982) Leukoencephalopathy after inhaling "heroin pyrolysate." *Lancet* **2**, 1233.

Hexachlorobenzene

Henry A. Peters
Derek J. Cripps
Ayhan Göcmen
George T. Bryan

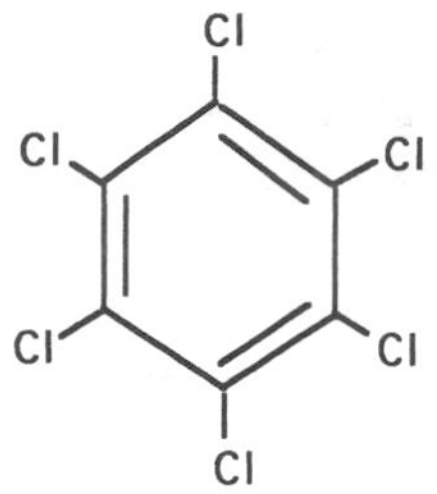

HEXACHLOROBENZENE
C_6Cl_6

Perchlorobenzene

NEUROTOXICITY RATING

Clinical

C   Peripheral neuropathy

C   Extrapyramidal syndrome

Experimental

A   Tremor, seizures

C   Neuropathy (chronic)

B   Behavioral teratogenicity

Hexachlorobenzene (HCB), formerly used as a seed fungicide, is a persistent pollutant that accumulates in the environment, in animals, and in humans. HCB disrupts the porphyrin-heme biosynthetic pathway, resulting in porphyria attended by photosensitivity, skin lesions, and liver pathology. Changes may also occur in the endocrine and immune systems, in renal function, and in reproductive and developmental parameters. HCB (like many other chlorinated aromatic hydrocarbons) elicits tremor and seizures in a range of laboratory species, and chronic neurological changes have been reported in HCB-exposed humans. The compound is classified as a possible human carcinogen (18).

General Toxicology

HCB forms colorless crystals (MP, 230°C) that are soluble in benzene, ether, and chloroform; the compound is insoluble in water. HCB is a stable, persistent compound with half-lives in soil, water, and air measured in years (2). Until 1965, HCB was widely employed as a fungicide on the seed of onions, sorghum, wheat, and other grains (18); it was also used to make fireworks, ammunition, and synthetic rubber (2). HCB is also a by-product in the manufacture of many other chlorinated chemicals (18), and is found in waste streams of chloralkali and wood-preserving plants (2).

In the U.S. population, annual HCB uptake from ingestion of food is estimated to be 1 µg/kg body weight (2). HCB is retained in body fat for years, and a large portion of stored HCB may be found in breast milk (2). The U.S. Agency for Toxic Substances and Disease Registry has derived an acute oral Minimum Risk Level* (MRL) of 0.008 mg/kg/day on the basis of developmental neurotoxic effects in rats, an intermediate MRL of 0.0003 mg/kg/day based on ovarian changes in monkeys, and a chronic oral MRL of 0.00002 mg/kg/day based on a rat liver study (2). There is no U.S. Occupational Safety and Health Standard for HCB.

HCB is moderately well absorbed by the intestinal tract *via* the lymphatic system; only a small portion enters the hepatic portal circulation. It is slowly metabolized to pentachlorophenol by the hepatic cytochrome P-450 system (CYP3A1, CYP3A2 isoforms); conjugated with glutathione to form pentachlorothiophenol; or dechlorinated to pentachlorobenzene, tetrachlorobenzene, and less-chlorinated benzenes, which are excreted in urine. Minor metabolites of HCB include tri- and tetrachlorophenols, and tetrachlorohydroquinone. Urine also contains pentachloroanisole and the *N*-acetylcysteine derivative of HCB (2). HCB is poorly excreted in urine but is excreted in sweat (to cause chloracne) and in maternal milk. Fecal excretion of HCB is enhanced with oral intake of mineral oil (29).

HCB induces porphyria characterized by increased enzyme activity of δ-aminolevulinic acid (δ-ALA) synthase, which controls the rate of porphyrin production, and decreased activity of uroporphyrinogen decarboxylase, which converts uroporphyrinogen III to coproporphyrinogen III. Marked inhibition of uroporphyrinogen decarboxylase precedes the porphyrinogenic effects of HCB. Detailed analysis of this subject is available (2).

---

*An estimate of the daily human exposure to a hazardous substance that is likely without appreciable risk of adverse noncancer health effects over a specified duration of exposure. MRLs are derived using the no-observed-adverse-effect level/uncertainty factor approach.

Animal Studies

HCB has a low acute oral toxicity in laboratory species (>1000–10,000 mg/kg body weight) (30). The rat subcutaneous LD_{50} is >2500 mg/kg; the rabbit dermal LD_{50} is >2000 mg/kg. Signs of acute intoxication include ataxia, weakness, paralysis, tremor, convulsions, and death (30). Rats given a single dose of 400 or 600 mg/kg HCB in corn oil showed no CNS, PNS, or skeletal muscle changes 14 days later (24). A single intraperitoneal dose of 1000 mg/kg increased δ-ALA synthase within 15 h (33); daily dosing triggered increased activity of liver enzymes (δ-ALA, γ-glutamyl transferase), hepatomegaly and hepatic cell degeneration, with increased urinary porphobilinogen, δ–ALA, and porphyrins (1,25).

Changes referable to the nervous system are also reported in animals treated with HCB for prolonged periods. Various laboratory species repeatedly dosed with HCB display hyperexcitability (9). Mice given 26 mg/kg/day for up to 17 weeks developed severe tremors prior to death (16). Muscle fasciculation and constant tremors were reported in rats treated with 50 mg/kg/day for 4–8 weeks (20,23). Male Wistar rats given oral doses of 317 or 427 mg/kg/day for up to 4 weeks showed a markedly decreased thyroid T_4 uptake into cerebrospinal fluid and brain in the absence of neurological signs (35). Rats fed 800 ppm HCB for 20 weeks exhibited mildly reduced sciatic nerve conduction velocity with no evidence of denervation. Animals fed 150 ppm for 2 years showed prolonged conduction times (31%) and electrophysiological evidence of muscle denervation (fibrillations and chronic repetitive discharges) (31). Adult male SPF pigs fed 50 mg/kg/day for 90 days exhibited tremors, panting, and an unsteady gait (10). Dogs reportedly showed a dysrhythmic electroencephalogram after oral doses of 50 mg/kg/day for 21 days (32). Female rhesus monkeys given oral doses of 64 mg/kg/day for 60 days showed severe tremors and muscular weakness, and marked lethargy and weakness at 128 mg/kg/day (22).

HCB may be a behavioral teratogen in Sprague-Dawley rats (15). Offspring of Sprague-Dawley rats exposed *in utero* to 2.5 or 25 mg/kg/day showed increased exploratory behavior or hyperactivity at 19–20 days of age, but there was no change in learning ability, locomotor activity, or exploratory activity at 60–100 days of age (15). Litters of female rats fed 20 or 100 mg/kg/day during gestation developed convulsions, tremor, and progressive weakness (6).

In Vitro Studies

HCB partly uncoupled oxidative phosphorylation in liver mitochondria, an effect attributed to the action of endogenously formed pentachlorophenol (34).

Human Studies

Human experience with HCB intoxication, while limited, shows a clear-cut relationship with the appearance of porphyria, specifically an acquired form of porphyria cutanea tarda (5).

Chloracne and porphyrinuria were observed in workers at a Norwegian hydroelectric plant involved in chlorine production; mean blood levels dropped from 30.40 ppb in 1976 to 13.54 ng/g HCB in 1988 (72 people) after the introduction of improved conditions and procedures (O.C. Bockman, personal communication, 1995).

Between 1944 and 1960, in southeastern Turkey, an estimated 3000–4000 people developed porphyria of varying severity after ingestion of bread prepared from grain treated with HCB (2 kg/1000 kg wheat) (12). Commercial fungicides containing 20% HCB had been imported from Europe in 1954 to mix with wheat seed for the control of a wheat fungus. Treated seed arrived too late for planting and, instead, was used to replace edible stores of wheat as bread or bulgar (5). Estimated HCB doses were 0.05–0.2 g/day (0.7–2.9 mg/kg/day for a 70-kg person) (4), although total dosage would have varied with eating habits, age, and chance. Sporadic cases of porphyria in this part of Turkey first occurred in 1955 and became more common until 1958 when the probable relationship with HCB exposure was recognized (3). Use of HCB in the affected area ceased in 1959.

The estimated interval between commencement of HCB ingestion and appearance of clinical symptoms attributed to HCB intoxication was approximately 6 months (13). Affected individuals developed porphyria, hyperpigmentation, hypertrichosis, fragile skin, bullae, and hirsuitism. The condition was termed *porphyria turcica* (PT). A survey of PT conducted between 1958 and 1963 found that most patients (83%) were aged 6–15 years; 5% of patients were under 5 years of age (11). The mortality rate of children (under the age of 1 year) of lactating mothers was extremely high. Maternal milk contained a high concentration of HCB (28). Analysis of human milk from HCB-exposed women and unexposed controls revealed values of 0.51 ppm and 0.07 ppm, respectively (14). After 1956, some offspring failed to thrive and developed localized cutaneous annular erythema, pink sores (*pembre yara*), on light-exposed hands and legs. An estimated 1000 children died over 2 years with malnourishment, diarrhea, respiratory infections, weakness, tremors, and occasional convulsions (3,7,19). In some villages, there were no children between 2 and 4 years of age (8,26,27).

Among survivors, 280 patients were followed-up between 1977 and 1995 (8,26,27). Most had continued to live in the endemic area. Average age was 41.5 years (at time of first examination), with mean onset of disease at 10.1 years of age, and mean duration of acute and subacute symptoms of 2.1 years. Dermatological and orthopedic abnormalities had persisted into adulthood. The most common clinical features were painless distal arthritis (69.1%); small hands (65.8%); skin hyperpigmentation (61%); large scars, usually on the cheeks, arms, and dorsal surface of the hands (84.6%); enlarged thyroid glands (34.5%); pinched facies (38.6%); and decreased stature. Porphyrin excretion, particularly uroporphyrin in urine and stools, was increased in 17 patients 20–30 years after disease outbreak (8).

Initial symptoms reported by most porphyric patients consisted of weakness; inability to handle utensils, rise from a squat, or climb stairs; loss of appetite; photosensitivity with erythema; and red or brown urine. Children were often so weak they had to be carried, and abdominal colic or pain was present in one-third of those who failed to gain weight. While the combination of abdominal pain, photosensitivity, porphyria, and weakness are features of certain hereditary porphyrias, including acute intermittent porphyric neuropathy (5), there are no reports of objective neurological examination in the early phases of HCB-associated PT. Thirty-five years after the acute onset of PT, neurological findings among 280 survivors (*vide supra*) included complaints of weakness (60%) and paresthesias (53%), distal sensory shading to pinprick (51%), and myotonia (44%) on forearm contraction but not on thenar percussion. Twenty-nine percent (1977–1981) and, later, 44% (1981–1995) displayed cogwheeling at the elbows, wrists, and neck, in addition to reduced or loss of associated movements. Although these findings raise the possibility of extrapyramidal dysfunction, patients lacked the following signs of parkinsonism: bradykinesia, resting tremor, loss of static reflexes, decreased power of phonation, start hesitation, and involvement of postural reflexes.

The neurological deficits are difficult to interpret. Weakness, tremor, and convulsions, constant features of acute HCB intoxication in laboratory species, are described in pembre yara infants who all died within 2 years of birth (13,14,28). Only 2 of 280 surviving PT patients developed *grand mal* seizures, no more than would be expected in a comparable population. Although peripheral neuropathy may occur in acute intermittent porphyria (17), insufficient data are available from human and animal studies to reach the conclusion that HCB induces peripheral neuropathy. Electrophysiological evidence of slowed sciatic nerve fiber conduction and paramyotonia in rats orally treated with HCB for 2 years is of uncertain significance because rats characteristically display marked pathological changes in sciatic nerves with advanced age. The mildly decreased sciatic nerve conduction times in rats treated with high doses

of HCB are unsupported by morphological evidence of nerve fiber damage. Psychiatric disorder, a feature of acute intermittent porphyria, is not described in subjects exposed to HCB, since only 2 of 280 patients were diagnosed as having schizophrenia.

The origin of changes suggestive of tardive extrapyramidal dysfunction in PT is obscure, although magnetic resonance imaging in non–HCB-related porphyria has revealed reversible multifocal cerebral lesions (attributed to transient ischemia) during attacks of acute porphyria (21). Additional considerations are the presence in PT patients of malnutrition and thyroid disease, both of which are potentially associated with CNS and PNS effects. Furthermore, before HCB was introduced in southeastern Turkey, a mercury-containing seed dressing was used to prevent the formation of rust or bunt on seed grain; this was regularly eaten during times of food shortage during late winter and spring. While mercury-treated seed was said to be dusted off prior to making bread, and no cases of mercury intoxication are reported in the population, mercury intoxication in other settings has been associated with sensory neuropathy, motor weakness, and tardive basal ganglia dysfunction.

Toxic Mechanisms

Although mechanistic evidence is lacking, the acute neurotoxic effects (tremor, seizures) of HCB in animals are characteristic features of organochlorine compounds that interfere with the normal flux of sodium and potassium ions across the axonal membrane.

REFERENCES

1. Adjarov D, Ivanov E, Keremidchiev D (1982) Gamma-glutamyl transferase: A sensitive marker in experimental hexachlorobenzene intoxication. *Toxicology* **23**, 73.
2. ATSDR (1996) *Toxicological Profile for Hexachlorobenzene (update)*. Agency for Toxic Substances and Disease Registry (ATSDR), U.S. Public Health Service.
3. Cam S (1959) Cutaneous porphyria related to hexachlorobenzene intoxication. *Saglik Dergisi* **32**, 315.
4. Cam S, Nigogosyan G (1963) Acquired toxic porphyria cutanea tarda due to hexachlorobenzene: Report of 348 cases caused by this fungicide. *J Amer Med Assn* **183**, 88.
5. Cripps DJ (1986) Porphyria: Genetic and acquired. In: *Hexachlorobenzene: Proceedings of an International Symposium*. Oxford University Press, New York p. 549.
6. Cripps DJ (1990) Transplacental and mammary absorption of hexachlorobenzene: Experimental pembre yara porphyria in neonates. *Mol Aspects Med* **11**, 81.
7. Cripps DJ, Peters HA, Göcmen A *et al.* (1981) Experimental pembre yara. *J Invest Dermatol* **76**, 223.

8. Cripps DJ, Peters HA, Göcmen A, Dogramaci I (1984) Porphyria turcica due to hexachlorobenzene. A 20 to 30 year follow-up study on 204 patients. *Brit J Dermatol* **111**, 413.

9. De Matteis F, Prior BE, Rimington C (1961) Nervous and biochemical disturbances following hexachlorobenzene intoxication. *Nature* **191**, 363.

10. Den Tonkelaar EM, Verschuuren HG, Bankovska J *et al.* (1978) Hexachlorobenzene toxicity in pigs. *Toxicol Appl Pharmacol* **43**, 147.

11. Dogramaci I (1964) Porphyrias and porphyrin metabolism with special reference to porphyria in childhood. *Adv Pediat* **13**, 11.

12. Dogramaci I, Düzgünes O, Ergene T, Göcmen A (1962) A possible genetic factor in the etiology of porphyria turcica. *Turk J Pediat* **4**, 193.

13. Göcmen A, Peters HA, Cripps DJ *et al.* (1986) Porphyria turcica: Hexachlorobenzene-induced porphyria. In: *Hexachlorobenzene: Proceedings of an International Symposium.* Oxford University Press, New York p. 567.

14. Göcmen A, Peters HA, Cripps DJ *et al.* (1989) Hexachlorobenzene episode in Turkey. *Biomed Environ Sci* **2**, 36.

15. Goldey ES, Taylor DH (1992) Developmental neurotoxicity following premating maternal exposure to hexachlorobenzene in rats. *Neurotoxicol Teratol* **14**, 15.

16. Hahn ME, Gasiewicz TA, Linko P *et al.* (1988) The role of the Ah locus in hexachlorobenzene-induced porphyria. Studies in congenic C57BL/6J mice. *Biochem J* **254**, 245.

17. Hierons R (1957) Changes in the nervous system in acute porphyria. *J Pathol Bacteriol* **71**, 495.

18. IARC (1979) *Monograph on the Evaluation of the Carcinogenic Risk of Chemicals to Humans: Some Halogenated Hydrocarbons. Vol 20.* International Agency for Research on Cancer (IARC), Lyon, France p.155.

19. Kantemir I, Giner S, Kayaalp O (1960) Investigations with hexachlorobenzene and organic mercury compounds. *Turk Hig Tecr Biyol Derg* **20**, 19.

20. Kennedy SW, Wigfield DC (1990) Dose-response relationships in hexachlorobenzene-induced porphyria. *Biochem Pharmacol* **40**, 1381.

21. King PH, Bragdon AC (1991) MRI reveals multiple reversible cerebral lesions in an attack of acute intermittent porphyria. *Neurology* **41**, 1300.

22. Knauf V, Hobson W (1979) Hexachlorobenzene ingestion by female rhesus monkeys: Tissue distribution and clinical symptomatology. *Bull Environ Contam Toxicol* **21**, 243.

23. Koss G, Seubert S, Seubert A *et al.* (1978) Studies on the toxicology of hexachlorobenzene: III. Observations in a long-term experiment. *Arch Toxicol* **40**, 285.

24. Lecavalier PR, Chu I, Villeneuve D *et al.* (1994) Combined effects of mercury and hexachlorobenzene in the rat. *J Environ Sci Health* **B29**, 951.

25. Ockner RK, Schmid R (1961) Acquired porphyria in man and rat due to hexachlorobenzene intoxication. *Nature* **189**, 499.

26. Peters H, Cripps D, Göcmen A *et al.* (1987) Turkish epidemic hexachlorobenzene porphyria: A 30-year study. *Ann N Y Acad Sci* **514**, **183**.

27. Peters HA, Göcmen A, Cripp DJ *et al.* (1982) Epidemiology of hexachlorobenzene-induced porphyria in Turkey: Clinical and laboratory follow-up after 25 years. *Arch Neurol* **39**, 744.

28. Peters HA, Johnson SAM, Cam S *et al.* (1966) Hexachlorobenzene-induced porphyria: Effect of chelation on the disease, porphyrin and metal metabolism. *Amer J Med Sci* **251**, 314.

29. Rozman K, Rozman T, Greim H (1981) Enhanced fecal elimination of stored hexachlorobenzene from rats and rhesus monkeys by hexadecane or mineral oil. *Toxicology* **22**, 33.

30. Strik JJTWA (1986) Subacute toxicity of hexachlorobenzene. In: *Hexachlorobenzene: Proceedings of an International Symposium.* Oxford University Press, New York p. 356.

31. Sufit RF, Hodach, Arends S *et al.* (1986) Decreased conduction velocity and pseudomyotonia in hexachlorobenzene-fed rats. In: *Hexachlorobenzene: Proceedings of an International Symposium.* Oxford University Press, New York p. 361.

32. Sundlof SF, Hansen LG, Koritz GD *et al.* (1982) The pharmacokinetics of hexachlorobenzene in male beagles: Distribution, excretion, and pharmacokinetics model. *Drug Metab Disposition* **10**, 371.

33. Sweeney GD, Janigan D, Mayman D, Lai H (1971) The experimental porphyrias—a group of distinctive metabolic lesions. *S Afr J Lab Clin Med* **17**, 68.

34. Trenti T, Ventura E, Ceccarelli D, Masini A (1986) Functional derangement of liver mitochondria from hexachlorobenzene-treated rats. In: *Hexachlorobenzene: Proceedings of an International Symposium.* Oxford University Press, New York p. 329.

35. van Raaij JAGM, Frijters CMG, Wong Yen Kong L (1994) Reduction of thyroxine uptake into cerebrospinal fluid and rat brain by hexachlorobenzene and pentachlorophenol. *Toxicology* **94**, 197.

Hexachlorophene

Mitchell Steinschneider

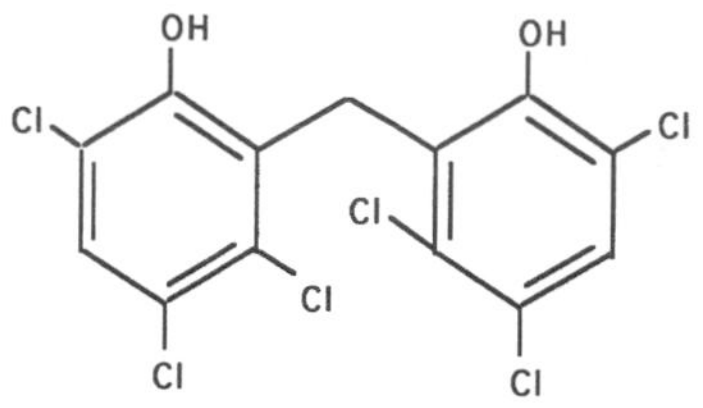

HEXACHLOROPHENE
$C_{13}H_6Cl_6O_2$

2,2′-Methylenebis[3,4,6-trichlorophenol]

NEUROTOXICOLOGY RATING

Clinical

A   Leukoencephalopathy

A   Peripheral neuropathy

B   Teratogenicity

Experimental

A   Leukoencephalopathy (myelinic edema)

A   Peripheral neuropathy (myelinic edema)

Hexachlorophene is a poorly soluble white powder synthesized from 2,4,5-trichlorophenol; the preparations may contain minute amounts of the toxic compound 2,3,7,8-tetrachlorodibenzo-p-dioxin (5,18). Hexachlorophene was used as an antimicrobial agent at high concentrations (3% solution) and as a cosmetic preservative at lower concentrations (<1%) (18). Effective against gram-positive bacteria, the agent was a popular additive for a range of topically applied products. Infants and premature babies were routinely bathed in 3% hexachlorophene-containing solutions. Its use has been markedly curtailed for several decades since the discovery of its toxicity to myelin. Soaps containing hexachlorophene are presently available only by prescription, and the compound is used to induce intramyelinic edema experimentally (1).

General Toxicology

Hexachlorophene is absorbed through the skin, gut, and mucous membranes (18). It circulates in the plasma bound to albumin, is metabolized by the liver, and is excreted in the bile. The primary targets of hexachlorophene toxicity are the brain and peripheral nerves, where it produces a vacuolar myelinopathy. Retinal photoreceptor cells are also damaged by hexachlorophene.

Animal Studies

Animal models have demonstrated that even short-term exposure to hexachlorophene may be lethal (3). Death is preceded by lethargy, paralysis, tachypnea, and hyperthermia (15,18). Vacuolar myelinopathy occurs in rats within a week of eating a diet containing hexachlorophene (15).

Prolonged exposure to hexachlorophene produces extensive white matter vacuolation that imparts a spongiform appearance to the brain (1,3,8,14). Pathological changes of this type even occur in rats exposed to daily dermal application of products that contain 3% hexachlorophene (3,17). Immature rats are more susceptible than older animals and may die after repeated exposures to these products (17). Peripheral myelin involvement also occurs after prolonged exposure (11). Intramyelinic vacuoles, formed from the splitting of myelin sheaths at the intraperiod lines, are characteristic of this disorder. There may be degeneration of photoreceptor and retinal ganglion cells (18). Teratogenic effects, with malformations of the brain, eye, and urogenital and skeletal systems, have also been described after vaginal administration of hexachlorophene to pregnant rats (18).

Human Studies

Toxicity develops after topical application of hexachlorophene (18). In 1972, 224 babies and children in France were poisoned, and 18% died, from administration of a talc powder that accidentally contained hexachlorophene at a concentration of 6.3% (9). Symptoms included an ulcerative rash, hyperthermia, and diarrhea. Children exhibited signs of increased intracranial pressure, seizures, paresis, and varying stages of mental status alterations that included coma and subsequent death. The same talc powder was applied to the skin of baby baboons, producing nearly identical results. The brains of four children (two neonates with congenital ichthyosis and two burned young children), who died after hexachlorophene exposure from repeated skin baths, contained extensive vacuolar degeneration in the white matter of the cerebrum and cerebellum (10). In two large histopathological studies of babies and children, premature infants of very low birth weight (<1400 g) and with greater exposure to hexachlorophene were more likely to exhibit vacuolar white matter changes (12,16). These lesions were primarily in the reticular formation and in the most heavily myelinated long tracts of the brainstem. While neurotoxicity has also been seen after oral exposure, systemic signs such as hyperthermia, hypotension, and gastrointestinal distress predominate (18). No specific treatment is available (18).

The carcinogenic potential of hexachlorophene is suggested by case reports of lymphoma in healthcare personnel after many years of occupational dermal exposure (5). However, these findings are not supported by the experimental failure of hexachlorophene to promote brain tumors in rat pups first treated *in utero* with the brain tumor initiator N-ethylnitrosourea (14).

A controversial report suggests that frequent washing with hexachlorophene-containing soaps is teratogenic (4). Severe congenital malformations were observed in 25 of 460 babies born to hospital personnel who repeatedly washed with hexachlorophene, while no malformations were noted in 233 babies of similarly employed mothers who did not use the compound. While serious methodological concerns cast doubt on the results of this study, the absorption of hexachlorophene through the skin and placenta argues against its use in pregnant women (6,7).

Toxic Mechanisms

Hexachlorophene binds nonspecifically to myelin (11). Intoxication leads to increased water content of the brain, diffuse white matter edema, decreased myelin formation in the immature animal, and vacuolar degeneration of myelin (1,2,8,18,19). White matter edema is intramyelinic and results from separation of myelin lamellae (18). Axons are spared but may be damaged if intoxication continues or is more intense (18). Despite the disruption of myelin, no changes in its chemical composition are produced by hexachlorophene (2). The specific toxic mechanism of hexachlorophene-induced myelin degeneration is unknown (8). Biochemical effects of hexachlorophene include mitochondrial dysfunction and the uncoupling of oxidative phosphorylation, and the inhibition of protein and lipid synthesis in nerves studied *in vitro* (11,15,18). The hyperthermia associated with hexachlorophene intoxication may reflect the uncoupling of oxidative phosphorylation (18). An elevation of blood and brain ammonia in association with degeneration of hepatocytes has also been observed in mice (13).

REFERENCES

1. Andreas K (1993) Efficacy of cerebroprotective substances in the management of functional disorders induced by the cytotoxic brain edema-producing substance hexachlorophene. *Naunyn-Schmied Arch Pharmacol* **347**, 79.
2. Cammer W, Rose AL, Norton WT (1975) Biochemical and pathological studies of myelin in hexachlorophene intoxication. *Brain Res* **98**, 547.
3. Gaines TB, Kimbrough RD, Linder RE (1973) The oral and dermal toxicity of hexachlorophene in rats. *Toxicol Appl Pharmacol* **25**, 332.
4. Halling H (1979) Suspected link between exposure to hexachlorophene and malformed infants. In: *Health Effects of Halogenated Aromatic Hydrocarbons. Vol 320*. Nicholson WJ, Moore JA eds. New York Academy of Science, New York p.426.
5. Hardell L, Eriksson M (1992) Non-Hodgkin lymphoma and previous exposure to hexachlorophene: A case report. *J Occup Med* **34**, 849.
6. Hill LM (1984) Effects of drugs and chemicals on the fetus and newborn (second of two parts). *Mayo Clin Proc* **59**, 755.
7. Källén B (1978) Hexachlorophene teratogenicity in humans disputed. *J Amer Med Assn* **240**, 1585.
8. Kung M-P, Nickerson PA, Sansone FM et al. (1989) Effect of chronic exposure to hexachlorophene on rat brain cell specific marker enzymes. *Neurotoxicology* **10**, 201.
9. Martin-Bouyer G, Lebreton R, Toga M et al. (1982) Outbreak of accidental hexachlorophene poisoning in France. *Lancet* **1**, 91.
10. Mullick FG (1973) Hexachlorophene toxicity—human experience at the Armed Forces Institute of Pathology. *Pediatrics* **51**, 395.
11. Pleasure D, Towfighi J, Silberberg D, Parris J (1974) The pathogenesis of hexachlorophene neuropathy: In vivo and in vitro studies. *Neurology* **24**, 1068.
12. Powell H, Swarner O, Gluck L, Lampert P (1973) Hexachlorophene myelinopathy in premature infants. *J Pediat* **82**, 976.
13. Prasad GV, Rajendra W, Indira K (1987) Brain ammonia metabolism in hexachlorophene-induced encephalopathy. *Bull Environ Contam Toxicol* **38**, 561.
14. Purves D, Dayan A (1992) A preliminary investigation of promotion of brain tumours by hexachlorophene in Sprague-Dawley rats transplacentally exposed to N-ethylnitrosourea. *Neuropathol Appl Neurobiol* **18**, 259.
15. Rose AL, Wisniewski HM, Cammer W (1975) Neurotoxicity of hexachlorophene: New pathological and biochemical observations. *J Neurol Sci* **24**, 425.
16. Shuman RM, Leech RW, Alvord EC Jr (1974) Neurotoxicity of hexachlorophene in the human: I. A clinicopathologic study of 248 children. *Pediatrics* **54**, 689.
17. Shuman RM, Leech RW, Alvord EC Jr (1975) Neurotoxicity of topically applied hexachlorophene in the young rat. *Arch Neurol* **32**, 315.
18. Towfighi J (1980) Hexachlorophene. In: *Experimental and Clinical Neurotoxicology*. Spencer PS, Schaumburg HH eds. Williams & Wilkins, Baltimore p. 440.
19. Yamamoto Y, Yoshikawa H, Nagano S et al. (1999) Myelin-associated oligodendrocytic basic protein is essential for normal arrangement of the radial component in central nervous system myelin. *Eur J Neurosci* **11**, 847.

2,4-Hexadiene-1-nitrile

John L. O'Donoghue

$$CH_3-CH=CH-CH=CH-C\equiv N$$

2,4-HEXADIENE-1-NITRILE
C_6H_7N

Sorbonitrile

NEUROTOXICITY RATING

Experimental

A   Olivary nucleus necrosis

2,4-Hexadiene-1-nitrile has had limited use as an intermediate in the synthesis of other chemicals. There are no current uses for this material; the last reported use was in 1983.

2,4-Hexadiene-1-nitrile is apparently rapidly absorbed from the gastrointestinal tract, as acute signs of toxicity appear within 1 h of dosing. Cyanide may be formed during metabolism of this material, as rats develop signs commonly associated with exposure to cyanide (alterations in respiration, bright red blood color, vasodilation, CNS depression). The CNS appears to be the primary target site for this material, although necrosis of lymphocytes is seen in the thymus.

Experimental results with 2,4-hexadiene-1-nitrile are limited to acute, single-dose toxicity studies. Single doses of 1600 or 3200 mg/kg are lethal to male and female rats within 24–48 h. Premorbid signs are limited to signs of acute CNS depression. In rats given 800 mg/kg, signs including gross ataxia, tremors, and posturing difficulties appear by the second day after dosing. In rats given 400 mg/kg and in animals given 800 mg/kg that did not develop clinical abnormalities shortly after exposure, exaggerated gaits developed after 11 days following exposure. Animals showing signs of delayed toxicity had a high-stepping gait with overextension of the limbs during walking, or a prancing gait.

Morphological lesions associated with single exposures to 2,4-hexadiene-1-nitrile were limited to neuronal necrosis in the inferior olivary nucleus complex. All regions of this complex were affected, but some sparing of the medial accessory nucleus was observed. Bodian silver impregnation of axons and histochemical staining for cytochrome oxidase did not reveal any other significant morphological changes in the brain.

Although the formation of cyanide may participate in the acute toxicity of 2,4-hexadiene-1-nitrile, it does not appear to play an obvious role in the development of the delayed CNS lesions, as the acute signs of toxicity disappear prior to the onset of longer term effects, cytochrome oxidase staining of the inferior olivary neurons was not altered except for cells that were obviously undergoing degeneration, and the lesions observed were not similar to those commonly associated with cyanide exposure.

There are no reported cases of human or domestic animal intoxication with this material.

REFERENCE

1. O'Donoghue JL (1985) In: *Neurotoxicity of Industrial and Commercial Chemicals, Vol 2.* O'Donoghue JL ed. CRC Press, Boca Raton, Florida p. 33.

Hexamethylmelamine

Herbert H. Schaumburg

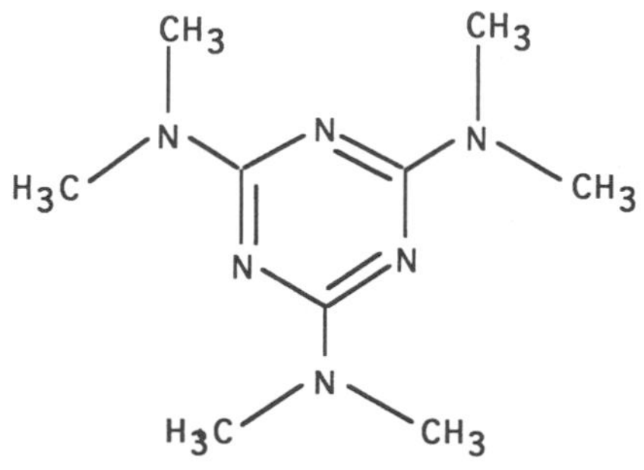

HEXAMETHYLMELAMINE
$C_9H_{18}N_6$

Altretamine; *N,N,N',N',N'',N''*-Hexamethyl-1,3,5-triazine-2,4,6-triamine; HMM

NEUROTOXICITY RATING

Clinical

B   Peripheral neuropathy

B   Acute encephalopathy (sedation, hallucinations, tremor)

Hexamethylmelamine (HMM) is a substituted melamine used in the chemotherapy of ovarian adenocarcinoma and bronchogenic carcinoma. Originally held to exert its therapeutic effect as an alkylator, more recent studies suggest the drug is an antimetabolite that inhibits DNA, RNA, and protein synthesis.

HMM is poorly soluble and is only administered orally. It is rapidly absorbed from the gastrointestinal tract, with 62% appearing in the liver in 24 h and 95% within 72 h. HMM is rapidly demethylated in the liver by the mixed function oxidase system to active methylmelamine derivatives and formaldehyde (2). The plasma half-life of the parent compound ranges from 2.9–10.2 h; the cerebrospinal fluid concentration is 6% of the plasma concentration. Most treatment regimens utilize a dose of 4–12 mg/kg for 14–21 days, with cycles repeated at 28- to 42-day intervals. Prolonged (3-month) therapy is associated with a high incidence of gastrointestinal and neurological toxicity.

The principal toxicities of HMM are gastrointestinal and neurological; myelotoxicity (leukopenia, thrombocytopenia) is mild and rarely dose-limiting. Gastrointestinal reactions appear in about 50%; they include anorexia, nausea, diarrhea, and abdominal cramps.

There are no detailed neurological evaluations of HNN neurotoxicity and no reports of electrodiagnostic or imaging studies in these cases; all reports are gleaned from descriptions of patients in oncology drug trials. Both the CNS (acute encephalopathy) and PNS (sensory polyneuropathy) manifestations of HMM neurotoxicity have been reversible in all reported instances. The incidence of neurotoxicity is 20% overall but increases in proportion to drug dose and treatment duration. At low levels of 12 mg/kg/day, neurological findings do not appear until after 100 days, while at levels of 32 mg/kg/day, signs appeared within 2 weeks (4,5). Dysfunction in the CNS and PNS generally appears in concert. Reports of CNS reactions include ataxia, depression, somnolence, hallucinations, and tremor of uncertain nature. Peripheral neuropathy is heralded by acral paresthesias and unsteady gait; findings include hyporeflexia, stocking-and-glove distribution of sensory loss (pin and position sense), and mild distal weakness. A report that describes amelioration of the neuropathy by concurrent administration of pyridoxine is unconvincing (2). No report describes nerve conduction studies or biopsies, and there are no appropriate experimental animal studies of HMM neuropathy. Signs of both CNS and PNS dysfunction dissipate within 3 weeks of discontinuing HMM therapy (1,3,6).

REFERENCES
1. Bergevin PR, Tormey DC, Blom J (1973) Clinical evaluation of hexamethylmelamine (NSC-13875). *Cancer Chemother Rep* **57**, 51.
2. Louis J, Louis NB, Linman JW *et al.* (1967) The clinical pharmacology of hexamethylmelamine: Phase I study. *Clin Pharmacol Ther* **8**, 55.
3. Stolinsky DC, Bateman JR (1973) Further experience with hexamethylmelamine (NSC-13875) in the treatment of carcinoma of the cervix. *Cancer Chemother Rep* **57**, 497.
4. Stolinsky DC, Bogdon DL, Solomon J (1972) Hexamethylmelamine (NSC-18375) alone and in combination with 5-(3,3-dimethyltriazeno) imidazole-4-carboxamide (NSC-45388) in the treatment of advanced cancer. *Cancer* **30**, 654.
5. Wilson WL, Schroeder JM, Bisel HF *et al.* (1969) Phase II study of hexamethylmelamine (NSC-13875). *Cancer* **23**, 132.
6. Vergote I, Himmelmann A, Frankendal B *et al.* (1992) Hexamethylmelamine as second-line therapy in platin-resistant ovarian cancer. *Gynecol Oncol* **47**, 282.

n-Hexane, Metabolites, and Derivatives

Anthony P. DeCaprio

$$CH_3CH_2CH_2CH_2CH_2CH_3$$

n-HEXANE

C_6H_{14}

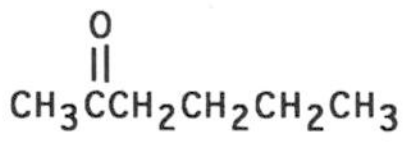

$$CH_3\overset{\overset{\displaystyle O}{\|}}{C}CH_2CH_2CH_2CH_3$$

2-HEXANONE
METHYL-*n*-BUTYL KETONE

$C_6H_{14}O$

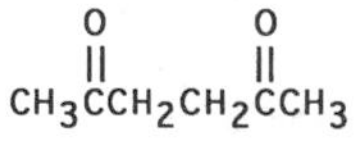

$$CH_3\overset{\overset{\displaystyle O}{\|}}{C}CH_2CH_2\overset{\overset{\displaystyle O}{\|}}{C}CH_3$$

2,5-HEXANEDIONE
$C_6H_{14}O_2$

n-Hexane
2-Hexanone; Methyl-*n*-butyl ketone
2,5-Hexanedione

NEUROTOXICITY RATING
Clinical
A   Peripheral neuropathy
C   Extrapyramidal syndrome
Experimental
A   Peripheral neuropathy

n-Hexane is a widely used hydrocarbon solvent derived from cracking of petroleum and from natural gas liquids

(5,35). It is typically present in motor fuels at 1–9 vol%. Discussion of n-hexane neurotoxicity necessarily includes consideration of two related compounds, methyl-n-butyl ketone (MBK) and 2,5-hexanedione (2,5-HD). Although rarely used today in pure form, MBK may still be present in some ketone-based solvent mixtures. It also occurs as a by-product of wood pulping and various petroleum processes and as a naturally occurring component of certain foods (5). 2,5-HD is an intermediate for organic synthesis and may also be a minor product of intermediary metabolism in mammalian systems. As discussed below, both compounds are key metabolites of n-hexane and are involved in the neurotoxic mechanism.

n-Hexane, MBK, and 2,5-HD are all colorless, low-molecular-weight liquids. n-Hexane is relatively volatile and only slightly soluble in water. MBK is moderately soluble in water and has a sharp, acetone-like odor. 2,5-HD is completely miscible with water and possesses a somewhat sweet odor.

n-Hexane is currently employed in a variety of industrial and commercial processes, including rubber, adhesive, ink, and paint manufacturing, and in the extraction of vegetable oils for human consumption (35). It has seen increasing usage in recent years as a replacement for benzene in solvent applications, with 1987 U.S. production of 386,500 tons. n-Hexane is typically present in mixed solvent products, such as petroleum ether and Stoddard solvent, in a wide range of concentrations. "Commercial grade hexane" consists of a mixture of primarily C_6 alkanes containing 20%–80% n-hexane. MBK was previously widely employed as one of a number of commercially important monoketonic solvents, along with methyl ethyl ketone (MEK) and methyl isopropyl ketone. Typical use was for solubilization of nitrocellulose, inks, paint and varnish materials, and as a component of cleaning solvents. Minor amounts of 2,5-HD are used in synthetic organic chemistry as a precursor for various heterocyclic systems.

The Americal Conference of Governmental Industrial Hygienists Threshold Limit Value (TLV) for n-hexane in occupational exposure is 50 ppm (180 mg/m³) in air, while the U.S. Occupational Safety and Health Administration Permissible Exposure Limit (PEL) is 500 ppm. The TLV for MBK is 5 ppm (20 mg/m³) in air, with a PEL of 100 ppm. The U.S. National Institute for Occupational Safety and Health has recommended a lowering of the TLV for MBK to 1 ppm. No regulatory standards are available for 2,5-HD.

General Toxicology

The toxicology, metabolism, and proposed mechanisms of action of n-hexane, MBK, and 2,5-HD have been reviewed in a number of comprehensive articles (5,13,35,47,58,72).

n-Hexane is rapidly absorbed via inhalation in experimental animals and humans. In rats, steady-state levels in blood occur within 10–30 min after the beginning of exposure to air concentrations of up to 92,000 ppm (6,8). Pulmonary retention in humans varies from 15%–30% over a wide range of exposure concentrations (45,77). Dermal absorption of n-hexane in guinea pigs is relatively slow, a finding also suggested by results with a single human volunteer (35). MBK is well absorbed by the inhalation, dermal, and oral routes in humans and experimental animals. Exposure of human volunteers to either 100 ppm MBK for 4 h or 10 or 50 ppm for 7.5 h resulted in respiratory uptake of 75%–92% (21). The dermal absorption rate of MBK in two human volunteers was found to be 4.8 and 8.0 µg/min/cm² (21). Peak serum levels of MBK were noted at 2 h in rats administered 200 mg/kg per os (p.o.) (20). Rapid absorption of MBK following intraperitoneal (i.p.) injection to rodents also occurs. 2,5-HD is readily absorbed following dermal application in hens, with peak plasma levels at 4 h and 90% of a 50-mg dose absorbed after 24 h (73). Many studies have also shown facile absorption of 2,5-HD by the oral and intraperitoneal routes.

n-Hexane is widely distributed to tissues following inhalation exposure. Exposure of rats to 50,000 ppm for 4 h resulted in steady-state levels of n-hexane in blood, spleen, kidney, brain, and adrenal, with the latter two organs showing the highest levels (8). In contrast, no plateau was reached in liver, where levels continued to increase up to 10 h of exposure. In another study, steady-state n-hexane concentrations were observed in tissues, including liver, from rats exposed to 500–10,000 ppm n-hexane for 6 h (6). In two separate studies, sciatic nerve was found to have the highest levels of n-hexane following a 6-h inhalation exposure in rats (6,9). n-Hexane is also widely distributed to both maternal and fetal tissues in pregnant rats exposed by inhalation.

Tissue distribution of both MBK and 2,5-HD is widespread, an expected result based on the high water solubility of these agents. Radiolabeled MBK was found in liver, kidney, and brain of rats administered a single oral dose of 200 mg/kg (20). Rapid distribution of 2,5-HD to liver, spinal cord, and brainstem occurred following an i.p. dose of 7.5 mmol/kg in rats (14). Extensive distribution of 2,5-HD was also noted in hens after a single dermal application of 50 mg/kg (73).

Numerous studies in laboratory animals and humans have examined the metabolism of n-hexane, MBK, and 2,5-HD, and have demonstrated common metabolic pathways. These pathways, although complex, are qualitatively similar among species and involve a sequence of hydroxylation and dehydrogenation reactions (Fig. 11). Hydroxylation of

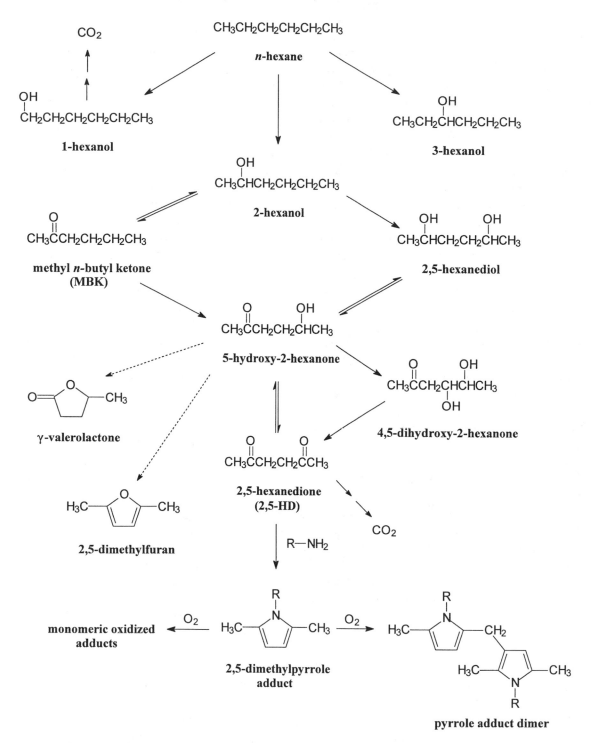

FIGURE 11. Biotransformation and macromolecular binding reactions of *n*-hexane, MBK, and 2,5-HD in mammalian systems. Dashed arrows indicate uncertainty in the actual pathway of formation. R—NH$_2$ represents protein amine side chain.

n-hexane occurs primarily in the liver *via* cytochrome P-450–mediated transformation, while cytoplasmic dehydrogenases reversibly oxidize hydroxylated metabolites to the corresponding ketones. Most of the hydroxylated products are excreted in urine as glucuronides and, possibly, sulfate esters. As discussed below, the ultimate neurotoxic end metabolite of both *n*-hexane and MBK is 2,5-HD.

Early studies in guinea pigs demonstrated formation of both 5-hydroxy-2-hexanone (5H2H) and 2,5-HD in serum following a single i.p. dose of 250 mg/kg (22). 2-Hexanol was detected in urine from guinea pigs 1 day after a single i.p. dose of 50 mg *n*-hexane per kilogram body weight (12). MBK and 1- and 2-hexanol can also be identified in urine from rats administered *n*-hexane by the i.p. route, and inhalation exposure to *n*-hexane results in formation of 1-, 2-, and 3-hexanol, MBK, 5H2H, and 2,5-HD in rats, rabbits, and monkeys (6,9,24,34,49). 1-Hexanol can apparently enter intermediary metabolism and ultimately yield CO_2.

An additional metabolite of *n*-hexane and MBK is 4,5-dihydroxy-2-hexanone, which is excreted in urine as the glucuronide (24). Strong acid hydrolysis of urine prior to analytical determination by gas chromatography/mass spectrometry results in conversion of this derivative to 2,5-HD, a phenomenon that can result in overestimation of urinary 2,5-HD. Minor metabolites of *n*-hexane include 2-amino-1-hexanoic acid, pentanone, γ-valerolactone, 2,5-dimethylfuran, 2,5-dimethyl-2,3-dihydrofuran, and urea, although some of these may represent artifacts of analysis (22). In contrast to some published reports, 2,5-hexanediol has not been clearly demonstrated as a metabolite of *n*-hexane (or MBK) *in vivo*, although it was detected in guinea pig serum following single i.p. doses of either 2-hexanol or 5H2H (22). Consequently, it also is likely to be present at low levels following administration of the parent compounds.

Administration of MBK to rats, guinea pigs, and mice by the p.o. or i.p. routes results in the formation of 2-hexanol, 5H2H, and 2,5-HD in both blood and urine (12,20,22). $^{14}CO_2$ is present in expired breath from rats given single i.p. doses of 200 mg/kg ^{14}C-MBK (20). Inhalation exposure to MBK in rodents is also associated with formation of 5H2H and 2,5-HD. Exposure of rats (24), guinea pigs (22), and hens (73) to 2,5-HD by several routes results in formation of 5H2H, 4,5-dihydroxy-2-hexanone, and CO_2 as major metabolites.

Human metabolism of *n*-hexane and MBK appears to follow the same general pathways found in experimental animals, with some quantitative differences. Both CO_2 and 2,5-HD were reported as metabolites in human volunteers exposed to 50 or 100 ppm MBK for 7.5 h (21). Numerous studies have examined the formation of metabolites in workers exposed to either pure *n*-hexane or to various hexane-based solvents (24,45,50). Major human metabolites include 4,5-dihydroxy-2-hexanone and 2,5-HD, whereas 2-hexanol is typically present at substantially lower levels than in experimental animals.

In vitro metabolism of *n*-hexane and MBK has been investigated. Liver and lung microsomal fractions from rabbit, rat, and mouse metabolize *n*-hexane to 1-, 2-, and 3-hexanol (75), while MBK is converted to 2,5-HD by guinea pig microsomes (12). In contrast, only liver was capable of

transformation of 2-hexanol to 2,5-hexanediol and oxidation of alcohols to corresponding ketones (75). Several P-450 isozymes are implicated in *n*-hexane metabolism, with CYP-IIB1 mediating the critical activation pathway from *n*-hexane to 2-hexanol (75). Metabolism of *n*-hexane and MBK can also be observed in organotypic cord-ganglion-muscle cultures (76).

Elimination of *n*-hexane, MBK, and 2,5-HD occurs *via* exhalation of unmetabolized agent, volatile metabolites, and CO_2, and by urinary excretion of conjugated and unconjugated metabolites. Some species differences are apparent in the proportion of various metabolites excreted by different routes (21,49). A biphasic blood elimination curve was observed in rats following a single i.p. dose of 160 mg/kg MBK, with an α-phase $t_{1/2}$ of 10 min and β-phase $t_{1/2}$ of 7 h (2). Biphasic elimination was also found after a 132-mg/kg i.p. dose of *n*-hexane in guinea pigs (α-phase $t_{1/2}$ of 36 min and β-phase $t_{1/2}$ of 4 h) (12). Serum half-lives of 72–100 min were determined following i.p. doses of MBK, 2-hexanol, 2,5-hexanediol, 5H2H, or 2,5-HD in guinea pigs (22). Radiolabel from a 200 mg/kg p.o. dose of ^{14}C-MBK in rats was recovered primarily in exhaled breath (44%) and urine (40%) (20). Clearance of dermally absorbed ^{14}C-2,5-HD (50 mg/kg) in hens was tissue-dependent, with elimination $t_{1/2}$ values of 12 h (adipose tissue) to 71 h (muscle) (73). After 48 h, excretion of label was found distributed among expired air and combined urine and feces. Remaining label was apparently retained in tissue. Urinary-fecal metabolites included primarily 5H2H and 2,5-HD.

In rats, the major urinary metabolites of *n*-hexane are 2-hexanol, 4,5-dihydroxy-2-hexanone, and 2,5-HD (in that order), although in humans, the latter two compounds predominate (24). In both species, approximately 80%–90% of these metabolites are present in urine as glucuronide conjugates.

Relatively slower excretion of MBK is noted in humans, although the primary pathways of elimination (breath and urine) are similar (21). Extended blood and urinary clearance times and accumulation of 2,5-HD in blood have been reported in both experimental animals and humans following repeated exposure to *n*-hexane (34,45,49). End-of-shift urinary 2,5-HD levels (unconjugated) appear to correlate well with the duration and level of exposure in hexane-exposed workers (45). A biological exposure index for occupational *n*-hexane exposure has been determined based on urinary 2,5-HD levels.

Other commercially important alkane and alkanone solvents have also been examined for metabolic transformations analogous to those of *n*-hexane. A variety of hydroxylated and oxidized metabolites, including low levels of

2,5-heptanedione, is present in urine from rats exposed to *n*-heptane. Following 3-heptanone [ethyl *n*-butyl ketone (EBK)] exposure in rats, 6-hydroxy-3-heptanone and 2,5-heptanedione are detected in serum, although at only a fraction of the corresponding serum levels of 5H2H and 2,5-HD seen after equivalent exposures to MBK. 2,5-Heptanedione and small amounts of 2,5-HD were also detected in urine from rats given daily (5 days/week) doses of 1–2 g/kg of EBK p.o. (48). 2-Heptanone [methyl *n*-amyl ketone (MAK)] is metabolized to *n*-amyl alcohol and several unidentified compounds in rats and monkeys. Administration of 5-nonanone (single dose of 500 mg/kg p.o.) to rats results in formation of 5-nonanol, 2-hydroxy-5-nonanone, and 2,5-nonanedione in plasma. Urinary metabolites include MBK, 2,5-HD, 5H2H, 2,5-hexanediol, and 2-hexanol. These results suggest the presence of oxidation/decarboxylation pathways capable of converting longer chain ketones into neurotoxic metabolites.

The metabolism of *n*-hexane, MBK, and related solvents is subject to influence by prior or concurrent exposure to other agents. Early studies revealed that inhalation coexposure of rats to MBK and to the related, nonneurotoxic solvent MEK resulted in higher blood levels of MBK than with MBK exposure alone (2). Intraperitoneal exposure to MEK/MBK mixtures in guinea pigs also produces increased urinary excretion of 2-hexanol, 2,5-HD, and MBK as compared with MBK alone (12). Pretreatment of rats with MEK prior to *n*-hexane exposure leads to increased 2,5-HD concentration in several tissues, including sciatic nerve. Concurrent exposure to MEK enhances metabolic conversion of 3-heptanone to 2,5-heptanedione (48). Phenobarbital pretreatment can increase the metabolism of *n*-hexane and MBK to 2-hexanol and 2,5-HD in guinea pigs (12). Methyl *iso*-butyl ketone (MiBK) and propanol can also enhance metabolic conversion of *n*-hexane in experimental animals, while decreased clearance of 2,5-HD occurs with 2,5-HD/acetone mixtures. In contrast to these potentiating effects, decreased 2,5-HD formation occurs in rats with combined *n*-hexane/toluene exposure. As discussed below, altered metabolism is associated with changes in the neurotoxic potency of *n*-hexane and its derivatives.

The major toxic effects of *n*-hexane, MBK, and 2,5-HD include those on the CNS and PNS of experimental animals and humans, and on the testes of experimental animals. Exposure to high levels of *n*-hexane and MBK by inhalation results in typical signs of solvent overexposure, including respiratory depression, narcosis, convulsions, coma, and death (72). Lower and/or subchronic exposure induces distal axonopathy in both CNS and PNS nerve fibers. There is some evidence for damage to the respiratory epithelium from high-dose inhalation studies in rats.

Animal Studies

The neurotoxicity of *n*-hexane and its metabolites has been studied in a number of animal species (5,35,47,72). Early single-exposure inhalation studies of *n*-hexane in rats and mice revealed exposure-related increases in the severity of various acute CNS effects (72). Rats developed sedation, ataxia, light-to-deep anesthesia, seizures, respiratory arrest, and death when exposed to 2000–90,000 ppm *n*-hexane. Similar effects occur following inhalation exposure to high concentrations of MBK. Large acute p.o. or i.p. doses of 2,5-HD administered to rats produce analgesia and vacuolar axonal and neuron perikaryal degeneration.

In contrast to the acute CNS effects of *n*-hexane and MBK, distal axonopathy is the characteristic neurotoxic syndrome induced by repeated, prolonged exposure to these agents (72). In fact, acute toxicity investigations did not reveal the neurotoxic potential of these compounds; the phenomenon only emerged after reports of human effects from chronic exposures. Early animal studies examined neurotoxic effects in rats exposed to 200 ppm MBK (8 h/day, 5 days/week) for 6 weeks, 1300 ppm MBK (6 h/day, 5 days/week) for 4 months, or 400–600 ppm *n*-hexane (continuous exposure) for up to 23 weeks (61,71). Rats exposed to 1300 ppm MBK exhibited hindlimb foot drop after 3-month exposure, while *n*-hexane–exposed animals displayed an unsteady gait after 6-week exposure, and bilateral hindlimb neuromuscular weakness and paralysis thereafter. Neuropathological examination revealed a characteristic pattern of scattered, focal paranodal or internodal axonal swelling, corresponding thinning of myelin, and axonal degeneration in peripheral nerves. These swellings were typically located in distal (but not terminal) regions of long myelinated nerve fibers, in particular within the tibial nerve branches (61). CNS changes included axonal degeneration in the distal areas of both long ascending and descending fibers of the spinal cord. Prolonged exposure causes distal axonal degeneration in the distal optic tracts (lateral geniculate body) and fornix (mammillary body) (62). Electron microscopic studies demonstrated that the axonal swellings consisted of densely packed masses of neurofilaments with segregation of other axonal organelles (mitochondria, microtubules) into a discrete central zone. Similar changes were observed in cats given daily subcutaneous (s.c.) doses of MBK (150 mg/kg) for 8.5 months, and in rats administered 2,5-HD (mean dose of 340 mg/kg/day, s.c.) for up to 23 weeks (68). These neuropathological alterations are generally consistent with the neurotoxic syndrome termed "central-peripheral distal axonopathy" (69). In contrast, commercial hexane mixtures that do not contain *n*-hexane are without neurotoxic effects in rats.

Comprehensive studies have examined the temporal evolution of this neuropathy and the relative vulnerabilities of CNS and PNS nerve fibers. Distal axonal swellings are both multifocal and subterminal (69). Frank nerve fiber degeneration appears to occur along the entire length of a fiber distal to an axonal swelling. The most susceptible sites within the CNS appear to be the distal regions of large myelinated fibers within the dorsal spinocerebellar, gracile, cuneate, ventrolateral, and ventromedial tracts, while the tibial nerve branches to the calf muscle are affected earliest in the PNS (70). Similar clinical and neuropathological findings have been made in hens, dogs, and monkeys exposed to MBK or 2,5-HD, while mice appear to be relatively resistant to this neuropathy. Although axonal swellings in 2,5-HD neuropathy are usually localized to more distal regions of the nerve fiber, this pattern can be altered to favor more proximal sites with very large acute doses of 2,5-HD (27) or by administration of certain 2,5-HD analogues (vide infra, Toxic Mechanisms).

Other pathological aspects of this neuropathy have been examined. Neurofilament (NF) accumulation occurs in autonomic nerve fibers of rats at an early time point during exposure to 2,5-HD by i.p. injection. Extensive study of the development and fate of NF masses in optic and other CNS and PNS fibers from rats exposed to 2,5-hexanediol has been made. Formation of NF accumulations is an early event in optic nerve axons, and both the number and size of masses are time-dependent (37). Following cessation of exposure, NF swellings slowly disappear, without accompanying axonal degeneration. In contrast, NF masses are not cleared from, and degeneration is prominent in, other types of fibers, particularly long PNS axons (10). In the PNS, NF masses form on the proximal sides of nodes of Ranvier, followed by paranodal myelin retraction and demyelination. Paranodal demyelination is the correlate of slowed nerve conduction in this disorder. Changes in nodal membrane glycoprotein composition can occur in 2,5-HD–treated rats, as can a decreased rate of outgrowth of peripheral nerve fibers distal to a crush injury. Demyelination and cytoskeletal alterations within Schwann cells occur in rats following administration in the drinking water (1% solution) for up to 23 weeks, suggesting a possible common action of this agent on cytoplasmic filaments (72). Motor neuron cell body changes and decreases in numbers and volumes of cortical neurons are also present in 2,5-HD–treated rats.

Direct exposure of nerve fibers to 2,5-HD can reproduce some of the neuropathological changes noted after systemic exposure. Application of undiluted or aqueous 2,5-HD to exposed sciatic nerves in anesthetized rats for 45 min results in formation of characteristic giant axonal swellings, myelin

thinning, and axonal degeneration 4 days after treatment (52). Subperineural injection of 2,5-HD into rat sural nerves induces segregation of microtubules and mitochondria within a central axonal channel surrounded by disorganized NFs within 2 h of exposure (32). Such cytoskeletal alterations can occur as early as 30 sec following injection of 2,5-HD. These studies have provided strong evidence for a direct toxic action of 2,5-HD on the axonal compartment.

Electrophysiological and behavioral deficits are present in experimental animals following exposure to n-hexane or its metabolites. Monkeys and rats exposed chronically to 100 ppm MBK (6 h/day, 5 days/week, 10 months) exhibited prolonged nerve conduction velocity (NCV) in sciatic-tibial nerves and decreased evoked muscle action potentials (36). Abnormal neuromuscular transmission can occur after 2,5-HD exposure, prior to histopathological damage. Decreased response rates on a fixed-interval-schedule operant test were measured in rats by the second week of exposure to 1000 ppm MBK. The behavioral effects of prolonged 2,5-HD exposure in rats were examined using a functional observational battery (FOB) that included tests for CNS excitability, autonomic signs, and motor and sensory integration (63). Numerous alterations in various FOB parameters, particularly those testing motor function, were noted as early as 1 week of exposure.

The relative neurotoxic potency of n-hexane, MBK, 2,5-HD, and other n-hexane metabolites has been examined in experimental animals. 2-Hexanol exposure results in neurotoxic signs and neuropathological changes identical to those for 2,5-HD, while exposure to 1-hexanol is without significant effect. Administration of n-hexane and various hexane metabolites to rats for 90–120 days resulted in clinical neuropathy in all dose groups (38). However, the time to achieve an end point of severe hindlimb weakness (indicative of relative potency) decreased in the order: n-hexane, 2-hexanol, MBK, 2,5-hexanediol, 5H2H, and 2,5-HD. The degree of neuropathy also correlated well with the area under the curve for serum 2,5-HD for each compound. A similar order of potency is observed in hens.

On the basis of these and a number of other studies, it has been proposed that n-hexane and MBK are neurotoxic by virtue of their metabolic conversion to 2,5-HD, the actual toxic agent in this neuropathy. 2,5-HD is classified as a "γ-diketone" based upon the two-carbon spacing between carbonyl groups. Following characterization of 2,5-HD–induced neuropathy, it was proposed that other diketones might exhibit such neurotoxic properties (66), and extensive studies were conducted to investigate the structure–activity relationships for this class of compounds. Of a series of diketones tested for neurotoxicity in rats, only γ-diketones, including 2,5-HD, 2,5-heptanedione, and 3,6-

octanedione were found to induce the classic clinical signs and pathological changes associated with n-hexane neuropathy (66). In contrast, 2,3-butanedione, 2,3-hexanedione (α-diketones), 2,4-hexanedione, 2,4-pentanedione, and 3,5-heptanedione (β-diketones), 2,6-heptanedione (a δ-diketone), 2,7-octanedione (an ε-diketone), glutaraldehyde (a dialdehyde), and the diols 1,4-butanediol and 1,6-hexanediol were not neurotoxic. These studies provided strong evidence for the requirement for a γ-diketone structure in this neuropathy. Additional studies (*vide infra*, Toxic Mechanisms) have investigated the neurotoxic potency of deuterated 2,5-HD and several 2,5-HD derivatives substituted at the 3 and/or 4 positions with alkyl or acyl functions. Related alkanes and alkanones have also been tested for neurotoxic potential. Motor NCV deficits and peripheral nerve damage do not occur in n-pentane– or n-heptane–treated rats. Inhalation of MAK or EBK does not result in neurotoxic effects in experimental animal studies. The lack of n-heptane or heptanone neurotoxicity in these studies can be attributed to their low metabolic conversion to the known neurotoxic compound 2,5-heptanedione. In contrast, multiple, large oral doses (2 g/kg/day for 14 weeks) of EBK have been shown to induce a typical γ-diketone neuropathy in rats (48). The apparent neurotoxicity of commercial methyl n-heptyl ketone in rats is likely due to the presence of 5-nonanone and the metabolism of this component to 2,5-nonanedione, MBK, and 2,5-HD. Other related compounds that have been found not to induce a γ-diketone neuropathy include 2- and 3-methylpentane, methylcyclopentane, diisoamyl ketone, methyl isoamyl ketone, di-n-propyl ketone, MiBK, MEK, cyclohexane, cyclohexanone, and acetone.

Coexposure to mixtures of n-hexane, MBK, or 2,5-HD in combination with certain other solvents modifies the neurotoxic response in experimental animals. Rats exposed to mixtures of either MBK or n-hexane with MEK exhibit hindlimb weakness earlier and display more severe neuropathological changes than those exposed to each solvent alone. Large oral doses of MEK were also found to increase the neurotoxic potential of EBK (48). Enhanced neurophysiological changes are apparent in rats exposed to binary mixtures of n-hexane or MBK with MEK, methyl propyl ketone, MAK, MiBK, or methyl hexyl ketone. In contrast to the potentiating effects of these agents, concurrent toluene exposure appears to decrease the neurotoxicity of n-hexane. Although the mechanisms of these interactions are not fully understood, differential induction and/or inhibition of various n-hexane metabolic pathways, in addition to toxicokinetic changes, are likely to be involved.

Numerous experimental animal studies have been conducted to examine neurochemical and biophysical changes in n-hexane, MBK, and γ-diketone neuropathy, including the effects on energy metabolism, membrane function, axonal transport, and cytoskeletal proteins. These are discussed below (*see* Toxic Mechanisms).

In Vitro Studies

n-Hexane neuropathy has been investigated using a number of cell lines, including human fibroblasts, PtK1 cells, PtK2 cells, and neuroblastoma cells, and in primary and organotypic tissue culture models. Aggregation of vimentin-type, but not keratin-type intermediate filaments occurs in fibroblasts treated with 1–85 mM 2,5-HD for up to 21 days (23). Aggregation of NFs is found in mouse and human dorsal root ganglion cell cultures treated with 2,5-HD. In contrast, nonneurotoxic 2,4-HD and 1,6-hexanediol are without effect. Functional mouse spinal cord, dorsal root ganglia, and skeletal muscle organotypic culture preparations have proven valuable for studying the effects of n-hexane and n-hexane metabolites (76). In one experiment, mature cultures were treated with 2.8 mM of several compounds for up 6 weeks, with an additional 12–15 weeks of recovery. Exposure to n-hexane, 2-hexanol, 2,5-hexanediol, MBK, 5H2H, or 2,5-HD resulted in development of paranodal axonal swelling, myelin retraction, and, ultimately, fiber degeneration, suggesting that these cultures were capable of converting n-hexane and intermediate metabolites to 2,5-HD. Interestingly, the relative time to development of neuropathological changes appeared to be approximately equal for both 2,5-HD and MBK in this system. Potentiation of n-hexane neuropathy by coexposure to MEK can also be reproduced in this model. 2,4-HD treatment produced only nonspecific effects.

Human Studies

Human peripheral neuropathy has occurred following occupational exposure to n-hexane or MBK and after deliberate, repeated inhalation of solvent or adhesive materials containing n-hexane for recreational purposes ("gluesniffing" or "huffing") (5,35,47,72). Initial controlled, acute human exposures to n-hexane and MBK did not reveal this type of neurotoxicity but were associated with dizziness, sedation, and irritative effects. Japanese investigators were the first to report peripheral neuropathy following prolonged n-hexane exposure in poorly ventilated polyethylene laminating operations in the early 1960s (74). These were followed by similar cases among household sandal-making workers in Japan and furniture finishers in the United States (33). Instances of neuropathy in Italian shoemakers exposed to n-hexane-containing solvents had been reported as early as 1957, but these were generally attributed to triorthocresyl phosphate exposure. Ambient air levels of *n*-hexane and exposure durations in these cases were typically in the 500- to 2500-ppm range for 3–10 months, and toxic effects were both exposure-related and time-dependent.

Workers present with an insidious progression of a number of neuropathic signs and symptoms, including acral paresthesia, weakness in the lower limbs, foot-drop, and moderately to severely compromised tendon reflexes. These motor and sensory deficits are symmetrical and usually limited to the feet and hands (70). Other common symptoms included fatigue, weight loss, abdominal pain, and blurred vision. Muscle biopsy in several of these cases revealed atrophy, while peripheral nerve (sural) biopsies exhibited axonal swellings, focal demyelination, and some nerve degeneration. Smaller myelinated and unmyelinated axons were unaffected. Electron microscopy revealed motor end-plate abnormalities and NF accumulation within peripheral axons (33). Electrophysiological findings consisted of prolonged NCVs in median and ulnar nerves and decreased muscle-resting-potential amplitudes. Cerebrospinal fluid analyses were typically normal, as were the results of blood chemistry and hematology studies. Recovery of neurological function in these workers tended to be slow but generally complete over a period of 2–5 years.

These early cases prompted a lowering of the Japanese TLV for *n*-hexane from 500 ppm to 100 ppm (74). Despite regulatory controls, clusters and isolated outbreaks of *n*-hexane neuropathy in occupational exposure settings have continued to occur over the last two decades, and additional clinical and neurotoxicological characterization of this syndrome has been made. Specific evidence for CNS nerve fiber damage, either during exposure or following recovery of PNS function, has been obtained. Evoked potential (EP) deficits, consisting of increased latencies of patterned visual EPs and increased absolute latencies and central conduction times of somatosensory EPs were noted in *n*-hexane–exposed Taiwanese printers (11). Hyperreflexia has been observed in some workers long after cessation of exposure, a residual effect attributed to subclinical corticospinal tract damage.

Following cessation of *n*-hexane exposure in affected workers, a continued worsening of symptoms over a period of 2 months ("coasting") before true recovery takes place is commonly encountered (72). The mechanism of this phenomenon is unclear. Functional and electrophysiological measurements in mild to moderate neuropathy gradually return to normal over months to years, although recovery may be incomplete in severely affected individuals. In general, the pattern of clinical signs, neuropathological findings, and electrophysiological changes in affected humans is identical to that observed with experimentally induced *n*-hexane neuropathy in rats and other animal species. A report of progressive fatal parkinsonism in an individual exposed to solvents containing *n*-hexane likely represents chance concurrence or the presence of a nigrotoxic substance in the solvent mixture (51).

Numerous cases of *n*-hexane–induced peripheral neuropathy have also been reported in individuals as a result of deliberate inhalation of *n*-hexane–containing glues or solvents for psychotropic effects. Early examples of this phenomenon were described by Japanese investigators (28), but many such cases have since been reported in the literature from a number of industrialized nations (3). Typically, the liquid glue or solvent is poured into a plastic bag and repeatedly inhaled until no longer volatile, after which more product is added and the process continued. The acute effects of glue-sniffing include narcosis and euphoria; the latter has been attributed to the frequent presence of toluene in these products. The activity can be habit-forming, and reports of daily glue-sniffing sessions lasting up to 12 h in these individuals are common. Death from suffocation and acute cardiac arrhythmias during inhalation can occur.

Three characteristics distinguish the neuropathy associated with solvent abuse from that encountered in exposed workers; the intermittent but extremely high inhalation exposure levels, the severity of the resulting clinical manifestations, and the usual presence of other solvent components in the inhaled vapors. Affected individuals usually present with weight loss and rapid progression (weeks) of sensorimotor neuropathy affecting the arms and legs, sometimes rendering the patient paraplegic or quadriplegic (3). Signs of cranial nerve damage are not usually present. Occasional progression to respiratory paralysis and death have been reported. Following cessation of exposure, symptoms generally progress for a period of time, followed by slow, and sometimes incomplete, recovery (3). Peripheral nerve biopsies in these cases have revealed axonal degeneration, demyelination, and paranodal axonal swelling with NF accumulation, although biopsies in severe cases may only indicate fiber degeneration. Electrophysiological deficits are marked, with very slowed NCVs and decreased sensory nerve action potential amplitudes and increased distal latencies. There is one report that describes long-term follow-up of an individual with severe subacute neuropathy from inhalation abuse (65). After 1 year of abstinence, strength was normal and only slight impairment of acral sensation was present. Motor nerve conduction velocities remained diminished (peroneal motor conduction was 27 m/sec).

Although levels of *n*-hexane in inspired air during glue-sniffing have been reported as high as 44,000 ppm, *n*-hexane is seldom the only volatile component of these products. Peripheral neuropathy, under these exposure conditions, can be enhanced by the presence of MEK as a potentiating agent. A significant outbreak of glue-sniffing neuropathy took place among adolescents in Berlin when MEK was added to the formulation of a commonly abused *n*-hexane-containing adhesive (3). Neuropathy had not previously been reported in individuals inhaling the old formulation, which actually contained approximately twice the level of *n*-hexane as the newer one. Changes in composition resulting in increased *n*-hexane levels have also been associated with development of neuropathy in some epidemics, while continued sniffing of glues in which *n*-hexane had been replaced has been followed by recovery. Despite the presence of multiple solvent components in these products, the identification of *n*-hexane as the neurotoxic agent is not in doubt in view of the virtually identical neuropathic effects to those observed with pure *n*-hexane in human or experimental animal studies. In contrast, MBK is not a reported exposure factor in any published report of glue- or solvent-sniffing neuropathy.

Human neuropathy due to occupational MBK exposure was first encountered following a major outbreak at a vinyl-coated fabric printing facility in Ohio in 1973 (7). Ultimately, 86 workers out of 1157 tested subjects in the plant were diagnosed with a toxic peripheral neuropathy. Eleven of these cases were classified as moderate to severe with disabling neurological signs, 38 as mild with nondisabling signs, and 37 as subclinical with electrophysiological changes only. Weight loss was prominent in the highly affected group, in addition to symmetrical motor and sensory functional deficits in the extremities. Electrodiagnostic findings consisted of reduction in the number of motor unit potentials in distal muscles, the presence of positive waves and fibrillations, and decreased NCVs in the ulnar, peroneal, tibial, and sural nerves. Peripheral nerve biopsies were not performed in these studies. Despite the lack of neuropathological data, the clinical neurological picture and pattern of recovery in these workers were found to be essentially the same as those previously encountered for *n*-hexane–induced neuropathy.

A major epidemiological effort identified the cause of this neuropathy. *n*-Hexane was not used in the plant in any significant quantity. However, appearance of the cases was associated with substitution of a 1:9 MBK/MEK mixture for the previously used 1:9 MiBK/MEK mixture as an ink solvent in the printing department. Ambient air levels of MBK within the plant during this time period were measured at 2.3–156 ppm. Initial neuropathic complaints were noted approximately 5–6 months after this change was made. The most seriously affected individuals were those who operated the printing machines and who were the most heav-

ily exposed to MBK vapor for the longest periods of time. Cessation of use of MBK in the plant was followed by an absence of new cases and slow reversal of symptoms in affected workers. In addition, studies in a similar plant that did not employ MBK as a solvent did not reveal any cases of toxic peripheral neuropathy. On the basis of these findings, MBK was proposed as the neurotoxic agent. Although the clinical neuropathic syndrome was similar, the potency of MBK in causing neuropathy was apparently much greater than that of *n*-hexane, as judged by the lower levels of exposure, shortened time necessary for development of symptoms, and greater severity of neuropathy under occupational exposure conditions. However, coexposure to MEK may have potentiated the effects of MBK.

Since the 1974 Ohio investigation, there have been few reported cases of human MBK neuropathy. This is due to both a lowering of occupational TLVs for MBK in a number of countries and to the almost universal substitution of safer solvents for industrial processes. In contrast, *n*-hexane usage as a major, large-volume commercial solvent persists, and epidemiological reports of *n*-hexane–exposed workers have continued to appear. A study of 122 Italian shoemakers with peripheral neuropathy revealed an increased prevalence of symptoms in poorly ventilated smaller factories during the winter months and among female as opposed to male workers (1). Evidence indicating the potential for subclinical neuropathy in some *n*-hexane–exposed workers is also available, including statistical differences in the number of self-reported neurological symptoms, in conduction velocities recorded in peripheral nerve, and in other neurophysiological end points. Overt, clinical neuropathy was not apparent in any of these workers.

Differential diagnosis of *n*-hexane or MBK neuropathy is based upon clinical signs, the results of electrophysiological and nerve biopsy examination, and, most importantly, a history of solvent exposure in an occupational or solvent abuse setting. There is a useful set of clinicopathologic correlates for diagnosis of this form of toxic polyneuropathy, including gradual onset of symptoms; initial symptoms symmetrically oriented in the feet, lower legs, and hands, sensory loss of the "stocking-and-glove" type; motor weakness in the extremities; loss of ankle reflexes; and "coasting" followed by slow recovery (60). Occasionally, *n*-hexane neuropathy induced by glue-sniffing can resemble Guillain-Barré syndrome (a demyelinating neuropathy) because of the more rapid onset sometimes seen under this exposure scenario and markedly prolonged nerve conductions and conduction block in severe cases. Without a clear exposure history, peripheral neuropathy from other metabolic or toxic causes can be difficult to rule out. Lead neuropathy is not usually associated with peripheral sensory changes, while optic nerve changes are frequently seen in carbon disulfide– or methanol-induced neuropathies. Acrylamide exposure is frequently accompanied by ataxia and skin peeling on the palms of the hands, while parasympathetic activation is usually noted with organophosphate exposure. Lack of anemia effectively rules out peripheral neuropathy due to vitamin B_{12} deficiency. Peripheral nerve biopsy showing evidence of giant axonal swellings with NF accumulation suggests n-hexane neuropathy, although this finding is not always present in biopsy specimens. Nerve conduction velocity may be markedly reduced in n-hexane and MBK neuropathies from inhalation abuse and may erroneously suggest a primary demyelinating polyneuropathy.

Removal from exposure and the institution of supportive measures such as physical therapy are typically employed in cases of human n-hexane neuropathy. There is no specific therapy.

Toxic Mechanisms

The neurotoxic mechanism of action of n-hexane and, more specifically, the γ-diketones has been extensively studied since the first major outbreaks of human neuropathy in the early 1970s. Although a number of hypotheses have been proposed and many important aspects of the mechanism have been clarified, the molecular determinants and pathological significance of axonal NF accumulation and the ultimate mechanism of axonal degeneration remain unclear (13,30,58,72). Some have suggested that the neuropathological sequelae are the result of a specific, early molecular event, others have proposed multiple independent mechanisms to account for the various aspects of this neuropathy. Mechanistic hypotheses on γ-diketone neuropathy generally fall into two categories: those that propose neurofilaments as the critical target site and those that suggest direct effects on other axonal components or metabolic processes, such as axonal transport.

Early experiments revealed that MBK administration to rats resulted in impaired fast anterograde axoplasmic transport in proximal areas of sciatic nerve (42) and through axonal swellings in rat sciatic nerve induced by 2,5-hexanediol (27). Later in vivo and in vitro studies confirmed these findings, extended them to include deficits in fast retrograde axonal transport after 2,5-HD exposure, and demonstrated the lack of transport effects of nonneurotoxic diketones. In general, the results of such studies have been consistent with decreases in the rate and capacity of fast axoplasmic transport.

Since fast axonal transport is an energy-dependent process, numerous studies have examined in vitro effects of 2,5-HD exposure on various glycolytic and citric acid cycle enzymes (57). Glyceraldehyde-3-phosphate dehydrogenase (GAPDH) activity is inhibited by 2,5-HD in in vitro preparations, in rat brain homogenates, and in directly exposed rat desheathed sciatic nerve segments, although relatively high (millimolar) concentrations are required. GAPDH is required for normal fast transport. Inhibition of GAPDH is not apparent after exposure to nonneurotoxic 2,4-HD. Similar in vitro effects occur with the glycolytic enzymes enolase and phosphofructokinase, but not with lactate dehydrogenase, transketolase, or succinate dehydrogenase. Decreased adenosine triphosphate production in rat brain mitochondria exposed to 2,5-HD also occurs. Results of in vivo studies of axonal energy metabolism in n-hexane neuropathy have been mixed. One study reported GAPDH inhibition in sciatic nerve from 2,5-HD–treated rats with severe neuropathy (56). Other effects, including decreases in local glucose utilization, decreased sciatic nerve uptake of oxygen, and inhibition of brain mitochondrial respiration in 2,5-HD–treated animals have been reported. In contrast, the results of other studies have not been consistent with inhibition of glycolysis (26).

These axonal transport findings, along with the observations that 2,5-HD is the neurotoxic metabolite of n-hexane and MBK, and that this agent acts directly upon the axon, led to the hypothesis that the γ-diketones may inhibit axonal energy production, resulting in a disruption of fast anterograde transport of critical molecules into the distal axon (67). The long, large-diameter myelinated fibers were postulated to be most vulnerable owing to their presumably greater energy requirements. NF accumulation was suggested to be triggered by impaired energy availability, and to further aggravate the transport status by providing a physical blockade to anterograde transport. Although the hypothesis can explain certain aspects of the neuropathy, it is unclear whether transport alterations are the proximate cause of the neuropathological changes or a result of other axonal mechanisms in γ-diketone neuropathy. In addition, the relatively high concentrations required to produce effects on glycolysis and respiration, and the likely generalized effects of such energy deficits within the organism, are not consistent with the theory.

Other hypotheses propose that the neurofilament is the critical target site for the γ-diketones and that alterations in filament structure and metabolism ultimately lead to NF accumulation and distal axonal degeneration (17,30,58). Based on the observed incorporation of radiolabel from ^{14}C-MBK into brain protein in experimental animals, the direct action of 2,5-HD upon the axon, and the requirement for the γ-diketone structure, it was proposed that covalent binding of 2,5-HD to amine groups in NFs was the critical initial step in this neuropathy. The product of this reaction was suggested to be either a conjugated diimine

(29) or a 2,5-dimethylpyrrole adduct (19). The latter structure is now accepted as the primary γ-diketone/protein reaction product, and formation of this adduct in NF proteins is the basis of the "pyrrole hypothesis" of *n*-hexane, MBK, and 2,5-HD neuropathy.

Pyrrole adduct formation in model amines and proteins has been extensively studied *in vitro*. The reaction proceeds *via* nucleophilic attack of the ε-amine nitrogen of lysine on a carbonyl group of the diketone, with loss of water and formation of an intermediate imine. The second carbonyl group is rapidly attacked by the imine nitrogen, resulting in loss of another water molecule and cyclization to the 1,2,5-trisubstituted pyrrole adduct. Pyrrolylation of model amines, bovine serum albumin, ovalbumin, and ribonuclease A by various γ-diketones has been demonstrated *in vitro* under physiological conditions of temperature and pH (16,30,79). Pyrrole adduction in tissue protein following *in vivo* exposure to 2,5-HD in laboratory animals has also been reported. Adducts were detected in serum, liver, kidney, brain, and myelin protein from hens administered 70 or 200 mg/kg/day 2,5-HD, p.o., for up to 135 or 55 days, respectively (18). Similarly, dosing of rats with 2,5-HD led to pyrrole adduct formation in serum and red blood cell proteins (4,17).

There is strong evidence that diketone neuropathy requires a toxicant with both the γ-diketone structure (as discussed previously) and the ability to react with lysine ε-amines to form pyrrole adducts. 2,5-HD derivatives with methyl substitutions at the 3- and/or 4-positions form pyrroles more rapidly than the parent compound and are more potent neurotoxicants *in vivo*. Interestingly, as compared with the distal axonal swellings induced by 2,5-HD, 3-methyl-2,5-HD produces swellings localized to intermediate axonal regions, while 3,4-dimethyl-2,5-HD (DMHD) exposure results in proximal axonal swellings (4,44). In addition, the relatively higher neurotoxic potency of *d,l*- compared to *meso*-DMHD correlates with the increased rate of pyrrole formation *in vitro* of the former diastereomer (55). In contrast, the γ-diketone 3,3-dimethyl-2,5-HD is not neurotoxic (59). This derivative cannot form the pyrrole owing to the lack of a free hydrogen at the 3 position. An absolute requirement for pyrrole formation is also supported by the decreased neurotoxicity of D^{10}-2,5-HD, a derivative that forms the pyrrole at only one-third the rate of 2,5-HD (14).

Pyrrole adduction of axonal proteins, including the NF proteins, has been intensively studied. Adduct formation in axonal pad proteins was observed in rats administered 1.0% 2,5-HD or 0.1% DMHD in the drinking water for 3 weeks (4). Pyrroles were also detected in axonal cytoskeletal protein preparations (containing primarily NF proteins) from rats given 0.5% 2,5-HD in water for up to 8 weeks, and following i.p. administration of 2,5-HD or D^{10}-2,5-HD (2.5 or 3.5 mmol/kg/day) (14,17). In the former study, pyrroles were still present in axonal, but not serum proteins 9 weeks after cessation of exposure. Although evidence for pyrrole formation in NFs during 2,5-HD neuropathy is strong, relative adduct levels in individual axonal cytoskeletal proteins following *in vivo* exposure to various γ-diketones have not been reported.

In vitro studies have also examined pyrrole formation in the NF proteins. Using a native rat NF model system, it was demonstrated that, following short-term incubation with relatively high concentrations of ^{14}C-2,5-HD, covalently bound label was present primarily within the more peripherally oriented NF-M and -H subunit proteins as compared with the NF-L "core" subunit (15). Within the M and H proteins, label was further localized to the carboxyl-terminal "tail" domains of these proteins. Only a small percentage of available lysines in the H and M proteins was found to be adducted by this treatment, suggesting that pyrrole formation in these proteins may be selective. Similar studies have confirmed the greater reactivity of the NF-H and -M proteins under physiological conditions (39), although substantial labeling of NF-L can also occur under certain experimental regimens.

Several proposals have been made that directly link pyrrole adduct formation in the NF proteins with the pathological NF alterations that are seen in this neuropathy. It was proposed that decreased NF solubility within the axoplasm, resulting from formation of hydrophobic pyrrole adducts, might alter their transport or metabolism (18). Based upon the relatively high reactivity of the NF-M and -H subunits, this hypothesis was modified to propose physicochemical changes in NF–NF or NF–microtubule (MT) interactions as a result of pyrrole adduction in the "tail" domains of these proteins (17). These regions extend out from the core of the filament and are thought to be responsible for interfilament association within the axoplasm. It was further suggested that modification of only a few critical lysines in these domains might be sufficient to initiate axonal cytoskeletal reorganization (15). Such reorganization had previously been proposed to account for the observed direct action of 2,5-HD on the axon (32). Neutralization of positive charge within the NF protein tail domains (*via* pyrrole adduction) might be sufficient to disrupt cytoskeletal interactions and alter NF transport (58). These alterations are not mutually exclusive, and pyrrole adduction may result in multiple physicochemical effects on NFs.

Once formed, pyrrole adducts can undergo additional, oxidative reactions to yield secondary, cross-linked derivatives. These reactions can be attributed to the well-known susceptibility of alkylpyrroles to auto-oxidation. This phenomenon is minimized under argon or nitrogen and in the presence of free-radical scavengers. Pyrrole auto-oxidation and cross-linking are likely to be free radical–mediated processes, and the major cross-linking structure appears to be a methylene bridge between C-2 of one pyrrole ring and C-3 of a second ring (79). Although cross-linking is a major pathway of pyrrole auto-oxidation under physiological conditions, stable, non–cross-linked products are also possible (79).

Covalent cross-linking of pyrrolylated proteins was first reported following *in vitro* studies with 2,5-HD under oxidative conditions (16,30). When purified model proteins are exposed to γ-diketones under air, prolonged incubation results in formation of high-molecular-weight polymeric protein, visualized as material that fails to migrate in sodium dodecyl sulfate polyacrylamide gel electrophoresis. Cross-linking of NF proteins is prominent following *in vitro* exposure to γ-diketones under physiological conditions (15,17). Covalent cross-linking of red blood cell spectrin, brain tubulin, and NF proteins also occurs in rats exposed to γ-diketones. In NFs, both intramolecular and intermolecular cross-linking occurs, and the NF-M and -H subunits seem particularly susceptible to this reaction (40). γ-Diketones also cross-link invertebrate NFs and other mammalian intermediate filament proteins, including glial fibrillary acidic protein and vimentin.

It is unclear whether pyrrole formation itself is sufficient to cause neuropathy or whether secondary autoxidative cross-linking is also required. The original proposal, that the critical molecular lesion in γ-diketone neuropathy is pyrrole-mediated NF cross-linking, was a process suggested to result in alterations in NF transport and paranodal NF accumulation (30). Correlations between the rate of auto-oxidative cross-linking for pyrroles formed by various diketones and their *in vivo* neurotoxic potential have been reported (4,55). Hyperbaric oxygen treatment during 2,5-HD intoxication in rats, a regimen postulated to enhance auto-oxidative NF cross-linking, produces a more rapid onset of neuropathy than 2,5-HD alone, although the difference is small (54). The strongest evidence for a requirement for NF cross-linking in the mechanism comes from examination of 3-acetyl-2,5-HD (AcHD). This γ-diketone forms pyrroles that are not susceptible to auto-oxidative cross-linking, owing to the presence of the deactivating acetyl substituent on the pyrrole ring. When administered to rats, AcHD reportedly pyrrolylated red blood cell globin more rapidly than seen with 2,5-HD, did not cross-link tissue protein, and did not appear to be neurotoxic (25). However, relative pyrrole adduct levels at the presumed critical target site (*i.e.*, the neurofilament) for AcHD as compared

with 2,5-HD have not been reported. These data are critical for the further evaluation of the cross-linking hypothesis.

The precise mechanisms by which NF pyrrole adduction and/or cross-linking could lead to NF accumulation and axonal degeneration have not been elucidated. Most hold changes in NF transport characteristics to be the first step in this process. The results of investigations of NF transport in γ-diketone neuropathy have been conflicting. NFs are transported along the axon within the "slow" component (SCa) of axoplasmic flow, at a net rate of about 0.5–1.0 mm/day. Current theory suggests that the NF network consists of moving and stationary phases, with a dynamic exchange continuously occurring along the length of the axon (46).

Early studies reported slowing of NF transport following DMHD intoxication in rats through axonal swellings in peripheral nerve (31). In contrast, 2,5-HD intoxication appears to result in acceleration of NF transport in optic and sciatic nerve fiber areas proximal to axonal swellings, resulting in a net decrease in NF content within these regions (43,78). This acceleration is not consistent with a NF cross-linking–based mechanism and has been attributed to a primary disruption of cytoskeletal interactions due to pyrrole adduction. Alternatively, it has been suggested to represent a secondary response of the axon to injury, unrelated to adduct formation (53). Observations of a decreased phosphorylation state of NF proteins as a result of 2,5-HD exposure may also be relevant to alterations in their transport rate (78). During development of mammalian nerve fibers, hypophosphorylated NFs, with accelerated rates of transport, are characteristic of the immature axon. How such changes in NF transport ultimately result in cytoskeletal disorganization, NF aggregation, and axonal degeneration is not clear.

Other mechanisms that postulate critical target sites other than the neurofilament have also been proposed for γ-diketone neuropathy. 2,5-HD exposure in rats induces changes in red blood cell and myelin membrane microviscosity (72), and decreased sterologenesis (26). Covalent binding of 2,5-HD to microtubule-associated protein 2 occurs *in vivo* (39). Inhibition of NF-associated protein kinases or activation of phosphatases by γ-diketones has also been proposed to account for decreased NF phosphorylation levels in this neuropathy (76). Some evidence is available that distal axonal degeneration can occur in the absence of NF accumulation, suggesting that independent mechanisms underlie these phenomena (41,64). However, any hypothesis that proposes target sites other than the neurofilament in γ-diketone neuropathy must also account for the well-supported observation that the pyrrole-forming reaction is absolutely required in the mechanism.

REFERENCES

1. Abbritti G, Siracusa A, Cianchetti C *et al.* (1976) Shoemakers' polyneuropathy in Italy: The aetiological problem. *Brit J Ind Med* **33**, 92.

2. Abdel-Rahman MS, Hetland LB, Couri D (1976) Toxicity and metabolism of methyl *n*-butyl ketone. *Amer Ind Hyg Assn J* **37**, 95.

3. Altenkirch H, Mager J, Stoltenburg G, Helmbrecht J (1977) Toxic polyneuropathies after sniffing a glue thinner. *J Neurol* **214**, 137.

4. Anthony DC, Boekelheide K, Anderson CW, Graham DG (1983) The effect of 3,4-dimethyl substitution on the neurotoxicity of 2,5-hexanedione. II. Dimethyl substitution accelerates pyrrole formation and protein crosslinking. *Toxicol Appl Pharmacol* **71**, 372.

5. Arlien-Søborg P (1992) *Solvent Neurotoxicity*. CRC Press, Boca Raton, Florida.

6. Baker TS, Rickert DE (1982) Dose-dependent disposition of *n*-hexane in F-344 rats after inhalation exposure. *Fund Appl Toxicol* **2**, 226.

7. Billmaier D, Allen N, Craft B *et al.* (1974) Peripheral neuropathy in a coated fabrics plant. *J Occup Med* **16**, 665.

8. Bohlen P, Schlunegger UP, Lauppi E (1973) Uptake and distribution of hexane in rat tissues. *Toxicol Appl Pharmacol* **25**, 242.

9. Bus JS, White EL, Gillies PJ, Barrow CS (1981) Tissue distribution of *n*-hexane, methyl *n*-butyl ketone, and 2,5-hexanedione in rats after single or repeated inhalation exposure to *n*-hexane. *Drug Metab Disposition* **9**, 386.

10. Cavanagh JB, Bennetts RJ (1981) On the pattern of changes in the rat nervous system produced by 2,5-hexanediol: A topographical study by light microscopy. *Brain* **104**, 297.

11. Chang YC (1987) Neurotoxic effects of *n*-hexane on the human central nervous system: Evoked potential abnormalities in *n*-hexane polyneuropathy. *J Neurol Neurosurg Psychiat* **50**, 269.

12. Couri D, Abdel Rahman MS, Hetland LB (1978) Biotransformation of *n*-hexane and methyl *n*-butyl ketone in guinea pigs and mice. *Amer Ind Hyg Assn J* **39**, 295.

13. DeCaprio AP (1985) Molecular mechanisms of diketone neurotoxicity. *Chem-Biol Inter* **54**, 257.

14. DeCaprio AP, Briggs RG, Jackowski SJ, Kim JCS (1988) Comparative neurotoxicity and pyrrole-forming potential of 2,5-hexanedione and perdeuterio-2,5-hexanedione in the rat. *Toxicol Appl Pharmacol* **92**, 75.

15. DeCaprio AP, Fowke JH (1992) Limited and selective adduction of carboxyl-terminal lysines in the high molecular weight neurofilament proteins by 2,5-hexanedione *in vitro*. *Brain Res* **586**, 219.

16. DeCaprio AP, Olajos EJ, Weber P (1982) Covalent binding of a neurotoxic *n*-hexane metabolite: Conversion of primary amines to substituted pyrrole derivatives by 2,5-hexanedione. *Toxicol Appl Pharmacol* **65**, 440.

17. DeCaprio AP, O'Neill EA (1985) Alterations in rat axonal cytoskeletal proteins induced by *in vitro* and *in vivo* 2,5-hexanedione exposure. *Toxicol Appl Pharmacol* **78**, 235.

18. DeCaprio AP, Strominger NL, Weber P (1983) Neurotoxicity and protein binding of 2,5-hexanedione in the hen. *Toxicol Appl Pharmacol* **68**, 297.

19. DeCaprio AP, Weber P (1980) *In vitro* studies on the amino group reactivity of a neurotoxic hexacarbon solvent. *Pharmacologist* **22**, 222.

20. DiVincenzo GD, Hamilton ML, Kaplan CJ, Dedinas J (1977) Metabolic fate and disposition of C-14-labeled methyl *n*-butyl ketone in the rat. *Toxicol Appl Pharmacol* **41**, 547.

21. DiVincenzo GD, Hamilton ML, Kaplan CJ *et al.* (1978) Studies on the respiratory uptake and excretion and the skin absorption of methyl *n*-butyl ketone in humans and dogs. *Toxicol Appl Pharmacol* **44**, 593.

22. DiVincenzo GD, Kaplan CJ, Dedinas J (1976) Characterization of the metabolites of methyl *n*-butyl ketone, methyl isobutyl ketone, and methyl ethyl ketone in guinea pig serum and their clearance. *Toxicol Appl Pharmacol* **36**, 511.

23. Durham HD, Pena SDJ, Carpenter S (1983) The neurotoxins 2,5-hexanedione and acrylamide promote aggregation of intermediate filaments in cultured fibroblasts. *Muscle Nerve* **6**, 631.

24. Fedtke N, Bolt HM (1987) The relevance of 4,5-dihydroxy-2-hexanone in the excretion kinetics of *n*-hexane metabolites in rat and man. *Arch Toxicol* **61**, 131.

25. Genter St.Clair MB, Amarnath V, Moody MA *et al.* (1988) Pyrrole oxidation and protein cross-linking as necessary steps in the development of γ-diketone neuropathy. *Chem Res Toxicol* **1**, 179.

26. Gillies PJ, Norton RM, Bus JS (1981) Inhibition of sterologenesis but not glycolysis in 2,5-hexanedione-induced distal axonopathy in the rat. *Toxicol Appl Pharmacol* **59**, 287.

27. Gold BG (1987) The pathophysiology of proximal neurofilamentous giant axonal swellings: Implications for the pathogenesis of amyotrophic lateral sclerosis. *Toxicology* **46**, 125.

28. Goto I, Matsumara M, Inoue N *et al.* (1974) Toxic polyneuropathy due to glue sniffing. *J Neurol Neurosurg Psychiat* **37**, 848.

29. Graham DG (1980) Hexane neuropathy: A proposal for the pathogenesis of a hazard of occupational exposure and inhalant abuse. *Chem-Biol Inter* **32**, 339.

30. Graham DG, Anthony DC, Boekelheide K *et al.* (1982) Studies of the molecular pathogenesis of hexane neuropathy. II. Evidence that pyrrole derivatization of lysyl residues leads to protein crosslinking. *Toxicol Appl Pharmacol* **64**, 415.

31. Griffin JW, Anthony DC, Fahnestock KE *et al.* (1984) 3,4-Dimethyl-2,5-hexanedione impairs the axonal transport of neurofilament proteins. *J Neurosci* **4**, 1516.

32. Griffin JW, Fahnestock KE, Price DL, Cork LC (1983) Cytoskeletal disorganization induced by local application of β,β′-iminodipropionitrile and 2,5-hexanedione. *Ann Neurol* **14**, 55.

33. Herskowitz A, Ishii N, Schaumburg H (1971) *n*-Hexane neuropathy. A syndrome occurring as a result of industrial exposure. *N Engl J Med* **285**, 82.

34. Howd RA, Bingham LR, Steeger TM *et al.* (1982) Relation between schedules of exposure to hexane and plasma levels of 2,5-hexanedione. *Neurobehav Toxicol Teratol* **4**, 87.

35. IPCS (1991) Environmental Health Criteria 122: *n*-Hexane. World Health Organization, Geneva.

36. Johnson BL, Setzer JV, Lewis TR, Anger WK (1977) Effects of methyl *n*-butyl ketone on behavior and the nervous system. *Amer Ind Hyg Assn J* **38**, 567.

37. Jones HB, Cavanagh JB (1982) The early evolution of neurofilamentous accumulations due to 2,5-hexanediol in the optic pathways of the rat. *Neuropathol Appl Neurobiol* **8**, 289.

38. Krasavage WJ, O'Donoghue JL, DiVincenzo GD, Terhaar CJ (1980) The relative neurotoxicity of methyl *n*-butyl ketone, *n*-hexane and their metabolites. *Toxicol Appl Pharmacol* **52**, 433.

39. Lanning CL, Wilmarth KR, Abou-Donia MB (1994) *In vitro* binding of [^{14}C]2,5-hexanedione to rat neuronal cytoskeletal proteins. *Neurochem Res* **19**, 1165.

40. Lapadula DM, Irwin RD, Suwita E, Abou Donia MB (1986) Cross-linking of neurofilament proteins of rat spinal cord *in vivo* after administration of 2,5-hexanedione. *J Neurochem* **46**, 1843.

41. LoPachin RM, Lehning EJ, Stack EC *et al.* (1994) 2,5-Hexanedione alters elemental composition and water content of rat peripheral nerve myelinated axons. *J Neurochem* **63**, 2266.

42. Mendell JR, Sahenk Z, Saida K *et al.* (1977) Alterations of fast axoplasmic transport in experimental methyl *n*-butyl ketone neuropathy. *Brain Res* **133**, 107.

43. Monaco S, Autilio-Gambetti L, Lasek RJ *et al.* (1989) Experimental increase in neurofilament transport rate: Decreases in neurofilament number and in axon diameter. *J Neuropathol Exp Neurol* **48**, 23.

44. Monaco S, Wongmongkolrit T, Shearson CM *et al.* (1990) Giant axonopathy characterized by intermediate location of axonal enlargements and acceleration of neurofilament transport. *Brain Res* **519**, 73.

45. Mutti A, Falzoi M, Arfini G *et al.* (1984) *n*-Hexane metabolism in occupationally exposed workers. *Brit J Ind Med* **41**, 533.

46. Nixon RA (1992) Slow axonal transport. *Curr Opin Cell Biol* **4**, 8.

47. O'Donoghue JL (1985) Alkanes, alcohols, ketones, and ethylene oxide. In: *Neurotoxicity of Industrial and Commercial Chemicals. Vol 2.* O'Donoghue JL ed. CRC Press, Boca Raton, Florida p. 61

48. O'Donoghue JL, Krasavage WJ, DiVincenzo GD, Katz GV (1984) Further studies on ketone neurotoxicity and interactions. *Toxicol Appl Pharmacol* **72**, 201.

49. Perbellini L, Amantini MC, Brugnone F, Frontali N (1982) Urinary excretion of *n*-hexane metabolites: A comparative study in rat, rabbit, and monkey. *Arch Toxicol* **50**, 203.

50. Perbellini L, Brugnone F, Pavan I (1980) Identification of the metabolites of *n*-hexane, cyclohexane, and their isomers in men's urine. *Toxicol Appl Pharmacol* **53**, 220.

51. Pezzoli G, Strada O, Silani V *et al.* (1996) Clinical and pathobiological features of hydrocarbon-induced parkinsonism. *Ann Neurol* **40**, 922.

52. Politis MJ, Pellegrino RG, Spencer PS (1980) Ultrastructural studies of the dying-back process. 5. Axonal neurofilaments accumulate at sites of 2,5-hexanedione application: Evidence for nerve fibre dysfunction in experimental hexacarbon neuropathy. *J Neurocytol* **9**, 505.

53. Pyle SJ, Amarnath V, Graham DG, Anthony DC (1993) Decreased levels of the high molecular weight subunit of neurofilaments and accelerated neurofilament transport during the recovery phase of 2,5-hexanedione exposure. *Cell Motility Cytoskel* **26**, 133.

54. Rosenburg CK, Anthony DC, Szakal-Quin G *et al.* (1987) Hyperbaric oxygen accelerates the neurotoxicity of 2,5-hexanedione. *Toxicol Appl Pharmacol* **87**, 374.

55. Rosenberg CK, Genter MB, Szakal-Quin G *et al.* (1986) *d,l*- versus *meso*-3,4-Dimethyl-2,5-hexanedione: A morphometric study of the proximo-distal distribution of axonal swellings in the anterior root of the rat. *Toxicol Appl Pharmacol* **87**, 363.

56. Sabri MI (1984) Further observations on the *in vitro* and *in vivo* effects of 2,5-hexanedione on glyceraldehyde-3-phosphate dehydrogenase. *Arch Toxicol* **55**, 191.

57. Sabri MI, Moore CL, Spencer PS (1978) Studies on the biochemical basis of distal axonopathies. I. Inhibition of glycolysis by neurotoxic hexacarbon compounds. *J Neurochem* **32**, 683.

58. Sayre LM, Autilio Gambetti L, Gambetti P (1985) Pathogenesis of experimental giant neurofilamentous axonopathies: A unified hypothesis based on chemical modification of neurofilaments. *Brain Res Rev* **10**, 69.

59. Sayre LM, Shearson CM, Wongmongkolrit T *et al.* (1986) Structural basis of gamma-diketone neurotoxicity: Nonneurotoxicity of 3,3-dimethyl-2,5-hexanedione, a gamma-diketone incapable of pyrrole formation. *Toxicol Appl Pharmacol* **84**, 36.

60. Schaumburg HH (1985) A tale of two solvents: The neurology of *n*-hexane and toluene. In: *The Toxicology of Petroleum Hydrocarbons*. MacFarland HN, Holdsworth CE, MacGregor JA *et al.* eds. American Petroleum Institute, Washington, DC p. 328.

61. Schaumburg HH, Spencer PS (1976) Degeneration in central and peripheral nervous system produced by pure *n*-hexane: An experimental study. *Brain* **99**, 183.

62. Schaumburg HH, Spencer PS (1978) Environmental hydrocarbons produce degeneration in cat hypothalamus and optic tract. *Science* **199**, 200.

63. Shell L, Rozum M, Jortner BS, Ehrich M (1992) Neurotoxicity of acrylamide and 2,5-hexanedione in rats evaluated using a functional observational battery and pathological examination. *Neurotoxicol Teratol* **14**, 273.

64. Sickles DW, Pearson JK, Beall A, Testino A (1994) Toxic axonal degeneration occurs independent of neurofilament accumulation. *J Neurosci Res* **39**, 347.

65. Smith AG, Albers JW (1997) *n*-Hexane neuropathy due to rubber cement sniffing. *Muscle Nerve* **20**, 1445.

66. Spencer PS, Bischoff MC, Schaumburg HH (1978) On the specific molecular configuration of neurotoxic aliphatic hexacarbon compounds causing central-peripheral distal axonopathy. *Toxicol Appl Pharmacol* **44**, 17.

67. Spencer PS, Sabri MI, Schaumburg HH, Moore CL (1979) Does a defect of energy metabolism in the nerve fiber underlie axonal degeneration in polyneuropathies? *Ann Neurol* **5**, 501.

68. Spencer PS, Schaumburg HH (1975) Experimental neuropathy produced by 2,5-hexanedione—a major metabolite of the neurotoxic industrial solvent methyl *n*-butyl ketone. *J Neurol Neurosurg Psychiat* **38**, 771.

69. Spencer PS, Schaumburg HH (1977) Ultrastructural studies of the dying-back process. III. The evolution of experimental peripheral giant axonal degeneration. *J Neuropathol Exp Neurol* **36**, 276.

70. Spencer PS, Schaumburg HH (1977) Ultrastructural studies of the dying-back process. IV. Differential vulnerability of PNS and CNS fibers in experimental central-peripheral distal axonopathies. *J Neuropathol Exp Neurol* **36**, 300.

71. Spencer PS, Schaumburg HH, Raleigh RL, Terhaar CJ (1975) Nervous system degeneration produced by the industrial solvent methyl *n*-butyl ketone. *Arch Neurol* **32**, 219.

72. Spencer PS, Schaumburg HH, Sabri MI, Veronesi B (1980) The enlarging view of hexacarbon neurotoxicity. *CRC Crit Rev Toxicol* **7**, 279.

73. Suwita E, Nomeir AA, Abou-Donia MB (1987) Disposition, pharmacokinetics, and metabolism of a dermal dose of [^{14}C]2,5-hexanedione in hens. *Drug Metab Disposition* **15**, 779.

74. Takeuchi Y (1993) *n*-Hexane polyneuropathy in Japan—a review of *n*-hexane poisoning and its preventive measures. *Environ Res* **62**, 76.

75. Toftgård R, Haaparanta T, Eng L, Halpert J (1986) Rat lung and liver microsomal cytochrome P-450 isozymes involved in the hydroxylation of *n*-hexane. *Biochem Pharmacol* **35**, 3733.

76. Veronesi B, Peterson ER, Bornstein MB, Spencer PS (1983) Ultrastructural studies of the dying-back process. VI. Examination of nerve fibers undergoing giant axonal degeneration in organotypic culture. *J Neuropathol Exp Neurol* **42**, 153.

77. Veulemans H, VanVlem E, Janssens H et al. (1982) Experimental human exposure to *n*-hexane. *Int Arch Occup Environ Health* **49**, 251.

78. Watson DF, Fittro KP, Hoffman PN, Griffin JW (1991) Phosphorylation-related immunoreactivity and the rate of transport of neurofilaments in chronic 2,5-hexanedione intoxication. *Brain Res* **539**, 103.

79. Zhu M, Spink DC, Yan B et al. (1994) Formation and structure of crosslinking and monomeric pyrrole autoxidation products in 2,5-hexanedione-treated amino acids, peptides, and protein. *Chem Res Toxicol* **7**, 551.

CASE REPORT

A 22-year-old female worked long hours in a small, poorly ventilated factory. She handled rags saturated with a solution containing n-*hexane and inhaled large amounts of* n-*hexane vapor for 2 years before developing anorexia, weight loss, and a cramping sensation in the hands. Two weeks later, she noticed cramping in the calves and an unsteady gait that was improved by the use of high-heeled boots. Two months later, her legs felt much weaker and she noted a sensation of numbness of the toes. These symptoms steadily increased in intensity over the next 2 months until she was unable to walk to work, when she was admitted to a hospital. Neurological examination revealed no abnormalities of cranial nerves or mental status. There was diffuse, symmetrical, distal, flaccid weakness of all extremities. The intrinsic muscles of the hands and dorsiflexors of the feet were 2/5 on the U.K. Medical Research Council (MRC) scale. Proximal limb muscles were 3/5 MRC scale, and abdominal muscles were 3/5 MRC scale. The vital capacity was normal. No tendon reflexes could be elicited. There was a moderate to severe loss of pin sensation in a stocking-and-glove distribution, with only a slight diminution in position and vibration sense. After 4 months in this state, she gradually began to improve, was discharged from the hospital, and steadily regained strength over the next 18 months. Since that time, she noticed no further improvement of strength and began to walk again, but in an abnormal fashion. Neurological examination, 2 years after discharge from the hospital, revealed that she walked with a slow, stiff-legged, waddling gait; could stand on a narrow base; and Romberg's sign was not present. Rapid alternating movements of the upper extremity were performed well, as were finger-to-nose movements. Distal and proximal upper-extremity muscles were 4/5 MRC scale, distal lower-extremity muscles were 4/5 MRC scale. Many large, proximal lower-extremity muscle groups were 4/5 MRC scale (hamstrings, glutei, quadriceps). She was unable to rise from a chair without using her hands for support, and unable to sit up from a supine position without rolling to one side and using her upper extremities for assistance. There was a moderate diminution of pinprick and touch sensation below the ankle and wrist, but position and vibration sensation were normal. The tendon reflexes were 2 in the upper extremities and 3 in the lower extremities. Babinski's sign was present bilaterally. There was increased resistance to rapid movement of the lower extremities, with a spastic catch.*

This patient demonstrated many of the features usually associated with toxic axonal neuropathies. However, she developed a neuropathy of unusual severity with quadriparesis and near-total paralysis of the distal extremities because of the prolonged, high-level exposure to n-hexane. The motor impairment was far more severe than the sensory loss. This has been a consistent feature, along with an early loss of the Achilles reflex, in the majority of cases of n-hexane neuropathy. Several cases with extreme degrees of n-hexane distal axonopathy have, upon recovery, demonstrated lower extremity spasticity. Spasticity reflects damage to the corticospinal tracts in the CNS. These signs of CNS disease were initially masked by the peripheral neuropathy and only emerged when the nerves regenerated.*

Histrionicotoxins

Alexander Storch
Albert C. Ludolph

HISTRIONICOTOXIN D
$C_{19}H_{29}NO$

Gephyrotoxin; [1R-(1α,3aβ,5aα,6α(Z),9aα)]-Dodecahydro-6-(2-penten-4-ynyl)pyrrolo[1,2-a]-quinoline-1-ethanol

NEUROTOXICITY RATING
Experimental
A   Nicotinic receptor-gated channel blocker

Histrionicotoxins represent a class of compounds with a unique spiropiperidine ring system and side chains with acetylenic, olefinic, and allenic groups. Histrionicotoxin and dihydroisohistrionicotoxin were isolated from skin extracts of the Colombian arrow poison frog *Dendrobates histrionicus*, and the chemical structures were elucidated in 1971 (7). Several histrionicotoxins were subsequently isolated and structurally defined (3,4). Extensive studies of skin extracts of neotropical frogs revealed that histrionicotoxins occur in all genera of the family Dendrobatidae (except *Minyobates*), and in the Madagascan frogs *Mantella aurantiaca* and *M. madagascariensis* (family Ranidae, subfamily Mantellinae) (6). The histrionicotoxins are stored in cutaneous granule glands and secreted under stress. Physical and chemical properties are described by Daly (3).

Histrionicotoxins have little mammalian toxicity. After subcutaneous (s.c.) injection into white mice (5 mg/kg), slight difficulties of locomotion and hypersensitivity to touch develop and persist for more then 3 h; recovery is gradual (7). Dihydrohistrionicotoxin (5 mg/kg), applied s.c. into mice, induces piloerection, prostration, and tachycardia for 5 h, followed by slow recovery (7). At a dose of 40 μg/mouse (s.c.), dihydrohistrionicotoxin had virtually no detectable effect (5).

Histrionicotoxins suppress cholinergic signal transmission in *in vitro* preparations of frog and murine neuromuscular junctions, *Torpedo* electroplax, and insect motoneuron (3,8,10,11). Binding, fluorescence, and pharmacological studies with histrionicotoxin derivatives showed that they are noncompetive inhibitors of muscular and neuronal nicotinic acetylcholine receptors and bind within the pore of the receptor–channel complex (1,3,9). Furthermore, histrionicotoxins are noncompetitive muscarinergic antagonists in neural cell lines, probably by interaction at a nonreceptor site (3). There are reports suggesting that histrionicotoxins bind competitively to the antagonistic binding site of atrial muscarinic acetylcholine receptors (2,3). In addition, histrionicotoxins are weak blockers of the voltage-dependent sodium channel in a manner reminiscent of local anesthetics, and they reduce conductances of the potassium channel in a time- and concentration-dependent manner. Structure–activity profiles of the histrionicotoxins at the various action sites are different (3). There are no reports of toxicity in humans.

REFERENCES

1. Albuquerque EX, Adler, M, Spivak CE, Aguayo L (1980) Mechanism of nicotinic channel activation and blockade. *Ann N Y Acad Sci* **358**, 204.

2. Cremo C, Schimerlik MI (1983) Histrionicotoxin and alkylguanidine interactions with the solubilized and membrane-bound muscarinic acetylcholine receptor from porcine atria. *Arch Biochem Biophys* **224**, 506.

3. Daly JW (1982) Alkaloids of neotropical poison frogs (*Dendrobatidae*). *Prog Chem Org Nat Prod* **41**, 206.

4. Daly JW (1995) The chemistry of poisons in amphibian skin. *Proc Nat Acad Sci USA* **92**, 9.

5. Daly JW, Brown GB, Mensah-Dwumah M (1978) Classification of skin alkaloids from neotropical poison-dart frogs (*Dendrobatidae*). *Toxicon* **16**, 163.

6. Daly JW, Highet RJ, Myers CW (1984) Occurrence of skin alkaloids in non-dendrobatid frogs from Brazil (Bufonidae), Australia (Myobatrachidae) and Madagascar (Mantellinae). *Toxicon* **22**, 905.

7. Daly JW, Karle I, Myers CW *et al.* (1971) Histrionicotoxins: Roentgen-ray analysis of the novel allenic and acetylenic spiroalkaloids isolated from a Colombian frog, *Dendrobates histrionicus. Proc Nat Acad Sci USA* **68**, 1870.

8. Glavinovic M, Henry JL, Kato G *et al.* (1974) Histrionicotoxin: Effects on some central and peripheral excitable cells. *Can J Physiol Pharmacol* **52**, 1220.

9. Johnson DA, Nuss JM (1994) The histrionicotoxin-sensitive ethidium binding site is located outside of the transmembrane domain of the nicotinic acetylcholine receptor: A fluorescence study. *Biochemistry* **33**, 9070.

10. Lapa AJ, Albuquerque EX, Sarvey JM *et al.* (1975) Effects of histrionicotoxin on the chemosensitive and electrical properties of skeletal muscle. *Exp Neurol* **47**, 558.

11. Mensah-Dwumah M, Daly JW (1978) Pharmacological activity of alkaloids from poison-dart frogs (*Dendrobatidae*). *Toxicon* **16**, 189.

Holothurins and Holotoxins

Peter S. Spencer

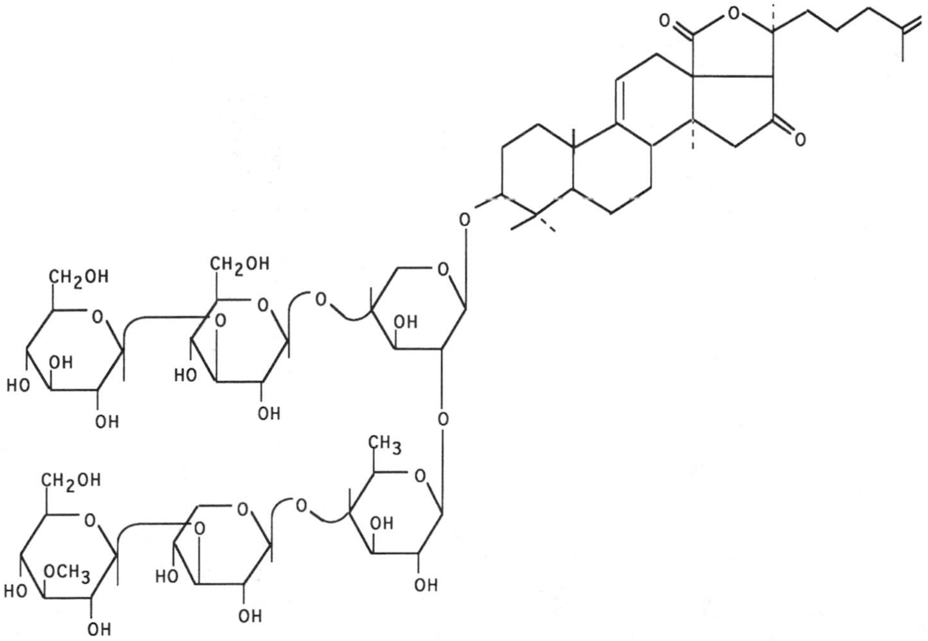

HOLOTOXIN

NEUROTOXICITY RATING

Experimental

B   Neuromuscular blockade (holothurin)

Holothurins and holotoxins are glycosidic triterpene saponins isolated from sea cucumbers (Holothurioidea) that inhabit tropical and subtropical waters and coral reefs (1). Holothurinogen is the prototypical aglycone (8). Holothurin A and B, which differ from each other mainly in the carbohydrate moiety, are found in the genera *Holothuria* and *Actinopyga* (9); they are toxic to invertebrates, fish, and mammals, and have antifungal and antiparasitic properties (11). Holotoxins are found in *Stichopus japonicus* (Far Eastern trepang), which is a highly valued food item (9).

The intravenous mouse LD_{100} for crude holothurin is 0.2 mg/animal; other routes require smaller amounts of the toxin (9). Toxicity is said to result from both hemolysis and irreversible blockade of neuromuscular transmission (3,6). Triterpene glycosides reportedly "inhibit" both Na^+, K^+-adenosine triphosphatase (ATPase) and Ca^{2+}, Mg^{2+}-ATPase (4). Holothurin A increases the resting sodium permeability of the squid axon in a tetrodotoxin-insensitive manner (2). Holothurin A stimulates calmodulin-deficient 3′,5′-phosphodiesterase in bovine brain tissue (10).

The visceral, toxin-containing liquids secreted by these echinoderms are primarily toxic to their prey. They may irritate human skin and mucous membranes but do not cause neurological disease (9).

The detergent properties of holothurins cause membrane disruption. Holothurin A forms a complex with cholesterol in artificial membranes (5); four toxin molecules are incorporated into *de novo* membrane channels measuring approximately 2.5 nm in diameter (7). Cholesterol-free liposomes are not lysed by these saponins (12).

REFERENCES

1. Chanley JD, Mezzetti T, Sobotka H (1966) The holothurinogenins. *Tetrahedron* **22**, 1857.
2. de Groof RC, Narahashi T (1976) The effects of holothurin A on the resting membrane potential and conductance of squid axon. *Eur J Pharmacol* **36**, 337.
3. Friess SL (1972) Mode of action of marine saponins on neuromuscular tissues. *Fed Proc* **31**, 1146
4. Gorshkov BA, Gorschkova IA, Stonik VA, Elyakov GB (1982) Effect of marine glycosides on adenosinetriphosphatase activity. *Toxicon* **20**, 655.
5. Likhatzkaya GN, Yarovaya TP, Rudnev VS et al. (1985) Formation of the complex between holothurin A triterpene glycoside and cholesterol in liposomal membranes. *Biophysica* **30**, 358.
6. Nigrelli RF, Jakowska S (1960) Effects of holothurin, a steroid saponin from the Bahamanian sea cucumber (*Actinopyga agassizii*) on various biological systems. *Ann NY Acad Sci* **90**, 884.
7. Popov AN, Rovin YG, Likhatskaya GN et al. (1982) Peculiarities of the action of triterpene glycoside holothurin A on bilayer lipid-sterol membrane. *Dokl Akad Nausk USSR* **264**, 987.
8. Russell FE (1967) Pharmacology of animal venoms. *Clin Pharmacol Ther* **8**, 849.
9. Stonig VA, Elyakov GB (1988) Structure and biologic activities of sponge and sea cucumber toxins. In: *Handbook of Natural Toxins. Vol 3. Marine Toxins and Venoms.* Tu AT ed. Marcel Dekker, New York p. 107.
10. Vig PJ, Mehrotra BD, Desaiah D (1990) Holothurin: an activator of bovine brain 3′,5′-phosphodiesterase. *Res Commun Chem Pathol Pharmacol* **67**, 419.
11. Walker MJA (1977) Coelenterate and echinoderm toxins: Mechanisms and actions. In: *Handbook of Natural Toxins. Vol 3. Marine Toxins and Venoms.* Tu AT ed. Marcel Dekker, New York p. 279.
12. Yu BS, Jo IH (1984) Interaction of sea cucumber saponins with multilamellar liposomes. *Chem Biol Interact* **52**, 185.

Hydralazine

Glen Kisby

HYDRALAZINE
$C_8H_8N_4$

1(2*H*)-Phthalazinone hydrazone; 1-Hydrazinophthalazine

NEUROTOXICITY RATING

Clinical

B   Peripheral neuropathy (pyridoxine deficiency)

Hydralazine is a white to off-white, odorless, crystalline powder that is used commercially as the hydrochloride salt for the treatment of moderate to severe hypertension (12), chronic congestive heart failure (5), pre-eclampsia and eclampsia (16), and more recently in conjunction with antineoplastic agents to enhance tumor cytotoxicity (4). Long-term treatment of patients with hydralazine induces a syndrome in humans similar to lupus erythematosus.

Hydralazine is an antihypertensive agent that acts by direct relaxation of vascular smooth muscle (10). The incidence of adverse effects with hydralazine therapy is high. Headache, palpitation, anorexia, nausea, dizziness, and sweating are common. In animals, the predominant side effects induced by toxic levels of hydralazine hydrochloride are anemia and a drug-induced lupus erythematosus.

Oral doses ranging from 20–120 mg/kg hydralazine hydrochloride have been reported to produce a low incidence of cleft palate and minor bone malformations (2). The deleterious effect of hydralazine on bones may be caused by the drug's inhibition of collagen synthesis. Hydralazine inhibits the hydroxylation steps in collagen synthesis and collagen secretion in *in-vitro* studies of chick tibia (21).

Hydralazine is eliminated rapidly in urine, the main route of excretion (>70% of absorbed dose); feces represent a minor route of excretion (<10%) in humans. Hydralazine undergoes extensive metabolism by acetylation, the major pathway for hydralazine clearance (23,32,33). Acetylation, *via* hepatic N-acetyl transferase of hydralazine, is subject to slow or rapid acetylation, a genetic polymorphism (9). The plasma half-life of hydralazine ranges from 2.0–7.8 h in both rapid and slow acetylators. However, plasma concentrations following intravenous administration are similar in both groups (23) and lower in rapid than in slow acetylators following oral administration (23,32). Slow acetylators can be identified by their higher plasma levels and rapid acetylators by their lower plasma concentrations after oral intake of hydralazine.

Acetyl hydrazine [1-(2-acetylhydrazino)phthalazine] is reportedly the major metabolite in rats, guinea pigs, and pigeons (8). Excretion of hydralazine and its metabolites is rapid (75% of administered drug in the urine in 24 h) in rats and rabbits. Several metabolites have been detected in rat and rabbit urine including 1-hydralazine-O-glucuronide (40%–50%), N-acetyl-1-hydrazine (25%–30%), and unchanged hydralazine (15%) (19). The actual acetylation metabolite was 3-methyl-S-triazolo(3,4-a)phthalazine (11).

A single subcutaneous injection of hydrazine and its derivatives were given alone and in combination with pyridoxine hydrochloride to Swiss mice (27). The convulsive, toxic, and lethal effects of the hydrazine derivatives were successfully prevented by administering pyridoxine hydrochloride before and/or after injection. Similar studies with slow and rapid N-acetylator rabbits demonstrate that N-acetylation of hydrazine derivatives (*e.g.*, hydralazine, isoniazid) is an important detoxication step to prevent hydrazine-induced CNS toxicity (13). The genetic background of animals is therefore an important factor in determining the susceptibility to hydralazine-induced neurotoxicity.

The neurotoxic effects of hydralazine are reversible with discontinuation of the drug or pyridoxine treatment and, therefore, have not been evaluated *in vitro*. In contrast, numerous *in vitro* studies with hydralazine have been conducted to investigate drug-induced lupus erythematosus (14), genotoxic properties (7,18,30), and metabolism to free radicals (26,29,31).

Aside from occasional headache early during the course of hydralazine treatment, there have been no reports of CNS toxicity. Occasional instances of peripheral neuropathy have occurred (15,20,22). In one report, a 61-year-old well-nourished Japanese male developed difficulty in walking, numbness, and weakness of both lower extremities following daily administration of hydralazine (150 mg) for 1 month (28). His neurological symptoms were aggravated when the dosage was increased to 300 mg daily. The symptoms subsided, as in previous studies (15,20,22), following a course of reduced dosage and/or withdrawal of hydralazine with pyridoxine supplementation. The neurological effects of hydralazine were remarkable given that most (88.5%) Japanese are rapid acetylators. Following a challenge dose of isoniazid, the patient was determined to be a slow acetylator.

Hydralazine-induced peripheral neuropathy is probably mediated by pyridoxine (vitamin B_6) deficiency (1,15,17, 22). Presumably, hydralazine reacts with pyridoxine to form a hydrazine-pyridoxal hydrazone that inactivates the coenzyme and facilitates its urinary excretion (22). Cornish (6) demonstrated that only primary hydrazines react with pyridoxal phosphate and produce neurotoxicity. Nonnervous tissue toxicity of hydralazine, like that of other hydrazine derivatives, is probably mediated through the production of free radicals and reactive oxygen species (3,24,25).

REFERENCES

1. Argov S, Mastaglia FL (1979) Drug-induced peripheral neuropathies. *Brit Med J* 1, 663.

2. Association of the British Pharmaceutical Industry (1979) Data Sheet Compendium, 1979–80. Pharmind Publications Ltd, Apresoline, London.

3. Augusto O, Du Plessis LR, Weingrill CLV (1985) Spin-trapping of methyl radical in the oxidative metabolism of 1,2-dimethylhydrazine. *Biochem Biophys Res Commun* 126, 853.

4. Chaplin DJ (1989) Hydralazine-induced tumor hypoxia: A potential target for cancer chemotherapy. *J Nat Cancer Inst* 81, 618.

5. Cohn JN, Johnson G, Ziesche S *et al.* (1991) A comparison of enalapril with hydralazine-isosorbide dinitrate in the treatment of chronic congestive heart failure. *N Engl J Med* 325, 303.

6. Cornish HH (1969) The role of vitamin B_6 in the toxicity of hydrazines. *Ann N Y Acad Sci* 166, 136.

7. De Flora S, Zanacchi S, Bennicelli C *et al.* (1982) *In vivo* and *in vitro* genotoxicity of three antihypertensive hydrazine derivatives (hydralazine, dihydralazine, and endralazine). *Environ Mutagen* 4, 605.

8. Douglass CD, Hogan R (1959) A metabolite of 1-hydrazinophthalazine (hydralazine). *Proc Soc Exp Biol Med* **100**, 446.

9. Evans DAP (1968) Genetic variations in the acetylation of isoniazid and other drugs. *Ann N Y Acad Sci* **151**, 723.

10. Gilman AG, Goodman LS, Gilman A (1980) Hydralazine. In: *Goodman and Gilman's The Pharmacological Basis of Therapeutics. 6th Ed.* Macmillan, New York p. 799.

11. Haegele KD, Skrdlant HB, Robie NW *et al.* (1976) Determination of hydralazine and its metabolites by gas chromatography-mass spectrometry. *J Chromatogr* **126**, 517.

12. Harvey SC (1975) Cardiovascular drugs. In: *Remington's Pharmaceutical Sciences. 15th Ed.* Osol A ed. Mack Publishing Co, Easton, Pennsylvania.

13. Hein DW, Weber WW (1984) Relationship between *N*-acetylator phenotype and susceptibility toward hydralazine-induced lethal central nervous system toxicity in the rabbit. *J Pharmacol Exp Ther* **228**, 588.

14. Hofstra AH (1994) Metabolism of hydralazine: Relevance to drug-induced lupus. *Drug Metab Rev* **26**, 485.

15. Kirkendall WM, Page EB (1958) Polyneuritis occuring during hydralazine therapy. *J Amer Med Assn* **167**, 427.

16. Kirshon B, Wasserstrum N, Cotton DB (1991) Should continuous hydralazine infusions be utilized in severe pregnancy-induced hypertension? *Amer J Perinatol* **8**, 206.

17. Koch-Weser J (1976) Hydralazine. *N Engl J Med* **295**, 320.

18. Mathison BH, Murphy SE, Shank RC (1994) Hydralazine and other hydrazine derivatives and the formation of DNA adducts. *Toxicol Appl Pharmacol* **127**, 91.

19. McIsaac WM, Kanda M (1964) The metabolism of 1-hydrazinophthalazine. *J Pharmacol Exp Ther* **143**, 7.

20. Moyer JH (1953) Hydralazine (apresoline) hydrochloride. *Arch Intern Med* **91**, 419.

21. Rapaka RS, Parr RW, Liu T-Z, Bhatnagar RS (1977) Biochemical basis of skeletal defects induced by hydralazine: Inhibition of collagen synthesis and secretion in embryonic chicken cartilage *in vitro*. *Teratology* **15**, 185.

22. Raskin NH, Fishman RA (1965) Pyridoxine-deficiency neuropathy due to hydralazine. *N Engl J Med* **273**, 1182.

23. Reidenberg MM, Drayer D, DeMarco AL, Bello CT (1973) Hydralazine elimination in man. *Clin Pharmacol Ther* **14**, 970.

24. Sinha BK (1983) Enzymatic activation of hydrazine derivatives. *J Biol Chem* **258**, 796.

25. Sinha BK, Motten AG (1982) Oxidative metabolism of hydralazine. Evidence for nitrogen centered radicals formation. *Biochem Biophys Res Commun* **105**, 1044.

26. Sinha BK, Patterson MA (1983) Free radical metabolism of hydralazine binding and degradation of nucleic acids. *Biochem Pharmacol* **32**, 3279.

27. Toth B, Erickson J (1977) Reversal of the toxicity of hydrazine and analogues by pyridoxine hydrochloride. *Toxicology* **7**, 31.

28. Tsujimoto G, Horai Y, Ishizaki T, Itoh K (1981) Hydralazine-induced peripheral neuropathy seen in a Japanese slow acetylator patient. *Brit J Clin Pharmacol* **11**, 622.

29. Weglarz L, Bartosz G. (1991) Hydralazine stimulates production of oxygen free radical in Eagle's medium and cultured fibroblasts. *Free Radical Biol Med* **11**, 149.

30. Williams GM, Mazue G, McQueen CA (1980) Genotoxicity of the antihypertensive drugs hydralazine and dihydralazine. *Science* **210**, 329.

31. Yamamoto K, Kawanishi S (1991) Free radical production and site-specific DNA damage induced by hydralazine in the presence of metal ions or peroxidase/hydrogen peroxide. *Biochem Pharmacol* **41**, 905.

32. Zacest R, Koch-Weser J (1972) Relation of hydralazine plasma concentration to dosage and hypotensive action. *Clin Pharmacol Ther* **13**, 420.

33. Zimmer H, McManus J, Novinson T *et al.* (1970) A major metabolite of 1-hydrazinophthalazine. *Arzneim Forsch* **20**, 1586.

Hydrazine

Glen Kisby

$$H_2N — NH_2$$

HYDRAZINE
H_4N_2

NEUROTOXICITY RATING

Clinical

A   Acute encephalopathy (agitation, seizures, sedation, tremor)

B   Peripheral neuropathy

Experimental

A   Seizure disorder

Hydrazine is a clear, colorless hygroscopic liquid used primarily in the manufacture of rocket propellants; lesser amounts are used in the manufacture of agricultural chemicals (*e.g.*, maleic hydrazide), plastic foams, soldering fluxes, herbicides (*e.g.*, 3-amino-1,2,4-triazole), and medicinals (*e.g.*, the antitubercular agent isoniazid), and in the treatment of boiler water (corrosion inhibitor) (24). The hydrazine derivative 1,1-dimethylhydrazine is used to combine gases, to develop photographs, as an intermediate in chemical synthesis (a strong reducing agent), and to regulate plant growth. 1,2-Dimethylhydrazine is used as a research chemical to study colon carcinogenesis and has no known commercial use. Hydrazine is acutely toxic to the liver, kidney, and CNS and has been reported to increase the incidence of tumors in liver and lung of rodents (17).

Inhalation, oral, and dermal studies in animals indicate that hydrazines are rapidly absorbed into the blood. Hydrazine and its derivatives are rapidly absorbed (*via* passive diffusion) through the skin of animals and can be detected in femoral blood within 30 sec (18,19). The half-life (indwelling catheters) of 16–64 mg/kg hydrazine in rats is 0.74–26.9 h (22). After absorption, hydrazines are readily distributed to tissues without preferential accumulation at any specific site. *In vitro* and *in vivo* studies demonstrate that hydrazines are metabolized by several enzymatic and nonenzymatic pathways. Hydrazines are rapidly metabolized by rat liver microsomes *in vitro* and require oxygen, reduced nicotinamide adenine dinucleotide phosphate, and active enzyme for maximal activity. Cytochrome P-450 inducers (*e.g.*, phenobarbital, rifampicin) or inhibitors (*e.g.*, metyrapone, piperonyl butoxide) which increase or decrease the metabolism of hydrazine attenuate or potentiate its toxicity, respectively. In one study, people with a slow-acetylator genotype were found to be unusually susceptible to the toxic effects of hydrazine (2). Hydrazine was shown to accumulate in the plasma of slow-acetylator patients treated with isoniazid or the antihypertensive agent hydralazine when compared with patients with a rapid-acetylator genotype.

No information is available on the excretion of hydrazine by the inhalation, dermal, or oral route in humans. Forty-eight hours after a 1-h exposure to 10–500 ppm hydrazine, 8%–29 % of the dose was excreted in the urine of rats as unchanged hydrazine, acetyl hydrazine, and diacetyl hydrazine (10). Higher concentrations (19%–46%) were found in the urine of rats administered a single oral dose of 2.9–81 mg/kg hydrazine (13). A single dermal exposure to 96–480 mg/kg hydrazine and 300–1800 mg/kg 1,1-dimethylhydrazine resulted in low concentrations (70 μg/ml and 600 μg/ml, respectively) of the agents in the urine of dogs (18,19). Findings from these limited animal studies indicate that hydrazine and its metabolites are excreted principally in the urine and expired air. Furthermore, hydrazines are readily cleared from the body and, therefore, levels in various tissues are usually not detectable after 24 h.

Studies of the neurological effects of hydrazines and derivatives in animals are limited to those that received the agent by inhalation or transdermally. Inhalation studies indicate that hydrazines are neurotoxic to animals. After 3 days of intermittent exposure to 25 ppm 1,1-dimethylhy-drazine, dogs developed depression, ataxia, salivation, emesis, and seizures. These effects were not observed in dogs exposed to 5 ppm for 26 weeks. Tonic convulsions were noted in one of eight dogs exposed continuously to 1 ppm hydrazine for 6 months (8), but were not observed in any dogs exposed to 0.2 ppm. Tremors were observed occasionally in rats and mice exposed continuously to 75 ppm 1,1-dimethylhydrazine (16). Mild convulsions were noted in 3 of 13 dogs receiving a single dermal dose of 300–1800 mg/kg 1,1-dimethylhydrazine (18). Similarly, convulsions were noted in 3 of 25 dogs administered a single dermal dose of 96–480 mg/kg hydrazine (18). In contrast to inhalation exposure, large dermal exposures to hydrazine or its derivatives are needed to induce CNS neurotoxicity.

There are no known *in vitro* studies examining the neurotoxic properties of hydrazine or its derivatives. However, there are numerous *in vitro* studies examining the metabolism, genotoxicity, and production of free radicals from hydrazine and its derivatives.

Human exposure to hydrazine and its derivatives usually occurs in the workplace during its manufacture or in the vicinity of aerospace facilities, industrial facilities, or hazardous waste sites where contamination has been detected. Humans may also be exposed to small amounts of these chemicals through use of tobacco products.

The liver and CNS are the primary targets in humans following inhalation, oral, and dermal exposures to hydrazine and 1,1-dimethylhydrazine. Inhalation exposure to hydrazine is limited to several case studies. Acute exposure to an undetermined concentration of a hydrazine/1,1-dimethylhydrazine mixture in air resulted in trembling, twitching, clonic movements, hyperactive reflexes, and weakness in two subjects (5,24). Nausea, vomiting, and tremors were observed in a worker exposed to undetermined levels of hydrazine in air once a week for 6 months (20). Difficulties in concentration, comprehension, memory, and task performance, as well as changes in mood status, were noted in a technician occupationally exposed to an undetermined concentration of hydrazine in air (15). Slow gradual improvement was noted in one case after the individual was removed from exposure. Although limited, these studies suggest that inhalation exposure to hydrazine and 1,1-dimethylhydrazine can adversely affect the human CNS.

Ingestion of hydrazine (estimated between a mouthful and a cupful) resulted in several neurological effects, including episodes of violent behavior, ataxia, coma, convulsions, hypesthesia of the hands, and paresthesia of the arms and legs (14). Confusion, lethargy, restlessness, paresthesia, and neurogenic atrophy were reported in a 24-year-old male who swallowed a mouthful of hydrazine (7).

Hydrazine has been used as a chemotherapeutic agent in cancer patients. Neurological side effects were observed in some cancer patients (4%–50%) treated with 0.2–0.7 mg/kg/day hydrazine sulfate for intermediate durations. For the most part, the neurological effects were relatively mild (lethargy, nausea, vomiting, dizziness, excitement, insomnia); however, two studies reported paresthesia, sensorimotor abnormalities, and "polyneuritis" (6,11). The appearance of more serious effects in these two studies may be related to increased exposure duration. For example, peripheral nerve effects developed only in patients receiving uninterrupted treatment with hydrazine for 2–6 months. The treatment duration used in two separate studies (3,21), which was <2 months in both, may have been sufficiently short to prevent the development of more serious neurological effects. A limitation to the significance of these findings was the poor health of these patients prior to hydrazine exposure; some of the observed effects may therefore be attributable to the underlying disease. Taken together, however, these studies suggest that the nervous system is a target of hydrazine in humans after oral exposure.

Dermal exposure to hydrazines is limited to two case studies. A man who suffered burns during an industrial hydrazine explosion became comatose 14 h after the explosion (9). Rapid recovery from the coma was facilitated by pyridoxine treatment. Another man who suffered burns during an industrial 1,1-dimethylhydrazine explosion exhibited narcosis and abnormal electroencephalogram within 40 h of exposure (4); recovery was also facilitated by pyridoxine treatment. Several months after the incident, the worker developed peripheral nerve dysfunction.

There are at least two general mechanisms by which hydrazine and its derivatives can induce toxicity: a methylcarbonium ion intermediate or free radicals. The first mechanism involves the reaction of a methylcarbonium hydrazine or 1,1-dimethylhydrazine with endogenous α-keto acids such as vitamin B_6 (pyridoxine). Hydrazones of pyridoxine are formed with hydrazine or 1,1-dimethylhydrazine; the inactivated metabolites are excreted, thereby producing a pyridoxine deficiency and neurological effects. Pyridoxine has been successfully used in treating neurological manifestations in humans exposed to hydrazine or 1,1-dimethylhydrazine (4,9). Moreover, pyridoxine in some cases can abolish the lethal and neurological effects induced in animals treated with hydrazine and 1,1-dimethylhydrazine.

The second mechanism involves the generation of free radical intermediates. Free radicals have been detected during the metabolism of hydrazines *in vitro* (1,12). *In vitro* studies demonstrate that glutathione is an effective scavenger of free radicals produced by the metabolism of 1,1-dimethylhydrazine and 1,2-dimethylhydrazine (23). Interestingly, agents such as disulfiram that inhibit the bioactivation of hydrazine derivatives by cytochrome P-450 2E1 are equally effective as free-radical scavengers in protecting tissue from cytotoxicity. The exact role of free-radical intermediates in hydrazine-induced neurotoxicity is not known.

REFERENCES

1. Augusto O, Du Plessis LR, Weingrill CLV (1985) Spin-trapping of methyl radical in the oxidative metabolism of 1,2-dimethylhydrazine. *Biochem Biophys Res Commun* **126**, 853.
2. Blair IA, Tinoco RM, Brodie MJ (1985) Plasma hydrazine concentrations in man after isoniazid and hydralazine administration. *Hum Toxicol* **4**, 195.
3. Chlebowski RT, Herber D, Richardson B (1984) Influence of hydrazine sulfate on abnormal carbohydrate metabolism in cancer patients with weight loss. *Cancer Res* **44**, 857.
4. Dhennin C, Vesin L, Feauvequx J (1988) Burns and the toxic effects of a derivative of hydrazine. *Burns* **2**, 130.
5. Frierson WB (1965) Use of pyridoxine HCl in acute hydrazine and UDMH intoxication. *Ind Med Surg* 650.
6. Gershanovich ML, Danova LA, Kondratyev VB (1976) Clinical data on the antitumor activity of hydrazine sulfate. *Cancer Treatment Rep* **7**, 933.
7. Harati Y, Niakan E (1986) Hydrazine toxicity, pyridoxine therapy, and peripheral neuropathy. *Ann Intern Med* **5**, 728.
8. Haun CC, Kinkead ER (1973) Chronic inhalation toxicity of hydrazine. U.S. Department of Commerce, Springfield, VA.
9. Kirklin JK, Watson M, Bondoc CC (1976) Treatment of hydrazine-induced coma with pyridoxine. *N Engl J Med* **17**, 938.
10. Llewellyn BM, Keller WC, Olson CT (1986) Urinary metabolites of hydrazine in male Fischer 344 rats following inhalation or intravenous exposure. *AAMRL-TR-86-025.*
11. Ochoa M, Wittes RE, Krakoff IH (1975) Trial of hydrazine sulfate (NSC-150014) in patients with cancer. *Cancer Chemother Rep* **59**, 1151.
12. Ortiz de Montellano PR, Augusto O, Viola F, Kunze KL (1983) Carbon radicals in the metabolism of alkyl hydrazines. *J Biol Chem* **258**, 8623.
13. Preece NE, Forrow S, Ghatineh S (1992) Determination of hydrazine in biofluids by capillary gas chromatography with nitrogen-sensitive or mass spectrometric detection. *J Chromatogr Biomed Appl* **573**, 227.
14. Reid FJ (1965) Hydrazine poisoning. *Brit Med J* **5472**, 1246.
15. Richter ED, Gal A, Bitchatchi E (1992) Residual neurobehavioral impairment in a water technician exposed to hydrazine-containing mixtures. *Isr J Med Sci* **28**, 598.

16. Rinehart WE, Donait E, Green EA (1960) The sub-acute and chronic toxicity of 1,1-dimethylhydrazine vapor. *Ind Hyg J* **122**, 207.

17. Shank RC (1983) Evidence for indirect genetic damage as methylation of DNA guanine in response to cytotoxicity. In: *Developments in the Science and Practice of Toxicology*. Hayes AW, Schnell RC, Miya TS eds. Elsevier, Amsterdam p. 145.

18. Smith EB, Clark DA (1971) Absorption of unsymmetrical dimethylhydrazine (UDMH) through canine skin. *Toxicol Appl Pharmacol* **18**, 649.

19. Smith EB, Clark DA (1972) Absorption of hydrazine through canine skin. *Toxicol Appl Pharmacol* **21**, 186.

20. Sotaniemi E, Hirvonen J, Isomaki H (1971) Hydrazine toxicity in the human. *Ann Clin Res* **3**, 30.

21. Spremulli E, Wampler GL, Regelson W (1979) Clinical study of hydrazine sulfate in advanced cancer patients. *Cancer Chemother Pharmacol* **3**, 121.

22. Springer DL, Krivak BM, Broderick DJ (1981) Metabolic fate of hydrazine. *J Toxicol Environ Health* **8**, 21.

23. Tomasi A, Albano E, Botti B (1987) Detection of free radical intermediates in the oxidative metabolism of carcinogenic hydrazine derivatives. *Toxicol Pathol* **15**, 178.

24. U.S. Department of Health and Human Services (1994) *Toxicological Profile for Hydrazines: Draft for Public Comment*. Life Systems, Inc, Atlanta, Georgia.

Hydrogen Sulfide

D. Gary Rischitelli
Herbert H. Schaumburg

H$_2$S

Sulfereted hydrogen; Hydrosulfuric acid; Sulfur hydride; Sewer gas; Stink damp; Sour gas

NEUROTOXICITY RATING

Clinical

A Acute encephalopathy (CNS depression, respiratory arrest)

B Olfactory syndrome

C Chronic encephalopathy (cognitive dysfunction)

Experimental

B Developmental perturbation (cerebellum)

B Reversible hippocampal dysfunction

Hydrogen sulfide (H$_2$S) is a colorless gas at room temperature. More than 90% of atmospheric hydrogen sulfide comes from natural sources (volcanoes, swamps, and bacterial decay). Occupational exposures are a significant source, however, the U.S. National Institute for Occupational Safety and Health estimating in 1977 that 125,000 workers in 73 industries had potential exposures to hydrogen sulfide (4).

Hydrogen sulfide can be released during drilling, mining, smelting, and other chemical manufacturing or metallurgy processes. Petroleum and natural gas extraction and processing are frequent sources of exposure, and there is a high fatality rate in some oil and natural gas fields. Hydrogen sulfide in lethal concentrations may be the major component of some "sour" natural gas fields, and is a particular hazard for workers because of its steep dose-response effect, its olfactory paralysis, and its rapid "knockdown effect" (4,6).

Hydrogen sulfide is also a by-product of many industrial and natural chemical reactions that involve the intentional or unintentional decomposition of sulfur-containing proteins. It presents a particular danger in confined spaces such as sumps, sewers, sewage-treatment facilities, fishing and agricultural storage facilities, slaughterhouses, and tanneries. The disgusting ("rotten egg") odor of hydrogen sulfide is common near sewage-treatment facilities and swine-containment pens. Significant exposures can also occur in viscose rayon production and in pulp and paper mills. Hydrogen sulfide gas may be liberated whenever sulfur-containing compounds react with an acid, a potential source of large-scale accidental releases (4,6). It is flammable and explosive in air and reactive with metals, acids, and oxidizing agents. One of its thermal degradation products is highly toxic sulfur oxide (4).

Inhalation is the primary route of human exposure. Hydrogen sulfide is heavier than air and accumulates in low-lying areas such as sewers, tanks, and holds. It is characterized by rapid alveolar-capillary exchange; rapid uptake and distribution to the brain, liver, kidneys, pancreas, and small intestine; and rapid metabolism by oxidation, methylation, and reaction with metallo- or disulfide-containing proteins. Metabolism is followed by rapid excretion as free sulfate or conjugated sulfate in the urine (12).

High-level exposure to hydrogen sulfide is associated with serious systemic and nervous system toxicity. The 1991 U.S. 8-h time-weighted Threshold Limit Value is 10 ppm (14 mg/m³); the Short-Term Exposure Limit is 15 ppm (21 mg/m³). There can be severe acute effects on the olfactory, ocular, respiratory, and nervous systems at increasing concentrations. Ocular effects include intense conjunctival injection, ocular pain, blurred vision, blepharospasm, lacrimation, photophobia, keratoconjunctivitis ("gas eye"), and halo formation from the vesiculation of the cornea (10). Respiratory effects include mucous membrane irritation, rhinitis, pharyngitis, tracheobronchitis, coughing, dyspnea, and pulmonary edema. Acute effects on the central nervous system (CNS) include drowsiness, fatigue, dizziness, headache, weakness, spasms, agitation, staggering, delirium, coma, seizure, and death.

The odor threshold for hydrogen sulfide is 0.01–0.3 ppm; at 1–5 ppm the odor is moderately offensive and may cause nausea, lacrimation, and headache. Levels of 20–50 ppm produce a very strong odor, keratoconjunctivitis, and pulmonary irritation. Levels between 150 and 200 ppm cause fatigue, anxiety, and loss of the sense of smell; the loss of olfaction compounds the hazard, since exposed persons may be unaware of subsequent lethal levels. With exposure to 500 ppm, pulmonary edema appears, followed by gradual loss of consciousness. Abrupt, transient episodes of loss of consciousness with subsequent amnesia ("knockdowns") may occur at this level (2). Exposure to levels of 1000 ppm or greater may cause sudden death following only a few breaths.

Hydrogen sulfide is a mitochondrial toxin that inhibits cytochrome aa_3 (more potently than cyanide) and leads to histotoxic hypoxia. It also has direct cytotoxicity by disrupting disulfide bonds in macromolecules. Although the critical target enzyme is cytochrome oxidase, with the consequent disruption of electron transport, its "knockdown effect" may in part be the result of other CNS mechanisms such as a direct inhibitory effect on CNS respiratory centers. The effect of high-dose hydrogen sulfide poisoning resembles asphyxiation, and most of the neurological sequelae in individuals who have survived high-level exposure mimic signs displayed by patients recovering from cerebral anoxia.

Direct measurements of brain sulfide levels in animals have demonstrated that small amounts of hydrogen sulfide are present in the normal mammalian nervous system, where it may act as an endogenous neuromodulator. These studies also demonstrated the selective uptake of sulfide by the brainstem where endogenous CNS levels of sulfide were the lowest. Lethality occurred at less than twice the endogenous levels with a steep dose-response relationship. The highest levels were detected in synaptosomal and mitochondrial fractions (20). Hydrogen sulfide is produced endogenously in the brain from L-cysteine by the action of

cystathionine β-synthetase (CBS). CBS is highly expressed in the hippocampus. Physiological concentrations of H_2S selectively enhance N-methyl-D-aspartate receptor-mediated responses and may facilitate the induction of hippocampal long-term potentiation (1).

Other experimental animal studies suggest that the lethal effect of hydrogen sulfide may also involve direct inhibition of CNS respiratory centers. There is a substantial effect upon brainstem amino acid levels following sulfide administration. Although no change in amino acid levels in cortex, striatum, or hippocampus were detected, there were measurable declines in aspartate and glycine in the cerebellum and elevation of aspartate, glutamate, glutamine, γ-aminobutyric acid (GABA), glycine, taurine, and alanine in the brainstem (9). Other biochemical effects of sulfide include monoamine oxidase inhibition [which is reversed in vitro by dithiothreitol (21)] and elevated catecholamine and serotonin (5-HT) levels in the hippocampus, striatum, and brainstem. Changes in catecholamine and 5-HT levels in brainstem may contribute to a loss of central respiratory drive (22).

Experimental perinatal and developmental animal studies indicate that developing cerebellar Purkinje cells display abnormal cytoarchitecture following systemic exposure to hydrogen sulfide. Exposure to low levels of hydrogen sulfide results in alteration of Purkinje cell architecture, and alteration in amino acid and monoamine neurotransmitter levels in the developing rat brain. Monoamine transmitter levels were elevated but gradually returned to control levels after exposure ceased. The most marked effect was in the hippocampus (13,14). Exposure to hydrogen sulfide also altered amino acid levels in the brains of rat pups exposed to low levels in utero. Reduced levels of aspartate, glutamate, and GABA were observed in the cerebellum, and reduced levels of aspartate and GABA in the cerebrum (7).

Prolonged low-level hydrogen sulfide exposure to rats also causes alterations in hippocampal electroencephalographic activity. Low-dose exposure to hydrogen sulfide resulted in increased theta activity in the hippocampal electroencephalogram (EEG), and repeated exposures resulted in a cumulative effect that took up to 2 weeks for recovery. The neocortical EEG was unaffected (15).

Two large-scale studies have been reported of workers' compensation claimants in Alberta, Canada. The first described 221 cases with 14 fatalities (6%) in 1977; 74% of those affected were initially unconscious, but few permanent neurological effects were documented. There was, however, no report of neuropsychological testing and no reported follow-up (3). A second series of 250 cases in Alberta, Canada, was reported in 1985. The death rate (2.8%) was significantly lower than observed in the first study (probably due to improved access to medical care). Other acute effects reported included unconsciousness (54%), headache (26%), dysequilibrium (21.6%), "neuropsychological" effects (8%), and convulsions (5%) (2).

Two reports describe workers overcome while cleaning hot-spring reservoirs in Taiwan. Three of seven workers died. Presence of pulmonary edema on admission was noted to be a grave prognostic sign (5). One published report describes persistent exertional dyspnea and abnormal lung volumes and CO diffusion capacity following an acute hydrogen sulfide exposure. Mild pulmonary fibrosis was attributed to a delayed effect of hydrogen sulfide exposure (11).

Six patients who lost consciousness after hydrogen sulfide exposure were reexamined 5 or more years after the event for evidence of persistent neuropsychological impairment. Patients whose exposure exceeded 5 min showed persistent impairment. Memory and motor function were most affected (19). One shipyard worker in the group who was exposed for 20 min was initially comatose for 2 days, improved, but 3 days later again became comatose for a month. He woke up amnesic, blind, and with impaired hearing and spastic tetraparesis. He improved over 1 month. A 5-year follow-up showed persistent motor, memory, mood, and visual impairment (18). There is also one reported case of an oil worker treated and released after hydrogen sulfide exposure. The following day he was readmitted with nausea, vomiting, diarrhea, and urinary incontinence. He developed leg shaking, dizziness, sweating, trouble sleeping, and nightmares. Three years later, follow-up testing showed abnormal reaction time; impaired balance, memory, and learning; and mood disturbance (8).

Mass exposure to hydrogen sulfide was described at a beachfront construction site in 1995. Thirty-seven individuals working at the site or living nearby were evaluated at a hospital; six were admitted and one died at the scene. One worker who arrived comatose with generalized seizures received a course of hyperbaric oxygen therapy. He reportedly had permanent cognitive and linguistic deficits, impaired memory, decreased auditory attention, and impaired visual memory and learning (17).

These case reports suggest that most individuals recover fully, but chronic CNS sequelae have been described following hydrogen sulfide "knockdowns." Cerebral anoxia, seizure, or head trauma often accompanies hydrogen sulfide exposures. Data are largely from case reports or case series; conclusive studies are lacking. Descriptions of permanent CNS effects from repeated low-level exposures are even less well described.

Acute high-level human exposure is clearly associated with serious CNS dysfunction; it can cause a postexposure syndrome that is indistinguishable from anoxic encephalopathy. Cognitive dysfunction, tremor, and gait instability are prominent findings (8,17–19). Repeated "knockdowns" resulting from exposures to nonlethal levels have been described in oil-field workers; these are generally unaccompanied by neurological dysfunction. There is no convincing report that describes persistent cognitive dysfunction following repeated low-level exposures to hydrogen sulfide. The efficacy of recommended antidotes is unproven (16).

REFERENCES

1. Abe K, Kimura H (1996) The possible role of hydrogen sulfide as an endogenous neuromodulator. *J Neurosci* **16**, 1066.
2. Arnold I, Dufresne R, Alleyne B, Stuart P (1985) Health implications of occupational exposures to hydrogen sulfide. *J Occup Med* **27**, 373.
3. Burnett WW, King EG, Grace M, Hall WF (1977) Hydrogen sulfide poisoning: Review of five years' experience. *Can Med Assoc J* **117**, 1277.
4. Deng JF (1992) Hydrogen sulfide. In: *Hazardous Materials Toxicology: Clinical Principles of Environmental Health*. Sullivan JB, Krieger GR eds. Williams & Wilkins, Baltimore p. 711.
5. Deng JF, Chang SC (1987) Hydrogen sulfide poisonings in hot spring reservoir cleaning: Two case reports. *Amer J Ind Med* **11**, 447.
6. Guidotti TL (1994) Occupational exposure to hydrogen sulfide in the sour gas industry: Some unresolved issues. *Int Arch Occup Environ Health* **66**, 153.
7. Hannah RS, Hayden LJ, Roth SH (1989) Hydrogen sulfide exposure alters the amino acid content in developing rat CNS. *Neurosci Lett* **99**, 323.
8. Kilburn K (1993) Case report: Profound neurobehavioral deficits in an oil field worker overcome by hydrogen sulfide. *Amer J Med Sci* **306**, 301.
9. Kombian SB, Warenycia MW, Mele FG, Reiffenstein RJ (1988) Effects of acute intoxication with hydrogen sulfide on central amino acid transmitter systems. *Neurotoxicology* **9**, 587.
10. Luck J, Kaye SB (1989) An unrecognized form of hydrogen sulphide keratoconjunctivitis. *Brit J Ind Med* **46**, 748.
11. Parra O, Monso E, Gallego M, Morera J (1991) Inhalation of hydrogen sulfide: A case of subacute manifestations and long term sequelae. *Brit J Ind Med* **48**, 286.
12. Reiffenstein RJ, Hulber WC, Roth SH (1992) Toxicology of hydrogen sulfide. *Annu Rev Pharmacol Toxicol* **32**, 109.
13. Roth SH, Skrajny B, Reiffenstein RJ (1995) Alteration of the morphology and neurochemistry of the developing mammalian nervous system by hydrogen sulfide. *Clin Exp Pharmacol Physiol* **22**, 379.
14. Skrajny B, Hannah RS, Roth SH (1992) Low concentrations of hydrogen sulfide alter monoamine levels in the

developing rat central nervous system. *Can J Physiol Pharmacol* **70**, 1515.

15. Skrajny B, Reiffenstein RJ, Sainsbury RS, Roth SH (1996) Effects of repeated exposures of hydrogen sulfide on rat hippocampal EEG. *Toxicol Lett* **84**, 43.

16. Smith RP (1997) Editorial commentary—sulfide poisoning. *Clin Toxicol* **35**, 305.

17. Snyder JW, Safir EF, Summerville GP, Middleberg RA (1995) Occupational fatality and persistent neurological sequelae after mass exposure to hydrogen sulfide. *Amer J Emerg Med* **13**, 199.

18. Tvedt B, Edland A, Skyberg K, Forberg O (1991) Delayed neuropsychiatric sequelae after acute hydrogen sulfide poisoning: Affection of motor function, memory, vision and hearing. *Acta Neurol Scand* **84**, 348.

19. Tvedt B, Skyberg K, Aaserud O *et al.* (1991) Brain damage caused by hydrogen sulfide: A follow-up study of six patients. *Amer J Ind Med* **20**, 91.

20. Warenycia MW, Goodwin LR, Benishin CG *et al.* (1989) Acute hydrogen sulfide poisoning: Demonstration of selective uptake of sulfide by the brainstem by measurement of brain sulfide levels. *Biochem Pharmacol* **38**, 973.

21. Warenycia MW, Goodwin LR, Francom DM *et al.* (1990) Dithiothreitol liberates non-acid labile sulfide from brain tissue of H₂S-poisoned animals. *Arch Toxicol* **64**, 650.

22. Warenycia MW, Smith KA, Blashko CS *et al.* (1989) Monoamine oxidase inhibition as a sequel of hydrogen sulfide intoxication: Increases in brain catecholamine and 5-hydroxytryptamine levels. *Arch Toxicol* **63**, 131.

Hydrophiidae Toxins

Albert C. Ludolph

NEUROTOXICITY RATING

Clinical

A Neuromuscular transmission syndrome

A Myopathy (necrotizing)

Experimental

A Neuromuscular transmission dysfunciton (receptor binding)

The venom of all sea snakes (family Hydrophiidae, subfamilies Hydrophinae and Laticaudae) is a mixture of proteinaceous neurotoxic and myotoxic compounds (5,10). In comparison to land snakes, sea snake venom carries only low levels of enzymatic activities, with the exception of phospholipase A and hyaluronidase in some species. Procoagulant and hemorrhagic enzymes are absent. Venoms of the genera *Acalyptophis, Aipysurus, Astrotia, Disteria, Emydocephalus, Enhydrina, Hydrophis, Kerilia, Lapemis, Laticauda, Microcephalophis, Pelamis,* and *Praescutata* are toxic to mice, and postsynaptic neurotoxins have been detected in most species (14). Neurotoxic compounds—of which the group of erabutoxins from *Laticauda semifasciata* are the best described (*see* Erabutoxin, this volume) —uniformly bind to the acetylcholine receptor at the neuromuscular junction; there is a strong relationship between the LD₅₀ of the respective toxin and its affinity for this receptor (14). In addition to these postsynaptic neurotoxins, a phospholipase A is present in Hydrophiidae venom; in some species (such as *Laticauda* spp.), this may also have a postsynaptic effect (3). Studies of phospholipase A activity from *Enhydrina schistosa* venom demonstrate myotoxicity (1,2,4,14); one report claims that venom of *E. schistosa* decreases oxygen uptake and induces swelling of muscle mitochondria (12). Phospholipase A from *E. schistosa* also inhibits Ca^{2+} uptake into the sarcoplasmic reticulum (7).

The distribution of sea snakes is restricted to the tropical and subtropical Pacific Ocean and Indian Ocean; the Atlantic Ocean has no sea snakes. Most sea snakes inhabit coastal marine waters; only one species of Hydrophiidae lives in a freshwater lake of the Philippines (14). Sea snake bites are rare; they occur most frequently when fishermen handle their catch (8.9). Divers and swimmers may also be bitten (13). Sea snake venom is more toxic than venom from kraits or cobras but, in comparison to other snakes, these animals only inject a small amount of the toxin. Therefore, only about 20% of sea snake bites are associated with clinical manifestations (9); however, 50% of the symptomatic victims may die without treatment (8,9,13,14). Since the fangs of sea snakes are short, bites often occur without pain or local reaction; some are initially unaware of an eventually fatal bite. Absent local pain may help distinguish sea snake bites from other injuries, such as those from fish spine stings. Diplopia, facial and bulbar weakness (including trismus), and generalized weakness develop within 2 h of the bite. Severe cases progress to generalized paralysis and life-threatening respiratory failure (8,9,13,14). Since venom components are myotoxic, muscle movements are painful and myoglobinuria occurs (8,9,13). Increased plasma creatine kinase levels (11), myoglobinuria, and the associated danger of renal failure and hyperkalemia may be present (13,14).

If clinical symptoms follow a history of swimming or wading within the preceding 2 days (6,13), the intravenous use of antivenin (*Enhydrina schistosa* Antivenom, Commonwealth Serum Lab., Parkville, VIC, Australia) is recommended, although its use may be complicated by serum sickness. This antivenin is effective against the toxic effect of bites of each member of the family Hydrophiidae. If a sea snake bite is suspected, careful observation of the patient is mandatory. First aid consists of the application of pressure/immobilization to slow the development of potentially life-threatening complications (6,13). These first aid measures should only be removed when the patient is at an institution where full ventilatory support, circulation support, and antivenin can be administered (6,13). Antivenin administration may be beneficial up to 48 h after the bite.

REFERENCES

1. Fohlman J, Eaker D (1977) Isolation and characterization of a lethal myotoxic phospholipase A from the venom of the common sea snake *Enhydrina schistosa* causing myoglobinuria in mice. *Toxicon* **15**, 385.

2. Geh SL, Toh HT (1978) Ultrastructural changes in skeletal muscle caused by a phospholipase A₂ fraction isolated from the venom of a sea snake, *Enhydrina schistosa*. *Toxicon* **16**, 633.

3. Harvey AL, Tamiya N (1980) Role of phospholipase A activity in the neuromuscular paralysis produced by some components isolated from the venom of the sea snake, *Laticauda semifasciata*. *Toxicon* **18**, 65.

4. Lind P, Eaker D (1981) Amino acid sequence of a lethal myotoxic phospholipase A₂ from the venom of the common sea snake (*Enhydrina schistosa*). *Toxicon* **19**, 11.

5. McDowell SB (1972) The genera of sea-snakes of the *Hydrophis* group (serpents: Elapidae). *Trans Zool Soc Lond* **32**, 189.

6. Mebs D (1992) *Gifttiere. Ein Handbuch für Biologen, Toxikologen, Ärzte, Apotheker.* Wissenschaftliche Verlagsgesellschaft, Stuttgart.

7. Ng RH, Howard BD (1980) Mitochondria and sarcoplasmatic reticulum as model targets for neurotoxic and myotoxic phospholipase A2. *Proc Natl Acad Sci USA* **77**, 1346.

8. Reid HA (1956) Sea-snake bite research. *Trans Roy Soc Trop Med Hyg* **50**, 417.

9. Reid HA (1975) Epidemiology of sea snake bites. *J Trop Med Hyg* **78**, 106.

10. Smith MA (1926) *Monograph of the Sea-snakes* (Hydrophiidae). British Musem, London.

11. Sutherland SK (1983) *Australian Animal Toxins.* Oxford University Press, Melbourne.

12. Taub AM, Elliott WB (1964) Some effects of snake venoms on mitochondria. *Toxicon* **2**, 87.

13. Tu AT, Fulde G (1987) Sea snake bite. *Clin Dermatol* **5**, 118.

14. Tu AT (1988) Sea snakes and their venoms. In: *Handbook of Natural Toxins. Vol 3. Marine Toxins and Venoms.* Tu AT ed. Marcel Dekker, New York p. 424.

6-Hydroxydopamine

Hans Georg Baumgarten
Zarko Grozdanovic

6-HYDROXYDOPAMINE
$C_8H_{11}NO_3$

2,4,5-Trihydroxyphenylethylamine

NEUROTOXICITY RATING
Experimental
A   Dopaminergic neuronopathy
A   Adrenergic neuronopathy

6-Hydroxydopamine (6-OH-DA) was originally synthesized in 1959 (38,39); the authors suggested that 6-OH-DA might be a naturally occurring oxidation product/metabolite of its congener dopamine. Systemic administration of 6-OH-DA caused a long-lasting depletion of noradrenaline from sympathetically innervated organs (28,32,42). The mechanism(s) of long-term action of 6-OH-DA remained unresolved until the discovery of its destructive action on peripheral and central noradrenergic preterminal axons and axon terminals (4,13,46,47,49,51,52).

6-Hydroxydopamine is the prototype of a class of compounds designated as "neurotoxic transmitter analogues" or, more commonly, as "catecholamine or catecholaminergic neurotoxins." This formulation emphasizes the structural similarity to dopamine and noradrenaline; it also implies that 6-OH-DA shares physicochemical properties, transport-site affinity, intraneuronal disposition, and enzymatic processing with its congeners dopamine and noradrenaline. In contrast to noradrenaline and dopamine, 6-OH-DA is toxic to neurons that synthesize and release dopamine and noradrenaline (*i.e.*, vertebrate CNS and PNS noradrenergic and dopaminergic neurons). Subtypes of noradrenaline and of dopamine (and also of adrenaline) neurons differ in their sensitivity to 6-OH-DA (Table 26).

Metabolism and Toxic Mechanisms

When exposed to air at pH 7.4 and ambient temperature, 6-OH-DA is rapidly oxidized to its corresponding 2,5-*p*-quinone (Fig. 12) *via* semiquinone radical intermediates. Auto-oxidation of dopamine proceeds at a much lower rate because its redox potential is higher ($E_{1/2}$ +0.24 V) than that of 6-OH-DA ($E_{1/2}$ −0.09 V) (15,16). Intramolecular side chain cyclization of the *p*-quinone of 6-OH-DA results in the formation of the *p*-quinoneimine of 5,6-dihydroxyindoline (aminochrome 1), which rearranges to yield 5,6-dihydroxyindole (an intermediate in melanogenesis). Upon oxidation, 5,6-dihydroxyindole is transformed into its corresponding *p*-quinoneimine (aminochrome 2) *via* semiquinone radical intermediates (5). An analogous sequence of auto-oxidation and slow intramolecular cyclization holds for dopamine under comparable conditions (2). The process of auto-oxidation of 6-OH-DA and that of dopamine results in the production of secondary reaction products [*i.e.*, reduced oxygen species and free radicals (peroxide ion; superoxide ion; singlet oxygen; hydroxyl radical)], the nature

and relative proportion of which significantly influence the oxidation of the original compounds and their auto-oxidation products (9,18,29). The direct reaction of oxygen with 6-OH-DA is relatively slow. During this initial reaction, superoxide and the semiquinone radical of 6-OH-DA are formed. Once formed, the superoxide radical speeds the oxidation of 6-OH-DA. The semiquinone of 6-OH-DA interacts with molecular oxygen to regenerate the superoxide radical. In concert, these radical intermediates are the driving forces in the free-radical catalysis and speeding of the auto-oxidation of 6-OH-DA. The presence or absence of catalysts [transition metal redox systems (*e.g.*, Fe^{2+}/Fe^{3+}; Cu^+/Cu^{2+}; Mn^{2+}/Mn^{3+}), organic redox pairs (*e.g.*, ascorbate/dehydro-ascorbate; preoxidized dopamine or 6-OH-DA)] significantly modify the speed of formation and the type and relative proportion of the radical species formed during the (auto)oxidation process (10).

Once redox cycling occurs in the presence of appropriate catalysts, the speed of formation of electrophilic quinoidal intermediates is significantly enhanced. In the presence of metal redox pairs (*e.g.*, of Fe^{2+}/Fe^{3+}), hydrogen peroxide (the main reduction product of O_2 during the auto-oxidation of 6-OH-DA and of 5,6-dihydroxyindole) undergoes a Fenton-type reaction to yield the highly cytotoxic species $OH^{\cdot}$ that is capable of hydroxylating and damaging proteins, lipids, and carbohydrates *in vivo*. These *in vitro* findings suggest interdigitating mechanisms of cytotoxicity of 6-OH-DA (and of dopamine) *in vivo*: radical attack on susceptible structures/components of cells and covalent nucleophilic addition reactions by electrophilic quinoidal species formed from either 6-OH-DA or dopamine. Studies in model systems (native serum albumin in solution) show that

TABLE 26. Neuronal/Extraneuronal Factors Influencing the Selectivity/Efficiency of 6-OH-DA

Neuronal	Extraneuronal
Maturity of neurons	Maturity of nonneuronal cells (particularly of the blood-brain barrier cellular substrates)
Transporter affinity and rate of transport of neurotoxins (uptake I) in relation to competitors	Transporter affinity and rate of transport of toxins (uptake II) in relation to competitors
Capacity to metabolize toxins (MAO, mixed function oxidase, conjugase)	Capacity to metabolize toxins (MAO, COMT)
Intraneuronal oxidation catalysis (enzymatic, nonenzymatic)	Intracellular oxidation catalysis
Redox state	Redox state
Capacity to detoxify radicals (SH-pool; glutathione transferase; glutathione peroxidase; superoxide dismutase; peroxidase; concentration of radical scavengers, *e.g.*, noradrenaline, dopamine, α-tocopherol, β-carotene)	Capacity to detoxify radicals (SH-pool; glutathione transferase; glutathione peroxidase; superoxide dismutase, peroxidase; concentration of radical scavengers, *e.g.*, noradrenaline, dopamine, α-tocopherol, β-carotene)
Degree of vascularization; diffusion conditions/clearance rate for neurotoxins	
Re-expression of neuroplasticity programs (*i.e.*, growth-promoting genes; release of catastrophy signals)	Induction of neurotrophin expression in glial cells

Based on reviews in references 2, 21, 22, and 36.

MAO, monoamine oxidase; COMT, catechol-*o*-methyl-transferase; SH, sulfhydryl.

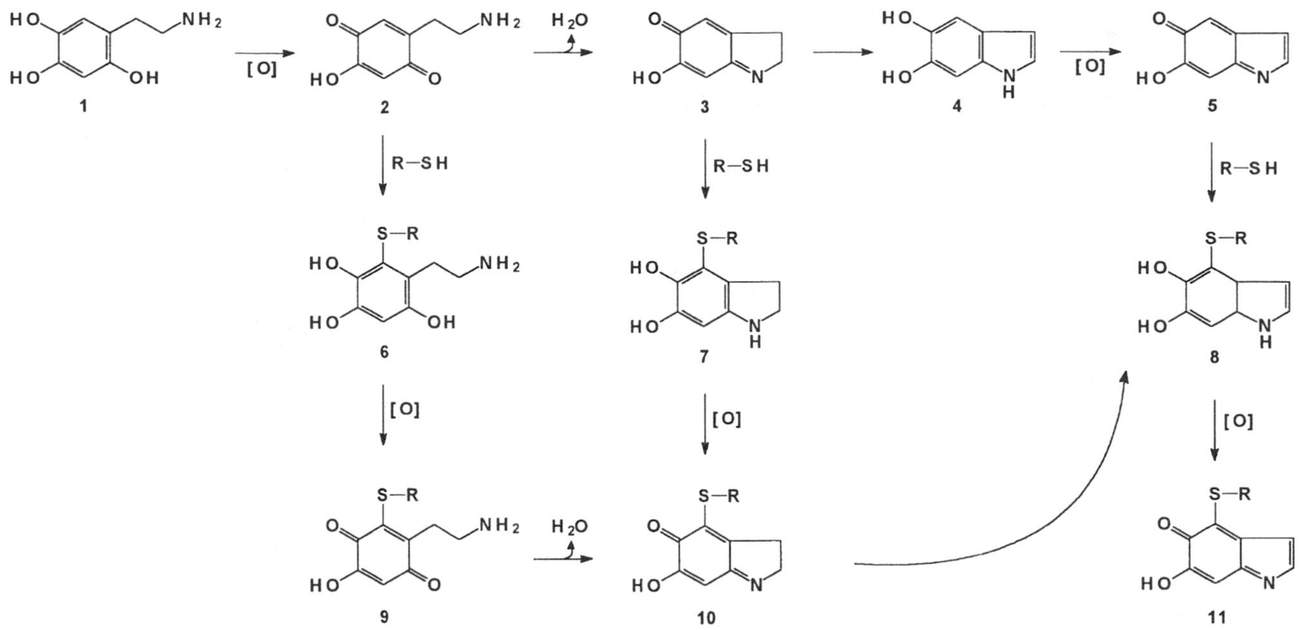

FIGURE 12. Autoxidation pathways of 6-hydroxydopamine and mode of reaction of its oxidation products with SH-nucleophiles. [O] autoxidation; R, alkyl, aryl; R-SH sulfhydryl nucleophile; **1**, 2,4,5-trihydroxyphenylethylamine ("6-hydroxydopamine," 6-OH-DA); **2**, p-quinone of 6-OH-DA; **3**, aminochrome 1; **4**, 5,6-dihydroxyindole; **5**, aminochrome 2; **6**, 2,4,5-trihydroxy-6-S-(R)-phenylethylamine; **7**, 5,6-dihydroxy-4-S-(R)-indoline; **8**, 5,6-dihydroxy-4-S-(R)-indole; **9**, p-quinone oxidation product of adduct **6**; **10**, p-quinoneimine oxidation product of adduct **7**; **11**, p-quinoneimine oxidation product of adduct **8**. [Modified from Borchardt et al. (5).]

oxidation products of 6-OH-DA expose and attack sulfhydryl (SH) groups in proteins leading to their arylation and to cross-linking of protein monomers to polymeric high-molecular-weight products (35,37). Intramolecular cyclization of the p-quinone of 6-OH-DA to 5,6-dihydroxyindole is not required for this protein arylating capacity of 6-OH-DA. Indeed, the rate of nucleophilic reactivity of the p quinone of 6-OH-DA to, for example, cysteine or glutathione (GSH), is many times higher than its readiness to undergo intramolecular cyclization to form indoline and indole species (1,48). The abundance of SH-nucleophiles in biological systems makes it unlikely that cyclization to indolic structures from 6-OH-DA (and from dopamine) will occur *in vivo* unless specific conditions are maintained with the exclusion of SH-nucleophiles. Using GSH *in vitro*, 2,4,5-trihydroxy-6-S-(glutathionyl)phenylethylamine was formed during the auto-oxidation of 6-OH-DA (29). The identical product has been isolated from rat brain after intracerebroventricular injection of 6-OH-DA. An analogous pathway holds for dopamine auto-oxidation. Following an initial lag period during which oxygen radicals and hydrogen peroxide are formed, dopamine oxidation proceeds autocatalytically *via* semiquinones to yield the corresponding o-quinone. The o-quinone of dopamine reacts much more rapidly with SH-nucleophiles (cysteine, GSH) than with its side-chain amino function (resulting in intramolecular cy-

clization). These concepts of the chemical properties of quinoidal auto-oxidation products of dopamine are consistent with the presence of 5-S-cysteinyl-dopamine in human brain tissue (34).

Provided that conditions allow cyclization of the p-quinone of 6-OH-DA or of the o-quinone of dopamine to occur, dihydroxyindoles are formed that are easily auto-oxidized to quinoidal species; these avidly undergo addition reactions with nonprotein and protein nucleophiles resulting in extensive cross-linking of proteins. At this point of the reaction cascade, the auto-oxidation pathways of 6-OH-DA, of dopamine, and of 5,6-dihydroxytryptamine (5,6-DHT) converge and undergo nucleophilic addition reactions with nonoxidized o-dihydroxyindoles to yield melanoid polymer products. No evidence for the incorporation of radioactivity into the melanin-rich fraction of heart tissue homogenates from mice injected with ^{3}H-6-OH-DA [given intravenously (i.v.) at a dose of 1–3 mg/kg body weight] was found (21); this confirms the concept that intramolecular cyclization of the 2,5-p-quinone of 6-OH-DA does not occur to any significant degree *in vivo*. The extensive covalent binding of radioactivity (perchloric acid extraction-resistant activity) to proteins of mouse heart after *in vivo* administration of ^{3}H-6-OH-DA is therefore mediated by nonindolic oxidation products/metabolites of 6-OH-DA. An important proportion of this radioactivity recovered from the mouse heart represents activity accumulated by active transport into the noradrenergic nerves *via* the desipramine-sensitive membrane transporter. Dopamine formed endogenously in neurons of the substantia nigra pars compacta may behave differently from 6-OH-DA, as suggested by the high content of melanin in the dopaminergic neurons of several species. This implies that slow oxidation and cyclization of dopamine to indolequinones may occur in a sulfhydryl-deficient and protected vesicular compartment of these cells.

Animal Studies
Anatomical and Pharmacological Studies

The stage of development/maturity of noradrenaline and dopamine neurons significantly modifies their sensitivity to 6-OH-DA. Immature catecholaminergic neurons of the developing PNS and CNS are particularly sensitive to direct toxic attack of 6-OH-DA and may be destroyed acutely, in contrast to mature neurons, which may undergo slow retrograde degeneration. Table 26 depicts the graded sensitivity of various central/peripheral types of noradrenaline, dopamine, and adrenaline neurons. It is evident from the ranking of sensitivity to 6-OH-DA that the surface–volume relationship of axons *vs.* cell bodies is a further modifier of the graded toxin sensitivity. Relatively more 6-OH-DA is incorporated into the axon terminals than into neuronal perikarya, assuming an equal density of transporter molecules per unit membrane area at the somatodendritic and terminal portion of the neuron. Certain subtypes of dopamine neurons (*e.g.*, the tuberoinfundibular dopamine neurons within the arcuate nucleus that project to the close-by median eminence) are resistant to 6-OH-DA, as are the so-called small intensely fluorescent paraneurons (SIF-cells) in sympathetic ganglia. The short noradrenergic neurons of the pelvic ganglia appear to be less sensitive to 6-OH-DA than long noradrenergic neurons of the sympathetic chain ganglia that innervate visceral organ structures of the thoracic cavity and the head (*e.g*, the heart and the iris). The former resprout more avidly and reinnervate the denervated target more rapidly and completely than the conventional long adrenergic neurons. These observations suggest that the degree of axonal branching and the total length of the axonal tree in a given neuron is a modifier of its toxin sensitivity, and that different types of adult catecholamine neurons seem to differ in their neuroplasticity (*i.e.*, growth potential). However, factors other than properties of the neurons themselves modify the toxin sensitivity of different types of catecholamine neurons. Among these factors are the capillary density of a given target organ and the rate of clearance of the extracellular fluid, properties of the extra-cellular matrix, the shielding of neurons by glia/satellite cells, and uptake and metabolism of 6-OH-DA by nonneuronal cells (*cf.* Table 27).

Doses lower than 0.5 mg/kg, given i.v. to adult cats or rats, result in temporary depletion of noradrenaline from sympathetic nerves (44); that is, at very low doses, 6-OH-DA may be handled as a false neurotransmitter similar to its nontoxic isomer 3,4,5-trihydroxyphenylethylamine ("5-hydroxydopamine"). Since 6-OH-DA has little intrinsic agonist activity at receptor sites, it acts mainly as an indirect sympathomimetic agent on noradrenaline receptors and effector systems. When given systemically to adult rats, mice, or cats at doses ranging from 1–250 mg/kg i.v. (either a single dose or repeated at daily or weekly intervals), 6-OH-DA causes dose-related long-lasting decreases of noradrenaline in various peripheral target organs that reflect degeneration of noradrenergic axon terminals (25,43,45). There is a decreasing order of susceptibility to the axodestructive potential of 6-OH-DA in noradrenergic axon terminals of different organs (cardiac ventricles > salivary gland > whole heart > iris > nictitating membrane > spleen > cardiac atria > blood vessels > vas deferens). Species differences in the molar potency of 6-OH-DA as a chemical sympathectomy-inducing agent are also known; the cat noradrenergic nerves are more vulnerable than those of the mouse or rat. Since the noradrenergic cell bodies and preterminal axons are resistant to the acute toxic actions of 6-OH-DA in adult animals, axonal sprouting, regrowth of axons and, eventually, partial or even near-complete regeneration of denervated targets may occur in a time-dependent fashion (30). The

TABLE 27. Graded Sensitivity of Different Types of Peripheral and Central Catecholamine Neurons Toward the Toxic Action of 6-OH-DA (Decreasing Order of Sensitivity)

Terminals and axons of immature sympathetic neurons

Terminals and axons of immature central LC neurons and the lateral tegmental NA neurons

Terminals and axons of adult "long" sympathetic neurons (perikarya in the para- and prevertebral ganglia)

Terminals and axons of adult central LC neurons

Terminals and axons of lateral tegmental NA neurons

Terminals and axons of adult central nigrostriatal and mesocortical DA neurons

Perikarya of immature sympathetic NA neurons

Perikarya of immature central NA neurons, in particular those of the LC

Terminals and axons of "short" adrenergic sympathetic neurons innervating the pelvic viscera

Terminals and axons of central A neurons and of central 5-HT neurons; perikarya of LC and of lateral tegmental NA neurons

Based on reviews in references 6, 8, 10, 14, 22, 23–25, 36, 43–45, 53 55.

LC, locus ceruleus; NA, noradrenaline; DA, dopamine; 5-HT, 5-hydroxytryptamine.

speed and degree of recovery by axonal sprouting depends on the extent of initial damage to sympathetic axon terminals and to the preterminal axons from which regrowth of axons and terminals will occur. Organs innervated by short adrenergic neurons of the pelvic viscera and targets harboring preterminal axon bundles that escape acute damage by 6-OH-DA—perivascular axon bundles of large arteries in, for example, the mesentery—are more rapidly and more completely reinnervated than organs that have lost their preterminal axon supply in addition to their axon terminals (*e.g.*, the iris or atrium). Sprouting and regeneration of 6-OH-DA–axotomized sympathetic neurons can be accelerated and improved by systemic administration of nerve growth factor (3), the presence of which is required for normal development of sympathetic nervous system during ontogeny. Compensatory changes occur following 6-OH-DA treatment in sympathetic ganglia, in adrenal medulla, and in target organ structures. The most important changes are reductions in the expression of transmitter phenotype-related enzymes at the expense of increases in mRNA synthesis for proteins involved in sympathetic axonal growth (cytoskeletal proteins, growth associated proteins, growth factor receptors), increased synthesis of phenylethanol-amine-N-methyltransferase in chromaffin cells, and postsynaptic-type supersensitivity responses in target cells (23,25).

Neonatal administration of high single or repeated doses of 6-OH-DA [100 mg/kg, intraperitoneally (i.p.) or subcutaneously (s.c.)] results in profound destruction of axon terminals in almost all sympathetically innervated organs of the rat and a partial loss of sympathetic ganglion cells in pre- and paravertebral ganglia. This immediate postnatal treatment is followed by persistent deficits in the density of sympathetic adrenergic innervation in many peripheral target organs, with the exception of those innervated by organ-close short adrenergic neurons located in the pelvic plexus (19,36). The same dose of 6-OH-DA (100 μg/g i.p. or s.c.) administered repeatedly during the first few days after birth selectively lesions the projections of the pontine locus ceruleus (LC) of the rat without causing acute destruction of the noradrenaline-containing cell bodies (36) thus allowing for compensatory sprouting of the lesioned preterminal axons within the dorsal tegmental bundle that harbors the ascending axons of the LC. This form of lesioning of the central noradrenaline projections of the LC results in compensatory hyperinnervation of LC-close brainstem areas and of the cerebellum, and a relative deficit in reinnervation of distantly located telecephalic targets (*e.g.*, basal ganglia and cortex). Thus, the same postnatal systemic dose of 6-OH-DA that causes subtotal destruction of the postganglionic sympathetic innervation in peripheral

targets and that induces a lifetime dystrophic effect on the sympathetic neurons in pre- and paravertebral ganglia, also damages telencephalic and spinal projections of the locus ceruleus. This occurs because of the immaturity of the blood-brain barrier for 6-OH-DA and a high toxin sensitivity of the developing central noradrenergic axons of the LC. Selective lesions of the LC in developing animals can be accomplished by injections of 6-OH-DA (20–80 μg free base) into the fourth ventricle [commonly termed "intracisternal" (i.c.) injection (6)], by infusing small amounts of 6-OH-DA (4 μg at three different cannula placements) into the LC (27) *via* stereotaxically implanted cannulas or by electrolytic destruction of the LC, either uni- or bilaterally (23). When high doses of 6-OH-DA (100 μg or more) are injected into the lateral or fourth ventricle of neonatal rats, dopaminergic projections (nigrostriatal and mesolimbic) to the forebrain are damaged in addition to the noradrenergic ascending and descending LC projections (6,8). The selectivity of 6-OH-DA for DA systems can be improved by pretreating animals with blockers of noradrenaline transport (*e.g.*, desipramine).

In adult animals, 6-OH-DA must be injected into the cerebrospinal fluid compartment or directly into the brain parenchyma for lesioning of noradrenaline and/or dopamine projection systems because the blood-brain barrier prevents systemic 6-OH-DA from reaching the central catecholaminergic systems. In adult rodents, injection of 50 μg 6-OH-DA into the lateral or fourth ventricle causes a moderate depletion of noradrenaline content without significant effects on brain dopamine concentration (6,23). Brain dopamine levels are moderately affected after 100 μg 6-OH-DA concomitant with proportionally larger decreases in brain noradrenaline content. Doubling or tripling of these moderately effective doses produces dose-related increases in brain noradrenaline and dopamine depletion (23,25). When 6-OH-DA is injected into the lateral ventricle of adult rats at doses higher than 200 μg (free base), nonspecific damage in ventricle-close brain regions (septum, striatum, hypothalamus, hippocampus) is noted in Fink-Heimer stained sections (17). There is a rank order of sensitivity for noradrenaline depletion by 6-OH-DA in representative brain regions (hippocampus > spinal cord > cerebellum > neocortex > hypothalamus > thalamus > midbrain > striatum > lower brainstem). The rank order of sensitivity for dopamine depletion in representative brain regions (striatum > amygdala > nucleus accumbens > hippocampus > midbrain > lower brainstem > hypothalamus > cortex) following stereotaxic infusion of 200 μg 6-OH-DA (with or without pretreatment of the animals with desipramine) into the lateral ventricle of rats thus differs from that measured for noradrenaline (11,25,33).

The intracerebral route of administration of 6-OH-DA has been used as an alternative to the intrathecal approach. However, considerable disagreement exists concerning the degree of nonspecific damage inflicted on noncatecholaminergic structures of the brain. While one study has found that intracerebrally administered 6-OH-DA caused restricted nonspecific damage to brain structures surrounding the tip of the injection cannula (50), others have obtained results indicative of a purely nonspecific lesion (31,50). 6-OH-DA will produce rather selective lesions in catecholaminergic neurons of the substantia nigra in a dose-related fashion within an area peripheral to a central zone facing the tip of the injection cannula in which indiscriminate destruction of brain tissue is apparent (20). Within dosage limits of 1–8 μg, 6-OH-DA can be used as a selective neurotoxin to interrupt catecholaminergic pathways by intracerebral lesion paradigms. Selective and profound ablation of noradrenergic and dopaminergic projections to the forebrain of the rat was obtained by infusing low doses of 6-OH-DA (2 μg) bilaterally into the ascending tegmental noradrenergic pathways (the dorsal and ventral tegmental bundle) and the substantia nigra, respectively (6). Application of 6-OH-DA into the dorsal and ventral tegmental catecholamine fiber bundles reduced noradrenaline levels throughout representative forebrain areas without affecting regional dopamine levels, whereas administration of 6-OH-DA into the substantia nigra reduced dopamine and noradrenaline levels to a comparable degree.

Behavioral Studies

The application of 6-OH-DA to experimental animals has assisted in the development of various models of CNS disease involving catecholamine neurons [Parkinson's syndrome; aggression dyscontrol and self-injurious behavior; attention deficit hyperactivity disorder (7,40,41)]. Sequential lesioning of catecholaminergic and serotonergic neurons with 6-OH-DA and 5,7-dihydroxytryptamine (5,7-DHT), the most versatile "serotonergic neurotoxin" (2), in developing animals has provided experimental medicine with developmentally founded models of neuropsychiatric diseases that become manifest in the human at childhood or adolescence [e.g., attention-deficit hyperactivity disorder (26)]. In most instances, these models simulate only selected neuropathological aspects of diseases.

Rats lesioned as neonates show aggressivity, self-biting, and self-injurious behavior when challenged with L-dopa or apomorphine at adulthood. By contrast, rats lesioned as adults show head nodding and paw treading (stereotyped behavior). Animals lesioned as neonates do not exhibit extrapyramidal signs even when their nigrostriatal projections are completely destroyed. They are refractory to doses of dopamine receptor antagonists (neuroleptics), which cause prolonged inactivity in controls, whereas those lesioned at adult age may become akinetic, adipsic, and aphagic and must temporarily be supported by intragastric tube feeding to help them survive. Adult rats subjected to partial destruction of their nigrostriatal projections are highly sensitive to moderate doses of neuroleptics and may become severely akinetic. Animals lesioned at birth are more active than intact animals of comparable age, and they are deficient in certain learning tasks. To rule out a participation of injured noradrenergic projections in such deficits, animals have to be pretreated with desipramine to prevent uptake of 6-OH-DA into noradrenergic axons and their varicose terminals.

Animals lesioned as neonates have been considered models of attention-deficit-hyperactivity disorder. Apart from changes in dopamine receptor sensitivity (vide infra), such animals have only residual amounts of dopamine in their striata at 4 months of age (1% compared to age-matched controls), but the levels of serotonin are increased above control as are those of 5-hydroxyindoleacetic acid, the major monoamine oxidase metabolite of serotonin (8). This finding indicates that serotonergic neurons sprout to hyperinnervate the dopaminergically denervated striata. Such animals spend more time in locomotion than nonlesioned controls and less time in immobility. In such animals, amphetamine reduces the time spent in locomotor activity and increases that spent in immobility, which is the opposite of responses seen in controls. When postnatally 6-OH-DA–lesioned rats receive a single intracerebroventricular dose of 5,7-DHT at adulthood (75 μg at 10 weeks), which destroys part of their serotonergic axons in the striatum (and probably elsewhere), their spontaneous locomotor activity is greatly enhanced (26). Neurochemical and immunohistochemical studies in rats lesioned after birth or at adulthood with 6-OH-DA reveal similarities in the preference of 6-OH-DA toxicity for dopamine neurons in the lateral portions of the substantia nigra and a relative sparing of neurons located in medial aspects of the substantia nigra and the ventral tegmental area (8). Dopamine neurons escaping the toxic actions of 6-OH-DA in neonatally treated animals and in those treated as adults give rise to dopaminergic projections innervating the medial and ventral portions of the striatum and nucleus accumbens. Therefore, differences in the susceptibility of dopaminergic neurons to the toxicity of 6-OH-DA at various stages of development do not account for the differences in spontaneous and drug-induced behavior noted in either group of animals. However, differential adaptation of D_1 and D_2 receptors lesioned at the different time points seems to contribute to differences in the behavioral responses to D_1 and D_2 agonists.

Neonatal 6-OH-DA destruction of nigrostriatal dopaminergic projections in the rat induces latent sensitization of dopamine D_1 receptor agonist–elicited, orally related behaviors such as sniffing, licking, grooming, head nodding, paw-treading, and "taffy pulling" (24). When the D_1 agonist is given repeatedly, a gradual supersensitization of the D_1 receptors, known as priming, becomes apparent (12). L-Dopa, a mixed D_1/D_2 agonist, is likewise capable of priming and thus of agonist-induced enhancement of behavioral responsivity. Concomitant with the increasing sensitization of the D_1 receptors by repeated challenge with agonists, unusual behaviors appear in the neonatally lesioned animals: self-biting and self-mutilation (8,12). Because of these phenomena, neonatally 6-OH-DA–lesioned rats are considered animal models of self-mutilative behavior, as seen in patients with Lesch-Nyhan syndrome (7). The D_1 receptor antagonist SCH 23390 attenuates almost all of these agonist-induced behaviors. Haloperidol, a D_2 antagonist, is not effective in preventing self-mutilative behavior. The selective D_1 agonist SKF 38393 elicits this behavior in about 50% of the lesioned rats; L-dopa is more effective, and the combination of the D_2 agonist quinpirole and SKF 38393 induces self-mutilation in almost all rats (8).

REFERENCES

1. Adams RN, Murrill E, McCreery R et al. (1972) 6-Hydroxydopamine, a new oxidation mechanism. *Eur J Pharmacol* **17**, 287.

2. Baumgarten HG, Zimmermann B (1992) Neurotoxic phenylalkylamines and indolealkylamines. In: *Handbook of Experimental Pharmacology. Vol 102: Selective Neurotoxicity.* Herken H, Hucho F eds. Springer-Verlag, Berlin, Heidelberg p. 225.

3. Bjerre B, Björklund A, Mobley W (1973) A stimulatory effect by nerve growth factor on the regrowth of adrenergic nerve fibres in the mouse peripheral tissues after chemical sympathectomy with 6-hydroxydopamine. *Z Zellforsch* **146**, 15.

4. Bloom FE, Algeri S, Gropetti A et al. (1969) Lesions of central norepinephrine terminals with 6-OH-dopamine: Biochemistry and fine structure. *Science* **166**, 1284.

5. Borchardt RT, Burgess SK, Reid JR et al. (1977) Effects of 2- and/or 5-methylated analogues of 6-hydroxydopamine on norepinephrine- and dopamine-containing neurons. *Mol Pharmacol* **13**, 805.

6. Breese GR (1975) Chemical and immunochemical lesions by specific neurotoxic substances and antisera. In: *Handbook of Psychopharmacology. Vol 1: Biochemical Principles and Techniques in Neuropharmacology.* Iversen LL, Iversen SD, Snyder SH eds. Plenum Press, New York p. 137.

7. Breese GR, Criswell HE, Duncan GE et al. (1990) A dopamine deficiency model of Lesch-Nyhan disease— the neonatal-6-OH-DA-lesioned rat. *Brain Res Bull* **25**, 477.

8. Breese GR, Criswell HE, Johnson KW et al. (1994) Neonatal destruction of dopaminergic neurons. *Neurotoxicology* **15**, 149.

9. Cohen G, Heikkila RE (1974) The generation of hydrogen peroxide, superoxide radical, and hydroxyl radical by 6-hydroxydopamine, dialuric acid, and related cytotoxic agents. *J Biol Chem* **249**, 2447.

10. Cohen G, Werner P (1994) Free radicals, oxidative stress, and neurodegeneration. In: *Neurodegenerative Diseases.* Calne DB ed. WB Saunders Co, Philadelphia p. 139.

11. Commins DL, Shaugnessy RA, Axt KJ et al. (1989) Variability among brain regions in the specificity of 6-hydroxydopamine (6-OH-DA)-induced lesions. *J Neural Transm* **77**, 197.

12. Criswell H, Mueller RA, Breese GR (1989) Priming of D_1-dopamine receptor responses: Long-lasting behavioral supersensitivity to a D_1-dopamine agonist following repeated administration to neonatal 6-OH-DA-lesioned rats. *J Neurosci* **9**, 125.

13. Descarries L, Beaudet A, DeChamplain J (1975) Selective deafferentiation of rat neocortex by destruction of catecholamine neurons with intraventricular 6- hydroxydopamine. In: *Chemical Tools in Catecholamine Research I.* Jonsson G, Malmfors T, Sachs S eds. North-Holland, Amsterdam p. 101.

14. Finch CE, Day JR (1994) Molecular biology of aging in the nervous system: A synopsis of the levels of mechanisms. In: *Neurodegenerative Diseases.* Calne DB ed. WB Saunders Co, Philadelphia p. 33.

15. Graham DG (1978) Oxidative pathways for catecholamines in the genesis of neuromelanin and cytotoxic quinones. *Mol Pharmacol* **14**, 633.

16. Graham DG, Tiffany SM, Bell WR Jr et al. (1978) Autoxidation versus covalent binding of quinones as the mechanism of toxicity of dopamine, 6-hydroxydopamine, and related compounds toward C1300 neuroblastoma cells *in vitro. Mol Pharmacol* **14**, 644.

17. Hedreen J (1975) Increased non-specific damage after lateral ventricle injection of 6-OH-DA compared with fourth ventricle injection in rat brain. In: *Chemical Tools in Catecholamine Research I.* Jonsson G, Malmfors T, Sachs S eds. North-Holland, Amsterdam p. 91.

18. Heikkila R, Cabbat FS (1977) Chemiluminescence from 6-hydroxydopamine: Involvement of hydrogen peroxide, the superoxide radical and the hydroxyl radical, a potential role for singlet oxygen. *Res Commun Chem Pathol Pharmacol* **17**, 649.

19. Jacobowitz DM (1975) Long-term effect on peripheral adrenergic nerves of 6-hydroxydopamine injected into newborn rats. In: *Chemical Tools in Catecholamine*

Research I. Jonsson G, Malmfors T, Sachs S eds. North-Holland, Amsterdam p. 153.

20. Javoy F, Agid Y, Glowinsky J *et al.* (1974) Biochemical and morphological changes after mechanical or chemical degeneration of the dopaminergic nigro-neostriatal pathway. In: *Dynamics of Degeneration and Growth in Neurons.* Fuxe K, Olson L, Zotterman Y eds. Pergamon Press, New York p. 85.

21. Jonsson G (1976) Studies on the mechanisms of 6-hydroxydopamine cytotoxicity. *Med Biol* **54**, 406.

22. Jonsson G (1980) Chemical neurotoxins as denervation tools in neurobiology. *Annu Rev Neurosci* **3**, 169.

23. Kostrzewa RM (1989) Neurotoxins that affect central and peripheral catecholamine neurons. In: *Neuromethods 12: Drugs as Tools in Neurotransmitter Research.* Boulton AA, Baker GB, Juorio AV eds. Humana Press, Totowa, New Jersey p. 1.

24. Kostrzewa RM (1995) Dopamine receptor supersensitivity. *Neurosci Biobehav Rev* **19**, 1.

25. Kostrzewa RM, Brus R, Kalbfleisch JH *et al.* (1994) Proposed animal model of attention deficit hyperactivity disorder. *Brain Res Bull* **34**, 161.

26. Kostrzewa RM, Jacobowitz DM (1974) Pharmacological actions of 6-hydroxydopamine. *Pharmacol Rev* **26**, 199.

27. Lanfumey L, Arluison M, Adrien J (1981) Destruction of noradrenergic cell bodies by intracerebral 6-hydroxydopamine in the newborn rat. *Brain Res* **214**, 445.

28. Laverty R, Sharman DE, Vogt M (1965) Action of 2,4,5-trihydroxyphenyl-ethylamine on the storage and release of noradrenaline. *Brit J Pharmacol* **24**, 549.

29. Liang Y-O, Wightman RM, Plotsky P *et al.* (1975) Oxidative interactions of 6-hydroxydopamine with CNS constituents. In: *Chemical Tools in Catecholamine Research I.* Jonsson G, Malmfors T, Sachs S eds. North-Holland, Amsterdam p. 15.

30. Lorez HP, Kuhn H, Bartholini G (1975) Degeneration and regeneration of adrenergic nerves in mesenteric blood vessels, iris and atrium of the rat after 6-hydroxydopamine injection. *J Neurocytol* **4**, 157.

31. Poirier LJ, Langelier P, Roberge A *et al.* (1972) Nonspecific histopathological changes induced by intracerebral injection of 6-hydroxydopamine (6-OH-DA). *J Neurol Sci* **16**, 401.

32. Porter CC, Totaro JA, Stone CA (1963) Effect of 6-hydroxydopamine and some other compounds on the concentration of norepinephrine in the hearts of mice. *J Pharmacol Exp Ther* **140**, 308.

33. Reader TA, Gauthier P (1984) Catecholamines and serotonin in the rat central nervous system after 6-OH-DA, 5,7-DHT and p-CPA. *J Neural Transm* **59**, 207.

34. Rosengren E, Linder-Eliasson E, Carlsson A (1985) Detection of 5-S-cysteinyldopamine in human brain. *J Neural Transm* **63**, 247.

35. Rotman A, Daly JW, Creveling CR (1976) Oxygen-dependent reaction of 6-hydroxydopamine, 5,6-dihydroxytryptamine, and related compounds with proteins *in vitro*: a model for cytotoxicity. *Mol Pharmacol* **12**, 887.

36. Sachs C, Jonsson G (1975) Mechanisms of action of 6-hydroxydopamine. *Biochem Pharmacol* **24**, 1.

37. Saner A, Thoenen H (1971) Model experiments on the molecular mechanism of action of 6-hydroxydopamine. *Mol Pharmacol* **7**, 147.

38. Senoh S, Witkop B (1959) Non-enzymatic conversions of dopamine to norepinephrine and trihydroxyphenylethylamines. *J Amer Chem Soc* **81**, 6222.

39. Senoh S, Witkop B (1959) Formation and rearrangements of aminochromes from a new metabolite of dopamine and some of its derivatives. *J Amer Chem Soc* **81**, 6231.

40. Shaywitz BA, Klopper JH, Yager RD *et al.* (1976) Paradoxical response to amphetamine in developing rats treated with 6-hydroxydopamine. *Nature* **261**, 153.

41. Shaywitz BA, Yager RD, Klopper JH (1976) Selective brain dopamine depletion in developing rats: An experimental model of minimal brain dysfunction. *Science* **191**, 305.

42. Stone CA, Stavorski JM, Ludden CT *et al.* (1963) Comparison of some pharmacological effects of certain 6-substituted dopamine derivatives with reserpine, guanethidine and metaraminol. *J Pharmacol Exp Ther* **142**, 147.

43. Thoenen H (1972) Chemical sympathectomy: A new tool in the investigation of the physiology and pharmacology of peripheral and central adrenergic neurons. In: *Perspectives in Neuropharmacology.* Snyder SH ed. Oxford University Press, New York p. 302.

44. Thoenen H, Tranzer JP (1968) Chemical sympathectomy by selective destruction of adrenergic nerve endings with 6-hydroxydopamine. *Naunyn-Schmied Arch Exp Pathol Pharmakol* **261**, 271.

45. Thoenen H, Tranzer JP (1973) The pharmacology of 6-hydroxydopamine. *Annu Rev Pharmacol* **13**, 169.

46. Tranzer JP, Thoenen H (1967) Ultramorphologische Veränderungen der sympathischen Nervenendigungen der Katze nach Vorbehandlung mit 5- und 6-Hydroxy-Dopamin. *Naunyn-Schmied Arch Pharmakol Exp Pathol* **257**, 343.

47. Tranzer JP, Thoenen H (1968) An electron microscopic study of selective acute degeneration of sympathetic nerve terminals after administration of 6-hydroxydopamine. *Experientia* **24**, 155.

48. Tse DCS, McCreery RL, Adams RN (1976) Potential oxidative pathways of brain catecholamines. *J Med Chem* **19**, 37.

49. Ungerstedt U (1968) 6-Hydroxydopamine induced degeneration of central monoamine neurons. *Eur J Pharmacol* **5**, 107.

50. Ungerstedt U (1971) Histochemical studies on the effect of intracerebral and intraventricular injections of 6-hydroxydopamine on monoamine neurons in the rat

brain. In: *6-Hydroxydopamine and Catecholamine Neurons*. Malmfors T, Thoenen H eds. North- Holland, Amsterdam p. 101.

51. Uretsky NJ, Iversen LL (1969) Effects of 6-hydroxydopamine on noradrenaline-containing neurons in the rat brain. *Nature* **221**, 557.

52. Uretsky NJ, Iversen LL (1970) Effects of 6-hydroxydopamine on catecholamine-containing neurones in the rat brain. *J Neurochem* **17**, 269.

53. Zigmond MJ, Hastings TG (1998) Neurochemical responses to lesions of dopaminergic neurons: implications for compensation and neuropathology. *Adv Pharmacol* **42**, 788.

54. Zigmond MJ, Hastings TG, Abercrombie ED (1992) Neurochemical responses to 6-hydroxydopamine and L-dopa therapy: Implications for Parkinson's disease. *Ann N Y Acad Sci* **648**, 71.

55. Zigmond MJ, Stricker EM (1989) Animal models of parkinsonism using selective neurotoxins: Clinical and basic implications. *Intern Rev Neurobiol* **31**, 1.

α-Hydroxytoluene

Peter S. Spencer

$$C_6H_5 \cdot CH_2OH$$

Benzyl alcohol; Benzenemethanol; Phenylcarbinol

NEUROTOXICITY RATING

Clinical

A   Radiculopathy (intrathecal)

B   Intraventricular hemorrhage (neonate, intravascular)

Experimental

A   Radiculopathy (intrathecal, axonal degeneration)

α-Hydroxytoluene (benzyl alcohol) is the most abundant volatile agent in the common mushroom (*Agaricus bisporus*) (4). Benzyl alcohol is used in concentrations up to 2% as a Gram-positive bacteriostatic compound. Concentrations up to 5% or more are employed when benzyl alcohol is used as a solubilizer. The substance also serves as a preservative in foods and cosmetics (18).

Benzyl alcohol is a clear, colorless, oily, refractive liquid with a slightly aromatic odor; it is soluble in water and miscible with alcohol. The alcohol oxidizes slowly in air to produce the toxic aldehyde, benzaldehyde, and benzoic acid. Benzaldehyde may also be produced during autoclaving (18).

Benzyl alcohol is the major hydroxylation product of toluene metabolism, comprising >99% of total metabolites formed in rats (3). Benzaldehyde formed through the action of alcohol dehydrogenase is the primary metabolite of benzyl alcohol in adult and neonatal CD-1 mice (17). In human neonates, benzyl alcohol is rapidly oxidized to benzoic acid, although large doses may result in the detection of serum benzaldehyde (15). Benzoic acid is conjugated with glycine in the mitochondrial fraction of the liver and kidney to form hippuric acid (15). Benzyl alcohol has free-radical-quenching properties *in vitro*, while benzaldehyde induces generation of reactive oxygen species and may represent the neurotoxic metabolite of toluene (16).

Pure benzyl alcohol is a dermal irritant and should be handled with care. Ingestion or inhalation reportedly causes nausea, vomiting and diarrhea, headache and central nervous system depression (18).

Parenteral toxicity studies have been performed with mice, rats, cats, dogs, and monkeys (7,14). In rats, intravenous benzyl alcohol (94%) was 23 times more acutely toxic than intravenous ethyl alcohol (95%) (14). Cats given two subcutaneous injections of 100 ml 1.5% benzyl alcohol or two 1.5-ml injections of reagent-grade benzyl alcohol developed ataxia, hyperesthesia, muscle fasciculation of the head and ears, and slight depression (7). Intracarotid injection of 0.9% benzyl alcohol did not cause any significant effects on the electroencephalogram, electrocardiogram, blood pressure, heart rate, or respiration of anesthetized dogs (14). Intracisternal injection of 4.5% and 7% benzyl alcohol produced rigid extension of the forelimbs followed by the hindlimbs; this suggested a direct action on medullary nuclei because motor neurons regulating the forelimbs lie more superficially. Intracisternal injection of a higher concentration (9%) of benzyl alcohol proved fatal for immature dogs, while adult animals displayed transient respiratory arrest (8). Rat lumbar spinal roots exposed intrathecally to aqueous 1.5% benzyl alcohol (bacteriostatic water) developed conduction block, with incomplete reversibility of A-fiber potentials after wash-out. Treatment of rat cauda equina for 7 days with 0.9% or 1.5% bacteriostatic water or saline resulted in scattered demyelination and nerve degeneration, respectively; no changes were seen in animals that received intrathecal injections of comparable quantities of distilled water (9,12).

Acute-onset and delayed neurotoxicity has been reported after introduction of benzyl alcohol into human cerebrospinal fluid (12). A 64-year-old man with lymphomatous meningitis received two intrathecal injections of cytosine arabinoside in distilled water without ill effects. A third intrathecal injection of cytoskine arabinoside in 1.5% bacteriostatic water resulted within 10 minutes in complete flaccid areflexic paraplegia and total anesthesia below the groin. Muscle activity began to return from proximal to distal regions within 15 min of saline irrigation, with return of full power and sensation within 30 min. Postmortem examination of well-preserved lumbosacral nerve roots showed perineurial and endoneural fibrosis, together with large numbers of remyelinated nerve fibers (12). Benzyl alcohol was present in the injectate in 7 of 20 other cases of paraparesis associated with intrathecal injection of cytarabine or methotrexate. Neurological changes occurred immediately in four cases and, in the other three, 6 to 48 h after administration. One patient experienced only transient effects; two recovered with 1.5 to 2.5 h; one did not improve, one made a partial recovery, and another took 5 days to recover (18).

During 1981 and 1982, two centers in the United States attributed 20 deaths of low-birth-weight neonates (<1250 g birth weight) to benzyl alcohol in solutions used to flush umbilical intravascular catheters and, in some cases, to reconstitute medications (6,10,11). The neonates suffered from a syndrome featured by gasping respiration, metabolic acidosis, seizures, neurological deterioration, hepatic and renal abnormalities, and eventual cardiovascular collapse and death. The U.S. Food and Drug Administration (FDA) advised against the use of benzyl alcohol in flushing solutions and in fluids used to dilute or reconstitute medicines for the newborn (2). A survey by the U.S. Centers for Disease Control subsequently revealed that, prior to the FDA warning, 20 of 29 hospitals responding to a survey had routinely used solutions containing benzyl alcohol in the care of the newborn. In one hospital, a comparison of the course of neonates (<1000 g) prior to and following withdrawal of benzyl alcohol revealed significant decreases in both mortality rate (80.7% to 45.7%) and incidence of grade III/IV intraventricular hemorrhage (from 49% to 19%) (13). Discontinuation of solutions containing benzyl alcohol was temporally associated with a dramatic reduction in the incidence of cerebral palsy and developmental delay (5). Controlled studies to assess the role of benzyl alcohol in the neonatal gasping syndrome were not performed (1).

REFERENCES

1. American Academy of Pediatrics (1983) Benzyl alcohol: toxic agent in neonatal use. *Pediatrics* **72**, 356.
2. Anonymous (1982) Benzyl alcohol may be toxic to newborns. *FDA Drug Bull* **12**, 10.
3. Backes WL, Sequeira DJ, Cawley GF, Eyer CS (1993) Relationship between hydrocarbon structure and induction of P450; effects on protein levels and enzyme activities. *Xenobiotica* **23**, 1353.
4. Beier RC (1990) Natural pesticides and bioactive components in foods. *Rev Environ Contam Toxicol* **113**, 47.
5. Benda GI, Hiller JL, Reynolds JW (1986) Benzyl alcohol toxicity: Impact on neurologic handicaps among surviving very low birth weight infants. *Pediatrics* **77**, 507.
6. Brown WJ, Buist NRM, Gepson HT *et al.* (1982) Fatal benzyl alcohol poisoning in a neonatal intensive care unit. *Lancet* **1**, 1250.
7. Cullison RF, Menard PD, Buck WB (1983) Toxicosis in cats from use of benzyl alcohol in lactated Ringer's solution. *J Amer Vet Med Assn* **182**, 61.
8. DeLand FH (1973) Intrathecal toxicity studies with benzyl alcohol. *Toxicol Appl Pharmacol* **25**, 153.
9. Feasby TE, Hahn AF, Gilbert JJ (1983) Neurotoxicity of bacteriostatic water. *N Engl J Med* **308**, 966.
10. Gershanik JJ, Boccler F, Ensley H *et al.* (1982) The gasping syndrome and benzyl alcohol poisoning. *N Engl J Med* **307**, 1384.
11. Gershanik JJ, Boccler F, George W *et al.* (1981) The gasping syndrome: benzyl alcohol (BA) poisoning. *Clin Res* **29**, 895.
12. Hahn AF, Feasby TE, Gilbert JJ (1983) Paraparesis following intrathecal chemotherapy. *Neurology* **33**, 1032.
13. Hiller JL, Benda GL, Rahatzad M *et al.* (1986) Benzyl alcohol toxicity: Impact on mortality and intraventricular hemorrhage among very low birth weight infants. *Pediatrics* **77**, 500.
14. Kimura ET, Darby TD, Krause RA, Brondyk HD (1971) Parenteral toxicity studies with benzyl alcohol. *Toxicol Appl Pharmacol* **18**, 60.
15. LeBel M, Ferron L, Masson M *et al.* (1988) Benzyl alcohol metabolism and elimination in neonates. *Dev Pharmacol Ther* **11**, 347.
16. Mattia CJ, LeBel CP, Bondy SC (1991) Effects of toluene and its metabolites on cerebral reactive oxygen species generation. *Biochem Pharmacol* **42**, 879.
17. McCloskey SE, Gershanik JJ, Lertora JJ *et al.* (19860 Toxicity of benzyl alcohol in adult and neonatal mice. *J Pharm Sci* **75**, 702.
18. Reynolds JEF (1996) *Martindale. The Extra Pharmacopoeia. 31st Ed.* London, Royal Pharmaceutical Society, p. 1119.

Hymenoxys richardsonii

Helge Völkel
Albert C. Ludolph

NEUROTOXICITY RATING

Clinical

B   Seizure disorder (cattle)

Hymenoxys richardsonii (Colorado rubberweed; family Compositae) is a cause of livestock loss in Colorado, New Mexico, and Arizona, U.S.A. (4). Since sheep and goats consume the plant during food shortages, poisoning is most frequent in spring and late autumn when other forage is reduced. Cattle are poisoned less frequently, as they find the plant unpalatable (2). Each part of the perennial plant is toxic, including leaves and stem. Symptoms include salivation, anorexia, depression, signs of abdominal distress, weakness, and respiratory compromise. Tremors and seizures are rare. Metabolic abnormalities include hypolipidemia and hypoglycemia (9).

Sesquiterpene lactones are the suspected cause of *H. richardsonii* poisoning (1). Hymenovin (hymenoxon), one of the sesquiterpene lactones present in *H. richardsonii*, is believed to be a major determinant of toxicity (3); however, feeding the compound to sheep did not cause neurological dysfunction (7). Possible muscle tremors and seizures are secondary to hypoglycemia.

The toxic effects of sesquiterpene lactones are possibly related to their highly reactive functional groups (8) and their ability to deplete hepatic glutathione levels (5). Hymenoxon inhibited state-3 respiration of mouse hepatic mitochondria, stimulated state-4 respiration, enhanced adenosine triphosphatase activity in the presence of Mg^{2+} and caused mitochondrial swelling (6). There is presently no evidence for human neurotoxicity of *Hymenoxys* spp.

REFERENCES

1. Ahmed AA, Spring O, Abd El-Razek M *et al.* (1995) Sesquiterpene lactones and other constituents from *Hymenoxys richardsonii* and *H. subintegra*. *Phytochemistry* 39, 1127.
2. Cheeke PR, Schull LR (1985) *Natural Toxicants in Feeds and Poisonous Plants*. AVI Publishing Company, Westport, Connecticut.
3. Ivie GW, Witzel DA, Herz W *et al.* (1976) Isolation of hymenovin from *Hymenoxys richardsonii* (pingue) and *Dugaldia hoopesi* (orange sneezeweed). *J Agr Food Chem* 24, 681.
4. Kingsbury JM (1964) *Poisonous Plants of the United States and Canada*. Prentice-Hall, Englewood Cliffs, New Jersey p. 409.
5. Merrill JC, Kim HL, Safe S *et al.* (1988) Role of glutathione in the toxicity of the sesquiterpene lactones hymenoxon and helenalin. *J Toxicol Environ Health* 23, 159.
6. Narasimham TR, Kim HL, Safe SH (1989) Effects of sesquiterpene lactones on mitochondrial oxidative phosphorylation. *Gen Pharmacol* 20, 681.
7. Rowe LD, Kim HL, Camp BJ (1980) The antagonistic effect of L-cysteine in experimental hymenoxon intoxication in sheep. *Amer J Vet Res* 41, 484.
8. Sylvia VL, Kim HL, Norman JO, Busbee DL (1987) The sesquiterpene lactone hymenoxon acts as a bifunctional alkylating agent. *Cell Biol Toxicol* 3, 39.
9. Witzel DA, Rowe LD, Clark DE (1974) Physiopathologic studies on acute *Hymenoxys odorata* (bitterweed) poisoning in sheep. *Amer J Vet Res* 35, 931.

Hypoglycine

Peter S. Spencer

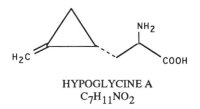

HYPOGLYCINE A
C₇H₁₁NO₂

[*S*-(*R**,*S**)]-α-Amino-2-methylenecyclopropane-propanoic acid; 2-Methylenecyclopropanealanine; Hypoglycin A

NEUROTOXICITY RATING

Clinical

A   Hepatic encephalopathy

Experimental

A   Hepatic encephalopathy

Hypoglycin A (hypoglycine) and hypoglycin B (γ-glutamyl hypoglycine) are water-soluble toxins and teratogens isolated from seed of the fruit of the ackee tree, *Blighia sapida*, a native of west Africa. Ackee was imported into the West Indies in the eighteenth century; thereafter, the inner portion (arilli) of the cooked ripe fruit became a staple of the Jamaican diet. *B. sapida* is also found in other islands in the Caribbean (outer Antilles), in Central America, and in southern Florida (10,19,23). Hypoglycine is found in related plants such as the common sycamore (*Acer pseudoplatinatus*) and, together with its lower homologue, methylenecyclopropylglycine, in seed of fruit of the litchi (*Litchi chinensis*) (12,19). These agents are not directly neurotoxic; rather, they induce hepatic encephalopathy reminiscent of Reye's syndrome (16). Ingestion of unripe seed, mostly by children, rapidly triggers a disorder featured by severe hypoglycemia, vomiting, seizures, coma, and death. Up to 5000 deaths are estimated to have occurred between the years 1886 and 1950 (14). Cases attributed to ackee poisoning have also been reported from Côte d'Ivoire (7). The metabolic basis for the condition, known as Jamaican vomiting sickness, has been extensively reviewed (19).

Naturally occurring hypoglycine, an L-amino acid, is a mixture of diastereoisomers at C4 with a slight excess of the *R* form (32). Concentrations up to 1% of wet weight are found in the arilli and seed of the unripe ackee fruit; the hypoglycine content drops as the fruit ripens (5). Arilli also contain up to 2.7% dry weight of glutamic acid (1). Importation of canned ackee arilli into the United States was banned in 1972 by the U.S. Food and Drug Administration.

General Toxicology

Hypoglycine is structurally related to leucine and metabolized by enzymes involved in the catabolism of leucine to isovaleryl-coenzyme A (CoA) (19). Hypoglycine is metabolized in the cytosol to methylene cyclopropylpyruvate and, after diffusion into the mitochondrial matrix where it is oxidatively decarboxylated, to methylene cyclopropylacetyl-CoA (MCPA), which is reponsible for most of the metabolic effects of hypoglycine. MCPA also reacts with glycine to form MCPA-glycine (19). MCPA inhibits isovaleryl-CoA dehydrogenase and causes the accumulation of large amounts of isovaleric acid and 2-methylbutyric acid in the blood of hypoglycine-treated animals (24). Animals excrete large amounts of *N*-isovalerylglycine, butyrylglycine, MCPA-glycine, adipate and, in addition, a number of unusual medium-chain dicarboxylic acids (21). Large quantities of glutaric acid are excreted along with adipic, suberic, and sebacic acids (19).

Animal Studies

The rat LD$_{50}$ for hypoglycine is 90–100 mg/kg body weight (23). Oral or parenteral administration of hypoglycine to fasted animals induces hypoglycemia. This has been described in the guinea pig (most sensitive), rabbit, monkey, dog, cat, mouse, and hamster (least senstive) (6,19). Hypoglycemia appears within 2–7 h of dosing and lasts for many hours (19). Onset of toxicity depends upon the formation of MCPA and the development of hypoglycemia and organic acidemia (19); peak plasma concentrations of MCPA occur 1–4 h after administration of hypoglycine (19,21). Vomiting, behavioral depression, coma, and death are seen in hypoglycine-treated cats and dogs. Ablation of the medullary emetic center abolishes hypoglycine-induced vomiting in cats but not the delayed toxic effects (4). Cats and rats develop an organic aciduria, and rats become hypothermic (19). Hypoglycine-induced hypoglycemia, organic acidemia, and hypothermia are blocked in rats receiving large intraperitoneal doses of glycine (2). Intravenous sodium bicarbonate attenuated some of the effects of feline hypoglycine toxicity (4). Riboflavin protected rats and mice from hypoglycine toxicity (11,26). Male rats fed 0.5% clofibrate for 1–2 months were protected against the toxic, hypoglycemic, and hypothermic effects of hypoglycine (25).

Pregnant rats given several daily doses of hypoglycine (15–30 mg/kg/day) have a high incidence of fetal malformations (17). Hypoglycin B also exhibits experimental teratogenic properties in rats (18).

Human Studies

Hypoglycine is one of several agents (pentanoate, valproate, salicylate) that produces a Reye's-like syndrome characterized by hepatic encephalopathy with fatty infiltration of the liver due to mitochondrial dysfunction (16). The historical background and clinical features of human ackee poisoning have been reviewed (8,20,23). Cases are now rarely reported in Jamaica (19); most occur between December and March. Children between ages 2 and 10 are most frequently affected; cases are not seen among babies. Signs of chronic malnutrition and those attributed to thiamine and riboflavin deficiency are common (8). Humans with ackee poisoning display up to 20 times the normal concentrations of volatile plasma fatty acids, significantly lower than those found in hypoglycine-treated rats and cats (22,23).

Two clinical variants of ackee poisoning are described in children and milder forms occur in adults (8); these presumably reflect different degrees of toxicity and individual susceptibility. One (acute) is characterized by sudden onset of foaming at the mouth, "twitching" of the limbs, collapse, convulsions, coma, and death, all of which occur over a span of a few hours. The second (subacute) is characterized by an abrupt onset of vomiting and generalized weakness.

Body temperature may be subnormal. Apparent recovery may occur after several hours only to be interrupted by another attack of vomiting. Convulsions, seen in about 85% of cases, are expressed in forms that vary from twitching of the limbs to tonic muscle spasms lasting several minutes. Some patients become unconscious with restlessness and irritation; others enter a state of deep coma and die. The clinical course is said to span 10 hours to a few days (23). Adults reportedly are less severely affected after ingestion of ackee fruit; they become excitable, restless, and apprehensive, with alternate periods of drowsiness. Nystgamus, ptosis, rolling of the eyes, intention tremor, ataxia, and increased deep tendon jerks are reported (8,23).

Pathological findings include marked hepatic changes consisting of fatty infiltration, depletion of glycogen granules, and nuclear fragmentation. Swelling of liver mitochondria is evident in hypoglycine-treated rats. In human cases, zymogen granules are absent in the pancreas, and islets of Langerhans may be prominent. Edema and hyperemia are present in the lungs, cerebrum, and meninges. Interstitial edema is also evident in the heart and connective tissues. Lipid droplets are seen in heart and kidney (23).

Intravenous administration of glucose is the first priority in ackee poisoning (19); prompt treatment may lead to a satisfactory clinical outcome (9,20). Treatment efficacy is unrelated to the severity of hypoglycemia; however, the outcome becomes less favorable with increasing intervals between onset of coma and administration of glucose (23). Favorable results obtained in experimental animal studies have suggested additional methods to treat ackee poisoning: (a) repeated administration of glycine (200 mg/kg body weight) every few hours, (b) riboflavin (50–200 mg) every 8 hours, and (c) sodium bicarbonate (19). Their application to humans would be experimental.

Mechanisms

Hypoglycine and other agents that cause hepatic encephalopathies comparable to Reye's syndrome produce similar biochemical manifestations: hypoglycemia due to impaired glyconeogenesis, accumulation of fatty acids, fatty acyl CoAs, and acyl carnitines, with depletion of free CoA and carnitine. Accumulated products may further perturb mitochondrial dysfunction, exacerbate impaired β-oxidation, uncouple oxidative phophorylation and increase mitochondrial permeability with consequent mitochondrial swelling (16). Both hypoglycemia and organic acidemia contribute to the toxic effects of hypoglycine; their relative importance depends on the species (19).

Gluconeogenesis and glucose utilization are severely impaired in hypoglycine-treated rats (15). Hypoglycine metabolites inhibit glyconeogenesis by antagonizing activation of pyruvate carboxylase by acetyl CoA (in the mitochondrial matrix) and by decreasing the ratio of reduced to oxidized nicotinamide adenine dinucleotide in the cytosol (19). Methylenecyclopropylglycine (12) also induces hypoglycemia. Hypoglycine interferes with the oxidation of fatty acids, the concentration of which increases in serum (13,19). Several acyl-CoA dehydrogenases are inactivated *in vivo*; MCPA-CoA inactivates medium-chain acyl CoA, butyryl CoA, isovaleryl CoA, and 2-methylbutyryl-CoA dehydrogenases *in vitro* (19).

REFERENCES

1. Addae JI, Melville GN (1988) A re-examination of the mechanism of ackee-induced vomiting sickness. *W Indian Med J* 37, 6.
2. Al-Basam SS, Sherratt HSA (1981) The antagonism of the toxicity of hypoglycin by glycine. *Biochem Pharmacol* 30, 2817.
3. Baldwin JE, Adlington RM, Bebbington D, Russell AT (1992) Assymetric total synthesis of the individual diastereoisomers of hypoglycin A. *J Chem Soc Chem Commun* 17, 1249.
4. Borrison H, Pendleton J, McCarthy LE (1974) Central vs. systemic neurotoxicity of hypoglycin (ackee toxin) and related substances in the cat. *J Pharmacol Exp Ther* 190, 327.
5. Chase GW, Landen WO, Gelbaum LT, Soliman AG (1989) Ion-exchange chromatographic determination of hypoglycin in canned ackee fruit. *J Assn Off Anal Chem* 72, 374.
6. Chen KK, Anderson RC, McCowen MC, Harris PN (1957) Pharmacologic action of hypoglycin A and B. *J Pharmacol Exp Ther* 121, 272.
7. Founge S, Naho Y, Declume C (1986) Étude expérimental de la toxicité des arilles de Blighia sapida (Sapindaceae) en rapport avec l'intoxication des enfants de Katiola (Côte-d'Ivoire). *Ann Pharmacol Fr* 44, 509.
8. Hill KR (1952) The vomiting sickness of Jamaica: A review. *W Indian Med J* 1, 243.
9. Hill KR, Bras G, Clearkin KP (1955) Acute toxic hypoglycaemia occurring in the vomiting sickness of Jamaica. *W Indian Med J* 4, 91.
10. Lynch SJ, Larson E, Daughty DD (1961) A study of the edibility of ackee (*Blighia sapida*) fruit of Florida. *Proc Fla St Hort Soc* 64, 281.
11. Marley J, Sherratt HSA (1973) The apparent failure of L-carnitine to prevent the hypoglyaemia and hypothermia caused by hypoglycin or by pent-2-enoic acid in mice. *Biochem Pharmacol* 22, 281.
12. Melde K, Buettner H, Boschert W *et al.* (1989) Mechanism of hypoglycaemic action of methylenecyclopropylglycine. *Biochem J* 259, 921.

13. McKerns KW, Bird HH, Kaleita BS *et al.* (1960) Effects of hypoglycin on certain aspects of glucose and fatty acid metabolism in the rat. *Biochem Pharmacol* **3**, 305.

14. Mitchell JC (1974) The posthumous misfortune of Captain Bligh of the "Bounty". Hypoglycemia from *Blighia*. *Diabetes* **23**, 919.

15. Osmundsen H, Billington D, Taylor J, Sherratt HSA (1978) The effects of hypoglycin on glucose metabolism in the rat. A kinetic study *in vivo* and [U-^{14}C, 2-^{3}H]glucose. *Biochem J* **170**, 337.

16. Osterloh J, Cunnigham W, Dixon A, Combest D (1989) Biochemical relationships between Reye's and Reye's-like metabolic and toxicologic syndromes. *Med Tox Adv Drug Exp* **4**, 272.

17. Persaud TVN (1967) Foetal abnormalities caused by the active principle of the fruit of *Blighia sapida* (ackee). *W Indian Med J* **16**, 193.

18. Persaud TVN (1973) Mechanism of teratogenic actions of hypoglycin A. *Experientia* **27**, 414.

19. Sherratt HSA (1995) Jamaican vomiting sickness. In: *Handbook of Clinical Neurology*. Vinken PJ, Bruyn GW eds. *Intoxications of the Nervous System. Pt II*. De Wolff FA ed. Revised Series 21, Vol **65**, Elsevier, Amsterdam p. 79.

20. Stuart KL (1975) Vomiting sickness of Jamaica. In: *Hypoglycin*. Kean EA ed. Academic Press, New York p. 39.

21. Tanaka K (1972) On the mode of action of hypoglycin A. III. Isolation and identification of *cis*-4-decene-1,10-dioic, *cis*, *cis*-4,7-decadiene-1,10-dioic, *cis*-4-octene-1,8-dioic, glutaric and adipic acids, *N*-(methylenecyclopropyl)acetyglycine, and *N*-isovalerylglycine from urine of hypoglycin A treated rats. *J Biol Chem* **247**, 7465.

22. Tanaka K (1975) Branched pentanoic acidemia and medium chain dicarboxylic aciduria induced by hypoglycin A: Inhibition of several short chain acyl CoA dehydrogensaes. In *Hypoglycin*. Kean EA ed. Academic Press, New York p. 67.

23. Tanaka K (1979) Jamaican vomiting sickness. In: *Handbook of Clinical Neurology. Intoxications of the Nervous System. Pt II. Vol 37*. Vinken PJ, Bruyn GW eds. Elsevier, Amsterdam p. 511.

24. Tanaka K, Isselbacher KJ, Shih V (1972) Isovaleric and alpha-methylbutyric acidemias induced by hypoglycin A: Mechanisms of Jamaican vomiting sickness. *Science* **175**, 69.

25. Van Hoof F, Hue L, Vamecq J, Sherratt HS (1985) Protection of rats by clofibrate against the hypoglycemic and toxic effects of hypoglycin and pent-4-enoate. An ultrastructural and biochemical study. *Biochem J* **229**, 387.

26. Von Holt CL, Von Holt C (1959) Biochemie des Hypoglycin A. I. Die Wirkung des Riboflavins auf den Hypoglycine effects. *Biochem Z* **331**, 422.

Iberiotoxin

Albert C. Ludolph

Albert C. Ludolph

NEUROTOXICITY RATING

Experimental

A Ion channel dysfunction (Ca^{2+}-activated potassium channel)

Iberiotoxin (IbTx) is a selective K$^+$-channel toxin of the venom of the scorpion *Buthus tamulus* (2). It is a 37-amino-acid peptide with 68% homology with charybdotoxin (ChTx) (2) and a molecular weight of 4.3 kDa. In contrast to ChTx, which also blocks intermediate- and small-conductance K$^+$ channels, IbTx selectively blocks high-conductance Ca^{2+}-activated K$^+$ channels in muscle and neuroendocrine tissue (2). IbTx does not block voltage-dependent K$^+$ channels of T lymphocytes, an effect of ChTx. IbTx binds to the external mouth of the Ca^{2+}-activated K$^+$ channel in muscle through a bimolecular reaction that blocks ion flux through the channel (1,3). Chimeric peptides have defined the toxin-channel interactions of IbTx and ChTx, respectively (4). IbTx decreases both the probability of channel opening and its mean open time, resulting in nonconducting states that may last for minutes. Periods of normal channel activity (3) may interrupt the quiescent state. IbTX is used as an experimental tool to study the high-conductance Ca^{2+}-activated K$^+$ channel.

It is most unlikely that IbTx neurotoxicity contributes to the toxic, sometimes lethal, effects of the sting of *B. tamalus*, since the agent represents <1% of the protein in *Bu-thus* venom (2). Experimental injection of a high dosage of *B. tamalus* venom into rats induces a reduction of blood pressure that is followed by hypertension (5). The animal dies of respiratory failure, but overt neurotoxic effects are not seen (5). IbTx increases *in vivo* acetylcholine release at the neuromuscular junction; this may be due to delayed inactivation of Na$^+$ channels (5).

REFERENCES

1. Candia S, Garcia ML, Latorre R (1992) Mode of action of iberiotoxin, a potent blocker of the large-conductance Ca^{2+}-activated K$^+$ channel. *Biophys J* 63, 583.
2. Galvez A, Gimenez-Gallego G, Reuben JP *et al.* (1990) Purification and characterization of a unique, potent, peptidyl-probe for the high-conductance calcium-activated potassium channel from the venom of the scorpion *Buthus tamulus*. *J Biol Chem* 265, 11083.
3. Giangiacomo KM, Garcia ML, McManus OB (1992) Mechanisms of iberiotoxin block of the large-conductance calcium-activated potassium channel from bovine aortic smooth muscle. *Biochemistry* 31, 6719.
4. Giangiacomo KM, Sugg EE, Garcia-Calvo M *et al.* (1993) Synthetic charybdotoxin-iberiotoxin chimeric peptides define toxin binding sites on calcium-activated and voltage-dependent potassium channels. *Biochemistry* 32, 2363.
5. Rowan EG, Vatanpour H, Furman BL *et al.* (1992) The effects of Indian red scorpion *Buthus tamalus* venom *in vivo* and *in vitro*. *Toxicon* 30, 1157.

Ibotenic Acid

Albert C. Ludolph

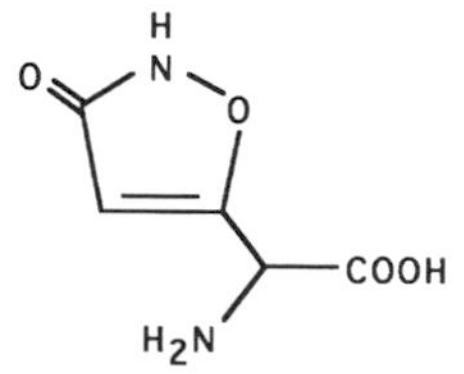

Albert C. Ludolph

IBOTENIC ACID
C$_5$H$_6$N$_2$O$_4$

α-Amino-2,3-dihydro-3-oxo-5-isoxazoleacetic acid

NEUROTOXICITY RATING

Clinical

A Acute encephalopathy (sedation, myoclonic seizures)

Experimental

A Excitotoxin

Ibotenic acid is a naturally occuring isoxazole amino acid with a MW of 158.11. The colorless crystal has a MP of 151°–152°C (anhydrous) and 144°–146°C (monohydrate). Structurally, the compound is a five-membered saturated ring containing one nitrogen and one oxygen linked to a quaternary amine. The neurotoxin is present in mushrooms of the genus *Amanita*, such as *A. muscaria*, *A. regalis*, *A. pantherina*, *A. cothurnata*, *A. gemmata*, and *Tricholoma muscarium* (1); its name is derived from the Japanese word for *A. strobiliformis*—*ibotengutake*—the mushroom from which ibotenic acid was first isolated (8). *Amanita* spp. may contain between 0.05% and 0.1% ibotenic acid (4). Accidental and deliberate intoxications with mushrooms of the species *Amanita* occur. The major use of ibotenic acid is as an experimental tool in neurobiology.

Muscimol, the decarboxylation product of ibotenic acid, is also present in mushrooms containing ibotenic acid; *in vivo*, the effects of muscimol can not be distinguished from those of ibotenic acid. Isoxazoles are resistant to cooking, readily absorbed by the gastrointestinal tract, and excreted by the kidneys. Ibotenic acid is also an insecticide (8).

Ibotenic acid has structural and functional similarities to the excitatory neurotransmitter glutamate (2). It has potent excitatory properties at mammalian CNS neurons (5,7); the compound is estimated to be approximately eight times more active than glutamate and equipotent to *N*-methyl-D-aspartate (NMDA) in provoking activity of cat spinal interneurons and Renshaw cells (3). The depression following ibotenate-induced excitation is likely to be induced by its *in vivo* metabolite, a muscimol-like γ-aminobutyric acid agonist (3). Effects of ibotenic acid on NMDA receptors are nonselective (6).

The intravenous LD_{50} of ibotenic acid in rats and mice is 42 and 15 mg/kg body weight; the respective total oral doses are 129 and 38 mg (9). Dosed animals appear sedated. Electroencephalography shows sharp waves and spikes, and animals die from cardiovascular reactions and respiratory failure (9). Human volunteers develop signs consistent with muscimol and *Amanita* poisoning, including ataxia, myoclonic jerks, somnolence, and euphoria or dysphoria (9).

In summary, although it is likely that ibotenic acid plays a role in the clinical manifestations of *Amanita* poisoning, its effects in humans (and experimental animals) cannot be separated from those induced by other compounds present in *Amanita* spp., in particular muscimol.

REFERENCES

1. Chilton WS, Ott J (1976) Toxic metabolites of *Amanita pantherina, A. cothurnata, A. muscaria,* and other *Amanita* species. *Lloydia* **39**, 150.
2. Collingridge GL, Lester RA (1989) Excitatory amino acid receptors in the vertebrate central nervous system. *Pharmacol Rev* **41**, 143.
3. Curtis DR, Lodge D, McLennan H (1979) The excitation and depression of spinal neurons by ibotenic acid. *J Physiol* **291**, 19.
4. Eugster CH (1969) Chemie der Wirkstoffe aus dem Fliegenpilz, *Amanita muscaria. Fortschr Chem Org Naturstoffe* **27**, 261.
5. Johnston GAR, Curtis DR, Davies J, McCulloch RM (1974) Spinal interneurone excitation by conformationally restricted analogues of L-glutamic acid. *Nature* **248**, 804.
6. Krogsgaard-Larsen P, Hansen JJ (1992) Naturally occuring excitatory amino acids as neurotoxins and leads in drug design. *Toxicol Lett* **64–65**, 409.
7. McLennan H, Wheal HV (1978) A synthetic, conformationally restricted analogue of L-glutamic acid which acts as a powerful neuron excitant. *Neurosci Lett* **8**, 51.
8. Takemoto T, Nakajima T, Sakuma P (1964) Isolation of a flyicidal constituent "ibotenic acid" from *Amanita muscaria* and *Amanita pantherina. Yagugaku Zasshi* **84**, 1233.
9. Theobald W, Büch O, Kunz HA *et al.* (1968) Pharmakologische und experimental-psychologische Untersuchungen mit 2 Inhaltsstoffen des Fliegenpilzes (*Amanita muscaria*). *Arzneim Forsch* **18**, 311.

Ibuprofen

Herbert H. Schaumburg

IBUPROFEN
$C_{13}H_{18}O_2$

α-Methyl-4-(2-methylpropyl)benzeneacetic acid

NEUROTOXICITY RATING

Clinical

B Aseptic meningitis (hypersensitivity)

B Visual dysfunciton

Ibuprofen is a well-tolerated, nonsteroidal anti-inflammatory agent; it is one of a group of propionic acid–derived, aspirin-like agents available over-the-counter in North America. The anti-inflammatory properties of the propionic acid derivatives stem from inhibition of prostaglandin biosynthesis. Orally administered ibuprofen is rapidly absorbed; peak plasma concentrations are achieved within 2 h. It is extensively bound to plasma proteins and slowly passes into the synovial spaces, where it may remain as the plasma level declines. Ibuprofen is rapidly excreted in the urine as conjugates or as hydroxylated and carboxylated metabolites; high concentrations of free ibuprofen do not appear in the cerebrospinal fluid (CSF). Ibuprofen therapy is associated with few serious systemic side effects; gastrointestinal distress is experienced by about 15%, and occasional instances of thrombocytopenia occur.

Hypersensitivity meningitis is a rare complication of ibuprofen treatment. Originally described in individuals with autoimmune diseases, it is now apparent that it may appear in otherwise healthy individuals (5,7). The syndrome is characterized by fever, nuchal rigidity, headache, and CSF neutrophilic pleocytosis. A report of elevated intrathecal immune complexes in a healthy individual with this disorder suggests an antigen-specific humoral immune process confined to the CNS (2). Inhibition of prostaglandin synthesis does not appear to be the cause, since patients tolerate indomethacin therapy following ibuprofen-induced meningitis. Individuals with connective tissue disease receiving ibuprofen may develop a multifocal encephalopathic syndrome as well as meningitis (1).

Toxic amblyopia has been recognized as a complication of ibuprofen since 1971 (3). This rare syndrome is usually heralded by a sudden unilateral decrease in visual acuity to 20/60–20/80 and central scotomata. It usually appears within 3 weeks of therapy at conventional doses. Few instances are well studied, and the pathophysiology of this condition is unknown. One individual displayed diminished amplitudes of visual evoked potentials and increased conduction times that returned to normal 6 days after stopping the drug (4). Another had depressed contrast sensitivity (6).

REFERENCES

1. Agus B, Nelson J, Kramer N et al. (1990) Acute central nervous system symptoms caused by ibuprofen in connective tissue disease. *J Rheum* **17**, 1094.
2. Chez M, Sila CA, Ransohoff RM et al. (1989) Ibuprofen-induced meningitis: Detection of intrathecal IgG synthesis and immune complexes. *Neurology* **39**, 1578.
3. Collum LMT, Bowen DI (1971) Ocular side-effects of ibuprofen. *Brit J Ophthalmol* **55**, 472.
4. Hamburger HA, Beckman H, Thompson R (1984) Visual evoked potentials and ibuprofen (Motrin) toxicity. *Ann Ophthalmol* **16**, 328.
5. Lawson JM, Grady MJ (1985) Ibuprofen-induced aseptic meningitis in a previously healthy patient. *West J Med* **143**, 386.
6. Ridder WH 3d, Tomlinson A (1992) Effect of ibuprofen on contrast sensitivity. *Optom Vis Sci* **69**, 652.
7. Ruppert GB, Barth WF (1981) Tolmetin-induced aseptic meningitis. *J Amer Med Assn* **245**, 67.

Ifosfamide

Steven A. Sparr

IFOSFAMIDE
$C_7H_{15}Cl_2N_2O_2P$

N,3-Bis(2-chloroethyl)tetrahydro-2H-1,3,2-oxazaphosphorin-2-amine 2-oxide

NEUROTOXICITY RATING
Clinical

A Acute encephalopathy (sedation, seizures, ataxia)
B Cranial neuropathy

Ifosfamide, an analog of cyclophosphamide, is an oxazaphosphorine alkylating agent used to treat a wide variety of pediatric and adult tumors, including lung cancer, sarcomas, gynecological malignancies, germ-cell tumors, and lymphomas (2,4,20). The drug is derived from nitrogen mustard, whose cytotoxic actions were first elucidated prior to World War II (4) (*see* Mustard Warfare Agents and Related Substances, this volume); many derivatives that avidly alkylate DNA and induce cell death have since been developed. Drugs in this class used most commonly today include cyclophosphamide, melphalan, chlorambucil, and ifosfamide (4).

When ifosfamide was introduced in the 1970s, dosage was limited by bladder toxicity that is characterized by severe hemorrhagic cystitis and potential bladder malignancy (4). These side effects have been ameliorated by the coadministration of 2-mercapto-ethane sulfonate (MESNA), which is activated in the renal tubules and protects the kidney and bladder from toxicity of ifosfamide and its metabolites (4). However, use of higher dosages of ifosfamide is commonly associated with encephalopathy and seizures (5,7,16,19,21).

The cytotoxic potential of ifosfamide and related compounds is activated by hepatic formation of an intermediate with a highly reactive carbonium group; this avidly combines with guanine and other residues of DNA and can cross-link DNA residues or link them to proteins (4). Drug activation is accomplished by hydroxylation of the 4-carbon or the chloroethyl side chain, thereby creating an active phosphoamide mustard (2). The resulting damage to DNA can cause mispairing of nucleotides during DNA synthesis, and other disruption of DNA replication, ultimately leading to cell death by poorly understood mechanisms (4).

Ifosfamide is administered by intravenous or oral routes. Bioavailability of oral ifosfamide is >90% (20), and peak serum levels occur approximately 1 h following oral administration (20). At standard doses, elimination half-life is 5–6 h with both oral and intravenous routes, although there is great individual variation (2,20). At higher doses (3.8–5.0 g/m^2), drug half-life increases to approximately 16 h (2). Serum half-life shortens with successive drug administration, a phenomenon attributed to self-induction of drug metabolism (14,20). Since first-pass metabolism of ifosfamide by the liver is <5%, the half-life of the parent compound is long, which allows prolonged and continuous activation to active metabolites in the liver (20). The half-life of the principal 4-hydroxy metabolite is similar to that of the parent compound (2).

Early use of ifosfamide for treatment of neoplasms employed dosages >5 g/m^2; these were found to induce hemorrhagic cystitis and nephrotoxicity. Since the introduction of cotreatment with MESNA, dosages up to 8 g/m^2 infused over 24 h can be tolerated without the appearance of urotoxicity (2). MESNA does not interfere with the metabolism or efficacy of ifosfamide, but deactivates active metabolites of ifosfamide in the urine (2).

The other major dose-related systemic toxicity of ifosfamide is marrow suppression with leukopenia, anemia, and thrombocytopenia; this usually resolves a week after treatment is completed (2). Alopecia develops in the vast majority of patients treated with ifosfamide, as does nausea, which can be controlled with antiemetics in most cases (2).

CNS toxic effects of ifosfamide are frequent, often severe, and can limit drug use. Neurotoxic effects include changes in mental status ranging from drowsiness to coma, ataxia, seizures, facial spasms, tremors, and focal neurological signs (18). There are no animal models for these side effects.

Incidence of neurotoxicity, reported to be 5%–30% of patients treated (5,17,19,21), was as high as 50% in one series (14). Ifosfamide encephalopathy is characterized by altered mental status, ranging from mild lethargy to coma. Patients may experience agitation, visual or auditory hallucinations, and urinary incontinence (21); paranoid ideation, mutism (1), and extrapyramidal signs (1); as well as seizures, focal motor weakness, cerebellar signs, and cranial nerve palsies (18). Symptoms are usually self-limited, clearing 48–72 h after cessation of therapy (1), but persistent neuropsychological abnormalities (12) and even fatalities have been reported (15,21). A 3-month-old girl developed cerebral atrophy and developmental delay following ifosfamide therapy (3).

In one study of 18 consecutive cases, onset of encephalopathy ranged from 12–146 h (mean, 46 h) after onset of infusion (21). Mean duration was 3 days, but lasted more than 1 week in five patients, and left permanent residua in two.

Experience with 50 pediatric patients treated with a total of 113 5-day courses of ifosfamide/MESNA found 11 neurotoxic reactions (18). Of these, eight developed stupor or coma; one experienced generalized seizures; and individual patients exhibited aphasia, ataxia, deafness, and/or peripheral facial weakness.

A 61-year-old man treated with ifosfamide for adenocarcinoma of the lung and abdominal lymphoma developed confusion, myoclonus, blepharospasm, torticollis/opisthotonos, and chorea (1). Intravenous diphenhydramine abolished extrapyramidal posturing.

Neuropsychiatric side effects appeared in four of six patients receiving an oral dose of 2 g/m^2, but not in patients receiving half that dose.

Predisposing factors for CNS toxicity include dehydration, decreased renal function, previous cerebrovascular events or brain metastases, pelvic tumors, and decreased serum albumin (2,5). Based on serum creatinine, serum albumin and the presence or absence of pelvic disease, a nomogram was developed that was highly predictive of the development of severe neurotoxicity (1). It was used to exclude patients at risk from receiving treatment with ifosfamide. Another study using this nomogram found a sensivity of only 18% for predicting severe neurotoxicity (21). Coadministration of other chemotherapeutic agents, such as methotrexate, vincristine, vindesine, and etoposide, does not increase CNS toxicity (2). However, prior exposure to multiple courses of cisplatin has been shown to increase risk of neurotoxicity, especially when associated with renal tubular damage (10,18). There is a higher incidence of neurotoxicity in patients treated with oral (vs. intravenous) ifosfamide because nonrenal clearance of the drug is significantly diminished (14). A low incidence of neurotoxic reactions was reported in 87 pediatric patients treated for brain tumors with ifosfamide *every other day* (11).

Electroencephalogram (EEG) abnormalities were observed in serially examined patients who developed CNS toxicity (18). EEG abnormalities progressed from generalized slowing, to increasing delta activity, followed by high-voltage rhythmic delta (18). However, a similar evolution of EEG abnormalities was seen with a comparable frequency in patients who did not develop clinical neurotoxicity, although they occurred later in the course of therapy in those who remained asymptomatic. Thus, these EEG abnormalities are not specific for symptomatic CNS toxicity. One study claims that pretreatment EEGs were not predictive of development of neurotoxicity (16,17). Periodic triphasic waves (22) and spike-and-wave abnormalities (8) have been reported in patients with encephalopathy or seizures, suggesting that these abnormalities are more specific for symptomatic CNS toxicity.

The mechanism of CNS toxicity of ifosfamide is unclear; based on several lines of evidence, the metabolite chloroacetaldehyde has been suggested as the causative agent (18). Chloroacetaldehyde is found in tenfold higher concentrations after metabolism of ifosfamide than cyclophosphamide, which does not have CNS toxicity (9,18). Chloroacetaldehyde is chemically similar to acetaldehyde, a neurotoxic metabolite of ethanol, and is degraded by the same enzyme, aldehyde dehydrogenase (9,18); it also has similarity to the sedative trichloroacetaldehyde (chloral hydrate) (9). Average serum levels of chloroacetaldehyde are elevated in patients who experience neurotoxicity relative to those who remain asymptomatic (9).

Two patients developed ifosfamide encephalopathy characterized by mutism, catatonia, and lip twitching; both had EEGs showing generalized slowing and sharp waves, and both responded promptly to intravenous diazepam (19). Within minutes of receiving diazepam, both began to speak and EEG patterns normalized. The EEG abnormalities were insufficient to qualify as nonconvulsant status epilepticus, in the authors' opinion; they proposed a distinct "diazepam-responsive encephalopathy." One woman displayed echolalia, perseveration, and upper-extremity myoclonus during ifosfamide/cisplatin therapy; she had diffuse slowing on EEG with superimposed synchronous periodic triphasic waves. The patient improved clinically and electroencephalographically with administration of intravenous diazepam. Although the EEG abnormalities did not meet electrographic criteria, the authors classified the acute encephalopathy as nonconvulsive status epilepticus.

There are several case reports of reversal of clinical and EEG abnormalities associated with ifosfamide encephalopathy following intravenous administration of methylene blue (6,13,23). The mechanism of action is unclear.

REFERENCES

1. Anderson NR, Tandon DS (1981) Ifosfamide extrapyramidal neurotoxicity. *Cancer* **68**, 72.
2. Brade WP, Herdrich K, Varini M (1985) Ifosfamide: Pharmacology, safety and therapeutic potential. *Cancer Treatment Rev* **12**, 1.
3. Brugger CS, Friedman HS, Tien R, Delong R (1994) Cerebral atrophy in an infant following treatment with ifosfamide. *Med Pediat Oncol* **23**, 380.
4. Chabner BA, Allegra CJ, Curt GA, Calabresi P (1996) Antineoplastic agents. In: *The Pharmacologic Basis of Therapeutics. 9th Ed.* Hardman JG, Goodman AG, Limbird LE eds. McGraw Hill, New York p. 1233.
5. Davies SM, Pearson AD, Craft AW (1989) Toxicity of high dose ifosfamide in children. *Cancer Chemother Pharmacol* **24**, S8.
6. Demandt M, Wandt H (1996) Successful treatment with methylene blue of ifosfamide-induced central nervous system effects. *Deut Med Wochenschr* **121**, 575.
7. Fleming RA (1997) An overview of cyclophosphamide and ifosfamide pharmacology. *Pharmacotherapy* **17**(5 Pt 2), 146S.
8. Gieron MA, Barak LS, Estrada J (1988) Severe encephalopathy associated with ifosfamide administration in two children with metastatic tumors. *J Neuro-oncol* **6**, 29.
9. Goren MP, Wright RK, Pratt CB, Pell FE (1986) Dechloroethylation of ifosfamide and neurotoxicity. *Lancet* **2**, 1219.
10. Goren MP, Wright RK, Pratt CB *et al.* (1987) Potentiation of ifosfamide neurotoxicity, hematotoxicity, and tubular nephrotoxicity by prior *cis*-diamminedichloroplatinum (II) therapy. *Cancer Res* **47**, 1457.
11. Heideman RL, Douglass EC, Langston JA *et al.* (1995) A phase II study of every other day high-dose ifosfamide in pediatric brain tumors: A Pediatric Oncology Group study. *J Neuro-oncol* **25**, 77.
12. Heim ME, Fiene R, Schick E *et al.* (1981) Central nervous system side effects following ifosfamide monotherapy of advanced renal carcinoma. *J Cancer Res Clin Oncol* **100**, 113.
13. Kupfer A, Aeschlimann C, Wermuth B, Cerny T (1994) Prophylaxis and reversal of ifosfamide encephalopathy with methylene-blue. *Lancet* **343**, 763.
14. Lind ML, Margison JM, Cerny T *et al.* (1989) Comparative pharmacokinetics and alkylating activity of fractionated intravenous and oral ifosfamide in patients with bronchogenic carcinoma, *Cancer Res* **49**, 753.
15. Meanwell CA, Blake AE, Blackledge G *et al.* (1985) Encephalopathy associated with ifosfamide/mesna therapy. *Lancet* **1**, 406.
16. Meanwell CA, Blake AE, Kelly KA *et al.* (1986) Prediction of ifosfamide/mesna associated encephalopathy. *Eur J Clin Oncol* **22**, 815.
17. Meanwell CA, Kelly KA, Blackledge G (1986) Avoiding ifosfamide/MESNA encephalopathy. *Lancet* **2**, 406.
18. Pratt CB, Green AA, Horowitz ME (1986) Central nervous system toxicity following the treatment of pediatric patients with ifosfamide/mesna. *J Clin Oncol* **4**, 1253.
19. Simonian NA, Gilliam FGF, Chiappa KH (1993) Ifosfamide causes a diazepam-sensitive encephalopathy. *Neurology* **43**, 2700.
20. Wagner T, Drings P (1986) Pharmacokinetics and bioavailability of oral ifosfamide. *Arzneim-forsch* **36**, 878.
21. Watkin SW, Husband DJ, Green JA, Warnius HM (1989) Ifosfamide encephalopathy: A reappraisal. *J Cancer Clin Oncol* **25**, 1303.
22. Wengs WJ, Talwar D, Bernard J (1993) Ifosfamide-induced nonconvulsive status epilepticus. *Arch Neurol* **50**, 1104.
23. Zulian GB, Tullen E, Maton B (1995) Methylene blue for ifosfamide-associated encephalopathy. *N Engl J Med* **332**, 1239.

β,β'-Iminodipropionitrile

Bruce G. Gold

β,β'-IMINODIPROPIONITRILE
$C_6H_9N_3$

Bis(2-cyanoethyl)amine

NEUTROTOXICITY RATING

Experimental

A Extrapyramidal dysfunction (acute dyskinesia)

A Peripheral neuropathy

β,β'-Iminodipropionitrile (IDPN) is a synthetic dimerous derivative of the natural compound β-aminopropionitrile (BAPN) present in the wild flat pea, *Lathyrus odoratus*. IDPN was first synthesized in the early 1930s (23). The MW of IDPN is 123.16. It is a clear liquid at room temperature; the BP is 205°C. The compound is highly soluble in water. It is readily oxidized and supplied in a brown bottle to protect it from exposure to UV light. Its use(s) is a trade secret.

IDPN is readily absorbed by oral administration (7) as well as intraperitoneal injection (6). Metabolism is largely *via* oxidative cleavage to cyanoacetic acid (CAA) and BAPN by cytochrome P-450–like α-C-hydroxylation (26). Excretion is largely *via* the kidney (31). BAPN is also hydrolyzed to β-alanine and CAA; although thiocyanate is present in the urine, it does not exceed 2% of the total dose administered (31).

Whether IDPN itself or a metabolite produces the neurotoxic effects is unknown. It has been suggested that IDPN is activated by flavin monooxygenase to N-hydroxy-IDPN, a more potent analog of IDPN (26). However, N-hydroxy-IDPN is not part of the metabolic pathway (8,9), and the N-hydroxy–substituted analog may appear more toxic simply by reducing hydrolysis (detoxification) of IDPN to BAPN and CAA (8). Also, the carboxyl group of β-alanine is formed by nitrile hydrolysis (8).

A single intraperitoneal injection of IDPN (1.5–2.0 g/kg) to a rat produces within 48 h a novel and permanent dyskinesia termed the "ECC (excitation, circling, and choreoathetosis) syndrome" (30) or "waltzing syndrome" (6). Several striking features are apparent, including excitement and motor hyperactivity, retropulsion and backward somersaulting, circling, head twitching, and overalertness and hyperalgesia (22). Similar behavioral changes (with the exception of backward somersaulting) can be induced in the cat by subchronic intraperitoneal injections of 50 mg/kg given at weekly intervals for 5 weeks (18); the maximum tolerated dose in this species is approximately 75 mg/kg, much lower than in the rat (B.G. Gold, unpublished observation). The precise mechanism of neurotoxicity is unknown. The pathogenesis of the profound behavioral changes has not been definitively determined. Possibilities include a dose-dependent degeneration of vestibular sensory hair cells (25) and an alteration in serotonergic pathways (2–4,10).

The major anatomical target for IDPN is larger caliber neurons in the brain, spinal cord, dorsal root ganglia, and peripheral nerves (6). Vestibular hair cells are also affected (25). The pathological hallmark of IDPN neuropathy is the massive accumulation of neurofilaments in the proximal portions of large axons producing giant axonal swellings. Development of axonal swellings is a strict function of the original axonal caliber and, thereby, the underlying neurofilament content in the axon (15). Despite the production of giant axonal swellings, no axonal degeneration ensues in the rat (20); rare degenerating fibers develop in the cat along with distal axonal swellings (18). The demonstration that aggregates of intermediate filaments can be induced in skin fibroblasts exposed to IDPN (11) shows this is not a unique attribute of neurofilaments; larger axons are probably vulnerable to IDPN because of their higher levels of neurofilament synthesis and transport.

Repeated exposure to IDPN leads to secondary demyelination and onion bulb formations (20,21). Prolonged (years) exposure produces axonal atrophy distal to proximal axonal swellings; this results from a permanent reduction in delivery of neurofilaments to the distal axon (7). Repeated injection in cats leads to production of distal as well as proximal axonal swellings (18). These changes do not appear to underlie the pathogenesis of the profound behavioral alterations (*vide supra*) since they are not observed following prolonged, low-dose administration.

There are no reports of controlled or uncontrolled exposures in humans.

The major pathological hallmark, neurofilament accumulations, arises from disruption of the relationship between neurofilaments and microtubules (16,27). This leads to a massive and selective impairment in slow axonal transport of the neurofilament triplet proteins (14,19,28,32). Cytoskeletal derangement appears to result from a direct action of the agent on the axon (17). One hypothesis (29) is that IDPN (or a metabolite) alters the chemical properties of neurofilament proteins, possibly *via* formation of neurofilament aggregation (1), thereby impairing their axonal transport.

Despite its low neurotoxic potential, the agent is of interest experimentally because of its ability to reproduce in animals the proximal giant axonal swellings seen in amyotrophic lateral sclerosis (ALS) (5,24). Although clearly not a model for ALS (since neurodegeneration does not ensue and axonal swellings develop in both motor and sensory neurons), motor neurons in IDPN-treated cats demonstrate electrophysiological changes reminiscent of the peculiar motor unit discharges observed in ALS patients (*see* 12).

IDPN-intoxicated cats and rats also demonstrate electrophysiological and morphological alterations in their neuronal cell bodies that are indistinguishable from those produced by nerve transection (axotomy) albeit in the absence of any axonal degeneration (13). This agent, therefore, provides a novel tool to decipher the signal mechanisms that initiate the neuronal cell body response to axonal injury.

REFERENCES

1. Anderson JP, Carroll Z, Smulowitz M, Lieberburg I (1991) A possible mechanism of action of the neurotoxic agent iminodiproprionitrile (IDPN): A selective aggregation of the medium and heavy neurofilament polypeptides (NF-M and NF-H). *Brain Res* 547, 353.

2. Cadet JL (1989) The iminodipropionitrile (IDPN)-induced dyskinetic syndrome: Behavioral and biochemical pharmacology. *Neurosci Biobehav Rev* 13, 39.

3. Cadet JL, Kuyatt B, Fahn S, De Souza EB (1987) Differential changes in ^{125}I-LSD-labeled 5-HT-2 serotonin receptors in discrete regions of brain in the rat model of persistent dyskinesias induced by iminodipropionitrile (IDPN): Evidence from autoradiographic studies. *Brain Res* 437, 383.

4. Cadet JL, Taylor E, Freed WJ (1988) The iminodipropionitrile (IDPN)-induced dyskinetic syndrome in mice: Antagonism by the calcium channel antagonist nifedipine. *Pharmacol Biochem Behav* 29, 381.

5. Carpenter S (1968) Proximal axonal enlargement in motor neuron disease. *Neurology* 18, 841.

6. Chou S-M, Hartmann HA (1964) Axonal lesions and waltzing syndrome after IDPN administration in rats: With a concept "axostasis". *Acta Neuropathol* 3, 428.

7. Clark AW, Griffin JW, Price DL (1980) The axonal pathology in chronic IDPN intoxication. *J Neuropathol Exp Neurol* 39, 42.

8. Denlinger RH, Anthony DC, Amarnath K *et al.* (1994) Metabolism of β,β'-iminodipropionitrile and deuterium-substituted analogs: Potential mechanisms of detoxification and activation. *Toxicol Appl Pharmacol* 124, 59.

9. Denlinger RH, Anthony DC, Amarnath V, Graham DG (1992) Comparison of location, severity, and dose response of proximal axonal lesions induced by β,β'-iminodipropionitrile and deuterium substituted analogs. *J Neuropathol Exp Neurol* 51, 569.

10. Diamond BI, Sethi K, Borison RL (1986) Serotonin modulation of hyperkinesia and phasic neck dystonia induced by iminodipropionitrile (IDPN) in rats. *Neurology* 36, 341.

11. Durham HD (1986) The effect of β,β'-iminodipropionitrile (IDPN) on cytoskeletal organization in cultured human skin fibroblasts. *Cell Biol Int Rep* 10, 599.

12. Gold BG (1987) The pathophysiology of proximal neurofilamentous giant axonal swellings: Implications for the pathogenesis of amyotrophic lateral sclerosis. *Toxicology* 46, 125.

13. Gold BG, Austin DR (1991) Regulation of aberrant neurofilament phosphorylation in neuronal perikarya III. Alterations following single and continuous β,β'-iminodipropionitrile administrations. *Brain Res* 563, 151.

14. Griffin JW, Anthony DC, Fahnestock KE *et al.* (1984) 3,4-Dimethyl-2,5-hexanedione impairs the axonal transport of neurofilament proteins. *J Neurosci* 4, 1516.

15. Griffin JW, Drucker N, Gold BG *et al.* (1987) Schwann cell proliferation and migration during paranodal demyelination. *J Neurosci* 7, 682.

16. Griffin JW, Fahnestock KE, Price DL, Cork LC (1983) Cytoskeletal disorganization induced by local application of β,β'-iminodipropionitrile and 2,5-hexanedione. *Ann Neurol* 14, 55.

17. Griffin JW, Fahnestock KE, Price DL, Hoffman PN (1983) Microtubule-neurofilament segregation produced by β,β'-iminodipropionitrile: Evidence for the association of fast axonal transport with microtubules. *J Neurosci* 3, 557.

18. Griffin JW, Gold BG, Cork LC *et al.* (1982) IDPN neuropathy in the cat: Coexistence of proximal and distal axonal swellings. *Neuropathol Appl Neurobiol* 8, 351.

19. Griffin JW, Hoffman PN, Clark AW *et al.* (1978) Slow axonal transport of neurofilament proteins: Impairment by β,β'-iminodipropionitrile administration. *Science* 202, 633.

20. Griffin JW, Price DL (1980) Proximal axonopathies induced by toxic chemicals. In: *Experimental and Clinical Neurotoxicology*. Spencer PS, Schaumburg HH eds. Williams & Wilkins, Baltimore p. 161.

21. Griffin JW, Price DL (1981) Demyelination in experimental β,β'-iminodipropionitrile and hexacarbon neuropathies: Evidence for an axonal influence. *Lab Invest* 45, 130.

22. Hartmann HA, Stick HF (1975) Psychopathologic symptoms induced by bis-beta-aminopropionitrile. *Science* 125, 445.

23. Hoffman KJ, Jacobi RS (1934) U.S. patent 1992,615. *Chem Abstr* 25, 5474.

24. Inoue K, Hirano A (1979) Early pathological changes in amyotrophic lateral sclerosis: Autopsy findings of a case of 10 months' duration. *Neurol Med Chir (Tokyo)* 11, 448.

25. Llorens J, Dememes D, Sans A (1994) The toxicity of IDPN on the vestibular system of the rat: New insights on its effects on behavior and neurofilament transport. *NeuroToxicology* 15, 643.

26. Morandi A, Gambetti P, Arora PK, Sayre LM (1987) Mechanism of neurotoxic action of β,β'-iminodipropionitrile (IDPN): N-Hydroxylation enhances neurotoxic potency. *Brain Res* 437, 69.

27. Papasozomenos SC, Autillio-Gambetti L, Gambetti P (1981) Reorganization of axoplasmic organelles following β,β'-iminodipropionitrile administration. *J Cell Biol* 91, 866.

28. Parhad IM, Griffin JW, Hoffman PN, Koves JF (1986) Selective interruption of axonal transport of neurofilament proteins in the visual system by β,β'-iminodipropionitrile (IDPN) intoxication. *Brain Res* 363, 315.

29. Sayre LM, Autilio-Gambetti L, Gambetti P (1985) Pathogenesis of experimental giant neurofilamentous axonopathies: A unified hypothesis based on chemical modifications of neurofilaments. *Brain Res Rev* 10, 69.

30. Selye H (1957) Lathyrism. Rev. *Rev Canad Biol* 16, 1.

31. Williams S, Brownlow EK, Heath H (1970) Studies on the metabolism of β,β'-iminodipropionitrile in the rat. *Biochem Pharmacol* 19, 2277.

32. Yokoyama K, Tsukita S, Ishikawa H, Kurokawa M (1980) Early changes in the neuronal cytoskeleton caused by β,β'-iminodipropionitrile: Selective impairment of neurofilament polypeptides. *Biomed Res* 1, 537.

Indolealkylamines

Albert C. Ludolph

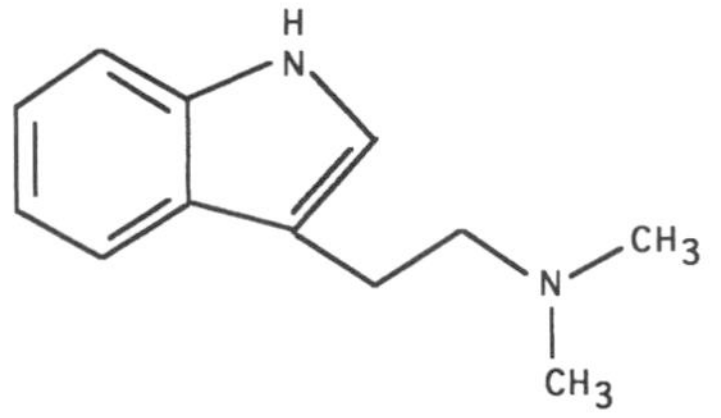

N,N-DIMETHYLTRYPTAMINE
$C_{12}H_{16}N_2$

N,N-Dimethyltryptamine; 3-[2-(Dimethylamino)ethyl]indole; DMT

NEUROTOXICITY RATING

Clinical

A   Psychobiological reaction (paranoia, anxiety)

B   Seizure disorder

Experimental

A   Serotonin agonist

All the indolealkylamines chemically resemble 5-hydroxytryptamine (5-HT; serotonin), and their agonistic action at the $5-HT_2$ and $5-HT_{1c}$ serotonin receptor subtypes likely accounts for their neurotoxicity. Some mushrooms (*Psilocybe* spp., *Panaeolus*, spp. *Gymnopilus* spp., and *Virola calophylla*) contain the indolealkylamines psilocybin and psilocin (3,6). The major effect of *N,N*-dimethyltryptamine (*N,N*-dimethyl-1*H*-indole-3-ethanamine),3-(2-(dimethylamino)ethyl)indole (DMT), and *N,N*-diethyltryptamine (DET), is a hallucinatory psychobiological reaction. Consumption of these plants was historically restricted to Mexican Indians (9) but, today, deliberate intake of mushrooms

for the hallucinogenic psilocybin syndrome (*mycetismus cerebralis*) is widespread (2,4) (for a more detailed description, *see* Psilocybin/Psilocin, this volume).

DMT is a naturally occuring indolealkylamine from *Anadenanthara* seeds. The compound has a MW of 188.26 and a MP of 44.6°–46.8°C. DMT is a controlled substance in the United States but, like DET, is readily synthesized. Parenteral administration of DMT induces the symptomatology of the psilocybin syndrome (7,8). Occasionally, seizures accompany the use of indolealkylamines (2,5); fatalities have not been reported. Panic and paranoia ("bad trips") may last up to 24 h. A comprehensive review on the experimental role of neurotoxic indolealkylamines and phenylalkylmines is available (1).

REFERENCES

1. Baumgarten HB, Zimmermann B (1992) Neurotoxic phenylalkylamines and indolealkylamines. In: *Selective Neurotoxicity*. Herken H, Hucho F eds. Springer-Verlag, Berlin p. 225.

2. Brust JCM (1993) *Neurological Aspects of Substance Abuse*. Butterworth-Heinemann, Boston, Massachusetts p. 149.

3. Guzman G (1983) The genus *Psilocybe*. *Beih Nova Hedwigia* 74, 1.

4. Lassen JF, Lassen NF, Skov J (1992) Unges brug af hallucinogene psilocybinholdige svampe. *Ugeskr Laeger* 154, 2678.

5. McCawley EL, Brummett RE, Dana GW (1962) Convulsions from *Psilocybe* mushroom poisoning. *Proc West Pharmacol Soc* 5, 27.

6. Ott J, Guzman G (1976) Detection of psilocybin in species of *Psilocybe, Panaeolus* and *Psatyrella. Lloydia* **39**, 258.

7. Rubin D (1967) Dimethyltryptamine—a do-it-yourself hallucinogenic drug. *J Amer Med Assn* **201**, 157.

8. Szara S, Rochland LH, Rosenthal D, Handlon JH (1966) Psychological effects and metabolism of *N,N*-dimethyltryptamine in man. *Arch Gen Psychiat* **15**, 320.

9. Wasson RG (1968) *Soma, Divine Mushroom of Immortality*. Harcourt Brace & World, New York.

Indomethacin

Steven A. Sparr

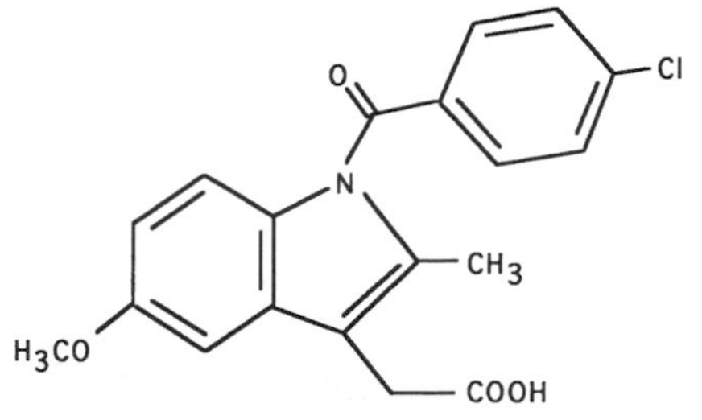

INDOMETHACIN
$C_{19}H_{16}ClNO_4$

1-(4-Chlorobenzoyl)-5-methoxy-2-methyl-1*H*-indole-3-acetic acid

NEUROTOXICITY RATING

Clinical

A   Headache

A   Acute encephalopathy (vertigo, confusion)

A   Psychobiological reaction (paranooia, depression)

B   Intracranial hemorrhage (neonatal)

B   Extrapyramidal syndrome (retrocollis)

Indomethacin, an indole 3-acetic acid derivative, was developed in the 1960s as a nonsteroidal anti-inflammatory drug (NSAID) (12). In common with many NSAIDs, indomethacin is thought to block cyclooxygenase and thereby inhibit prostaglandin synthesis (2,4,10). It also has been shown to inhibit polymorpholeukocyte motility, which further modulates the inflammatory response, and to inhibit platelet aggregation (10). Indomethacin also has antipyretic as well as analgesic activity and is useful in the management of nephrogenic diabetes insipidus (8). The drug is a potent anti-inflammatory used in a variety of rheumatological disorders, and is particularly effective in treating ankylosing spondylitis and exacerbations of gout (10). It is effective as an antipyretic, particularly in fevers associated with neoplasms, which may be mediated by a prostaglandin mechanism (10). Indomethacin is a potent analgesic and is useful in the management of migraine headaches (8). The drug is also used to suppress uterine contractions in labor and to close a patent ductus arteriosus in neonates, again by blocking prostaglandin synthesis (8,10). Although effective, its use is limited by a high incidence of side effects, especially gastrointestinal and neurological, which often limit toleration of the drug (8).

Indomethacin may be administered intravenously, orally, or rectally. It is rapidly absorbed from the gastrointestinal tract after oral administration; peak plasma levels occur about 2 h after ingestion (8). The drug is metabolized in the liver to inactive metabolites, although there is also enterohepatic recirculation of the drug (8). Usually <20% of an indomethacin dose is eliminated unchanged through the kidneys (8). Plasma half-life ranges from 2.6–11.2 h (10). The drug is highly protein-bound and has low penetrance into the cerebrospinal fluid, but high penetrance into synovial fluid (8,10).

Systemic side effects are primarily gastrointestinal, with nausea, abdominal pain, and dyspepsia in 3%–9% of patients treated (10). Gastrointestinal bleeding is frequent, and may be due to occult hemorrhage or to gastrointestinal or esophageal ulceration (8,10). Adverse hematological, dermatological, and renal side effects are seen in <1% of patients.

There are no animal models for direct toxicity of indomethacin on the CNS or PNS.

The most common neurotoxic reaction is headache, experienced by 10%–50% of patients on chronic therapy (10). Headache is usually diffuse and throbbing in quality, may be associated with vertigo or lightheadedness, and responds to dose reduction (10). In a survey of drug-induced headache conducted by the World Health Organization, indomethacin was the drug most frequently associated with this side effect, with 457 cases of nonspecific headache reported, and 18 cases of migraine (3). In an early study of the safety and efficacy of indomethacin for a mean of 33 weeks for various rheumalogical disorders, headache, often associated with vertigo or confusion, was a side effect in 19 of 137 patients treated (12). A similar incidence was found in a long-term study of patients treated with indomethacin for 2.5 years (7). Headache was the most common side effect, with an incidence of 46 of 202 treated patients. Another study suggested possible mechanisms for indomethacin-induced headache, including salt and water retention with increased intracranial fluid, and rebound cerebral vasodilatation after indomethacin-induced vasoconstriction (3).

Altered mental status has been described in patients taking indomethacin (3,6,11–13). Four of 137 patients developed depression, one developed seizures and became comatose while treated with indomethacin (12). The first case of frank psychosis was reported in 1977 (3); a 65-year-old woman with rheumatoid arthritis developed paranoid ideation and visual and olfactory hallucinations after 2 years of indomethacin treatment. Her symptoms remitted with cessation of the drug. Another patient experienced similar symptoms after her first dose of indomethacin (10). Paranoid psychosis, however, did not appear with rechallenge. An 83-year-old woman became delusional 6 days after starting indomethacin treatment and responded to neuroleptics and withdrawal of the drug (13). A 61-year-old woman had an episode of depersonalization and depression after beginning indomethacin for gout (11). A review of the literature explored the unproven "Horrobin hypothesis" that prostaglandin E_1 deficiency may be implicated in schizophrenia, mania, and depression. The causes of indomethacin-induced psychosis remain speculative.

Intraventricular hemorrhage has been observed in 3%–9% of premature infants treated with indomethacin for patent ductus arteriosis (10). Although this complication is seen with prematurity alone, and not necessarily related to the use of the drug, caution should be observed in premature infants with all drugs that impede platelet aggregation. Doppler studies of cerebral hemodynamics in premature infants treated with intravenous indomethacin for patent ductus artertiosus demonstrated decreased cerebral blood flow and a corresponding increase in cerebral vascular impedance when injections of 0.2 mg/kg indomethacin were infused over a 5-min period, but not when given over 20 min (4). The clinical significance of these changes is unclear, but rapid drug infusion is not recommended.

Other neurotoxic experiences with indomethacin are recorded in single case reports. A 51-year-old man developed retrocollis and oculogyric crisis while being treated for gout with indomethacin and azapropazone (14). Symptoms lasted about an hour, recurred when he took both drugs again, and disappeared after discontinuing them. The authors noted that the U.S. Committee on Safety of Medicines had received nine case reports of extrapyramidal reactions associated with indomethacin therapy, although details were not provided.

A single case of pseudotumor cerebri was described in a 10-year-old girl with Bartter's syndrome while treated with indomethacin (9). A 70-year-old man developed progressive leg weakness and paresthesias of the extremities after initiating indomethacin treatment for arthritis (5). Slowing of motor conduction velocities with normal sensory latencies was present; symptoms abated with cessation of the drug. The authors reported three other cases, two with predominantly motor and one with predominantly sensory neuropathic signs and symptoms while on indomethacin; electrodiagnostic studies were not performed.

REFERENCES

1. Ashmark H, Lundberg PO, Olsson S (1989) Drug-related headache. *Headache* **29**, 441.
2. Biscarini L (1992) Anti-inflammatory analgesics and drugs used in gout. In: *Meyler's Side Effects of Drugs. 12th Ed.* Dukes MNG ed. Elsevier Science Publishers BV, Amsterdam p. 181.
3. Carney MWP (1977) Paranoid psychosis with indomethacin. *Brit Med J* **2**, 994.
4. Colditz P, Murphy D, Rolfe P, Wilkinson AR (1989) Effects of infusion rate of indomethacin on cerebrovascular responses in preterm infants. *Arch Dis Child* **64**, 8.
5. Eade OE, Acheson ED, Cuthbert MF, Hawkes CH (1975) Peripheral neuropathy and indomethacin. *Brit Med J* **2**, 667.
6. Gotz V (1978) Paranoid psychosis with indomethacin. *Brit Med J* **1**, 49.
7. Hart FD, Boardman PL (1965) Indomethacin and phenylbutazone: A comparison. *Brit Med J* **2**, 1281.
8. Insel PA (1996) Analgesic-antipyretic and antiinflammatory agents and drugs employed in the treatment of gout. In: *The Pharmacologic Basis of Therapeutics. 9th Ed.* Hardman JG, Goodman AG, Limbird LE eds. McGraw Hill, New York p. 617.
9. Konomi H, Imai M, Nehei K *et al.* (1978) Indomethacin causing pseudotumor cerebri in Bartter's syndrome. *N Engl J Med* **298**, 855.
10. McEvoy GK (1995) *American Hospital Formulary Service Drug Information.* American Society of Health System Pharmacists p. 1315.
11. Schwartz JI, Moura RJ (1983) Severe depersonalization and anxiety associated with indomethacin. *Southern Med J* **76**, 679.
12. Thompson M, Percy JS (1966) Further experiences with indomethacin in the treatment of rheumatic disorders. *Brit Med J* **1**, 80.
13. Tollefson GD, Garvey MJ (1982) Indomethacin and prostaglandins: Their behavioral relationships in an acute toxic psychosis. *J Clin Psychopharm* **2**, 62.
14. Wood N, Pall HS, Williams AC, Dieppe C (1988) Extrapyramidal reactions to anti-inflammatory drugs. *J Neurol Neurosurg Psychiat* **51**, 731.

Interferon-α

Herbert H. Schaumburg

NEUROTOXICITY RATING

Clinical

B   Acute encephalopathy (fatigue, headache, lethargy, delirium, ataxia, stupor)

B   Chronic encephalopathy (cognitive dysfunction, mania)

B   Myasthenia gravis

Interferons (IFNs) are naturally occurring cytokines. Three types of IFNs (α, β, and γ) have found wide clinical use in treating malignant, viral, granulomatous, and immunologically mediated diseases. IFNs have dissimilar structural and antigenic features and have different therapeutic domains. Both naturally occurring and recombinant IFN preparations are available. Although synthesized in the periphery, IFNs have ready access to selected areas of the mammalian CNS (4).

Only IFN-α has been associated with serious neurotoxicity. IFN-β, used in treatment of relapsing multiple sclerosis (3), is allegedly associated with depression. Physicians are warned, by the manufacturer, of risk of suicide when administering IFN-β to individuals with pre-existent depression. This association seems questionable, since severe depression is common in patients with untreated multiple sclerosis and these individuals are at risk of suicide.

IFN-α is used as purified leukocyte or lymphoblastoid human IFN, or as recombinant preparations, and is administered *via* subcutaneous, intramuscular or intravenous routes. Clinical indications for IFN-α include hairy cell leukemia, Kaposi's sarcoma, malignant melanoma, chronic myelogenous leukemia, and chronic active hepatitis B and C. Regardless of dose, all experience, soon after administration, a flu-like syndrome with fever, arthralgia, chills, and headache; this is usually transient and most patients develop tolerance. Dose-limiting side effects include bone marrow suppression, cardiotoxicity, and thyroid dysfunction (5,6).

Acute and chronic CNS side effects are common, generally dose-related, and may be debilitating. Acute, transient CNS reactions usually accompany the flu-like syndrome; they appear even at low doses of 1–2 million units/day. The most common symptoms are malaise, headache, mild memory disorder, vertigo, and somnolence. Severe CNS reactions are common following doses of 10–20 million units/day; symptoms include confusion, visual hallucinations, delirium, and stupor (5,6).

A randomized controlled clinical trial of the neurologic impact of low-dose adjuvant IFN-α in patients with malignant melanoma metastatic to regional lymph nodes after radical surgery identified a small number with a significant degree of action tremor. Anxiety states were more marked in the IFN-α, but there were no between-group differences on cognitive testing (2).

Persistent, dose-limiting CNS reactions may appear following 3 months of treatment in those receiving low-level therapy of 1–2 million units/day (5,6). Behavioral changes include depression with psychomotor slowing, irritability, mania, and aggressiveness (7). Cognitive dysfunction accompanies the psychiatric symptoms; cognitive signs and symptoms include poor attention, memory loss, poor reading, and visuospatial disorientation. The behavioral and psychiatric signs have been attributed to frontal lobe dysfunction (5,6). This notion is supported by the appearance of diffuse frontal slow-wave changes in electroencephalographic recordings from some of the affected individuals. Seizures may rarely develop in individuals receiving prolonged high doses.

Myasthenia gravis during interferon alpha therapy has been described in nine case reports (1). Patients display elevated levels of anti-acetyl choline receptor antibodies and may require pyridostigmine therapy. This condition is suggested to result from alpha interferon-induced autoantibodies against the postsynaptic neuromuscular membrane, and may be analogous to myasthenia gravis associated with penicillamine therapy.

REFERENCES

1. Batocchi AP, Evoli A, Servidea S et al. (1995) Myasthenia gravis during interferon alpha therapy. *Neurol* 45, 382.
2. Caraceni A, Gangeri L, Martini C et al. (1998) Neurotoxicity of interferon-alpha in melanoma therapy: results from a randomized controlled trial. *Cancer* 83, 482.
3. Ebers GC, Oger J et al. (1997) The multiple sclerosis PRISMS study: Prevention of relapses and disability by Interferon B-1a subcutaneously in multiple sclerosis. *Ann Neurol* 42, 986.
4. Pan W, Banks WA, Kastin AJ (1997) Permeability of the blood-brain and blood-spinal cord barriers to interferons. *J Neuroimmunol* 76, 105.
5. Quesada JR, Talpaz M, Rios A et al. (1986) Clinical toxicity of interferons in cancer patients: A review. *J Clin Oncol* 4, 234.
6. Sriskandan K, Garner P, Watkinson J et al. (1986) A toxicity study of recombinant interferon-gamma given by intravenous infusion to patients with advanced cancer. *Cancer Chemother Pharmacol* 18, 63.
7. Valentine AD, Meyers CA, Kling MA (1998) Mood and cognitive side effects of interferon-alpha therapy. *Semin Oncol* 25(1 Suppl 1): 39.

Iodoacetate

Albert C. Ludolph
Peter S. Spencer

$C_2H_3IO_2$

Iodoacetic acid

NEUROTOXICITY RATING
Experimental
A Myopathy

Iodoacetate (IAA), a sulfhydryl-oxidizing agent, is used experimentally to block glyceraldehyde phosphate dehydrogenase (GAPDH) activity *in vivo* and *in vitro* (3). IAA has been used in a series of *in-vitro* experiments to block fast axonal transport in peripheral nerve (5,8). The relation between energy depletion and excitotoxicity has been studied in the chick retina using IAA and cyanide (10–12). IAA-induced neuronal damage in chick retina is predominantly mediated by N-methyl-D-aspartate receptors (12). Intrastriatal administration of IAA produced a lesion that was attenuated by removal of the corticostriatal glutamatergic input; this is consistent with an excitotoxic process triggered by IAA-induced tissue energy compromise. Lesions were accompanied by increased production of hydroxy free radicals and a small increase in lactate, as visualized by *in-vivo* magnetic resonance imaging (6). IAA has also been used to produce experimental myopathy (1). After injection of IAA into the rat aorta, muscle GAPDH was reduced to 10% of control levels, and mild degeneration of muscle fibers occurred (4,7).

IAA is more potent than potassium cyanide or arsenate in compromising neuronal viability *in vitro*. Whereas cyanide and arsenate in concentrations up to 10 mM produced only partial neuronal degeneration, application of 0.1 mM IAA for 5 min to 8-day-old preparations of rat cortical or hippocampal CA1 neurons resulted in inhibition of energy metabolism and protein synthesis, with a calcium-independent activation of neuronal death after 3–24 h. Inhibition of protein synthesis and neuronal degeneration were prevented by treatment with vitamin E, a free-radical scavenger (9). *In-vitro* treatment of hippocampal neurons with IAA and pyruvate produced partial depletion of adenosine triphosphate (1).

No cases of human iodoacetate toxicity are known.

REFERENCES

1. Brorson JR, Schumacker PT, Zhang H (1999) Nitric oxide acutely inhibits neuronal energy production. The Committees on Neurobiology and Cell Physiology. *J Neurosci* **19**, 147.
2. Brumback RA (1980) Iodoacetate inhibition of glyceraldehyde-3-phosphate dehydrogenase as a model of human myophosphorylase deficiency (McArdle's disease) and phosphofructokinase deficiency (Tarui's disease). *J Neurol Sci* **48**, 383.
3. Cori GP, Slein PW, Cori GF (1948) Crystalline D-glyceraldehyde-3-phosphate dehydrogenase from rabbit muscle. *J Biol Chem* **173**, 605.
4. Furukuwa N, Sugie H, Tsurui S *et al.* (1992) A biochemical study of animal model with defective muscle glycolysis, induced by iodoacetate administration. *No To Hattatsu* **24**, 342.
5. Ochs S, Smith CB (1971) Fast axoplasmic transport in mammalian nerve *in vitro* after block of glycolysis with iodoacetic acid. *J Neurochem* **8**, 833.
6. Matthews RT, Ferrante RJ, Jenkins BG (1997) Iodoacetate produces striatal excitotoxic lesions. *J Neurochem* **69**, 285.
7. Ruff RL, Weissman J (1991) Iodoacetate-induced contracture in rat skeletal muscle: Possible role of ADP. *Amer J Physiol* **5**, 2828.
8. Sabri MI, Ochs S (1971) Inhibition of glyceraldehyde-3-phosphate dehydrogenase in mammalian nerve by iodoacetic acid. *J Neurochem* **8**, 1509.
9. Uto A, Dux E, Kusumoto M, Hossmann KA (1995) Delayed neuronal death after brief histotoxic hypoxia *in vitro*. *J Neurochem* **64**, 2185.
10. Zeevalk GD, Nicklas WJ (1990) Chemically induced hypoglycemia and anoxia: Relationship to glutamate-mediated toxicity in retina. *J Pharmacol Exp Ther* **253**, 1285.
11. Zeevalk GD, Nicklas WJ (1991) Mechanisms underlying initiation of excitotoxicity associated with metabolic inhibition. *J Pharmacol Exp Ther* **257**, 870.
12. Zeevalk GD, Nicklas WJ (1997) Contribution of glial metabolism to neuronal damage caused by partial inhibition of energy metabolism in retina. *Exp Eye Res* **65**, 397.

Iohexol and Other Radiographic Contrast Agents

George Lantos

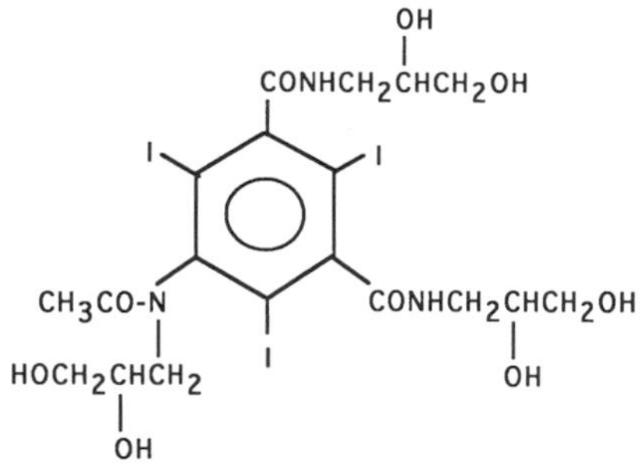

IOHEXOL

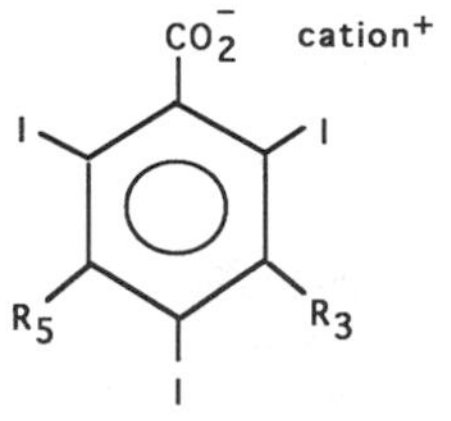

for TRIIODOBENZOATE DERIVATIVES

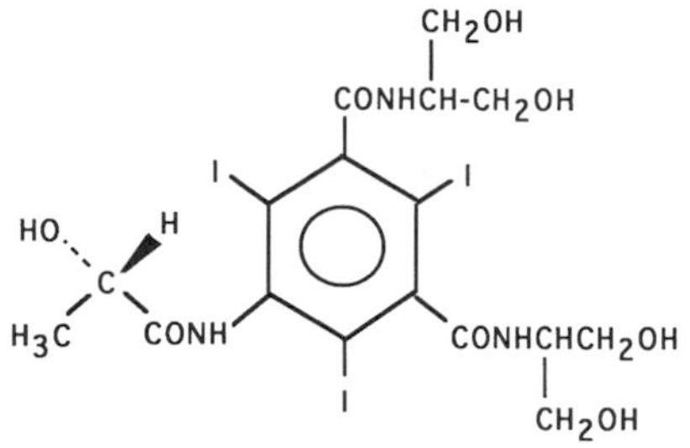

IOPAMIDOL

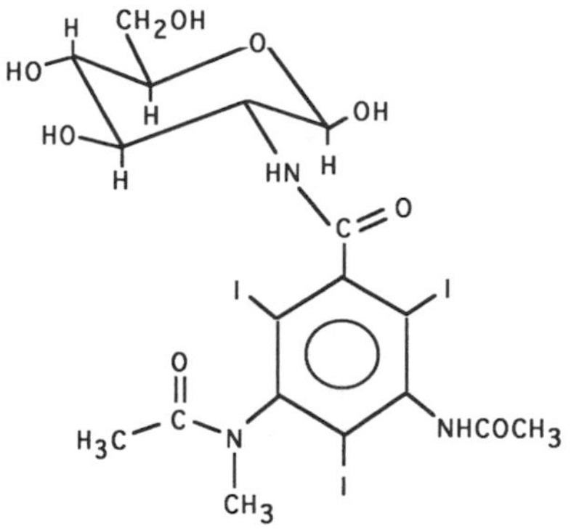

METRIZAMIDE

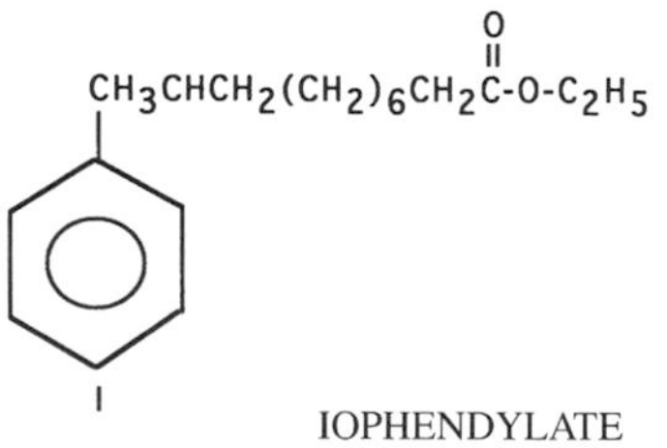

IOPHENDYLATE

NEUROTOXICITY RATING

Clinical

A Arachnoiditis (intrathecal administration)

B Seizure disorder

Contrast agents are used extensively in the everyday practice of radiology. Contrast materials are used to improve radiological diagnosis by increasing the difference in signal either between normal anatomical structures or between pathological and surrounding normal tissues. In x-ray studies, including radiography, angiography, and x-ray computed tomography (CT), the "signal" is related to the ability of the anatomical structures in the region of interest to attenuate an x-ray beam. The degree of attenuation of the x-ray beam is proportional to the electron density (and therefore the physical density) of the tissues, and iodinated contrast agents are introduced to alter these attenuation properties (5,6,21,38). Iodinated contrast agents are not used in magnetic resonance imaging (MRI).

Triiodobenzoic Acid Derivatives

Starting with acetrizoate, several derivatives of triiodobenzoic acid were introduced in the early 1950s as radiographic contrast agents. Diatrizoate (3-acetamido-2,4,6 triiodobenzoate) has probably been the most widely used; others include iothalamate and metrizoate (Table 28). These compounds are all ionic, monomeric molecules. Indications for use of these agents include intra-arterial injection for cerebral and peripheral angiography, intravenous injection for CT and urography, and intracavitary injection for studies such as cystography and pyelography. Sodium and methyl glucamine (meglumine) are the most commonly employed cations (10). Because of their ionic nature and the concentration required for a suitable radiographic contrast effect, these agents have osmolalities five to ten times that of normal serum (10).

The triiodobenzoates are largely excreted by the kidney. About 98% is excreted by glomerular filtration, with very small amounts undergoing excretion and reabsorption by

TABLE 28. Common Triiodobenzoic Acid Derivatives

Year Introduced	Generic Name	Chemical Name	R3	R5	Brand Name	Cation
1950	Acetrizoate	3-Acetamido-2,4,6-triiodobenzoate	$-NHCOCH_3$	$-H$	Urokon	Na^+
1954	Diatrizoate	3,5-Diacetamido-2,4,6-triiodobenzoate	$-NHCOCH_3$	$-NHCOCH_3$	Hypaque	Na^+
					Renograffin	Meglumine
					Renovist	Na^+
					Hypaque-M	Meglumine
1962	Iothalamate	5-Acetamido-2,4,6-triiodo-N-methylisophthalmate	$-CONHCH_3$	$-NHCOCH_3$	Conray	Meglumine
					Conray-400	Na^+
1974—USA	Metrizoate	2,4,6-triiodo-5-(N-methylacetamido)benzoate	$-NHCOCH_3$	$-NCH_3COCH_3$	Isopaque 280	Meglumine
1961—Europe						Ca^{2+}
					Isopaque 440	Meglumine
						Na^{2+}
						Ca^{2+}
						Mg^{2+}

the renal tubules (7,35). Part of the remainder (0.5%–2%) can be recovered from the feces (3).

The neurotoxic effects of contrast materials can be divided into two main categories: increase in permeability of the brain vessels as a consequence of their high osmolality, and direct toxic effects on CNS tissue once the substance gains access to the CNS. Under normal circumstances, most of the CNS is protected from the chemotoxic effects of ionic and water-soluble intravascular contrast materials by the presence of an intact blood-brain barrier (BBB) (9). However, the high osmolality of diatrizoate and similar contrast materials can cause a BBB breach by inducing both increased pinocytosis and actual shrinkage of brain endothelial cells. This was first demonstrated with Diodrast (4); similar effects occur with diatrizoate and the other triiodobenzoate derivatives (40). It is likely that BBB lesions alone, without passage of contrast into the brain parenchyma, can cause neurological complications (34).

The osmotic effects of these contrast agents on the brain are obviously greater with direct arterial injection than with intravenous injection. In clinical cerebral angiography, an iodine concentration of about 300 mg iodine per milliliter is needed for optimal visualization of the cerebral arteries. The ionic triiodobenzoate compounds have an osmolality in the range of 1.1–2.2 osm/kg, compared with normal plasma osmolality of 0.29. Osmolalities in this range can open the BBB in animals (33). Clinical studies have demonstrated breakdown of a normal BBB is manifest by seizures, cortical blindness, and other clinical sequelae, as well as abnormal CT contrast enhancement in brain vascular territories following cerebral angiography (25,28).

Contrast agents can gain access to the brain in regions where a BBB is normally absent, including the area postrema in the floor of the fourth ventricle, choroid plexus, pineal gland, and neurohypophysis. Certain side effects such as nausea and vomiting, bradycardia, and hyperthermia are likely due to direct neuronal toxicity as contrast material penetrates the BBB in the brainstem and hypothalamus (23). Absence or destruction of the BBB is also the hallmark of many inflammatory and neoplastic diseases of the CNS. Penetration of the CNS by radiographic contrast agents traversing a damaged or absent BBB is a phenomenon critical for diagnosis (11,12), but the presence of contrast agent in the CNS is responsible for the chemotoxic side effects. One study early in the CT era demonstrated that patients given contrast in the course of diagnosis of ischemic lesions fared worse than a control group not receiving contrast material (22). With other pathology, seizures have been reported in up to 15% of patients with metastases (30) and up to 16% of patients with glioblastomas (31) undergoing intravenous injection of contrast for CT.

For this group of triiodobenzoate derivatives (Table 28), each new anion synthesized appears to be better tolerated than earlier ones. For example, iothalamate is associated with less neurotoxicity than diatrizoate (8,40). However, the cation used also has an influence on the neurotoxicity. Although the cations yield no diagnostic information because they have no effect on the x-ray beam, they contribute half the number of particles in solution and, therefore, half the osmolality. In addition, the meglumine cation is associated with less toxicity than the sodium cation for this group of triiodobenzoic acid–derived contrast agents (40), presumably because the meglumine ion causes less in the way of excitatory effects than sodium (13).

Nonionic Contrast Agents

A decisive advance was made in reducing the BBB toxicity of intravascular contrast agents by reducing their hypertonicity. The first clinically useful nonionic, low-osmolality agent was metrizamide. The nonionic nature of these compounds means that there are fewer particles in solution for a given degree of radiopacity. One index of the radiopacity of contrast media in relation to their osmolality is the ratio of iodine atoms divided by the number of particles in solution. The triiodobenzoate derivatives considered in the previous section have an iodine ratio of three iodine atoms for each two particles in solution, or 1.5:1. Because they are nonionic, metrizamide, iohexol, and iopamidol have a ratio of 3:1, permitting solutions of lower osmolality for similar degrees of radiopacity. Less frequently used nonionic monomers include ioversol, iopromide, and ioxilan. Nonionic dimers have been synthesized but are not widely used; these compounds are ratio-6 molecules (*e.g.*, iotrol and iodixanol). One combination ionic-nonionic dimer has been synthesized and marketed (ioxaglate); with six iodines and two particles per molecule, it is a ratio-3 molecule.

Although the nonionic compounds have molecular weights nearly double those of the triiodobenzoate derivatives, they have similar clinical pharmacological properties (16,27).

Metrizamide is not stable in solution and was provided by the manufacturer as a lyophylized powder that needed to be mixed with saline shortly prior to use. While this inconvenient feature was not decisive for the small volumes (up to 20 ml) injected for myelography, the necessity of reconstituting a solution of this agent represented a serious practical impediment to the use of metrizamide for larger-volume examinations such as urography, angiography, and CT scanning. For this reason, as well as the toxicological profiles (including generalized seizures and arachnoiditis), metrizamide is no longer used. Iohexol is by far the most commonly used agent for myelography, while both iohexol and iopamidol are commonly used for angiography, urography, and CT scanning.

Water-soluble agents, which contrast with the insoluble iophendylate, represented a major advance in myelography because of the fine, detailed examination they permit of the spinal cord and nerve roots. Other water-soluble agents had been tried in myelography, including the ionic meglumine iocarmate and meglumine iothalamate, but their use was limited to the lumbar region because of their epileptogenic and spasmogenic effects (29,36). Local toxicity with the use of these ionic agents for myelography is the rather high incidence of arachnoiditis, both with Conray (2) and Dimer-X (1). Although large doses of both metrizamide and iohexol cause arachnoiditis in monkeys (15), this complication is very rare with clinical doses. Headache, nausea, and vomiting are the most common side effects following myelography with these nonionic agents. The incidence of these reactions is greatest with metrizamide and the least with iohexol (17,24,42).

Iophendylate

Iophendylate is a mixture of ethyl esters of isomeric iodophenylundecylic acids containing about 30% firmly bound organic iodine. It was developed in the 1940s for myelography (37). It is not miscible with cerebrospinal fluid (CSF), has better cohesive properties, and is considerably less viscous than iodized poppy seed oil Lipiodol, which it replaced in the 1940s. Although it is no longer routinely used for this purpose, iophendylate is considered here because occasional patients still present with signs and symptoms of chronic arachnoiditis as a complication of iophendylate.

Inflammatory effects on the meninges were noted soon after the introduction of iophendylate (39). Inflammation has been demonstrated in experimental animals (19). The irritant effects appear to be potentiated by the presence of blood in the subarachnoid space (18) and possibly by the presence of starch glove-powder as well (41). CSF studies have revealed that iophendylate produces a modest lymphocytosis and a prolonged elevation of CSF total protein and IgG (9). The exact rate of development of arachnoiditis following clinical myelography with iophendylate is difficult to determine with certainty because of the confounding effects of subsequent surgery.

Although it is not miscible with CSF, iophendylate is slowly resorbed. The rate of absorption is about 1 ml/year, but this rate is variable (32). Because of the long-term toxicity of iophendylate, it was the practice in the United States to remove as much as possible after a myelogram (20).

The localized lumbar arachnoiditis associated with iophendylate myelography (and lumbar disc surgery) is characterized by back and/or leg pain. Signs of radiculopathy are inconstant, including loss of tendon reflexes, weakness, and sensory loss; these are frequently bilateral. However, iophendylate may reach the intracranial subarachnoid space following examination of the craniocervical junction or while the patient is recumbent, occasionally resulting in cranial nerve palsies and hydrocephalus due to obstruction of the fourth ventricular outlets (26).

REFERENCES

1. Ahlgren P (1973) Long term effects after myelography with water soluble contrast media: Conturex, Conray meglumine 282 and Dimer-X. *Neuroradiology* 6, 206.
2. Autio E, Suolanen J, Norrback S, Salis P (1972) Adhesive arachnoiditis after myelography with meglumine iothalamate (Conray). *Acta Radiol* 12, 17.

3. Blaufox MD, Sanderson DR, Tauxe WN *et al.* (1963) Plasmatic diatrizoate-I-131 disappearance and glomerular filtration in the dog. *Amer J Physiol* **204**, 536.

4. Broman T, Olson O (1948) The tolerance of cerebral blood vessels to a contrast medium of the Diodrast group. An experimental study of the effect on the blood-brain barrier. *Acta Radiol* **30**, 32.

5. Brooks B (1924) Intra-arterial injection of sodium iodide. *J Amer Med Assn* **82**, 1016.

6. Cameron DF (1918) Aqueous solutions of potassium and sodium iodide as opaque mediums in roentgenology: Preliminary report. *J Amer Med Assn* **70**, 754.

7. Cattell WR (1970) Excretory pathways for contrast media. *Invest Radiol* **5**, 473.

8. Conventional or low-osmolality: Picking the right contrast media (1991) *Diagn Imaging* **20**, 47.

9. Ferry DW, Gooding R, Standefer JC, Wiese GM (1973) Effect of Pantopaque myelography on cerebrospinal fluid fractions. *J Neurosurg* **38**, 167.

10. Fischer HW (1986) Catalog of intravascular contrast media. *Radiology* **159**, 561.

11. Gado MH, Phelps ME, Coleman RE (1975) An extravascular component of contrast enhancement in cranial computed tomography. Part I. The tissue-blood ratio of contrast enhancement. *Radiology* **117**, 589.

12. Gado MH, Phelps ME, Coleman RE (1975) An extravascular component of contrast enhancement in cranial computed tomography. Part II. Contrast enhancement and the blood-tissue barrier. *Radiology* **117**, 595.

13. Gonsette RE (1987) Cerebral complications of angiography and computed tomography. In: *Complications in Diagnostic Imaging*. Ansell G, Wilkins RA eds. Oxford, Blackwell.

14. Harnish PP, Hagberg DJ (1988) Contrast media-induced blood-brain barrier damage: Potentiation by hypertension. *Invest Radiol* **23**, 463.

15. Haughton VM, Ho KG, Lipman BT (1982) Experimental study of arachnoiditis from iohexol. *Amer J Neuroradiol* **3**, 375.

16. Hoey GB, Smith KR (1984) Chemistry of X-ray contrast media. In: *Radiocontrast Agents*. Sovak M ed. Springer-Verlag, New York.

17. Holder JC, Binet EF, Kido DK *et al.* (1984) Iohexol lumbar myelography: Clinical study. *Amer J Neuroradiol* **5**, 399.

18. Howland WJ, Curry JL (1966) Experimental studies of Pantopaque arachnoiditis. *Radiology* **87**, 253.

19. Jager R (1950) Irritant effects of iodated vegetable oils on the brain and spinal cord when divided into small particles. *Arch Neurol Psychiat* **64**, 715.

20. James F (1971) Toal, U.S. Court of Appeals for the Second Circuit, decided February 10, 1971. *N Y Law J* March 4.

21. Kassabian MK (1907) *Roentgen Rays and Electrotherapeutics with Chapters on Radium and Phototherapy*. JB Lippincott Co, Philadelphia.

22. Kendall BE, Pullicino P (1980) Intravascular contrast injection in ischaemic lesions. II. Effect on prognosis. *Neuroradiology* **19**, 241.

23. Lalli AF (1980) Contrast media reactions: Data analysis and hypothesis. *Radiology* **134**, 1.

24. Lamb J (1985) Iohexol *vs.* iopamidol for myelography. *Invest Radiol* **20**, 37.

25. Lantos G (1989) Cortical blindness due to osmotic disruption of the blood-brain barrier by angiographic contrast material: CT and MR studies. *Neurology* **39**, 567.

26. Mason MS, Raff J (1962) Complications of Pantopaque myelography. *J Neurosurg* **19**, 302.

27. McClennan BL (1990) Ionic and nonionic iodinated contrast media: Evaluation and strategies for use. *Amer J Neuroradiol* **155**, 225.

28. Numaguchi Y, Fleming MS, Hasuo K *et al.* (1984) Blood-brain barrier disruption due to cerebral arteriography: CT findings. *J Comput Assist Tomogr* **8**, 936.

29. Oftedal ST, Kayed K (1973) Epileptogenic effects of water-soluble contrast media: an experimental investigation in rabbits. *Acta Radiol* **335**, 45.

30. Pagani JJ, Hayman LA, Bigelow RH *et al.* (1983) Diazepam prophylaxis of contrast-media induced seizures during computed tomography of patients with brain metastases. *Amer J Neuroradiol* **4**, 67.

31. Pagani JJ, Hayman LA, Bigelow RH *et al.* (1984) Prophylactic diazepam in prevention of contrast media-associated seizures in glioma patients undergoing cerebral computed tomography. *Cancer* **54**, 2200.

32. Ramsey GHS, French JD, Strain WH (1945) Myelography with ethyliodophenylundecylate (Pantopaque). *NY J Med* **45**, 1209.

33. Rapaport SL, Fredericks WR, Ohno K, Pettigrew KD (1980) Quantitative aspects of reversible osmotic opening of the blood-brain barrier. *Amer J Physiol* **238**, 421.

34. Sage JI, Van Uitert RL, Duffy TE (1984) Early changes in blood-brain barrier permeability to small molecules after transient cerebral ischemia. *Stroke* **15**, 46.

35. Saxton HM (1969) Urography. *Brit J Radiol* **42**, 346.

36. Skalpe IO (1973) Myelography with metrizamide, meglumine iothalamate and meglumine iocarmate: An experimental investigation in cats. *Acta Radiol* **335**, 57.

37. Strain WH, Plati JT, Warren SL (1942) Iodinated organic compounds as contrast media for radiographic diagnosis. I. Iodinated aracyl esters. *J Amer Chem Soc* **64**, 1436.

38. Swick M (1929) Darstellung der Niere und Harnwege in röntgenbild durch intravenose Einbringung eines neuen kontrastoffes: des Uroslectans. *Klin Urochenschr* **8**, 2087.

39. Tarlov IM (1945) Pantopaque meningitis disclosed at operation. *J Amer Med Assn* **129**, 1014.

40. Velaj R, Drayer B, Albright R, Fram E (1985) Comparative neurotoxicity of angiographic contrast media. *Neurology* **35**, 1290.

41. Williams AG, Seigel RS, Kornfield M, Whorton JA (1984)

Experimental production of arachnoiditis with glove powder contamination during myelography. *Amer J Neuroradiol* 3, 121.

Ipomoea Spp.

Matthias W. Riepe

NEUROTOXICITY RATING

Clinical

A Psychobiological reaction (hallucinations)

Ipomoea species (family Convolvulaceae) of sweet potato have partially replaced wheat flour in Latin America (4). Polynesian and Mexican traditional medicines use this species for the treatment of infectious diseases (8,11); it has also have been used as a herbicide in Mexico (10). Seeds of *Ipomoea* spp. are used as hallucinogens in the United States.

Several tetrasaccharides, cyanidin glycosides, and alkaloids have been isolated from *Ipomoea* spp. (2,9,13,17,18). The alkaloids of the indolizidine and nortropane classes are glycosidase inhibitors. *N-trans-* and *N-cis-*Feruloyltyramines in *I. aquatica* and *I. pes-caprae* (L.) inhibit prostaglandin synthetase and arachidonate 5-lipoxygenase (12,16). Of the many alkaloids present in morning glory seeds, the most psychoactive appears to be *d*-lysergic acid amide (14) (*see* Lysergide, this volume).

In sheep, *Ipomoea* spp. toxicity is characterized by limb paresis with knuckling of the fetlocks (3). Histological examination of brain tissue from sheep poisoned by *Ipomoea* spp. (Weir vine) show lesions similar to those in animals poisoned by the swainsonine-containing poison peas (*see* Swainsonine, this volume) of Australia and the locoweeds of North America (9). Weir vine toxicosis, a lysosomal storage disorder, has been reported in goats fed *I. carnea* under uncontrolled and experimental conditions (6).

In humans, acute effects include nausea, vomiting, diarrhea, and paresthesias of the limb (15). Ingestion of seeds produces psychosis and visual and tactile hallucinations (5,7). Flashbacks may occur (5).

Aqueous extracts of *Ipomoea* exert a vasorelaxant effect *in vitro* (4). Aqueous extracts of *I. fistulosa* cause depolarizing neuromuscular blockade (1).

REFERENCES

1. Abdelhaadi AA, Elkheir YM, Hassan T, Mustafa AA (1986) Neuromuscular blocking activity of a crude aqueous extract of *Ipomoea fistulosa*. *Clin Exp Pharmacol Physiol* 13, 169.

2. Abou-Chaar CI, Digenis GA (1966) Alkaloids of an *Ipomoea* seed commonly known as Kaladana in Pakistan. *Nature* 212, 618.

3. Bourke CA (1995) The clinical differentiation of nervous and locomotor disorders of sheep in Australia. *Aust Vet J* 72, 228.

4. Cardenas H, Kalinowski J, Huaman Z, Scott G (1993) Nutritional evaluation of sweet potato cultivars *Ipomoea batata* (L.) Lam used in bread as partial substitute of wheat flour. *Arch Latinoamer Nutr* 43, 304.

5. Cohen S (1964) Suicide following morning glory seed ingestion. *Amer J Psychiat* 120, 1024.

6. de Balogh KK, Dimande AP, van der Lugt JJ et al. (1999) A lysosomal storage disease induced by *Ipomoea carnea* in goats in Mozambique. *J Vet Diagn Invest* 11, 266.

7. Flach C (1967) A case of morning-glory-(*Ipomoea*)-seed psychosis. *Nord Psykiatr Tidsskr* 21, 313.

8. Locher CP, Burch MT, Mower HF et al. (1995) Antimicrobial activity and anti-complement activity of extracts obtained from selected Hawaiian medicinal plants. *J Ethnopharmacol* 49, 23.

9. Molyneux RJ, McKenzie RA, O'Sullivan BM, Elbein AD (1995) Identification of the glycosidase inhibitors swainsonine and calystegine B2 in Weir vine (*Ipomoea* sp. Q6 [aff. calobra]) and correlation with toxicity. *J Nat Prod* 58, 878.

10. Pereda-Miranda R, Mata R, Anaya AL et al. (1993) Tricolorin A, major phytogrowth inhibitor from *Ipomoea* tricolor. *J Nat Prod* 56, 571.

11. Perusquia M, Mendoza S, Bye R et al. (1995) Vasoactive effects of aqueous extracts from five Mexican medicinal plants on isolated rat aorta. *J Ethnopharmacol* 46, 63.

12. Pongprayoon U, Baeckstrom P, Jacobsson U et al. (1991) Compounds inhibiting prostaglandin synthesis from *Ipomoea pes-caprae*. *Planta Med* 57, 515.

13. Reynolds WF, Yu M, Enriquez RG et al. (1995) Isolation and characterization of cytotoxic and antibacterial tetrasaccharide glycosides from *Ipomoea* stains. *J Nat Prod* 58, 1730.

14. Rice WB, Genest K (1965) Acute toxicity of extracts of morning glory seeds in mice. *Nature* 207, 302.

15. Spoerke DG, Hall AH (1990) Plants and mushrooms of abuse. *Emerg Med Clin N Amer* 8, 579.

42. Witwer G, Cacayorin ED, Bernstein AD et al. (1984) Iopamidol and metrizamide for myelography. Double blind clinical trial. *Amer J Neuroradiol* 5, 403.

16. Tseng CF, Iwakami S, Mikajiri A *et al.* (1992) Inhibition of *in vitro* prostaglandin and leukotriene biosyntheses by cinnamoyl-beta- phenethylamine and *N*-acyldopamine derivatives. *Chem Pharm Bull Tokyo* **40**, 396.

17. Weber JM, Ma TS (1976) Microchemical investigation of medicinal plants. XIV. Identification of the alkaloids in the leaves of *Ipomoea violacea* using preparative thin layer chromatography and solid probe mass. *Mikrochim Acta* **2–3**, 227.

18. Weber JM, Ma TS (1976) Microchemical investigation of medicinal plants. XV. Quantitation of total alkaloid content in leaves of *Ipomoea violacea* (Morning Glory) *via* spectrophotofluorimetry. *Mikrochim Acta* **6**, 581.

Isoflurane

Herbert H. Schaumburg

$$C_3H_2ClF_5O$$

2-Chloro-2-(difluoromethoxy)-1,1,1-trifluoroethane

NEUROTOXICITY RATING

Clinical

B   Malignant hyperthermia syndrome

Isoflurane, an isomer of enflurane, is a widely used anesthetic agent. Its safety and low level of metabolism (~ 0.2%) have suggested its prolonged use as a sedative or bronchodilator for patients in status asthmaticus (4).

Isolated case reports describe isoflurane-associated malignant hyperthermia, a well-known hereditary acute metabolic myopathy. The myopathy is characterized by sudden onset of diffuse and sustained muscle contractions along with hyperthermia and circulatory collapse during the course of anesthetic administration (2). It has been described with many commonly used inhalation anesthetics (especially following halothane/succinylcholine combination). Isoflurane alone can precipitate this reaction in a susceptible individual (3). In contrast to enflurane (1), isoflurane is rarely associated with generalized seizures. Its pathogenesis is unclear.

REFERENCES

1. Fahy LT (1987) Delayed convulsions after day case anesthesia with enflurane. *Brit J Anesth* **59**, 1173.
2. Isaacs H, Barlow MB (1973) Malignant hyperthermia. *J Neurol Neurosurg Psychiat* **36**, 228.
3. Johannesson G, Veel T, Rogstadius J (1987) Malignant hyperthermia during isoflurane anesthesia. A case report. *Acta Anesth Scand* **31**, 231.
4. Levy WJ (1984) Clinical anesthesia with isoflurane. *Brit J Anesth* **56**, 101s.

Isoniazid

J. Michael Schröder

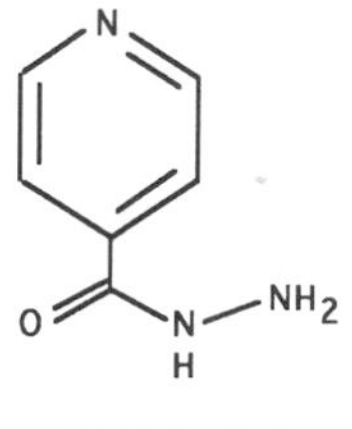

ISONIAZID
$$C_6H_7N_3O$$

Isonicotinoylhydrazine; Isonicotinic acid hydrazide

NEUROTOXICITY RATING

Clinical

A   Peripheral neuropathy

A   Seizure disorder

Experimental

A   Peripheral neuropathy

A   Acute leukoencephalopathy (vacuolar)

Isoniazid (INH), the hydrazide of isonicotinic acid, is used in the treatment of active tuberculosis and for prophylaxis (51). It is an odorless, white, crystalline powder soluble in water at a concentration of 1:10. INH is synthesized from γ-picoline, which is converted by permanganate oxidation into isonicotinic acid. This is esterified by ethyl alcohol and concentrated sulfuric acid; condensation of the ester with hydrazine gives the required hydrazide.

Discovery of INH, one of the cheapest and most effective antituberculosis drugs, was fortuitous (5). In 1945, nicotinamide was found to have tuberculostatic action; examination of compounds related to nicotinamide indicated that many pyridine derivatives showed tuberculostatic activity. Because the thiosemicarbazones were already known to inhibit *Mycobacterium tuberculosis*, the thiosemicarbazone of isonicotinaldehyde was synthesized and studied. The starting material for this synthesis was the methyl ester of isonicotinylhydrazine, a compound that proved to be more effective than any known tuberculostatic agent. The beneficial effect of INH in experimental animals was demonstrated in 1950 (20). The first trials with INH were carried out on humans with tuberculosis in 1951, when the dramatic effects of oral isoniazid medication became apparent.

General Toxicology

INH is readily absorbed following oral or parenteral administration. Its bioavailability is decreased in 50% of patients when taken with a high-carbohydrate or a high-lipid diet (60). Peak plasma concentrations of $1-7$ μg/ml develop $1-2$ h after oral ingestion and fall to 50% or less after 6 h. After acetylation in the liver, 75%–95% of a dose of INH is excreted in the urine within 24 h. There is marked genetic heterogeneity in humans with regard to the rate of INH acetylation. Patients who are slow acetylators (*vide infra*) will accumulate INH in serum and thus have an increased risk of side effects. The half-life of the drug may also be prolonged by hepatic or renal insufficiency. INH is water-soluble and diffuses readily into all body fluids; substantial levels are present in the cerebrospinal fluid (CSF) (35). In the dog, INH levels in CSF have been found to be 60%–70% of blood levels 3 h after dosing (35). INH crosses the placenta, and concentrations in milk are similar to those in plasma.

In humans, the primary route of INH metabolism is by acetylation. The enzyme responsible, N-acetyltransferase, is located in the soluble fraction of liver cells (39). Individuals can be divided into two groups depending on their ability to acetylate INH. Slow acetylation is an autosomal recessive trait; these individuals maintain high blood levels of INH longer than the more rapid acetylators, who are homozygous or heterozygous for the rapid-acetylation gene (19,39). A gene dose effect can be shown but is of little clinical significance. In general, the concentration of active INH in

the circulation of rapid inactivators is about 20%–50% of that in slow activators. Patients who inactivate the drug slowly tend to develop polyneuropathy and other signs of INH toxicity more often than rapid acetylators, but reversal of infections is usually more rapid (19). There is a racial distribution of acetylate phenotypes: almost 100% of Inuit (Eskimos), 90% of Japanese, and 50% of Europeans are rapid acetylators.

Between 50% and 70% of a dose of INH is excreted in the urine in 24 h, part being present unchanged. The main products in humans are acetylisoniazid and isonicotinic acid, small quantities of isonicotinic acid conjugates (probably isonicotinyl hydrazones), and traces of N-methyl isoniazid. Hydrolysis of INH results in the formation of isonicotinic acid and acetylhydrazine (2). Hydrazine was also detected as a breakdown product in the urine and in the plasma of slow acetylators taking 200 mg of INH daily (4). Hydrazine is a known mutagen, carcinogen, and hepatotoxin in laboratory animals (*see* Hydrazine, this volume). It undergoes a reaction in plasma with α-ketoacids to form the corresponding azines. Acetylhydrazine appears more important than hydrazine for the pathogenesis of isoniazid-induced liver damage (4). The metabolism of hydrazine involves oxidation, generating N_2 gas (26). In children, no correlation is found between any clinical or biochemical indicator of liver dysfunction and hydrazine production (17). The quantity of drug administered plays a role in determining its mode of inactivation (39). With a dose of 5 mg/kg, the primary metabolic reaction is acetylation; at 10 mg/kg, isonicotinyl-hydrazone fractions are formed, mainly present as pyruvic and ketoglutaric hydrazones. These latter substances also occur at higher concentrations in slow acetylators.

The customary daily dose of INH is $3-5$ mg/kg, taken as two or three equally divided doses. Higher doses are recommended in certain circumstances, for instance, in tuberculous meningitis, $25-30$ mg/kg/day. INH is not recommended for use in pregnant women because the metabolite hydrazine is teratogenic and carcinogenic in rats and mice after long-term administration (4).

The incidence of toxic side effects is related to duration of dose and the acetylation status of the individual. When the daily dose is 3 mg/kg, the incidence is 1%, but this rises to 15% when the total daily dose reaches 10 mg/kg.

INH interferes with the compounds of the vitamin B_6 group (pyridoxine, pyridoxal, and pyridoxamine), which exert their physiological effects after being phosphorylated to form coenzymes (23). Specifically, INH inhibits pyridoxal phosphokinase, the enzyme that phosphorylates pyridoxal to yield the active coenzyme. In addition, as a hydrazine, it also chelates with pyridoxal phosphate; this chelate inhibits pyridoxal phosphokinase more actively than INH alone—93% inhibition as against 42% (32,34). The differential sensitivity of the two actions of INH is 100–1000 times in favor of its inhibition of pyridoxal phosphokinase.

INH also interacts with certain drugs. It potentiates acetaminophen and halothane hepatotoxicity, presumably through its inducer effect on the microsomal cytochrome P-450 2E1 fraction of isoenzymes (59). INH, at a daily dose of 300 mg, inhibits the clearance of chlorzoxazone by 58%, and the formation of acetaminophen thioether metabolites. In anesthetized rats, INH potentiates the hypotensive effect of the vasodilator hydralazine and transforms the accompanying reflex tachycardia to bradycardia (54).

INH Activity on Mycobacteria

The effect of INH on the tubercle bacillus is related to concentration and duration of exposure. At low concentrations, it is bacteriostatic; at higher concentrations, it is bactericidal. The primary drug effect is considered to be inhibition of synthesis of mycolic acids (40,56). These important components of the cell wall of mycobacteria are long-chain α-branched β-hydroxy fatty acids substituted at the α-position with a long aliphatic side chain. The mycolic acid–synthesizing system is inhibited by very low concentrations of INH, and gross morphological changes of the cell wall can be observed within 24 h of exposure. Since the effect on mycolic acid synthesis is reversible, concentrations of the drug must be maintained long enough to kill the organism.

INH Resistance

There are newly emergent INH-resistant strains of *M. tuberculosis* that account for as many as 26% of the bacterial isolates. In 25%–50% of INH-resistant strains, drug resistance is associated with a loss of catalase and peroxidase activities; both are encoded by the *katG* gene. These activities are thought to participate in the drug sensitivity mechanism by converting INH into its biologically active form, which then acts on its intracellular target. Five of nine strains with INH resistance had one or more missense mutations and a common G → T transversion in codon 463, causing replacement of arginine with leucine and loss of a NciI or MspI restriction site (13). Another 20%–25% of INH-resistant clinical isolates displayed missense mutations within the mycobacterial *inhA* gene (1). This was mediated by substitution of alanine for serine 94 in the InhA protein, the drug's primary target (16). The three-dimensional structures of wild-type and mutant InhA suggest that drug resistance is directly related to a perturbation in the hydrogen-bonding network that stabilizes binding of reduced nicotinamide adenine dinucleotide (16).

Loss of catalase activity by mutation of the *katG* gene and mutation of *inhA* had a cumulative effect on INH resistance; on the other hand, mutation of the *katG* gene reduced virulence of *Mycobacterium bovis*, whereas the *inhA* gene had no effect on virulence (55).

Animal Studies

Table 29 gives the LD$_{50}$ for acute dosing with INH. Dogs and young birds are particularly sensitive to INH. There is little difference in toxicity between orally or systemically administered INH. All species show the same general signs of acute toxicity. Chronic intoxication causes an axonal neuropathy in rats and a vacuolar leukoencephalopathy in dogs and birds.

Peripheral Neuropathy

A peripheral neuropathy similar to that seen in humans occurs in rats after either a large single dose of INH (1000–2000 mg/kg) or chronic lower dosages (250 mg/kg/day, or 0.25% of the diet). Neuropathy is characterized by distal axonal degeneration of sensory and motor nerve fibers (10,12,21,24,25,37,44–48). The extent and time of onset of degeneration are dose-dependent. Axonal regeneration rapidly follows nerve fiber degeneration, even in animals still exposed; after subchronic intoxication, nerves show a mixture of degeneration and regeneration (12,42,44,46,48). Axonal regeneration appears in lumbar ventral roots within 10 days of cumulative dosing, about 5 days after the onset of nerve fiber degeneration (24).

TABLE 29. LD$_{50}$ Doses of Isoniazid

Species	Dose (mg/kg)
Dog	Oral (50)
	Oral (100)
Duckling	Intraperitoneal (57)
Man	Oral (80–150)
Monkey	Oral (320)
Rabbit	Intravenous (165)
Mouse	Oral (140–190)
	Subcutaneous (282)
	Intraperitoneal (132)
	Intravenous (153)
Rat	Oral (1400)
	Oral (2000)

[From Blakemore (5).]

With a single high dose of INH (2000 mg/kg), the medial plantar nerve shows the highest proportion of degenerating nerve fibers, while fewer are found in the more proximal, posterior tibial nerve (24). The mixed nerve to the head of the gastrocnemius contains a higher percentage of degenerating fibers than the predominantly sensory sural nerve. Within the spinal roots, less degeneration appears adjacent to the spinal cord, even in severely affected animals. Sensory roots are not as severely affected as motor roots, although this observation is based on the evaluation of very few rats (24) and was not confirmed by another study (46). Within the spinal cord, axonal degeneration is initially limited to the rostral portion of gracile tracts and only when peripheral nerve degeneration is extensive (24). At 4 weeks, there are many degenerated fibers in the dorsal tracts of the spinal cord, even at the lumbar level (47). Chromatolysis of ventral motor neurons, but not the neurons of the dorsal root ganglia, was detected 7 days after a single large dose of INH (24). Following 7 days of 650 mg/kg INH, lumbar spinal ganglia showed chromatolysis, dilated components of the endoplasmic reticulum, and a displaced nucleus, suggesting a retrograde reaction to distal axotomy (47). Once axonal degeneration has commenced, the changes are indistinguishable from those of wallerian degeneration (10,25,46,49). Studies of nerves prior to the onset of axonal degeneration revealed focal periaxonal swelling similar to that seen in CNS fibers (6,24,25). This was associated with focal accumulations of axonal organelles, particularly smooth endoplasmic reticulum (37). These swellings did not distend the myelin sheath but appeared to compress the axon. Schwann cell abnormalities include paranodal retraction, proliferation of smooth endoplasmic reticulum to form whorls, cell swelling, and mitochondrial enlargement. Nerve growth factor receptor mRNA (NGFR-mRNA) expression in Schwann cells appears to correlate with sites of axonal perturbation (41). In distal regions of INH- and acrylamide-intoxicated rats, NGFR-mRNA is elevated 2 days prior to histological signs of axonal degeneration.

Degeneration of unmyelinated axons is also seen in rat nerves. The most frequent change is a loss of microtubules and neurofilaments with swelling or shrinkage of axons (45).

Intraneural edema is a prominent feature (25,46). The blood-nerve barrier, following 6 daily doses of 600 mg/kg INH, was severely disrupted at 9 days, and occasional erythrodiapedesis was evident (46).

Central Nervous System

Several studies have examined the effects on chicks and ducklings fed a diet containing INH (9,29,30). At high doses (0.15%), chicks develop seizures; at lower doses, tremor and ataxia appear before convulsions. Birds are not protected from the CNS effects by concurrent feeding with pyridoxol, niacin, or arginine and glutamic acid (9).

Histological changes are largely restricted to CNS white matter; they are especially prominent in the cerebellar roof nuclei. The PNS is unaffected. White matter lesions appear as intense myelin sheath vacuolation (30). Myelin sheaths are also lost (9,30) and there is reactive astrocytosis. The extracellular space was enlarged, but studies with colloidal thorium dioxide (Thorotrast) indicated breakdown in permeability of cerebral blood vessels only in two animals with advanced lesions (30). Vascular changes are also seen in advanced lesions (29).

The dog is the most sensitive species to the CNS effects of INH. This may result from failure to acetylate INH due to an absence of the acetylation enzyme; dogs cannot acetylate sulfonamides (5). There have been two studies on the CNS changes following oral dosing with INH: one examined clinical signs and the histology of CNS degeneration following prolonged dosing (35), and the other described morphological changes induced by both acute high doses and chronic low doses of INH (6). The canine clinical signs are similar to those seen with acute toxicity in humans (35). Maximal signs occurred 1–2 h after dosing and ranged from excitement to twitching and jerking movements. Seizures appeared at dosages above 20 mg/kg/day; these were often triggered by auditory or visual stimulation.

The intensity of CNS lesions reflects both the dose and duration of exposure to INH. In high-dose animals (20–40 mg/kg), white matter vacuolation is most marked in the thalamus, midbrain, medulla oblongata, and cerebellum; chronic, low-dosed animals (15 mg/kg for over 45 days) have more severe changes in the subcortical and hippocampal white matter. Vacuoles arise within the myelin sheath from separation of the intraperiod lines. Vacuolation also reflects swelling of the cytoplasm of the internal oligodendrocyte tongue, distention of the periaxonal space, and focal axonal swelling. In both high- and low-dose animals, there was focal swelling of myelinated and unmyelinated CNS axons. Astrocytic hypertrophy was prominent with prolonged dosing (6,35).

In Vitro Studies

Some *in vitro* studies have addressed clinical drug sensitivity testing of *Mycobacterium tuberculosis* (1,13,16,55); others have focued on INH-induced lupus (27) and INH hepatotoxicity (15,26,38,53).

Human Studies

Peripheral neuropathy is the most common chronic toxic effect and occurs in 17% of patients receiving 6 mg/kg of INH daily; with higher dosages, the incidence of neuropathy increases. CNS syndromes are rare and usually associated with higher doses of INH. Acute and chronic toxic effects of INH show a different clinical spectrum. The main signs following (suicidal) acute poisoning are acidosis, seizures, and coma.

Acute Neurotoxicity

Ingestion of 6–10 g of INH in a single dose is associated with severe toxicity and significant mortality. As little as 1.5 g of INH in a single dose may induce minor toxicity, while 15 g or more is often fatal without appropriate therapy (5). After ingestion of larger amounts of INH, the patient is usually asymptomatic for 30 min to 2 h; this is followed by nausea, vomiting, slurred speech, dizziness, and anticholinergic effects (dilated pupils, photophobia, tachycardia). Severe poisoning may produce seizures, hypotension, cyanosis, and death. Patients may display acidosis, fever, hypotension, and oliguria or anuria (18). Between 80 and 150 mg/kg of INH usually results in severe seizures with a high likelihood of fatality (34). In children, afebrile seizures developed following 14.3–99.3 mg/kg INH and could be controlled only after parenteral pyridoxine (50). INH lowers the seizure threshold to photic stimulation; spontaneous convulsions are reported in 1%–3% of tuberculosis patients receiving drug doses of 14 mg/kg/day or 14 mg/kg twice weekly (14). Seizures following an overdose of INH are common and often refractory to standard treatment strategies (50). The prevalence of INH overdose is now so high that it is recommended that pyridoxine be administered to all patients with repeated seizures refractory to conventional doses of benzodiazepines (52).

Gastrointestinal signs of acute poisoning include diffuse abdominal pain, nausea, vomiting, and abdominal distress following acute overdosage with over 5 mg/kg/day. The clinical and pathological signs of liver damage resemble viral hepatitis. Bridging or multilobular necrosis, or both, may be present (18). Recurrent pancreatitis induced by INH has been recorded in a single case (11).

Antinuclear antibodies may appear during treatment, but these disappear when dosing ceases. These antibodies may be associated with drug-induced lupus erythematosus. Lupus may appear when INH is used for long-term therapy; it is seen more commonly in patients of the slow-acetylator phenotype (4).

Histopathological changes associated with acute INH neurotoxicity in humans have not been documented.

Chronic Neurotoxicity

Peripheral neuropathy is a dose-related chronic effect. It is more likely to occur in malnourished individuals, those with chronic alcoholism, and in slow acetylators. An incidence of 2% is expected with commonly used INH dosages (3–5 mg/kg/day). With high doses of INH, neuropathic symptoms often appear within 3–5 weeks. In patients receiving conventionally low doses of INH therapy, symptoms do not usually appear until 6 months. Symptoms include numbness and tingling of the lower extremities and, occasionally, of the hands and fingers. Frequently, there is also muscle aching that is made worse by exercise. Optic neuropathy and blindness occurred in three cases, despite drug withdrawal (8; cf. 33). Ataxia and weakness are uncommon. Cerebellar ataxia has been described in only five adult cases (7) and one child (31). If neuropathic symptoms are mild, recovery is rapid; however, if dosing continues and signs progress, resolution of symptoms takes considerably longer (up to 1 year). The syndrome can be prevented in most cases by daily administration of pyridoxine (100 mg).

Postmortem studies have detected axonal degeneration in distal peripheral nerves with associated denervation atrophy of muscle, as well as axonal degeneration in the dorsal columns of the spinal cord (5,28). Quantitative studies of sural nerve biopsies from nine cases of INH neuropathy disclosed degeneration of both myelinated and unmyelinated axons, as well as evidence of degeneration and regeneration of axons (36). There appears to be a close clinicopathological correlation between clinical manifestations and the pattern of denervation present in the sural nerve (10,21,36,42,46).

Toxic Mechanisms

The convulsions of acute INH toxicity likely stem from inhibition of both glutamate decarboxylase and the synthesis of γ-aminobutyric acid (GABA) (22,57). Glutamate decarboxylase employs pyridoxal phosphate as a cofactor. There is evidence that GABA levels in the brain are lowered in INH toxicity. In rats, INH (250 mg/kg) caused a rapid and sustained decrease in the extracellular levels of GABA and, during this period, convulsions of increasing severity were observed (3). Basal levels of glutamine, taurine, aspartate, and glutamate were unchanged by INH. Convulsions were prevented by sodium valproate.

INH produces a marked increase in urinary excretion of B_6 and its metabolites. Substances such as ethanol, which increase the utilization of phosphorylated B_6, increase an individual's susceptibility to INH-associated seizures. The exact mechanism of induction of convulsions in INH toxicity is unclear; administration of pyridoxine in sufficiently large doses has a protective effect and should be used in treatment of acute toxicity (18).

In species that develop CNS changes following INH intoxication, the main cells affected appear to be oligodendrocytes (5). The lesions observed, both in distribution and nature, are very similar to those induced by feeding biscyclohexanone oxaldihydrazone (Cuprizone) in mice. An additional feature common to these two compounds is the observation that the pathological changes cannot be prevented by simultaneous administration of pyridoxine or nicotinamide, even when high doses of these compounds are used. With INH, it cannot be determined which enzyme systems within the oligodendrocyte are primarily affected to bring about myelin vacuolation and, with higher doses, oligodendrocyte degeneration. Lesions induced by hydrazine monoamine oxidase inhibitors and those induced by INH are similar; it has been suggested the lesions may have a common pathogenesis (43,58).

Astrocytic change, rather than myelin vacuolation, is the predominant alteration in avian species and dogs treated with high doses of isoniazid. The changes are those of swelling and metabolic hypertrophy; both are nonspecific in nature and reflect the need for increased metabolism by these cells. Observations on avian species (29) treated with high doses suggest that INH may have a primary effect on astrocytes as well as on oligodendrocytes.

The pathogenesis of INH large-fiber distal axonopathy is unclear. The organelles primarily affected within the axons are thought to be the mitochondria (46) or axoplasmic reticulum (37). Multiplicity of lesions at the site of the node of Ranvier would result in a distal accentuation of axonal loss by wallerian degeneration of all affected nerve fibers. The perikarya of peripheral motor and sensory neurons appear to be resistant to the toxic drug effect; they display only retrograde reactions secondary to degeneration of the peripheral axon. The morphological and clinical features are consistent with a "dying back" type of neuropathy.

REFERENCES

1. Banerjee A, Dubnau E, Quemard A *et al.* (1994) InhA, a gene encoding a target for isoniazid and ethionamide in *Mycobacterium tuberculosis. Science* **263**, 227.
2. Benson WM, Stefko PL, Roe MD (1952) Pharmacologic and toxicologic observation on hydrazine derivatives of isonicotinamide (Rimifon, Marsilid). *Amer Rev Tubercul* **65**, 376.
3. Biggs CS, Pearce BR, Fowler LJ, Whitton PS (1994) Effect of isonicotonic acid hydrazide on extracellular amino acids and convulsions in the rat: Reversal of neurochemical and behavioural deficits by sodium valproate. *J Neurochem* **63**, 2197.
4. Blair IA, Mansilla Tinoca R, Brodi MJ *et al.* (1985) Plasma hydrazine concentration in man after isoniazid and hydralazine administration. *Hum Toxicol* **4**, 195.
5. Blakemore WF (1980) Isoniazid. In: *Experimental and Clinical Neurotoxicology.* Spencer PS, Schaumburg HH eds. Williams & Wilkins, Baltimore p. 476.
6. Blakemore WF, Palmer AC, Noel PRB (1972) Ultrastructural changes in isoniazid-induced brain oedema in the dog. *J Neurocytol* **1**, 263.
7. Blumberg EA, Gil RA (1990) Cerebellar syndrome caused by isoniazid. *DICP: Ann Pharmacother* **24**, 829.
8. Boulanouar A, Abdallah E, el Bakkali M *et al.* (1995) Severe toxic optic neuropathies caused by isoniazid. Apropos of 3 cases. *J Fr Ophthalmol* **18**, 183.
9. Carlton WW, Kreutzberg G (1966) Isonicotinic acid hydrazide-induced spongy degeneration of the white matter in the brains of Peking ducks. *Amer J Pathol* **48**, 91.
10. Cavanagh JB (1967) On the pattern of changes in peripheral nerves produced by isoniazid intoxication in rats. *J Neurol Neurosurg Psychiat* **30**, 26.
11. Chan KL, Chan HS, Lui SF, Lai KN (1994) Recurrent acute pancreatitis induced by isoniazid. *Tubercle Lung Dis* **75**, 383.
12. Chua CL, Ohnishi A, Tateishi J, Kuroiwa Y (1983) Morphometric evaluation of degenerative and regenerative changes in isoniazid-induced neuropathy. *Acta Neuropathol* **60**, 183.
13. Cockerill FR 3rd, Uhl JR, Temesgen Z *et al.* (1995) Rapid identification of a point mutation of the *Mycobacterium tuberculosis* catalase-peroxidase (katG) gene associated with isoniazid resistance. *J Infect Dis* **171**, 240.
14. Davadatta S (1965) Isoniazid-induced encephalopathy. *Lancet* **2**, 440.
15. Delaney J, Timbrell JA (1994) Modulation of hydrazine toxicity *in vitro* using various inhibitors and inducers of cytochrome P-450 2E1. *Human Exp Toxicol* 292.
16. Dessen A, Quemard A, Blanchard JS *et al.* (1995) Crystal structure and function of the isoniazid target of *Mycobacterium tuberculosis. Science* **267**, 1638.
17. Donald PR, Seifart HI, Parkin DP, van Jaarsveld PP (1994) Hydrazine production in children receiving isoniazid for the treatment of tuberculosis meningitis. *Ann Pharmacother* **28**, 1340.
18. Ellenhorn MJ, Barceloux DG (1988) Isoniazid. In: *Medical Toxicology.* Ellenhorn MJ, Barceloux DG eds. Elsevier, New York p. 364.
19. Evans DAP, Manley KA, McKusick VA (1960) Genetic control of isoniazid metabolism. *Brit Med J* **2**, 485.
20. Grunberg E, Titsworth EH (1953) Preliminary note on the effect of isoniazid and ipsoniazid in murine leprosy. *Amer Rev Tubercul* **67**, 674.
21. Hildebrand J, Joffroy A, Coërs C (1968) Myoneural changes in experimental isoniazid neuropathy. Electrophysiological and histological study. *Arch Neurol* **19**, 60.

22. Holtz P, Palm D (1964) Pharmacological aspects of vitamin B6. *Pharmacol Rev* **16**, 113.

23. Isler O, Brubacher G (1988) Vitamin B6. In: *Vitamine II. Wasserlösliche Vitamine.* Isler O, Brubacher G, Ghisla S, Kräutler B eds. Georg Thieme, Stuttgart, New York p. 193.

24. Jacobs JM, Miller RH, Cavanagh JB (1979) The distribution of degenerative changes in INH neuropathy: Further evidence for focal axonal lesions. *Acta Neuropathol* **48**, 1.

25. Jacobs JM, Miller RH, Whittle A, Cavanagh JB (1979) Studies on the early changes in acute isoniazid neuropathy in the rat. *Acta Neuropathol* **47**, 85.

26. Jenner AM, Tibrell JA (1994) Influence of inducers and inhibitors of cytochrome P450 on the hepatotoxicity of hydrazine *in vivo*. *Arch Toxicol* **68**, 349.

27. Jiang X, Khursigara G, Rubin RL (1994) Transformation of lupus-inducing drugs to cytotoxic products by activated neutrophils. *Science* **266**, 810.

28. Klinghardt EW (1954) Experimentelle Nervenfaserschädigungen durch Isonicotinsäurehydrazid und ihre Bedeuntung für die Klinik. *Verh Deut Ges Inn Med* **60**, 764.

29. Kreutzburg GW, Carlton WW (1967) Pathogenetic mechanism of experimentally-induced spongy degeneration. *Acta Neuropathol* **9**, 175.

30. Lampert AW, Schochet SS (1968) Electron microscopic observations on experimental spongy degeneration of the cerebellar white matter. *J Neuropathol Exp Neurol* **27**, 210.

31. Lewin PK, McGreal D (1993) Isoniazid toxicity with cerebellar ataxia in a child. *Can Med Assn J* **148**, 49.

32. McCormick DB, Snell EE (1959) Pyridoxal kinase of human brain and its inhibition by hydrazine derivatives. *Proc Nat Acad Sci USA* **45**, 1371.

33. Meyer-König E (1973) Ultrastruktur due glia und Axonschädigung durch 6-aminonicotinamid (6-An) am Sehnerv der Ratte. *Acta Neuropathol* **26**, 155.

34. Nelson LG (1964) Grand mal seizures following overdose with isoniazid. *Amer Rev Resp Dis* **90**, 248.

35. Noel PRB, Worden AN, Palmer AC (1967) Neuropathologic effects and comparative toxicity for dogs of isonicotinic acid hydrazide and its methanosulfonate derivative. *Toxicol Appl Pharmacol* **30**, 337.

36. Ochoa J (1970) Isoniazid neuropathy in man. *Brain* **93**, 891.

37. Ohnishi A, Lee Chua C, Kuroiwa Y (1985) Axonal degeneration distal to the site of accumulation of vesicular profiles in the myelinated fiber axon in experimental isoniazid neuropathy. *Acta Neuropathol* **67**, 195.

38. Omar RF, Rahimtula AD (1993) Possible role of iron-oxygen complex in 4(S)-4-hydroxyorchratoxin a formation by rat liver microsomes. *Biochem Pharmacol* **46**, 2073.

39. Peters JH, Miller KS, Brown P (1965) Studies on the metabolic basis of genetically determined capacities for isoniazid inactivation. *J Pharmacol Appl Ther* **150**, 298.

40. Quemard A, Maeres S, Sut A *et al.* (1995) Certain properties of isoniazid inhibition of mycolic acid synthesis in cell-free systems of *M. aurm* and *M. avium*. *Biochim Biophys Acta* **1254**, 98.

41. Robertson MD, Toews AD, Bouldin TW *et al.* (1995) NGFR-mRNA expression in sciatic nerve: a sensitive indicator of early stages of axonopathy. *Brain Res Mol Brain Res* **28**, 231.

42. Schlaepfer WW, Hager H (1964) Ultrastructural studies of INH-induced neuropathy in rats. Repair and regeneration. *Amer J Pathol* **45**, 679.

43. Schneider H, Cervos-Navarro J (1974) Acute gliopathy in spinal cord and brain stem induced by 6-aminonicotinamide. *Acta Neuropathol* **27**, 11.

44. Schröder JM (1968) Die Hyperneurotisation Büngnerscher Bänder bei der experimentellen Isoniazid-Neuropathie: Phasenkontrast- und elektronenmikroskopische Untersuchungen. *Virch Arch* **1**, 131.

45. Schröder JM (1970) Die Feinstruktur markloser (remakscher) Nervenfasern bei der Isoniazid-Neuropathie. *Acta Neuropathol* **15**, 156.

46. Schröder JM (1970) Zur Pathogenese der Isoniazid-Neuropathie. I. Eine feinstrukturelle Differenzierung genüber der Wallerschen Degeneration. *Acta Neuropathol* **16**, 301.

47. Schröder JM (1970) Zur Pathogenese der Isoniazid-Neuropathie. II. Phasenkontrast- und elektronenmikroskopische Untersuchungen am Rückenmark, an den Spinalganglien und Muskelspindeln. *Acta Neuropathol* **16**, 324.

48. Schröder JM (1970) Zur Feinstruktur und quantitativen Auswertung regenerierter peripherer Nervenfasern. *Proc VIth Int Cong Neuropathol* Masson et Cie, Paris, p. 628.

49. Sea CP, Peterson RG (1975) Ultrastructure and biochemistry of myelin after isoniazid-induced nerve degeneration in rats. *Exp Neurol* **48**, 252.

50. Shah BR, Santucci K, Sinert R, Steiner P (1995) Acute isoniazid neurotoxicity in an urban hospital. *Pediatrics* **95**, 700.

51. Stead WW (1995) Management of health care workers after inadvertant exposure to tuberculosis: A guide for the use of preventive therapy. *Ann Intern Med* **122**, 906.

52. Sullivan EA, Geoffroy P, Weisman R *et al.* (1998) Isoniazid poisonings in New York City. *J Emerg Med* **16**, 57.

53. van der Walt BJ, van Zyl JM, Kriegler A (1994) Different oxidative pathways of isonicotinic acid hydrazide and its meta-isomer, nicotinic acid hydrazide. *Int J Biochem* **26**, 1081.

54. Vidrio H (1994) Potentiation of cardiovascular responses to hydralazine by diverse hydrazine derivatives. *J Pharmacol Exp Ther* **271**, 171.

55. Wilson TM, de Lisle GW, Collins DM (1995) Effect of inhA and katG on isoniazid resistance and virulence of *Mycobacterium bovis*. *Mol Microbiol* **15**, 1009.

56. Winder FG, Collins PB (1970) Inhibition by isoniazid of synthesis of mycolic acids in *Mycobacterium tuberculosis*. *J Gen Microbiol* **63**, 41.
57. Wood JD, Peesker SJ (1972) Correlation between changes in GABA metabolism and isonicotinic hydrazide-induced seizures. *Brain Res* **45**, 489.
58. Worden AN, Palmer AC, Noel PRB, Mawdesley-Thomas LE (1967) Lesions in the brain of the dog induced by pro-longed administration of monoamine oxidase inhibitors and isoniazid. *Proc Eur Soc Study Drug Toxic* **8**, 149.
59. Zand R, Nelson SD, Slattery JT *et al.* (1993) Inhibition and induction of cytochrome P-450 2E1-catalyzed oxidation by isoniazid in humans. *Clin Pharmacol Ther* **54**, 142.
60. Zent C, Smith P (1995) Study of the effect of concomitant food on the bioavailability of rifampicin, isoniazid and pyrazinamide. *Tubercle Lung Dis* **76**, 109.

Isopropanol

Herbert H. Schaumburg

$$C_3H_8O$$

2 Propanol; Isopropyl alcohol

NEUROTOXICITY RATING

Clinical

A Acute encephalopathy (ataxia, confusion, stupor)

Isopropanol is widely used as household rubbing alcohol and in the manufacture of windshield deicers, resins, perfumes, and lacquers; it is also an occasional ethanol substitute. Orally administered isopropanol is rapidly absorbed; dermal absorption is negligible, but significant inhalation exposure in children occurs with repeated sponging for fever (4). Approximately 80% of ingested isopropanol is slowly metabolized to acetone by alcohol dehydrogenase; the remaining 20% is excreted unchanged by the kidneys and lungs, with small amounts resecreted into the stomach (3). Pronounced systemic effects (vomiting, hypotension, hematemesis) and encephalopathy are associated with serum concentrations exceeding 400 mg/dl. The most severe toxic effects of isopropanol—cardiac and CNS depression—are attributed to persistently elevated serum levels of acetone and isopropanol; ketosis without lactic acidosis is characteristic of this condition. Treatment consists of continuous gastric lavage and general support in mild cases; hemodialysis is used for hypotensive or comatose individuals (6).

Ataxia, confusion, and stupor develop within 10 h of ingestion of >150 ml of isopropanol. Coma, miosis, absent tendon reflexes, and hypothermia characterize extreme instances of intoxication. Compared to ethanol intoxication, the duration of isopropanol encephalopathy is prolonged due to the slower metabolism of isopropanol and the contribution of the acetone metabolite. Isopropanol is the offending agent and, in contrast to methanol intoxication, nothing is gained by using another alcohol to compete for alcohol dehydrogenase and thereby prevent formation of a toxic metabolite. For this reason, ethanol is not given to alleviate CNS isopropanol toxicity as it is following methanol ingestion (6).

Experimental studies have been conducted by industry to assess the neurotoxic potential of isopropanol in developing and mature rodents (1,2,5). There was no evidence of developmental neurotoxicity in the offspring of dams given up to 1200 mg/kg/day by gavage from gestation day 6 through postnatal day 21 (1). Mature rodents exposed by inhalation showed no effects at 500 ppm, sedation at 5000 ppm, and narcosis at 10,000 ppm (5). Repeated exposure of female rats to 5000 ppm produced reversible increases in motor activity (2).

REFERENCES

1. Bates HK, McKee RH, Bieler GS *et al.* (1994) Developmental neurotoxicity evaluation of orally administered isopropanol in rats. *Fundam Appl Toxicol* **22**, 152.
2. Burleigh-Flayer H, Gill M, Hurley J *et al.* (1998) Motor activity effects in female Fischer 344 rats exposed to isopropanol for 90 days. *J Appl Toxicol* **18**, 373.
3. Daniel DR, McAnalley BH, Garriott JC (1983) Isopropyl alcohol metabolism after acute intoxication in humans. *J Anal Toxicol* **5**, 110.
4. Garrison RF (1953) Acute poisoning from use of isopropyl alcohol in tepid sponging. *J Amer Med Assn* **152**, 317.
5. Gill MW, Burleigh-Flayer HD, Strother DE *et al.* (1995) Isopropanol: acute vapor inhalation neurotoxicity study. *J Appl Toxicol* **15**, 77.
6. Lacouture PG, Wason S, Abrams A *et al.* (1983) Acute isopropyl alcohol intoxication: Diagnosis and management. *Amer J Med* **75**, 680.

Isoxazololes

Matthias Riepe

MUSCIMOL
$C_4H_6N_2O_2$

5-(Aminomethyl)-3(2H)-isoxazolone; Muscimol

NEUROTOXICITY RATING

Clinical

A   Psychobiological reaction (euphoria, delirium, sedation)

Experimental

A   Seizure disorder

Isoxazololes are structural analogues of γ-aminobutyric acid (GABA). Depending on the side chain of the 3-isoxazolol or 5-isoxazolol ring, these substances are either partial GABA agonists (muscimol: 5-aminomethylisoxazol-3-ol; THIP: 4,5,6,7-tetrahydroisoxazolo[5,4-c]pyridin-3-ol, THAZ: 5,6,7,8-tetrahydro-4H-isoxazolo[4,5-d]azepin-3-ol; isomuscimol: 3-aminomethylisoxazol-5-ol), partial GABA antagonists (iso-THIP: 4,5,6,7-tetrahydroisoxazolo[3,4-c]pyridin-5-ol; iso-THAZ: 5,6,7,8-tetrahydro-4H-isoxazolo[3,4-d]azepin-5-ol) or glial-selective GABA-uptake inhibitors (THPO: 4,5,6,7-tetrahydroisoxazolo[4,5c]pyridin-3-ol) (3,25). Values computed by the Hartree-Fock *ab initio* molecular orbital method show that the 3-isoxazolol ring mimics the carboxylic function of GABA. The analysis also shows that the larger electronic delocalization within the 5-isoxazolol ring causes the antagonist character (3). Structure–activity relationships for several analogs have been studied in detail (4,15,16). For a discussion of naturally occuring isoxazololes, *see* Ibotenic Acid and *Amanita* spp., this volume.

The profile of clinical effects of isoxazololes reflects their structural diversity. For example, THIP is an analgesic of potency comparable to that of morphine (5,13,14) and has a weak anxiolytic effect (7,12). The idea of using the GABAergic mechanism of isoxazololes in antiepileptic therapy has not been successful (21). The main CNS toxic effects are sedation, somnolence, and unsteadiness of gait (10). By contrast, the 3-isoxazolol amino acid (RS)-2-amino-3-(3-hydroxy-5-methylisoxazol-4-yl) propionic acid (AMPA) and the isomeric compound (RS)-2-amino-3-(3-hydroxy-4-methyl-isoxazol-5-yl)propionic acid (4-methylhomoibotenic acid) are potent agonists at the AMPA subtype of central excitatory amino acid receptors (6).

Upon intramuscular injection, THIP reaches peak plasma concentrations within 1 h of application (14,20). Mean

half-time is <2 h (14). THIP and THPO enter the brain poorly after systemic administration, but their thio analogues cross the blood-brain barrier readily (17,25). THIP is excreted as a THIP-O-glucuronide but not as a THIP-N-glucuronide (1). A high-performance liquid chromatographic method for detection of THIP in serum has been described (19). THPO is metabolized to a considerable extent in the liver (24). In the brain, metabolites of THPO correspond to only ~ 8% of the parent compound 30 min after administration of the drug intramuscularly in mice (24).

Intraperitoneal administration of 5–10 mg/kg of THIP induces transient bilaterally synchronous spikes and waves in rats (9). Muscimol and THIP enhance the duration of spontaneous *petit mal*–like seizures in a dose-dependent fashion in seizure-prone animals (27). THIP induces analgesia, as well as sedation and loss of righting reflex. Recovery upon single application of 100 μM/kg is complete, and no adverse effects are noted in rodents (5).

THIP produces a syndrome of bradykinesia, dystonia, ataxia, myoclonus, sedation, and decreased responsiveness in monkeys (*Cercopithecus aethiops*) chronically pretreated with haloperidol. Hallucinatory-like behavior is markedly aggravated by THIP (11).

Like muscimol in humans, THIP at an oral dose of 60–120 mg/day causes unsteadiness of gait, diminishes attention to sensory stimuli, and induces somnolence (10,22). In a group of patients with chronic pain of malignant origin, 5–30 mg THIP intramuscularly induces sedation, dizziness, euphoria, nausea, and blurred vision in up to to 80% of the patients (14). THIP (up to 20 mg) does not lead to changes in respiratory function, or in plasma cortisol, prolactin, or glucose, suggesting an analgesic action independent of opiate receptors (18,26). In patients with anxiety disorders, 5–20 mg THIP three times a day for 2 weeks in a single-blind study, with placebo conditions preceding and following the active drug period, the anxiolytic effects of THIP appeared to be weak and occurred at or close to dose levels that induce sedation and undesirable side effects. As with other GABA agonists and GABA-mimetic drugs, side effects included giddiness, depersonalization, poor concentration, and transitory delirious states (12). Cellular energy demand is increased upon application of THIP in humans (22). While clinical and electroencephalographic monitoring shows a sedative effect and sleepiness after THIP administration, glucose metabolism is paradoxically increased in gray matter structures, which are known to have a high density of $GABA_A$ receptors (22). THIP causes a dose-dependent decrease of regional cortical blood flow and, in one study, was used as an alternative test for hemispheric dominance (23).

Repeated administration of THIP induces the development of tolerance to its antinociceptive effect beginning between day 3 and day 5 of administration. This alteration was not present after acute treatment with THIP and was specific for α_2-adrenergic receptors; α_1- and β-adrenergic, muscarinic and GABA receptors were unchanged in THIP-tolerant mice (2,8).

REFERENCES

1. Andersen JV, Dalgaard L, Hansen SH (1989) Enzymic synthesis of two glucuronides of the hydroxyisoxazole GABA-agonist, THIP, and the *in vivo* glucuronidation of THIP in rat. *Xenobiotica* **19**, 1399.
2. Andree T, Kendall DA, Enna SJ (1983) THIP analgesia: Cross tolerance with morphine. *Life Sci* **32**, 2265.
3. Boulanger T, Vercauteren DP, Durant F, Andre JM (1987) 3- and 5- Isoxazolol zwitterions: An *ab initio* molecular orbital study relating to GABA agonism and antagonism. *J Theor Biol* **127**, 479.
4. Byberg JR, Labouta IM, Falch E *et al.* (1987) Synthesis and biological activity of a GABA$_A$ agonist which has no effect on benzodiazepine binding and of structurally related glycine antagonists. *Drug Des Deliv* **1**, 261.
5. Cheng SC, Brunner EA (1985) Inducing anesthesia with a GABA analog, THIP. *Anesthesiology* **63**, 147.
6. Christensen IT, Ebert B, Madsen U *et al.* (1992) Excitatory amino acid receptor ligands. Synthesis and biological activity of 3-isoxazolol amino acids structurally related to homoibotenic acid. *J Med Chem* **35**, 3512.
7. Corbett R, Fielding S, Cornfeldt M, Dunn RW (1991) GABA-mimetic agents display anxiolytic-like effects in the social interaction and elevated plus maze procedures. *Psychopharmacology* **104**, 312.
8. Costa LG, Murphy SD (1984) Antinociceptive effect of the GABA-mimetic 4,5,6,7-tetrahydroisoxazolo [5,4-c]pyridin-3-ol (THIP): Chronic treatment increases alpha-2 adrenoceptors in the mouse brain. *J Pharmacol Exp Ther* **229**, 386.
9. Fariello RG, Golden GT (1987) The THIP-induced model of bilateral synchronous spike and wave in rodents. *Neuropharmacology* **26**, 161.
10. Foster NL, Chase TN, Denaro A *et al.* (1983) THIP treatment of Huntington's disease. *Neurology* **33**, 637.
11. Gerlach J, Bjorndal N, Christensson E (1984) Methylphenidate, apomorphine, THIP, and diazepam in monkeys: Dopamine-GABA behavior related to psychoses and tardive dyskinesia. *Psychopharmacology* **82**, 131.
12. Hoehn SR (1983) Effects of THIP on chronic anxiety. *Psychopharmacology* **80**, 338.
13. Johnston GA (1992) GABA$_A$ agonists as targets for drug development. *Clin Exp Pharmacol Physiol* **19**, 73.
14. Kjaer M, Nielsen H (1983) The analgesic effect of the GABA-agonist THIP in patients with chronic pain of ma-

lignant origin. A phase-1-2 study. *Brit J Clin Pharmacol* **16**, 477.
15. Krogsgaard-Larsen P, Falch E (1981) GABA agonists. Development and interactions with the GABA receptor complex. *Mol Cell Biochem* **38**, 129.
16. Krogsgaard-Larsen P, Hjeds H, Curtis DR *et al.* (1982) Glycine antagonists structurally related to muscimol, THIP, or isoguvacine. *J Neurochem* **39**, 1319.
17. Krogsgaard-Larsen P, Mikkelsen H, Jacobsen P *et al.* (1983) 4,5,6,7-Tetrahydroisothiazolo [5,4-c]pyridin-3-ol and related analogues of THIP. Synthesis and biological activity. *J Med Chem* **26**, 895.
18. Lindeburg T, Folsgard S, Sillesen H *et al.* (1983) Analgesic, respiratory and endocrine responses in normal man to THIP, a GABA-agonist. *Acta Anesthesiol Scand* **27**, 10.
19. Madsen SM (1983) Quantitative determination of the gamma-aminobutyric acid agonist, 4,5,6,7-tetrahydroisoxazolo[5,4-c]pyridin-3-ol, in serum by high-performance liquid chromatography. *J Chromatogr* **274**, 209.
20. Madsen SM, Lindeburg T, Folsgard S *et al.* (1983) Pharmacokinetics of the gamma-aminobutyric acid agonist THIP (Gaboxadol) following intramuscular administration to man, with observations in dog. *Acta Pharmacol Toxicol Copenh* **53**, 353.
21. Petersen HR, Jensen I, Dam M (1983) THIP: A single-blind controlled trial in patients with epilepsy. *Acta Neurol Scand* **67**, 114.
22. Peyron R, Cinotti L, Le BD *et al.* (1994) Effects of GABA$_A$ receptors activation on brain glucose metabolism in normal subjects and temporal lobe epilepsy (TLE) patients. A positron emission tomography (PET) study. Part II: The focal hypometabolism is reactive to GABA$_A$ agonist administration in TLE. *Epilepsy Res* **19**, 55.
23. Roland PE, Friberg L (1988) The effect of the GABA-A agonist THIP on regional cortical blood flow in humans. A new test of hemispheric dominance. *J Cereb Blood Flow Metab* **8**, 314.
24. Schousboe A, Hjeds H, Engler J *et al.* (1986) Tissue distribution, metabolism, anticonvulsant efficacy and effect on brain amino acid levels of the glia-selective gamma-aminobutyric acid transport inhibitor 4,5,6,7-tetrahydroisoxazolo[4,5-c]pyridin-3-ol in mice and chicks. *J Neurochem* **47**, 758.
25. Schousboe A, Larsson OM, Wood JD, Krogsgaard-Larsen P (1983) Transport and metabolism of gamma-aminobutyric acid in neurons and glia: Implications for epilepsy. *Epilepsia* **24**, 531.
26. Valentin N, Bank MO (1983) Respiratory effect of THIP, a GABA-agonistic analgesic, during halothane anaesthesia. *Acta Anaesthesiol Scand* **27**, 366.
27. Vergnes M, Marescaux C, Micheletti G *et al.* (1984) Enhancement of spike and wave discharges by GABA-mimetic drugs in rats with spontaneous petit-mal-like epilepsy. *Neurosci Lett* **44**, 91.

Janthitrems

Albert C. Ludolph

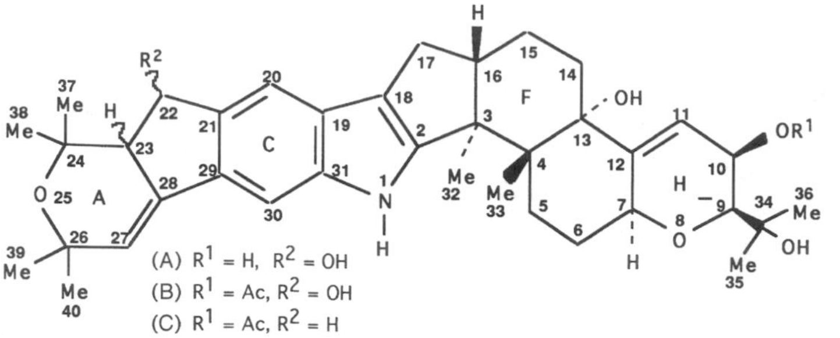

(A) $R^1 = H$, $R^2 = OH$
(B) $R^1 = Ac$, $R^2 = OH$
(C) $R^1 = Ac$, $R^2 = H$

JANTHITREM A
$C_{37}H_{47}NO_6$
JANTHITREM B
$C_{37}H_{47}NO_5$
JANTHITREM C
$C_{37}H_{47}NO_4$

Janthitrem A
Janthitrem B
Janthitrem C

NEUROTOXICITY RATING

Experimental

A Tremor

Janthitrems A, B, and C are tremorgenic mycotoxins produced by *Penicillium janthinellum* (2). These tremorgenic strains were isolated from pastures associated with outbreaks of ovine ryegrass staggers in New Zealand (3). Janthitrems A, B, and C have a MW of 601, 585, and 569, respectively; janthitrems E, F, and G have a MW of 603, 645 and 629, and formulas of $C_{37}H_{49}NO_6$, $C_{39}H_{51}NO_7$, and $C_{39}H_{51}NO_6$, respectively (1,4). Janthitrems display purple-blue fluorescence when irradiated with long-wave ultraviolet light. A detailed description of the isolation, analytical procedures, and structure of janthitrems is available (5). Tremors and hypersensitivity to touch and sound appeared in mice receiving an intraperitoneal injection of 200 μg of janthitrem B in 0.1 ml of propylene glycol (3) (*see also* Penitrems and Other Tremorgens, this volume).

REFERENCES

1. DeJesus AE, Steyn PS, Van Heerden FR, Vleggaar R (1984) Structure elucidation of the janthitrems: Novel tremorgenic mycotoxins from *Penicillium janthinellum* isolates from ryegrass pastures. *J Chem Soc Perkins Trans* 1, 697.

2. Frisvad JC (1989) The connection between the Penicillia and Aspergilli and mycotoxins with special emphasis on misidentified isolates. *Arch Environ Contam Toxicol* 18, 452.

3. Gallagher RT, Latch GCM, Keogh RG (1980) The janthitrems: Fluorescent tremorgenic toxins produced by *Penicillium janthinellum* isolates from ryegrass pastures. *Appl Environ Microbiol* 39, 272.

4. Lauren DS, Gallagher RT (1982) High-performance liquid chromatography of the janthitrems: Fluorescent tremorgenic mycotoxins produced by *Penicillium janthinellum*. *J Chromatogr* 150, 248.

5. Steyn PS, Vleggaar R (1985) Tremorgenic mycotoxins. *Fortschr Chem Org Naturst* 48, 1.

JSTX-3

Nobufumi Kawai

JSTX-3

$C_{27}H_{47}O_6N_7$

NEUROTOXICITY RATING

Experimental

A   Anticonvulsant

A   Glutamate receptor blockade (AMPA receptor)

Joro spider toxin (JSTX) contains a group of closely homologous toxins with MWs of 600–700 (1,3,11). Common to all of these compounds is a 2,4-dihydroxyphenylacetyl asparaginyl cadaverine moiety connected to a polyamine.

JSTX-3, a major component of the venom of the Japanese and East Asian Joro spider, *Nephilia clavata*, is an antagonist at glutamate receptors of invertebrate and vertebrate neurons. In particular, synthetic JSTX-3 toxin produces a selective, voltage-dependent blockage of Ca^{2+}-permeable AMPA (α-amino-3-hydroxy-5-methyl-4-isoxazole propionic acid) receptors in cultured rat hippocampal neurons (9).

The blocking action of JSTX at glutamate receptors was first investigated in the lobster, since neuromuscular transmission of crustacea is similar to that of insects, the prey of spiders. At the lobster synapse, JSTX irreversibly blocks glutamate and excitatory postsynaptic potentials (EPSPs), the latter with an EC_{50} as low as 10 nM, but the toxin mixture fails to affect resting membrane conductance and inhibitory postsynaptic potentials (1,15). Pharmacological studies reveal that JSTX preferentially blocks quisqualate receptors; aspartate-induced responses are less sensitive (10,13). At the squid giant synapse, JSTX blocks postsynaptic potentials, while presynaptic and antidromic action potentials are unaltered. The action of JSTX is therefore confined to the postsynaptic membrane (14).

Synthesis of JSTX-3 (6) and other analogs (20) paved the way for structure–activity studies. Dihydroxyphenylacetyl asparagine fails to block the crustacean glutamate receptor, but suppressive activity is acquired by the addition of a polyamine chain. 2,4-Dihydroxyphenylacetyl asparaginylspermine and 2,4-dihydoxyphenylacetyl asparaginylcadverine are, respectively, approximately 10 and 100 times less potent than JSTX-3 as glutamate-receptor blockers. Autoradiographic studies show that radiolabel from ^{125}I-JSTX-3 is concentrated in synaptic boutons of lobster muscle (18).

In mammals, biotinylated JSTX-3 concentrates in glutamate receptor-rich regions of the cerebellum and hippocampus of rat brain (19). JSTX-3 blocks EPSPs and iontophoretically induced glutamate potentials in CA1 pyramidal neurons in slice preparations of guinea pig hippocampus (17). Non–N-methyl-D-aspartate receptor-mediated synaptic currents are preferentially blocked by JSTX-3 (16). Intracerebroventricular injection of the toxin in mice prevents convulsions induced by quisqualate. Administration of the toxin by this route inhibited memory retrieval in a step-through test, but there was no effect on acquisition or consolidation of memory (8). In mice, JSTX-3 is unlikely to cross the blood-brain barrier, since peripheral injection precipitates no obvious changes in the behavior.

Clarification of the site of action of JSTX-3 has been provided by studies examining the action of the toxin at glutamate subunits expressed in the plasma membrane of *Xenopus* oocytes (4). Glutamate currents induced by receptors encoded by GluR1 and GluR3 genes are blocked by submicromolar concentrations of JSTX-3, whereas receptors formed by subunits containing GluR2 are insensitive to the agent. Further studies have shown that a single amino acid position regulates the blockade induced by JSTX-3; toxin activity is lost by substitution of arginine for glutamine in the second transmembrane domain of GluR1 or GluR3.

Glutamate-receptor antagonists similar to JSTXs have been found in the venom of other spiders of the Araneid family (12). Effective components in the venom of *Argiope lobata* are named argiopin (5) or argiotoxins. Argiopin and argiotoxins show a large degree of homology with JSTXs in having a chromophore group coupled to asparagine and aliphatic polyamines. Similar types of polyamine toxins have been isolated from the venom of *Argiope aurantia* (2); these share a common hydrophilic, basic domain consisting of arginine, apolyamine, and aspargine connected to an aromatic moiety. Some of these toxins have been synthesized and shown to have a paralytic effect on insects. Like JSTX-3, argiotoxin exhibits a subunit-specific block of glutamate-receptor channels expressed in homomeric and heteromeric configuration in *Xenopus* oocytes (7).

REFERENCES

1. Abe T, Kawai N, Miwa A (1983) Effects of a spider toxin on the glutaminergic synapse of lobster muscle. *J Physiol-London* **339**, 243.

2. Adams ME, Carney RL, Enderlin FE *et al.* (1987) Structure and biological activities of three synaptic antagonists from orb weaver spider venom. *Biochem Biophys Res Commun* **148**, 678.

3. Aramaki Y, Ysuhara T, Higashijima T *et al.* (1986) Chemical characterization of spider toxin, JSTX and NSTX. *Proc Jpn Acad* **62**, 359.

4. Blaschke M, Keller BU, Rivosecchi R *et al.* (1993) A single amino acid determines the subunit-specific spider toxin block of α-amino-3-hydroxy-5-methylisoxazole-4-propionate/kainate receptor channels. *Proc Nat Acad Sci USA* **90**, 6528.

5. Grishin EV, Volkova TM, Arseniev AS *et al.* (1986) Structure-function characterization of argiopin-anion channel blocker from the venom of spider *Argiope lobata*. *Bioorg Khim* **12**, 1121.

6. Hashimoto Y, Endo Y, Shudo K *et al.* (1987) Synthesis of spider toxin (JSTX-3) and its analogs. *Tetrahedron Lett* **28**, 3511.

7. Herlitz S, Raditsch M, Ruppersberg JP *et al.* (1993) Argiotoxin detects molecular differences in AMPA receptor channels. *Neuron* **10**, 1131.

8. Himi T, Saito H, Kawai N, Nakajima T (1990) Spider toxin (JSTX-3) inhibits the convulsions induced by glutamate agonists. *J Neural Transm* **80**, 95.

9. Iino M, Koike M, Isa T, Ozawa S (1996) Voltage-dependent blockage of Ca(2+)-permeable AMPA receptors by Joro spider toxin in cultured rat hippocampal neurones. *J Physiol (Lond)* **496**, 431.

10. Kawai N (1991) Neuroactive toxins of spider venoms. *J Toxicol-Toxin Rev* **10**, 131.

11. Kawai N, Miwa A, Abe T (1982) Spider venom contains specific receptor blocker of glutaminergic synapses. *Brain Res* **247**, 169.

12. Kawai N, Miwa A, Abe T (1983) Specific antagonism of the glutamate receptor by an extract from the venom of the spider *Araneus ventricosus*. *Toxicon* **21**, 438.

13. Kawai N, Nakajima T (1993) Neurotoxins from spider venoms. In: *Natural and Synthetic Neurotoxins*. Harvey A ed. Academic Press, New York p. 319.

14. Kawai N, Yamagishi S, Saito M, Furuya K (1983) Blockade of synaptic transmission in the squid giant synapse by a spider toxin (JSTX). *Brain Res* **278**, 346.

15. Miwa A, Kawai N, Saito M *et al.* (1987) Effect of a spider toxin (JSTX) on excitatory postsynaptic current at neuromuscular synapse of spiny lobster. *J Neurophysiol* **58**, 319.

16. Sahara Y, Robinson HPC, Miwa A, Kawai N (1991) A voltage-clamp study of the effects of Joro spider toxin and zinc on excitatory synaptic transmission in CA1 pyramidal cells of the guinea pig hippocampal slice. *Neurosci Res* **10**, 200.

17. Saito M, Sahara Y, Miwa A, Shimazaki K *et al.* (1989) Effects of a spider toxin (JSTX) on hippocampal CA1 neurons *in vitro*. *Brain Res* **481**, 16.

18. Shimazaki K, Hagiwara K, Hirata Y *et al.* (1988) An autoradiographic study of binding of iodinated spider toxin to lobster muscle. *Neurosci Lett* **84**, 173.

19. Shimazaki K, Hirata Y, Nakajima T, Kawai N (1990) A histochemical study of glutamate receptor in rat brain using biotinyl spider toxin. *Neurosci Lett* **114**, 1.

20. Shudo K, Endo Y, Hashimoto Y (1987) Newly synthesized analogues of the spider toxin block the crustacean glutamate receptor. *Neurosci Res* **5**, 82.

Kaliotoxin

Albert C. Ludolph

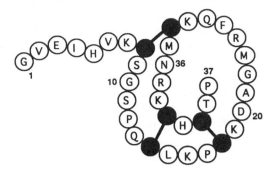

KALIOTOXIN

NEUROTOXICITY RATING

Experimental

A   Ion channel dysfunction (certain potassium channels)

Kaliotoxin (KTX), used as an experimental neurotoxin, is a minor component (<0.5%) of the venom of the scorpion *Androctonus mauretanicus mauretanicus*. The 38-amino-acid, single-chain, 4-kDa truncated peptide has a 44% sequence homology with charybdotoxin (ChTX) and iberiotoxin (IbTX) and a 52% homology with noxiustoxin (NTX) (1), three other compounds from scorpion venom that also act at Ca^{2+}-activated or voltage-gated K^+ channels. Complete KTX has an α-helix and a β-sheet linked by two disulfide bonds, and a folding pattern similar to that of related toxins (1,4). KTX potently and dose-dependently blocks high-conductance Ca^{2+}-activated K^+ channels, but does not affect voltage-gated K^+ channels or Ca^{2+} currents in molluscan neurons (*Helix pomatia*) or sympathetic neurons in the celiac ganglion of the rabbit (2). Studies with rat brain synaptosomes (6) revealed that KTX also interacts with voltage-gated K^+ channels, specifically Kv1.1 and Kv1.3 channels (5). It is suggested that the arrangement IbTX-ChTX-KTX-NTX reflects a decreasing affinity for Ca^{2+}-activated K^+ channels and an increasing affinity for voltage-gated K^+ channels (6). The highly conserved 26–32 sequence of KTX may be the core of the binding site at the outer face of the channel (6). The three-dimensional structure of KTX has been determined (3,4).

Intracerebroventricular injection of the synthesized compound into mice caused paralysis and yielded an LD_{50} of 24 ng, but KTX was not toxic by subcutaneous injection of amounts up to 200 μg (6). Since KTX is only a minor part of the venom of *Androctonus mauretanicus mauretanicus*, it is unlikely this K^+ channel toxin plays a major role in the human toxicity of this scorpion.

REFERENCES

1. Aiyar J, Withka JM, Rizzi JP *et al.* (1995) Topology of the pore-region of a K^+ channel revealed by the NMR-derived structures of scorpion toxins. *Neuron* **15**, 1169.
2. Crest M, Jacquet G, Gola M *et al.* (1992) Kaliotoxin, a novel peptidyl inhibitor of neuronal BK-type Ca^{2+}-activated K^+ channels characterized from *Androctonus mauretanicus mauretanicus*. *J Biol Chem* **267**, 1640.
3. Fernandez I, Romi R, Szendeffy S *et al.* (1994) Kaliotoxin (1-37) shows structural differences with related potassium channel blockers. *Biochemistry* **33**, 14256.
4. Gairi M, Romi R, Fernandez I *et al.* (1997) 3D structure of kaliotoxin: is residue 34 a key for channel selectivity? *Pept Sci* **3**, 314.
5. Legros C, Martin-Eauclaire MF, Cattaert D (1998) The myth of scorpion suicide: are scorpions insensitive to their own venom? *Exp Biol* **201**, 2625.
6. Romi R, Crest M, Gola M *et al.* (1993) Synthesis and characterization of kaliotoxin. Is the 26-32 sequence essential for potassium recognition? *J Biol Chem* **268**, 26302.

Kallstroemia hirsutissima

Alexander Storch
Albert C. Ludolph

NEUROTOXICITY RATING

Clinical

B   Hindlimb weakness (cattle, goats)

The plant *Kallstroemia hirsutissima* (carpet weed) grows on the ground like a carpet and is found in North America from Colorado to Arizona, Kansas to central Texas, and on into Mexico. It causes hindlimb weakness in sheep, goats, and cattle.

Cows that ingest large amounts of *K. hirsutissima* developed hindlimb weakness that progressed to complete paralysis in 8–14 days; the forelegs were unaffected (1). Some affected cows died, probably from exposure to the sun. Weakness was largely reversible within 2 weeks, after the cows had been moved from pastures containing the plant (1). One report describes abnormal hindlimb somatosensory-evoked responses in goats with weakness of the hindlegs after eating *K. hirsutissima* and administration of haloxon as an anthelmintic (1.4 times the therapeutic dose) (2). Since haloxon (an organophosphate compound) can produce a distal axonopathy, the significance of this report is uncertain.

Administration of high doses of carpet weed (~ 86% of the body weight) to sheep produced hindlimb weakness af-ter several weeks on the diet. Feeding the plant to one heifer (1.0%–1.5% body weight daily over 4 weeks) produced an unsteady gait (1).

REFERENCES
1. Mathews FP (1944) The toxicity of *Kallstroemia hirsutis-sima* (carpet weed) for cattle, sheep, and goats. *J Amer Vet Med Assn* **105**, 152.
2. Wilson RD, Witzel DA, Verlander JM (1982) Somatosensory-evoked response of ataxic Angora goats in suspected haloxon-delayed neurotoxicity. *Amer J Vet Res* **43**, 2224.

Kalmia latifolia

Albert C. Ludolph

NEUROTOXICITY RATING

Clinical

A   Ion channel syndrome (sodium channel)

Experimental

A   Ion channel dysfunction (sodium channel)

Kalmia latifolia (mountain laurel, calico bush, mountain ivy, ivy bush, spoon wood) is a cause of human intoxication. Grayanotoxins, in particular grayanotoxin I (andromedotoxin), are responsible for the symptoms (*see* Grayanotoxins, this volume). These toxins bind to site 2 on sodium channels and cause increased resting permeability but no significant inactivation of the channel (1,4). They also shift the membrane potential conductance curve toward the direction of hyperpolarization (1,4). Human poisonings are reported after ingestion of plants (children) or contaminated honey. The clinical symptomatology is consistent with the effects of a channel toxin. Symptoms include circumoral and distal-extremity paresthesia and numbness, burning of the mouth, generalized muscle weakness; with higher doses, somnolence, coma, and possibly seizures are part of the clinical picture (2,3,5). Gastrointestinal (vomiting, diarrhea, nausea) and cardiac (bradycardia, hypotension) dysfunction also occur (2,3,5). Gastrointestinal lavage may be necessary and life-supportive measures, particularly for cardiac complications, may be indicated. Symptoms commence 30–180 min after ingestion and may last up to 24 h.

REFERENCES
1. Catterall WA (1980) Neurotoxins that act on voltage-sensitive sodium channels in excitable membranes. *Annu Rev Pharmacol Toxicol* **20**, 15.
2. Gössinger H, Hruby K, Haubenstock A (1983) Cardiac arrhythmias in a patient with grayanotoxin-honey poisoning. *Vet Hum Toxicol* **25**, 328.
3. Lampe KF (1988) Rhododendrons, mountain laurel, and mad honey. *J Amer Med Assn* **259**, 2009.
4. Strichartz G, Rando T, Wang GK (1987) An integrated view of the molecular toxinology of sodium channel gating in excitable cells. *Annu Rev Neurosci* **10**, 237.
5. Sutlupinar N, Mat A, Satganoglu Y (1993) Poisoning by toxic honey in Turkey. *Arch Toxicol* **67**, 148.

Karwinskia humboldtiana

Roy O. Weller

KARWINSKIA HUMBOLDTIANA
C$_{32}$H$_{32}$O$_8$

7-[3′,4′-Dihydro-7′,9′-dimethoxy-1′,3′-dimethyl-10′-hydroxy-1′*H*-naphtho(2′,3′-c′)[pyran-5′-yl]-3,4-dihydro-3-methyl-3,8,9-trihydroxy-1(2*H*) anthracenone; (T-544)

NEUROTOXICITY RATING

Clinical

A   Peripheral neuropathy

Experimental

A   Peripheral neuropathy (axonal—systemic administration; demyelinating—local administration)

A   Neuronopathy (*in vitro*)

Karwinskia humboldtiana (buckthorn, coyotillo, tullidora, capulín tullidor, capulín cimarrón) grows as a shrub in Mexico and the southwestern United States.

T-544 (Tullidinol) is one of four principal neurotoxic agents (T-544, T-514, T-516, T-496) derived from the stone, seed, and roots of *K. humboldtiana* (family Rhamnaceae) (8). *K. humboldtiana* is a spineless shrub 1–7 m in height, with leaves 3–8 cm long and small five-petaled yellow-green flowers clustered in the axials of the leaves. The flaccid paralysis and fatal consequences of eating the 1-cm-long brown-black fruit and leaves of this plant were recorded in 1789 by D. Francisco Xavier Clavijero in his *Historia de la Antigua o Baja California* (*see* 20). He also described how the sweet fruit pulp could be eaten (once the stones and seeds had been removed) without apparent ill effect.

The genus *Karwinskia* consists of about 15 species of trees and shrubs and, apart from *K. humboldtiana*, ingestion of other species, such as *K. johnstonii* (Fernandez) has resulted in flaccid paralysis (1). Cases of intoxication are most common in cattle, sheep, and children (1,17,21). The isolated toxins comprise some 2% of the dried fruit and seeds of *K. humboldtiana*; they are contained in yellow powders, insoluble in water but soluble in glacial acetic acid and vegetable oils, such as sesame and peanut oils (15).

Cases of naturally occurring intoxication follow oral ingestion of the fruit, but little is known about the metabolism, distribution, or excretion of the toxins. Damage occurs to the PNS and CNS (2–5) and to the liver (9), cardiac and skeletal muscle (6), and kidney (13). Inflammation of mucous membranes of the stomach also occurs following ingestion of the fruit and leaves.

Many animal species are affected by *K. humboldtiana*, including snakes, frogs, pigs (20), goats (2), sheep, chickens, guinea pigs, horses, cattle, man, cats, rats, rabbits (21), and monkeys (14). Susceptibility among various species differs; cattle are most readily affected, but twice the cattle dose is required to poison sheep, and four times the dose to poison chickens. Short-term exposure by oral administration of dried fruit, stones, or seeds results in hindlimb weakness after 6–8 days, with rapid extension of the weakness to the forelimbs (2–5,12). As weakness increases, animals are unable to rise from the ground. Autonomic disturbances have not been observed, and animals remain alert with good appetite and bowel function. There is decrease in limb reflexes, with little impairment of pain sensation (2). Conduction velocities in the sciatic nerves of goats, 9 days after administration of the toxic fruit (0.5 g/kg ground fruit), were reduced to 34–39 m/sec (normal, 53–55 m/sec) indicating the presence of segmental demyelination (3,4). Conduction velocities at 3–6 days were normal. Pathological studies in animals with flaccid limb paresis revealed segmental demyelination and axonal degeneration (12). Chromatolysis has been reported in anterior horn cells, and axonal swelling and degeneration in the long tracts of the spinal cord in goats (5) and monkeys (14). Swollen axons were also found in the white matter of the cerebellum of goats with clinical signs of cerebellar damage (5). No studies of long-term administration of the toxins have been reported.

Oral administration of toxins to cats results in preferential involvement of motor nerves (11) and alteration in fast axonal transport (19). Similarly, oral administration of fruit or purified toxin to rats results in axonal degeneration of intramuscular nerves in a "dying-back" pattern (18).

Intraperitoneal injection of purified toxins in sesame oil in mice resulted in splayed hindlegs after 6 days and death 1–7 days after injection (8). Injections of toxin in sesame oil into rat sciatic nerves produced paresis in the injected leg 5–7 days later, with maximum weakness 10–20 days after injection (16); signs of recovery were present 25 days after injection. Pathologically, there was extensive segmental demyelination with little axonal degeneration; remyelination occurred in animals showing clinical recovery and was present as early as 12 days after injection (16). Electron microscopy showed that Schwann cells phagocytosed the oil, and segmental demyelination occurred without the presence of lymphocytes or macrophages, suggesting that demyelination was due to a direct effect of the toxin on Schwann cells. The oil remained within Schwann cells for at least 3 weeks, but there is no indication how long the toxins remained active.

Uncontrolled exposure to *K. humboldtiana* is of economic importance in relation to the poisoning of livestock in areas of Mexico and Texas where the plant is prevalent (6,7). Goats, cattle, sheep, and pigs develop a flaccid quadriparesis following ingestion of the fruit from plants in their grazing pastures. If large amounts are eaten, the animals may die within 24 h, before they develop neurological signs. In less severe cases, there is progressive weakness of the legs associated with incoordination and ataxia (6), a syndrome known as "limberleg." Finally, animals are unable to rise from the recumbent position and die. If the animal survives, recovery begins after 3 weeks or more but may not be complete for several months, or even 2 years. The prognosis is poor, as cattle and sheep fall into ditches and are unable to climb out. Pathological studies on a group of monkeys (*Macaca fuscata*) accidentally poisoned with *K. humboldtiana* (14) revealed wallerian degeneration and segmental demyelination in the sciatic and radial nerves, with axonal degeneration in the dorsal columns of the spinal cord and astrocytosis in the gracile nuclei.

In vitro studies in which cultures of mouse spinal cord and dorsal root ganglia were treated with *K. humboldtiana* toxins for 48 h to 14 days revealed axonal degeneration consistent with an abnormality in neuronal metabolism (10).

The most famous description of exposure of humans to *K. humboldtiana* fruit is that of 106 soldiers in 1918. Many were affected by fever, cramps, headache, diarrhea, and dyspnea. Some were disabled 14 months later, and 10% of the affected soldiers died (20,22). The majority of human cases of accidental exposure to *K. humboldtiana* toxins occurs in children (1,17,20,21). Symptoms present 5–20 days after ingestion of fruit, with malaise and slow onset of flaccid quadriparesis and bulbar weakness 24–72 h later (21). Weakness begins in the lower limbs and progresses over 14–72 h to involve the upper limbs. Dyspnea, dysphagia, and dysarthria follow. Those who ingest a large amount of the fruit may die before the onset of neurological signs. In patients who survive, dysphagia, anxiety, dyspnea, insomnia, difficulty in micturition, and cramps are usually present for 1–2 weeks. Pain is uncommon, the patient remains mentally alert, and appetite is unimpaired. On examination, there is usually no loss of temperature, touch, or pain sensation, although discrete distal sensory defects have been described. Tendon reflexes are reduced. Recovery occurs over 3–12 months in the reverse order to the onset of symptoms. In the most severe cases, recovery takes longer and muscle wasting and contracture may occur. In less severely affected individuals, recovery may be complete.

Diagnosis depends upon the history of ingestion of the fruit and the exclusion of other causes of acute neuropathy, such as Guillain-Barré syndrome and poliomyelitis (17,20).

Traditional treatments included wrapping the paralyzed limbs in the stomachs of freshly killed cattle. The daily administration of 25–50 mg thiamine hydrochloride intramuscularly and 50 mg orally resulted in improvement in affected children (20), and similar improvement has been seen in experimental animals (20). In most cases, patients are supported through the acute stages and the neuropathy resolves spontaneously.

Pathological studies in man (22) have revealed segmental demyelination in peripheral nerves with some axonal swelling and chromatolysis in anterior horn cells of the spinal cord.

In vitro studies suggest that *K. humboldtiana* causes uncoupling of oxidative phosphorylation (23) similar to that seen with triethyltin and hexachlorophene.

REFERENCES

1. Arellano Cervantes E, Mendoza Cruz JF, De Jesus D, Chavez F (1994) Intoxicación por *Karwinskia johnstonii* Fernandez: Estudio de 12 pacientes. *Bol Med Hosp Infant Mex* **51**, 105.
2. Charlton KM, Claborn LD, Pierce KR (1971) A neuropathy in goats caused by experimental coyotillo (*Karwinskia humboldtiana*) poisoning: Clinical and neurophysiological studies. *Amer J Vet Res* **32**, 1381.
3. Charlton KM, Pierce KR (1970) A neuropathy in goats caused by experimental coyotillo (*Karwinskia humboldtiana*) poisoning: III. Distribution of lesions in peripheral nerves. *Pathol Vet* **7**, 420.
4. Charlton KM, Pierce KR (1970) A neuropathy in goats caused by experimental coyotillo (*Karwinskia humboldtiana*) poisoning: IV. Light and electron microscopic lesions in peripheral nerves. *Pathol Vet* **7**, 420.
5. Charlton KM, Pierce KR, Storts RW *et al.* (1970) A neuropathy in goats caused by experimental coyotillo (*Karwinskia humboldtiana*) poisoning: V. Lesions in the central nervous system. *Pathol Vet* **7**, 435.

6. Dewan ML, Henson JB, Dollahite JW, Bridges CH (1965) Toxic myodegeneration in goats produced by feeding mature fruits from the coyotillo plant (*Karwinskia humboldtiana*). *Amer J Pathol* **46**, 215.

7. Dominguez XA, Temblador S, Cedillo LME (1976) Estudio químico de la raíz de la tullidora (*Karwinskia humboldtiana* Zucc.). *Rev Latinoamer Quimica* **7**, 46.

8. Dreyer DL, Arai I, Bachman CD *et al.* (1975) Toxins causing non-inflammatory paralytic neuronopathy. Isolation and structure elucidation. *J Amer Chem Soc* **97**, 4985.

9. Garza-Ocanas L, Jiang T, Acosta D *et al.* (1994) Comparison of the hepatotoxicity of toxin T-514 of *Karwinskia humboldtiana* and its diastereoisomer in primary liver cell cultures. *Toxicon* **32**, 1287.

10. Heath JW, Ueda S, Bornstein MB *et al.* (1982) Buckthorn neuropathy *in vitro*: Evidence for a primary neuronal effect. *J Neuropathol Exp Neurol* **41**, 204.

11. Hernandez-Cruz A, Munoz-Martinez EJ (1984) Tullidora (*Karwinskia humboldtiana*) toxin mainly affects fast conducting axons. *Neuropathol Appl Neurobiol* **10**, 11.

12. Izquierdo AE, Nieto D (1965) Aspectos neuropatológicos de la intoxicación con *Karwinskia humboldtiana*. Estudio experimental. *Gac Med Mex* **95**, 163.

13. Jaramillo Juarez F, Ortiz GG, Rodriguez Vazquez ML *et al.* (1995) Renal failure during acute toxicity produced by tullidora ingestion (*Karwinskia humboldtiana*). *Gen Pharmacol* **26**, 649.

14. Joiner GN, Russell LH, Bush DE *et al.* (1975) A spontaneous neuropathy of free-ranging Japanese macaques. *Lab Anim Sci* **25**, 232.

15. Kim HL, Camp BJ (1972) Isolation of a neurotoxic substance from *Karwinskia humboldtiana* Zucc. (Rhamnaceae). *Toxicon* **10**, 83.

16. Mitchell J, Weller RO, Evans H *et al.* (1978) Buckthorn neuropathy; effects of intraneural injection of *Karwinskia humboldtiana* toxins. *Neuropathol Appl Neurobiol* **4**, 85.

17. Montoya Cabrera MA, López Martín G, Hernández Zamora A (1982) Intoxicación por *Karwinskia humboldtiana*. Conceptos actuales. *Rev Med Inst Mex Seguro Soc* **20**, 707.

18. Munoz-Martinez EJ, Cueva J, Joseph-Nathan P (1983) Denervation caused by tullidora (*Karwinskia humboldtiana*). *Neuropathol Appl Neurobiol* **9**, 121.

19. Munoz-Martinez EJ, Massieu D, Ochs S (1984) Depression of fast axonal transport produced by tullidora. *J Neurobiol* **15**, 375.

20. Padron-Puyou F (1951) Estudio clínico-experimental de la parálisis por *Karwinskia humboldtiana* ("tullidora") en niños. *Gac Med Mex* **81**, 299.

21. Padron-Puyou F, Velazquez T (1956) Patología experimental y clínica de la parálisis por *Karwinskia humboldtiana*. *Rev Mex Pediat* **25**, 225.

22. Pozo Del EC (1965) Los efectos paralizantes de la "Tullidora" estudios clinicos y experimentales. (Comentario al trabajo aspectos neuropathologicos de la intoxicación con *Karwinskia humboldtiana* estudio experimental). *Gac Med Mex*, **95**, 179.

23. Wheeler MH, Camp BJ (1971) Inhibitory and uncoupling actions of extracts from *Karwinskia humboldtiana* on respiration and oxidative phosphorylation. *Life Sci* **10**, 41.

CASE REPORT

A 4-year-old Mexican boy ingested an unknown number of fruits from a coyotillo bush. A few hours later, he presented with nausea, diffuse abdominal pain, and pasty stools. The symptoms resolved spontaneously, and he remained asymptomatic for 10 days when he developed paralysis, ascending from the lower limbs to involve the upper limbs and resulting in a claw-like deformity of the hands. There was no disturbance of consciousness, but he suffered progressive difficulty with breathing and short periods of apnea, which required assisted ventilation. Electromyography suggested demyelination in the peripheral nerves, but there was no abnormality of the cerebrospinal fluid (CSF). After a week, spontaneous respiration returned, and his neurological symptoms began to resolve in descending order, starting in the arms. He was left with residual weakness in the lower limbs for which he received rehabilitation. The source of the fruit was definitely identified as Karwinskia humboldtiana.

Comment. The latent period before the onset of symptoms is similar to Guillain-Barré syndrome but the cranial nerves are not affected, and there is no change in the CSF. [Kindly supplied by Dr. M.A. Montoya Cabrera (17), and Dr. Laura Chávez Macías, México.]

Lead, Inorganic

Deborah A. Cory-Schlecta
Herbert H. Schaumburg

NEUROTOXICITY RATING

Clinical

A Peripheral neuropathy (axonal)

A Acute encephalopathy (seizures, papilledema)

B Chronic encephalopathy (cognitive dysfunction)

Experimental

A Peripheral neuropathy (demyelinating)

A Acute encephalopathy (neonatal)

Inorganic lead (Pb) is a venerable hazard; lead colic and weakness were known to Hippocrates and Roman physicians. While lead-ore mining and processing commenced in antiquity, epidemics of lead poisoning were first recognized in the eighteenth century, usually associated with use of lead as an adulterant in alcoholic beverages (*e.g.*, the "Devonshire cyder colic of 1767"). By the nineteenth century, most workers in the lead trades could expect to develop effects of some sort, and the women who dipped articles into lead glazes had a stillbirth rate approaching 60%. Environmental and body-burden levels steadily increased in North America until the mid 1980s, when blood levels began a modest decline attributable to the removal of lead from paint, gasoline, and domestic cans (47). While disabling neurotoxicity associated with high levels of circulating inorganic lead is now rare in North American medical practice, it appears likely that many inner-city children still experience cognitive dysfunction associated with modest body burdens. Despite a formidable scientific effort to understand lead toxicity (more than 300 manuscripts a year), the mechanisms of lead-induced nervous system damage remain elusive. Although organic (tetraethyl and tetramethyl) lead compounds can contribute to the environmental pool of inorganic lead, their neurotoxic effects differ (*see* Lead, Organic, this volume).

Lead metal is a gray-white substance with a low MP (327.4°C), an atomic number of 82, and an atomic weight of 207.2. Its density is 11.2 g/ml. It is soft, malleable, and resists corrosion. Lead is obtained from roasting the ore (galena) in which lead occurs as the sulfide. Mining operations contribute lead sulfide, smelters contribute lead oxide, and pigment manufacture contributes the carbonates and chromates. Organic lead (tetraethyl) in gasoline eventually adds to the environmental pool of inorganic lead. Tetraethyl lead is converted in part to halogenated lead during combustion by combining with halogenated hydrocarbon additives; subsequently, halogen loss occurs with the formation of lead sulfate or lead oxide.

Lead is now so ubiquitous in air, water, and soil that it is even difficult to achieve a lead-free environment in experimental laboratories devoted to its study. The principal route of exposure for the average healthy person is oral (in food and beverages); inspired air constitutes about one-half of the lead consumed orally. Lead content of food is extremely variable, but there is almost no lead-free food item; the average adult diet contains 150 μg/day. Environmental sources account for lead exposure in the air and the diet. For adults, occupational sources of lead neurotoxicity have included several industries: mining, smelting, storage batteries, pigments, ink, ceramics, automobile radiator repair, high-temperature cutting of old metal structures, and firing ranges. Consumption of illicit "moonshine" whiskey condensed in automobile radiators has caused small epidemics in the southern United States, and occasional individual cases have arisen from exotic sources (cocktail glasses, missile silos). Young children and infants are especially vulnerable to ingested lead in paint flakes and dust in and around older inner-city dwellings. Children and adolescents in some rural areas in the United States have developed encephalopathy from sniffing leaded gasoline.

The 1991 time-weighted Threshold Limit Value is 0.15 mg/m^3, for inorganic lead compounds in air, dust, or fumes. The U.S. Environmental Protection Agency (EPA) community air standard is 1.5 μg/m^3, computed as a quarterly average. The EPA standard for lead in drinking water is 50 μg/l (50 ppb). There are no standards to regulate lead concentrations in dust or soil.

General Toxicology

Humans are exposed to inorganic lead primarily by inhalation or ingestion; cutaneous absorption is less significant. Approximately 50% of large particles of inhaled lead are deposited in the lung and about half of the deposited lead appears in the blood. Gastrointestinal absorption is affected by age, physical state of food, and nutritional factors. Adults absorb 10%–15% of ingested lead, children about 40%. Absorption is greater from liquid foods and beverages, and is greater in calcium- and iron-deficiency states as well as after a period of fasting. A pediatric diet low in calcium enhances gastrointestinal uptake of lead. Inorganic lead readily crosses the placenta in humans and laboratory animals; umbilical cord blood contains approximately the same level as maternal blood. Transfer begins at the end of the first trimester and continues until birth; maternal lead burden may decrease during pregnancy, suggesting that maternal lead is transferred to the fetus or excreted in some way.

The total body burden of inorganic lead is subdivided into three pools: (a) Blood, bone marrow, and soft tissues (rapid-exchange pool); (b) skin, muscle, and trabeculated bone (intermediate-exchange pool) and (c) dense bone and teeth (slow-exchange pool).

Blood is the vehicle of transport and distribution, wherein 95% of circulating lead is bound to erythrocytes. The small plasma fraction is the source of deposited tissue stores. Blood levels are good indicators only of recent exposure, but generally only account for 2% of the body burden. Levels vary with age. Children under 7 years have higher lead levels than adolescents, probably reflecting bone growth and deposition. In 1994, the U.S. mean blood level of all persons aged 1–74 was 2.8 μg/dl; in non-Hispanic black children, it was 5.6 μg/dl (47). Twenty-one percent of non-Hispanic black children had levels >10 μg/dl, the currently acceptable upper limit for children. The World Health Organization has proposed that 40 μg/dl and 30 μg/dl be considered the maximal tolerable levels in unexposed adult males and females, respectively. Since transplacental fetal toxicity may occur at levels of 10–20 μg/dl, women of childbearing age should maintain blood levels below 20 μg/dl. The American Conference of Governmental Industrial Hygienists Biological Exposure Index is 50 μg/dl; this is the biological exposure index that represents the level in a specimen from an exposed worker corresponding to inhalation exposure at the Threshold Limit Value. The maximum permitted for an exposed worker is 60 μg/dl for males and 30 μg/dl for females. Levels between 70 and 80 μg/dl may be associated with symptoms of encephalopathy; intervention should be strongly considered at a level of 70 μg/dl. Children are considered to need environmental intervention at levels in excess of 25 μg/dl, and to require chelation therapy if levels exceed 45 μg/dl (7). Studies in early childhood suggest that even levels in excess of 10 μg/dl may have a subtle detrimental effect on subsequent cognitive development (51).

Lead accumulates steadily until age 60; bone accounts for about 90% of the total body-burden. The soft-tissue pool is mostly in the liver and kidneys. Lead appears to enter the brain readily at blood levels encountered in adult and immature laboratory animals (13). Normally, brain and muscle contain relatively little lead. Within brain, lead appears to be widely distributed (60). Subcellular distribution studies indicate selective distribution within nuclei and in mitochondria. Intranuclear inclusion bodies containing lead are found in many tissues in lead intoxication. Studies suggest that the cellular lead uptake in epithelial cells is *via* calcium channels, and calcium acts as a competitive inhibitor of lead uptake (14,56).

Lead is not metabolized. Absorbed lead is excreted primarily by the kidneys and unabsorbed lead appears in the feces. The half-life of lead in bone is measured in decades; the half-life in soft tissues is about 30–40 days. The half-life in blood reflects that of the erythrocyte (approximately 35 days). Bone lead declines with age, presumably reflecting bone resorption.

An elevated body burden in currently lead-exposed subjects will usually be indicated by an elevated blood level. Urine levels following a chelating challenge with ethylenediaminetetraacetic acid (EDTA) are used to determine an elevated soft tissue pool from past exposure. An unexposed person will excete <634 μg/24 h. In individuals with normal blood levels, excretion of >1 g/24 h following a 2-g intravenous (i.v.) EDTA challenge indicates a dangerous body burden from past exposure. In adults with current exposure, excretion of >2 g/24 h is common.

Lead intoxication has profound effects upon the hematological system. Microcytic anemia results from two causes: depression of heme synthesis and shortened erythrocyte lifespan. Lead inhibits δ-aminolevulinic acid dehydratase (ALA-D) and increases circulating δ-aminolevulinate by virtue of a negative feedback control. Blood levels of ALA-D activity have a negative exponential correlation with blood levels of lead. ALA-D activity serves as one of the most useful biochemical indicators of early lead intoxication; inhibition takes place at blood lead levels between 20 and 40 μg/dl. The no-effect level of inhibition of ALA-D is between 10 and 20 μg/dl. Blood and urine levels of coproporphyrin III and free erythrocyte protoporphyrin (FEP) are elevated. FEP combines with zinc in the blood to form zinc protoporphyrin (ZPP); measurement of blood ZPP is considered a good indicator of chronic lead intoxication.

There are two forms of lead toxicity on the kidney. Reversible renal tubular destruction with Fanconi's syndrome may accompany acute exposure to lead in children; lead-containing intranuclear inclusion bodies in proximal tubule cells are characteristic of this disorder. Chronic lead intoxication in adults may produce an irreversible, disabling, chronic interstitial nephropathy characterized by vascular sclerosis, tubule cell atrophy, interstitial fibrosis, and glomerular sclerosis.

Reproductive effects occur in both sexes. Males experience oligospermia and women become less fertile. An increased incidence of spontaneous abortion and stillbirths has long been associated with occupational lead exposure.

Animal Studies

The effects of short- and long-term lead exposure on laboratory animals vary with dose, duration, species, and age. Exposure at early stages of development (pre- and postnatal) is often more devastating than long-term exposure in the mature animal. Most studies utilize oral ingestion of powdered lead or its salts in maternal milk, water, food, or gavage. Inhalation studies are rare. In general, experimental studies confirm clinical experience in humans that exposure to high levels of lead causes encephalopathy in the young and neuropathy in adults.

Short Term Exposure—Central Nervous System

Rodents have been extensively used in studies of short-term lead encephalopathy. Suckling rats exposed to extremely high levels of lead in maternal milk and food become paraplegic at 3 weeks and usually die (46). Their brains display macroscopic discoloration and swelling of the cerebellum. There are extensive hemorrhages and pronounced edema throughout the CNS, especially in cerebellum and spinal cord. Hemorrhages are associated with a striking capillary vasculopathy wherein dilated capillaries are lined with necrotic endothelial cells. Postnatal rats and rabbits display similar changes if high lead levels are administered in a more controlled manner before 20 days of age (36). Subsequent studies of the temporal sequence of the development of these changes in suckling rats employed oral gavage to administer lead (49). This achieved blood levels in excess of 1800 μg/dl, moderate elevations of lead in forebrain (228 μg/100 g), and very high levels (1223 μg/100 g) in the cerebellum. Petechial hemorrhages in the brain were apparent (with absence of clinical signs) and extensive hemorrhages appeared by 5 days; edema fluid accumulated later. Golgi preparations demonstrated that the endothelial buds were most sensitive to lead, and ultrastructural studies disclosed changes in interendothelial capillary junctions. A combined morphological and uptake study of the effect of lead on brain capillaries suggested that the endothelial cells were *not* altered despite accumulations of parenchymal edema fluid (28). Tracer studies with horseradish peroxidase have shown increased permeability of these capillaries. The edema and clinical signs in rats can be diminished by lead chelation but not by corticosteroids. Suckling mice display less pronounced edema and capillary junctions appear unaffected. This may reflect the intolerance of the dam for a diet with more than 1% lead carbonate. Newly weaned monkeys orally dosed with lead acetate and vitamin D develop an encephalopathy with pronounced edema in the cerebellum and subcortical white matter without changes in endothelial cells (19). Experimental intoxication of calves causes an encephalopathy similar to that seen in uncontrolled exposure of mature cows (*vide infra*). Calves displayed multifocal neuronal necrosis in the cortex. Capillary changes temporally mirrored the development of encephalopathy: the initial stage featured dilated capillaries; the intermediate stage, swollen endothelial cells; and, eventually, striking endothelial cell hypertrophy and proliferation were apparant. Studies of the chicken embryo and of immature chicks noted endothelial changes and parenchymal edema (30). In sum, there is disparity between the studies that demonstrate obvious endothelial necrosis and studies that fail to detect these major capillary changes. It is claimed the latter studies indicate a functional change in the endothelial state rather than cell necrosis (14). Furthermore, *in vitro* studies that indicate selective astrocyte vulnerability to lead suggest that perturbation of the astrocyte–endothelial cell relationship in a newborn plays a role in the loss of the barrier function normally expressed by brain endothelial cells. Taken in concert, the results of the morphological and tracer studies indicate that dysfunction of developing capillaries is a primary mechanism of the encephalopathy in immature animals treated with large lead doses in the short term.

While neuronal degeneration is not a prominent feature in suckling animals, and survivors appear to improve with few vascular abnormalities, there are distinct effects on subsequent brain development, especially in the cerebellum (48). There are fewer mitoses in the cerebellar external granule cell layer and an increased number of pyknotic neurons. Purkinje cell development is slowed, pyramidal cell dendritic numbers and synaptic density are reduced, and brain growth is retarded (32,33). Suckling rats dosed at somewhat lower levels for 15 days (blood levels of 250 μg/dl) displayed a smaller mossy fiber zone and granule cell layer.

Mature rats, guinea pigs, rabbits, dogs, and monkeys do not develop light histological abnormalities of the CNS following short-term lead exposure, although rats may have generalized seizures during dosing (12).

There have been no definitive studies of neurophysiology, neurochemistry, or behavior in animals subjected to short-term, high-level lead exposure. The PNS of mature and immature animals appears unaffected by short-term exposure.

Prolonged Exposure—Central Nervous System

Prolonged-exposure studies have predominantly used immature rats or primates treated with either moderately high levels (30–200 μg/dl) or low levels (20–30 μg/dl) of inorganic lead. Prolonged exposure of mature animals causes little significant structural or functional CNS change. The immature rodent given low levels of lead has been extensively used as a model to establish a neurobiological basis for the cognitive and behavioral changes reported in urban children with environmental exposure.

Subtle changes in rate of synaptogenesis and glial development have each been reported following intermediate and long-term, low-level lead exposure in rats and monkeys. An ultrastructural study of rat pups treated prenatally and postnatally describes 50% inhibition of the normal increase in synaptic density of parietal cortex by day 15; by day 21, the synaptic density was equal to controls (39). Blood levels were high at birth, 80 μg/dl, and 30 μg/dl at 15 days. Animals dosed only postnatally had elevated blood lead levels but displayed no morphological abnormalities.

A meticulous correlative study of morphological and biochemical events associated with low-level prenatal lead exposure of rat pups (blood levels 15–50 μg/dl), lasting from day of conception to postnatal day 20, detected no abnormalities in cerebellar morphogenesis; there was a persistent increase in the rate of DNA biosynthesis in lead-exposed rats (29). There was also a significant impairment of desialylation of neural cell adhesion molecules (N-CAM) when the blood levels exceeded 20 μg/dl (20,21,50). Since the developmental sialation state of N-CAMs is believed to regulate cell–cell interaction, fiber outgrowth, and synapse formation, its impairment by low-level lead may be a critical facet in the subtle dysfunction of the immature nervous system in prenatal lead exposure.

The lack of a low-level lead effect on early cerebellar structuring is a striking contrast to the inhibition of cerebellar cell proliferation described in short-term exposures to higher levels of inorganic lead.

Exposure of rat pups for 20 days to high (encephalopathic) levels of lead in the mother's milk produced paraparesis and a severe reduction in the size of the hippocampal mossy fiber layer that was still apparent in animals allowed to recover for 40 days (1).

Monkeys exposed from birth to age 9 years to intermediate lead levels (350–600 ppm in diet with blood levels 51–74 μg/dl) displayed a dose-dependent increase in glial fibrillary acid protein–positive radial glia and star-shaped vimentin-positive astrocytes in the hippocampus. This was interpreted as a lead-induced developmental delay of astrocytic differentiation (15). The monkeys also showed dose-related cognitive and behavioral abnormalities.

Prolonged or lifetime exposures to high levels of lead (blood level >300 μg/dl) are associated with degeneration of the cochlear nerve and necrosis of retinal photoreceptors (44).

Electrophysiological studies indicate that both visual and auditory evoked responses are slowed by lead (44). Latencies of peak II brainstem auditory evoked potentials were increased in monkeys exposed to moderately high doses of lead. Both decreased amplitude and increased latencies of rod photoreceptor potentials have been described. Decreased amplitude, increased latency, as well as decreased absolute sensitivity of rod α-wave and β-wave of the electroretinogram, decreased rod flicker sensitivity, and altered rod dark adaptation, have all been observed in rats with peak blood lead levels of 19 μg/dl at weaning. These effects appear to reflect direct effects of lead on rods. Defects in scotopic visual function are reported in monkeys and rats (44).

A series of studies indicates that lead exposure alters mechanisms of energy metabolism. Specifically, prenatal exposures resulting in blood lead levels of 36 μg/dl were associated with reduced cytochrome content in cerebral cortex and a possible uncoupling of energy metabolism. The reduction in cytochrome content was reversible, suggesting a developmental delay rather than a permanent alteration (59).

Lead exposure has been reported to alter the function of a wide variety of neurotransmitter systems, as indicated by altered kinetics and receptor population parameters. These changes have been reported for dopaminergic, noradrenergic, serotonergic, opiate, γ-aminobutyric acid (GABA)ergic, glutamatergic, and cholinergic systems (55,58,61). For any given neurotransmitter system, results with respect to the exact nature of the effects of lead have sometimes been contradictory. These apparent inconsistencies no doubt reflect differences in critical aspects of the investigations, including developmental periods of exposure and lead doses. Since most neurotransmitter systems show their primary development postnatally in the rodent (from birth to 21 days of age), it should not be surprising that lead exposures carried out prenatally might have different outcomes from those associated with postnatal exposures, or those based on postweaning or adult exposures—periods when development is largely completed. Even when comparisons can be made within a particular developmental period, it is clear that effects on neurotransmitter systems are not necessarily linearly related to lead exposure level, and that biphasic concentration-effect curves can be observed (57,61).

Studies fail to suggest a particular vulnerability of any one neurotransmitter system during lead exposure. Several lines of evidence point to changes in dopaminergic systems consistent with a decrease in dopamine release and availability that may be presynaptic in origin. Such evidence includes the reduced ability of dopamine agonists to prevent the increase in dopamine produced by γ-butyrolactone, as well as decreased levels of dopamine and metabolites, and decreased dopamine turnover. Some of these changes have been noted at blood lead concentrations in the range of 32–36 μg/dl, levels within the range of current concern. Furthermore, changes in dopamine function are evidenced in a behavioral context in lead-treated animals, based on alterations both in discriminability of dopamine agonists in drug- discrimination paradigms, and in their impact on a variety of behavioral baselines (22,23).

It appears that dopaminergic (DA) function is differentially affected by lead in the two terminal dopamine projection areas, striatum and nucleus accumbens (23). Changes in opposing directions are frequently observed, differences that may reflect regional variance in parameters of dopaminergic function. Under some conditions, nucleus accumbens appears to be preferentially sensitive to lead (59,61).

Opioid peptides and related behavioral end points are likewise modified by lead exposure. Changes in both μ and δ receptor levels have been noted. GABAergic neurotransmitter systems display apparent region-specific differences in response to lead. For example, increases in GABA synthesis and decreases in GABA binding occur in the striatum, while the converse pattern has been observed in the cerebellum (59). A relatively uniform finding, both *in vivo* and *in vitro*, is a lead-induced decline in evoked acetylcholine release and diminished cholinergic function. There is a selective reduction in choline acetyltransferase activity of 30%–40% in the septum and hippocampus of rats treated from gestational day 16 through postnatal day 28 and exhibiting blood lead concentrations in the range of only 20 μg/dl (8).

Effects of lead on glutamatergic systems include changes in glutamine synthetase activity, and alterations in binding of *N*-methyl-D-aspartate (NMDA) and of the noncompetitive antagonist MK-801 (22,23). *In vivo* studies describe, at blood lead concentrations ranging from approximately 14–38 μg/dl, inhibition of long-term potentiation, thought to be a cellular substrate of learning and memory processes dependent upon NMDA receptor activation (3,35). Furthermore, alterations in learning accuracy as well as discriminability of stimulus properties produced by the noncompetitive antagonist MK-801 are attenuated by lead exposure, consistent with the reported inhibition of MK-801 binding. In contrast, the accuracy impairments and the discriminability of the stimulus properties engendered by NMDA are potentiated by lead exposure, providing evidence for a role of the glutamatergic system in lead-induced learning impairments.

Results of animal studies are claimed to support the cognitive impairments suggested by group IQ decrements in pediatric longitudinal studies and to demonstrate such behavioral manifestations at approximately the same blood lead concentrations. Lead-related cognitive defects have been reported, in rodents and in nonhuman primates; these are based on various behavioral baselines, such as repeated learning of response sequences, fixed-interval schedule-controlled behavior, transition behavior on concurrent schedules of reinforcement, and acquisition as well as reversal discrimination learning at blood lead concentrations as low as 11–15 μg/dl (22). Several studies have attempted to document that these deficits represent direct effects of lead on cognitive function, rather than arising indirectly from changes in other behavioral functions. For example, in one such study, lead-exposed rats exhibited accuracy impairments only under conditions where learning a response sequence was required. A previously learned response sequence requiring the same sensory, motor, and motivational processes was not affected by lead. These studies suggest that simple learning paradigms are less sensitive to disruption by lead than more complex learning situations. Evidence for changes in memory function in experimental animal studies is not compelling.

The suggestion that lead exposure causes hyperactivity in children prompted investigations of motor activity levels in experimental animal studies. These studies have produced conflicting results, with virtually equivalent numbers of studies reporting increased activity levels, unchanged activity levels, and decreased activity levels.

Prolonged Exposure—Peripheral Nervous System

There is considerable species variation in susceptibility in experimental lead neuropathy. Adult baboons do not develop neuropathy after a year of high-level dosing, while guinea pigs display a mixture of segmental demyelination and axonal degeneration (34). Most experimental neuropathy studies have been conducted with mature rats; these animals reliably develop a demyelinating neuropathy after 35 days of high-level dosing associated with blood levels in excess of 300 μg/dl (32). Endoneurial lead is first detected on day 7 and segmental demyelination between days 25 and 35. Dysfunction of the blood-nerve barrier follows, with significant endoneurial fluid accumulations from about day 50 (41,42,64). It is now clear that lead has a direct toxic effect on Schwann cells, and one experiment that utilized radioactive lead suggests a direct effect on the myelin membrane (63).

In Vitro Studies

In conjunction with *in vivo* evidence, *in vitro* studies likewise indicate that lead interferes with chemically mediated synaptic transmission. The prevailing hypothesis is that lead exerts its impact presynaptically. First, lead inhibits Ca^{2+}

entry through calcium channels, thus decreasing evoked release. Studies of peripheral adrenergic synapses, for example, suggest a blockade of noradrenaline release. There is a similar decrease in acetylcholine release from presynaptic terminals at neuromuscular junctions. The second effect of lead is to increase the frequency of basal neurotransmitter release. Once lead enters cells, it can increase basal release through interactions with calcium-mediated processes (27). Intracellular lead can directly stimulate transmitter release (55,58), and these effects occur at lead concentrations 100–1000 times lower than Ca^{2+} concentrations.

Numerous *in vitro* studies address other possible lead–calcium interactions. Lead is known to serve as an effective substrate for the erythrocyte Ca^{2+} pump. There is evidence that lead modifies intracellular Ca^{2+} homeostasis (56). For example, lead has been shown to substitute for calcium in calcium-calmodulin–dependent processes, such as the activation of phosphodiesterase, a calcium-calmodulin–dependent enzyme that terminates the action of cyclic adenosine monophosphate (27).

Mitochondrial respiration is inhibited by lead *in vitro*; such effects have been described in cerebrum and cerebellum of immature as well as adult rats exposed to lead. While these effects were observed at high lead concentrations (50 μM) in the first case, the latter study reported changes at pathophysiologically more relevant levels of 5 μM (8).

Measured electrophysiologically, lead exposure reduces the responsiveness of neurons to external stimulation. Numerous studies have examined the impact of lead on voltage-sensitive, ion-specific membrane channels, particularly those permeable to sodium, potassium, or calcium. The combined evidence indicates that lead is, among the heavy metals, one of the most potent inhibitors of voltage-sensitive calcium channels, an effect noted in both vertebrates and invertebrates. There is evidence to suggest that lead inhibits all calcium channel types within a given cell with little difference in potency, but different cell types may exhibit substantial differences in lead concentration-dependence (4). The neuronal nicotinic receptor–mediated ion channel is the most sensitive among ion channels; it is blocked by lead at concentrations of only 20 nM (43) but activated rather than inhibited at much higher concentrations (21 μM EC_{50}). In contrast, serotonin receptor–mediated ion current exhibited an EC_{50} of 50 μM, and glutamatergic NMDA receptor complex ion channel inhibition has been reported at an EC_{50} of 10 μM (2).

In addition to changes in neurotransmitter release and ion channel function, *in vitro* studies indicate that lead inhibits long-term potentiation. These effects parallel reports of inhibited long-term potentiation *in vivo* in lead-exposed rats. *In vitro* lead-induced changes in long-term potentiation have been reported at concentrations of 5–10 μM and above, although some evidence suggests these effects may not be mediated directly *via* the NMDA receptor complex (31).

Lead has been found to substitute for calcium in the activation of protein kinase C (PKC), a phenomenon that occurs in the picomolar range (27). These effects are considered controversial in part because of the extremely low lead concentrations at which they were observed. Moreover, a subsequent study examining the effects of lead on highly purified PKC subtypes found lead to be a potent inhibitor of all three subtypes but with IC_{50} values of 2–10 μM (40). The inhibition, moreover, did not appear to be due to competition with calcium and was totally reversible.

In vitro studies of lead in a model system of dorsal root ganglion cells utilizing morphometry to monitor neurite outgrowth and myelination indicate that lead produces a complete inhibition of myelination (62).

Human Studies

Most cases of clinically evident childhood and adult plumbism result from exposures lasting weeks to months (chronic/subchronic). Terms such as "acute lead encephalopathy" are misleading; the condition does not have an acute onset and it follows prolonged exposure. The term "acute lead poisoning" should properly be restricted to instances of sudden ingestion of large quantities of lead; in practice, this only occurs in laboratory animals.

The three human neurotoxic conditions associated with lead are overt encephalopathy, subclinical encephalopathy and peripheral neuropathy. The first two are largely encountered in childhood, the third is almost always an adult condition. Table 30 depicts the relationship between some clinical phenomena and blood lead levels.

TABLE 30. Relationship Between Concentration of Pb in Blood (PbB) and Onset of Clinical Findings

PbB (μ/dl)	Effect
10–20	Developmental toxicity: IQ↓, hearing↓, growth↓
20–30	Hemoglobin synthesis↓
40–70	Nephropathy, anemia, nerve conduction changes
70–100	Neuropathy, encephalopathy in children
100–120	Encephalopathy in adults

Overt "Acute" Lead Encephalopathy

This disorder is now rare in north America. The incidence of lead poisoning is at its highest between 12 and 35 months of age. Pica is common, and its history can be elicited in at least one-half of cases. Symptoms develop insidiously, first becoming apparent in late summer in about 80% of instances. This is perhaps a consequence of increased lead absorption in the presence of vitamin D and actinic rays at that time. Even before a child comes to the attention of a physician, there is usually a prodromal period of several weeks or months during which the subject is pale, irritable, listless and lacking an appetite. Epigastric pain, vomiting and constipation are common. These nonspecific symptoms are often interrupted by the sudden onset of a series of generalized convulsions or depression of consciousness.

Seizures are common and resistant to anticonvulsant therapy. They may be followed by hemiplegia or other neurological sequelae.

On physical examination, the child with lead encephalopathy has all the signs of increased intracranial pressure. These include papilledema, a bulging fontanelle, and separation of the sutures, indicated by a tympanitic note or a cracked-pot sound on percussion of the skull (Macewen's sign). Less frequently, patients develop cerebellar ataxia and paralysis of the sixth and seventh cranial nerves. Nuchal rigidity is fairly common and may be related to tonsillar herniation.

Peripheral neuropathy is a far less common form of lead poisoning in children. In contrast to adults, children develop footdrop early, and the legs are usually more involved than the arms. A lead line is rarely seen in children. When present it takes the form of a bluish black line at the margin of the gums or at the anus, the result of the deposition of lead sulfide.

Anemia usually accompanies neurological symptoms. Red cells in peripheral blood and bone marrow may show basophilic stippling; the presence of a large percentage of such cells is almost invariable in chronic poisoning due to inorganic lead, although not in poisoning with organic (tetraethyl) lead. This finding, however, is not specific for lead intoxication.

Many patients have deranged renal tubular function. This may result in glycosuria and a generalized aminoaciduria and, less commonly, in hypophosphatemia and radiological evidence of renal rickets.

Cerebrospinal fluid (CSF) is under increased pressure in lead encephalopathy. Pleocytosis is common, and most patients have cell counts of 10–60. The CSF protein content is usually elevated.

Radiological findings are characteristic. Most prominent is the presence of a dense, radiopaque band at the metaphyses of numerous long bones. Less commonly, there are radiopaque particles within the gastrointestinal tract, evidence of a recent plaster ingestion.

The brain in acute lead encephalopathy is usually, but not invariably, swollen, with flattened gyri, narrowed sulci, and sometimes collapsed ventricles. The cut surfaces may reveal vascular congestion or occasional petechiae in the gray and white matter. The most conspicuous microscopic findings are related to blood vessels. There is an amorphous, acidophilic, periodic acid–Schiff (PAS)–positive exudate (presumably, protein-rich edema) around vessels in the brain, spinal cord, and leptomeninges. This proteinaceous exudate is also often pooled beneath the pia mater of the cortex. Perivascular, PAS-positive globules and basophilic, mineralized concretions within vessel walls are also frequent. Extravasated erythrocytes are found around some vessels. The capillaries are often conspicuous due to proliferation and/or swelling of their endothelial cells; some capillaries are necrotic and may contain thrombi. Such vascular morphological changes and perivascular exudates have been found throughout the entire neuraxis, optic nerve, retina, and leptomeninges, but are most conspicuous in the cerebrum and cerebellum. Foci of astrocytic proliferation are frequent in white and gray matter, and especially in the molecular layer of the cerebrum and cerebellum. The white matter may appear edematous on microscopic examination. Scattered throughout the brain in some but not all cases is a variable number of necrotic neurons. Besides the acute changes just described, the cerebellum often displays more chronic changes. Prominent among these chronic changes are focal atrophy and gliosis of cerebellar folia due to loss of Purkinje cells and neurons of the internal granular layer.

Several points must be emphasized after this general and idealized description of the gross and neurocytopathology of lead encephalopathy. First, some cases of lead encephalopathy have no recognizable pathological alterations, either macroscopically or microscopically. There is no constant or pathognomonic lesion in lead encephalopathy. Second, the cause of death is not apparent in most cases. Although cerebral swelling is usually lethal if it precipitates uncal and tonsillar herniation, the cerebral swelling described in lead encephalopathy is rarely associated with this phenomenon. A pathogenetic mechanism other than cerebral swelling and herniation must be the basis of death in the majority of fatal cases of lead encephalopathy.

Peripheral Neuropathy

Lead neuropathy usually occurs in the context of a systemic illness, which may be acute, subacute, or chronic. The typical clinical triad is that of abdominal pain and constipation, anemia, and neuropathy. The abdominal colic is thought to be due to an effect of ingested lead on gastrointestinal mobility, although this has never been demonstrated directly. Anemia is probably always present in cases with clinically demonstrable neuropathy.

Typically, in adults, the upper limbs are involved more commonly than the lower limbs. Lead neuropathy is motor and commonly devoid of sensory symptoms or signs. Tenderness of the nerves is not present, although the joints can be painful and the muscles tender. If sensory changes are present, they are overshadowed by weakness, which characteristically appears to affect the radial nerves, although other nerves are involved. The wristdrop of lead neuropathy is not necessarily symmetrical. There is some question that, in earlier times, this was seen more frequently in housepainters as an occupational disease not only associated with the use of leaded paints but also as part of an occupational trauma to the radial nerve itself or to the deep branch in the forearm (deep radial nerve or posterior interosseous nerve).

In typical cases of wristdrop from lead neuropathy, the weakness commences with the proximal extensors of the middle and ring fingers, with later involvement in the index and little fingers, followed by weakness of extension of the thumb. With more involvement, the extensors of the wrist then become weak. The weakness and atrophy are often not confined to the distribution of the radial nerve and can include the thenar muscles, especially the abductor pollicis brevis, and to a lesser extent the interossei.

At times, the weakness of the upper limbs may involve the limb muscles supplied by the C5 and C6 nerve roots; rarely, the proximal muscles of the shoulder girdle are affected. Weakness in the lower limbs is usually manifest as footdrop, indicating involvement of the peroneal nerve or L5 root, although this is more apt to be found in children than in adults. The few electrophysiological studies in severe lead neuropathy describe denervation accompanied by small-amplitude motor responses without prolonged conduction times.

Most electrophysiological reports suggest there are minor abnormalities of nerve conduction in workers with blood lead levels in the region of 50–140 μg/dl. Different authors employed different techniques and, therefore, comparison of findings is difficult. No difference was found in the maximal motor or sensory nerve conduction velocity when lead-exposed workers were compared with age-matched controls (17). However, there was a statistically significant decrease in the ratio of the amplitude of the compound muscle action potential of the extensor digitorum brevis muscle when stimulated at the knee compared with the ankle. This im-

plied some minor degree of conduction block or dispersion without fiber loss between these points. The study did not address the possibility that the subjects may have incurred an occupationally-related low-grade traumatic peroneal palsy. These workers appeared to have had very significant lead exposure. Seven of the 14 had lead levels >120 μg/dl, seven had hemoglobin values <12 g/dl, and three had lead lines on the iv gums.

One study examined a group composed of 26 storage battery factor workers with blood lead levels <70 μg/dl (54). Compared with the controls, there was a slight but significant slowing of maximal motor conduction velocity for the ulnar and median nerves and of the conduction velocity of the slower motor fibers. Although they were relatively reduced, the values were still within the normal range. Sensory conduction parameters were normal. Another study examined a group of 20 workers with maximal blood lead levels of 70–140 μg/dl (16). Minor abnormalities of nerve conduction were found that were considered of doubtful clinical significance. Motor conduction velocity in the median nerve was reduced by a mean of 5.5 m/sec relative to controls, which was highly significant in statistical terms, although both groups remained within the laboratory's normal range. Abnormalities of sensory conduction to a similar degree were demonstrated.

Most studies have not established any correlation between blood lead level and reduction of nerve conduction velocity.

The neuropathology of human lead neuropathy is poorly characterized; this is due to the inadequacy and contradictory findings of many of the early pathological studies. One can only conclude that lead damages peripheral nerves and that the histopathological change is mainly wallerian degeneration. Segmental demyelination has never been described in humans, in striking contrast to rats, in which primary demyelination is characteristic. Early descriptions also included degenerative changes in spinal roots and in anterior horn cells. These reports have fueled continuing speculation concerning a role of lead in the pathogenesis of amyotrophic lateral sclerosis (11). At present, most hold that lead is not a factor in this condition.

Subclinical Encephalopathy

Recognition that subclinical lead poisoning, without encephalopathy, could nevertheless engender permanent neurological sequelae in children, including behavioral disturbances, became evident from studies undertaken in the United States in the late 1940s and 1950s. They revealed that such children had poor academic achievement, intellectual and sensory-motor deficits, and other behavioral problems.

Clinic and smelter studies were followed by population-based cross-sectional epidemiological studies relating lead exposure to changes in cognitive functions evaluated primarily by standardized intelligence and other psychometric tests (IQ tests). These efforts relied on measures of either blood lead or tooth lead to assign exposure classifications to subjects and included a wider range of blood lead concentrations than was typical of the clinic or smelter studies (57). Like the smelter- and clinic-based studies, though, the ability to interpret and compare findings across these studies was hindered by significant variations in methodology, including differences in the specific potential confounders of IQ score. Nevertheless, even when important confounding factors, including parental intelligence and social demographic measures, were included in the statistical modeling, many of these studies still reported an inverse association between measures of lead exposure and intelligence test scores. Such effects were registered at 25–30 μg/dl blood lead levels.

Subsequent prospective epidemiological studies eliminated many of the methodological limitations of the clinical cross-sectional studies. These investigations, many of which are ongoing in populations both in the United States and abroad, share common elements of design, including: pre- or perinatal subject recruitment; longitudinal assessment of blood lead beginning antenatally or at birth; use of similar instruments for determination of cognitive function; and assessments of such functions in infancy, late pre-school age and, where possible, during the school-age years. A more uniform set of findings has emerged with respect to later preschool and school-age assessments, where lead-related deficits in cognitive functions, as indicated by changes in IQ scores and other psychometric indices, have been much more routinely observed (5). This has been attributed in part to the fact that more precise measurement of such functions can be obtained in older children. The specific threshold for lead-induced alterations in intelligence test scores is not yet known, but in the Boston cohort, the mean blood lead level for the cohort was only 7.0 μg/dl and the decrement in intelligence test score relevant to a blood lead range of approximately 4–14 μg/dl (6). In a Cincinnati-based cohort in which socioeconomic status was considerably lower, decrements of 7 IQ points were noted at blood lead levels of ≥20 μg/dl (25,26). Toxicokinetic factors may well account for the absence of comparable effects in two of the prospective studies. A Cleveland cohort comes from a population base comprising 50% alcoholic pregnancies, and interactions between lead and alcohol are well known.

Changes in cognitive functions related to lead have also been described in studies of occupationally lead-exposed workers. As has been the case with pediatric studies, the occupational studies have largely utilized standardized intelligence tests as their primary measure of cognitive function. A problem with this approach, however, is that tests of this type make concurrent demands on multiple behavioral functions. Therefore, delineation of specific behavioral impairments produced by lead cannot easily be surmised. Computerized neurobehavioral test batteries show that occupational exposures resulting in blood lead levels of ≥40 μg/dl produced a general slowing of sensory-motor reaction time, as well as mild impairment of attention, verbal memory, and linguistic processing. When these behavioral functions were evaluated longitudinally (*i.e.*, three times over an 8-month period), the slowing of sensory-motor reaction time persisted, was unaffected by practice, and was not evident when the cognitive demands of the task were low. The second study also revealed difficulties in recall of incidental information. Other studies of occupationally exposed populations report significantly poorer performance on psychometric tests such as the Wisconsin Adult Intelligence Scale, with deficits noted in cognitive tasks, visual-motor tasks, and verbal reasoning ability. A recent report suggests that older individuals are more susceptible to the CNS effects of chronic lead exposure (10).

Sensory function changes in response to lead exposure in humans parallel those described in experimental animal studies (45). Changes in auditory thresholds have been reported at blood lead levels of 70 μg/dl in occupationally exposed workers. Recently, small but systematic elevations of hearing thresholds with increasing lead levels have been reported in children. Two studies described such effects in children whose blood lead values were only 10 μg/dl (52,53). In conjunction with these findings, brainstem auditory evoked potentials have been found to be impaired in lead-exposed pediatric and occupationally exposed populations. In studies of children, such effects were found to be linearly or curvilinearly related to blood lead in the range of values of 6–59 μg/dl. Disturbances of auditory function may contribute to reports of changes in speech perception (45). The anatomical and cellular bases of the auditory effects of lead remain to be fully determined, since little information is available regarding any lead-induced changes in auditory nerve morphology or cochlear microphonics.

Lead exposure also impairs visual function (44). It is well known that lead poisoning in humans is associated with visual system pathology and symptoms. These can include blindness, optic atrophy, amblyopia, and scotomata. Moreover, the electroretinogram is altered in lead-exposed workers. Disturbances in pattern-reversal visual evoked potentials (PREP) have been noted in some studies of lead-exposed workers and children, but not in others. This is attributed to the fact that the PREP response is mediated by cones, which appear to be far less susceptible than rods to the impact of lead.

Diagnosis

Three different measures are used in the diagnosis of elevated lead burden. In clinical diagnosis, blood lead and erythrocyte protoporphyrin are the first indices. Currently, the U.S. Centers for Disease Control and Prevention define a blood lead level of 10 $\mu g/dl$ as elevated in children and the U.S. Environmental Protection Agency defines levels of 10–15 $\mu g/dl$ as levels of concern. Erythrocyte protoporphyrin levels above 35 $\mu g/dl$, when combined with an elevated blood lead reading, are considered additional evidence of elevated lead burden (38).

Further evaluation of the extent of elevated lead body burden is sometimes carried out using diagnostic chelation with CaEDTA, or a procedure also known as the CaEDTA or lead mobilization test. In this procedure, three doses of 25 ng/kg CaEDTA, a chelating agent that binds metals (including lead) and accelerates their excretion, is administered at 8-h intervals. The amount of lead excreted in urine is measured over some subsequent time interval, typically 24 h. If the amount of lead excreted exceeds 500 μg, the patient is considered to have plumbism and would generally qualify for a full course of chelation treatment.

The efficacy and safety of the CaEDTA diagnostic test are uncertain because of recent reports that, at least in rats, this specific protocol can actually increase the concentrations of lead in brain (18,24). The mechanism of this effect appears to be a mobilization of lead from bone by CaEDTA and its subsequent redistribution, *via* the plasma lead compartment, to soft tissue target organs such as the brain.

Since >90% of the lead body burden is "stored" in bone, a measurement of the bone lead concentration provides the most accurate assessment of the total extent of lead exposure. An emerging technology of x-ray fluorescence is suggested as a noninvasive measure of bone lead levels. Studies suggest relationships between results of CaEDTA diagnostic tests and x-ray fluorescence outcomes. It is unclear whether this technology will replace CaEDTA diagnostic testing for several reasons. Questions remain about the various forms of x-ray fluorescence, the exact pools of bone lead tapped by these measures, and the absolute sensitivity of the techniques. Moreover, the technology may never be sufficiently available for wide-scale application to potentially exposed populations.

Treatment

Until recently, treatment for elevated lead burden and lead poisoning relied almost exclusively on CaEDTA. Treatment typically consists of a 5-day course of chelation, with CaEDTA administered intravenously by slow drip or sometimes intramuscularly, and sometimes in conjunction with British antilewisite (BAL). Succimer (DMSA), an orally administered analog of dimercaprol, is used in chelation therapy in children (*vide infra*). Repeat courses of treatment are not implemented more than 2–5 days following a previous course of CaEDTA. CaEDTA can reverse mortality in cases of acute lead encephalopathy and can, at least temporarily, reverse some of the symptoms and biochemical effects of acute lead poisoning, including colic, basophilic stippling, and the inhibition of red blood cell ALA-D. Although many earlier studies suggested that CaEDTA could reverse the behavioral sequelae that were residual consequences of high-level lead exposure, these studies generally suffered from the absence of any sham-treated groups to control for the intervention procedures *per se*. A more recent study reported a lack of effect of CaEDTA in altering a cognitive index score (51).

The July 1995 American Academy of Pediatrics treatment guidelines for lead-exposed children are as follows (7):

1. Chelation treatment is not indicated in patients with blood lead levels of <25 $\mu g/dl$, although environmental intervention should occur (9).
2. Patients with blood lead levels of 25–45 $\mu g/dl$ need aggressive environmental intervention but should not routinely receive chelation therapy, because no evidence exists that chelation avoids or reverses neurotoxicity at these blood levels. If blood lead levels persist in this range, despite repeated environmental study and abatement, some patients may benefit from (oral) chelation therapy by enhanced lead excretion.
3. Chelation therapy is indicated in patients with blood lead levels between 45 and 70 $\mu g/dl$. In the absence of clinical symptoms suggesting encephalopathy (*e.g.*, obtundation, headache, and persistent vomiting), patients may be treated with succimer at 30 mg/kg/day for 5 days, followed by 20 mg/kg/day for 14 days. Children may need to be hospitalized for the initiation of therapy to monitor for adverse effects and institute environmental abatement. Discharge should be considered only if the safety of the environment after hospitalization can be guaranteed. An alternate regimen would be to use $CaNa_2EDTA$ as inpatient therapy at 25 mg/kg/day for 5 days. Before chelation with either agent is begun, if an abdominal radiograph shows that enteral lead is present, bowel decontamination may be considered as an adjunct to treatment.

4. Patients with blood levels >70 µg/dl or with clinical symptoms suggesting encephalopathy require inpatient chelation therapy using the most efficacious parenteral agents available. Lead encephalopathy is a life-threatening emergency that should be treated using contemporary standards for intensive care treatment of increased intracranial pressure, including appropriate pressure monitoring, osmotic therapy, and drug therapy in addition to chelation therapy. Therapy is initiated with intramuscular dimercaprol (BAL) at 25 mg/kg/day divided into six doses. The second dose of BAL is given 4 h later, followed immediately by intravenous CaNa₂EDTA at 50 mg/kg per day as a single dose infused during several hours or as a continuous infusion. Current labeling of CaNa₂EDTA does not support the intravenous route of administration, but clinical experience suggests that it is safe and more appropriate in the pediatric population. The hemodynamic stability of these patients, as well as changes in neurological status that may herald encephalopathy, needs to be closely monitored. Adequate hydration should be maintained to ensure renal excretion.

5. Therapy should be continued for a minimum of 72 h. After this initial treatment, two alternatives are possible: (a) parenteral therapy with two drugs (CaNa₂EDTA and BAL) may be continued for a total of 5 days; or (b) therapy with CaNa₂EDTA alone may be continued for a total of 5 days. If BAL and CaNa₂EDTA are used for the full 5 days, a minimum of 2 days with no treatment should elapse before considering another 5-day course of treatment. In patients with lead encephalopathy, parenteral chelation should be continued with both drugs until they are clinically stable before therapy is changed.

6. After chelation therapy, a period of re-equilibration of 10–14 days should be allowed, and another blood lead concentration should be obtained. Subsequent treatment should be based on this determination, following the categories represented above.

Toxic Mechanisms

While the toxic mechanism(s) of lead are not yet known, much of the focus has been on calcium-mediated events and, more recently, on changes in second-messenger systems. Lead can activate calmodulin-dependent phosphodiesterase and calmodulin inhibitor–sensitive potassium channels. It is postulated that the concentration-dependent biphasic effect of lead on neurotransmission could be explained first by a competitive block of voltage-sensitive calcium ion channels, a phenomenon that would explain the inhibition of synaptic transmission that follows depolarization of presynaptic terminals (27). The subsequent increase in small-amplitude postsynaptic discharge is accounted for by entry of lead into the nerve terminal and its subsequent action as a calcium agonist.

It has been argued, however, that the changes in calmodulin-independent protein kinase C, because they occur in the picomolar range, are more biologically relevant in a mechanistic context than the activation of calmodulin, which requires high nanomolar levels of lead (37).

REFERENCES

1. Alfano DP, LeBoutillier JC, Petit TL (1982) Hippocampal mossy fiber pathway development in normal and postnatally lead-exposed rats. *Exp Neurol* **75**, 308.
2. Alkondon M, Costa ACS, Radhakrishnan V *et al.* (1990) Selective blockade of NMDA-activated channel currents may be implicated in learning deficits caused by lead. *FEBS Lett* **261**, 124.
3. Altmann L, Sveinsson K, Wiegand H (1991) Long term potentiation in rat hippocampal slices is impaired following acute lead perfusion. *Neurosci Lett* **128**, 109.
4. Audesirk G (1993) Electrophysiology of lead intoxication: Effects on voltage-sensitive ion channels. *Neurotoxicology* **14**, 137.
5. Baghurst PA, McMichael AJ, Wigg N *et al.* (1992) Environmental exposure to lead and children's intelligence at the age of seven years. *N Engl J Med* **327**, 1279.
6. Bellinger D, Sloman J, Leviton A *et al.* (1991) Low-level lead exposure and children's cognitive function in the preschool years. *Pediatrics* **87**, 219.
7. Berlin CM, Gorman RL, May DG *et al.* (1995) Treatment guidelines for lead exposure in children. *Pediatrics* **96**, 155.
8. Bielarczyk H, Tomsig JL, Suszkiw JB (1994) Perinatal low-level lead exposure and the septohippocampal cholinergic system: Selective reduction of muscarinic receptors and cholineacetyl-transferase in the rat septum. *Brain Res* **643**, 211.
9. Binder S, Matte T (1993) Childhood lead poisoning. The impact of prevention. *J Amer Med Assn* **269**, 1679.
10. Bleecker ML, Lindgren KN, Ford DP (1997) Differential contribution of current and cumulative indices of lead dose to neuropsychological performance by age. *Neurology* **48**, 639.
11. Boothby JA, deJesus PV, Rowland LP (1974) Reversible forms of motor neuron disease. *Arch Neurol* **31**, 18.
12. Bouldin TW, Mushak P, O'Tuama LA, Krigman MR (1975) Blood-brain barrier dysfunction in acute lead encephalopathy: A reappraisal. *Environ Health Perspect* **12**, 81.
13. Bradbury MWB, Deane R (1993) Permeability of the blood-brain barrier to lead. *Neurotoxicology* **14**, 131.
14. Bressler JP, Goldstein GW (1991) Mechanisms of lead neurotoxicity. *Biochem Pharmacol* **41**, 479.
15. Buchheim K, Noack S, Stoltenburg G *et al.* (1994) Developmental delay of astrocytes in hippocampus of rhesus monkeys reflects the effects of pre- and postnatal chronic low level lead exposure. *Neurotoxicology* **15**, 665.

16. Buchthal F, Behse F (1979) Electrophysiology and nerve biopsy in men exposed to lead. *Brit J Ind Med* **36**, 135.

17. Catton MJ, Harrison MJG, Fullerton PM, Kazantzis G (1970) Subclinical neuropathy in lead workers. *Brit Med J* **2**, 80.

18. Chisolm JJ Jr (1987) Mobilization of lead by calcium disodium edetate, a reappaisal. *Amer J Dis Children* **141**, 1266.

19. Clasen RA, Hartman JF, Coogan PS *et al.* (1974) Experimental acute lead encephalopathy in the juvenile rhesus monkey. *Environ Health Perspect* **7**, 175.

20. Cookman GR, Hemmens SE, Keane GJ *et al.* (1988) Chronic low level lead exposure precociously induces rat glial development *in vitro* and *in vivo*. *Neurosci Lett* **86**, 33.

21. Cookman GR, King W, Regan CM (1987) Chronic low-level lead exposure impairs embryonic to adult conversion of the neural cell adhesion molecule. *J Neurochem* **49**, 399.

22. Cory-Slechta DA (1995) Relationships between lead-induced learning impairments and changes in dopaminergic, cholinergic and glutamatergic neurotransmitter system functions. *Annu Rev Pharmacol Toxicol* **35**, 391.

23. Cory-Slechta DA, Pounds JG (1994) Lead neurotoxicity. In: *Handbook of Neurotoxicology: II. Effects and Mechanisms*. Chang LW, Dyer RS eds. Marcel Dekker, New York p. 61.

24. Cory-Slechta DA, Weiss B, Cox C (1987) Mobilization and redistribution of lead over the course of calcium disodium edetate chelation therapy. *J Pharmacol Exp Ther* **243**, 804.

25. Dietrich KN, Berger OG, Succop PA *et al.* (1993) The developmental consequences of low to moderate prenatal and postnatal lead exposure: Intellectual attainment in the Cincinnati lead study cohort following school entry. *Neurotoxicol Teratol* **14**, 37.

26. Dietrich KN, Succop PA, Berger OG, Keith RW (1992) Lead exposure and the central auditory processing abilities and cognitive development of urban children: The Cincinnati lead study cohort at 5 years of age. *Neurotoxicol Teratol* **14**, 51.

27. Goldstein GW (1993) Evidence that lead acts as a calcium substitute in second messenger metaboism. *Neurotoxicology* **14**, 97.

28. Goldstein GW, Asbury AK, Diamond I (1974) Pathogenesis of lead encephalopathy. *Arch Neurol* **31**, 382.

29. Hasan F, Cookman GR, Kean GJ *et al.* (1989) The effect of low level lead exposure on the postnatal structuring of the rat cerebellum. *Neurotoxicol Teratol* **11**, 433.

30. Hirano A, Kochen JA (1973) Neurotoxic effects of lead in the chick embryo. Morphologic studies. *Lab Invest* **29**, 659.

31. Hori N, Busselberg D, Matthews MR *et al.* (1993) Lead blocks LTP by an action not at NMDA receptors. *Exp Neurol* **119**, 192.

32. Krigman MR, Bouldin TW, Mushak P (1980) Lead. In: *Experimental and Clinical Neurotoxicology*. Spencer PS, Schaumburg HH eds. Williams & Wilkins, Baltimore p. 490.

33. Kriegman MR, Druse MJ, Traylor TD *et al.* (1974) Lead encephalopathy in the developing rat: Effect on cortical ontogenesis. *J Neuropathol Exp Neurol* **33**, 671.

34. Lampert PW, Schochet SS (1968) Demyelination and remyelination in lead neuropathy. *J Neuropathol Exp Neurol* **27**, 527.

35. Lasley SM, Polan-Curtain J, Armstrong DL (1993) Chronic exposure to environmental levels of lead impairs *in vivo* induction of long term potentiation in rat hippocampal dentate. *Brain Res* **614**, 347.

36. Lorenzo AV, Gewortz M, Averill D (1978) CNS lead toxicity in rabbit offspring. *Environ Res* **17**, 131.

37. Markovac J, Goldstein GW (1988) Lead activates protein kinase C in immature rat brain microvessels. *Toxicol Appl Pharmacol* **96**, 14.

38. Markowitz ME, Rosen JF (1991) Need for the lead mobilization test in children with lead poisoning. *Pediat Pharmacol Ther* **119**, 305.

39. McCauley PT, Bull RJ, Tonti AP (1982) The effect of prenatal and postnatal lead exposure on neonatal synaptogenesis in rat cerebral cortex. *J Toxicol Environ Health* **10**, 639.

40. Murakami K, Feng G, Chen SG (1993) Inhibition of brain protein kinase C subtypes by lead. *J Pharmacol Exp Ther* **264**, 757.

41. Myers RR, Powell HC, Shapiro HM *et al.* (1980) Changes in endoneurial fluid pressure, permeability, and peripheral nerve ultrastructure in experimental lead neuropathy. *Ann Neurol* **8**, 392.

42. Ohnishi A, Dyck PJ (1981) Retardation of Schwann cell division and axonal regrowth following nerve crush in experimental lead neuropathy. *Ann Neurol* **10**, 469.

43. Oortgiesen M, Leinders T, Van Kleef RGDM *et al.* (1993) Differential neurotoxicological effects of lead on voltage-dependent and receptor-operated ion channels. *Neurotoxicology* **14**, 87.

44. Otto DA, Fox DA (1993) Auditory and visual dysfunction following lead exposure. *Neurotoxicology* **14**, 191.

45. Otto DA, Robinson G, Bauman S *et al.* (1985) 5 Year follow-up study of children with low to moderate lead absorption: Electrophysiological evaluation. *Environ Res* **38**, 168.

46. Pentschew A, Garro F (1966) Lead encephalomyelopathy of the suckling rat and its implication on the porphyrinopathic nervous diseases. *Acta Neuropathol* **6**, 266.

47. Pirkle JL, Brody DJ, Gunter EW *et al.* (1994) The decline in blood lead levels in the United States. The National Health and Nutrition Examination Surveys (NHANES). *J Amer Med Assn* **272**, 284.

48. Press MF (1976) Purkinje cell development and synaptogenesis in lead poisoned neonatal rats. *J Cell Biol* **70**, 40a.

49. Press MF (1977) Lead encephalopathy in neonatal long-Evans rats: Morphologic studies. *J Neuropathol Exp Neurol* **36**, 169.

50. Regan CM (1993) Neural cell adhesion molecules, neuronal development and lead toxicity. *Neurotoxicology* **14**, 69.

51. Ruff HA, Bijur PE, Markowitz M *et al.* (1993) Declining blood lead levels and cognitive changes in moderately lead-poisoned children. *J Amer Med Assn* **269**, 1641.

52. Schwartz J, Otto DA (1987) Blood lead, hearing thresholds, and neurobehavioral development in children and youth. *Arch Environ Health* **42**, 153.

53. Schwartz J, Ottto DA (1991) Lead and minor hearing impairment. *Arch Environ Health* **46**, 300.

54. Seppäläinen AM, Tola S, Hernberg S, Kock B (1975) Subclinical neuropathy at "safe" levels of lead exposure. *Arch Environ Health* **30**, 180.

55. Shao Z, Suszkiw JB (1991) Ca^{2+}-surrogate action of Pb^{2+} on acetylcholine release from rat brain synaptosomes. *J Neurochem* **56**, 568.

56. Simons TJB (1993) Lead-calcium interactions in cellular lead toxicity. *Neurotoxicology* **14**, 77.

57. Slomianka L, Rungby J, West MJ *et al.* (1989) Dose-dependent bimodal effect of low-level lead exposure on the developing hippocampal region of the rat: A volumetric study. *Neurotoxicology* **10**, 177.

58. Tomsig JL, Suszkiw JB (1990) Pb^{2+}-induced secretion from bovine chromaffin cells: Fura-2 as a probe for Pb^{2+}. *Amer J Physiol-Cell Physiol* **259**, C762.

59. U.S. Environmental Protection Agency. (1986) Air Quality Criteria for Lead. Report No. EPA-600/8-83/028dF. Environmental Criteria and Assessment Office, U.S. Environmental Protection Agency, Research Triangle Park, North Carolina.

60. Widzowski DV, Cory-Slechta DA (1994) Homogeneity of regional brain lead concentrations. *Neurotoxicology* **15**, 295.

61. Widzowski DV, Finklestein JN, Pokora MJ *et al.* (1994) Time course of postnatal lead-induced changes in dopamine receptors and their relationship to changes in dopamine sensitivity. *Neurotoxicology* **15**, 294.

62. Windebank AJ (1986) Specific inhibition of myelination by lead *in vitro*; comparison with arsenic, thallium and mercury. *Exp Neurol* **94**, 203.

63. Windebank AJ, Dyck PJ (1985) Localization of lead in rat peripheral nerve by electron microscopy. *Ann Neurol* **18**, 197.

64. Windebank AJ, McCall JT, Hunder HG, Dyck PJ (1980) The endoneurial content of lead related to the onset and severity of segmental demyelination. *J Neuropathol Exp Neurol* **39**, 692.

Lead, Organic

Herbert H. Schaumburg

$$C_8H_{20}Pb$$

Tetraethyl lead; Tetraethyl plumbane

NEUROTOXICITY RATING

Clinical

A   Acute encephalopathy (hallucinations, tremor)

B   Cerebellar syndrome (abuse)

Experimental

A   Acute encephalopathy (seizures, coma)

Since tetraethyl lead (TTEL) is now little used as a fuel additive in North America, organic lead compounds constitute only a minor fraction of the total lead exposure of the general population. Two groups are at risk for organolead intoxication: workers who clean old petroleum storage tanks and persons who deliberately sniff petroleum vapors containing TTEL.

Tetraalkyl leads are rapidly converted in the liver to trialkyl leads and eventually to inorganic lead. Trialkyl lead compounds are lipophilic, they bind strongly to hemoglobin and readily penetrate the CNS. Degradation of trialkyl lead eventually occurs as a mixed-oxidase function of the liver and can be accelerated by prior treatment with phenobarbital.

Experimental animals repeatedly dosed at high levels (100 mg/kg) develop tremor and may have generalized seizures, coma, and death. Postmortem CNS changes include widespread necrosis of cortical and brainstem neurons (5). Rats given a single dose of 20–25 mg/kg display swollen, eosinophilic hippocampal and brainstem neurons. Some hippocampal neurons only had accumulations of lysosomal dense bodies that were cleared in recovered animals (6). Weanling rats given a daily gavage of 0.05–1.0 mg/kg/day, 5 days/week for 91 days, showed dose-related nerve fiber degeneration confined to the spinal cord (10).

More than 160 fatal human cases of TTEL intoxication are reported (3,4). Symptoms of an encephalopathy may commence within hours of a large oral dose (8) or after weeks of working as a tank cleaner. Initial symptoms in industrial cases include headache, vomiting, irritability, and insomnia. Some develop delusions, hallucinate, and attempt suicide. There are no characteristic neurological or physical findings. Most display an intention tremor and are ataxic before coma appears. Symptoms are similar in gasoline sniffers, but onset is more insidious because of chronicity and intermittent exposure. In addition, gasoline sniffers may have a confusing neurological profile that also includes prominent cerebellar dysfunction from effects of chronic exposure to hydrocarbon solvents. Chronic inorganic lead poisoning from sniffing gasoline may cause irreversible dementia and cerebellar ataxia (9). There are few postmortem studies that adequately depict CNS morphology (1,8). Most describe widespread, nonspecific degeneration in cerebral and cerebellar cortical neurons; in industrial cases, recovery once begun is rapid and few have symptoms after 6 weeks.

Laboratory diagnosis depends upon demonstration of elevated blood alkyl-lead levels. Fecal and urinary levels are also raised. Erythrocyte δ-aminolevulinic acid dehydratase levels are depressed in organolead as with inorganic lead intoxication (2).

There is no satisfactory treatment. Chelation is ineffectual in the industrial cases but has been of modest benefit in gasoline sniffers (7).

REFERENCES

1. Bini L, Bollea G (1947) Fatal poisoning by lead benzine. *J Neuropathol Exp Neurol* **6**, 271.
2. Bondy SC (1986) The effect of organolead and tin compounds on δ-aminolevulinic acid synthetase. *Neurochem Res* **11**, 1653.
3. Grandjean P (1984) Organolead exposures and intoxications. In: *Biological Effects of Organolead Poisoning.* Grandjean P, Grandjean EC eds. CRC Press, Boca Raton, Florida p. 227.
4. Keenlyside RA (1984) The gasoline-sniffing syndrome. In: *Biological Effects of Organolead Poisoning.* Grandjean P, Grandjean EC eds. CRC Press, Boca Raton, Florida p. 219.
5. Niklowitz WJ (1974) Ultrastructural effects of acute tetraethyl lead poisoning on nerve cells in the rabbit brain. *Environ Res* **8**, 17.
6. Nolan CC, Brown AW (1989) Reversible neuronal damage in hippocampal pyramidal cells with triethyllead: The role of astrocytes. *Neuropathol Appl Neurobiol* **15**, 441.
7. Seshia S, Rajani KR, Boeck RL, Chow PN (1978) Neurological manifestations of chronic leaded gasoline sniffing. *Dev Med Child Neurol* **20**, 323.
8. Stasik M, Byczkowska Z, Szendzikowski S, Fiedorvczuk Z (1969) Acute tetraethyl lead poisoning. *Arch Toxicol* **24**, 283.
9. Valpey R, Sumi M, Michael K *et al.* (1978) Acute and chronic progressive encephalopathy due to gasoline sniffing. *Neurology* **28**, 507.
10. Yagminas AP, Little PB, Rousseaux CG *et al.* (1992) Neuropathologic findings in young male rats in a subchronic oral toxicity study using triethyl lead. *Fundam Appl Toxicol* **19**, 380.

Leiurotoxin

Albert C. Ludolph

```
     1              5                  10
Ala-Phe-Cys-Asn-Lau-Arg-Met-Cys-Gln-Leu-Ser
              15                 20
Cys-Arg-Ser-Leu-Gly-Leu-Leu-Gly-Lys-Cye-Ile
              25                 30
Gly-Asp-Lys-Cys-Glu-Cys-Val-Lys-His-NH2
```

LEIUROTOXIN

Scyllatoxin

NEUROTOXICITY RATING

Experimental

A Ion channel dysfunction (Ca^{2+}-activated potassium channel)

Leiurotoxin I from the venom of the scorpion *Leiurus quinquestriatus hebraeus* is a basic peptide that selectively inhibits small-conductance Ca^{2+}-activated K^+ channels. The 3400-Da peptide, representing <0.02% of the venom protein, inhibits binding of apamine to rat brain synaptosomal membranes (4). Apamine and leiurotoxin I have similar pharmacological effects; they attenuate the slow hyperpolarization that follows an action potential in skeletal muscle cells in culture and inhibit epinephrine-induced relaxation of guinea pig taenia coli (1). Binding sites for the 31-amino-acid peptide have been demonstrated in brain and a human cell line (2,6); two arginines (Arg6 and Arg13) are responsible for the binding of leiurotoxin to the K^+ channel (6). Leiurotoxin in a concentration of 20 nM has no effect on currents in hippocampal CA1 neurons (5). Leuritoxin-containing scorpion venom also harbors similar-sized leiuropeptides I, II and III, which lack significant insect and mammalian toxicity (3).

REFERENCES

1. Auguste P, Hugues M, Grave B *et al.* (1990) Leiurotoxin I (scyllatoxin), a peptide ligand for Ca^{2+}-activated K^+ chan-

nels. Chemical synthesis, radiolabeling, and receptor characterization. *J Biol Chem* **265**, 4753.

2. Auguste P, Hugues M, Mourre C *et al.* (1992) Scyllatoxin, a blocker of Ca²⁺-activated K⁺ channels: Structure-function relationships and brain localization of the binding sites. *Biochemistry* **31**, 648.
3. Buisine E, Wieruszeski JM, Lippens G *et al.* (1997) Characterization of a new family of toxin-like peptides from the venom of the scorpion *Leiurus quinquestriatus hebraeus*. 1H-NMR structure of leiuropeptide II. *Pept Res* **49**, 545.
4. Chicchi GG, Gimenez-Gallego G, Ber E *et al.* (1988) Purification and characterization of a unique, potent inhibitor of apamin binding from *Leiurus quinquestriatus hebraeus* venom. *J Biol Chem* **263**, 10192.
5. Goh JW, Kelly ME, Pennefather PS *et al.* (1992) Effect of charybdotoxin and leiurotoxin I on potassium currents in bullfrog sympathetic ganglion and hippocampal neurons. *Brain Res* **591**, 165.
6. Gossen D, Gesquiere J-C, Tastenoy M *et al.* (1991) Characterization and regulation of the expression of scyllatoxin (leiurotoxin I) receptors in the human neuroblastoma cell line NB-OK1. *FEBS Lett* **2**, 271.

Leptinotoxin H

Albert C. Ludolph

LPTx; β-Leptinotarsin-h

NEUROTOXICITY RATING

Experimental

A   Ion channel dysfunction (calcium channel)

Leptinotoxin-h (LPTx) is a 57-kDa peptide found in the hemolymph of the beetle *Leptinotarsa haldemani* (Colorado potato beetle) (1,2,5). The peptide increases presynaptic transmitter release in the presence of extracellular Ca²⁺. This effect has been demonstrated for transmitter release in various preparations of rat, mouse, cow, and guinea pig (5), especially for acetylcholine release from mammalian brain synaptosomes (2) and at the neuromuscular junction (4). LPTx also induces cholinergic transmitter release from elasmobranch (*Ommata discopyge*) electric organ synaptosomes (6). LPTx has no effect on the frog neuromuscular junction (5). It is suggested that leptinotarsin opens voltage-sensitive presynaptic calcium channels (3).

REFERENCES

1. Augustine GJ, Charlton MP, Smith SJ (1987) Calcium action in synaptic transmitter release. *Ann Rev Neurosci* **10**, 633.
2. Crosland RD, Hsiao TH, McClure WO (1984) Purification and characterization of beta-leptinotarsin-h, an activator of presynaptic calcium channels. *Biochemistry* **14**, 734.
3. Harvey AL (1990) Presynaptic effects of toxins. *Int Rev Neurobiol* **32**, 201.
4. McClure WO, Abbott BC, Baxter DE *et al.* (1980) Leptinotarsin: A presynaptic neurotoxin that stimulates release of acetylcholine. *Proc Nat Acad Sci USA* **77**, 1219.
5. Miljanich GP, Yeager RE, Hsiao TH (1988) Leptinotarsin-d, a neurotoxic protein, evokes transmitter release from, and calcium influx into, isolated electric organ nerve terminals. *J Neurobiol* **19**, 373.
6. Yeager RE, Yoshikami D, Rivier J *et al.* (1987) Transmitter release from presynaptic terminals of electric organ: Inhibition by the calcium channel antagonist omega Conus toxin. *J Neurosci* **7**, 2390.

Levamisole

Herbert H. Schaumburg

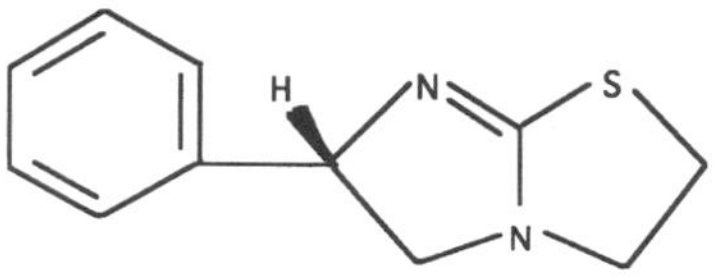

LEVAMISOLE
$C_{11}H_{12}N_2S$

(S)-2,3,5,6-Tetrahydro-6-phenylimidazo[2,1-*b*]thiazole

NEUROTOXICITY RATING

Clinical

A   Leukoencephalopathy (multifocal)

Experimental

A   CNS perivascular cuffing

Levamisole, an imidazole, was initially developed for treatment of intestinal nematodes; it has been superceded by more effective anthelmintics. Currently, levamisole is employed as an immunomodulator in oncological disease to restore immune responsiveness in patients with depressed immune function (1,7). It is generally administered in conjunction with antineoplastic agents. Systemic adverse reactions are minor and uncommon; agranulocytosis may accompany chronic therapy.

Several case reports support an association between combined levamisole–5-fluorouracil adjuvant cancer therapy and multifocal inflammatory leukoencephalopathy (2,4). A primary role for levamisole in the pathogenesis of this disorder is supported by a recent report of reversible multifocal leukoencephalopathy temporally linked to commencement and cessation of levamisole monotherapy in a patient with malignant melanoma (3). Since all instances of this disorder occur in concert with systemic malignancy, this may be a requisite predisposition for the drug-induced disorder. General surveys of adverse effects in individuals without systemic malignancy describe rare instances of insomnia and a "hyperalert state" (5). Three children with rheumatoid arthritis had generalized seizures while taking levamisole.

Administration of high doses of levamisole to dogs produces transient, diffuse, perivascular mononuclear cell cuffing throughout the CNS; there are no clinical findings and no damage to adjacent nervous system tissue (6). The pathogenesis and significance of these changes are unclear.

REFERENCES

1. Hirshaut I, Kesselheim H, Pinsky CM et al. (1978) Levamisole as an immunoadjuvant: Phase I study and application in breast cancer. Cancer Treatment Rep 62,1693.
2. Hook CC, Kimmel DW, Kvols LK et al. (1992) Multifocal inflammatory leukoencephalopathy with 5-fluorouracil and levamisole. Ann Neurol 31, 262.
3. Kimmel DW, Eelco FM, Wijdicks MD, Rodriguez M (1995) Multifocal inflammatory leukoencephalopathy associated with levamisole therapy. Neurology 45, 374.
4. Kimmel DW, Schutt AJ (1993) Multifocal leukoencephalopathy: Occurrence during a 5-fluorouracil and levamisole therapy and resolution after discontinuation of chemotherapy. Mayo Clin Proc 68, 363.
5. Symoens J, Veys E, Mielants M et al. (1978) Adverse reactions of levamisole. Cancer Treatment Rep 62, 1721.
6. Vandevelde M, Boring JC, Hoff EJ et al. (1978) The effect of levamisole on the canine central nervous system. J Neuropathol Exp Neurol 37, 165.
7. Wanebo HJ, Hilal EY, Pinsky CM (1978) Randomized trial of levamisole in patients with squamous cancer of the head and neck: A preliminary report. Cancer Treatment Rep 62, 1693.

Levodopa

John D. Rogers

LEVODOPA
$C_9H_{11}NO_4$

(—)-3-(3,4-Dihydroxyphenyl)-L-alanine

NEUROTOXICOLOGY RATING

Clinical

A   Extrapyramidal syndrome (dyskinesia)

A   Psychobiological reaction (hallucinations, paranoia)

Levodopa, the precursor of dopamine, was introduced in 1970 as a dramatic advance in treatment for idiopathic Parkinson's disease (PD); it remains the single most effective agent for this CNS disorder (4). Levodopa ameliorates, in most instances, all of the cardinal disabling features of PD: tremor, bradykinesia, rigidity, and gait disturbance. Levodopa is usually administered in combination with an inhibitor of peripheral decarboxylase (carbidopa, bensarazide) to prevent the drug's conversion to dopamine in the gastrointestinal tract and other peripheral sites. There are two benefits of combination therapy; one is the elimination of debilitating systemic toxicity of dopamine (vomiting, hypotension), the other is guaranteeing that an adequate level of circulating levodopa enters the CNS. The most commonly prescribed form of levodopa is a tablet containing 25 mg of carbidopa and 100 mg of levodopa (25/100 tablet). Generally, one 25/100 dose three times daily will initially ameliorate tremor and rigidity and provide adequate inhibition of peripheral decarboxylase activity. Sustained-release forms of carbidopa/levodopa may provide a smoother delivery of levodopa and lessen the peaks and troughs in blood levels held responsible, in part, for fluctuating clinical signs (the disabling "wearing off" and "on-off" phenomena). The current treatment of PD no longer depends upon levodopa alone. Generally the initial mild manifestations are treated with monoamine oxidase type B (MAO-B) inhibitor (selegiline); later, carbidopa/levodopa is introduced. Dopamine receptor agonists (pergolide, bromocriptine) are commonly added when levodopa doses have reached high levels, usually late in the disease (22). Major complications of PD and/or side effects of levodopa therapy often emerge after 3–5 years; management then becomes a formidable problem (3). For this reason, many clinicians delay commencement of levodopa treatment as long as possible.

Ingested levodopa is rapidly absorbed from the small intestine by an active transport system. Plasma concentrations peak between 0.5 and 2 h of dosing; the half-life is 1–3 h. The rate of gastrointestinal absorption is slowed by eating, especially by high-protein meals, since there is competition with other dietary amino acids for absorption sites. Levodopa entry into the CNS is an active process mediated by an amino acid carrier, another site of competition with dietary amino acids. Levodopa is converted, in the brain, into dopamine primarily by decarboxylation in the presynaptic terminals of dopaminergic neurons in the neostriatum. The released dopamine is either metabolized at the postsynaptic site by MAO and catechol-O-methyl-transferase, or is transported back into the presynaptic terminal (reuptake) (23).

In normal animals, levodopa administration has not demonstrated neurotoxicity (8,15,16,18). In rats with partial lesions of the nigral system, the addition of levodopa potentiates cell death (2).

In vitro studies of the possible effects of levodopa upon catecholaminergic neurons have been encouraged by the suggestion that prolonged levodopa therapy may actually accelerate the natural history of PD (12).

The toxicity of levodopa has been demonstrated in several cell lines, including fetal mesencephalic cells, neuroblastoma, fetal fibroblasts, pheochromocytoma PC-12 cells, neostriatal synaptosomes, as well as cerebellar and sympathetic neurons (5,9,24,26). Oxidation of levodopa generates toxic free radical species including superoxide, hydrogen peroxide, semiquinones, and quinones (6,7); these can induce membrane lipid peroxidation and rupture (11), as well as inhibition of the mitochondrial electron-transport chain (14,19). Rat mesencephalic cell cultures incubated with levodopa for 48 h display reduction of the number of tyrosine hydroxylase neurons and decreased ^{3}H-dopamine uptake (10). Toxicity is relatively specific for dopamine neurons. Cultured chick sympathetic neurons undergo apoptosis when treated with levodopa (24). Rat ventral tegmental neurons previously exposed to 6-hydroxydopamine undergo apoptosis when exposed to chronic levodopa therapy (2). The hydroxyl radical, which can be produced in the presence of ferrous iron (relatively abundant in the basal ganglia), is linked to neuronal toxicity (11). Measuring hydroxyl radical production with microdialysis in awake rats after systemic levodopa therapy demonstrated a dose-dependent increase in hydroxyl radical, which paralleled the rate of dopa catabolism (20). Treatment with deprenyl and antioxidants in vitro partially prevents the biological and morphological characteristics of levodopa neurotoxicity including chromatin condensation, membrane blebbing, and internucleosomal DNA fragmentation (1). Dopamine-induced programmed cell death can be blocked by treatment with antioxidants (13,21) and vector-driven expression of the proto-oncogene bcl-2, which inhibits apoptosis (25).

Human adverse reactions to levodopa usually appear in the late stages of PD after prolonged drug therapy. As the nigrostriatal system loses its ability to reuptake exogenously derived dopamine, the buffering capacity fails and there is a loss of the ability to compensate for fluctuations in plasma levels of levodopa. Thus, motor function begins to fluctuate dramatically with each dose and rigidity occurs at the end of the dosing interval; this is the "wearing-off effect." Increasing the dose to high levels causes dyskinesias; eventually, a state is reached wherein each dose provokes dyskinesias that are abruptly followed by a prolonged period of no beneficial effect (the "on-off" phenomenon).

Another distressing side effect is the appearance of hallucinations, confusion, and paranoia. This adverse reaction is especially common among the elderly and persons with pre-existent cognitive impairment. These symptoms may respond to antipsychotic medication; clozapine, an atypical neuroleptic not associated with parkinsonism, is currently used.

There are no convincing human clinical studies to support the suggestion (12) that levodopa-induced neurotoxicity participates in the evolution of PD (17).

REFERENCES

1. Ahlskog JE, Uitti RJ, Low PA (1996) Levodopa and deprenyl treatment on peripheral indices of oxidant stress in Parkinson's disease. *Neurology* **46**, 796.
2. Blunt SB, Jenner P, Marsden CD (1993) Suppressive effects of L-dopa on dopamine cells remaining in the ventral tegmental area of rats previously exposed to the neurotoxin 6-hydroxy dopamine. *Movement Disord* **8**, 129.
3. Calne DB (1993) Treatment of Parkinson's disease. *N Engl J Med* **329**, 1021.
4. Cotzias GC, Papavasiliou PS, Gellene R (1969) Modification of parkinsonism—chronic treatment with L-dopa. *N Engl J Med* **280**, 337.

5. Fahn S (1996) Is levodopa toxic? *Neurology* **47**, S184.

6. Graham DG (1978) Oxidative pathways for catecholamines in the genesis of neuromelanin and cytotoxic quinones. *Mol Pharmacol* **14**, 633.

7. Graham DG, Tiffany SM, Bell WR *et al.* (1978) Autooxidation versus covalent binding of quinones as the mechanism of toxicity of dopamine, 6-hydroxydopamine, and related compounds toward c1300 neuroblastoma cells *in vitro*. *Mol Pharmacol* **14**, 644.

8. Hefti F, Melamed E, Bhawan J, Wurtman RJ (1981) Long term administration of levodopa does not damage dopamine neurons in the mouse. *Neurology* **31**, 1194.

9. Mena MA, Pardo B, Casarejos MJ *et al.* (1992) Neurotoxicity of levodopa on catecholamine-rich neurons. *Movement Disord* **7**, 22.

10. Mytilineou C, Han SK, Cohen G (1993). Toxic and protective effects of L-dopa on mesencephalic cell cultures. *J Neurochem* **61**, 1470.

11. Olanow CW (1993) A radical hypothesis for neurodegeneration. *Neuroscience* **16**, 439.

12. Olanow CW (1990) Oxidation reactions in Parkinson's disease. *Neurology* **3**, 32.

13.. Pardo B, Mena MA, Casarejos MJ *et al.* (1995) Toxic effects of L-dopa on mesencephalic cell cultures: Protection with anti-oxidants. *Brain Res* **682**, 133.

14. Pardo B, Mena MA, de Yebenes JG (1995) L-Dopa inhibits complex IV of the electron transport chain in catecholamine-rich human neuroblastoma NB69 cells. *J Neurochem* **64**, 576.

15. Perry TL, Yong VW, Ito M (1984) Nigrostriatal dopamine neurons remain undamaged in rats given high doses of L-dopa and carbidopa chronically. *J Neurochem* **43**, 990.

16. Quinn N, Parkes D, Janota I, Marsden CD (1986) Preservation of the substantia nigra and locus coeruleus in a patient receiving levodopa (2 kg) plus decarboxylase inhibitor over a four year period. *Movement Disord* **1**, 65.

17. Rajput AH, Fenton ME, Dhand A (1996) Is levodopa toxic to non-degenerating substantia nigra cells? Clinical evidence. *Neurology* **46**, A371.

18. Reches A, Fahn S (1982) Chronic dopa feeding of mice. *Neurology* **32**, 684.

19. Schapira AH, Mann VM, Cooper JM *et al.* (1990) Anatomic and disease specificity of NADH CoQ1 reductase (complex 1) deficiency in Parkinson's disease. *J Neurochem* **55**, 2142.

20. Smith TS, Parker WD, Bennet JP (1994) L-Dopa increases nigral production of hydroxyl radicals *in vivo*: Potential L-dopa toxicity? *Neuroreport* **5**, 1009.

21. Walkinshaw G, Waters CM (1995) Induction of apoptosis in catecholamine PC12 cells by L-dopa. Implications for the treatment of Parkinson's disease. *J Clin Invest* **6**, 2458.

22. Weiner WJ, Nausieda PA, Klawans HL (1978) The effects of levodopa, lergotrile, and bromocriptine on brain iron, manganese and copper. *Neurology* **28**, 734.

23. Wichtmann T, Delong MR (1993) Pathophysiology of parkinsonian motor abnormalities. *Adv Neurol* **60**, 53.

24. Ziv I, Melamed E, Nardi N *et al.* (1994) Dopamine induces apoptosis-like cell death in cultured sympathetic neurons—a possible novel pathogenic mechanism in Parkinson's disease. *Neurosci Lett* **170**, 136.

25. Ziv I, Offen D, Barzilai A *et al.* (1995) The proto-oncogene Bcl-2: A novel cellular protective mechanism against dopamine toxicity—possible implications for Parkinson's disease. *Neurology* **45**, 427S.

26. Ziv I, Zilkha-Falb R, Offen D *et al.* (1997) Levodopa induces apoptosis in cultured neuronal cells—a possible accelerator of nigrostriatal degeneration in Parkinson's disease? *Movement Disord* **12**, 17.

Lidocaine and Related Local Anesthetics

Michael W. Kalichman

Henry C. Powell

LIDOCAINE
$C_{14}H_{22}N_2O$

2-(Diethylamino)-N-(2,6-dimethylphenyl)acetamide

NEUROTOXICITY RATING

Clinical

B   Peripheral neuropathy

Experimental

A   Axonal degeneration (local administration)

Local anesthetics are unusual therapeutic agents since they are valued for one of their adverse effects upon the nervous tissue, the blockade of nerve conduction. Clinical use of local anesthetics is occasionally associated with unwanted effects. Intravenous overdose can cause cardiac arrest, seizures, and cerebral depression (27). Spinal or epidural local anesthetic administration is associated with long-lasting neurological deficits (45). Focal peripheral nerve degeneration can follow near-nerve injection of local anesthetics for peripheral nerve blocks (38). All of these unintended neurotoxicities are rare and most are acutely reversed with clearance of the local anesthetic. There are few instances in which use of local anesthetics is associated with persistent neurological deficits, specifically those likely to result from degeneration of nerve fibers (summarized in Table 31).

The local anesthetic molecule consists of an aromatic lipophilic portion with an ester or amide linkage to a hydrophilic portion. Most local anesthetics are tertiary amines in which a terminal nitrogen is bonded to two alkyl groups and is able to accept a hydrogen ion to form a cationic species. Some local anesthetics are secondary amines in which one of the alkyl groups is replaced by hydrogen. Cocaine, an ester-linked agent extracted from the coca plant (*Erythroxylum coca*) in 1860 (reviewed in 16), was the first local anesthetic to be introduced into modern medicine. By the beginning of the 20th century, several other ester-linked local anesthetics had been synthesized, including procaine (reviewed in 16,95). In the search for more diverse agents, an alternative line of local anesthetics was synthesized around an amide linkage beginning in the 1940s. Among these agents was lidocaine. Lidocaine is one of the most widely used, and a prototypical example, of the local anesthetics.

As with most local anesthetics, lidocaine in solution is present in both charged and uncharged forms. The dissociation constant (pKa) defines the relative proportions of local anesthetic base and cation that are present at a given pH. Uncharged, local anesthetics are highly lipid soluble and readily penetrate cell membranes. Although the charged cations do not readily pass through plasma membranes, it is the charged local anesthetic that is believed to interact with the axoplasmic aspect of voltage-dependent Na^+ gates to interrupt nerve conduction and thereby cause local anesthesia (12,66,91). Once the uncharged local anesthetic has diffused across the axolemma, a new equilibrium defined by its pKa results in charged cations that block the Na^+ gates (24,67) and block nerve conduction by interrupting the flow of inorganic ions (Na^+, K^+) through transmembrane ion channels.

The binding of local anesthetics to lipids and proteins determines diffusion from the site of injection, duration of action, and the potential for toxicity. Increased lipid solubility of the local anesthetic agent results in slower effects because the low water solubility impedes diffusion to membrane barriers, but the stronger affinity for membrane sites favors a longer duration of action. The proportion of lipid-soluble (uncharged) local anesthetic is closely related to pH. A decrease in pH favors the cation—the form responsible for binding to anionic channel receptors, but which is much less effective than the uncharged species in crossing cellular, membrane, and connective tissue barriers.

The primary use of local anesthetics is to produce analgesia by interrupting nerve fiber conduction. The ability to render nerve and muscle inexcitable has also made local anesthetics useful as antiarrhythmics and anticonvulsants. The antiarrhythmic properties of local anesthetics were recognized early in their clinical history (59); lidocaine was found to be particularly useful as an antiarrhythmic drug (33). For systemic effects, local anesthetics are normally injected into the bloodstream. The etiology of systemic analgesia appears to be inhibition of multisynaptic transmission rather than blockade of peripheral nerve impulse conduction (17,103). The anticonvulsant property is not now in routine clinical use (6).

Local anesthetics are available as creams, ointments, and injectable solutions. Depending on concentration and uses, most are regulated as prescription drugs, although some agents are available in over-the-counter preparations. All of

TABLE 31. Clinical Incidence of Long-Lasting Neurotoxic Sequelae Associated with Local Anesthetic Administration

Local Anesthetic Block	Number of Anesthetic Blocks	Neurotoxicity	Incidence	References
Spinal	65,304	Motor or sensory deficits	0.04%	50
Epidural	55,686	Transient or permanent paralysis	0.11%	17
Epidural	45,783	Motor or sensory deficits	0.09%	50
Brachial plexus	1100	Transient paresis	0.4%	8
Brachial plexus	300	Paresthesias, loss of motor function	5.7%	69
Brachial plexus	106	Persistent neurological symptoms	4%	113
Brachial plexus	476	Pain	1.5%	10
Wrist, metacarpal	49	Loss of sensation	14%	9

these preparations are regulated by the U.S. Food and Drug Administration.

General Toxicology

Exposure to local anesthetics is the result of intentional administration, usually to minimize or prevent painful sensation. Although local anesthetics are sometimes administered systemically for analgesia or as antiarrhythmic agents, such uses produce intravascular concentrations too low to cause serious neurotoxicity. By contrast, adverse effects may result when these agents are used to block a nerve or nerve plexus, after spinal or epidural injection, topical (skin, mucosa) application, or intramuscular injection, and in subcutaneous infiltration. In these cases, there is potential for high focal concentration of the local anesthetic agent in close proximity to the population of nerve fibers to be anesthetized. Although connective tissue barriers do slow the rate of local anesthetic entry to nerve, the impact of this delay on onset or extent of anesthesia is minimal (21,48).

An important factor regulating movement of local anesthetics across membrane barriers is the relative proportion of charged and uncharged species. The uncharged, lipid-soluble, local anesthetic much more readily crosses plasma membranes. At a given tissue pH, this proportion can be easily predicted; however, injection of a large bolus of local anesthetic or topical application could overload local buffering systems, resulting in ambient pH approximating that of the injected solution. This pH, typically lower than physiological pH, increases the proportion of charged local anesthetic, decreasing its transmembrane passage and anesthetic efficacy.

Diffusion of the anesthetic away from the site of administration is the primary factor limiting the depth of local anesthesia and potential for local toxicity. In clinical practice, local anesthetics tend to be injected in sufficiently high concentration to guarantee that the onset of anesthesia will be rapid and the duration of analgesia will be long-lasting, despite diffusion. Distribution of local anesthetics away from or into tissues is primarily governed by regional blood flow. The local anesthetics move down their concentration gradient and can readily cross vessel walls to enter the circulation (90). The importance of blood flow as the prime mechanism for removing local anesthetics from the site of administration is exemplified by the difference between subarachnoid and epidural anesthesia. Because of poorer perfusion, subarachnoid anesthesia requires less local anesthetic and lasts longer than epidural anesthesia (11). To limit absorption and loss of anesthetic effect, epinephrine is often added to clinical preparations of local anesthetics, thereby reducing local blood flow and loss of local anesthetic to vascular absorption.

Like other highly lipid-soluble agents, systemic local anesthetics distribute, or partition, into more poorly perfused tissues, such as fat, only after initial distribution to the more highly perfused tissues, including brain, heart, liver, and kidneys. This initial flow dependent distribution is quite rapid. Lidocaine, for example, after entering the venous system, distributes out of the vascular space with a half-life of <2 min (5). After initial losses due to distribution into highly perfused tissues, the steady state rate of clearance in an adult male is 0.85 l/kg/h with a half-life of approximately 1.6 h and a volume of distribution on the order of 1.3 l/kg; binding of lidocaine to plasma protein is in the range of 51%–70% (16). It is noteworthy for systemic toxicity of local anesthetics that percentage plasma protein binding decreases with high concentrations of local anesthetic. This means that the available (unbound) drug increases even more than might be predicted based on the total dose administered.

The metabolism of local anesthetics can be subdivided into the hydrolysis of esters by circulating esterases and hepatic degradation of amide-linked agents, including lidocaine. The distinction between esters and amides is important to both anesthetic and neurotoxic effects of local anesthetic agents. The local concentration of amide- and ester-linked agents is limited by diffusion and blood flow, which can transport the local anesthetic to other body sites, including the liver; however, ester-linked agents can theoretically be degraded at the site of injection by local esterases. Metabolism of ester-linked local anesthetics is primarily extrahepatic and is catalyzed by plasma esterases that hydrolyze these agents into their constituent parts, aromatic acids and amino alcohols. Amide-linked agents also undergo hydrolysis, but a necessary first step is dealkylation to convert tertiary amines to secondary amines. This dealkylation is catalyzed by microsomal enzymes localized to the endoplasmic reticulum of liver cells. Lidocaine, an amide-linked agent, is specifically an aminoacyl amide.

The primary site of lidocaine metabolism is the liver. Because the long-term clearance of lidocaine from blood is determined virtually entirely by hepatic metabolism, lidocaine clearance is proportional to hepatic blood flow and is independent of its blood concentration. The primary mechanism of lidocaine (diethylglycine xylidide) catabolism is two successive de-ethylations to form monoethylglycine xylidide (MEGX) and then glycine xylidide (GX). Hydrolysis of MEGX or GX yields xylidine and N-ethylglycine or glycine, respectively. Hydroxylation of the xylidine results in the major product of lidocaine metabolism, 4-hydroxy-2,6-xylidine, which is excreted in the urine. The MEGX and GX metabolites of lidocaine are significant in that they retain some anesthetic activity, can be present in levels comparable to residual plasma levels of lidocaine, and can contribute to systemic convulsive toxicity (1,7,16).

Animal Studies

Because of the nature of the clinical use of local anesthetics, virtually all relevant experimental studies are best described as short-term, controlled exposures (i.e., single injections of a known concentration of local anesthetic). In one of the earliest such studies, in 1939, evidence of degeneration was found after a single intraneural injection of the ester-linked local anesthetic procaine (71). However, subsequent studies found that perineural injection of up to 5% procaine resulted in no observable injury (53). Although it is expected that the risk of nerve injury should be greater with intraneural than with perineural injection, these early histopathological studies did not have the benefit of techniques either to deliver volumes of fluid into nerves without causing mechanical trauma (57,84), or to visualize fine structural changes with electron microscopy. Unfortunately, because some early studies lacked adequate controls, comparisons of different doses and drugs, and sensitive histopathological measures of nerve injury, the available data are often ambiguous. For both perineural and subarachnoid injections,

diverse and sometimes conflicting conclusions about potential causes for nerve injury have included mechanical damage (31,85); additives (32,100,101); some, but not all, local anesthetics (4,76); or all local anesthetics (30,56). These data are best reconciled by noting that both mechanical injury and any chemical agent—in sufficient concentration—are expected to have neurotoxic sequelae.

One of the first recent controlled studies employed electron microscopy to examine the effects of five different local anesthetics after intraneural and extraneural administration (30). At concentrations well within the range of those used clinically, no damage was noted following extraneural injection, but intraneural injections of 50–100 μl caused nerve fiber injury characterized by degeneration of axons and myelin, and breakdown of the blood-nerve barrier. Taken together with subsequent reports, it is clear that, in animal models, local anesthetics have neurotoxic potential and can cause long-lasting nerve injury (41,42,49,65). Furthermore, the dose range that elicits anesthesia may possibly also elicit neurotoxic effects (40).

The nerve microenvironment is severely disrupted within 2 days of perineural injection. The nerve fascicle is swollen with edematous endoneurial fluid and the endoneurium exhibits other characteristics of inflammation, including extravasation of hematogenous inflammatory cells and increased numbers of fibroblasts and macrophages. Increased permeability of the blood-nerve barrier is observed both immediately and at 2 days after local anesthetic injection (30,41,65). Whether this is a cause or a consequence of the accumulation of endoneurial fluid is not yet clear. A prominent sign of cytotoxicity is the intracellular accumulation of lipid droplets in cells of the perineurial sheath, fibroblasts, macrophages, endothelial cells, and Schwann cells (41). The Schwann cells containing lipid droplets are much more common in myelinated than unmyelinated fibers (42,73). By 7 days, cell proliferation is evident in Schwann cells, endothelial cells, and pericytes (73). Both axonal degeneration and myelin loss secondary to wallarian degeneration are typically observed at the site of local anesthetic-induced injury.

The neurotoxic effects of continuous or repeated injection of local anesthetics are less well studied but also known to be associated with nerve injury. Rats were injected with 1 ml of 0.5% bupivacaine adjacent to the sciatic nerve twice daily for up to 7 days (54). In addition to a significant inflammatory response, there was evidence for some myelin damage and a reduction in the compound action potential elicited by electrical stimulation of the nerve. Although the dose of bupivacaine (5 mg/rat) employed in this experiment was substantially greater than 5 mg in a 70-kg human, it should be noted that the local concentrations following tissue injection are likely to have been comparable. The importance of local concentration for local neurotoxicity, rather than systemic dose, is emphasized by another study in which lidocaine was injected thrice daily for 3 days into a perineural cuff (49). By injecting various concentrations (1%–4%) in decreasing volumes (400 μl to 200 μl), the authors partially dissociated the effect of dose from concentration. Only the highest concentration, 4% lidocaine, nearly abolished toe twitch in response to electrical stimulation of the nerve and caused widespread axonal degeneration.

2-Chloroprocaine, but not sodium bisulfite [an antioxidant that was added to the commercial preparation (Nesacaine-CE) of 2-chloroprocaine], is an *in vivo* cause of neurotoxicity (43). This contrasts with the *in vitro* demonstration that sodium bisulfite, and not 2-chloroprocaine, is responsible for irreversible conduction block (31). Two differences between *in vivo* and *in vitro* preparations may explain this inconsistency. First, an *in vitro* preparation does not exhibit rapid dilution and diffusion, which occurs following *in vivo* local anesthetic injection. *In vitro* bathing of a nerve in an anesthetic (or additive) concentration comparable to that injected *in vivo* actually represents a continuous immersion of the nerve in a concentration as high or higher than that occurring *in vivo*. Second, an *in vitro* preparation does not utilize a blood supply for oxygenation or removal of toxins. Thus, *in vitro* nerve experiments cannot address the possibility that a local anesthetic might interrupt a nerve's blood supply and cause ischemic injury to the nerve.

Experimental studies of spinal cord anesthesia have demonstrated that additives used in local anesthetic preparations can be neurotoxic. They have also helped to diminish concern that the local anesthetics themselves are a potential cause of nerve injury. In rabbits, subarachnoid injections of 2-chloroprocaine did not cause hindlimb paralysis, while sufficient (? excessive) doses of sodium bisulfite induced irreversible paralysis in 12 of 14 rabbits (100). Unfortunately, it is difficult to be sure that the cause of injury was solely the bisulfite (1.2–2.4 mg) because the study did not include control injections of volumes of vehicle (0.6–1.2 ml) comparable to those used with bisulfite. Following several studies implicating bisulfite as a neurotoxin, the commercial preparation was modified to include ethylenediaminetetraacetic acid (EDTA) in place of bisulfite. Because of additional reports of Nesacaine neurotoxicity, the effects of disodium EDTA were tested in a rabbit model of subarachnoid injection and the EDTA was found to produce hindlimb tetanic contractions (101).

Although several tests of subarachnoid local anesthetics have failed to reveal neurotoxicity, other studies provide evidence that injury is a function of the agent, the dose, and the duration of exposure. A commercial preparation of 2-chloroprocaine (containing bisulfite) induced hindlimb paralysis following subarachnoid administration in 7 of 20 dogs, but no adverse sequelae developed with saline, bupivacaine, or normal saline at low pH (75). Testing of several local anesthetics at concentrations well within the range of clinical use disclosed no evidence of neurological deficits, nor was histopathological damage significantly different from that of controls following intrathecal injections in rats (2). However, with more prolonged exposures through continuous subarachnoid infusions of bupivacaine, lidocaine, and 2-chloroprocaine in rats, both abnormal histology and paralysis were associated with lidocaine and 2-chloroprocaine (56). Little evidence of injury was found following intrathecal injections of clinical concentrations of local anesthetics, or bisulfite, in rabbits (76); however, at concentrations exceeding those used clinically, both functional and structural deficits were observed with bisulfite, tetracaine, bupivacaine, and lidocaine. Nerve injury was characterized by axonal degeneration in the cauda equina, marked necrosis of the central cord in some animals, and subpial vacuolation. In general, histopathology was correlated with deficits in neurological function.

Because some clinical reports of local anesthetic neurotoxicity implicate lidocaine solutions used for continuous spinal anesthesia (19,81), intrathecal infusion in the rat was done to test the effects of three different local anesthetics (20). At 6 days after infusion, tail-flick latency, a measure of sacral sensory deficit, was significantly increased by 5% lidocaine as compared to bupivacaine, tetracaine, and saline. These data provide additional support for the argument that concentrations at the high end of clinical use carry at least a small risk of neurotoxicity.

One potential effect of local anesthetic neurotoxicity is disruption of axonal transport. The rapid (<2 days) appearance of nerve-fiber injury following perineural local anesthetic injection (65) implicates rapid transport (~400 mm/day) rather than slow transport (a few millimeters per day). Local anesthetics can inhibit rapid axonal transport; for lidocaine, this may occur at clinical doses (23). However, lidocaine blockade of fast transport apparently is reversible and does not correlate with relative potency for local anesthesia (22,55) or, by extension, with neurotoxicity (40).

Another possible mechanism of local anesthetic neurotoxicity is interruption of nutritive nerve blood flow. Lidocaine, bupivacaine, procaine, and cocaine topically applied to rat sciatic nerve reduced nerve blood flow as measured by laser Doppler flowmetry (39,70). The magnitude of blood flow reductions (>50%), the duration (4 h), and their correlation with subsequent nerve injury assayed at 2 days, are all consistent with injury (39). Since laser Doppler flowmetry does not distinguish between endoneurial and epineurial blood flow, further studies are needed to assess the locus of changes.

Studies of spinal or subarachnoid injection of lidocaine concentrations of up to 2% in dogs or cats revealed no change or an *increased* spinal cord blood flow (18,47,72). One study of *epidural* lidocaine in dogs described a significant reduction in spinal cord blood flow at 30 min (61). The authors attributed this effect to either an autoregulatory response to a decreased metabolic need or to vasoconstriction caused by lidocaine. The possibility of such an epidural effect on spinal cord blood flow is particularly significant in light of clinical reports of long-lasting neurological deficits following epidural anesthesia with accidental subarachnoid delivery of local anesthetic.

In Vitro Studies

Many specific mechanisms and effects of local anesthetics can be studied in tissue homogenates or isolated nerves. Although such preparations allow experimental control of variables that might confound *in situ* studies, *in vitro* experiments are not subject to the effects of local anesthetics on nerve blood flow or the buffering and dilution that occur *in vivo*.

From the perspective of axonal action-potential conduction, the difference between therapeutic and toxic effects of local anesthetics is defined by the extent to which conduction block is reversed by removing the local anesthetic. The mechanisms by which local anesthetics reversibly inhibit nerve conduction have largely been determined with *in vitro* models, including isolated axons of invertebrates, or with whole mammalian nerve. Until recently, it was assumed that the *in vitro* concentrations needed to produce irreversible conduction block were many times higher than that necessary to produce anesthesia (*e.g.*, 87). Belief in the relative safety of local anesthetics was further supported by a series of *in vitro* studies with isolated rabbit vagus nerve in which the additive rather than the local anesthetic was implicated as the neurotoxic agent in Nesacaine-CE (34). In these studies, the local anesthetic, 2-chloroprocaine, was shown to produce a reversible conduction block unless it was combined with the additive sodium bisulfite, and a low pH. In the case of low pH, conduction block was not reversible over a period of 5 days despite repeated washing with buffer. The rationale was made more plausible since the accumulation of sulfuric acid derived from metabolism of the bisulfite would lower pH. This notion is seriously challenged by subsequent *in vivo* evidence that rat sciatic nerve is susceptible to injury from 2-chloroprocaine, but

not sodium bisulfite, even at four times its clinical concentration (43).

Two *in vitro* studies have demonstrated that concentrations of local anesthetics only slightly higher than those used clinically can produce irreversible conduction block. In one study, exposure of isolated frog sciatic nerve to lidocaine for 15 min resulted in a nonreversible block that persisted despite washing for as long as 3 h (3); in the other, irreversible conduction block was produced by tetracaine in isolated rat sciatic nerve (58). Furthermore, *in vitro* exposure to local anesthetics has produced demyelination as well as loss of axonal cytoskeletal components (13,58). These *in vitro* data demonstrate the potential neurotoxic effects of local anesthetics and provide evidence for nerve damage without ischemia.

In isolated aortic rings, four different local anesthetics were found to inhibit endothelium-dependent vasodilation (36). The inhibition was inferred to be after receptor-mediated stimulation of endothelial cells, but before activation of smooth muscle guanylate cyclase. This *in vitro* result has not yet been verified *in vivo*. To explain local anesthetic-induced ischemia, it would be necessary to assume that vasodilation mediated by endothelium-derived relaxing factor (EDRF) is the primary protective mechanism. *In vitro* studies have addressed three possible effects of local anesthetics on nerve-blood flow: EDRF, cytoplasmic calcium (particularly in smooth cells), and vasoactive prostaglandin metabolites.

Another possible cause of local anesthetic-mediated contraction and vasoconstriction is increased smooth muscle intracellular calcium. Although local anesthetics impede calcium influx (37,89) and might therefore *protect* against vasoconstriction, local anesthetics *in vitro* inhibit various membrane proteins, including those responsible for calcium uptake in sarcoplasmic reticulum and mitochondria (25,26,52,86,92,98,99). Inhibiting the reuptake of calcium could maintain high cytoplasmic concentrations and cause persistent smooth muscle contraction.

Prostaglandin metabolites are potent vasodilators and vasoconstrictors. Phospholipase A_2 is the initial enzyme essential for cleaving arachidonic acid, the precursor for most prostaglandins, from membrane phospholipids. *In vitro*, local anesthetics can inhibit phospholipase A_2 (14,35,50,96, 102); the relative potency for inhibition parallels relative potency for local anesthesia.

Human Studies

Despite the frequent, worldwide use of local anesthesia, reports of injury are few and there are no prospective studies. Reviews of nerve-block anesthesia have reported 1.5%–

13.2% incidence of neurological complications (9,62,104). This incidence challenges the notion that local anesthetic use carries almost no neurotoxic risk (16,60). There are two obvious explanations for this discrepancy. One is that the standard clinical use of local anesthetics consists of a single exposure; and even if localized mild loss of sensory or motor-function occurred, the normal regenerative capacity of the PNS would resolve the deficit. The other is that long-lasting deficits associated with peripheral nerve blocks and spinal-epidural anesthesia may be easily attributed to either surgical trauma or an underlying neuropathy. One report of an unplanned experiment supports the notion that the local anesthetic caused nerve injury. In this study, a clinic that had performed wrist and metacarpal blocks, without untoward sequelae, switched to the local anesthetic bupivacaine (8). Persistent loss of sensation appeared in 7 of 49 patients; nerve injury may reflect the concentration (0.25%–0.5%) of bupivacaine. If the local anesthetic were potentially neurotoxic, then the risk of neurotoxicity should have been greater with increasing concentration. The proposed use of higher concentrations to increase the speed of anesthesia should be pursued with caution (88).

CNS toxicity has the potential to be far more severe than the temporary loss of function to peripheral nerve fibers. High intravascular concentrations of local anesthetics can cause generalized seizures or trigger episodes of status epilepticus. Any persistent neurological deficits result from the convulsions, not the local anesthetic, especially since arterial concentrations of local anesthetics high enough to cause convulsions (<30 μg/ml 0.003%) (60) are far lower than concentrations useful for regional anesthesia (0.25%–5.0%) (79). For these reasons, long-lasting injury to the CNS and PNS presumably does not follow from high systemic concentrations.

Injury to the CNS is plausible following local injection of high concentrations of local anesthetic for spinal or epidural anesthesia. Reviews of case reports and studies prior to 1950 indicate an incidence of 0.01%–0.5% for neurological complications from spinal anesthesia (46,94). While spinal anesthesia places the anesthetic directly in contact with spinal nerves, epidural anesthesia places it outside of dura/arachnoidal barriers protecting the CNS. Although the risk of injury might be expected to be less with epidural than spinal anesthesia, epidural anesthesia makes use of much larger anesthetic volumes, higher concentrations of local anesthetic, and the anesthetic agent may accidentally be inserted into the subarachnoid space. In 1969, a review of 32,718 published cases of epidural anesthesia reported a 0.02% permanent and 0.1% transient loss of motor function (15). Subsequent studies of (a) long-lasting nerve injury with epidural Nesacaine-CE (2-chloroprocaine) (63,74,77),

(b) continuous spinal anesthesia with 5% lidocaine (78,80,81,83), (c) 16,000 cases of epidural anesthesia with 3% incidence of paresthesia or local anesthetic toxicity (93), and (d) both epidural and spinal anesthesia (45) provide continuing evidence of a small but clear risk of injury associated with spinal and epidural anesthesia.

The incidence is so low (0.09%) for spinal anesthesia and epidural anesthesia (0.05%) that the neurotoxicity associated with spinal anesthesia is disputed (16,60). The issue is clouded by the known toxicity of some local anesthetic additives, such as calcium disodium edetate and bisulfite (100,101), and because of the complications of this type of anesthesia (hematoma, arachnoiditis, trauma, infarction, or abscess) (28,69,97).

After the initial reports of long-lasting nerve-root injury associated with 5% epidural lidocaine, some attributed the injury to the unintended pooling of a high anesthetic concentration delivered continuously. A description of lumbosacral radiculopathy in ten patients subsequent to *single* subarachnoid injections of 5% lidocaine or 37 mg tetracaine (83) challenges this notion.

The clinical use of high concentrations of lidocaine injected in the subarachnoid region, in combination with decreased vascularization in the cauda equina region of the spinal column (68), favors the hypothesis that persistent neurological deficits in conjunction with spinal anesthesia might also be a consequence of ischemia. This position is challenged by one report that intraspinal tetracaine actually protects against spinal-cord ischemic injury in rabbits (10), and humans have not developed the vascular myelopathy syndrome.

Toxic Mechanisms

The biochemical and physiological mechanisms by which local anesthetics cause nerve injury are uncertain. Since the order of potency for local anesthesia is similar to that for producing local anesthetic-induced nerve injury, the most likely possibilities should include properties that account for this factor.

The evidence of widespread cellular injury in models of local anesthetic neuropathy suggests that injury is caused either by a nonspecific mechanism, such as ischemia, or by something common to diverse cell types. One possibility is that local anesthetics impede synthesis of adenosine triphosphate by inhibiting oxidative phosphorylation. Specifically, it is known that local anesthetics inhibit cellular respiration and electron transport (*e.g.*, 29,34) and, although toxic concentrations are higher than those typical of clinical local anesthesia, the relative order of potency is the same as that for anesthesia (and therefore neurotoxicity). Inhibition of cellular respiration could be a direct cause of toxicity to cells of the endoneurium or, by stressing endothelial cells and smooth muscle, it could result in vascular collapse and nerve ischemia.

Experimental models of local anesthetic neurotoxicity suggest that injury may be, in part, caused by an ischemic mechanism. Local anesthetics are known to decrease nerve blood flow (64); the magnitude and duration of blood flow reduction are consistent with ischemic injury (39). If ischemia is the physiological basis for local anesthetic-induced nerve injury, then local anesthetics presumably decrease regional blood flow either by aggregation of formed vascular elements or constriction of blood vessels. Accumulation of cytoplasmic calcium in smooth muscle of arteriolar vessels would favor vasoconstriction. Although local anesthetics inhibit a variety of membrane proteins, including calcium channels, this mechanism would diminish, not increase, smooth muscle contraction; however, local anesthetics inhibit reuptake of calcium by pumps present in membranes of mitochondria and sarcoplasmic reticulum (25,26,52,86, 92,98,99). In sum, local anesthetics could cause vasoconstriction by inhibiting calcium reuptake and favoring continued smooth muscle contraction.

Another mechanism by which local anesthetics could alter nerve blood flow is by inhibiting the synthesis of prostaglandins, many of which are potent vasomediators. The first step in prostaglandin synthesis is catalyzed by the enzyme phospholipase A_2, which is inhibited by local anesthetics with the same order of potency as for local anesthesia (51,82). In the only reported study of the effects of a local anesthetic on nerve prostaglandin metabolites, the synthesis of both a vasodilator (prostacyclin) and a vasoconstrictor (thromboxane A_2) was reduced at the time of cocaine-reduced nerve blood flow (44). The magnitude of reduction in vasodilator synthesis was much greater than that of the vasoconstrictor, resulting in a ratio favoring vasoconstriction, and possibly ischemia. The proposal that local anesthetics inhibit prostaglandin synthesis, and therefore blood flow, was further supported by demonstrating that perineural indomethacin (a prostaglandin-synthesis inhibitor) also reduces nerve blood flow (44).

Although the targets of local anesthetic neurotoxicity include all of the cells of the nerve microenvironment, deficits in nerve conduction are most directly caused by toxicity to axons or Schwann cells. It is now clear that local anesthetics can induce irreversible block of nerve conduction *in vitro* (3), implying direct toxicity to the axon without invoking ischemic mechanisms of injury. It is possible that high concentrations of local anesthetics, independent of effects on nerve blood flow, directly damage axons. One measure of local anesthetic injury is inhibition of rapid axoplasmic transport. Local anesthetics do inhibit rapid axonal transport both *in vitro* and *in vivo* (22,23,55); however, the order of potency for this effect does not parallel that for local anesthesia or nerve injury.

Schwann cells also have a role in mediating normal sensory and motor conduction. Although local anesthetics nonspecifically injure Schwann cells of both myelinated and unmyelinated fibers, the responses of these two populations of axon-ensheathing cells is distinct (42,73). Both types of cells accumulate cytoplasmic lipid droplets, but these inclusions are far more frequent in Schwann cells of myelinated fibers than in those of unmyelinated fibers. The accumulation of abnormal quantities of lipid likely is a toxic reaction, but does not indicate degeneration or disintegration. Conversely, disintegration of cytoplasm, plasma membrane, and basal lamina is seen in both types of Schwann cells, but is far more frequent in Schwann cells of unmyelinated fibers.

In summary, neurotoxic concentrations of local anesthetics are expected to have diverse biochemical effects, many of which are likely to be factors in defining the characteristics of nerve injury. Ischemia appears the most likely basis for injury. Ischemia (vasoconstriction) may stem from (a) inhibition of cellular respiration resulting in failure of normal autoregulatory mechanisms in the endothelial and smooth muscle cells of nutritive vessels; (b) accumulation of cytoplasmic calcium because of inhibition of intracellular calcium pumps; and (c) disruption in prostaglandin metabolism favoring the accumulation of vasoconstrictors.

REFERENCES

1. Arthur GR (1987) Pharmacokinetics of local anesthetics. In: *Local Anesthetics*. Strichartz GR ed. *Handb Exp Pharmacol* 81, 165.
2. Bahar M, Cole G, Rosen M *et al.* (1984) Histopathology of the spinal cord after intrathecal cocaine, bupivacaine, lignocaine and adrenaline in the rat. *Eur J Anaesth* 1, 293.
3. Bainton CR, Strichartz GR (1994) Concentration dependence of lidocaine-induced irreversible conduction loss in frog nerve. *Anesthesiology* 81, 657.
4. Barsa J, Batra M, Fink BR *et al.* (1982) A comparative *in vivo* study of local neurotoxicity of lidocaine, bupivacaine, 2-chloroprocaine, and a mixture of 2-chloroprocaine and bupivacaine. *Anesth Analg* 61, 961.
5. Benowitz N, Forsyth RP, Melmon KL *et al.* (1974) Lidocaine disposition kinetics in monkey and man. 1. Prediction by a perfusion model. *Clin Pharmacol Ther* 16, 87.
6. Bernhard CG, Bohm E (1965) *Local Anaesthetics as Anticonvulsants. A Study on Experimental and Clinical Epilepsy.* Almqvist & Wiksell, Stockholm.
7. Blumer J, Strong JM, Atkinson AJ (1973) The convulsant potency of lidocaine and its *N*-dealkylated metabolites. *J Pharmacol Exp Ther* 186, 31.

8. Born G (1984) Neuropathy after bupivacaine (Marcaine) wrist and metacarpal nerve blocks. *J Hand Surg-Am* **9A**, 109.

9. Brand, L, Papper EM (1961) A comparison of supraclavicular and axillary techniques for brachial plexus blocks. *Anesthesiology* **22**, 226.

10. Breckwoldt WL, Genco CM, Connolly RJ et al. (1991) Spinal cord protection during aortic occlusion: Efficacy of intrathecal tetracaine. *Ann Thorac Surg* **51**, 959.

11. Burm AGL, van Kleef JW, Vermeulen NPE et al. (1988) Pharmacokinetics of lidocaine and bupivacaine following subarachnoid administration in surgical patients: Simultaneous investigation of absorption and disposition kinetics using stable isotopes. *Anesthesiology* **69**, 584.

12. Butterworth JF, Strichartz GR (1990) Molecular mechanisms of local anesthesia: A review. *Anesthesiology* **72**, 711.

13. Byers MR, Fink BR, Kennedy RD et al. (1973) Effects of lidocaine on axonal morphology, microtubules, and rapid transport in rabbit vagus nerve *in vitro*. *J Neurobiol* **4**, 125.

14. Cejtin HE, Parsons MR, Wilson L (1990) Cocaine use and its effect on umbilical artery prostacyclin production. *Prostaglandins* **40**, 249.

15. Dawkins CJM (1969) An analysis of the complications of extradural block. *Anaesthesia* **24**, 554.

16. de Jong RH (1994) *Local Anesthetics*. Mosby, St. Louis, Missouri.

17. de Jong RH, Nace RA (1968) Nerve impulse conduction during intravenous lidocaine injection. *Anesthesiology* **29**, 22.

18. Dohi S, Matsumiya N, Takeshima R et al. (1984) The effects of subarachnoid lidocaine and phenylephrine on spinal cord and cerebral blood flow in dogs. *Anesthesiology* **61**, 238.

19. Drasner K, Rigler ML, Sessler DI et al. (1992) Cauda equina syndrome following intended epidural anesthesia. *Anesthesiology* **77**, 582.

20. Drasner K, Sakura S, Chan VW et al. (1994) Persistent sacral sensory deficit induced by intrathecal local anesthetic infusion in the rat. *Anesthesiology* **80**, 847.

21. Fink BR, Cairns AM (1984) Diffusional delay in local anesthetic block *in vitro*. *Anesthesiology* **61**, 555.

22. Fink BR, Kennedy RD, Hendrickson AE et al. (1972) Lidocaine inhibition of rapid axonal transport. *Anesthesiology* **36**, 422.

23. Fink BR, Kish SJ (1976) Reversible inhibition of rapid axonal transport *in vivo* by lidocaine hydrochloride. *Anesthesiology* **44**, 139.

24. Frazier DT, Narahashi T, Yamada M (1970) The site of action and active form of local anesthetics. II. Experiments with quaternary ammonium compounds. *J Pharmacol Exp Ther* **171**, 45.

25. Garcia-Martin E, Gonzalez-Cabanillas S, Gutierrez-Merino C (1990) Modulation of calcium fluxes across synaptosomal plasma membrane by local anesthetics. *J Neurochem* **55**, 370.

26. Garcia-Martin E, Gutierrez-Merino C (1986) Local anesthetics inhibit the Ca^{2+}, Mg^{2+}-ATPase activity of rat brain synaptosomes. *J Neurochem* **47**, 668.

27. Garfield JM, Gugino L (1987) Central effects of local anesthetic agents. *Local Anesthetics*. Strichartz GR ed. *Handb Exp Pharmacol* **81**, 253.

28. Gaudin P, Lefant D (1991) Paraplegie après anesthesie peridurale pour chirurgie vasculaire. *Ann Fr Anesth Reanim* **10**, 468.

29. Geddes IC, Quastel JH (1956) Effects of local anaesthetics on respiration of rat brain cortex *in vitro*. *Anesthesiology* **17**, 666.

30. Gentili F, Hudson AR, Hunter D, Kline DG (1980) Nerve injection injury with local anesthetic agents: a light and electron microscopic, fluorescent microscopic, and horseradish peroxidase study. *Neurosurgery* **6**, 263.

31. Gissen AJ, Datta S, Lambert D (1984a) The chloroprocaine controversy. I. A hypothesis to explain the neural complications of chloroprocaine epidural. *Reg Anesth* **9**, 124.

32. Gissen AJ, Datta S, Lambert D (1984b) The chloroprocaine controversy. II. Is chloroprocaine neurotoxic? *Reg Anesth* **9**, 135.

33. Harrison DC, Sprouse JH, Morrow AG (1963) The antiarrhythmic properties of lidocaine and procaine amide: Clinical and physiologic studies of their cardiovascular effects in man. *Circulation* **28**, 486.

34. Haschke RH, Fink BR (1975) Lidocaine effects on brain mitochondrial metabolism *in vitro*. *Anesthesiology* **42**, 737.

35. Hendrickson HS, van Dam-Micras MC (1976) Local anesthetic inhibition of pancreatic phospholipase A_2 action on lecithin monolayers. *J Lipid Res* **17**, 399.

36. Johns RA (1989) Local anesthetics inhibit endothelium-dependent vasodilation. *Anesthesiology* **70**, 805.

37. Kai T, Nishimura J, Kobayashi S et al. (1993) Effects of lidocaine on intracellular Ca^{2+} and tension in airway smooth muscle. *Anesthesiology* **78**, 954.

38. Kalichman MW (1995) Neurotoxicity of local anesthetics. In: *Handbook of Clinical Neurology*. Vinken PJ, Bruyn GW eds. Vol 65, revised series 21, *Intoxications of the Nervous System Part II*, de Wolff FA vol ed. Elsevier, Amsterdam p. 419.

39. Kalichman MW, Lalonde AW (1991) Experimental nerve ischemia and injury produced by cocaine and procaine. *Brain Res* **565**, 34.

40. Kalichman MW, Moorhouse DF, Powell HC et al. (1993) Relative neural toxicity of local anesthetics. *J Neuropathol Exp Neurol* **52**, 234.

41. Kalichman MW, Powell HC, Myers RR (1988) Pathology of local anesthetic-induced nerve injury. *Acta Neuropathol* **75**, 583.

42. Kalichman MW, Powell HC, Myers RR (1989) Quantitative histologic analysis of local anesthetic-induced injury to rat sciatic nerve. *J Pharmacol Exp Ther* **250**, 406.

43. Kalichman MW, Powell HC, Reisner LS *et al.* (1986) The role of 2-chloroprocaine and sodium bisulfite in rat sciatic nerve edema. *J Neuropathol Exp Neurol* **45**, 566.

44. Kalichman MW, Sanicolas MT, Jorge MC, Roux L (1994) Effects of cocaine on blood flow and prostaglandin metabolites in rat sciatic nerve. *Amer J Physiol* **266**, H2515.

45. Kane RE (1981) Neurologic deficits following epidural or spinal anesthesia. *Anesth Analg* **60**, 150.

46. Kennedy F, Effron AS, Perry G (1950) The grave spinal cord paralyses caused by spinal anesthesia. *Surg Gynecol Obstet* **91**, 385.

47. Kozody R, Swartz J, Palahniuk RJ *et al.* (1985) Spinal cord blood flow following subarachnoid lidocaine. *Can Anaesth Soc J* **32**, 472.

48. Kristerson L, Nordenram Å, Nordqvist P (1965) Penetration of radio-active local anaesthetic into peripheral nerve. *Arch Int Pharmacodyn* **157**, 148.

49. Kroin JS, Penn RD, Levy FE *et al.* (1986) Effects of repetitive lidocaine infusion on peripheral nerve. *Exp Neurol* **94**, 166.

50. Kunze H, Bohn E, Vogt W (1974) Effects of local anaesthetics on prostaglandin biosynthesis *in vitro*. *Biochim Biophys Acta* **360**, 260.

51. Kunze H, Nahas N, Traynor JR *et al.* (1976) Effects of local anaesthetics on phospholipases. *Biochim Biophys Acta* **441**, 93.

52. Kurebayashi N, Ogawa Y, Harafuji H (1982) Effect of local anesthetics on calcium activated ATPase and its partial reaction with fragmented sarcoplasmic reticulum from bullfrog and rabbit skeletal muscle. *J Biochem* **92**, 915.

53. Kuschke HJ, Kuschke M (1955) Polarisationsoptische Untersuchung zur Frage morphologischer Veranderungen an der Markscheide peripherer Nerven durch Novocain. *Arch Exp Pathol Pharmakol* **224**, 378.

54. Kyttä J, Heinonen E, Rosenberg PH *et al.* (1986) Effects of repeated bupivacaine administration on sciatic nerve and surrounding muscle tissue in rats. *Acta Anaesthesiol Scand* **30**, 625.

55. Lavoie PA (1982) Block of fast axonal transport *in vitro* by the local anesthetics dibucaine and etidocaine. *J Pharmacol Exp Ther* **223**, 251.

56. Li DR, Bahar M, Cole G *et al.* (1985) Neurological toxicity of the subarachnoid infusion of bupivacaine, lignocaine or 2-chloroprocaine in the rat. *Brit J Anaesth* **57**, 424.

57. Löfström B (1969) Clinical evaluation of local anesthetics. *Clin Anesth* **2**, 19.

58. Mateu L, Luzzati V, Villegas GM *et al.* (1992) Order-disorder phenomena in myelinated nerve sheaths. IV. The disordering effects of high levels of local anaesthetics on rat sciatic and optic nerves. *J Mol Biol* **226**, 535.

59. Mautz FR (1936) Reduction of cardiac irritability by the epicardial and systemic administration of drugs as a protection in cardiac surgery. *J Thorac Surg* **5**, 612.

60. Michenfelder JD, Steen PA (1979) Neural toxicity of local and general anesthetics. In: *Handbook of Clinical Neurology*. Vinken PJ, Bruyn GW eds. Elsevier/North-Holland Biomedical Press, Amsterdam p. 401.

61. Mitchell P, Goad R, Erwin CW *et al.* (1989) Effect of epidural lidocaine on spinal cord blood flow. *Anesth Analg* **68**, 312.

62. Moberg E, Dhunér K-G (1951) Brachial plexus block analgesia with Xylocaine. *J Bone Joint Surg* **33-A**, 884.

63. Moore DC, Spierdijk J, vanKleef JD *et al.* (1982) Chloroprocaine neurotoxicity: Four additional cases. *Anesth Analg* **61**, 155.

64. Myers RR, Heckman HM (1989) Effects of local anesthesia on nerve blood flow: Studies using lidocaine with and without epinephrine. *Anesthesiology* **71**, 757.

65. Myers RR, Kalichman MW, Reisner LS *et al.* (1986) Neurotoxicity of local anesthetics: Altered perineurial permeability, edema, and nerve fiber injury. *Anesthesiology* **64**, 29.

66. Narahashi T, Frazier DT (1975) Site of action and active form of procaine in squid giant axons. *J Pharmacol Exp Ther* **194**, 506.

67. Narahashi T, Frazier DT, Yamada M (1970) The site of action and active form of local anesthetics. I. Theory and pH experiments with tertiary compounds. *J Pharmacol Exp Ther* **171**, 32.

68. Parke WW, Gammell K, Rothman RH (1981) Arterial vascularization of the cauda equina. *J Bone Joint Surg* **63**, 53.

69. Parnass SM, Schmidt KJ (1990) Adverse effects of spinal and epidural anaesthesia. *Drug Safety* **5**, 179.

70. Partridge BL (1991) The effects of local anesthetics and epinephrine on rat sciatic nerve blood flow. *Anesthesiology* **75**, 243.

71. Pizzolato P, Mannheimer W (1961) *Histopathologic Effects of Local Anesthetic Drugs and Related Substances*. Charles C Thomas, Springfield, Illinois.

72. Porter SS, Albin MS, Watson WA *et al.* (1985) Spinal cord and cerebral blood flow responses to subarachnoid injection of local anesthetics with and without epinephrine. *Acta Anaesthesiol Scand* **29**, 330.

73. Powell HC, Kalichman MW, Garrett RS *et al.* (1988) Selective vulnerability of unmyelinated fiber Schwann cells in nerves exposed to local anesthetics. *Lab Invest* **59**, 271.

74. Ravindran RS, Bond VK, Tasch MD *et al.* (1980) Prolonged neural blockade following regional analgesia with 2-chloroprocaine. *Anesth Analg* **59**, 447.

75. Ravindran RS, Turner MS, Muller J (1982) Neurologic effects of subarachnoid administration of 2-chloroprocaine-

CE, bupivacaine, and low pH normal saline in dogs. *Anesth Analg* 61, 279.

76. Ready LB, Plumer MH, Haschke RH *et al.* (1985) Neurotoxicity of intrathecal local anesthetics in rabbits. *Anesthesiology* 63, 364.

77. Reisner LS, Hochman BN, Plumer MH (1980) Persistent neurologic deficit and adhesive arachnoiditis following intrathecal 2-chloroprocaine injection. *Anesth Analg* 59, 452.

78. Rigler ML, Drasner K, Krejcie TC *et al.* (1991) Cauda equina syndrome after continuous spinal anesthesia. *Anesth Analg* 72, 275.

79. Ritchie JM, Greene NM (1990) Local anesthetics. In: *The Pharmacological Basis of Therapeutics. 8th Ed.* Gilman AG, Rall TW, Nie AS eds. Pergamon Press, Elmsford, New York p. 311.

80. Ross BK, Coda B, Heath CH (1992) Local anesthetic distribution in a spinal model: A possible mechanism of neurologic injury after continuous spinal anesthesia. *Reg Anesth* 17, 69.

81. Schell RM, Brauer FS, Cole DJ *et al.* (1991) Persistent sacral nerve root deficits after continuous spinal anaesthesia. *Can J Anaesth* 38, 908.

82. Scherphof GL, Scarpa A, van Toorenenbergen A (1972) The effect of local anesthetics on the hydrolysis of free and membrane-bound phospholipids catalyzed by various phospholipases. *Biochim Biophys Acta* 270, 226.

83. Schneider M, Ettlin T, Kaufmann M *et al.* (1993) Transient neurologic toxicity after hyperbaric subarachnoid anesthesia with 5% lidocaine. *Anesth Analg* 76, 1154.

84. Selander D, Brattsand R, Lundborg G *et al.* (1979) Local anesthetics: Importance of mode of application, concentration and adrenaline for the appearance of nerve lesions. An experimental study of axonal degeneration and barrier damage after intrafascicular injection or topical application of bupivacaine (Marcain). *Acta Anaesthesiol Scand* 23, 127.

85. Selander D, Dhuner KG, Lundborg G (1977) Peripheral nerve injury due to injection needles used for regional anesthesia. An experimental study of the acute effects of needle point trauma. *Acta Anaesthesiol Scand* 21, 182.

86. Sidek HM, Nyquist-Battie C, Vanderkooi G (1984) Inhibition of synaptosomal enzymes by local anesthetics. *Biochim Biophys Acta* 801, 26.

87. Skou JC (1954) Local anaesthetics. II. The toxic potencies of some local anesthetics and of butyl alcohol, determined on peripheral nerves. *Acta Pharmacol* 10, 292.

88. Smith BE, Siggins D (1988) Low volume, high concentration block of the sciatic nerve. *Anaesthesia* 43, 8.

89. Spedding M, Berg C (1985) Antagonism of Ca^{2+}-induced contractions of K^+-depolarized smooth muscle by local anaesthetics. *Eur J Pharm* 108, 143.

90. Steffenson JL, Shnider SM, de Lorimier AA (1970) Transarterial diffusion of lidocaine. *Anesthesiology* 32, 459.

91. Strichartz GR, Ritchie JM (1987) The action of local anesthetics on ion channels of excitable tissues. In: *Local Anesthetics*. Strichartz GR ed. *Handbook Exp Pharmacol* 81, 21.

92. Suko J, Winkler F, Scharinger B *et al.* (1976) Aspects of the mechanism of action of local anesthetics on the sarcoplasmic reticulum of skeletal muscle. *Biochim Biophys Acta* 443, 571.

93. Tanaka K, Watanabe R, Harada T *et al.* (1993) Extensive application of epidural anesthesia and analgesia in a university hospital: Incidence of complications related to technique. *Reg Anesth* 18, 34.

94. Thorsén G (1947) Neurological complications after spinal anaesthesia and results from 2493 follow-up cases. *Acta Chir Scand* 95, 1.

95. Vandam LD (1987) Some aspects of the history of local anesthesia. *Local Anesthetics*. Strichartz GR ed. *Handb Exp Pharmacol* 81, 1.

96. Vanderhoek JY, Feinstein MB (1979) Local anesthetics, chlorpromazine and propranolol inhibit stimulus-activation of phospholipase A_2 in human platelets. *Mol Pharmacol* 16, 171.

97. Veselis RA (1990) Ischemic neuropathy presenting as prolonged epidural anesthesia. *Reg Anesth* 15, 264.

98. Volpi M, Sha'afi RI, Epstein PM *et al.* (1980) Antagonism of calmodulin by local anesthetics, mepacrine, and propranolol. *Ann N Y Acad Sci* 356, 441.

99. Volpi M, Sha'afi RI, Feinstein MB (1981) Antagonism of calmodulin by local anesthetics. Inhibition of calmodulin-stimulated calcium transport of erythrocyte inside-out membrane vesicles. *Mol Pharmacol* 20, 363.

100. Wang BC, Hillman DE, Spielholz NI *et al.* (1984) Chronic neurological deficits and Nesacaine-CE—an effect of the anesthetic, 2-chloroprocaine, or the antioxidant, sodium bisulfite? *Anesth Analg* 63, 445.

101. Wang BC, Li D, Hiller JM *et al.* (1992) Lumbar subarachnoid ethylenediaminetetraacetate induces hindlimb tetanic contractions in rats: Prevention by $CaCl_2$ pretreatment; observation of spinal nerve root degeneration. *Anesth Analg* 75, 895.

102. Wilschut JC, Regts J, Westenberg H *et al.* (1976) Hydrolysis of phosphatidylcholine liposomes by phospholipases A_2. Effects of the local anesthetic dibucaine. *Biochim Biophys Acta* 433, 20.

103. Woolf CJ, Wiesenfeld-Hallin Z (1985) The systemic administration of local anaesthetics produces a selective depression of C-afferent fibre evoked activity in the spinal cord. *Pain* 23, 361.

104. Woolley EJ, Vandam LD (1959) Neurological sequelae of brachial plexus nerve block. *Ann Surg* 149, 53.

Lincomycin

Steven Herskovitz

LINCOMYCIN
$C_{18}H_{34}N_2O_6S$

(2S-*trans*)-Methyl 6,8-dideoxy-6-[[(1-methyl-4-propyl-2-pyrrolidinyl)carbonyl]amino]-1-thio-D-erythro-α-D-galacto-octopyranoside

NEUROTOXICITY RATING

Clinical

A Neuromuscular transmission syndrome

Experimental

A Neuromuscular transmission dysfunction (pre- and postsynaptic)

Lincomycin is an antibiotic produced by an actinomycete, *Streptomyces lincolnensis* (4). Clindamycin, the 7-deoxy, 7-chloro derivative, is more active, has fewer side effects, and has supplanted lincomycin. The mechanism of action of lincomycin involves binding to the 50 S subunit of bacterial ribosomes and suppression of protein synthesis. The agents' antibacterial spectrum includes Gram-positive species and some anaerobes. Neurotoxicity is manifest as neuromuscular blockade.

Lincomycin is rapidly absorbed after the usual 500 mg oral dose and reaches peak levels in 2–4 h. Gastrointestinal absorption is only partial (20%–35%). Intravenous infusion of 600 mg over 2 h produces therapeutic concentrations for 14 h. Distribution is widespread to most tissues. Concentrations are insignificant in the cerebrospinal fluid of normal individuals and reach approximately 40% of the plasma level in patients with meningitis. The half-life is about 5 h. The bile is an important route of excretion; urinary excretion is limited and variable. Important systemic side effects with standard doses include diarrhea and occasionally pseudomembranous colitis (4,5). Inadvertant high-dose, rapid infusions may be associated with hypotension, arrythmias, and cardiac arrest (2).

Lincomycin administered intravenously to chickens at 200 mg/kg produces immediate ataxia, wing-sagging, ptosis, and body relaxation, similar to the effects of *d*-tubocurarine; higher doses are lethal (12). In rabbit sciatic nerve–gastrocnemius muscle preparations, lincomycin at 12.5–50 mg/kg results in dose-related depression of neuromuscular transmission with high-frequency stimulation (11,12). The effect is much weaker with lower stimulation frequencies. This nondepolarizing competitive blockade is partially antagonized by edrophonium, but not by neostigmine or calcium. In isolated mouse phrenic nerve–hemidiaphragm preparations, neuromuscular blockade produced by lincomycin is only partially reversed by calcium, but readily reversed by 3,4-diaminopyridine (9).

In humans, standard or even high doses of lincomycin alone do not cause significant neuromuscular blockade (1,6). Lincomycin augments a partial pancuronium neuromuscular blockade in anesthetized subjects (1). This effect is brief and is antagonized by neostigmine and 4-aminopyridine. Reports of clinical neuromuscular blockade with lincomycin result from potentiation of the effects of *d*-tubocurarine, pancuronium, or magnesium; the effects may be prolonged (hours) (1,3,8). There is a variable response to neostigmine.

The mechanism of action of lincomycin likely involves both pre- and postsynaptic sites. *In vitro* studies show reduction in miniature end-plate potential amplitude and frequency, decrease in end-plate sensitivity to acetylcholine, and decrease in evoked transmitter release (7,10). A direct depressant effect on muscle has also been suggested (13).

REFERENCES

1. Booij LHDJ, Miller RD, Crul JF (1978) Neostigmine and 4-aminopyridine antagonism of lincomycin-pancuronium neuromuscular blockade in man. *Anesth Analg* 57, 316.

2. Daubeck JL, Daughety MJ, Petty C (1974) Lincomycin-induced cardiac arrest: A case report and laboratory investigation. *Anesth Analg* 53, 563.

3. Duignan NM, Andrews J, Williams JD (1973) Pharmacologic studies with lincomycin in late pregnancy. *Brit Med J* 3, 75.

4. Goodman LS, Gilman A (1975) *The Pharmacological Basis of Therapeutics. 5th Ed*. Macmillan, New York.

5. Keller H (1992) Miscellaneous antibiotics. In: *Meyler's Side Effects of Drugs. 12th Ed*. Dukes MNG ed. Elsevier, Amsterdam p. 659.

6. Novak E, Vitti TG, Chodos DJ *et al*. (1971) Lincomycin administered by intravenous infusion to normal volunteers. Part I: Tolerance. *J Clin Pharmacol* 11, 46.

7. Rubbo JT, Gergis SD, Sokoll MD (1977) Comparative neuromuscular effects of lincomycin and clindamycin. *Anesth Analg* 56, 329.

8. Samuelson RJ, Giesecke AH, Kallus FJ *et al.* (1975) Lincomycin curare interaction. *Anesth Analg* 54, 103.

9. Singh YN, Harvey AL, Marshall IG (1978) Antibiotic-induced paralysis of the mouse phrenic nerve-hemidiaphragm preparation, and reversibility by calcium and neostigmine. *Anesthesiology* 48, 418.

10. Singh YN, Marshall IG, Harvey AL (1979) Depression of transmitter release and postjunctional sensitivity during neuromuscular block produced by antibiotics. *Brit J Anaesth* 51, 1027.

11. Straw RN, Hook JB, Williamson HE, Mitchell CL (1965) Neuromuscular blocking properties of lincomycin. *J Pharm Sci* 54, 1814.

12. Tang AH, Schroeder LA (1968) The effect of lincomycin on neuromuscular transmission. *Toxicol Appl Pharmacol* 12, 44.

13. Wright JM, Collier B (1976) Characterization of the neuromuscular block produced by clindamycin and lincomycin. *Can J Physiol Pharmacol* 54, 937.

Lithium

Klaus Windgassen

Li

NEUROTOXICITY RATING

Clinical

A   Cerebellar syndrome (acute and chronic)

A   Acute encephalopathy

B   Benign intracranial hypertension

B   Extrapyramidal syndrome

B   Neuromuscular transmission syndrome

C   Peripheral neuropathy

C   Myopathy

Experimental

A   Myopathy (necrotizing)

A   Neuromuscular transmission dysfunction

Lithium (Li), the lightest element in the alkali metal group, has an atomic weight of 6.94. Only the lithium ion (Li^+) is stable in an aqueous solution. The physiological serum lithium concentration is 0.004 mmol/l (28,31).

Water-soluble lithium salts, primarily lithium carbonate, but also acetate, sulfate, and others, are widely used therapeutically in the treatment and prevention of affective psychoses. In a Danish region with a population of *ca.* 372,000, lithium salts are used to treat 1.5 per 1000; comparable figures are likely in other industrialized nations (60).

General Toxicology

The water-soluble lithium salts are absorbed rapidly and almost completely in the intestinal tract; the bioavailability and course of the absorption phase depend on the anion of the lithium salt and, in the case of lithium-based drugs, on the galenic preparation. Absorption is independent of the gastric hydrogen ion concentration. Distribution is gradual and corresponds to a two-compartment model; distribution volume approximates 50%–90% of the body weight. Serum concentrations are subject to substantial interindividual variation. Lithium crosses the placenta, appears in breast milk, and is primarily eliminated by renal excretion; only 1%–2% is discharged in feces or perspiration. Lithium undergoes glomerular filtration in the kidney; about 75% is reabsorbed in the proximal tubule. The clearance rate is 10–40 ml/min; this is reduced in renal insufficiency, negative sodium balance, and old age.

Depending on the duration and level of lithium exposure and individual disposition, lithium may act on virtually all organs, especially the thyroid, kidney, heart, and reticuloendothelial system. Gastrointestinal complaints are frequent with initial lithium dosing (especially with serum levels >0.8 mmol/l). Abnormalities of the skin or integumentary appendages are reported in rare cases. The target organ for therapeutic lithium administration is the CNS; neurological side effects are frequent at the onset of lithium therapy. Neurotoxic effects appear with serum lithium levels of >1.5–2.0 mmol/l, and serum levels of 3.0–3.5 mmol/l are life-threatening.

Animal Studies

Six of 15 mice survived intraperitoneal injections of 12.9 mEq/kg/day Li^+ (as lithium chloride) for 30 days (24). The lowest tissue concentration was found in the liver (0.8 mEq/kg); high lithium concentrations were recorded in kidneys (2.2 mEq/kg), salivary glands (2.2 mEq/kg), skeletal muscles (2.7 mEq/kg), and bones (2.5 mEq/kg). Tissue concentration in the brain (1.2 mEq/kg) was approximately equivalent to that in blood (1.4 mEq/kg). Clear-cut differences in lithium concentration exist among various brain areas in rats; lithium concentration is highest (twice as high as in serum or in most other brain areas) in white matter (13).

In one study, a daily dosage of 100 mg (equal to 2.7 mmol/kg) of lithium carbonate was administered *per os* to rats for 15, 30, 60, and 90 days (30). Light microscopy of striated muscle showed fiber necrosis; electron microscopy revealed Z-band streaming, mitochondrial aggregations, and abnormally enlarged mitochrondria. Rats treated with varying doses of lithium chloride over a 15-day period showed a mean serum level of 2.00 mEq/l in the group receiving the highest drug dose (44). In this study, lithium had no significant effect on nerve conduction velocity (NCV); long-term nontoxic doses administered to rats induced no abnormalities when compared with untreated animals (12). These animals were subsequently treated for 7 days with a toxic dosage of lithium (2×2.5 mmol/kg/day); NCV decreased, but changes were reversible 1 week after cessation of exposure. In dogs, lithium significantly prolonged both pancuronium bromide- and succinylcholine-induced neuromuscular blockade (43).

Human Studies

In a study of healthy volunteers (17), NCV was significantly decreased (though still within the normal range) and the duration of potentials slightly increased after increasing lithium dosages administered over 7 days (starting with 12 mval on day 1 and increasing by 6-mval increments to 36 mval). A decrease in NCV with long-term lithium medication has been documented in patients with affective psychosis (9,14,17,34,42). However, clinical manifestations of peripheral neuropathy have not appeared.

Electroencephalography (EEG) recordings have revealed a decrease of mean frequencies and an increase in θ and δ activity and amplitude. In particular, after long-term lithium intake, varying focal changes and paroxysmal spike-and-wave activity appear (19,55). There is no correlation between the extent of EEG changes and serum lithium concentration; EEG changes correlate with onset of neurotoxic symptoms. These changes are detected from 1 week to 1 month after lithium exposure (25,35). In toxic dosages, lithium induces generalized seizures (*vide infra*).

Fine hand tremor (8–10 Hz) is common in the initial phase of lithium medication (3,58,59,61). Tremor has a higher incidence rate in patients receiving lithium combined with neuroleptics, especially with antidepressants, than in those receiving lithium alone (16). Older patients are more often affected (59).

Acute lithium intoxication is rare (47); 95% of affected patients have neurotoxic symptoms (15, 18). Initial symptoms are apathy and sluggishness, followed by disturbances of consciousness (delirium or stupor, coma). Frequent neurological manifestations are coarse tremor, fasciculations, myoclonus, and muscle twitching. Less common are muscular hypertonicity, hyperreflexia, parkinsonism, choreoathetoid dyskinesia, dysarthria, ataxia, downbeat nystagmus, gaze palsy, and generalized seizures (18,50,51). Lithium can potentiate neuromuscular blockade induced by pancuronium and succinylcholine; these anesthetic agents should be used with caution in patients receiving lithium (7,20).

Even when serum levels are identical, neurotoxic symptoms may vary substantially (16). However, serum lithium levels reported in intoxicated patients are difficult to compare, since intervals between last lithium intake and blood test are often unknown. It is suggested that abnormal CNS tissue may have a diminished capacity for lithium removal, resulting in "islands of high lithium concentration, influencing the surrounding (normal) brain and giving rise to the specific phenomenon of lithium neurotoxicity at normal lithium levels" (27). Pre-existing EEG abnormalities, combined medication with neuroleptics, and rapid increase of dosage may be additional risk factors. Since brain uptake and discharge of lithium are substantially slower than the changes in serum level, and tissue concentrations in some brain regions are twice as high as that in serum, the clinical picture may continue to deteriorate even after lithium is discontinued (15,18,38,47). The estimated rate of persistent neurological sequelae following acute intoxication is 10% (18).

Chronic (years) lithium treatment may be accompanied by neurological dysfunction despite normal blood levels (46). Findings include cerebellar disturbances, truncal ataxia, broad-based ataxic gait, dyskinesia, dysarthria, head and hand tremor, and nystagmus (including downbeat nystagmus). Computed tomography and magnetic radiologic imaging may show cerebellar atrophy after chronic lithium intoxication (4,23,53,57). Detailed neuropathological examinations are few (44). Studies have reported damage to cerebellar granule and Purkinje cells, gliosis in the dentate nucleus, the inferior olives, and the red nucleus, and cytoplasmic inclusions in the cells of cranial nerve nuclei (36,40). An especially detailed postmortem report describes intracytoplasmic vacuoles in cerebellar white matter and loss of Purkinje cells (45). Isolated reports of peripheral neuropathy and myopathy are unconvincing (5,8,10,26,37-39,49,54,56,57).

Papilledema during lithium therapy (with serum levels within the therapeutic range) was first described in 1978 (33); subsequent case reports suggest pseudotumor cerebri is the cause. These cases have occurred almost exclusively in overweight women.

Toxic Mechanism

Mechanisms underlying the therapeutic and neurotoxic effects of lithium are unclear. Lithium ions have complex effects on neurotransmission and cell metabolism. For example, lithium influences cholinergic and aminergic transmitter systems as well as γ-aminobutyric acid–related and peptidergic processes. The second messenger system is one site of postsynaptic action (1). Lithium affects the phosphoinositide (PI) system, which plays a key role in intracellular signal transduction. When the transmitter is bound to the receptor, membrane-based phosphatidylinositol 4,5-bisphoshate (PIP_2) is hydrolyzed to inositol 1,4,5-triphosphate (IP_3) and diacylglycerol (DAG). IP_3 acts as a second messenger and releases calcium ions at the endoplasmic reticulum, which, in turn, activates a protein kinase by means of calmodulin. DAG activates protein kinase C. IP_3 is metabolized to inositol in several pathways, finally *via* inositol monophoshate. PIP_2 is resynthesized from inositol and the CDP-DAG form from DAG (*via* PI and PIP). Some enzymes involved in the breakdown of IP_3 into inositol are inhibited by lithium; this includes inhibition of the inositol monophosphate phosphatase, which results in a reduced hydrolysis of IP_1 to inositol. An elevated IP_1 concentration and a reduced inositol concentration are found in brains of lithium-treated rats. While negligible after low lithium doses, changes are clear-cut after treatment with toxic doses (48). It is unclear whether lithium-induced inositol depletion also leads to a critical decline in phosphoinositide synthesis and, thus, to a relevant disturbance of the second-messenger system.

Lithium changes seizure thresholds of cholinomimetics. Muscarinic agonists in subconvulsive doses trigger limbic seizures when animals have been pretreated with lithium (21,22,41,52). There is a concomitant decrease in myoinositol and an increase in inositol monophosphate; this is approximately tenfold those levels found after administration of either lithium or pilocarpine alone. The proconvulsive effect of lithium can be partially alleviated by inositol; when rats are given intraventricular injections of myoinositol, convulsive activity induced by administering LiCl (3 mEq/kg) and pilocarpine (20 or 30 mg/kg) is significantly reduced (prolonged latency and less-pronounced convulsion) (29). In contrast, convulsions triggered by a very high dose (200 mg/kg) of pilocarpine alone (*i.e.*, without pretreatment with LiCl) cannot be suppressed with intraventricular inositol administration. These findings suggest a pathogenetic role for lithium-induced inositol depletion. In contrast, the mortality rate after lithium administration in toxic doses could not be reduced by intraventricular inositol injection (6); lethal and convulsive lithium effects accordingly seem to be based on different biochemical principles.

Lithium does not appear to affect the phosphoinositide system by enzyme induction alone. For instance, studies on ^{3}H-glutamic-pyruvic transaminase binding (2) suggest that lithium also inhibits the activation of G proteins. Chronic lithium treatment also influences G-protein mRNA and protein concentrations (11,32), but the mechanisms underlying these effects are unknown.

Editors' Note: Experimental mutation of the astroglial GLT-1 glutamate transporter, in particular serine-440 to glycine, has been recently reported to enable lithium ions (as well as sodium ions) to drive net influx of acidic amino acids (62).

REFERENCES

1. Allison JH, Stewart MA (1971) Reduced brain inositol in lithium-treated rats. *Nature New Biol* **233**, 267.
2. Avissar S, Schreiber G, Danon A, Belmaker RH (1988) Lithium inhibits adrenergic and cholinergic increases in GTP binding in rat cortex. *Nature* **331**, 440.
3. Bech P, Thomsen J, Prytz S *et al.* (1979) The profile and severity of lithium-induced side effects in mentally healthy subjects. *Neuropsychobiology* **5**, 160.
4. Bejar JM (1985) Cerebellar degeneration due to acute lithium toxicity. *Clin Neuropharmacol* **8**, 371.
5. Bell AJ, Cole A, Eccleston D, Ferrier IN (1993) Lithium neurotoxicity at normal therapeutic levels. *Brit J Psychiat* **162**, 689.
6. Bersudsky Y, Vinnitsky I, Ghelber D *et al.* (1993) Mechanism of lithium lethality in rats. *J Psychiat Res* **27**, 415.
7. Borden H, Clarke MT, Katz H (1974) The use of pancuronium bromide in patients receiving lithium carbonate. *Can Anaesth Soc J* **21**, 78.
8. Brust JCM, Hammer JS, Challenor Y *et al.* (1979) Acute generalized polyneuropathy accompanying lithium poisoning. *Ann Neurol* **6**, 360.
9. Chang Y-C, Lin H-N, Deng H-C (1990) Subclinical lithium neurotoxicity: Correlation of neural conduction abnormalities and serum lithium levels in manic-depressive patients with lithium treatment. *Acta Neurol Scand* **82**, 82.
10. Chang Y-C, Yip P-K, Chiu Y-N, Lin H-N (1988) Severe generalized polyneuropathy in lithium intoxication. *Eur Neurol* **28**, 39.
11. Colin SF, Chang H-C, Mollner S *et al.* (1991) Chronic lithium regulates the expression of adenylate cyclase and Gi-protein subunit in rat cerebral cortex. *Proc Nat Acad Sci USA* **88**, 10634.
12. Ebara T, Nakayama K, Otsuki S, Watanabe S (1981) Effects of lithium on rat tail nerve conduction velocity. *Int Pharmacopsychiat* **16**, 129.
13. Edelfors S (1975) Distribution of sodium, potassium and lithium in the brain of lithium-treated rats. *Acta Pharmacol Toxicol* **37**, 387.

14. Eisenstädter A, Seiser A, Brainin M (1989) Neurotoxizität bei Langzeit-Lithiumtherapie: Eine elektroneurographische Studie. *Wien Klin Wochenschr* **101**, 166.

15. El-Mallakh RS (1986) Acute lithium neurotoxicity. *Psychiat Develop* **4**, 311.

16. Emilien G, Maloteaux JM (1996) Lithium neurotoxicity at low therapeutic doses. Hypotheses for causes and mechanism of action following retrospective analysis of published case reports. *Acta Neurol Belg* **96**, 281.

17. Girke W, Krebs F-A, Müller-Oerlinghausen B (1975) Effects of lithium on electromyographic recordings in man. *Int Pharmacopsychiat* **10**, 24.

18. Hansen HE, Amdisen A (1978) Lithium intoxication. *Quart J Med* **47**, 123.

19. Helmchen H, Kanowski S (1971) EEG-Veränderungen unter Lithium-Therapie. *Nervenarzt* **42**, 144.

20. Hill GE, Wong KC, Hodges MR (1976) Potentiation of succinylcholine neuromuscular blockade by lithium carbonate. *Anesthesiology* **44**, 439.

21. Hirvonen MR, Paljarri L, Naukkarinen A *et al.* (1990) Potentiation of malaoxon-induced convulsions by lithium: Early neuronal injury, phosphoinositide signaling and calcium. *Toxicol Appl Pharmacol* **104**, 276.

22. Honchar MP, Olney JW, Sherman WR (1983) Systemic cholinergic agents induce seizures and brain damage in lithium-treated rats. *Science* **220**, 323.

23. Jacome DE (1987) Cerebellar syndrome in lithium poisoning. *J Neurol Neurosurg Psychiat* **50**, 1722.

24. Jernigan HM, Schrank GD, Kraus LM (1978) Lithium chloride and dilithium carbamyl phosphate: Lithium distribution and toxicity in mice. *Toxicol Appl Pharmacol* **44**, 413.

25. Johnson G, Maccario M, Gershon S, Korein J (1970) The effects of lithium on electroencephalogram, behavior and serum electrolytes. *J Nerv Ment Dis* **151**, 273.

26. Julien J, Vallat JM, Lagueny A (1979) Myopathy and cerebellar syndrome during acute poisoning with lithium carbonate. *Muscle Nerve* **2**, 240.

27. Kemperman CJF, Gerdes JH, De Rooij J, Venkens LM (1989) Reversible lithium neurotoxicity at normal serum level may refer to intracranial pathology. *J Neurol Neurosurg Psychiat* **52**, 679.

28. Klaus R (1971) Flammenphotometrische Lithium-Bestimmung im Serum. *Z Klin Chem Klin Biochem* **9**, 107.

29. Kofman O, Sherman WR, Katz V, Belmaker RH (1993) Restoration of brain myo-inositol levels in rats increases latency to lithium-pilocarpin seizures. *Psychopharmacology* **110**, 229.

30. Kumamoto T, Fukuhara N, Hirahara H, Wakabayashi M (1981) Morphological studies on the skeletal muscles and peripheral nerves of rats intoxicated with lithium carbonate. *Clin Neurol* **21**, 16.

31. Lang W, Herrman (1965) Eine Methode zur flammenpho-

tometrischen Lithiumbestimmung im Serum. *Z Ges Exp Med* **139**, 200.

32. Li PP, Tam Y-K, Young LT, Warsh JJ (1991) Lithium decreases Gs-, Gi-1 and Gi-2 alpha subunits mRNA levels in rat cortex. *Eur J Pharmacol* **206**, 165.

33. Lobo A, Pilek E, Stokes PE (1978) Papilledema following therapeutic dosages of lithium carbonate. *J Nerv Ment Dis* **166**, 526.

34. Manocha M, Chokroverty S, Nora R (1984) Peripheral and central neural conduction in patients on chronic lithium therapy. *Muscle Nerve* **7**, 575.

35. Müller-Oerlinghausen B, Bauer H, Girke W *et al.* (1977) Impairment of vigilance and performance under lithium treatment. Studies in patients and normal volunteers. *Pharmacopsychiatry* **10**, 67.

36. Naramoto A, Koizumi N, Itoh N, Shigematsu H (1993) An autopsy case of cerebellar degeneration following lithium intoxication with neuroleptic malignant syndrome. *Acta Pathol Jpn* **43**, 55.

37. Neil JF, Himmelhoch JM, Licata SM (1976) Emergence of myasthenia gravis during treatment with lithium carbonate. *Arch Gen Psychiat* **33**, 1090.

38. Newman PK, Saunders M (1979) Lithium neurotoxicity. *Postgrad Med J* **55**, 701.

39. Pamphlett RS, Mackenzie RA (1982) Severe polyneuropathy due to lithium intoxication. *J Neurol Neurosurg Psychiat* **45**, 656.

40. Peiffer J (1981) Clinical and neuropathological aspects of long-term damage to the central nervous system after lithium medication. *Arch Psychiatr Nervenkr* **231**, 41.

41. Persinger MA, Makarec K, Bradley JC (1988) Characteristics of limbic seizures evoked by peripheral injections of lithium and pilocarpine. *Physiol Behav* **44**, 27.

42. Presslich O, Mairhofer E, Opgenoorth E, Schuster P (1981) Maximale motorische Nervenleitgeschwindigkeit unter Lithium. In: *Current Perspectives in Lithium Prophylaxis.* Berner P, Lenz G, Wolf R eds. Karger, Basel, München, Paris, London, New York p. 121.

43. Reimherr FW, Hodges MR, Hill G, Wong KC (1977) Prolongation of muscle relaxant effects by lithium carbonate. *Amer J Psychiat* **134**, 205.

44. Samples JR, Seybold ME (1977) The electrophysiological effects of lithium in the rat. *Int Pharmacopsychiat* **12**, 160.

45. Schneider JA, Mirra SS (1994) Neuropathologic correlates of persistent neurologic deficit in lithium intoxication. *Ann Neurol* **36**, 928.

46. Schou M (1984) Long-lasting neurological sequelae after lithium intoxication. *Acta Psychiat Scand* **70**, 594.

47. Schou M, Hansen HE, Thomsen K, Vestergaard P (1989) Lithium treatment in Aarhus. 2. Risk of renal failure and of intoxication. *Pharmacopsychiatry* **22**, 101.

48. Sherman WR, Munsell LY, Gish BG, Honchar MP (1985) Effects of systematically administered lithium on phos-

phoinositide metabolism in rat brain, kidney, and testis. *J Neurochem* **44**, 798.

49. Slonim R, McLarty B (1985) Sixth cranial nerve palsy—unusual presenting symptom of lithium toxicity. *Can J Psychiat* **30**, 443.

50. Smith SJM, Kocen RS (1988) A Creutzfeldt-Jakob like syndrome due to lithium toxicity. *J Neurol Neurosurg Psychiat* **51**, 120.

51. Spatz R, Kugler J, Greil W, Lorenzi E (1978) Das Elektroenzephalogramm bei der Lithium-Intoxikation. *Nervenarzt* **49**, 539.

52. Terry JB, Padzernik TL, Nelson SR (1990) Effect of LiCl pretreatment on choliomimetic-induced seizures and seizure-induced brain edema in rats. *Neurosci Lett* **114**, 123.

53. Tesio L, Porta GL, Messa E (1987) Cerebellar syndrome in lithium poisoning: A case of partial recovery. *J Neurol Neurosurg Psychiat* **50**, 235.

54. Uchigata M, Tanabe H, Hasue I, Kurihara M (1981) Peripheral neuropathy due to lithium intoxication. *Ann Neurol* **9**, 414.

55. Ulrich G, Scheuler W, Müller-Oerlinghausen B (1983) Zur visuell-morphologischen Analyse des hirnelektrischen Verhaltens bei Patienten mit manisch-depressiven und schizo-affektiven Psychosen unter Lithiumprophylaxe. *Fortschr Neurol Psychiat* **51**, 24.

56. Unger J, Decaux G, L'Hermite M (1982) Rhabdomyolysis, acute renal failure, endocrine alterations and neurological sequelae in a case of lithium selfpoisoning. *Acta Clin Belg* **37**, 216.

57. Vanhooren G, Dehaene I, Van Zandycke M *et al.* (1990) Polyneuropathy in lithium intoxication. *Muscle Nerve* **13**, 204.

58. Vestergaard P, Amdisen A, Schou M (1980) Clinically significant side effects of lithium treatment. *Acta Psychiat Scand* **62**, 193.

59. Vestergaard P, Poulstrup I, Schou M (1988) Prospective studies on a lithium cohort. Tremor, weight gain, psychological complaints. *Acta Psychiat Scand* **78**, 434.

60. Vestergaard P, Schou M (1989) Lithium treatment in Aarhus. 1. Prevalence. *Pharmacopsychiatry* **22**, 99.

61. Volk J, Müller-Oerlinghausen B (1986) Time course of AMP-documented side-effects in patients under long-term lithium treatment. *Pharmacopsychiatry* **19**, 286.

62. Zhang Y, Kanner BI (1999) Two serine residues of the glutamate transporter GLT-1 are crucial for coupling the fluxes of sodium and the neurotransmitter. *Proc Natl Acad Sci USA* **96**, 1710.

Lobeline

John C.M. Brust

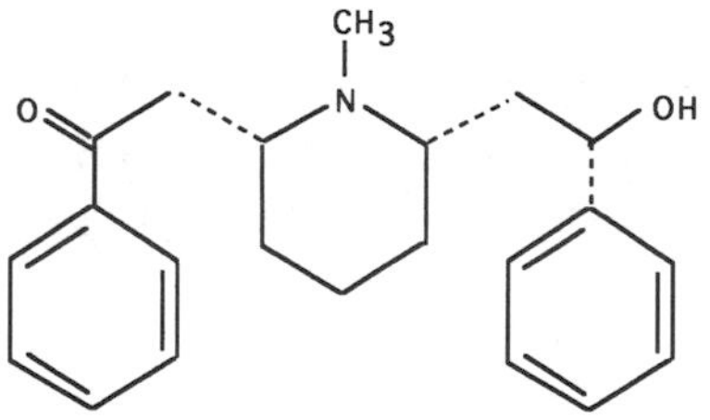

LOBELINE
$C_{22}H_{27}NO_2$

[2R-[2α,6α(S*)]]-2-[6-(2-Hydroxy-2-phenylethyl)-1-methyl-2-piperidinyl]-1-phenylethanone

NEUROTOXICITY RATING

Clinical

A   Acute encephalopathy (nicotinic effect on CNS and PNS)

The Indian tobacco plant, *Lobelia inflata*, contains alkaloids—lobeline, lobelanine, and lobelanidine—with weak nicotine-like actions (2). Although the plant also contains atropine and scopolamine, lobeline accounts for most of *Lobelia*'s effects (1,3). Popular during the nineteenth century as an emetic and an expectorant, it is today smoked as a marijuana substitute, drunk as lobelia tea, or taken as capsules of the powdered drug. It is marketed as tablets, lozenges, and chewing gum as a nicotine substitute that is claimed to help tobacco addicts stop smoking.

Like nicotine, lobeline has biphasic actions on autonomic ganglia and the CNS; low doses are stimulatory and high doses are depressant (*see* Nicotine, this volume). Following low doses, there is bronchodilation and increased respiration; higher levels cause headache, nausea, and vomiting, limiting its popularity as a euphoriant. Overdose causes sweating, tachycardia, hypotension, seizures, coma, and fatal respiratory depression (1,3).

REFERENCES

1. Lewin NA, Howland MA, Goldrank LR (1990) Herbal preparations. In: *Toxicologic Emergencies. 4th Ed.* Goldfrank LR, Flomenbaum NE, Lewin NA *et al.* eds. Appleton & Lange, Norwalk Connecticut p. 587.

2. Taylor P (1990) Agents acting at the neuromuscular junc-

tion and autonomic ganglia. In: *The Pharmacological Basis of Therapeutics*. 8th Ed. Gilman AG, Ral T, Nies AS, Taylor P eds. Pergamon Press, New York p. 166.

3. Tyler VE (1993) *The Honest Herbal. A Sensible Guide to the Use of Herbs and Related Remedies*. 3rd Ed. Pharmaceutical Products Press (Haworth Press), New York p. 205.

Lophotoxin and Other Gorgonian Toxins

Albert C. Ludolph

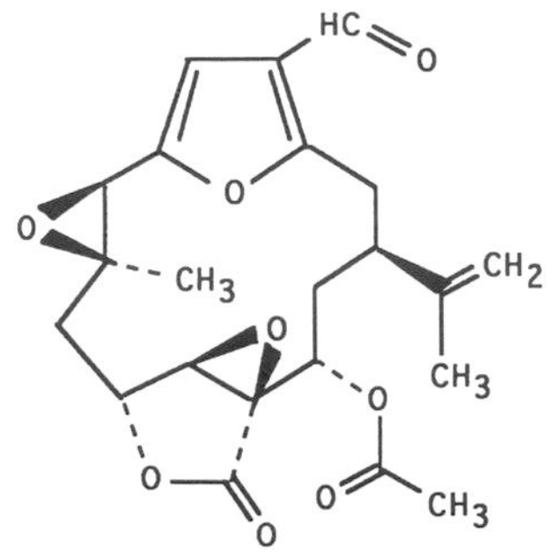

LOPHOTOXIN
$C_{22}H_{24}O_8$

[1R-(1R*,2S*,4S*,10R*,12R*,14R*,15R*)]-2-(Acetyloxy)-12-methyl-4-(1-methylethenyl)-17-oxo-11,16,18,19-tetraoxapentacyclo[12.2.2.1^{6,9}.0^{1,15}.0^{10,12}]nonadeca-6,8-diene-7-carboxaldehyde

NEUROTOXICITY RATING

Clinical

A Neuromuscular transmission syndrome

Experimental

A Neuromuscular transmission dysfunction

Lophotoxin is an ichthyotoxic diterpene lactone from the Pacific gorgonian (soft) coral (sea fans and whips, *Lophogorgia* spp.) (7). The compound serves as a defense mechanism for these animals. Lophotoxin is a potent antagonist at both neuronal and muscle nicotinic channels; it binds covalently at the acetylcholine receptor. Structurally, the molecule is a small, uncharged cyclic diterpene with furanoaldehyde and α,β-epoxy-γ-lactone groups. It is suggested that the lactone carbonyl serves as a hydrogen acceptor, and the C7 carbon is responsible for the specific binding to the acetylcholine receptor α-subunit (3). The compound has a MW of 416.43; at room temperature, lophotoxin forms white needles with a MP of 164°–166°C (7).

Eupalmerin acetate (EUAC), 12,13-bisepieupalmerin (BEEP), and eunicin (EUNI)—diterpeneoids from Carribean *Eunicea* spp.—also block the function of the acetylcholine receptor; however, their effects differ from lophotoxin, since they are reversible, noncompetitive inhibitors (6).

Lophotoxin covalently binds to the acetylcholine receptor of vertebrate muscle, prevents its activation by acetylcholine, and produces an irreversible neuromuscular blockade (4,5). Covalent binding is achieved by interaction of lophotoxin with Tyr190 on the α-subunit of the receptor (1–3,10). Effects are reversed by high concentrations of *d*-tubocurarine (9); 300 μmol tubocurarine protects against binding of 3 μmol of lophotoxin at the specific α-subunit. With similar affinity and specifity, lophotoxin also binds to and blocks nicotinic receptors in frog autonomic ganglia and chick ciliary ganglion (8,9). Subcutaneous injection of lophotoxin into mice is followed by ataxia, paralysis, and severe respiratory depression resulting in death; the LD$_{50}$ is 8.0 μg/g (7). There are no reports of neurotoxic effects in humans.

REFERENCES

1. Abramson SN, Culver P, Kline T *et al.* (1988) Lophotoxin and related coral toxins covalently label the alpha-subunit of the nicotinic acetylcholine receptor. *J Biol Chem* 263, 18568.

2. Abramson SN, Li Y, Culver P, Taylor P (1989) An analog of lophotoxin reacts covalently with Tyr190 in the alpha-subunit of the nicotinic acetylcholine receptor. *J Biol Chem* 264, 12666.

3. Abramson SN, Trischman JA, Tapiolas DM *et al.* (1991) Structure/activity and molecular modeling studies of the lophotoxin group of irreversible nicotinic receptor antagonists. *J Med Chem* 34, 1798.

4. Culver P, Jacobs RS (1981) Lophotoxin: A neuromuscular acting toxin from the sea whip (*Lophorgorgia rigida*). *Toxicon* 19, 825.

5. Culver P, Fenical W, Taylor P (1984) Lophotoxin irreversibly inactivates the nicotinic acetylcholine receptor by preferential association at one of the two primary agonist sites. *J Biol Chem* 259, 3763.

6. Eterovic VA, Hann RM, Ferchmin PA *et al.* (1993) Diterpenoids from Caribbean gorgonians act as noncompetitive inhibitors of the nicotinic acetylcholine receptor. *Cell Mol Neurobiol* 13, 99.

7. Fenical W, Okuda RK, Bandurragga MM *et al.* (1981) Lo-

photoxin: A novel neuromuscular toxin from Pacific sea whips from the genus *Lophorgorgia*. *Science* **212**, 1512.

8. Langdon RB, Jacobs RS (1985) Irreversible autonomic actions by lophotoxin suggest utility as a probe for both C6 and C10 nicotinic receptors. *Brain Res* **359**, 233.

9. Sorenson EM, Culver P, Chiapinelli VA (1987) Lophotoxin: Selective blockade of nicotinic transmission in au-

tonomic ganglia by a coral neurotoxin. *Neuroscience* **20**, 875.

10. Tornoe C, Holden-Dye L, Garland C *et al.* (1996) Lophotoxin-insensitive nematode nicotinic acetylcholine receptors. *J Exp Biol* **199**, 2161.

Lovastatin

Herbert H. Schaumburg

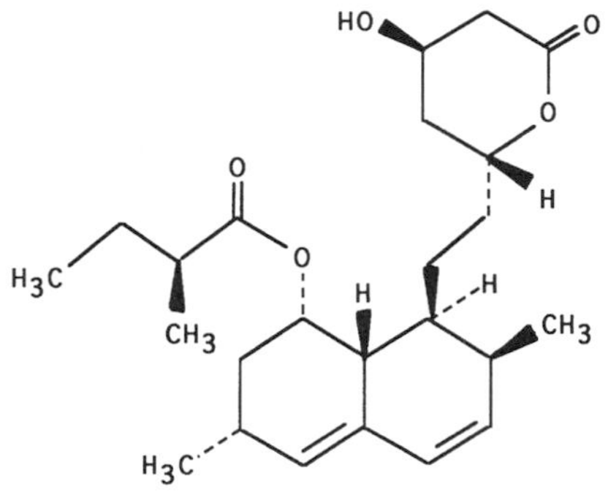

LOVASTATIN
$C_{24}H_{36}O_5$

[1S-[1α(R*),3α,7β,8β(2S*,4S*)-8aβ]]-2-Methylbutanoic acid 1,2,3,7,8,8a-hexahydro-3,7-dimethyl-8-[2-tetrahydro-4-hydroxy-6-oxo-2H-pyran-2-yl)ethyl]-1-naphthalenyl ester

NEUROTOXICITY RATING

Clinical

A Myopathy

B Peripheral neuropathy

Experimental

A Myopathy (necrotizing)

Lovastatin, a microbial-derived hydroxymethylglutaryl coenzyme A (HMG-CoA)–reductase inhibitor, is widely used for control of hyperlipoproteinemia. HMG-CoA–reductase inhibitors block the hepatic synthesis of cholesterol, thereby initiating compensatory reactions that lead to a reduction in plasma levels of low-density lipoprotein. Systemic adverse effects are rare, minor, and almost never lead to a discontinuation of therapy. Mild elevations in serum transaminase levels occur in 2%, and jaundice may develop if transaminase elevations increase and persist (1).

Toxic myopathy, cholesterol-lowering-agent myopathy (CLAM), is the most serious side effect of lovastatin therapy; it occurs in 2% of patients treated for longer than 3 months (2). Asymptomatic elevations of plasma levels of

the muscle isoenzyme of creatine phosphokinase appear in 11% of patients receiving lovastatin; this is not an absolute indication for stopping the drug; the appearance of proximal weakness is. Most instances of myopathy develop in individuals who are concurrently receiving other medication, especially immunosuppressive agents or gemfibrozil. Generally, weakness and myalgia appear about 6–9 months following commencement of conventional doses of 60 mg/day. Electrodiagnostic findings include fibrillation potentials, myotonia, and polyphasic potentials (2). Muscle biopsy discloses a nonspecific pattern of type ll atrophy, with little fiber necrosis and no inflammation. Mild or moderately disabled individuals make a satisfactory recovery, and some may receive another course of therapy at lower doses. Rarely, rapid-onset necrotizing myopathy and rhabdomyolysis develop. Experimental animal studies have demonstrated myotonia in rabbits and necrotic changes in fast-twitch muscles of rats (4,5); none of these studies clearly suggests the pathogenesis of lovastatin myopathy. One report describes four persons treated with conventional doses who developed a sensorimotor polyneuropathy that improved following withdrawal of the drug (3).

REFERENCES

1. Dujovne CA, Chremos AN, Pool JL *et al.* (1991) Expanded clinical evaluation of lovastatin (EXCEL) study results: IV. Additional perspectives on the tolerability of lovastatin. *Amer J Med* **91**, 25S.

2. London SF, Gross KF, Ringel SP (1992) Cholesterol-lowering agent myopathy (CLAM). *Neurology* **41**, 1159.

3. Phan T, McLeod JG, Pollard JD *et al.* (1994) Peripheral neuropathy associated with simvastatin. *J Neurol Neurosurg Psychiat* **58**, 625.

4. Sonoda Y, Gotow T, Kuriyama M *et al.* (1994) Electrical myotonia of rabbit skeletal muscles by HMG-CoA reductase inhibitors. *Muscle Nerve* **17**, 891.

5. Waclawik A, Lindal S, Engel A (1993) Experimental lovastatin myopathy. *J Neuropathol Exp Neurol* **52**, 542.

Lupinus Spp.

Thomas Meyer
Albert C. Ludolph

LUPININE
$C_{10}H_{19}NO$

Lupinine; [1*R*-*trans*]-Octahydro-2*H*-quinolizine-1-methanol

NEUROTOXICITY RATING

Clinical

B   Acute encephalopathy (cattle—agitation, seizures, coma)

Members of the genus *Lupinus* (family Leguminosae) serve as food and feed for livestock in agriculturally marginal regions. The herbaceous perennials often grow from a creeping root and may reach 12–30 inches in height. Blue, purple, white, magenta, or bicolored pea-like flowers are seen in early summer and are followed by pea-like pods. Leaves, mature fruit, seeds, and stems are potentially toxic. Some species contain substantial amounts of quinolizidine alkaloids and are considered poisonous. Death from toxic lupins is well documented in livestock. In addition to an intoxication by quinolizidines, poisoning by fungal (*Phomopsis leptostromiformis*) infection, especially with sweet lupins, such as *L. albus* and *angustifolius*, is a potential second cause of toxicosis.

Lupin consumption has been fatal in cattle, goats, horses, and sheep, especially when animals consume large quantities of lupin pods over short periods of time. Acutely intoxicated animals appear irritable and agitated, and develop muscle twitching, seizures, and coma (11). In some, severe dyspnea may develop rapidly. Death results from respiratory paralysis after repeated seizures (7). The clinical picture appears to be species-specific: horses develop respiratory dysfunction, labored convulsions, and trembling; cattle display convulsions, torticollis, and trembling; and in sheep, CNS depression, dyspnea, coma, convulsions, and death occur.

A teratogenic syndrome ("crooked calf disease") has been attributed to maternal ingestion of lupins. Malformations, which are predominantly characterized by arthrogryposis, occurred in cows; the responsible alkaloid is thought to be anagyrine (9,16).

Low-alkaloid lupins are consumed by humans in parts of South America and Asia; there are several reports of lupin toxicity (10). Symptoms appear within hours of ingestion; they include nausea, mydriasis, visual disturbances, ataxia, progressive weakness, coma, and respiratory arrest (8,15). Recovery usually occurs within a day. Oral intake of bitter lupins in a dosage of 11–46 mg/kg of mixed alkaloids was lethal for three adults and induced a serious intoxication in two other individuals. After the oral ingestion of water that was used to remove the bitter taste from lupin seeds, an individual developed an anticholinergic syndrome that subsided spontaneously after 48 h (13).

Quinolizidine alkaloids are held responsible for the toxicity of lupins; the compounds are found in bicyclic, tricyclic, and tetracyclic forms (6,8,14).

The fungus *Phomopsis leptostromiformis* is another cause for intoxications in animals following consumption of lupins. The cyclic hexapeptides phomopsin A and B have been isolated from a fungus culture on lupin seed. If these cultures are administered to experimental animals (sheep, pigs and young rats) (5), signs of toxicity can be produced. Pigs develop hindlimb weakness. Sheep show changes in liver, kidney, adrenal cortex, kidney, and striate muscle. The syndrome is associated with decreased α-tocopherol levels in the liver, but cannot be ameliorated by antioxidants (4). Spongiform pathology in brainstem myelin has been reported; it is uncertain how these findings are causally related to the liver disease (3). Phomopsin inhibits microtubule assembly with an IC_{50} of 2.4 μmol (12). Lupinosis induced by these fungi is primarily a hepatic disease, but also affects muscle (1,2). Subcutaneous injection of selenomethionine and vitamin E is reported to prevent lupinosis-associated myopathy in sheep (17).

REFERENCES

1. Allen JG (1981) An evaluation of lupinosis in cattle in Western Australia. *Aust Vet J* **57**, 212.
2. Allen JG, Dolling MJ, Ellis TM *et al.* (1984) Effects of feeding lupin seed naturally infected with *Phomopsin leptostromiformis* to sheep and pigs. *Aust Vet J* **61**, 178.
3. Allen JG, Nottle FK (1979) Spongy transformation of the brain in sheep with lupinosis. *Vet Rec* **104**, 31.
4. Allen JG, Randall AG (1993) The clinical biochemistry of experimentally produced lupinosis in the sheep. *Aust Vet J* **70**, 283.
5. Culvenor CC, Beck AB, Clark M *et al.* (1977) Isolation of toxic metabolites of *Phomopsis leptostromiformis* responsible for lupinosis. *Aust J Biol Sci* **30**, 269.
6. Gardiner MR (1967) Lupinosis. *Adv Vet Sci* **11**, 85.

7. Gardner CA, Bennetts HW (1956) *The Toxic Plants of Western Australia.* Western Australian Newspapers, Perth.

8. Hatzold T (1982) *Chemische und chemisch-technische Untersuchungen zur Beurteilung von Lupinen (L. mutabilis) als Nahrungsmittel für den Menschen. Schwerpunkt: Lipid- und Alkaloidfraktionen.* Promotion, Justus-Liebig Universität Gießen.

9. Keeler RF (1976) Lupin alkaloids from teratogenic and non-teratogenic lupins. III. Identification of anagyrine as the probable teratogen by feeding trials. *J Toxicol Environ Health* **1**, 87.

10. Keeler RF (1989) Quinolizidine alkaloids in range and grain lupins. In: *Toxicants of Plant Origin. Vol I. Alkaloids.* Cheeke PR ed. CRC Press Inc. Boca Raton, Florida p. 133.

11. Kingsbury JM (1964) *Poisonous Plants of the United States and Canada.* Prentice-Hall, Englewood Cliffs, New Jersey.

12. Li Y, Kobayashi H, Tokiwa Y *et al.* (1992) Interaction of phomopsin A with porcine brain tubulin. Inhibition of tubulin polymerization and binding at a rhizoxin binding site. *Biochem Pharmacol* **43**, 219.

13. Luque MR, Gutierrez-Rave M, Infante MF (1991) Acute poisoning by lupine seed debittering water. *Vet Hum Toxicol* **33**, 265.

14. Petersson DS, Ellis ZL, Harris DJ, Spadek ZE (1987) Acute toxicity of the major alkaloids of cultivated *Lupinus angustifolius* seed to rats. *J Appl Toxicol* **7**, 51.

15. Schmidlin-Meszaros J (1973) Eine Nahrungsmittelvergiftung mit Lupinenbohnen. *Mitt Geb Lebensmitelunters Hyg* **64**, 194.

16. Shupe JL, Binns W, James LF, Keeler RF (1968) A congenital deformity in calves induced by the maternal consumption of lupin. *Aust J Agr Res* **19**, 335.

17. Smith GM, Allen JG (1997) Effectiveness of alpha-tocopherol and selenium supplements in preventing lupinosis-associated myopathy in sheep. *Aust Vet J* **75**, 341.

Lysergide

Arnold E. Merriam

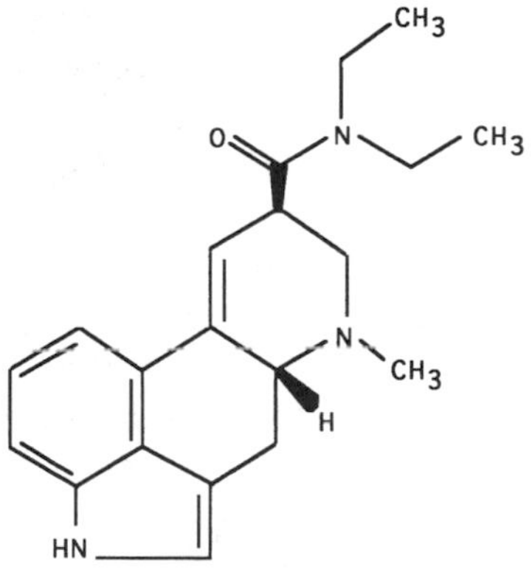

LYSERGIDE
$C_{20}H_{25}N_3O$

9,10-Didehydro-N,N-diethyl-6-methylergoline-8β-carboxamide; LSD

NEUROTOXICITY RATING

Clinical

A   Psychobiological reaction (hallucinations, euphoria)

B   Psychobiological reaction (posthallucinogenic perceptual disorder)

Lysergic acid diethylamide (LSD) is rapidly absorbed after oral administration and is widely distributed. The plasma half-life is 7 min in the mouse, 100 min in the macaque, and about 3 h in man. LSD crosses the blood-brain barrier easily; the target organ is the brain, where it exerts complex interactions with serotonergic and catecholaminergic systems and induces profound alterations in perception, mood, and judgment at a concentration of 0.5 ng/g of brain tissue. LSD metabolites include 2-oxo-LSD and 2-oxo-3-hydroxy-LSD (13). There is no established clinical utility for LSD, although its use was briefly advocated some decades ago as an adjunct to verbal psychotherapy. It has, however, been in continuous illicit use since the 1950s.

Humans on LSD experience mydriasis, increased blood pressure, tachycardia, piloerection, elevated body temperature, tremor, and hyperreflexia—all signs of catecholaminergic stimulation. LSD also induces severe perceptual distortion and hallucinations, predominantly of a visual nature. Alterations of mood are usually of a positive nature, but severe dysphoria and fear can also be precipitated, sometimes in the company of grossly delusional thinking. The effects decline over a period of several hours and usually largely disappear within 12 h.

Animal studies provide abundant evidence that LSD perturbs serotoninergic neurotransmission. Animals may be trained to recognize LSD administration; this learned discrimination can be blocked by the administration of specific 5-HT$_2$ antagonists (12). In rats, LSD administration disrupts bar-press responding; this effect can also be reversed by 5-HT$_2$ antagonists (8). Chronic administration of LSD to rats leads to persistently increased brain serotonin turnover (4) and causes 5-HT$_2$ receptor density to drop, an effect that persists after an 8-day continuous infusion (7).

Evidence from radioligand-binding studies for cortical serotonin-binding sites in rat brain homogenates indicates a correlation of 5-HT$_2$–binding affinity with behavioral measures characteristic of hallucinogens (5). LSD has also been shown to activate 5-HT$_{1c}$ receptors, a subtype structurally and functionally similar to the 5-HT$_2$ subtype, in cultured choroid-plexus epithelial cells (11).

Tolerance to the acute somatic and psychological effects of LSD develops rapidly. In a study of the effects of daily administration of LSD for up to 22 days, human volunteers were given a test dose of 180 mg, followed by a schedule of increasing doses culminating in a final repeat dose of 180 mg. The results were graphically described by the experimenter (6):

> When this dose was given prior to chronic intoxication, the patient became extremely anxious and felt that he was being shocked with electricity. His body seemed to shrink and enlarge. His hands appeared to have extra fingers. People and objects changed size, shape, and color. The walls were a flickering mass of shadows and colors. He felt that he would die or would become permanently insane. Blood pressure was elevated to 60 mm. of mercury; pupils were maximally dilated; knee jerks were very hyperactive; spontaneous tremors of large muscle groups were observed, and ankle clonus could be elicited. After recovery from this severe reaction, the patient wished to drop out of the experiment but, after considerable persuasion, agreed to continue. He was started on 50 mg of LSD once daily, and this dose was increased until he again received 180 mg of LSD on the 22nd day. At this time he had no subjective effects, sat quietly, read, and watched television. His reflex, pupillary, and blood pressure changes were minor.

When LSD ingestion results in an acute toxic psychiatric disturbance, the situation is best managed by the administration of benzodiazepine tranquilizers in a protected and quiet environment until the effects wane.

While numerous cases of prolonged psychotic disorders following LSD ingestion have been reported, the question of whether the psychopathology represents a lasting toxic effect of LSD or, instead, the emergence of another disorder (*e.g.*, schizophrenia), is almost impossible to determine; most cases of persistent psychosis following LSD use have been in young recreational users in whom the ostensible psychiatric toxicity appeared at an age when idiopathic schizophrenia also commonly first manifests itself. Furthermore, premorbid diathesis is difficult to evaluate retrospectively, and the chemical identity of the hallucinogen ingested cannot be conclusively determined. Despite these pitfalls, some have concluded on epidemiological grounds that there is sufficient evidence to indicate that LSD can precipitate persistent psychosis (3). In a comparison of cerebrospinal fluid concentrations of the serotonin metabolite 5-hydroxyindoleacetic acid (5-HIAA) between a group of patients suffering from LSD-induced acute psychosis and a group with non–drug-related psychoses, the former exhibited evidence of diminished central 5-HIAA formation. The differences, which were present prior to and during neuroleptic treatment, provide evidence of a neurotoxic etiology of the psychotic illnesses experienced by the LSD group (2).

The other persistent psychiatric manifestation alleged to result from LSD neurotoxicity is the so-called posthallucinogen perceptual disorder, consisting of recurrent intermittent visual hallucinations lasting many years following cessation of LSD use. These are variously described as geometric visual phenomena, fleeting misperceptions in peripheral areas of the visual fields, color flashes, and afterimagery. Some investigators have found evidence of persistent visual anomalies in past LSD users, including decreased critical flicker-fusion thresholds and abnormal dark adaptation (1).

While the toxic mechanism of LSD is likely related to perturbations of serotonergic neurotransmission, the precise route by which this occurs has not been conclusively identified. Investigators continue to unravel LSD's role as an agonist as well as an antagonist at different serotonin receptor subtypes (9,10), with the aim of better understanding neurotoxic hallucinogenesis.

REFERENCES

1. Abraham HD, Wolf E (1988) Visual function in past users of LSD: Psychophysical findings. *J Abnormal Psychol* 97, 443.
2. Bowers MB (1972) Acute psychosis induced by psychotomimetic drug abuse. *Arch Gen Psychiat* 27, 440.
3. Breakey W, Goodell H, Lorenz P, McHugh R (1974) Hallucinogenic drugs as precipitants of schizophrenia. *Psychol Med* 4, 225.
4. Diaz J, Juttunen MO (1971) Persistent increase in brain serotonin turnover after chronic administration of LSD in the rat. *Science* 174, 62.
5. Glennon RA, Titeler M, McKenney JD (1984) Evidence for 5-HT2 involvement in the mechanism of action of hallucinogenic agents. *Life Sci* 35, 2505.
6. Isbell H, Belleville RE, Fraser HF *et al.* (1956) Studies on lysergic acid diethylamide (LSD-25). *AMA Arch Neurol Psychiat* 76, 468.
7. King W, Ellison G (1989) Long-lasting alterations in behavior and brain neurochemistry following continuous

low-level LSD administration. *Pharmacol Biochem Behav* **33**, 69.

8. Mokler DJ, Stoudt KW, Rech RH (1985) The 5HT2 antagonist pirenperone reverses disruption of FR-40 by hallucinogenic drugs. *Pharmacol Biochem Behav* **22**, 677.

9. Pierce PA, Peroutka SJ (1990) Antagonist properties of d-LSD at 5-hydroxytryptamine2 receptors. *Neuropsychopharmacology* **3**, 503.

10. Sadzot B, Baraban JM, Glennon RA *et al.* (1989) Hallucinogenic drug interactions at human brain 5-HT₂ receptors: Implications for treating LSD-induced hallucinogenesis. *Psychopharmacology* **98**, 495.

11. Sanders-Bush E, Breeding M (1991) Choroid plexus epithelial cells in primary culture: A model of 5-HT$_{1c}$ receptor activation by hallucinogenic drugs. *Psychopharmacology* **105**, 340.

12. Winter JC, Rabin RA (1988) Interactions between serotonergic agonists and antagonists in rats trained with LSD as a discriminative stimulus. *Pharmacol Biochem Behav* **30**, 617.

13. Verstraete AG, Van de Velde EJ (1999) 2-Oxo-3-hydroxy-LSD: an important LSD metabolite? *Acta Clin Belg Suppl* **1**, 94.

Lysolecithin

Thomas W. Bouldin

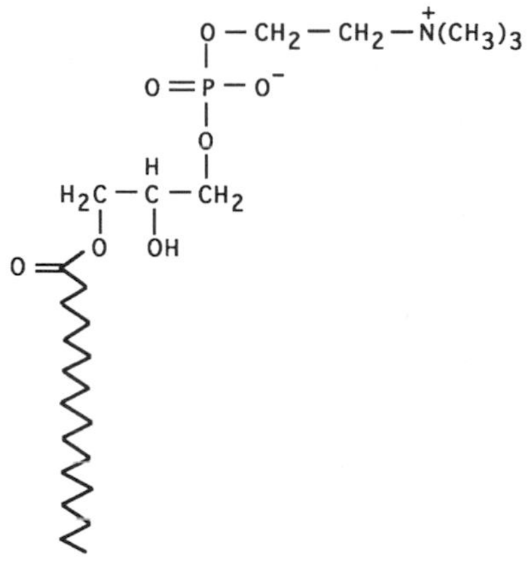

LYSOLECITHIN
C$_{26}$H$_{54}$NO$_7$P

Lysophosphatidyl choline; LPC

NEUROTOXICITY RATING

Experimental

A CNS demyelination (local injection)

A PNS demyelination (local injection)

Lysolecithin (LPC) is the lysophosphatide produced when phospholipase A₂ catalyzes the hydrolysis of phosphatidyl choline (lecithin). Phospholipase A₂ and LPC are normally found in trace amounts within nerve tissue (15). LPC is a potent natural detergent and has a wide variety of membrane-altering properties, including cytolysis (22). It completely solubilizes brain myelin *in vitro* and causes demyelination *in vivo* when injected into the white matter of the

CNS or into peripheral nerve (6,10,12). The demyelination is rapid and self-limited, and is quickly followed by remyelination (13,20). These synchronized phases of demyelination and remyelination have made LPC a popular agent for producing experimental models of demyelination and remyelination in the CNS and PNS. There are no recorded cases of toxicity in humans from exogenously derived LPC, but it has been suggested that endogenously derived LPC may have a role in the pathogenesis of a number of disease states (8,22).

The absorption, distribution, and excretion of exogenously derived LPC are unknown. The concentration of LPC normally present in nerve tissue is controlled by the phosphatidyl–choline deacylation/lysophosphatidyl–choline reacylation cycle and by lysophosphatidyl–choline deacylation (15). It has been suggested these enzyme systems also neutralize exogenously derived LPC (8,12). Cell membranes are the primary target of LPC; low concentrations of LPC cause a variety of membrane perturbations ranging from altered ionic permeability and activation of membrane-bound enzymes, to cytolysis (8,22). The CNS and PNS are the organs principally involved when LPC is administered to laboratory animals (10,12). LPC-induced hemolysis of erythrocytes has been a principal model for *in vitro* studies (22).

Demyelination begins within 30 min after 0.2 μl of a 1% solution of LPC is injected into mouse peripheral nerve *in vivo* (12). Myelin breakdown starts at Schmidt-Lanterman incisures and adjacent to nodes of Ranvier, and then spreads to involve the entire internode (9,12). The process typically affects whole internodes, and only a small percentage of fibers shows demyelination restricted to paranodal regions (20). The myelin undergoes vesicular degeneration morphologically, with the sheath splitting primarily at the intraperiod lines (12). Myelin breakdown products are composed initially of strands of 4 to 6 nm repeat material; later, this material breaks down into disorganized lamellated fragments (12). Axons are completely demyelinated within 2–4 days (5,9,12); myelin debris is phagocytosed by infiltrating macrophages (5,9,21). Despite the intense breakdown of myelin sheaths, supporting Schwann cells show no evidence of cell injury or necrosis during the phase of demyelination (9,12). Axons develop LPC-induced spontaneous evoked action potentials and depolarization immediately after exposure, but do not show morphological abnormalities during the demyelinating process (20). Only a very small number of myelinated fibers shows wallerian-type axonal degeneration; this pathological change cannot be attributed entirely to the trauma of intraneural injection, because rare degenerating fibers are also found in models in which LPC has been topically applied to the nerve (21). One rat study suggests that LPC also causes degeneration of unmyelinated axons (16). Schwann cell proliferation begins 2–3 days after onset of demyelination, and Schwann cells reach maximum numbers between days 15 and 25 (14). Proliferating Schwann cells arise from demyelinating internodes and from unmyelinated fibers (9). PNS remyelination begins as early as 6 days after injection in the rat, 7 days in the mouse, and 12 days in the frog (5,9,19). As with other models of primary demyelination and remyelination, short internodal lengths characterize regions of restored myelin (5).

LPC produces demyelination in the CNS when injected into brain or spinal cord *in vivo* (1,10). The demyelinating process is similar to that in the PNS, except for greater destruction of glial cells and axons and later onset of remyelination (1,2,8). In cats, 2.0–2.5 μl of a 1% solution of LPC produced degeneration of glial cells and myelin 30 min after intraspinal injection (2). By 24 h, there were many completely demyelinated axons and a few axons undergoing wallerian-type axonal degeneration. Seven days after injection, the lesion showed demyelinated axons, myelin-debris-filled macrophages, and an absence of astrocytes and oligodendrocytes in the center of the lesion. A similar progression of LPC-induced demyelination is found in the rat, except that axonal degeneration is less common (1,2). Remyelinated fibers are numerous by 1 month after injection; axons in the center of the lesion are myelinated by oligodendrocytes while those at the periphery are ensheathed by Schwann cells (1,2). Remyelinated internodes have foreshortened internodal lengths, like their counterparts in the PNS (2).

LPC has been used to produce demyelination of CNS and PNS tissue *in vitro* (3,17). Remyelination occurs in cultured nervous system tissue following LPC-induced demyelination (18).

LPC produces demyelination in a wide range of species, including frog, mouse, rat, rabbit, cat, and monkey (1–5,7,9–16,19–21). There does not appear to be a hierarchy of vulnerability to LPC-induced demyelination among different species, although species-specific variations in the amount of associated axonal degeneration and time of onset of remyelination are reported (2,5). Advanced age is associated with impaired remyelination in the CNS of the rat (7).

The pathogenesis of LPC-induced demyelination is incompletely known. Several lines of evidence suggest demyelination is not simply due to the potent detergent properties of LPC (8,15). Related molecules with much less detergent action also produce demyelination (15); the LPC molecule, not its products of catabolism, appears to be responsible for demyelination (15). It has been speculated that injection of LPC triggers a sequence of metabolic events at the level of the cell membrane (8). These events may include activation of phospholipase A_2 and increased permeability of the Schwann cell membrane to Ca^{2+} (8).

REFERENCES

1. Blakemore WF (1976) Invasion of Schwann cells into the spinal cord of the rat following local injections of lysolecithin. *Neuropathol Appl Neurobiol* 2, 21.
2. Blakemore WF, Eames RA, Smith KJ et al. (1977) Remyelination in the spinal cord of the cat following intraspinal injections of lysolecithin. *J Neurol Sci* 33, 31.
3. Chiu SY, Schwarz W (1987) Sodium and potassium currents in acutely demyelinated internodes of rabbit sciatic nerves. *J Physiol* 391, 631.
4. Dousset V, Brochet B, Vital A et al. (1995) Lysolecithin-induced demyelination in primates: Preliminary *in vivo* study with MR and magnetization transfer. *Amer J Neuroradiol* 16, 225.
5. Dugandzija-Novakovic S, Koszowski AG, Levinson SR, Shager P (1995) Clustering of Na$^+$ channels and node of Ranvier formation in remyelinating axons. *J Neurosci* 15, 492.
6. Gent WLG, Gregson NA, Gammack DB, Raper JH (1964) The lipid protein unit in myelin. *Nature* 204, 553.
7. Gibson J, Blakemore WF (1993) Failure of remyelination in areas of demyelination produced in the spinal cord of old rats. *Neuropathol Appl Neurobiol* 19, 173.
8. Gregson NA (1989) Lysolipids and membrane damage: Lysolecithin and its interaction with myelin. *Biochem Soc Trans* 17, 280.
9. Griffin JW, Stocks EA, Fahnestock K et al. (1990) Schwann cell proliferation following lysolecithin-induced demyelination. *J Neurocytol* 19, 367.

10. Hall SM (1972) The effect of injections of lysophosphatidylcholine into white matter of the adult mouse spinal cord. *J Cell Sci* **10**, 535.

11. Hall SM (1984) The effects of multiple sequential episodes of demyelination in the sciatic nerve of the mouse. *Neuropathol Appl Neurobiol* **10**, 461.

12. Hall SM, Gregson NA (1971) The *in vivo* and ultrastructural effects of injection of lysophosphatidylcholine into myelinated peripheral nerve fibers of the adult mouse. *J Cell Sci* **9**, 769.

13. Hall SM, Gregson NA (1974) The effects of mitomycin C on remyelination in the peripheral nervous system. *Nature* **252**, 303.

14. Hall SM, Gregson NA (1975) The effects of mitomycin C on the process of remyelination in the mammalian peripheral nervous system. *Neuropathol Appl Neurobiol* **1**, 149.

15. Low PA, Schmelzer JD, Yao JK *et al.* (1983) Structural specificity in demyelination induced by lysophospholipids. *Biochim Biophys Acta* **754**, 298.

16. Mitchell J, Caren CA (1982) Degeneration of non-myelinated axons in the rat sciatic nerve following lysolecithin injection. *Acta Neuropathol* **56**, 187.

17. Morrison LR, Zamecnick PC (1950) Experimental demyelination by means of enzymes, especially the toxin of *Clostridium welchii. Arch Neurol Psychiat* **63**, 367.

18. Périer O (1965) Démyélination de cultures de tissu nerveux central par la lysolécithine. *Acta Neurol Psychiat Belg* **65**, 78.

19. Shrager P (1988) Ionic channels and signal conduction in single remyelinating frog nerve fibres. *J Physiol* **88**, 695.

20. Smith KJ, Hall SM (1980) Nerve conduction during peripheral demyelination and remyelination. *J Neurol Sci* **48**, 201.

21. Stoll G, Li CY, Trapp BD, Griffin JW (1993) Expression of NGF- receptors during immune-mediated and lysolecithin-induced demyelination of the peripheral nervous system. *J Neurocytol* **22**, 1022.

22. Weltzien HU (1979) Cytolytic and membrane-perturbing properties of lysophosphatidylcholine. *Biochim Biophys Acta* **559**, 259.

Maitotoxin

Albert C. Ludolph

NEUROTOXICITY RATING

Clinical

A Ion channel syndrome

Experimental

A Ion channel dysfunction

Ciguatoxin, scaritoxin, and maitotoxin (MTX) are the marine compounds held responsible for ciguatera poisoning, although the role of MTX is disputed (8). Like ciguatoxin, MTX is produced by the marine dinoflagellate *Gambierdiscus toxicus*, and accumulates in the marine food chain in fish in tropical coral reefs. It is infrequently detected in tropical fish and is likely not as important clinically as ciguatoxin. Different strains of the dinoflagellate produce distinct maitotoxins with specific physiological effects (5). In contrast to ciguatoxin, the polyether and highly polar substance MTX (MW of the disodium salt, 3424) (16) is soluble in water, unlikely to cross cellular membranes, and often detected in herbivorous (algae-eating) fish. The name maitotoxin is derived from the Tahitian name of the fish (*maito* for surgeon fish, *Ctenochaetus striatus*) from which this chemical was originally isolated (15). Its structure is partly elucidated; it contains a chain with more than 100 carbons, many small ether rings, 21 methyl groups, numerous tertiary amine groups, two sulfate esters, and a basic nitrogen (4). Fish harboring the toxin do not become ill.

When injected intraperitoneally into mice, the LD_{50} of MTX is as low as 0.13 μg/kg body weight. Signs of murine poisoning are similar to those produced by ciguatoxin; they include diarrhea, reduced locomotor activity, convulsions, and hypothermia. MTX acts on many cell types, including muscle cells and neurons. MTX dose-dependently increases Ca^{2+} entry into a wide range of cultured cells at concentrations as low as 100 pM to 30 nM; however, the precise mechanism of Ca^{2+} influx is controversial and may differ among cell types (3,4,9,12,14). The relative contribution of L-type and N-type voltage-gated Ca^{2+} channels and the mobilization of Ca^{2+} from intracellular stores to the consistent, large intracellular increase of Ca^{2+} concentration, is unknown (9,12,14). Other biological, largely Ca^{2+}-dependent effects are stimulation of neurotransmitter and hormone release, stimulation of phosphoinositide breakdown; and contraction of smooth, cardiac, and skeletal muscle (4).

In striatal neurons, MTX stimulates calcium influx and release of γ-aminobutyric acid (GABA). Ca^{2+} only incompletely abolishes the effect on GABA, indicating that transmitter release is not solely calcium-dependent (11). If 1 mmol extracellular Ca^{2+} ions are present in rat brain synaptosomal preparations, MTX causes an increase of intracellular Ca^{2+} levels and concentration-dependently depolarizes synaptosomal membranes; this is unaffected by the presence of tetrodotoxin (13). MTX also increases permeability of Ca^{2+} channels at presynaptic terminals at the neuromuscular junction, thereby increasing presynaptic acetylcholine release; this effect can be delayed by tetrodotoxin, which suggests the involvement of voltage-dependent Na^+ channels (6).

Since MTX may be a component of the acute and chronic symptomatology of human ciguatera poisoning, nifedipine is recommended to counteract the effects of maitotoxin (2,7,10). However, since MTX might interact with opiates, opiate treatment of ciguatera poisoning is avoided (1).

REFERENCES

1. Brown CK, Shepherd SM (1992) Marine trauma, envenomations, and intoxications. *Emerg Med Clin N Amer* 10, 385.
2. Calvert GM, Hryhorczuk DO, Leikin JB (1987) Treatment of ciguatera fish poisoning with amitriptyline and nifedipine. *Clin Toxicol* 25, 423.
3. Glossmann H, Striessnig J (1990) Molecular properties of calcium channels. *Rev Physiol Biochem Pharmacol* 114, 1.
4. Gusovsky F, Daly JW (1990) Maitotoxin: A unique pharmacological tool for research on calcium-dependent mechanisms. *Biochem Pharmacol* 39, 1633.
5. Holmes MJ, Lewis RJ (1994) Purification and characterisation of large and small maitotoxins from cultured *Gambierdiscus toxicus*. *Nat Toxins* 2, 64.
6. Kim YI, Login IS, Yasumoto T (1985) Maitotoxin activates quantal transmitter release at the neuromuscular junction: Evidence for elevated intraterminal Ca^{2+} in the motor nerve terminal. *Brain Res* 346, 357.
7. Lange WR, Snyder FR, Fudala PJ (1992) Travel and ciguatera fish poisoning. *Arch Intern Med* 152, 2049.
8. Lewis RJ, Holmes MJ (1993) Origin and transfer of toxins involved in ciguatera. *Comp Biochem Physiol C* 106, 615.
9. Meucci O, Grimaldi M, Scorziello A *et al.* (1992) Maitotoxin-induced intracellular calcium rise in PC12 cells: Involvement of dihydropyridine-sensitive and omega-conotoxin-sensitive calcium channels and phosphoinositide breakdown. *J Neurochem* 59, 679.
10. Miller DM (1991) *Ciguatera Seafood Toxins*. CRC Press, Boca Raton, Florida.
11. Pin J-P, Yasumoto T, Bockaert J (1988) Maitotoxin-evoked gamma-aminobutyric acid release is due not only to opening of calcium channels. *J Neurochem* 50, 1227.

12. Soergel DG, Yasumoto T, Daly JW, Gusovsky F (1992) Maitotoxin effects are blocked by SK&F 96365, an inhibitor of receptor-mediated calcium entry. *Mol Pharmacol* **41**, 487.

13. Taglialatella M, Canzoniero LM, Fatatis A *et al.* (1990) Effect of maitotoxin on cytosolic Ca^{2+} levels and membrane potential in purified rat brain synaptosomes. *Biochim Biophys Acta* **1026**, 126.

14. Takahashi M, Tatsumi M, Ohizumi Y, Yasumoto T (1983) Calcium channel-activating function of maitotoxin, the most potent marine toxin known, in clonal rat pheochromocytoma cells. *J Biol Chem* **258**, 10944.

15. Yasumoto T, Hashimoto Y, Bagnis R *et al.* (1971) Marine toxins from the Pacific. IX. Toxicity of surgeon fishes. *Bull Jap Soc Sci Fisheries* **37**, 724.

16. Yokoyoma A, Murata M, Oshima Y *et al.* (1988) Some chemical properties of maitotoxin, a putative calcium channel agonist isolated from a marine dinoflagellate. *J Biochem* **104**, 184.

Mamba Snake Venom

Albert C. Ludolph

NEUROTOXICITY RATING

Clinical

A Neuromuscular transmission syndrome

Experimental

A Muscarinic and nicotinic receptor blockade

Mamba snake venom (*Dendroaspis angusticeps, polylepis, viridis, jamesoni*) contains a mixture of neurotoxic compounds including postsynaptic α-neurotoxins, dendrotoxins, fasciculins, and muscarinic toxins (2). Effects at the neuromuscular junction include acetylcholinesterase inhibition (fasciculins) and increased presynaptic release of acetylcholine (dendrotoxins); together with the high acetylcholine content of mamba toxin (6–24 mg/g), these effects are synergistic and enhance neurotoxicity and lethality (4,5). Some of these toxins are discussed elsewhere (*see* Fasciculins, Dendrotoxin, this volume).

Toxins that facilitate neuromuscular transmission are a characteristic component of mamba venom. The four known fasciculins (*see* Fasciculins, this volume) bind to a peripheral regulatory anionic site of acetylcholinesterase in a noncompetitive and irreversible manner (2). The dendrotoxins comprise the second group of facilitatory neurotoxins and are present in most mamba venoms (with the exception of *Dendroaspis jamesoni*); they inhibit voltage-dependent K^+ channels in motor nerve terminals and facilitate acetylcholine release at the neuromuscular junction (2,5). Postsynaptic toxins present in mamba venom bind to and block nicotinic acetylcholine receptors. The muscarinic toxins present in mamba venom are small (7 kDa) proteins that selectively bind to muscarinic cholinergic receptors and may constitute up to 1% of the venom protein (1,3).

About twelve muscarinic toxins have been isolated. M1 toxin binds noncompetitively and with high affinity to the M_1 muscarinic receptor subtype. MTx1 and MTx2 show high affinity for both muscarinic M_1 and M_3 receptors; little is known about the receptor selectivity of MTx3 and MTx4. Dpα and Dpβ are also muscarinic agonists displaying similiar affinity for both the M_1 and M_2 receptor subtypes. The last two agonists, DpMTx and DvMTX, are selective muscarinic agonists present in the venom of some mamba species; these agonists also show affinity for the M_1 muscarinic receptor subtype.

Clinically, mamba bites may not provoke a major local reaction. If neurotoxins are injected by the bite, clinical symptoms appear within minutes to hours. Clinical signs of impairment of neuromuscular transmission (ptosis, ophthalmoplegia, bulbar symptoms, or generalized weakness) dictate administration of antivenin.

REFERENCES

1. Adem A, Karlsson E (1985) Mamba venom toxins that bind to muscarinic cholinergic receptors. *Toxicon* **23**, 551.

2. Hawgood B, Bon C (1991) Snake venom presynaptic toxins. In: *Handbook of Natural Toxins. Vol 5. Reptile Venoms and Toxins.* Tu AT ed. Marcel Dekker, New York p. 3.

3. Jerusalinsky D, Harvey AL (1994) Toxins from mamba venoms: Small proteins with selectivities for different subtypes of muscarinic acetylcholine receptors. *TIPS* **15**, 424.

4. Karlsson E, Cervenansky, Jolkkonen M (1990) Chemistry of mamba toxins. *Toxicon* **28**, 154.

5. Tu AT (1994) Neurotoxins from snake venoms. In: *Handbook of Neurotoxicology.* Chang LW, Dyer RS eds. Marcel Dekker, New York p. 637.

Mandaratoxin

Albert C. Ludolph

NEUROTOXICITY RATING

Experimental

A   Neuromuscular transmission syndrome (lobster)

Mandaratoxin (MDTX) is a basic, single-chain protein from the hornet (*Vespa mandarinia*) with a MW of *ca.* 20,000 (1). MDTX lacks enzymatic activity and is not hemolytic. In lobster, nanomolar concentrations of the heat-labile compound irreversibly blocks the excitatory post-synaptic potential of the neuromuscular junction. This effect is observed with the resting conductance of the post-synaptic membrane remaining unchanged; in contrast, sodium currents of the presynaptic nerve fiber are reduced (1).

REFERENCES

1. Abe T, Kawai N, Niwa A (1982) Purification and properties of a presynaptically acting neurotoxin, mandaratoxin, from hornet (*Vespa mandarinia*). *Biochemistry* **21**, 1693.

Manganese

Nai-Shin Chu
Chin-Chang Huang
Donald B. Calne

NEUROTOXICITY RATING

Clinical

A   Extrapyramidal syndrome (parkinsonism)

Experimental

A   Dopamine depletion in striatum

A   Extrapyramidal dysfunction (chorea, parkinsonism)

Manganese (Mn), recognized as an element in 1771 by the Swedish chemist Scheele, is the twelfth most abundant element in the earth's crust. Eight million tons of Mn are extracted annually. Mn dioxide is the most common form found in Mn-rich ore, and over 90% of Mn dioxide is used in the production of ferromanganese alloys and other industrial products. The industrial use of Mn is mainly in steelmaking and as an alloying element (21). Mn dioxide is an essential part of a dry-cell battery, the second most important use for Mn. Manganese compounds are also used in the production of artificial flavors and fragrances, paints, glazes, varnishes, chemicals for coloring glasses and tiles, and electronic parts. As a powerful oxidizing agent, potassium permanganate is used in purifying drinking water, treating waste water, and removing waste odor. A widely used agricultural fungicide, maneb, contains Mn. Another important application for Mn is an organic compound, methylcyclopentadienyl manganese tricarbonyl, used as an octane booster and antiknock agent in gasoline (7).

Mn is an essential trace element in the metabolism of all living organisms including humans (21). It is a natural component of most foods. High concentrations of Mn are present in nuts, grains, and beverages such as tea. Estimation of the daily requirement of Mn varies considerably, ranging from 0.035 mg/kg to 3.5 mg/kg (21). Mn deficiency in humans has not been reported.

Excessive exposure to Mn, mainly occupational *via* inhalation, may cause clinical disorders affecting primarily the CNS and the lungs (11,17,20,21). Although there is an increased incidence of pneumonia, bronchitis, and nonspecific pulmonary disease with impaired ventilatory function, the major target of Mn toxicity is the CNS. Manganism, or manganese poisoning, was not recognized until 1837, when a peculiar syndrome was reported in five miners working in a manganese ore-crushing plant in France (8). These miners exhibited limb tremor, muscle weakness, whispering speech, salivation, and a bent posture while walking. This parkinsonian-like "manganese crusher's disease" appeared only 20 years after publication of Parkinson's classic paper "*An Essay on Shaking Palsy.*" Almost a century passed before a relationship was established between occupational exposure, clinical syndrome, and basal ganglia pathology (9). Subsequently, several hundred cases of chronic Mn poisoning were reported not only from miners but also from industrial workers (17). Rare cases have occurred in agricultural workers exposed to maneb, patients receiving long-term total parenteral nutrition, persons drinking contaminated well water, and one case following ingestion of potassium permanganate solution mistakenly given by a pharmacist (6,17). With improved working conditions and enforced protective measures, chronic manganism is rare nowadays.

The World Health Organization has tentatively recommended a Time-Weighted Average (TWA) occupational exposure limit of 0.3 mg/m³ for respirable particles (25). The U.S. National Institute of Occupational Safety and Hygiene recommends a TWA exposure limit of 1 mg/m³. The time-weighted Threshold Limit Value currently adopted by the American Conference of Governmental Industrial Hygienists is 5 mg/m³; reduction to 0.2 mg/m³ is under consideration (1). These values will probably need to be modified as more epidemiological studies become available.

General Toxicology

Although gastrointestinal absorption from foods is the main route of Mn intake, pulmonary absorption of Mn dust is the main route of human loading leading to manganism. For pulmonary absorption, the size of Mn dust particles is critical; particles of 2–4 μm are maximally absorbed (16). Gastrointestinal absorption of Mn occurs in the small intestine; the metal utilizes the same carrier system as iron. Three to five per cent of ingested Mn is absorbed (21).

Mn has several valence states; divalent and trivalent Mn are biologically most active (21). Once Mn is absorbed into the circulation, Mn^{2+} is bound to plasma α_2-macroglobulin, while Mn^{3+} is bound to transferrin. Mn^{2+} is transformed to Mn^{3+} in the liver, where approximately 97% of Mn is cleared and excreted into the bile prior to its systemic circulation. The half-time of this clearance is 1–2 min. Absorbed Mn is rapidly distributed mainly to the liver, pancreas, and kidney (17). A small amount of Mn is distributed to the brain, muscle, and bone. Within the CNS, Mn is highly concentrated in the striatum, particularly the globus pallidus (17).

Metabolic studies using radioactive tracers have revealed that accelerated excretion of Mn associated with an overload and a higher turnover rate of Mn is found only in healthy working miners with current exposure, but not in normal control subjects nor in patients with the neurological syndrome who were no longer working with Mn (17). These findings suggest that high tissue concentrations of Mn are linked to recent exposure to Mn but not necessarily to neurological disease. This conclusion accords with autopsy findings showing that the overall concentration of Mn in the brain is not elevated in patients with chronic Mn poisoning (26). On the other hand, recent magnetic resonance imaging (MRI) studies on Mn-intoxicated humans and monkeys with neurological signs have shown an increased Mn content in the basal ganglia. The presumed accumulation of Mn in this region decreased or disappeared after cessation of exposure (10,18).

Animal Studies

In 1955, investigators demonstrated that Mn accumulated preferentially in mitochondria and suggested that Mn neurotoxicity is due to an impairment of oxidative metabolism (16). In the brain, Mn accumulates preferentially in the mitochondrial fraction of the rat striatum. Activity of brain succinate dehydrogenase and adenosine triphophatase is inhibited in Mn-treated rats. Monkeys treated with Mn showed a depletion of dopamine in the striatum and more than a tenfold increase in brain content of Mn, with the highest content found in the globus pallidus and putamen. Severe neuronal loss and gliosis are also observed mainly in the globus pallidus. Injection of Mn into one caudate in rats results in predominantly ipsilateral turning, and bilateral injection produces severe bradykinesia (3). Long-term intoxication in monkeys has been shown to produce choreic or choreoathetoid types of movement, tremor, clumsiness of movement, rigidity, and ataxia (3). A recent experimental animal study has demonstrated that repeated systemic administration of Mn chloride to primates causes a parkinsonian syndrome. Histopathological findings in these animals included gliosis and mineralization (iron, aluminum) of globus pallidus and substantia nigra, without depletion of neurons (19). Thus, Mn-induced parkinsonism spares the nigrostriatal pathways and can be distinguished from Parkinson's disease by clinical findings and lack of dopa responsiveness.

Mn, injected into the rat striatum, reduces concentrations of dopamine, γ-aminobutyric acid (GABA), and substance P, and produces lesions similar to those produced by injection of a N-methyl-D-aspartate (NMDA) excitotoxin (4); lesions are prevented by the NMDA antagonist MK-801. Thus, Mn neurotoxicity involves a NMDA receptor-mediated process presumably by impairing oxidative energy metabolism.

In Vitro Studies

Mn is reported to inhibit synaptosomal uptake of dopamine, norepinephrine, serotonin, glutamate, and GABA (2). Mn activates Ca^{2+} influx and inhibits Ca^{2+} efflux from brain mitochondria. Mn has a role as an enzyme cofactor in mitochondrial superoxide dismutase, and mitochondria have an active system to concentrate Mn (2). Mn also greatly enhances the oxidation of dopamine to its semiquinone and quinone. This process may generate hydrogen peroxide when dopamine is being oxidized *via* monoamine oxidase.

Human Studies

Most published cases of human manganism are due to exposure to MnO_2 (6). Human manganism is well documented, but there is a slightly different clinical presentation between miners and industrial workers (17).

The onset of manganism is usually insidious but may be acute or subacute following exposure to Mn dust for several months to several years, depending upon the level of exposure, size of Mn particles, and individual susceptibility (17). Initial symptoms are often nonspecific and may include asthenia, restlessness, lumbago, muscle stiffness or cramp, apathy, anorexia, somnolence, and disturbed sexual activity. In miners, psychomotor excitement may be the presenting symptom; this is characterized by compulsive acts, delusions, and hallucinations, and is referred to as "*locura manganica*," manganese madness, in the mining villages of northern Chile.

This general or psychiatric initial phase is followed in a few months by the appearance of progressive extrapyramidal symptoms including hypokinesia, fixed gaze, masked face, monotonous speech, clumsiness of movement, loss of dexterity, micrographia, tremor, dystonia, abnormal gait, and postural instability (6,17). Inability to walk backward because of severe retropulsion is usually quite prominent. Some patients have a "cock gait," with a tendency to walk on the metatarsophalangeal joints with slight elevation of arms. While tremor at rest is unusual, a fine postural hand tremor and a tremor of the tongue and lips are common. Although festination may be seen, a stamping gait is more common. When gait disturbance and postural instability are severe, patients may resort to walking aids or be confined to a wheelchair.

Neurological manifestations of intoxication may become permanently established within 1–2 years following clinical onset of disease. Previous reports are unclear as to whether established cases remain stationary, improve with time, or progress slowly after cessation of exposure. A recent long-term follow-up on five well-documented cases of manganism indicates an overall progression of symptoms (14). Gait difficulty, postural instability, dystonia, dexterity, writing, and speech tend to worsen while tremor and rigidity tend to improve. One report describes a late-life movement disorder in miners who were asymptomatic while exposed 5 years previously (12).

The neuropathological hallmark of human manganism is degeneration of the basal ganglia (9,26), particularly the globus pallidus, with relative sparing of the substantia ni-

gra. In the pallidum, the median segment is preferentially damaged (9). Positron emission tomography (PET) scans have shown normal fluorodopa uptake *unlike* the reduction of uptake in patients with Parkinson's disease; this suggests the presence of intact dopaminergic nigrostriatal projections in manganism (24). PET studies with the D_2 receptor ligand raclopride suggest some reduction in raclopride uptake (22). These findings are in accord with the major pathology being in the striatum, involving structures downstream from the dopaminergic nerve endings.

Deposition of Mn, usually asymptomatic, appears in MRI examinations of the striatum of patients with cirrhosis of the liver (23). Chronic hepatic encephalopathy with elevated blood levels of Mn and pallidal MRI hyperintensity is thought to be related to Mn intoxication (13). Furthermore, extrapyramidal and psychiatric symptoms in chronic hepatic encephalopathy bear some similarities to manganism. The efficacy of treating human manganism with edetic acid, L-dopa, 5-hydroxytryptophan, and para-aminosalicylic acid is difficult to ascertain mainly due to a lack of controlled studies and long-term follow-up. Response to L-dopa is at best mild to moderate and transient (14). Noticeable in long-term L-dopa therapy is an absence of side effects such as dyskinesia, on-off phenomenon, and mental changes (14). Other antiparkinsonian drugs including trihexyl phenidyl, bromocriptine, and amantadine are also ineffective. A double-blind, placebo-controlled study further demonstrated L-dopa failure in manganism (15).

Toxic Mechanisms

The primary mechanism of Mn neurotoxicity is unknown. Perhaps the most important and yet still unresolved issue is the kinetic mechanism that determines the regional distribution of Mn in the CNS (1,5). Such mechanisms may have a central role in the pathogenesis of manganism and other metal-accumulation diseases, such as Hallervorden-Spatz disease and Wilson's disease, because the patterns of regional accumulation of metals and clinical features are strikingly similar among these three clinical conditions.

MRI studies on patients and monkeys currently exposed to Mn for weeks to months showed preferential uptake of Mn in globus pallidus and to a lesser extent in putamen, subthalamus, and midbrain tegmentum (10,18). The abnormal signal intensities from these areas decrease or subside after cessation of Mn administration (10,18). The normal brain content of Mn in patients with manganism suggests that permanent parkinsonism from Mn intoxication may be the sequela of the initial phase of Mn intoxication. In animal studies, an increase of Mn levels in the basal ganglia is associated with a decrease in dopamine concentration, suggesting a displacement of dopamine from its storage sites by Mn, followed by a decrease in the rate of dopamine synthesis possibly by a reduction in cofactor level (2,3).

Why the pallidum is selectively vulnerable to Mn is unknown. Several mechanisms of Mn neuronal toxicity have been proposed (2,4): (a) Mn enhances the formation of reactive oxygen species (*e.g.*, superoxide, hydroxyl radical, hydrogen peroxide, and quinones); (b) Mn causes a decrease in tissue levels of protective thiol; (c) Mn decreases glutathione peroxidase and catalase contents; (d) Mn generates high-valence Mn species that have direct toxicity on neuronal membranes; and (e) Mn impairs oxidative metabolism resulting in NMDA receptor-mediated excitotoxicity. These actions of Mn presumably may generate significant oxidative stress leading to neuronal death.

REFERENCES

1. American Conference of Governmental Industrial Hygienists (ACGIH) (1992) Threshold limit values for chemical substances and physical agents and biological exposure indices. ACGIH, Cincinnati.

2. Aschner M, Aschner JL (1991) Manganese neurotoxicity: Cellular effects and blood-brain barrier transport. *Neurosci Biobehav Rev* **15**, 333.

3. Barbeau A (1984) Manganese and extrapyramidal disorders. *Neurotoxicology* **5**, 13.

4. Brouillet EP, Shinobu L, McGarvey U *et al.* (1993) Manganese injection into the rat striatum produces excitotoxic lesions by impairing energy metabolism. *Exp Neurol* **120**, 89.

5. Calne DB, Chu NS, Huang CC *et al.* (1994) Manganism and idiopathic parkinsonism: Similarities and differences. *Neurology* **44**, 1583.

6. Chu NS, Olanow CW, Calne DB (1995) Manganese neurotoxicity. In: *Handbook of Neurotoxicology.* Chang LW, Deyer RS eds, Marcel Dekker, New York p. 91.

7. Cooper WC (1984) The health implications of increased manganese in the environment resulting from the combustion of fuel additives: A review of the literature. *J Toxicol Environ Health* **14**, 23.

8. Couper J (1837) On the effects of black oxide of manganese when inhaled into the lungs. *Brit Ann Med Pharmacol* **1**, 41.

9. Edsall DL, Wilbur FP, Drinker CK (1919) The occurrence, course and prevention of chronic manganese poisoning. *J Ind Hyg* **1**, 183.

10. Ejima A, Imamura T, Nakamura S *et al.* (1992) Manganese intoxication during total parenteral nutrition. *Lancet* **2**, 426.

11. Feldman RG (1994) Manganese. In: *Handbook of Clinical Neurology. Vol 64.* Vinken PJ, Bruyn GW eds. *Intoxications of the Nervous System. Pt 1.* de Wolff FA ed. Elsevier Science BV, Amsterdam p. 303.

12. Hauser RA, Zesiewicz TA, Rosemurgy AS *et al.* (1994) Manganese intoxication and chronic liver failure. *Ann Neurol* **36**, 871.

13. Hochberg F, Miller G, Valenzuela R *et al.* (1996) Late motor deficits in Chilean manganese miners: A blinded control study. *Neurology* **47**, 788.

14. Huang CC, Lu CS, Chu NS *et al.* (1993) Progression after chronic manganese exposure. *Neurology* **43**, 1479.

15. Lu CS, Huang CC, Chu NS, Calne DB (1994) Levodopa failure in chronic manganism. *Neurology* **44**, 1660.

16. Maynard LS, Cotzias GC (1955) The partition of manganese among organs and intracellular organelles of the rat. *J Biochem Chem* **214**, 489.

17. Mena I (1979) Manganese poisoning. In: *Handbook of Clinical Neurology. Vol 36.* Vinken PJ, Bruyn GW eds. Elsevier/North Holland, Amsterdam p. 217.

18. Newland MC, Ceckler TL, Kordower JH *et al.* (1989) Visualizing manganese in the primate basal ganglia with magnetic resonance imaging. *Exp Neurol* **106**, 251.

19. Olanow MD, Good PF, Shinotoh H *et al.* (1996) Manganese intoxication in the rhesus monkey: A clinical, imaging, pathologic and biochemical study. *Neurology* **46**, 492.

20. Roels H, Lauwerys R, Buchet JP *et al.* (1987) Epidemiological survey among workers exposed to manganese: Effects on lung, central nervous system, and some biological indices. *Amer J Ind Med* **11**, 307.

21. Saric M (1986) Manganese. In: *Handbook of Toxicology of Metals.* Friberg I, Nordberg GI, Vouk V eds. Elsevier, Amsterdam p. 354.

22. Shinotoh H, Snow BJ, Chu NS *et al.* (1997) Presynaptic and postsynaptic dopaminergic function in patients with manganese intoxication: A positron emission tomography study. *Neurology* **48**, 1053.

23. Spahr L, Butterworth RF, Fontaine S *et al.* (1996) Increased blood manganese in cirrhotic patients: Relationship to pallidal magnetic resonance signal hyperintensity and neurological symptoms. *Hepatology* **24**, 1116.

24. Wolters EC, Huang CC, Clark C *et al.* (1989) Positron emission tomography in manganese intoxication. *Ann Neurol* **26**, 647.

25. World Health Organization (1981) Environmental health criteria #17: Manganese. WHO, Geneva p. 1.

26. Yamada M, Ohno S, Okayasu I *et al.* (1986) Chronic manganese poisoning: A neuropathological study with determination of manganese distribution in the brain. *Acta Neuropathol* **70**, 273.

Margatoxin

Albert C. Ludolph

NEUROTOXICITY RATING

Experimental

A   Ion channel dysfunction (certain potassium channels)

Margatoxin (MgTX) is a 39-amino-acid peptide that was purified from the venom of the New World scorpion *Centruroides margaritatus* and then synthesized by a solid-phase technique (1). The three-dimensional structure of the compound has been determined by nuclear magnetic resonance spectroscopy (4). It has a 79% sequence identity with noxiustoxin (NxTX). MgTX is a member of a group of scorpion toxins—charybdotoxin (ChTX), iberiotoxin, NxTX, kaliotoxin, and leiurotoxin—that selectively interact with K^+ channels. The compound blocks voltage-sensitive K^+ channels of human T lymphocytes ($K_v1.3.$) with a 20-fold greater potency relative to that of ChTX (3). In brain, MgTX acts *via* voltage-sensitive K^+ channels to inhibit binding of ChTX to synaptic membranes and to modulate dopamine and acetylcholine release in striatum (2,5).

REFERENCES

1. Bednarek MA, Bugianesi RM, Leonard RJ, Felix JP (1994) Chemical synthesis and structure-function studies of margatoxin, a potent inhibitor of voltage-dependent potassium channel in human T lymphocytes. *Biochem Biophys Res Commun* **198**, 619.
2. Fischer HS, Saria A (1999) Voltage-gated, margatoxin-sensitive potassium channels, but not calcium-gated, iberiotoxin-sensitive potassium channels modulate acetylcholine release in rat striatal slices. *Neurosci Lett* **263**, 208.
3. Garcia-Calvo M, Leonard RJ, Novick J *et al.* (1993) Purification, characterization, and biosynthesis of margatoxin, a component of *Centruroides margaritatus* venom that selectively inhibits voltage-dependent potassium channels. *J Biol Chem* **268**, 18866.
4. Johnson BA, Stevens SP, Williamson JM (1994) Determination of the three-dimensional structure of margatoxin by 1H, 13C, 15N triple-resonance nuclear magnetic resonance spectroscopy. *Biochemistry* **333**, 15061.
5. Saria A, Seidl CV, Fischer HS (1998) Margatoxin increases dopamine release in rat striatum *via* voltage-gated K^+ channels. *Eur J Pharmacol* **343**, 193.

Measles Vaccine

Neil L. Rosenberg

NEUROTOXICITY RATING

Clinical

C   Acute encephalopathy

C   Ototoxicity

The first measles vaccine, licensed in 1961, used formalin-inactivated virus; this was replaced in 1963 with a live-attenuated virus vaccine (5). In recent years, a high-titer measles vaccine (Edmonston-Zagreb vaccine) has been used outside North America (16). Increased mortality among female recipients has occurred and, although effective, this vaccine is no longer used (1,6,8,16). The increased mortality was attributed to diarrhea, malaria, or malnutrition (6). No increase in incidence of subacute sclerosing panencephalitis (SSPE), an illness associated with measles, followed these vaccinations (4,7,11,12). There has been a strong inverse relationship between measles vaccine and SSPE (7,12).

Adverse reactions to measles vaccine are uncommon; they are generally attributed to acute allergic reactions (3). Neurological disorders are rare; most common is a nonspecific encephalopathy, usually associated with fever (5). Because the association is so rare, the relationship between measles vaccine and encephalopathy is uncertain.

In addition to encephalopathy, anecdotal reports describe parkinsonism (2), hearing loss (9), delayed measles encephalitis (10), disseminated measles occurring in a child with a congenital immunodeficiency (13), toxic shock syndrome (14), and Mucha-Habermann disease (15).

REFERENCES

1. Aaby P, Samb B, Simondon F *et al.* (1991) Child mortality after high-titre measles vaccines in Senegal: The complete data set. *Lancet* **338**, 1518.
2. Alves RS, Barbosa ER, Scaff M (1992) Postvaccinal parkinsonism. *Movement Disord* **7**, 178.
3. Caffarelli C, Cavagni G, Deriu FM, Zambelloni GF (1994) Adverse reactions to measles immunisation. *Brit Med J* **309**, 808.
4. Cho CT, Lansky LJ, D'Souza BJ (1973) Panencephalitis following measles vaccination. *J Amer Med Assn* **224**, 1299.

5. Fenichel GM (1982) Neurological complications of immunization. *Ann Neurol* **12**, 119.

6. Halsey NA (1993) Increased mortality after high titer measles vaccines: Too much of a good thing. *Pediat Infect Dis J* **12**, 462.

7. Halsey NA, Modlin JF (1991) Subacute sclerosing panencephalitis. *Pediat Neurol* **7**, 151.

8. Holt EA, Moulton LH, Siberry GK, Halsey NA (1993) Differential mortality by measles vaccine titer and sex. *J Infect Dis* **168**, 1087.

9. Hulbert TV, Larsen RA, Davis CL, Holtom PD (1991) Bilateral hearing loss after measles and rubella vaccination in an adult. *N Engl J Med* **325**, 134.

10. Kim TM, Brown HR, Lee SH *et al.* (1992) Delayed acute measles inclusion body encephalitis in a 9-year-old girl: Ultrastructural, immunohistochemical, and *in situ* hybridization studies. *Mod Pathol* **5**, 348.

11. Landrigan PJ, Witte JJ (1973) Neurologic disorders following live measles virus vaccination. *J Amer Med Assn* **223**, 1459.

12. Modlin JF, Jabbour JT, Witte JJ, Halsey NA (1977) Epidemiologic studies of measles, measles vaccine, and subacute sclerosing panencephalitis. *Pediatrics* **59**, 505.

13. Monafo WJ, Haslam DB, Roberts RL *et al.* (1994) Disseminated measles infection after vaccination in a child with a congenital immunodeficiency. *J Pediat* **124**, 273.

14. Phadke MA, Joshi BN, Warerkar UV, Diwan MP (1991) Toxic shock syndrome: An unforeseen complication following measles vaccination. *Indian Pediat* **28**, 663.

15. Torinuki W (1992) Mucha-Habermann disease in a child: Possible association with measles vaccination. *J Dermatol* **19**, 253.

16. Weiss R (1992) Measles battle loses potent weapon. *Science* **258**, 546.

Mechlorethamine

Herbert H. Schaumburg

H3C — N
/CH2 — CH2 — Cl
\CH2 — CH2 — Cl

MECHLORETHAMINE
C5H11Cl2N

Nitrogen mustard; 2-Chloro-N-(2-chloroethyl)-N-methylethanamine

NEUROTOXICITY RATING

Clinical

A Acute encephalopathy (hallucinations, stupor)

A Cerebral necrosis (local administration)

B Ototoxicity

Experimental

A Acute encephalopahty

A Cerebral necrosis (local administration)

Mechlorethamine (ME) is an alkylating chemotherapy agent; it exerts its primary effect on dividing cells by alkylating pyrimidine and purine bases which prevents replication of DNA and causes cell death. ME was the first nitrogen mustard to be introduced and is the most reactive of the drugs in this class. Originally indicated for many hematological malignant conditions, ME is now only used as a component of the MOPP (mechlorethamine, Oncovin, procarbazine, prednisone) regimen for Hodgkin's disease and as a topical treatment for mycosis fungoides.

ME is a highly reactive, unstable substance and dangerous to use because of its vesicant properties (similar to mustard gas); the administrator must take care to avoid skin or mucous membrane contact while promptly dissolving the powder and then rapidly infusing ME intravenously. Once administered, it is cleared from the blood within seconds; as a consequence, its clinical pharmacokinetics are undescribed. Cellular uptake of nitrogen mustard is by active transport; the natural substrate for this active carrier system is thought to be choline. It is given by intravenous administration in dosages of 6–12 mg/m² on days 1 and 8 of the 28-day cycles of each course of MOPP treatment. A dose of 0.4 mg/kg was administered when ME was used as a single agent.

ME has considerable systemic toxicity. It is severely myelosuppressive and the myelosuppression becomes more severe with continuing cycles. This forms the rationale for attempts to use ME as a pretreatment for bone marrow transplant recipients (7). Nausea and vomiting follow every administration and last about 2 h. ME, like other alkylating agents, blocks reproductive function and causes oligospermia. It can be fetotoxic and should not be used in the first trimester of pregnancy. Local perfusion-site thrombophlebitis is common, and venous access becomes a problem in repeated treatment cycles.

There are experimental animal studies on the effects of nitrogen mustards on the mammalian CNS (*see also* Mustard Warfare Agents and Related Substances, this volume). Administration of several β-chlorethamines to mice caused a "waltzing syndrome" of hyperactive behavior that included circular running and choreic head bobbing (6). Histopathological examination, utilizing only paraffin-embedded tissues, disclosed nonspecific changes of uncertain relationship to ME toxicity, namely, eosinophilia and shrinkage of Purkinje cells in the cerebellar vermis and multifocal gliosis in the brainstem. The other study utilized carotid injections of 1–4 mg/kg of ME in nine cats and two monkeys in an attempt to duplicate the carotid-injection studies in humans with brain tumors (5). Animals treated with a dose of ME developed severe focal neurological signs—sometimes hemiplegia—within a day of administration. Animals on a low drug dose displayed mild transitory findings. The electroencephalogram displayed slow-wave foci within minutes of injection; this reversed in the low-dose animals. The low-dose animals displayed low voltage over the perfused hemisphere after about 10 days. Multifocal zones of edema and petechial hemorrhage were found in the ipsilateral hemisphere in high-dose animals terminated 2 days following treatment. Recovered low-dose animals who survived longer displayed multifocal small-vessel occlusion and corresponding areas of necrosis; changes were more intense on the perfused side but a few scattered lesions were present in the contralateral hemisphere as well.

With doses customarily used for chemotherapy, either as a single agent or as part of the MOPP regimen, nonspecific reactions, such as headache and malaise, have been loosely attributed to a CNS effect (7). There is one report of hemiplegia, coma, fever, and cerebrospinal fluid pleocytosis 2 weeks following two conventional doses of ME in a patient with Hodgkin's disease (2). The patient improved rapidly following ventricular drainage. Postmortem examination 4 years later disclosed only multifocal zones of cortical neuronal loss and gliosis. Although temporally linked, the relationship of these findings to ME therapy is unclear.

Intracarotid injection of ME has been performed in an attempt to perfuse cerebral neoplasms directly with the agent and avoid exposure of bone marrow. This procedure has caused unacceptable neurological morbidity and has been fatal in some instances (1,5). One patient survived with a progressive encephalopathy for 7 weeks; at autopsy, the larger part of the perfused hemisphere and part of the contralateral hemisphere showed extensive demyelination and gliosis. Another patient who died shortly after treatment had scattered petechial hemorrhages and massive edema (5). The authors concluded that the normal CNS is vulnerable to the necrotizing effect of ME, and that the parenchymatous necrotic lesion can continue to expand for weeks after drug treatment. It is possible that the effects of ME on the CNS reflect, in part, a direct toxic effect on small arterioles and venules; occlusive lesions were seen in the CNS vessels of some of the acute experimental animals following carotid injection. The human lesion is not a large cerebral infarct from carotid occlusion; angiograms after intracarotid injections have shown the large cerebral vessels to be patent in cases of postperfusion encephalopathy (1).

A syndrome of immediate and delayed encephalopathy has occurred in individuals pretreated with ME before receiving bone marrow transplantation (7). The immediate syndrome of hallucinations, confusion, headache, and tremor appeared within 4 days of ME dosages between 0.3 and 2.0 mg/kg; these findings cleared after 11 days. Five months later, some of the patients developed personality change, confusion, seizures, and cognitive impairment. Postmortem findings included diffuse gliosis in subcortical white matter and, in subependymal regions, diffuse neuronal loss, and a striking increased number of small blood vessels in the subcortical white matter; the authors suggest these findings may reflect ischemic lesions from a diffuse vascular injury (7). They were impressed by the uniformity of the histological abnormalities and their resemblance to findings in experimental animals. Neurotoxicity appeared to increase with age and ME dose and was more common in patients given additional procarbazine or cyclophosphamide.

Signs attributed to peripheral nerve dysfunction may appear in extremities undergoing isolated perfusion with ME for local tumors; these patients have not had systematic neurological evaluation (3).

Hearing loss, tinnitus, and vestibulopathy have appeared in patients receiving high levels of systemic therapy (4).

REFERENCES

1. Ariel IM (1961) Intra-arterial chemotherapy for metastatic cancer to the brain. *Amer J Surg* **102**, 647.
2. Bethlenfalvay NC, Bergin JJ (1972) Severe cerebral toxicity after intravenous nitrogen mustard therapy. *Cancer* **29**, 366.
3. Conrad ME, Crosby WH (1960) Massive nitrogen mustard therapy in Hodgkin's disease with protection of bone marrow by tourniquets. *Blood* **16**, 1089.
4. Creech O, Ryan RF, Krementz ET (1961) Regional chemotherapy of isolated perfusions in the treatment of melanoma of the extremities. *Plast Reconstr Surg* **28**, 333.
5. French JD, West PM, von Amerongen FK, Magoun HW (1952) Effects of intracarotid administration of nitrogen mustard on normal brain and brain tumors. *J Neurosurg* **9**, 379.
6. Goldin A, Noe HA, Landing BH *et al.* (1948) A neurological syndrome induced by administration of some chlorinated tertiary amines. *J Pharmacol Exp Ther* **94**, 249.
7. Sullivan KM, Storb R, Shulman HM *et al.* (1982) Immediate and delayed neurotoxicity after mechlorethamine preparation for bone marrow transplantation. *Ann Intern Med* **97**, 182.

Mefloquine

Steven A. Sparr

MEFLOQUINE
$C_{17}H_{17}ClF_6N_2O$

DL-Erythro-α-2-piperidyl-2,8-bis(trifluoromethyl)-
4-quinolinemethanol

NEUROTOXICITY RATING

Clinical

A Psychobiological reaction (confusion, hallucinations, psychosis)

A Seizure disorder

B Extrapyramidal dysfunction (akathisia)

Mefloquine is a quinoline-methanol derivative developed at the U.S. Walter Reed Army Institute of Research for treatment of drug-resistant malaria, particularly chloroquine-resistant *Plasmodium falciparum* malaria. The mechanism of action is unknown. It is a blood schizonticide but is inactive against latent tissue forms of *P. vivax* (18) and the sexual form (gametocytes) of *P. falciparum* (6).

Clinical testing of the drug began in 1972. Early clinical trials in patients with *P. falciparum* malaria demonstrated cure rates of 96.7% (pooled data from 17 trials involving 854 patients) (20). The drug proved to be highly effective for chemoprophylaxis of travelers to areas endemic for drug-resistant strains; it is considered the drug of choice for this purpose by the U.S. Centers for Disease Control and Prevention (10). In 1993, 2–4 million Americans and Europeans had received the drug as prophylaxis and 10,000 for treatment of malaria (13).

Mefloquine is usually well tolerated, although there is a high incidence of mild side effects (47%–90% in adults and 57%–61% in children), primarily nausea, vomiting, diarrhea, dizziness, and skin rashes (13). The major neurological toxicities of the drug are dizziness or vertigo, which are usually mild and self-limited, and acute neuropsychiatric disturbances, encephalopathy and seizures, which are rare, especially when the drug is used as prophylaxis. A single case of paresthesias possibly induced by mefloquine has been reported (11).

Mefloquine is well absorbed after oral ingestion. Parenteral administration is contraindicated due to severe local reactions (18). Absorption peaks in 0.3–2.0 h (20) but, because of extensive enterohepatic circulation, plasma levels do not peak until 17 h (18). The drug is 99% protein-bound in serum. Concentration in erythrocytes is substantially higher than that in plasma (13). Urinary excretion of mefloquine is very low (<5%), and the major excretory route is through biotransformation and biliary-fecal elimination (18). The main metabolite of mefloquine is 2,8-trifluoromethyl-quinoline-4-carboxylic acid; this is detectable in plasma 4 h after ingestion and, after a few days, plasma levels exceed that of the parent compound (20). Terminal half-life of elimination of mefloquine is exceedingly long (15–33 days; mean, 21.4 days), which allows for weekly dosing in prophylactic use (20).

The recommended dose of mefloquine for prophylaxis of adult travelers is 250 mg weekly beginning 1 week prior to arrival and concluding 4 weeks after leaving the endemic area (13). A single dose of 1250–1500 mg is recommended for therapy of chloroquine-resistant or multidrug-resistant *P. falciparum* for nonimmune individuals, or 750–1000 mg for patients living in endemic areas and presumed to be semi-immune (13). Combination therapy using mefloquine with sulfadoxine and pyrimethamine was initially advocated to reduce the emergence of drug-resistant strains; this recommendation was abandoned when clinical trials showed no therapeutic advantage and increased toxicity of combination therapy as opposed to mefloquine alone (13). Due to possible neurological and psychiatric side effects, the drug is not recommended for patients with histories of psychiatric disorders, epilepsy, or cardiac conduction abnormalities.

There are no animal studies showing neurotoxicity.

Adverse effects are common (47%–90% in adults, and 57%–61% in children) but are usually mild and self-limited, consisting of gastrointestinal complaints (nausea, epigastric pain, diarrhea), headache, dizziness, dermatitis, or asymptomatic bradycardia (13).

Dizziness or vertigo, often ill-defined ("giddiness"), was reported in over 80% of patients treated for malaria with doses of mefloquine ranging from 750–1000 mg (17). All seven patients treated for malaria in one study developed lightheadedness, difficulty concentrating, dizziness or vertigo withing 6 h of receiving mefloquine 15 mg/kg (12). Symptoms were disabling in three patients and lasted up to 2 weeks. Symptoms were not correlated with serum levels of mefloquine or its major metabolite. Pooled data from 11 early clinical trials of mefloquine for treatment of malaria (20) showed an overall 15% incidence of dizziness after treatment. Specialized studies conducted at the U.S. Walter Reed Army Institute of Research, including vestibular testing (caloric stimulation, orthokinetic nystagmus), audiometry, and electroencephalography (20), revealed no abnormalities in patients receiving mefloquine. The pathogenesis of dizziness is obscure.

Neuropsychiatric disturbances, including confusion, psychosis, and seizures, have been reported in patients receiving mefloquine for treatment of malaria. In early clinical trials (11 trials involving 479 patients), four such cases were reported (20), and single cases of encephalopathies were subsequently observed in later trials (3,4,6,7).

Five cases of "acute brain syndrome" were reported in patients treated for malaria with mefloquine (14). All had generalized seizures 2–21 days after treatment was initiated. Two patients were comatose and required intubation. Electroencephalograms in two indicated diffuse encephalopathy. High levels of mefloquine were found in serum and cerebrospinal fluid (CSF) of two patients, whereas the major metabolite was absent from CSF. One had normal serum levels of mefloquine but detectable levels of the major metabolite in the CSF. Three had been treated with quinine before or after receiving mefloquine, thus suggesting possible synergy of the two drugs in causing encephalopathy. The authors suggested that since toxicity was better correlated with levels of mefloquine than with those of its principal metabolite, and given that metabolite penetrates the blood-brain barrier poorly, neuropsychiatric toxicity is likely due to the parent compound.

Two individuals developed acute psychosis with confusion, visual hallucinations, and aggressive behavior when treated for malaria with mefloquine (15). Symptoms cleared in 2–3 days. Whereas one patient with borderline psychosis developed pyschiatric symptomatology after taking mefloquine, none of a series of 20 prospectively treated patients without prior psychiatric illness was similarly affected (8). The authors suggested that premorbid psychiatric disorders were a risk factor in the development of neuropsychiatric toxicity. These initial reports of neuropsychiatric complications were confined to patients recieving mefloquine as treatment for malaria. Acute psychosis has appeared in a patient receiving prophylactic treatment (2).

A German experience with mefloquine-associated neuropsychiatric side effects showed that, over a 2-year period, 12 patients had been reported with symptoms ranging from mild (headache, dizziness, vertigo, asthenia) to severe (seizures, psychosis, disturbance of consciousness, hallucinations, depression, anxiety neurosis) after taking the drug (19). Of these patients, four were receiving prophylactic

therapy, while eight were receiving treatment for malaria. Symptoms began 1–2 days after initiation of treatment, lasted a median of 6 days, and did not correlate with serum levels of mefloquine. Seven patients had received prior therapy with other antimalarial drugs. Based on manufacturer's sales data and a survey of travelers, the authors estimated the incidence of neuropsychiatric complication due to mefloquine to be 1 per 215 in patients treated for malaria and 1 per 13,000 in those receiving prophylaxis.

Forty percent of neuropsychiatric side effects occur after the first dose of mefloquine and approximately 30% of serious neurotoxicity could be averted if patients discontinued the medication once prodromal symptoms appeared (16).

Three cases of transient akathesia and mutism after emerging from general anesthesia were reported in Americans serving in Somalia who received mefloquine prophylaxis (5).

A single case of status epilepticus was reported in a 5-year-old receiving prophylactic mefloquine therapy (1). The child was found to have high serum and CSF levels of the drug.

A single case was reported of painful paresthesias affecting upper and lower extemities, which were intermittent but severe, and which resolved 3 weeks after discontinuing mefloquine (11). Nerve conduction velocities were normal in this patient.

The mechanism of neurotoxicity of mefloquine is unknown. Inhibition of acetylcholinesterase by mefloquine has been demonstrated *in vitro*; the resulting increased cholinergic activity is proposed to contribute to the CNS, gastrointestinal, and cardiac toxicities of the drug (9).

REFERENCES

1. Ajana F, Fortier B, Martinot A *et al.* (1990) Mefloquine prophylaxis and neurotoxicity. Report of a case. *Sem Hop Paris* **66**, 918.
2. Bjorkman A (1989) Acute psychosis following mefloquine prophylaxis. *Lancet* **2**, 865.
3. De Souza JM, Sheth UK, De Oliveira RMG *et al.* (1985) A phase I clinical trial of Fansimef (mefloquine plus sulfadoxine-pyriethamine) in Brazilian male subjects. *Bull WHO* **63**, 611.
4. Ekue JMK, Ulrich AM, Rwabwogo-Atenyi J, Sheth UK (1983) A double blind comparative clinical trial of mefloquine and chloroquine in symptomatic falciparum malaria. *Bull WHO* **61**, 713.
5. Gullahorn GM, Bohman HR, Wallace MR (1993) Anaesthesia emergence delerium after mefloquine prophylaxis. *Lancet* **341**, 632.
6. Harinasuta T, Bunnag D, Lasserre R *et al.* (1985) Trials of mefloquine in vivax and of mefloquine plus "Fansidar" in falciparum malaria. *Lancet* **1**, 885.

7. Harinasuta T, Bunnag D, Wernsdorfer WH (1983) A phase II clinical trial of mefloquine in patients with chloroquine-resistant falciparum malaria. *Bull WHO* **61**, 299.

8. Held T, Trautmann M, Weinke T, Mravak S (1991) A prospective clinical trial of the treatment of falciparum malaria with mefloquine, with special reference to neuropsychiatric side effects. *Trans Roy Soc Trop Med Hyg* **85**, 444.

9. Lim LY, Go ML (1985) The anticholinesterase activity of mefloquine. *Clin Exp Pharmacol Physiol* **12**, 527.

10. Lobel HO, Lackritz EM, Campbell CC (1991) Malaria, mefloquine, madness, and mosquito nets. *J Amer Med Assn* **265**, 2808.

11. Olson PE, Kennedy CA, Morte PD (1992) Paresthesias and mefloquine prophylaxis. *Ann Intern Med* **117**, 1058.

12. Patchen LC, Campbell CC, Williams SB (1989) Neurologic reactions after a therapeutic dose of mefloquine. *N Engl J Med* **321**, 1415.

13. Palmer KJ, Holliday SM, Brogden RN (1993) Mefloquine: A review of its antimalarial activity, pharmacokinetic properties and therapeutic efficacy. *Drugs* **45**, 430.

14. Rouveix B, Bricaire F, Michon C et al. (1989) Mefloquine and acute brain syndrome. *Ann Intern Med* **110**, 577.

15. Stuiver PC, Ligtheim RJ, Gould TJLM (1989) Acute psychosis after mefloquine. *Lancet* **2**, 282.

16. Sturchler D, Handschin J, Kaiser D et al. (1990) Neuropsychiatric side effects of mefloquine. *N Engl J Med* **322**, 1752.

17. Tin F, Hlaing N, Lasserre R (1992) Single-dose treatment of falciparum malaria with mefloquine: Field studies with different doses in semi-immune adults and children in Burma. *Bull WHO* **60**, 913.

18. Tracy JM, Webster LT (1996) Drugs used in the chemotherapy of protozoal infections. In: *Goodman and Gilman's The Pharmacological Basis of Therapeutics. 9th Ed.* Hardman JG, Gilman AG, Limbird LE eds. McGraw-Hill, New York p. 987.

19. Weinke T, Trautmann M, Held T et al. (1991) Neuropsychiatric side effects of mefloquine. *Amer J Trop Med Hyg* **45**, 86.

20. World Health Organization (1984) Advances in malaria chemotherapy. *WHO Tech Ser* **711**, 101.

Meperidine

John C.M. Brust

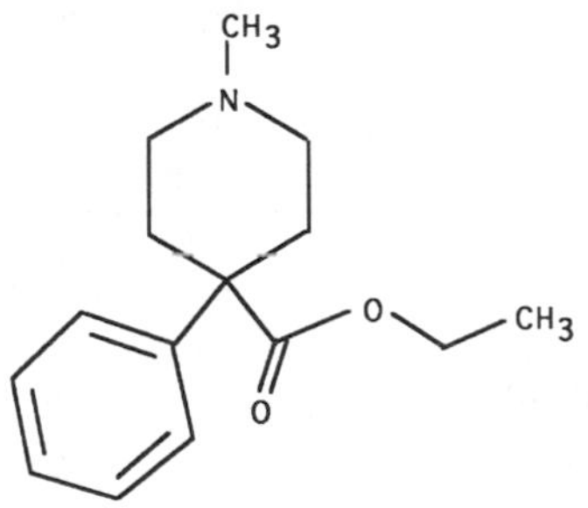

MEPERIDINE
$C_{15}H_{21}NO_2$

1-Methyl-4-phenyl-4-piperidinecarboxylic acid ethyl ester;
Ethyl-1-methyl-4-phenylpiperidine-4-carboxylate

NEUROTOXICITY RATING

Clinical

A Acute encephalopathy (coma, apnea)

A Physical dependence and withdrawal

B Seizure disorder (myoclonic and generalized)

C Chronic encephalopathy (long-term behavioral or cognitive disturbance)

Experimental

A Acute encephalopathy (coma)

Meperidine is a synthetic opiate, structurally unlike morphine, that produces morphine-like effects. It is available as a pill or a syrup for oral use and in solution for parenteral use. Originally introduced as a "nonaddicting analgesic," its ready availability soon led to addiction among physicians and nurses; today, it is an occasional street drug (1,7). It is classified by the U.S. Food and Drug Administration as a Schedule II agent ("high potential for abuse, currently accepted medical use").

Well absorbed orally, meperidine has considerable first-pass metabolism in the liver, and oral analgesic doses are therefore double parenteral doses. Oral administration produces analgesic effects beginning within 15 min, peaking in about 2 h, and subsiding gradually over several hours. Subcutaneous administration produces more rapid analgesia. Liver disease increases bioavailability, and ethanol decreases it. Older patients have less protein binding and higher plasma concentrations of meperidine (4).

Symptoms of meperidine intoxication are similar to those of morphine or heroin, but constipation and urinary retention are less pronounced. In addition, a meperidine metabolite, normeperidine, causes CNS excitation, with tremor, muscle twitches, agitation, delirium, hallucinations, myoclonus, or seizures (2,3).

Normeperidine's usual half-life of 15–20 h is greatly prolonged in patients with renal failure, sickle-cell disease, and cancer. When meperidine is combined with a monoamine oxidase inhibitor, excitatory symptoms are exacerbated, and fatal respiratory depression has been reported (6). Phenothiazines greatly enhance meperidine-induced sedation. Tolerance develops to meperidine effects (although not to the excitatory actions of normeperidine), and the drug's abuse liability is comparable to that of other opiate agonists. Symptoms of withdrawal begin within 3 h of the last dose, peak at 8–12 h, and decline over 4 or 5 days. Craving and muscle spasms can be intense, but mydriasis, nausea, vomiting, and diarrhea are encountered less often than in withdrawal from other opiates.

Acute meperidine neurotoxicity (orofacial dyskinesia, arm flexion, leg stiffness) was described in a 6-week-old male with possible changes in basal ganglia resulting from perinatal hypoxemia (8), and parkinsonism was reported in an elderly man who had received large doses of meperidine (5); in both cases, symptoms cleared after the drug was withdrawn.

The physiological mechanisms of meperidine intoxication, withdrawal and dependence, are presumably similar to those underlying the effects of other opioid agonists and involve stereospecific CNS neuronal receptors. In addition, the meperidine metabolite normeperidine causes direct CNS excitation by mechanisms not as yet understood.

REFERENCES
1. Brust JCM (1993) *Neurological Aspects of Substance Abuse*. Butterworth-Heinemann, Stoneham, Massachusetts p. 16.
2. Hershey LA (1983) Meperidine and central neurotoxicity. *Ann Intern Med* **98**, 548.
3. Hochman MS (1983) Meperidine-associated myoclonus and seizures in long-term hemodialysis patients. *Ann Neurol* **14**, 593.
4. Jaffe JH, Martin WR (1990) Opioid analgesics and antagonists. In: *The Pharmacological Basis of Therapeutics. 8th Ed.* Gilman AG, Rall TW, Nies AS, Taylor P eds. Pergamon Press, New York p. 485.
5. Lieberman AN, Goldstein M (1985) Reversible parkinsonism related to meperidine. *N Engl J Med* **312**, 509.
6. Meyer D, Halfin V (1981) Toxicity secondary to meperidine in patients on monoamine oxidase inhibitors: A case report and critical review. *J Clin Psychopharmacol* **1**, 319.
7. Rasor WW, Oreocrft HJ (1955) Addiction to meperidine (Demerol) hydrochloride. *J Amer Med Assn* **157**, 654.
8. Saneto RP, Fitch JA, Cohen BH (1996) Acute neurotoxicity of meperidine in an infant. *Pediatr Neurol* **14**, 339.

3-Mercaptopropionic Acid

Peter S. Spencer

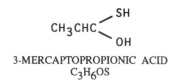

3-MERCAPTOPROPIONIC ACID
C₃H₆OS

NEUROTOXICITY RATING

Experimental

A   Convulsant

3-Mercaptopropionic acid (MPA) is an experimental convulsant; the agent competitively inhibits activity of glutamic acid decarboxylase (GAD) [EC. 4.1.1.1.15], the enzyme responsible for synthesis of the inhibitory neurotransmitter γ-aminobutyric acid (GABA) (2). 3-MPA reduces stimulus-evoked GABA release without affecting the release process (5).

Whole-brain GABA levels of adult mice decreased by 15% within 2 min of intraperitoneal (i.p.) administration of 100 mg/kg 3-MPA; the GABA concentration remained stable from 2–4 min postinjection (4). Regional brain GABA levels of guinea pigs treated i.p. with 195 mg/kg 3-MPA were reduced approximately one-third first in the cerebellum (15 min postinjection) and, subsequently, in the hypothalamus (30 min), medulla-pons (60 min), and cerebral cortex (90 min) (1).

3-MPA–induced brain GAD inhibition and decreased GABA release are associated with the induction of clonic-tonic seizures (3,6). Seizure latency was longer in 12-day-old rats than in 90-day-old animals treated with 3-MPA (70 mg/kg i.p.) (6). In mature, ventilated rats, 3-MPA–induced status epilepticus was associated with spongiform degeneration of neurons and astrocytes in the substantia nigra (8). Unilateral administration of 3-MPA into the rat caudate-putamen produced GABA-sensitive dyskinesia (7).

REFERENCES
1. Alsip NL, DiMicco JA (1992) Time course of 3-mercaptopropionic acid on GABA levels in different brain regions in guinea pigs: Possible relationship with associated cardiovascular changes. *Neurochem Res* **17**, 443.

2. Davies MF, Esplin B, Capek R (1983) GABA-mediated responses are not selectively depressed by 3-mercaptopropionic acid in the spinal cord. *Can J Physiol Pharmacol* **61**, 174.

3. Folbergrova J (1977) Cerebral energy reserves of mice during seizures induced by 3-mercaptopropionic acid. *Neuroscience* **2**, 315.

4. Gomes C, Trolin G (1982) GABA turnover in mouse brain: Agreement between the rate of GABA accumulation after aminooxyacetic acid and the rate of disappearance after 3-mercaptopropionic acid. *J Neural Transm* **54**, 265.

5. Kihara M, Amano H, Misu Y, Kubo T (1989) Release of [³H]- and endogenous GABA from slices of the rat medulla oblongata: Modification by 3-mercaptopropionic acid, ni-

pecotic acid and diaminobutyric acid. *Arch Int Pharmacodyn Ther* **298**, 50.

6. Netopilova M, Drsata J, Haugvicova R *et al.* (1997) Inhibition of glutamate decarboxylase activity by 3-mercaptopropionic acid has different time course in the immature and adult rat brains. *Neurosci Lett* **226**, 68.

7. Toth E, Lajtha A (1988) 3-Mercaptopropionic acid administration into the caudate-putamen of the rat provokes dyskinesia. *Pharmacol Biochem Behav* **29**, 525.

8. Towfighi J, Kofke WA, O'Connell BK (1989) Substantia nigra lesions in mercaptopropionic acid induced status epilepticus: A light and electron microscopic study. *Acta Neuropathol* **77**, 612.

Mercury and Mercury Compounds

M. Anthony Verity

Ted A. Sarafian

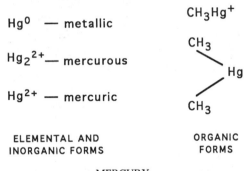

Human exposure to mercury occurs in the form of elemental mercury vapor, inorganic mercury with varied oxidation states of the metal, and organic mercurials such as methyl mercury. Elemental and organic mercury cause very different forms of neurotoxicity. Microepidemics of methyl mercury poisoning have occurred in Japan and Iraq.

Inorganic Mercury

NEUROTOXICITY RATING

Clinical

A   Cerebellar syndrome (tremor, ataxia)

A   Psychobiological reaction (anxiety, personality changes, memory loss)

B   Peripheral neuropathy (motor and sensory-motor)

B   Visual dysfunction

B   Chronic encephalopathy (dementia)

Experimental

A   Granule cell degeneration

A   Dorsal root ganglion cell degeneration

General Toxicology

Inorganic mercurials are absorbed following inhalation or ingestion and, in the case of creams, through the skin. Eighty percent of inhaled mercury vapor is absorbed by the lung and converted to Hg^{2+} intracellularly by catalase oxidation (47). Hg^{2+} has a minor gastrointestinal absorption but a major fecal excretion. Hg^0 readily crosses cell membranes, including the blood-brain barrier. Autoradiographic studies show that inorganic mercury does not penetrate the blood-brain barrier but accumulates in areas such as the pituitary gland and area postrema where the anatomical barrier is normally absent. Intracellular Hg^{2+} and Hg^0 are bound to glutathione (GSH) and cysteine. Inorganic mercury from muscular nerve terminals gains access to spinal and brainstem motor neurons *via* retrograde axonal transport (4).

Animal Studies

Experimental studies in which rats were exposed to inorganic mercury salts have revealed granule cell loss in the cerebellum and degeneration of dorsal root ganglion cells associated with ribosome disaggregation from rough endoplasmic reticulum (17,18,37).

Human Studies

Mercury exposure occurs in workers associated with glass cutting and in the manufacture of scientific instruments, in dental personnel, and following release of mercury vapor

(Hg^0) from amalgam tooth fillings (54). Maternal-fetal transfer of amalgam mercury has demonstrated greater mercury concentrations in fetal tissues when the source of exposure was Hg^0 rather than mercuric salt (26). The threshold for occupational mercury vapor toxicity averages an exposure >0.1 mg/m^3. Signs and symptoms include weight loss, finger tremor, insomnia, and nervousness. A threshold limit of mercury concentration in urine of 50 $\mu g/g$ creatinine has been obtained for workers chronically exposed to mercury vapor. The clinical and pathological features of human neurotoxicity from inorganic mercury have been recently reviewed (39).

Early clinical features of toxicity include psychological disturbances such as memory loss, increased excitability, insomnia, and personality changes (19). Continued exposure produces intention tremor, visual field constriction (58) and, rarely, a subacute motor neuropathy resembling the Guillain-Barré syndrome (69,71). Symptomatic polyneuropathy is not associated with inorganic mercury intoxication. There are two reports of asymptomatic sensory neuropathy following occupational exposure (2,3).

One report describes two patients with dementia with cerebellar granule cell loss following mercurous chloride ingestion (25). Brain mercury levels in selected cases varied from 6–9 $\mu g/g$ (14), 5–34 $\mu g/g$ (65), and 106 $\mu g/g$ (70). Treatment includes immediate cessation of exposure when poisoning is suspected. Chelation therapy with dimercaprol or penicillamine is required to prevent nephrotoxicity or neurotoxicity following acute or chronic mercury vapor exposure. Newer derivatives of dimercaprol, including 2,3-dimercaptosuccinic acid, appear promising.

Toxic Mechanisms (*see* Organic Mercury)

CASE REPORT

A 70-year-old man worked in a factory that manufactured temperature gauges for marine engines. He pumped liquid mercury under high pressure into these instruments, then cut and melted the connecting tubes between the pump and the filed gauges. He also cleaned the mercury-filled apparatus and mopped up spills. After 27 years of this employment, he gradually developed progressive "nervousness" and tremor over 6 months. There was no history of alcoholism or family history of tremor.

General physical examination was unremarkable, aside from gingival pigmentation. Mental status, visual fields, cranial nerve function, strength, sensation, and reflexes were normal. There was a marked tremor of the outstretched hands, with occasional coarse jerks. The tremor became more severe on intentional movement. Resting

tremor was not present. The eyelids were tremulous on closure. Occasional spontaneous jerks occurred in the legs. His gait was mildly broad based and unsteady, and he was unable to walk in tandem. Handwriting was severely impaired, and his signature was illegible. He could not lift a glass of water without spilling most of it.

Routine laboratory studies were unremarkable, as were computed tomography, electroencephalogram, electromyogram, and nerve conduction studies. Cerebrospinal fluid was acellular, with a glucose content of 71 mg/dl and 400 μg/l. He was given two 10-day courses, 3 weeks apart, of N-acetyl-penicillamine, 250 mg, four times daily. The tremor improved markedly after the first course and abated further after the second. Toward the end of the second course, he suffered pruritus, facial swelling, and epigastric pain. Despite this reaction, N-acetyl-penicillamine therapy was continued for 4 days, and he was given diphenylhydramine 75 mg/day once it was established that complete blood count, SMA-12, electrocardiogram, and upper gastrointestinal series were normal. These side effects resolved 10 days after chelation therapy was completed.

Three months after treatment, the tremor was negligible. He could drink a glass of water normally, his handwriting was nearly normal, and his gait was unremarkable. [from Markowitz and Schaumburg (48)]

Comment

This patient displayed several of the usual features of inorganic mercury intoxication: insidious onset of symptoms, tremor, and gingival disease. There was a typical history of occupational exposure and he made a satisfactory recovery.

Examination of 20 other workers in the same factory revealed urine mercury levels in excess of 150 mg/l in five individuals. None had clinical signs of mercury intoxication.

Organic Mercury

NEUROTOXICITY RATING
Clinical
A Visual dysfunction
A Cerebellar syndrome
A Peripheral neuropathy
A Chronic encephalopathy (cognitive change)
A Teratogenicity
Experimental
A Peripheral neuropathy (dorsal root ganglion degeneration)
A Cerebellar granule cell degeneration
A Calcarine cortex degeneration
A Neuroteratogen

Methyl mercury is used in the manufacture of paper, in the chloralkali industry, and in other chemical production. Human exposure usually results from ingestion of fish obtained from water contaminated with industrial effluents containing methyl mercury (30).

General Toxicology

The organomercurials, especially methyl mercury, are potent neurotoxicants. Greater than 90% of the ingested dose of methyl mercury is absorbed from the gastrointestinal tract. Methyl mercury is bound primarily to hemoglobin with further binding to intracellular GSH (51). Methyl mercury is distributed throughout the body and readily traverses placental and blood-brain barriers. The concentration of organomercurials in fetal brain is higher than in maternal tissue (56).

Brain influx and efflux of methyl mercury is dependent upon high-affinity sulfhydryl-group binding and is similar to that found in kidney and liver. Methyl mercury enters the cerebral capillary endothelium as the L-cysteine complex and is translocated at the neutral amino acid barrier site (5). Brain and nerve uptake is similar to that in kidney; here, γ-glutamyl transpeptidase has an important role, since it allows for the interactive cycling of cysteine, GSH, and methyl mercury (31,52).

Numerous factors influence the metabolism of methyl mercury and its disposition; these include genetic differences in hemoglobin (acting as the principal carrier molecule) and other plasma protein sulfhydryl groups, intestinal flora, nutritional state, and species variation in renal excretion mechanisms (32,72). Biotransformation by demethylation occurs in the brain of primates (46).

Animal Studies

Experimental animal studies have revealed spasticity, seizures, and abnormal swimming behavior following exposure to 6 mg/kg methyl mercury. Similarly, decreases in exploratory behavior and spontaneous locomotor activity were found in mice exposed prenatally to methyl mercury at 8 mg/kg. Moderate brain concentrations (3–11 ppm) in nonhuman primates have been associated with retarded visual system development, disturbed social behavior, abnormal reflexes, and retarded motor development.

Experimental methyl mercury neurotoxicity in adult rats is associated with early degeneration of dorsal root ganglia (16,18,19,37). Neuronal changes include degranulation of the rough endoplasmic reticulum prior to morphological changes in mitochondria or other organelles. In rabbits and monkeys, neuron chromatolysis, gliosis, and status spongiosus are observed in the calcarine cortex (11); there is variable cerebellar pathology, including preferential loss of granule cells with relative sparing of Purkinje cells (17,37).

The developing nervous system of animals and humans is particularly sensitive to organomercurials. Microencephaly and hypoplasia of the corpus callosum may be seen grossly. Neuronal proliferation and migration are principal targets of methyl mercury in the neonate. Neurotoxicity is characterized by abnormalities in mitosis, ribosome dissolution, and loss of microtubules (23). Abnormalities of neuronal migration are seen in the human brain (24).

Human Studies

The hazard of exposure to organic mercury is demonstrated by a report of a case of fatal dimethyl mercury intoxication in a scientist following transdermal exposure (12). The patient, a 48-year-old chemist, was transferring liquid dimethyl mercury in a fume hood and spilled a few drops on her disposable latex gloves. The material apparently permeated the gloves and seeped into her skin within seconds. A severely toxic dose of 100–200 mg of mercury requires absorption of <0.1 ml of liquid (density, 3 g/ml). Three months later, she experienced episodes of nausea and vomiting. Five months after exposure, she developed unsteady gait, slurred speech, and decline in vision and hearing. Whole-blood level of mercury was 4000 μg/l; the usual toxic threshold is 50 μg/l, and the normal level is <10 μg/l. Three weeks later she was cognitively impaired and became comatose; she died less than 1 year after exposure. As a result of this incident, it is urged that dimethyl mercury be handled with extreme caution and only when using two layers of gloves (one layer should be a resistant laminate, the other a neoprene or nitrile heavy-duty glove).

Miniepidemics of methyl mercury intoxication occurred (1953–56) following exposure to industrial effluents in Minamata and Niigata, Japan (49). Subsequent episodes have occurred in Iraq following ingestion of fungicide-treated seed (10), and in the United States (55). Methyl mercury is deposited in growing hair, which allows for assessment of prior mercury exposure. Analysis of hair samples from Niigata revealed the lowest mercury concentration at the onset of symptoms of 50 μg/g. The outbreak in Iraq demonstrated a lowest threshold body burden of 25 mg methyl mercury associated with the onset of paresthesias. Treatment includes identification of the route of methyl mercury intake and acceleration of clearance by dialysis and with the aid of chelating agents. Dimercaprol (British antilewisite) is contraindicated in methyl mercury poisoning because of accelerated mercury uptake into the brain. Although 2,3-dimercapto-1-propanesulfonic acid

(DMPS) has proved more effective as a chelator, clinical improvement was not clearly related to the reduction of mercury.

The epidemic of Minamata disease affected fishermen and their families living around Minamata Bay in southwestern Kyushu, Japan; methyl mercuric sulfide was isolated from toxic shellfish in the bay. Clinical manifestations included sensory paresthesias, ataxia, constriction of visual fields, tremor, and impairment of speech and hearing (36,56). The first autopsy, performed in August 1956, revealed pathological features similar to autopsy cases of organic mercury poisoning reported previously (35). Histopathological changes were especially severe in the cerebrum and cerebellum, with sparing of the hypothalamus, substantia nigra, and red nucleus (66). The calcarine cortex revealed atrophy and nerve cell degeneration, especially in the depths of sulci, with associated gliosis and perivascular macrophage aggregation. The cerebellum was involved in all cases, especially the vermis and lateral hemispheres, with sparing of the deep dentate nucleus and white matter. Granule cell loss of the central type began adjacent to the Purkinje cell layer, which was usually spared. Spinal cord changes were minimal apart from symmetrical "demyelination" of the cortical tracts. No major change was found in the optic nerve or retina in eight cases examined. Abnormalities in peripheral nerves were variable. Some authors have described degeneration of posterior columns and dorsal root ganglion cells with abnormalities in posterior roots and sensory nerve fiber degeneration. Sural nerve biopsies from eight patients revealed minor degenerative changes associated with some increase in small myelinated fibers (interpreted as regeneration) (27). The early, severe limb paresthesia commences distally and progresses in a proximal direction, eventually involving the entire extremity and even the face and tongue. These symptoms and the limb ataxia likely reflect an early effect upon the dorsal root and trigeminal sensory ganglion. One electrophysiological study failed to detect changes in peripheral nerves and suggested that the paresthesia may reflect CNS dysfunction (44). A summary of the principal differences in the neuropathology of congenital/early infantile Minamata disease and that of adult-onset poisoning is presented in Table 32.

Toxic Mechanisms

The primary molecular target(s) of methyl mercury and/or demethylated mercury species are likely to be sulfhydryl ligands in critical membrane sites or enzyme complexes. Methyl mercury induces disturbances in membrane biophysical properties, Ca^{2+} homeostasis, neurotransmitter metabolism, energy potential, and other neurochemical parameters. The reader is referred to reviews on other mechanistic aspects of mercurial toxicity (7,19). The pattern and severity of neurotoxicity ultimately depend upon numerous factors, including age, state of neural development, and the presence or absence of blood-brain or blood-nerve barriers.

Abnormalities *in vivo* and *in vitro* have been detected in monoaminergic, cholinergic, and γ-aminobutyric acid transmitter systems. Preferential changes in dopamine synthesis and release have been observed (13,53). *In vitro* studies have revealed both methyl mercury inhibition and stimulated release of dopamine or norepinephrine from synaptosomes (13,41). These results may be explained in terms of disrupted energy status or in terms of Ca^{2+} influx/efflux. Methyl mercury affects presynaptic transmission manifested electrophysiologically as an increase in miniature end-plate potential frequency (8,9,38). Alterations in Ca^{2+} flux or release from mitochondrial stores have been coupled to changes in acetylcholine release from synaptosomes (45). Therefore, changes in Ca^{2+} homeostasis may underlie the disturbances in neurotransmitter metabolism capable of accounting for the behavioral neurotoxicity, and evidence can be provided to support a role for methyl mercury in disturbed Ca^{2+} homeostasis. Increased neurotransmitter leakage is Ca^{2+}-dependent (7,13), and Ca^{2+} uptake

TABLE 32. Comparison of the Neuropathology Following Fetal/Early Infantile and Adult Exposure to Methyl Mercury

	Fetal/Early Infantile	Adult
Microencephaly	++	−
Cerebral neuron degeneration		
Generalized	++	+
Localized	−	++
Cortical neuron dysplasia	++	−
Cerebellar dysplasia and degeneration	+	++
Hypoplasia of corpus callosum	+	−
Peripheral neuropathy	−	+

into PC-12 cells and synaptosomes is inhibited at voltage-dependent channels (63); methyl mercury increases cellular and synaptosomal Ca^{2+} uptake (40,59,67,68) and disrupts mitochondrial Ca^{2+} sequestration (28,40).

A reduction in adenosine triphosphate (ATP) is closely associated with the dose–response progression in the methyl mercury–induced decline of protein synthesis in cell- and membrane-lined systems (20,42,60). The inhibition of protein synthesis *in vitro* is more sensitive in synaptosomes, cerebellar granule cell cultures, and granule cell suspensions than in cell-free reconstituted systems (20–22,42). It is likely that cell-free inhibition occurring in the presence of a regenerating energy system is due to direct inhibition of select enzymes of translation (*vide infra*) while inhibition in intact cell systems is a reflection of the shift in ATP/adenosine diphosphate (ADP) ratio. Observations have shown a suppressive influence on translation exerted by subtle increases in ADP or monophosphate (34). The rate of initiation is highly sensitive to ADP/ATP and guanosine diphosphate/guanosine triphosphate ratios but relatively indifferent to the absolute levels of either the adenosine or guanosine diphosphate. These biochemical observations explain the morphological finding of ribosome dissolution early in toxicity. The ribosomal disaggregation is not due to a direct mercurial effect on the integrity of the endoplasmic reticulum (22). Evidence for a mercurial effect on ATP synthesis and energy charge stems from multiple sources: inhibition of ATP regeneration was observed in reticulocyte translation (42), and methyl mercury inhibits mitochondrial respiration, oxidative phosphorylation, and ATP production (20,28,40,64).

Apart from the energy-charge modulation of protein synthesis initiation, methyl mercury inhibits peptide elongation. Specifically, *in vivo* and *in vitro*, methyl mercury inhibits selective aminoacyl-tRNA synthetases (22,29). Moreover, *in vivo* methyl mercury significantly suppresses aminoacyladenylate synthesis from all amino acids, suggesting a more fundamental linkage to an ATP defect that is not dependent upon the selective inhibition of tRNA synthetases.

Arrested mitotic activity following methyl mercury exposure has been noted by numerous investigators (50,57,73). Such action results from the disassembly of microtubules at the mitotic spindle (50). Methyl mercury reacts with sulfhydryl groups on tubulin monomers, inhibits the assembly process, and also causing depolymerization. Blockade of microtubule-dependent fast axoplasmic transport has been associated with depolymerization of reassembled microtubules by methyl mercury (1). Dendrite hypoplasia in the developing cerebellum may reflect a mercurial-induced inhibition of neuritogenesis that is

known to be dependent upon the posttranslational modification of tubulin. The mechanism of mercurial-induced tubulin depolymerization is unclear; however, observations relating to the role of microtubule-associated protein 2 (MAP-2) are relevant. Protein kinase C (PKC)–mediated phosphorylation of MAP-2 inhibits its ability to induce tubulin polymerization (33). Therefore, an increased potential for phosphorylation may be expected to block tubulin polymerization. Such an increase in phosphorylation was observed in cerebellar granule neurons in culture after treatment with 1 μM methyl mercury for 24 h (61). Subsequent studies (59) demonstrated that methyl mercury increased intracellular Ca^{2+} and inositol phosphate; this suggested that second-messenger–mediated activation of protein kinases may be the mechanism underlying mercurial-induced stimulation of protein phosphorylation. While methyl mercury had no direct stimulatory effect on PKC partially purified from adult rat brain, stimulation of intracellular activity could result from observed elevations of inositol phosphate and Ca^{2+}. Quantitative two-dimensional polyacrylamide gel electrophoresis studies revealed increased phosphorylation of numerous protein species but especially of 58-kDa and 68- to 75-kDa proteins allied to β-tubulin and *tau* factor. It is possible that the microtubule depolymerization may be directly coupled to a PKC-activated phosphorylation of associated proteins.

Methyl mercury treatment of astrocytes *in vitro* causes a breakdown of the transmembrane K^+ gradient and inhibition of energy-dependent, Na^+-dependent glutamate uptake (6,15). Increased extracellular glutamate would be expected to trigger neuronal degeneration by an excitotoxic mechanism (*see* Chapter 1).

Other biochemical abnormalities, such as enhanced lipoperoxidation and oxidative injury, have been described (43,62). A role for free-radical mechanisms in methyl mercury neurotoxicity has been supported by observations that antioxidant systems are partially successful in protecting against mercurial toxicity.

REFERENCES

1. Abe T, Haga T, Kurokawa M (1975) Blockage of axoplasmic transport and depolymerization of reassembled microtubules by methyl mercury. *Brain Res* 86, 504.
2. Albers JW, Cariender D, Levine SP *et al.* (1982) Asymptomatic sensorimotor polyneuropathy in workers exposed to elemental mercury. *Neurology* 32, 1168.
3. Albers JW, Kallenbach LR, Fine LG *et al.* (1988) Neurological abnormalities associated with remote occupational elemental mercury exposure. *Ann Neurol* 24, 651.
4. Arvidson B (1992) Inorganic mercury is transported from muscular nerve terminals to spinal and brain stem motor neurons. *Muscle Nerve* 15, 1089.

5. Aschner M, Clarkson TW (1988) Uptake of methyl mercury in the rat brain: Effects of amino acids. *Brain Res* **462**, 31.

6. Aschner M, Eberle NB, Miller K, Kimelberg HK (1990) Interactions of methyl mercury with rat primary astrocyte cultures: Inhibition of rubidium and glutamate uptake and induction of swelling. *Brain Res* **530**, 245.

7. Atchison WD, Hare MF (1994) Mechanisms of methyl mercury-induced neurotoxicity. *FASEB J* **8**, 622.

8. Atchison WD, Joshi U, Thornburg JE (1986) Irreversible suppression of Ca^{2+} entry into nerve terminals by methyl mercury. *J Pharmacol Exp Ther* **238**, 618.

9. Atchison WD, Narahashi T (1982) Methyl mercury induced depression of neuromuscular transmission in the rat. *Neurotoxicology* **3**, 37.

10. Bakir F, Damluji S, Amin-Zaki L et al. (1973) Methyl mercury poisoning in Iraq. *Science* **181**, 230.

11. Berlin M, Grant CA, Hellberg J et al. (1975) Neurotoxicity of methyl mercury in squirrel monkeys. *Arch Environ Health* **30**, 340.

12. Blayney MB, Winn JS, Nierenberg DW (1997) Handling dimethylmercury. *Chem Eng News* May 12, p. 7.

13. Bondy SC, Anderson CL, Harrington ME, Prasad KN (1979) The effects of organic and inorganic lead and mercury on neurotransmitter high-affinity transport and release mechanisms. *Environ Res* **19**, 102.

14. Brigatti L (1949) Mercury levels in human organs with and without mercury exposure. *Med Lab* **40**, 233.

15. Brookes N (1988) Specificity and reversibility of the inhibition by $HgCl_2$ of glutamate transport in astrocyte cultures. *J Neurochem* **50**, 1117.

16. Cavanagh JB, Chen FC-K (1971) Amino acid incorporation in protein during the "silent phase" before organomercury and β-bromophenylacetylurea neuropathy in the rat. *Acta Neuropathol* **19**, 216.

17. Chang LW (1979) Pathological effect of mercury poisoning. In: *Biogeochemistry of Mercury*. Nriagu JO ed. Elsevier, New York p. 519.

18. Chang LW, Hartmann HA (1972) Ultrastructural studies of the nervous system of mercury intoxication. I. Pathologic changes in the nerve cell bodies. *Acta Neuropathol* **20**, 122.

19. Chang LW, Verity MA (1995) Mercury neurotoxicity: Effects and mechanisms. In: *Handbook of Neurotoxicology*. Chang LW, Dyer RS eds. Marcel Dekker, New York p. 31.

20. Cheung M, Verity MA (1981) Methyl mercury inhibition of synaptosome protein synthesis: Role of mitochondrial dysfunction. *Environ Res* **24**, 286.

21. Cheung MK, Verity MA (1983) Experimental methyl mercury neurotoxicity: Similar *in vivo* and *in vitro* perturbation of brain cell-free protein synthesis. *Exp Mol Pathol* **38**, 230.

22. Cheung MK, Verity MA (1985) Experimental methyl mercury neurotoxicity: Locus of mercurial inhibition of brain protein synthesis *in vivo* and *in vitro*. *J Neurochem* **44**, 1799.

23. Choi BH (1991) Effects of methyl mercury on neuroepithelial germinal cells in the developing telencephalic vesicles of mice. *Acta Neuropathol* **81**, 359.

24. Choi BH, Lapham LW, Amin-Zaki L, Saleem T (1978) Abnormal neuronal migration, deranged cerebro-cortical organization, and diffuse white matter astrocytosis of human fetal brain: A major effect of methyl mercury poisoning *in utero*. *J Neuropathol Exp Neurol* **37**, 719.

25. Davis LE, Wands JR, Weiss SA et al. (1974) Central nervous system intoxication from mercurous chloride laxatives. *Arch Neurol* **30**, 428.

26. Drasch G, Schupp I, Hofl H et al. (1994) Mercury burden of human fetal and infant tissues. *Eur J Pediat* **153**, 607.

27. Eto K, Takeuchi T (1977) Pathologic changes of human sural nerves in Minamata disease (methyl mercury poisoning). *Virchows Arch Cell Path* **23**, 109.

28. Hare MF, Atchison WD (1992) Comparative action of methyl mercury and divalent inorganic mercury on nerve terminal and intraterminal mitochondrial membrane potentials. *J Pharmacol Exp Ther* **261**, 166.

29. Hasegawa K, Omata S, Sugano H (1988) *In vivo* and *in vitro* effects of methyl mercury on the activities of amino acyl-tRNA synthetases in rat brain. *Arch Toxicol* **62**, 470.

30. Hecky RE, Ramsey DJ, Bodaly RA, Strange NE (1991) Increased methyl mercury contamination in fish in newly formed fresh water reservoir. In: *Advances in Mercury Toxicology*. Suzuki T, Imura N, Clarkson T eds. Plenum Press, New York p. 33.

31. Hirayama K (1980) Effect of amino acids on brain uptake of methyl mercury. *Toxicol Appl Pharmacol* **55**, 318.

32. Hirayama K, Yasutake A, Inouye M (1987) Effect of sex hormones on the fate of methyl mercury and on glutathione metabolism in mice. *Biochem Pharmacol* **36**, 1919.

33. Hoshi M, Akiyama T, Schinohara Y et al. (1988) Protein kinase C–catalyzed phosphorylation of the microtubule-binding domain of microtubule-associated protein-2 inhibits its ability to induce tubulin polymerization. *Eur J Biochem* **174**, 225.

34. Hucul JA, Henshaw EC, Young DA (1985) Nucleoside diphosphate regulation of overall rates of protein biosynthesis acting at the level of initiation. *J Biol Chem* **260**, 15585.

35. Hunter D, Russell DS (1954) Focal cerebral and cerebellar atrophy in a human subject due to organic mercury compounds. *J Neurol Neurosurg Psychiat* **17**, 235.

36. Igata A (1991) Epidemiological and clinical features of Minamata disease. In: *Advances in Mercury Toxicology*. Suzuki T, Imura N, Clarkson T eds. Plenum Press, New York p. 439.

37. Jacobs JM, Carmichael N, Cavanagh JB (1975) Ultrastructural changes in the dorsal root and trigeminal gan-

glia of rats poisoned with methyl mercury. *Neuropathol Appl Neurobiol* **1**, 1.

38. Juang MS, Yonemura K (1975) Increased spontaneous transmitter release from pre-synaptic nerve terminal by methyl mercuric chloride. *Nature* **256**, 211.

39. Kark RAP (1994) Clinical and neurochemical aspects of inorganic mercury investigation. In: *Investigations of the Nervous System. Vol 64.* DeWolfe FA ed. *Handbook of Clinical Neurology.* Vinken PJ, Bruyn GU eds. Elsevier/North-Holland, Amsterdam p. 367.

40. Kauppinen RA, Komulainen H, Taipale H (1989) Cellular mechanisms underlying the increase in cytosolic free calcium concentration induced by methyl mercury in cerebrocortical synaptosomes from guinea pig. *J Pharmacol Exp Ther* **248**, 1248.

41. Komulainen H, Tuomisto J (1982) Effects of heavy metals on monoamine uptake and release in brain synaptosomes and blood platelets. *Neurobehav Toxicol Teratol* **4**, 647.

42. Kuznetsov DA, Zavijalov NV, Govorkov AV, Ivanov-Snaryad AA (1986) Methyl mercury-induced combined inhibition of ATP regeneration and protein synthesis in reticulocyte lysate cell-free translation system. *Toxicol Lett* **30**, 267.

43. LeBel CP, Ali SF, Bondy SC (1992) Deferoxamine inhibits methyl mercury-induced increases in reactive oxygen species formation in rat brain. *Toxicol Appl Pharmacol* **112**, 161.

44. LeQuesne PM, Damlujl SF, Rustam H (1974) Electrophysiological studies of peripheral nerves in patients with organic mercury poisoning. *J Neurol Neurosurg Psychiat* **37**, 1974.

45. Levesque PC, Hare MF, Atchison WD (1992) Inhibition of mitochondrial Ca^{2+} release diminishes the effectiveness of methyl mercury to release acetylcholine from synaptosomes. *Toxicol Appl Pharmacol* **115**, 11.

46. Lind B, Friberg L, Nylander M (1988) Preliminary studies on methyl mercury biotransformation and clearance in the brain of primates. II. Demethylation of mercury in brain. *J Trace Elem Exp Med* **1**, 49.

47. Lorscheider FL, Vimy MJ, Summers AO (1995) Mercury exposure from "silver" tooth fillings: Emerging evidence questions a traditional dental paradigm. *FASEB J* **9**, 504.

48. Markowitz M, Schaumburg HH (1980) Successful treatment of inorganic mercury neurotoxicity with N-acteyl-penicillamine despite an adverse reaction. *Neurology* **30**, 1000.

49. McAlpine D, Araki S (1959) Minamata disease. Late effects of an unusual neurological disorder caused by contaminated fish. *Arch Neurol* **1**, 522.

50. Miura K, Suzuki K, Imura N (1978) Effects of methyl mercury on mitotic mouse glioma cells. *Environ Res* **17**, 453.

51. Naganuma A, Koyama Y, Imura N (1980) Behavior of methyl mercury in mammalian erythrocytes. *Toxicol Appl Pharmacol* **54**, 405.

52. Naganuma A, Oda-Urano N, Tanaka T, Imura N (1988) Possible role of hepatic glutathione in transport of methyl mercury into mouse kidney. *Biochem Pharmacol* **37**, 291.

53. Omata S, Hirakawa E, Daimaon Y *et al.* (1982) Methyl mercury-induced changes in the activities of neurotransmitter enzymes in nervous tissues of the rat. *Arch Toxicol* **51**, 285.

54. Patterson JE, Weissberg B, Dennison PJ (1985) Mercury in human breath from dental amalgam. *Bull Environ Contam Toxicol* **34**, 459.

55. Pierce PE, Thompson JF, Likosky WH *et al.* (1972) Alkyl mercury poisoning in humans. Report of an outbreak. *J Amer Med Assn* **220**, 1439.

56. Reuhl KR, Chang LW (1979) Effects of methyl mercury on the development of the nervous system: A review. *Neurotoxicology* **1**, 21.

57. Rodier PM, Aschner M, Sager PR (1984) Mitotic arrrest in the developing CNS after prenatal exposure to methyl mercury. *Neurobehav Toxicol Teratol* **6**, 379.

58. Rosen E (1950) Mercurialism. *Amer J Ophthalmol* **33**, 1287.

59. Sarafian TA (1993) Methyl mercury increases intracellular Ca^{2+} and inositol phosphate levels in cultured cerebellar granule neurons. *J Neurochem* **61**, 648.

60. Sarafian TA, Cheung MK, Verity MA (1984) *In vitro* methyl mercury inhibition of protein synthesis in neonatal cerebellar perikarya. *Neuropathol Appl Neurobiol* **10**, 85.

61. Sarafian T, Verity MA (1990) Altered patterns of protein phosphorylation and synthesis caused by methyl mercury in cerebellar cell culture. *J Neurochem* **55**, 922.

62. Sarafian T, Verity MA (1991) Oxidative mechanisms underlying methyl mercury neurotoxicity. *Int J Devel Neurosci* **9**, 147.

63. Shafer TJ, Atchison WD (1991) Methylmercury blocks N- and L-type Ca^{2+} channels in nerve growth factor-differentiated pheochromocytoma (PC12) cells. *J Pharmacol Exp Ther* **258**, 149.

64. Sone N, Larsstuvold MK, Kagawa Y (1977) Effect of methyl mercury on phosphorylation, transport and oxidation in mammalian mitochondria. *J Biochem* **82**, 859.

65. Takahata N, Hayashi H, Watanabe S, Anso T (1970) Accumulation of mercury in the brains of two autopsy cases with chronic inorganic mercury poisoning. *Folia Psychiatr Neurol* **24**, 59.

66. Takeuchi T (1968) Pathology of Minamata disease. In: *Minamata Disease.* Kutsuma M ed. Study Group of Minamata Disease, Kumamoto University, Japan p. 141.

67. Verity MA, Brown WJ, Cheung M (1975) Organic mercurial encephalopathy: *In vivo* and *in vitro* effects of methyl mercury on synaptosomal respiration. *J Neurochem* **25**, 759.

68. Verity MA, Sarafian T, Pacifici EHK, Sevanian A (1994) Phospholipase A_2 stimulation by methyl mercury in neuron culture. *J Neurochem* **62**, 705.

69. Vroom FQ, Greer M (1972) Mercury vapor intoxication. *Brain* **95**, 305.
70. Wands JR, Weiss SW, Yardley JH, Maddrey WC (1974) Chronic inorganic mercury poisoning due to laxative abuse. A clinical and ultrastructural study. *Amer J Med* **57**, 92.
71. Windebank AJ (1993) Metal neuropathy. In: *Peripheral Neuropathy. Vol 12. 3rd Ed.* Dyck PJ, Thomas PK,

Griffin JW *et al.* eds. WB Saunders Co, Philadelphia p. 1549.
72. Yasutake A, Hirayama K (1986) Strain difference in mercury excretion in methyl mercury-treated mice. *Arch Toxicol* **59**, 99.
73. Zucker RM, Elstein KH, Easterling RE, Massaro EJ (1990) Flow cytometric analysis of the mechanism of methyl mercury cytotoxicity. *Amer J Pathol* **137**, 1187.

Mescaline

John C.M. Brust

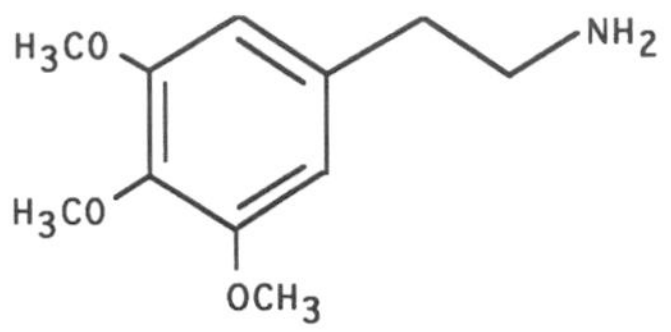

MESCALINE
$C_{11}H_{17}NO_3$

3,4,5-Trimethoxyphenethylamine

NEUROTOXICITY RATING

Clinical

A   Psychobiological reaction (hallucinations, psychosis)

C   Chronic encephelopathy

Experimental

A   Serotonin agonist

Mescaline, named after the Mescalaro Apaches, is present in the peyote cactus (*Lophophora williamsii*) and the San Pedro cactus (*Trichocercus pachanoi*), which are indigenous to Mexico and the southwestern United States (6). Native Americans have used these plants for thousands of years to induce visions in religious ceremonies. The concentration of mescaline is higher in peyote than in the easier-to-find San Pedro cactus, and so peyote is more highly prized. Either the raw peyote plant itself or dried powdered cactus "buttons" are eaten. In the United States, peyote is still used by some Native Americans in religious ceremonies (3).

During the nineteenth century, the neurologist S. Weir Mitchell enthusiastically described the psychic effects of mescaline (10); subsequent writers such as Havelock Ellis and Aldous Huxley promoted it as a means to self-transcendence and cosmic revelation. Infrequently abused as a street drug, mescaline is currently sold either as peyote buttons ("tops," "moon," "cactus," "mesc") or, as synthetic powdered mescaline, in capsules or dissolved in water

(3,14). It is taken orally or as an enema. One peyote button contains about 45 mg mescaline; synthetic mescaline usually comes in doses of 200–500 mg (8). Most alleged street mescaline, however, is really lysergic acid diethylamide (LSD) or phencyclidine. Mescaline is classified by the U.S. Food and Drug Administration as a Schedule I drug ("high potential for abuse, no medical use"). In most people, about 5 mg/kg of mescaline produces the desired psychic effects, which then persist for about 12 h.

Mescaline is classified as an "LSD-like" drug, and its mechanism of action is presumed to be that of LSD, namely agonism or partial agonism at serotonin [5-hydroxytryptamine (5-HT)] receptors (especially the 5-HT_{1c} and 5-HT_2 types) at various levels of the neuraxis (1,9,12). Like serotonin itself, LSD and mescaline inhibit 5-HT–containing neurons of the midbrain dorsal raphe nuclei as well as cerebral neurons onto which dorsal raphe neurons project (9). These actions are blocked by the 5-HT_2–selective inhibitor ritanserin. Somatic effects, sympathomimetic in nature, are perhaps related to enhancement of locus ceruleus activation by peripheral stimuli (11).

Animal studies of LSD-like drugs require end points other than altered perception. In spiders, mescaline disrupts web-spinning (4). Animals trained to discriminate mescaline from saline generalize to other LSD-like drugs as well as to drugs with both LSD-like and amphetamine-like effects (*e.g.*, 3,4-methylenedioxyamphetamine) but not to amphetamine itself (7).

Differences between mescaline and other hallucinogens have been described. For example, in cats, LSD and psilocybin reportedly inhibited neurons in the brainstem raphe nuclei; mescaline did not (16). In rats, LSD down-regulates 5-HT_2 receptors in cerebral cortex, but mescaline does not (2).

Animals do not self-administer mescaline (17). They rapidly develop tolerance to mescaline, with cross-tolerance to

LSD and psilocybin. Withdrawal signs are not observed (13).

LSD is 4000 times as potent as mescaline and its hallucinogenic effects in humans begin sooner after ingestion. With the possible exception of more frequent vomiting after mescaline (the reason for administration as an enema), the clinical effects of LSD and mescaline are identical, and even experienced users cannot tell them apart. The earliest symptoms, within minutes of ingestion, include dizziness, sleepiness, weakness, blurred vision, paresthesias, chilliness, headache, nausea, and either euphoria or anxiety. After 2–3 h, visual illusions appear, with altered body image, micropsia, macropsia, and a heightened awareness of sensory input. Afterimages are prolonged (palinopsia), and there may be synesthesias (stimuli in one modality producing perception in another). Hallucinations then develop, progressing from complex geometric shapes to vivid beautiful or grotesque formed images. Subjective time is strikingly prolonged, and depersonalization is accompanied by a sense of loss of control. Concentration on inner feelings and the seemingly cosmic significance of the experience can lead to a mute state resembling catatonia. Memories intrude vividly, and events seem to occur in the wrong order. Mystical elation may alternate with anxiety or paranoia, but insight is usually preserved. Somatic symptoms and signs include fever, increased blood pressure, tachycardia, piloerection, and mydriasis with preserved pupillary reactivity. There may be tremor and ataxia.

Subjective effects begin to wane after 6–12 h, with waves of progressively shorter recurrence. Tolerance develops after 3–4 days of use but is no longer present after 3–4 days of abstinence. There is cross-tolerance of mescaline to LSD and psilocybin but not to amphetamine or δ-9-tetrahydrocannabinol. There is no withdrawal syndrome.

Like LSD, mescaline can produce marked paranoia or panic following intended dosage. Also, such adverse reactions carry the risk of morbidity and mortality—self-mutilation and fatal accidents. Mescaline overdose can cause hypertension, hyperthermia, seizures, and coma, but fatal overdose has not been documented (3,15).

As with LSD, the weight of evidence is against lasting neurobehavioral abnormalities as a consequence of mescaline. Reports of chromosomal breakage in leukocytes of LSD users led to a study of Mexican Huichol Indians, generations of whom had used peyote; no chromosomal abnormalities were found (5).

Like LSD and psilocybin, mescaline appears to produce most, if not all, of its powerful subjective effects by agonist or partial-agonist actions at serotonin 5-HT$_{1C}$ and 5-HT$_2$ receptors at several levels of the central nervous system.

Permanent neurobehavioral or neurophysiological abnormalities have not been documented.

REFERENCES

1. Appel JB, Callahan PM (1989) Involvement of 5HT receptor subtypes in the discriminative stimulus properties of mescaline. *Eur J Pharmacol* **159**, 41.

2. Buchholtz NS, Zhou DF, Freedman DX, Potter WZ: (1990) Lysergic acid diethylamide (LSD) administration selectively down-regulates serotonin-2 receptors in rat brain. *Neuropsychopharmacology* **3**, 137.

3. Brust JCM (1993) *Neurological Aspects of Substance Abuse.* Butterworth-Heineman, Stoneham, Massachusetts p. 149.

4. Christiansen A, Baum R, Witt PN (1962) Changes in spider webs brought about by mescaline, psilocybin, and an increase in body weight. *J Pharmacol Exp Ther* **136**, 31.

5. Cohen MM, Shiloh Y (1977–1978) Genetic toxicology of lysergic acid diethylamide (LSD-25). *Mutat Res* **47**, 183.

6. Farnsworth NR (1968) Hallucinogenic plants. *Science* **162**, 1086.

7. Glennon RA (1991) Phenylalkylamine stimulants, hallucinogens, and designer drugs. In: *Problems of Drug Dependence, 1990.* Harris I ed. National Institute on Drug Abuse Research Monograph 105, DHHS, Rockville, Maryland p. 154.

8. Jaffe JH (1990) Drug addiction and drug abuse. In: *The Pharmacological Basis of Therapeutics. 8th Ed.* Gilman AG, Rall TW, Nies AS, Taylor P eds. Pergamon Press, New York p. 522.

9. McKenna DJ, Nazarali AJ, Hoffman AJ *et al.* (1989) Common receptors for hallucinogens in rat brain: A comparative autoradiographic study using ^{125}I-LSD and ^{125}I-DOL, a new psychotomimetic radioligand. *Brain Res* **476**, 45.

10. Mitchell SW (1896) Remarks on the effects of *Anhalonium lewinii* (the mescal button). *Brit Med J* **2**, 1625.

11. Rasmussen K, Aghajanian GK (1986) Effect of hallucinogens on spontaneous and sensory-evoked locus coeruleus activity in the rat: Reversal by selective 5-HT$_2$ antagonists. *Brain Res* **385**, 395.

12. Sanders-Bush E, Burris KD, Knoth K (1988) Lysergic acid diethylamide and 2,5-dimethoxy-4-methyl-amphetamine are partial agonists at serotonin receptors linked to phosphoinositide hydrolysis. *J Pharmacol Exp Ther* **246**, 924.

13. Schlemmer RF, David JM (1986) A primate model for the study of hallucinogens. *Pharmacol Biochem Behav* **24**, 381.

14. Schwartz RH (1988) Mescaline: A survey. *Amer Fam Physician* **37**, 122.

15. Teitelbaum DT, Wingeleth DC (1977) Diagnosis and management of recreational mescaline self-poisoning. *J Anal Toxicol* **1**, 36.

16. Trulson ME, Heym J, Jacobs BL (1981) Dissociations between the effects of hallucinogenic drugs on behavior and

raphe unit activity in freely moving cats. *Brain Res* **215**, 275.

17. Yokel RA (1987) Intravenous self-administration: Response rates, the effects of pharmacological challenges, and drug preference. In: *Method of Assessing the Reinforcing Properties of Abused Drugs*. Bozarth MA, ed. Springer-Verlag, New York p. 1.

Methadone

John C.M. Brust

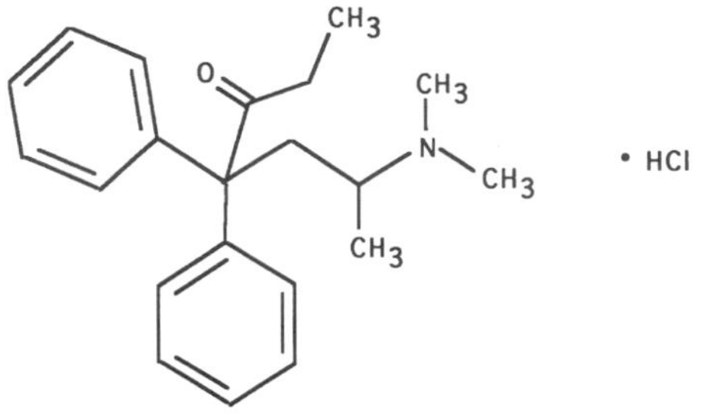

METHADONE HYDROCHLORIDE
$C_{21}H_{28}ClNO$

6-Dimethylamino-4,4-diphenyl-3-heptanone hydrochloride

NEUROTOXICITY RATING

Clinical

A Acute encephalopathy (coma, apnea)

A Physical dependence and withdrawal

C Chronic encephalopathy (cognitive disturbance)

C Teratogenicity

Experimental

A Opioid agonist

Methadone is a synthetic opioid agonist. Although its structure does not resemble that of morphine, it produces very similar effects. Classified by the U.S. Food and Drug Administration as a Schedule II drug ("high potential for abuse, currently accepted medical use"), it is available in the United States as a tablet and in solution for either oral or parenteral use. Methadone is a potent analgesic appropriate for moderate to severe pain (13); it is also used to prevent or reverse opiate-withdrawal symptoms and as long-term maintenance therapy to treat heroin addiction (3,11). For nonhospitalized patients, methadone detoxification or maintenance is available only in federally certified treatment programs.

The introduction of methadone maintenance therapy during the 1960s was soon followed by the agent's appearance as a street drug. Some illicit users take it orally as self-therapy (including supplementation of inadequate prescribed dosage). Others inject it as a heroin substitute.

Accidental poisoning by children ingesting "take-home" methadone led to requirements in many treatment centers that the drug be taken only on-site (1).

Methadone is well absorbed from the gastrointestinal tract; it is detected in plasma within 30 min of ingestion and reaches a peak concentration after about 4 h. For analgesia, the usual starting dose is 5–15 mg orally and 5–10 mg parenterally. Analgesia begins 10–30 min after parenteral administration and 30–60 min after oral administration. For heroin detoxification, 20 mg is given once or twice daily with subsequent tapering titrated to symptoms. For maintenance therapy, oral doses are gradually increased to 80–120 mg daily, a dose usually necessary to saturate CNS receptors and block the effects of injected heroin (2,7). In most subjects, a blood methadone level of 200 $\mu g/ml$ is required for such blockade; in some, unusually high doses are necessary to achieve such levels (6,14).

The half-life of methadone is 1–1.5 days. It is mostly metabolized in the liver; metabolic products are detectable in the urine for days to weeks after last use, the result of slow release from extravascular binding sites that maintains low concentrations in the blood. Despite methadone's longer half-life, its duration of analgesic action (4–5 h) differs little from that of morphine (9).

Studies with animals and human volunteers demonstrate that methadone intoxication, withdrawal, and abuse potential are qualitatively similar to that produced by morphine or heroin, but with differences in severity and duration. Methadone overdose causes the same triad of coma, respiratory depression, and miosis, and close observation is especially necessary, for symptoms of intoxication are likely to recur as the much shorter acting antagonist nalaxone wears off. Methadone withdrawal produces milder but more protracted symptoms than those associated with heroin or morphine abstinence. Controversial are claims that neonatal opiate-withdrawal symptoms are more severe in offspring of mothers receiving methadone maintenance therapy than in those exposed *in utero* to heroin (10).

Whereas parenteral methadone abusers, like heroin users, tend to be dysphoric between doses and to "nod" or otherwise behave dysfunctionally following injection, most patients receiving oral methadone maintenance treatment are behaviorally and cognitively normal, even after many years; decreased male libido and sexual performance are common (5). *In utero* methadone exposure appears to have no long-term adverse neurobehavioral effect (4,10), although birth-weight was lower in monkeys exposed *in utero* to methadone than in controls (8). Supratherapeutic doses of methadone (40 mg/kg/day, from gestation days 8–18) retarded the intrauterine growth of mice but, in contrast to cocaine (30 mg/kg/day), did not disrupt their neocortical development (12).

The physiological mechanisms of methadone intoxication, withdrawal, and dependence appear to be the same as those of morphine, heroin, and other opiate agonists (*see* Morphine and Related Opiates, this volume).

REFERENCES

1. Aronow R, Paul SD, Wooley PV (1972) Childhood poisoning: An unfortunate consequence of methadone availability. *J Amer Med Assn* **219**, 321.
2. Bell J, Bowron P, Lewis J, Batey R (1990) Serum levels of methadone in maintenance clients who persist in illicit drug use. *Brit J Addict* **85**, 1599.
3. Brust JCM (1993) *Neurological Aspects of Substance Abuse.* Butterworth-Heinemann, Stoneham, Massachusetts p. 16.
4. Chiriboga C (1993) Fetal effects. *Neurol Clin* **11**, 707.
5. Cicero TJ, Bell RD, Wiest WG *et al.* (1975) Function of the male sex organs in heroin and methadone users. *N Engl J Med* **292**, 882.
6. D'Aunno T, Vaughn TE (1992) Variations in methadone treatment practices. Results from a national study. *J Amer Med Assn* **267**, 253.
7. Dele VP (1988) Implications of methadone maintenance for theories of narcotic addiction. *J Amer Med Assn* **260**, 3025.
8. Hein PR, Schatorje J, Frencken HJ (1988) The effect of chronic methadone treatment on intrauterine growth of the cynomolgus monkey (*Macaca fascicularis*). *Eur J Obstet Gynecol Reprod Biol* **27**, 81.
9. Jaffe JH, Martin WR (1990) Opioid analgesics and antagonists. In: *The Pharmacological Basis of Therapeutics. 8th Ed.* Gilman AG, Rall TW, Nies AS, Taylor P eds. Pergamon Press, New York p. 485.
10. Kaltenbach K, Finnegan LP (1987) Perinatal and developmental outcome of infants exposed to methadone *in utero*. In: *Problems of Drug Dependence, 1986.* Harris LS ed. National Institute on Drug Abuse Research Monograph 76, DHHS, Rockville, Maryland p. 276.
11. Kreek MJ (1979) Methadone in treatment: Physiological issues. In: *Handbook on Drug Abuse.* Dupont RI, Goldstein A, O'Donnell J eds. U.S. Government Printing Office, Washington, DC p. 57.
12. Nassogne MC, Gressens P, Evrard P, Courtoy PJ (1998) In contrast to cocaine, prenatal exposure to methadone does not produce detectable alterations in the developing mouse brain. *Brain Res Dev Brain Res* **110**, 61.
13. Ripamonti C, Zecca E, Bruera E (1997) An update on the clinical use of methadone for cancer pain. *Pain* **70**, 109.
14. Tennant FS (1987) Inadequate plasma concentration in some high dose methadone patients. *Amer J Psychiat* **144**, 1349.

Methanol

Albert C. Ludolph

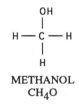

METHANOL
CH₄O

Methyl alcohol

NEUROTOXICITY RATING

Clinical

A Optic neuropathy (axonal degeneration, primary demyelination)

A Extrapyramidal syndrome (putaminal necrosis)

A Visual dysfunction

B Retinopathy (edema)

Experimental

A Optic neuropathy

Methyl alcohol (methanol), also known as wood alcohol, was produced by wood distillation and fractionation after its discovery in the early nineteenth century. Other synonyms used were Columbian spirit, eagle spirit, Manhattan spirit, pyroxylic spirit, colonial spirit, Hastings spirit, and *Lion d'Or* (5). Prior to the late nineteenth century, the odor and taste of wood alcohol was effective in preventing consumption by humans. Human poisonings greatly increased during the first part of the twentieth century once wood alcohol could be inexpensively deodorized (64).

Methanol is long known as a potential human neurotoxicant (vision, basal ganglia), and the well-characterized syndrome of acute poisoning is based on descriptions of individual human reactions and mass poisonings (5,47). Methanol is now widely used as an industrial solvent (*e.g.,* in the production of formaldehyde, methyl chloride, and acetic acid). It serves as an antifreeze ingredient, denaturant, and paint remover. Since methanol has an octane rating of between 106 and 115, and a high energy content, it is considered a possible future automotive fuel.

Methanol is a colorless liquid with a BP of 64.7°C, a MP of −97.8°C, and a MW of 32.04. It is miscible with water and nonpolar solvents such as alcohols, ketones, esters, halogenated hydrocarbons, and benzene.

The most frequent route of intoxication is ingestion of unexpectedly high proportions of methanol in ethanol-containing liquids; for example, in the early 1950s, there was an epidemic of 323 cases of methanol poisoning in Atlanta, Georgia, caused by adulterated contraband whisky (5). The number of intoxications increases during times when ethanol is not available or prohibited and methanol is used as a substitute. Outbreaks of methanol poisonings occurred during Prohibition in the United States and among civilians and soldiers during World War II (5,10,46). Some poisonings are related to suicide attempts. Inhalation of high vapor concentrations or percutaneous absorption of methanol liquids may also cause acute poisoning; convincing evidence for associated neurological disease is lacking.

The Threshold Limit Value (TLV) set by the American Conference of Governmental Industrial Hygienists for methanol exposure (averaged over an 8-h workday) is 260 mg/m^3 (12). The U.S. National Institute for Occupational Safety and Health standard for a 5-min exposure to methanol vapor is 1050 mg/m^3 or 800 ppm.

The existence of a normal body burden of methanol and formate may confound conclusions from experience with *chronic* methanol intoxication; diet and normal metabolic processes contribute to endogenous formate and methanol production. The mean blood methanol level in healthy subjects is 0.73 mg/l (range, 0.32–2.61) (56); a mean of 0.25 μg/l (range, 0.06–0.45) can be measured in the breath (15). In the body, methanol is produced by methyltransferases (19); typical dietary sources are fresh fruits and vegetables, fruit juices, and fermented beverages (18). The sweetener aspartame is also a source of methanol (59,60). Mean blood levels for formate range from 3–19 mg/l (3,59,60); significant dietary sources are honey, fruit syrups, and roasted coffee (29).

General Toxicology

Ingested or inhaled methanol is rapidly absorbed; it is then distributed throughout the body in direct relation to the water content of organs and tissues (53). Methanol is also readily absorbed through the skin. The rate of absorption from all routes is similar in all mammalian species (61).

Small amounts of ingested methanol are excreted unchanged in urine and breath; the majority is metabolized by the liver. Elimination from the blood is much slower than for ethanol; the half-life is 1 day for high doses (blood levels >300 mg/dl) and approximately 2–3 h for low doses (<2–10 mg/dl) (29,61,63). Less than 10% of the ingested compound leaves the body unaltered through the kidneys or lungs (29). Since there is no active renal excretion mechanism, the concentration of methanol in urine is directly proportional to that in blood; similarly, the small amount of methanol that leaves the body through diffusion *via* the lungs reflects the blood concentration. The major part of methanol (>90%) is metabolized by hepatic alcohol dehydrogenase to formaldehyde. Formaldehyde is subsequently oxidized to formate, the metabolite most likely to be responsible for the neurotoxic effects. Formate levels will generally increase if generation exceeds metabolic removal. In the final step, formate is converted to carbon dioxide by a tetrahydrofolate-dependent reaction: this metabolic pathway saturates with higher methanol concentrations in contrast to excretion by lungs and kidneys.

Some aspects of methanol metabolism have important consequences for (a) the pathogenesis of the human intoxication, and (b) the differential vulnerability of species to the neurotoxic effects of methanol (61,63). While the conversion of methanol to formaldehyde is mediated by alcohol dehydrogenase in nonhuman primates, a catalase-peroxidation system is primarily responsible for this metabolic step in rats (61). The rate of methanol conversion is similar in both species; differential susceptibility to methanol neurotoxicity is not explained by these disparate mechanisms of oxidation (61). Formaldehyde is oxidized to *S*-formylglutathione by a nicotinamide adenine dinucleotide (NAD)–dependent formaldehyde dehydrogenase, then converted by a thiolase to formate. This rapid, irreversible metabolic step depends on the presence of reduced glutathione. In nonhuman primates and rats, the detoxification of formate is achieved by oxidation to carbon dioxide through a folate-dependent pathway in the liver. First, formate forms a complex with tetrahydrofolate, then conversion to 10-formyltetrahydrofolate by formyltetrahydrofolate synthetase takes place. The next reaction uses phosphorylated NAD as a hydrogen acceptor, is catalyzed by formyltetrahydrofolate dehydrogenase and results in the conversion of 10-formyltetrahydroformate to carbon dioxide. Since this tetrahydrofolate-dependent metabolic pathway is used more efficiently by rodents (maximal rate of oxidation, 75 mg/kg/h) than by primates (maximal rate of oxidation, 35 mg/kg/h) (37), differences in metabolic clearance of formate are likely the major cause of the species differences observed in methanol neurotoxicity (13,28,61). Stated otherwise, formate does not accumulate in rats, since the rate-limiting step for methanol metabolism is not formate oxidation (as in primates) but formate generation. Formate oxidation again is critically dependent on tetrahydrofolate concentrations in the liver which, in turn, are dependent on dietary supply and vitamin B_{12}–dependent generation of S-adenosylmethionine—a precursor of tetrahydrofolate. The nutritional supply of vitamin B_{12} and folate likely influences susceptibility to the neurotoxic effects of methanol in all primates (61). Conversely, chemical inhibition of S-adenosylmethionine synthesis or folate deficiency predisposes rodents and primates to the neurotoxic effects of methanol. Finally, in humans, a minor amount of formate is directly excreted by the kidneys; excretion reaches its maximum after 1–2 days and may persist up to 10 days after ingestion.

The major target organ of methanol toxicity is the CNS, especially the optic nerves; isolated reports of possible peripheral nerve toxicity may reflect pre-existing neuropathy from ethanol (2,5,27,40,47). Since formate interrupts the synthesis of chemical energy, pancreatic structures and the heart are also potential targets of toxicity. It is unclear whether clinically observed alterations such as "pancreatitis," increased blood glucose, and electrocardiogram abnormalities are directly related to the toxic effects of methanol/formate or are secondary. Muscle aching and tenderness in the back and legs are part of the clinical picture (54).

Animal Studies

There have been repeated attempts to reproduce the selective vulnerability of ocular and basal ganglia structures by controlled studies in experimental animals. Comprehensive studies of experimental methanol toxicity in various animal species were first performed in 1901. Unequivocal changes occurred only in the primate (7). Species differences in metabolism of methanol are now understood to be the cause for this early observation. Since methanol is more efficiently metabolized in nonprimate species such as dogs, rabbits, rats, and mice, the toxic metabolite formate does not accumulate, and the narcotic properties of methanol dominate the response in these species. These animals do not develop the "delayed" acidosis that is characteristic and causally related to primate and human neurotoxicity (13,63). The significance of some experimental rat studies that reported neurobehavioral effects after chronic exposure to oral doses of methanol or vapors is unclear (for review, see 13,29). However, if folate regeneration is reduced by inhibition of 5-methyl-tetrahydrofolate homocysteine methyltransferase (methionine synthetase), tetrahydrofolate levels in the liver and formate oxidation decrease, the susceptibility of rats to methanol increases and animals become acidotic (for review, see 13). This inhibition can be achieved by subanesthetic concentrations of nitrous oxide, which inactivates vitamin B_{12}, a necessary cofactor of methionine synthetase (13). In this model, animals develop signs of intoxication after the typical latency, accumulate formate, and develop uncompensated metabolic acidosis. Electrophysiological studies showed evidence of reduced retinal function during the intoxication (13). The same effect can be achieved by a folate-deficient diet (35).

Since the metabolism of methanol is unique to primates, only experimental studies in subhuman species reproduce the salient features of the human intoxication. The pig may be an alternative: this animal may be equally or even more susceptible to the neurotoxic effects of methanol, since it has been shown that this species' ability to dispose of formate is even more limited and slower than that of monkeys (36). The Yucatan micropig appears to be especially sensitive to methanol, since it possesses the lowest hepatic folate level of any animal species studied (62).

The neurotoxic effects of methanol have been compared among various species and a unique susceptibility of rhesus macaques noted (21). Although the lethal dosage for macaques was 10 times higher than that for humans, the primate was two to three times more susceptible than other species, such as mice, rats, rabbits, and dogs (21,23). Even more important, only macaques developed the typical syndrome of toxicity after an initial asymptomatic latent period of 12–24 h; this syndrome included the development of severe acidosis and ocular damage. Ethanol and bicarbonate are effective in attenuating the neurological deficits (9,20,22,42,50,51). Monkeys pretreated with nitrous oxide or a folate-deficient diet show an increased susceptibility to the neurotoxic effects of methanol (61). It is unclear if prolonged exposure to small doses of methanol affects primates; the available studies failed to show a convincing neurotoxic effect (for review, see 29).

Neuropathological study of optic nerves from primates intoxicated with methanol revealed intra-axonal swelling in the anterior segment (4); axonal mitochondria were swollen and microtubules were disrupted. Oligodendroglia were also swollen (4,26,37,38). Retina and ganglion cells were unremarkable. Functional and structural deficits of the retina and optic nerve were produced in rodents made sensitive by pretreatment with nitrous oxide (44). Neuropathological alterations included generalized retinal edema and vacuolation of photoreceptors and retinal pigment epithelium. Swelling and disruption of mitochondria were apparent in the optic nerve.

In Vitro Studies

Formate inhibits the activity of cytochrome oxidase *in vitro*, with inhibition constants of 5 and 30 mM (45,46). It also inhibits succinate–cytochrome-*c* reductase *in vitro* (46). Since these concentrations are encountered in the blood, vitreous humor, and cerebrospinal fluid of methanol-poisoned humans and nonhuman primates (38,41,57), inhibition of mitochondrial energy metabolism is likely to have a role in the pathogenesis of methanol-induced tissue damage.

Human Studies

Methanol poisoning in humans is usually accidental; there are no reports of controlled exposures. Comparison of individual dosages in mass intoxications (such as the Atlanta poisoning) indicate individual susceptibility (5). In the Atlanta poisoning, one victim reportedly died from intake of 15 ml, while another person survived ingestion of 500 ml without sequelae (5). An intake of 0.3–1.0 g/kg is considered the minimum lethal dose for untreated cases (29).

The use of wood alcohol as an adulterant in alcoholic beverages has often led to mass poisonings. Today, large-scale episodes of intoxication are restricted to countries where methanol is an inexpensive alternative intoxicant to ethanol (55). In the United States in 1987, 1601 cases of methanol poisonings were reported to the American Association of Poison Control Centers (34). Only a few cases of formalin ingestion are reported in the literature (8). Formalin contains ~37% formaldehyde and 12%–15% methanol and its toxicity is similar to that of methanol; the pharmacokinetics of the toxic compounds differ (8).

Acute methanol intoxication after uncontrolled exposures in humans is characterized by an initial short CNS depression that is milder than after ethanol ingestion. An asymptomatic latent period of 12–24 h follows. In rare cases, latencies of minutes to one hour or more than 48 h are described. Gastrointestinal disturbances such as nausea, vomiting, and occasionally diarrhea are prominent in the early phase. Violent upper abdominal pain, possibly indicative of pancreatic involvement, is common. Dyspnea is rare and correlates poorly with acidosis (5). The skin of the intoxicated patient appears cool, although cardiovascular function and, in particular, blood pressure are normal. Early visual symptoms are common in the conscious patient; they include photophobia, cloudy or diminished vision or even early loss of light perception, perception of dancing spots, flashes, or a sense of brightness (5,6). Complete bilateral blindness may develop within hours or gradually over several days. Neurological examination discloses dilated and poorly reacting pupils even in the absence of visual deficits. Ophthalmoscopic findings include hyperemia of the optic disc and mild to severe retinal edema (5). The correlation between funduscopic results and the severity of the visual defects is inconsistent. Visual field defects are common; initially, there are cecocentral or central scotomata that may develop into a complex deficit. Other symptoms in methanol-intoxicated patients include headache, dizziness, amnesia, and generalized weakness. Later, somnolence and coma, rarely delirium, develop; these more severe stages of intoxication are accompanied by generalized seizures, increased muscle tone (rigidity), (transitory) pyramidal signs and, in some cases, opisthotonus (5). The development of bradycardia is an ominous sign and, in the latest stages of poisoning, patients develop rigor or tonic contractions of extremities, and opisthotonus. Respiration ceases after agonal gasping.

The major finding in methanol intoxication is severe metabolic acidosis with a profound decrease in serum bicarbonate levels, lactate and pyruvate elevations, and reduced blood pH. Correction of acidosis by bicarbonate may result in hypokalemia. Ketonemia, a decrease of urine pH, and acetonuria accompany this picture. Blood chemistry may show increased glucose levels, and serum amylase is often increased, indicating pancreatic involvement. Electrocardiograms are often abnormal; however, it is uncertain whether abnormalities are related to hypokalemia (induced by correction of acidosis) or are part of an effect of the metabolic inhibitor formate on the energy-dependent heart muscle.

If the patient survives the acute intoxication and regains consciousness, neurological sequelae are usually confined to the ocular and extrapyramidal systems. Partial or even complete recovery from visual disturbances is the rule, although central scotomata frequently persist. In rare cases, visual acuity may temporarily improve but secondarily deteriorate for unknown reasons (5,47). Blindness is associated with pallor of the optic disc. Prognosis of retinal damage appears to be dependent on rapid reversal of acidosis. The longer the initial visual deficits exist, the poorer the prognosis (31).

Extrapyramidal findings include rigidity, akinesia, and dystonia. They are less common sequelae than visual dysfunction (32). Symmetrical putaminal necrosis is a hallmark of methanol poisoning (2,16,25,27,32,33,52). One report describes pseudobulbar palsy in a few patients (55) and, in an hypoxic case, necrosis of spinal anterior horn cells was documented pathologically and electrophysiologically (40). Spasticity, including hyperreflexia, clonus, and extensor plantar responses, have appeared weeks after the acute event (25,33,40,47). Tremor and cog-wheeling are rare (32,52). Putaminal necrosis is readily demonstrated in severe cases by computed tomography and magnetic resonance imaging. Rigor and akinesia may improve spontaneously during the months after the acute event. L-Dopa has a limited therapeutic effect (32).

In a retrospective study of 30 patients suffering an acute intoxication, blood pH was lower in those patients who died or had neurological deficits (basal ganglia damage, optic atrophy) compared with those who survived without sequelae (1). The rate of complications, however, was independent of methanol blood levels. This suggests major differences in individual susceptibility and a pathogenetic role of formate. The factors that influence individual susceptibility are unknown; however, it is likely that the amount of ethanol ingested with methanol, and the folate and vitamin B_{12} status of the victim, combine to influence the outcome of the intoxication.

It is unclear whether chronic continuous or repeated low-level exposure to methanol has any effect on the CNS. Most reports are from the old literature (for review, see 29) and are poorly documented. In contrast to cases of acute poisonings, no neuropathological findings have been associated with chronic, low-level methanol poisonings. Epidemiological studies on health effects of chronic low-level methanol exposure are unconvincing (for review, see 29).

Histopathological studies of postmortem specimens from intoxicated humans show congestion, edema, and hemorrhage in many organs, including the pancreas. Neuropathological evaluation discloses global bilateral necrosis of putaminal structures affecting both neurons and glia (40,47). Putaminal necrosis was found in 41 of 124 patients with methanol poisoning; the lateral, basal, and caudal parts of the putamen are affected predominantly (47). More widespread lesions have been reported (40): in one patient, changes were not confined to the putamen; changes were seen in the frontocentral white matter—widespread neuronal damage was described in cerebrum, cerebellum, brainstem, and spinal cord. In one large series of autopsies of human methanol poisoning, postmortem artifacts were indistinguishable from specific changes (47). The results of histological examinations of the eyes of affected individuals are controversial, since the many observations of damage to retinal ganglion cells appear to represent nonspecific artifact (6,17,26). One postmortem study clearly demonstrated "demyelination" of retrolaminar optic nerve (58).

Diagnosis of methanol poisoning relies on a history of exposure; typical clinical complaints include "delayed hangover," gastrointestinal disturbances, and blurring of vision. Rapid diagnosis is critical, since early treatment is recommended to prevent neurotoxicity. In the emergency room, useful laboratory aids are the detection of methanol or formate, or both, in blood or urine in combination with a severe metabolic acidosis and an increase of pancreatic enzymes. Ethylene glycol intoxication can result in a similar clinical picture, and differential diagnosis may only be possible by the determination of blood levels (11).

Current treatment of the acute intoxication focuses on four approaches:

1. Gastric lavage with 3% sodium bicarbonate is appropriate. Since methanol is rapidly absorbed, this attempt is often late.
2. Early correction of the severe metabolic acidosis with intravenous bicarbonate (1,24) to maintain a blood pH >7.35. Serum pH, bicarbonate, and CO_2 levels should be monitored. Hypokalemia may develop during restoration of acid balance.
3. Intravenous administration of ethanol to retard the metabolism of methanol via formaldehyde to formate (by alcohol dehydrogenase). Blood levels of 0.1% ethanol should be obtained and maintained during treatment. An initial dose of 1 g ethanol per kilogram body water is recommended (~45 g in a 70-kg patient). For maintenance of blood levels, 7–10 g ethanol normally is administered per hour. However, in chronic alcoholics, this dose must be increased up to two- to threefold. During ethanol treatment, repeated measurements of glucose levels are necessary to avoid the development of hypoglycemia.
4. Hemodialysis is commonly employed to remove methanol and formate from body fluids (1,14,30,39,49). Hemodialysis will not only decrease methanol but also ethanol levels, and therefore increase ethanol demands. Blood methanol levels have been used as criteria for treatment with hemodialysis; however, there has been no correlation with outcome (1,24,48,49). Peritoneal dialysis is less effective than hemodialysis.

It is unclear how helpful these treatments are if administered after the acute phase. Some regimens include the administration of folic acid and vitamin B_{12} to reduce formate levels by maximum synthesis of tetrahydrofolate. 4-Methylpyrazole, a potent inhibitor of alcohol dehydrogenase, is suggested as an alternative to ethanol therapy.

Toxic Mechanisms

Methanol is metabolized by alcohol dehydrogenase to formaldehyde and formate, which inhibits the mitochondrial enzyme cytochrome oxidase (complex IV of the mitochondrial chain) at concentrations detected in experimental nonhuman primate and human methanol poisonings (45,46). This results in an interruption of aerobic adenosine triphosphate (ATP) production and leads to lactate accumulation and metabolic acidosis. There is no convincing evidence that formaldehyde toxicity plays a major role in the pathogenesis of methanol-induced damage, since its half-life is extremely short (43), and experiments in nonhuman primates provide some evidence that formate alone can produce the characteristic ocular lesions observed in methanol toxicity (38). In these experiments, blood pH was maintained within normal limits, indicating the independence of ocular lesions from *systemic* acidotic conditions. It is unclear how acute and radical interruption of chemical energy production by formate leads to the characteristic selective destruction of retinal and basal ganglia structures. It is possible that excitotoxicity has a role (*see* Chapter 1). The biochemical mechanisms of formate detoxification strongly suggest that dietary or metabolically induced folate and vitamin B_{12} deficiencies may increase the individual susceptibility to methanol intoxication. However, supporting data in humans are not available, not even in the form of case reports.

REFERENCES

1. Anderson TJ, Shuaib A, Becker WJ (1989) Methanol poisoning: Factors associated with neurologic complications. *Can J Neurol Sci* **16**, 432.
2. Aquilonius SM, Askmark H, Enoksson P *et al.* (1978) Computerised tomography in severe methanol intoxication. *Brit Med J* **1**, 929.
3. Baumann K, Angerer J (1979) Occupational chronic exposure to organic solvents. VI. Formic acid concentration in blood and urine as an indicator of methanol exposure. *Int Arch Occup Environ Health* **42**, 241.
4. Baumbach GL, Cancilla PA, Martin-Amat G *et al.* (1977) Methyl alcohol poisoning. IV. Alterations of the morphological findings of the retina and optic nerve. *Arch Ophthalmol* **95**, 1859.
5. Bennett IL, Cary FH, Mitchell GL, Cooper MN (1953) Acute methyl alcohol poisoning: A review based on experiences in an outbreak of 323 cases. *Medicine* **32**, 431.
6. Benton CD Jr, Calhoun FP Jr (1953) The ocular effects of methyl alcohol poisoning. Report of a catastrophe involving 320 persons. *Amer J Ophthalmol* **36**, 1677.
7. Birch-Hirschfeld A (1901) Experimentelle Untersuchungen zur Pathogenese der Methylalkoholamblyopie. *Arch Ophthalmol* **52**, 358.
8. Burkhart KK, Kulig KW (1990) Formate levels following a formalin ingestion. *Vet Hum Toxicol* **32**, 135.
9. Clay KL, Murphy RC, Watkins WD (1975) Experimental methanol toxicity in the primate: Analysis of metabolic acidosis. *Toxicol Appl Pharamcol* **34**, 49.
10. Cooper JR, Kini MM (1962) Biochemical aspects of methanol poisoning. *Biochem Pharmacol* **11**, 405.
11. DaRoza R, Henning RJ, Sunshine I, Sutheimer C (1984) Acute ethylene glycol poisoning. *Crit Care Med* **12**, 1003.
12. Documentation of the Threshold Limit Values and Biological Exposure Indices, 5th ed. (1985) American Conference of Government Industrial Hygienists Inc. Cincinnati, Ohio 372.
13. Eells JT (1991) Methanol-induced visual toxicity in the rat. *J Pharmacol Exp Ther* **257**, 56.
14. Ekins BR, Rollins DE, Duffy DP *et al.* (1985) Standardized treatment of severe methanol poisoning with ethanol and hemodialysis. *West J Med* **142**, 337.
15. Eriksen SP, Kulkarni AB (1963) Methanol in normal human breath. *Science* **141**, 639.
16. Erlanson P, Fritz H, Hagstem KE *et al.* (1965) Severe methanol intoxication. *Acta Med Scand* **117**, 393.
17. Fink WH (1943) The ocular pathology of methyl alcohol poisoning. *Amer J Ophthalmol* **26**, 694.
18. Francot P, Geoffrey P (1956) Le methanol dans les jus de fruits, les boissons, fermentées, les alcohols et spiriteux. *Rev Ferment Ind Aliment* **11**, 279.
19. Gagnon C, Heisler S (1979) Protein carboxyl-methylation: Role in exocytosis and chemotaxis. *Life Sci* **25**, 993.
20. Gilger AP, Farkas IS, Potts AM (1959) Studies on the visual toxicity of methanol. X. Further observations on the ethanol therapy of acute methanol poisoning in the monkey. *Amer J Ophthalmol* **48**, 153.
21. Gilger AP, Potts AM (1955) Studies on the visual toxicity of methanol. V. The role of acidosis in experimental methanol poisoning. *Amer J Ophthalmol* **39**, 63.
22. Gilger AP, Potts AM, Farkas IS (1956) Studies on the visual toxicity of methanol. IX. The effect of ethanol on methanol poisoning in the rhesus monkey. *Amer J Ophthalmol* **42**, 244.
23. Gilger AP, Potts AM, Johnson AV (1952) Studies on the visual toxicity of methanol. II. The effect of parenterally administered substances on the systemic toxicity of methyl alcohol. *Amer J Ophthalmol* **35**, 113.
24. Gonda A, Gault H, Churchill D *et al.* (1978) Hemodialysis for methanol intoxication. *Amer J Med* **64**, 749.
25. Guggenheim MA, Couch JR, Weinberg W (1971) Motor dysfunction as a permanent complication of methanol ingestion. *Arch Neurol* **24**, 550.
26. Hayreh MS, Hayreh SS, Baumbach GL *et al.* (1977) Methyl alcohol poisoning. III. Ocular toxicity. *Arch Ophtalmol* **95**, 1851.
27. Henze T, Scheidt P, Prange HW (1986) Die Methanol-Intoxikation. Klinische, neuropathologische und computertomografische Befunde. *Nervenarzt* **57**, 658.
28. Johlin FC, Fortman CS, Nghiem DD, Tephly TR (1987) Studies on the role of formic acid and folate-dependent enzymes in human methanol poisoning. *Mol Pharmacol* **31**, 557.
29. Kavet R, Nauss KM (1990) The toxicity of inhaled methanol vapors. *Crit Rev Toxicol* **21**, 21.
30. Keyvan-Larijarni H, Tannenberg AM (1974) Methanol intoxication. *Arch Intern Med* **134**, 293.
31. Krolman GM, Pidde WJ (1968) Acute methyl alcohol poisoning. *Can J Ophthalmol* **3**, 270.
32. LeWitt PA, Martin SD (1988) Dystonia and hypokinesis with putaminal necrosis after methanol intoxication. *Clin Neuropharmacol* **11**, 161.
33. Ley CO, Gali FG (1983) Parkinsonian syndrome after methanol intoxication. *Eur Neurol* **22**, 405.

34. Litovitz TL (1988) Acute exposure to methanol and fuels: A prediction of ingestion incidence and toxicity. *Proceedings of the Methanol Health Safety Workshop.*

35. Makar AB, Tephly TR (1976) Methanol poisoning in the folate-deficient rat. *Nature* **261**, 715.

36. Makar AB, Tephly TR, Sahin G, Osweiler G (1990) Formate metabolism in young swine. *Toxicol Appl Pharmacol* **105**, 315.

37. Martin-Amat G, McMartin KE, Hayreh SS *et al.* (1978) Methanol poisoning: Ocular toxicity produced by formate. *Toxicol Appl Pharmacol* **45**, 201.

38. Martin-Amat G, Tephly TR, McMartin KE *et al.* (1977) Methyl alcohol poisoning: Development of ocular toxicity in methyl alcohol poisoning using the rhesus monkey. *Arch Ophthalmol* **95**, 1847.

39. McCoy HG, Cipolle RJ, Ehlers SM *et al.* (1979) Severe methanol poisoning. *Amer J Med* **67**, 804.

40. McLean DR, Jacobs H, Mielke BW (1980) Methanol poisoning: A clinical and pathological study. *Ann Neurol* **8**, 161.

41. McMartin KE, Ambre JJ, Tephly TR (1980) Methanol poisoning in human subjects: Role of formic acid accumulation in the metabolic acidosis. *Amer J Med* **68**, 414.

42. McMartin KE, Makar AB, Martin-Amat G *et al.* (1975) Methanol poisoning. I. The role of formic acid in the development of metabolic acidosis in the monkey and the reversal by 4-methylpyrazole. *Biochem Med* **13**, 319.

43. McMartin KE, Martin-Amat G, Noker PE, Tephly TR (1979) Lack of role for formaldehyde in methanol poisoning in the monkey. *Biochem Pharmacol* **28**, 645.

44. Murray TG, Burton TC, Rajani C *et al.* (1991) Methanol poisoning. A rodent model with structural and functional evidence for retinal involvement. *Arch Ophthalmol* **109**, 1012.

45. Nicholls P (1975) Formate as an inhibitor of cytochrome *c* oxidase. *Biochem Biophys Res Commun* **67**, 610.

46. Nicholls P (1976) The effect of formate on cytochrome *aa*3 and on electron transport in the intact respiratory chain. *Biochim Biophys Acta* **430**, 13.

47. Orthner H (1950) *Die Methylalkoholvergiftung.* Springer-Verlag, Berlin.

48. Osterloh J, Pond S, Grady S, Becker CE (1986) Serum formate concentrations in methanol intoxication as a criterion for hemodialysis. *Ann Intern Med* **104**, 200.

49. Pappas SC, Silverman M (1982) Treatment of methanol poisoning with ethanol and hemodialysis. *Can Med Assn J* **126**, 1391.

50. Potts AM (1955) The visual toxicity of methanol. VI. The clinical aspects of experimental methanol poisoning treated with base. *Amer J Ophthalmol* **39**, 86.

51. Potts AM, Praglin J, Farkas L *et al.* (1955) Studies on the visual toxicity of methanol: VIII. Additional observations on methanol poisoning in the primate test object. *Amer J Ophthalmol* **40**, 76.

52. Riegel H, Wolf G (1966) Schwere neurologische Ausfälle als Folge einer Methylalkoholvergiftung. *Fortschr Neurol Psychiatr* **34**, 346.

53. Rowe VK, McCollister SB (1985) Alcohols. In: *Patty's Industrial Hygiene and Toxicology, 3rd Ed.* Clayton GD, Clayton FE eds. Wiley, New York p. 4527.

54. Schneck SA (1979) Methyl alcohol. In: *Handbook of Clinical Neurology.* Vinken PJ, Bruyn GW eds. Elsevier, Amsterdam p. 351.

55. Scrimgeour EM (1980) Outbreak of methanol and isopropanol poisoning in New Britain, Papua, New Guinea. *Med J Aust* **2**, 36.

56. Sedivec V, Mraz M, Flek J (1981) Biological monitoring of persons exposed to methanol vapors. *Int Arch Occup Environ Health* **48**, 257.

57. Sejersted OM, Jacobsen D, Ovrebo S, Jansen H (1983) Formate concentrations in plasma from patients poisoned with methanol. *Acta Med Scand* **213**, 105.

58. Sharpe JA, Hostovsky M, Bilbao JM, Rewcastle NB (1982) Methanol optic neuropathy: A histopathological study. *Neurology* **32**, 1093.

59. Steginck LD (1984) Aspartame metabolism in humans: Acute dosing studies. In: *Aspartame: Physiology and Biochemistry.* Steginck LD, Filer LJ Jr eds. Marcel Dekker, New York p. 509.

60. Steginck LD, Brummel MC, McMartin K *et al.* (1981) Blood methanol concentrations in normal adult subjects administered abuse doses of aspartame. *J Toxicol Environ Health* **7**, 281.

61. Tephly TR (1991) The toxicity of methanol. *Life Sci* **48**, 1031.

62. Tephly TR, Green MD, Gamble J (1992) Formate metabolism in micropigs. *Toxicol Appl Pharmacol* **116**, 142.

63. Tephly TR, McMartin KE (1984) Methanol metabolism and toxicity. In: *Aspartame: Physiology and Biochemistry.* Steginck LD, Filer LJ Jr eds. Marcel Dekker, New York p. 111.

64. Wood CA, Buller F (1904) Poisoning by wood alcohol. Cases of death and blindness from Columbian spirits and other methylated preparations. *J Amer Med Assn* **43**, 972, 1058, 1117, 1213, 1289.

CASE REPORT

A 21-year-old schizophrenic woman tried to commit suicide by repeated ingestion of methanol of unknown purity. She did not take neuroleptics. Reportedly, the first dosage of 30 ml methanol and a second of 50 ml (2 days later) had no effect. Seven days later, the patient drank 150 ml of the compound and slept for 2–3 h. On awakening, the patient suffered nausea, severe vomiting, and dizziness. Forty-eight hours after the acute ingestion, she was admitted to a hospital where she was somnolent and displayed "tremors" and horizontal nystagmus. Methanol and a severe metabolic acidosis were detected in the blood (pH, 7.11; P_{CO_2},

8.0 mm Hg; P_{O_2}, 131 mm Hg; bicarbonate, 2.4 mmol/l). Treatment was immediately initiated with bicarbonate, ethanol, and hemodialysis. Visual impairment was not detected. After 5 days, the patient appeared physically and mentally slow; hypomimia was noticed. A neurologist found severe generalized rigidity, a slight tremor (high frequency, no typical resting tremor), akinesia, hypersalivation, and micrographia. Muscle reflexes were brisk and dyspraxia was suspected. Intravenous amantadine (subsequently shown to be a N-methyl-D-aspartate antagonist) improved the clinical picture within hours. An oral L-dopa therapeutic regimen was started and had a positive

effect on signs and symptoms but did not completely abolish them. Two computed tomography scans (7 days and 3 weeks after the acute event) showed bilateral selective putaminal necrosis. Three weeks after the acute intoxication, latencies of visual evoked potentials, sural nerve action potentials, and conduction velocities were completely normal. Electrophysiological examination of peroneal nerve conduction revealed no abnormalities. L-Dopa medication was stopped 2 months after the intoxication. Neurological examination uncovered minor signs of a residual akinetic-rigid picture but, 1 month later, neurological signs and symptoms had completely disappeared.

Methaqualone

John C.M. Brust

METHAQUALONE
$C_{16}H_{14}N_2O$

2-Methyl-3-o-tolyl-4(3H)-quinazolinone

NEUROTOXICITY RATING
Clinical

A   Acute encephalopathy (hallucinations, coma)

A   Physical dependence and withdrawal

B   Seizure disorder

B   Peripheral neuropathy

Methaqualone, until its withdrawal from the U.S. market in the 1980s, was promoted as a sedative-hypnotic. It also possesses anticonvulsant, antispasmodic, local anesthetic, antitussive, and antihistamine actions. During the 1970s, it became a popular recreational drug among young people in the United States, West Germany, Japan, and Britain (6). (A British commercial preparation also contained antihistamine.) Users of methaqualone ("Canadian blues," "quacks," "sopars," "qualudes," "ludes") often take the drug orally with wine or soft drinks in "juice bars" ("luding out") (7,10). Some report that it causes a "high" resembling that of heroin and without barbiturate-like sedation; others use the drug as a "downer" following cocaine intoxication.

In the 1980s, production and distribution of methaqualone became illegal in the United States; abuse declined, but illegally produced or imported methaqualone remains available (12). Abusers take daily oral doses of 75 mg to 2 g. "Counterfeit" methaqualone pills sold on the street contain unpredictable quantities of other drugs, including barbiturates, benzodiazepines, and phencyclidine.

Oral methaqualone is rapidly absorbed from the gastrointestinal tract (2). Nearly all is metabolized in the liver to 4'-hydroxymethaqualone and its N-oxide; the role of these metabolites in some of methaqualone's toxic effects is uncertain. The elimination half-life of methaqualone is 10–40 h. It induces hepatic P-450 and uridine diphosphate (UDP)-glucuronyl-transferase activity.

Methaqualone-induced sedation, which has an unclear mechanism but is comparable to that induced by short-acting barbiturates, is preceded by dizziness and paresthesias, and there may be anxiety, excessive dreaming, and somnambulism (8). "Hangover" is common. Taken with ethanol, methaqualone can cause marked synergistic CNS depression. Overdose, however, can cause excitement rather than sedation, progressing to delirium, hallucinations, pyramidal signs, myoclonus, seizures, coma, and death (14,15). Methaqualone is less likely than barbiturates to cause respiratory depression or shock. There may be elevated prothrombin time and bleeding (9). A man with seizures and coma after taking methaqualone with diphenhydramine had methaqualone blood levels much lower than expected, suggesting synergism with the antihistamine (3). In another report, methaqualone caused muscular hyperactivity requiring treatment with curare (1). A major cause of mortality in methaqualone abusers (who are often adolescents) is accident, especially involving motor vehicles (4,16).

Treatment of severe overdose is supportive and includes hemoperfusion through activated charcoal or cation-exchange resins. A tendency to congestive heart failure contraindicates forced diuresis (13).

Methaqualone use can lead to physical dependence, with withdrawal symptoms resembling barbiturate abstinence, including delirium tremens (5). Peripheral neuropathy lasting months or years has been described in methaqualone abusers (9,11). Although anecdotal, some cases are temporally correlated to a convincing degree.

REFERENCES

1. Abboud RT, Freedman MT, Rogers RM, Daniele RP (1974) Methaqualone with muscular hyperactivity necessitating the use of curare. *Chest* **65**, 204.
2. Brown SS, Goenechiea S (1973) Methaqualone: Metabolic, kinetic, and clinical pharmacologic observations. *Clin Pharmacol Ther* **14**, 314.
3. Coleman JR, Barone JA (1981) Abuse potential of methaqualone-diphenhydramine combination. *Amer J Hosp Pharm* **38**, 160.
4. Editorial (1981) Methaqualone abuse implicated in injuries and death nationwide. *J Amer Med Assn* **246**, 813.
5. Ewart RBL, Priest RG (1967) Methaqualone addiction and delirium tremens. *Brit Med J* **3**, 92.
6. Falco M (1976) Methaqualone misuse: Foreign experience and United States drug control policy. *Int J Addict* **11**, 597.
7. Fishburne PM, Abelson HI, Cisin I (1980) National Survey on Drug Abuse: Main Findings: 1979. U.S. Dept Hlth Human Services Publication No (ADM) 80-976, Washington, DC.
8. Gerald MC, Schwirian PM (1973) Non-medical use of methaqualone. *Arch Gen Psychiat* **28**, 627.
9. Hoaken PCS (1975) Adverse effects of methaqualone. *Can Med Assn J* **112**, 685.
10. Inaha DS, Gay GR, Newmeyer JA, Whitehead C (1973) Methaqualone abuse. "Luding out." *J Amer Med Assn* **224**, 1505.
11. Marks P (1974) Methaqualone and peripheral neuropathy. *Practitioner* **212**, 721.
12. O'Malley PM, Bachman JG, Johnson LD (1988) Period, age, and cohort effects on substance use among young Americans: A decade of change, 1976–86. *Amer J Public Health* **78**, 1315.
13. Pascarelli EF (1973) Methaqualone abuse: The quiet epidemic. *J Amer Med Assn* **224**, 1512.
14. Sanderson JH, Cowdell RH, Higgins G (1966) Fatal poisoning with methaqualone and diphenhydramine. *Lancet* **2**, 803.
15. Wallace MR, Allen E (1968) Recovery after massive overdose of diphenhydramine and methaqualone. *Lancet* **2**, 1247.
16. Wetli CV (1983) Changing patterns of methaqualone abuse. *J Amer Med Assn* **249**, 621.

Methionine Sulfoximine

Mohammad I. Sabri

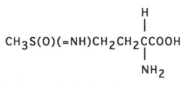

METHIONINE SULFOXIMINE
$C_5H_{12}N_2O_3S$

2-Amino-4-(*S*-methylsulfonimidoyl) butanoic acid

NEUROTOXICITY RATING

Experimental

A   Seizure disorder

Methionine sulfoximine (MSO) is a centrally acting neurotoxic amino acid isolated from the fresh seed of *Cnestis palala* (Lour.) Merr. (4,14,19). A potent convulsant, MSO has been used as an experimental epileptic agent (5,11, 22,25). The LD_{50} for MSO in mice is 218 mg/kg by intraperitoneal injection (23,26). Mice injected with 100 mg/kg of MSO exhibit facial twitching, spreading of hindlimbs, incontinence of urine, and repeated head bobbing prior to convulsive activity (25). Seizures occur 3–6 h after intoxication and are characterized by frequent generalized convulsions, followed by an inconstant quiescent interictal period. The "convulsive period" lasts for about 6 h and is followed by ataxia, weakness, and general recovery.

Morphological effects of MSO intoxication are restricted to astrocytes (2,11,22) and CNS axonal terminals (3,25). Ultrastructural changes have been described in the rat motor sensory cerebral cortex (25). In the preconvulsive period, a slight decrease in electron density of some glial processes was observed, especially in the vicinity of blood vessels. After 15–30 min of onset of convulsions, a slight increase in glial cytosol translucency was seen. One hour after the onset of seizures, enlarged and edematous glial processes containing glycogen granules were found. Two hours after the onset of seizures, "swollen" axon terminals containing a decreased number of vesicles were seen in animals showing the most severe seizure activity. These terminals are similar to those seen in hypoxic states induced by ouabain administration (25). At later stages of MSO intoxication, no axonal terminal abnormalities were seen (22). Neonatal rats given high doses (400–600 mg/kg) of MSO did not exhibit any convulsions for up to 7 days. However, glial alterations similar to those produced in adults were observed. Small daily doses of MSO administered to adult rabbits, either intravenously or intracerebroventricularly, cause rigid hindlimb paralysis with histological changes in the sciatic nerve, cerebellum, and spinal cord (14).

Morphological alterations confined to astrocytes have been described 7 h after MSO administration, during the convulsive period (11). Astrocytic changes included cytoplasmic enlargement, proliferation of mitochondria and rough endoplasmic reticulum, development of cisternal and saccular smooth endoplasmic reticulum, clumping of nuclear chromatin, and accumulation of glycogen. The latter occurred to a greater extent in astrocytic processes in the vicinity of blood vessels.

Ultrastructural changes in mouse cerebral cortex were examined 24 and 48 h after MSO injection (22). At these time points, qualitative and quantitative changes were similar. Massive accumulation of glycogen granules was seen throughout astrocytic processes and cell bodies. Some of the pathological changes in astrocytes during the preconvulsive and convulsive periods occurred earlier and to a greater extent in astrocyte cell processes (11); these then appeared to "spread" into the cell soma (22).

MSO inhibits glutamine synthetase and glutamate transferase *in vivo* (18). The effects of MSO on glycogen, ammonia, and related metabolites have been studied in mouse brain (6). Adenosine triphosphate and lactate levels were unchanged. However, increased glycogen and glucose concentrations were found in cerebrum and cerebellum. Glycogen levels were increased in both areas 1 h after MSO administration (before seizure activity). Levels of ammonia were increased in cerebrum and cerebellum 3–6 h after intoxication (at the onset of the convulsive period). Increased cerebellar ammonia occurred as early as 2 h after administration (prior to the convulsive period). The ammonia concentrations in the cerebral cortex prior to seizure activity were not determined.

Alterations in glycogen and glucose metabolism may be involved in the accumulation of glycogen in astrocytes following MSO intoxication (3). In the preconvulsive and convulsive periods, there is decreased activity of mouse brain fructose-1,5-biphosphatase, which is utilized in glyconeogenesis (13). During seizure activity, a 50% reduction in the active form of glycogen phosphorylase activity occurs. Methionine can prevent convulsions induced by MSO; in the presence of methionine, the effects of MSO on glycogen, glucose, and ammonia levels are diminished, but not abolished.

Several workers have proposed that MSO exerts its toxic effects by inhibiting glutamine synthetase (10,11,22,25). This enzyme converts glutamate plus ammonia to glutamine. Accumulation of ammonia and glutamate may be involved in morphological and convulsive alterations observed with MSO intoxication. After 2 and 4 days of MSO treatment, arterial glutamine concentrations were reduced to 55%, while arterial ammonia concentrations increased by 70% (12). Ultrastructural changes in astrocytes following MSO intoxication resemble those seen in experimental conditions in which levels of plasma ammonia are increased (2,15,16,20,21). Mitochondrial disorganization in the axons and astrocytic swellings are also reported. Increased brain ammonia concentrations are seen in the mouse cerebellum and cerebrum during convulsive activity. However, it is not known if brain ammonia levels cause the behavioral alterations induced by MSO. No measurement of ammonia levels has been made in the cerebral cortex prior to the convulsive period. Early, preconvulsive increases in cerebellar ammonia have been found, and these may be related to the observed disturbances in gait and coordination. The convulsive episodes in MSO intoxication might be due to a diminished capacity of astrocytes to take up excess potassium from the extracellular fluid; astrocytes normally have a role in the regulation of the extracellular milieu of CNS neurons (10). Astrocyte dysfunction in MSO intoxication might result in increased potassium ion concentrations in the vicinity of neurons causing subsequent membrane depolarization. Alternatively, it has been proposed that the increased glutamate/glutamine ratio may induce seizures because glutamate is an excitatory neurotransmitter (25). *In vitro* studies have shown that treatment of striatum with MSO increases the neurotoxic effects of kainate and N-methyl-D-aspartate (17).

Local infusion of MSO into the dorsal raphe nucleus induces hypothermia in rats, showing thereby the involvement of 5-hydroxytryptamine (5-HT) and γ-aminobutyric acid type-B receptors (8,10). The mechanism initiating hypothermia following MSO administration appears to be linked to a slow 5-HT turnover, at the level of raphe nuclei (7,9). Treatment of rats with a subacute dose (150 mg/kg) of MSO shows that activity of γ-glutamyl transpeptidase was suppressed in all the brain regions except the cerebral cortex and cerebellum of 90-day-old animals (24). While older animals showed convulsions and succumbed to the toxic effects of MSO, younger animals had wobbly gait and splayed legs but recovered from the toxic effects of the drug.

Editors' Note: Readers are encouraged to refer to Nitrogen Trichloride, this volume.

REFERENCES

1. Cole M, Rutherford RB, Smith FO (1972) Experimental ammonia encephalopathy in the primate. *Arch Neurol* **26**, 130.

2. DeRobertis E, Sellinger OZ, Arnaiz GRDL *et al.* (1967) Nerve endings in methionine sulfoximine convulsive rats, a neurochemical and ultrastructural study. *J Neurochem* **14**, 81.

3. Diemer NH (1975) Size and density of oligodendroglial nuclei in rats with CCl₄-induced liver disease. *Neurobiology* **5**, 197.

4. Exposito I, Sanz B, Porras A *et al.* (1994) Effects of apomorphine and L-methionine sulphoximine on the release of excitatory amino acid neurotransmitters and glutamine in the striatum of the conscious rat. *Eur J Neurosci* **6**, 287.

5. Folbergrova J (1973) Glycogen and glycogen phosphorylase in the cerebral cortex of mice under the influence of methionine sulfoximine. *J Neurochem* **20**, 547.

6. Folbergrova J, Passoneau JV, Lowry OH *et al.* (1969) Glycogen, ammonia and related metabolites in the brain during seizures evoked by methionine sulfoximine. *J Neurochem* **16**, 191.

7. Ginefri-Gayet M, Gayet J (1992) Involvement of serotonin receptors in methionine sulfoximine-induced hypothermia in the rat. *Eur J Pharmacol* **217**, 85.

8. Ginefri-Gayet M, Gayet J (1992) Possible link between brain serotonin metabolism and methionine sulfoximine-induced hypothermia and associated behavior in the rat. *Pharmacol Biochem Behavior* **43**, 173.

9. Ginefri-Gayet M, Gayet J (1993) Hypothermia induced by infusion of methionine sulfoximine into the dorsal raphe nucleus of the rat: Involvement of 5-HTIA and GABA_B receptors. *Eur J Pharmacol* **235**, 189.

10. Guttierrez JA, Norenberg MD (1975) Alzheimer II astrocytosis following methionine sulfoximine. *Arch Neurol* **32**, 123.

11. Guttierrez JA, Norenberg MD (1977) Ultrastructural study of methionine sulfoximine-induced Alzheimer type II astrocytes. *Amer J Pathol* **86**, 285.

12. Heeneman S, Dejong CH, Deutz NE (1994) Effects of methionine sulphoximine treatment on renal amino acid and ammonia metabolism in rats. *Eur J Physiol* **427**, 524.

13. Hevor TK, Gayct J (1978) Fructose-1,6-biphosphatase and phosphofructokinase activation in the brain of mice submitted to methionine sulfoximine. *Brain Res* **150**, 210.

14. Kallaras C, Anogianakis G, Apostolakis M *et al.* (1994) Ultrastructural alterations of the rabbit sciatic nerve, spinal cord and cerebellum, following methionine sulphoximine administration. *Histol Histopathol* **9**, 105.

15. Kline DG, Chun BK, Doberneck RC, Rutherford RB (1966). Encephlopathy in graded portocaval shunts. *Ann Surg* **164**, 1003.

16. Kline DG, Crook JN, Nance FC (1971) Eck fistula encephalopathy: Long term studies in primates. *Ann Surg* **173**, 97.

17. Kollegger H, McBean GJ, Tipton KF (1991) The inhibition of glutamine synthetase in rat corpus striatum *in vitro* by methionine sulfoximine increases the neurotoxic effects of kainate and N-methyl-D-aspartate. *Neurosci Lett* **130**, 95.

18. Lamar C, Sellinger OZ (1965) The inhibition *in vivo* of cerebral glutamine synthetase and glutamine transferase by methionine sulfoximine. *Biochem Pharm* **14**, 489.

19. Murakoshi I, Sekine T, Maeshima K *et al.* (1993) Absolute configuration of L-methionine sulfoximine as a toxic principle in *Cnestis palala* (Lour.) Merr. *Chem Pharmaceut Bull* **41**, 388.

20. Norenberg MD, Lapham LW (1974) The astrocytic response in experimental portal-systemic encephalopathy: An electron microscopic study. *J Neuropathol Exp Neurol* **33**, 422.

21. Norenberg MD, Lapham LW, Nichols FA *et al.* (1974) An experimental model of hepatic encephalopathy. *Arch Neurol* **31**, 106.

22. Phelps CH (1975) An ultrastructural study of methionine sulfoximine-induced glycogen accumulation in astrocytes of the mouse cerebral cortex. *J Neurocytol* **4**, 479.

23. Politis MJ, Schaumburg HH, Spencer PS (1980) Neurotoxicity of selected chemicals: In *Experimental and Clinical Neurotoxicology*. Spencer PS, Schaumburg HH eds. Williams & Wilkins, Baltimore p. 613.

24. Rao VL, Murthy CR (1991) Variations in the effects of L-methionine-DL-sulfoximine on the activity of cerebral gamma-glutamyl transpeptidase in rats as a function of age. *Neurosci Lett* **126**, 13.

25. Rizzuto N, Gonatas NK (1974) Ultrastructural study of methionine sulfoximine in developing and adult rat cerebral cortex. *J Neuropathol Exp Neurol* **33**, 237.

26. Swinyard EA, Chin L, Cole FR *et al.* (1957) Anticonvulsant properties of L-glutamine and L-asparagine in mice and rats. *Proc Soc Exp Biol Med* **94**, 12.

Methohexital Sodium

Albert C. Ludolph

METHOHEXITAL SODIUM
$C_{14}H_{17}N_2NaO_3$

1-Methyl-5-(1-methyl-2-pentynyl)-5-(2-propenyl)-
2,4,6(1H,3H,5H)-pyrimidinetrione sodium salt

NEUROTOXICITY RATING

Clinical

B   Seizure disorder

Methohexital sodium is an ultra-short-acting barbiturate that is clinically administered intravenously for brief surgical procedures that require potent and rapidly reversible anesthesia. The compound is also used in the presurgical evaluation of epileptics, since it reliably activates an epileptic focus, is of major help in the correct lateralization of epileptic activity (12), and is believed to be a strong predictor for a positive outcome of the surgical procedure (4,12).

Methohexital has the characteristic structure of a barbiturate with a methyl group at position R3. After a single injection, anesthesia is induced for 5–7 min; the half-life of the compound is 3.9 ± 2.1 h (3). Methohexital is widely distributed after intravenous injection and reaches plasma concentrations of 3.5–11 μg/ml. The highly lipophilic substance is initially rapidly taken up by the brain, but then redistributed into less vascularized tissues such as muscle and fat; this leads to a decline of CNS drug concentration and awakening of the patient (3). Methohexital is metabolized by the liver; <1% of the compound is excreted in the urine (3).

Neurological side effects of methohexital include the presence of restlessness (6.7% in a large series) and excitation (0.5%) (6). Seizures are rarely but consistently reported (8,11). There are also two reports on the provocation of generalized seizures during the use of methohexital for anesthesia *shortly before* the use of electroconvulsive therapy (ECT) (1,2). In one of the cases, the patient was concomitantly treated with the selective serotonin-reuptake blocker paroxetine, which might have played an additional facilitating role (2). In contrast, in a study of 39 patients, seizure duration was not significantly increased after me-

thohexital anesthesia during ECT if compared with propofol (7), and convulsions are even shortened after higher dosages (9). This is consistent with results of studies in experimental rodents: in these animals, methohexital shortened the duration of ECT-associated seizures by 42% (5). It is controversial whether provocation of spontaneous seizures by methohexital is limited to patients with a history of epilepsy; however, methohexital should not be given to this group of patients if no specific indication exists.

In epileptic patients, the activation of electroencephalographic (EEG) abnormalities at the site of the epileptic focus shortly after injection is used as a diagnostic tool; however, the provocation of seizures during this procedure is an exceptional event (4,10,12). The mechanism by which methohexital induces spiking in the EEG is unknown; it may be related to depression of inhibitory circuits (4).

REFERENCES

1. Constantino JN, Hasna Z, Bezirganian J (1992) Spontaneous seizure activity as a complication of unilateral electroconvulsive therapy: A case report and brief review of the literature. *J Nerv Ment Dis* **180**, 398.
2. Folkerts H (1995) Spontaneous seizure after concurrent use of methohexital anesthesia for electroconvulsive therapy and paroxetine: A case report. *J Nerv Ment Dis* **183**, 115.
3. Hudson RJ, Stanski DR, Burch PG (1983) Pharmacokinetics of methohexital and thiopental in surgical patients. *Anesthesiology* **59**, 215.
4. Hufnagel A, Burr W, Elger CE *et al.* (1992) Localization of the epileptic focus during methohexital-induced anesthesia. *Epilepsia* **33**, 271.
5. Lunn RJ, Savageau MM, Beatty WW *et al.* (1981) Anesthetics and electroconvulsive therapy seizure duration: Implications for therapy from rat model. *Biol Psychiat* **16**, 1163.
6. MacDonald D (1980) Methohexitone in dentistry. *Aust Dent J* **25**, 335.
7. Matters RM, Beckett WG, Kirkby KC, King TE (1995) Recovery after electroconvulsive therapy: Comparison of propofol with methohexitone anaesthesia. *Brit J Anesth* **75**, 297.
8. Metriyakool K (1981) Seizures induced by methohexital. *Anaesthesia* **35**, 718.
9. Miller AL, Faber RA, Hatch JP, Alexander HE (1985) Factors affecting amnesia, seizure duration, and efficacy in ECT. *Amer J Psychiat* **142**, 692.
10. Paul R, Harris R (1970) A comparison of methohexitone and thiopentone in electrocorticography. *J Neurol Neurosurg Psychiat* **33**, 100.

11. Rockoff MA, Goudsouzian NG (1981) Seizures induced by methohexital. *Anesthesiology* **54**, 333.

12. Stefan H, Wieser HG (1987) Presurgical epileptological intensive evaluation. In: *Presurgical Evaluation of Epileptics. Basics, Techniques, Implications.* Elger CE, Wieser eds. Springer-Verlag, Heidelberg p. 146.

Methotrexate

Raul Francisco Valenzuela
Fred H. Hochberg

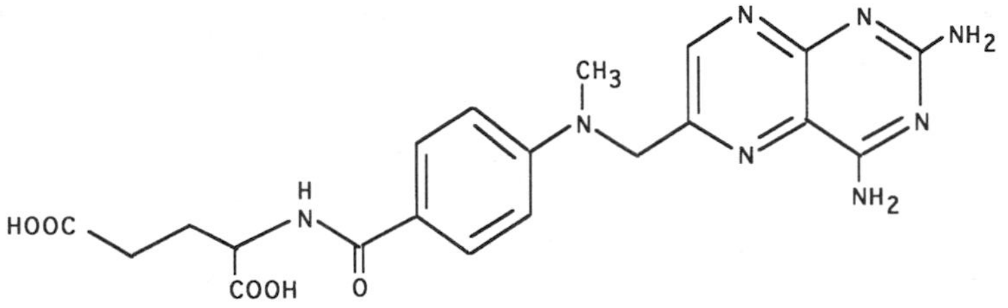

METHOTREXATE
$C_{20}H_{22}N_8O_5$

N-[4-[[2,4-Diamino-6-pteridinyl)methyl]-methylamino]benzoyl]-L-glutamic acid

NEUROTOXICITY RATING

Clinical

A Acute encephalopathy (confusion, somnolence, seizures)

A Myelopathy (intrathecal administration)

A Aseptic meningitis (hydrocephalus, intrathecal administration)

A Leukoencephalopathy (systemic or intrathecal administration)

B Chronic encephalopathy (cognitive dysfunction)

Experimental

A Leukoencephalopathy (necrotizing)

A Acute encephalopathy (sedation)

Methotrexate (MTX) is a synthetic antimetabolite (specifically an antifolate) widely used in several chemotherapy regimens. It is a weak organic acid with pKa values of 4.84 and 5.51 and therefore has limited solubility at acid pH (6). MTX exerts its cytotoxic effect by inhibition of the enzyme dihydrofolate reductase and blockade of thymidilate and purine biosynthesis, and is cell-cycle selective for cells in S-phase. As a single chemotherapeutic agent, the drug is curative for trophoblastic tumors. It is used as a component of combination regimens for several other malignancies, including non-Hodgkin's lymphoma, acute lymphoblastic leukemia, breast cancer, and osteogenic sarcoma. Very high doses of MTX given intravenously, followed by rescue with reduced folates (Leucovorin), have been used for osteogenic sarcoma, childhood acute leukemia, and primary CNS lymphoma. MTX is administered into the lumbar or ventricular cerebrospinal fluid spaces (with or without concomitant radiotherapy) for prophylactic treatment of the CNS in leukemias and non-Hodgkin's lymphomas, and for the palliative treatment of cancer of the meninges. In these instances, the preservative-free drug (in lactated Ringer's solution or diluted in spinal fluid) is frequently administered into the ventricles or subarachnoid spaces of the brain *via* a catheter in continuity with an Ommaya reservoir. MTX in low doses, usually by mouth, is also used in the management of some cases of psoriasis and severe rheumatoid arthritis.

MTX is readily absorbed from the gastrointestinal tract through a saturable active transport system. At increasing doses above 30 mg/m², the efficiency of the system decreases with progressively lower proportions of the drug being absorbed (5). Peak plasma levels occur 1–2 h after oral intake. After intravenous administration, it is rapidly distributed to total body water with a half-life of 0.75 ± 0.11 h (15). In the setting of pleural effusion, ascites, or brain edema, the MTX accumulating within a "third space" may leach into the circulation at an unexpectedly slow rate, prolonging the half-life of the drug, extending the duration of "rescue" and accounting for unexpected sources of clinical neurotoxicity. With these exceptions, MTX is loosely bound to serum albumin and can be easily displaced by other drugs. Cellular uptake of MTX depends on a saturable active transport system; once inside the malignant cell, the drug is trapped by addition of multiple glutamate moieties that slow cellular efflux (15). The polyglutamate derivatives are potent inhibitors of the enzyme dihydrofolate reductase and also of thymidilate synthetase.

Disappearance from plasma follows a biexponential curve with half-lives of 2 and 10 h, respectively (17). More than 90% of MTX is eliminated unchanged through the kidney. The 10% eliminated through the bile is of importance only in the setting of renal impairment or in the setting of "ileal-loop" kidney drainage into the intestinal tract. Metabolism plays no significant role in MTX excretion. Renal excretion in the monkey involves active tubular secretion that can be blocked with probenecid, salicylates, and nonsteroidal anti-inflammatory drugs; in the dog, there is a bidirectional tubular transport with reabsorption and secretion—the reabsorption can be competitively inhibited by folic acid, resulting in increased excretion (6). Cholestyramine binds MTX substantially, and oral administration of this drug to rats has resulted in improved clearance from serum and from bile, as well as reduced toxicity after intraperitoneal injection of MTX (8). Penetration into the cerebrospinal fluid (CSF) is slow, resulting in levels between 1/1000 and 1/30 of the corresponding plasma concentrations. Levels of MTX in spinal fluid can exceed 10 μmol after high-dose intravenous or direct subarachnoid administration. Elimination from this compartment may take days (if the CSF is loculated) and is accomplished mainly by bulk-flow kinetics dependent on CSF circulation and reabsorption. Reliable estimates of drug concentration cannot be made in the setting of hydrocephalus, elevated spinal fluid protein concentration, loculated collections of spinal fluid, or after radiation therapy has been provided. There is also an active transport system (1). After intrathecal administration of MTX, therefore, the CSF may constitute an endogenous reservoir that slowly releases the drug to plasma. Unexpectedly late high plasma levels of MTX may ensue.

The most common systemic toxicities of MTX involve tissues with rapidly dividing cells: myelosuppression, mucositis, and diarrhea can be avoided with opportune administration of reduced folates. Other adverse effects include a reversible pneumonitis with features of hypersensitivity reaction. Acute reversible elevations of liver enzymes occur often during treatment at very high doses; hepatic fibrosis has been associated with chronic oral administration. Renal failure, which follows very-high-dose treatment, results from intratubular MTX precipitation. This can be avoided by adequate hydration, maintained urinary output (>100 ml/h is suggested) and urine alkalinization (>pH 7 is suggested) (12).

Mechanisms underlying the neurotoxic effects of MTX are unclear; probably these are multiple and involve altered glucose metabolism, altered folate metabolism, and altered neurotransmitter synthesis by reduced availability of tetra-

hydrobiopterin, an essential cofactor for the hydroxylation of catecholamines (11,16). The astrocyte seems to be especially sensitive to MTX; astrocyte dysfunction may result in indirect damage to other cells, since these glial cells may play a regulatory or supplementary role in blood-brain barrier function, and in the uptake and metabolism of glucose and some neurotransmitters (4).

The effects of short-term exposure (2 weeks or less) to MTX have been studied in the rat. Continuous 24-h intravenous infusion >2.5 mg/kg produced a picture that resembled acute high-dose MTX-associated encephalopathy in humans. The animals, lethargic with reduced spontaneous activity and diminished startle to loud noise, exhibited electroencephalographic high-voltage delta waves in the absence of biochemical evidence of systemic toxicity. The cerebral glucose metabolism, determined by an autoradiographic method, was reduced in a dose-dependent manner (11). There were no differences in ammonia levels when compared with controls infused with normal saline.

Morphological studies have been made after short-term MTX infusion by intraperitoneal (one to three doses of 10 or 100 mg/kg over 24 h) or intraventricular (single dose of 1, 3, or 5 mg/kg) routes. Reversible changes were noted after high doses. The earliest change occurred after 2 or more intraperitoneal injections of 10 mg/kg. These consisted of increased numbers of Alzheimer type II astrocytes with clumped and peripherally marginated nuclear chromatin. There were no liver alterations, nor was there evidence of hypoxic or ischemic change. With increased dose intensity, features of white matter change emerged: increased Alzheimer type II cells were noted along with microglial hyperplasia, spongy change in the neuropil, focal white matter necrosis with proportional loss of myelin and axons, scattered swollen axons, and occasional neuronal necrosis. Endothelial cells were spared. Corresponding ultrastructural changes included pleomorphism and condensation of mitochondria, membrane-bound vacuoles, distended Golgi complexes, and hydropic swelling of astrocyte perikarya and their processes. At higher MTX doses, there was neuronal necrosis, loss of axons in necrotic areas, and focal accumulations of membranous dense bodies with dissolution of neurofilaments and microtubules in swollen axons. The oligodendrocytes showed dense cytoplasm and dilated Golgi complexes, and there was prominent splitting of myelin lamellae; endothelial cells had a normal appearance (4). The early, reversible astrocytic changes probably correlated with the acute encephalopathy, while the more severe changes with necrosis and axonal disruption are related to the chronic leukoencephalopathy in humans.

Myelopathy with demyelination of white matter tracts has been induced by intrathecal MTX in the rabbit (2). A rat model of behavioral change has been utilized to study delayed effects of CNS therapy for childhood lymphoblastic leukemia. Male rats treated at 17 and 18 days of age with 1000 cGy of cranial irradiation plus 2 mg/kg of MTX and 18 mg/kg of prednisolone showed a male-specific change in behavior. Rats treated at 18 days of age with 1000 cGy of cranial radiotherapy alone did not show any change (9). The effects of MTX alone were not studied.

In humans, MTX (30–60 mg/m^2) is not associated with neurotoxicity when administered *via* intravenous injection or oral intake. High-dose treatments (>1 g/m^2) can produce an acute or subacute encephalopathy in up to 20% of patients. The syndrome usually becomes apparent within 24 h; it is characterized by confusion, somnolence, headaches and, less frequently, by seizures and transient focal neurological deficits. Computed tomography (CT) fails to show changes, but the electroencephalogram shows slow waves. Blood chemistry studies are normal except for increased plasma phenylalanine. The toxic mechanism is unknown, but studies with positron emission tomography using fluorodeoxyglucose and rubidium isotopes have demonstrated depression of cerebral glucose metabolism and increased passage of rubidium from blood to brain indicating blood-brain barrier dysfunction (10). Lacking specific treatment, the syndrome is transient, reversible within 72 h, and may not recur with rechallenge.

Five syndromes follow intrathecal or intraventricular MTX administration:

1. An acute myelopathy within minutes to hours of administration.
2. Subacute myelopathic changes occurring after repetitive spinal or ventricular administration.
3. A chronic demyelinating encephalopathy usually in the setting of postirradiation MTX administration.
4. Localized necrotizing and edematous white matter changes in proximity to ventricular catheter sites of MTX administration.
5. Subtle neuropsychiatric changes in the setting of prior irradiation.

Acute Myelopathy

Within minutes to hours of lumbar subarachnoid or ventricular MTX administration, there may appear a devastating acute transverse myelopathy. Acute or subacute paraplegia with sensory abnormalities develops. Spinal magnetic resonance imaging (MRI) may show diffuse cord swelling, increased signal intensity, and gadolinium enhancement. The process, likely vascular or necrotizing, is usually irreversible, but some patients have recovered completely. The value of systemic steroid therapy is doubtful. Uncertain is

the role of the MTX diluent (examples may involve either unsuspected use of MTX with alcohol preservative or the use of autologous CSF as a diluent). Autopsy studies demonstrate diffuse coagulative necrosis of the spinal cord (18). Intrathecal or intraventricular administration may produce a chemical meningitis. This uncommon complication appears within 24 h of the injection with fever, headaches, nuchal rigidity, and CSF leukocytosis; it resolves spontaneously, but steroids can also be helpful. The short latency between injection and the syndrome helps differentiate between methotrexate intoxication or bacterial meningitis resulting from contamination during the procedure.

Subacute Myelopathy

Repetitive injections of MTX into the lumbar CSF increase the risk of damage to the white matter of the spinal cord or the nerve roots. This risk increases with increasing frequency of treatments (such as continuous infusions or injections three times a week), with increased cumulative MTX doses (>150 mg), with concomitant administration of intrathecal or high-dose systemic cytarabine, and with prior or concomitant spinal radiotherapy. Pareses from damage to lumbar or cranial nerve roots are accompanied by neck stiffness, headaches, and vomiting and a proliferation of activated lymphocytes in the CSF. The protein concentration often rises, but diminished glucose concentrations are uncommon. The process is usually irreversible and is a contraindication to further administration of MTX by the subarachnoid route.

Chronic Leukoencephalopathy

Delayed and progressive necrotizing leukoencephalopathy is a well-known complication of intrathecal or intraventricular MTX treatments and, less frequently, of intravenous high-dose administration. The risk is increased with higher cumulative doses (usually >40 g/m^2); with associated cranial irradiation, especially when radiotherapy precedes or is simultaneous with the chemotherapy; with patient age under 5 years; in the setting of known leptomeningeal disease rather than as part of CNS prophylactic treatment; and with obstruction of CSF flow. The syndrome, appearing during therapy, may be delayed for more than 8 months, and then progressively worsens. Death follows usually within a few months, although in some patients the condition seems to stabilize transiently. First symptoms are subtle changes in memory and intellect, accompanied by blunting of personality and speech. The motor dysfunction is often punctuated by myoclonic jerks involving the pharyngeal and peripheral muscles. Abnormal gait and extremity ataxia with spasticity are followed by sphincter disorders and seizures. The CSF contains elevated concentrations of protein with lymphocytes and histiocytes. The CT scan shows white-matter hypodensities and patchy contrast enhancement followed by subcortical calcifications and dilated ventricles. Similar changes appear on MRI with extensive T2 abnormalities of the periventricular white matter. The electroencephalogram exhibits frontal slow waves. Examination of the brain reveals multiple coalescent foci of coagulation necrosis especially affecting the white matter in a perivascular pattern. Vascular lesions, inconstantly present, consist of a calcific microangiopathy affecting small arterioles. Their walls are hyalinized, with notable endothelial proliferation and fibrinoid necrosis. The white matter reveals nerve fiber damage with axonal swelling (13,14).

Localized White Matter Changes

Patients receiving MTX *via* intraventricular catheters may develop focal leukoencephalopathic changes around the catheter tip. These changes often progress to involve the white matter along the catheter shaft as well. On microscopic examination, these changes are identical to the necrotizing leukoencephalopathy noted above. Since catheters are commonly inserted through nondominant frontal or occipital craniotomy holes, clinical presentations first involve slowness of motor function, and apraxias of speech or visual difficulties. MRI or CT of the brain reveals large pericatheter hypodensities with or without contrast enhancement. This toxicity involves CSF backflow around the catheter resulting in exposure of surrounding tissue to concentrations of MTX approximating tens to hundreds of microgram equivalents. The same effect may result from a malposition of the condition (7).

Subtle Neuropsychiatric Syndromes

There is epidemiological evidence that long-term neuropsychological changes may accompany intrathecal MTX when the agent is administered in close temporal proximity to cranial irradiation. These therapies, used as prophylactic CNS treatment for leukemia or lymphoma, result in changes primarily in nondominant hemispheric functions. Lower scores in neuropsychological tests that measure these functions appear in populations studied even after controlling for age, socioeconomic status, age at diagnosis, months since onset and cessation of treatment, time missed from schooling, and presence/type of CNS cancer. The use of intrathecal or systemic MTX without radiotherapy was not associated with these findings, although this effect cannot be completely excluded (3).

REFERENCES

1. Balis FM, Poplack DG (1989) Central nervous system pharmacology of antileukemic drugs. *Amer J Pediat Hematol Oncol* **11**, 74.

2. Burch PA, Grossman SA, Reinhard CS (1988) Spinal cord penetration of intrathecally administered cytarabine and methotrexate: A quantitative autoradiographic study. *J Nat Cancer Inst* **90**, 1211.

3. Butler RW, Hill JM, Steinherz PG et al. (1994) Neuropsychologic effects of cranial irradiation, intrathecal methotrexate, and systemic methotrexate in childhood cancer. *J Clin Oncol* **12**, 2621.

4. Gregorios JB, Gregorios AB, Mora J et al. (1989) Morphologic alterations in rat brain following systemic and intraventricular methotrexate injection: Light and electron microscopic studies. *J Neuropathol Exp Neurol* **48**, 33.

5. Henderson ES, Adamson RH, Oliverio VT (1965) The metabolic fate of tritiated methotrexate II. Absorption and excretion in man. *Cancer Res* **25**, 1018.

6. Huang KC, Wenczac BA, Yong KL (1979) Renal tubular transport of methotrexate in the rhesus monkey and dog. *Cancer Res* **39**, 4843.

7. Lemann W, Wiley RG, Posner JB (1988) Leukoencephalopathy complicating intraventricular catheters: Clinical, radiographic and pathologic study of 10 cases. *J Neurooncol* **6**, 67.

8. McAnena OJ, Ridge JA, Daly JM (1987) Alteration of methotrexate metabolism in rats by administration of an elemental liquid diet II. Reduced toxicity and improved survival using cholestyramine. *Cancer* **59**, 1091.

9. Mullenix PJ, Kernan WJ, Tassinari MS (1990) An animal model to study toxicity of central nervous system therapy for childhood acute lymphoblastic leukemia: Effects on behavior. *Cancer Res* **50**, 6461.

10. Phillips PC, Dhawan V, Strother SC et al. (1987) Reduced cerebral glucose metabolism and increased brain capillary permeability following high-dose methotrexate chemotherapy: A positron emission tomographic study. *Ann Neurol* **21**, 59.

11. Phillips PC, Thaler HT, Berger CA et al. (1986) Acute high-dose methotrexate neurotoxicity in the rat. *Ann Neurol* **20**, 583.

12. Pitman SW, Parker LM, Tattersall MHN et al. (1975) Clinical trial of high-dose methotrexate (NSC-740) with citrovorum factor (NSC-3590)—toxicologic and therapeutic observations. *Cancer Chemother Rep* **6**, 43.

13. Robain O, Dulac O, Dommergues JP et al. (1984) Necrotising leukoencephalopathy complicating treatment of childhood leukemia. *J Neurol Neurosurg Psychiat* **47**, 65.

14. Rubinstein LJ, Herman MM, Long TF, Wilbur JR (1975) Disseminated necrotizing leukoencephalopathy: A compli-

cation of treated central nervous system leukemia and lymphoma. *Cancer* **35**, 291.

15. Schilsky RL (1992) Antimetabolites. In: *The Chemotherapy Source Book*. Perry MC ed. Williams & Wilkins, Baltimore p. 301.

16. Silverstein FS, Johnston MV (1986) A model of methotrexate encephalopathy: Neurotransmitter and pathologic abnormalities. *J Child Neurol* **1**, 351.

17. Stoller RG, Hande KR, Jacobs SA *et al.* (1977) Use of plasma pharmacokinetics to predict and prevent methotrexate toxicity. *N Engl J Med* **297**, 630.

18. Watterson J, Toogood I, Nieder M *et al.* (1994) Excessive spinal cord toxicity from intensive central nervous system directed therapies. *Cancer* **74**, 3034.

Methoxyflurane

Herbert H. Schaumburg

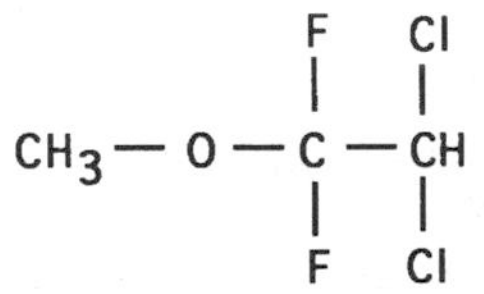

METHOXYFLURANE
$C_3H_4Cl_2F_2O$

2,2-Dichloro-1,1-difluoro-1-methoxyethane

NEUROTOXICITY RATING
Clinical

B Neuromuscular transmission syndrome

Methoxyflurane, the most potent of the hydrocarbon inhalation anesthetics, is seldom used because of potential renal dysfunction. Methoxyflurane is metabolized to a greater extent than other volatile anesthetics; its principal metabolites are two nephrotoxic agents, oxalic acid and fluoride.

CNS and cardiovascular depression are the principal neurotoxic effects of methoxyflurane, similar to those associated with halothane and enflurane. There is an unusually thorough report of repeated occurrences of a myasthenia gravis syndrome in an anesthetist that is clearly related to use of methoxyflurane (1). Controlled administration of methoxyflurane to this individual reproduced the syndrome; weakness was rapidly ameliorated by anticholinesterase medication. It is suggested that this individual had subclinical myasthenia gravis disclosed by the effect of methoxyflurane on the neuromuscular junction (2).

REFERENCES
1. Elder BF, Beal H, DeWald W, Cobb S (1971) Exacerbation of subclinical myasthenia gravis by occupational exposure to an anesthetic. *Anesth Analg* **50**, 383.

2. Waud BE (1977) Neuromuscular blocking agents. In: *Current Problems in Anesthesia and Critical Care Medicine*. Brunner EA ed. Year Book Medical Publishers, Chicago p. 5.

β-N-Methylamino-L-Alanine

Glen Kisby

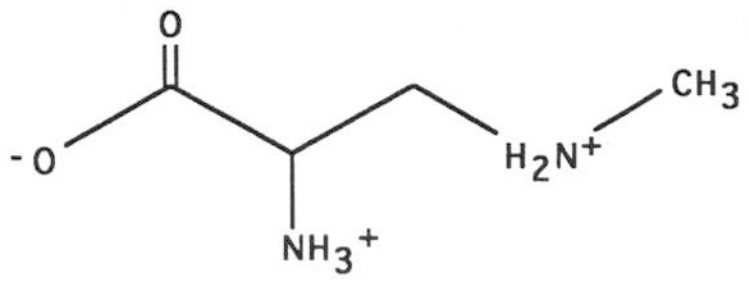

β-N-METHYLAMINO-L-ALANINE
$C_4H_{11}N_2O_2$

(+)-β-Methyl-α,β-diaminopropionic acid; BMAA

NEUROTOXICITY RATING
Experimental

A Cerebellar degeneration (rats)

A Motor system dysfunction (primates)

B Excitotoxin

This neurotoxic amino acid was originally isolated from seed of the false sago palm (*Cycas circinalis*, L.) (39), which is used by the Chamorro people of Guam for food and medicine. The predominant form isolated from the cycad plant is the L-isomer (39). The L-isomer is more neurotoxic than the racemate (±), and the synthetic D-isomer is not neurotoxic (40). The concentration of "free" BMAA in the seed of various cycad plant species ranges from 0.29–1.61 mg/g dry weight of the female gametophyte (7). Low levels of BMAA (>0.005% w/w) have also been detected by mass spectrometry (10) and high-performance liquid chromatography fluorescence (15) in Guamanian cycad flour prepared in a traditional manner by Chamorros. Cited levels may underestimate the exact concentration of BMAA; toxin levels increase when seed extracts are acidified with hydrochloric acid (6,24) (G. Kisby, unpublished data). The source of this BMAA is unknown, but failure to detect the agent in cycad (*Cycas media*, R.Br.) plant protein hydrolyzed with methanesulfonic acid (G. Kisby, unpublished data) suggests that BMAA is not incorporated into protein, but may be chelated. BMAA is a potent chelator of divalent metal ions like copper and zinc (23), and cycad flour samples processed on Guam may contain significant levels of zinc (8). The coordination chemistry of the BMAA chelate is similar to that of 2,3-diaminopropionic acid; BMAA forms quaternary nitrogen complexes with copper or zinc in aqueous solutions. BMAA and metal complexes are more stable than corresponding neurotransmitter amino acids (*e.g.*, L-glutamate).

Cycads are used for food (*e.g.*, flour) and/or medicine (*e.g.*, oral tonics, poultices) by certain western Pacific populations, notably the Chamorros of Guam, formerly the Japanese of the Kii peninsula of Japan, and the Auyu people of Iran Jaya, Indonesia. Oral and dermal absorption of BMAA are therefore primary routes of exposure to humans. BMAA is a nonprotein amino acid which, at physiological pH (7.4), exists predominately (~51%) in the β-protonated neutral zwitterion form with smaller fractions of the α-protonated (~8%) and tripolar cation (~10%) forms (35). BMAA reacts with physiological bicarbonate to produce β- and α-carbamates (31%) (22). β-Carbamate, the predominant form under physiological conditions (37°C, pH 7.4) (21), is essential for expression of the excitotoxic property of BMAA in nervous tissue (41,42).

Raw cycad seed is either taken orally (p.o.) or applied topically for medicinal purposes, while cycad flour is used in the preparation of food (37). Studies with rats (9) and primates (8) indicate the bioavailability of BMAA by the oral route is just as efficient (80%) as the parenteral route. The half-life ($t_{1/2}$) of BMAA in various rodent tissues ranges from 0.45–0.7 day (9). Less than 10% of BMAA injected into rodents is recovered unchanged in the urine and feces 7 days later, an indication that the neurotoxic amino acid

accumulates in tissue and/or is metabolized. BMAA accumulates rapidly (15–60 min) in toxin-treated (>1.0 mM) mouse cerebral cortical explant tissue (15,16) and is metabolized *in vitro* by purified rat brain microsomes and mitochondria (15).

BMAA is widely distributed in the CNS of rats administered a bolus injection of the amino acid (100 mg/kg, intravenously) (11). The highest concentration of BMAA is found in the pons, thalamus, and cerebellum, and the lowest levels in the spinal cord, cerebral cortex, and cerebrospinal fluid (CSF). A similar CNS distribution was found in adult Sprague-Dawley rats administered an intracarotid injection of ^{14}C-BMAA (2 μCi/100 μl for 30 sec), with the highest concentration in brain tissue ipsilateral to the injected radiolabeled neurotoxin (13). Some brain regions (*e.g.*, hippocampus) had relatively higher levels of BMAA than those previously reported (11). BMAA gains access to rodent CNS tissue by the large neutral amino acid (LNAA) carrier (25) of the blood-brain barrier (35), an unexpected finding considering the substrate requirements for the LNAA carrier: (a) a free carboxyl group, (b) an unsubstituted (charged α-amino group), and (c) a bulky neutral side chain. BMAA is transported across the rodent blood-brain barrier in a sodium-independent manner with a transfer rate (V_{max}) of 1.6 ± 0.3 × 10^{-3} μmol/sec/g; transport is inhibited by excess amounts of L-leucine, L-lysine, L-glutamate, or methylaminoisobutyric acid (35). Various factors like age, diet, and disease, which are known to increase the blood-brain transport of LNAAs (35), conceivably could influence the blood-brain transport of BMAA, a consideration of toxicological importance given that cycad products were heavily consumed during times of privation (*e.g.*, World War II on Guam) (44).

Unlike other excitant neurotoxins, BMAA is rapidly transported by nervous tissue *in vitro* (16); this is dependent on sodium and protein concentration, pH, and temperature, an indication that the neurotoxin may be transported like other amino acid neurotransmitters. BMAA accumulation is more pronounced in mouse cortical explant tissue than rat cortical astrocytes (16), suggesting a preferential neuronal uptake of the toxin.

Since BMAA may be rapidly transported into neural tissue, the fate of intracellularly accumulated toxin may be important in characterizing its neurotoxic properties. Because BMAA lacks the characteristic dicarboxylic acid structure of glutamate and is a weak glutamate agonist, its neurotoxic properties may be attributable to the production of a metabolite (37). BMAA has been proposed to undergo metabolism by L-amino acid oxidase to ammonia and β-methylaminopyruvate (12), but enzyme activity is low in peripheral organ tissue and almost nonexistent in brain tissue (M.W. Anderson, personnel communication). The availability of radiolabeled BMAA provided an opportunity to characterize the metabolism of this neurotoxin both *in vivo* and *in vitro*. The presence of at least six radioactive peaks was determined in the urine of young male rats (111–140 g) administered unlabelled BMAA [1.8 μmol/g/day, intraperitoneally (i.p.)] for 6 days followed by 1 μCi of ^{14}C-BMAA (*specific activity* 41 μCi/mmol) from day 7 onward (30). Although most of the radioactive peaks were not identified, it was proposed that one metabolite was α-acetamido-β-methylaminopropionic acid based upon chromatographic and chemical analysis (sensitive to acylase I) of a urine sample. A previous report noted that BMAA is not metabolized *in vitro* by rodent liver, muscle, kidney, or brain tissue (11). Other *in vitro* studies demonstrate that BMAA is metabolized by rodent brain microsomes (15).

BMAA has been proposed (15) to be N-demethylated to formaldehyde *via* brain mixed function oxidases in a manner comparable to the N-methylated compound aminopyrine (20,28,29). Formaldehyde is a genotoxin (3,13) that can react with cellular macromolecules or can be further metabolized to formic acid, which depletes energy stores (17). Several studies demonstrate that mouse (28), rat (15), and human (29) brain tissue aminopyrine-N-demethylase activity is even higher than hepatic levels. BMAA is metabolized by mouse cortical explant tissue and purified rat brain microsomes and mitochondria (15). Moreover, the cytochrome P-450 inhibitors SKF 525A and piperonyl butoxide inhibited (25%–60%) cerebral microsomal N-demethylation of BMAA (1.6 mM) and aminopyrine (1.6 mM). Taken together, these studies demonstrate that BMAA is metabolized by rodent brain and peripheral organ tissue, but the role of these metabolite(s) in relationship to BMAA neurotoxicity is unknown.

The neurotoxic properties of BMAA have been examined in rodents (18,26,27,33,34,40) and primates (37). Investigators who worked previously on the structurally related plant (*Lathyrus sativus*) excitant amino acid, β-N-oxalylamino-L-alanine, found that primates heavily intoxicated with purified BMAA (300 mg/kg/day for up to 13 months) gradually developed signs of pyramidal, extrapyramidal, and behavioral dysfunction associated with chromatolysis of Betz cells and occasional large anterior horn cells (37). Postsynaptic vacuolation and neuronal necrosis of the type associated with acute glutamate-like excitotoxic damage was absent, suggesting that extracellular concentrations of BMAA were low (36). Serum and cerebrospinal fluid from one animal had micromolar and nanomolar concentrations, respectively. While the clinical and pathological picture of chronic primate BMAA neurotoxicity had features reminiscent of the cycad-associated western Pacific

amyotrophic lateral sclerosis (ALS) and parkinsonism-dementia complex, the experimental disorder differed from the human disease in that the primate disorder did not progress once treatment with BMAA ceased (36). In addition, there was also no correlation between the concentration of BMAA in Chamorro cycad flour and the age-adjusted incidence of ALS on Guam (45).

The neurotoxic effect of BMAA in rodents is different from that seen in comparably treated primates. Young Wistar rats (~85 g) administered BMAA (500–2000 mg/kg) or DL-BMAA (350–4000 mg/g, i.p.) displayed delayed-onset ataxia and dystonia, with selective cerebellar degeneration of stellate, basket, Purkinje, and Golgi cells, but not granule cells or other CNS tissue (34). All the damaged cells were γ-aminobutyric acid (GABA)ergic, and there is preliminary evidence indicating that BMAA may be taken up into cells by a GABA transporter (15).

In contrast to rats, mice appear to be refractory to BMAA. CD-1 mice treated p.o. with 250–1000 mg/kg/day for 11 weeks showed no behavioral, neuropathological (cerebellum not reported), or neuropharmacological changes, except for a reduction in CNS glycine levels (26). In separate studies, CD-1 mice administered BMAA (100 mg/kg, p.o.) for 45 days also failed to develop evidence of BMAA neurotoxicity (G. Kisby, unpublished data). The concentration of BMAA (0.1–0.5 mM; non–saline-perfused) in the brains of these animals reportedly approached those (0.5 mM) that routinely elicited neuronal degeneration in mouse cortical explants treated with BMAA (32). Injection of BMAA into mice, rats, and rabbits by an intracerebroventricular (i.c.v.) or intrastriatal route was reproducibly neurotoxic in a dose- and time-dependent manner (33). Intrastriatal injections in rats and rabbits damaged the entire striatum but did not trigger behavioral changes in rats or rabbits. Infusion i.c.v. consistently elicited irritability, excitability, seizures, and death. Pathological changes involved neurons, glial cells, and endothelial cells, a pattern that differed from that of a classic excitotoxic lesion but which may have reflected the large concentration of the neurotoxin. Mice exhibited hyperexcitability, jumping fits, and a delayed-onset whole-body shake/wobble after i.c.v. injection of BMAA; this was attenuated in a dose-dependent manner by systemic pretreatment with N-methyl-D-aspartate (NMDA) antagonists (32).

Taken together, these studies suggest that BMAA behaves as a weak, atypical NMDA-like excitant neurotoxin at high concentrations after i.c.v. injection. At lower concentrations, BMAA may be preferentially transported and accumulate or be metabolized in brain tissue to produce its chronic effects. The presence of chromatolytic and nuclear chromatin changes in Betz cells and the absence of excitotoxic lesions in primates heavily dosed with BMAA (37) suggest that mechanisms other than excitotoxicity are responsible for the agent's chronic neurotoxic effects.

The acute neurotoxic properties of BMAA have been examined *in vitro* using organotypic CNS explants (24,32), neuronal cultures (4,19,41–43), and CNS tissue slices (4,5,38). In mouse cord and cortex explants, BMAA stereospecifically (L- *vs.* D-isomer) elicited an excitotoxic pattern of damage consisting of postsynaptic vacuolation and dark shrunken cells (24,32). Unlike the more acutely potent *Lathyrus sativus* toxin, β-N-oxalylamino-L-alanine, the postsynaptic vacuolation and neuronal degeneration elicited by BMAA was attenuated in a concentration-dependent manner by selective antagonists for the NMDA receptor and ion channel (32). Furthermore, *in vitro* neurotoxicity of BMAA was potentiated by physiological concentrations of bicarbonate (41,42), which forms a stable adduct with the α-amino group of the toxin. High concentrations of BMAA [>300 μM (30)] (in the presence or absence of bicarbonate) are needed to displace ligands for the NMDA-, α-amino-3-hydroxy-5-methyl-4-isoxazole-, or kainate-preferring receptors, indicating that the receptor-mediated acute excitotoxic effects of BMAA may be different from its chronic effects (37).

BMAA has been shown to interact with both NMDA and non–NMDA-type excitatory amino acid receptors. At low *in vitro* concentrations and in the presence of $NaHCO_3$, BMAA is selectively toxic to NADPH-diaphorase-containing neurons; these cells are selectively vulnerable to non–NMDA-type agonists (41). BMAA also precipitates seizures and postsynaptic vacuolation in CNS tissue *in situ* and *in vitro*, respectively; these events are markedly attenuated by the NMDA receptor antagonists 7-amino-phosphonoheptanoate and MK-801 (32,33,37,43). D-BMAA may be a stereospecific modulator of NMDA receptor function by acting as an agonist at the strychnine-insensitive glycine modulatory site of the NMDA receptor (1). In the presence of $NaHCO_3$, BMAA activates currents in hippocampal neurons *in vitro*; these are antagonized by 6-cyano-7-nitroquinozaline-2,3-dione, but not 2-amino-5-phosphonovaleric acid (2). BMAA is more potent in displacing ^3H-glutamate than ^3H-(+/−)-3,2-carboxypiperazin-4-yl-propyl-1-phosphonic acid, an NMDA-type antagonist, suggesting an interaction at non–NMDA-type receptors (4).

The principal route by which humans come into contact with BMAA is through oral or topical application of cycad seed preparations. The relative risk to humans from BMAA-induced neurotoxicity is probably low because of several factors: (a) raw cycad seed and cycad flour both contain low levels of the neurotoxin (7,10,15), (b) BMAA is poorly transported across the blood-brain barrier (9,11), (c) large concentrations are needed to induce neurotoxicity in animals and cultured nervous tissue (31,32), and (d) primates require serial large doses of BMAA to express neurological compromise (36). Taken together, these studies indicate that BMAA is a low-potency neurotoxin.

Findings from *in vitro* and *in vivo* studies suggest that BMAA may have two possible mechanisms of toxicity: (a) activation of NMDA and non-NMDA (metabotropic) receptors (acute toxicity) and (b) depletion of energy metabolism and/or alkylation of intracellular macromolecules (chronic neurotoxicity). While there is ample experimental evidence from *in vivo* and *in vitro* studies that BMAA activates glutamate receptors to induce excitotoxic damage to nervous tissue, the failure to detect a similar pattern of neuropathology in brain tissue of primates chronically treated with BMAA suggests that alternative mechanisms exist for its chronic effects. One possibility is that BMAA is transported into nervous tissue and bioactivated to a toxic metabolite. Preliminary studies indicate that BMAA is taken up by a GABA transporter (15). Recent studies indicate that BMAA competes with GABA for its uptake and generates currents during its transport into frog oocytes overexpressing a GABA transporter (GAT1; C. Allen, personal communication). BMAA is metabolized by brain mixed-function oxidases (*e.g.*, aminopyrine N-demethylase) to formaldehyde (15), a known genotoxin (3,13) that can react with cellular macromolecules or deplete energy stores through its metabolite, formic acid (17). These findings indicate that BMAA is transported into nervous tissue and bioactivated to a toxic metabolite. The role of these metabolite(s) in nervous tissue and their relationship to BMAA-induced chronic neurotoxicity is unknown.

REFERENCES

1. Allen CN, Omelchenko I, Ross SM, Spencer PS (1995) The neurotoxin, β-N-methylamino-L-alanine (BMAA) interacts with the strychnine-insensitive glycine modulatory site of the N-methyl-D-aspartate receptor. *Neuropharmacology* **34**, 651.

2. Allen CN, Spencer PS, Carpenter DO (1993) β-N-methylamino-L-alanine in the presence of bicarbonate is an agonist at non-N-methyl-D-aspartate-type receptors. *Neuroscience* **54**, 567.

3. Bolt HM (1987) Experimental toxicology of formaldehyde. *J Cancer Res Clin Oncol* **113**, 305.

4. Copani A, Cononico PL, Catania MV *et al.* (1991) Interaction between β-N-methylamino-L-alanine and excitatory amino acid receptors in brain slices and neuronal cultures. *Brain Res* **558**, 79.

5. Copani A, Canonico PL, Nicoletti F (1990) β-N-Methylamino-L-alanine (L-BMAA) is a potent agonist of 'metabotropic' glutamate receptors. *Eur J Pharmacol* **181**, 327.

6. Dossaji SF (1974) *The Distribution of Azoxyglycosides, Amino Acids and Biflavanoids in the Order Cycadales: Their Taxonomic, Phylogenetic and Toxicological Significance.* Doctoral Thesis, University of Texas, Austin.

7. Duncan MW, Crowley JS, Jones SM *et al.* (1989) Quantification of the putative neurotoxin 2-amino-3-(methylamino)-propanoic acid (BMAA) in cycadales: Analysis of the seeds of some members of the family Cycadaceae. *Anal Toxicol* **13**, 169.

8. Duncan MW, Marini AM, Watters R *et al.* (1992) Zinc, a neurotoxin to cultured neurons, contaminates cycad flour prepared by traditional Guamanian methods. *J Neurosci* **12**, 1523.

9. Duncan MW, Markey SP, Weick BG *et al.* (1991) 2-Amino-3-(methylamino)propanoic acid (BMAA) bioavailability in the primate. *Neurobiol Aging* **13**, 333.

10. Duncan MW, Steele JC, Kopin IJ, Markey SP (1990) 2-Amino-3-(methylamino)-propanoic acid (BMAA) in cycad flour: An unlikely cause of amyotrophic lateral sclerosis and parkinsonism-dementia of Guam. *Neurology* **40**, 767.

11. Duncan MW, Villacreses NE, Pearson PG *et al.* (1991) 2-Amino-3-(methylamino)-propanoic acid (BMAA) pharmacokinetics and blood-barrier permeability in the rat. *J Pharmacol Exp Ther* **258**, 27.

12. Hashmi M, Anderson MW (1991) Enzymatic reaction of β-N-methylaminoalanine with L-amino acid oxidase. *Biochim Biophys Acta* **1074**, 36.

13. Heck Hd'A, Casanova M, Starr TB (1990) Formaldehyde toxicity—new understanding. *Crit Rev Toxicol* **20**, 397.

14. Kisby GE, Gold BG, Austin DR *et al.* (1993) DNA damage in rodent brain tissue induced by cycad toxins. *Soc Neurosci Abstr* **19**, 196.

15. Kisby GE, Nottingham V, Kayton R *et al.* (1992) Brain metabolism of β-N-methylamino-L-alanine (BMAA) and protection of excitotoxicity by GABA-uptake inhibitors. *Soc Neurosci Abstr* **18**, 82.

16. Kisby GE, Ross SM, Spencer PS *et al.* (1992) Cycasin and BMAA: Candidate neurotoxins for western Pacific amyotrophic lateral sclerosis/parkinsonism-dementia complex. *Neurodegeneration* **1**, 73.

17. Liesivuori J, Savolainen H (1991) Methanol and formic acid toxicity: Biochemical mechanisms. *Pharmacol Toxicol* **69**, 157.

18. Lindstrom H, Luthman J, Mouton P *et al.* (1990) Plant-derived neurotoxic amino acids (β-N-oxalylamino-L-alanine and β-N-methylamino-L-alanine): Effects on central monoamine neurons. *J Neurochem* **55**, 941.

19. Manzoni OJJ, Prezeau L, Bockaert J (1991) β-N-Methylamino-L-alanine is a low affinity agonist of metabotropic glutamate receptors. *NeuroReport* **2**, 609.

20. Marietta MP, Vessel ES, Hartmann RD *et al.* (1979) Characterization of cytochrome P-450 dependent aminopyrine N-demethylase in rat brain: Comparison with hepatic aminopyrine N-demethylation. *J Pharmacol Exp Ther* **208**, 271.

21. Myers TG, Nelson SD (1990) Neuroactive carbamate adducts of β-N-methylamino-L-alanine and ethylenediamine. *J Biol Chem* **265**, 10193.

22. Nunn PB, O'Brien P (1989) The interaction of β-N-methylamino-L-alanine with bicarbonate: A ^{1}H-NMR study. *FEBS Lett* **251**, 31.

23. Nunn PB, O'Brien P, Pettit LD, Pyburn SI (1989) Complexes of zinc, copper, and nickel with the nonprotein amino acid L-α-amino-β-methylaminopropionic acid: A naturally occurring neurotoxin. *J Inorgan Biochem* **37**, 175.

24. Nunn PB, Seelig M, Spencer PS (1987) Stereospecific acute neuronotoxicity of "uncommon" plant amino acids linked to human motor-system disease. *Brain Res* **410**, 375.

25. Olendorf WH (1971) Brain uptake of radiolabeled amino acids, amines, and hexoses after arterial injection. *Amer J Physiol* **221**, 1629.

26. Perry TL, Bergeron C, Biro AJ, Hansen S (1989) β-N-Methylamino-L-alanine. Chronic oral administration is not neurotoxic to mice. *J Neurol Sci* **94**, 173.

27. Polsky FI, Nunn PB, Bell EA (1972) Distribution and toxicity of α-amino-β-methylaminopropionic acid. *Fed Proc* **31**, 1473.

28. Ravindranath V, Anandatheerthavarada HK (1989) High activity of cytochrome P-450-linked aminopyrine N-demethylase in mouse brain microsomes, and associated sex-related difference. *Biochem J* **261**, 769.

29. Ravindranath V, Anandatheerthavarada HK (1990) Preparation of brain microsomes with cytochrome P450 activity using calcium aggregation method. *Anal Biochem* **187**, 310.

30. Reece DM, Nunn PB (1989) Synthesis of ^{14}C-labelled L-α-amino-β-methylaminopropionic acid and its metabolism in the rat. *Biochem Soc Trans* **17**, 203.

31. Ross SM, Roy DN, Spencer PS (1989) β-N-Oxalylamino-L-alanine action of glutamate receptors. *J Neurochem* **53**, 710.

32. Ross SM, Seelig M, Spencer PS (1987) Specific antagonism of excitotoxic action of 'uncommon' amino acids assayed in organotypic mouse cortical cultures. *Brain Res* **425**, 120.

33. Ross SM, Spencer PS (1987) Specific antagonism of behavioral action of "uncommon" amino acids linked to motor-system diseases. *Synapse* **1**, 248.

34. Seawright AA, Brown AW, Nolan CC, Cavanagh JB (1990) Selective degeneration of cerebellar cortical neurons caused by cycad neurotoxin, L-β-methylaminoalanine (L-BMAA), in rats. *Neuropathol Appl Neurobiol* **16**, 153.

35. Smith QR, Nagura H, Takada Y, Duncan MW (1992) Facilitated transport of the neurotoxin, β-N-methylamino-L-alanine, across the blood-brain barrier. *J Neurochem* **58**, 1330.

36. Spencer PS, Kisby GE, Ludolph AC (1991) Slow toxins, biologic markers, and long-latency neurodegenerative disease in the western Pacific region. *Neurology* **41**, 62.

37. Spencer PS, Nunn PB, Hugon J *et al.* (1987) Guam amyotrophic lateral sclerosis-parkinsonism-dementia linked to a plant excitant neurotoxin. *Science* **237**, 517.

38. Stewart GR, Olney JW, Pathikonda M, Snider WD (1991) Excitotoxicity in the embryonic chick spinal cord. *Ann Neurol* **30**, 758.

39. Vega A, Bell EA (1967) α-Amino-β-methylaminopropionic acid, a new amino acid from seeds of *Cycas circinalis*. *Phytochemistry* **6**, 759.

40. Vega A, Bell A, Nunn PB (1968) The preparation of L- and D-α-amino-β-methylaminopropionic acids and the identification of the compound isolated from *Cycas circinalis* as the L-isomer. *Phytochemistry* **7**, 1885.

41. Weiss JH, Choi DW (1988) β-N-Methylamino-L-alanine neurotoxicity: Requirement for bicarbonate as a cofactor. *Science* **241**, 973.

42. Weiss JH, Christine CW, Choi DW (1989) Bicarbonate dependence on glutamate receptor activation by β-N-methylamino-L-alanine: Channel recording and study with related compounds. *Neuron* **3**, 321.

43. Weiss JH, Koh J-Y, Choi DW (1989) Neurotoxicity of β-N-methylamino-L-alanine (BMAA) and β-N-oxalylamino-L-alanine (BOAA) on cultured cortical neurons. *Brain Res* **497**, 64.

44. Whiting MG (1963) Toxicity of cycads. *Econ Bot* **17**, 271.

45. Zhang ZX, Anderson DW, Mantel N, Román GC (1996) Motor neuron disease on Guam: Geographic and familial occurence, 1965–85. *Acta Neurol Scand* **94**, 51.

Methyl Bromide

Steven Herskovitz

CH_3Br

Monobromomethane

NEUROTOXICITY RATING

Clinical

A Acute encephalopathy (confusion, seizures, coma)

A Peripheral neuropathy

A Optic neuropathy

Experimental

A Acute encephalopathy (coma, seizures)

A Cerebellar granule cell degeneration

Methyl bromide is a colorless, nonflammable gas used as an insecticidal fumigant in agriculture. It has also been used as a refrigerant; a solvent for the extraction of oils from nuts, seeds, and flowers; an industrial methylating agent; and a component in fire extinguishers. It is odorless in low concentrations and has a chloroform-like odor at high concentrations. When used for fumigation, it usually contains chloropicrin as a lacrimatory warning agent. Short-term, high-dose toxic exposure results in a reversible but potentially fatal encephalopathy; prolonged, low-level exposure is associated with a peripheral neuropathy.

Methyl bromide is absorbed through the lungs, gastrointestinal tract, and probably skin (1,10). Most toxic exposures are from inhalation. It is highly lipid soluble and widely distributed. There is rapid metabolism in the liver to the bromide ion, and no accumulation of methyl bromide in the body. The half-life of the bromide ion is 12 days in humans. The maximum allowable inhalation concentration of methyl bromide in the United States is 5 ppm.

Short-term inhalation exposures in animals, including rats, rabbits, and guinea pigs, show various dose-dependent neurological and behavioral manifestations including inactivity, drowsiness, gait disturbance, excitation, tremor, spasms, paralysis, or seizures (1,11). Histologically, rats show dose-dependent cerebellar granule cell and cerebral cortical degeneration (11). Acute, fatal exposure in a dog caused edema of the cerebral cortex (15).

Prolonged exposures in rats, rabbits, and monkeys produce a similar array of clinical manifestations at varying doses and exposure periods (1,6). With 500 ppm exposure at 6 h/day, 3 days/week for 3–8 weeks, rats showed necrosis of the caudate-putamen and neuronal atrophy and pallor of the neuropil in caudate, putamen, thalamus, and cingulate cortex (7). In one rabbit study of 65 ppm for 1 month, a significant decrease in sciatic and ulnar nerve conduction velocities was observed (2).

In humans, acute exposure is heralded by mucosal irritation, followed in several hours by malaise, nausea, and vomiting (1,13). There may be headache, dizziness, and gastrointestinal and pulmonary symptoms. Mild exposures may evolve no further. Almost invariably, a latent period of several to many hours occurs before the onset of visual symptoms, dysarthria, ataxia, myalgias, numbness, paresis, confusion, delirium, psychosis, drowsiness, tremor, myoclonus, seizures (including status epilepticus), and death. Symptom onset can be quite sudden, without a prodrome indicative of toxic exposure. Clinical features may be reversible in mild intoxication; in severe cases, they can be permanent. Additional features may include dermatological lesions and renal failure. The few postmortem neuropathological studies have followed acute, high-dose exposures. Findings include cerebral edema, petechial hemorrhage, cell loss in the cerebral and cerebellar cortex, changes in dentate and various brainstem nuclei, or lesions in the inferior colliculi and mammillary bodies microscopically similar to those seen in Wernicke's encephalopathy (1,9,13,15).

The clinical manifestations of prolonged human exposure overlap to some degree with those of acute toxicity; the syndrome is a mixture of peripheral neuropathy, pyramidal and cerebellar dysfunction, and neuropsychiatric disturbances. Clinical descriptions of peripheral neuropathy are few (3,12); they suggest that a distal, sensorimotor polyneuropathy develops following over 3–7 months of exposure. Initial symptoms are acral paresthesias, eventually pain, and ataxia then appears. The cerebrospinal fluid is normal. In the one recent case with electrophysiological and biopsy studies, electromyography indicates a distal, predominantly motor axonopathy; sural biopsy showed loss of predominantly large myelinated fibers (3). Clinical recovery may be complete over 6–8 months (12). In one acute fatal case, postmortem examination revealed neuronal loss in dorsal root ganglia and axonal degeneration in nerve roots and proximal nerve segments (15). Optic neuropathy is infrequent and may be irreversible. Defective color vision may be an early sign of toxic exposure (3,4).

The mechanism of neurotoxicity is unclear. It appears to be related to methyl bromide itself, rather than to its hydrolysis product methanol, or to the bromide ion (1,13,14). A suggested mechanism is the direct disruption of cellular membranes related to the high lipid solubility of methyl bromide. One hypothesis invokes *in vivo* and *in vitro* evidence that methyl bromide may cause enzyme inhibition by alkylating sulfhydryl groups (1,13). Methyl bromide depletes brain glutathione in the rat (5); in cell culture, cytotoxicity is reduced in the presence of glutathione (14).

Editors' Note: A role for methylglutathione metabolites (methanethiol and formaldehyde) has been suggested on the basis of findings in two individuals with comparable acute occupational exposure to methyl bromide: one with normal erythrocyte glutathione transferase activity experienced severe neurotoxicity, while the second lacked detectable enzyme activity and had only mild symptoms (8). The authors note that if methylglutathione metabolites are the ultimate toxic species, treatment with *N*-acetylcysteine could have a toxifying rather than a detoxifying effect (8) (*see also* Methyl Chloride, this volume).

REFERENCES

1. Alexeeff GV, Kilgore WW (1983) Methyl bromide. *Residue Rev* **88**, 101.
2. Anger WK, Setzer JV, Russo JM *et al.* (1981) Neurobehavioral effects of methyl bromide inhalation exposures. *Scand J Work Environ Health* **7**, 40.
3. Cavalleri F, Galassi G, Ferrari S *et al.* (1995) Methyl bromide induced neuropathy: A clinical, neurophysiological, and morphological study. *J Neurol Neurosurg Psychiat* **58**, 383.
4. Chavez CT, Hepler RS, Straatsma BR (1985) Methyl bromide optic neuropathy. *Amer J Ophthalmol* **99**, 715.
5. Davenport CJ, Ali SF, Miller FJ *et al.* (1992) Effect of methyl bromide on regional brain glutathione, glutathione-S-transferases, monoamines, and amino acids in F344 rats. *Toxicol Appl Pharmacol* **112**, 120.
6. Eustis SL, Haber SB, Drew RT, Yang RSH (1988) Toxicology and pathology of methyl bromide in F344 rats and B6C3F1 mice following repeated inhalation exposure. *Fund Appl Toxicol* **11**, 594.
7. Furuta A, Hyakudo T, Ohnishi A *et al.* (1993) Neurotoxicity of methyl bromide—neuropathologic evaluation—preliminary study. *Sangyo Ika Daigaku Zasshi* **15**, 21.
8. Garnier R, Rambourg-Schepens MO, Muller A, Hallier E (1996) Glutathione transferase activity and formation of macromolecular adducts in two cases of acute methyl bromide poisoning. *Occup Environ Med* **53**, 211.
9. Hauw JJ, Escourolle R, Baulac M *et al.* (1986) Postmortem studies on posthypoxic and post-methyl bromide intoxication: Case reports. *Adv Neurol* **4**, 201.
10. Herzstein J, Cullen MR (1990) Methyl bromide intoxication in four field-workers during removal of soil fumigation sheets. *Amer J Indust Med* **17**, 321.
11. Hurtt ME, Morgan KT, Working PK (1987) Histopathology of acute toxic responses in selected tissues from rats exposed by inhalation to methyl bromide. *Fund Appl Toxicol* **9**, 352.
12. Kantarjian AD, Shaheen AS (1963) Methyl bromide poisoning with nervous system manifestations resembling polyneuropathy. *Neurology* **13**, 1054.
13. Moses H, Klawans HL (1979) Bromide intoxication. In: *The Handbook of Clinical Neurology*. Vinken PJ, Bruyn GW eds. Elsevier, Amsterdam p. 291.
14. Nishimura M, Umeda M, Ishizu S, Sato M (1980) Effect of methyl bromide on cultured mammalian cells. *J Toxicol Sci* **5**, 321.
15. Squier MV, Thompson J, Rajgopalan B (1992) Case report: Neuropathology of methyl bromide intoxication. *Neuropathol Appl Neurobiol* **18**, 579.

Methyl Chloride

Peter S. Spencer

CH_3Cl

Chloromethane

NEUROTOXICITY RATING

Clinical

A   Acute encephalopathy

A   Cerebellar syndrome

Experimental

A   Cerebellar granule cell degeneration

Methyl chloride (MeCl) was formerly used in North America and Europe as a refrigerant for domestic and commercial units; accidental leakage of these units resulted in 200 cases of severe acute MeCl intoxication between 1914 and 1950 (3,9,19). Occupational poisoning has also resulted from use of MeCl as a methylating agent in the production of synthetic rubber (7) and as a blowing agent in the manufacture of plastic foams (16). Occupational experience with MeCl has revealed the potential for toxic effects on the brain, visual system, kidneys, liver, bone marrow, cardiovascular system, respiratory system, and intestinal tract (14). Neurological dysfunction may be selective (1); detailed neuropathological assessment of the CNS and PNS is unavailable.

MeCl is a colorless gas. The BP is $-24°C$; it compresses to a colorless liquid of ethereal odor and sweet taste. A 1996 Threshold Limit Value of 50 ppm MeCl in workroom air has been set by the American Conference of Governmental Industrial Hygienists.

MeCl is conjugated by the erythrocyte glutathione-S-transferase isoenzyme class theta (GSTT), which is encoded by the GSTT-1 gene. The conjugation status of an individual is determined by GSTT-1 polymorphism. Of 208 healthy males and females from the southern and central parts of Sweden, 11.1% lacked *in-vitro* conjugation activity (nonconjugators), 46.2% had intermediate activity, and 42.8% had high activity (20). A recent study using a polymerase chain reaction assay classified 34 of 40 individuals as GSTT-1 positive; only 15% were "nonconjugators" (10).

Monohalogenated methanes, including MeCl, methyl bromide (MeBr), and methyl iodide (MeI), are mutagenic and carcinogenic compounds (21). However, in contrast to the response of MeI- or MeBr-treated rats and mice, which undergo systemic DNA methylation with formation of specific DNA adducts (3-methyladenine, 7-methyladenine, O^6-methylguanine), methylation of DNA bases is *not* observed in rats and mice treated with ^{14}C-MeCl by inhalation (4). Male mice develop renal tumors, but only at concentrations (1000 ppm) high enough to deplete target-tissue glutathione (GSH) and cause secondary DNA damage (4). Cytochrome P-450 1E1 in mouse kidney oxidizes MeCl to formaldehyde; activity is higher in males, and this gender selectively develops renal tumors (6). Microsomes from the kidney of male and female rats, both of which are refractory to MeCl-induced renal tumors, failed to catalyze the formation of detectable concentrations of formaldehyde (6).

Lethal effects were reported in early experimental studies of rats, mice, guinea pigs, and rabbits exposed to 2000–4000 ppm MeCl 6 h/day for 1–3 weeks (17). The lethal effect on B6C3F1 mice of a single, 6-h inhalation exposure to 2500 ppm was blocked by prior treatment with L-buthionine-S,R-sulfoximine (BSO), an inhibitor of GSH synthesis. Daily BSO pretreatment protected mice from renal toxicity and cerebellar damage in B6C3Fl male mice exposed to 1500 ppm MeCl 6 h/day, 5 days/week for 2 weeks (5). Female C57BL/6 mice exposed to this regimen developed focal and diffuse malacia of the inner granule cell layer of the cerebellum, notably in the ventral paraflocculus; these changes preceded the appearance, and were therefore judged to be independent of, renal pathology (8). Ultrastructural examination revealed early changes in granule cell heterochromatin followed by nuclear condensation and edematous swelling of perikaryal cytoplasm (8). Degeneration of cerebellar granule cells was reported in female C57BL/6 mice exposed for 11 days to either 100 ppm MeCl continuously (22 h/day) or 400 ppm intermittently (5.5 h/day); no pathological changes were observed in mice exposed to 50 ppm continuously or 150 ppm intermittently. No-observable-effect levels for both exposure regimens were nearly proportionate to exposure concentration times duration, but the dose–response curve was much steeper for mice exposed continuously to MeCl (11).

Dogs and monkeys acutely exposed to high levels of MeCl develop cumulative neurological effects that eventuate in convulsions and prolonged coma (17). Chronic effects in rodents, cats, and dogs include convulsive seizures, hyperactive reflexes, and stiff, unsteady gait (18).

Reports of controlled 3-h exposures to 100 ppm or 200 ppm MeCl suggest no effects on coordination, time discrimination, or dual-task performance (2).

A worksite study examined 122 workers exposed to MeCl (2–70 ppm) in the manufacture of foam products and 49 unexposed controls (13). Mean postshift breath concentration of MeCl-exposed workers was 0.4–80 ppm.

Neurological examination could not distinguish the two groups; electroencephalographic activity was generally normal. Behavioral assessment showed that the MeCl-exposed group had increased tremor, prolonged reaction time, and impaired performance on a dual task (2,13).

Early experience with gross overexposure to MeCl gas has been reviewed (1). Severe acute intoxication results in rapid-onset nausea and weakness followed by convulsions and coma, pupillary dilatation, cyanosis, and death (9). Brain edema may be present postmortem (1).

With less intense MeCl exposures (*ca.* 500 ppm for several hours), a characteristic pattern of progressively intensifying illness develops over 1 or more days (7). Symptoms begin with dizziness, nausea, and vomiting. Anorexia is marked and sleep patterns are disrupted. Blurred vision is a common complaint, and acral paresthesias are occasionally reported. Examination reveals a dull, lethargic individual with reduced attention span and impaired recent memory. Breath may have a sweet odor. Speech is slurred, and a staggering gait may be evident. Cerebellar signs are present; reflexes are hypoactive or absent. Tachycardia is common and, occasionally, body temperature is mildly elevated.

Repeated exposures to lower concentrations of MeCl results in a milder syndrome that gradually develops over days or weeks; it begins with fatigue, staggering gait, weakness, giddiness, anorexia, nausea and vomiting, blurred vision, and paresthesias (1).

Frontal electroencephalographic abnormalities, including diffuse theta waves, sometimes with irregular or absent alpha waves, were reported in individuals chronically exposed to MeCl and, possibly, to other substances (15).

Neurological abnormalities may persist for up to 10 weeks after cessation of exposure, with anorexia, gait ataxia, intention tremor, emotional instability, and insomnia (9,16).

The mechanism of MeCl neurotoxicity is unknown. Some of the effects have been linked to potential MeCl metabolites, including methanol and formate (19). Methanol was not found in the blood of MeCl-treated animals (17). Formate was reported in human urine after severe intoxication (9) but was not found in humans or animals by other investigators (7,18). However, formate is present in urine of mice exposed to MeCl; moreover, formate concentration is increased by subsequent treatment with chloramine which, *in vitro*, inhibits the enzyme activity of N10-formyl tetrahydrofolate dehydrogenase. Simultaneous exposure of a human subject to MeCl and chloramine resulted in severe metabolic acidosis and permanent blindness (12). Formic acid and formate are respectively held responsible for these effects in methanol intoxication (*see* Methanol, this volume). Mitochondrial function is a potential target in meth-

anol and monohalomethane toxicity (*see also* Methyl Iodide, and Methyl Bromide, this volume).

REFERENCES

1. Allen N (1979) Solvents and other industrial organic compounds. In: *Handbook of Clinical Neurology, Vol 36. Intoxications of the Nervous System. Pt 1.* Vinken PJ, Bruyn GW eds. North-Holland, Amsterdam p. 361.
2. Anger WK, Johnson B (1985) Chemicals affecting behavior. In: *Neurotoxicity of Industrial and Commercial Chemicals. Vol 1.* O'Donoghue JL ed. CRC Press, Boca Raton, Florida p. 51.
3. Baker AB, Tichy FY (1953) The effects of the organic solvents and industrial poisonings on the central nervous system. *Ass Res Nerv Ment Dis* **32**, 671.
4. Bolt HM, Gansewendt B (1993) Mechanisms of carcinogenicity of methyl halides. *Crit Rev Toxicol* **23**, 237.
5. Chellman GJ, White RD, Norton RM, Bus JS (1986) Inhibition of the acute toxicity of methyl chloride in male B6C3Fl mice by glutathione depletion. *Toxicol Appl Pharmacol* **86**, 93.
6. Dekant W, Frieschmann C, Speerschneider P (1995) Sex, organ and species specific bioactivation of chloromethane by cytochrome P4502E1. *Xenobiotics* **25**, 1259.
7. Hansen H, Weaver NK, Venable FS (1953) Methyl chloride intoxication. *Arch Indust Hyg* **8**, 328.
8. Jiang XZ, White R, Morgan KT (1985) An ultrastructural study of lesions induced in the cerebellum of mice by inhalation exposure to methyl chloride. *Neurotoxicology* **6**, 93.
9. Kegel AH, McNally WE, Pope AS (1929) Methyl chloride poisoning from domestic refrigerators. *J Amer Med Assn* **93**, 353.
10. Kempkes M, Wiebel FA, Golka K *et al.* (1996) Comparative genotyping and phenotyping of glutathione S-transferase GSTT1. *Arch Toxicol* **70**, 306.
11. Landry TD, Quast JF, Gushow TS, Mattsson JL (1985) Neurotoxicity of methyl chloride in continuously versus intermittently exposed female C57BL/6 mice. *Fund Appl Toxicol* **5**, 87.
12. Minami M, Inagaki H, Katsumata M *et al.* (1993) Inhibitory action of chloramine on formate-metabolizing system. Studies suggested by an unusual case record. *Biochem Pharmacol* **45**, 1059.
13. Repko JD, Jones PD, Garcia LS, Schnweider EJ (1977) *Behavioral and Neurological Effects of Methyl Chloride.* U.S. Department of Health, Education and Welfare, Washington, DC Publ No. 77-155.
14. Repko JD, Lasley SM (1979) Behavioral, neurological, and toxic effects of methyl chloride: A review of the literature. *CRC Crit Rev Toxicol* **6**, 283.
15. Roth B, Deutschova K (1964) The effect of chronic exposure to industrial poisons on the electroencephalogram in man. *Cesk Neurol* **27**, 40.

16. Scharnweber HC, Spears GN, Cowles SR (1974) Chronic methyl chloride intoxication in six industrial workers. *J Occup Med* **16**, 112.

17. Smith WW, von Oettingen WF (1947) The acute and chronic toxicity of methyl chloride. I. Mortality resulting from exposure to methyl chloride in concentrations of 4000 to 300 parts per million. *J Indust Hyg* **29**, 47.

18. Smith WW, von Oettingen WF (1947) The acute and chronic toxicity of methyl chloride. II. Symptomatology of animals poisoned with methyl chloride. *J Indust Hyg* **29**, 123.

19. Van Raalte HG, van Velzen, HG (1945) Methyl chloride intoxication. *Ind Med* **14**, 707.

20. Warholm M, Alexandrie AK, Hogberg J *et al.* (1994) Polymorphic distribution of glutathione transferase activity with methyl chloride in human blood. *Pharmacogenetics* **4**, 307.

21. Xu DG, He HZ, Zhang GG *et al.* (1993) DNA methylation of monohalogenated methanes of F344 rats. *J Tongji Med Univ* **13**, 100. [German]

Methylene Chloride

Richard D. Stewart
Herbert H. Schaumburg

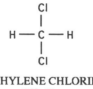

METHYLENE CHLORIDE
CH_2Cl_2

Dichloromethane

NEUROTOXICITY RATING

Clinical

A   Acute encephalopathy (sedation, coma)

C   Chronic encephalopathy

C   Peripheral neuropathy

Experimental

A   Acute encephalopathy (sedation, coma)

Methylene chloride (MC) is synthetically produced either by chlorination of methane or from hydrochloric acid and methanol. MC is a colorless liquid at room temperature and evaporates rapidly. MC has a mild, sweet odor, detectible at 200 ppm. At high temperatures, such as those encountered with molten metal, MC vapor mixed with oxygen may form phosgene. MC is widely used in industry as a degreasing agent, refrigerant, aerosol propellant, and paint remover, and as a multipurpose solvent in adhesives and paints. It is also a constituent of household and marine paint removers. Air concentrations ranging from 732–7030 mg/m³ have been observed when paint removers are used in an enclosed space (20). The time-weighted Threshold Limit Value set by the American Conference of Governmental Industrial Hygienists in 1991 is 50 ppm (175 mg/m³). MC causes CNS depression following high-level inhalation exposure. It is uncertain if prolonged low-level exposure can cause permanent cognitive dysfunction.

MC is readily absorbed through the lungs and gastrointestinal tract; 70% of inhaled MC is absorbed by humans (6). Exercise and obesity increase absorption (5). Rapid evaporation limits the risk of dermal absorption unless MC becomes trapped under rubber gloves or multiple layers of clothing (31). Experimental animal studies indicate that inhaled MC is rapidly distributed to the liver, kidneys, cerebral white matter, and subcutaneous adipose tissue (4). MC is lipophilic; transient storage in fat and slow sustained release occur for several hours following exposure. There is no bioaccumulation of MC or its metabolites.

MC is metabolized by two pathways: one is oxidation by microsomal cytochrome P-450 mixed-function oxidase (MFO) with formation of carbon monoxide (10). The other utilizes glutathione-*S*-transferase (GST) to form carbon dioxide (24). The MFO pathway appears to be the preferred route of metabolism at low levels of inhalation exposure (<500 ppm). Controlled studies of humans exposed to a range of 50–200 ppm of MC disclosed a steady rise in blood carboxyhemoglobin to levels of 1.9% (50 ppm) and 6.8% (200 ppm) after termination at 7.5 h (20). Exposure to levels of 986 ppm for 2 h causes an increase in carboxyhemoglobin saturation to a mean level of 10.1%, and levels remain elevated to 3.1% for 17 h following exposure (28). Controlled studies of individuals working indoors with paint removers containing MC describe levels ranging between 5% and 10%, sufficient for subjects to experience angina pectoris or cardiovascular disease (29). Two reports of uncontrolled exposures to MC in paint removers describe carbon monoxide levels of 26%, 46%, and 50% with few clinical symptoms (7,15). These reports are suspect: it is extremely unlikely to be able to walk normally with a COHb of 46% to 50%, a level indicative of severe hypoxia.

At levels exceeding 500 ppm, saturation of the enzymatic pathways commences in humans and in experimental animals; proportionally more MC is excreted unchanged in expired air and urine as air levels rise. In one study, 20 healthy adults of both sexes were exposed to MC vapor concentrations of 0, 50, 100, 250, and 500 ppm for periods of 1, 3, and 7 h for 2–5 days in a controlled-environment chamber (30). Exposure to 100 ppm for 7 h resulted in a COHb of 4.7% rising to 5.4% 2 h postexposure; exposure to 250 ppm for 7 h resulted in a COHb of 7.9% rising to 8.8% 2 h postexposure; and exposure to 500 ppm for 7 h resulted in a COHb of 10.7% rising to 11.7% 2 h postexposure. With each successive increase in vapor concentration, less COHb was formed. Rats exposed to 1500 ppm produced no more COHb than when exposed to 1000 ppm (18). Professional paint removers exposed to MC vapor concentrations ranging from 1000–1200 ppm for 8 h had maximum COHb saturations of 13%–17%, indicating that the metabolic pathway for the formation of COHb is saturable.

Two additional factors affect exposure to MC. One is obesity, which is associated with sustained release of endogenous MC and elevated levels of carboxyhemoglobin for hours following exposure. The other is smoking; one controlled industrial study of MC-exposed workers demonstrated carboxyhemoglobin levels as high as 14% in exposed smokers (21). Coadministration of certain other substances (toluene, methanol, or ethanol) reduces the formation of carboxyhemoglobin (3).

Experimental animal studies have demonstrated malignant lung and liver neoplasms in several species (19). Limited animal studies suggest slight fetotoxicity at high levels (26).

Acute high-level exposure in humans causes corneal and upper-respiratory-tract irritation, skin irritation, and cardiac arrhythmias. Extreme chronic exposure (30 years) has not been associated with cardiovascular disease or increased mortality (13). One human study indicates a possible association between MC and pancreatic carcinoma (12). The U.S. Environmental Protection Agency considers MC to be a probable human carcinogen.

The acute nervous system effects of high-level exposure (>1000 ppm) in laboratory animals include reduction of random-eye-movement sleep and prolongation of latencies of both visual and brainstem auditory evoked potentials (23,31). It is suggested that, in the rat, there is a narrow margin between the inhalation levels associated with anesthesia and the fatal level of 16,000–19,000 ppm.

Two unconvincing reports describe slowed nerve conduction in rats following chronic MC exposure (11,22). There have been no experimental morphological studies of either chronic low-level or acute high-level exposures that have utilized contemporary histopathological techniques. A biochemical study of 3-month, 210- to 700-ppm exposure to MC analyzed levels of S-100 protein, glial fibrillary acid protein, and DNA content of several areas of the rodent CNS (25). The authors claim evidence of astroglial reaction. Furthermore, they conclude that carbon monoxide alone could not account for all of the changes; MC itself, or a metabolite, is claimed to have a role.

Controlled human studies disclose that exposure to levels up to 200 ppm for 4 h has little effect on performance; likewise, exposure for 30 min to levels ranging from 800–3470 ppm is without consequence (9). A dose-related decline in psychomotor performance appears at levels of 300–800 ppm inhaled for 4 h (7). Accidental acute high-level exposure exceeding 6000 ppm is associated with CNS depression; air levels that produce human anesthesia or fatality are undetermined (17). Blood levels of carboxyhemoglobin have not been markedly elevated in instances of extremely high-level exposure, even those associated with loss of consciousness or fatality.

Epidemiological studies of neuropsychological status and nerve conduction of workers exposed to levels of 75–100 ppm for up to 10 years failed to disclose findings significantly different from controls (2). A study of aircraft mechanics exposed for 20 years to levels ranging from 100–800 ppm also showed no evidence of MC-associated neurotoxicity (16).

There is one case report of dementia and another with peripheral neuropathy following chronic (years) exposure. Both are unconvincing: the dementia case features neither detailed neurological evaluations nor follow-up examinations (1); the neuropathy cases failed to improve following withdrawal, and the author expresses reservations about a causal relationship with methylene chloride (14).

REFERENCES

1. Barrowcliff DF, Knell AJ (1979) Cerebral damage due to endogenous chronic carbon monoxide poisoning caused by exposure to methylene chloride. *J Soc Occup Med* **29**, 12.
2. Cherry N, Venables H, Waldron HA *et al.* (1981) Some observations on workers exposed to methylene chloride. *Brit J Ind Med* **38**, 351.
3. Ciuchta HP, Savell GM, Spiker RC Jr (1979) The effect of alcohols and toluene upon methylene chloride-induced

carboxyhemoglobin in the rat and monkey. *Toxicol Appl Pharmacol* **49**, 347.

4. DiVincenzo GD, Hamilton ML (1975) Fate and disposition of [^{14}C]methylene chloride in the rat. *Toxicol Appl Pharmacol* **32**, 385.

5. DiVincenzo GD, Kaplan CJ (1981) Effect of exercise or smoking on the uptake, metabolism, and excretion of methylene chloride vapor. *Toxicol Appl Pharmacol* **59**, 141.

6. DiVincenzo GD, Kaplan CJ (1981) Uptake, metabolism, and elimination of methylene chloride vapor by humans. *Toxicol Appl Pharmacol* **59**, 130.

7. Fagin J, Bradley J, Williams D (1980) Carbon monoxide poisoning secondary to inhaling methylene chloride. *Brit Med J* **281**, 1461.

8. Fodor GG, Winneke G (1971) Nervous system disturbances in men and animals experimentally exposed to industrial solvent vapors. In: *Proceedings of Second International Clean Air Congress.* Englund HM ed. Academic Press, New York p. 238.

9. Gamberale F, Annwall G, Hultengren M (1975) Exposure to methylene chloride. II. Psychological functions. *Scand J Work Environ Health* **1**, 95.

10. Gargas ML, Clewell HJ, Anderse ME (1986) Metabolism of inhaled dihalomethanes *in vivo*: Differentiation of kinetic constants for two independent pathways. *Toxicol Appl Pharmacol* **82**, 211.

11. Glatzel W, Tietze K, Gutewort R *et al.* (1987) Interaction of dichloromethane and ethanol in rats: Toxicokinetics and nerve conduction velocity. *Alcohol Clin Exp Res* **11**, 450.

12. Hearne FT, Grose F, Pifer JW *et al.* (1987) Methylene chloride mortality study: Dose-response characterization and animal model comparison. *J Occup Med* **29**, 217.

13. Hearne FT, Pifer JW, Grose F (1990) Absence of adverse mortality effects in workers exposed to methylene chloride: An update. *J Occup Med* **32**, 234.

14. Konietzko H (1981) Polyneuropathien durch organische Loesemittel. *Arbeitsmed Sozial Praeventimed* **16**, 247.

15. Langehenning PL, Seeler RA, Berman E (1976) Paint removers and carboxyhemoglobin. *N Engl J Med* **295**, 1137.

16. Lash A, Becker CE, So Y *et al.* (1991) Neurotoxic effects of methylene chloride: Are they long lasting in humans? *Brit J Ind Med* **48**, 418.

17. Manno M, Rugge M, Cocheo V (1992) Double fatal inhalation of dichloromethane. *Hum Exp Toxicol* **11**, 540.

18. McKenna MJ, Zempel JA, Braun WH (1982) The pharmacokinetics of inhaled methylene chloride in rats. *Toxicol Appl Pharmacol* **65**, 1.

19. National Toxicology Program (1986) Toxicology and carcinogenesis studies of dichloromethane (methylene chloride) (CAS no 75-09-2) in F344/N Rats and B6C3F1 Mice (inhalation studies) TR-306. Department of Health and Human Services (National Institutes of Health) Pub. No. 86-2562. Washington, DC, U.S. Government Printing Office.

20. Otson R, Williams DT, Bothwell PD (1981) Dichloromethane levels in air after application of paint removers. *Amer Ind Hyg Assn J* **42**, 56.

21. Ott MG, Skory LK, Holder BB *et al.* (1983) Health evaluation of employees occupationally exposed to methylene chloride. *Scand J Work Environ Health* **9**, 31.

22. Pankow D, Gutewort R, Ponsold W *et al.* (1979) Effect of dichloromethane on the sciatic motor conduction velocity of rats. *Experientia* **35**, 373.

23. Rebert CS, Matteucci MJ, Pryor GT (1989) Acute effects of inhaled dichloromethane on the EEG and sensory-evoked potentials of Fischer-344 rats. *Pharmacol Biochem Behav* **34**, 619.

24. Reitz RH, Mendrala AL, Guengerich FP (1980) *In vitro* metabolism of methylene chloride in human and animal tissues; use in physiologically based pharmacokinetic models. *Toxicol Appl Pharmacol* **97**, 230.

25. Rosengren LE, Kjellstrand P, Aurell A *et al.* (1986) Irreversible effects of dichloromethane on the brain after long-term exposure: A quantitative study of DNA and the glial cell marker proteins S-100 and GFA. *Brit J Ind Med* **43**, 291.

26. Schwetz BA *et al.* (1975) The effect of maternally inhaled trichloroethylene, perchloroethylene, methyl chloroform and methylene chloride on embryonal and fetal development in mice and rats. *Toxicol Appl Pharmacol* **32**, 84.

27. Stewart RD, Dodd HC (1964) Absorption of carbon tetrachloride, trichloroethylene, tetrachloroethylene, methylene chloride, and 1,1,1-trichloroethane through the human skin. *Amer Ind Hyg Assn* **25**, 439.

28. Stewart RD, Fisher TN, Hosko MJ *et al.* (1972) Experimental human exposure to methylene chloride. *Arch Environ Health* **25**, 342.

29. Stewart RD, Hake CL (1976) Paint-remover hazard. *J Amer Med Assn* **235**, 398.

30. Stewart RD, Hake CL, Forster HV *et al.* (1974) Methylene chloride: Development of a biologic standard for the industrial worker by breath analysis. National Institute for Occupational Safety and Health Report: NTIS #PB 83245860/LL.

31. Winneke G (1982) Acute behavioral effects of exposure to some organic solvents—psychological aspects. *Acta Neurol Scand* **66**, 117.

3,4-Methylenedioxymethamphetamine

William Slikker Jr.
Herbert H. Schaumburg

MDMA
$C_{11}H_{15}NO_2$

MDMA; Ecstasy; Adam; N,α-Dimethyl-1,3-benzodioxole-5-ethanamine

NEUROTOXICITY RATING

Clinical

A   Acute encephalopathy (tremor, hallucination, ataxia)

A   Seizure disorder

B   Autonomic syndrome (hyperthermia, myonecrosis)

B   Chronic encephalopathy

C   Psychobiological reaction (chronic psychosis)

Experimental

A   Serotonergic axonopathy

A   Hyperactivity

The initial chemical synthesis of MDMA was in 1912 (33). The drug was originally prepared as an anorectic agent but was never marketed for this purpose.

MDMA forms salts with several acids and, as such, is a white solid at room temperature. It is soluble in water and has a bitter taste (33). The $(+)$-(S)-isomer and the $(-)$-(R)-isomer exhibit somewhat different pharmacological and metabolic profiles. Since the 1970s, MDMA and congener methylenedioxyamphetamine (MDA) have been used in psychoanalysis (38); MDMA was for a time, legally available in the United States for psychiatric use as a conversation enhancer and promoter of introspection. Because of the abuse potential as a street drug and reported neurotoxicity, the U.S. Drug Enforcement Administration placed MDMA in Schedule I status in 1986 (10).

General Toxicology

Bioavailability of MDMA is high regardless of route of administration, and absorption rate constants are similar for the two enantiomers of MDMA (12,20,34).

The volume of distribution for MDMA in the rat is large and variable (1.1–5.8 liters) but does not vary between enantiomers (11). Studies with ^{3}H-MDMA indicate peak concentrations of total radioactivity are achieved within 30 min of oral (p.o.) administration and are eliminated by 24 h (2). Subcutaneous (s.c.) injection of 20 mg/kg of MDA (a behaviorally active dose) along with 0.5 μCi of ^{3}H-MDA resulted in peak brain levels (36 μg/g brain tissue) within 50 min of injection into the rat (40). As with MDMA, no regional variation in brain distribution was observed.

The biotransformation pathways of MDMA include N-demethylation, O-dealkylation, deamination, and conjugation (O-methylation, O-glucuronidation, and/or O-sulfation) (23). MDA, 4-hydroxy-3-methoxymethamphetamine, 3,4-dihydroxymethamphetamine, and 4-hydroxy-3-methoxyamphetamine are found in rat brain supernatants incubated with MDMA (Fig. 13). The similarities of the plasma and brain metabolic profiles for MDMA indicate that these metabolites may penetrate the blood-brain barrier in the unconjugated form. Alternatively, brain metabolism may contribute significantly to the brain concentration of these metabolites (23).

2,4,5-Trihydroxymethamphetamine (THM) has been identified as an *in vivo* metabolite of MDMA in the rat (24). Unlike other MDMA metabolites, including 6-hydroxy-MDMA, this trihydroxy product (THM) exhibits potent neurotoxicity when administered by intracerebroventricular injection. The enzyme believed to be responsible for the O-dealkylation of 6-hydroxy-MDMA to THM is cytochrome P-450 2D1 in rat. The human orthologue of this enzyme (P-450 2D6) is present in the brain.

After intravenous (i.v.) administration of racemic MDMA (20 mg/kg) to the rat, an average of 40.5% was excreted in the urine as the enantiomers of MDMA and MDA (11). After s.c. administration of MDMA (10 mg/kg) to the rat, an average of 22.6% was excreted in the urine and <1% in the feces (25) as MDMA and MDA. In the mouse, a larger percent was excreted in the urine (53.6%) and <2% in the feces as MDMA and MDA enantiomers (25). Terminal plasma elimination half-lives were not significantly different for the enantiomers: 2.5 ± 0.8 h for $(-)$-(R)-MDMA and 2.2 ± 0.8 h for $(+)$-(S)-MDMA in the rat. There was no evidence of nonlinear pharmacokinetics (11).

The serotonergic neurotransmitter system within the CNS is reported to be the main target of MDMA (9,15,36). The effect of MDMA on serotonergic nerve terminals, as evidenced by decrements in 5-hydroxytryptamine (5-HT) content and uptake sites, is most dramatic on rostral brain structures (*e.g.*, frontal cortex, hippocampus and striatum) rather than caudal structures (*e.g.*, brainstem) (34).

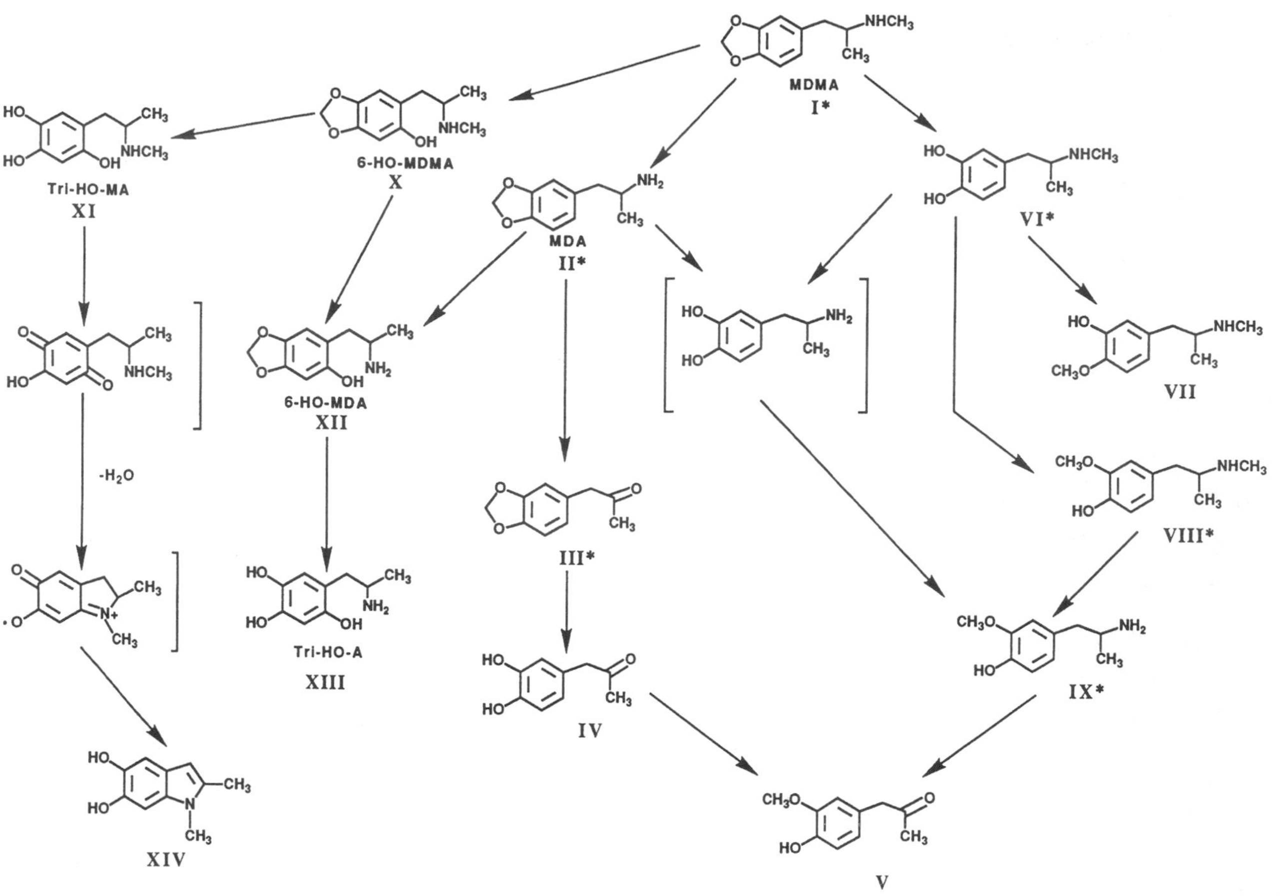

FIGURE 13. Metabolic pathways of MDMA in the rat: I = MDMA; II = MDA; III = 3,4-(methylenedioxy-phenyl)-acetone; IV = 3,4-dihydroxyphenyl-acetone; V = (4-hydroxy-3-methoxyphenyl) acetone; VI = 3,4-dihydroxymethamphetamine; VII = 3-hydroxy-4-methoxymethamphetamine; VIII = 4-hydroxy-3-methoxymethamphetamine; IX = 4-hydroxy-3-methoxymethamphetamine; X = 6-hydroxy-MDMA (6-OH-MDMA); XI = 2,4,5-trihydroxy-methamphetamine (Tri-HO-MA, THM); XII = 6-hydroxy-MDA (6-HO-MDA); XIII = 2,4,5-trihydroxyamphetamine (Tri-HO-A); XIV = 5,6-dihydroxy-2-dimethylindole. Compounds identified with an asterisk have been found in rat brain tissue after administration of MDMA or recovered from rat brain supernatant (10,000 × g) incubated with MDMA. Compounds in brackets are postulated intermediates and have not been identified. Compounds IV–IX are primarily excreted as glucuronide and sulfate conjugates in the urine (19,23–25).

Animal Studies

Single high-dose, short-term studies resulting in lethality in 50% of animals over a 24-h period have been reported as the mean (95% confidence level): mouse, intraperitoneally (i.p.), 97 [89–106] mg/kg; rat, i.p., 49 [46–52] mg/kg; guinea pig, i.p., 98 [88–111] mg/kg; dog, i.v., 14 [8–23] mg/kg, and monkey (rhesus), i.v., 22 [17–28] mg/kg (9). Single, low-dose studies in the rat resulted in significant reductions of tryptophan hydroxylase (rate-limiting enzyme for 5-HT synthesis) at 3 h after administration of 10 mg/kg MDMA (36).

Short-term, single-dose-response studies in the rat indicate that, at 1 week after administration, 20 or 40 mg/kg MDMA p.o. produced significant decreases in 5-HT concentrations in frontal cortex, hippocampus, and caudate putamen, whereas 10 mg/kg had no effect (7). Both devel-

opmental age and body temperature have been demonstrated to modulate MDMA-induced effects. Prenatal, multidose studies and neonatal single-dose studies up to postnatal day (PND) 10 indicate resistance to MDMA-induced alteration of 5-HT regional brain concentrations compared to PND 40, 70, or 150 rats (unpublished observations). When adult rats were placed in a cold environment (10°C), rectal temperatures were reduced and so were the MDMA-induced effects on the 5-HT brain concentrations. When the rats were placed in a warm environment (33°C), rectal temperatures were increased, as were MDMA-induced effects on 5-HT concentrations (6).

Multiple-dose, short-term studies (two doses a day for 4 days) have demonstrated lasting MDMA-induced reductions (1 week to 4 months) in several 5-HT neurotransmitter biomarkers (5-HT content, 5-HT uptake sites, tryptophan hydroxylase, immunohistochemical staining of serotonergic innervation) in several different species (rat, mouse, squirrel monkey, and rhesus monkey) (1,3,15, 28,29,32,35). The MDMA-induced serotonergic alterations increased with dose, tended to plateau at higher doses, were approximately equivalent regardless of route of administration [s.c., i.p., intramuscular (i.m.), p.o.] and exhibited differential species sensitivity (monkey > rat > mouse) (14). Two studies reported selective damage to central serotonergic terminals in the monkey (3,30).

Prolonged exposure studies with MDMA are less common but include multiple or escalating dose studies in the dog and rat (13) and monkey (12). In the dog, daily doses of up to 15 mg/kg MDMA administered p.o. for 28 days resulted in dose-related behavioral changes, reduced weight gain, testicular atrophy, and prostatic hyperplasia (13). In the rat, daily doses of up to 100 mg/kg MDMA administered orally for 28 days resulted in clinical signs (e.g., hyperactivity, excitability, salivation), reduced weight gain, and decreased urinary pH, blood urea nitrogen and glucose. Neither species exhibited brain lesions as assessed by routine histological procedures (i.e., hematoxylin and eosin) (13). In rhesus monkeys performing a battery of behavioral tasks, MDMA administered i.m. twice daily for 14 consecutive days at each of an escalating series of doses from 0.1–20 mg/kg resulted in behavioral disruption of the motivation task at lower doses (1.75 mg/kg) than the other behavioral tasks (short-term memory and attention, time estimation, learning or color and position discrimination, 20 mg/kg). Repeated exposure to each escalating dose of MDMA produced behavioral tolerance to MDMA's disruptive effects on task performance, and tolerance was also evident as the dose increased. After a several-month non-drug period, however, acute dose–response curves for MDMA-induced behavioral effects were significantly shifted to the right, suggesting a long-lasting (>20 months) residual decrease in MDMA sensitivity (12). It is unclear, however, if such tolerance to MDMA is related to the observed decreases in turnover and uptake sites of 5-HT in the hippocampus of these monkeys, although data from rodent studies support this hypothesis (35,39).

In Vitro Studies

In vitro studies with MDMA have been conducted to elucidate metabolic pathways and define mechanisms. Many of the metabolites of MDMA (Fig. 13) were first identified from in-vitro liver or brain preparations (23). The predominantly constitutive isozymes responsible for MDMA oxidate metabolism (demethylenation) were described in vitro (22), and evidence that MDMA needs to be metabolized to

be toxic also was derived, in part, from in vitro experiments (16).

In vitro studies have shown that either MDMA uptake or its interaction with the Na^+-dependent serotonin transporter is responsible, at least in part, for both vesicular release of 5-HT and blockade of 5-HT reuptake (31). In vitro studies to define a specific receptor to mediate MDMA-induced effects have been confounded, however, both by the releasing and uptake-blocking properties of the agent, and the artifactual binding of ^{3}H-MDMA to glass fiber filter paper (37).

Human Studies

There are no published controlled human studies of MDMA (18).

The uncontrolled use of MDMA, known as "Ecstasy" or "Adam," has been reviewed (5). A similar drug, 3,4-methylenedioxyethamphetamine (MDEA), is known as "Eve." Available as powders or pills, they are usually taken orally in group sessions; typically 100 mg is followed by supplemental doses of 40 mg, up to several hundred milligrams over 30–120 min. Infrequently, MDMA is taken intranasally or parenterally; compulsive use rarely if ever occurs. Desired effects include "enhanced communication, empathy, or understanding"; euphoria or ecstasy; and "transcendental or religious experiences." Perceptual changes include vivid color enhancement, illusions, and hallucinations (visual, tactile, auditory, olfactory, or gustatory); visual hallucinations are either formed or unformed, and polyopia has been reported (3). Undesirable side effects include anxiety, tremor, muscle tightness, jaw clenching, diaphoresis, profuse salivation, blurred vision, ataxia, tachycardia, hypertension, and nausea. Mydriasis and horizontal or vertical nystagmus are seen. Effects usually disappear within 24 h, but users have reported jaw tightness, blurred vision, fatigue, nausea, anxiety, depression, or insomnia lasting days or even weeks, and "flashbacks" have occurred. Tolerance may develop more rapidly to MDMA's desirable effects than to its undesirable effects (8).

Case reports have documented acute clinical symptoms associated with the ingestion of extremely large doses of MDMA. Common, sometimes life-threatening features of these cases include elevated core body temperature (40°–43.3°C), tachycardia (160–180 beats/min), muscle rigidity, tachyrhythmia, rhabdomyolysis, disseminated intravascular coagulation, seizures, panic, and delirium. This syndrome resembles heat stroke. The most important step in the management of these patients is rapid cooling. Forced diuresis should be established to enhance myoglobin clearance and prevent acute renal failure.

A recent controlled study of abstinent users of MDMA found a deficit in visual and verbal memory, and that higher average monthly doses of MDMA were associated with greater decrements in memory function (4). Cerebrospinal fluid levels of 5-hydroxyindoleacetic acid, an indirect measure of central 5-HT function, were associated with poor memory performance, suggesting that MDMA-induced brain 5-HT neurotoxicity may account for memory impairment in MDMA users.

Toxic Mechanisms

There is general agreement concerning the initial actions of MDMA upon the serotonergic neurotransmitter system. *In vitro*, microdialysis and *in vivo* results agree that MDMA releases 5-HT, blocks its reuptake, and inhibits tryptophan hydroxylase in serotonergic nerve terminals in the CNS (15,17,31). In the long-term (3 h to several months), MDMA treatment results in serotonin–uptake site depletion and immunohistochemical evidence of nerve terminal destruction (30). There is also general agreement that MDMA itself is not the neurotoxic agent (2,26), and that 5-HT uptake blockers can decrease MDMA toxicity (32). Although a complete toxic mechanism has yet to be defined, at least three major hypotheses are under study.

The bioactivation hypothesis (may also underlie the other two mechanisms) states that MDMA is metabolized to a toxic intermediate analogous to the potent catecholaminergic neurotoxin, 6-hydroxydopamine (19). This MDMA metabolite has been postulated to be 2,4,5-trihydroxymethamphetamine (THM, Fig. 13). THM has been demonstrated, 5 days after its intracerebroventricular administration, to decrease cortical striatal and hippocampal tryptophan hydroxylase activity and 5-HT concentrations in a dose-related manner. Because THM also decreased dopamine content and tyrosine hydroxylase activity—effects not usually induced by systemic administration of MDMA —other bioactivated compounds, not THM, may actually be involved. The mechanism of action of THM or related compound(s) may be similar to that of 6-hydroxydopamine, which involves the generation of quinones, hydrogen peroxide, and reactive radicals (21). Other hypotheses, however, involving the down-regulation of genomic function or decreased cellular energy exacerbated by heat stress, cannot be ruled out (5).

Manipulations of the dopaminergic neurotransmitter system have been shown to modify MDMA-induced toxicity, and, therefore, the hypothesis was developed that the dopaminergic system plays a role in MDMA toxicity (15). 5-HT$_2$ receptor antagonists exert a protective effect when administered along with MDMA, presumably because these agents block serotonergic neurotransmission (27). Therefore, two different but related hypotheses of MDMA-induced toxicity involve the enhanced functioning of the dopamine and/or serotonergic neurotransmitter systems. Recently, however, results from studies of MDMA in developing animals and in animals under strict temperature control have raised additional questions concerning the neurotoxic mechanisms of MDMA and demonstrated that both age and body temperature are major determinants in the outcome of MDMA exposure (6,7). These data add credence to the hypothesis that metabolic activation and subsequent free radical production are central to the mechanism of MDMA-induced neurotoxicity.

REFERENCES

1. Ali SF, Scallet AC, Newport GD *et al.* (1989) Persistent neurochemical and structural changes in rat brain after oral administration of MDMA. *Res Commun Alcohol Subs Abus* **10**, 225.
2. Ali SF, Tandon P, Tilson HA *et al.* (1990) Intracerebral and oral administration of methylenedioxymethamphetamine (MDMA): Distribution and neurochemical alterations in rat brain. *Eur J Pharmacol* **183**, 450.
3. Battaglia GS, Yeh SY, O'Hearn ME *et al.* (1987) 3,4-Methylenedioxyamphetamine (MDA) and 3,4-methylenedioxymethamphetamine (MDMA) destroy serotonin terminals in rat brain: Quantification of neurodegeneration by measurement of [^{3}H] paroxetine-labeled serotonin uptake sites. *J Pharmacol Exp Ther* **243**, 911.
4. Bolla KI, McCann UD, Ricaurte GA (1998) Memory impairment in abstinent MDMA ("Ecstasy") users. *Neurol* **51**, 1532.
5. Bowyer JR, Holson RR (1995) Methamphetamine and amphetamine neurotoxicity. In: *Handbook of Neurotoxicology*. Chang L, Dyer R eds. Marcel Dekker, New York p. 845.
6. Broening HW, Bacon L, Slikker W Jr (1994) Age modulates the long-term but not the acute effects of the serotonergic neurotoxicant 3,4-methylenedioxymethamphetamine. *J Pharmacol Exp Ther* **271**, 1.
7. Broening HW, Bowyer JF, Slikker W Jr (1995) Age dependent sensitivity of rats to the long term effects of the serotonergic neurotoxicant (+)-3,4-methylenedioxymethamphetamine (MDMA) correlates with the magnitude of MDMA-induced hyperthermia. *J Pharmacol Exp Ther* **275**, 325.
8. Brust JCM (1993) *Neurological Aspects of Substance Abuse*. Butterworth-Heinemann, Boston p. 70.
9. Davis WM, Hatoum HT, Waters IW (1987) Toxicity of MDA (3,4-methylenedioxyamphetamine) considered for relevance to hazards of MDMA (Ecstasy) abuse. *Alcohol Drug Res* **7**, 123.
10. Federal Register (1986) **51**, 36552.

11. Fitzgerald RL, Blanke RV, Poklis A (1990) Stereoselective pharmacokinetics of 3,4-methylenedioxymethamphetamine in the rat. *Chirality* **2**, 241.

12. Frederick DL, Ali SF, Slikker W Jr *et al.* (1995) Behavioral and neurochemical effects of chronic methylenedioxymethamphetamine (MDMA) treatment in rhesus monkeys. *Neurotoxicol Teratol* **17**, 531.

13. Frith CH, Chang LW, Lattin DL *et al.* (1987) Toxicity of methylenedioxymethamphetamine (MDMA) in the dog and the rat. *Fund Appl Toxicol* **9**, 110.

14. Gaylor DW, Slikker W JR (1990) Risk assessment for neurotoxic effects. *Neurotoxicology* **11**, 211.

15. Gibb JW, Stone D, Hanson GR (1990) MDMA: Historical Perspectives. In: *The Neuropharmacology of Serotonin*. Whitaker-Azmitia PM, Peroutka SJ eds. N Y Acad Sci, New York p. 601.

16. Gollamudi R, Ali SF, Lipe G *et al.* (1989) Influence of inducers and inhibitors on the metabolism *in vitro* and neurochemical effects *in vivo* of MDMA. *Neurotoxicology* **10**, 455.

17. Gough B, Ali SF, Slikker W Jr, Holson RR (1991) Acute effects of 3,4-methylenedioxymethamphetamine (MDMA) on monoamines in rat caudate. *Pharmacol Biochem Behav* **39**, 619.

18. Grob CS (1994) MDMA research update: The Harbor-UCLA project. *MAPS* **4**, 2.

19. Johnson M, Elayan I, Hanson GR *et al.* (1992) Effects of 3,4-dihydroxymethamphetamine and 2,4,5-trihydroxymethamphetamine, 2 metabolites of 3,4-methylenedioxymethamphetamine. *J Pharmacol Exp Ther* **261**, 447.

20. Kleven MS, Woolverton WL, Seiden LS (1989) Evidence that both intragastric and subcutaneous administration of methylenedioxymethamphetamine (MDMA) produce serotonin neurotoxicity in rhesus monkeys. *Brian Res* **488**, 121.

21. Kostrzewa RM, Jacobowitz DM (1974) Pharmacological actions of 6-hydroxydopamine. *Pharmacol Rev* **26**, 199.

22. Kumagai Y, Wickham KA, Schmitz DA, Coh AK (1991) Metabolism of methylenedioxyphenyl compounds by rabbit liver preparations. *Biochem Pharmacol* **42**, 1061.

23. Lim HK, Foltz RL (1988) *In vivo* and *in vitro* metabolism of 2,3-(methylenedioxy)methamphetamine in the rat: Identification of metabolites using an ion trap detector. *Chem Res Toxicol* **1**, 370.

24. Lim HK, Foltz RL (1991) Ion trap tandem mass spectrometric evidence for the metabolism of 3,4-(methylenedioxy)methamphetamine to the potent neurotoxins 2,4,5-trihydroxymethamphetamine and 2,4,5-trihydroxyamphetamine. *Chem Res Toxicol* **4**, 626.

25. Lim HK, Seng S, Chei DM, Foltz FL (1992) Comparative investigation of disposition of 3,4-(methylenedioxy)methamphetamine (MDMA) in the rat and the mouse of a capillary gas chromatography-mass spectrometry assay based on perfluorotributylamine-enhanced ammonia positive ion chemical ionization. *J Pharmaceut Biomed Anal* **10**, 657.

26. Molliver ME, O'Hearn E, Battaglia G, DeSouza EB (1986) Direct intracerebral injection of MDA and MDMA does not produce serotonin neurotoxicity. *Soc Neurosci Abstr* **12**, 336.3.

27. Nash JF (1990) Ketanserin pretreatment attenuates MDMA-induced release in the striatum as measured by *in vivo* microdialysis. *Life Sci* **47**, 2401.

28. Ohearn E, Battaglia G, DeSouza EB *et al.* (1988) Methylenedioxyamphetamine (MDA) and methylenedioxymethamphetamine (MDMA) cause selective ablation of serotonergic axon terminals in forebrain: Immunocytochemical evidence for neurotoxicity. *J Neurosci* **8**, 2877.

29. Ricaurte GA, DeLanney LE, Irwin I, Langston JW (1988) Toxic effects of MDMA on central serotonergic neurons in the primate: Importance of route and frequency of drug administration. *Brain Res* **446**, 165.

30. Ricurte GA, Forno LS, Wilson MA *et al.* (1988) 3,4-Methylenedioxymethamphetamine selectively damages central serotonergic neurons in the subhuman primate. *J Amer Med Assn* **260**, 51.

31. Rudnick G, Wall SC (1992) The molecular mechanisms of "ecstasy" [3,4-methylenedioxymethamphetamine (MDMA)]: Serotonin transporters are targets for MDMA-induced serotonin release. *Proc Nat Acad Sci USA* **89**, 1817.

32. Schmidt CJ (1987) Neurotoxicity of the psychedelic amphetamine, methylenedioxymethamphetamine. *J Pharmacol Exp Ther* **240**, 1.

33. Shulgin AT (1986) The background and chemistry of MDMA. *J Psycho Drugs* **18**, 291.

34. Slikker W Jr, Ali SF, Scallet AC *et al.* (1988) Neurochemical and neurohistological alterations in the rat and monkey produced by orally administered methylenedioxymethamphetamine (MDMA). *Toxicol Appl Pharmacol* **94**, 488.

35. Slikker W Jr, Paule MG, Broening HW (1995) Role of serotonergic systems in behavioral toxicity. In: *Neurotoxicology: Approaches and Methods*. Chang L, Slikker W Jr eds. Academic Press, New York p. 371.

36. Stone DM, Merchant KM, Hanson GR, Gibb JW (1987) Immediate and long-term effects of 3,4-methylenedioxymethamphetamine on serotonin pathways in brain of rat. *Neuropharmacology* **26**, 1677.

37. Wang SS, Ricaurte GA, Peroutka SJ (1987) [³H]3,4-Methylenedioxymethamphetamine (MDMA) interactions with brain membranes and glass fiber filter paper. *Eur J Pharmacol* **138**, 439.

38. Yensen R, DiLeo FB, Rhead JC *et al.* (1976) MDA-assisted psychotherapy with neurotoxic outpatients: A pilot study. *J Nerv Ment Dis* **163**, 233.

39. Zacny JP, Virus RM, Woolverton WL (1990) Tolerance and cross-tolerance to 3,4-methylenedioxymethamphet-

amine (MDMA), methamphetamine and methylenedioxy-amphetamine. *Pharmacol Biochem Behav* **35**, 637.

40. Zaczek R, Hurt S, Culp S, DeSouza EB (1989) Characterization of brain interactions with methylenedioxyam-phetamine and methylenedioxymethamphetamine. In: *National Institute on Drug Abuse Research Monograph, Pharmacology and Toxicology: Amphetamine Related Drugs.* Rockville, Maryland p. 223.

Methyl Ethyl Ketone

Herbert H. Schaumburg

$$CH_3 - C - CH_2 - CH_3$$
$$\underset{O}{\overset{\|}{}}$$

METHYL ETHYL KETONE
C_4H_8O

2-Butanone

NEUROTOXICITY RATING

Clinical

A   Acute encephalopathy (narcosis, coma)

A   Potentiation of γ-diketone neuropathy

C   Peripheral neuropathy

Experimental

A   CNS depression

A   Potentiation of γ-diketone neuropathy

Methyl ethyl ketone (MEK) is a volatile hydrocarbon solvent used in paint, glue, paint removers, printing ink, rubber cement, and resins. MEK is rapidly absorbed by the lungs, less well following ingestion. MEK can be recognized at 25 ppm by its irritating, acetone-like odor. It has a long half-life compared to that of other ketones; following intraperitoneal injection, the serum half-life is 270 minutes. The biotransformation and metabolism of MEK are poorly understood; following inhalation exposure, 3-hydroxy-2-butanone and 2,3-butanediol both appear in the urine. There are no serious systemic effects associated with industrial exposure to MEK; long-term occupational exposure to levels of 100–200 ppm is associated with ocular irritation, nose and throat discomfort, and dermatitis. The time-weighted Threshold Limit Value set by the American Conference of Governmental Industrial Hygienists in 1991 is 200 ppm (590 mg/m³).

Rats exposed to 200 ppm displayed no abnormalities in behavioral testing (4). Inhalation of 6000 ppm of MEK for 8 h daily for 7 weeks caused no gross behavioral impairment; animals died of pneumonia (2). Guinea pigs inhaling 10,000 ppm rapidly displayed signs of nose and eye irritation and were unconscious after 5 h.

MEK alone does *not* cause peripheral neuropathy in laboratory animals (10) but potentiates the neuropathies produced by *n*-hexane, methyl *n*-butyl ketone and 2,5-hexanedione (3,6,9). MEK potentiation of *n*-hexane neuropathy is manifest in an earlier onset of signs of hindlimb weakness; in addition, lower concentrations of *n*-hexane are required to produce the same degree of peripheral neuropathy when administered along with MEK (3).

There are no reports of controlled human exposures that have produced CNS dysfunction. A woman who ingested a large volume of MEK became comatose and had a severe metabolic acidosis; her plasma concentration of MEK was 13.2 mmol/l and MEK was also present in the urine. She recovered following correction of the metabolic abnormality (8).

Reports of peripheral neuropathy from MEK have all been instances wherein there was either coexposure to neurotoxic hydrocarbons or detailed analysis of the contents of the solvent was not performed (5,7). An epidemic of unusually severe glue-sniffing peripheral neuropathy in Berlin in 1973 occurred following the addition of MEK to a *n*-hexane containing solvent (1). This phenomenon suggested the potentiating effect of MEK, an hypothesis that was subsequently confirmed by experimental animal studies (*see also n*-Hexane, Metabolites, and Derivatives, this volume).

REFERENCES

1. Altenkirch H, Mager J, Stoltenburg G, Helmbrecht J (1977) Toxic polyneuropathies after sniffing a glue thinner. *J Neurol* **214**, 137.

2. Altenkirch H, Wagner HM, Stoltenburg-Didinger G, Steppat R (1982) Potentiation of hexacarbon neurotoxicity by methyl ethyl ketone and other substances: Clinical and experimental aspects. *Neurobehav Toxicol Teratol* **4**, 623.

3. Altenkirch H, Wagner HM, Stoltenburg G, Spencer PS (1982) Nervous system responses of rats to subchronic inhalation of *n*-hexane and *n*-hexane + methyl-ethyl-ketone mixtures. *J Neurol Sci* **57**, 209.

4. Dick RVB, Setzer JV, Taylor BJ *et al.* (1989) Neurobehavioral effects of short duration exposures to acetone and methyl ethyl ketone. *Brit J Ind Med* **46**, 111.

5. Dyro FM (1978) Methyl ethyl ketone polyneuropathy in shoe factory workers. *Clin Toxicol* **13**, 371.

6. O'Donoghue JL, Krasavage WJ, DiVincenzo GO, Katz GV (1984) Further studies on ketone neurotoxicity and interactions. *Toxicol Appl Pharmacol* **72**, 201.

7. Oh SJ, Kim JM (1976) Giant axonal swelling in "Huffer's" neuropathy. *Arch Neurol* 33, 583.
8. Ropelman PG, Kalfayan PY (1983) Severe metabolic acidosis after ingestion of butanone. *Brit Med J* 286, 21.
9. Saida K, Mendell JR, Weiss HS (1976) Peripheral nerve changes induced by methyl *n*-butyl ketone and potentiation by methyl ethyl ketone. *J Neuropathol Exp Neurol* 35, 207.
10. Spencer PS, Schaumburg HH (1976) Feline nervous system response to chronic intoxication with commercial grades of methyl *n*-butyl ketone, methyl isobutyl ketone, and methyl ethyl ketone. *Toxicol Appl Pharmacol* 37, 301.

3,3′-Methyliminobis(N-methylpropylamine)

Peter S. Spencer

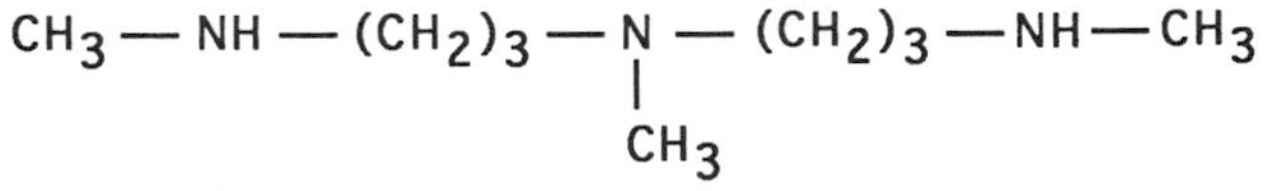

$$CH_3 - NH - (CH_2)_3 - N - (CH_2)_3 - NH - CH_3$$
$$|$$
$$CH_3$$

3,3′-METHYLIMINOBIS(N-METHYLPROPYLAMINE)
$C_9H_{23}N_3$

3,3′-Bis(methylamino)-N-methyldipropylamine

NEUROTOXICITY RATING

Experimental

B   Acute encephalopathy

3,3′-Methyliminobis(N-methylpropylamine) (MIMPA) is a clear, colorless, water-soluble, oily liquid. Systemic treatment of rodents induces regional, insulin-independent brain damage, especially in areas lacking a blood-brain barrier (1,2). 1,4,7-Trimethyldiethylenetriamine, a somewhat related compound, caused mild lesions. Other polyamines, including nine triamines and two tetramines, failed to induce damage at the doses tested (2).

Subcutaneous (s.c.) injection of MIMPA (800 mg/kg) proved fatal in 10 of 14 rats; 0 of 15 died within the same period (48 h) after receiving 400 mg/kg s.c. Smaller MIMPA dosages were required for lethality when the compound was administered after neutralization with 10% acetic acid. One to 2 days following injection, symmetrical zones of perivascular edema or necrosis were noted in hypothalamus and medulla oblongata adjacent to the median eminence and area postrema, respectively. Lesions began in the arcuate nuclei and more lateral neuropil of the hypothalamus, and in the hypoglossal, dorsal vagal and gracile nuclei, and nuclei of the solitary tracts of the lower medulla. More severe lesions featured necrosis of arcuate, ventromedial, dorsomedial, and paraventricular nuclei of the hypothalamus, medullary nuclei, and contiguous reticular formation. Anterior, middle, and posterior hypothalamic necrosis was seen in the most severely affected animals. Occasional rats exhibited focal lesions of cerebellum, hippocampus, olfactory bulb, liver, or proximal renal tubules (2,3).

REFERENCES

1. Brown DF, McGuirk JP, Larsen SP, Minter SD (1991) The effect of alloxan-induced diabetes on triamine lesions in the ventromedial hypothalamus. *Physiol Behav* 49, 41.
2. Levine S, Sowinski R (1982) Hypothalamic and medullary lesions caused by an aliphatic triamine unrelated to gold thioglucose. *J Neuropathol Exp Neurol* 41, 54.
3. Nochlin D, Levine S (1982) Ultrastructure of hypothalamic and medullary lesions caused by an aliphatic triamine. *J Neuropathol Exp Neurol* 41, 233.

Methyl Iodide

Peter S. Spencer

$$CH_3I$$

Monoiodomethane; Iodomethane

NEUROTOXICITY RATING

Clinical

A   Acute encephalopathy

A   Chronic encephalopathy

A   Cerebellar syndrome

Experimental

A   Olfactory epithelial toxin

Methyl iodide is used as a methylating agent in chemical syntheses; as a light-sensitive etching agent for electronic circuits; and as a high-refractive-index aid in light microscopy (9). In the past, it was used in pest control and as a fire extinguisher. ^{11}C-Methyl iodide is employed in nuclear medicine in the synthesis of short-acting radiolabels for study of CNS receptors and other structures by positron emission tomography (*e.g.*, 14).

Methyl iodide (MeI) is a colorless, highly volatile liquid with a pungent odor; it turns brown on exposure to light. In the United States, the Threshold Limit Value and Short-Term Exposure Limit are 12 and 30 mg/m^3, respectively. Subacute MeI poisoning results from workplace exposures in the range of 100–150 mg/m^3 (15). Methods to prevent exposure to MeI vapors include adequate respiratory protection, including a self-contained breathing apparatus provided with a full face piece and operated in a positive-pressure mode (15). Cotton overalls, fluorocarbon rubber gloves, and splash-proof safety goggles should be worn if skin contact is possible (15).

The oral LD$_{50}$ for MeI in rats is 76 mg/kg body weight. Narcosis, congestion of lungs, and damage to the liver, kidney and olfactory epithelium are seen in acutely intoxicated rodents (8,11,16,21,24). MeI, like another halogenated halomethane (methyl bromide), has mutagenic and carcinogenic potential (5). MeI-treated rats and mice undergo systemic DNA methylation with formation of specific DNA adducts (3-methyladenine, 7-methyladenine, O^6-methylguanine) (25). The N'-methyl iodide salt and the bis-N'-methyl iodide salt of diazene dicarboxylic acid (N'-methyl piperazide) are potent muscle-depolarizing agents (10).

MeI conjugates with glutathione (GSH) largely nonenzymatically to form methylglutathione (13); it is then transformed by transpeptidases into S-methylcysteine. Further metabolism generates methanethiol; this is oxidized to formaldehyde and hydrogen sulfide, which are oxidized to formate and sulfate, respectively (3,18,20).

MeI appears preferentially to target mitochondrial (not cytosolic) GSH in neural cells *in vitro* . The 5-min ED$_{50}$ for MeI-induced GSH depletion is 0.2 mM and 0.5 mM for glial and mixed (neurons + glia) murine CNS cultures, respectively (6,7). Loss of mitochondrial GSH after 2-h MeI treatment of primary cultures of fetal mouse cerebrocortical cells correlated with leakage of lactate dehydrogenase (cell-injury marker) 24 h after exposure. Provided that at least 50% of mitochondrial GSH was preserved, MeI-induced damage was preventable by treatment with antioxidants and N-acetyl-L-cysteine, a GSH precursor. MeI-induced depletion of mitochondrial GSH correlated with reduction of mitochondrial metabolic activity, as indicated by reduction of 3-[4,5-dimethylthiazol-2-yl]-2,5-diphenyltetrazolium bromide (6).

Only 11 cases of human MeI poisoning are reported in the literature (15). Most reports describe 30- to 40-year-old men who developed neurological and tardive psychiatric disease after exposure to MeI vapors during synthesis or occupational use of the chemical (1,2,4,12,15,17). Onset of neurological symptoms may be delayed for a few hours to a few days, and repeated exposure may give rise to recurrent attacks of neurological dysfunction; cerebellar and oculomotor deficits are common (15). Multiple sclerosis was not totally excluded in one individual with recurrent neurological manifestations (15). An adult female who developed a chemical burn after handling MeI experienced no reported systemic effects (23).

Blurred vision and unsteadiness of gait may manifest during MeI exposure (2). Vertigo, ataxia, diplopia, headache, dysarthria, and tremor develop sometime later. Agitation, confusion, hallucinations, delusions, and delirium may follow. Electroencephalographic abnormalities may appear and then disappear, or persist (4,19). A cerebellar, pyramidal or parkinsonian syndrome (one case only) may develop (2,19). Subsequent clinical improvement may be interrupted by psychiatric disease that persists for many months: manifestations include a cognitive deficit, personality deficits, hypochrondria, depression, insomnia, and paranoid ideation (2,4,17,19). One individual who experienced episodic giddiness and sleepiness while working with MeI, upon re-exposure developed drowsiness, ataxia, dysarthria, strabismus, twitching of the extremities, and vomiting; coma developed and the individual died 8 days after exposure. Postmortem examination revealed congestion of all organs (12). Another individual self-administered MeI (14 g in 6 ml) by intravenous injection; [MeI]$_{serum}$ 3 h later was approximately 60 mg/ml (22). He became drowsy, agitated, hypotensive, and hyperthermic; metabolic acidosis and hyperleukocytosis were present. Treatment by hemoperfusion with N-acetylcysteine was followed by complete recovery within 5 days (22). Note that therapeutic use of N-acetylcysteine has been questioned because GSH conjugation may be a toxifying, rather than a detoxifying, step in MeI metabolism (15).

The mechanism of MeI neurotoxicity has not been established. Formaldehyde appears to be an indicator of MeI metabolism in mouse cerebral cultures, but semicarbazide, an agent that protects against formaldehyde-producing toxicants, failed to protect neural and glial cells from MeI-induced toxicity *in vitro* (7). Interruption of oxidative phosphorylation by formate or hydrogen sulfide metabolites are other possibilities (15).

REFERENCES

1. Anatovskaia VS, Iaschenko VI (1967) Klinkie porazhenia nernoi sistey iodistym metalou. *Vrach Delo* 6, 147.
2. Appel GB, Galen R, O'Brien J, Schoenfeldt R (1981) Methyl iodide intoxication. A case report. *Ann Intern Med* 82, 534.
3. Barnsley EA, Young L (1965) Biochemical studies of toxic agents: The metabolism of iodomethane. *Biochem J* 95, 77.

4. Baselga-Monte M, Estadella-Botha S, Quer-Brossa D, Forenells-Martinez E (1965) Intoxicacion professional por yoduro de metilo. *Med Lav* **56**, 592.

5. Bolt HM, Gansewendt B (1993) Mechanisms of carcinogenicity of methyl halides. *Crit Rev Toxicol* **23**, 237.

6. Bonnefoi MS (1992) Mitochondrial glutathione and methyl iodide-induced neurotoxicity in primary neural cell cultures. *Neurotoxicology* **13**, 401.

7. Bonnefoi MS, Davenport CJ, Morgan KT (1991) Metabolism and toxicity of methyl iodide in primary dissociated neural cell cultures. *Neurotoxicology* **12**, 33.

8. Buckell M (1950) The toxicity of methyl iodide. I. Preliminary survey. *Brit J Ind Med* **7**, 122.

9. Budavari S (1996) *The Merck Index. 12th Ed.* Merck & Co. Whitehouse Stn, New Jersey p. 6167.

10. Carlen PL, Kosower EM, Werman R (1976) Diamide acts intracellularly to enhance transmitter release: The differential permeation of diamide, DIP, DIP+1 and DIP+2 across the nerve terminal membrane. *Brain Res* **117**, 277.

11. Chamberlain MP, Lock EA, Reed CJ (1998) Investigations of the pathways of toxicity of methyl iodide in the rat nasal cavity. *Toxicology* **129**, 169.

12. Garland A, Camps FE (1945) Methyl iodide poisoning. *Brit J Ind Med* **2**, 209.

13. Hallier E, Deutschmann S, Reichel *et al.* (1990) A comparative investigation of the metabolism of methyl bromide and methyl iodide in human erythrocytes. *Int Arch Occup Environ Health* **62**, 221.

14. Hara T, Koasaka N, Shinoura N, Kondo T (1997) PET imaging of brain tumor with [methyl-^{11}C]choline. *J Nucl Med* **38**, 842.

15. Hermouet C, Garnier R, Efthymiou M, Fournier P (1996) Methyl iodide poisoning: report of two cases. *Amer J Ind Med* **30**, 759.

16. Irish DD (1963) Halogenated hydrocarbons. I. Aliphatic. In: *Patty's Industrial Hygiene and Toxicology. Vol 2B. 3rd Ed.* Clayton GD, Clayton FE eds. John Wiley, New York p. 3442.

17. Jacquet A (1901) Ueber Brommethylvergiftung. *Deut Arch Klin Med* **71**, 370.

18. Johnson MK (1966) Studies on glutathione S-alkyltransferase in the rat. *Biochem J* **98**, 44.

19. Kiec E, Stasik M (1966) Klinica zatrucia jodkiem metylu. *Med Pr* **17**, 243.

20. Kornbrust KS, Bus JS (1983) The role of glutathione and cytochrome P450 in the metabolism of methyl chloride. *Toxicol Appl Pharmacol* **67**, 246.

21. Reed CJ, Gaskell BA, Banger KK, Lock EA (1995) Olfactory toxicity of methyl iodide in the rat. *Arch Toxicol* **70**, 51.

22. Robertz-Vaupel GM, Bierl R, von Unruh G (1991) Intravenöse Methyliodidintoxikation—Detoxikation durch Hämoperfusion. *Anästhesiol Intensivmed Notfallmed Schmerzher* **26**, 44.

23. Skutilova J (1975) Akutni poskozcni metyljodidem. *Prac Lek* **27**, 341.

24. Torkelson TR, Rowe VK (1981) Halogenated aliphatic hydrocarbons containing chlorine, bromine and iodine. In: *Patty's Industrial Hygiene and Toxicology. 3rd Ed. Vol 2B.* Clayton GD, Clayton DE eds. John Wiley, New York p. 3346.

25. Xu DG, He HZ, Zhang GG *et al.* (1993) DNA methylation of monohalogenated methanes of F344 rats. *J Tongji Med Univ* **13**, 100. [German]

Methyllycaconitine

Albert C. Ludolph

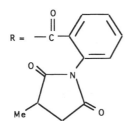

METHYLLYCACONITINE

NEUROTOXICITY RATING

Clinical

A Neuromuscular transmission syndrome (cattle)

Experimental

A Neuromuscular transmission dysfunction (postsynaptic neuromuscular blockade)

Methyllycaconitine is a norditerpenoid alkaloid and potent insecticide found in the seeds of *Delphinium* spp. (larkspur). It is used as a selective probe for CNS nicotinic receptors and is likely to have a role in larkspur poisoning, a neuromuscular disease observed in cattle feeding on *Delphinium* spp. (3,7). The chemistry, methods of isolation, characterization, and synthesis of diterpenoids in *Delphinium* have been reviewed (6).

Experimentally, methyllycaconitine is used to distinguish between α-bungarotoxin binding sites in rat brain and muscle. Since the compound inhibits (^{125}I) α-bungarotoxin binding to rat brain membranes with a K_i of 1.4×10^{-9} M, but binding to frog and human muscle extracts with a K_i of only 10^{-5} to 10^{-6} M, its selectivity for the CNS protein is of experimental importance (8). In cultured fetal rat hippocampal neurons, picomolar concentrations of methyllycaconitine inhibit acetylcholine-induced currents (2). The antagonism was shown to be specific, reversible, concentration-dependent, but voltage-independent (2), and possibly competitive (2).

Methyllycaconitine is present in some *Delphinium* spp., which cause cattle poisoning in parts of the western United States (6). The precise concentration of methyllycaconitine in the diverse *Delphinium* spp. is unknown, although analysis of *D. bicolor* and *nuttallium* revealed the presence of as much as 50%–70% methyllycaconitine of the total amount of alkaloid identified (6). The intravenous LD_{50} for mice is 3.2 mg/kg body weight indicating that methyllycaconitine may be the most toxic compound present in larkspur. In the rat nerve-diaphragm preparation, methyllycaconitine has a curare-like effect (1). Oral intake of larkspur by cattle dose-dependently induces a syndrome (larkspur toxicosis) of weakness that may progress to generalized paralysis; it is accompanied by increased salivation and possibly constipation (5,6). Sensory nerve function is normal even during severe intoxication (6). Intravenous administration of methyllycaconitine to calves produces a neuromuscular block (4). Sheep and horses show a higher tolerance to larkspur than cattle (6). Intravenous administration of physostigmine to steers influenced the clinical manifestations therapeutically, indicating that neuromuscular dysfunction is a major cause of the syndrome (7).

REFERENCES

1. Aiyar VN, Benn MH, Hanna T *et al.* (1979) The principal toxin of *Delphinium brownii* Rydb., and its mode of action. *Experientia* **35**, 1367.
2. Alkondon M, Pereira EF, Wonnacott S, Albuquerque EX (1992) Blockade of nicotinic currents in hippocampal neurons defines methyllycaconitine as a potent and specific receptor antagonist. *Mol Pharmacol* **41**, 802.
3. Davies AR, Hardick DJ, Blagbrough IS *et al.* (1999) Characterisation of the binding of [³H]methyllycaconitine: a new radioligand for labelling alpha 7-type neuronal nicotinic acetylcholine receptors. *Neuropharmacology* **38**, 679.
4. Nation PN, Benn MH, Roth SH, Wilkens JL (1982) Clinical signs and studies of the site of action of purified larkspur alkaloid methyllycaconitine, administered parenterally to calves. *Can Vet J* **23**, 264.
5. Olsen JD (1978) Tall larkspur poisoning in cattle and sheep. *J Amer Vet Med Assn* **173**, 762.
6. Olsen JD, Manners GD (1989) Toxicology of diterpenoid alkaloids in rangeland larkspur (*Delphinium* spp.). In: *Toxicants of Plant Origin. Vol 1. Alkaloids.* Cheeke PR ed. CRC Press, Boca Raton, Florida p. 291.
7. Pfister JA, Gardner DR, Panter KE (1999) Larkspur (*Delphinium* spp.) poisoning in livestock. *Nat Toxins* **8**, 81.
8. Ward JM, Cockcroft VB, Lunt GG *et al.* (1990) Methyllycaconitine: A selective probe for neuronal α-bungarotoxin binding sites. *FEBS Lett* **270**, 45.

Methyl Methacrylate

Steven Herskovitz

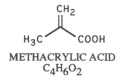

METHACRYLIC ACID
$C_4H_6O_2$

2-Methyl-2-propenoic acid; α-Methylacrylic acid

NEUROTOXICITY RATING

Clinical

A Peripheral neuropathy (local administration)
B Peripheral neuropathy (systemic)

Experimental

B Peripheral neuropathy (local administration)

Methyl methacrylate (MMA), the methyl ester of α-methylacrylic acid, is used extensively for fabricating acrylic plastics for prosthetic dentistry and as a bone cement in reconstructive orthopedic surgery. MMA monomer is a colorless, volatile liquid, an ester of methylacrylic acid that polymerizes to form polymethyl methacrylate, a rigid polymer. Prolonged cutaneous exposure to MMA monomer can result in a local sensory neuropathy; generalized, axonal, sensorimotor peripheral neuropathy is rare.

MMA is an irritant and may result in toxicity by inhalation of vapors, swallowing, or skin and mucous membrane contact. It is readily absorbed through the skin, and rubber gloves are an ineffective barrier (14). The characteristic penetrating odor is appreciable at low concentrations. The occupational permissible level as set by the U.S. Occupational Safety and Health Administration is an 8-h Time-Weighted Average of 100 ppm, a level difficult to exceed in the operating room. MMA gains access to the venous circulation within minutes during hip arthroplasties but is rapidly cleared; the lungs and peripheral capillary beds are effective filters (1,6,11,15). Exact toxic levels in humans and their relationship to clinical features are not established.

Direct immediate or delayed physical nerve injury may result from the use of MMA in reconstructive prosthetic hip surgery. Aside from traction injury during the procedure, sciatic neuropathy can be the result of inadvertent encasement of the nerve by MMA, delayed erosion into the nerve by a sharp spur of MMA, or following thermal injury during the polymerization process (4).

Animals, like humans, develop skin sensitization from topical MMA (7). After 4 weeks of topical exposure to MMA for 3 h daily, motor conduction studies in rat tail show reduced amplitudes and unchanged conduction velocities, suggesting axonal degeneration from a local neurotoxic effect (13). Degenerative features are seen on electron microscopy in some unmyelinated nerves in the papillary dermis of exposed rat tails (7). Other studies have suggested "demyelination" in vitro, or depression of action potentials in isolated desheathed nerve (7). Little is known of generalized neurotoxic responses to cutaneous or inhalation exposure.

During simulated hip arthroplasties in dogs, 0.5% of the total amount of MMA monomer used was detected in the blood. In intravenous injection experiments, amounts 30–40 times larger than those that probably reach the blood in human hip replacement, were required to produce pulmonary dysfunction (6). In another animal study, intravenous injection of 10 mg/ml or higher doses resulted in transient hypotension, pulmonary hemorrhage, and cardiac depression; concentrations measured during human hip replacement were 1 mg/dl or less (1). Similar clinical effects occur occasionally in humans during hip replacement, including hypoxia, hypotension and, rarely, cardiac arrest; these effects are poorly correlated with dose, and it is difficult to exclude possible contributing roles of air or fat emboli, platelet aggregation, and neurogenic reflexes (10,11).

Human cutaneous exposure to MMA is most common in dental technicians or orthopedic surgeons who mix or mold the resin with their fingers. In addition to allergic contact dermatitis, paresthesias appear in the fingertips and persist for several weeks to months after the dermatitis has subsided (5,7). In a Finnish questionnaire study of dental technicians, 34% reported dermatitis, and 25% reported possible local neuropathic symptoms in areas with frequent exposure to MMA (7). Digital sensory nerve conduction studies showed significant reduction in some conduction velocities and amplitudes predominantly in the dominant hand compared to controls (7,9). There was no correlation with dermatitis.

There is only one well-documented report of a generalized sensorimotor peripheral neuropathy in association with MMA (3). A 58-year-old dental prosthetic technician with 30 years of heavy occupational cutaneous and inhalational exposure to MMA monomer, and no other apparent etiology, presented with gradually progressive, diffuse, bilateral, distal sensory and motor dysfunction, beginning in the thumb and index finger of the dominant hand. Nerve conduction studies and needle electromyography were consistent with an axonal polyneuropathy, and sural biopsy showed a moderately severe axonopathy with loss of large-diameter myelinated and unmyelinated fibers. Increased numbers of neurofilaments were present in a few axons, resembling changes seen with acrylamide neuropathy.

The mechanism of neurotoxicity is not established. MMA reacts with sulfhydryl groups, which are important in the axonal transport of macromolecules, and may thereby affect the integrity of the distal axon (8,12). Free-radical scavengers protected cortical neurons in vitro from the toxic effects of MMA (2).

REFERENCES

1. Bright DS, Clark HG, McCollum DE (1972) Serum analysis and toxic effects of methylmethacrylate. Surg Forum 23, 455.
2. Chen MS, Wu JN, Yang SN et al. (1998) Free radicals are involved in methylmethacrylate-induced neurotoxicity in human primary neocortical cell cultures. Chin J Physiol 31, 203.
3. Donaghy M, Rushworth G, Jacobs JM (1991) Generalized peripheral neuropathy in a dental technician exposed to methyl methacrylate monomer. Neurology 41, 1112.
4. Edwards MS, Barbaro NM, Asher SW, Murray WR (1981) Delayed sciatic palsy after total hip replacement: Case report. Neurosurgery 9, 61.
5. Fisher AA (1979) Paresthesia of the fingers accompanying dermatitis due to methylmethacrylate bone cement. Contact Derm 5, 56.
6. McLaughlin RE, DiFazio CA, Hakala M et al. (1973) Blood clearance and acute pulmonary toxicity of methylmethacrylate in dogs after simulated arthroplasty and intravenous injection. J Bone Joint Surg 55, 1621.
7. Rajaniemi R (1986) Clinical evaluation of occupational toxicity of methylmethacrylate monomer to dental technicians. J Soc Occup Med 36, 56.
8. Savolainen H (1982) Neurotoxicity of industrial chemicals and contamitants: Aspects of mechanisms and effects. Arch Toxicol 5, 71.
9. Seppäläinen AM, Rajaniemi R (1984) Local neurotoxicity of methyl methacrylate among dental technicians. Amer J Ind Med 5, 471.
10. Svartling N (1988) Detection of embolized material in the right atrium during cementation in hip arthroplasty. Acta Anaesthesiol Scand 32, 203.

11. Svartling N, Pfäffli P, Tarkkanen (1985) Methacrylate blood levels in patients with femoral neck fractures. *Arch Orthop Trauma Surg* **104**, 242.

12. Tanii H, Hashimoto K (1982) Structure-toxicity relationship of acrylates and methacrylates. *Toxicol Lett* **11**, 125.

13. Verkkala E, Rajaniemi R, Savolainen H (1983) Local neurotoxicity of methylmethacrylate monomer. *Toxicol Lett* **18**, 111.

14. Waegemaekers THJM, Seutter E, den Arend JACJ, Malten KE (1983) Permeability of surgeons' gloves to methyl methacrylate. *Acta Orthop Scand* **6**, 790.

15. Weissman BN, Sosman JL, Braunstein EM *et al.* (1984) Intravenous methyl methacrylate after total hip replacement. *J Bone Joint Surg* **66**, 443.

MPTP and Analogs

Donato A. Di Monte
J. William Langston

MPTP
$C_{12}H_{15}N$

1-Methyl-4-phenyl-1,2,3,6-tetrahydropyridine

NEUROTOXICITY RATING

Clinical

A   Extrapyramidal syndrome (parkinsonism)

Experimental

A   Extrapyramidal dysfunction (parkinsonism; substantia nigra degeneration)

The neurotoxicant 1-methyl-4-phenyl-1,2,3,6-tetrahydropyridine (MPTP) was identified in 1983 as the contaminant of synthetic illicit drugs that caused the abrupt onset of parkinsonian signs in young drug addicts (27).

MPTP is commercially available as a hydrochloride salt. In this form, MPTP is a white, odorless powder (MP, 241°–243°C) that is soluble in water. Because of its toxicity to humans, special precautions must be taken for its use and disposal. MPTP solutions should be treated with a 50% excess of commercial bleach before disposal (60).

MPTP has been extensively used for research purposes. The clinical, neuropathological, and neurochemical features of MPTP-induced toxicity are very similar to those observed in idiopathic parkinsonism, (a) raising the possibility that MPTP-like toxins may play a role in the etiology of Parkinson's disease, and (b) providing a valuable experimental tool for the development of *in-vitro* and *in-vivo* models of nigrostriatal degeneration.

General Toxicology

Because of its lipophilic structure, MPTP is not only rapidly distributed throughout body tissues but also crosses the blood-brain barrier. Once in the CNS, however, MPTP does not cause neurotoxicity unless it is activated to its fully oxidized metabolite, 1-methyl-4-phenylpyridinium (MPP^+). This metabolism occurs in two steps: first, MPTP is oxidized to the intermediate 1-methyl-4-phenyl-2,3-dihydropyridinium ($MPDP^+$) and then $MPDP^+$ is converted to MPP^+. The first step is catalyzed by the enzyme monoamine oxidase (MAO) type B (9), while the conversion of $MPDP^+$ to MPP^+ is likely to occur *via* auto-oxidation (59). The critical role played by MPP^+ in MPTP toxicity is demonstrated by findings showing that (a) MAO B inhibitors completely protect against MPTP toxicity both *in vivo* and *in vitro* (16,22,29), and (b) MPP^+ itself causes toxic effects similar to those seen after systemic administration of MPTP (3). On the other hand, systemically administered MPP^+ does not cross the blood-brain barrier; therefore, MPP^+-induced neurotoxicity only occurs when this pyridinium compound is directly injected into the brain. Thus, conversion of MPTP to MPP^+ in peripheral tissue can be considered a detoxification pathway, since peripherally generated MPP^+ is relatively "inert" from the point of view of inducing CNS damage.

Nigrostriatal dopaminergic neurons represent the primary target of MPP^+ toxicity. However, they are unlikely to be the site for MPTP bioactivation to MPP^+. Immunocytochemical studies show that dopamine-containing neuronal groups do not express MAO B, whereas this enzyme is located within serotonergic neurons and astrocytes (30). MPTP neurotoxicity is not significantly affected when serotonergic neurons are lesioned (33), thus leaving astrocytes as the most likely cells that generate MPP^+ in the CNS. Once MPP^+ is produced within glial cells, it can reach the extracellular space by at least two mechanisms: (a) it is released from damaged astrocytes as a consequence of cell membrane disruption (18,59); and (b) despite its charged chemical structure, it possesses enough lipid solubility to cross undamaged astrocyte membranes (18). A third mechanism could also account for the presence of MPP$^+$ in the extracellular space: MAO-generated MPDP$^+$ could cross astrocyte membranes in the form of the lipophilic free base 1,2-MPDP and then undergo auto-oxidation to MPP$^+$ (18).

The fate of MPP$^+$ in the extracellular space represents a critical step in the mechanism of action of MPTP that explains at least in part the selectivity of this neurotoxicant. It seems likely that MPP$^+$ would be cleared from the CNS with only minor neurotoxic effects if it were not recognized as a substrate by the catecholamine uptake system (24). MPP$^+$ can therefore be accumulated into dopaminergic neurons where it reaches high enough concentrations and persists long enough to cause irreversible damage. The importance of the active uptake of MPP$^+$ in relation to MPTP neurotoxicity is demonstrated by studies showing that dopamine-uptake blockers are capable of preventing the neurotoxic effects of MPTP in rodents (34,50). The effectiveness of uptake blockers against MPTP neurotoxicity in the monkey model is less clear (26,54), possibly due to the different regimens of administration of these agents by different groups of investigators.

Active uptake of MPP$^+$ into dopaminergic neurons does not completely explain MPTP selectivity, however. For example, it cannot explain why dopaminergic neurons are particularly vulnerable to MPTP toxicity as compared to other neurons that also express catecholaminergic-uptake sites. It has been suggested that the presence of neuromelanin may be another mechanism contributing to MPTP selectivity toward the nigrostriatal dopaminergic system. MPP$^+$ binds with high affinity to neuromelanin and could therefore be selectively sequestered within neuromelanin-containing neurons of the substantia nigra (13). At least three lines of evidence support a relevant role for neuromelanin in MPTP neurotoxicity. First, chloroquine, a compound able to displace MPP$^+$ from neuromelanin-binding sites, has been shown to attenuate neurotoxic effects of MPTP in primates (12). Second, injection of synthetic neuromelanin enhanced MPTP-induced dopaminergic neurotoxicity in rodents (35). On the other hand, animal species that do not have a melanized substantia nigra (e.g., aged mice) appear to be susceptible to the neurotoxic effects of MPTP.

Animal Studies

Research on the effects and mechanism of action of MPTP has involved a remarkable variety of animal models, ranging from the medicinal leech to monkeys. A 1984 report first documented the observation that certain strains of mice, particularly C57BL/6 mice, were more sensitive than other rodents to the neurotoxic effects of MPTP (21). These animals have since become the most widely used rodent model for MPTP studies, providing a great body of valuable information. There is little doubt, however, that when one compares the behavioral, neuropathological and neurochemical features of MPTP toxicity with those of idiopathic parkinsonism, the most reliable animal model is the non-human primate. For example, parkinsonian signs such as bradykinesia, postural abnormalities, and tendency to freeze are consistent effects of MPTP neurotoxicity in monkeys (14), while MPTP causes relatively nonspecific behavioral changes in rodents. Thus, the comparison of neuropathological and neurochemical features between MPTP-induced and idiopathic parkinsonism in the following paragraphs relates primarily to findings in the primate model.

The main neuropathological feature of idiopathic parkinsonism is a degeneration of neuromelanin-containing neurons in the pars compacta of the substantia nigra, with the lateral and ventral cell groups being most severely affected. Degeneration of pigmented noradrenergic neurons of the locus ceruleus is also typically observed. Another neuropathological hallmark is the presence of eosinophilic inclusions first described in 1912 by F.H. Lewy and since called Lewy bodies. These cytoplasmic inclusions are observed not only in the substantia nigra and the locus ceruleus but also in sites such as the dorsal motor nucleus of the vagus, the nucleus basalis of Meynert, and the sympathetic ganglia. They are not specific for Parkinson's disease and are thought to be indicative of an ongoing degenerative process.

MPTP-induced parkinsonism is characterized by a marked destruction of neurons in the zona compacta of the substantia nigra (4,28). The distribution of lesions within this area appears to depend upon the severity of injury and the duration of survival of exposed animals (19). In animals surviving for more than 6 weeks, the middle and lateral cell groups seem to be more severely affected, thus resembling the pattern of neuronal degeneration in idiopathic parkinsonism. Another similarity between the MPTP model and Parkinson's disease concerns the involvement of the locus ceruleus; nerve cell loss has been reported to occur in this area of the brain in older squirrel monkeys after a protracted MPTP regimen (20). Although eosinophilic intraneuronal inclusions have been observed in monkeys exposed to MPTP, they cannot be considered classic Lewy bodies because of significant histopathological differences (14,19). It has been hypothesized that MPTP-induced inclusions may represent Lewy bodies at an early stage (so-called "pre-Lewy bodies") and that differences between inclusions in MPTP and idiopathic parkinsonism may result from the acute vs. more chronic type of neuronal degeneration. This hypothesis has yet to be proved, and therefore the absence of typical Lewy bodies remains the most evident neuropathological distinction between MPTP neurotoxicity and Parkinson's disease.

Dopamine is the neurotransmitter used by pigmented neurons which project their axons from the zona compacta of the substantia nigra into the striatum. It is not surprising, therefore, that degeneration of these neurons in Parkinson's disease as well as in MPTP neurotoxicity leads to depletion of dopamine in the nigrostriatal pathway. The pattern and time course of MPTP-induced dopamine depletion have been elucidated in the monkey model and appear to differ significantly in the substantia nigra and the striatum. In the substantia nigra of squirrel monkeys, dopamine levels fall to <50% of the initial values just 24 h after systemic MPTP exposure and remain decreased for at least 10 days (23). This dopamine depletion is accompanied by reduced levels of the dopamine metabolites dihydroxyphenylacetic acid (DOPAC) and homovanillic acid (HVA). In the striatum, no decrease in dopamine levels is measured at 1 and 3 days after MPTP injection to squirrel monkeys, and actually dopamine values in the putamen are increased in MPTP-treated vs. untreated animals (23). Then, after 5 days of MPTP exposure, a dramatic dopamine depletion occurs in both the caudate and the putamen and persists for at least several days (23). Striatal levels of DOPAC and HVA are consistently reduced from 1–10 days after MPTP injection.

The reason(s) for the different time course of dopamine depletion in the substantia nigra and striatum remain to be elucidated and may include different responses of cell bodies and nerve terminals to MPTP injury. It is possible, for example, that a "paralysis" of dopamine release from nerve terminals in the striatum may result from an initial damage to cell bodies in the substantia nigra, leading to unchanged or increased striatal dopamine levels. The pattern of MPTP-induced dopamine depletion is also likely to reflect tissue features characteristic of the nigrostriatal pathway of primates. Indeed, striatal dopamine depletion in the rodent model (i.e., in mice) occurs within hours of systemic administration of MPTP, and dopamine levels remain below initial values during the following days and weeks (7,26). Understanding the different mechanisms of MPTP-induced neurochemical changes in the primate and the rodent models may help to explain the greater sensitivity of monkeys to MPTP neurotoxicity (26).

It has been reported that, in idiopathic Parkinson's disease, the loss of dopamine is significantly greater in the putamen than in the caudate (25). Whether a similar regional pattern occurs in MPTP neurotoxicity has often been debated. It seems likely, however, that the controversial results reported by different research groups (23,44) are due to variations in MPTP dose, route, and regimen of adminis-

tration in the different monkey models. However, the finding that dopamine levels in the putamen are more severely depleted than in the caudate of squirrel monkeys injected with MPTP (23) bears significant implications in bringing the MPTP model even closer to idiopathic parkinsonism. This regional pattern of MPTP neurotoxicity is further indicated by data showing a more extensive loss of ^{3}H-mazindol binding sites in the putamen as compared to the caudate of squirrel monkeys (36).

Although dopamine depletion represents the most dramatic and consistent neurochemical feature of MPTP toxicity, several reports suggest the involvement of other neurotransmitter systems, such as the noradrenergic system (45). This is not surprising in view of the pathological findings of extranigral MPTP damage (e.g., to the locus ceruleus) and the possible alterations of nondopaminergic systems in Parkinson's disease.

In Vitro Studies

Several in vitro models have been used to evaluate and clarify molecular aspects of MPTP toxicity. The role of the mitochondrial enzyme MAO B in MPTP bioactivation has been determined in mitochondrial preparations (9). Mitochondria have also been used to discover and characterize the ability of MPP${}^+$ to block mitochondrial respiration, a property that is likely to underlie its cytotoxic effects (see Toxic Mechanisms vide infra) (40). Synaptosomal preparations have provided valuable information concerning the uptake of MPP${}^+$ into nerve terminals and the metabolic changes following this active accumulation (55). Mesencephalic neuronal cultures have helped characterize the selective cytotoxic effects of MPP${}^+$ toward dopaminergic neurons (37), while glial cultures have allowed detailed study of the metabolic pathways of MPTP biotransformation (17). Studies with adrenal chromaffin cells have suggested that sequestration of MPP${}^+$ by chromaffin vesicles may protect against its cytotoxicity (48), and findings with preparations of brain microvessels support the concept that peripheral metabolism of MPTP prevents its access into the CNS and the consequent neurotoxic effects (49).

This brief review emphasizes the wide range of information obtained using in vitro models. By elucidating the mechanism of action of MPTP, these studies have shed light on molecular processes that are likely to be of more general neurotoxicological relevance, such as the role of MAO B in the bioactivation of neurotoxins. Furthermore, in vitro studies with MPTP/MPP${}^+$ have provided valuable models of dopaminergic degeneration. For example, the efficacy of potential therapeutic agents (e.g., neurotrophic factors) against dopaminergic cell death can now be tested in MPP${}^+$-treated mesencephalic cultures (42).

Human Studies

Although it is estimated that approximately 400 intravenous narcotics users were exposed to MPTP, a frank parkinsonian syndrome was observed in only seven subjects. A number of reasons can explain this numerical discrepancy, including degree of exposure (*i.e.*, number of doses) and, perhaps, greater vulnerability of the dopaminergic system of the affected population. Affected individuals rapidly developed a clinical syndrome virtually indistinguishable from idiopathic Parkinson's disease (27). This syndrome included not only all the major parkinsonian features (*i.e.*, tremor, rigidity, bradykinesia, and postural instability), but also more subtle signs of the disease such as hypomimia, micrographia, and seborrhea. MPTP patients responded to L-dopa treatment and actually developed the same side effects as those seen in patients with idiopathic parkinsonism (*e.g.*, end-of-dose "wearing off" and peak-dose dyskinesia). A significant reduction in levels of HVA, a major dopamine metabolite, was measured in the cerebrospinal fluid of severely affected MPTP patients (5). Furthermore, positron emission tomography (PET) scanning using ^{18}F-fluorodopa as the tracer revealed a similar reduction in nigrostriatal radioactivity in MPTP-exposed subjects as compared to parkinsonian patients (6).

Three patients affected with MPTP-induced parkinsonism have undergone bilateral fetal mesencephalic grafting. Transplantation of fetal dopamine-rich neuronal tissue has been reported to exert functional effects in experimental animal models as well as in patients with Parkinson's disease (2,31). An initial report evaluating the effects of mesencephalic grafting in two of the three MPTP patients revealed significant motor function improvement and increased striatal uptake of fluorodopa at 1 and 2 years postoperatively in both patients (58). This positive response to implantation of dopamine-rich mesencephalic tissue further supports the view that the clinical effects of MPTP result from the selective damage of the nigrostriatal dopaminergic system.

Toxic Mechanisms

MPTP-induced neurotoxicity is the consequence of a seemingly concerted sequence of pharmacological and biochemical events, some of which have previously been discussed. Briefly, (a) MPTP crosses the blood-brain barrier by virtue of its lipophilic structure; (b) in the brain, MPTP is converted to its toxic metabolite MPP$^+$ *via* MAO B localized within glial cells; (c) MPP$^+$ is released from astrocytes into the extracellular space; and (d) dopaminergic neurons actively accumulate MPP$^+$ through their catecholamine-uptake system. The final step of this sequence is neuronal cell death, but the ultimate mechanism by which MPP$^+$ induces cytotoxicity is still a matter of debate.

It was initially suggested that MPP$^+$ could induce the formation of oxygen radicals leading to cytotoxicity *via* a condition of oxidative stress. Experimental evidence supporting this hypothesis has been controversial, however, and most likely the contribution of oxidative stress to MPP$^+$-induced toxicity is only secondary (15). The search for a toxic property of MPP$^+$ that could directly link its intracellular presence to cytotoxicity led to the finding that MPP$^+$ is able to interfere with mitochondrial function. MPP$^+$ has been shown to be accumulated into mitochondria *via* the mitochondrial transmembrane potential (46,52). High concentrations of intramitochondrial MPP$^+$ are able to inhibit the flow of electrons through the respiratory chain; the site of MPP$^+$ inhibition appears to be the same as the classic complex I inhibitor rotenone (40). Blockade of electron flow may lead to oxygen radical formation that could then contribute to the cytotoxic effects of MPP$^+$ (10). However, the most serious consequence of complex I inhibition by MPP$^+$ is likely to be an impairment of oxidative phosphorylation with depletion of cellular energy supplies in the form of adenosine triphosphate (ATP). Indeed, cytotoxicity caused by both MPTP and MPP$^+$ *in vitro* has been clearly correlated with ATP depletion (16,59). Furthermore, it has been shown that the addition of substrates for glycolysis-dependent ATP production can delay MPTP/MPP$^+$-induced cell death (16). A decrease in ATP has also been documented in mice after exposure to MPTP; this decrease selectively occurs in the striatum and ventral mesencephalon, and its time course seems to parallel the accumulation and clearance of MPP$^+$ in these areas of the mouse brain (8).

Impairment of mitochondrial function by MPP$^+$ could also account for the involvement of excitotoxicity in the cascade of MPTP-induced neurotoxic events. Although studies using N-methyl-D-aspartate (NMDA) receptor antagonists as protective agents against MPTP have generated conflicting results (7,56,57), there are reasons to suspect that they play a role in neurotoxicity. For example, increased extracellular levels of excitatory amino acids (EAAs) and/or increased sensitivity of EAA receptors seem probable in view of the following: depletion of energy supplies is likely to affect the uptake and inactivation of EAAs, leading to their accumulation in the synaptic cleft; and, membrane depolarization due to ATP depletion could relieve the voltage-dependent Mg^{2+} block of NMDA channels, resulting in increased receptor sensitivity. Thus, impaired mitochondrial function and excitotoxicity are likely to be linked, and the effects of EAAs may play a role in MPTP neurotoxicity as a consequence of MPP$^+$-induced ATP depletion.

MPTP Analogs

Many MPTP analogs have been synthesized and tested both *in vitro* and *in vivo* in order to identify the molecular properties that would predictively underlie neurotoxicity. These structure–activity studies first focused on the relationship between neurotoxicity of MPTP analogs and their ability to be oxidized by MAO. Several compounds were found to be good substrates for either MAO A or MAO B or both (61). This metabolic activation appeared to be necessary, but not sufficient, however, to predict the neurotoxic effects of MPTP analogs. For example, 1-methyl-4-(2',6'-dimethylphenyl)-1,2,3,6-tetrahydropyridine was found to be metabolized by MAO at significantly higher rates than MPTP, but did not cause significant reduction in striatal dopamine levels after systemic administration to mice (61). Thus, other properties besides being a MAO substrate are necessary for MPTP analogs to become neurotoxic; knowledge of the events underlying the action of MPTP has helped to identify the critical factors. Such factors include the ability of MPP^+ analogs to (a) function as substrates for the dopamine-uptake system, and (b) interfere with mitochondrial respiration. Cultured mesencephalic neurons were used to show a correlation between selective neurotoxicity of MPP^+ analogs and uptake into dopaminergic neurons (51); also, compounds with high affinity for the dopamine-uptake system did not exert neurotoxic effects unless they were also potent inhibitors of mitochondrial respiration. This correlation between respiratory chain inhibition and neurotoxicity of $MPTP/MPP^+$ analogs has been emphasized in a number of reports (47,53). It is noteworthy, however, that extremely potent mitochondrial inhibitors (*i.e.*, 4'-alkylated analogs of MPP^+), which lack affinity for the uptake system, did not target dopaminergic neurons but caused a nonselective damage of neurons in culture (51). Thus, structure–activity studies with $MPTP/MPP^+$ analogs have emphasized the need for at least three critical molecular properties that would make these compounds selectively neurotoxic: (a) MAO activation of the pyridine derivative to the corresponding pyridinium metabolite, (b) active uptake by dopaminergic neurons, and (c) inhibition of oxidative phosphorylation after accumulation into mitochondria.

The search for compounds structurally similar to MPTP that could be formed endogenously within the CNS has pointed to tetrahydroisoquinolines (TIQs) and tetrahydro-β-carbolines (TBCs) as possible endotoxins. These compounds could be formed in the brain *via* spontaneous Pictet-Spengler cyclization of catecholamines and tryptamine. TIQs have been detected in the human brain and, in particular, in the brain of patients with Parkinson's disease (41). They have been reported to decrease dopamine and tyrosine hydroxylase levels in the nigrostriatal pathway of monkeys after prolonged administration (38), although these findings have not been confirmed by other investigators (43). TBCs have also been detected in mammalian brain (32). *N*-Methylated derivatives of TBCs have been shown to possess biochemical properties similar to MPP^+ (*e.g.*, inhibition of mitochondrial respiration) as well as dopaminergic neurotoxicity (1,32,52). Thus, *N*-methylation has been suggested to be a toxification route for potential endogenous toxins (11).

Both TIQs and TBCs seem to be similar to MPTP in their requirement for activation to the corresponding quinolinium and carbolinium metabolites to become neurotoxic. Although controversial data have been reported concerning the ability of TIQs to be metabolized by MAO (39,52), it appears that TIQs and TBCs are not substrates or are very poor substrates for MAO. It is possible, therefore, that lack of dramatic neurotoxicity following systemic administration of TIQs or TBCs is the consequence of a limited production of the corresponding toxic metabolites. Hence, detection of quinolinium and carbolinium compounds in mammalian brain, as well as evaluation of possible metabolic pathways for the production of these MPP^+-like agents, is a critical area for investigation (11,32). Findings from these studies may provide evidence in favor of an etiological role of TIQs and/or TBCs in Parkinson's disease.

REFERENCES

1. Albores R, Collins MA, Neafsey EJ *et al.* (1990) Mitochondrial respiratory inhibition by *N*-methylated β-carboline derivatives structurally resembling *N*-methyl-4-phenylpyridine (MPP^+). *Proc Nat Acad Sci USA* **87**, 9368.
2. Bankiewicz KS, Plunkett RJ, Jacobowitz DM *et al.* (1990) The effect of fetal mesencephalon implants on primate MPTP-induced parkinsonism. Histochemical and behavioral studies. *J Neurosurg* **72**, 231.
3. Bradbury AJ, Costall B, Domeney AM *et al.* (1986) 1-Methyl-4-phenylpyridine is neurotoxic to the nigrostriatal dopamine pathway. *Nature* **319**, 56.
4. Burns RS, Chiueh CC, Markey SP *et al.* (1983) A primate model of parkinsonism: Selective destruction of dopaminergic neurons in the pars compacta of the substantia nigra by N-methyl-4-phenyl-1,2,3,6-tetrahydropyridine. *Proc Nat Acad Sci USA* **80**, 4546.
5. Burns RS, Lewitt PA, Ebert MH *et al.* (1985) The clinical syndrome of striatal dopamine deficiency. Parkinsonism induced by 1-methyl-4-phenyl-1,2,3,6-tetrahydropyridine (MPTP). *N Engl J Med* **312**, 1418.
6. Calne DB, Langston JW, Martin WRW *et al.* (1985) Positron emission tomography after MPTP: Observations relating to the cause of Parkinson's disease. *Nature* **317**, 246.

7. Chan P, Langston JW, Di Monte DA (1993) MK-801 temporarily prevents MPTP-induced acute dopamine depletion and MPP⁺ elimination in the mouse striatum. *J Pharmacol Exp Ther* **267**, 1515.

8. Chan P, Langston JW, Irwin I et al. (1993) 2-Deoxyglucose enhances 1-methyl-4-phenyl-1,2,3,6-tetrahydropyridine (MPTP)-induced ATP loss in the mouse brain. *J Neurochem* **61**, 610.

9. Chiba K, Trevor AJ, Castagnoli N Jr (1984) Metabolism of the neurotoxic tertiary amine, MPTP, by brain monoamine oxidase. *Biochem Biophys Res Commun* **120**, 574.

10. Cleeter MWJ, Cooper JM, Schapira AHV (1992) Irreversible inhibition of complex I by 1-methyl-4-phenylpyridinium: Evidence for free radical involvement. *J Neurochem* **58**, 786.

11. Collins MA, Neafsey EJ, Matsubara K et al. (1992) Indole-N-methylation of beta-carbolines: The brain's bioactivation route to toxins in Parkinson's disease? *Ann N Y Acad Sci* **648**, 263.

12. D'Amato RJ, Alexander GM, Schwartzman RJ et al. (1987) Evidence for neuromelanin involvement in MPTP-induced neurotoxicity. *Nature* **327**, 324.

13. D'Amato RJ, Lipman ZP, Snyder SH (1986) Selectivity of the parkinsonian neurotoxin MPTP: Toxic metabolite MPP⁺ binds to neuromelanin. *Science* **231**, 987.

14. Di Monte DA, Langston JW (1993) MPTP-induced parkinsonism in non-human primates. In: *Current Concepts in Parkinson's Research*. Schneider JS, Gupta M eds. Hogrefe/Hans Huber Science Publishing, Frankfurt p. 159.

15. Di Monte DA, Smith MT (1988) Free radicals, lipid peroxidation and 1-methyl-4-phenyl-1,2,3,6-tetrahydropyridine (MPTP)-induced parkinsonism. *Rev Neurosci* **2**, 67.

16. Di Monte DA, Wu EY, DeLanney LE et al. (1992) Toxicity of 1-methyl-4-phenyl-1,2,3,6-tetrahydropyridine in primary cultures of mouse astrocytes. *J Pharmacol Exp Ther* **261**, 44.

17. Di Monte DA, Wu EY, Irwin I et al. (1991) Biotransformation of 1-methyl-4-phenyl-1,2,3,6-tetrahydropyridine in primary cultures of mouse astrocytes. *J Pharmacol Exp Ther* **258**, 594.

18. Di Monte DA, Wu EY, Irwin I et al. (1992) Production and disposition of 1-methyl-4-phenylpyridinium in primary cultures of mouse astrocytes. *Glia* **5**, 48.

19. Forno LS, DeLanney LE, Irwin I et al. (1993) Similarities and differences between MPTP-induced parkinsonism and Parkinson's disease. Neuropathologic considerations. *Adv Neurol* **60**, 600.

20. Forno LS, Langston JW, DeLanney LE et al. (1986) Locus ceruleus lesions and eosinophilic inclusions in MPTP-treated monkeys. *Ann Neurol* **20**, 449.

21. Heikkila RE, Hess A, Duvoisin RC (1984) Dopaminergic neurotoxicity of 1-methyl-4-phenyl-1,2,3,6-tetrahydropyridine in mice. *Science* **224**, 1451.

22. Heikkila RE, Manzino L, Cabbat FS et al. (1984) Protection against the dopaminergic neurotoxicity of 1-methyl-4-phenyl-1,2,5,6-tetrahydropyridine by monoamine oxidase inhibitors. *Nature* **311**, 467.

23. Irwin I, DeLanney LE, Forno LS et al. (1990) The evolution of nigrostriatal neurochemical changes in the MPTP-treated squirrel monkey. *Brain Res* **531**, 242.

24. Javitch JA, D'Amato RJ, Strittmatter SM et al. (1985) Parkinsonism-inducing neurotoxin, N-methyl-4-phenyl-1,2,3,6-tetrahydropyridine: Uptake of the metabolite N-methyl-4-phenyl-pyridine by dopamine neurons explains selective toxicity. *Proc Nat Acad Sci USA* **82**, 2173.

25. Kish SJ, Shannak K, Hornykiewicz O (1988) Uneven pattern of dopamine loss in the striatum of patients with idiopathic Parkinson's disease. *N Eng J Med* **318**, 876.

26. Langston JW (1995) MPTP as it relates to the etiology of Parkinson's disease. In: *Etiology of Parkinson's Disease*. Ellenberg JH, Koller WC, Langston JW eds. Marcel Dekker, New York p. 367.

27. Langston JW, Ballard PA, Tetrud JW et al. (1983) Chronic parkinsonism in humans due to a product of meperidine analog synthesis. *Science* **219**, 979.

28. Langston JW, Forno LS, Rebert CS et al. (1984) Selective nigral toxicity after systemic administration of 1-methyl-4-phenyl-1,2,3,6-tetrahydropyridine (MPTP) in the squirrel monkey. *Brain Res* **292**, 390.

29. Langston JW, Irwin I, Langston EB et al. (1984) Pargyline prevents MPTP-induced parkinsonism in primates. *Science* **225**, 1480.

30. Levitt P, Pintar JE, Breakefield XO (1982) Immunocytochemical demonstration of monoamine oxidase B in brain astrocytes and serotonergic neurons. *Proc Nat Acad Sci USA* **79**, 6385.

31. Lindvall O, Brundin P, Widner H et al. (1990) Grafts of fetal dopamine neurons survive and improve motor function in Parkinson's disease. *Science* **247**, 574.

32. Matsubara K, Collins MA, Akane A et al. (1993) Potential bioactivated neurotoxicants, N-methylated β-carbolinium ions, are present in human brain. *Brain Res* **610**, 90.

33. Melamed E, Pikarski E, Goldberg A et al. (1986) Effect of serotonergic, corticostriatal and kainic acid lesions on the dopaminergic neurotoxicity of 1-methyl-4-phenyl-1,2,3,6-tetrahydropyridine (MPTP) in mice. *Brain Res* **399**, 178.

34. Melamed E, Rosenthal J, Cohen O et al. (1985) Dopamine but not norepinephrine or serotonin uptake inhibitors protect mice against neurotoxicity of MPTP. *Eur J Pharmacol* **116**, 179.

35. Melamed E, Soffer D, Rosenthal J et al. (1987) Effect of intrastriatal and intranigral administration of synthetic neuromelanin on the dopaminergic neurotoxicity of MPTP in rodents. *Neurosci Lett* **83**, 41.

36. Moratalla R, Quinn B, DeLanney LE et al. (1992) Differential vulnerability of primate caudate-putamen and striosome-matrix dopamine systems to the neurotoxic

effects of 1-methyl-4-phenyl-1,2,3,6-tetrahydropyridine. *Proc Nat Acad Sci USA* **89**, 3859.

37. Mytilineou C, Cohen G (1984) 1-Methyl-4-phenyl-1,2,3,6-tetrahydropyridine destroys dopamine neurons in explants of rat embryo mesencephalon. *Science* **225**, 529.

38. Nagatsu T, Yoshida M (1988) An endogenous substance of the brain, tetrahydroisoquinoline, produces parkinsonism in primates with decreased dopamine, tyrosine hydroxylase and biopterin in the nigrostriatal regions. *Neurosci Lett* **87**, 178.

39. Naoi MS, Matsuura S, Parvez T *et al.* (1989) Oxidation of *N*-methyl-1,2,3,4-tetrahydroiso-quinoline into the *N*-methyl-isoquinolinium ion by monoamine oxidase. *J Neurochem* **52**, 653.

40. Nicklas WJ, Vyas I, Heikkila RE (1985) Inhibition of NADH-linked oxidation in brain mitochondria by 1-methyl-4-phenyl-1,2,3,6-tetrahydropyridine. *Life Sci* **36**, 2503.

41. Niwa T, Takeda N, Kaneda N *et al.* (1987) Presence of tetrahydroisoquinoline and 1-methyl-tetrahydroisoquinoline in parkinsonian and normal human brain. *Biochem Biophys Res Commun* **144**, 1084.

42. Park T, Mytilineou C (1992) Protection from 1-methyl-4-phenylpyridinium (MPP⁺) toxicity and stimulation of regrowth of MPP⁺-damaged dopaminergic fibers by treatment of mesencephalic cultures with EGF and basic FGF. *Brain Res* **599**, 83.

43. Perry TL, Jones K, Hansen S (1988) Tetrahydroisoquinoline lacks dopaminergic nigrostriatal neurotoxicity in mice. *Neurosci Lett* **85**, 101.

44. Pifl C, Schingnitz G, Hornykiewicz O (1988) The neurotoxin MPTP does not reproduce in the rhesus monkey the interregional pattern of striatal dopamine loss typical of human idiopathic Parkinson's disease. *Neurosci Lett* **92**, 228.

45. Pifl C, Schingnitz G, Hornykiewicz O (1991) Effects of 1-methyl-4-phenyl-1,2,3,6-tetrahydropyridine on the regional distribution of monoamines in the rhesus monkey. *Neuroscience* **44**, 591.

46. Ramsay RR, Singer TP (1986) Energy-dependent uptake of *N*-methyl-4-phenylpyridinium, the neurotoxic metabolite of 1-methyl-4-phenyl-1,2,3,6-tetrahydropyridine, by mitochondria. *J Biol Chem* **261**, 7585.

47. Ramsay RR, Youngster SK, Nicklas WJ *et al.* (1989) Structural dependence of the inhibition of mitochondrial respiration and of NADH oxidase by 1-methyl-4-phenylpyridinium (MPP⁺) analogs and their energized accumulation by mitochondria. *Proc Nat Acad Sci USA* **86**, 9168.

48. Reinhard JF, Diliberto EJ, Viveros OH *et al.* (1987) Subcellular compartmentalization of 1-methyl-4-phenylpyridinium with catecholamines in adrenal medullary chromaffin vesicles may explain the lack of toxicity to adrenal chromaffin cells. *Proc Nat Acad Sci USA* **84**, 8160.

49. Riachi NJ, Harik SI, Kalaria RN *et al.* (1988) On the mechanisms underlying 1-methyl-4-phenyl-1,2,3,6-tetrahydropyridine neurotoxicity. II. Susceptibility among mammalian species correlates with the toxin's metabolic patterns in brain microvessels and liver. *J Pharmacol Exp Ther* **244**, 443.

50. Ricaurte GA, Langston JW, DeLanney LE *et al.* (1985) Dopamine uptake blockers protect against the dopamine depleting effects of 1-methyl-4-phenyl-1,2,3,6-tetrahydropyridine (MPTP) in the mouse striatum. *Neurosci Lett* **59**, 259.

51. Saporito MS, Heikkila RE, Youngster SH *et al.* (1992) Dopaminergic neurotoxicity of 1-methyl-4-phenylpyridinium analogs in cultured neurons: Relationship to dopamine uptake system and inhibition of mitochondrial respiration. *J Pharmacol Exp Ther* **260**, 1400.

52. Sayre LM (1989) Biochemical mechanism of action of the dopaminergic neurotoxin 1-methyl-4-phenyl-1,2,3,6-tetrahydropyridine (MPTP). *Toxicol Lett* **48**, 121.

53. Sayre LM, Wang F, Arora PK *et al.* (1991) Dopaminergic neurotoxicity *in vivo* and inhibition of mitochondrial respiration *in vitro* by possible endogenous pyridinium-like substances. *J Neurochem* **57**, 2106.

54. Schultz W, Scarnati E, Sundstrom E *et al.* (1986) The catecholamine uptake blocker nomifensine protects against MPTP-induced parkinsonism in monkeys. *Exp Brain Res* **63**, 216.

55. Scotcher KP, Irwin I, DeLanney LE *et al.* (1990) Effects of 1-methyl-4-phenyl-1,2,3,6-tetrahydropyridine and 1-methyl-4-phenylpyridinium ion on ATP levels of mouse brain synaptosomes. *J Neurochem* **54**, 1295.

56. Sonsalla PK, Nicklas WJ, Heikkila RE (1989) Role for excitatory amino acids in methamphetamine-induced nigrostriatal dopaminergic toxicity. *Science* **243**, 398.

57. Turski L, Bressler K, Rettig KJ *et al.* (1991) Protection of substantia nigra from MPP⁺ neurotoxicity by *N*-methyl-D-aspartate antagonists. *Nature* **349**, 414.

58. Widner H, Tetrud J, Rehncrona S *et al.* (1992) Bilateral fetal mesencephalic grafting in two patients with parkinsonism induced by 1-methyl-4-phenyl-1,2,3,6-tetrahydropyridine (MPTP). *N Engl J Med* **327**, 1556.

59. Wu EY, Langston J, Di Monte DA (1992) Toxicity of the 1-methyl-4-phenyl-2,3-dihydropyridinium and 1-methyl-4-phenylpyridinium species in primary cultures of mouse astrocytes. *J Pharmacol Exp Ther* **26**, 225.

60. Yang SC, Markey SP, Bankiewicz KS *et al.* (1988) Recommended safe practices for using the neurotoxin MPTP in animal experiments. *Lab An Sci* **38**, 563.

61. Youngster SK, Sonsalla PK, Sieber B-A *et al.* (1989) Structure-activity study on the mechanism of 1-methyl-4-phenyl-1,2,3,6-tetrahydropyridine (MPTP)-induced neurotoxicity. I. Evaluation of the biological activity of MPTP analogs. *J Pharmacol Exp Ther* **249**, 820.

Methylxanthines

Albert C. Ludolph

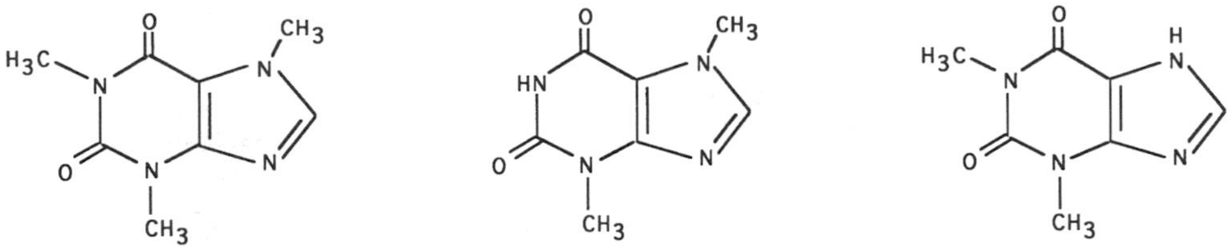

CAFFEINE
$C_8H_{10}N_4O_2$

THEOBROMINE
$C_7H_8N_4O_2$

THEOPHYLLINE
$C_7H_8N_4O_2$

Caffeine
   1,3,7-Trimethylxanthine
Theobromine
   3,7-Dimethylxanthine
Theophylline
   1,3-Dimethylxanthine

NEUROTOXICITY RATING

Clinical

A Psychobiological reaction
A Seizure disorder
A Physical dependence and withdrawal

Experimental

A Locomotor stimulation

The closely related alkaloids caffeine (from *Coffea arabica*, but also present in tea, mate leaves, and cola nuts), theophylline (from *Thea sinensis*), and the less potent theobromine (from the seeds of *Theobroma cacao*) are widely used centrally acting stimulants. Theophylline is employed therapeutically to relax bronchial smooth muscles in asthma, and caffeine is a component of some migraine medications and drug mixtures used to treat common colds. Methylxanthines are present in popular beverages such as tea, coffee, cola-flavored drinks (to which caffeine is added), cocoa, and chocolate (theobromine). Methylxanthines reduce drowsiness and fatigue, improve mood, and increase work capacity; however, arithmetic skills and delicate muscular coordination can be impaired (2).

Caffeine has a MW of 194.19, a MP of 238°C, and can be dissolved in water. Both theophylline and theobromine have a MW of 180.17; their MPs are 270°–274° and 357°C, respectively, and both are preferentially soluble in hot water. Solubility is increased if salts or complex double salts of each of the compounds are formed (21).

Methylated xanthines are readily absorbed after parenteral administration or from the gastrointestinal tract. Food intake and sleep slow but do not reduce their absorption. Caffeine is more readily absorbed than theophylline (plasma peaks after 1 and 2 h, respectively). Specific sustained-release preparations of theophylline exist to slow absorption for their use as bronchodilators in pulmonology; this might complicate the clinical profile of an intoxication. The blood concentration of caffeine after two to three cups of coffee (170–250 mg caffeine) reaches 12 mg/l (20); in comparison a cup of tea contains about 50 mg of caffeine and 1 mg of theophylline. After absorption, methylxanthines are bound to plasma proteins and distributed into all compartments of the body. In comparison, caffeine reaches greater concentrations in the cerebrospinal fluid and in brain than theophylline. Elimination of methylxanthines occurs in the liver, and <15% (5%) of theophylline (caffeine) can be detected in the urine. After caffeine intake, peak serum levels are reached after 30–60 min and its half-life in plasma is 3–7 h in adults; the half-life of theophylline is 8–9 h. Young children eliminate theophylline at a twofold rate; the elimination rate is much lower in premature infants (21). The half-life of caffeine increases during pregnancy. Genetic factors greatly influence the rate of elimination of methylxanthines. For theophylline, inhibition of hepatic microsomal cytochrome P-450–metabolizing enzymes by other drugs, such as oral contraceptives, histamine-receptor antagonists, certain antibiotics, and allopurinol, are factors that increase serum levels and promote neurotoxicity (9). Exogenous factors influence the elimination of caffeine (18); smoking increases elimination.

Methylxanthines not only stimulate the CNS (including the medullary respiratory center), but also have effects on smooth and skeletal muscles, the heart, gastric secretion, and the kidneys (21). There are three major pharmacological effects of methylxanthines (21): (a) they inhibit cyclic nucleotide phosphodiesterases, which results in an increase of cyclic adenosine monophosphate; (b) they are antagonists of adenosine (A_1 and A_2) receptors; and (c) they have a number of direct and indirect effects on intracellular Ca^{2+} concentrations.

Administration of caffeine to rats increases locomotor activity (12); tolerance for this effect develops. In drug-discrimination studies, generalization of this behavioral effect of caffeine extends to all methylxanthines (15). Caffeine reduces ischemic damage in rodents, possibly by up-regulation of adenosine receptors (26).

In humans, neurological side effects of caffeine occur after ingestion of doses exceeding 1 g or 15 mg/kg, which result in plasma concentrations >30 μg/ml. A psychobiological reaction ("caffeinism") with nervousness and restlessness, headache, anxiety and fear, tremor, and insomnia is the hallmark of the neurotoxic response after high doses. These symptoms may be more readily induced in patients suffering from panic attacks (5). Dosage increase is followed by ocular dyskinesias, dysesthesias, myalgia, "restless legs," tinnitus, scotomata and, finally, toxic delirium; exceptionally, seizures appear (5,14,16,17,21). Six cases of abnormal sleepiness induced by caffeine have been documented (19). Coma, seizures, and death were observed after intravenous administration of 400 mg and 3.2 g caffeine, respectively (9). The lethal dose for oral caffeine in adults reportedly is 5–10 g (3,7,8,11,25,27). The therapeutic concentration of theophylline in plasma should not exceed 20 μg/l (9); when plasma levels are higher than 40 μg/ml after oral or parenteral theophylline administration, symptoms of caffeine consumption appear. Generalized or focal seizures occur more frequently with theophylline than during caffeine intoxication (4). Susceptibility to seizures may increase during long-term treatment with theophylline, which possibly explains the loose dose–response relationship. Patients with pre-existing disorders of the CNS and older individuals (1,6,10,22) are more likely to experience neurotoxic side effects. Cases of status epilepticus in patients treated with comparatively high doses of theophylline and electroconvulsive therapy occur (9).

Withdrawal symptoms may appear after caffeine dosages as low as 235 mg/day (mean value) (23). The typical symptoms include headache, yawning, drowsiness, irritability, difficulty concentrating, muscle pain, dysphoria, depression, diarrhea, and nausea (13,21).

Theophylline is also used in preterm infants to prevent apnea and sudden-infant-death syndrome (21). In premature newborns, biotransformation of theophylline is slowed, resulting in increased susceptibility to its neurotoxic effects (24).

Treatment of methylxanthine intoxication includes gastric lavage; charcoal; and respiratory, cardiac, and blood pressure support. Seizures should be treated with benzodiazepines. In some cases of theophylline-induced seizures, treatment by conventional means may be difficult and general anesthesia may be required. If sustained-release preparations of theophylline have caused the intoxication, the use of activated charcoal is recommended. It is unclear whether hemodialysis or hemoperfusion are adequate methods to treat theophylline intoxication (9).

The mechanism of neurotoxicity is partly explained by the increased release of catecholamines from the adrenal glands; seizures may reflect an antagonistic effect at benzodiazepine receptors (18). It is also suggested that theophylline-induced seizures may be linked to vitamin B_6 deficiency (9).

REFERENCES

1. Aitken ML, Martin TR (1987) Life-threatening theophylline toxicity is not predictable in serum levels. *Chest* **91**, 10.
2. Arnaud MJ (1987) The pharmacology of caffeine. *Prog Drug Res* **31**, 273.
3. Banner W, Czajka PA (1980) Acute caffeine overdose in a neonate. *Amer J Dis Child* **134**, 495.
4. Burkle WS, Gwizdala CJ (1981) Evaluation of "toxic" theophylline concentrations. *Amer J Hosp Pharm* **38**, 1164.
5. Charney DS, Heninger GR, Jatlow PI (1985) Increased anxiogenic effects of caffeine in panic disorders. *Arch Gen Psychiat* **42**, 233.
6. Covelli HD, Knodel AR, Heppner BT (1985) Predisposing factor to apparent theophylline-induced seizures. *Ann Allergy* **54**, 411.
7. DiMaio VJM, Garriott JC (1974) Lethal caffeine poisoning in a child. *Forensic Sci Int* **3**, 275.
8. Eisele JW, Reay DT (1980) Deaths related to coffee enemas. *J Amer Med Assn* **244**, 1608.
9. Ellinwood EH, Rockwell EJK (1992) Central nervous system stimulants and anorectic agents. In: *Meyler's Side Effects of Drugs. 12th Ed.* Dukes MNG ed. Elsevier, Amsterdam p. 1.
10. Emmerman CL, Devlin C, Connors AF (1990) Risk of toxicity in patients with elevated theophylline levels. *Ann Emerg Med* **19**, 643.
11. Garriott JC, Simmons LM, Poklis A, Mackell MA (1985) Five cases of fatal overdose from caffeine-containing "look-alike" drugs. *J Anal Toxicol* **9**, 141.
12. Holtzman SG, Finn IB (1988) Tolerance to behavioral effects of caffeine in rats. *Pharmacol Biochem Behav* **29**, 411.
13. Hughes JR, Higgins ST, Bickel WK *et al.* (1991) Caffeine self-administration, withdrawal, and adverse effects among coffee drinkers. *Arch Gen Psychiat* **48**, 611.
14. Lutz EG (1978) Restless legs, anxiety and caffeinism. *J Clin Psychiat* **39**, 693.
15. Mumford GK, Holtzman SG (1991) Quantitative differences in the discriminative stimulus effects of low and high doses of caffeine in the rat. *J Pharmacol Exp Ther* **258**, 857.
16. Myers MG (1988) Caffeine and cardiac arrhythmias. *Chest* **94**, 4.
17. Myers MG (1988) Effects of caffeine on blood pressure. *Arch Intern Med* **148**, 115.

18. Pentel P (1984) Toxicity of over-the-counter stimulants. *J Amer Med Assn* **18**, 98.
19. Regestein QR (1989) Pathologic sleepiness induced by caffeine. *Amer J Med* **87**, 586.
20. Robertson D, Frolich SC, Carr RK *et al.* (1978) Effects of caffeine on plasma renin activity, catecholamines and blood pressure. *N Engl J Med* **298**, 181.
21. Serafin WE (1995) Drugs used in the treatment of asthma. In. *Goodman and Gilman's The Pharmacological Basis of Therapeutics. 9th Ed.* Hardman JG, Limbird LE, Molinoff PB, Ruddon RW eds. McGraw Hill, New York p. 659.
22. Shannon M, Lovejoy FH (1990) The influence of age *vs.* peak serum concentration on life-threatening events after chronic theophylline intoxication. *Arch Intern Med* **150**, 2045.
23. Silverman K, Evans SM, Strain EC, Griffiths RR (1992) Withdrawal syndrome after the double-blind cessation of caffeine consumption. *N Engl J Med* **327**, 1110.
24. Srinivasan G, Singh J, Cattamanchi G *et al.* (1983) Plasma glucose changes in pre-term infants during oral theophylline therapy. *J Pediat* **103**, 473.
25. Sullivan JL (1980) Caffeine poisoning in an infant. *J Pediat* **90**, 1022.
26. Sutherland GR, Peeling J, Lesiuk HJ *et al.* (1991) The effects of caffeine on ischemic neuronal injury as determined by magnetic resonance imaging and histopathology. *Neuroscience* **42**, 171.
27. Turner JE, Cravey RH (1977) A fatal ingestion of caffeine. *Clin Toxicol* **10**, 341.

Methysergide

Herbert H. Schaumburg

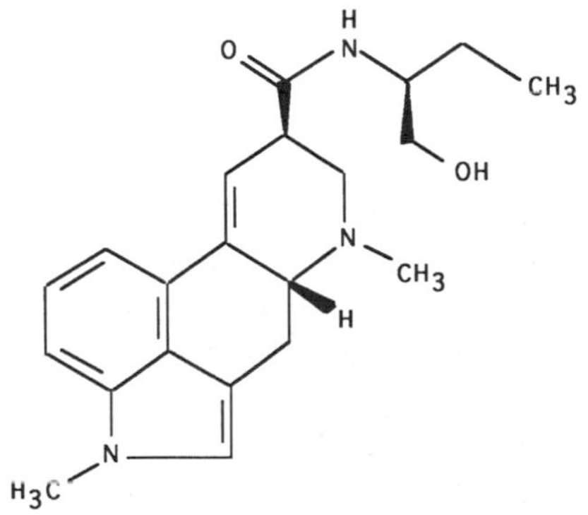

METHYSERGIDE
$C_{21}H_{27}N_3O_2$

[8β(S)]-9,10-Didehydro-*N*-[1-(hydroxymethyl)propyl]-1,6-dimethylergoline-8-carboxamide

NEUROTOXICITY RATING

Clinical

B   Acute encephalopathy (insomnia, anxiety)

Methysergide, a lysergic acid–derived serotonin antagonist, was formerly widely used in the prophylaxis of migraine headache; serious adverse reactions, especially retroperitoneal fibrosis, now limit its employment to recalcitrant cases. Methysergide is rapidly absorbed from the gastrointestinal tract and its principal metabolite, methylergonovine, is widely distributed. The locus of action is likely CNS serotonergic neurons, not peripheral vessels. Methysergide is primarily a serotonin type 2 (5-HT2) antagonist; it also acts as a partial agonist at 5-HT1 receptors (3,4). The most common adverse effect, appearing in 10% of cases, is peripheral vasoconstriction; the most serious is retroperitoneal or endocardial fibrosis (2). Fibrosis is dose-related, occurs in <1% of patients, and generally recedes after treatment ceases.

Neurotoxic effects are uncommon; <0.5% experience insomnia, anxiety, impaired concentration, and depression (1). Rarely, frightening dreams, confusion, and hallucinations appear; this unusual reaction is suggested to reflect the lysergic acid moiety of methysergide.

REFERENCES

1. Curran DA, Hinterberger H, Lance JW (1967) Methysergide. *Res Clin Stud Headache* **1**,74.
2. Graham J (1967) Cardiac and pulmonary fibrosis during methysergide therapy for headache. *Amer J Med Sci* **254**, 1.
3. Liston H, Bennett L, Usher B Jr, Nappi J (1999) The association of the combination of sumatriptan and methysergide in myocardial infarction in a premenopausal woman. *Arch Intern Med* **159**, 511.
4. Silberstein SD (1998) Methysergide. *Cephalalgia* **18**, 421.

Metoclopramide

Steven A. Sparr

METOCLOPRAMIDE
$C_{14}H_{22}ClN_3O_2$

4-Amino-5-chloro-N-[2-(diethylamino)ethyl]-2-methoxybenzamide

NEUROTOXICITY RATING

Clinical

A Extrapyramidal syndrome (dystonia, parkinsonism, dyskinesias)

Experimental

A D_2 dopamine receptor blockade

Metoclopramide, a benzamide derivative, is used as an antiemetic and for disorders of gastric motility. The drug selectively blocks both D_2 dopamine receptors (centrally and in the gut) (8) and central serotonin 5-HT_3 receptors (32). Antiemetic activity may be due to blockade of both of these receptors in the chemoreceptor trigger zone in the medulla oblongata. The drug is a potent antiemetic and is useful in treating cancer patients receiving chemotherapy (23). In the gut, metoclopramide increases gastric and small-bowel (but not large-bowel) motility, relaxes the pyloric sphincter, and increases resting tone in the lower esophageal sphincter (8). The mechanism by which metoclopramide effects these changes in the gut is not well understood, but it appears to be mediated by enhanced cholinergic activity in that the effects are blocked by anticholinergic drugs (although not by vagotomy). Metoclopramide has been particularly effective in treating diabetic gastroparesis, delayed gastric-emptying disorders, and esophageal reflux. The drug's antagonism of serotonin has been useful in the treatment of migraine (32), although it failed to show efficacy in one placebo-controlled trial (11).

Metoclopramide is usually well tolerated, although the high incidence of extrapyramidal side effects limits its use. Newer agents, such as the prokinetic agent cisapride (13,26), and the antiemetics domperidone, perphenizine, and odansetron (6,12,28,34), may be better tolerated.

Metoclopramide may be administered by oral or intravenous routes. Oral doses are rapidly and completely ab-

sorbed. There is extensive first-pass metabolism by the liver that reduces its bioavailability by up to 75% (8). Peak plasma concentrations can vary up to fivefold for a given dose due to individual variations in first-pass metabolism (4). The drug is excreted in the bile after conjugation in the liver or excreted unchanged by the kidney. Half-life of the medication is 2.5–5.0 h, up to 14 h in patients with renal failure (30), and also prolonged in patients receiving higher dosages (4). In serum, metoclopramide is about 30% protein-bound, primarily to albumin; this may contribute to toxicity in patients with hypoalbuminemic states (30).

Due to its dopamine-blocking activity, metoclopramide can cause increased secretion of prolactin from the pituitary, leading to galactorrhea, amenorrhea, or impotence (8). It also elevates plasma aldosterone levels, possibly by 5-HT_4 receptor antagonism (33). Tongue edema, or "blue tongue sign," has been reported with metoclopramide (1).

Metoclopramide has serious extrapyramidal side effects; acute dystonic reactions, parkinsonism, akathisia, tardive dyskinesia, as well as other less commonly reported extrapyramidal syndromes. There are no animal models for these side effects, although an acute dystonic reaction with ataxia, torticollis, and opisthotonos has been reported in a macaw after receiving metoclopramide for vomiting (21).

Acute dystonic reactions have been frequently observed, particularly in chemotherapy patients receiving high-dose intravenous metoclopramide for prevention of nausea and vomiting (3,5,15,17,19,24,27,35). These reactions include torticollis, retrocollis, opisthotonos, oculogyric crisis, trismus, respiratory dyskinesia, and hypertonicity of the limbs. Fever may accompany dystonia (mechanism unclear) and abates with discontinuation of the drug (35). Onset may follow a single dose or appear after prolonged treatment (15). Dystonia usually subsides with cessation of treatment, although it may be prolonged, especially in patients with renal failure (15).

Children are very susceptible to dystonic side effects, especially when treated with dosages exceeding 0.5 mg/kg/day; casual use of the drug is discouraged in pediatric practice (3). Adolescents and young adults (under age 30) are also at increased risk. There was an overall incidence of 3.1% dystonic reactions in 452 patients receiving high-dose metoclopramide, whereas the incidence was 27.3% in patients under age 30 (19). Dystonic reactions in a group of 2557 prospectively evaluated patients receiving first-time treatment with oral metoclopramide had an incidence of 1:572 in those over age 30, but 1:81 in those younger (5).

A male predominance of dystonic reactions of 1.5- to 2-fold higher was found in one study (10), whereas female predominance was noted in another (27), and no sex differences were found in a third study (5). Patients with renal failure are at particular risk because of decreased excretion of the drug and lower protein binding of the drug due to hypoalbuminemia, leading to higher serum levels and prolonged drug half-life (15,27). Consequently, dosing should be decreased by 60% in patients with severe renal impairment. Patients with acquired immunodeficiency syndrome may also be at increased risk for acute dystonic reactions, possibly because of the high frequency of basal ganglia infections seen in this group (17,27).

Treatment of acute dystonic reaction with cessation of metoclopramide, and with antihistamines, anticholinergics, or benzodiazipines, usually leads to rapid resolution, although fatalities have been reported (24,25). Pretreatment with diphenhydramine has been recommended for younger patients with history of dystonic reactions who require metoclopramide at high dose (19).

Parkinsonian signs of bradykinesia, rigidity, and resting tremor have been frequently reported in patients receiving metoclopramide (4,15,18), especially in subjects over age 40 and those receiving prolonged therapy. Given the dopamine receptor-blocking properties of the drug, these side effects are not unexpected. One study found an incidence of parkinsonism of 0.2% in a group of 2557 patients that was prospectively followed after the initiation of oral therapy, all occurring in patients over age 40 (incidence of 0.4% in this group) (4). In this study, patients with known Parkinson's disease were at particular risk for drug exacerbation, especially with doses over 60 mg daily. Patients with renal failure are at very high risk for drug-induced parkinsonism; as metoclopramide is not well dialyzed, dialysis patients are not spared this side effect (4,31). One group claims clinical features that differentiated this disorder from idiopathic Parkinson's disease: (a) acute or subacute onset, (b) bilateral signs at onset, (c) postural tremor, and (d) association with oral-bucchal dyskinesias (18). Nevertheless, parkinsonian signs are frequently not recognized as drug-induced. One study surveying medication use in Medicaid recipients in New Jersey, USA, found that patients using metoclopramide were three times more likely than age-matched controls to receive antiparkinsonian medications (2). With discontinuation of metoclopramide, drug-induced parkinsonism usually abates, although it may take up to a year for the patient to return to baseline function (18).

Akathisia, a symptom complex that includes agitation, restlessness, difficulty concentrating, and spasmodic movements of the lower extremities, has been reported especially after intravenous metoclopramide (5,9,10,16,19,22). Incidence of akathisia was 1 in 320 in a prospective study of patients on oral metoclopramide (5), whereas an incidence of 20%–25% has been reported after intravenous administration (10,19). Children and young adults are at increased risk (22). Treatment with anticholinergics may relieve the symptoms (9).

Tardive dyskinesia is a late complication of chronic metoclopramide use; it appears after months to years of treatment, even if the dosage is kept within recommended guidelines (10,15,22,27,30,36). One report describes seven patients, all over age 65, treated with metoclopramide for 14–48 months who developed oral-bucchal dyskinesias after cessation of the drug. Symptoms persisted for at least 15 months in some, and may be irreversible. Two similar cases have been described, both in patients with diabetes mellitus and renal impairment (30). One report reviews 11 cases, all woman over age 70, treated for over 2 years prior to onset (36); in the majority, tardive dyskinesia developed while the patients were still receiving metoclopramide treatment, and only in a minority did the onset occur after cessation of the drug. As with other dopamine receptor-blocking agents that cause tardive dyskinesia, the postulated mechanism of tardive dyskinesia is receptor hypersensitivity due to prolonged blockade (22).

Other neurological side effects have been reported less frequently. These include restless leg syndrome (31), disordered sleep patterns and insomnia (29), depression with suicidal ideation (7), and delayed neuroleptic malignant syndrome after cessation of metoclopramide (20). A single instance of acute onset of chorea appeared in a patient with a family history of Huntington's disease after receiving metoclopramide (14).

REFERENCES

1. Alroe C, Bowen P (1989) Metoclopramide and prochlorperazine: "The blue-tongue sign." *Med J Australia* 150, 724.
2. Avorn J, Gurwitz JH, Bohn RL (1995) Increased incidence of levodopa therapy following metoclopramide use. *J Amer Med Assn* 274, 1780.
3. Ayers Al, Dawson KP (1980) Acute dystonic reactions in childhood to drugs. *N Z Med J* 92, 464.
4. Bateman DN, Davies DS (1979) Pharmacokinetics of metoclopramide. *Lancet* 1, 166.
5. Bateman DN, Darling WM, Boys R, Rawlins MD (1989) Extrapyramidal reactions of metoclopramide and prochlorperazine. *Quart J Med* 71, 307.
6. Billet AE, Sallan SE (1994) Antiemetics in children receiving cancer chemotherapy. *Support Cancer Care* 2, 279.
7. Bottner RK, Tullio CJ (1985) Metoclopramide and depression. *Ann Intern Med* 103, 482.

8. Brunton LL (1996) Agents affecting gastrointestinal water flux and motility; emesis and antiemetics; bile acids and pancreatic enzymes. In: *The Pharmacological Basis of Therapeutics. 9th Ed.* Hardman JG, Goodman AG, Limbird LE eds. McGraw-Hill, New York p. 932.

9. Caldwell C, Rains G, McKiterick K (1987) An unusual reaction to preoperative metoclopramide. *Anesthesiology* **67**, 854.

10. Casey DE (1983) Metoclopramide side effects. *Ann Intern Med* **98**, 673.

11. Coppola M, Yealy DM, Leibold RA (1995) Randomized, placebo-controlled evaluation of prochlorperazine versus metoclopramide for emergency department treatment of migraine headache. *Ann Emerg Med* **26**, 541.

12. DeSilva PH, Darvish AH, McDonald SM *et al.* (1995) The efficacy of prophylactic ondansetron, droperidol, perphenazine, and metoclopramide in the prevention of nausea and vomiting after major gynecological surgery. *Anesth Analg* **81**, 139.

13. Fumagalli I, Hammer B (1994) Cisapride versus metoclopramide in the treatment of functional dyspepsia. *Scand J Gastroenterol* **29**, 33.

14. Giroud M, Fabre JL, Putelat R *et al.* (1982) Can metoclopramide reveal Huntington's chorea? *Lancet* **2**, 1153.

15. Grimes JD, Hassan MN, Preston DN (1982) Adverse neurologic effects of metoclopramide. *Can Med Assn J* **126**, 23.

16. Hamilton FA (1989) Metoclopramide-induced akathisia. *Milit Med* **152**, 585.

17. Hollander H, Golden J, Mendelson T, Cortland D (1985) Extrapyramidal symptoms in AIDS patients given low-dose metoclopramide or chlorpromazine. *Lancet* **2**, 1186.

18. Indo T, Ando K (1982) Metoclopramide-induced parkinsonism. *Ann Neurol* **39**, 494.

19. Kris MG, Tyson LB, Gralla RJ *et al.* (1983) Extrapyramidal reactions with high-dose metoclopramide. *N Engl J Med* **309**, 433.

20. LeCouteur DG, Kay T (1995) Delayed neuroleptic syndrome following cessation of prolonged therapy with metoclopramide. *Aust N Z J Med* **25**, 261.

21. Massey JG (1993) Adverse drug reaction to metoclopramide hydrochloride in a macaw with proventricular dilation syndrome. *J Amer Vet Med Assn* **203**, 542.

22. Patel M, Louis S (1986) Long-term neurologic complications of metoclopramide. *N Y State J Med* **86**, 210.

23. Poka R, Hernadi Z, Juhasz B, Lampe B (1993) Comparison of four antiemetic regimens for the treatment of cisplatin-induced vomiting. *Int J Gynecol Obstet* **42**, 19.

24. Pollera CF, Cognetti F, Nardi M, Mazza D (1984) Sudden death after acute dystonic reaction to high-dose metoclopramide. *Lancet* **2**, 460.

25. Reasbeck P, Hossenbocus A (1979) Death following dystonic reaction to oral metoclopramide. *Brit J Clin Pract* **133**, 31.

26. Robinson M (1995) Prokinetic therapy for gastroesophageal reflux disease. *Amer Fam Physician* **52**, 957.

27. Rodgers C (1992) Extrapyramidal side effects of antiemetics presenting as psychiatric illness. *Gen Hosp Psychiat* **14**, 192.

28. Rust M (1995) Intravenous administration of ondansetron versus metoclopramide for the prophylaxis of postoperative nausea and vomiting. *Anaesthesist* **44**, 288.

29. Saxe TG (1983) Metoclopramide side effects. *Ann Intern Med* **98**, 674.

30. Sewell DD, Yoshinobu BH, Caligiuri MP, Jeste DV (1992) Metoclopramide-associated tardive dyskinesia in hemodialysis patients with diabetes mellitus. *Gen Hosp Psychiat* **14**, 416.

31. Sirota RA, Kimmel PL, Trichtinger MD *et al.* (1986) Metoclopramide-induced Parkinsonism in hemodialysis patients. *Arch Intern Med* **146**, 2070.

32. Skews A (1993) Application of metoclopramide specificity in migraine attacks therapy. *Headache* **34**, 439.

33. Sommers DK, Snyman JR, Van Wyk M (1993) Effects of metoclopramide, odansetron and granisetron on aldosterone secretion in man. *Eur J Clin Pharmacol* **44**, 337.

34. Tsvaris N, Charalambidis G, Ganas N *et al.* (1995) Ondansetron versus metoclopramide as antiemetic treatment during cisplatin-based chemotherapy. *Acta Oncol* **34**, 243.

35. Wandless I, Evans JG, Jackson M (1980) Fever associated with metoclopramide-induced dystonia. *Lancet* **1**, 1255.

36. Wilholm BE, Mortimer O, Boetius G, Haggstrom JE (1984) Tardive dyskinesia associated with metoclopramide. *Brit Med J* **288**, 545.

Metrizamide

Steven Herskovitz

METRIZAMIDE
$C_{18}H_{22}I_3N_3O_8$

2-[[3-(Acetylamino)-5-(acetylmethylamino)-
2,4,6-triiodobenzoyl]amino]-2-deoxy-D-glucose

NEUROTOXICITY RATING

Clinical

A Acute encephalopathy (seizures, headache, delirium)

A Aseptic meningitis

Experimental

A Arachnoiditis

A Seizure disorder

Metrizamide is a triiodinated, nonionic, water-soluble contrast agent derived from metrizoic acid and bound to glucosamine. Because of reduced viscosity and toxicity, methrizamide mostly supplanted the iodinated contrast media such as iophendylate (Pantopaque) for conventional myelography and ventriculography; it has now been replaced in human and veterinary medicine by newer and safer nonionic agents, iopamidol and iohexol (18,20) (*see* Iohexol, this volume). Metrizamide neurotoxicity includes headaches, aseptic meningitis, encephalopathy, seizures, asterixis, myoclonus, and arachnoiditis.

Metrizamide is completely miscible with cerebrospinal fluid (CSF) and reabsorbed from the subarachnoid space *via* the cranial and spinal arachnoid granulations (average half-life is 9.3 h) (6). It can be detected in the blood after 15 min, reaches maximum serum concentration at 2 h, and is excreted unchanged mostly in the urine after 1–3 days. Recommended concentrations range from 170–300 mg of iodine per milliliter with a total iodine load of under 3 g.

Rats given intracisternal metrizamide develop dose-dependent electroencephalographic (EEG) abnormalities, including epileptiform patterns (1). Phenothiazines are reported to increase the risk of seizures in rabbits (11). In monkeys, myelographic and histological evidence of arachnoiditis is observed after metrizamide myelography, but only at concentrations higher than those in standard clinical use (13). Arachnoiditis is characterized by fibrous changes with minimal inflammation. Laboratory animal studies show that metrizamide—a small, water-soluble molecule—penetrates from CSF into the extracellular space of the brain and spinal cord, probably by simple diffusion (6).

Metrizamide stimulates protein and collagen production when fibroblasts are exposed to the drug *in vitro* (8). Treatment of rat hippocampus slice preparations with metrizamide elicits a depression of electrical activity characterized by hyperpolarization of the resting membrane potential (5). Fresh metrizamide solution is highly toxic to glial cells, and less toxic to neurons in mixed cultures; when refrigerated for 2 weeks, it is highly toxic to neurons (15).

Neurotoxic effects occur in as many as 53%–77% of patients after intrathecal metrizamide (6). The incidence correlates with the intracranial concentration, with patient positioning resulting in intracranial spillage, and with the procedure performed. Incidence is higher in cervical as compared with lumbar and thoracic myelography (6). Neurological dysfunction may correlate with the dependent position of the head. The hemisphere or lobe experiencing the highest concentration of contrast agent is most affected. For example, the left lateral decubitus position may eventuate in aphasia, while cortical blindness may result from pooling in the occipital poles in the supine position (17).

Headache is the most common side effect after intrathecal metrizamide, similar to post–lumbar puncture headache, but with a substantially higher incidence (average, >40%) (6,10). There may be associated nausea and vomiting. A chemical meningitis with meningeal irritation and hyperthermia occurs in up to 5% of patients. Seizures are rare and most commonly are generalized; occasionally seizures are focal, epilepsia partialis continua, partial complex, or nonconvulsive status epilepticus. Most seizures occur within 4 h of metrizamide administration, are usually single, and tend to be associated with intracranial spillage and large doses of the contrast agent. EEG abnormalities, usually diffuse or focal slow waves and occasionally epileptiform discharges, occur in up to 35% of patients within the first 24 h. Potentiation of metrizamide-induced seizures by phenothiazines is suggested (6).

Acute encephalopathy, from subtle to severe, is common. Encephalopathy commences within the first 24 h and usually abates over 2–3 days (6). Metrizamide encephalopathy is a protean condition; its manifestations include drowsiness, inattention, depression, anxiety, insomnia, nightmares, delirium, psychosis, mania, and hallucinations. In some instances, subtle cognitive deficits are not apparent except with neuropsychological testing. There may be asterixis or multifocal myoclonus (3,6,7) accompanied by triphasic EEG waves (9,19). Rarely, focal features such as aphasia, cortical blindness, or stuttering speech appear (3,6,17,21).

Signs of spinal cord dysfunction include transient micturition difficulties, reflex changes, spinal segmental myoclonus, and rarely, persistent myelopathy (6). Paresthesias and pain, both radicular and nonradicular, are frequent. Chronic adhesive arachnoiditis occurs with older myelographic contrast agents but rarely follows standard clinical use of metrizamide unless the patients have had prior myelography with other contrast agents, intervening surgical procedures, or prior arachnoiditis (6,12,14). A single case resembling Guillain-Barré syndrome following metrizamide myelography is described (14).

One postmortem study, performed 11 days after intraventricular metrizamide, described perivascular mononuclear inflammatory infiltrates limited to the ventricles (2). Computed tomography can demonstrate either generalized or focal penetration of metrizamide into the brain parenchyma in some cases (17).

A metabolic mechanism of neurotoxicity is suggested by the demonstration that metrizamide is a competitive inhibitor of mammalian brain hexokinase, an enzyme central to the regulation of cerebral glucose metabolism (4,6,16). An alternative mechanism posits inhibition of glucose membrane-specific carrier systems.

REFERENCES

1. Adams MD, Hopkins RM, Ferrendelli JA (1988) A rat EEG model for evaluating contrast media neurotoxicity. *Invest Radiol* **23**, S217.
2. Auer RN, Fox AJ, Kaufman JCE (1982) The histologic effect of intraventricular injection of metrizamide. *Arch Neurol* **39**, 60.
3. Bertoni JM, Schwartzman RJ, Van Horn G, Partin J (1981) Asterixis and encephalopathy following metrizamide myelography: Investigations into possible mechanisms and review of the literature. *Ann Neurol* **9**, 366.
4. Bertoni JM, Steinman CG (1982) Competitive inhibition of brain hexokinase by metrizamide. *Neurology* **32**, 320.
5. Bryan RN, Hershkowitz N (1984) Neuronal effects of water-soluble contrast agents. *Invest Radiol* **19**, 329.
6. Buchman AS, Klawans HL, Russell EJ (1987) Metrizamide and its neurologic complications. *Clin Neuropharmacol* **10**, 1.
7. Chehrazi B, Virapongse C (1981) Transient encephalopathy and asterixis following metrizamide myelography. Case report. *J Neurosurg* **55**, 826.
8. Cheung HS, Johansen JG, Haughton VM, Nichols TR (1985) *In vitro* testing for the risk of arachnoiditis from myelographic contrast media. *Invest Radiol* **20**, 472.
9. Drake ME, Erwin CW (1984) Triphasic EEG discharges in metrizamide encephalopathy [Letter]. *J Neurol Neurosurg Psychiat* **47**, 324.
10. Gelmers HJ (1979) Adverse side effects of metrizamide in myelography. *Neuroradiology* **18**, 119.
11. Gonsette RE, Brucher JM (1977) Potentiation of Amipaque epileptogenic activity by neuroleptics. *Neuroradiology* **14**, 27.
12. Hansen EB, Fahrenkrug A, Praestholm J (1978) Late meningeal effects of myelographic contrast media with special reference to metrizamide. *Brit J Radiol* **51**, 321.
13. Haughton VM, Eldevik OP, Ho KC et al. (1978) Arachnoiditis from experimental myelography with aqueous contrast media. *Spine* **3**, 65.
14. Kelley RE, Daroff RB, Sheremata WA, McCormick JR (1980) Unusual effects of metrizamide lumbar myelography. Constellation of aseptic meningitis, arachnoiditis, communicating hydrocephalus, and Guillain-Barré syndrome. *Arch Neurol* **37**, 588.
15. Kormano M, Frey H (1980) Toxicity of x-ray contrast media in cell cultures. *Invest Radiol* **15**, 68.
16. Simon JH, Ekholm SE, Morris TW, Fonte DJ (1987) Further support for the glucose hypothesis of metrizamide toxicity. The effect of metrizamide and glucose analogue-free contrast media on hexokinase. *Invest Radiol* **22**, 137.
17. Smirniotopoulos JG, Murphy FM, Schellinger D et al. (1984) Cortical blindness after metrizamide myelography. Report of a case and proposed pathophysiologic mechanism. *Arch Neurol* **41**, 224.
18. Torvik A, Walday P (1995) Neurotoxicity of water-soluble contrast media. *Acta Radiol Suppl* **399**, 221.
19. Vincent FM, Zimmerman JE (1980) Metrizamide encephalopathy. *Ann Neurol* **7**, 494.
20. Widmer WR, Blevins WE, Jakovljevic S et al. (1998) A prospective clinical trial comparing metrizamide and iohexol for equine myelography. *Vet Radiol Ultrasound* **39**, 106.
21. Witwer G, Cacayorin ED, Bernstein AD et al. (1984) Iopamidol and metrizamide for myelography: Prospective double-blind clinical trial. *Amer J Roentgenol* **143**, 869.

Metronidazole

Steven Herskovitz

METRONIDAZOLE
$C_6H_9N_3O_3$

1-(2-Hydroxyethyl)-2-methyl-5-nitroimidazole

NEUROTOXICITY RATING

Clinical

A   Acute encephalopathy (lethargy, confusion)

A   Cerebellar syndrome

A   Peripheral neuropathy

Experimental

A   Seizure disorder

A   Cerebellar degeneration (Purkinje cells)

A   "Wernicke-like" mesencephalic lesions

Metronidazole is a nitroimidazole derivative used to treat protozoal and some bacterial infections, and in Crohn's disease. Specifically, it is indicated in treatment of trichomoniasis, amebiasis, giardiasis, and anaerobic bacterial infections and, more recently, is included in a regimen for *Helicobacter pylori* infection. It has also been used as a radiosensitizer. Neurotoxic effects include encephalopathy, cerebellar dysfunction, and peripheral neuropathy.

Metronidazole has excellent bioavailability, with maximum plasma levels 1–4 h after oral intake. It is widely distributed in tissues and fluids, including cerebrospinal fluid. Binding to plasma proteins is <20%. The elimination half-life averages 8 h. There is extensive metabolism in the liver before renal excretion; about 20% of the dose is excreted unchanged in the urine (3,8,14,19).

In animal experiments, long-term high-dose metronidazole in dogs produces Purkinje cell lesions and seizures (16). In rats, very large doses cause behavioral changes; histological lesions appear in brainstem and cerebellum similar to those of Wernicke's encephalopathy (21). Long-term studies with lower doses, approximating those used in humans, fail to show degenerative changes in the CNS and PNS (4). ^{14}C-Labeled metronidazole accumulates in the cerebellum and hippocampus of mice (13).

The most common side effects of metronidazole therapy are headache, nausea, dry mouth, and a metallic taste; occasionally, vomiting, diarrhea, or abdominal discomfort occur. A disulfuram-like effect can follow alcohol ingestion.

Suicidal overdoses, up to 15 g, have caused nausea, vomiting, and ataxia; doses from 3.6–19.5 g have been tolerated without significant morbidity.

Neurotoxicity following prolonged therapy is related to cumulative dose and duration of treatment. Most instances received weeks to months of therapy. Reversible CNS dysfunction includes lethargy, disorientation, confusion, dysarthria, and cerebellar ataxia (1,11). Chronic high doses may result in seizures (7,10). One study of 37 patients receiving high-dose metronidazole as a radiosensitizer reported a 25% incidence of dizziness, tremors, ataxia, and confusion (20).

A predominantly sensory polyneuropathy may follow large, cumulative doses (4–6,12,15). A case report of limb ataxia and absent sensory nerve action potentials suggests that, in some instances, this may represent a sensory neuronopathy (9). A maximum daily dose of 800 mg is well tolerated in terms of objective neurotoxicity in controlled trials of patients with Crohn's disease (17). Clinical features of the neuropathy include distal paresthesias, pain, little or no motor weakness, glove-and-stocking sensory loss and occasionally absent ankle jerks. Symptoms and signs usually improve or resolve within weeks or months after treatment ceases, but occasionally can persist for years (5). Nerve conduction studies suggest sensory axonal degeneration with low-amplitude or absent sensory potentials and minimal, if any, involvement of motor fibers.

Sural nerve biopsies in several reports of patients with sensory polyneuropathy, including teased fiber studies and electron microscopy, demonstrate primary axonal pathology with degeneration of both myelinated and unmyelinated fibers (4,9,15,18). There are no human postmortem reports. Magnetic resonance imaging in a single case with encephalopathy and ataxia showed reversible T2-weighted hyperintensities in the cerebellum, supratentorial white matter, and corpus callosum (1).

The mechanism of neurotoxicity is unknown. Suggested mechanisms include inhibition of neuronal protein synthesis by binding to RNA (4), and thiamine antagonism (2).

REFERENCES

1. Ahmed A, Loes DJ, Bressler EL (1995) Reversible magnetic resonance imaging findings in metronidazole-induced encephalopathy. *Neurology* 45, 588.

2. Alston TA (1985) Neurotoxicity of metronidazole. *Ann Intern Med* 103, 161. [Letter]

3. Andersson KE (1981) Pharmacokinetics of nitroimidazoles. Spectrum of adverse reactions. *Scand J Infect Dis Suppl* 26, 60.

4. Bradley WG, Karlsson IJ, Rassol CG (1977) Metronidazole neuropathy. *Brit Med J* **2**, 610.

5. Boyce EG, Cookson ET, Bond WS (1990) Persistent metronidazole-induced peripheral neuropathy. *DICP Ann Pharmacother* **24**, 19.

6. Coxon A, Pallis CA (1976) Metronidazole neuropathy. *J Neurol Neurosurg Psychiat* **39**, 403.

7. Frytak S, Moertel CG, Childs DS, Albers JW (1978) Neurologic toxicity associated with high-dose metronidazole therapy. *Ann Intern Med* **88**, 361.

8. Gilman AG, Rall TR, Nies AS, Taylor P (1990) *The Pharmacological Basis of Therapeutics. 8th Ed.* Pergamon Press, New York p. 1002.

9. Hahn AF, Feasby TE (1989) Metronidazole neuropathy— a sensory neuronopathy. *Neurology* **39**, 289.

10. Halloran TJ (1982) Convulsions associated with high cumulative doses of metronidazole. *Drug Intell Clin Pharmacol* **16**, 409.

11. Kusumi RK, Plouffe JF, Wyatt RH, Fass RJ (1980) Central nervous system toxicity associated with metronidazole therapy. *Ann Intern Med* **93**, 59.

12. Learned-Coughlin S (1994) Peripheral neuropathy induced by metronidazole. *Ann Pharmacother* **28**, 536.

13. Placidi GF, Masouka D, Alcaraz A *et al.* (1970) Distribution and metabolism of ^{14}C-metronidazole in mice. *Arch Int Pharmacodyn Ther* **188**, 168.

14. Ralph ED (1983) Clinical pharmacokinetics of metronidazole. *Clin Pharmacokinet* **8**, 43.

15. Said G, Goasguen J, Laverdant C (1978) Neuropathy in long term treatment with metronidazole. *Rev Neurol* **134**, 515.

16. Scharer K (1972) Selective alterations of Purkinje cells in the dog after oral administration of high doses of nitroimidazole derivatives. *Verh Deut Ges Pathol* **56**, 407.

17. Stahlberg D, Barany F, Einarsson K *et al.* (1991) Neurophysiologic studies of patients with Crohn's disease on long-term treatment with metronidazole. *Scand J Gastroenterol* **26**, 219.

18. Takeuchi H, Yamada A, Touge T *et al.* (1988) Metronidazole neuropathy: A case report. *Jpn J Psychiat Neurol* **42**, 291.

19. Tester-Dalderup CBM (1992) Metronidazole and related compounds. In: *Meyler's Side Effects of Drugs. 12th Ed.* Dukes MNG ed. Elsevier, Amsterdam p. 705.

20. Urtasun RC, Rabin HR, Partington J (1983) Human pharmacokinetics and toxicity of high-dose metronidazole administered orally and intravenously. *Surgery* **93**, 145.

21. von Rogulja P, Kovac W, Schmid H (1973) Metronidazole encephalopathy in rats. *Acta Neuropathol* **25**, 36.

Misonidazole

Steven Herskovitz

$$C_7H_{11}N_3O_4$$

1-(2-Nitro-1-imidazolyl)-3-methoxy-2-propanol

NEUROTOXICITY RATING

Clinical

A   Peripheral neuropathy

B   Acute encephalopathy (lethargy, confusion, seizures)

Experimental

A   "Wernicke-like" brainstem lesions

A   Peripheral neuropathy

Misonidazole, a 2-nitroimidazole compound, is a hypoxic cell radiosensitizer used to sensitize radioresistant tumor cells. Neurotoxicity consists of a dose-limiting, predominantly sensory peripheral neuropathy and, at high doses, encephalopathy.

Misonidazole is lipophilic, with high oral bioavailability, little plasma protein binding, and uniform equilibration between plasma and cerebrospinal fluid (15). Absorption rate is variable, with median values for peak plasma concentration of 1.5–2 h. The mean half-life, about 12 h, is independent of dose and not altered by repeated administration. There is good tissue penetration. Five to 20% is excreted unchanged and the balance undergoes hepatic metabolism. Hepatic microsomal enzyme induction with phenytoin reduces misonidazole half-life by 25%, but does not appear to protect against neurotoxicity (6). The metabolite desmethylmisonidazole also appears to be neurotoxic (11).

Prolonged exposure to misonidazole in rats produces distal axonal degeneration, most severe in the sensory terminals of intrafusal fibers, and edema in dorsal root ganglia (5). In the CNS, spongy changes progress to necrosis and petechiae in the lateral and superior vestibular nuclei, superior olives, cochlear nuclei, and cerebellar roof nuclei. Changes in brainstem auditory evoked potentials correlate with histopathological findings (3). These changes show topographic and pathological similarities to those seen in thiamine-deficient rats. Somewhat analogous findings occur in short-term experiments in mice exposed to desmethyl-misonidazole; tremors and seizures also occur (1).

Intravenous administration of misonidazole is reported to damage the brain selectively. Male Sprague-Dawley rats were treated intravenously with 100–400 mg/kg misonidazole once daily, 5 days per week, for 2 weeks. Animals treated with the high dose had abnormal behavior (ataxia, tremor, circling, head jerking) during and immediately following treatment. Neuropathological study of these animals on day 16 and 44 revealed necrosis and gliosis in the cerebellum and medulla oblongata. No microscopic changes were detected in sampled peripheral nerves (4).

High doses of nitroimidazoles in humans can produce CNS toxicity, including encephalopathy with lethargy, confusion, and seizures (2,12). The incidence of peripheral neuropathy in human studies is related to the total dose and fractionation schedule. It occurs frequently at a total dose of >18 g (14). Thirty-nine percent of patients receiving 11 g/m² developed neuropathy (8–10). Clinical features are those of a predominantly sensory polyneuropathy affecting distal legs more than arms. Pain is common. There is distal limb impairment of touch, pain, vibration, and position senses. Tendon reflexes tend to be preserved (8,9), but not invariably (7). Improvement, sometimes incomplete, occurs over months after treatment is discontinued. Nerve conduction studies are consistent with an axonal polyneuropathy; sural nerve amplitudes are most prominently affected (7,8). Sural nerve biopsies display axonal degeneration of predominantly large fibers, with secondary demyelination (8).

Studies of nitroimidazole neurotoxicity in cultured neuronal cell lines suggest that the mechanism may be disruption and degradation of the neurofilament lattice (13). Other postulated mechanisms include impaired membrane transport from reactions with sulfhydryl groups, and inhibition of protein synthesis (7). Although thiamine antagonism is suggested by the pathological features, the administration of thiamine does prevent neuropathy in animals or humans (2,5).

REFERENCES

1. Chao CF, Subjeck JR, Johnson RJ (1983) Behavioral and ultrastructural studies of desmethylmisonidazole-induced neurotoxicity in mice. *Brit J Radiol* 56, 27.

2. Dische S, Saunders MI, Lee ME *et al.* (1977) Clinical testing of the radiosensitizer Ro-07-0582: Experience with multiple doses. *Brit J Cancer* 35, 567.

3. Edwards MS, Powers SK, Baringer RA *et al.* (1983) Evoked potentials in rats with misonidazole neurotoxicity. I. Brain stem auditory evoked potentials. *J Neuro-oncol* 1, 115.

4. Graziano MJ, Henck JW, Meierhenry EF, Gough AW (1996) Neurotoxicity of misonidazole in rats following intravenous administration. *Pharmacol Res* 33, 307.

5. Griffin JW, Price DL, Keuthe DO, Goldberg AM (1979) Neurotoxicity of misonidazole in rats. I. Neuropathology. *Neurotoxicology* 1, 299.

6. Jones DH, Bleehen NM, Workman P, Smith NC (1983) The role of microsomal enzyme inducers in the reduction of misonidazole neurotoxicity. *Brit J Radiol* 56, 865.

7. Mamoli B, Wessely P, Kogelnik HD *et al.* (1979) Electroneurographic investigations of misonidazole polyneuropathy. *Eur Neurol* 18, 405.

8. Melgaard B, Hansen HS, Kamieniecka Z *et al.* (1982) Misonidazole neuropathy: A clinical, electrophysiological, and histological study. *Ann Neurol* 12, 10.

9. Melgaard B, Kohler O, Sand Hansen H *et al.* (1988) Misonidazole neuropathy. A prospective study. *J Neuro-oncol* 6, 227.

10. Paulson OB, Melgaard B, Hansen HS *et al.* (1984) Misonidazole neuropathy. *Acta Neurol Scand Suppl* 100, 133.

11. Sasai K, Shibamoto Y, Takahashi M *et al.* (1990) Pharmacokinetics of 2-nitroimidazole hypoxic cell radiosensitizers in rodent peripheral nervous tissue. *Int J Radiat Biol* 57, 971.

12. Saunders ME, Dische S, Anderson P, Flockhart IR (1978) The neurotoxicity of misonidazole and its relationship to dose, half-life and concentration in the serum. *Brit J Cancer Suppl* 37, 268.

13. Stevenson MA, Calderwood SK, Coleman CN (1989) Effects of nitroimidazoles on neuronal cells in vitro. *Int J Radiat Oncol Biol Phys* 16, 1225.

14. Urtasun RC, Chapman JD, Feldstein ML *et al.* (1978) Peripheral neuropathy related to misonidazole: Incidence and pathology. *Brit J Cancer Suppl* 37, 271.

15. Workman P (1980) Pharmacokinetics of hypoxic cell radiosensitizers. A review. *Cancer Clin Trials* 3, 237.

Mitotane

Herbert H. Schaumburg

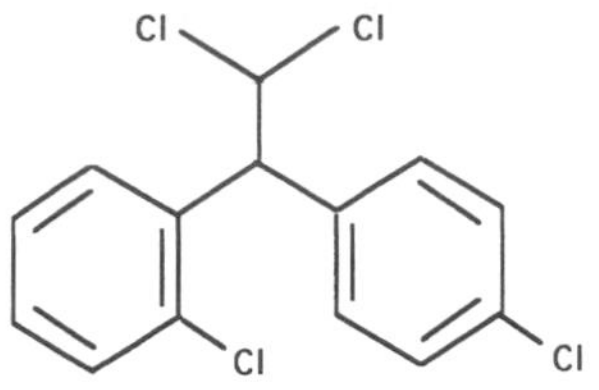

MITOTANE
$C_{14}H_{10}Cl_4$

1-Chloro-2-[2,2-dichloro-1-(4-chlorophenyl)ethyl]benzene

NEUROTOXICITY RATING

Clinical

B   Acute encephalopathy (lethargy, confusion)

Mitotane is a polychlorinated diphenyl compound, structurally similar to the insecticide dichlorodiphenyltrichloroethane (DDT), that is used to treat adrenal adenocarcinoma. The drug is cytotoxic to the mitochondria of normal adrenal cortex; it blocks 11-β hydroxylation of adrenal steroids, decreases production of cortisol, and inhibits glucose-6-phosphate dehydrogenase. Oral absorption is extremely variable, and studies have failed to establish consistent dose–response data for efficacy or toxicity. Therapy is best adjusted to plasma levels; the minimum effective plasma level is 10 μg/ml. More than 60% of ingested mitotane is eliminated unchanged in the urine and stool; the remainder is stored in fat and is released gradually for weeks following withdrawal (4). The drug is orally administered daily in gradually increasing doses until 9–10 g/day is reached or a minimal effective plasma level is established. Treatment generally lasts for 2–3 months.

The principal adverse systemic effects are gastrointestinal disturbances, which appear in 10% of cases dosed over 8 g/day; they include nausea, anorexia, and diarrhea.

Encephalopathic signs appear in about 40% of cases receiving doses >8 g/day. All recover completely once the dose is lowered (1,2). Repeated neurological evaluation is suggested in individuals receiving doses in excess of 8 g/day (5). The most common neurotoxic reaction is somnolence and lethargy. Dizziness, vertigo, headache, tremor, and confusion are also described (6). All reports of neurotoxicity are in the oncological literature; there has been no systematic or electrodiagnostic evaluation of these cases by neurologists. One report describes retinal hemorrhage in a patient receiving mitotane (3).

REFERENCES

1. Brennan MF (1987) Adrenocortical carcinoma. *Can J Clin* **37**, 348.
2. Danowski TS, Sarver ME, Moses C, Bonessi JV (1964) *o,p'*-DDD therapy in Cushing's syndrome and in obesity with cushingoid changes. *Amer J Med* **37**, 235.
3. Fraunfelder FT, Meyer SM (1983) Ocular toxicity of antineoplastic agents. *Amer Acad Ophthal* **90**, 1.
4. Gutierrez, Crooke ST (1980) Mitotane (*o,p'*-DDD). *Cancer Treat Rev* **7**, 49.
5. Hutter AM, Kayhoe DE (1966) Adrenal cortical carcinoma. *Amer J Med* **41**, 581.
6. Samaan NA, Hickey RC (1987) Adrenal cortical carcinoma. *Semin Oncol* **14**, 292.

MMR Vaccine

Neil L. Rosenberg

NEUROTOXICITY RATING

Clinical

C   Peripheral neuropathy (Guillain-Barré syndrome)
C   Optic neuritis
C   Seizure disorder

Immunization against measles (M), mumps (M), and rubella (R) has been carried out with a combined vaccine in North America since 1975 (9). All three components are live, attenuated viruses, and all separately cause adverse reactions. MMR vaccine is safe and associated with a high rate of seroconversion, suggesting efficacy (7). Some adverse effects associated with the combined MMR vaccine differ from those ascribed to the individual components.

Controlled trials of MMR vaccine have found the frequency of side effects to be between 0.5% and 4%; mild, self-limited respiratory and gastrointestinal symptoms and lymphadenopathy are the most common reactions (4,5,10, 18). Side effects are less common if children 4 years and older are immunized (4). A randomized controlled trial (10) found that mild, self-limited increases in lymphadenopathy, fever, and rash were higher in the immunized group. Six children became ill enough to be hospitalized. None had neurological complications; all recovered completely (10).

Other generalized systemic reactions following MMR vaccination have been hypersensitivity reactions (8,13,24). Some investigators have administered MMR vaccine in full dosage without complication (18). Most recommend skin testing to the MMR vaccine and subsequent graded injections in children with a positive test to minimize the risk of serious allergic reaction (24). The virus is grown in chick embryo fibroblasts; children with egg hypersensitivity may develop an acute allergic reaction to MMR vaccination (8,24). Other cases of allergic reactions to MMR vaccine may be related to gelatin rather than egg protein components (13).

Anecdotal reports of reactions include pancreatitis (1), joint and limb symptoms (3), thrombocytopenia or thrombocytopenic purpura (6,17,20), seizures (11), optic neuritis (12), aseptic meningitis (14,23), Guillain-Barré syndrome (15,19), seizures and hemiplegia (21), and sensorineural hearing loss (16,22). Joint and limb symptoms are likely related to the rubella component (3) and cases of aseptic meningitis related to the mumps component (14,23). Rare instances of sensorineural hearing loss are likely secondary to the mumps or measles components (16), but may also be chance occurrences (2). Guillain-Barré syndrome has been suggested as a possible complication of MMR vaccine (19), but only one case report suggests a temporal association (15). Single reports of seizures and hemiplegia (21) and optic neuritis (12) appear to be random events and not causally linked to MMR immunization.

A retrospective cohort study of seizures following MMR immunization was conducted among 18,364 children who received either MMR or MR immunizations in the first 3 years of life (11). One hundred children had seizures sometime during the 3-year follow-up period, but no encephalopathies appeared. Only four had febrile seizures during the first 14 days following immunization, compared with 72 in the 30 days or more interval. The increase in febrile seizures during the 7- to 14-day interval is likely related to the fever that occurs following MMR immunization.

REFERENCES

1. Adler JB, Mazzotta SA, Barkin JS (1991) Pancreatitis caused by measles, mumps, and rubella vaccine. *Pancreas* 6, 489.
2. Anonymous (1992) Meningitis associated with measles-mumps-rubella vaccines. *Wkly Epidemiol Rec* 67, 301.
3. Benjamin CM, Chew GC, Silman AJ (1992) Joint and limb symptoms in children after immunization with measles, mumps, and rubella vaccine. *Brit Med J* 304, 1075.
4. Benjamin CM, Silman AJ (1991) Adverse reaction and

mumps, measles and rubella vaccines. *J Public Health Med* 13, 32.
5. Chen RT, Moses JM, Markowitz LE, Orenstein WA (1991) Adverse events following measles-mumps-rubella and measles vaccinations in college students. *Vaccine* 9, 297.
6. Drachtman RA, Murphy S, Ettinger LJ (1994) Exacerbation of chronic idiopathic thrombocytopenic purpura following measles-mumps-rubella immunization. *Arch Pediatr Adolesc Med* 148, 326.
7. Edees S, Pullan CR, Hull D (1991) A randomized single blind trial of a combined mumps-measles-rubella vaccine to evaluate serological response and reactions in the UK population. *Public Health* 105, 91.
8. Fasano MB, Wood RA, Cooke SK, Sampson HA (1991) Egg hypersensitivity and adverse reactions to measles, mumps, and rubella vaccine. *J Pediat* 120, 878.
9. Fenichel GM (1982) Neurological complications of immunization. *Ann Neurol* 12, 119.
10. Freeman TR, Stewart MA, Turner L (1993) Illness after measles-mumps-rubella vaccination. *Can Med Assn J* 149, 1669.
11. Griffin MR, Ray WA, Mortimer EA *et al.* (1991) Risk of seizures after measles-mumps-rubella immunization. *Pediatrics* 88, 881.
12. Kazarian EL, Gager WE (1978) Optic neuritis complicating measles, mumps, and rubella vaccination. *Amer J Ophthalmol* 86, 544.
13. Kelso JM, Jones RT, Yunginger JW (1993) Anaphylaxis to measles, mumps, and rubella vaccine mediated by IgE to gelatin. *J Allerg Clin Immunol* 91, 867.
14. Miller E, Goldacre M, Pugh S *et al.* (1993) Risk of aseptic meningitis after measles, mumps, and rubella vaccine in UK children. *Lancet* 341, 979.
15. Morris K, Rylance G (1994) Guillain-Barré syndrome after measles, mumps, and rubella vaccine *Lancet* 343, 60.
16. Nabe-Nielsen J, Walter B (1988) Unilateral deafness as a complication of the measles, mumps, and rubella vaccination. *Brit Med J* 297, 489.
17. Nieminen U, Peltola H, Syrjala MT *et al.* (1993) Acute thrombocytopenic purpura following measles, mumps and rubella vaccination. A report on 23 patients. *Acta Paediat* 82, 267.
18. Peltola H, Heinonen OP (1986) Frequency of true adverse reactions to measles-mumps-rubella vaccine: A double-blind, placebo-controlled trial in twins. *Lancet* 1, 939.
19. Rees J, Hughes R (1994) Guillain-Barré syndrome after measles, mumps and rubella vaccine. *Lancet* 343, 733.
20. Rejjal AL, Britten G, Nazer H (1993) Thrombocytopenic purpura following measles-mumps-rubella vaccination. *Ann Trop Paediat* 13, 103.
21. Sackey AH, Broadhead RL (1993) Hemiplegia after measles, mumps, and rubella vaccination. *Brit Med J* 306, 1169.

22. Stewart BJ, Prabhu PU (1993) Reports of sensorineural deafness after measles, mumps, and rubella immunisation. *Arch Dis Child* **69**, 153.
23. Tesovic G, Begovac J, Bace A (1993) Aseptic meningitis after measles, mumps, and rubella vaccine. *Lancet* **341**, 1541.
24. Trotter AC, Stone BD, Laszlo DJ, Georgitis JW (1994) Measles, mumps, rubella vaccine administration in egg-sensitive children: Systemic reactions, during vaccine desensitization. *Ann Allergy Asthma Immunol* **72**, 25.

Mojave Toxin

Albert C. Ludolph

NEUROTOXICITY RATING

Clinical

A   Neuromuscular transmission syndrome

B   Myopathy (necrotizing)

Experimental

A   Neuromuscular transmission dysfunction

Mojave toxin (MoTX) is a potent neurotoxin and protein complex (MW, 22,000) from the venom of the North American rattle snake *Crotalus scutulatus scutulatus* (3). Structurally homologous to crotoxin (4), this heterodimeric polypeptide is a presynaptic (β-) neurotoxin that inhibits acetylcholine release and also has myotoxic effects. Like crotoxin, MoTX consists of two nonidentical subunits (basic and acidic) which by themselves are comparatively nontoxic. The strongly basic subunit B shows phospholipase activity. Like the subunits of crotoxin, component A increases the efficiency of component B by preventing its binding to sites (*i.e.*, erythrocytes) other than its major effector site, the presynaptic membrane of the neuromuscular junction (5). Both the basic (1) and the acidic subunit of MoTX (2) have been sequenced; both show major similarities to the corresponding chain from the crotoxin complex.

The presynaptic inhibition caused by MoTX has a time course typical for β-neurotoxins (5): an initial brief decrease of contraction that lasts only a few minutes is followed by facilitation of acetylcholine release and then—in a final stage—a decline of transmitter release that eventually results in complete neuromuscular blockade. The LD_{50} for this presynaptic toxin in mice is 52 μg/kg after intravenous administration (6). MoTX also has a direct myotoxic effect that is caused by the phospholipase A_2 (7). In primary rat muscle cell cultures and clonal muscle cell lines, exposure to MoTX or its basic subunit prevented fusion of primary myoblasts to myotubes (11). Binding studies with purified MoTX revealed a noncompetitive interaction with ^{3}H-nitrendipine binding to dihydropyridine receptors in rat brain but no interference with binding in Na^+- and Cl^--

channel assays, indicating the presence of a selective effect of the toxin on Ca^{2+} channels (10). There is evidence that MoTX increases capillary membrane permeability by increasing the release of histamine (8).

Clinically, the bite of the North American rattlesnake is, in most but not all cases, associated with local pain and followed by local necrosis. In contrast to bites of the South American rattlesnake, *C. durissus terrificus*, bites by *C. scutulatus scutulatus* less often cause myotoxicity and cranial nerve palsies (*i.e.*, other signs and symptoms indicative of failure of neuromuscular transmission) (9). Instead, coagulopathy and hypovolemia dominate the clinical picture and may lead to cerebral complications such as hemorrhage. The application of antivenom is indicated if, during the observation period, evidence of envenomation is obtained. "Prophylactic" administration (without evidence of envenomation) of antivenom is not recommended. The effect of antivenoms against presynaptic neurotoxins has, in contrast to postsynaptic neurotoxins, no immediate effect on signs of neurotoxicity, but eliminates the toxin from the circulation.

REFERENCES

1. Aird SD, Kruggel WG, Kaiser II (1990) Amino acid sequence of the basic subunit of Mojave toxin from the venom of the Mojave rattlesnake (*Crotalus s. scutulatus*). *Toxicon* **28**, 669.
2. Bieber AL, Becker RR, McParland R *et al.* (1990) The complete sequence of the acidic subunit from Mojave toxin determined by Edman degradation and mass spectrometry. *Biochim Biophys Acta* **1037**, 413.
3. Bieber AL, Mills JP, Ziolkowski C, Harris J (1990) Rattlesnake neurotoxins—biochemical and biological aspects. *J Toxicol Toxin Rev* **9**, 285.
4. Cate RL, Bieber AL (1978) Purification and characterization of Mojave (*Crotalus scutulatus scutulatus*) toxin and its subunits. *Arch Biochem Biophys Acta* **400**, 178.
5. Hawgood B, Bon C (1991) Snake venom presynaptic toxins. In: *Handbook of Natural Neurotoxins. Vol. 5. Reptile*

Venoms and Toxins. Tu AT ed. Marcel Dekker, New York p. 3.

6. Ho CL, Lee CY (1982) Presynaptic actions of Mojave toxin isolated from the Mojave rattlesnake (*Crotalus scutulatus*) venom. *Toxicon* 21, 301.

7. Mebs D, Ownby CL (1990) Myotoxic components of snake venoms: Their biochemical and biological activities. *Pharmacol Ther* 48, 223.

8. Miller RA, Tu AT (1989) Factors in snake venoms that increase capillary permeability. *J Pharm Pharmacol* 41, 792.

9. Minton SA (1990) Neurotoxic snake envenoming. *Semin Neurol* 10, 52.

10. Valdes JJ, Thompson RG, Wolff VL *et al.* (1989) Inhibition of calcium channel dihydropyridine receptor binding by purified Mojave toxin. *Neurotoxicol Teratol* 11, 129.

11. Ziolkowski C, Bieber AL (1992) Mojave toxin affects fusion of myoblast and viability of myotubes in cell cultures. *Toxicon* 30, 733.

Morphine and Related Opiates

John C.M. Brust

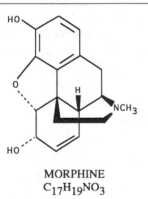

MORPHINE
C₁₇H₁₉NO₃

$(5\alpha,6\alpha)$-7,8-Didehydro-4,5-epoxy-17-methylmorphinan-3,6-diol

NEUROTOXICITY RATING

Clinical

A   Acute encephalopathy (sedation, coma)

A   Physical dependence and withdrawal

C   Chronic encephalopathy (cognitive dysfunction)

Experimental

A   Acute encephalopathy (CNS depression)

A   Physical dependence and withdrawal

Opium is obtained from the poppy, *Papaver somniferum*, which is indigenous to the Middle East and Southeast Asia (2,6). Milky fluid from the unripe seed capsules is dried to make powdered opium, which contains a number of pharmacologically active alkaloids, including the opiate agonists morphine and codeine.

Classified by the U.S. Food and Drug Administration as a Schedule II drug ("high potential for abuse, currently accepted medical use"), morphine is a potent analgesic commercially available in parenteral, oral, and suppository preparations. It is used to treat severe pain and in the management of cardiogenic pulmonary edema. Also legally available is a number of opiate analgesics with chemical structures similar to morphine (Table 33). Of these, codeine, hydrocodone, and hydromorphone are prescribed for cough suppression as well as analgesia, sometimes combined with other analgesics, antihistamines, or expectorants. Commercially available opium alkaloid mixtures include the antidiarrheal paregoric and an opium-belladonna mixture used to treat ureteral colic (6). The major active ingredient of opium is morphine. Legal opiate products are variably classified as Schedule II or Schedule III ("lower potential for abuse than Schedule II"). Diacetylmorphine (heroin) as well as opioid agonists with chemical structures unlike morphine (*e.g.*, meperidine, fentanyl, and methadone) are discussed elsewhere.

Although in most parts of the world heroin is the opiate of choice for recreational use, morphine, hydromorphone, and related legally available opiates are sometimes abused. In some countries opium itself is taken recreationally, often by smoking.

Opiates are readily absorbed from the gastrointestinal tract, nasal mucosa, and lungs, and after subcutaneous or intramuscular administration. First-pass metabolism by the liver reduces the bioavailability of oral preparations, requiring higher doses but providing longer duration of action. (Codeine, oxycodone, and levorphanol have less first-pass metabolism than other opiates and therefore a higher oral-to-parenteral dosage ratio.) Highly lipophilic agents such as hydromorphone or codeine cross the blood-brain barrier faster than less lipid-soluble agents (*i.e.*, morphine), but all morphine-like opiates act promptly after intravenous administration. The plasma half-life of morphine-like opi-

TABLE 33. Opium, Morphine, and Chemically Related Opiates

Drug	FDA Schedule	Indications	Preparations
Powdered opium	II	Pain	p.r.
Camphorated tincture of opium (paregoric)	III	Diarrhea	p.o.
Morphine	II	Pain	Parenteral, p.o., p.r.
Hydromorphone	II	Pain, cough	Parenteral, p.o., p.r.
Oxymorphone	II	Pain	Parenteral, p.r.
Oxycodone	II	Pain	p.o.
Levorphanol	II	Pain	Parenteral, p.o.
Hydrocodone	III	Pain, cough	p.o.
Codeine	III	Pain, cough	Parenteral, p.o.

FDA, U.S. Food and Drug Administration; p.r., *per rectum*; p.o., *per os*.

ates is about 3 h, and their duration of action is about 3–4 h (3,6). Conjugated with glucuronic acid and largely excreted in urine, they are detectable in urine for up to several days after the last dose.

Opioid agonists act at stereospecific receptors—classified as mu, delta, and kappa, each with several subtypes—in the CNS and PNS (8). Indirectly affected is a large number of CNS neurotransmitter systems, including the dopaminergic "reward circuit," which runs from the midbrain ventral tegmental area to the nucleus accumbens and the medial prefrontal cortex (9,10).

An enormous amount of research has addressed the relationship between opiate effects—analgesia, sedation, respiratory depression, nausea, constipation, hypothermia, cough suppression, miosis, euphoria (in animals, reinforcement or reward-seeking), and physical dependence—and actions at particular brain regions or receptors, as well as interactions with endogenous opioid peptides (β-endorphin, the enkephalins, and the dynorphins). In laboratory animals, morphine and related opiates are strongly reinforcing. Animal studies have also shown that opiate-induced reward-seeking and physical dependence are dissociable (1,7), but the goal of an opiate analgesic devoid of addictive liability remains elusive.

Taken in intended dosage, morphine and related opiates produce a constellation of effects (Table 34). Analgesia is more to deep burning pain than to pinprick; threshold to pain perception and ability to tolerate pain are both increased. There is drowsiness, difficulty concentrating, and usually euphoria, but some users develop fear or anxiety. Psychotomimetic effects and visual hallucinations are unusual. Miosis may be so marked that the light reflex—which opiates do not interrupt—is difficult to discern. Respiratory depression can be a problem in patients with decreased respiratory reserve (*e.g.*, emphysema, kyphoscoliosis, or obesity). Constipation is the result of gastrointestinal hypertonicity and decreased propulsion.

Electroencephalographic slowing occurs as in normal sleep, but less time is spent in the rapid-eye-movement phase. High doses produce electroencephalographic irritability, but myoclonus or seizures are rare, even with a severe overdose. Production of antidiuretic hormone, prolactin, and calcitonin is increased; adrenocorticotropic hormone, luteinizing hormone, and growth hormone production are decreased, and repeated use leads to reduced libido (5).

Parenterally, opioid agonists produce a "rush," an ecstatic feeling lasting about a minute and compared to orgasm (but usually referred to the abdomen). There follows either a more prolonged euphoric "nodding," with alternating dozing and sudden awakening, or "drive," with garrulous hyperactivity (2).

Rapid and marked tolerance develops to analgesia, euphoria, and respiratory depression; for continuous pain control, hundreds or even thousands of milligrams of morphine may be required daily. There is less tolerance for smooth muscle effects, such as miosis or constipation.

TABLE 34. Acute Effects of Morphine and Related Opiates

Analgesia
Drowsiness
Euphoria or dysphoria
Respiratory depression
Miosis
Nausea, vomiting
Dryness of the mouth
Pruritis
Sweating
Suppression of the cough reflex
Hypothermia
Postural hypotension
Constipation
Biliary tract spasm
Reduced gastric acid secretion
Urinary retention
Suppression of rapid-eye-movement sleep

TABLE 35. Treatment of Opiate Overdose

Ventilatory support
   If hypotension does not respond promptly to ventilation, i.v. fluids (Pressors are rarely needed)
Consider prophylactic intubation
   If respiratory depression, naloxone 2 mg i.v., i.m., or s.c., repeated as needed up to 10–20 mg; if no
     respiratory depression, naloxone 0.4 mg i.v., i.m., or s.c., repeated as needed (For children, the initial
     dose of naloxone is 0.1 mg/kg)
Hospitalization and close observation, with additional naloxone as needed
   Consider overdose with other drugs, especially cocaine and ethanol

i.v., intravenously; i.m., intramuscularly; s.c., subcutaneously.

Overdose produces the triad of coma, pinpoint pupils, and respiratory depression; treatment includes ventilatory support and the opioid receptor antagonist naloxone (Table 35). Higher-than-usual doses of naloxone are often required for codeine poisoning. Hypotension usually responds quickly to correction of hypoxia and administration of fluids, but some patients have concomitant noncardiogenic pulmonary edema (the basis of which is uncertain), and so fluids should be given cautiously (4).

Recreational opiate users develop both psychic dependence [a psychic drive (craving), such that drug procurement becomes a daily preoccupation (*i.e.*, addiction)] and physical dependence (physical symptoms and signs when the drug is withdrawn or its effect blocked by a specific antagonist). Psychic and physical dependence are dissociable. For example, patients receiving morphine for days or weeks in a hospital setting may with abstinence experience physical discomfort yet little or no craving. Conversely, opiate abusers may crave the drug while taking it in doses too low to produce physical withdrawal symptoms.

The symptoms and signs of opiate withdrawal are highly disagreeable but rarely dangerous (Table 36) (2). Hallucinations, seizures, or delirium are not part of the clinical picture. A few hours after the last dose, there is irritability and anxiety and then weakness, lacrimation, sweating, and yawning. A few hours of restless sleep may follow, from which the subject awakens feeling worse than ever, with achiness, mydriasis, tachycardia, piloerection ("cold turkey"), anorexia, nausea, diarrhea, abdominal cramps, fever, hot flashes, sweating alternating with chills, cough with clear sputum, and muscle spasms of the back and limbs ("kicking the habit"). Recreational users experience craving out of proportion to these symptoms, which may be compared to a bad case of "the flu." With morphine and related opiates, symptoms peak at 24–72 h and usually last 7–10 days.

"Protracted abstinence" is more subtle: several weeks of increased pulse, blood pressure, temperature, and carbon dioxide sensitivity are followed by up to several months of pulse, blood pressure, temperature, and carbon dioxide sensitivity below predependence levels. The relevance of such changes to prolonged craving is uncertain.

Symptoms of opiate abstinence are usually prevented or relieved by oral methadone 20 mg once or twice daily, with subsequent tapering titrated to symptoms. Such treatment is available to ambulatory patients only through federally approved drug-treatment programs.

In contrast to adults, newborns of opiate-dependent mothers develop potentially fatal withdrawal signs, including myoclonus and seizures (which can be difficult to distinguish from nonepileptic jitteriness) (Table 37). Treatment is usually with titrated doses of methadone or paregoric, although some workers recommend nonopiates such as phenobarbital. Careful comparative studies are lacking (2).

Other than producing psychic and physical dependence, morphine and related opiates do not have long-term adverse consequences on the adult CNS or PNS. Whether lasting neurobehavioral abnormalities can result from *in utero* exposure is controversial (*see* Methadone and Heroin, this volume).

TABLE 36. Symptoms and Signs of Opiate Withdrawal

Drug craving
Irritability, anxiety
Tearing
Rhinorrhea
Sweating
Yawning
Myalgia
Mydriasis
Piloerection
Anorexia, nausea, and vomiting
Diarrhea
Hot flashes
Fever
Tachypnea
Productive coughing
Tachycardia
Hypertension
Abdominal cramps
Muscle spasms
Erection, orgasm

TABLE 37. Neonatal Opiate Withdrawal Manifestations

Irritability
Tremor, jitteriness
Increased muscle tone and tendon reflexes
Screaming
Sneezing
Yawning
Tearing
Sweating
Skin pallor or mottling
Fever
Tachypnea and respiratory distress
Tachycardia
Vomiting
Diarrhea
Myoclonus, seizures?

Acute and chronic effects of morphine and related opiates are the result of actions at specific opioid receptors in the CNS and PNS. Analgesia is likely mediated through receptors in the spinal cord, the midbrain periaqueductal gray matter, and limbic structures.

Emotional effects, including dependence, are the result of actions on the limbic system, especially the nucleus accumbens and the prefrontal cortex, as well as, perhaps, the locus ceruleus. Sedation follows inhibition of the midbrain reticular formation and cerebral cortex, and respiratory depression follows inhibition of brainstem respiratory centers. As with other drugs, the precise physiological basis of psychic and physical dependence is unknown.

REFERENCES

1. Bozarth MA, Wise RA (1984) Anatomically distinct opiate receptor fields mediate reward and physical dependence. *Science* 224, 514.
2. Brust JCM (1993) *Neurological Aspects of Substance Abuse.* Butterworth-Heinemann, Stoneham, Massucchusetts p. 16.
3. Chan GLC, Matzke GR (1987) Effects of renal insufficiency on the pharmacokinetics and pharmacodynamics of opioid analgesics. *Drug Intell Clin Pharm* 21, 773.
4. Goldfrank LR, Bresnitz EA (1990) Opioids. In: *Toxicologic Emergencies.* 4th Ed. Goldfrank LR, Flomenbaum NE, Lewin NA *et al.* eds. Appleton & Lange, Norwalk, Connecticut p. 433.
5. Grossman A (1988) Opioids and stress in man. *J Endocrinol* 119, 377.
6. Jaffe JH, Martin WR (1990) Opioid analgesics and antagonists. In: *The Pharmacological Basis of Therapeutics.* 8th Ed. Gilman AG, Rall TW, Nies AS, Taylor P eds. Pergamon Press, New York p. 485.
7. Koob GF, Bloom FE (1988) Cellular and molecular mechanisms of drug dependence. *Science* 242, 715.
8. Loh HH, Smith AP (1990) Molecular characterization of opioid receptors. *Ann Rev Pharmacol Toxicol* 30, 123.
9. Wise RA (1989) Opiate reward: Sites and substrates. *Neurosci Biobehav Rev* 13, 129.
10. Yuan XR, Madamba S, Siggins GR (1992) Opioid peptides reduces synaptic transmission in the nucleus accumbens. *Neurosci Lett* 134, 223.

Mumps Vaccine

Neil L. Rosenberg

NEUROTOXICITY RATING

Clinical

B   Aseptic meningitis (Urabe Am9 vaccine)

In the past, meningitis was associated with the Urabe Am9 mumps vaccine (2,4–7,9,11,12). The only other established complication of mumps vaccine is parotitis (8,10).

Mumps infection formerly was a common cause of meningitis and encephalitis (11). During mumps epidemics, the frequency of meningitis approximated 1 per 1000 cases of clinical mumps. Since introduction of the measles-mumps-rubella (MMR) vaccination programs, mumps is rare, and meningitis and encephalitis are virtually unknown (*see* MMR Vaccine, this volume).

Some cases of meningitis were linked to Urabe Am9 mumps vaccination and the mumps component of the MMR vaccine (1,2,5,6,9,12). Most cases were in the United Kingdom (1,2,5) and Japan (7,9,11), where the mumps vaccine component utilized the Urabe Am9 mumps virus strain. Viral and molecular studies of mumps vaccine–associated meningitis show linkage with the Urabe Am9 strain (4,5,7,9,12).

The United States, Canada, and Scandinavia now use the Jeryl Lynn B mumps virus strain, which is not meningitogenic (3,11).

REFERENCES

1. Anonymous (1992) Meningitis associated with measles-mumps-rubella vaccines. *Wkly Epidemiol Rec* 67, 301.
2. Begg N (1993) Reporting of vaccine-associated mumps meningitis. *Arch Dis Child* 68, 526.

3. Black S, Scheinfield H, Ray P *et al.* (1997) Risk of hospitalization because of aseptic meningitis after measles-mumps-rubella vaccination in one to two year old children: An analysis of the Vaccine Safety Datalink (VSD) project. *Pediatr Inf Dis J* **16**, 500.

4. Brown EG, Furesz J, Dimock K *et al.* (1991) Nucleotide sequence analysis of Urabe mumps vaccine strain that caused meningitis in vaccine recipients. *Vaccine* **9**, 840.

5. Colville A, Pugh S (1992) Mumps meningitis and measles, mumps, and rubella vaccine. *Lancet* **340**, 786.

6. Ehrengut W (1989) Mumps vaccine and meningitis. *Lancet* **2**, 751.

7. Fujinaga T, Motegi Y, Tamura H, Kuroume T (1991) A prefecture-wide survey of mumps meningitis associated with measles, mumps and rubella vaccine. *Pediat Infect Dis J* **10**, 204.

8. Mihaly I, Budai J, Gero A, Kukan E (1994) Acute parotitis in children previously vaccinated against mumps. *Orvosi Hetilap* **135**, 287.

9. Mori I, Torii S, Hammamoto Y *et al.* (1991) Virological evaluation of mumps meningitis following vaccination against mumps. *J Jpn Assn Infect Dis* **65**, 226.

10. Nakayama T, Oka S, Komase K *et al.* (1992) The relationship between the mumps vaccine strain and parotitis after vaccination. *J Infect Dis* **165**, 186.

11. Peltola H (1993) Mumps vaccination and meningitis. *Lancet* **341**, 994.

12. Sugiura A, Yamada A (1991) Aseptic meningitis as a complication of mumps vaccination. *Pediat Infect Dis J* **10**, 209.

Mustard Warfare Agents and Related Substances

Peter S. Spencer
Jeffrey L. Daniels
Glen Kisby

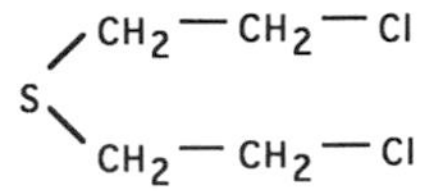

AGENT HD
$C_4H_8Cl_2S$

1,1′-Thiobis[2-chloroethane]; bis(β-Chloroethyl)sulfide; Yperite; Yellow cross; HS; H; Agent H

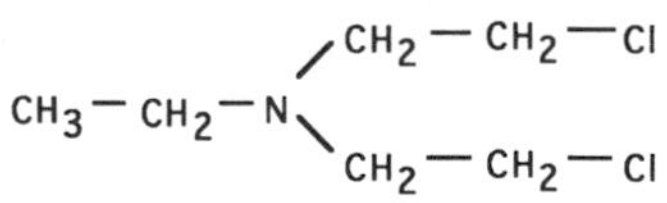

HN-1
$C_6H_8Cl_2N$

2,2′-Dichloro-N-ethyldiethylamine; Ethyl-bis(β-chloroethyl)amine; HN-1

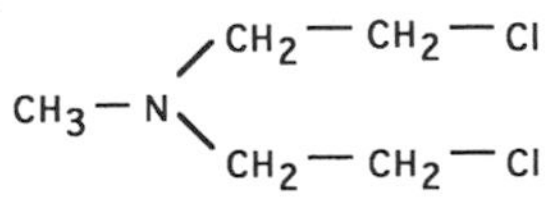

MECHLORETHAMINE
$C_5H_{11}CL_2N$

2,2′-Dichloro-N-methyldiethylamine; Methyl-bis(β-chloroethyl)amine; HN-2; Mechlorethamine (as hydrochloride)

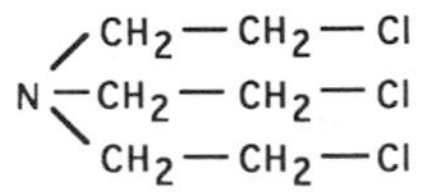

TRIMUSTINE
$C_6H_{12}Cl_3N$

2,2′,2″-Trichloroethylamine; tris(β-Chloroethyl)amine; HN-3; Trimustine (as hydrochloride)

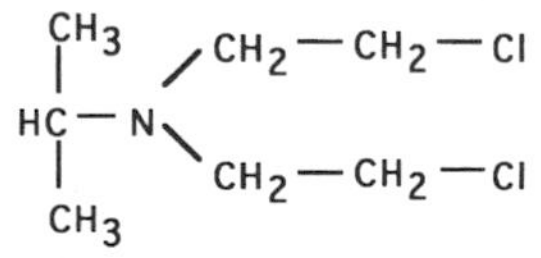

TL 301
$C_7H_{15}Cl_2N$

2,2′-Dichloro-N-isopropyldiethylamine; Isopropylbis (β-chloroethyl)amine; TL 301

NEUROTOXICITY RATING (MUSTARDS)
Clinical

A   Acute encephalopathy

A   Cerebral necrosis (local administration)

Experimental

A   Acute encephalopathy (hyperexcitability, seizures)

Warfare agents of this chemical class historically include both nitrogen mustard compounds and the much more widely deployed sulfur mustard (mustard gas). While the potent vesicant properties of mustard gas dominate the acute toxic actions of this agent, large doses of nitrogen and sulfur mustards also elicit a poorly understood acute encephalopathy in animals and humans. Symptoms relating to brain function reportedly are prominent among survivors of mustard gas attack, and a number of those exposed to sulfur mustard develop psychological dysfunction.

Sulfur mustard may have been synthesized by Despretz in 1822 (59). Distilled sulfur mustard was known as early as the late 1880s as a by-product of the dye industry. Germany was the first country to develop sulfur mustard for offensive use during World War I. Britain and France continued limited production of mustard gas after World War I. By 1925, production of sulfur mustard had begun in Italy and the Soviet Union, and, by 1928, in Japan. Huge quantities of mustard gas were produced (but not used) by both Germany and Allied Forces during World War II. Throughout the Cold War, the Soviet Union and United States developed large weaponized stockpiles of mustard gas and nerve agents; the June 1990 Bilateral Destruction Agreement between the two countries requires both states to stop producing chemical weapons and to reduce their respective chemical-weapon stockpiles to no more than 5000 agent tons by the end of 2002. The United States began to destroy its stockpiles by controlled incineration of chemical weapons at facilities on Johnson Atoll and at the Tooele Ordnance Depot, Utah; incineration is planned at five other sites in the continental United States and is expected to continue until at least 2007. Destruction of weapon stockpiles is required by the international chemical weapons convention* (ratified by the United States Senate in 1997); this pact, signed by 167 nations (excluding Libya, Iraq, and North Korea), also requires signatories never to develop, produce, or acquire such weapons. In the 1990s, the United Nations destroyed a large stockpile of chemical weapons developed by Iraq; this nation also reportedly assisted Sudan and Libya to become self-sufficient (by 2000) in the production and weaponization of mustard gas and nerve agent (9).

Sulfur mustard ("mustard gas") was first used offensively by Germany against the British near Ypres, Belgium, on July 12, 1917 (45,46). Mustard gas was responsible in World War I for nearly 100,000 deaths (approximately 1.3% of total deaths) and approximately 1.2 million nonfatal casualties, including approximately 400,000 Russians and half that number each of German, French, and British

soldiers, among others (45,60). It also claimed the lives of a few children exposed to mustard shells that exploded on former World War I battlefields (26,27). Sulfur mustard is alleged to have been used against the Afghans by the British in 1919, and by the Germans and Poles against each other in 1939 (59). The substance is reported to have been used against Moroccans by the French and Spanish in 1925; against Ethiopians by the Italians after 1935; by the Japanese against China after 1934 and ending by 1944; by Iraq against the Kurds in 1965; by Egyptians in Yemen in 1965; by the Vietnamese in Cambodia and Laos between 1976 and 1980; and by Armenians against Azerbaijanis in 1992 (12,59,64,74). During the Iraq-Iran War in the early and mid-1980s, heavy casualties reportedly resulted from Iraq's large-scale offensive use of mustard gas and nerve agents (89). From 1995 onward, Sudanese Armed Forces reportedly used mustard canisters against the Sudan's People's Liberation Army near Juba, southern Sudan and, in 1997, mustard gas was reportedly used by the Sudanese government in bombing raids in the eastern part of the country (9).

Sulfur mustard has also been released nonoffensively during and following wartime activity. In December 1943, release of mustard gas from a U.S. military vessel sunk in a German air-raid killed hundreds of seamen and over 1000 Italian civilians in the nearby city of Bari, Italy (1,23). In January and February 1991, during the Gulf War, aerial bombing by Coalition forces damaged munitions containing mustard gas at Muhammadiyat, Ukhaydir, and possibly other sites in Iraq (61,62). Mustard agent was reportedly detected by Czech units north of King Khalid Military City, Saudi Arabia, on January 24, 1991, and a U.S. soldier is said to have received a mustard burn when exploring a captured bunker in southern Iraq on March 1, 1991 (38,61). Fisherman working in the North Sea have been periodically exposed to sulfur mustard leaking from tens of thousands of tons of German shells dumped by Allied forces in the late 1940s near the islands of Christians, Denmark, and Grotland, Sweden (68,72).

Nitrogen mustards (HN-1, HN-2, and HN-3) were synthesized in the mid-1930s and not generally stockpiled during World War II (68). They are irritant and vesicant liquids with poor water solubility and a faint, fishy odor. The hydrochlorides of HN-2 and HN-3 serve as antineoplastic drugs. Clinical use of nitrogen mustards (see Mechlorethamine, this volume) and their derivatives (see Ifosfamide, this volume) in the treatment of neoplastic disease began in 1942 (20).

Physicochemical Properties

Sulfur mustard is prepared by treating either ethylene with sulfur chloride or β,β-dihydroxyethyl sulfide with hydrogen

---

*Titled: Convention on the Prohibition of Development, Production, Stockpiling and Use of Chemical Weapons and on their Destruction.

chloride gas. The letter H signifies sulfur mustard produced by a process (Levinstein) that results in 20%–30% impurities (mostly sulfur) (68). Contaminants in commercial products produce a yellow-brown color and sweet, garlic, or onion odor (41,72). Pure sulfur mustard is a colorless, odorless, oily liquid with a molecular weight of 159.08. Boiling point is 215°–217°C (with decomposition); the freezing point is 13°–14°C. Sulfur mustard vapor is 5.4 times heavier than air; vapor pressure is 0.11 mm Hg at 25°C. The compound is stable at normal temperatures and pressures (72), but vapor may explode if exposed to fire or munitions detonation (flash point 105°C). Vapor and liquid forms of sulfur mustard are readily soluble in oils, fats, and organic solvents; water solubility is slight (0.092 g/100 g at 22°C). In aqueous solution, sulfur mustard hydrolyzes to form thiodiglycol and hydrochloric acid (57). However, under certain conditions, bulk sulfur mustard can persist in water and soil for years (65,69). Several methods are available for the qualitative and quantitative analysis of mustards in soil, water, air, urine, and tissue samples (72). Gas chromatography–mass spectrometry (GC-MS) and GC-tandem MS were used in the 1990s to detect sulfur mustard and its hydrolysis product, thiodiglycol, in soil samples collected from a Kurdish village of Birjinni, Iraq (8).

General Toxicology

Sulfur and nitrogen mustards are absorbed both from skin and mucosal surfaces. Penetration of skin by these lipophilic compounds is proportional to temperature and varies principally as a function of agent volatility. Human skin absorbs approximately 20% of an applied dose of sulfur mustard; half binds to skin and half is distributed systemically (63). Intravenous sulfur mustard rapidly disappears from the circulation (71). Body distribution of sulfur mustard in a fatally exposed Iranian patient revealed the following hierarchical concentrations in tissues: fat from the thigh > brain (10.7 mg/kg) > abdominal skin > kidney > spleen > liver > lung (0.8 mg/kg), with marginally higher concentrations in cerebrospinal fluid (1.9 mg/l) than in blood (1.1 mg/l) (15). Small amounts of radioactivity from ^{14}C-labeled monofunctional sulfur mustard administered subcutaneously or applied topically to the skin of nude mice was detected in the brain (and other organs) after 1 h and increased progressively after 24 h (35). HN-2 also enters the brain and spinal cord of intravenously treated mice (76).

Sulfur mustard appears to undergo oxidation to form the sulfone, possibly *via* a sulfoxide (14), which may be conjugated by glutathione and cysteine (72). Metabolism also proceeds *via* hydrolysis to form thiodiglycol and then thiodiglycolic acid, followed by conjugation by glucuronide,

sulfate, or glycine. Monofunctional hemimustards are other possible metabolites (72). Human excretion of radiolabel from intravenous ^{35}S-sulfur mustard peaks at 12 h, is present in a reduced amount at 24 h, and is complete by 48 h (14,72).

Mustards undergo intramolecular cyclization in polar solvents (such as water) to form an intermediate cyclic onium cation and a free chloride anion; sulfur mustard forms a sulfonium cation, nitrogen mustard an immonium cation. While most sulfur mustard in aqueous solution is converted to thiodiglycol and hydrochloric acid, the cyclic intermediate is also available to alkylate various nucleophiles (72), including key cellular macromolecules (protein, RNA and, especially, DNA). The sulphonium ion produces adducts at the N^7 position of guanine and the N^3 position of adenine; the immonium ion, however, only forms N^7 alkylguanine. N^7 adducts may form on two adjacent guanines (to produce an intrastrand cross-link) or at two guanines on opposite nucleic acid strands (10). Other work shows that all nitrogens and oxygens in DNA bases can be alkylated by mustards (59,72). Cells in early S phase (DNA synthesis) and in late G_1 phase (interphase) are especially sensitive to the effects of mustard alkylation (40,58). Cross-linkage of DNA strands blocks normal replication of DNA and interferes with synthesis and mitosis.

DNA adducts formed by mustard gas are detectable by multiple methods, including an electrochemical technique (6,39) using antibodies directed at the N^7 adduct (79). DNA adducts produced by sulfur and nitrogen mustard can be detected with high sensitivity (one adduct per 10^7–10^8 nucleotides) using the technique of ^{32}P-postlabeling/two-dimensional thin-layer chromatography (56,90,92). Femtomole amounts of the principal HN-2 guanine mono-DNA adduct, N-(2-hydroxyethyl)-N-[2-(7-guaninyl)ethyl]-methylamine (GMOH), can be rapidly (5 min) assayed in neural and other tissues by high-performance liquid chromatography with electrochemical detection (34). Levels of GMOH, the only DNA adduct detected in neuronal cells treated *in vitro* with 0.1–1 μmol HN-2 for 24 h, are approximately twofold higher in postmitotic neurons (rat granule cells) than in comparably treated, dividing human SY5Y neuroblastoma cells (34).

DNA alkylation appears to result in cytotoxicity. DNA damage (in skin cells) is thought to activate the chromosomal enzyme poly(ADP ribose) polymerase, which consumes available oxidized nicotine adenine dinucleotide (NAD^+) as substrate for adenosine diphosphate (ADP) ribosylation (58). Depletion of cellular NAD^+ is proposed to disrupt glycolysis, perturb energy metabolism, and cause cell death (50,58).

Mustards also appear to induce tissue damage by a free-radical mechanism. Single subcutaneous injection of a sublethal dose of sulfur mustard results in biochemical markers of oxidative stress and a significant increase in brain lipid peroxidation (17). Mustards deplete cytoplasmic glutathione and thereby increase cellular oxyradicals and electrophiles (72). Both monofunctional and bifunctional sulfur mustard are proposed to induce an oxidative stress response, with biochemical indices of lipid peroxidation and depleted glutathione in the murine brain, liver, and lung (17,18,81). Only 0.01% of the administered dose of ^{14}C-labeled monofunctional sulfur mustard reaches the brain of nude mice treated topically or subcutaneously with sulfur mustard (35), but this may be sufficient to induce lipid peroxidation (18). Activity of superoxide dismutase, which catalyzes the dismutation of two molecules of superoxide anion into hydrogen peroxide and oxygen, is significantly depressed in white blood cells, platelets, spleen, and brain of mice 24 h after topical treatment with sulfur mustard $(0.5 \times LD_{50})$ (32).

Animal Studies

Mustards have mutagenic, carcinogenic, and teratogenic properties. The International Agency for Research on Cancer considers sulfur mustard a Group 1 carcinogen. Single intraperitoneal injection of 1 mg/g body weight on days 12 and 14 of gestation induces malformation of the feet and head (cleft palate and exencephalia) and disrupted eye and brain development of mice (53). Other animal studies show that nitrogen mustards are potent teratogens (13,24,54,66).

The lowest lethal inhalation concentration of sulfur mustard for mice is an integrated concentration equal to 1890 $(mg \cdot min)/m^3$ for a 10-min exposure. Mice exposed to HN-2 at 2–3 LC_{50} develop severe agitation, ataxia, and incoordination that resolves within 48 h. Similarly treated rats develop comparable neurological manifestations but die after 40 h (22). Mice receiving a comparable dose by the subcutaneous route show depression, incoordinated movements, severe tremors, overreaction to stimuli, dullness, diarrhea, and retropulsive movements (2). Mice treated with subconvulsive doses of HN-3 develop progressive muscular weakness, diarrhea, coldness, hyperexcitability and overactivity, retropulsive movements, tremors and incoordination, prostration, failure of respiration, and terminal convulsions thought to be related to anoxia (2). Hyperirritability and loss of coordination remain for 2–4 weeks in mice given 0.1 mg HN-2.HCl (mechlorethamine) and, in a few instances, abnormalities of posture and movement are noted among 30-day survivors (49). "Nerve cell shrinkage" is reported in the neocortex, pyriform cortex, hippocampus, cerebellum, and medulla oblongata of treated mice (49). Rabbits given 20 mg/kg HN-2 intrave-

nously develop (after 5–15 min) marked incoordination accompanied by brief convulsive running movements, salivation, urination, defecation, lacrimation, bronchorrhea, and miosis (22). Dogs exposed to sulfur mustard develop systemic effects (vomiting, diarrhea, hyperexcitability, heart changes) and local effects on the eyes, skin, and respiratory tract (44). Mustards induce injury to lymphatic tissue, spleen, bone marrow, and the epithelium of the small intestine, and delayed death 3–6 days later. Large doses administered parenterally induce rapidly appearing neurological symptoms: convulsions, depression, incoordination, irritability, tremors, weakness, and dyspnea, with death after 1–40 h varying with dose (22).

Controlled experiments with dogs conducted during the 1940s showed that intravenous injection of dichloroethylsulfide induces (after 10–20 min) hypersalivation followed by diarrhea, vomiting, and an increased breathing rate. The animal becomes hyperexcitable and the gait unsteady. Spasmodic, tetanic contractions of muscle appear and increase until convulsions and opisthotonus supervene. The pulse slows, blood pressure falls, and the animal becomes comatose and dies after approximately 24 h. Prior to death, a normal heart rate resumes and vagal blockade can be demonstrated. Dogs given subcutaneous or intramuscular injection of a lethal dose of dichloroethylsulfide in olive oil develop, after a latent period, copious salivation; hyperexcitability and convulsions; diarrhea; slow and irregular heart beat that becomes rapid before death; muscle weakness; and, finally, coma and death (80). Other early research involving mice, rats, rabbits, and dogs noted that parenteral administration of large doses $(5–10 \times LD_{50})$ of sulfur and nitrogen mustards induced "neurologic manifestations consisting of convulsions, depression, loss of coordination, irritability, tremors, weakness, dyspnea, evidence of parasympathomimetic activity—salivation, lacrimation with red tears, defecation, and urination—and terminal respiratory paralysis" (22).

Rats treated with HN-1 or HN-2 intravenously or by inhalation of vapor sometimes developed after 3–4 days increased irritability, abnormalities of posture and movement, progressing in severe cases to involve vestibular and cochlear mechanisms. Survivors showed hyperirritability persisting for weeks; pathological examination "showed extensive demyelination of the peripheral nerves in half of the animals" (2). Contemporary studies are unavailable.

Cats and monkeys treated with a single intracarotid injection of 0.25–1 mg/kg HN-2 develop various CNS effects ranging from transient electroencephalographic changes to marked hemiparesis, cerebral edema, and death. Signs usually develop within a day of drug administration but, occasionally, are delayed for as long as 6 days. Neuropathological examination of longer-term survivors reveals brain changes greater on the injected side but present elsewhere in a patchy distribution: varicose degenerated vessels, large numbers of perivascular phagocytes, chronic neuronal degeneration, areas of myelin loss, and cortical astrogliosis (19). CNS changes in topically treated cats and rabbits are described below (*see* later under Case Report).

Human Studies

Sulfur Mustard

The 50% lethal inhalation dose of sulfur mustard (1500 mg·min/m^3) is measured as the amount of mustard gas inhaled per unit time [L(C$_t$)$_{50}$], a value that varies directly with the rate of ventilation. Volatilized sulfur mustard also penetrates the skin: the 50% lethal percutaneous dose is 10,000 mg·min/m^3 (12). In the United States, the maximum permissible airborne workplace concentration of sulfur mustard is 0.003 mg/m^3 for an 8-h Time-Weighted Average (TWA) over a 40-h work week (78). For the general U.S. population, the 72-h TWA is 0.0001 mg/m^3 with a ceiling of 0.003 mg/m^3 (77).

Humans exposed to the vapor of mustard gas notice only a faint characteristic odor. The latent period to onset of signs and symptoms (usually a few hours) varies with the dose received and with individual susceptibility (80). Bradycardia appears early in intoxication, tachycardia later (70). The local symptoms initially consist of smarting of the eyes giving way to intense, burning eye pain, with excessive lacrimation, blepharospasm, and photophobia. Rhinorrhea, sneezing, throat irritation, dry cough, and hoarse voice appear; the latter may be the first sign of exposure (68). Exposed skin areas develop a painless erythema, comparable to sunburn, followed by an itching and burning sensation (80). Other areas of the body, especially where the skin is thin and richly supplied with sweat glands, are similarly affected. Over a period of 24–48 h, affected areas become edematous, darkened (increased melanization), and blistered. Blisters are dome-like and contain clear or yellowish fluid; they heal slowly and, after exfoliation, are replaced by areas of hypopigmentation. If death does not supervene as a result of airway irritation, sloughing, bronchopneumonia, or intercurrent infection, many casualties will have recovered by 6 weeks or longer.

Clinical and laboratory findings are reported for 233 Iranian soldiers aged 15–60 years (mean = 24 years) who were exposed to sulfur mustard in 1986 during the Iraq-Iran conflict. Some of the symptoms and signs were interpreted by the authors as indicative of cholinergic stimulation (4). While exposure to other warfare chemicals (*i.e.*, nerve agents) was not excluded, plasma (butyryl) cholinesterase

activity was not reduced. The most common clinical findings (including symptoms) related to the respiratory tract (95%), eyes (92%), skin (83%), CNS (83%), digestive tract (68%), and cardiovascular system (58%). Listed under CNS manifestations were headache (61%), insomnia (47%), generalized pain (30%), anxiety (27%), restlessness and agitation (12%–13%), confusion and depression (7%–8%), and convulsions (2.5%).

Other indications of neurological involvement may be apparent in patients with severe sulfur mustard intoxication (4,26,27,70); however, it is unclear whether this represents a direct neurotoxic effect or results from hypoxia related to seizures, coma, and/or CNS vascular damage. The latter may include "intense capillary and venular engorgement with hemorrhages in the white substance and degeneration of the endothelium," and "congested meninges and diffuse petechial hemorrhages" (25,73,84). Clinical manifestations are heralded by "intellectual dullness or stupidity, headache, oppression in the region of the stomach, nausea or vomiting, malaise, and great languor and exhaustion. In many cases these symptoms may not be noticed, and the local symptoms [presumably, skin and mucous membrane irritation] first attract attention" (51,80). Others have noted "apathy and somnolence interrupted by states of excitement, tremor, and in some cases deep coma with or without terminal paralysis." (84). Two children had abnormal muscular activity, and a third showed alternating agitation and coma, after accidental exposure to a large amount of airborne sulfur mustard. Two died 3–4 h after exposure (26). As noted above, muscle spasms, hyperexcitability, convulsions, and coma are also described in dogs given massive doses of sulfur mustard (22).

Upon recovery, some victims of sulfur mustard poisoning reportedly develop a state of functional neurosis with depression, persistent conjunctivitis, and photophobia (46). Follow-up of 1500 cases of mustard poisoning acquired on a World War I battlefield revealed that 125 men "failed at first to respond normally"; in 19, symptoms of "effort syndrome [not defined] persisted in spite of graduated exercise. In 14 of those men, the symptoms were due to other conditions or had existed before the [First World] war, and only 5 were directly due to gas" (80).

Soldiers exposed to mustard gas in World War I appear to have been at increased risk for cancer of the lung and pleura (11). During World War II, at least 4000 U.S. military personnel served as human experimental subjects who were repeatedly exposed to mustard gas or Lewisite (dichloro[*trans*-2-chlorovinyl]arsine; *see* Arsenic, this volume) in laboratory and field studies designed to assess methods of protection (59). The Institute of Medicine, Washington, DC (a nongovernmental American organization), found a causal relationship between experimental exposure to mustard gas and a number of health disorders: respiratory and skin cancer, leukemia, chronic respiratory diseases, recurrent eye diseases, bone marrow depression and immunosuppression, psychological disorders, and sexual dysfunction (59). Some U.S. soldiers (92% volunteers) exposed to mustard gas in controlled settings during World War II were judged to have full (17%) or subdiagnostic (33%) lifetime posttraumatic stress disorder when evaluated decades later; risk was related to the number of exposures (67). Clinical follow-up of U.S. Army volunteers who received skin burns from mustard gas reported no significant frequency of adverse health effects or cancer when studied by questionnaire approximately two decades later (55). Interview of 257 U.S. soldiers and surviving spouses or relatives approximately 50 years after repeated experimental exposure of the veterans to mustard gas and Lewisite generated frequent reports of neurological diseases* and psychological difficulties†; no analysis of their frequency relative to a comparable control population was carried out (59). Airway compromise and tardive respiratory and skin malignancy, but not neurological illness, is reported in civilians occupationally exposed to sulfur mustards and other warfare chemicals (52,85–87).

Nitrogen Mustard

Intracarotid injection of mechlorethamine may trigger immediate seizures, coma, and death, with autopsy evidence of neuronal degeneration and gliosis (3). Intravenous injection using standard doses (0.4 mg/kg body weight as single agent), or in combination with other antineoplastic drugs, rarely shows neurotoxicity (7,91). In one report, however, 14 patients with aplastic anemia or malignancy developed one or more immediate neurological abnormalities: confusion or disorientation ($n = 6$), severe generalized headaches ($n = 6$), auditory or visual hallucinations ($n = 4$), lethargy ($n = 4$), tremors ($n = 3$), paraplegia ($n = 1$), *grand mal* seizures ($n = 1$) and vertigo ($n = 1$). Thirteen patients survived more than 60 days: 6 of 6 whose previous acute toxic response had resolved then developed delayed-onset (70–284 days) changes that lasted for 5–90 days. Clinical manifestations consisted of confusion, somnolence, personality changes, dementia, focal motor seizures, and hydrocephalus, with electroencephalograms that revealed diffuse slowing. Postmortem, the brains showed neuronal degeneration with increased vascularity, gliosis, and perivascular fibrosis.

---

*Neurological problems included multiple sclerosis and amyotrophic lateral sclerosis, abnormal sensory disturbances, Alzheimer's disease, paralysis and weakness, and chronic pain, among others.
†Psychological difficulties included chronic depression or anxiety, nervousness, and tenseness.

Neurotoxicity appeared to increase with age and with mechlorethamine dose, and was more common in patients given additional procarbazine or cyclophosphamide (75).

Decontamination and Treatment

Human exposure to sulfur mustard is likely to be encountered in warfare and as a result of terrorist activity. Exposure might also occur in association with the destruction of chemical weapons which, in some cases (*e.g.*, Umatilla Ordnance Depot, Oregon, USA), will take place close to sizeable civilian populations. The greatest risk appears to be mishap during the loading for transportation of warheads from storage sites to customized, explosion-proof incineration facilities. Incineration is expected to destroy >99.99%.

Detailed information on the decontamination and treatment of patients with mustard poisoning is available elsewhere (16,68,72). Appropriately protected responders should remove the patient's contaminated clothing, cut away and discard contaminated hair, and clean the skin and remaining hair with 0.5% sodium hypochlorite solution followed 3–4 min later with water. Intravenous sodium thiosulfate (500 mg/kg) may be administered within minutes of exposure in an attempt to bind circulating mustard and reduce its systemic effects. Atropine (0.4–0.8 mg) is recommended to control eye pain and the early nausea and vomiting associated with systemic sulfur mustard poisoning (83). Hemodialysis has been of no benefit in sulfur mustard intoxication (88). Lost fluid should be replaced. Frequent hematologic evaluations are required (especially for nitrogen mustards, which depress bone marrow function); the patient should be isolated against infection and antibiotics used vigorously if indicated (16).

Therapeutic intervention for the acute neurotoxic effects of lethal doses of mustards appears not to have been addressed. While mechanisms are poorly understood, the combination of cholinergic actions and hyperexcitability in humans and animals suggests, *a priori*, that anticholinergic drugs and antiglutamatergic drugs might ameliorate the neurological changes associated with severe mustard intoxication; however, such therapeutic approaches are *not* part of the present treatment armamentarium.

Mechanisms of Acute Neurotoxicity

Reports of early animal studies note that sulfur mustard (H) and HN-2 produce CNS cholinergic actions as well as peripheral stimulation of muscarinic and nicotinic pathways (22). Mustards reportedly inhibit cholinesterase activity in serum, liver, and diaphragm, but not the acetylcholinesterase activity of erythrocytes or brain (83). Supra-LD_{50} parenteral doses of mustards induce in animals a picture of "neurologic injury" characterized by "convulsions, depression, loss of coordination, irritability, tremor, weakness, dyspnea, and evidence of parasympathomimetic activity." "Neurologic injury" is also observed in animals exposed by inhalation or intravenous administration of HN-1 or HN-2; the injury appeared after 3–4 days in the absence of other signs of systemic intoxication, and survivors displayed hyperirritability that persisted for weeks (22). Small doses of HN-3 were found to have a "parasympathicolytic action," as judged by the "paralysis of cardiac vagal fibers" and "antagonism toward parasympathomimetic drugs." A similar parasympathicolytic action was opined in severe intoxication with H, HN-2, or TL 301. The "paralytic action" of HN-2 and HN-3 is associated with a progressive, irreversible muscular weakness leading to death within hours (22).

Compounds related to nitrogen mustard and hemimustard also induce hyperexcitability and seizures in laboratory animals after large doses (Table 38) (2). Methyl-2-chloroethyl-ethylenimonium (chlorimine of HN-2) has striking cholinergic effects on the autonomic nervous system, sympathetic ganglia, and striated muscle (31). Methyl-2-hydroxyethyl-ethylenimonium (hydroximine of HN-2) is a less potent cholinergic agent; its principal effect is to produce a neurological disorder characterized by ataxia, incoordination, tremors, and muscular weakness (31). β-Chloroethylamines are positive or negative for the induction in mice of a "waltzing syndrome" characterized by hyperactivity, retropulsion, choreic head movement, running in circles, incoordination, poor balance, poor righting reflex, and uncoordinated swimming pattern (Table 39). Histopathological examination of paraffin sections disclosed nonspecific changes, namely, eosinophilia and shrinkage of Purkinje cells in the cerebellar vermis and multifocal gliosis in the brainstem (21).

Nitrogen mustard derivatives of choline (choline mustard aziridinium and ethylcholine aziridinium) and certain hemicholinium mustard derivatives (hemicholinium mustard-9) have been used as experimental tools to examine inhibition of high-affinity choline transport mechanisms *in vitro* and *in vivo* (Fig. 14) (29,47). A cholinotoxic action of choline mustard aziridinium and ethylcholine aziridinium (AF64A) results from the selective transport of the agents into nerve terminals equipped with the high-affinity choline carrier followed by irreversible inhibition of enzymes that use choline as substrate (5). Acetylcholinesterase activity is not affected by AF64A treatment (43). The degeneration process induced by these compounds, which eventually involves axon, soma and dendrites (82), should therefore proceed in a retrograde direction from nerve terminal to cell body (29). Systemic AF64A treatment of rodents with an opened

TABLE 38. Acutely Neurotoxic Compounds Related to Nitrogen Mustards

Ethyl-β-chloroethyl-β-hydroxyethyl picrylsulfonate
Ethyl-β-hydroxyethyl-ethylimonium chloride
Methyl-β-chloroethyl-ethylenimonium picrylsulfonate
Methyl-β-chloroethyl-β-hydroxyethylamine hydrochloride
Methyl-β-acetoxyethyl-β-chloroethylamine
Methyl-β-chloroethyl-ethylenimonium picrylsulfonate
Methyl-β-chloroethyl-β-hydroxyethylamine
Methyl-β-hydroxyethyl-ethylenimonium picrylsulfonate
N,N'-diethyl-N,N'-bis(β-chloroethyl)-piperazinium dichloride
Disodium bis(β-thiosulfatethyl)methylamine
Vinyl-β-[bis(β-chloroethyl)amino]ethyl sulfone
N,N,N',N'-Tetrakis-β-chloroethyl)-ethylenediamine dihydrochloride

[From Anslow *et al.* (2).]

blood-brain barrier results in cholinotoxic effects in vulnerable regions such as the hippocampus, especially the ventral portion and CA3 subfield (28,37). Toxin-treated animals display secondary changes in other central neurotransmitter systems, impaired learning acquisition, and other memory deficits. AF64A also causes a selective impairment of cho-

TABLE 39. Chlorinated Tertiary Amines Positive and Negative for the Waltzing Syndrome

Positive
Dimethyl-β-chloroethylamine hydrochloride
Diethyl-β-chloroethylamine hydrochloride
Dipropyl-β-chloroethylamine hydrochloride
Methyl-ethyl-β-chloroethylamine hydrochloride
Methyl-n-propyl-β-chloroethylamine hydrochloride
Ethyl-n-propyl-β-chloroethylamine hydrochloride
β-Chloroethyl-piperidine hydrochloride
β-Chloroethyl-morpholine hydrochloride

Transient Effects
Ethyl-β-chloroethyl-γ-chloro-n-propylamine hydrochloride
N-N'-(β-Chloroethyl)-1,4-piperazine hydrochloride

Negative
Dimethyl-β-hydroxyethylamine hydrochloride
Diethyl-β-hydroxyethylamine hydrochloride
β-Hydroxyethylpiperidine hydrochloride
β-Hydroxyethylmorpholine hydrochloride
β-Chloroethylamine hydrochloride
Ethyl-β-chloroethylamine hydrochloride
Methyl-β-chloroethylamine hydrochloride
Propyl-β-chloroethylamine hydrochloride
Dibenzyl-β-chloroethylamine hydrochloride
Di-(p-chloro)-β-chloroethylamine hydrochloride
Di-(p-methoxybenzyl)-β-chloroethylamine hydrochloride
Dimethyl-β-bromoethylamine hydrobromide
Phenyl-β-bromoethamine hydrobromide
Dimethyl-β-phenyl-β-chloroethylamine hydrochloride
Diethyl-γ-trichloro-n-propylamine hydrochloride
Diethyl-ε-trichloro-pentylamine hydrochloride
N-N'-Ethyl-N,N'-(β-chloroethyl)-ethylenediamine hydrochloride
β-Chloroethyl-trimethylammonium chloride
Choline chloride

[From Goldin *et al.* (21).]

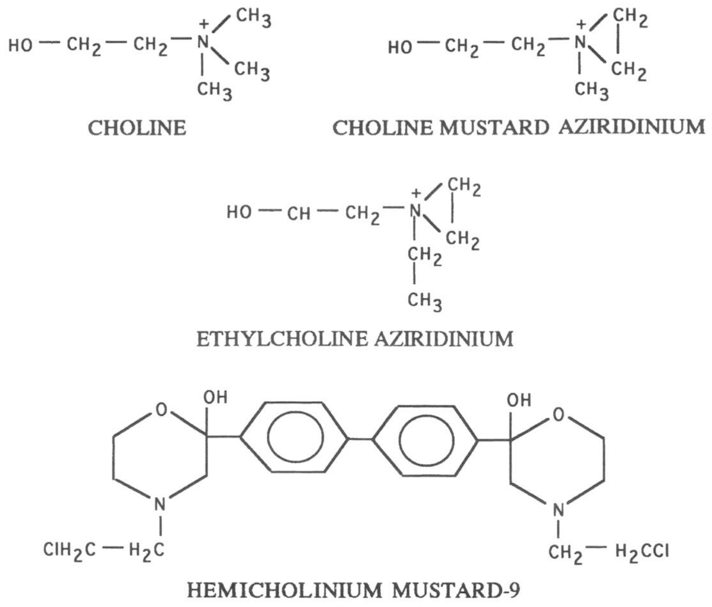

FIGURE 14. Structural relations of choline and choline mustards. [From Hörtnagl and Hanin (29).]

linergic transmission in the peripheral autonomic and somatic neuromuscular system (30,42,48). Larger doses of AF64A produce cholinospecific and nonspecific brain damage in rats (36,82).

REFERENCES

1. Alexander SF (1947) Medical report of the Bari Harbor mustard casualties. *Mil Surg* **101**, 1.

2. Anslow WP Jr, Karnovsky DA, Val Jager B, Smith HW (1947) The toxicity and pharmacological action of the nitrogen mustards and certain related compounds. *J Pharmacol Exp Ther* **91**, 224,

3. Ariel IM (1961) Intra-arterial chemotherapy of metastatic cancer to the brain. *Amer J Surg* **102**, 647.

4. Balali-Mood M, Navaeian A (1986) Clinical and paraclinical findings in 233 patients with sulfur poisoning. In: *Proceedings of the 2nd World Congress on New Compounds in Biological Warfare.* Heyndrickx B ed. Ghent, Belgium p. 464.

5. Barnes DM, Hanin I, Erickson LC (1988) Cytotoxic and DNA-damaging effects of AF64A in cholinergic and noncholinergic human cell lines. *Fed Proc* **47**, 1749.

6. Benschop HP, Moes GWH, Fidder A *et al.* (1989) Immunochemical detection of mustard gas adducts with DNA: Identification of adducts. *Proc Med Def Biosci Rev* 1.

7. Bethlenfalvay NC, Bergin JJ (1972) Severe cerebral toxicity after intravenous nitrogen mustard therapy. *Cancer* **29**, 366.

8. Black RM, Clarke RJ, Read RW, MT Reid (1994) Application of gas chromatography-mass spectrometry and gas chromatography-tandem mass spectrometry to the analysis of chemical warfare samples, found to contain residues of the nerve agent sarin, sulfur mustard and their degradation products. *J Chromatogr A* **662**, 301.

9. Bodansky Y (1998) *The Iraqi WMD Challenge. Myth and Reality.* Task Force Report, February 10, Task Force on Terrorism & Unconventional Warfare, U.S. House of Representatives, Washington, DC.

10. Brooks P, Lawley PD (1961) The reaction of mono- and difunctional alkylating agents with nucleic acids. *Biochem J* **80**, 496.

11. Case RAM, Lea AJ (1955) Mustard gas poisoning, chronic bronchitis and lung cancer. An investigation into the possibility that poisoning by mustard gas in the 1914–1918 war might be a factor in production of neoplasia. *Brit J Prev Med* **9**, 62.

12. Compton JAF (1987) *Military Chemical and Biological Agents. Chemical and Toxicological Properties.* Telford Press, Caldwell, New Jersey.

13. Danforth CH, Center E (1954) Nitrogen mustard as a teratogenic agent in the mouse. *Proc Soc Exp Biol Med* **86**, 705.

14. Davison C, Rozman RS, Smith PK (1961) Metabolism of bis-β-chloroethyl sulfide (sulfur mustard gas). *Biochem Pharmacol* **7**, 65.

15. Drasch G, Kretschmer E, Kauert G, von Meyer L (1987) Concentrations of mustard gas [bis(β-chloroethyl)sulfide] in the tissues of a victim of a vesicant exposure. *J Forensic Sci* **32**, 1788.

16. Ellenhorn MJ (1997) *Ellenhorn's Medical Toxicology: Diagnosis and Treatment of Human Poisoning. 2nd Ed.* Williams & Wilkins, Baltimore p. 1293.

17. Elsayed NM, Omaye ST, Klain GJ et al. (1989) Response of mouse brain to a single subcutaneous injection of the monofunctional sulfur mustard, butyl 2-chloroethyl sulfide (BCS). Toxicology 58, 11.

18. Elsayed NM, Omaye ST, Klein GJ, Korte DW Jr (1992) Free radical-mediated lung response to the monofunctional sulfur mustard butyl 2-chloro-ethyl sulfide after subcutaneous injection. Toxicology 72, 153.

19. French JD, West PM, Von Amerongen FK, Magoun HW (1952) Effects of intracarotid administration of nitrogen mustard on normal brain and brain tumors. J Neurosurg 9, 378.

20. Gilman A, Philips FS (1992) The biological actions of therapeutic applications of the β-chlorethyl amines and sulfides. Science 103, 409.

21. Goldin A, Noe HA, Landing BH et al. (1948) A neurological syndrome induced by administration of chlorinated tertiary amines. J Pharmacol Exp Ther 94, 249.

22. Graef I, Karnofsky DA, Val Jager B et al. (1948) The clinical and pathologic effects of the nitrogen and sulfur mustards in laboratory animals. Amer J Pathol 24, 1.

23. Harris R, Paxman J (1982) A Higher Form of Killing: The Secret Story of Chemical and Biological Warfare. Hill & Wang, New York.

24. Haskin D (1948) Some effects of nitrogen mustard on the development of external body form in the fetal rat. Anat Rec 102, 493.

25. Heitzmann O (1921) Ueber Kampfgasvergiftungen. VIII. Die pathologischanatomischen Veränderungen nach Vergiftung mit Dichloräthylsulfide unter Berücksichtigung der Tierversuche. Erste Teil: Ergebnisse der Tierversuche. Zeit Ges Exp Med 13, 484. Zweiter Teil: Veranderungen beim Menschen. Ibid 491.

26. Heully F, Gruninger M (1956) Collective intoxication caused by the explosion of a mustard gas shell. Ann Med Legal 36, 195. [French]

27. Hobbs FB (1944) A fatal case of mustard gas poisoning. Brit Med J ii, 306.

28. Hörtnagl H, Berger ML (1989) Subregional differences of cholinergic deficit in rat hippocampus induced by ethylcholine aziridinium ion (AF64A). J Neurochem 52, S94.

29. Hörtnagl H, Hanin L (1992) Toxins affecting the cholinergic system. In: Selective Neurotoxicity. Herken H, Hucho F eds. Springer-Verlag, Berlin p. 294.

30. Hoyle CHV, Moss HE, Burnstock G (1986) Ethylcholine mustard aziridinium (AF64A) impairs cholinergic neuromuscular transmission in the guinea-pig ileum and urinary bladder, and cholinergic neuromodulation in the enteric nervous system of the guinea-pig distal colon. Gen Pharmacol 17, 543.

31. Hunt CC, Philips FS (1940) The acute pharmacology of methyl-bis(2-chloroethylamine) (HN2). J Pharmacol Exp Ther 95, 131.

32. Husain K, Dube SN, Sugendran K et al. (1996) Effect of topically applied sulfur mustard on antioxidant enzymes in blood cells of body tissues of rats. J Appl Toxicol 16, 245.

33. Janokovich L (1938) Beiträge zur Histologie der experimentallen Senfgas vergiftung. Int Kongr Gericht Soz Med Verhand, Bonn.

34. Kisby GE, Springer N, Spencer PS (1999) In vitro neurotoxic and DNA-damaging properties of nitrogen mustard (HN2). J Appl Toxicol in press.

35. Klain GJ, Bonner SJ, Omaye ST (1988) Skin penetration and tissue distribution of [14C]butyl 2-chloroethyl sulfide in the rat. J Toxicol-Cutan Ocul Toxicol 7, 255.

36. Kozlowski MR, Arbgast RE (1986) Specific toxic effects of ethylcholine nitrogen mustard on cholinergic neurons in the basal forebrain of the rat: A new animal model of Alzheimer's disease. Neurosci Lett 102, 125.

37. Laganiere S, Marinko M, Corey J et al. (1990) Sector-dependent neurotoxicity of ethylcholine aziridinium (AF64A) in the rat hippocampus. Neuropharmacology 29, 961.

38. Lederberg J (1994) Report of the Defense Science Board Task Force on Persian Gulf War Health Effects. Office of the Under Secretary of Defense for Acquisition and Technology, U.S. Department of Defense, Washington, DC.

39. Ludlum DB, Austin-Ritchie P, Hagopian M et al. (1994) Detection of sulfur mustard-induced DNA modifications. Chem-Biol Interact 91, 39.

40. Ludlum DB, Papirmeister B (1986) DNA modification by sulfur mustards and nitrosoureas and repair of these lesions. In: Mechanisms of DNA Damage and Repair. Simic AL ed. Plenum, New York p. 119.

41. MacNaughton MG, Brewer JH (1994) Environmental Chemistry and Fate of Chemical Warfare Agents. Southwest Research Institute, San Antonio, Texas.

42. Mantione CR, DeGroat WC, Fisher A, Hanin I (1983) Selective inhibition of peripheral cholinergic transmission in the cat produced by AF64A. J Pharmacol Exp Ther 255, 616.

43. Mantione CR, Zigmond MJ, Fisher A, Hanin I (1983) Selective presynaptic cholinergic neurotoxicity following intrahippocampal AF64A injection in rats. J Neurochem 41, 251.

44. Marshall EK Jr (1926) Physiological action of dichloroethyl sulphide (mustard gas). In: The Medical Department of the United States Army in the World War. Vol XIV. Medical Aspects of Gas Warfare. Weed FW ed. Government Printing Office, Washington, DC p. 369.

45. Maynard RL (1988) The Ethics of Chemical Warfare: An Historical Perspective. Royal College of Defence Studies, London.

46. Maynard RL (1993) Toxicology of chemical warfare agents. In: General and Applied Toxicology. Vol 2. Ballantyne B, Marrs T, Turner P eds. Stockton Press, New York p. 1253.

47. Maysinger D, Tagari PC, Cuello C (1986) Cholinergic and GABAergic neurotoxicity of some alkylating agents. *Biochem Pharmacol* **35**, 3583

48. McArdle J, Hanin I (1986) Acute *in vivo* exposure to ethylcholine aziridinium (AF64A) depresses the secretion of quanta from nerve terminals. *Eur J Pharmacol* **131**, 119.

49. McDonald TP, Asano M (1961) Effects of nitrogen mustard on the mouse brain. *Amer J Pathol* **38**, 695.

50. Meier HL, Gross CL, Papirmeister B (1984) The use of human models for validating the biochemical mechanism of mustard-induced injury and for developing and evaluating therapeutic regimens to prevent mustard gas incapacitation. *Proc Army Sci Conf.* West Point, New York [cited in ref. 72].

51. Moorhead TG (1919) The clinical results of poisoning by mustard gas. *Dublin J Med Sci* **147**, 1.

52. Morgenstern P, Koss FR, Alexander WW (1947) Residual mustard gas bronchitis; effects of prolonged exposure to low concentrations. *Ann Intern Med* **26**, 27.

53. Müller M, Skreb N (1964) Does nitrogen mustard mimic the x-ray effects in any case? *Experientia* **20**, 70.

54. Murphy ML, Del Moro A, Lacon C (1958) The comparative effects of five polyfunctional alkylating agents on the rat fetus, with additional notes on the chick embryo. *Ann N Y Acad Sci* **68**, 762.

55. National Research Council (1985) *Possible Long-Term Health Effects of Short-Term Exposure to Chemical Agents. Vol 3. Final Report. Current Health Status of Test Subjects.* National Academy Press, Washington, DC.

56. Niu T, Matijasevic Z, Austin-Ritchie P *et al.* (1996) A ^{32}P-postlabeling method for the detection of adducts in the DNA of human fibroblasts exposed to sulfur mustard. *Chem Biol Interact* **100**, 77.

57. Papiermeister B, Feister AJ, Robinson SI, Ford RD (1991) *Medical Defense Against Mustard Gas: Toxic Mechanisms and Pharmacological Implications.* CRC Press, Boca Raton, Florida p. 359.

58. Papiermeister B, Gross CL, Meier HL *et al.* (1985) Molecular basis for mustard-induced vesication. *Fund Appl Toxicol* **5**, S134.

59. Perchura CM, Rall DP (1993) *Veterans at Risk: The Health Effects of Mustard Gas and Lewisite.* National Academy Press, Washington, DC.

60. Prentiss AM (1937) *Chemicals in War.* McGraw Hill, New York.

61. Presidential Advisory Committee on Gulf War Veterans' Illnesses (1996) *Final Report.* U.S. Government Printing Office, Washington, DC.

62. Presidential Advisory Committee on Gulf War Veterans' Illnesses (1997) *Special Report.* U.S. Government Printing Office, Washington, DC.

63. Renshaw B (1946) Mechanisms in production of cutaneous injuries by sulfur and nitrogen mustards. In: *Chemical Warfare Agents and Related Chemical Problems. Vol 1.* U.S. Office of Scientific Research and Development, National Defense Research Committee, Washington, DC.

64. Riegle DW (1994) *U.S. Chemical and Biological Warfare-Related Dual Use Exports to Iraq and Their Possible Impact on the Health Consequences of the Persian Gulf War.* Committee Staff Report No. 3, Appendix B-9. Committee on Banking, Housing and Urban Affairs, U.S. Senate, Washington, DC.

65. Rosenblatt DH, Small MJ, Kimmell TA, Anderson AW (1995) *Agent Decontamination Chemistry Technical Report.* U.S. Army Test and Evaluation Command (TECOM) Technical Report Phase 1. Draft. Argonne National Laboratory, Wisconsin.

66. Sanyal MK, Kitchin KT, Dixon RL (1981) Rat conceptus development *in vitro*: Comparative effects of alkylating agents. *Toxicol Appl Phamacol* **57**, 14.

67. Schnurr PP, Friedman MJ (1996) Post-traumatic stress disorder among World War II mustard gas test participants. *Mil Med* **161**, 131.

68. Sidell F, Hurst CG (1992) Clinical considerations in mustard poisoning. In: *Chemical Warfare Agents.* Somani SM ed. Academic Press, London p. 52.

69. Small MJ (1984) *Compounds Formed from the Chemical Decontamination of HD, GB and VX and Their Environmental Fate.* Tech Rep 8304. AD A149515, U.S. Army Medical Bioengin Res Develop Lab, Fort Detrick, Fredrick, Maryland.

70. Smith HW (1943) *Review of the Literature on the Systemic Action of Mustard Gas.* Div 9, Office of Scientific Research and Development, National Defense Research Committee (New York University College of Medicine, New York).

71. Smith PK, Nadkarni MV, Trams EG, Davison C (1958) Distribution and fate of alkylating agents. *Ann N Y Acad Sci* **68**, 834.

72. Somani SM (1992) Toxicokinetics and toxicodynamics of mustard. In: *Chemical Warfare Agents.* Somani SM ed. Academic Press, London p. 13.

73. Stewart M (1918) *Report on Cases of Poisoning by "Mustard Gas" (Dichloroethylsulphide), with Special Reference to the Histological Changes and to Alterations in the Leucocyte Count.* Report No. 17, Chemical Warfare Medical Committee, London.

74. Stockholm International Peace Research Institute (1971) *The Problem of Chemical and Biological Warfare: A Study of the Historical, Technical, Military, Legal, and Political Aspects of Chemical and Biological Warfare and Possible Disarmament Measures. Vol 1. The Rise of Chemical and Biological Weapons.* Almqvist & Wiksell, Stockholm.

75. Sullivan KM, Storb R, Shulman HM *et al.* (1982) Immediate and delayed neurotoxicity after mechlorethamine preparation for bone marrow transplantation. *Ann Intern Med* **97**, 182.

76. Tubarao E, Bulgini MJ (1968) Cytotoxic and antifungal agents: Their body distribution and tissue affinity. *Nature* **218**, 395.

77. U.S. Army Environmental Hygiene Agency (1989) *Occupational Health Guidelines for the Evaluation and Control of Occupational Exposures to Mustard Agents H, HD, and HT.* USAEHA Tech Guide TG 173, U.S. Army Environmental Hygiene Agency (USAEHA), Aberdeen Proving Ground, Maryland.

78. U.S. Department of Health and Human Services (1988) *Final Recommendation for Protecting the Health and Safety Against Potential Adverse Effects of Long-Term Exposure to Low Doses of Agents: GA, GB, VX, Mustard Agent (H, HD, HT), and Lewisite (L).* Fed Regist **53**, 8504.

79. Van der Schans GP, Scheffer AG, Mars-Groenendijk RH, et al. (1994) Immunochemical detection of adducts of sulfur mustard to DNA of calf thymus and human white blood cells. *Chem Res Toxicol* **7**, 408.

80. Vedder EB (1925) *The Medical Aspects of Chemical Warfare.* Williams & Wilkins, Baltimore.

81. Vijayaraghavan R, Sugendran K, Pant K et al. (1991) Dermal intoxication of mice with bis(2-chloroethyl) sulfide and the protective effect of flavinoids. *Toxicology* **69**, 35.

82. Villani L, Contestabile A, Migani P et al. (1986) Ultrastructural and neurochemical effects of the presumed cholinergic toxin AF64A in the rat interpeduncular nucleus. *Brain Res* **379**, 223.

83. Vojvodic V, Milosavljevic Z, Boskovic B, Bojanic N (1985) The protective effect of different drugs in rats poisoned by sulfur and nitrogen mustards. *Fund Appl Toxicol* **5**, S160.

84. Von den Velden (1921) Uber Kampfgasvergiftungen. X. Klinik der Erkrankungen nach Dichlordäthylsulfidvergiftung. *Zeit Ges Exp Med* **14**, 1.

85. Wada S, Nishimoito Y, Miyanshji S (1968) Mustard gas is a cause of respiratory neoplasm in man. *Lancet* i, 1161.

86. Wada S, Nishimoito Y, Miyanshji S et al. (1962) Review of Okuno-jima poison gas factory regarding occupational environment. *Hiroshima J Med Sci* **11**, 75.

87. Wada S, Nishimoito Y, Miyanshji S et al. (1962) Malignant respiratory tract neoplasms related to poison gas exposure. *Hiroshima J Med Sci* **11**, 81.

88. Willems JL (1989) Clinical management of mustard gas casualties. *Ann Med Milit Belg* **3**, S1.

89. Wormser U (1991) Toxicology of mustard gas. *Trends Pharmacol Sci* **120**, 164.

90. Yu D, Niu TQ, Austin-Ritchie P, Ludlum DB (1994) A ^{32}P-postlabeling method for detecting unstable N^7-substituted deoxyguanosine adducts in DNA. *Proc Nat Acad Sci USA* **91**, 7232.

91. Zaniboni A, Simoncini E, Marpicati P et al. (1988) Severe delayed neurotoxicity after accidental high-dose nitrogen mustard. *Am J Hematol* **27**, 304.

92. Zhou GH, Teicher BA, Frei E III (1996) Postlabeling detection of DNA adducts of antitumor alkylating agents. *Cancer Chemother Pharmacol* **38**, 71.

CASE REPORT

The following historical description (from 1933) highlights CNS and PNS changes in a case of oral sulfur mustard intoxication; most, perhaps all, of the neuropathological changes may be ascribed to the effects of hypoxia and postmortem autolysis. The accompanying description of CNS changes in cats and rabbits raises the possibility of neurotoxicity.

[A] young man in a state of inebriation drank 5 cc. of mustard gas [sulfur mustard] with suicidal intention. After 8 min, he vomited and collapsed unconscious with urination and defecation. He recovered from collapse and the stomach was twice lavaged and rinsed with permanganate, but the activity of his heart deteriorated and he died after 5 h. [Autopsy revealed hyperemia of laryngeal, tracheal and pharyngeal mucosa.] The gastric mucosa was gelatinous, turgid and very inflamed. There was only slight inflammation of the intestinal mucosa. The meningeal membranes were injected ... Histological examination revealed no marked changes in the gastointestinal tract. The kidneys showed cloudy swelling of the tubules with pale nuclear staining and the liver [exhibited] very finely dispersed fat at the peripheral lobes. Serious alterations were observed only in the central nervous system where the ganglia of the brain, spinal cord and sympathetic system showed degeneration and dissolution of nerve cells ... Nissl bodies were demonstrable only occasionally in the ganglion cells of the pons and medulla oblongata. Nerve cells generally showed either shrinking or hyperchromasia with disappearance of the nucleus and nuclear vesicle, the edges of the homogenized cell becoming lace-like; or, alternatively, in some regions of the brain and in the cortex, edematous swelling of the nerve cells with the appearance of fissures and vacuoles which displaced the disintegrating cytoplasm, the nuclei become pycnotic and the cells disintegrating to shadowy residues. This latter type of changes was observed also in the basal ganglia and in Ammon's horn. Other types of pathological changes were observed in the olivary nucleus, the Purkinje cells of the cerebellum and the sympathetic ganglia of the neck and chest. In the latter instance entirely normal ganglion cells disappeared, the majority being in a state of disintegration. These changes were missed in large part in preparations stained with eosin or Van Gieson and were clearly demonstrable only in Nissl preparations."

"In rabbits intoxicated orally by "fractions of a drop" of mustard gas dissolved in oil or alcohol and introduced into the stomach by tube it was found that severe changes occurred in the gastrointestinal tract and in the central nervous system, the latter resembling those described above in the human case. In a cat which received a total of 10 drops of mustard over a period of 5 months the cells of the cortex, basal ganglia, pons and medulla were reduced to degenerate shadows and a numerical reduction of the Purkinje cells of the cerebellum was objectively evident." (33).

Muzolimine

Herbert H. Schaumburg

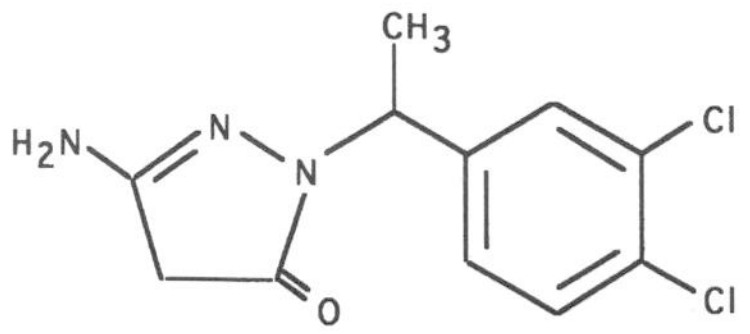

MUZOLIMINE
$C_{11}H_{11}Cl_2N_3O$

5-Amino-2-[1-(3,4-dichlorophenyl)ethyl]-2,4-dihydro-3*H*-pyrazol-3-one

NEUROTOXICITY RATING

Clinical

B   Peripheral neuropathy

B   Myelopathy

Muzolimine, a pyrazolon derivative, is a long-duration loop-diuretic with a pattern of excreted metabolites similar to that of furosemide (1). The drug was introduced in Europe in 1987 and withdrawn after 2 years because of severe neurological adverse effects (2,4).

Rapid-onset peripheral neuropathy, spastic paraparesis, and myelopathy developed in 5 of 28 patients with renal insufficiency who were treated with muzolimine for periods exceeding 3 months; none was receiving clioquinol or other agents associated with myelopathy (2). Postmortem study of two cases revealed myelin loss in the posterior and lateral columns of the spinal cord and multifocal demyelination in peripheral nerves (4). Magnetic resonance imaging in some cases has depicted multifocal white-matter lesions in the cerebral hemispheres. Serum B_{12} and folic acid determinations were normal, and there was no evidence of inflammatory reaction in the postmortem lesions that suggested an immune basis for this condition.

The neurotoxic properties of muzolimine and a number of other drugs with neurotoxic potential have been investigated in relation to vitamin B_6 metabolism. Drugs were tested for their inhibitory effect on erythrocyte pyridoxal kinase [EC. 2.7.1.35] and their ability to react chemically with substrates for this enzyme. Theophylline, which has the potential to induce seizures (*see* Methylxanthines, this volume), was judged to be a true pyridoxal kinase inhibitor. Isoniazid, a drug associated with seizures and peripheral neuropathy (*see* Isoniazid, this volume), fell into a second class of drugs that blocked enzyme activity by forming covalent complexes with the enzyme's substrates pyridoxal or pyridoxal-5'-phosphate. A third group of drugs "inhibited" enzyme activity using pyridoxal but not pyridoxamine as substrate; this group included muzolimine and D-penicillamine, both of which have been linked to the induction of peripheral neuropathy (*see* Penicillamine, this volume) (3). The neurotoxic effects of muzolimine might therefore be mediated by its reactivity with a substrate required for pyridoxal kinase activity.

REFERENCES

1. Berg KJ, Jorstad S, Tromsdal A (1976) Studies on the clinical pharmacology of a new potent diuretic Bay g 2821. *Pharmatherapeutica* 1, 319.
2. Gilli M, Papurello D, Cutin IC *et al.* (1989) Azione neurotossica della muzolimina ad alte dosi in pazienti uremica. *Minerva Urol Nefrol* 41, 215.
3. Laine-Cessac P, Cailleux A, Allain P (1997) Mechanisms of the inhibition of human erythrocyte pyridoxal kinase by drugs. *Biochem Pharmacol* 54, 863.
4. Pohlmann-Eden B, Rerlit P, Maibach EA, Gretz N (1991) Muzolimine-induced severe neuromyeloencephalopathy: report of seven cases. *Acta Neurol Scand* 83, 41.

Myristica fragrans

Frank Bretschneider
Albert C. Ludolph

MYRISTICIN
$C_{11}H_{12}O_3$

Nutmeg; *Nux moschata*; Myristicin (major oil constituent); 4-Methoxy-6-(2-propenyl)-1,3-benzodioxole

NEUROTOXICITY RATING

Clinical

B Psychobiological reaction (euphoria, confusion, visual hallucinations)

Nutmeg, the seed of *Myristica fragrans*, contains 25%–40% of fatty oils (nutmeg butter), 8%–15% of volatile oils, and 45%–60% of structural materials including cellulose (23,24). Nutmeg was used in India and Arab countries as a spice and as a remedy but was unknown to the Greeks and Romans. In the Middle Ages, nutmeg was introduced into Europe by Arab merchants and, later, by Portuguese and Dutch traders. European physicians of the Middle Ages prescribed nutmeg for a wide range of maladies. The end of the nineteenth century saw a brief popularity in the wake of a rumor that nutmeg is an effective abortifacient. Intoxication due to psychotropic effects of nutmeg was frequent around the end of the 19th century. In recent years, the use of nutmeg as a psychotropic agent was popularized after mention of the phenomenon in the autobiography of the American Malcolm X (21). Nutmeg preparations have been used as an alternative for cannabis, mescaline, or lysergic acid diethylamide (LSD). In the search for the medicinally active constituents, it was found that the nuts no longer had any action after removal of the volatile oil; the volatile oil and its constituents were thus implicated. 3-Methoxy-4,5-methylenedioxyallylbenzene (myristicin), 3,4,5-trimethoxyallylbenzene (elemicin), and 4,5-methylenedioxyallylbenzene (safrole) have been identified as constituting ~80% of the group of allylbenzene derivatives in the volatile oil. In early descriptions of natural products, the name "myristicin" referred to the solids that crystallized from old samples of nutmeg oil on prolonged standing (10).

Nutmeg and mace are both products of the same tree, *Myristica fragrans* Houtt., the economically important member of the family Myristicaceae (11,36). The nutmeg tree has male and female flowers that resemble lily-of-the-valley; they are pale yellow with a strong scent of nutmeg. The fruit of the tree is similar to an apricot. Within the husk is the seed, the nutmeg of commerce, enclosed in a deep-brown shining seed coat. Over this lies a crimson network, the arillus (39). The arillus, when dried, is known in commerce as mace and used as a spice.

The essential oil of mace and nutmeg are obtained by steam distillation. It contains the active principles for the supposed pharmacological effects. Myristicin, the major component of the volatile oil of nutmeg and mace, has usually been isolated from natural oils by fractional distillation, as it is crystallized with difficulty, even at very low temperatures. Myristicin is a clear, mobile, colorless oil. It has a faintly aromatic odor due to inefficiencies of vacuum distillation (32). The physical properties of myristicin as isolated from oil of nutmeg must allow for the presence of the contaminant elemicin (30).

Nutmeg is commonly added to custards, puddings, pies, and eggnog. Mace is used in soups, sauces, and pastries. Both spices are important ingredients of frankfurters and other meat products, pickles, and tomato ketchup. The fixed oil of nutmeg (nutmeg butter) is used as an ingredient of certain soaps, hair tonics, and perfumes, and was formerly used as a poultice for arthritis (25,39). Essential oil of nutmeg and mace (volatile oil) has been widely used as a flavoring agent for perfumes and dentifrices (14).

The therapeutic applications of nutmeg were first catalogued by Arab physicians as early as the seventh century BC, principally as a remedy for disorders of the digestive system. It was also considered beneficial in such diverse conditions as kidney disease, pain, and lymphatic aliments. It was even described as an aphrodisiac (6,37), and Yemenite men still consume it to increase virility. In India, nutmeg is still used as an analgesic and sedative by folk-medicine practitioners and also has religious significance (12,13,36,39). At the end of the 1800s, a rumor spread in England and America that nutmeg could induce an overdue menstruation and induce abortion (38).

The drug is generally ground, stirred into a drink, and taken in a quantity of 5–30 g. It is assumed that terpene hydrocarbons, which are constituents of nutmeg and volatile oil promote the absorption of the allylbenzene derivatives by irritating the gastrointestinal tract (17). Since the psychotropic component(s) and the mechanism of action of nutmeg are unknown (*vide infra*), data relating to pharmacokinetics, metabolism, and excretion are limited. Probable derivatives of myristicin and elemicin are 3-methoxy-4,5-dimethylene-dioxyamphetamine (MMDA) and 3,4,5-trimethoxyamphetamine (TMA), respectively, both of which are psychoactive compounds related to amphetamine, with effects similar to LSD (20). The metabolism of myristicin was investigated in rat liver and revealed an amination of myristicin's and elemicin's side chains (propene) after perfusion of the liver (4).

Most reports suggesting that nutmeg has psychoactive properties stem from its recreational use by prisoners. Visual and auditory hallucinations, floating sensations, and separation of limb and body typify most prison tales (19,27,39).

The psychotomimetic action of nutmeg, which begins to take effect 2–5 h after ingestion, allegedly ranges from a slight change in consciousness to very intense hallucinations. Whereas visual hallucinations are much less common than with LSD or mescaline intoxication, distinct alterations occur in the perception of time and space. Visual hallucinations are claimed to involve distortions of space, color, and time. Inappropriate apprehension, anxiety, and fear of impending death are common. Reports describe a feeling of soaring and of dissociation of the limbs from the body. Systemic side effects include nausea, headache, dry mouth, epigastric burning, increased pulse rate, palpitations, and a giddy feeling. All symptoms of nutmeg intoxication usually disappear after 12–48 h. The intoxication is often followed by heavy sleep. For a period of several days, there may be headaches and spells of dizziness. An occasional aftereffect is a lasting aversion to the taste and/or smell of nutmeg (1,2,17,29,32). Nutmeg and synthetic myristicin inhibit monoamine oxidase in animals (2). The supposed interactions with prostaglandins may be responsible for the anti-inflammatory and antidiarrheal effects of myristicin (9,22).

The hallucinogenic activity of nutmeg and related agents has been tested in mice during short-term controlled exposures (34). Studies have attempted to validate behavioral tests as useful indices of hallucinogenic activity (5,35). Only the head-twitching test (8) showed the expected increase in frequency after intraperitoneal injections of mescaline and LSD-25, whereas application of myristicin and elemicin (up to 80 mg/kg body weight essential oil) did not induce this effect. 1-Δ9-Trans-tetrahydrocannabinol (THC) in the dosage of 1.5 mg/kg body weight—which is known to be psychotomimetic in man (16,18)—had no effect on the frequency of head twitching (34). A ligroin extract of nutmeg (without myristicin, elemicin, safrole, or eugenol) was found to cause a significant increase in the duration of light and deep sleep in young chickens (28,29). Myristicin and elemicin disrupted rope-climbing and bar-pressing performances of rats. Catatonia and decreased motor activity were seen in mice after intraperitoneal injection of 40 and 20 mg/kg body weight of myristicin and elemicin, respectively. The effects were dose-dependent. These components were shown to have 33%–65% and 16%–32% of the potency of THC. The drug effects appeared about 2–4 min after injection; animals displayed dyspnea, writhing, and distention of the posterior paws. These effects disappeared 10–15 min after the injections (7).

Long-term experiments (7) showed the development of tolerance to myristicin and elemicin after 30 days of drug exposure (*vide supra*) but no cross-tolerance to THC. The actions of myristicin, elemicin, and THC therefore seem to differ.

Myristicin, the most abundant and active fraction of nutmeg, was tested in humans for psychotropic activity; only 60% of the subjects tested displayed symptoms that were "suggestive" of psychotropic effects (26). A controlled trial in 42 first-year psychology students to examine psychological effects of 6 g ground nutmeg given in a single oral dose *vs.* placebo showed no effect (3). In another study, 10 prisoners were given excessive amounts of nutmeg; two exhibited toxic psychosis (40).

The mechanism of action of nutmeg and mace as psychotropic agents and their active principles are poorly understood. No controlled study in humans demonstrates a psychotropic or hallucinogenic effect of nutmeg. It must be concluded that since nutmeg's hallucinogenic effects are only a manifestation of general toxicity and since its levels of intoxication are "extremely variable," nutmeg is not a specific hallucinogen in the usual sense of the word, but is best termed a "pseudohallucinogen" (26). Animal studies support this view, since any behavioral effects occurred after a period of intoxication (7). It has been been suggested that, *in vivo*, nutmeg components may be aminated to the corresponding hallucinogenic amines [*e.g.*, myristicin to MMDA and elemicin to TMA or to mescaline (33)], which could be the cause of psychotropic effects (4,17,31–33). Therefore, it is possible that myristicin *per se* is not the form in which the substance is found in nature. This natural form may then be either the actual toxicant in the instance of human ingestion, or may generate the active product *in vivo*. These speculations are in accord with the inability to imitate nutmeg intoxication with synthetic myristicin (32).

REFERENCES

1. Abernethy MK, Becker LB (1992) Acute nutmeg intoxication. *Amer J Emerg Med* 10, 429.

2. Anon (1984) The pharmacology of nutmeg. *Lawrence Rev Nat Prod* **5**, 13.

3. Beattle RT (1968) Nutmeg as a psychoactive agent. *Brit J Addict* **63**, 105.

4. Braun U, Kalbhen DA (1972) Nachweis der Bildung psychotroper Amphetamin-Derivate aus Inhaltsstoffen der Muskatnuß. *Deut Med Wochenschr* **97**, 1614.

5. Brimblecombe RW (1963) Effects of psychotropic drugs on open-field behavior in rats. *Psychopharmacologia* **4**, 139.

6. Burkill IH (1935) *Dictionary of the Economic Products of the Malay Peninsula. 2nd Ed.* Crown Agents, London.

7. Cesario de Mello A, Carlini EA (1973) Behavioral observations on compounds found in nutmeg. *Psychopharmacologia* **31**, 349.

8. Corne SJ, Pickering RW (1967) A possible correlation between drug-induced hallucinations in man and a behavioural response in mice. *Psychopharmacologia* **11**, 65.

9. Dietz WH Jr, Stuart MJ (1976) Nutmeg and prostaglandins. *N Engl J Med* **294**, 503.

10. Fluckinger FA (1874) *Pharm J* **5**, 136.

11. Forrest EF, Heacock RA (1972) Nutmeg and mace, the psychotropic spices from *Myristica fragrans*. *Lloydia* **35**, 440

12. Gimlette JD (1930) *The Medical Book of Malayan Medicine.* Garden Bulletin, Straits Settlement, Singapore.

13. Greenberg S, Ortiz EL (1983) *The Spice of Life.* Amaryllis Press, New York.

14. Guenther E (1952) *The Essential Oils. Vol 5.* D. van Nostrand, Princeton, New Jersey.

15. Hallstrom H, Thuvander A (1997) Toxicological evaluation of myristicin. *Nat Toxins* **5**, 186.

16. Isbell H, Gorodetzky CW, Jasinski D *et al.* (1967) Effects of (−)Δ9-trans-tetrahydrocannabinol in man. *Psychopharmacologia* **11**, 528.

17. Kalbhen DA (1971) A contribution to the chemistry and pharmacology of nutmeg. *Angew Chem Int Ed* **10**, 370.

18. Karniol IG, Carlini EA (1973) Comparative studies in man and in laboratory animals on Δ8- and Δ9-trans-tetrahydrocannabinol. *Pharmacology* **9**, 115.

19. Lewis WH, Elvin-Lewis MPF (1977) *Medical Botany.* Wiley, New York p. 408.

20. Mack RB (1982) Toxic encounters of the dangerous kind. *North Carol Med J* **43**, 439.

21. Malcolm X, Haley A (1964) The Autobiography of Malcolm X. Grove Press, New York.

22. Ozaki Y, Soedigdo S, Wattimena YR, Suganda AG (1988) Antiinflammatory effect of mace, aril of *Myristica fragrans* Houtt., and its active principles. *Jpn J Pharmacol* **49**, 155.

23. Power FB, Salway J (1907) The constituents of oil of nutmeg. *J Chem Soc* **91**, 2037.

24. Power FB, Salway J (1907) The constituents of the expressed oil of nutmeg. *J Chem Soc* **93**, 1653.

25. Ridley HN (1912) *Spices.* Macmillan, London.

26. Rumphius GE (1741–1755) *Herbarium Amboinense. Vol 2.* Amsterdam.

27. Schulze RG (1976) Nutmeg as an hallucinogen. *N Engl J Med* **295**, 174.

28. Sherry CJ, Burnett RE (1977) Enhancement of ethanol-induced sleep by whole oil of nutmeg. *Experientia* **34**, 492.

29. Sherry CJ, Ray LE, Herron RE (1982) The pharmacological effects of a ligroin extract of nutmeg (*Myristica fragrans*). *J Ethnopharmacol* **6**, 61.

30. Shulgin AT (1963) Composition of the myristicin fraction from oil of nutmeg. *Nature* **197**, 379.

31. Shulgin AT (1964) 3-Methoxy-4,5-methylenedioxyamphetamine, a new psychotomimetic agent. *Nature* **201**, 1120.

32. Shulgin AT (1966) Possible implication of myristicin as a psychotropic substance. *Nature* **210**, 380.

33. Shulgin AT, Sargent T, Naranjo C (1967) The chemistry and psychopharmacology of nutmeg and of several related phenylisopropylamines. In: *Ethnopharmacologic Search for Psychoactive Drugs.* Efron DH, Holmsted B, Kline NS eds. U.S. Government Printing Office, Washington, DC p. 202.

34. Silva MTA, Calil M (1974) Screening hallucinogenic drugs: Systematic study of three behavioral tests. *Psychopharmacologia* **42**, 163.

35. Smythies JR, Johnston VS, Bradley RJ (1969) Behavioural models of psychosis. *Brit J Psychiat* **115**, 55.

36. van Gils C, Cox PA (1994) Ethnobotany of nutmeg in the Spice islands. *J Ethnopharmacol* **42**, 117.

37. Warburg 0 (1897) Die Muskatnuß. Leipzig.

38. Weil AT (1965) Nutmeg as a narcotic. *Econ Bot* **19**, 194.

39. Weil AT (1971) Nutmeg as a psychoactive drug. *J Psychodelic Drugs* **3**, 72.

40. Weiss G (1960) Hallucinogenic and narcotic-like effects of powdered *Myristica* (nutmeg). *Psychiat Quart* **34**, 346.

Nalidixic Acid

Steven A. Sparr

NALIDIXIC ACID
C₁₂H₁₂N₂O₃

3-Carboxy-1-ethyl-7-methyl-1,8-naphthyridin-4-one

NEUROTOXICITY RATING

Clinical

A Seizure disorder

A Visual dysfunction (diplopia, blurring)

A Acute encephalopathy (hallucinations, sedation, coma)

A Benign intracranial hypertension (pseudotumor cerebri)

Experimental

A Seizure disorder

Nalidixic acid, a quinolone derivative, is a synthethic antibiotic available since the 1960s for the treatment of urinary tract and gastrointestinal bacterial infections due to drug-susceptible organisms. Given the rapid development of bacterial resistance and frequent toxicity, nalidixic acid has been largely replaced by fluorinated quinolone antibiotics, such as ciprofloxacin and ofloxacin (11).

The quinolones inhibit bacterial enzyme DNA gyrase, an enzyme that prevents supercoiling of DNA strands during replication. Since the enzyme is not found in eukaryotic cells, this class of drug is selectively cidal to susceptible bacteria (11). Specifically, nalidixic acid is effective against many gram-negative urinary pathogens, including most *Proteus* spp., Enterobacteriaceae, and *Escherichia coli*. In addition, nalidixic acid is effective against several gastrointestinal bacterial pathogens, such as *Salmonella* and *Shigella* (11).

The drug is usually well tolerated but has the potential to cause severe neurological side effects. This, coupled with frequent development of drug resistance, has led to declining use.

Nalidixic acid is rapidly and almost completely absorbed after oral administration, with peak plasma levels 1–3 h after ingestion (11). The drug and its principal hydroxy metabolite are highly protein-bound. Nalidixic acid penetrates poorly into body tissues and the CNS. The drug is metabolized in the liver to hydroxynalidixic acid, which has an-

tibacterial potency similar to that of the parent compound, and to glucuronic acid conjugates. It is also metabolized in the kidney to a dicarboxylic acid derivative (1). Nalidixic acid and metabolites are excreted in the urine (urinary half-life of 6 h). Serum half-life is 1–6 h, depending on the method of determination, and is markedly prolonged to 21 h in patients with severe renal failure (1). About 4% of the drug is excreted unchanged in the feces.

The primary toxic effects of nalidixic acid are neurological. Neurological side effects include pseudotumor cerebri, visual disturbances, seizures, toxic encephalopathy, coma with metabolic acidosis, and a variety of nonspecific neurological symptoms (1). Other reported side effects include photosensitivity reaction; nausea, vomiting, and abdominal pain; hematological disorders, including hemolytic anemia in patients with glucose-6-phosphate dehydrogenase deficits; and hyperglycemia and hepatotoxicity (1).

Animal models have been developed for the proconvulsive effects of nalidixic acid and other quinolone antibiotics. Nalidixic acid has been shown to lower the threshold of mice to electroshock-induced seizures; this effect was completely blocked by MK-801 (dizocilpine), an open-channel N-methyl-D-aspartate antagonist (17). Nalidixic acid may therefore trigger seizures by promoting excitatory amino acid transmission.

In a review of toxic reaction to urinary tract antibiotics, the Australian Drug Evaluation Committee reported an incidence of convulsions in three patients of an estimated 200,000 courses of treatment with nalidixic acid (2). Seizures have occurred in patients with pre-existing cerebrovascular disease, parkinsonism, or epilepsy; however, one case of generalized seizures developed in a 31-year-old woman with no prior neurological history and coincident moderate hyperglycemia 2 days after commencing treatment with nalidixic acid (6). Seizures, electroencephalographic abnormalities, and hypergylcemia resolved with cessation of drug usage. Seizures have been reported with toxic overdose of nalidixic acid (3).

There have been numerous reports of intracranial hypertension with nalidixic acid therapy, particularly in infants and children (4,5,8,10,13,15,16). Signs of increased intracranial pressure in infants may be subtle and restricted to bulging fontanelles. In a review of 22 previously described cases of intracranial hypertension due to nalidixic acid— all in children under the age of 12—there is a report of an illustrative case of a 16-year-old with chronic pyelonephritis who developed headache, diplopia, and visual obscurations 2 days after commencing treatment with nalidixic acid (7).

On examination, she had bilateral papilledema, unilateral paresis of the fourth and sixth cranial nerves, and unilateral lower-extremity weakness. She had a normal computed tomography scan of the brain and elevated opening pressure on lumbar puncture with normal cerebrospinal fluid protein and cell count. An electroencephalogram (EEG) showed left-sided slowing. All clinical and EEG abnormalities resolved with discontinuation of the drug. In all reported cases, abnormalities disappeared with cessation of therapy.

Toxic psychosis and coma have been described following even a single dose of nalidixic acid. After a 2-g dose, a 28-year-old woman developed dimming of vision, paresthesias, and headache; she lapsed into a coma 3 h after ingestion (8). She had elevated serum levels of nalidixic acid and its hydroxy metabolite. Despite symptoms suggestive of increased intracranial pressure, she had a normal opening pressure on lumbar puncture; there was no metabolic acidosis and the patient recovered fully in several hours. Another individual developed coma and severe metabolic acidosis following ingestion of 28 g of nalidixic acid; with supportive care, the patient recovered over several days (14). A 46-year-old woman with interstitial nephritis developed metabolic acidosis, hallucinations, convulsions, and coma 4 days after initiating therapy with nalidixic acid (12). Speculation has been given to the relative roles in the causation of coma and mental status changes of high serum levels of nalidixic acid and its metabolites *vs.* induction of acid-base disturbances.

Visual changes associated with nalidixic acid therapy include blurred vision, decreased visual acuity, diplopia, and photophobia (1). Disturbances of color perception have also been described (9). These symptoms resolve with discontinuation of therapy.

Other, less-specific neurological side effects of nalidixic acid therapy are dizziness, headache, drowsiness, insomnia, paresthesias, and depression (1,2); all respond to cessation of therapy.

REFERENCES

1. *American Hospital Formulary Service Drug Information* (1995) McEvoy GK ed. American Society of Health System Pharmacists, 510.
2. Australian Drug Evaluation Committee (1972) Adverse effects of drugs commonly used in the treatment of urinary tract infection. *Med J Australia* 1, 435.
3. Beal G, Busuttil R, Gaildry ML, Guran P (1976) Acute nalidixic acid poisoning in children. *Arch Fr Pediatr* 35, 416.
4. Cohen DN (1973) Intracranial hypertension and papilledema associated with nalidixic acid therapy. *Amer J Ophthalmol* 76, 680.
5. Deonna T, Guignard JP (1974) Acute intracranial hypertension after nalidixic acid administration. *Arch Dis Child* 49, 743.
6. Fraser AG, Harrower ADB (1977) Convulsions with hyperglycaemia associated with nalidixic acid. *Brit Med J* 177, 1518.
7. Gedroyc W, Shorvon SD (1982) Acute intracranial hypertension and nalidixic acid therapy. *Neurology* 32, 212.
8. Granstrom G, Berndt S (1984) Unconsciousness after one therapeutic dose of nalidixic acid. *Acta Med Scand* 216, 237.
9. Haut J, Haye C, Legras M *et al.* (1972) Color perception disorders after nalidixic acid absorption. *Bull Soc Ophtalmol Fr* 72, 147.
10. Leu GE, Burlea M, Circo E, Pita PT (1982) Acute benign intracranial hypertension with spontaneous recovery. *Rev Pediatr Obstet Ginecol Pediatr* 31, 253.
11. Mandell GL, Petrie WA (1996) Antimicrobial agents. In: *The Pharmacologic Basis of Therapeutics. 9th Ed.* Hardman JG, Goodman AG, Limbird LE eds. McGraw-Hill, New York p. 1057.
12. Mobbs JP, Balant L, Revillard C, Favre H (1977) Effets secondaires de l'acide nalidixique chez une patiente atteinte d'insuffisance renale sévere. *Schweiz Med Wochenschr* 107, 300.
13. Mukherjee A, Dutta P, Lahiri M *et al.* (1990) Benign intracranial hypertension after nalidixic acid overdose in infants. *Lancet* 335, 1602.
14. Nogue S, Bertran A, Mas A *et al.* (1979) Metabolic acidosis and coma due to an overdose of nalidixic acid. *Intens Care Med* 5, 141.
15. Rao KG (1974) Pseudotumor cerebri associated with nalidixic acid. *Urology* 4, 204.
16. Riyaz A, Aboobacker CM, Sreelatha PR (1998) Nalidixic acid-induced pseudotumour cerebri in children. *Indian Med Assn* 96, 308.
17. Williams PD, Helton DR (1991) The proconvulsive activity of quinolone antibiotics in an animal model. *Toxicol Lett* 58, 23.

Naphthalene

John D. Rogers

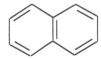

NAPHTHALENE
C$_{10}$H$_8$

NEUROTOXICOLOGY RATING

Clinical

B Acute encephalopathy (headache, seizures, sedation, coma)

Experimental

A Retinal degeneration (photoreceptors)

An antiseptic and anthelmintic, naphthalene also serves as a moth repellent and insecticide. Naphthalene is also used in the manufacture of dyes, synthetic resins, solvents, and motor fuels.

Human poisoning may occur by skin absorption, inhalation, and ingestion. Symptoms and signs of toxicity include nausea, vomiting, headache, diaphoresis, hematuria, hemolytic anemia, hepatic failure, seizures, and coma (1,2).

Animal studies have focused on the cataractogenic and retinotoxic effects of naphthalene (6); the latter is characterized by degeneration of photoreceptors accompanied by reaction and proliferation of retinal pigment epithelium, followed by subsequent subretinal neovascularization (4). In a rabbit lens culture system and in *in-vivo* rat studies, naphthalene caused lens opacity (3); cataract formation can be modified by concomitant administration of an aldose reductase inhibitor (5,6).

REFERENCES

1. Bastani JB, Blose IL (1976) Neuropsychiatric studies of drinkers of denatured alcohol. *Dis Nerv Syst* **37**, 683.
2. Kleinfeld M, Messite J, Swencicki R (1972) Clinical effects of chlorinated naphthalene exposure. *J Occup Med* **14**, 377.
3. Lubek BM, Kubow S, Basu PK *et al.* (1989) Cataractogenicity and bioactivation of naphthalene derivatives in lens culture and *in vivo*. *Lens Eye Toxic Res* **6**, 203.
4. Orzalesi N, Migliavacca L, Miglior S (1994) Subretinal neovascularization after naphthalene damage to the rabbit retina. *Invest Ophthalmol Vis Sci* **35**, 696.
5. Siegel E, Wason S (1986) Mothball toxicity. *Pediat Clin N Amer* **33**, 369.
6. Tao RV, Takahashi Y, Kador PF (1991) Effect of aldose reductase inhibitors on naphthalene cataract formation in the rat. *Invest Ophthalmol Vis Sci* **32**, 1630.

1-Naphthylacetyl Spermine

Nobufumi Kawai

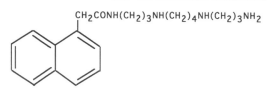

NAPHTHYLACETYL SPERMINE
C$_{22}$H$_{34}$N$_4$O

NEUROTOXICITY RATING

Experimental

A Glutamate receptor blocker (Ca^{2+}-permeable AMPA type)

1-Naphthylacetyl spermine (Naspm) is a synthesized analog of a spider toxin (Joro spider toxin, JSTX). At the crustacean neuromuscular synapse, Naspm blocks excitatory postsynaptic potentials and glutamate potentials with an EC$_{50}$ of 10 μmol. The potency is 1.0–1.5 orders less than JSTX-3, but the effect is reversible (2,4) (*see* JSTX-3, this volume).

In cultured hippocampal neurons, Naspm (100 μmol) reversibly blocks both kainate- and quisqualate-activated currents in a noncompetitive manner. Noise analysis of quisqualate- and kainate-induced currents shows that single-channel conductances are reduced, whereas the mean time constants are increased by Naspm. The results indicate that Naspm exerts its blocking action on non–N-methyl-D-aspartate (NMDA) receptor channels through effects on both single-channel conductance and kinetics (7).

In the mammalian CNS, Naspm suppresses glutamatergic transmission in the pontine reticular formation (8). Excitatory postsynaptic potentials in Purkinje cells, evoked by stimulation of parallel fibers in rat cerebellar slices, are effectively blocked by Naspm, but the responses evoked by climbing-fiber stimulation are unaffected (1).

Naspm is effective in inhibiting convulsions of rats (3). Intraventricular injection (5–20 μg) blocks quisqualate-induced epileptic discharges in the rat dorsal hippocampus. Pretreatment with Naspm inhibits quisqualate-induced hippocampal discharges and generalized tonic-clonic seizures in a dose-dependent manner. The agent has no effect on seizures mediated by NMDA receptors.

Patch recordings from CA1 pyramidal neurons in gerbil hippocampal slices revealed that Naspm depresses the excitatory postsynaptic currents (EPSCs) mediated by non-NMDA receptor channels. Naspm (50–200 μmol) reduced EPSC amplitude to 60%–90% of control. A further reduction of EPSCs occurred with the addition of 6-cyano-7-nitroquinoxaline-2,3-dione (CNQX), a competitive antagonist of the glutamate receptor. Conversely, when CNQX was applied first, no further depression of EPSCs was obtained upon addition of Naspm, indicating that Naspm blocks a fraction of the CNQX-sensitive non-NMDA receptor-mediated currents.

In a gerbil model of ischemia, CA1 pyramidal neurons were selectively damaged after transient forebrain ischemia by 5-min occlusion of the carotid arteries (5). Twenty-four to 36 h after ischemia, a great majority of postischemic CA1 pyramidal neurons elicited Ca^{2+}-dependent EPSCs with a slow time course (9). Naspm depressed these slow EPSCs in postischemic neurons more strongly than those in control neurons. Analysis of single-channel currents by outside-out patch-clamp recording from ischemic CA1 neurons revealed that Naspm blocks a subpopulation of α-amino-3-hydroxy-5-methylisoxazole-4-propionate (AMPA) and kainate-induced single-channel currents. Since the excitatory postsynaptic currents in CA1 neurons following ischemia are mediated by Ca^{2+}-permeable, non-NMDA receptor-mediated conductances (10), this indicates that Naspm is effective in blocking abnormal EPSCs, which may induce Ca^{2+} accumulation leading to delayed neuronal death after transient ischemia (*see also* 6).

REFERENCES

1. Ajima A, Hensch T, Kado RT, Ito M (1991) Differential blocking action of Joro spider toxin analog on parallel fiber and climbing fiber synapses in cerebellar Purkinje cells. *Neurosci Res* **12**, 281.
2. Asami T, Kagechika H, Hashimoto Y *et al.* (1989) Acylpolyamines mimic the action of Joro spider toxin (JSTX) on crustacean muscle glutamate receptors. *Biomed Res* **10**, 185.
3. Kanai H, Ishida N, Nakajima T, Kato M (1992) An analogue of Joro spider toxin selectively suppresses hippocampal epileptic discharges induced by quisqualate. *Brain Res* **581**, 161.
4. Kawai N (1991) Spider toxin and pertussis toxin differentiate post- and presynaptic glutamate receptors. *Neurosci Res* **12**, 3.
5. Kirino T (1982) Delayed neuronal death in the gerbil hippocampus following ischemia. *Brain Res* **239**, 57.
6. Koike M, Iino M, Ozawa S (1997) Blocking effect of 1-naphthyl acetyl spermine on Ca(2+)-permeable AMPA receptors in cultured rat hippocampal neurons. *Neurosci Res* **29**, 27.
7. Sahara Y, Robinson HPC, Miwa A *et al.* (1990) Blocking mechanisms of a JSTX analogue on kainate and quisqualate-activated currents in cultured hippocampal neurons. *Jpn J Physiol* **40**, S10.
8. Shimamura M, Fuwa T, Tanaka I (1990) Crossed forelimb extension produced in thalamic cats by injection of putative transmitter substances into the paralemniscal pontine reticular formation. *Brain Res* **524**, 282.
9. Tsubokawa H, Oguro K, Masuzawa T, Kawai N (1994) Ca^{2+}-dependent non-NMDA receptor-mediated synaptic currents in ischemic CA1 hippocampal neurons. *J Neurophysiol* **71**, 1190.
10. Tsubokawa H, Oguro K, Masuzawa T *et al.* (1995) Effects of a spider toxin and its analogue on glutamate-activated currents in the hippocampal CA1 neuron after ischemia. *J Neurophysiol* **74**, 218.

Naproxen

Herbert H. Schaumburg

NAPROXEN
$C_{14}H_{14}O_3$

(S)-6-Methoxy-α-methyl-2-naphthaleneacetic acid

NEUROTOXICITY RATING

Clinical

A Ototoxicity

A Aseptic meningitis

B Peripheral neuropathy

C Chronic encephalopathy

Naproxen is a well-tolerated, nonsteroidal anti-inflammatory agent. It is one of a group of propionic acid-derived, aspirin-like agents available over-the-counter in North America. The anti-inflammatory properties of the propionic acid derivatives stem from their ability to inhibit prostaglandin biosynthesis. Orally administered naproxen is rapidly absorbed; peak concentrations in plasma are achieved within 2–4 h. Plasma half-life is 14 h, much greater than that of other propionic acid derivatives; it may be twofold increased in the elderly, and this may require dose adjustment. The drug is extensively bound to plasma proteins and slowly passes into synovial spaces where it may remain as the plasma level declines. Naproxen is rapidly excreted in urine as the glucuronide or as other conjugates. Naproxen therapy is associated with few serious systemic side effects: gastrointestinal distress is experienced by about 10%; serious renal impairment and agranulocytosis are rare (5).

Side effects of naproxen include tinnitus and transient hearing loss. Sudden sensorineural hearing loss may accompany naproxen therapy at conventional doses. Impaired renal function or autoimmune disease may have been contributing factors in some instances. Recovery has been variable. Permanent sensorineural hearing loss is reported in a healthy individual who had only a brief course of naproxen (4). One report suggests the ototoxic lesion is in the outer layer of the cochlear hair cells commencing in the basal turns, analogous to the site of dysfunction caused by ethacrynic acid (1).

Aseptic meningitis is a major CNS adverse effect of nonsteroidal anti-inflammatory agents, especially in instances of impaired immunity. There is only one report of recurrent bouts of naproxen-induced aseptic meningitis; it occurred in a patient with lupus erythematosus (7).

Peripheral neuropathy is described in a patient with psoriatic arthritis receiving hydroxychloroquine and naproxen (6). Sensory symptoms commenced in the hands, unusual for a toxic distal axonopathy, and eventually involved all distal limbs. Symptoms and electrodiagnostic evidence of dysfunction improved following removal from therapy and reappeared when naproxen was again instituted. Despite

the presence of a connective tissue disease and an agent associated with neuropathy (hydroxychloroquine) in this case, the exacerbation of findings clearly linked to naproxen is reason to consider this as a possible, albeit unproven, neurotoxic effect. This notion is somewhat supported by allegations of an indomethacin sensory neuropathy characterized by initial symptoms in the upper limbs (2).

Cognitive decline in elderly arthritic patients receiving naproxen therapy for variable times is reported in one cross-sectional study; however, formal cognitive tests were not performed (3). A subsequent prospective study of 12 elderly patients receiving 750 mg/day of naproxen for 3 weeks demonstrated no cognitive decline (8). The conclusions of this report must be considered strongly because a complete battery of cognitive tests was administered to each subject, both at study commencement and termination.

REFERENCES

1. Chapman B (1982) Naproxen and sudden hearing loss. *J Laryngol Otol* **96**, 133.
2. Eade OE, Acheson ED, Cuthbert MF, Hawkes CH (1975) Peripheral neuropathy and indomethacin. *Brit Med J* **2**, 66.
3. Goodwin JS, Regan M (1982) Cognitive dysfunction associated with naproxen and ibuprofen in the elderly. *Arthritis Rheum* **25**, 103.
4. McKinnon BJ, Lassen LF (1998) Naproxen-associated sudden sensorineural hearing loss. *Mil Med* **163**, 792.
5. O'Brien WM, Bagby GF (1984) Rare adverse reactions to nonsteroidal antiinflammatory drugs. *J Rheumatol* **12**, 785.
6. Rothenberg RJ, Sufit RL (1987) Drug-induced peripheral neuropathy in a patient with psoriatic arthritis. *Arthritis Rheum* **30**, 221.
7. Weksler BB, Lehany AM (1991) Naproxen-induced recurrent aseptic meningitis. *Drug Intel Clin Pharmacol* **25**, 1183.
8. Wysenbeek AJ, Klein Z, Nakar S, Mane R (1988) Assessment of cognitive function in elderly patients treated with naproxen. A prospective study. *Clin Exp Rheumatol* **6**, 399.

Neosurugatoxin

Albert C. Ludolph

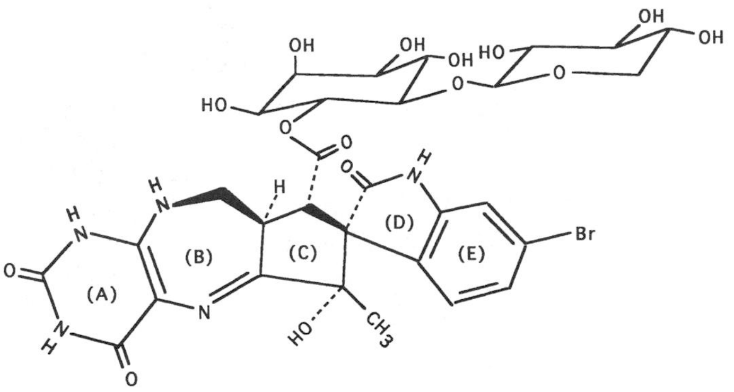

NEOSURUGATOXIN
$C_{33}H_{34}N_5O_{15}Br$

NEUROTOXICITY RATING

Experimental

A   Nicotinic antagonist

Surugatoxin and neosurugatoxin (NSTX) are glycosides from the Japanese ivory mollusc, *Babylonia japonica*, named after the Suraga bay where the compounds were first detected (7,8). *B. japonica* may also be contaminated with tetrodotoxin. The heat-labile colorless powder neosuruga-toxin is unstable under alkaline conditions, has a MW of 802, and is 100-fold more potent than suragatoxin (7), which was isolated earlier. In 1981, investigators obtained 4 mg of powder from 20 kg of shellfish (7).

Studies of the experimental neurotoxicity of NSTX showed that the compound competitively blocks nicotinic neurotransmission in autonomic ganglia of the rat (3) but no effect was seen under physiological conditions on neuromuscular transmission (5,6,9). However, at higher concentrations, a response characteristic of a competitive nicotinic antagonist has been described at the postsynaptic receptor (6). Concentrations used to show effects in the CNS were about 1% of those that influenced neuromuscular transmission: At 70–80 nM, the compound has a selective effect on CNS nicotinic receptors, since it inhibits binding of ^{3}H-nicotine to nicotinic sites in rat brain (5,9), but does not interfere with ^{125}I-α-bungarotoxin binding or muscarine binding (2,5). Several functional studies have also demonstrated the selectivity of this effect of NSTX on nicotinic CNS receptors (4). It has also been reported that neosurugatoxin blocks nicotinic acetylcholine receptors in both insect and nematode (1,8).

Toxin levels in *B. japonica* vary seasonally and may be the product of bacterial contamination. Symptoms of human poisoning by contaminated ivory shells include the presence of a gastrointestinal syndrome with nausea, vomiting, diarrhea, and also mydriasis, amblyopia, bladder disturbances, and even impairment of consciousness. The intoxication is reversible.

REFERENCES

1. Bai D, Sattelle DB (1993) Neosurugatoxin blocks an alpha-bungarotoxin-sensitive neuronal nicotinic acetylcholine receptor. *Arch Insect Biochem Physiol* **23**, 161.
2. Billiar RB, Kalash J, Romita V *et al.* (1988) Neosurugatoxin: CNS acetylcholine receptors and luteinizing hormone secretion in ovariectomized rats. *Brain Res Bull* **20**, 315.
3. Brown DA, Garthwaite J, Hayashi E, Yamada S (1976) Action of surugatoxin on nicotinic receptors in the superior cervical ganglion of the rat. *Brit J Pharmacol* **58**, 157.
4. Chiappinelli VA (1993) Neurotoxins acting on acetylcholine receptors. In: *Natural and Synthetic Neurotoxins*. Harvey A ed. Academic Press, London p. 65.
5. Hayashi E, Yamada S (1975) Pharmacological studies on surugatoxin, the toxic principle from Japanese ivory mollusc (*Babylonia japonica*). *Brit J Pharmacol* **53**, 207.
6. Hong SJ, Tsuji K, Chang CC (1992) Inhibition by neosurugatoxin and omega-conotoxin of acetylcholine release and muscle and neuronal nicotinic receptors in mouse neuromuscular junction. *Neuroscience* **48**, 727.
7. Kosuge T, Tsuji K, Hirai K (1982) Isolation of neosurugatoxin from the Japanese ivory shell, *Babylonia japonica*. *Chem Pharm Bull* **30**, 3255.
8. Tornoe C, Bai D, Holden-Dye L *et al.* (1995) Actions of neurotoxins (bungarotoxins, neosurugatoxin and lophotoxins) on insect and nematode nicotinic acetylcholine receptors. *Toxicon* **33**, 411.
9. Yamada S, Isogai M, Kagawa Y *et al.* (1985) Brain nicotinic acetylcholine receptors. Biochemical characterization by neosurugatoxin. *Mol Pharmacol* **28**, 120.

Nereistoxin and Related Compounds

William R. Kem

NEREISTOXIN
C5H11NS2

4-*N,N*-Dimethylamino-1,2-dithiolane

NEUROTOXICITY RATING

Experimental

A Nicotinic receptor antagonist

Nereistoxin (NTX) occurs in a marine worm (*Lumbriconereis heteropoda*) found along the coast of Japan. Although this toxin was initially isolated in the 1930s (9), fisherman had known for a long time that the animal is toxic because they sometimes suffered respiratory depression, headaches, and nausea when using the worm as bait (7). Flies that consume the flesh of this worm quickly die. The structure of NTX was reported almost 30 years later (10). Many analogs of NTX have been synthesized for use as agricultural insecticides (5). NTX is a unique compound because it possesses a ring containing a disulfide bond (4).

Cartap, Bancol, and Padan are the commercial insecticidal forms of NTX in which the disulfide bond is replaced with 2 thiocarbamoyl, benzenesulfonyl, or thioester groups, respectively. These thiol-protecting groups can be hydrolyzed to yield the reduced form of NTX, which then spontaneously oxidizes upon contact with air to NTX. The pesticidal and toxic actions of these commercial insecticides are largely due to their conversion to nereistoxin within the organism.

NTX is a nicotinic receptor antagonist. In contrast with most insecticides, NTX depresses insect motor activity prior to paralysis (11,15). The toxin is a particularly effective insecticide on lepidopteran (moths and butterflies) larvae such as the rice stem borer, an economically important pest in Asian countries with large rice plantings (14).

A relatively small lipophilic molecule, NTX readily enters the CNS and other tissues of insects and vertebrates. Little is known about the biotransformation and mode of excretion of NTX. The toxic actions of NTX upon vertebrates are primarily due to its ability to act as an antagonist at skeletal muscle nicotinic receptors (1–3). The major target organ is the skeletal muscle neuromuscular synapse, and vertebrate species die from peripheral respiratory depression. The mouse LD_{50} for nereistoxin is 118 mg/kg, while

the rat LD_{50} is 420 mg/kg. The corresponding values for Cartap are 165 and 250 mg/kg, respectively (6).

The commercial insecticides apparently have little effect upon mammalian nicotinic receptors unless they are metabolized to NTX (7). This is the likely basis for the long latency between administration and onset of effects in animals.

Administration of a relatively low dose of NTX causes peripherally induced respiratory depression at the neuromuscular junction, while higher dosage (10 mg/kg) additionally causes a variety of CNS effects. Tonic convulsions accompanied by electroencephalographic seizure discharges were observed in the cat (1). Mono- and polysynaptic reflexes were inhibited in the cat spinal cord, and ventral root neuron activity increased when tremors appeared. Signs of autonomic excitation, including enhancement of intestinal motility, lacrimation, salivation, and tachycardia (small doses) or bradycardia (larger doses), have been observed at high doses (7,10,12).

Several *in-vitro* electrophysiological studies of NTX have been reported. In the frog sartorius-phrenic nerve preparation, NTX reduced the sensitivity of the muscle postsynaptic membrane to nerve stimulation or iontophoretically applied acetylcholine (ACh) (2). No depolarizing action of NTX was reported. However, some depression of presynaptic function was observed; namely, a decrease in quantal content (the number of packets of neurotransmitter released per nerve action potential) and a decrease in miniature endplate potential frequency. These changes in presynaptic activity were relatively minor in comparison to the curare-like muscle relaxant action on the skeletal muscle membrane.

Electrophysiological observations were combined with radioligand binding to investigate the action of NTX on three different neuromuscular preparations (3): frog sartorius, rat phrenic nerve-diaphragm muscle, and electric organ from *Torpedo californica*. At 0.1 mM, NTX caused an initial postsynaptic depolarization of about 20 mV at the frog neuromuscular junction, indicating a weak partial agonist action. Since the extrajunctional membrane was not depolarized, this effect was likely mediated through the postsynaptic membrane receptors. No significant presynaptic action of NTX was observed. While NTX was able to block the binding of radiolabeled ACh and α-bungarotoxin to the ACh-recognition sites on the *Torpedo* receptor with a K_I of 0.15 mM, it did not interfere with the binding of radiolabeled histrionicotoxin, which binds to another site within the nicotinic-receptor ion channel. The rat diaphragm preparation was almost 100 times less sensitive to

NTX than the frog neuromuscular junction. The curarimimetic effect of NTX was difficult to reverse in both preparations, even after 2 h of washing with physiological saline.

It has been proposed that NTX becomes covalently attached to one or more sulfhydryl groups within the nicotinic receptor ACh recognition site (3). This hypothesis seems plausible, since it is known that there is a disulfide bond in the α-subunit of the ACh recognition site that can be reduced and even alkylated by bromoacetylcholine. In addition, blockade of nicotinic receptors in several *in vitro* preparations is very difficult to reverse by washing with saline, further suggesting that covalent bond attachment by NTX to the receptor occurs (13,16).

No human studies of NTX intoxication have been reported. Pharmacological treatment of humans exposed to NTX and its insecticidal forms can be expected to rely upon enhancement of peripheral neuromuscular cholinergic function by administration of acetylcholinesterase inhibitors like physostigmine and neostigmine. Several strategies for treating NTX intoxication were tested on experimental animals, including acetylcholinesterase inhibitors, muscarinic and nicotinic agonists, and disulfide-bond-reducing agents. Physostigmine and neostigmine were found to be most effective, as predicted for a compound like NTX that acts primarily like a competitive antagonist, similar to tubocurarine, gallamine, and other nondepolarizing muscle relaxants (1,12). Muscarinic and nicotinic agonists were not effective in restoring skeletal muscle function, and the ameliorating effects of the disulfide reductants were only temporary. Although the action of NTX on CNS sites is not so clear, one should probably administer physostigmine rather than neostigmine because of the greater ability of the former compound to pass across the blood-brain and blood-spinal barriers.

Editors' Note: Receptor blockade induced by NTX (100 μM, 2–10 min) is reproduced by dithiothreitol (2 mM, 20 min) in the intact chick ciliary ganglion, suggesting that NTX acts both as an antagonist and a reducing agent at nicotinic receptors (16,17). The receptor-reducing action of NTX appears to be due to an unidentified NTX metabolite, such as dihydronereistoxin (17). A new gas chromatography-mass spectrometry method for the detection of NTX in human serum was applied to a patient who attempted suicide with a herbicide containing 4% cartap hydrochloride, an analogue of NTX. Serum [NTX] in this individual ranged from 0.09–2.69 μg/ml (8).

REFERENCES

1. Chiba S, Nagawa Y (1971) Effects of nereistoxin and its derivatives on the spinal cord and motor nerve terminals. *Jpn J Pharmacol* 21, 175.

2. Deguchi T, Narahashi T, Haas HG (1971) Mode of action of nereistoxin on the neuromuscular transmission in the frog. *Pestic Biochem Physiol* 1, 196.

3. Eldefrawi AT, Bakry NM, Eldefrawi ME *et al.* (1979) Nereistoxin interaction with the acetylcholine receptor-ionic channel complex. *Mol Pharmacol* 17, 172.

4. Hashimoto Y, Okaichi T (1960) Some chemical properties of nereistoxin. *Ann N Y Acad Sci* 90, 667.

5. Konishi K (1968) New insecticidally active derivatives of nereistoxin. *Ag Biol Chem* 32, 678.

6. Konishi K (1970) Synthesis of nereistoxin and related compounds. *Ag Biol Chem* 34, 935.

7. Nagawa Y, Saji Y, Chiba S, Yu T (1971) Neuromuscular blocking actions of nereistoxin and its derivatives and antagonism by sulfhydryl compounds. *Jpn J Pharmacol* 21, 185.

8. Namera A, Watanabe T, Yashiki M *et al.* (1999) Simple and sensitive analysis of nereistoxin and its metabolites in human serum using headspace solid-phase microextraction and gas chromatography-mass spectrometry. *Chromatogr Sci* 37, 77.

9. Nitta S (1934) Über Nereistoxin, einen giftigen Bestandteil von *Lumbriconereis heteropoda* Marenz (Eunicidae). *Yakagaku Zasshi* 54, 648.

10. Okaichi T, Hashimoto Y (1962) The structure of nereistoxin. *Ag Biol Chem* 26, 224.

11. Sattelle DB, Harrow ID, David JA *et al.* (1985) Nereistoxin: Actions on a CNS acetylcholine receptor/ion channel in the cockroach *Periplaneta americana*. *J Exp Biol* 118, 37.

12. Schopp RT, DeClue RT (1980) Paralytic properties of 4-N,N-dimethylamino-1,2-dithiolane (Nereistoxin). *Arch Int Pharmacodyn* 248, 166.

13. Sherby SM, Eldefrawi AT, David JA *et al.* (1986) Interactions of charatoxins and nereistoxin with the nicotinic acetylcholine receptors of insect CNS and *Torpedo* electric organ. *Arch Insect Biochem Physiol* 3, 431.

14. Tomizawa C, Kazano H (1979) Environmental fate of rice paddy pesticides in a model ecosystem. *J Environ Sci Health B-Pestic* 14, 121.

15. Tomizawa M, Otsuka H, Miyamoto T *et al.* (1995) Pharmacological characteristics of insect nicotinic acetylcholine receptor with its ion channel and the comparison of the effect of nicotinoids and neonicotinoids. *J Pestic Sci* 20, 57.

16. Xie Y, Lane WV, Loring RH (1993) Nereistoxin: A naturally occurring toxin with redox effects on neuronal nicotinic acetylcholine receptors in chick retina. *J Pharmacol Exp Ther* 264, 689.

17. Xie Y, McHugh T, McKay J *et al.* (1996) Evidence that a nereistoxin metabolite, and not nereistoxin itself, reduces neuronal nicotinic receptors: studies in the whole chick ciliary ganglion, on isolated neurons and immunoprecipitated receptors. *J Pharmacol Exp Ther* 276, 169.

Nicotine

John C.M. Brust

NICOTINE
$C_{10}H_{14}N_2$

β-Pyridyl-α-N-methylpyrrolidine

NEUROTOXICITY RATING

Clinical

A   Acute encephalopathy (tremor seizures, agitation, coma)

A   Physical dependence and withdrawal

B   Encephalomalacia (occlusive, hemorrhagic)

Experimental

A   Nicotinic stimulation and blockade

A   Acute encephalopathy (agitation, tremor)

A natural alkaloid present in leaves of the tobacco plant (*Nicotiana tabacum*), as well as in other *Nicotiana* and *Datura* species, nicotine is the addicting substance of tobacco (1,13,16). Its complex pharmacological actions include both excitatory and inhibitory effects on autonomic ganglia, muscle, and the CNS. Most nicotine addicts are cigarette smokers, but cigars, pipes, and "smokeless tobacco" (snuff or chewing) also deliver addicting quantities of nicotine (2). Since 1964, when the first of several reports by the United States Surgeon General described the health consequences of smoking, the prevalence of cigarette smoking has steadily declined, from two-thirds of adults to currently less than one-third (4,19). On the other hand, in an apparent response to promotional assaults targeted at children (7), nearly 20% of American high-school seniors are regular smokers, and "smokeless tobacco" has become increasingly popular among adolescents. It is claimed that the addictive potency of nicotine indirectly accounts for over 400,000 annual deaths in the United States—20%–25% of American mortality, and the major cause of preventable death in the industrialized world (3).

A colorless, bitter-tasting liquid, nicotine is used industrially and is present in some insecticides. Its therapeutic use—in chewing gum, skin patches, or nasal spray—is to assist smoking cessation.

Nicotine is readily absorbed through the oral or gastrointestinal mucosa, the skin, and the lung. Suspended on the hydrocarbon "tars" of cigarette smoke, it reaches the brain within 8 sec of inhalation. Similar amounts of nicotine are delivered to the brain by smokeless tobacco, cigars, and pipe tobacco; these forms of tobacco are more alkaline than cigarette tobacco, allowing greater absorption from the oral mucosa (2,3). Most American cigarettes contain about 9 mg of nicotine, of which 1 mg is absorbed during smoking. The elimination half-life of nicotine following inhalation or parenteral administration is about 2 h; with continuous smoking, there is accumulation. Most nicotine is metabolized in the liver, and the major metabolite, cotinine, has a half-life of 10–27 h. Pharmacologically inactive, cotinine is detectable in the urine for several days after smoking cessation. Nicotine is excreted in the milk of lactating mothers who smoke.

Nicotine causes nausea and vomiting by actions at both vagus nerve afferents and the medullary chemoreceptor trigger zone. It reduces appetite, and both reduced caloric intake and increased energy expenditure contribute to weight loss (15). Nicotine stimulates release of vasopressin.

Nicotine's pharmacological effects are biphasic: low doses stimulate nicotinic receptors; higher doses block them (21). CNS and PNS effects are complex. For example, heart rate may be increased or decreased depending on actions at sympathetic or parasympathetic ganglia at chemoreceptors of the carotid and aortic bodies, at medullary centers, and in the adrenal medulla. Human smokers and dogs receiving nicotine intravenously usually experience increased heart rate and blood pressure.

Nicotine initially stimulates the CNS. Low doses produce improved concentration and work performance; toxic doses induce tremor and then seizures, and very high doses cause CNS depression and respiratory failure. The electroencephalogram may show an alerting response. In muscle, stimulation is quickly overcome by inhibition, and toxic doses of nicotine cause paralysis.

Rodents, dogs, and monkeys self-administer nicotine, but its reinforcing properties are less powerful than those of cocaine (18,20). In tests of stimulus discrimination, animals generalize to nicotinic agonists but not to other drugs of abuse. As with other drugs, the limbic dopaminergic "reward circuit" [midbrain ventral tegmental area (VTA) to nucleus accumbens and medial prefrontal cortex] is crucial in nicotine reinforcement (5). Low doses of systemic nicotine release dopamine in the nucleus accumbens, nicotine injected directly into the VTA increases locomotion, and lesions of the nucleus accumbens block nicotine self-administration. Withdrawal after chronic administration in animals produces impaired attention and task performance, decreased heart rate and blood pressure, and slower frequencies on the electroencephalogram; however, except for jaw clenching in monkeys, a predictable prominent abstinence syndrome is not observed.

Human smokers experience increased alertness followed by relaxation, and they titrate nicotine intake to favor one phase or the other. Total smoking tends to decrease or increase as the nicotine content of tobacco rises or falls. Intravenous nicotine produces euphoria in smokers but not in nonsmokers, suggesting "sensitization" or "reverse tolerance" (10). Tolerance develops to dizziness, nausea, and vomiting, but not to tremor or increased heart rate and blood pressure. Rapid acquisition and loss of tolerance are reflected in the tendency of the first cigarette of the day to produce the greatest subjective arousal. Abstinence in nicotine addicts produces irritability, anxiety, depression, difficulty concentrating, drowsiness, fatigue, insomnia, headache, and reduced heart rate and blood pressure. Infrequently there is sweating, nausea, constipation, or diarrhea (12). The intense craving that occurs is not only out of proportion to other symptoms but often outlasts them by months or years. Most smokers who quit gain weight.

Some of the medical consequences of smoking (e.g., chronic obstructive pulmonary disease and cancer) are the result of exposure to substances in tobacco other than nicotine. In the case of coronary artery disease and stroke, nicotine may directly contribute; potential mechanisms include vasoconstriction, effects on platelets and fibrinogen, and accelerated atherosclerosis secondary to endothelial damage and influences on serum lipoproteins (3,6,17)

The rationale for treating nicotine addiction with nicotine gum or skin patches is that other toxic substances in tobacco are thereby eliminated. Intermittent therapy is recommended because potential problems attributable to nicotine itself remain, including coronary artery disease and stroke. Such treatment requires psychological support to be effective (22,23). Clonidine reduces nicotine craving, but its effectiveness decreases with time (8).

Acute nicotine poisoning occurs in small children who ingest tobacco. There is nausea, vomiting, salivation, lacrimation, tachypnea, hypertension, tachycardia, abdominal pain, diarrhea, sweating, headache, miosis, agitation, delirium, fasciculations, and weakness. Symptoms progress to bradycardia, hypotension, mydriasis, seizures, coma, and fatal respiratory arrest. Treatment includes gastric lavage, activated charcoal, ventilatory and blood-pressure support, atropine for parasympathetic overstimulation, and anticonvulsants for seizures (9).

Cigarette smoking during pregnancy leads to fetal growth retardation and spontaneous abortion. Low Apgar scores are associated with heavy maternal smoking, and some studies have found adverse effects on later child development, including IQ. As with other drugs, confounders include poor prenatal care, other substance abuse, and inadequate parenting. Whether smoking during pregnancy carries a risk of teratogenicity is controversial. Nicotine could contribute to the adverse effects of maternal smoking through placental vasoconstriction or through trophic effects on the developing brain (3,14).

Also controversial is whether smoking—and by implication nicotine—exerts a protective effect on the development of Parkinson's disease or Alzheimer's disease (11).

Through complex actions at CNS and PNS cholinergic receptors, nicotine can be fatally neurotoxic in overdose and is powerfully addicting when used in intended doses. It seems likely that nicotine's addictive liability accounts, in part, indirectly for the mortality and morbidity—vascular disease, pulmonary disease, and cancer—that afflict tobacco users, and by direct actions on blood vessels, it may contribute to myocardial infarction and stroke.

REFERENCES

1. Benowitz NL (1988) Pharmacologic aspects of cigarette smoking and nicotine addiction. *N Engl J Med* **319**, 1318.
2. Benowitz NL, Porchet H, Sheiner L, Jacob P III (1988) Nicotine absorption and cardiovascular effects with smokeless tobacco use: Comparison with cigarettes and nicotine gum. *Clin Pharmacol Ther* **44**, 23.
3. Brust JCM (1993) *Neurological Aspects of Substance Abuse*. Butterworth-Heinneman, Stoneham, Massachusetts p. 253.
4. Centers for Disease Control (1991) Cigarette smoking among adults—United States. *Morb Mortal Wkly Rep* **40**, 757.
5. Clarke PBS, Fu DS, Jakubovic A, Fibiger HC (1988) Evidence that mesolimbic dopaminergic activation underlies the locomotor stimulant action of nicotine in rats. *J Pharmacol Exp Ther* **246**, 701.
6. Dempsey RJ, Moore RW (1992) Amount of smoking independently predicts carotid artery atherosclerosis severity. *Stroke* **23**, 693.
7. DiFranza JR, Richards JW, Paulman PM *et al.* (1991) RJR Nabisco's cartoon camel promotes Camel cigarettes to children. *J Amer Med Assn* **266**, 3149.
8. Glassman AH, Stetner F, Walsh BT *et al.* (1988) Heavy smokers, smoking cessation, and clonidine. *J Amer Med Assn* **259**, 2863.
9. Goldfrank LR, Melinek M, Weisman RS (1990) Nicotine. In: *Toxicologic Emergencies. 4th Ed.* Goldfrank LR, Flomenbaum NE, Lewin NA *et al.* eds. Appleton & Lange, Norwalk, Connecticut p. 613.
10. Henningfield JE, Miyasato K, Jasinski DR (1983) Cigarette smokers self-inject intravenous nicotine. *Pharmacol Biochem Behav* **248**, 127.
11. Hofman A, van Duijn CM (1990) Alzheimer's disease,

Parkinson's disease, and smoking. *Neurobiol Aging* **11**, 295.

12. Hughes JR, Gust SW, Skoog K *et al.* (1991) Symptoms of tobacco withdrawal. *Arch Gen Psychiat* **48**, 52.

13. Jaffe JH (1990) Tobacco smoking and nicotine dependence. In: *Nicotine Psychopharmacology. Molecular, Cellular and Behavioral Aspects.* Wonnacot S, Russell MAH, Stolerman IP eds. Oxford University Press, Oxford p. 1.

14. Kunhert DB (1991) Drug exposure to the fetus. The effect of smoking. In: *Methodological Issues in Controlled Studies in Effects of Prenatal Exposure to Drug Abuse.* Kilbey MM, Ashgar K eds. National Institute on Drug Abuse Research Monograph 114, Department of Health and Human Services, Rockville, Maryland p. 1.

15. Perkins KA, Epstein LH, Marks BL *et al.* (1989) The effect of nicotine on energy expenditure during light physical activity. *N Engl J Med* **320**, 898.

16. Schelling TC (1992) Addictive drugs: The cigarette experience. *Science* **255**, 430.

17. Shinton R, Beevers G (1989) Meta-analysis of relation between cigarette smoking and stroke. *Brit Med J* **298**, 789.

18. Stolerman IP (1990) Behavioral pharmacology of nicotine in animals. In: *Nicotine Psychopharmacology. Molecular,*

Cellular, and Behavioral Aspects. Wonnacot S, Russell MAH, Stolerman IP eds. Oxford University Press, Oxford p. 278.

19. Surgeon General (1988) *The Health Consequences of Smoking. Nicotine Addiction.* (Office of Smoking and Health, eds.) Department of Health and Human Services, Centers for Disease Control Publ No 88-8406. U.S. Government Printing Office, Washington, DC.

20. Swedberg MDB, Henningfield JE, Goldberg SR (1990) Nicotine dependency: Animal studies. In: *Nicotine Psychopharmacology. Molecular, Cellular, and Behavioral Aspects.* Wonnacot S, Russell MAH, Stolerman IP eds. Oxford University Press, Oxford p. 38.

21. Taylor P (1990) Agents acting at the neuromuscular junction and autonomic ganglia. In: *The Pharmacological Basis of Therapeutics. 8th Ed.* Gilman AG, Rall TW, Nies AS, Taylor P eds. Pergamon Press, New York p. 166.

22. Tonnesen P, Fryd V, Hansen M *et al.* (1988) Effect of nicotine chewing gum in combination with group counseling on the cessation of smoking. *N Engl J Med* **318**, 15.

23. Tonnesen P, Norregaard J, Simonsen K, Sawe U (1991) A double-blind trial of 16-hour transdermal nicotine patch in smoking cessation. *N Engl J Med* **325**, 311.

Nifedipine

Steven A. Sparr

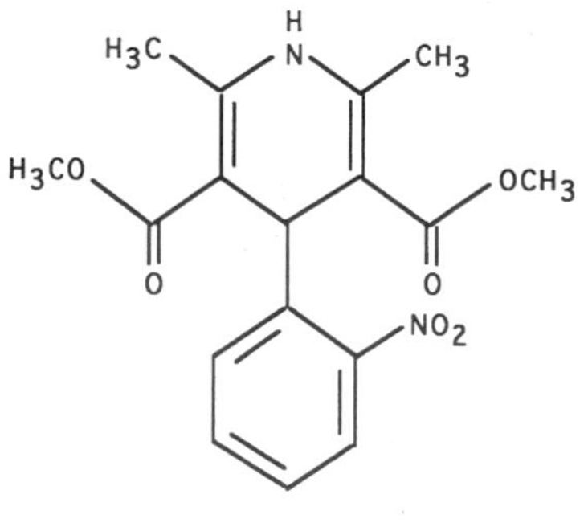

NIFEDIPINE
$C_{17}H_{18}N_2O_6$

1,4-Dihydro-2,6-dimethyl-4-(2-nitrophenyl)-3,5-pyridine-dicarboxylic acid dimethyl ester

NEUROTOXICOLOGY RATING

Clinical

A   Headache

B   Encephalomalacia (retinal ischemia)

B   Psychobiological reaction (depression)

Experimental

A   Ion channel dysfunction (L-type calcium channels)

Nifedipine, a dihydropyridine derivative, is a member of a class of drugs that acts by blocking the entry of calcium into cells of vascular smooth muscle and myocardium, the so-called calcium channel blockers. The drug has been used as an antihypertensive agent, as an antianginal agent, for migraine prophylaxis and treatment of primary pulmonary hypertension (16,18,19). The major effect of nifedipine on vascular smooth muscle is to inhibit Ca^{2+} flow through L-type voltage-dependent calcium channels. At higher concentration, the drug can also interfere with inward calcium current through receptor-mediated channels and with release of intracellular calcium stores from sarcoplasmic reticulum (16). The net effect of inhibition of calcium flux into the cytosol of the vascular smooth muscle cell is to inhibit muscle contraction, causing dilatation of peripheral and coronary arteries. In the heart, calcium channel antagonists inhibit the slow inward calcium current that contributes to the plateau phase of cardiac muscle depolarization, producing negative inotropic effects. Some calcium channel blockers, such as verapamil, also slow the recovery rate of the slow calcium channel, leading to decreased heart rate and slowing of conduction through the atrioventricular node; nifedipine does not have this property and thus has little effect on heart rate and atrioventricular nodal conduction (16). The drug is usually well tolerated, with headache and dizziness the only frequently experienced neurological side effects. Additional neurological side effects have been documented in case reports.

Nifedipine is well absorbed after oral administration, with 90% taken up from the gastrointestinal tract when the drug is taken with food (2). However, due to extensive first-pass metabolism by the liver, only 45%–75% of the drug reaches the systemic circulation (2). Peak plasma levels occur 30 min to 2 h after oral ingestion. The drug is 96% bound to plasma proteins (16). Nifedipine is metabolized in the liver to inactive metabolites that are primarily excreted in the urine. Half-life ranges from 2–5 h, and is as high as 7 h in patients with cirrhosis (2). The drug may also be administered sublingually for more rapid onset of action in hypertensive emergencies (6).

Nifedipine is usually well tolerated, although myocardial infarction, congestive heart failure, and ventricular arrhythmias have been reported; it is unclear if these complications are due to nifedipine or to underlying cardiac disease. Nifedipine can cause hypotension that is usually mild and well tolerated (2). Peripheral edema occurs in 10%–30% of patients, probably due to vasodilation of precapillary arterioles (2). Cases of phenytoin toxicity have been reported in patients after initiation of concomitant nifedipine therapy, possibly due to induction of diminished hepatic metabolism of phenytoin (2).

There are no animal models demonstrating direct neurotoxic effects of nifedipine.

The most frequent neurological symptoms associated with nifedipine therapy are headache and dizziness, experienced by up to 25% of patients (2). In a report from the World Health Organization Collaboration Center for International Drug Monitoring, nifedipine was implicated in causing headache in 434 patients, surpassed only by indomethacin in their series (3). Drug-related migraine headaches were reported in 13 cases (3). The authors suggested that the mechanism of headache production was peripheral vasodilation; they noted that headache was less commonly seen with less potent vasodilatory calcium channel blockers (3).

There are isolated case reports of cerebrovascular events associated with nifedipine therapy (7,8,15,16). One report describes two patients: one, a 72-year-old man with prior history of atrial fibrillation who developed aphasia and right hemiparesis on two occasions shortly after taking nifedipine; the other, a 67-year-old woman who had a syncopal spell with symptoms of drowsiness and vertigo after she regained consciousness (14).

In a study of the efficacy of sublingual nifedipine in 30 patients with hypertensive emergencies, one patient developed aphasia and hemiparesis that worsened 15 min following nifedipine administration (6). A 32-year-old woman had rupture of a posterior communicating artery aneurysm after her second dose of oral nifedipine (7). It was speculated that vasodilation of the cerebral circulation caused increased blood flow through the aneurysmal vessel and also increased wall stress, leading to rupture of the aneurysm. A 67-year-old male patient with angina developed ischemia of the left retina, confirmed by ophthalmoscopy and tangent screen testing, after increasing the nifedipine dose from 10 mg *q.i.d.* to 20 mg *q.i.d* (15). After the first dose of 20 mg, he experienced loss of visual acuity in the left eye, which improved, but this recurred with rechallenge of that dose. The authors speculated that the patient had an atherosclerotic left ophthalmic artery that did not dilate with nifedipine, whereas the remainder of the cerebral circulation responded to the medication, causing a "steal" phenomenon.

Myoclonus with dystonic features was described in a 35-year-old man treated with nifedipine for asthma, on the assumption the drug may prevent histamine-induced bronchoconstriction (4). Ten days after initiating therapy, the patient developed involuntary head movements and myoclonic twitching of the limbs. Symptoms resolved after 24 h. Similar symptoms have been reported with verapamil therapy (8,11).

A 62-year-old developed agitation and akathisia that responded to cessation of the drug (1). Akathisia has also been reported in a patient taking diltiazem (10), another calcium channel blocker. The author speculated these effects may be due to drug-induced depletion of the enzyme dopamine-β-hydroxylase (1).

Four patients developed depression during the first week of nifedipine therapy (5,9). Symptoms were resistant to tricyclic antidepressants but resolved within a week of discontinuing the drug. The authors suggested that nifedipine may blunt the effects of norepinephrine in neuronal transmission that depend on "second messenger"–induced calcium uptake. A similar case was reported (4). No significant disturbances of mood were present in a series of patients who received extensive serial neuropsychometric testing while on nifedipine (16).

Subtle impairments of cognition in an elderly population treated with nifedipine were detected in one study (17). Designed as a double-blind crossover study, with serial neuropsychometric testing, 31 hypertensive patients over the age of 65 were treated with nifedipine and atenolol, a β-blocker. Patients treated with nifedipine demonstrated a 9% decrease in recall score on the Buschke selective-reminding test and worsened on their scores on the digit-symbol test.

There were no significant differences in performance on other neuropsychological tests, including those that measure verbal fluency, abstract reasoning, or psychomotor ability. The authors concluded that nifedipine can cause subtle learning and memory impairments in the elderly.

Severe muscle cramping in the lower extremities and occasionally in the upper extremities was observed in three patients with ischemic cardiac disease treated with nifedipine (12). Symptoms resolved after discontinuing the drug, and recurred in two patients rechallenged with the drug.

Muscle fatigue is common in patients treated with calcium channel blockers (17) although, in patients without underlying neuromuscular disease, electrophysiological testing remains normal (13). A single case of muscle strength deterioration was reported in a patient with Lambert-Eaton syndrome after the subject started treatment with verapamil (13), another calcium channel blocker.

Sleep disturbances have been associated with nifedipine treatment (2). As with all purported CNS side effects of nifedipine, the underlying mechanism is unknown.

REFERENCES

1. Ahmad S (1984) Nifedipine-induced acute psychosis. *J Amer Geriat Soc* **32**, 408.
2. *American Hospital Formulary Service Drug Information* (1995), McEvoy GK ed. American Society of Health System Pharmacists p. 1116.
3. Ashmark H, Lundberg PO, Olsson S (1989) Drug-related headache. *Headache* **29**, 441.
4. De Medina A, Biasini O, Rivera A, Sampera A (1986) Nifedipine and myoclonic dystonia. *Ann Intern Med* **104**, 125.
5. Eccleston D, Cole AJ (1990) Calcium channel blockade and depressive illness. *Brit J Psychiat* **156**, 889.
6. Ellrodt AG, Ault MJ, Reidinger MS, Murata HH (1985) Efficacy and safety of sublingual nifedipine in hypertensive emergencies. *Amer J Med* **79**, 19.
7. Gill JS, Zezulka AV, Horrocks PM (1986) Rupture of a cerebral aneurysm associated with nifedipine treatment. *Postgrad Med J* **62**, 1029.
8. Hicks CB, Abraham K (1985) Verapamil and myoclonic dystonia. *Ann Intern Med* **103**, 154.
9. Hullett FJ, Potkin SG, Levy AB, Ciasca R (1988) Depression associated with nifedipine-induced calcium channel blockade. *Amer J Psychiat* **145**, 1277.
10. Jacobs MB (1983) Diltiazem and akathesia. *Ann Intern Med* **99**, 794.
11. Jacobsen FM, Sack DA, James SP (1987) Delirium induced by verapamil. *Amer J Psychiat* **144**, 248.
12. Keidar S, Binenboim C, Palant A (1982) Muscle cramps during treatment with nifedipine. *Brit Med J* **285**, 1241.
13. Krendel DA, Hopkins LC (1986) Adverse effect of verapamil in a patient with the Lambert-Eaton syndrome. *Muscle Nerve* **9**, 519.
14. Nobile-Orazio E, Sterzl R (1981) Cerebral ischaemia after nifedipine treatment. *Brit Med J* **283**, 948.
15. Pitlick S, Manor KS, Lipshitz I et al. (1983) Transient retinal ischaemia induced by verapamil. *Brit Med J* **287**, 1845.
16. Robertson RM, Robertson D (1996) Drugs used for the treatment of myocardial ischemia. In: *The Pharmacologic Basis of Therapeutics. 9th Ed.* Hardman JG, Goodman AG, Limbird LE eds. McGraw-Hill, New York p. 759.
17. Skinner MH, Futterman A, Morrissette D et al. (1992) Atenolol compared with nifedipine: Effect on cognitive function and mood in elderly hypertensive patients. *Ann Intern Med* **116**, 615.
18. Vacek JL (1984) Nifedipine and primary pulmonary hypertension. *Ann Intern Med* **100**, 459.
19. van Zwieten PA (1998) The pharmacological properties of lipophilic calcium antagonists. *Blood Press Suppl* **2**, 5.

Nitrobenzene

John L. O'Donoghue

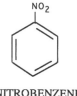

NITROBENZENE
C₆H₅NO₂

Nitrobenzol; Oil of mirbane; Essence of mirbane

NEUROTOXICITY RATING

Clinical

B   Acute encephalopathy (sedation, confusion)

C   Peripheral neuropathy

Experimental

A   Cerebellar degeneration (myelinic vacuolation)

Nitrobenzene is a volatile, oily, pale yellow to colorless liquid. An almond-like odor has led to its use in soaps, polishes, leather dressings, and paint solvents where it serves to mask other odors. It is also used as a solvent and chemical intermediate in the manufacture of explosives, aniline, benzidine, benzidine and aniline-based dyes, acetaminophen, and other chemicals.

Toxic effects of primary concern in the workplace are methemoglobinemia, hemolytic anemia, and liver toxicity. A Threshold Limit Value of 1 ppm with a skin notation has been adopted by the American Conference of Governmental Industrial Hygienists to prevent methemoglobinemia and related effects (1). Nitrobenzene is readily absorbed through the skin and by other routes of exposure. At exposure concentrations of 1 or 5.5 ppm, half of an absorbed dose in humans could be due to percutaneous absorption (13). It is retained in the body following exposure. Among a group of human volunteers who inhaled nitrobenzene at 6 ppm for 6 h, 73%–87% of the inhaled dose was retained and, 100 h after a single 1-h exposure, a nitrophenol metabolite was still present in the urine (14). Nitrobenzene is metabolically reduced to p-nitrophenol and conjugated with glucuronide or sulfuric acid (3). Nitrobenzene can also undergo nitroreduction to nitrosobenzene and/or phenylhydroxylamine. Other metabolites that have been identified in experimental animals include aniline, nitrophenols, aminophenols, 4-hydroxyanilide, 4-hydroxyacetanilide sulfate, 4-nitrophenyl sulfate, and 3-nitrophenyl sulfate (3). p-Nitrophenol and p-aminophenol have been identified in the urine of humans exposed to nitrobenzene (8,14). In one case of intoxication with nitrobenzene, a woman excreted these two metabolites for 2 weeks after exposure; clinical signs (including headache, nausea, vertigo, and numbness of the legs) resolved as the concentrations of the metabolites decreased in urine (8). The metabolism of nitrobenzene depends on species and animal strain; route of exposure may play a significant role in its toxicity (11). Metabolism by intestinal bacteria plays an important role in the metabolism of nitrobenzene; in germ-free rats, methemoglobinemia is not produced by nitrobenzene exposure (3,15). The role of metabolism in nitrobenzene-induced neurotoxicity in experimental animals has not been investigated.

Signs of cerebellar and vestibular impairment predominate in animals treated with nitrobenzene. Acute signs of CNS damage include nystagmus, opisthotonos, loss of righting reflexes, tremor, paralysis, and coma (2,12,16). Cerebellar Purkinje cell degeneration has been described in dogs, chickens, and pigeons exposed to nitrobenzene; however, this effect may be secondary or related to anoxia (2). The more common lesion associated with nitrobenzene is focal malacia or extensive focal vacuolization in the cerebellar peduncle of rats (4,12) and the medulla oblongata of rats and rabbits (10).

Sensitivity to the neurotoxic effects of nitrobenzene varies according to the species and strain of animal tested and the route of exposure. Mice and Sprague-Dawley rats exposed to 10–125 ppm nitrobenzene vapor for 6 h/day, 5 days/ week, for 2 weeks showed signs of altered respiration and prostration after 2–4 days of exposure, and increased mortality (11). At 125 ppm nitrobenzene, mice and rats had perivascular hemorrhages in the cerebellar peduncles. Fischer 344 (F344) rats exposed under identical conditions did not develop similar cerebellar lesions or hepatic and pulmonary effects observed in mice and Sprague-Dawley rats (11).

The resistance of F344 rats to nitrobenzene-induced cerebellar damage can be overcome by gavage administration. Among groups of F344 rats given 50–450 mg/kg nitrobenzene orally, one animal treated with 450 mg/kg had microscopic cerebellar lesions (4). Gavage administration of nitrobenzene also produced hepatic and testicular lesions in F344 rats; similar lesions were not observed in F344 rats that had inhaled nitrobenzene (4,11).

Light and electron microscopic observations of cerebellar lesions induced in male F344 rats by single oral doses of 550 mg/kg nitrobenzene revealed petechial hemorrhages in the brainstem and cerebellum, and malacia in the cerebellum and cerebellar peduncles within 48 h of dose administration (12). Malacia was attributed to the accumulation of fluid within unidentified membrane-bound tissue components. Less affected areas were characterized by fluid accumulation within myelin sheaths.

Neurotoxicity similar to that observed in experimental animals has not been observed in humans intoxicated with nitrobenzene. Methemoglobinemia and its associated hematological effects, and hepatotoxicity, are the primary concerns associated with human exposure to nitrobenzene (3). Occupational exposure levels have primarily been set to avoid hematological effects. Severe headache, nausea, vertigo, confusion and coma, suggesting CNS involvement; and general weakness, parathesias, hyperalgesia, and "polyneuritis," suggesting peripheral nerve involvement, have been reported in nitrobenzene-intoxicated humans (2,5–9,17). These signs and symptoms are typically transitory in nature and resolve on removal of exposure. Following lethal nitrobenzene exposures, edema, hemorrhage, and softening in the brain have been observed, but it is not clear if these lesions were comparable to those seen in the rat studies (2).

The mechanism of action of nitrobenzene on the nervous system of experimental animals has not been studied in detail. While nitrobenzene is a well-recognized inducer of methemoglobinemia, this abnormal state does not appear to play a role in the induction of brain lesions, as sodium nitrate can induce similar levels of methemoglobinemia without brain damage (4). Regional accumulation of nitrobenzene in the brain also does not appear to play a role in CNS toxicity, as the small amounts of nitrobenzene that pass through the blood-brain barrier do not show increased accumulation in areas of malacia (12). The importance of intestinal or hepatic metabolism for the development of cerebellar pathology is indicated by the observation of cerebellar lesions in F344 rats given nitrobenzene orally and the absence of CNS effects when nitrobenzene is inhaled. The presence of cerebellar lesions in mice and Sprague-Dawley rats after inhalation suggests that the formation of active metabolites in the liver or enterohepatic circulation of metabolites is greater in these animals than in the F344 rat.

There are no mechanistic data related to neurotoxicity in humans. The observation that headache, nausea, vertigo, general weakness, and numbness of the legs disappeared in a patient intoxicated with nitrobenzene as nitrobenzene metabolites disappeared from the urine suggests a role for *p*-nitrophenol and/or *p*-aminophenol in causing these signs and symptoms (8).

REFERENCES

1. American Conference of Governmental Industrial Hygienists (1992) Nitrobenzene. In: *Documentation of the Threshold Limit Values. Vol I. 6th Ed.* Cincinnati, Ohio p. 305.
2. Beauchamp RO, Irons RD, Rickert DE *et al.* (1982) A critical review of the literature on nitrobenzene. *Crit Rev Toxicol* 11, 33.
3. Benya TJ, Cornish HH (1994) Aromatic nitro and amino compounds. In: *Patty's Industrial Hygiene and Toxicology. 4th Ed.* Clayton GD, Clayton FE eds. Wiley, New York p. 1016.
4. Bond JA, Chism JP, Rickert DE, Popp JA (1981) Induction of hepatic and testicular lesions in Fischer-344 rats by single oral doses of nitrobenzene. *Fund Appl Toxicol* 1, 389.
5. Carter FW (1936) An unusual case of poisoning, with some notes on non-alkaloid organic substances. *Med J Australia* 2, 558.
6. Donovan WM (1920) The toxicity of nitrobenzene with report of a fatal case. *J Amer Med Assn* 74, 1647.
7. Hamilton A (1919) Industrial poisoning by compounds of the aromatic series. *J Ind Hyg* 1, 200.
8. Ikeda M, Kita A (1964) Excretion of *p*-nitrophenol and *p*-aminophenol in the urine of a patient exposed to nitrophenol. *Brit J Ind Med* 21, 210.
9. Larens L, Bierme R, Jorda MF *et al.* (1974) Acute, toxic methemoglobinemia from accidental ingestion of nitrobenzene. *Eur J Toxicol* 17, 12.
10. Matsumara H, Yoshida T (1959) Experimental studies of nitrobenzol poisoning. *Kyusho J Med Sci* 10, 259.
11. Medinsky MA, Irons RD (1985) Sex, strain and species differences in the response of rodents to nitrobenzene vapors. In: *The Toxicity of Nitroaromatic Compounds.* Rickerts DE ed. Hemisphere Publishing, New York p. 35.
12. Morgan KT, Gross EA, Lyght O, Bond JA (1985) Morphologic and biochemical studies of a nitrobenzene-induced encephalopathy in rats. *Neurotoxicology* 6, 105.
13. Piotrowski J (1967) Further investigations on the evaluation of exposure to nitrobenzene. *Brit J Ind Med* 24, 60.
14. Salmowa J, Piotrowski J, Neuhorn U (1963) Evaluation of exposure to nitrobenzene. Absorption of nitrobenzene vapour through the lungs and excretion of *p*-nitrophenol in urine. *Brit J Ind Med* 20, 41.
15. Reddy BG, Pohl LR, Krisha G (1976) The requirement of the gut flora in nitrobenzene-induced methemoglobinemia in rats. *Biochem Pharmacol* 25, 1119.
16. Smith RP, Alkaitis AA, Shafer PR (1967) Chemically induced methemoglobinemias in the mouse. *Biochem Pharmacol* 16, 317.
17. Stifel RE (1919) Methemoglobinemia due to poisoning by a shoe dye. *J Amer Med Assn* 72, 395.

Nitrofurantoin

Herbert H. Schaumburg

NITROFURANTOIN
$C_8H_6N_4O_5$

1-[[(5-Nitro-2-furanyl)methylene]amino]-2,4-imidazolidinedione

NEUROTOXICITY RATING

Clinical

A   Peripheral neuropathy

Experimental

B   Peripheral neuropathy

Nitrofurantoin is a water-soluble, synthetic hydantoin derivative used for prevention and treatment of urinary tract infections. Its antibacterial activity is dependent on the presence of a nitro group in the 5 position of the furan ring (7). Drug-sensitive bacteria contain a reductase flavoprotein that converts nitrofurantoin to its active form (16). The drug is reduced more rapidly in bacteria than mammalian cells, thus accounting for its selective antimicrobial activity; this results either from inhibition of acetyl coenzyme A (CoA) synthesis from pyruvate, or from an action on bacterial DNA that delays replication (3). An acidic urine enhances the drug's antimicrobial action. Except for *Escherichia coli*, relatively few urinary tract pathogens are highly susceptible; most species of *Proteus*, *Enterobacter*, and *Klebsiella* are refractory. Bacteria that are susceptible rarely become resistant during therapy.

Introduced in 1952, nitrofurantoin soon became a mainstay of urinary antimicrobial therapy. Early enthusiasm stemmed from the ready achievement of persistent high drug concentrations in the urine with only modest tissue and plasma levels. Because of serious pulmonary and PNS toxicity, its use is now restricted to prophylaxis and treatment of susceptible *E. coli* infections.

Nitrofurantoin is rapidly and completely absorbed from the gastrointestinal tract. Renal excretion of unchanged drug is also swift, the circulatory half-life is only 30 min. The drug is excreted by both glomerular filtration and by tubular secretion, and there is considerable reabsorption in the distal tubule in acid urine (27). For an average dosage of 200 mg/day, the urine concentration approaches 20 μg/ml and the plasma concentration ranges from 1.8–2.2 μg/ml; only the urine reaches the bacteriostatic level of 7.5 μg/ml. The rate of nitrofurantoin excretion falls in individuals with poor glomerular filtration; it shows a linear relationship with creatinine clearance. Because the drug is so rapidly eliminated by the kidney, high plasma levels and nervous system toxicity are unlikely in individuals with normal renal function. In the presence of impaired glomerular filtration, the urine concentrations fall below the therapeutic range, and plasma concentrations rise to a level associated with adverse reactions (>5.0 μg/ml) (20).

Nitrofurantoin treatment has been associated with considerable systemic toxicity. The most common adverse reaction is a dose-related upper-gastrointestinal-distress syndrome with nausea and vomiting (6). More serious are acute pulmonary hypersensitivity syndrome, chronic pulmonary vasculitis-pneumonitis, immune-mediated chronic active hepatitis, megaloblastic anemia related to folate depletion, and hemolytic anemia from glucose-6-phosphate dehydrogenase deficiency (11,22). There is an unexplained geographic discrepancy in type of adverse reaction; pulmonary and hepatic complications predominate in Scandinavia, while peripheral neuropathy is the most common reaction in the United Kingdom (19).

Experimental animal studies, limited to short-term high-level doses, suggest that nitrofurantoin causes an axonal neuropathy (1,2,10). These studies are not definitive; none has utilized perfusion fixation with contemporary histopathological methods or modern neurophysiological techniques. Dosage ranging from 20–100 mg/kg daily to rats results in plasma levels of 3–15 μg/ml. Subtle axonal changes are detectable after only 2 days in high-dose animals; after 10 days, there is axonal shrinkage with myelin collapse and focal axonal swelling. Electrophysiological measurements in one study include alterations in chronaxy after 2 days that steadily worsened (1).

Human peripheral neuropathy of the distal axonopathy type has been clearly associated with nitrofurantoin therapy for 40 years; over 140 cases are described in 59 reports (3–5,8,9,13–15,23–25,28,29). Isolated instances of cerebellar dysfunction and benign intracranial hypertension have also occurred during nitrofurantoin therapy; they may be coincidental (9,17).

There are several characteristic features of nitrofurantoin neuropathy; it is most common in the elderly, in females, and in individuals with renal dysfunction. Neuropathy does not bear a strong relationship to dose or duration; it may appear between 7 and 336 days of commencement of therapy; cumulative doses range from 1.4–67.0 g. In 16%, neuropathy appeared after therapy had ceased. Renal dysfunction is not a requisite for neuropathy; in one-third of reported cases, renal function was normal. For example, 7 of 14 normal volunteers developed abnormally slowed or diminished nerve conduction velocities; all had blood levels below 2 μg/ml (27).

Nitrofurantoin neuropathy is heralded clinically by paresthesias of the distal lower limbs. Characteristically, there is rapid onset and progression of severe weakness followed by muscle wasting. The speed of progression of muscle weakness is almost unique among the toxic neuropathies and may suggest an erroneous diagnosis of acute demyelinating polyradiculoneuropathy (28). The severity of neuropathy is not obviously dose-related. Nitrofurantoin neuropathy carries a poor prognosis once weakness appears; if medication is continued after commencement of weakness, an incapacitating, poorly reversible neuropathy is almost inevitable. In one review of 100 cases, 34 experienced total regression of symptoms, 45 partial regression, 13 no change, and 8 died (23). Recovery is related to severity of neuropathy and unrelated to dose.

Histopathological examination of sural nerve biopsies in only one series has utilized meticulous, contemporary techniques, including ultrastructural study (28). It describes widespread acute axonal degeneration with no distinctive features or abnormalities of blood vessels; in two specimens, there were no surviving myelinated fibers. Axonal changes are also described in paraffin-embedded specimens from biopsies in some of the initial reports. An autopsy report of a patient with a severe neuropathy describes axonal degeneration in peripheral nerves, and in posterior more than anterior spinal nerve roots. Alterations in the dorsal root ganglia and chromatolytic changes in anterior horn cells are also noted (12).

Nerve conduction studies also indicate an axonal neuropathy. These studies disclose absent distal limb sensory potentials, and motor conduction velocities that are either decreased or unobtainable because a compound action potential cannot be evoked (28). Electromyography reveals denervation potentials in the majority of cases with weakness.

One report suggests that subclinical diabetic neuropathy may predispose to nitrofurantoin neurotoxicity (26).

The toxic mechanism underlying nitrofurantoin neuropathy is unclear. The mechanism most favored is inhibition of synthesis of acetyl CoA by furan derivatives; an *in vitro* study demonstrates the ability of nitrofurantoin to inhibit the formation of acetyl CoA from pyruvate (18). One experimental study suggests that accumulation of metabolites such as semicarbizides, which can produce polyneuropathy in rats, may be a contributing factor (10). Inhibition of glutathione reductase is suggested to account for the hepatotoxicity of nitrofurantoin (21); there are no reports on the response of nervous system glutathione reductase to nitrofurantoin.

REFERENCES

1. Behar A, Rachmilewitz E, Rahamimoff R *et al.* (1965) Experimental nitrofurantoin polyneuropathy in rats. *Arch Neurol* 13, 160.
2. Behar AJ, Livni N, Soffer D (1977) Fine structure of sciatic nerves in nitrofurantoin neuropathy induced in rats. *Neurotoxicology* 4, 13.
3. Bell DM (1961) Neuropathy associated with furaltadone. *J Amer Med Assn* 176, 808.
4. Collings H (1960) Polyneuropathy associated with nitrofurantoin therapy. *Arch Neurol* 3, 656.
5. De Fine Olivarius B (1956) Polyneuropathy during treatment with nitrofurantoin. *Ugeskr Laeger* 16, 55.
6. Delaney RA, Miller DA, Gerbino PD (1977) Adverse effects resulting from nitrofurantoin administration. *Amer J Pharm* 149, 26.
7. Dodd ME, Stillman NB (1944) The *in vitro* bacteriostatic action of some simple furan derivatives. *J Pharmacol Exp Ther* 82, 11.
8. Ellis FG (1962) Acute polyneuritis after nitrofurantoin therapy. *Lancet* 2, 1136.
9. Graebner RW, Herskowitz A, Augusta G (1973) Cerebellar toxic effects from nitrofurantoin. *Arch Neurol* 29, 257.
10. Klinghardt GW (1970) Experimentelle Unterschungen zur Aetiology der Polyneuropathie durch Nitrofurane und zur Histopathologie der Neuromyopathie durch Chloroquinidiphosphat. *Beitr Neurochir* 16, 55.
11. Koch-Weser J, Sidel V (1971) Adverse reactions of nitrofurantoin. *Arch Intern Med* 128, 399.
12. Lhermitte F, Fritel D, Cambier J *et al.* (1963) Polynévrites au cours de traitements par la nitrofurantoine. *Presse Med* 71, 767.
13. Loughridge L, Belf MB (1962) Peripheral neuropathy due to nitrofurantoin. *Lancet* 2, 1133.
14. Martin WJ, Corbin KB, Utz DC (1962) Paresthesia during treatment with nitrofurantoin. *Proc Mayo Clin* 37, 288.
15. Mather BS (1963) Acute polyneuritis after nitrofurantoin therapy. *Med J Australia* 1, 330.
16. McCarra DR, Reuvers A, Kaiser C (1970) Mode of action of nitrofurazone. *J Bacteriol* 104, 1126.
17. Mushet GR (1977) Pseudotumor and nitrofurantoin therapy. *Arch Neurol* 34, 257.
18. Paul MF, Paul HE, Kopko F *et al.* (1954) Inhibition by furacin of citrate formation in testis preparation. *J Biol Chem* 206, 491.
19. Penn RG, Griffin JP (1982) Adverse reactions to nitrofurantoin in the United Kingdom, Sweden, and Holland. *Brit Med J* 284, 399.
20. Roelsen E (1964) Polyneuritis after nitrofurantoin therapy: A survey and report of two new cases. *Acta Med Scand* 175, 145.
21. Sachs J, Geer T, Noell P *et al.* (1962) Effect of renal function on urinary recovery of orally administered nitrofurantoin. *N Engl J Med* 278, 1032.
22. Silva JM, McGirr L, O'Brien PJ (1991) Prevention of nitrofurantoin-induced cytotoxicity in isolated hepatocytes by fructose. *Arch Biochem Biophys* 289, 313.
23. Toole JF, Gergen JA, Hayes DM *et al.* (1968) Neural effects of nitrofurantoin. *Arch Neurol* 18, 680.
24. Toole JF, Parrish ML (1973) Nitrofurantoin polyneuropathy. *Neurology* 23, 554.
25. Wagner H, Thiele KG (1968) Polyneuropathie unter der behandlung mit nitrofurantoin. *Munch Med Wochenschr* 110, 591.
26. White WT, Harrison L, Dumas J (1984) Nitrofurantoin unmasking peripheral neuropathy in a type 2 diabetic patient. *Arch Intern Med* 144, 821.
27. Willett RW (1963) Peripheral neuropathy due to nitrofurantoin. *Neurology* 13, 344.
28. Woodruff MN, Malvin RL, Thompson IM (1961) The renal transport of nitrofurantoin. Effect of acid-base balance upon its excretion. *J Amer Med Assn* 175, 1132.
29. Yiannikas C, Pollard JD, McLeod JG (1981) Nitrofurantoin neuropathy. *Aust N Z J Med* 11, 400.

Nitrogen Trichloride

John L. O'Donoghue

NITROGEN TRICHLORIDE
NCl₃

Nitrogen chloride; Chlorine nitride; Agene; Trichloramine; Trichlorine nitride

NEUROTOXICITY RATING

Experimental

A Acute encephalopathy (canine agitation, seizures)

A Multifocal cortical necrosis

Nitrogen trichloride is an oily, yellow, unstable liquid that can be detonated by impact at temperatures above 60°C. It has a pungent odor and is a lachrimator and mucous membrane irritant (7). It has been used primarily to bleach wheat (prohibited in the United States since 1950) and fumigate citrus fruit. Small amounts of nitrogen trichloride may be present as a residual chloramine in chlorinated water.

Feeding nitrogen trichloride–bleached bread or biscuits has been associated since the 1920s with a clinical condition in dogs referred to as canine hysteria, fright disease, or running fits (6,8,13). Affected dogs suddenly appear frightened with wild, unnatural facial expressions. The dogs are frequently seen to run about in an uncontrolled manner, eventually becoming exhausted and depressed. Episodes of running may be followed by development of ataxia and incoordination. Running fits may be initiated or followed by convulsions. The condition has been reproduced in dogs, rabbits, and ferrets by feeding nitrogen trichloride–treated wheat flour or injecting protein extracts of treated flour (9). Humans, cats, monkeys, and guinea pigs are resistant to the toxic effects of nitrogen trichloride–treated flour (8).

Neuropathological lesions associated with ingestion of nitrogen trichloride–treated wheat include necrosis of the deep layers of the cerebral cortices, the subcortical arcuate fibers, and the hippocampus (4,5). Degenerative changes in the cerebellar Purkinje cells, basket cells, and their processes have been described. The similarity between nitrogen trichloride–induced lesions and anoxia has led to speculation that the lesions observed are due to anoxia or interference with oxidative processes in the brain (6).

Methionine sulfoximine has been identified as the agent in nitrogen trichloride–treated wheat that is responsible for the clinical disease (1). Rats and mice fed methionine sulfoximine developed cerebrocortical necrosis and necrosis of the thalamus and hypothalamus (4). Methionine sulfoximine induces seizures in experimental animals and is an antagonist of methionine and glutamine (2,3,10,11) (*see* Methionine Sulfoximine, this volume).

Editors' Note: It has been proposed that the widespread use of nitrogen trichloride to bleach flour in the first half of the 20th century is related to an increased level of human neurodegenerative disease in the second half (12). The hypothesis is based on the principle that cells in the nervous system are sensitive to reductions of glutathione and glutamine that would be expected from the metabolic effects of methionine sulfoxamine. Decreased glutamine synthesis would act to increase free glutamate and ammonia (both have neurotoxic potential), while decreased glutathione would reduce antioxidant defenses on which nerve cells are dependent (11). There is no direct evidence in support of this interesting proposal.

REFERENCES

1. Bentley HR, McDermott EE, Whitehead JK (1950) Action of nitrogen trichloride on proteins: A synthesis of the toxic factor from methionine. *Nature* **165**, 735.

2. Folbergrova J (1973) Glycogen and glycogen phosphorylase in the cerebral cortex of mice under the influence of methionine sulfoximine. *J Neurochem* **20**, 547.

3. Guttierrez JA, Norenberg MD (1977) Ultrastructural study of methionine sulfoximine-induced Alzheimer type II astrocytes. *Amer J Pathol* **86**, 285.

4. Hicks SP, Coy MA (1958) Pathologic effects of antimetabolites. Convulsions and brain lesions caused by sulfoximine and their variation with genotype. *Arch Pathol* **65**, 378.

5. Innes JRM, Saunders LZ (1962) *Comparative Neuropathology*. Academic Press, New York.

6. Lewey FH (1950) Neuropathological changes in nitrogen trichloride intoxication in dogs. *J Neuropathol Exp Neurol* **9**, 396.

7. Massin N, Bohadana AB, Wild P (1998) Respiratory symptoms and bronchial responsiveness in lifeguards exposed to nitrogen trichloride in indoor swimming pools. *Occup Environ Med* **55**, 258.

8. Mellanby E (1946) Diet and canine hysteria. *Brit Med J* **2**, 885.

9. Newell GW, Erickson TC, Gilson WE et al. (1949) The effect of feeding agene-treated food materials to experimental animals and human beings. *Trans Amer Assn Cereal Chem* **7**, 1.

10. Phelps CH (1975) An ultrastructural study of methionine sulfoximine-induced glycogen accumulation in astrocytes of the mouse cerebral cortex. *J Neurocytol* **4**, 479.

11. Rizzuto N, Gonatas NK (1974) Ultrastructural study of methionine sulfoximine in developing and adult cerebral cortex. *J Neuropathol Exp Neurol* **33**, 237.
12. Shaw CA, Bains JS (1998) Did consumption of flour bleached by the agene process contribute to the incidence of neurological disease? *Med Hypotheses* **51**, 477.
13. Silver ML (1949) Canine epilepsy caused by flour bleached with nitrogen trichloride. *J Neuropathol Exp Neurol* **8**, 441.

3-Nitropropionic Acid and Related Compounds

Fengsheng He
Albert C. Ludolph

$$CH_2 - COOH$$
$$|$$
$$CH_2$$
$$|$$
$$NO_2$$

3-NITROPROPIONIC ACID
$C_3H_5NO_4$

NEUROTOXICITY RATING

Clinical

A   Acute encephalopathy (headache, seizures, sedation, coma)

A   Extrapyramidal syndrome (choreoathetosis, dystonia)

Experimental

A   Succinyl dehydrogenase inhibition

A   Striatal neuronopathy

A   Extrapyramidal dysfunction (dystonia)

3-Nitropropionic acid (3-NPA) is a plant toxin and mycotoxin. The neurotoxic effects of 3-NPA are similar to those associated with related aliphatic nitrocompounds, including 3-nitropropanol (3-NPOH), 1-phenyl-2-nitroethane, and 1-(4′-hydroxyphenyl)-2-nitroethane. In nature, 3-NPA may occur as the glucose ester (karakin, coronillin, corynocarpin, hiptagin), whereas NPOH is most commonly found as a glycoside (miserotoxin; 3-nitro-1-propyl-β-D-glucopyranoside).

3-NPA is a colorless crystalline solid with a MP of 66.7°–67.5°C (57,58), whereas 3-nitropropanol is a liquid with a BP of 85°C at 2 mm Hg (31). High-performance liquid chromatography (HPLC) permits fast quantitative detection of minute amounts of 3-NPA, 3-nitropropanol, and miserotoxin (30,34). Other methods of isolation and identification include colorimetry, thin-layer chromatography, paper chromatography, and gas chromatography (28,29). There are no pharmaceutical or commercial uses of 3-NPA. Its potential as an "antihypertensive" drug has been explored in rabbits (8), and its use as a forest herbicide in the biological control of weeds has been suggested (11).

There are no regulations for the control of human or animal exposure to 3-NPA or related compounds.

The most significant source of nitrocompounds in nature is higher plants. The presence of 3-NPA in *Astragalus* spp. (milk vetches, locoweeds, poison vetches) is of economic importance, since intoxication with this legume genus is a significant cause of livestock loss on the western North American continent. Here, 14%–22% of *Astragalus* spp. contain neurotoxic nitrocompounds (47,55). Neurotoxic *Astragalus* spp. are also found in South America, Europe, and Asia (52), and cattle poisoning has also been reported in regions outside the United States and Canada (43,49). Other significant sources of aliphatic nitrocompounds are the genera *Coronilla*, *Indigofera*, and *Lotus*; the Malpiaghazeae; the Corynocarpaceae; and the Violaceae (31). The apparently less frequently occurring aliphatic nitrocompounds, 1-phenyl-2-nitroethane and 1-(4′-hydroxyphenyl)-2-nitroethane, were detected in five and three higher plant species, respectively (31).

The medical significance of *fungal* synthesis of 3-NPA has been recognized (18,26). This was stimulated by the discovery that consumption of moldy sugar cane containing the cosmopolitan fungal *Arthrinium* spp. was associated with striatal necrosis in rural Chinese children. *A. sacchari*, *A. saccharicola*, and *A. phaeospermum* were found to produce 3-NPA, and data strongly indicate that this compound is the cause of the human disease. However, the production of 3-NPA is not limited to *Arthrinium* species, and systematic surveys on toxin synthesis in fungi have not been done. Several reports identified 3-NPA as a fungal product in the 1950s: 3-NPA is a major metabolite of *Penicillium atrovenetum* (13,40,58), *Aspergillus flavus* (7,13,57) and *A. oryzae* (35), and *Streptomyces* spp. (2). The fungus *Melanconis thelebola*, which damages trunk and branches of *Alder* spp., produces 3-NPA as a metabolite (11). In screening experiments in North America, HPLC analysis revealed the presence of 3-NPA on molded breads, most likely due to contamination with *Aspergillus* species (A.C. Ludolph *et al.*, unpublished data). In China, human food poisoning by mycotoxins was already suspected in the early twentieth century (51,59); classical features of mycotoxicoses were observed (9), and the pattern of clinical signs and symptoms and neuropathological damage seem to be complementary to relatively recent reports from northern China (18,20,25). In the 1960s, studies in Japan tried to define the potential impact of 3-NPA as a food contaminant (21,24). Although no human cases of poisoning were described, the results clearly demonstrated that strains of fungi were able to produce significant amounts of the toxin on cheese curds, soy beans, peanuts, traditionally fermented foods, and cycad *miso*. Taken together, the plant toxin 3-NPA is clearly a compound of worldwide significance in veterinary neurology; in contrast, reports of fungal neurotoxicity in humans presently are restricted to China.

General Toxicology

There are no reports on normal levels of 3-NPA or related nitrocompounds in the human. In the rumen of animals, ester conjugates of 3-NPA are enzymatically hydrolyzed by esterases, whereas a β-glucosidase generates NPOH from glycosides. In nonruminants, glycosides are not hydrolyzed (32). 3-NPA and NPOH are rapidly absorbed by the gastrointestinal tract (32,33), and the alcohol is immediately converted to 3-NPA by alcohol dehydrogenase (37).

After absorption, 3-NPA is metabolized to nitrites by glucose and amino acid oxidases (38). Since nitrites oxidize hemoglobin, increased methemoglobin levels are a feature of 3-NPA intoxication. The formation of methemoglobin does not participate in the neurological consequences of intoxication. Specifically, administration of methylene blue has no influence on the outcome of poisonings in the majority of species, indicating that 3-NPA—not nitrite—causes the motor behavioral signs (56).

Since the CNS is the principal target of aliphatic nitrocompounds, their effects have been predominantly studied in this tissue. 3-NPA is a suicide inhibitor of the Krebs cycle enzyme succinate dehydrogenase (SDH), an effect of the agent that can be demonstrated throughout the brain of systemically intoxicated animals (14,15; A.C. Ludolph *et al.*, unpublished data). SDH activity is also drastically reduced in heart and liver mitochondria after 3-NPA administration (14). The effect of 3-NPA on other highly energy-dependent tissues, such as striated muscles and pancreatic islets, is unknown. Whether 3-NPA also has a direct vasodilating effect on vessels, independent of its effect on mitochondrial enzymes, is unclear. In studies on precontracted rabbit aortic rings, 3-NPA allegedly induced relaxation; it also led to a mild consistent decrease of arterial blood pressure in renal hypertensive dogs (8). In other studies of the acutely 3-NPA–intoxicated rat, continuous intra-arterial monitoring clearly revealed that blood pressure remained stable and even showed a tendency to increase in most animals (16,17; A.C. Ludolph *et al.*, unpublished data).

Animal Studies

Field observations of several species of domestic animals poisoned by *Astragalus* spp. indicate neurotoxic effects in-

duced by 3-NPA. Typical signs of acute intoxication of cattle, sheep, and horses are dyspnea, cyanosis, frequent urination, and weakness or paralysis of hindquarter muscles (23,53,56). The chronic disease ("roaring disease," "cracker heels," "knocking disease") may develop after smaller doses of the toxin and a silent period of more than 2–3 weeks (22,23). Typically, labored and rapid respiration develops in the affected animal; this is accompanied by general body weakness, beginning in the pelvic limbs, knuckling of the fetlocks, goose stepping, and knocking together of the hindlimbs when walking (22). Later, weakness of hindlimbs or even loss of control of this part of the body develops; visual impairment is described in one report (22).

Uncontrolled exposures in nonlaboratory animals demonstrate a significant species dependency of 3-NPA neurotoxicity. With acute exposure, large farm animals reduce their food intake and develop posterior weakness and paralysis, staggering gait and incoordination, head extension, possibly blindness, and hyperpnea (23,45,46,54,56). Chronic exposure of cattle, sheep, meadow voles, and pigs (22,23,46) causes posterior limb weakness and "interference of hind limbs when walking," stiffness of gait, incoordination, and knuckling of fetlocks. Stiff front legs are described in sheep. The globus pallidus of one cow fed *Astragalus* spp. revealed moderate spongy vacuolation in the white matter, and "wallerian degeneration in the spinal cord and severe wallerian degeneration and loss of nerve fibers in the sciatic nerve" (23). An experimental feeding trial with *Coronilla* spp. performed in Hungary revealed degeneration of Purkinje cells in coypu stocks (43).

Acute responses to 3-NPA are comparable in rats and mice (3,14–17): somnolence develops after a dose-dependent, symptom-free interval. The treated animal then becomes hyperactive and unsteady, stereotyped paddling movements appear, and the animal may roll over repeatedly. In the last stage, intoxicated animals are recumbent and display stiffened limbs.

In 17- to 29-g mice, single or repeated injections of 120 mg/kg body weight of 3-NPA induced uniform inhibition of SDH activity in all areas of the brain. This was followed by selective and symmetrical damage of the lateral parts of the caudate-putamen, the globus pallidus, the entopeduncular nucleus, and the pars reticulata of the substantia nigra (14,15). Lesions of midbrain, medulla oblongata, and spinal tract damage (preferentially myelin) were part of the picture. In a study of 200- to 720-g rats, a single injection of 30 mg/kg body weight or 10 mg/kg body weight for 1–4 days consistently produced selective bilateral symmetrical lesions of the caudate-putamen (16,17). If a comparatively larger dosage was used, hippocampal structures, thalamus, and the roof of the fourth ventricle were also affected; white matter tracts were most significantly damaged in the internal capsule. Neuropathological alterations were comparable in both species and consisted of nuclear pyknosis and chromatin clumping, increased cytoplasmic lucency, severe cellular swelling or shrinkage, and swelling of mitochondria and dendritic processes. In rats, oligendrocyte changes were minor, but astrocytes were swollen and showed chromatin clumping. Monitoring of blood gases revealed a metabolic acidosis that decompensated during the third stage of the intoxication.

The toxic effect of 3-NPA is greater in older animals (6; A.C. Ludolph et al., unpublished data) and, under certain defined and dose-dependent conditions, the pattern of vulnerability induced bears remarkable similarities to Huntington's disease (3,4). After acute striatal or systemic 3-NPA injection, proton-chemical-shift magnetic resonance imaging (MRI) disclosed that lactate increases in vivo in the striatum of the rat. Levels of adenosine triphosphate (ATP) decline and concentrations of markers of striatal projection neurons and aspiny interneurons decrease (3). Chronic systemic administration of 3-NPA (1 month) to rats produces selective lesions in the striatum similar to the pattern of tissue vulnerability in Huntington's disease (3). The chronic regimen caused lesions confined to the striatum and relative sparing of NADPH-diaphorase interneurons. This is consistent with an excitotoxic process mediated by the N-methyl-D-aspartate (NMDA) glutamate receptor subtype. Ablation of the glutamatergic corticostriatal pathway reduced the degree of striatal damage induced by 3-NPA.

Repeated 3-NPA treatment of primates produced a chronic model of 3-NPA toxicity (5,12). Some of the macaques (and baboons) spontaneously developed dystonia and choreoathetosis; others exhibited the same extrapyramidal symptoms after apomorphine challenge (5). Studies of histochemical and immunocytochemical markers in primate tissue demonstrated a profile of neuronal degeneration in the caudate and putamen closely resembling that seen in Huntington's disease (12).

In Vitro Studies

SDH inhibition, ATP depletion, neuroprotection by excitatory amino acid receptor antagonists, and changes of membrane-channel activity induced by 3-NPA–related energy depletion have been demonstrated in in vitro studies.

Human Studies

Ingestion of sugar cane infested with a 3-NPA–producing fungus has resulted in severe illness that may eventuate in a permanent movement disorder. Intoxications in China are reported predominantly from the northern provinces of Hebei, Henan, Shandong, and Liaoning (18,25). The implicated sugar cane is harvested in southern provinces, transported and stored in the north, where it is marketed in the winter or spring. Improper storage of cane promotes growth of mold. Disease outbreaks typically occur in January, February, and March. From 1972–1989, 884 intoxications were reported mainly in children; the oldest patient was aged 27 years. Eighty-eight patients reportedly died from the accidental intake of contaminated sugar cane. The disparity between the selective involvement of children and the greater sensitivity of older animals to 3-NPA is unresolved.

Human intoxication with mildewed sugar cane reportedly follows a stereotyped time course: 15 min to 8 h after consumption of the sugar cane, patients may complain of headache and dizziness; this is consistently followed by nausea, vomiting, and other gastrointestinal disturbances (abdominal pain, and diarrhea). Initial clouding of consciousness often leads to coma and is accompanied by seizures (sometimes even status epilepticus), and visual and visuomotor deficits such as horizontal or vertical nystagmus, double vision, and forced upward gaze. Extensor plantar reflexes appear and, during coma, opisthotonus and decerebrate rigidity may be observed. White blood cell counts and cerebrospinal fluid remain normal, and signs of infection (fever and nuchal rigidity) are consistently absent. Antibiotic treatment has no effect. Among those patients who survive (90%), signs and symptoms of acute intoxication usually last 3–7 days, the longest being 20 days; 50% of the patients recover completely. Results of autopsies are reported in three patients (25), but details on the histopathology of the nervous system are unavailable; only the diagnoses "cerebral edema," "hernia cerebri," and "congestion of the brain" are mentioned. After regaining consciousness, some patients are unable to speak or move voluntarily and suffer from urinary and fecal incontinence. One-quarter of patients develops a self-limited, irreversible, and severely incapacitating movement disorder 11–60 days after the initial symptoms. This disorder features choreoathetotic and dystonic components affecting the facial musculature, speech, neck, and extremity muscles. Dystonia usually appears in severely affected patients with coma of more than 3 days duration at the acute stage of intoxication, suggesting that the frequency of neurological defects may be related to the duration of coma (18). Computed tomography scans and MRI of the brains of patients with dystonia show bilateral symmetrical lesions of the putamen and, less frequently, the globus pallidus (18). Visual evoked potentials were delayed in two patients with dystonia (18). Biopsy of caudate tissue adjacent to a lesion during intrastriatal transplantation of adrenal medulla showed shrinkage of neurons, vacuolation of astrocytes and oligodendroglia, degeneration of axons and myelin, and edematous changes within capillary endothelial cells (48).

These epidemiological and clinical observations strongly suggest that food contamination by the fungal toxin 3-NPA is the cause of the disease. This link is supported by several studies (18,25,26). Sugar cane samples associated with intoxications contained fungous hyphae, mostly *Arthrinium*; extracts thereof induced "circular movements," limb paralysis, and death in mice, and similar motor behavioral changes appeared in treated cats, while convulsions were seen in dogs. *Arthrinium* fungi dominated the poisonous samples; the great majority caused signs identical to those seen after application of the juice. Intragastric intubation of condensed *Arthrinium* culture in rats at a 3-NPA dose of 40 mg/kg, three times a day, also induced bilateral striatal necrosis.

Chemotaxonomy of the toxigenic *Arthrinium* spp. revealed that *A. sacchari*, *A. saccharicola*, and *A. phaeospermum* were responsible for toxin production. High levels of 3-NPA (285–6660 μg/g) in poisonous sugar cane samples have been identified by thin layer chromatography (20,25). There are no data on the dose–effect relationship.

Specific treatment is unavailable for patients intoxicated with 3-NPA. Anticonvulsants have been ineffective. Intrastriatal transplantation of autogenous adrenal medulla with delayed dystonia has not produced improvement.

Pathogenetic Mechanisms

Several studies have partially elucidated the pathogenesis of the neurotoxicity of 3-NPA. The principal effect of 3-NPA is suicide inhibition of the mitochondrial enzyme SDH *in vitro* and *in vivo* (1,10,15; A.C. Ludolph *et al.*, unpublished data), and the consequent irreversible inhibition of Krebs cycle and complex II activity. Effects with apparently less impact on pathogenesis are reversible inhibition of fumarase and aspartase—an enzyme not present in humans (39)—isocitrate lyase (44), and acetylcholinesterase (36). In rats, SDH inhibition is uniform in both lesioned and morphologically intact areas of the brain. In mouse cortical explants and hippocampal slices of the rat, SDH inhibition results in a reduction of cellular nucleotide levels (27). In hippocampal neurons *in vitro*, this is followed by an increase of potassium conductance due to opening of ATP-dependent channels (42). After this phase of hyperpolarization, the cell gradually depolarizes and excitotoxic mechanisms contribute to the early phase of depolarization; this can be blocked or temporarily reversed by antagonists to glutamate receptors (42). Glutamate antagonists also attenuate morphological damage induced by 3-NPA in mouse explants *in vitro* (27). Prior decortication to remove the corticostriatal glutamatergic input protects vulnerable neurons (3,6). In the late agonal phase of ATP depletion, failure of ion pumps appears to be a limiting factor (41). It is suggested that glutamate receptor activation is caused by the inability of the energy-deficient cell to maintain a stable membrane potential by functioning ion pumps. Since the energy-dependent pumps lose their function, the cell depolarizes, the voltage-dependent magnesium block of the NMDA glutamate receptor subtype is relieved, and ions enter the cell *via* its associated channel (19). Later, in energy-deficiency states, the energy-dependent high-affinity uptake for glutamate is reduced, extracellular glutamate increases, and NMDA *and* non-NMDA receptors are activated (60,61). The resulting increase of intracellular calcium can cause neuronal death. This hypothetical cascade of events presents opportunities for pharmacological intervention. There are other factors that may have a role, including lactate accumulation, acidosis, generation of free radicals, and dosage of 3-NPA.

Editor's Note: Recent studies with mice suggest the convulsant and proconvulsant actions of 3-NPA are mediated by non-NMDA receptors (50).

REFERENCES

1. Alston TA, Mela L, Bright HJ (1977) 3-Nitropropionate, the toxic substance of *Indigofera*, is a suicide inactivator of succinate dehydrogenase. *Proc Nat Acad Sci USA* **74**, 3767.
2. Anzai K, Suzuki S (1960) A new antibiotic bovinocidin, identified as β-nitropropionic acid. *J Antibiot* **13**, 133.
3. Beal MF, Brouillet E, Jenkins BG *et al.* (1993) Neurochemical and histologic characterization of striatal excitotoxic lesions produced by the mitochondrial toxin 3-nitropropionic acid. *J Neurosci* **13**, 4181.
4. Bossi SR, Simpson JR, Isacson O (1993) Age dependence of striatal neuronal death caused by mitochondrial dysfunction. *NeuroReport* **4**, 73.
5. Brouillet E, Hantraye P, Dolan R *et al.* (1993) Chronic administration of 3-nitropropionic acid induced selective striatal degeneration and abnormal choreiform movements in monkeys. *Soc Neurosci Abstr* **19**, 409.
6. Brouillet E, Jenkins BG, Hyman BT *et al.* (1993) Age-dependent vulnerability of the striatum to the mitochondrial toxin 3-nitropropionic acid. *J Neurochem* **60**, 356.
7. Bush MT, Touster O, Brockman JE (1951) The production of beta-nitropropionic acid by a strain of *Aspergillus flavus*. *J Biol Chem* **188**, 685.
8. Castillo C, Valencia I, Reyes G, Hong E (1993) 3-Nitropropionic acid obtained from *Astragalus* species has vasodilator and antihypertensive properties. *Drug Develop Res* **28**, 183.
9. Ciegler A, Burmeister HR, Vesonder HF (1983) Poisonous fungi: Mycotoxins and mycotoxicosis. In: *Fungi Pathogenic for Humans and Animals*. Howard DH ed. Marcel Dekker, New York p. 413.

10. Coles CJ, Edmondson DE, Singer TP (1979) Inactivation of succinate dehydrogenase by 3-nitropropionate. *J Biol Chem* **254**, 5161.

11. Evidente A, Capretti P, Giordano F, Surico G (1992) Identification and phytotoxicity of 3-nitropropionic acid produced *in vitro* by *Melanconis thelebola*. *Experientia* **48**, 1169.

12. Ferrante RJ, Hantraye P, Brouillet E *et al.* (1993) Striatal pathology of impaired mitochondrial metabolism in primates profiles Huntington's disease. *Soc Neurosci Abstr* **19**, 408.

13. Frisvad JC (1989) The connection between the Penicillia and Aspergilli and mycotoxins with special emphasis on misidentified isolates. *Arch Environ Contam Toxicol* **18**, 452.

14. Gould DH, Gustine DL (1982) Basal ganglia degeneration, myelin alterations, and enzyme inhibition induced in mice by the plant toxin 3-nitropropionic acid. *Neuropathol Appl Neurobiol* **8**, 377.

15. Gould DH, Wilson MP, Hamar DW (1985) Brain enzyme and clinical alterations induced in rats and mice by nitroaliphatic toxicants. *Toxicol Lett* **27**, 83.

16. Hamilton BF, Gould DH (1987) Nature and distribution of brain lesions in rats intoxicated with 3-nitropropionic acid: a type of hypoxic (energy deficient) brain damage. *Acta Neuropathol* **72**, 286.

17. Hamilton BF, Gould DH (1987) Correlation of morphologic brain lesions with physiologic alterations and blood-brain barrier impairment in 3-nitropropionic acid toxicity in rats. *Acta Neuropathol* **74**, 67.

18. He F, Zhang S, Zhang C *et al.* (1990) Mycotoxin induced encephalopathy and dystonia in children. In: *Basic Science in Toxicology*. Volans GN, Sims J, Sullivan FM, Turner P eds. Taylor & Francis, London p. 596.

19. Henneberry RC, Novelli A, Cox JA, Lysko PG (1989) Neurotoxicity at the N-methyl-D-aspartate receptor in energy-compromised neurons: An hypothesis for cell death in aging and disease. *Ann N Y Acad Sci* **568**, 225.

20. Hu W (1986) The isolation and structure identification of a toxic substance, 3-nitropropionic acid, produced by *Arthrinium* from mildewed sugarcanes. *Chin J Prev Med* **20**, 321.

21. Iwasaki T, Koskowski FV (1973) Production of β-nitropropionic acid in foods. *J Food Sci* **38**, 1162.

22. James LF (1983) Neurotoxins and other toxins from *Astragalus* and related genera. In: *Handbook of Natural Toxins. Vol 1*. Keeler RF, Tu AT eds. Marcel Dekker, New York p. 445.

23. James LF, Hartley J, Williams MC, Van Kampen KR (1980) Field and experimental studies in cattle and sheep poisoned by nitro-bearing *Astragalus* or their toxins. *J Amer Vet Res* **41**, 377.

24. Kinosita R, Ishiko T, Sugiyama S *et al.* (1968) Mycotoxins in fermented food. *Cancer Res* **28**, 2296.

25. Liu X, Luo X, Hu W (1992) Studies on the epidemiology and etiology of moldy sugarcane poisoning in China. *Biomed Environ Sci* **5**, 161.

26. Ludolph AC, He F, Spencer PS *et al.* (1991) 3-Nitropropionic acid—exogenous animal neurotoxin and possible human striatal toxin. *Can J Neurol Sci* **18**, 492.

27. Ludolph AC, Seelig M, Ludolph AG *et al.* (1992) Cellular energy deficits and excitotoxic lesions induced by 3-nitropropionic acid *in vitro*. *Neurodegeneration* **1**, 155.

28. Majak W, Bose RJ (1974) Chromatographic methods for the isolation of miserotoxin and detection of aliphatic nitro compounds. *Phytochemistry* **13**, 1005.

29. Majak W, Cheng K-J, Muir AD, Pass MA (1985) Analysis and metabolism of nitrotoxins in cattle and sheep. In: *Plant Toxicology*. Seawright AA, Hegarty MP, James LF, Keeler RF eds. Queensland Poisonous Plants Committee, Yeerongpilly p. 446.

30. Majak W, McDiarmid RE (1990) Detection and quantitative determination of 3-nitropropionic acid in bovine urine. *Toxicol Lett* **50**, 213.

31. Majak W, Pass MA (1990) Aliphatic nitrocompounds. In: *Toxicants of Plant Origin. Vol II. Glycosides*. Cheeke PR ed. CRC Press, Boca Raton, Florida p. 143.

32. Majak W, Pass MA, Madryga FJ (1983) Toxicity of miserotoxin and its aglycone (3-nitropropanol) to rats. *Toxicol Lett* **19**, 171.

33. Majak W, Pass MA, Muir AD, Rode LM (1984) Absorption of 3-nitropropanol (miserotoxin aglycone) from the compound stomach of cattle. *Toxicology* **23**, 9.

34. Muir AD, Majak W (1984) Quantitative determination of of 3-nitropropionic acid and 3-nitropropanol in plasma by HPLC. *Toxicol Lett* **20**, 133.

35. Nakamura S, Shimoda C (1954) Studies on an antibiotic substance oryzacidin, produced by *Asp. oryzae*. Part 5. Existence of 3-nitropropionic acid. *J Agr Chem Soc Jpn* **28**, 909.

36. Osman MY (1982) Effect of β-nitropropionic acid on rat brain acetylcholinesterase. *Biochem Pharmacol* **31**, 4067.

37. Pass MA, Muir AD, Majak W, Yost GS (1985) Effect of alcohol and aldehyde dehydrogenase inhibitors on the toxicity of 3-nitropropanol in rats. *Toxicol Appl Pharmacol* **78**, 310.

38. Porter DJT, Bright HJ (1980) 3-Carbanionic substrate analogues bind very tightly to fumarase and aspartase. *J Biol Chem* **255**, 4772.

39. Porter DJT, Voet JG Bright HJ. (1980) Nitroalkanes as reductive substrates for flavoprotein oxidases. *Z Naturforsch* **27**, 1052.

40. Raistrick H, Stössl A (1958) Studies in the biochemistry of micro-organisms. 104. Metabolites of *Penicillium atrovenetum* G. Smith: β-nitropropionic acid, a major metabolite. *Biochem J* **68**, 647.

41. Riepe MW, Hori N, Ludolph AC, Carpenter DO (1995) Failure of neuronal ion exchange, not potentiated excitation, causes excitotoxicity after inhibition of oxidative phosphorylation. *Neuroscience* **64**, 91.

42. Riepe M, Hori N, Ludolph AC *et al.* (1992) Inhibition of

energy metabolism by 3-nitropropionic acid activates ATP-sensitive potassium channels. *Brain Res* **586**, 61.

43. Salyi G, Sztojkov V, Hilbertne Miklovics M (1988) A nutria tarka koronafürt (*Coronilla varia L.*) okozta mergezese. *Magy Allatorv Lapja* **43**, 313.

44. Schloss JV, Cleland WW (1982) Inhibition of isocitrate lyase by 3-nitropropionate, a reaction-intermediate analogue. *Biochemistry* **21**, 4420.

45. Shenk JS, Risius ML, Barnes RF (1974) Weanling meadow vole responses to crownvetch forage. *Agron J* **66**, 386.

46. Shenk JS, Wangsness PJ, Leach RM *et al.* (1976) Relationship between beta-nitropropionic acid content of crownvetch and toxicity in nonruminant animals. *J Anim Sci* **42**, 616.

47. Stermitz FR, Lowry WT, Norris FA *et al.* (1972) Aliphatic nitrocompounds from *Astragalus* species. *Phytochemistry* **11**, 1117.

48. Sun YL, Li B, Qu BQ *et al.* (1993) Ultrastructural studies of the caudate nucleus in toxic cerebropathy. *Chin J Neurol Psychiat* **74**, 229.

49. Tarazona JV, Sanz F (1987) Aliphatic nitrocompounds in *Astragalus lusitanicus* Lam. *Vet Human Toxicol* **29**, 437.

50. Urbanska EM, Blaszczak P, Saran T *et al.* (1999) AMPA/kainate-related mechanisms contribute to convulsant and proconvulsant effects of 3-nitropropionic acid. *Eur J Pharmacol* **370**, 251.

51. Verhaart WJC (1938) Symmetrical degeneration of the neostriatum in Chinese infants. *Arch Dis Child* **13**, 225.

52. Williams MC, Barneby RC (1977) The occurrence of nitrotoxins in Old World and South American *Astragalus* (Fabeaceae). *Brittonia* **29**, 310, 327.

53. Williams MC, James LF (1978) Livestock poisoning from nitro-bearing *Astragalus*. In: *Effects of Poisonous Plants on Livestock*. Keeler RF, Van Kampen KR, James LF eds. Academic Press, New York 379.

54. Williams MC, James LF, Bleak AT (1976) Toxicity of introduced nitro-containing *Astragalus* to sheep, cattle, and chicks. *J Range Manage* **28**, 260.

55. Williams MC, Parker R (1974) Distribution of organic nitrites in *Astragalus*. *Weed Sci* **22**, 259.

56. Williams MC, Van Kampen KR, Norris FA (1969) Timber milk vetch poisoning in chickens, rabbits, and cattle. *Amer J Vet Res* **30**, 2185.

57. Wilson BJ (1971) Miscellaneous *Aspergillus* toxins. In: *Microbial Toxins*. Vol. 6. *Fungal Toxins*. Ciegler A, Kadis S, Ajl SJ eds. Academic Press, New York p. 257.

58. Wilson BJ (1971) Miscellaneous *Penicillium* toxins. In: *Microbial Toxins*. Vol. 6. *Fungal Toxins*. Ciegler A, Kadis S, Ajl SJ eds. Academic Press, New York p. 475.

59. Woods AH, Pendleton L (1925) Fourteen simultaneous cases of an acute degenerative striatal disease. *Arch Neurol Psych* **13**, 549.

60. Zeevalk GD, Nicklas WJ (1990) Chemically induced hypoglycemia and anoxia: Relationship to glutamate receptor-mediated toxicity in retina. *J Pharmacol Exp Ther* **253**, 1285.

61. Zeevalk GD, Nicklas WJ (1991) Mechanisms underlying initiation of excitotoxicity associated with metabolic inhibition. *J Pharmacol Exp Ther* **257**, 870.

Nitroprusside

Herbert H. Schaumburg

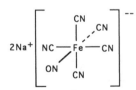

SODIUM NITROPRUSSIDE
Na₂[Fe(CN)₅NO]

Pentakis(cyano-C)nitrosylferrate(2−) disodium; Sodium nitroprussiate; Nitroferricyanide

NEUROTOXICITY RATING
Clinical
A Encephalomalacia
B Acute encephalopathy
Experimental
A Neuronopathy (*in vitro*)

Sodium nitroprusside is a powerful vasodilator used primarily to treat hypertensive crises. It is rapidly metabolized by smooth muscle to nitric oxide, which activates guanylate cyclase with the formation of cyclic guanosine monophosphate and subsequent vasodilation. Nitroprusside dilates both arterioles and venules; systemic vascular hypotension results from a combination of venous pooling and diminished arterial resistance. The drug is available as an intravenous solution, is dangerous to use, and should only be administered by skilled individuals. Following infusion, the hypotensive response is almost immediate and disappears within 3 min of withdrawal. Nitroprusside is rapidly reduced to cyanide and nitric oxide (NO). Cyanide is further metabolized to thiocyanate by the liver. The mean elimination time for thiocyanate is 3 days by individuals with normal liver function.

Experimental studies have examined the *in vitro* effects

of nitroprusside on cultured rat embryos, cerebellar granule cells, and hippocampal slices (1,3,6). Apoptosis appeared in the embryonic neurons (1) and nonspecific neuronal necrosis in the other preparations (3,6). These effects have been attributed to energy depletion resulting from NO-induced inhibition of glyceraldehyde-3-phosphate dehydrogenase (5). The immature rat brain was not affected by direct injection of nitroprusside into the hippocampus (2).

Humans receiving nitroprusside for acute hypertensive situations do not experience serious nervous system toxicity other than the effects of hypoperfusion. Individuals with renal or hepatic compromise receiving repeated infusions of nitroprusside for 2 days or longer may display toxic manifestations: nausea, fatigue, anorexia, and mild confusion; severely affected patients may develop a toxic psychosis (4).

REFERENCES

1. Lee QP, Park HW, Thayer J et al. (1996) Apoptosis induced in cultured rat embryos by intra-amniotically microinjected sodium nitroprusside. *Teratology* **53**, 21.

2. Maragos WF, Silverstein FS (1994) Resistance to nitroprusside neurotoxicity in perinatal rat brain. *Neurosci Lett* **172**, 80.

3. Satoh S, Murayama T, Nomura Y (1996) Sodium nitroprusside stimulates noradrenaline release from rat hippocampal slices in the presence of dithiothreitol. *Brain Res* **733**, 167.

4. Schulz V (1984) Clinical pharmacokinetics of nitroprusside, cyanide, thiosulphate and thiocyanate. *Clin Pharmacokinet* **9**, 239.

5. Yasuda M, Fujimori H, Panhou H (1998) NO depletes cellular ATP contents via inactivation of glyceraldehyde-3-phosphate dehydrogenase in PC12 cells. *J Toxicol Sci* **23**, 389.

6. Yu O, Chuang DM (1996) Inhibition of excitatory amino acid-induced phosphoinositide hydrolysis as a possible mechanism of nitroprusside neurotoxicity. *J Neurochem* **66**, 346.

Nitrosoureas

Glen Kisby

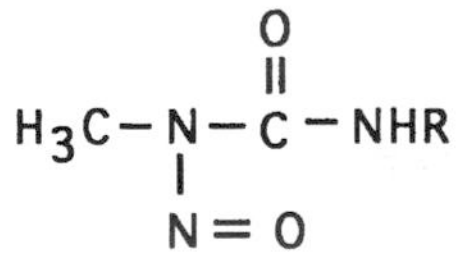

N-Methylnitrosourea (MNU)   R = methyl
N-Ethylnitrosourea (ENU)   R = ethyl
Streptozotocin   R = 2-substituted glucose

ALKYLNITROSOUREAS

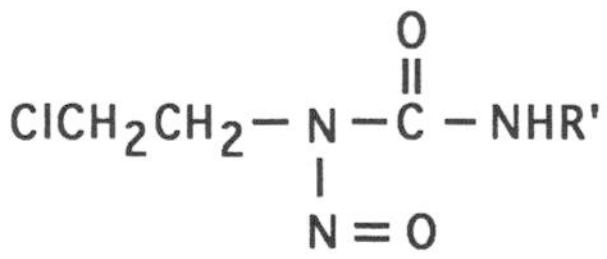

BCNU (Carmustine)   R' = -CH₂CH₂Cl

CCNU (Lomustine)   R' =

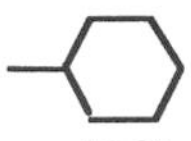

Methyl-CCNU (Semustine)   R' =

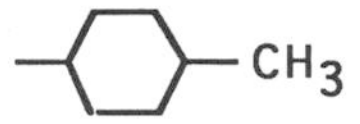

Chlorozotocin   R' = 2-substituted glucose

CHLOROETHYLNITROSOUREAS

NEUROTOXICITY RATING

Clinical

A Acute encephalopathy

Experimental

A Neurocarcinogen

Chemotherapeutic agents are widely used, usually in conjunction with radiation therapy, for the management of tumors. Historically, alkylating agents (*e.g.*, nitrogen mustards) were the first chemotherapeutic agents developed between World War I and World War II for the treatment of lymphomasarcomas (15). Presently, there are five general categories of alkylating chemotherapeutic agents: (a) nitrogen mustards, (b) the ethylinimines, (c) the alkyl sulfonates, (d) the triazenes, and (e) the nitrosoureas. Nitrosoureas belong to the clinically most active group of chemotherapeutic agents for brain tumors because they readily cross the blood-brain barrier (15). A serious complication of nitrosourea chemotherapy is the development of neurotoxicity. Nitrosoureas may induce neurotoxicity by several general mechanisms including: (a) a direct drug-related toxic effect on the nervous system; (b) a drug-induced metabolic encephalopathy; (c) a drug-induced intracranial hemorrhage or infection (due to coagulopathy or myelosuppression); or (d) a psychological effect of the agent (38).

Nitrosoureas can generally be classified (based upon structure) into two categories: (a) the 2-chloroethylnitrosoureas [*e.g.*, BCNU (carmustine), CCNU (lomustine), methyl-CCNU (semustine), PCNU (1-(2-chloroethyl)-3-(2,6-dioxo-3-piperidyl)-1-nitrosourea), ACNU (1-[4-amino-2-methyl-5-pyrimidinyl]methyl-3-[2-chloroethyl]-3-nitrosourea) hydrochloride, and MCNU 7-(methyl 6-[3-(2-chloroethyl-3-nitrosoureido]-6-deoxy-alpha-D-glucopyranoside) (54); and (b) the alkylnitrosoureas [*e.g.*, streptozotocin, N-methylnitrosourea (NMU), ethylnitrosourea (ENU)]. Chloroethylnitrosoureas are clinically effective in the management of tumors, while alkylnitrosoureas are experimental agents used predominantly in cancer research. Alkylnitrosoureas produce pronounced adverse effects (*e.g.*, myelosuppression), limiting their usefulness in antitumor therapy. The therapeutic action of nitrosoureas is related to their interaction with DNA; therapeutic efficacy is compromised in tumors capable of repairing nitrosourea-induced DNA damage (1).

BCNU is a light yellow powder at 4°C; it melts to an oily liquid at 27°C and is stable in the anhydrous state. BCNU is synthesized commercially from a solution of 1,3-bis(2-chloroethyl)urea and formic acid (23). It is slighly soluble in water (4 mg/ml) and 50% ethanol (150 mg/ml), and highly soluble in lipids. BCNU is sensitive to oxidation and hydrolysis, forming alkylating and carbamoylating intermediates. It has a half-life of 24 h in a 0.9% sodium chloride solution (pH 6.0) at room temperature. BCNU is usually administered intravenously in dosages of 100–200 mg/m^2 given by infusion over a period of ~1 h, and it is not repeated for 6 weeks. This dosing regimen is also used for other chloroethylnitrosoureas (*e.g.*, CCNU, methyl-CCNU). The dose of BCNU and other chloroethylnitrosoureas is reduced by 25%–50% when used in combination with other chemotherapeutics.

CCNU, unlike BCNU, is usually administered orally even though both compounds are rapidly absorbed across the gastrointestinal tract. Streptozotocin, like BCNU, is administered either intravenously or intra-arterially in dosages of 500–1500 mg/m^2 once a week for 4 weeks. Streptozotocin is usually used in combination with other chemotherapeutic agents to reduce their adverse effects (inhibition of glutathione).

NMU, a representative alkylnitrosourea, was first prepared by Bruning in 1889 by the reaction of sodium nitrite with an aqueous solution of methylurea and nitrate (42). NMU and other alkylnitrosoureas are produced primarily in small quantities for research purposes. NMU and related nitrosamides can be formed *in vivo* following the consumption of food products containing methylurea (proteins) and sodium nitrite (cured or smoked meat) (22,31). Both alkylnitrosoureas and chloroethylnitrosoureas are highly reactive compounds that demonstrate different reaction rates with various biologically important nucleophiles including proteins and nucleic acids. NMU and other alkylnitrosoureas are sensitive to humidity and light and subject to decomposition to a diazoalkane (*e.g.*, diazomethane, diazoethane) in alkaline solutions (22). The half-life of NMU and other alkylnitrosoureas in physiological solutions at room temperature (~20°C) is pH-dependent with a greater stability in acidic (*e.g.*, pH 4.0, $t_{1/2}$ 190–125 h) than in alkaline (*e.g.*, pH 9.0, $t_{1/2}$ 0.03–0.05 h) environments.

NMU decomposes at physiological pH to produce the cyanate ion, which can carbamoylate cellular proteins. The cyanate ion has been suggested to be responsible for the *in vitro* toxic effects of NMU on cell cultures (30).

Nitrosoureas undergo spontaneous decomposition under physiological conditions to produce a diazonium hydroxide, bifunctionally alkylating chloroethylcarbonium ions, carbamoylating isocyanates (chloroethylnitrosoureas), or cyanates (alkylnitrosoureas) (2,30). Of these metabolites, the diazonium hydroxide and chloroethylcarbonium ions are the predominant chemical species responsible for inducing DNA damage (cross-links) in brain tissue (4). These adducts are likely responsible for the neuro-oncogenic properties of nitrosoureas (6).

General Toxicology

Because of their high lipid solubility, the chloroethylnitrosoureas BCNU (parental) and CCNU (oral) readily cross (*via* passive diffusion) the blood-brain barrier and have therapeutic efficacy for brain tumors. Some 40 min after injection, BCNU is no longer an effective antitumor agent (8), and a few minutes after administration no unchanged BCNU can be detected in plasma (37). Alkylnitrosoureas like the chloroethylnitrosoureas are rapidly absorbed and undetectable in the blood of rats 15 min after an intravenous injection of 100 mg/kg NMU (51).

Following parental (intraperitoneal or subcutaneous) or oral administration, chloroethylnitrosoureas (40,49) and alkylnitrosoureas (29) are rapidly distributed to most tissues, including brain and cerebrospinal fluid. Peak metabolite levels are seen within 1–6 h of oral or parenteral chloroethylnitrosourea administration, and the distribution is widespread to brain and other organs (*e.g.*, liver, kidney, lungs). Metabolites have been detected in the cerebrospinal fluid of patients within minutes of an intravenous injection of a chloroethylnitrosourea. The plasma half-life of BCNU is 34 h after oral administration and 67 h after intravenous injection.

In addition to its spontaneous decomposition, chloroethylnitrosoureas may be denitrosated enzymatically to a corresponding urea (20). BCNU is a substrate for glutathione S-transferases (19) and significantly reduces glutathione levels in liver but not lung of injected mice. The antineoplastic activity of chloroethylnitrosoureas and alkylnitrosoureas is related to the formation of the alkylating intermediates, chloroalkyl carbonium ion and diazoxide hydroxide, respectively. Nitrosourea-induced cytotoxicity is triggered by the reaction of these intermediates with nucleosides and nucleic acids to form monofunctional and cross-linked DNA adducts.

Urine is the major route by which chloroethylnitrosoureas are eliminated in humans. About 50%–77% of an administered radiolabeled dose of a chloroethylnitrosourea is recovered in the urine 24–48 h after dosing (49). Urinary excretion does not vary with route of administration. Cerebrospinal fluid levels are 30% of plasma levels, and metabolites are the predominant form. About 80% of a radiolabeled chloroethylnitrosourea is recovered in the urine of chloroethylnitrosourea-dosed animals (40). Excretion of chloroethylnitrosoureas in humans is similar to that in monkeys and dogs (11) but considerably slower than in mice (35,36).

The highly reactive nature of nitrosoureas towards biologically relevant nucleophiles (e.g., nucleic acids) is the mechanism by which these agents induce their antineoplastic effects in humans (chloroethylnitrosoureas) and genotoxic (mutagenic, teratogenic, and carcinogenic) properties in animals. Alkylnitrosoureas, such as NMU, are direct alkylating agents that need no bioactivation to alkylate nucleic acids in vitro or in vivo. Alkylnitrosoureas produce predominantly monofunctional adducts like N^7-alkylguanine (~69%), O^6-alkylguanine (~3%–6%), and alkylphosphate triesters (~12%) (44). The chloroethylnitrosoureas bind to DNA and produce predominantly bifunctional adducts like interstrand and intrastrand cross-links, and carbamoylated proteins. These DNA adducts have been detected in a number of tissues including brain, lung, kidney, liver, intestine, thymus, and spleen from various species (mice, rats, hamsters, minipigs) dosed with nitrosoureas. One of these DNA adducts, O^6-alkylguanine, is slowly repaired (16,18,26,36) in nervous tissue of nitrosourea-treated animals, suggesting that DNA repair in the nervous system is poor or inefficient. The persistence of these DNA adducts in the nervous tissue of alkylnitrosourea-treated animals is the mechanism by which these agents are proposed experimentally to induce

neurogenic tumors in animals. However, alkylation of nervous tissue DNA by alkylnitrosoureas does not always induce neurogenic tumors. Both glial and neuronal DNA have been found to be alkylated to the same extent by NMU but only glial tumors are formed (27). Therefore, differences in the proliferative capacity of nervous tissue cell types (i.e., mitotic vs. postmitotic) (25) are likely to determine the nature of alkylnitrosourea-induced neurogenic tumors.

In contrast to alkylnitrosoureas, chloroethylnitrosoureas strongly carbamoylate cellular proteins. It has been shown that the carbamoylation of cellular proteins can result in either activation or inactivation of chloroethylnitrosourea. BCNU reacts with cellular glutathione to produce an S-carbamoylated glutathione (GSH) derivative that is genotoxic and mutagenic in vitro (50). Whether S-carbamoylated derivatives of chloroalkylnitrosoureas contribute to their in vivo cytotoxicity is unknown. Alternatively, certain chloroalkylnitrosoureas inactivate glutathione reductase and reduce intracellular glutathione pools, increasing the sensitivity of tissues or cells to reactive oxygen species (i.e., free radicals). Low concentrations of N,N′-bis(trans-4-hydroxy-cyclohexyl)-N′-nitrosourea (BHCNU), a derivative of BCNU with predominant carbamoylating but low alkylating properties, depletes GSH levels to 40% of control values in human leukemia cells (7). The biological significance of GSH depletion by chloroethylnitrosoureas is uncertain given that it does not correlate with antitumor efficacy, chronic toxicity, or carcinogenic potential (12). However, the antitumor efficiency of chloroethylnitrosoureas against neurogenic tumors has been shown to be dependent on its DNA–DNA cross-linking properties in vitro (3).

Alkylnitrosoureas are used almost exclusively for research purposes, but there is one study from the former U.S.S.R. that examined its antitumor efficacy in humans (13). Almost all patients experienced severe nausea and vomiting, often accompanied by diarrhea, within 40 min of receiving the drug. Myelosuppression was significantly pronounced in NMU-treated patients, thereby limiting its clinical usefulness as an antitumor agent.

In contrast, the chloroethylnitrosoureas are used widely in the management of tumors and have produced a number of adverse effects. The chloroethylnitrosourea BCNU is a mild vesicant, producing local vein discomfort during infusion. Nausea and vomiting may be severe but usually are short-lived. Myelosuppression is delayed and cumulative; nadir blood counts occur 4–5 weeks following treatment and are worse with subsequent courses of therapy. Myelosuppression is at least partly linked to the carbamoylation of cellular proteins by BCNU (3). Pulmonary fibrosis is a serious late complication that occurs in <5% of patients with a cumulative dose of <1400 mg/m² BCNU (38); higher doses may induce pulmonary failure. Renal insufficiency, hepatotoxicity, and leukemia are uncommon late complications of nitrosoureas. Chloroalkylnitrosoureas administered by the intracarotid route also produce significant ocular toxicity: retinopathy, blindness, or ocular necrosis (10,32,34). Intracarotid infusions distal to the ophthalmic artery prevent chloroalkylnitrosourea-induced ocular toxicity.

Human Disease

Human exposure to alkylating agents, including nitrosamides (NNO), is widespread. Sources include dietary exposure to preformed NNO (5,21) or to precursors for endogenous nitrosation (33), tobacco-specific NNO (17), occupational exposure (e.g., in rubber and tire manufacturing) (52), and some chemotherapeutic agents (46).

The chloroethylnitrosoureas have little or no neurotoxicity at the usual intravenous dose (200 mg/m² or 80 mg/m²/day for 3 days). BCNU given intravenously causes dizziness, loss of equilibrium, and ataxia in 9% of 223 patients treated for solid tumors (43). At higher doses, however, neurotoxicity is a common side effect. Encephalopathy with confusion and seizures may follow high-dose (600–800 mg/m² or more) intravenous BCNU with autologous bone marrow transplantation (41). Intracarotid BCNU (usually, 100–200 mg/m²) will produce severe local pain in the ipsilateral face, eye, and head during infusion (39). Some patients become transiently confused and disoriented 4–24 h after BCNU infusion. A severe ipsilateral encephalopathy with seizures, hemiparesis, progressive neurologic deficits, and cerebral necrosis (pathologically similar to radiation necrosis) has followed intracarotid BCNU (53). Focal seizures occur immediately in some (~4%) patients, but the majority (~31%) experiences a delayed effect after BCNU infusion (53). Concurrent cranial radiotherapy and intracarotid BCNU may increase the risk of neurotoxicity. Drug streaming during intracarotid injections may produce extreme drug levels in branches where the drug has been channeled with subtherapeutic levels in other vessels.

Pronounced neurotoxicity has been demonstrated in patients with malignant gliomas after direct administration (e.g., via an investigational multiperforated Silastic basket) of chloroethylnitrosoureas to the brain (54). Twenty patients were administered ACNU (20 mg × 15 times) or MCNU (11 mg × 2 times). ACNU was well tolerated while MCNU induced marked brain edema. Adverse effects consisted of headache, nuchal stiffness, vomiting, motor weakness, and cranial nerve palsy for ACNU, and headache, vomiting, abnormal respiration, and arrhythmia for MCNU. Neuropathological changes included spongy degeneration and reactive gliosis of adjacent white matter, occlusion of neighboring arteries, and demyelination of cranial nerves in patients treated with ACNU, while patients treated with MCNU exhibited focal brain necrosis. Differences in the neurotoxic profile of these two chloroethylnitrosoureas are probably related to differences in blood-brain transport.

Animal Studies

Neurogenic tumors are the most consistent neurotoxic effect of alkylnitrosoureas in treated (>5 mg/kg) animals. Analysis of a large number of nervous tissue tumors demonstrates that glial cells and Schwann cells are the main targets. Alkylnitrosourea-induced CNS tumors are predominantly oligodendrogliomas, astrocytomas, mixed gliomas, and ependymomas, while malignant neurinomas (schwannomas) are found in the PNS (55). Age and species are two factors that contribute to the susceptibility of animals to alkylnitrosourea-induced neurogenic tumors. Young animals are more susceptible to neurogenic tumors than adult animals, and rodents are more susceptible than higher organisms (e.g., primates). Furthermore, there is a regional susceptibility of brain tissue to alkylnitrosourea-induced neurogenic tumors. At lower drug doses (1 mg/kg or less), however, alkylnitrosoureas are predominantly cytotoxic and not neurogenic. In one study, a late-onset degenerative disease in the cerebellum was produced in the offspring of mice exposed to a single dose of NMU (1 mg/kg) on day 16 of gestation (47). The animals developed a mild ataxia, as evidenced by compromised performance on a motor coordination task, in addition to quantitative evidence of degenerative changes characterized by Purkinje cell loss and disrupted folial organization. Examination of nervous tissue from these animals revealed a delayed expression of abnormal morphology and function. A late-onset progressive retinal degeneration beginning at 4 weeks of age was also seen in the offspring of these mice (48).

DNA damage is proposed to be the key event in triggering nitrosourea-induced neurogenic tumors in animals (45). Studies in both neonatal (16,28) and young adult rats (26) using radiolabelled NMU (N-^{14}C-methyl-N-nitrosourea) demonstrate significant DNA damage in the nervous system. The predominant adduct detected in brain tissue DNA and RNA is N^7-methylguanine (7-mG). Brain DNA also contained O^6-alkylguanine (12% of 7-mG), while cytoplasmic RNA had half as much as brain DNA. Moreover, the removal (or repair) of O^6-alkylguanine is significantly slower in rodent brain than in corresponding liver tissue (9). Human brain cells also appear to be particularly inefficient at repairing damage induced by alkylnitrosoureas or ultraviolet light (14). It is this inefficient repair of DNA damage that may be responsible for alkylnitrosourea-induced cerebellar degeneration seen in NMU-treated mice (47).

While the predominant effect of alkylnitrosoureas on the animal's nervous system is related to their carcinogenic properties, these agents also perturb neurotransmitter synthesis and metabolism. Significant changes in the level of brain monoamine neurotransmitters [norepinephrine (NE), dopamine (DA)] and their metabolites [5-hydroxytryptamine (5-HT), vanillylmandelic acid (VMA), dihydroxyphenyl acetic acid (DOPAC), homovanillic acid (HVA), 5-hydroxyindoleacetic acid (5-HIAA), dihydroxyphenylalanine (DOPA)] have been found in brain tissue from CD-1 mice treated with ENU (24). Brain monoamine levels and their metabolites were measured in brain tissue from young male CD-1 mice treated intraperitoneally with ENU (0, 2, 8, or 32 mg/kg) twice a week for 3 weeks. Elevated levels of NE and 5-HT were found in the hypothalamus and striatum and 5-HIAA in various brain regions. In addition, NE was elevated in the cerebral cortex, medulla oblongata, and cerebellum of treated animals. The NE metabolite VMA was decreased in several brain regions to nondetectable levels. Neuropathological examination of the brain tissue from ENU-treated animals was unremarkable. Tryptophan hydroxylase activity was increased in the hypothalamus and striatum, dopa decarboxylase activity was elevated in the cerebral cortex, and monoamine oxidase activity was unchanged when mice were treated with low-dose ENU. The concomitant alteration in enzyme activity and elevated brain monoamine levels indicate that ENU interferes with brain monoamine metabolism. Alkylating agents (*e.g.*, alkylnitrosoureas) may perturb monoamine neurotransmitter metabolism in the nervous system through their reaction with nucleic acids or by altering the transport mechanism for monoamine precursors or metabolites (24).

REFERENCES

1. Aamdal S, Gerard B, Bohman T, D'Incalci M (1992) Sequential administration of dacarbazine and fotemustine in patients with disseminated malignant melanoma—an effective combination with unexpected toxicity. *Eur J Cancer* 28, 447.

2. Ali-Osman F (1989) Quenching of DNA cross-link precursors of chloroethylnitrosoureas and attenuation of DNA interstrand cross-linking by glutathione. *Cancer Res* 49, 5258.

3. Ali-Osman F, Giblin J, Berger M *et al.* (1985) Chemical structure of carbamoylating groups and their relationship to bone marrow toxicity and antiglioma activity of bifunctionally alkylating and carbamoylating nitrosoureas. *Cancer Res* 45, 4185.

4. Ali-Osman F, Rairkar A, Young P (1995) Formation and repair of 1,3-bis-(2-chloroethyl)-1-nitrosourea and cisplatin induced total genomic DNA interstrand crosslinks in human glioma cells. *Cancer Biochem Biophys* 14, 231.

5. Bianchini F, Montesano R, Shuker DEG *et al.* (1993) Quantification of 7-methyldeoxyguanosine using immunoaffinity purification and HPLC with electrochemical detection. *Carcinogenesis* 14, 1677.

6. Bilzer T, Reifenberger G, Wechsler W (1989) Chemical induction of brain tumors in rats by nitrosourea: molecular biology and neuropathology. *Neurotoxicol Teratol* 11, 551.

7. Chresta CM, Crook TR, Souhami RL (1990) Depletion of cellular glutathione by N,N'-bis(trans-4-hydroxycyclohexyl)-N'-nitrosourea as a determinant of sensitivity of K562 human leukemia cells to 4-hydroperoxycyclophosphamide. *Cancer Res* 50, 4067.

8. Connors TA, Hare JR (1975) Studies of the mechanisms of action of the tumour-inhibitory nitrosoureas. *Biochem Pharmacol* 24, 2133.

9. Craddock VM, Henderson AR, Gash S (1984) Repair and replication of DNA in rat brain and liver during foetal and post-natal development, in relation to nitroso-alkylurea induced carcinogenesis. *J Cancer Res Clin Oncol* 108, 30.

10. Defer G, Fauchon F, Schaison M *et al.* (1991) Visual toxicity following intra-arterial chemotherapy with hydroxyethyl-CNU in patients with malignant gliomas. *Neuroradiology* 33, 432.

11. DeVita VT, Denham C, Davison JD, Oliverio VT (1967) The physiological disposition of the carcinostatic 1,3-bis(2-chloroethyl)-1-nitrosourea (BCNU) in man and animals. *Clin Pharmacol Ther* 8, 566.

12. Eisenbrand G (1984) Anticancer nitrosoureas: investigations on antineoplastic, toxic and neoplastic activities. In: *N-Nitroso Compounds: Occurrence, Biological Effects and Relevance to Human Cancer.* O'Neill IK, Von Borstel RC, Miller CT *et al.* eds. Oxford University Press, New York p. 695.

13. Emanuel NM, Vermel EM, Ostrovskaya LA, Korman NP (1974) Experimental and clinical studies of the antitumour activity of 1-methyl-1-nitrosourea (NSC 23909). *Cancer Chemother Rep* 58, 135.

14. Gibson-D'Ambrosio RE, Leong Y, D'Ambrosio SM (1983) DNA repair following ultraviolet and N-ethyl-N nitrosourea treatment of cells cultured from human fetal brain, intestine, kidney, liver and skin. *Cancer Res* 43, 5846.

15. Gilman AG, Goodman LS, Gilman A (1980) *Goodman and Gilman's The Pharmacological Basis of Therapeutics.* Macmillan, New York.

16. Goth R, Rajewsky MF (1974) Persistence of O^6-ethylguanine in rat brain DNA: Correlation with nervous system-specific carcinogenesis by ethylnitrosourea. *Proc Nat Acad Sci USA* 71, 693.

17. Hecht SS, Hoffman D (1988) Tobacco-specific nitrosamines, an important group of carcinogens in tobacco and tobacco smoke. *Carcinogenesis* 9, 875.

18. Heyting C, Van Der Laken CJ, Raamsdonk WV, Pool CW (1983) Immunohistochemical detection of O^6-ethyldeoxyguanosine in the rat brain after *in vivo* applications of N-ethyl-N-nitrosourea. *Cancer Res* 43, 2935.

19. Hill DL (1976) N,N'-bis(2-Chloroethyl)-N-nitrosourea (BCNU), a substrate for glutathione (GSH) S-transferase. *Proc Amer Assn Cancer Res* 17, 56 (abstr).

20. Hill DL, Kirk MC, Struck RF (1975) Microsomal metabolism of nitrosoureas. *Cancer Res* 35, 296.

21. Hotchkiss JH (1989) Preformed N-nitroso compounds in foods and beverages. In: *Cancer Surveys: Nitrate, Nitrite and Nitrosocompounds in Human Cancer. 8th Ed.* Forman D, Shuker D eds. Oxford University Press, Oxford p. 322.

22. IARC (1978) *IARC Monographs on the Evaluation of Carcinogenic Risk of Chemicals to Humans: N-Nitroso Compounds. Vol 17.* International Agency for Research on Cancer Working Group, Lyon, October 10–15, 1977.

23. IARC (1981) *IARC Monographs on the Evaluation of Carcinogenic Risk of Chemicals to Humans: Some Antineoplastic and Immunosuppressive Agents. Vol 26.* International Agency for Research on Cancer Working Group, Lyon, October 14–20, 1980.

24. Jayasekara S, Sharma RP, Drown DB (1992) Effects of N-ethyl,N-nitrosourea on monoamine concentrations and metabolizing enzymes in mouse brain regions. *Eur J Pharmacol* 228, 37.

25. Kleihues P, Cooper HK, Bucheler J *et al.* (1979) Mechanism of perinatal tumor induction by neuro-oncogenic alkylnitrosoureas and dialkyltriazenes. *Nat Cancer Inst Monogr* 51, 227.

26. Kleihues P, Magee PN (1973) Alkylation of rat brain nucleic acids by N-methyl-N-nitrosourea and methyl methanesulphonate. *J Neurochem* 20, 595.

27. Kleihues P, Magee PN, Cox JA, Mathias AP (1973) Reaction of N-methyl-N-nitrosourea with DNA of neuronal and glial cells *in vivo*. *FEBS Lett* 32, 105.

28. Kleihues P, Margison GP (1974) Carcinogenicity of N-methyl-N-nitrosourea: Possible role of excision repair of O^6-methylguanine from DNA. *J Natl Cancer Inst* 53, 1839.

29. Kleihues P, Patzschke K (1971) Verteilung von N-[^{14}C]-Methyl-N-nitrosoharnstoff in der Ratte nach systemischer applikation. *Z Krebsforsch* 75, 193.

30. Knox P (1976) Carcinogenic nitrosamides and cell cultures. *Nature* 259, 671.

31. Koestner A, Denlinger RH, Wechsler W (1975) Induction of neurogenic and lymphoid neoplasms by the feeding of threshold levels of methyl- and ethylnitrosourea precursors to adult rats. *Food Cosmet Toxicol* 13, 605.

32. Kupersmith MJ, Frohman LP, Choi IS (1988) Visual system toxicity following intra-arterial chemotherapy. *Neurology* 38, 284.

33. Leaf CD, Wishnok JS, Tannenbaum SR (1989) Mechanisms of endogenous nitrosation. In: *Cancer Surveys: Nitrate, Nitrite and Nitrosocompounds in Human Cancer. 8th Ed.* Forman D, Shuker D eds. Oxford University Press, Oxford p. 334.

34. Lennan RM, Taylor HR (1978) Optic neuroretinitis in association with BCNU and procarbazine therapy. *Med Pediatr Oncol* 4, 43.

35. Levin VA, Kabra PA, Freedman-Dove MA (1978) Relationship of 1,3-bis(2-chloroethyl)-1-nitrosourea (BCNU) and 1-(2-chloroethyl)-3-cyclohexyl-1-nitrosourea (CCNU) pharmacokinetics of uptake, distribution, and tissue/plasma partitioning in rat organs and intracerebral tumors. *Cancer Chemother Pharmacol* 1, 233.

36. Likhachev AJ, Ivanov MN, Bresil H *et al.* (1983) Carcinogenicity of single doses of N-nitroso-N-methylurea and N-nitroso-N-ethylurea in Syrian golden hamsters and the persistence of alkylated purines in the DNA of various tissues. *Cancer Res* 43, 829.

37. Loo TL, Dion RL, Dixon RL, Rall DP (1966) The antitumor agent, 1,3-bis(2-chloroethyl)-1-nitrosourea. *J Pharmacol Sci* 55, 492.

38. Macdonald DR (1991) Neurologic complications of chemotherapy. *Neurol Clin* 9, 955.

39. Madajewicz S, West CR, Park HC (1981) Phase II study—intraarterial BCNU therapy for metastatic brain tumors. *Cancer* 47, 653.

40. Oliverio VT (1973) Pharmacology of the nitrosoureas: An overview. *Cancer Treatment Rep* 3, 13.

41. Phillips GL, Wolff SN, Fay JW (1986) Intensive 1,3-bis(2-chloroethyl)-1-nitrosourea (BCNU) monochemotherapy and autologous marrow transplantation for malignant glioma. *J Clin Oncol* 4, 639.

42. Prager B, Jacobson P, Schmidt P *et al.* (1922) *Beilsteins Handbuch der Organischen Chemie.* Springer, Berlin.

43. Ramirez G, Wilson W, Grage T (1972) Phase II evaluation of 1,3-bis(2-chloroethyl)-1-nitrosourea (BCNU; NSC-409962) in patients with solid tumors. *Cancer Chemother Rep* 56, 787.

44. Richardson FC, Beauchamp RO Jr, Swenberg JA (1987) Properties and biological consequences of alkylpyrimidine deoxyribonucleosides. *Pharmacol Ther* 34, 181.

45. Robbiano L, Brambilla M (1987) DNA damage in the central nervous system of rats after *in vivo* exposure to chemical carcinogens: Correlation with the induction of brain tumors. *Teratogen Carcin Mut* 7, 175.

46. Schmahl D, Kaldor JM (1986) Carcinogenicity of alkylating cytostatic drugs. *IARC Sci. Publ. No. 78.* International Agency for Research on Cancer, Lyon.

47. Smith SB, Brown CB, Wright ME, Yielding KL (1987) Late-onset cerebellar degeneration in mice induced transplacentally by methylnitrosourea. *Teratogen Carcin Mut* 7, 449.

48. Smith SB, Yielding KL (1986) Retinal degeneration in the mouse: A model of progressive deterioration induced transplacentally by methylnitrosourea. *Exp Eye Res* 43, 791.

49. Sponzo RW, DeVita VT, Oliverio VT (1973) Physiologic disposition of 1-(2-chloroethyl)-3-cyclohexyl-1-nitrosourea (CCNU) and 1-(2-chloroethyl)-3-(4-methyl-cyclohexyl)-1-nitrosourea (Me CCNU) in man. *Cancer* 31, 1154.

50. Stahl W, Denkel E, Eisenbrand G (1988) Influence of glutathione on the mutagenicity of 2-chloroethylnitrosoureas: Mutagenic potential of glutathione derivatives formed from 2-chloroethylnitrosourease and glutathione. *Mutat Res* 206, 459.

51. Swann PF (1968) The rate of breakdown of methyl methanesulphonate dimethyl sulphate and *N*-methyl-*N*-nitrosourea in the rat. *Biochem J* 110, 49.

52. Tricker AR, Spiegelhalder B, Preussman R (1989) Environmental exposure to preformed nitroso compounds. In: *Cancer Surveys: Nitrate, Nitrite and Nitrosocompounds in Human Cancer*. Forman D, Shuker D eds. Oxford University Press, Oxford p. 251.

53. West CR, Avellanosa AM, Barua NR (1980) Phase II study on malignant gliomas of the brain treated with intraarterial BCNU in combination with vincristine and procarbazine. *Proc Amer Assn Cancer Res* 21, 482.

54. Yamashima T, Yamashita J, Shoin K (1990) Neurotoxicity of local administration of two nitrosoureas in malignant gliomas. *Neurosurgery* 26, 794.

55. Zeller WJ (1992) Neurotrophic carcinogenesis. In *Selective Neurotoxicity*. Herken H, Hucho F eds. Springer-Verlag, Berlin p. 193.

Nitrous Oxide

Stephen N. Scelsa

$$N \equiv N = O$$

NITROUS OXIDE
N_2O

Dinitrogen monoxide

NEUROTOXICITY RATING

Clinical

A Peripheral neuropathy

A Myelopathy

B Chronic encephalopathy (memory impairment)

Experimental

A Myelopathy (vacuolar)

A Vitamin B_{12} deficiency (methionine synthetase inhibition)

Nitrous oxide is an inorganic gas that constitutes about 0.00005% of the earth's atmosphere by volume (52). It is manufactured by thermal decomposition of ammonium nitrate and stored in cylinders under pressure in a gas:liquid equilibrium. N_2 is the principal impurity of the marketed product; other possible contaminants include NO_2, N, O_2, and CO_2. The liquid vaporizes at room temperature as it is released from the cylinder.

Nitrous oxide is colorless and has a minimally sweet taste and odor. It weighs more than air and is not flammable, although when combined with a flammable anesthetic, it actively supports combustion (32). The blood:gas partition coefficient of nitrous oxide is 0.47 at 37°C, which indicates relatively low solubility in blood. It has a similarly low oil:gas partition coefficient of 1.4 at 37°C.

Nitrous oxide is the oldest inhalational anesthetic in current use. The principal medical use of nitrous oxide is as an adjuvant anesthetic for many surgical procedures that require general anesthesia. Nitrous oxide has the appealing properties of rapid induction and reversibility; pleasant, mild odor; and relative respiratory and circulatory stability (9). However, it is typically combined with other agents because of its low anesthetic potency as suggested by a minimum alveolar concentration in humans of only 1.04 ± 0.10 atm absolute (23). Use of nitrous oxide allows for concentration reductions of the other more potent agents that have greater cardiovascular effects, lessening respiratory and circulatory depression while maintaining rapid induction and recovery. Nitrous oxide, often in combination with local anesthetics, is also administered frequently by dentists and dental surgeons to induce general anesthesia.

Nitrous oxide is commonly used in the food industry because of its neutral flavor, chemical inertness, moderately high water solubility, and bacteriostatic properties (17). Commercially, it is used as a propellant in whipped-cream dispensers. The automotive industry uses nitrous oxide as a source of injectable oxygen (24). Rocket fuel preparations utilize nitrous oxide in combination with carbon disulfide (52).

Nitrous oxide is not a controlled substance. The United States Pharmacopeia requires that manufactured preparations include at least 99% nitrous oxide by volume and not more than 0.001% carbon monoxide, 1 ppm of nitric oxide, 1 ppm of nitrogen dioxide, and 1 ppm of halogen (49). The U.S. National Institute for Occupational Safety and Health (NIOSH) has proposed 25 ppm as the maximal allowed time-weighted exposure per anesthetic administration for health care personnel (46); this has been criticized as unduly restrictive (46).

General Toxicology

Because of the low blood solubility of nitrous oxide, an alveolar-arterial pressure equilibrium is achieved rapidly. The rate of net gas uptake in adult men is rapid, approaching 1 l/min (32). As nitrous oxide is taken up by the pulmonary circulation, additional gas is pulled into the alveoli so that nitrous oxide is delivered to the lung faster than the minute ventilation rate. At higher inhaled gas concentrations, arterial tension increases more rapidly; this is known as the *concentration effect*. Because of its rapid uptake by the blood, nitrous oxide may increase the uptake of other gas anesthetics when given concurrently, a phenomenon known as the *second-gas effect*. The sudden substitution of air for nitrous oxide results in diffusion of nitrous oxide from blood to alveoli that causes a drop in alveolar and arterial oxygen tension. This phenomenon, termed *diffusional hypoxia*, may be avoided by oxygen supplementation during the recovery period. Since the blood:gas partition coefficient is much greater for nitrous oxide than for nitrogen, pockets of trapped gas in the body expand as administered nitrous oxide replaces nitrogen. As a consequence of this expansion, loops of bowel, emphysematous blebs, visceral cysts, an occluded middle ear cavity, or a pneumothorax may increase in pressure or size.

There is minimal or no appreciable metabolism of nitrous oxide in human tissue (32). Nitrous oxide is rapidly eliminated as an expired gas with minor diffusion through the skin. The rate of elimination, 987 ml/min at 1 min, is similar to the rate of uptake (10). Reductive metabolism of nitrous oxide *in vitro* to molecular nitrogen by human and rat intestinal bacteria has been reported (Fig. 15) (2). Transfer of a single electron has been postulated to result in hydroxide radical and nitrogen formation. The effects of nitrous oxide on hepatic enzyme induction are unclear, but are likely to be negligible (2).

$$N_2O \longrightarrow [N_2O^-] \longrightarrow OH + OH^- + N_2$$

FIGURE 15. Proposed reductive metabolism of nitrous oxide *in vitro* by rat and human intestinal bacteria. (Reproduced with permission from Miller RD, *Anesthesia*. Churchill Livingstone, New York, 1990.)

Assessment of the metabolic effects of nitrous oxide is complicated because a high dose can be given only at the expense of reducing oxygen delivery; therefore, it is difficult to separate the effects of hypoxia. Prolonged exposure may cause death (24); some deaths related to nitrous oxide use have been attributed to hypoxia.

Although nitrous oxide has mild, direct myocardial and respiratory depressant effects, these effects are rarely clinically significant (9). When used in combination with other inhalational agents, the mild myocardial depressant effect is mostly offset by secondary increases in circulating norepinephrine levels, increases in vascular smooth muscle responsiveness to epinephrine, and reductions in the quantity needed of other agents (32). When used alone, 40%–50% nitrous oxide causes decreases in inspiratory time, increases in the ventilatory rate, and decreases in the end-tidal carbon dioxide tension (40). These findings suggest that nitrous oxide is a mild respiratory stimulant. Although nitrous oxide causes no significant respiratory depression when used alone, it may augment the depressive effects of other agents (32). Additionally, the ventilatory response to hypoxia is decreased (32). Respiratory depression is predominantly a concern in patients with chronic obstructive pulmonary disease where respiratory drive is dependent on arterial oxygen tension. These patients may become hypoxic if given nitrous oxide without controlled respiration. In the presence of hypoventilation, diffusional hypoxia may occur for 30 min following cessation of nitrous oxide (10).

In the dog, nitrous oxide administration results in increased cerebral blood flow, diffuse electroencephalographic slowing and, unlike other inhalational agents, cerebral metabolic stimulation (43). Autoregulation and carbon dioxide responsiveness of the cerebral vasculature are generally maintained during nitrous oxide administration. However, in patients with intracranial pathology, nitrous oxide causes increased intracranial pressure and decreased cerebral perfusion pressure during induction (20); nitrous oxide induction should be avoided in this setting.

The euphoric effects of nitrous oxide have been attributed to activation of mesocortical dopaminergic projections and to interactions with opioid receptors (18,36). Increased levels of 3,4-dihydroxyphenylalanine in the cerebral cortex of rats reportedly suggests mesocortical dopaminergic activation. Similar increases in the pons and medulla oblongata have led to the suggestion that activation of the medullary dopaminergic system may be responsible for the nausea and vomiting sometimes associated with inhalation of higher concentrations of nitrous oxide. Following prolonged exposure of mice to 5000 ppm nitrous oxide, significant increases of norepinephrine, dopamine, and serotonin occur in the hypothalamus; these changes in neurotransmitters may be associated with behavioral effects of nitrous oxide exposure. Through direct and indirect actions with opioid receptors, nitrous oxide may produce analgesia, chemical dependence, and chemical tolerance (18). In rats and mice, tolerance to nitrous oxide may develop within 1–24 h; a similar effect is reported in humans (17).

Nitrous oxide increases muscle tone, particularly in combination with narcotics (9,14,27). While this may suggest that patients receiving nitrous oxide need increased doses of neuromuscular blocking agents, other studies demonstrate a mild facilitation of neuromuscular blockade when nitrous oxide is added to vecuronium or succinylcholine (13). The sole toxic effects of nitrous oxide on the gastrointestinal tract are mild postoperative nausea and vomiting, and, possibly mild elevations of serum bilirubin levels (9,26).

Nitrous oxide has the potential to cause deleterious effects on red blood cell production by interfering with vitamin B_{12} metabolism. In rats, exposure to 50% nitrous oxide reduces activity of the cytosol enzyme methionine synthetase by about 50% within 5 min (7,38). Methionine synthetase is a vitamin B_{12}–dependent enzyme involved in the synthesis of methionine and tetrahydrofolate (Fig. 16). Nitrous oxide may reduce methionine synthetase activity by oxidation of vitamin B_{12}, which in turn lessens availability of tetrahydrofolate and methionine (7). Decreased availability of tetrahydrofolate or methionine may lead to impaired DNA synthesis as reflected by decreased thymidylate synthetase activity in the rat (39). This indirect effect of nitrous oxide in rats on thymidylate synthetase is exaggerated by concomitant vitamin B_{12} deficiency (39). Chronic alcohol treatment does not enhance the degree of disturbed vitamin B_{12} metabolism in rats exposed to 60% nitrous oxide (12). Hemopoietic depression caused by nitrous oxide may be prevented by pretreatment with folinic acid (29). Abnormalities of vitamin B_{12} metabolism have also been shown in monkeys, although hematological parameters and bone marrow morphology were normal, highlighting interspecies differences in the toxic effects of nitrous oxide (33).

Similar disturbances of vitamin B_{12} metabolism have been demonstrated in humans. Megaloblastic change in the bone marrow occurred in eight of eight patients given 50% nitrous oxide for 24 h (1). During surgery, three of nine patients given 50% nitrous oxide for 5–12 h had megaloblastic bone marrow change and abnormalities of vitamin B_{12} metabolism (1). After 46 min of 70% nitrous oxide exposure, there is about a 50% decrease in methionine synthase activity in human liver (38). Prolonged exposure to nitrous oxide may result in aplastic anemia. However, recent studies show that exposure to 50%–70% nitrous oxide during routine surgery does not cause clinically significant alterations in hemopoiesis (25,51). Although transient laboratory abnormalities suggesting disturbed folate metabolism occur—namely, increases of urinary foriminoglutamic acid and decreases in the normal postoperative leukocytosis—such changes have little clinical relevance. Bone marrow stores are probably sufficient to overcome the transient depression of methionine synthetase activity. Despite these findings, some clinicians recommend that nitrous oxide be avoided in immunosuppressed patients because of possible effects on white blood cell production and function.

Teratogenicity has been demonstrated in rats exposed to nitrous oxide during organogenesis (16). Adverse gestational abnormalities include skeletal anomalies (*i.e.*, cervical ribs), visceral malformations, and fetal wastage. Teratogenicity has been attributed to the reduced availability of tetrahydrofolate or methionine attributable to methionine synthetase inhibition. While there is conflicting evidence in rats regarding the protection provided by folinic acid, a recent study suggests that nitrous oxide teratogenicity is due, in part, to decreased methionine and that methionine treatment prevents adverse reproductive effects (15). In addition, the sympathomimetic action of nitrous oxide may play

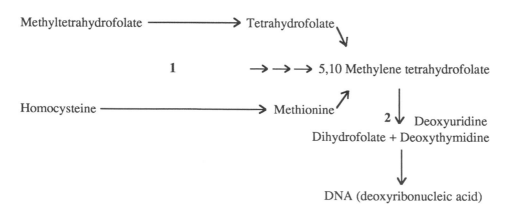

FIGURE 16. Vitamin B_{12}–dependent metabolic pathways affected by nitrous oxide exposure.

a role in the development of *situs inversus* (15). Female dental assistants exposed to nitrous oxide, but not other inhalational agents, had twice the rate of spontaneous abortions and 1.5 times the rate of congenital malformations compared to controls (6). The most frequent anomalies in children of female dental assistants exposed to various inhalational anesthetics were musculoskeletal in nature (6). Nitrous oxide therefore should be avoided during pregnancy and delivery.

Animal Studies

Animal studies show clear evidence of nitrous oxide neurotoxicity in some species but not in others. Monkeys exposed to about 30%–50% nitrous oxide for up to 8 weeks develop two types of clinical neurological deficits. Some demonstrate acute unsteadiness that is reversed by nitrous oxide cessation, while others show progressive irreversible ataxia that ultimately limits their ability to sit up and drink (33). Monkeys exposed to a continuous flow of 15% nitrous oxide show similar progressive ataxia beginning at about 10 weeks (45). Early signs include shaking of the limbs and transient inability to hold objects steadily. Animals subsequently develop progressive ataxia, with some fluctuation of clinical state, until they are unable to climb and hold bars. Ultimately, monkeys are unable to stand and breathing becomes difficult. Pathological examination demonstrates vacuolar demyelination and axonal degeneration of the posterior and lateral columns (33,45). Fatty macrophage accumulations are evident. These changes are identical to those observed in subacute combined degeneration of the spinal cord (45). Consistent with this are metabolic studies suggestive of impaired vitamin B_{12} metabolism. Peripheral nerves reportedly show severe demyelination, though detailed pathological descriptions are not given (45).

Rats exposed to intermittent, daily 70% nitrous oxide for 6 months exhibit no clinical neurological deficit and no functional abnormalities of nerve as measured by a variety of parameters, including caudal nerve conduction velocity, axonal content, and transport of acetylcholinesterase and dopamine-β-hydroxylase (8). In addition, rodents demonstrate no pathological abnormalities in terms of myelinated fiber number and size; teased myelinated fibers are also normal. Although it is not known whether continuous, rather than periodic, administration of nitrous oxide is neurotoxic to rats, the lack of neurotoxic effects in this study suggests there are significant interspecies differences in response to the agent.

Myelopathy develops in fruit bats with low dietary vitamin B_{12} intake and exposure to 50% nitrous oxide, 90 min daily for 8–10 weeks (34). Despite proposals that methyl group transfer is impaired by vitamin B_{12} deficiency, rates of protein and lipid methylation are not disturbed (34).

In Vitro Studies

Protein kinase C activity of growth cones isolated from neonatal rat forebrains is significantly depressed following a 6-h exposure of rats to 50%–70% nitrous oxide; protein composition is unaltered (42). Such an effect on protein phosphorylation (*i.e.*, inactivation of protein kinase C) may contribute to the neuroteratogenic effects of nitrous oxide.

Human Studies

Data concerning the neurotoxic effects of nitrous oxide in humans are largely limited to single case reports and small series. There are no reports in humans of controlled exposure to nitrous oxide that specifically examined possible neurotoxic effects. However, reports of uncontrolled exposures are many; some strongly suggest a dose–effect relationship. Neurological manifestations are stereotyped and unusual, and clinical improvement following cessation of nitrous oxide exposure is common (4,6,8,19,27,41).

Exposure can be divided into abuse of nitrous oxide anesthesia, abuse of whipped-cream dispensers, and occupational exposure. It seems unlikely that contaminants are responsible for the neurotoxic effects associated with nitrous oxide anesthesia, since nitrous oxide given as anesthetic is regulated and contains <1 ppm of other nitrogen compounds and halogens. Although nitrous oxide cartridges used to make whipped cream contain no significant impurities (36), the same cartridges dispensed through a standard whipped-cream dispenser show several contaminants, including phenol, trichloroethylene, and toluene, all of which have neurotoxic potential (41). This has suggested to some that contaminants may be responsible for the neurotoxicity ascribed to nitrous oxide in patients abusing whipped-cream dispensers. However, such an effect is unlikely, since a nearly identical neurological syndrome is associated with abuse of nitrous oxide anesthesia and heavy occupational exposures.

Patients with prolonged, heavy exposures (50%–80% concentrations for 10 min to 10 h, twice weekly to daily, for 3 months to 6 years) to nitrous oxide anesthesia develop a myeloneuropathy syndrome (19,27,31,50). A similar effect occurs following inhalation of between 24 and 200 cartridges of nitrous oxide delivered through a whipped-cream dispenser, twice weekly to daily for 3 months to a few years (21,37,41,47). Each cartridge dispenses about a

5-sec continuous stream of gas (41). The neurological disorder resembles subacute combined degeneration of the spinal cord, although features of peripheral nerve disease are frequently more apparent. Patients commonly present with acral paresthesias, often beginning in the legs, gait unsteadiness, and Lhermitte's sign (an electric-shock sensation down the spine or legs with neck flexion) (3,19,27,28, 41,50). Subsequently, hand clumsiness, leg weakness accentuated distally, impotence, bladder and bowel dysfunction, mood and concentration disturbances, and truncal numbness may develop (27). Symptoms usually begin during a period of prolonged nitrous oxide abuse, though by some reports, symptom onset is delayed 6–12 months after cessation of nitrous oxide (21,31). The reliability of such accounts is questionable. Early signs often include only distal diminution of touch and vibration perception and depressed reflexes in the legs (27). Later, a combination of myelopathic and neuropathic signs develops, including Babinski's signs, distal-greater-than-proximal weakness, more severe posterior column dysfunction, truncal sensory levels, hyper- or hypoactive reflexes in the legs, and gait ataxia (19,27,41).

Serum B_{12} levels have been reduced in 8 of 17 patients reported in the literature (3,27,31,47,50). Schilling tests are characteristically normal (21,27,47). Cerebrospinal fluid is typically normal, though there are isolated reports of mild protein elevation (3,21,27,28,37,47). Nerve conduction studies and electromyography are consistent with a predominantly distal, axonal, sensorimotor polyneuropathy (21,27,50). Somatosensory-evoked responses demonstrate prolonged or absent cortical potentials, more severe with tibial than median nerve stimulation (21,50). The presence of markedly prolonged cortical response latencies following tibial nerve stimulation, minimal slowing of distal tibial nerve conduction, and a normal median nerve evoked response may suggest myelopathic dysfunction. However, an alternative explanation is that the peripheral neuropathy affects the legs more than the arms. Mild abnormalities of visual-evoked responses in one of four patients has been reported to suggest foveal dysfunction (21).

There are no postmortem studies. Sural nerve biopsy in one patient showed a normal number of fibers; however, teased single-fiber preparations revealed abnormalities including myelin ovoid formation, axonal swellings, and focally denuded myelin; electron microscopy showed membranous whorls within Schwann cell cytoplasm (41). These are relatively nonspecific abnormalities consistent with mild axonal degeneration. Severe axonal degeneration was demonstrated in another patient (31). A third patient had a normal sural nerve biopsy, but biopsy of the gastrocnemius muscle revealed evidence of denervation (37).

Reports that detail the degree of nitrous oxide exposure

suggest that neurological manifestations are precipitated by or worsen as the dose of nitrous oxide is increased (21,41). Most patients improve clinically following cessation of nitrous oxide exposure (19,21,27,28,41). This may correlate with electrophysiological improvement (21).

A clinical presentation with features of both myelopathy and distal axonopathy is also rarely described in relation to occupational exposure, predominantly in dentists (19,27). The level of exposure necessary to cause myeloneuropathy in this setting is unclear, although two patient reports described exposures of 6–7 h daily or 2000 liquid pounds/ month over 28 years (19,27). A survey of 30,000 dentists and 30,000 dental assistants by mailed questionnaire suggests a dose-dependent increase in neuropathic symptoms in those exposed to nitrous oxide (4). This study shows a fourfold increase in the symptoms of numbness, tingling, or muscle weakness reported by heavily exposed dentists (>3000 h/10 years) and a threefold increase in the same symptoms reported by heavily exposed dental assistants as compared to dentists and dental assistants not exposed to nitrous oxide. Those with light exposure (<2999 h/10 years) to nitrous oxide show a less significant increase in these neuropathic symptoms. Although this study suggests a dose–effect relationship for the development of neuropathic symptoms, it is unclear if any patients had objective evidence of myelopathy or neuropathy. In addition, it is possible that some participants abused nitrous oxide.

Another study, which assessed neurological disability scores, nerve condition parameters, and quantitative sensory tests, shows no significant differences in these measures between ten dentists using >5 liter-h/week of nitrous oxide in their practice compared to nine dentists using <5 liter-h/ week (8). Estimates suggest that the dentists who used nitrous oxide more often (mean, 31 liter-h/week) were routinely exposed to ambient concentrations of 300–1200-plus ppm. Therefore, prolonged exposure to concentrations well above that recommended as safe for operating rooms (25 ppm) does not appear to be neurotoxic. However, data from rat studies suggest that significant inhibition of methionine synthetase—the proposed mechanism of nitrous oxide neurotoxicity (*vide infra*)—occurs between exposures of 400 and 1000 ppm (46). It is conceivable that nitrous oxide levels were insufficient to inhibit methionine synthetase and that higher levels of occupational exposure may result in myelopathy or peripheral neuropathy. Nitrous oxide levels >2000 ppm are reported in unscavenged dental offices (46), yet reports of myeloneuropathy associated with high occupational exposures are infrequent.

There are rare reports of patients with subclinical B_{12} deficiency developing myeloneuropathy following general anesthesia with nitrous oxide (22,35,44). Symptoms begin approximately 2 weeks to 2 months following 1.5–2 h of

50% nitrous oxide (22,44). Preoperative hematological abnormalities may include an elevated mean corpuscular volume or anemia. Relatively prolonged nitrous oxide anesthesia during surgery in normal patients apparently causes no significant neuropathic effects (26).

An encephalopathy, characterized by altered consciousness and mood, concentration and memory difficulties, and intellectual decline, may accompany myeloneuropathic dysfunction (3,48). This improves following cessation of nitrous oxide exposure. Healthy volunteers exposed to increasing doses of nitrous oxide (0%–49%) show prolonged P-300 latency and deterioration of continuous-performance test and symbol-digit test performance in a dose-dependent manner (11). The finger-tapping test is also abnormal. These test abnormalities suggest a deficit in psychomotor speed. A report of impaired audiovisual performance tasks after inhaled concentrations as low as 50 ppm led to the current NIOSH requirements; however, these findings have not been reproduced. More recent safety levels proposed, based on the degree of methionine synthetase inhibition in the rat, are 200 ppm for the mean concentration breathed by the anesthetist and 100 ppm at the periphery of the surgical suite (46).

Nitrous oxide–induced myeloneuropathy occurs most frequently in groups prone to chronic abuse of the drug. Myeloneuropathy due to nitrous oxide anesthesia abuse is most frequently described in dentists and dental surgeons. Both easy access and a greater prevalence of substance abuse (excluding alcohol) among dentists may explain this association (18). The prevalence of nitrous oxide abuse among dentists is unknown, although heavy exposure is reported in 1% of those polled, many of whom practiced self-administration (24). Individuals who abuse whipped-cream dispensers are characteristically young men and women in their twenties and thirties. Polydrug abuse is common (18). In the United States, recreational use of nitrous oxide is reported in 18% of dental students and 14% of medical students; the majority used whipped-cream cans or cartridges (24). Although use of nitrous oxide appears to be fairly common, severe abuse to the point of overt neurotoxicity is rare, even in high-risk groups (18). Occupational exposure is greater among dental surgeons than anesthesiologists, possibly because they more frequently apply anesthesia by mask and are less often protected by institutional regulations (46).

The diagnosis of nitrous oxide–induced myeloneuropathy should be entertained when a patient presents with onset over months to years of distal paresthesias, gait unsteadiness, and a combination of CNS and PNS signs. Confirmation requires sufficient exposure to produce the syndrome, and improvement should follow withdrawal of the drug. Tests demonstrating impaired vitamin B_{12} metabolism with normal

Schilling tests and electrophysiological studies showing a distal axonopathy are considered supportive. The differential diagnosis is limited, since few disorders clinically affect both the CNS and PNS. Possibilities include vitamin B_{12} deficiency (*i.e.*, pernicious anemia); vitamin E deficiency; Friedreich's ataxia; spinocerebellar ataxia type 2; and prolonged intoxications due to mercury, acrylamide, *n*-hexane, tri*ortho*cresylphosphate, and clioquinol. A longer course, more prominent ataxia, and nystagmus may favor the hereditary ataxias. Mercury intoxication typically has more significant cognitive manifestations. Though multiple sclerosis is often included in the differential, the presence of prominent lower motor neuron signs in nitrous oxide toxicity makes this diagnosis unlikely.

Withdrawal of nitrous oxide is the most important therapeutic intervention in patients with myeloneuropathy. A few anecdotal reports suggest patients also respond to B_{12} and methionine supplementation (3,47,50). Studies in monkeys support the use of methionine treatment (45).

Preventive measures may lessen the degree of occupational exposure to nitrous oxide. Local scavenging in a poorly ventilated operating room reduced nitrous oxide exposure by 75% (5). Such concentrations are often regarded as safe, although NIOSH regulations require concentrations below 25 ppm.

Toxic Mechanisms

There is considerable evidence suggesting that nitrous oxide exerts its neurotoxic effects through interference with vitamin B_{12} metabolism, although the precise mechanism is unknown. Both rat and human studies show that nitrous oxide inhibits methionine synthetase, an enzyme involved in the synthesis of methionine and tetrahydrofolate from the substrates homocysteine and methyl tetrahydrofolate (Fig. 15) (7,12,38). Oxidation of cobalt may underlie this inhibitory effect (7). Methionine and tetrahydrofolate are necessary precursors of a carbon donor, 5,10-methylenetetrahydrofolate, which allows conversion of deoxyuridine to deoxythymidine. Thymidine is an essential component of DNA. Methionine also serves as a methyl donor and is involved in the synthesis of many proteins.

Nitrous oxide reduces methionine synthetase activity rapidly in rats and humans, though more rapidly in the former (38). Recovery of enzyme activity, however, occurs more slowly than inactivation, at least in rats (38). As such, prolonged inactivation of methionine synthetase may underlie the neurotoxic effects of repeated nitrous oxide exposures.

It is unknown how reduced methionine synthetase activity leads to neurological dysfunction. Although reduced DNA synthesis is a likely mechanism of impaired hemopoiesis, this may not relate to the development of myeloneuropathy. Neural cells are less mitotically active than hematological cells, so they should be less vulnerable to impaired DNA metabolism. Additionally, the deoxyuridine suppression test, an indicator of impaired DNA synthesis due to methionine synthetase deficiency, was normal in one patient with myeloneuropathy (21). Impaired methylation reactions because of decreased methionine synthetase activity seems a more plausible mechanism of neurological toxicity. However, protein methylation is not disturbed in nitrous oxide–treated fruit bats with myelopathy (34).

A causative role of impaired vitamin B_{12} metabolism is strongly supported by the finding that pathological changes in the spinal cord of monkeys exposed to nitrous oxide are nearly identical to those associated with chronic vitamin B_{12} deficiency in humans (45). Furthermore, these changes and the associated clinical deficits are prevented by methionine treatment, suggesting that impaired methionine synthesis causes the neurological manifestations (45).

Editors' Note: Whereas occupational exposure to 50–55 ppm nitrous oxide was associated with reduced end-of-week reaction times among Italian operating room personnel, no neurobehavioral changes were detected at levels of 25 ppm nitrous oxide and 0.5 ppm isoflurane (30). The American Conference of Governmental Industrial Hygienists has adopted a 1999 Threshold Limit Value time-weighted average of 50 ppm.

REFERENCES

1. Amess JAL, Burkman JF, Rees GM et al. (1978) Megaloblastic hemopoiesis in patients receiving nitrous oxide. *Lancet* 2, 339.
2. Baden JM, Rice SA (1990) Metabolism and toxicity. In: *Anesthesia. 3rd Ed.* Miller RD ed. Churchill Livingstone, New York p. 142.
3. Blanco G, Peters HA (1983) Myeloneuropathy and macrocytosis associated with nitrous oxide abuse. *Arch Neurol* 40, 416.
4. Brodsky JB, Cohen EN, Brown BW et al. (1981) Exposure to nitrous oxide and neurologic disease among dental professionals. *Anesth Analg* 60, 297.
5. Carlson P, Lunqvist B, Hallen B (1983) The effect of local scavenging on occupational exposure to nitrous oxide. *Acta Anaesthesiol Scand* 27, 470.
6. Cohen EN, Brown BW, Wu ML et al. (1980) Occupational disease and chronic exposure to trace anesthetic gases. *J Amer Dent Assn* 101, 21.
7. Deacon R, Perry J, Lumb M et al. (1978) Selective inactivation of vitamin B_{12} in rats by nitrous oxide. *Lancet* 2, 1023.
8. Dyck PJ, Grina LA, Lambert EH et al. (1980) Nitrous oxide neurotoxicity studies in man and rat. *Anesthesiology* 53, 205.
9. Eger EI II, Lampe GH, Wauk LZ et al. (1990) Clinical pharmacology of nitrous oxide: An argument for its continued use. *Anesth Analg* 71, 575.
10. Einarsson S, Stenqvist O, Bengtsson A et al. (1993) Nitrous oxide elimination and diffusion hypoxia during normo- and hypoventilation. *Brit J Anaesth* 71, 189.
11. Estrin WJ, Moore P, Letz R, Wasch HH (1988) The P-300 event-related potential in experimental nitrous oxide exposure. *Clin Pharmacol Ther* 43, 86.
12. Everman BW, Koblin DD (1991) Aging, chronic administration of ethanol, and acute exposure to nitrous oxide: Effects on vitamin B_{12} and folate status in rats. *Mech Age Dev* 62, 229.
13. Fiset P, Balendren P, Bevan DR, Donati F (1991) Nitrous oxide potentiates vecuronium neuromuscular blockade in humans. *Can J Anesth* 38, 866.
14. Freund FG, Martin WE, Wong KC, Hornbein TF (1973) Abdominal-muscle rigidity induced by morphine and nitrous oxide. *Anesthesiology* 38, 358.
15. Fujinaga M, Baden JM (1994) Methionine prevents nitrous oxide-induced teratogenicity in rat embryos grown in culture. *Anesthesiology* 81, 184.
16. Fujinaga M, Baden JM, Mazze RI (1989) Susceptible period of nitrous oxide teratogenicity in Sprague-Dawley rats. *Teratology* 40, 439.
17. Gillman MA (1986) Nitrous oxide, an opioid addictive agent: review of the evidence. *Amer J Med* 81, 97.
18. Gillman MA (1992) Nitrous oxide abuse in perspective. *Clin Neuropharmacol* 15, 297.
19. Gutmann L, Johnson D (1981) Nitrous oxide-induced myeloneuropathy: Report of cases. *J Amer Dent Assn* 103, 239.
20. Henriksen HT, Balslev Jorgensen P (1973) The effect of nitrous oxide on intracranial pressure in patients with intracranial disorders. *Brit J Anaesth* 45, 486.
21. Heyer EJ, Simpson DM, Bodis-Wollner I, Diamond SP (1986) Nitrous oxide: Clinical and electrophysiologic investigation of neurologic complications. *Neurology* 36, 1618.
22. Holloway KL, Alberico AM (1990) Postoperative myeloneuropathy: A preventable complication in patients with B_{12} deficiency. *J Neurosurg* 72, 732.
23. Hornbein TF, Eger EI II, Winter PM et al. (1982) The minimum alveolar concentration of nitrous oxide in man. *Anesth Analg* 61, 553.
24. Jastak JT (1991) Nitrous oxide and its abuse. *J Amer Dent Assn* 122, 48.
25. Koblin DD, Tomerson BW, Waldman FM et al. (1990) Effect of nitrous oxide on folate and vitamin B_{12} metabolism in patients. *Anesth Analg* 71, 610.
26. Lampe GH, Wauk LZ, Donegan JH et al. (1990) Effect on outcome of prolonged exposure of patients to nitrous oxide. *Anesth Analg* 71, 586.
27. Layzer RB (1978) Myeloneuropathy after prolonged exposure to nitrous oxide. *Lancet* 2, 1227.
28. Layzer RB, Fishman RA, Schafer JA (1978) Neuropathy following abuse of nitrous oxide. *Neurology* 28, 504.

29. Lee JH, Sung CH, Moon SH *et al.* (1993) Folinic acid protection against hematopoietic depression induced by nitrous oxide in rats. *Anesth Analg* 77, 356.

30. Lucchini R, Belotti L, Cassitto MG *et al.* (1997) Neurobehavioral functions in operating theatre personnel: a multicenter study. *Med Lav* 88, 396.

31. Lunsford JM, Wynn MH, Kwan WH (1983) Nitrous oxide-induced myeloneuropathy. *J Foot Surg* 22, 222.

32. Marshall BE, Wollman H (1990) General anesthetics. In: *The Pharmacological Basis of Therapeutics. 8th Ed.* Gilman AG, Goodman LS, Rall TW, Murad F eds. Macmillan, New York p. 289.

33. McCann SR, Weir DG, Dinn J *et al.* (1979) Neurological damage induced by nitrous oxide in the monkey in the absence of any detectable haematological change. *Brit J Haematol* 43, 496.

34. McLoughlin JL, Cantrill RC (1986) Nitrous oxide induced vitamin B_{12} deficiency: Measurement of methylation reactions in the fruit bat (*Rousettus aegyptiacus*). *J Biochem* 18, 199.

35. McMorrow AM, Adams RJ, Rubenstein MN (1995) Combined system disease after nitrous oxide anesthesia: A case report. *Neurology* 45, 1224.

36. Murakawa M, Adachi T, Nakao S *et al.* (1994) Activation of the cortical and medullary dopaminergic systems by nitrous oxide in rats: A possible neurochemical basis for psychotropic effects and postanesthetic nausea and vomiting. *Anesth Analg* 78, 376.

37. Nieves MA (1980) Neuropathy after nitrous oxide abuse. *J Amer Med Assn* 244, 2264.

38. Nunn JF, Weinbren HK, Royston D (1988) Rate of inactivation of human and rodent hepatic methionine synthase by nitrous oxide. *Anesthesiology* 68, 213.

39. O'Leary PW, Combs MJ, Schilling RF (1985) Synergistic deleterious effects of nitrous oxide exposure and vitamin B_{12} deficiency. *J Lab Clin Med* 105, 428.

40. Royston D, Jordan C, Jones JG (1983) Effect of subanaesthetic concentrations of nitrous oxide on the regulation of ventilation in man. *Brit J Anaesth* 55, 449.

41. Sahenk Z, Mendell JR, Couri D, Nachtman J (1978) Polyneuropathy from inhalation of N_2O cartridges through a whipped-cream dispenser. *Neurology* 28, 485.

42. Saito S, Fujita T, Igarashi M (1993) Effects of inhalational anesthetics on biochemical events in growing neuronal tips. *Anesthesiology* 79, 1338.

43. Sakabe T, Kuramoto T, Inoue S, Takeshita H (1978) Cerebral effects of nitrous oxide in the dog. *Anesthesiology* 48, 195.

44. Schilling RF (1986) Is nitrous oxide a dangerous anesthetic for vitamin B_{12}-deficient subjects. *J Amer Med Assn* 255, 1605.

45. Scott JM, Wilson P, Dinn JJ, Weir DG (1981) Pathogenesis of subacute combined degeneration: A result of methyl group deficiency. *Lancet* 2, 334.

46. Sharer NM, Nunn JF, Royston JP, Chanarin I (1983) Effects of chronic exposure to nitrous oxide on methionine synthase activity. *Brit J Anaesth* 55, 693.

47. Stacy CB, Di Rocco A, Gould RJ (1992) Methionine in the treatment of nitrous-oxide-induced neuropathy and myeloneuropathy. *J Neurol* 239, 401.

48. Sternman AB, Coyle PK (1983) Subacute toxic delirium following nitrous oxide abuse. *Arch Neurol* 40, 446.

49. United States Pharmacopeial Convention (1991) In: *United States Pharmacopeia Dispensing Information-Volume III: Approved Drug Products and Legal Requirements.* United States Pharmacopeial Convention, Inc. Rockville, Maryland p. 185.

50. Vishnubhakat SM, Beresford HR (1991) Reversible myeloneuropathy of nitrous oxide abuse: Serial electrophysiological studies. *Muscle Nerve* 14, 22.

51. Waldman FM, Koblin DD, Lampe GH *et al.* (1990) Hematologic effects of nitrous oxide in surgical patients. *Anesth Analg* 71, 618.

52. Windholz M, Budavari S, Blometti R, Otterbein E (1983) *The Merck Index: An Encyclopedia of Chemicals, Drugs and Biologicals. 10th Ed.* Merck & Co, Rahway, New Jersey p. 863.

Noxiustoxin

Albert C. Ludolph
Peter S. Spencer

NEUROTOXICITY RATING

Experimental

A Ion channel dysfunction (certain potassium channels)

Noxiustoxin is a small basic protein (MW, 4.2 kDa) and K^+-channel toxin from the venom of the Mexican scorpion *Centruroides noxius*. (11). The 39-amino-acid single-chain peptide shows sequence homology with other scorpion neurotoxins such as kaliotoxin (KTX) and neurotoxins present in the venom of *Tityus serrulatus*, a Brazilian scorpion. Noxiustoxin adopts a α/β scaffold constituted of a three-stranded β-sheet (residues 2–3, 25–30, 33–38) linked to a helix (residues 10–20) through two disulfide bridges (4).

Experiments demonstrated that noxiustoxin reversibly blocks the delayed-rectifier K^+ current in squid giant axon (2,3). However, in these studies, inhibition was not complete, indicating the presence of one insensitive subtype of K^+ channel in this preparation or an incomplete blocking effect of the toxin. At higher concentrations, noxiustoxin inhibits T-tubular Ca^{2+}-activated K^+ channels of skeletal muscle incorporated in lipid bilayers (15). Noxiustoxin also blocks whole-cell K_{Ca} currents in bovine aortic endothelial cells (14). These results indicate that the effect of noxiustoxin on voltage-sensitive K^+ channels is not selective. By using the effect on bovine endothelial cells and several synthetic polypeptide fragments from noxiustoxin, it was shown that the N-terminal region of noxiustoxin is likely to recognize the K^+ channels (14). In rat brain synaptic membranes, noxiustoxin interferes with the binding of ^{125}I-charybdotoxin and dendrotoxin—a neurotoxin from the venom of the black mamba (7,16)—which shows that the voltage-sensitive K^+ channel blocked by noxiustoxin may also be sensitive to charybdotoxin and dendrotoxin. Noxiustoxin also facilitates acetylcholine release at the neuromuscular junction (8), and in the CNS it induces neurotransmitter release from synaptosomal preparations of mouse brain (13).

While there is a 48% similarity in the amino acid sequences of noxiustoxin and charybdotoxin (12), it is suggested that the K^+ channel-recognition site resides in the N-terminal region or β-sheet of the first (4–6,10,14) and the C-terminal region of the second peptide (6). Others have proposed multiple sites of potential noxiustoxin-channel interaction (1). Site-directed mutants of noxiustoxin indicate that residues K6, T8 at the amino end, and K28 and a tripeptide at the carboxyl end, are involved in the toxin's specific interactions with rat brain synaptosomal membranes and/or Kv1.1 K^+ channels expressed in *Xenopus laevis* oocytes (9).

Since noxiustoxin is a minor component of scorpion venom, it is unlikely to contribute to the symptomatology of human envenomation.

REFERENCES

1. Aiyar J, Withka JM, Rizzi JP *et al.* (1995) Topology of the pore-region of a K^+ channel revealed by the NMR-derived structures of scorpion toxins. *Neuron* **15**, 1169.

2. Carbone E, Prestipino G, Spadavecchia L *et al.* (1987) Blocking of the squid axon K^+ channel by noxius toxin, a toxin from the venom of the scorpion *Centruroides noxius*. *Pflugers Arch* **408**, 423.

3. Carbone E, Wanke E, Prestipino G *et al.* (1982) Selective blockage of voltage-dependent K^+ channel by a novel scorpion toxin. *Nature* **296**, 90.

4. Dauplais M, Gilquin B, Possani LD *et al.* (1995) Determination of the three-dimensional solution structure of noxiustoxin: analysis of structural differences with related short-chain scorpion toxins. *Biochemistry* **34**, 16563.

5. Gomez-Lagunas F, Olamendi-Portugal T, Zamudio FZ, Possani LD (1996) Two novel toxins from the venom of the scorpion *Pandinus imperator* show that the N-terminal amino acid sequence is important for their affinities towards Shaker B K^+ channels. *Membr Biol* **152**, 49.

6. Gurrola GB, Possani LD (1995) Structural and functional features of noxiustoxin: a K^+ channel blocker. *Biochem Mol Biol Int* **37**, 527.

7. Harvey AL, Marshall DL, Possani CD (1992) Dendrotoxin-like effect of noxiustoxin. *Toxicon* **30**, 1497.

8. Marshall DL, Harvey DL, Possani LD (1990) Noxiustoxin blocks neuronal potassium channels and facilitates the evoked release of acetylcholine. *Toxicon* **28**, 152.

9. Martinez F, Muñoz-Garay C, Gurrola G *et al.* (1998) Site directed mutants of Noxiustoxin reveal specific interactions with potassium channels. *FEBS Lett* **429**, 381.

10. Nieto AR, Gurrola GB, Vaca L, Possani LD (1996) Noxiustoxin 2, a novel K^+ channel blocking peptide from the venom of the scorpion *Centruroides noxius* Hoffmann. *Toxicon* **34**, 913.

11. Possani LD, Martin BM, Svendsen IB (1982) The primary structure of noxiustoxin: A K^+ channel blocking peptide, purified from the venom of the scorpion *Centruroides noxius* Hoffmann. *Carlsberg Res Commun* **47**, 285.

12. Sacile R, Ruggiero C, Ballestrero R *et al.* (1994) Secondary structure of noxiustoxin and charybdotoxin from hydropathy power spectra. *Biochem Biophys Res Commun* **201**, 186.

13. Sitges M, Possani LD, Bayon A (1986) Noxiustoxin, a short chain toxin from the Mexican scorpion *Centruroides noxius* induces transmitter release by blocking K^+ permeability. *J Neurosci* **6**, 1570.

14. Vaca L, Gurrola GB, Possani LD, Kunze DL (1993) Blockade of K_{Ca} channel with synthetic peptides from noxiustoxin: a K^+ channel blocker. *J Membrane Biol* **134**, 123.

15. Valdivia HH, Smith JS, Martin BM *et al.* (1988) Charybdotoxin and noxiustoxin, two homologous peptide inhibitors of the K^+ (Ca^{2+}) channel. *FEBS Lett* **226**, 280.

16. Vasquez J, Feigenbaum P, King VF *et al.* (1990) Characterization of high-affinity binding site for charybdotoxin in synaptic plasma mambranes from rat brain. Evidence for a direct association with an inactivating, voltage-dependent potassium channel. *Biol Chem* **265**, 15564.

Ochratoxins

Albert C. Ludolph
Peter S. Spencer

OCHRATOXIN A
$C_{20}H_{18}ClNO_6$

(R)-N-[(5-Chloro-3,4-dihydro-8-hydroxy-3-methyl-1-oxo-1H-2-benzopyran-7-yl)carbonyl]-L-phenylalanine

NEUROTOXICITY RATING

Experimental

A   Neuroteratogenicity

Ochratoxins are mycotoxins containing a chlorinated dihydroisocoumarin linked through a 7-carboxyl group to L-phenylalanine by an amide bond. The major toxin, ochratoxin A, also exists in the hydroxylated form; in contrast, its dechloro analog, ochratoxin B, is considered less toxic. Ochratoxin C is metabolized to ochratoxin A.

The group of ochratoxins (ochratoxin A, B, and C) is produced by various *Penicillium* and *Aspergillus* spp., which explains their wide natural occurrence in the environment, including food and feed. These compounds have nephrotoxic, hepatotoxic, teratogenic, carcinogenic, and immunosuppressive properties (7). The major target of ochratoxins in animals as well as in humans is the kidney, but they are also neuroteratogenic in animals.

Ochratoxins are found as food contaminants primarily produced by *Aspergillus* and *Penicillium* spp. (for details, *see* 7). As with other molds, the quantity of toxin produced by fungi is not only a function of the species or strain but also significantly dependent on specific environmental conditions, including substrate, temperature, and moisture. The long half-life of ochratoxin A in many edible animal species increases the potential health risks for humans.

Ochratoxins are absorbed from the entire gastrointestinal tract of various species: absorption is followed by enterohepatic cycling (10). After tightly binding to serum albumin, the toxins distribute into organs; in rats, the highest specific activity of the labeled compound is found in lung, liver, and kidney, whereas activity in muscle and brain is comparatively low (4). An elimination half-time of 840 h has been described in monkeys. Toxins are excreted in urine and feces as ochratoxin A, hydroxylated ochratoxin A, or as ochratoxin α-(7-carboxy-5-chloro-8-hydroxy-3,4-dihydro-3R-methylisocoumarin). In comparison to ochratoxin A, ochratoxin B is rapidly hydrolyzed and, consequently, less toxic.

The occurrence of ochratoxins in food has been widely reported, primarily in cereal grains, but also in beans, coffee, olives, and food products such as cheese, pork, milk, and bread. In Germany, blood ochratoxin A was detected in 50%–70% of healthy humans (1); similar but less striking results were reported from Poland, Yugoslavia, and Bulgaria. Although regulatory limits for ochratoxins have been set in some countries, their scientific basis is weak (11).

Oral intake of ochratoxin A was linked to Balkan endemic nephropathy and associated urinary system tumors. The pathological lesions of this nephropathy resemble those found in endemic porcine nephropathy (6), a condition characterized by impairment of proximal renal tubular function.

No neurotoxic effects of ochratoxin A are reported in humans or grazing animals. However, prenatal treatment of rats and mice results in microcephaly in neonates (8). Brains of orally treated rats show increased extracellular lactate dehydrogenase (LDH) in the ventral mesencephalon (VM), hippocampus, and striatum (4). Markers of cytotoxicity (level of LDH release and malondialdehyde) are also elevated in primary cultures of VM > cerebellum treated with ochratoxin A *in vitro* (2). Toxin-induced changes in brain cytotoxic markers, free amino acid levels, and necrotic cells, are reportedly blocked by concurrent treatment of rats with aspartame (N-L-α-aspartyl-L-phenylalanine 1-methyl ester), a structural relative of ochratoxin A (3). Other toxic effects of ochratoxin A include (a) inhibition of mitochondrial respiration, (b) inhibition of tRNA-synthetase accompanied by reduced protein synthesis, and (c) enhanced lipid peroxidation (5,9).

REFERENCES

1. Bauer J, Gareis M (1987) Ochratoxin A in der Nahrungsmittelkette. *Z Veterinarmed B* **34**, 613.
2. Belmadani A, Steyn PS, Tramu G *et al.* (1999) Selective toxicity of ochratoxin A in primary cultures from different brain regions. *Arch Toxicol* **73**, 108.
3. Belmadani A, Tramu G, Betbeder AM, Creppy EE (1998) Subchronic effects of ochratoxin A on young adult rat brain and partial prevention by aspartame, a sweetener. *Hum Exp Toxicol* **17**, 380.

4. Belmadani A, Tramu G, Betbeder AM *et al.* (1998) Regional selectivity to ochratoxin A, distribution and cytotoxicity in rat brain. *Arch Toxicol* **72**, 656.

5. Hohler D (1998) Ochratoxin A in food and feed: occurrence, legislation and mode of action. *Z Ernahrungswiss* **37**, 2.

6. Krogh P (1978) Casual associations of mycotoxic nephropathy. *Acta Pathol Microbiol Scand Suppl* **269**, 1.

7. Marquardt RR (1990) Ochratoxin A: an important western Canadian storage mycotoxin. *Can J Physiol Pharmacol* **68**, 991.

8. Miki T, Fukui Y, Uemura N, Takeuchi Y (1994) Regional difference in the neurotoxicity of ochratoxin A on the developing cerebral cortex in mice. *Brain Res Dev Brain Res* **82**, 259.

9. Monnet-Tschudi F, Sorg O, Honegger P *et al.* (1997) Effects of the naturally occurring food mycotoxin ochratoxin A on brain cells in culture. *Neurotoxicology* **18**, 831.

10. Sreemannarayana O, Frohlich AA, Vitti TG *et al.* (1988) Studies of the tolerance and disposition of ochratoxin A in young calves. *J Anim Sci* **66**, 1703.

11. Van Egmond HP (1991) Worldwide regulations for ochratoxin A. *Int Agency Res Cancer Sci Publ* 331.

Okadaic Acid

Peter S. Spencer

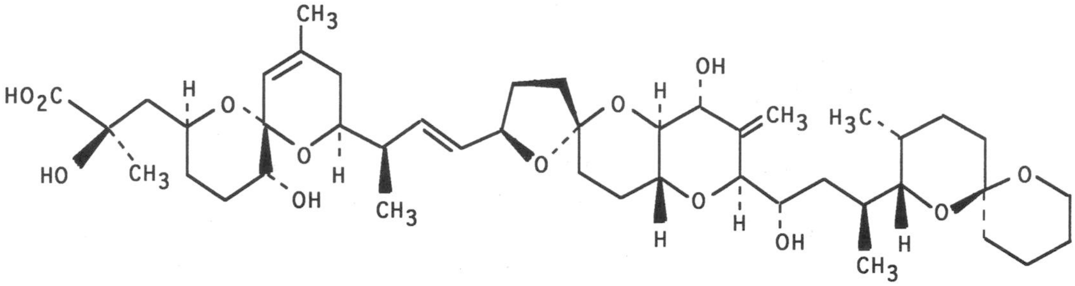

OKADAIC ACID
$C_{44}H_{68}O_{13}$

9,10-Deepithio-9,10-didehydroacanthifolicin; Halochondrine A

NEUROTOXICITY RATING

Experimental

A   Protein phosphatase inhibitor

Okadaic acid (OA) is an ionophoric polyether macrocarboxylic acid first isolated from two sponges, *Halichondria okadai*, which inhabits coastal Japan, and *H. melanodocia*, a Caribbean sponge found in the Florida Keys (USA) (19). OA is a member of one of three groups* of polyether toxins—the OA group comprises OA, dinophysistoxin-1 (DTX-1) and DTX-3—found in the digestive organ (hepatopancreas) of mussels and scallops; the toxins originate in dinoflagellates such as *Dinophysis fortii* (21), other *Dinophysis* spp. and *Prorocentrum* spp. Ingestion of OA-contaminated shellfish has resulted in outbreaks of diarrhetic shellfish poisoning (DSP) in many regions of the world, notably Europe (3). While neurotoxicity is not a feature of DSP, the selective protein-phosphatase inhibitory activity of OA provides an exceptionally useful tool for the experimental neuroscientist to probe cellular regulation (6). In addition to its contractile action on smooth muscles, OA exhibits neurotoxic, mutagenic, tumor-promoting, and immunosuppressive properties (3).

An estimated amount of 40 mg OA is required to induce gastrointestinal distress in humans (10). Diarrhea, nausea, vomiting, and abdominal pain dominate the illness resulting from ingestion of seafood contaminated with OA and related toxins. Symptoms commence within 30 min or a few hours of ingestion of the offending meal. DSP may be perceived by the subject as a severe illness, but hospitalization is usually not required (3). Recovery occurs spontaneously within a few days (22).

---

*The two other groups of toxins (which do not induce DSP symptoms) include polyether macrolides named *pectenotoxins* (mouse hepatotoxins) and sulfate toxins known as *yessotoxins* (mouse cardiac effects) (13,20,21).

Mice treated by intraperitoneal (i.p.) injection of extracts of contaminated mussels develop generalized weakness within 30 min to several hours (22). The oral lethal dose in mice is 16 times higher than the lethal i.p. dose (192 mg/kg body weight). Mice treated with DTX-1 (160 mg/kg) exhibit constant diarrhea and die within 24 h; postmortem examination reveals distention of the duodenum and upper portion of the small intestine (14,20). OA, DTX-1, and DTX-3 destroy and desquamate the intestinal mucous epithelium (19). Chickens and cats are less sensitive to the systemic effects of DSP toxins (3).

OA is a potent inhibitor of protein phosphatase-1 and protein phosphatase-2A, two of the major cytosolic protein phosphatases of mammalian cells. The toxin thus increases the phosphorylation of proteins and disrupts phosphorylation-regulated cellular functions. OA dramatically increases high-affinity glutamate uptake into rat striatal synaptosomes (16) and, *via* presynaptic mechanisms, increases release of neurotransmitter at the crayfish neuromuscular junction (18), the lobster (glutamatergic, γ-aminobutyric acidergic) neuromuscular junction, and the frog (cholinergic) neuromuscular junction (1). In rat cortical neurons and mouse cerebellar cells in culture, OA hyperphosphorylates the microtubule-associated protein tau by decreasing glutamate-induced, Ca^{2+}-dependent dephosphorylation (2,11). OA increases neurofilament fragmentation in dorsal root ganglion cultures (8,17) and inhibits nerve growth factor–directed neurite outgrowth in PC-12 cells (5). Low concentrations reversibly inhibit (0.5 nM) and arrest (1 nM) neurite outgrowth from embryonic dorsal root ganglion cells (9). Treatment of fetal rat hippocampal neurons *in vitro* with OA or calyculin A (another phosphatase inhibitor) causes retraction of neuritic processes and the appearance of focal neuritic dilatations containing vesicles (12). Persistent phosphorylation induced by OA (5–20 nM) kills cerebellar cells *in vitro* (4) by an apoptotic mechanism that is blocked by insulin-like growth factor-1 (7). Implantation of crystalline OA into sheep brain reportedly induced the formation of Alz-50-immunoreactive neurites (15).

The human and mammalian enteric toxicity of OA probably results from increased phosphorylation of proteins that regulate sodium secretion by intestinal cells or by enhanced phosphorylation of cytoskeletal elements that regulate ion permeability, thereby resulting in passive loss of fluid and resultant diarrhea (3). Binding of OA to the intestinal lining presumably reduces absorption and systemic circulation of this potent, lipophilic experimental neurotoxin.

REFERENCES

1. Abdul-Ghani M, Kravitz EA, Meiri H, Rahamimoff R (1991) Protein phosphorylation inhibitor okadaic acid enhances transmitter release at neuromuscular junctions. *Proc Nat Acad Sci USA* **85**, 1803.

2. Adamec E, Mercken M, Beerman ML *et al.* (1997) Acute rise in the concentration of free cytoplasmic calcium leads to dephosphorylation of the microtubule-associated protein tau. *Brain Res* **757**, 93.

3. Aune T, Yndestad M (1993) Diarrhetic shellfish poisoning. In: *Algal Toxins in Seafood and Drinking Water*. Academic Press, London p. 87.

4. Candeo P, Favaron M, Lengyel I (1992) Pathological phosphorylation causes neuronal death: effect of okadaic acid in primary culture of cerebellar granule cells. *J Neurochem* **59**, 1558.

5. Chiou JY, Westhead EW (1992) Okadaic acid, a protein phosphatase inhibitor, inhibits nerve growth factor-directed neurite outgrowth in PC12 cells. *J Neurochem* **59**, 1963.

6. Cohen P, Holmes CFB, Tsukitani Y (1990) Okadaic acid: A new probe for the study of cellular regulation. *Trends Biochem Sci* **3**, 98.

7. Fernandez-Sanchez MT, Garcia-Rodriguez A, Diaz-Trelles R, Novelli A (1996) Inhibition of protein phosphatases induces IGF-1-blocked neurotrophic-insensitive neuronal apopotosis. *FEBS Lett* **398**, 106.

8. Giasson BI, Cromlish JA, Athlan ES, Mushynski WE (1996) Activation of cyclic AMP-dependent protein kinase in okadaic acid-treated neurons potentiates neurofilament fragmentation and stimulates phosphorylation of Ser2 in the low-molecular-mass neurofilament subunit. *J Neurochem* **66**, 1207.

9. Giasson BI, Mushynski WE (1997) Okadaic acid reversibly inhibits neurite outgrowth in embryonic dorsal root ganglion neurons. *J Neurobiol* **32**, 193.

10. Hamano Y, Kinoshita Y, Tasumoto T (1985) Suckling mice assay for diarrhetic shellfish toxins. In: *Toxic Dinoflagellate*. Anderson DM, White AM, Badem DG eds. Elsevier, New York p. 383.

11. Ho DT, Shayan H, Murphy TH (1997) Okadaic acid induces hyperphosphorylation of tau independently of mitogen-activated protein kinase activation. *J Neurochem* **68**, 106.

12. Malchiodi-Albedi F, Petrucci TC, Picconi B *et al.* (1997) Protein phosphatase inhibitors induce modification of synapse structure and tau hyperphosphorylation in cultured rat hippocampal neurons. *J Neurosci Res* **48**, 425.

13. Murata M, Kumagi M, Lee JS, Yasumoto TY (1987) Isolation and structure of yessotoxin, a novel polyether compound implicated in diarrhetic shellfish poisoning. *Tetrahedron Lett* **28**, 5869.

14. Murata M, Shimatani M, Sugitani H *et al.* (1982) Isolation and structural elucidation of the causative toxin of the diarrhetic shellfish poisoning. *Bull Jpn Soc Sci Fish* **48**, 549.

15. Nelson PT, Saper CB (1996) Injections of okadaic acid, but not beta-amyloid peptide, induce Alz-50 immunoreactive dystrophic neurites in the cerebral cortex of sheep. *Neurosci Lett* 208, 77.

16. Pisano D, Samuel D, Nieoullon A, Kerkerian-Le Goff L (1996) Activation of the adenylate cyclase-dependent protein kinase pathway increases high affinity glutamate uptake into rat striatal synaptosomes. *Neuropharmacology* 35, 541.

17. Sacher MG, Athlan ES, Mushynski WE (1992) Okadaic acid induces the rapid and reversible disruption of the neurofilament network in rat dorsal root ganglion neurons. *Biochem Biophys Res Commun* 186, 524.

18. Swain JE, Robitaille R, Dass GR, Charlton MP (1991) Phosphatases modulate transmission and serotonin facilitation at synapses: Studies with the inhibitor okadaic acid. *J Neurobiol* 22, 855.

19. Tachibana K, Scheuer PJ, Tsukitani Y *et al.* (1981) Okadaic acid, a cytotoxic polyether from two marine sponges of the genus *Halichondria*. *J Amer Chem Soc* 103, 2469.

20. Terao K, Ito E, Oarada M *et al.* (1990) Histopathological studies on experimental marine toxin poisoning I. Ultrastructural changes in the small intestine and liver of suckling mice induced by dinophysistoxin-1 and pectenotoxin-1. *Toxicon* 24, 1141.

21. Yasumoto T, Murata M, Lee JS, Torigoe K (1989) Polyether toxins produced by dinoflagellates. In: *Mycotoxins and Phycotoxins '88*. Natori S, Hashimoto K, Ueno Y eds. Elsevier, Amsterdam p. 375.

22. Yasumoto T, Oshima Y, Yamaguchi M (1978) Occurrence of a new type of shellfish poisoning in the Tohoku district. *Bull Jpn Soc Sci Fish* 44, 1249.

Organic Solvent Mixtures

Herbert H. Schaumburg
Peter S. Spencer

NEUROTOXICITY RATING

Clinical

A   Acute encephalopathy

B   Chronic encephalopathy

More than twenty-five years have passed since the initial reports of behavioral changes in painters with chronic, low-level, occupational exposure to organic solvents. First described in the Scandinavian occupational literature, this "organic solvent syndrome" (OSS) has since been the focus of many epidemiological reports (1,3,5,6,11,13,18,19). Many of the early studies were seriously flawed by methodological difficulties including (*inter alia*) selection bias, poor choice of matching controls, avoidance of acute effects, lack of standardized neuropsychological assessment methods, and failure to define the type and levels of chemical exposure. The initial studies implied that the OSS was a world-wide phenomenon and a cause of irreversible CNS damage; it was widely held to be a symptomatic occupational disease and has been a cause of premature retirement in Scandinavia (12). Recent, more careful studies have challenged this notion and redefined the issues (3,5,11,18,19).

Organic solvents comprise a large variety of chemicals of very considerable economic and industrial importance. They are classified as aliphatic or aromatic hydrocarbons, halogenated aliphatic hydrocarbons, alcohols, ethers, esters, ketones, or glycol derivatives. They are used to dissolve fats, waxes, lacquers, resin, plastics, and other materials. They serve as degreasers, dry-cleaners, extractors, fuels, ink solvents, and components of paint and paint removers. Table 40 lists some of the chemical components implicated in the OSS.

Organic solvents are mostly volatile substances of low molecular weight. They and their metabolites have individually distinctive physico-chemical properties, toxicokinetics, and binding properties. Most organic solvents are highly lipophilic substances that, in liquid form, are readily absorbed by skin. Primary exposure in the occupational setting is usually by inhalation. Their ready absorption from the respiratory tract and CNS depressant effects led in former years to the use of some organic solvents (chloroform, trichloroethylene, methylene chloride) as anesthetics. As small, lipophilic molecules, organic solvents are rapidly distributed throughout the blood and readily enter the nervous system. Many organic solvents are metabolized in the liver to intermediate compounds, and some of these metabolites bind to tissue macromolecules in the nervous system. For example, 2,5-hexanedione, the water-soluble metabolite of *n*-hexane, binds to neurofilaments.

The distribution and fate of a number of radiolabeled organic solvents have been meticulously studied in mice exposed acutely to individual compounds by inhalation. Postmortem low-temperature whole-body autoradiography was used to capture and record the location of volatile and nonvolatile radiolabeled material (2). Well-perfused organs, such as the liver and kidneys, were rapidly and heavily radiolabeled immediately after inhalation exposure to organic solvents. With the notable exception of chloroform, the distribution of hydrocarbon solvents in the CNS (white matter) was governed by their respective lipid solubility values, and there was little or no evidence of the generation or retention of metabolites in the brain. Immediately following inhalation of ^{14}C-labeled benzene or ^{14}C-labeled-toluene, a very high level of volatile radioactivity was evident in the white matter of the brain and spinal cord, as well as the bone marrow and body fat; radioactivity had cleared from the CNS within 30 minutes of administration. In the case of ^{14}C-labeled *m*-xylene or styrene, volatile radioactivity was present in the CNS and spinal nerves up to 1 h after inhalation. Styrene was retained for a longer period of time in body fat than benzene, toluene or *m*-xylene. For [14]C-

labeled chloroform, there was pronounced uptake and retention of volatile radioactivity in the cerebellar cortex, meninges, and spinal nerves. Radioactivity from ^{14}C-labeled carbon tetrachloride also had a high affinity for fat and nervous tissue; high levels were still present in the brain 4 hours after inhalation. Radiolabeled trichloroethylene, which readily decomposes to dichloroacetylene (a compound causally associated with trigeminal neuropathy), was rapidly cleared from the brain within 30 minutes of inhalation exposure. By contrast, very little radioactivity was registered in the brain of animals administered ^{35}S-carbon disulfide, the unlabeled form of which is an established cause of psychosis and peripheral neuropathy, and a possible cause of tardive parkinsonism. These results emphasize the individual behaviors of specific chemical compounds within the class of organic solvents. Further information on these substances and those mentioned in the following paragraph is available elsewhere in this volume (listed under the names of specific compounds).

Entry of organic hydrocarbon solvents into the brain is generally associated with CNS depression, sometimes preceded (as in the case of imbibed ethanol) by a period of disinhibition. Short-term, high-level inhalation exposure to most organic solvents will produce transient headache and depressed consciousness (acute encephalopathy). Chronic low-level or high-level exposure to some (toluene, trichloroethylene, *n*-hexane, methyl *n*-butyl ketone) can cause serious degenerative change in specific areas of the central or peripheral nervous system, or both (17). 1,2-Diethylbenzene also produces a peripheral neuropathy in animals. Exposure to each of these four substances can produce symptomatic disease that is consistently characteristic for the compound and the dose. It is also likely that repeated multiyear, high-level (prenarcotic) occupational exposure to many of the agents in Table 40 can cause symptomatic, subtle, irreversible alterations in cognitive performance (15,19). It is suggested that some of the initial Scandinavian reports may have included house painters who had experienced such repeated, unprotected, prenarcotic exposures while utilizing the indoor spray-painting techniques employed in Denmark at that time (19). Proponents of the OSS claim that extreme prolonged, *very low-level* (below the Threshold Limit Value), daily occupational exposure to virtually any combination or single substance in this list can produce the syndrome.

The OSS has various other names. It has been called "painters syndrome", "psycho-organic syndrome", "solvent neurasthenic syndrome", or "chronic solvent encephalopathy". The OSS is generally held to be a two-stage illness (6). The first stage is a constellation of mild, reversible symptoms (headache, fatigue, impaired concentration); this

TABLE 40. Some Organic Solvent Chemicals[1] and Solvent Mixtures[2]

Acetone	Kerosene[6]
Benzene	Methanol
N-Butanol	Methyl *n*-butyl ketone
Butyl acetate	Methyl ethyl ketone
Chloromethane	Methyl isobutyl ketone
Cyclohexane	Naphtha (aromatic)[7]
Cyclohexanone	Perchloroethylene
Dichloromethane	Petroleum ether[8]
Diethyl ether	Propyl benzene
Diisobutyl ketone	Stoddard solvent[9]
Ethanol	Styrene
Ethyl acetate	1,1,1-Trichloroethane
Ethyl benzene	Trichloroethylene
Ethylene chloride	Trichloromethane
Ethylene glycol	Trimethylbenzene
N-Hexane	Toluene
Gasoline[3]	Turpentine
Isobutanol	VM & P naphtha[10]
Isopropanol	Xylene
Jet fuel, JP-4[4], JP-5[5]	White spirit[11]

[1]Commercial preparations vary in purity and contain other components as minor constituents.

[2]Mixtures are of variable content and are known by a range of titles that provide no information on the nature or proportion of the individual chemicals they contain. Illustrative information is given in the following footnotes.

[3]Paraffins, olefins, ethanol, aromatics.

[4]C_4-C_{14} *n*-alkanes (n = 11), isoalkanes (n = 23), cycloparaffins (n = 17) and aromatics (n = 24).

[5]*N*- and iso-paraffins (30.8%), total cycloparaffins (52.8%), total aromatics (15.9%), olefins (0.5%).

[6]Linear aliphatics, branched aliphatics, olefins, cycloparaffins, C_{10}-C_{16} aromatics (deodorized kerosene lacks benzene).

[7]Alkyl benzenes, cumene, toluene, xylenes.

[8]Principally *n*-pentane and *n*-hexane (also known as ligroin and petroleum distillate).

[9]VM & P: Varnish Makers' and Painters'. Paraffins, mono- and dicycloparaffins, olefins, alkylbenzenes.

[10]*m*-Xylene > *o*-xylene = *p*-xylene > diethylbenzene > other aromatics.

[11]C_7-C_8 paraffins, naphthenes, and aromatics (also known as mineral spirit and refined petroleum solvent).

stage appears in workers after approximately one year of exposure to very low levels (below the Scandinavian work levels) of organic solvent mixtures (9). The second stage follows 3-9 years of exposure; it is claimed to include irreversible, subtle neurological signs and symptoms including altered memory, attention and concentration; these occur in concert with personality changes of depression, apathy and irritability.

Only three (one British and two North American) of the many cross-sectional epidemiological studies of encephalopathy in workers with prolonged legal levels of exposure have incorporated the critical feature of industrial hygiene personal breathing zone sampling data into an exposure estimate (3,5,11); only the 1991 North American study included sampling over many years (3). None of these studies supports the notion that the OSS is a *symptomatic* condition at these acceptable levels of exposure. The 1991 North American study was multidisciplinary and is a landmark in the field; it featured longitudinal analysis of personal breathing space (7), careful neuropsychological testing (3), neuropsychiatric measures (4), and measurement of olfactory function (16). This study of 187 North American workers in paint manufacturing plants found no evidence of subjective symptoms of CNS or PNS disease. The abnormalities detected were all subclinical and slight; the authors state "the association of a psycho-organic syndrome with exposure to low-levels of solvent exposure was not supported by this study." Neuropsychological testing revealed small, exposure-related alterations in tests of sustained attention and concentration (digit-symbol substitution, serial digit learning, Trails A & B); no significant changes were detected in memory tests. Neuropsychiatric assessment, utilizing objective standardized measures, of subjective complaints failed to detect increased complaints of fatigue, decreased concentration, headache or poor memory. A measure of olfactory function (University of Pennsylvania Smell Identification Test) showed dose-related decrements in olfactory function in non-smokers in the highest exposure category.

A subsequent, meticulously controlled, long-term, cross-sectional epidemiological study of British brush painters (unfortunately, without breathing space analysis) found no increase in psychiatric symptoms (18);. significant, subclinical effects on cognitive function was found only in workers with more than 30 years of exposure. In addition, neither was a German cross-sectional study (that included some measures of workplace air solvent content) of brush painters with a median of 27 years of exposure able to detect symptomatic encephalopathy (19); nor was a careful North American study (featuring breathing zone analysis, neuropsychological testing, and quantitative sensory testing) of

painters exposed for 7 years mainly to *n*-hexane and isopropanol able to find evidence of peripheral neuropathy or encephalopathy (10,11).

In sum, contemporary painstaking studies indicate that prolonged (10-20 years) occupational exposure to permissible North American or European levels of organic solvent mixtures does not cause symptomatic CNS or PNS dysfunction. Such exposure possibly can be associated with mild, subclinical cognitive dysfunction in the form of psychomotor or attentional deficits, which have limited treatment options (20)

Prolonged maternal exposure to high levels of toluene is clearly teratogenic (*see* Toluene, this volume). A recent report suggests that other organic solvents may present a similar hazard. This report describes the results of a recent prospective, observational, controlled study of 125 pregnant women who were exposed occupationally to organic solvents and seen during the first trimester between 1987 and 1996 (8). Most subjects were factory workers, laboratory technicians, professional artists and graphic designers, and workers in the printing industry. The solvents most commonly involved were aliphatic and aromatic hydrocarbons, phenols, trichloroethylene, xylene, vinyl chloride and acetone; no information was given on the levels of exposure. Each study subject was matched to a pregnant woman (on age, gravidity, and smoking and drinking status) who was exposed to a nonteratogenic agent. Significantly more major malformations occurred among fetuses of women exposed to organic solvents than of controls. The relative risk was thirteen-fold (95% confidence interval, 1.8–99.5). Twelve malformations occurred among the babies of 75 women who reported they had had CNS symptoms temporally associated with their exposure; none was seen among 43 women who reportedly had been asymptomatic during exposure to organic solvents. While epidemiological studies of this type are limited by a number of factors— notably the lack of specific association between chemical type, exposure level, and outcome—it nevertheless seems prudent to minimize the exposure of women of childbearing age to organic solvents (8).

REFERENCES

1. Axelson O, Hane M, Hogstedt C (1976) A case-referent study on neuropsychiatric disorders among workers exposed to solvents. *Scand J Work Environ Health* **2**, 14.
2. Bergmann K (1983) Application and results of whole-body autoradiography in distribution studies of organic solvents. *CRC Crit Rev Toxicol* **12**, 59.
3. Bleecker ML, Bolla KI, Agnew J et al. (1991) Dose-related subclinical neurobehavioral effects of chronic exposure to low levels of organic solvents. *Amer J Ind Med* **19**, 715.

4. Bolla KI, Schwartz BS, Agnew J *et al.* (1990) Subclinical neuropsychiatric effects of chronic low-level solvent exposure in US paint manufacturers. *J Occup Med* 32, 671.

5. Cherry N, Hutchins H, Pace T *et al.* (1985) Neurobehavioral effects of repeated occupational exposure to toluene and paint solvents. *Brit J Ind Med* 42, 291.

6. Cranmer JM, Golberg L (1986) Neurobehavioral effects of solvents. *Neurotoxicology* 7, 1.

7. Ford DP, Schwartz BS, Powell S *et al.* (1991) A quantitative approach to the characterization of cumulative and average solvent exposure in paint manufacturing plants. *Amer Ind Hyg Assoc J* 52, 226.

8. Khattak S, K-Moghtader G, McMartin K *et al.* (1999) Pregnancy outcome following gestational exposure to organic exposure. A prospective controlled study. *J Amer Med Assn* 281, 1106.

9. Lindstrom K (1980) Changes in psychological performances of solvent-poisoned and solvent-exposed workers. *Amer J Ind Med* 1, 69.

10. Maizlish NA, Fine LJ, Albers JW *et al.* (1987) A neurological evaluation of workers exposed to mixtures of organic solvents. *Brit J Ind Med* 44, 14.

11. Maizlish NA, Langolf GD, Whitehead LW *et al.* (1985) Behavioral evaluation of workers exposed to mixtures of organic solvents. *Brit J Ind Med* 42, 579.

12. Mikkelsen S (1980) A cohort study of disability pension and death among painters with special regard to disabling

13. presenile dementia as an occupational disease. *Scand J Suc Med Suppl* 16, 34.

13. Morrow LA, Ryan CM, Hodgson MJ *et al.* (1990) Alterations in cognitive and psychological functioning after organic solvent exposure. *J Occup Med* 32, 444.

14. Seppalainen AM, Lindstrom K, Martelin T (1980) Neurophysiological and psychological picture of solvent poisoning. *Amer J Ind Med* 1, 31.

15. Schaumburg HH, Daffner KR, Grober E *et al.* (1993) Cognitive impairment and single photon emission computed tomography abnormality following occupational solvent exposure. *Ann Neurol* 34, 258.

16. Schwartz BS, Ford DP, Bolla KI *et al.* (1990) Solvent-associated decrements in olfactory function in paint manufacturing workers. *Amer J Ind Med* 18, 697.

17. Spencer PS, Schaumburg HH (1985) Organic solvent neurotoxicity. Facts and research needs. *Scand J Work Environ Health* 11 *Suppl* 1:53.

18. Spurgeon A, Gray CN, Sims J *et al.* (1992) Neurobehavioral effects of long-term occupational exposure to organic solvents—two comparable studies. *Amer J Ind Med* 22, 325.

19. Triebig G, Claus D, Csuzda I *et al.* (1988) Cross-sectional epidemiological study on neurotoxicity of solvents in paints and lacquers. *Int Arch Occup Environ Health* 60, 233.

20. White RF, Proctor SP (1997) Solvents and neurotoxicity. *Lancet* 349, 1239.

Organophosphorus Compounds

Marcello Lotti

OP

NEUROTOXICITY RATING

Clinical

A Cholinergic syndrome (nicotinic, muscarinic, CNS)

A Peripheral neuropathy (delayed)

A Neuromuscular transmission syndrome (junctional myopathy)

C Chronic encephalopathy (cognitive dysfunction)

Experimental

A Cholinergic dysfunction (nicotinic, muscarinic, CNS)

A Peripheral neuropathy (delayed)

Well over 20,000 compounds form a large and diverse family of chemicals collectively designated as organophospho-

rus compounds (OP) (60). Only the triesters of phosphoric acid are considered here. OPs can generally be denoted with the above structural formula, given by G. Schräder in 1937 when he described derivatives of phosphorus acids with insecticidal properties (91). R1 and R2 vary (*e.g.*, alcohols, amides) as well as the X moiety (*e.g.*, fluorine, phenoxy). Nomenclature of OPs is complex, and their classification may follow various schemes (36,60,81,90,91). Examples of classifications of OP esters are given in Table 41 and Figure 17. OPs other than anatoxin-a(s) (*see* Anatoxins, this volume) do not occur naturally.

Physicochemical characteristics of OPs vary. They may be solid, liquid, or gaseous; soluble in water, organic solvents, or both; corrosive or not, highly volatile or not; *etc.* All OPs are usually rapidly degraded by strong alkali (60,221).

The long inventory of applications of OPs, besides their

TABLE 41. Classification of Organophosphorus Esters*

General Formula:

$$R_1 \diagdown \underset{R_2 \diagup}{P} \diagup^{O(S)}_{\diagdown X}$$

A. Compounds where X = halogen or CN, CNS *etc.*

1. R1 = alkoxy, R2 = alkyl
   example:

   $$i\text{-}C_3H_7O \diagdown \underset{CH_3 \diagup}{P}\overset{O}{\overset{\|}{}}\!\!-F$$

   Sarin
   (isopropyl methylphosphonofluoridate),
   nerve gas

2. R1 and R2 = alkoxy
   example:

   $$i\text{-}C_3H_7O \diagdown \underset{i\text{-}C_3H_7O \diagup}{P}\overset{O}{\overset{\|}{}}\!\!-F$$

   DFP
   (diisopropyl phosphorofluoridate),
   laboratory chemical and drug

3. R1 = alkylamide, R2 = alkoxy
   example:

   $$(CH_3)_2N \diagdown \underset{C_2H_5O \diagup}{P}\overset{O}{\overset{\|}{}}\!\!-CN$$

   Tabun
   (ethyl *N*-dimethylphosphoroamidocyanidate),
   nerve gas

4. R1 and R2 = mono or dialkylamido
   example:

   $$i\text{-}C_3H_7NH \diagdown \underset{i\text{-}C_3H_7NH \diagup}{P}\overset{O}{\overset{\|}{}}\!\!-F$$

   Mipafox
   (*N,N'*-diisopropyl phosphorodiamidofluoridate),
   laboratory chemical

B. Compounds where X = alkyl, alkoxy, or aryloxy

1. Alkoxydialkyl or dialkoxyalkyl compounds
   example:

   $$CH_3O \diagdown \underset{CH_3O \diagup}{P}\overset{O}{\overset{\|}{}}\!\!-CHCCl_3$$
   $$\underset{OH}{|}$$

   Trichlorfon
   (dimethyl(2,2,2-trichloro-1-hydroxyethyl)phosphonate),
   insecticide and drug

2. Trialkoxy compounds and dialkoxy, aryloxy compounds
   example:

   $$CH_3O \diagdown \underset{CH_3O \diagup}{P}\overset{O}{\overset{\|}{}}\!\!-O-CH=CCl_2$$

   Dichlorvos
   (dimethyl 2,2-dichlorovinyl phosphate),
   insecticide

C. Thiol- and thiono-phosphorus compounds

1. Thiol compounds
   example:

   $$CH_3O \diagdown \underset{CH_3O \diagup}{P}\overset{O}{\overset{\|}{}}\!\!-S-CH-CH_2CH_2SC_2H_5$$

   Demeton-*S*-methyl
   (*S*-[2-(ethylthio)ethyl]dimethyl phosphorothioate),
   insecticide

2. Thiono compounds
   example:

   $$C_2H_5O \diagdown \underset{C_2H_5O \diagup}{P}\overset{S}{\overset{\|}{}}\!\!-O-\!\!\!\bigcirc\!\!\!-NO_2$$

   Parathion
   (diethyl *O*-(4-nitrophenyl)phosphorothioate),
   insecticide

TABLE 41. Classification of Organophosphorus Esters* (*Continued*)

3. Thiol-thiono compounds
   example:

$$CH_3O-\underset{CH_3O}{\overset{S}{\overset{\|}{P}}}-S-\underset{\underset{CH_2CO.OC_2H_5}{|}}{CHCO.OC_2H_5}$$

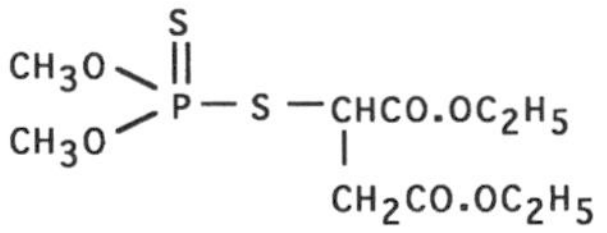

Malathion
(dimethyl *S*-(1,2-dicarboxylethyl)phosphorodithioate),
insecticide

D. Derivatives of pyrophosphorous acid and similar compounds

2. Thiono compounds
   example:

$$C_2H_5O-\underset{C_2H_5O}{\overset{S}{\overset{\|}{P}}}-O-\underset{}{\overset{S}{\overset{\|}{P}}}-\underset{OC_2H_5}{\overset{OC_2H_5}{}}$$

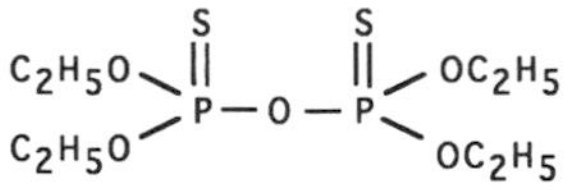

Sulfotepp
(tetraethyl thiodiphosphate),
insecticide

E. Compounds containing a quaternary nitrogen. Phosphorylcholines *etc.*

   example:

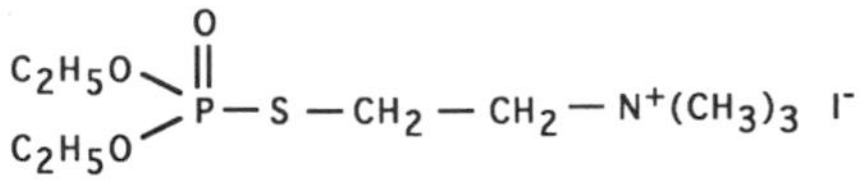

$$C_2H_5O-\underset{C_2H_5O}{\overset{O}{\overset{\|}{P}}}-S-CH_2-CH_2-N^+(CH_3)_3 \quad I^-$$

Ecothiophate
(diethyl-*S*-2-trimethyl-ammonium-ethyl-phosphorothioate iodide),
drug

---

*Nerve gases belong to group A; most commercial pesticides belong to groups B and C. [From Holmstedt (91).]

main uses as crop protection agents and growth regulators, include flame retardants, polymer additives, drugs, radiodiagnostic agents, metal extraction agents, corrosion inhibitors, emulsifiers, antistatic agents, complexing agents, phase-transfer and regular catalysts, ligand modifiers of catalysts, and warfare agents (60).

About 80 OPs are thought to be in use as pesticides, primarily as insecticides (221), though they are present in thousands of formulations and applied in almost infinite working and climatic conditions to a variety of crops. Information on global production and uses of OPs for crop protection is scarce. It has been estimated that fewer than 50 pesticides account for about 75% of all pesticides used in the world and several of these are OPs (178). Although they are progressively being replaced by less toxic chemicals, OPs are likely to continue to be the most important insecticides used in developing countries; demand for them was predicted to more than double during the 1990s (218).

Besides crop protection, OP pesticides are widely used in public health programs to control vector-borne diseases in tropical areas and worldwide in gardening.

OPs have been used and recommended as anticholinesterase drugs for treatment of a variety of disorders, although their acceptability has been established for only a few conditions. Ecothiophate (0.03%–0.25% solution) and, to a lesser extent, diisopropylphosphorofluorophosphate (DFP) (0.025%) (structures shown in Table 41), are used for local treatment of glaucoma either alone or in combination with other drugs (201). Trichlorfon has been successfully used for treatment of schistosomiasis (74,160).

OPs have also been used as warfare agents, and large amounts are thought to be stockpiled in arsenals worldwide. Three OPs were developed as nerve gases by the German army during the Second World War. The first was tabun followed by sarin (structures shown in Table 41) and soman (pynacolyl methyl phosphonofluoridate). In the

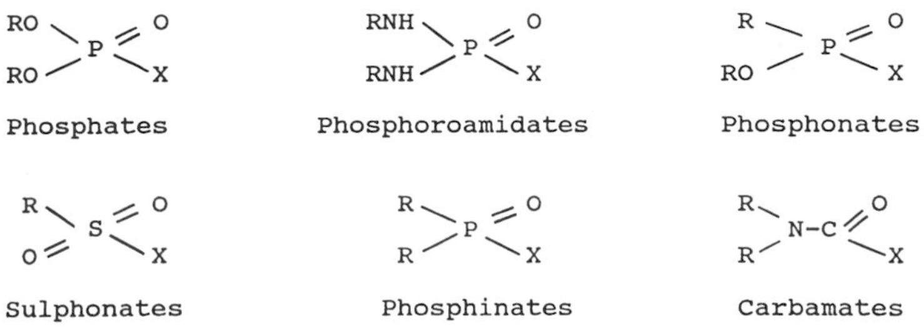

$$RO-\underset{RO}{\overset{}{P}}\overset{O}{\underset{X}{<}} \qquad RNH-\underset{RNH}{\overset{}{P}}\overset{O}{\underset{X}{<}} \qquad R-\underset{RO}{\overset{}{P}}\overset{O}{\underset{X}{<}}$$

Phosphates   Phosphoroamidates   Phosphonates

$$R-\underset{O}{\overset{}{S}}\overset{O}{\underset{X}{<}} \qquad R-\underset{R}{\overset{}{P}}\overset{O}{\underset{X}{<}} \qquad R-\underset{R}{\overset{}{N-C}}\overset{O}{\underset{X}{<}}$$

Sulphonates   Phosphinates   Carbamates

FIGURE 17. Chemistry of neuropathy target esterase (NTE) inhibitors.

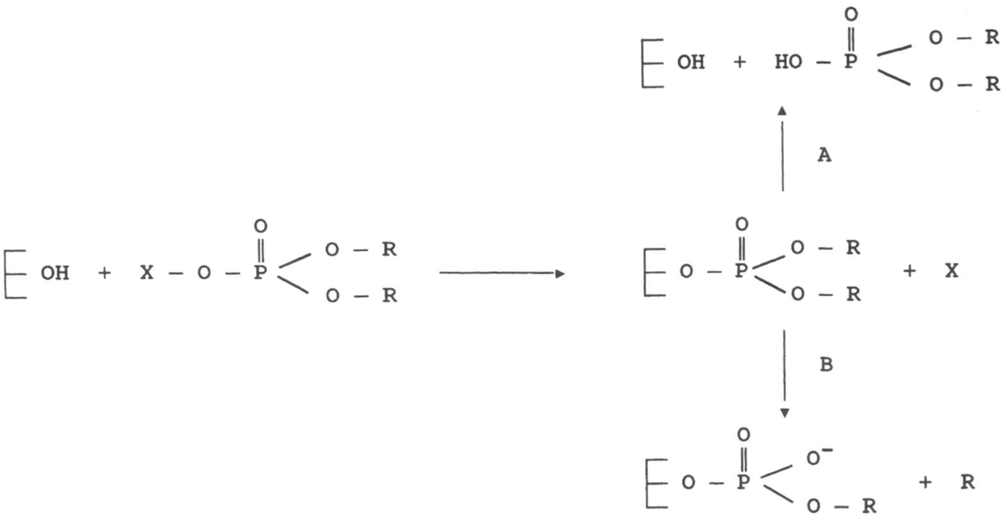

FIGURE 18. Schematic representation of biochemical interactions of OPs with esterases. OPs are substrates for esterases: reaction A occurs with A-esterases, leading to the hydrolysis of OPs, whereas reaction B causes irreversible inhibition of B-esterases through a nonenzymatic reaction called "aging."

1950s, another nerve gas, VX (*S*-[2-[bis(1-methylethyl)-amino]ethyl] *O*-ethyl methylphosphonothioate), was developed by Britain and the United States (*see* Sarin, other "Nerve Agents" and Their Antidotes, this volume). Sarin was recently used as a weapon of civilian terrorism in Japan (197).

Exposures to OP pesticides occur at workplaces, in food and drinking water, and in the environment. Several studies on workers spraying and applying OP insecticides assessed exposure to a variety of OPs, and they have been summarized (93). Exposure of the general population through food contamination is generally low if good agricultural practices are followed during OP applications. Such exposure may be estimated from the measurements of OP residues in most crops; these are regularly reported by various national authorities and by the Joint Food and Agriculture Organization (FAO)–World Health Organization Meeting on Pesticides Residues in Food (JMPR) (66). Exposures from contaminated drinking water and environmental air are usually very low, unless accidental. In some countries, OPs are used as an instrument of suicide (71).

OP pesticides are usually strictly regulated by governments throughout the world. Restrictions include formulations, packaging, labeling, licensing for use, and limitation of uses on certain crops, among others. Moreover, a code of conduct has been developed by the United Nations FAO, and agreed to by involved parties (producers, traders, regulatory bodies of member states, *etc.*), which regulates international distribution and use of pesticides (65). Indications of acceptable levels of exposure to OPs, both for occupational and food exposures, are usually given and up-

dated on a yearly basis by national and international bodies, for instance by the American Conference of Governmental Industrial Hygienists (ACGIH)(6) and by the JMPR (66), respectively. Table 42 reports Threshold Limit Values for occupational exposures to OPs and the corresponding acceptable daily intake of OPs, when they leave residues in food commodities. Of interest are the large differences between the limits for the two exposures, suggesting, at least in part, that different databases have been used to estimate such values.

General Toxicology

OPs are among the most extensively investigated class of chemicals in toxicology; huge numbers of research papers, books, book chapters, and reviews have been published over the last 40 years (3,7,14,38,58,64,88,90,91,102,104, 114,122,123,125,152,168,214).

Both the toxicodynamics (mechanism of action) and toxicokinetics (*e.g.*, distribution, metabolism) of OPs are largely explained by their biochemical characteristic of interacting with esterases and proteases (9). Figure 18 illustrates the biochemical reactions of OPs with the catalytic center of esterases. Esterases have been ranked into two main categories: those inhibited by OPs, B-esterases, representing potential targets for toxicity; and A-esterases, which hydrolyze OPs, thereby being involved in detoxification. OPs interact with either esterase as substrates: B-esterases after the formation of a Michaelis complex are phosphorylated and the reactivation is either very slow or it does not occur at all. A-esterases, on the contrary, hydro-

TABLE 42. Threshold Limit Values-Time Weighted Average (TLV-TWA) of Organophosphates Adopted by the American Conference of Governmental Industrial Hygienists (6) and Corresponding Acceptable Daily Intakes (ADI) Adopted by the Joint FAO/WHO Meeting on Pesticide Residues in Food (68)

Organophosphate	TWA (mg/m³)	ADI (mg/kg b.w.)
Azinphos-methyl	0.2	0.005
Chlorpyrifos	0.2	0.01
Diazinon	0.1	0.002
Dichlorvos	0.9	0.004
Dicrotophos	0.25	
Disulfoton	0.1	0.0003
EPN	0.5	
Ethion	0.4	0.002
Fenamiphos	0.1	0.0005
Fensulfothion	0.1	0.0003
Fenthion	0.2	0.001
Fonofos	0.1	
Malathion	10	0.02
Methyl demeton	0.5	0.0003
Methyl parathion	0.2	0.02
Mevinphos	0.092*	0.0015
Monocrotophos	0.25	0.0006
Naled	3	
Parathion	0.1	0.005
Phorate	0.05†	0.0002
Sulfotep	0.2	
Temephos	10	

*Short-Term Exposure Limit (STEL) = 0.27 mg/m³.   EPN: *O*-ethyl *O-p*-nitrophenyl phenylphosphonothioate.
†STEL = 0.2 mg/m³.

lyze OPs and their catalytic center is rapidly restored. Moreover, a further reaction might occur on phosphorylated B-esterases, a phenomenon called *aging*, involving the loss of an R group and leading to the formation of a negatively charged irreversibly phosphorylated enzyme. On a given enzyme, rates of reactions depend on the chemistry as well as on chirality of the inhibitor (48).

The interactions of several A- and B-esterases with a large number of OPs have been studied both *in vivo* and *in vitro*. Any given B-esterase is inhibited by various OPs at different rates. In addition, rates of reactivation and aging of phosphorylated enzymes are variable, depending on the phosphoryl residue that occupies the catalytic center. Therefore, the degree of inhibition of an esterase and its duration at the site depend both on the enzyme itself and on the chemistry of the OP. Table 43 illustrates the interaction of various OPs with B-esterase acetylcholinesterase (AChE). While OPs inhibit AChE at variable concentrations, both spontaneous reactivation and aging depend on the phosphoryl residue bound to the active site. As a result of AChE phosphorylation by different OPs, this residue can be the same.

Various A-esterases that hydrolyze OPs are known, but their biochemical classification is controversial (167,168). Some A-esterases display high substrate specificity, others do not. In many species, including humans, the largest amounts of A-esterases are in plasma, and they are thought to be relevant for OP detoxification (42,212).

Absorption of OPs occurs through the skin and the respiratory and gastrointestinal tracts, and depends on both OP chemistry and type of exposure. For instance, the main route of absorption is by inhalation for nerve gases, dermal for organophosphates in the workplace, and by ingestion in voluntary or accidental exposures. Table 44 shows differences between oral and dermal absorption for some OPs.

The distribution of OPs is variable. Blood half-lives are usually short, although plasma levels are, in some cases, maintained for several days (Fig. 19). After intravenous (i.v.) injection of several OPs in rats, the inhibition of brain AChE was shown to depend both on their power to inhibit the enzyme and on their water-lipid partition characteristics (166). Because of lipophilicity, high chemical reactivity, and large apparent volume of distribution of OPs, it is particularly important for the clinician to appreciate that plasma levels represent a minute fraction of body burden, the clearance from body compartments may vary substantially among OPs, and that redistribution might occur. The clinical course of poisoning by OPs (which are distributed to a significant extent in the fat) may be characterized by re-

TABLE 43. Interactions of Some OPs with Human AChE

Organophosphates		Inhibition (AChE I_{50} $10^{-6}M^{\dagger}$)		Phosphorylated AChE* Spontaneous Reactivation ($t_{1/2}$ h)	Aging ($t_{1/2}$ h)
CH_3O–$P(=O)$–O–$CH=CCl_2$ (CH_3O)	Dichlorvos	0.95	$[-O-P(=O)(OCH_3)(OCH_3)]$	0.85	3.9
CH_3O–$P(=O)$–S–$CH_2CO.NHCH_3$ (CH_3O)	Omethoate	140			
C_2H_5O–$P(=O)$–O–(pyridine, Cl,Cl,Cl) (C_2H_5O)	Chlorpyrifos-oxon	0.007	$[-O-P(=O)(OC_2H_5)(OC_2H_5)]$	58	41
C_2H_5O–$P(=O)$–O–$CH=CCl_2$ (C_2H_5O)	Diethyldichlorvos	0.41			
$i\text{-}C_3H_7O$–$P(=O)$–F ($i\text{-}C_3H_7O$)	DFP	0.83	$[-O-P(=O)(OC_3H_7\text{-}i)(OC_3H_7\text{-}i)]$	No reactivation at 6	4.6

*Human red blood cell AChE (220).
$\dagger$Concentration to inhibit 50% of human brain AChE (33,129).

AChE: Acetylcholinesterase
DFP: Diisopropylphosphorofluoridate

lapsing episodes of cholinergic toxicity, particularly at the time when treatment is discontinued (59).

Biotransformation of OPs is extremely complex and involves several metabolic systems in different organs. Although OP metabolism has been extensively investigated (38,64,152) and several single chemical reactions as well as metabolic pathways have been described, the entire metabolic profile of an OP in a given species is seldom completely understood. Most commercial pesticides are phosphorothioate esters; a general scheme of their main metabolic transformations is given in Figure 20.

OPs undergo oxidative desulfuration (reaction 1 in Fig. 20), leading to formation of the oxon analog, which is the actual substrate for A- and B-esterases. This key reaction of metabolic activation might be catalyzed by cytochrome P-450 or flavine-containing microsomal monooxygenases, or both, either in the liver (118,154) or in other organs including the nervous system (37). Rates of oxidation depend on the tissue, species, and chemistry of the OP. Table 45 shows examples of OPs undergoing oxidation catalyzed by rat and mouse liver.

OP hydrolysis (reactions 3 and possibly 2 in Fig. 20) is catalyzed by both microsomal oxygenases and A-esterases (154,167). Hydrolysis leads to detoxification because the resulting phosphate does not phosphorylate esterases. At least for some OPs and in some species, it is believed that hydrolysis by A-esterases is a most important mechanism for OP detoxification (212). For instance, it has been re-

TABLE 44. Dermal and Oral Absorption of Some Organophosphates in Mice

OP	MW	H_2O sol (ppm)	Oil/H_2O Coefficient	Time for Half Applied Dose to Penetrate (min) Dermal	Oral	Percentage Penetrated (in 60 min) Dermal	Oral
Malathion	330	145	56	129	33	25	89
Chlorpyrifos	350	2	1044	21	78	69	47
Parathion	292	24	1738	66	33	32	57

[From Guthrie and Hodgson (87).]

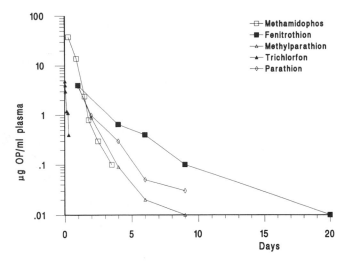

FIGURE 19. Plasma concentration decays of various OPs after single oral doses in man (159,160, and unpublished data from poisoning cases).

ported that intravenous injection of rabbit serum paraoxonase in rats increased the plasma levels of enzyme and protected animals from acute toxicity of paraoxon (the oxygen analog of parathion) and chlorpyrifos-oxon (structure in Table 43) (42). A-esterases are present in a variety of species and in several tissues. Human serum hydrolyzes several OPs including paraoxon, chlorpyrifos, tabun, DFP, pyrimiphos methyl-oxon, dichlorvos, soman (*see* Table 46) and *p*-nitrophenyl ethyl *n*-alkyl and phenyl alkyl phosphonates (167,168). Whether serum A-esterases represent effective protection from OP toxicity in humans remains to be ascertained. The most studied A-esterase is human serum paraoxonase, which hydrolyzes paraoxon and other OPs (79,80). Human serum paraoxonase has recently been cloned and sequenced (78); its high polymorphism (Fig. 21) suggests a possible variability of human responses to OPs, particularly after relatively low exposures such as those occurring in the working environment.

Other hydrolyzing enzymes, such as carboxylesterases acting at the carboxyl ester moiety of malathion (structure in Table 41), have been shown to provide substantial protection. The lack of these enzymes in insects justifies the selectivity of the insecticide malathion (116), and when these enzymes are inhibited by some OPs contained as impurities in certain malathion formulations (199,209), the toxicity of malathion sharply increases both in humans (13) and rats (8).

Reactions 4 and 5 in Figure 20 are catalyzed by P-450 monooxygenases, as well as by glutathione transferases, leading to aldehydes and glutathione conjugates, respectively, plus dealkylated or dearylated derivatives that are not phosphorylating agents (150,194,195). The relevance of these detoxifying reactions within the entire metabolic pathway varies among OPs. Figure 22 shows the decrease of glutathione (GSH) content of mouse liver after dosing with two homologous OPs. Although reduction of GSH was thought to reflect GSH conjugation, doubts have been raised about the overall relevance of this metabolic reaction at least for certain OPs and in some species (194).

Several oxidative reactions catalyzed by monooxygenases might occur at substituents of side groups of OPs; that is, sulfoxidation of thioethers (118) and cyclization of some triaryl-phosphates—the latter are thought to be relevant for metabolic activation and subsequent toxicity (102).

Given the complexity of OP metabolism and the interactions of OPs with esterases, it is not surprising that metabolic interactions among various OPs might occur, such as that described above between malathion and its OP impurities. Nevertheless, interactions are hardly predictable and information is, in this respect, only seldom available.

OPs are mainly excreted in urine either as parent compounds or as products of hydrolysis (dialkylphosphates and acidic groups). Percentage of doses and time course of excretion of each metabolite vary among OPs, dose ranges, and species (30). Figure 23 shows the time course of urinary excretion in humans of two main metabolites of parathion,

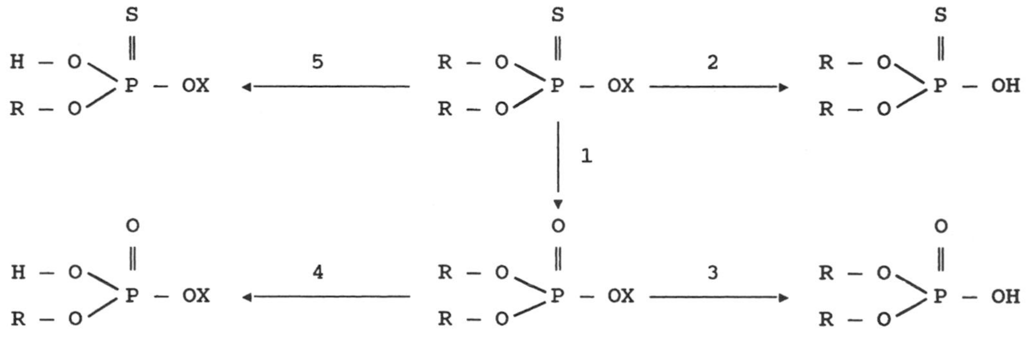

FIGURE 20. General scheme of biotransformation of dialkylphosphorothioate pesticides (150).

TABLE 45. Cholinesterase Inhibitors (P=O) formed when some Thiophosphate Insecticides (P=S) were Incubated with Rat and Mouse Liver Slices

Name	Structure	P=O Equivalent Accumulation/100 mg Liver/30 min	
		Rat	Mouse
Parathion		5.8	7.7
Azinphos-methyl		9.0	14.2
Malathion		Traces	6.4

[From Murphy (151).]

indicating that recovery of the administered dose is poor and time for peak excretion varies. Analytical methods for measuring OPs and their metabolites in human urine are poorly validated and often, when urinary metabolites are used for quantitative assessment of human exposure, the experimental design is inappropriate (153). Moreover, the very same metabolites (*i.e.*, dimethylphosphates) arise from several OPs, each possibly displaying a very different toxicity. Therefore, it is not surprising that no correlation is usually found between urinary levels of metabolites and cholinesterase inhibition when assessing human exposures (54). For these reasons, measurements of urinary metabolites, as suggested for biomonitoring of human exposures to OPs (100), are of little value, at best proving exposure.

Given the widespread distribution of the cholinergic system, effects of OPs on various organs have been described, reflecting consequences of the primary cholinergic toxicity. Some primary noncholinergic extranervous effects have been associated with OPs.

Certain trialkylphosphorothioates are potential impurities of P=S phosphorothioate pesticides and cause selective pulmonary toxicity to both bronchial and alveolar cells of rodents, in particular to the type 1 pneumocytes. The rea-

son for such selectivity is thought to be related to *in situ* metabolic reactions, leading to the formation of metabolite(s) toxic to the cell (52).

Certain ocular diseases have been associated with human exposures to OPs in Japan (Saku disease) (97), although other reports dispute these findings (94,163). Relevant literature (both case reports and experimental data) has been reviewed and experiments have been initiated to clarify the issue (29). Nevertheless, it should be noted that effects are not consistent among OPs, and it is not clear whether they are secondary to AChE inhibition or represent another toxicity.

OP-induced testicular toxicity has been produced in experimental animals after repeated dosing with tri-*o*-cresylphosphate (TOCP) (188) and after single doses of the OP herbicide amiprophos (92). Little or no information is available for other OPs.

OPs have alkylating properties and several positive mutagenic responses have been observed *in vitro* (149). However, these effects have rarely been detected *in vivo* because of the cholinergic toxicity of OPs and the relatively higher alkylating dose that would be needed. Consequently, it has been suggested that OPs are unlikely to cause either mu-

TABLE 46. Rate Constants of Soman Isomers' Enzymatic Hydrolysis by Human Serum

Soman	Isomer	Soman Rate Constant (m^{-1})
	C(+) P(−)	0.016
	C(−) P(+)	0.74
	C(−) P(−)	0.028
	C(+) P(+)	>1

[From De Bisschop *et al.* (45).]

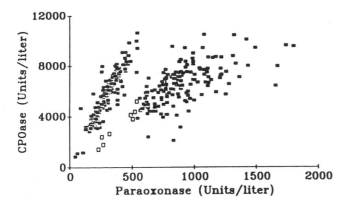

FIGURE 21. Paraoxonase and chlorpyrifos-oxonase in a Caucasian population. [Reproduced with permission from Furlong *et al.* (80).]

tations or cancer *in vivo* (216). There is one notable exception, namely dichlorvos, which was found to be weakly carcinogenic when given at high doses to experimental animals (39). The susceptibility of rodents to dichlorvos-induced cancer is likely related to their ability to tolerate very high doses of the chemical. In these species, dichlorvos has low toxicity probably because of the rapid spontaneous reactivation of AChE *in vivo* (169).

Numerous reports indicate that OPs may interfere with certain immune functions and speculate that they may be involved in the pathogenesis of a number of diseases, including infectious diseases and cancer (158,174,183). Despite the large number of immunological parameters that have been reported to be affected by OPs both *in vitro* and *in vivo*, either in the experimental animal or human, nothing has been substantiated experimentally, clinically, or epidemiologically. Cases of allergic dermatitis have been at-

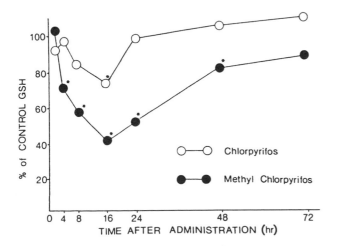

FIGURE 22. Hepatic glutathione (GSH) levels after administration of two homologous OPs to mice (nonlethal equitoxic doses i.p.). [Reproduced with permission from Sultatos *et al.* (195).]

tributed to several OPs (136), and anecdotal reports of OP-induced asthma occasionally appear (49).

Animal Studies

OP neurotoxicity has been observed in most species, either in controlled or uncontrolled exposures, and is characterized by two distinct syndromes; cholinergic overstimulation and delayed polyneuropathy.

OP cholinergic toxicity is related to inhibition of AChE at nerve endings and to the subsequent accumulation of acetylcholine. In general, there is a good correlation between acute toxicity (LD_{50}) of OPs and their ability to inhibit AChE *in vitro* (Fig. 24). Major differences in cholinergic toxicity have been observed across species (Table 47). The pharmacokinetics of OPs account in part for different susceptibility (214) although species-related differences in AChE sensitivity to inhibition also appear to be relevant (213). For practical purposes, the World Health Organization has ranked pesticides by hazard on the basis of acute oral and dermal toxicities of their formulations to rats (Table 48). However, the LD_{50} in animals should be regarded as a broad indication of cholinergic toxicity to humans, because, besides species differences, OP insecticides are manufactured and formulated in various ways and in many countries. Consequently, different procedures of synthesis, formulation, and storage influence the nature and amount of impurities in the formulated materials and, thus, their toxicity. It has been shown, for instance in the quoted case of malathion poisoning, that small amounts of impurities formed in various conditions of storage interfere with detoxification of the major ingredient in mammals, thereby potentiating its toxicity. Impurities may also be toxic in their own right, and when present in formulations where the major component has low toxicity, they represent the chemical species responsible for the overall toxicity of the material.

Age-related differences in the cholinergic toxicity of OPs have been detected, mainly between weanlings and adult animals. They seem to be related to changes in the developing metabolizing systems. However, since metabolism may cause activation and/or deactivation, as in the case of liver monooxygenases, it is difficult to predict toxicity differences with respect to development; in several reports, younger animals appear to be more sensitive to certain OPs (156). For instance, a progressive decrease in susceptibility to poisoning by parathion and methyl-parathion was reported when 1- to 40-day-old rats were studied. Increased detoxication of both parent compounds and active oxygen analogs, as well as the extensive binding to noncritical sites, were thought to account for the lower sensitivity of adult

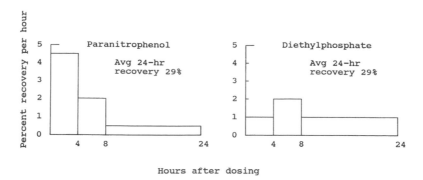

FIGURE 23. Average time course of urinary excretion of main metabolites of parathion in volunteers (147).

animals (18). Sex-related differences, although often reported, are probably not as important.

The clinical onset of cholinergic overstimulation varies from almost instantaneous to several hours after dosing animals with OPs; this depends on dosage, route of exposure, pharmacokinetics and pharmacodynamics of the OP, as well as on animal species. Table 49 shows the variability of onset and duration of cholinesterase inhibition in body compartments after dosing rats with different OPs.

The relationship between cholinergic symptoms and degree of AChE inhibition both in the CNS and PNS is influenced by several factors. In general, the nervous system compensates for substantial AChE inhibition. In most cases 50%–80% inhibition of AChE in the nervous system is needed before symptoms are noted, whereas 85%–90% is associated with severe toxicity and more than 90% with death. Therefore, the transition from an asymptomatic dose to a lethal one is often related with a three- to fivefold increase. Signs of cholinergic overstimulation include, in most species, a variety of muscarinic, nicotinic, and CNS signs such as lacrimation, chromodacryorrhea in rats, hypersalivation, bronchorrea and bronchoconstriction, urination and defecation, skeletal muscle fasciculation and twitching, ataxia, respiratory failure, convulsions, hypothermia, and death. Death is due to respiratory failure resulting from the combination of these effects. When assessing the relative importance of these symptoms in causing death, a clinical discrimination between primary effects on the CNS and those on the PNS is difficult (123).

Recovery from cholinergic toxicity depends on several

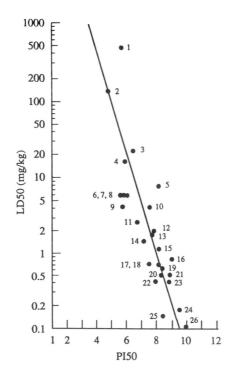

FIGURE 24. *In vivo* toxicity of some directly acting organophosphorus insecticides as related to their ability to inhibit acetylcholinesterase *in vitro*. Values used for calculating the regression line were those for 1, trichlorfon; 2, *O,O*-diethyl-4-chlorophenylphosphate; 3, *O,O*-diethyl-bis-dimethyl pyrophosphordiamide (sym); 4, TIPP; 5, *O,O*-diethylphosphostigmine; 6, isodemeton sulfoxide; 7, isodemeton; 8, isodemeton sulfone; 9, diisopropylphosphofluoridate; 10, diethylamidoethoxy-phosphoryl cyanide; 11, *O,O*-dimethyl-*O,O*-diisopropyl pyrophosphate (asym); 12, diethylamidomethoxy-phosphoryl cyanide; 13, tetramethyl pyrophosphate; 14, *O,O*-diethylphosphorylcyanidate; 15, *O,O*-dimethyl-*O,O*-diethyl pyrophosphate (asym); 16, soman; 17, tetraethylpyrophosphate; 18, *O*-isopropyl-ethylphosphonofluoridate; 19, tabun; 20, amiton; 21, diethylamido-isopropoxyphosphoryl cyanide; 22, *O,O*-diethyl-*S*-(2-diethylaminoethyl)phosphorothioate; 23, sarin; 24, *O,O*-diethyl-*S*-(2-triethylammoniumethyl)thiophosphate iodide; 25, echothiophate; 26, methylfluorophosphorylcholine iodide; 27, methylfluorophosphoryl-B-methylcholine iodide; 28, *O*-ethylmethylphosphorylthiocholine iodide; 29, methylfluorophosphorylhomo-choline iodide. The last three of these, which had LD_{50} values in the range of 0.03–0.07 mg/kg, are not shown on the graph. [Reproduced with permission from Gallo and Lawryk (81).]

TABLE 47. Species Differences in Acute Toxicities of some OP Insecticides

	Acute Oral LD_{50} (mg/kg)					
	Rat	**Mouse**	**Guinea Pig**	**Rabbit**	**Hen**	**Dog**
Dimethoate	500–680	60	550	500		
Methylparathion	6–24	20–33	1270	420		90
Phoxim	6000–7000	2000–3000	350–500	250–500	20	>1000

[From FAO/WHO (67); WHO (215 and 217).]

factors including the type of inhibitor (*i.e.*, pharmacokinetics and spontaneous reactivation *vs.* aging of AChE), dosage, and *de novo* synthesis of AChE in the nervous system, which has a half-life of about 5–7 days in most species. Recovery is usually complete within several hours. Exceptions include poisoning by dimethylphosphates, where recovery is usually faster because of the high rate of spontaneous reactivation of dimethylphosphorylated AChE (81) (*see* Table 43) and poisoning by long-lasting OPs when recovery is usually delayed for several days. Figure 25 shows an example of the different speed of AChE recovery in brain after single doses of two long-lasting isomers of methamidophos and its correlation with the duration of symptoms.

Acute manifestations of OP poisoning in primates are accompanied by marked desynchronization of the electroencephalogram (EEG). More severe toxicity causes slowing of the EEG followed by the development of spike-and-wave discharges that accompany clinical convulsions. The recovery from electrophysiological changes usually parallels that from clinical signs. However, computerized analysis of brain-wave topography from EEGs taken in monkeys 1 year after a single convulsive dose of an OP showed persistent changes. Controversy exists about the value of computerized analysis, caution in its use has been recommended, and the toxicological significance of these findings is obscure (123). High doses of OPs, when accompanied by clinical signs of cholinergic stimulation, cause a block of peripheral nerve conduction.

Neuropathology is nonspecific. Common features include vascular damage associated with increased permeability of the vessels. Other neuropathological findings are related either to the seizure activity and/or to the hypoxic status induced by lethal doses of OPs (123).

Neuromuscular pathology is observed when anti-AChE agents are given at doses causing muscle fasciculations. Several OPs have been shown to cause a myopathy in selected skeletal muscles, characterized by localized necrosis in the region of the neuromuscular junction. Myopathy occurs in

TABLE 48. Organophosphorus Pesticides and Risk of Cholinergic Syndrome*

Classification	Common Name
Extremely hazardous	Chlorfenvinphos, chlormephos, coumaphos, disulfoton, EPN, ethoprophos, fenamiphos, fensulfothion, fonofos, mephosfolan, mevinphos, parathion, parathion-methyl, phorate, phosfolan, phosphamidon, prothoate, sulfotep, terbufos
Highly hazardous	Azinphos ethyl, azinphos methyl, cadusafos, cythioate, demeton-*S*-methyl, demeton-*S*-methylsulphon, dichlorvos, dicrotophos, edifenphos, famphur, fenthion, fosfmethylan, heptenophos, isazofos, isofenphos, isoxathion, mecarbam, methamidophos, methidathion, monocrotophos, omethoate, oxydemeton-methyl, pirimiphos-ethyl, propaphos, propetamphos, thiometon, triazophos, vamidathion
Moderately hazardous	Chlorpyrifos, cyanophos, diazinon, dimethoate, dioxabenzophos, ethion, etrimfos, fenitrothion, formothion, metacrifos, naled, phentoate, phosalone, phosmet, phoxim, profenfos, prothiofos, pyraclofos, quinalphos
Slightly hazardous	Acephate, alkatox, azamethiophos, chlorpyrifos-methyl, iodofenphos, malathion, pirimiphos-methyl, pyridaphenthion, temephos, tetrachlorvinphos, trichlorfon

*WHO-recommended classification of pesticides by hazard (96). Based on acute oral and dermal toxicity in rats and the physical state of product or formulation, pesticides are ranked as follows:
  Extremely hazardous: 5 mg/kg or less if solid; 20 mg/kg or less if liquid
  Highly hazardous: 5–50 mg/kg if solid; 20–200 mg/kg if liquid
  Moderately hazardous: 50–500 mg/kg if solid; 200–2000 mg/kg if liquid
  Slightly hazardous: over 500 mg/kg if solid; over 2000 mg/kg if liquid
Compounds in use or being developed are reported (221).

TABLE 49. Onset and Duration of the Anticholinesterase Action of some Organophosphorus Compounds in Rats

Compound	Dose* (mg/kg body wt.)	Maximum Inhibition of Cholinesterase (%)			Time (h) to Maximum Inhibition	Time (h) to Complete Reversal
		Brain	Serum	Submaxillary Gland		
Demeton-*S*	1.0	85	80	75	3.0	120
Disulfoton	1.25	75	85	75	3.0	120
Azinphosmethyl	3.5	60	0	50	0.5	24
Trichlorfon	140.0	85	82	85	0.25	6
Octamethyl pyrophosphortetramide (OMPA)	5.0	0	85	88	2.0	144

*5/8 LD$_{50}$.
[From DuBois (55).]

a limited number of fibers of affected muscles. Necrosis is not observed in end-plate-free regions of the muscle, indicating that the myopathy reflects changes induced in the region of the end plate as a consequence of AChE inhibition. The mechanism of myopathy has been explored, although its contribution to the overall clinical picture of acute OP poisoning is undetermined (51).

When AChE is inhibited, an increased permeability of the blood-brain barrier has been observed (90). Since this may facilitate the access of chemicals to the brain (157), including oximes (72), the phenomenon has implications for the treatment of OP poisoning.

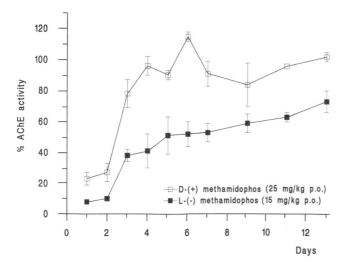

FIGURE 25. Time course of AChE inhibition in hen's brain after dosing with D-(+) or L-(−) methamidophos at doses causing similar inhibition on day 1. Differences are due to faster spontaneous reactivation of AChE when inhibited by D-(+) methamidophos. Symptoms lasted 2 days after D-(+) methamidophos, whereas after L-(−) methamidophos symptoms were detectable for up to 4–5 days. [Reproduced with permission from Lotti *et al.* (131).]

Single doses of certain OPs cause a central-peripheral distal sensory-motor axonopathy known as organophosphate-induced delayed polyneuropathy (OPIDP) (3,102,104,106, 122,125,170).

The molecular target is thought to be a protein in the nervous system called neuropathy target esterase (NTE). High inhibition of NTE (>70%) in the nervous system, measured within hours after dosing, correlates with the delayed onset of clinical signs of OPIDP 10–20 days later. Several OPs cause OPIDP and most available data have been summarized in key reviews (102,104,122). OPIDP is caused by certain, but not all, OPs, provided they inhibit NTE above the threshold. Among these, some are not anticholinesterases, like triarylphosphates, while others, (*e.g.*, pesticides) display both toxicities.

Doses causing OPIDP depend on the OP, the route of administration, the species and other factors (*e.g., see* Table 50 for the hen). However, from the practical point of view, it is important how the dose causing OPIDP compares with that causing cholinergic toxicity (129). This concept, represented numerically by the ratio LD$_{50}$/neurotoxic dose, allows comparisons of the potential of OPs to cause OPIDP. Thus a ratio LD$_{50}$/neurotoxic dose >1 discriminates OPs causing OPIDP at doses that do not cause cholinergic toxicity from those that cause OPIDP only if animals are treated against cholinergic symptoms (ratio <1). All commercial OP insecticides have a ratio of <1 and most have a ratio <0.1. Figure 26 shows that the relative potency of OPs in relation to the induction of OPIDP (LD$_{50}$/neurotoxic dose ratio) correlates with the *in vitro* ratio obtained measuring the power of inhibitors on corresponding molecular targets, AChE and NTE, respectively. Therefore, among NTE inhibitors, cholinergic toxicity is the limiting factor for OPIDP development.

Several species are sensitive to OPIDP, and the animal of choice for mechanistic studies and toxicity testing is the hen

TABLE 50. OPs causing Delayed Neuropathy in Humans—A Comparison with Experimental Data in the Hen

	Man				Hen		
Compound	No. of Cases	Circumstances	Cholinergic Toxicity	References	Neuropathic Dose* (mg/kg; route)	Cholinergic Toxicity	References
Chlorpyrifos	1	Suicide	+	123	90; p.o.	+	33
Dichlorvos	3	Suicide	+	206,211	200; s.c.	+	34
Isofenphos	3	Suicide	±	35,144,203	100; p.o.	+	219
Methamidophos	>20	Suicide & occupational	+	181	130 + 50 + 50; p.o.	+	109
Mipafox	2	Occupational	+	21	25; i.m.	+	101
TOCP	Thousands	Food contamination	–	95	175; p.o.	–	101
Trichlorfon	Several	Suicide	+	205	200 + 100; p.o.	+	101
Trichlornate	2	Suicide	+	99	310; p.o.	+	101

*Single dose.

–, no cholinergic toxicity; ±, mild cholinergic toxicity; +, severe cholinergic toxicity; p.o., orally; s.c., subcutaneously; i.m., intramuscularly.

TOCP: Tri-*o*-cresylphosphate.

(102). Rodents were believed to be resistant to OPIDP until it was shown that repeated doses of TOCP caused histopathological lesions in Long-Evans rats similar to those found in hens (207). Neuropathology in rats was related to brain and spinal cord NTE inhibition above the threshold (70%–80%) and was also obtained with single doses of TOCP (161). Neuropathology was also observed in mice after TOCP treatment, although the inhibition of NTE never exceeded 68% and some small differences in lesion distribution were observed relative to those seen in treated rats (209). As in the hen, the clinical expression of OPIDP in rats is age-dependent and correlates with body weight increases (141).

Characteristics of age-related sensitivity to OPIDP have been studied in hens (102). Although NTE specific activity in nervous tissue increases and the pool of phenyl valerate esterases (*see* later under Toxic Mechanisms) changes qualitatively with age, OPs affect NTE in chicks as in the hen (142). Very high doses of OPs cause mild and reversible OPIDP in chicks 20 days of age, but animals display spastic gait and not classical flaccid paralysis suggesting selective toxicity to the spinal cord (162). Two-week-old chicks develop spinal cord lesions without clinical signs of OPIDP; at 10 weeks of age, the initial lesions occur in spinal cord and precede development of those in peripheral nerve (76). Recovery depends on age and severity of clinical manifestations, being shorter in younger and less severely affected chicks. Why chicks are resistant to, and recover from, OPIDP is unknown. No sex-related sensitivity to OPIDP has been reported.

The clinical onset of OPIDP in the hen and in several species occurs 10–15 days after single doses. The period is inversely related to the dose and the severity of resulting OPIDP; clinical onset might occur as soon as 6–7 days after high doses (1,2,172). Full expression of clinical signs is usu-

ally complete within 3–4 days. However, if animals are severely paralyzed, access to food is hampered and the clinical condition evolves for several days. Clinical OPIDP develops only if NTE inhibition higher than 70% in the nervous tissue is detected soon after dosing (106,122). Although, for

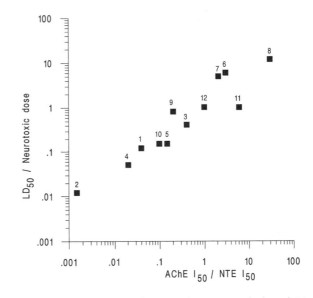

FIGURE 26. The relationship between the potency of selected OPs to cause OPIDP in hens and that to inhibit hen brain NTE *in vitro*. Since dose–effect relationships of OPs indicate that lethality and OPIDP might overlap, the neuropathic potency (neurotoxic dose and NTE I_{50}) is expressed relatively to LD_{50} *in vivo* and to AChE I_{50} *in vitro*. For compounds 1, 9, and 10, *in vitro* data were obtained with the oxon analogue. When the exact LD_{50} was not available, estimations were used. Compounds 1, 2, 3, 4, and 10 are currently used pesticides. Unless otherwise stated, data are from Lotti and Johnson (129). 1 = chlorpyrifos (33), 2 = L-(−) isomer of methamidophos (19,131), 3 = D-(+) isomer of methamidophos (19,131), 4 = dichlorvos, 5 = diethyl 2,2-dichlorovinylphosphate, 6 = di-*n*-butyl 2,2-dichlorovinyl phosphate (146), 7 = di-*n*-propyl 2,2-dichlorvinyl phosphate, 9 = leptophos, 10 = trichlornate, 11 = mipafox, 12 = DFP.

a given compound, there is a direct relationship between degree of NTE inhibition and severity of neurological compromise; this is not true if various OPs are compared (132). Certain OPs cause neuropathy with a corresponding NTE inhibition of about 70%, whereas others require much higher inhibition rates to cause mild neuropathy (Table 51).

OPIDP is characterized by flaccid paralysis of legs in hens and of posterior limbs in cats, rats, and other quadrupeds. In most severe cases, wings and anterior limbs are also affected. Mild ataxia is usually reversible within several weeks, but follow-up of most severe cases is hampered by the limited access to food of paralyzed animals. Based on studies in humans (148) and selective OPID spinal-cord lesions induced experimentally in hens (128), the development of spastic ataxia is expected if animals are kept alive long enough.

Histopathology of OPIDP has been described for several species (23,25,26,200,207). The morphological hallmark is axonal degeneration of motor and sensory fibers characterized by focal nerve varicosities and paranodal demyelination located in the distal but not terminal axons. There is no evidence of death of corresponding neurons, but varying degrees of chromatolysis occur in proportion to the severity of neuropathy. Ultrastructural studies show aggregation and accumulation of neurofilaments and neurotubules as well as proliferation of smooth endoplasmic reticulum, particularly in proximity to nodes of Ranvier (25,26,165). Lesions are distributed both in the CNS and PNS. In the CNS, although some brainstem nuclei and cerebellum are moderately affected, most lesions are found in the spinal cord. Degeneration is more prominent in the fasciculus gracilis and lateral funiculus of dorsal and ventral spinocerebellar tracts of cervical spinal cord and at lumbar levels of corticospinal tracts. In the PNS, nerve fiber vulnerability is directly related to axonal length and diameter with large-diameter and long fibers being more susceptible than small

and short ones. Lesions progress somatopetally. Minor differences in the distribution of lesions have been described for specific OP compounds (3), dosages, and species (209).

Electrophysiology of OPIDP reflects the underlying axonopathy (117). In general, nerve conduction velocities are slightly reduced, and electromyographic indices of denervation are prominent. Several experimental electrophysiological studies have been performed either during the development of or in clinically expressed OPIDP (12,173) and various parameters have been found to be affected. However, results are difficult to interpret and to compare uniformly, given the different experimental conditions (122).

Bicyclic OPs, such as certain 4-alkyl derivatives of 1-phospha-2,6-trioxabicyclo-[2.2.2] octane-1-oxide, cause seizures and death in mice within minutes of dosing. These effects are not related to AChE inhibition in brain and have been attributed to the γ-aminobutyric acid–antagonist characteristics of these OPs (17,28).

Prolonged exposure to OPs causes cholinergic toxicity if the threshold of AChE inhibition is reached. Animal studies demonstrated that prolonged exposure to OPs causes typical cholinergic patterns of behavioral and physiological changes followed by recovery toward pre-exposure values. The initial behavioral effects are related to AChE inhibition and consequently to an increase of acetylcholine (15). During the late phases of acute intoxication, and in states of subacute and chronic intoxication, behavior can return toward normal despite low enzyme activity (22). A number of mechanisms could be involved in the development of this tolerance (177), although not all OPs show a consistent pattern of cholinergic changes after repeated exposures (31,32).

All OPs currently used as pesticides have been tested in animals after prolonged exposures (up to 2 years in rodents); results on individual chemicals are regularly summarized in the JMPR monographs (66). However, the no-

TABLE 51. The Relationship between the Degree of Neuropathy Target Esterase (NTE) Inhibition caused by some OPs and the Development of OP-Induced Delayed Polyneuropathy (OPIDP) in Hens

Compound	Dose (mg/kg; route)	% NTE Inhibition in Peripheral Nerves	OPIDP
DFP	0.3; s.c.	50	–
	0.5; s.c.	70	±
	1.0; s.c.	90	+ +
Methamidophos	100; p.o.	80	–
	130 + 50 + 50; p.o.	90	±
Dichlorvos*	100; s.c.	70	–
	100; s.c.	90	+

*Two different batches.
–, no OPIDP; ±, mild OPIDP in some birds; +, OPIDP; + +, severe OPIDP; s.c. subcutaneously; p.o., orally.
DFP: Diisopropylphosphorofluoridate.
[From Caroldi and Lotti (34); Johnson et al. (109); Lotti et al. (127); and Lotti et al. (132).]

adverse-effect levels (NOAELs) have often been based on changes other than cholinesterase inhibition, that is, on body or organ weights, clinical biochemistry, or histopathology. Although statistically significant, some changes may be relevant, but others are of uncertain biological significance, such as the variation of a parameter other than erythrocyte AChE within its normal range. Moreover, the inhibition of plasma butyrylcholinesterase has no neurotoxic significance and should not be used to establish NOAELs. Rather, the measurement of brain AChE is indicated as the adverse effect to be considered (69,185).

Repeated dosing of experimental animals with certain OPs might also lead to OPIDP. Clinical, morphological, and physiological characteristics are the same as those observed after single doses. However, the delay in onset may be variable, probably depending on the time when threshold inhibition of NTE is reached. Repeated dosing with OP showed that the threshold of NTE inhibition (>70%) for OPIDP development is the same as after single doses. Repeated doses causing subthreshold NTE inhibition for several weeks do not cause tolerance to OPIDP when animals are challenged at the end of treatment with a neuropathic OP (130).

In Vitro Studies

Several studies have investigated OP toxicology *in vitro*. The biochemical mechanisms of OPs' interactions with various enzymes have been studied either on isolated enzymes or on tissue homogenates (*see*, for instance, Table 43) (9). Some of the results help in assessing the toxicological risk associated with OPs, based on the broad agreement between certain *in vitro* and *in vivo* data (Figs. 24 and 26). Several *in vitro* systems have been recently developed using cell lines of various origin (77,208), with the aim of better exploring the mechanisms of OP toxicities.

Moreover, *in vitro* studies have shown that OPs interact with acetylcholine receptors (62,63); however, it is difficult to assess the toxicological significance of such interactions because they seem to occur, in most cases, at OP concentrations that also inhibit AChE.

Human Studies

Whereas acute OP poisoning is relatively uncommon in the western world, it represents a major health problem in developing countries (14,71). The majority of cases in either area is due to suicide. In most case reports, evidence of poisoning is circumstantial; rarely has chemical analysis of the incriminated sample and/or the identification of the compound in body fluids been performed. Dose–response data are therefore seldom available. It is assumed that lethal

OP doses for humans are similar to those for animals (Table 48), but there is evidence that humans display a different sensitivity to certain OPs (19). Past studies on volunteers were aimed at assessing the maximal dose of a given OP that would not inhibit either plasma butyrylcholinesterase or erythrocyte AChE. Summaries of these results on individual OP pesticides can be traced in the JMPR monographs (66).

Clinical signs of acetylcholine excess observed in OP-intoxicated patients are ranked as follows (121,201):

Muscarinic—lacrimation, salivation, sweating, bronchorrhea, miosis, bronchoconstriction, abdominal cramp and diarrhea, bradycardia

Nicotinic—muscular weakness and fasciculation, tachycardia, hypertension

Central—anxiety, confusion, blurred vision, tremor, convulsions, respiratory depression, coma

These signs are observable in various combinations; the muscarinic ones usually appear first. The clinical picture of severe poisoning is dominated by respiratory failure due to a combination of the above effects.

The time between exposure and onset of symptoms varies with OP, route, and degree of exposure: within a few minutes after massive ingestion, or delayed for several hours with slowly absorbed OPs. EEG abnormalities can be detected at the onset of symptoms and are characterized by irregularities in rhythm, variation and increase in potential, and intermittent bursts of abnormally slow waves of elevated voltage similar to those seen in epilepsy. They usually persist for about a week when major symptoms have already disappeared (86).

Recovery from major cholinergic signs is almost complete within a few days and depends on type of inhibitor, dose, and treatment. Occasionally, symptomatology may last for several weeks owing to a slower than normal recovery of AChE, probably because of the slow elimination of inhibitors (58). The half-life of recovery of inhibited AChE in the nervous system is thought to be about 1 week, as in the experimental animal, whereas it was estimated to be about 1% a day in erythrocytes for the majority of OPs (88,155).

Histopathology of the nervous system performed at autopsy after fatal poisoning is unremarkable or nonspecific, unless severe hypoxia or convulsions occurred.

No significant neuropsychiatric sequelae were detected in a group of individuals after mild, moderate, and severe poisoning (198). However, other studies reported persistent behavioral changes as a result of acute poisoning. In one study, clinical and neuropsychological evaluation of subjects with previous acute poisoning indicated that cognitive functions were impaired when compared to a control group (179). However, the severity of past poisoning and whether some patients suffered brain hypoxia is unclear, and patients also had substantial exposure to organochlorine pesticides. In a further study, a persistent decrease in neuropsychological functions, including attention, memory, visuomotor, and motor performance was observed 1–2 years after acute poisoning (176). However, the severity of poisoning was again not stated and matched controls were subjects from the same area who were occupationally exposed to OPs but never poisoned. It might be argued that the reduced performance observed in past-poisoned subjects as compared with nonpoisoned controls was cause and not consequence of OP poisoning.

Diagnosis of OP poisoning is easy, based on history of exposure and on clinical observation of cholinergic overstimulation. For confirmatory purposes, measurement of erythrocyte AChE might be useful; however, it is of no value in assessing the course of OP poisoning because its correlation with AChE inhibition at nerve endings is not expected (121,135).

With timely and appropriate treatment, patients might survive large doses of OPs, and the reduction or disappearance of signs of cholinergic hyperstimulation can be achieved within hours. Treatment should be maintained for as long as necessary to avoid recurrence of symptoms. Therapy is both specific and symptomatic and it also involves decontamination, induction of vomiting, or gastric lavage (121). Administration of atropine (1–5 mg i.v. every 10–30 min) counteracts the muscarinic effects, whereas AChE reactivators, such as pralidoxime (2-PAM 1 g i.v. over 30 min every 8–12 h), reduce acetylcholine levels by restoring AChE activity.

The degree of atropinization, and therefore the dose of atropine, is assessed clinically and titrated against pupil size, heart rate, and dry skin. Full atropinization of the patient represents the key achievement of pharmacological treatment of OP poisoning, and very large doses of atropine may be required because patients are tolerant to its effects. Overatropinization rarely occurs, although normal oxygenation should be ensured before administering atropine because ventricular arrhythmias may develop in hypoxic patients. Moreover, it should be noted that atropine is not absolutely contraindicated in the symptomatic patient who has tachycardia (89), given the complex effects on the heart that are possibly produced by AChE inhibition at the cardiac level (16).

Oximes are drugs designed to exert a nucleophilic attack on the phosphorus of the enzyme–inhibitor complex, leading to the formation of an oxime–phosphate complex and to the restoration of AChE catalytic activity (24). However, oximes are active only when the phosphoryl–AChE complex has not undergone the aging reaction (see Fig. 18).

Therefore, it is believed that oximes may not be effective if they are administered several days after poisoning when most phosphorylated AChE may have aged. Nevertheless, in the case of poisoning by OPs (i.e., diethylphosphates) that form an inhibited AChE that reactivates relatively slowly, the administration of oximes for several days may stop the progress toward complete irreversible inhibition of AChE (108).

The optimal plasma maintenance concentration of 2-PAM is believed to be 4 mg/l.

Some clinical evidence casts some doubts on the effectiveness of pralidoxime when given in combination with atropine (50). The clinical outcome in a group of patients treated with atropine alone was similar to that in patients treated with atropine plus pralidoxime. Nevertheless, pralidoxime treatment should continue to be given to OP-intoxicated patients until more conclusive clinical evidence is available. Supportive treatment is symptomatic. Essential procedures include artificial ventilation and administration of centrally acting drugs such as diazepam, which sedates the patient and reduces convulsions. The combination of therapeutic procedures, as well as their sequence, depends on the severity of poisoning (121).

OPIDP is a rare disorder in humans, although epidemics of TOCP poisoning in the past caused thousands of cases, referred to as the Ginger-Jake paralysis (148).

Limited evidence suggests that OPIDP in humans also involves inhibition of NTE. The enzyme is found in circulating lymphocytes, thereby allowing measurement of its inhibition by OPs to mirror the effects on nervous system NTE. It was shown that inhibition of lymphocytic NTE measured soon after poisoning heralds the development of OPIDP in humans (120,122,133).

Several OPs have been associated with human OPIDP, after single or short-term exposures, although convincing clinical evidence supported by experimental data is available only for a few. Table 50 lists OPs for which there is sufficient evidence they caused OPIDP in humans; comparison with experimental data for the hen shows that the relationship between cholinergic toxicity and OPIDP is consistent across the two species. Chlorpyrifos seems to be an exception because several human cases of mostly motor neuropathy compatible with OPIDP were consistently observed after repeated exposures that caused either mild or no cholinergic manifestations (112). However, in contrast, a case of very mild sensory-motor neuropathy is reported in Table 50 occurring after a massive dose of chlorpyrifos causing severe cholinergic toxicity; this agrees with experimental data in hens. Moreover, in a series of patients severely poisoned with several different OPs, the sensory component of OPIDP, when it occurred, was never an isolated finding and, if present, was mild when compared to the motor deficit (144).

Ethyl 4-nitrophenyl phenylphosphonothionate (EPN) and leptophos are NTE inhibitors that cause OPIDP in hens (101) and probably in humans. An anecdotal report of OPIDP involved workers who had long-term occupational exposure to EPN and were also exposed during the release of EPN and other chemicals from an explosion and fire in an EPN-manufacturing facility (222). An outbreak of neurological disorders occurred in a plant manufacturing leptophos. Three subjects had signs compatible with OPIDP at medical examination and 6 on a retrospective study. Several subjects, however, had neurological signs unrelated to OPIDP; all were exposed to a variety of chemicals with neurotoxic potential, including n-hexane (223).

Although they are not NTE inhibitors and are always negative in the hen test, the pesticides omethoate, parathion, and mecarbam have been associated with OPIDP in man (68,102,122); however, toxicological evidence of the causative agents was lacking. Polyneuropathy compatible with OPIDP developed after a suicidal attempt with omethoate (44). However, in a subsequent report of a man who died of acute omethoate poisoning, no NTE inhibition was detected in postmortem nervous tissues (122). Parathion was associated with OPIDP after massive parathion and methanol poisoning (47). However, several cases of parathion poisoning have occurred and none resulted in OPIDP. Mecarbam was reported to cause OPIDP in humans, but nerve biopsy revealed segmental demyelination, which is not expected in OPIDP (189). It should be pointed out that neuropathic impurities may be present in commercial formulations, perhaps accounting for these discrepancies [e.g., ethyl bis-(4-nitrophenyl)phosphate, detected in parathion samples and found to inhibit NTE (105)].

Children are resistant to OPIDP (84) and, when affected, recover within a few months (180).

Symptoms of OPIDP begin 1–4 weeks after single doses when, as in the cases of pesticides, cholinergic symptoms have subsided (125). Cramping muscle pain in the legs is the usual initial complaint, followed by distal numbness and paresthesias. Progressive leg weakness occurs, together with depression of tendon reflexes. Symptoms may also appear in the arms and forearms. Sensory loss is often mild. Physical examination reveals distal symmetrical predominantly motor polyneuropathy, with wasting and flaccid weakness of distal limb muscles, especially in the legs. In severe OPIDP, quadriplegia with foot- and wristdrop are observed, as well as mild pyramidal signs. In time, there may be some functional recovery, but pyramidal and other signs of central neurological involvement may become more evident. The degree of pyramidal involvement determines the prognosis for functional recovery, and spastic ataxia may represent a permanent outcome of severe OPIDP (148). Objective evidence of sensory loss is usually slight or absent, although in the above-mentioned chlorpyrifos series of patients it was predominant.

Postmortem morphological studies performed after the Ginger-Jake episode described wallerian degeneration of peripheral nerve and CNS involvement, including changes in the fasciculus gracilis at the cervical level and in the corticospinal tracts at lumbar levels (11). Sural nerve biopsies, rarely performed in OPIDP, confirm a picture of axonal degeneration (99,133).

Electrophysiological evaluation reveals denervation of affected muscles with increased insertional activity, abnormal spontaneous activity (fibrillation potentials and positive sharp waves), and a reduced interference pattern; large polyphasic motor unit potentials may also be found after a few weeks. The compound muscle action potentials to supramaximal stimulation of motor nerves are reduced in amplitude, and terminal motor latencies are delayed; maximal motor conduction velocity is usually normal or slightly reduced (125).

Differential diagnosis is easy because in most patients there is evidence of a recent episode of cholinergic toxicity. In cases of OPIDP caused by nonanticholinesterase OPs, etiological diagnosis may be difficult and is mainly based on the evidence of exposure. There is no specific treatment for OPIDP.

Another form of OP toxicity, the intermediate syndrome, distinct from the cholinergic and delayed effects, has been described (182). Several cases have also been reported from retrospective analysis of previous reports. This toxicity is observed after exposures to several OPs including dimethoate, fenthion, methamidophos, monocrotophos (182), diazinon (210), parathion, methylparathion (48), demeton S-methyl sulfone (20), trichlorfon (113), and phosmet (85). Patients display paralysis of proximal limb muscles, neck flexors, motor cranial nerves, and respiratory muscles developing after the cholinergic phase. The onset is usually 1–4 days (182) after exposure, though it might be delayed up to 15 days (154), and severe symptoms usually last up to a week. Complete recovery occurs within 2 weeks (182), though a delay up to 30 days has been reported (85).

The syndrome is not a relapse of cholinergic toxicity, although on some occasions the two phenomena might be associated (46) and it is not responsive to atropine treatment. The development of the syndrome does not seem to depend on the OP involved nor on the initial severity of symptoms. Prolonged cholinergic overstimulation was observed in a series of patients who developed intermediate syndrome, although the significance of this association is unclear (46). Muscle necrosis was also ruled out.

Electrophysiological studies indicate that dysfunction at the neuromuscular junction is postsynaptic (20,85,182) and related to end-plate degeneration (85); as discussed before, this junctional myopathy has been shown to occur in the muscles of experimental animals subjected to OP-induced fasciculation (202). It remains to be explained why the intermediate syndrome develops in some patients only (estimates indicate in about 20% of acute OP poisonings), why clinical effects are evident on certain nicotinic junctions only, and why the delay in onset is variable. Treatment is symptomatic and artificial ventilation is life-saving. Caution was suggested in using 2-PAM because, in patients with postsynaptic dysfunction, reactivation of AChE and the subsequent decrease of acetylcholine might increase neuromuscular block and weakness. This was observed in a patient with postsynaptic block after OP exposure, when infusion of 2-PAM precipitated ventilatory weakness and required artificial ventilation (85).

Cholinergic effects caused by prolonged exposure to OPs are similar to those observed after short exposures. To prevent cholinergic toxicity after repeated occupational exposures to OPs, biological monitoring procedures have been developed based on measurement of AChE in red blood cells. Although interpretation of erythrocyte AChE inhibition after occupational exposure is complex (88,124), some practical indications are available (Table 52).

Over the years, the question has repeatedly arisen as to whether chronic exposures to OPs cause neuropsychiatric, behavioral, and electrophysiological changes without overt cholinergic toxicity, whether or not related to AChE inhibition. Behavioral effects of OP poisoning have been reviewed (119). Various parameters have not been found impaired during subacute low-level exposure (134) or in chronic exposures with normal blood cholinesterases (175). Schizophrenic and depressive reactions with severe memory impairment and difficulties in concentration were reported in workers exposed to OPs (82), but no evidence of exposure was given. Mental alertness was not impaired in an-

other study where the exposure was small enough not to produce clinical signs of cholinergic hyperstimulation (57). In a further study on volunteers, altered awareness correlated with substantial inhibition of whole-blood cholinesterase (27). A recent cross-sectional study assessed the neurophysiological performance of sheep-dip farmers (191, 192). Farmers performed significantly poorer than controls in tests to assess sustained attention and speed of information processing. However, the somewhat biased selection of workers, the retrospective assessment of exposure, and the dose–response relationship found only for one test, raise questions about the significance of the findings. In conclusion, there is no evidence that behavioral deficits occur in workers with asymptomatic exposures and in the absence of AChE inhibition.

EEG changes derived from a complex analysis of spectra have been reported in industrial workers who had repeated accidental exposures to sarin (56). Exposures caused symptoms and significant inhibition of erythrocyte AChE, but it is unclear if severe poisonings occurred. Changes, detected for up to 1 year after exposure, included increased beta activity, increased delta and theta slowing, decreased alpha activity, and increased amounts of rapid-eye-movement sleep. However, the significance of this computerized analysis of brainwave topography is undetermined (10). Similarly, minimal EEG disturbances were observed in another study, but exposure data were lacking and workers were also exposed to organochlorine pesticides (137). It is also unclear whether such persistent EEG changes were accompanied by changes in psychological or behavioral parameters. In another study that claimed a correlation between neuropsychological tests and EEG changes, data for the alleged exposure to OPs and the organochlorine pesticide dieldrin were unavailable, and EEG changes were different from those previously reported. Moreover, EEG data surprisingly indicated "selective" effects on the left frontal hemisphere (115).

It is concluded that toxic effects of repeated and prolonged exposures to OPs are the same as those after single or short exposures, and no toxicity is evident in the absence

TABLE 52. Biomonitoring of Occupational Exposures to Cholinesterase Inhibitors

RBC AChE (% Inhibition)*	Significance	Action
20–30	Evidence of exposure	Check hygienic conditions
30–50	Hazard	As above plus remove from exposure
50–60	Poisoning	As above plus hospitalization

*Calculated on pre-exposure values.
RBC, red blood cell. AChE: Acetylcholinesterase.
[From WHO (214).]

of cholinesterase inhibition (123). Moreover, little confidence is placed in existing descriptions of the behavioral effects of anticholinesterases in humans (53).

Given the anticholinesterase characteristics of OP pesticides, it is unlikely that long-term exposures cause delayed polyneuropathy without preceding cholinergic toxicity. However, minimal electrophysiological changes have been noted in peripheral nerves of workers reportedly exposed to a variety of OPs (98,171,193). Nevertheless, in other studies where exposure was better characterized, no changes were found (111,126). It has been suggested that exposures to the few OPs devoid of cholinergic toxicity could be monitored in exposed workers by measuring NTE activity in circulating lymphocytes (120,122). However, given the very rare exposures to OPs with little or no cholinergic toxicity, the difficulties of measuring lymphocytic NTE and the complexity of interpreting its inhibition, this test has limited practical value.

No reports are available of the intermediate syndrome after prolonged exposure to OPs. However, a single case report of postsynaptic block of muscarinic transmission after repeated exposure to OP suggests that the syndrome might also occur in particular circumstances of exposure (85).

Toxic Mechanisms

The molecular mechanism of cholinergic toxicity involves the interaction of OPs with AChE (75,201). AChE, an elongated molecular structure formed by heterologous subunits, is localized in the outer basal lamina of the synapse. A single gene encodes the catalytic subunits of AChE. The three-dimensional structure of AChE has been determined (196), and knowledge of interactions between AChE and OPs at the molecular level will probably be revised in light of this information. Figure 27 illustrates the interaction of the enzyme with its substrate acetylcholine and compares these to those with an inhibitor. Both substrate and inhibitor react covalently with the enzyme in essentially the same manner because acetylation of the serine residue in the active center of AChE is analogous to phosphorylation. However, in contrast with the acetylated enzyme, which rapidly gives acetic acid and restores the catalytic center, the phosphorylated enzyme is stable. Spontaneous reactivation of enzyme may require several hours (dimethoxy) or does not occur at all (secondary, such as DFP, or tertiary alkyl groups). The loss of one alkyl group, occurring through the nonenzymatic process of aging, further enhances the stability of the phosphorylated enzyme.

AChE's crystal structure reveals that the anionic moiety of AChE, thought to attract the quaternary nitrogen of the

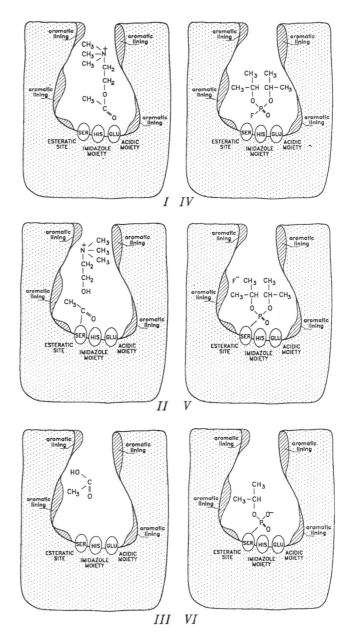

FIGURE 27. Schematic representation of interactions of the substrate acetylcholine (I–III) and the inhibitor diisopropylphosphofluoridate (DFP) (IV–VI) with the acetylcholinesterase active center. The atomic structure of acetylcholinesterase (AChE) was determined by x-ray analysis (196). The active site contains a Ser-His-Glu catalytic triad which lies near the bottom of a deep and narrow gorge that reaches halfway into the protein. Acetylcholine is drawn to the active site of the enzyme by an "aromatic guidance mechanism" of the positive charge on the nitrogen atom. Some of the 14 aromatic residues that line about 40% of the gorge interact with the quaternary nitrogen, providing an array of low-affinity binding sites. (I). The formation of an acetylenzyme on the serine residue also involves the imidazol and acidic moieties (II). Within milliseconds the acetylenzyme is hydrolyzed, resulting in the free enzyme and acetate (III). Phosphorylation of the active site by DFP is analogous to acetylation (IV, V). In contrast to acetylated enzyme, phosphorylated AChE is stable and when the aging reaction occurs, the enzyme is irreversibly inhibited (VI).

substrate, is misnamed because it contains at most one negative charge. It has been proposed instead that the quaternary moiety of acetylcholine binds chiefly through interactions with the aromatic residues that line the walls and floor of the gorge (Fig. 27). This aromatic lining will possibly explain further some of the biochemical characteristics of OP–AChE interactions.

When blocked by the phosphoryl residue, the serine group of the catalytic center is no longer able to participate in the hydrolysis of acetylcholine. Thus, the neurotransmitter accumulates, its action is enhanced and, given the widespread distribution of cholinergic neurotransmission, toxic effects of OPs will involve parasympathetic, sympathetic, and somatic motor components of the PNS, and also the CNS. The degree of increase of acetylcholine in brain tissue and the time course of accumulation may vary regionally (190).

The interaction of acetylcholine with either muscarinic or nicotinic receptors leads to various biochemical effects on second-messenger systems (41) and eventually to the toxic response.

Single doses of OPs do not affect brain muscarinic receptors (187), whereas repeated exposures may reduce both their density and affinity for specific ligands (61). Reduction in muscarinic receptors shows regional specificity (40), reflecting either differences in duration or intensity of cholinergic stimulation, or a selective access of the inhibitor. Reductions of high-affinity brain nicotine-binding sites have also been found after chronic cholinergic stimulation (43). Symptoms of excessive cholinergic stimulation are gradually reduced during chronic OP exposure, despite significant inhibition of AChE; the development of this tolerance has been in part associated with down-regulation of muscarinic receptors caused by prolonged AChE inhibition and acetylcholine stimulation (177).

AChE inhibitors have been shown to be able to interact directly with both nicotinic and muscarinic acetylcholine receptors (62,63,184). However, the toxicological significance of this direct interaction with receptors is unclear, as well as the possible additional action of AChE inhibitors as direct agonist and/or antagonists, although the postsynaptic effects of OPs, known as intermediate syndrome, may possibly be explained by this mechanism. It will also be significant if such interactions occur, at least for some OPs, at doses that would not inhibit AChE.

Other components of the cholinergic system are not directly affected by AChE inhibition. Choline acetyltransferase levels do not change after lethal doses of several OPs (186) and variable effects on choline levels have been reported (73). Given the interactions of the cholinergic system with other neurotransmitter systems, several noncholinergic biochemical effects have been associated with AChE inhibition (70,187).

The primary molecular event in OPIDP pathogenesis is thought to be the phosphorylation of NTE in the nervous system. Solubilization and purification of NTE have only recently been achieved. Biotinylated covalent inhibitors of proteases and esterases have been synthesized, among which is a potent inhibitor of NTE. A 155-kDa polypeptide was detected in brain microsomes by specific labeling with this inhibitor. Biotinylated NTE in labeled microsomes was then adsorbed on avidin-Sepharose and the subsequent elution yielded a fraction enriched in NTE. Essentially pure NTE was then obtained after separation from other biotinylated polypeptides (83).

The physiological function(s) of the protein NTE, which carries an esteratic site, as well as the chain of events that follow OP–NTE interactions, are unknown. Nevertheless, since the discovery of NTE, the 20-year-long mechanistic research on OPIDP has provided information that is summarized in several reviews (3,102,104,106,120,122, 125,214). Most of these results will be verified and expanded because purification of NTE only recently has been achieved.

NTE esteratic activity was identified by means of combined radiolabeled binding and enzymatic studies (102). After either *in vitro* or *in vivo* exposures of hen brain to radiolabeled DFP, some covalent binding sites were detected. About 80% of these sites, however, were affected by OPs that do not cause OPIDP. Moreover, 20% of the remaining binding sites were found to be affected by OPs causing OPIDP (~4% of total). These sites corresponded to an esteratic activity when several substrates were tested. Thus, NTE was defined, among nervous tissue esterases hydrolyzing the artificial substrate phenyl valerate, as the enzyme that is resistant to paraoxon (nonneuropathic inhibitor) and sensitive to mipafox (neuropathic inhibitor) (102–104).

NTE inhibition higher than 70% by neuropathic OPs, measured soon after dosing in hen brain, correlates with the appearance of OPIDP 2 weeks later. However, not all NTE inhibitors cause OPIDP, despite a relatively high inhibition of NTE. The chemical structure of NTE inhibitors is reported in Figure 17. It was believed that phosphates, phosphonates, and phosphoroamidates, if affecting more than 70% NTE, cause OPIDP because the inhibited NTE would undergo the aging reaction (*see* Fig. 18). Other NTE inhibitors such as carbamates, sulfonates, and phosphinates, cannot form, on chemical grounds, an aged inhibited NTE and therefore will not cause OPIDP. Strong support for this explanation derived from experiments showing that if sufficient non–aged inhibited NTE is formed in animals treated with OPs unable to produce neuropathy, then ani-

TABLE 53. Protection from and Promotion of OPIDP in Hens According to the Sequence of Dosing with Two NTE Inhibitors*

Treatment[†] (mg/kg; Route)		% NTE Inhibition[‡] X + SD (n)		Clinical Effect[§]
First	Second	After First Treatment	After Second Treatment	Median (Range) (n)
DFP (0.3; s.c.)	Vehicle	75 + 6(3)		1(1−1)(3)
PMSF (120; s.c.)	Vehicle	93 + 1(4)		0(0−0)(10)
PMSF (120; s.c.)	DFP (0.3; s.c.)		>93	0(0−0)(3)
DFP (0.3; s.c.)	PMSF (120; s.c.)		>93	8(4−8)(3)
DBDCVP (0.45; s.c.)	Vehicle	90 + 1(3)		3(1−6)(16)
Methamidophos (50; p.o.)	Vehicle	50		0(0−0)(3)
Methamidophos (50; p.o.)	DBDCVP (0.45; s.c.)		88	0(0−0)(4)
DBDCVP (0.45; s.c.)	Methamidophos (50; p.o.)		92	6(6−7)(5)

*Phenylmethanesulfonyl fluoride (PMSF) and methamidophos either protect from or potentiate diisopropylphosphofluoridate (DFP) and di-*n*-butyldichlorovinyl phosphate (DBDCVP) neuropathies depending on the sequence of dosing (132,139).

[†]First and second treatment given 24 h apart.

[‡]In brain and calculated from concurrent controls.

[§]Peak scores were assessed 14−20 days after treatment; severity was evaluated on a 0−8 point scale.

s.c., subcutaneously; p.o., orally.

OPIDP, organophosphate-induced delayed polyneuropathy.

NTE, Neuropathy target esterase.

mals are protected from a subsequent challenging dose of one that induces OPIDP (102,104,106). Therefore, it is difficult to maintain that NTE catalytic activity is essential for normal neuronal and axonal function, given the substantial inhibition of NTE observed in the absence of neuropathy after dosing with phosphinates, sulfonates, or carbamates. Mechanistic studies performed so far have exploited this enzymatic assay to assess quantitatively and qualitatively (by measuring the aging reaction) the effects of OPs on NTE, knowing however that the loss of esteratic activity is a surrogate to measure a still unknown effect (probably on the protein NTE itself) of neurotoxic OPs.

The relationship between the degree of NTE inhibition and the severity of clinical OPIDP varies among inhibitors (132). Examples of such differences are shown in Table 48. Moreover, protective NTE inhibitors are also found to cause neuropathy, though very mild and at extremely high doses causing almost complete NTE inhibition. These results challenge the idea that aging of inhibited NTE is absolutely necessary to trigger neuropathy. This conclusion is reinforced by findings that phosphoroamidates (including the classical OP neurotoxicant mipafox) also form an inhibited NTE that can be reactivated by electrophiles, suggesting that aging has not occurred (109,138). Therefore, the pathophysiological significance of OP-NTE interactions is unknown, aging of phosphorylated NTE is not essential for OPIDP development, and the severity of OPIDP seems to depend on the chemical structure attached to the NTE catalytic center (132).

The same chemicals that protect from OPIDP when given prior to a neuropathic OP may potentiate the neuropathy if given afterwards (127,164). The effect of potentiation is called promotion of OPIDP. The paradox of protection/promotion, in that opposite effects are produced with the same chemicals by varying only the sequence of dosing, is shown in Table 53. Both phenylmethanesulfonyl fluoride (PMSF) and methamidophos cause mild neuropathy when given at very high doses, causing more than 96% and 85% NTE inhibition, respectively (131,132). When they are given at lower doses, causing 40%−50% NTE inhibition, prior to neuropathy-inducing (neurotoxic) doses of another OP, they protect from OPIDP. However, when given at the same doses after neurotoxic OPs, they exaggerate OPIDP. These opposite outcomes are explained by considering that protection from and promotion of OPIDP are due to effects on distinct targets, NTE and an unknown target(s), respectively. It has been shown that promotion might occur without affecting NTE when a promoter is given before neurotoxic OPs, suggesting that the promotion site is other than NTE (140). When promoters affect NTE before dosing with a neurotoxic OP, they protect from OPIDP initiation and their effect on the promotion site is irrelevant. Conversely, when promoters are given afterwards, OPIDP is initiated and their effect on the promotion site exaggerates the clinical response.

Other axonopathies, including toxic (2,5-hexanedione) (139) and nontoxic neuropathies (nerve crush) (143) are potentiated by either pre- or postdosing with PMSF. Given the variety of promotable axonopathies, it seems that the effect of PMSF and methamidophos, and also of carbamates and phosphinates (107,127), is unspecific. Moreover, since promotion also occurs if the promoter is given several days before the neuropathic insult, it is concluded that promotion affects a target that is present in healthy axons, leading animals to commit themselves to an exaggerated response if and when a neurotoxic insult follows. Perhaps these results might be explained by an impairment of a repair mechanism(s) that maintains axonal homeostasis, although repeated dosing with a promoter did not cause neuropathy in the absence of a neuropathic insult (110).

Little is known about the cascade of biochemical and physiological events following NTE inhibition and preceding the clinical and morphological expression of OPIDP. Retrograde axonal transport is selectively affected very early (145), leading to an accumulation of NTE in distal parts of affected axons (122). However, the relationship between effects on NTE, reduction of axonal transport, accumulation of NTE, and clinical expression of OPIDP, is unknown.

Based on morphological evidence of axonal swelling, the hypothesis was advanced that OPIDP may be initiated by abnormal phosphorylation of cytoskeletal proteins (3,4). In TOCP-treated animals, increased protein kinase–mediated phosphorylation correlated with OPIDP. Moreover, a calcium-calmodulin–dependent increase in the *in vitro* phosphorylation of brain microtubules and spinal cord neurofilament protein was observed. Enhanced calmodulin binding and kinase-dependent phosphorylation of cytoskeletal proteins were also observed after DFP (5). However, it is not clear whether these effects represent the primary biochemical lesion in OPIDP or a secondary response, associated or not with OPIDP pathogenesis (122).

REFERENCES

1. Abou-Donia MB, Graham DG (1979) Delayed neurotoxicity of *O*-ethyl *O*-4-nitrophenyl phenylphosphonothioate: Toxic effects of a single oral dose on the nervous system of hens. *Toxicol Appl Pharmacol* 48, 57.

2. Abou-Donia MB, Graham DG, Timmons PR, Reichert BL (1979) Delayed neurotoxic and late acute effects of *S,S,S*-tributyl phosphorotrithioate in the hen: Effect of route of administration. *Neurotoxicology* 1, 425.

3. Abou-Donia MB, Lapadula DM (1990) Mechanisms of organophosphorus ester-induced delayed neurotoxicity: Type I and type II. *Annu Rev Pharmacol Toxicol* 30,405.

4. Abou-Donia MB, Lapadula DM, Suwita E (1988) Cytoskeletal proteins as targets for organophosphorus compound and aliphatic hexacarbon-induced neurotoxicity. *Toxicology* 49, 469.

5. Abou-Donia MB, Viana ME, Gupta RP, Anderson JK (1993) Enhanced calmodulin binding concurrent with increased kinase-dependent phosphorylation of cytoskeletal proteins following a single subcutaneous injection of diisopropyl phophorofluoridate in hens. *Neurochem Int* 22, 165.

6. ACGIH (1993) *1993–1994 Threshold Limit Values for Chemical Substances and Physical Agents and Biological Exposure Indices*. American Conference of Governmental Industrial Hygienists (ACGIH) Cincinnati, Ohio.

7. Aldridge WN (1989) Cholinesterase and esterase inhibitors and reactivation of organophosphorus inhibited esterases. In: *Design of Enzyme Inhibitors and Drugs*. Sandler M, Smith HJ eds. Oxford University Press, Oxford p. 294.

8. Aldridge WN, Miles JW, Mount DR, Verschoyle RD (1979) The toxicological properties of impurities in malathion. *Arch Toxicol* 42, 95.

9. Aldridge WN, Reiner E (1972) *Enzyme Inhibitors as Substrates*. North-Holland Publ Co, Amsterdam.

10. American Electroencephalographic Society (1987) Statement on the clinical use of quantitative EEG. *J Clin Neurophysiol* 4, 75.

11. Aring CD (1942) The systemic nervous affinity of triorthocresyl phosphate (Jamaican ginger palsy). *Brain* 65, 34.

12. Baker T, Lowndes HE (1980) Muscle spindle function in organophosphorus neuropathy. *Brain Res* 185, 77.

13. Baker EL, Zack M, Miles JW *et al.* (1978) Epidemic malathion poisoning in Pakistan malaria workers. *Lancet* i, 31.

14. Ballantyne B, Marrs TC (1992) *Clinical & Experimental Toxicology of Organophosphates and Carbamates*. Butterworth-Heinemann, Oxford.

15. Banks A, Russel RW (1967) Effects of chronic reductions in acetylcholinesterase activity on serial problem solving behavior. *J Comp Physiol Psychol* 64, 262.

16. Baskin SI, Whitmer MP (1992) Cardiac effects of anticholinesterase agents. In: *Clinical & Experimental Toxicology of Organophosphates and Carbamates*. Ballantyne B, Marrs TC eds. Butterworth-Heinemann, Oxford p. 135.

17. Bellet EM, Casida JE (1973) Bicyclic phosphorus esters: High toxicity without cholinesterase inhibition. *Science* 182, 1135.

18. Benke GM, Murphy SD (1975) The influence of age on the toxicity and metabolism of methylparathion and parathion in male and female rats. *Toxicol Appl Pharmacol* 31, 254.

19. Bertolazzi M, Caroldi S, Moretto A, Lotti M (1991) Interaction of methamidophos with hen and human acetylcholinesterase and neuropathy target esterase. *Arch Toxicol* 65, 580.

20. Besser R, Gutmann L, Dillmann U *et al.* (1989) End-plate dysfunction in acute organophosphate intoxication. *Neurology* 39, 561.

21. Bidstrup PL, Bonnel JA, Beckett AG (1953) Paralysis following poisoning by a new organic phosphorus insecticide (mipafox). *Brit Med J* 1, 1068.

22. Bignami G, Rosic N, Michalek H *et al.* (1975) Behavioral toxicity of anticholinesterase agents: Methodological,

neurochemical and neuropsychological aspects. In: *Behavioural Toxicology*. Weiss B, Laties VG eds. Plenum Press, London p. 155.

23. Bischoff A (1970) Ultrastructure of tri-ortho-cresyl phosphate poisoning in the chicken. II. Studies on spinal cord alterations. *Acta Neuropathol* 15, 142.

24. Bismuth C, Inns RH, Marrs TC (1992) Efficacy, toxicity and clinical use of oximes in anticholinesterase poisoning. In: *Clinical & Experimental Toxicology of Organophosphates and Carbamates*. Ballantyne B, Marrs TC eds. Butterworth-Heinemann, Oxford p. 555.

25. Bouldin TW, Cavanagh JB (1979) Organophosphorus neuropathy. I. A teased-fiber study of the spatio-temporal spread of axonal degeneration. *Amer J Pathol* 94, 241.

26. Bouldin TW, Cavanagh JB (1979) Organophosphorous neuropathy. II. A fine-structural study of the early stages of axonal degeneration. *Amer J Pathol* 94, 253.

27. Bowers MB Jr, Goodman E, Sim VM (1964) Some behavioral changes in man following anticholinesterase administration. *J Nerv Ment Dis* 138, 383.

28. Bowery NG, Collins JF, Hill RG (1976) Bicyclic phosphorus esters that are potent convulsants and GABA antagonists. *Nature* 261, 601.

29. Boyes WK, Tandon P, Barone S Jr, Padilla S (1994) Effects of organophosphates on the visual system of rats. *J Appl Toxicol* 14, 135.

30. Bradway DE, Shafik TM, Lores EM (1977) Comparison of cholinesterase activity, residue levels and urinary metabolite excretion of rats exposed to organophosphorus pesticides. *J Agr Food Chem* 25, 1353.

31. Bushnell PJ, Padilla SS, Ward T et al. (1991) Behavioural and neurochemical changes in rats dosed repeatedly with diisopropylfluorophosphate. *J Pharmacol Exp Ther* 256, 741.

32. Bushnell PJ, Pope CN, Padilla S (1993) Behavioral and neurochemical effects of acute chlorpyrifos in rats: Tolerance to prolonged inhibition of cholinesterase. *J Pharmacol Exp Ther* 266, 1007.

33. Capodicasa E, Scapellato ML, Moretto A et al. (1991) Chlorpyrifos-induced delayed polyneuropathy. *Arch Toxicol* 65, 150.

34. Caroldi S, Lotti M (1981) Delayed neurotoxicity caused by a single massive dose of dichlorvos to adult hens. *Toxicol Lett* 9, 157.

35. Catz A, Chen B, Jutrin I, Mendelson L (1988) Late onset isofenphos neurotoxicity. *J Neurol Neurosurg Psychiat* 51, 1338.

36. Chambers HW (1992) Organophosphorus compounds: An overview. In: *Organophosphates. Chemistry, Fate, and Effects*. Chambers JE, Levi PE eds. Academic Press, San Diego p. 3.

37. Chambers JE (1992) The role of target-site activation of phosphorothionates in acute toxicity. In: *Organophosphates. Chemistry, Fate, and Effects*. Chambers JE, Levi PE eds. Academic Press, San Diego p. 229.

38. Chambers JE, Levi PE (1992) *Organophosphates. Chemistry, Fate, and Effects*. Academic Press, San Diego.

39. Chan PC, Huff J, Haseman JK et al. (1991) Carcinogenesis studies of dichlorvos in Fischer rats and B6C3F1 mice. *Jpn J Cancer Res* 82, 157.

40. Churchill L, Pazdernik TL, Jackson JL et al. (1984) Topographical distribution of decrements and recovery in muscarinic receptors from rat brains repeatedly exposed to sublethal doses of Soman. *J Neurosci* 4, 2069.

41. Costa LG (1992) Role of second-messenger systems in response to organophosphorus compounds. In: *Organophosphates. Chemistry, Fate, and Effects*. Chambers JE, Levi PE eds. Academic Press, San Diego p. 271.

42. Costa LG, McDonald BE, Murphy SD et al. (1990) Serum paraoxonase and its influence on paraoxon and chlorpyrifos-oxon toxicity in rats. *Toxicol Appl Pharmacol* 103, 66.

43. Costa LG, Murphy SD (1983) [^{3}H]Nicotinic binding in rat brain: Alteration after chronic acetylcholinesterase inhibition. *J Pharmacol Exp Ther* 226, 392.

44. Curtes JP, Develay P, Hubert JP (1981) Late peripheral neuropathy due to an acute voluntary intoxication by organophosphorus compounds. *Clin Toxicol* 18, 1453.

45. De Bisschop HC, Mainil JG, Willems JL (1985) *In vitro* degradation of the four isomers of soman in human serum. *Biochem Pharmacol* 34, 1895.

46. De Bleecker J, Van den Neucker K, Colardyn F (1993) Intermediate syndrome in organophosphorus poisoning: A prospective study. *Crit Care Med* 21, 1706.

47. de Jager AEJ, van Weerden TW, Houthoff HJ, de Monchy JGR (1981) Polyneuropathy after massive exposure to parathion. *Neurology* 31, 603.

48. de Jong LPA, Benschop HP (1988) Biochemical and toxicological implications of chirality in anticholinesterase organophosphates. In: *Stereoselectivity of Pesticides. Biological and Chemical Problems*. Ariens EJ, van Rensen JJS, Welling W eds. Elsevier, Amsterdam p. 109.

49. Deschamps D, Questel F, Baud FJ et al. (1994) Persistent asthma after acute inhalation of organophosphate insecticide. *Lancet* 344, 1712.

50. De Silva HJ, Wijewickrema R, Senanayake N (1992) Does pralidoxime affect outcome of management in acute organophosphorus poisoning? *Lancet* 339, 1136.

51. Dettbarn WD (1992) Anticholinesterase-induced myonecrosis. In: *Clinical & Experimental Toxicology of Organophosphates and Carbamates*. Ballantyne B, Marrs TC eds. Butterworth-Heinemann, Oxford p. 167.

52. Dinsale D (1992) Pulmonary toxicity of anticholinesterases. In: *Clinical & Experimental Toxicology of Organophosphates and Carbamates*. Ballantyne B, Marrs TC eds. Butterworth-Heinemann, Oxford p. 156.

53. D'Mello GD (1993) Behavioural toxicity of anticholinesterases in humans and animals—a review. *Hum Exp Toxicol* 12, 3.

54. Drevenkar V, Radic Z, Vasilic Z, Reiner E (1991) Dial-

kylphosphorus metabolites in the urine and activities of esterases in the serum as biochemical indicies for human absorption of organophosphorus pesticides. *Arch Environ Contam Toxicol* **20**, 417.

55. DuBois KP (1963) Toxicological evaluation of the anti-cholinesterase agents. In: *Handbuch der Experimentellen Pharmakologie, Cholinesterases and Anticholinesterase Agents.* Koelle GB sub-ed. Springer Verlag, Berlin p. 833.

56. Duffy FH, Burchfiel JL, Bartles PH *et al.* (1979) Long term effects of an organophosphate upon the human electroencephalogram. *Toxicol Appl Pharmacol* **47**, 161.

57. Durham WF, Wolfe HR, Quinby GE (1965) Organophosphorus insecticides and mental alertness. Studies in exposed workers and in poisoning cases. *Arch Environ Health* **10**, 55.

58. Ecobichon DJ (1991) Toxic effects of pesticides. In: *Casarett & Doull's Toxicology. The Basic Science of Poisons.* 4th Ed. Amdur MO, Doull J, Klaassen CD ed. Pergamon Press, New York p. 565.

59. Ecobichon DJ, Ozere RL, Reid E, Crocker JFS (1977) Acute fenitrothion poisoning. *Can Med Assn J* **116**, 377.

60. Edmundson RS (1988) *Dictionary of Organophosphorus Compounds.* Chapman and Hall, London.

61. Ehlert FJ, Kokka N, Fairhurst AS (1980) Altered [³H]quinuclidinyl benzilate binding in the striatum of rats following chronic cholinesterase inhibition by diisopropylfluorophosphate. *Mol Pharmacol* **17**, 24.

62. Eldefrawi AT, Jett D, Eldefrawi ME (1992) Direct actions of organophosphorus anticholinesterases on muscarinic receptors. In: *Organophosphates. Chemistry, Fate, and Effects.* Chambers JE, Levi PE eds. Academic Press, San Diego p. 257.

63. Eldefrawi A, Manssour NA, Eldefrawi ME (1982) Insecticides affecting acetylcholine receptor interactions. *Pharmacol Ther* **16**, 45.

64. Eto M (1974) *Organophosphorus Pesticides: Organic and Biological Chemistry.* CRC Press, Boca Raton, Florida.

65. FAO (1990) *International Code of Conduct on the Distribution and Use of Pesticides.* Food and Agriculture Organization of the United Nations, Rome.

66. FAO/WHO (1962–1995) *Monographs on Pesticide Residues in Food.* Food and Agriculture Organization of the United Nations, Rome.

67. FAO/WHO (1983) *Joint Meeting on Pesticide Residues in Food: 1982 Evaluations.* Food and Agriculture Organization of the United Nations, Rome.

68. FAO/WHO (1987) *Joint Meeting of Pesticide Residues in Food. 1986.* Food and Agriculture Organization of the United Nations, Rome.

69. FAO/WHO (1988) *Joint Meeting on Pesticide Residues in Food. 1987 Evaluations.* Food and Agriculture Organization of the United Nations, Rome.

70. Fernando JCR, Hoskins BH, Ho IK (1984) A striatal serotonergic involvement in the behavioural effects of anticholinesterase organophosphates. *Eur J Pharmacol* **98**, 129.

71. Fernando R (1989) *Pesticides in Sri Lanka.* Friedrich-Ebert-Stiftung, Colombo.

72. Firemark H, Barlow CF, Roth LJ (1964) The penetration of 2-PAM C¹⁴ into brain and the effect of cholinesterase inhibitors on its transport. *J Pharmacol Exp Ther* **145**, 252.

73. Flynn CJ, Wecker L (1986) Elevated choline levels in brain. A non-cholinergic component of organophosphate toxicity. *Biochem Pharmacol* **35**, 3115.

74. Forsyth DM, Rashid C (1967) Treatment of urinary schistosomiasis with trichlorphone. *Lancet* **2**, 909.

75. Fukuto TR (1990) Mechanism of action of organophosphorus and carbamate insecticides. *Environ Health Perspect* **87**, 245.

76. Funk KA, Henderson JD, Liu CH *et al.* (1994) Neuropathology of organophosphate-induced delayed neuropathy (OPIDN) in young chicks. *Arch Toxicol* **68**, 308.

77. Funk KA, Liu CH, Wilson BV, Higgins RJ (1994) Avian embryonic brain reaggregate culture system. I. Characterization for organophosphorus compound toxicity studies. *Toxicol Appl Pharmacol* **124**, 149.

78. Furlong CE, Costa LG, Hassett C *et al.* (1993) Human and rabbit paraoxanases: Purification, cloning, sequencing, mapping and the role of polymorphism in organophosphate detoxification. *Chem-Biol Inter* **87**, 35.

79. Furlong CE, Richter RJ, Seidel SL, Motulsky AG (1988) Role of genetic polymorphism of human plasma paraoxonase/arylesterase in hydrolysis of the insecticide metabolites chlorpyrifos oxon and paraoxon. *Amer J Hum Genet* **43**, 230.

80. Furlong CE, Richter RJ, Seidel SL *et al.* (1989) Spectrophotometric assay for the enzymatic hydrolysis of the active metabolites of chlorpyrifos and parathion by plasma paraoxonase and arylesterase. *Anal Biochem* **180**, 242.

81. Gallo MA, Lawryk NJ (1991) Organic phosphorus pesticides. In: *Handbook of Pesticide Toxicology.* Hayes WJ Jr, Laws ER Jr eds. Academic Press, San Diego p. 917.

82. Gershon S, Shaw FH (1961) Psychiatric sequelae of chronic exposure to organophosphorus insecticides. *Lancet* **i**, 1371.

83. Glynn P, Read DJ, Guo R *et al.* (1994) Synthesis and characterization of a biotinylated organophosphorus ester for detection and affinity purification of a brain serine esterase: neuropathy target esterase. *Biochem J* **301**, 551.

84. Goldstein DA, McGuigan MA, Ripley BD (1988) Acute tricresylphosphate intoxication in childhood. *Hum Toxicol* **7**, 179.

85. Good JL, Khurana RK, Mayer RF *et al.* (1993) Pathophysiological studies of neuromuscular function in subacute organophosphate poisoning induced by phosmet. *J Neurol Neurosurg Psychiat* **37**, 841.

86. Grob D, Harvey AM, Langworthy OR, Lilienthal JL Jr (1947) The administration of diisopropyl fluorophos-

phate (DFP) to man. III. Effect on the central nervous system with special reference to the electrical activity of the brain. *Bull Johns Hopkins Hosp* **81**, 257.

87. Guthrie FE, Hodgson E (1987) Absorption and distribution of toxicants. In: *Modern Toxicology*. Hodgson E, Levi PE eds. Elsevier, New York p. 23.

88. Hayes WJ Jr, Laws ER Jr (1991) *Handbook of Pesticide Toxicology. Vols 1, 2, 3*. Academic Press, San Diego.

89. Heath AJW, Meredith T (1992) Atropine in the management of anticholinesterase poisoning. In: *Clinical & Experimental Toxicology of Organophosphates and Carbamates*. Ballantyne B, Marrs TC eds. Butterworth-Heinemann, Oxford p. 543.

90. Holmstedt B (1959) Pharmacology of organophosphorus cholinesterase inhibitors. *Pharmacol Rev* **11**, 567.

91. Holmstedt B (1963) Structure-activity relationship of the organophosphorus anticholinesterase agents. In: *Handbuch der Experimentellen Pharmakologie, Cholinesterases and Anticholinesterase Agents*. Koelle GB sub-ed. Springer-Verlag, Berlin p. 430.

92. Huang XS, Shu WA, Zu WC *et al.* (1979) Toxicity studies of the herbicide amiprophos. *Chekiang Univ School Med Bull* **8**, 63.

93. IARC (1991) *Monographs on the Evaluation of Carcinogenic Risks to Humans. Occupational Exposures in Insecticide Application and Some Pesticides. Vol 53*. Lyon.

94. Imai S (1986) A critical evaluation of "the strange disease of Saker". *Folia Ophthalmol Jpn* **37**, 1351.

95. Inoue N, Fujishiro K, Mori K, Matsuoka M (1988) Triorthocresyl phosphate poisoning—a review of human cases. *Sangyo Ika Daigaku Zasshi* **10**, 433.

96. IPCS (1992) *International Programme on Chemical Safety*. The WHO recommended classification of pesticides by hazard and guidelines to classification 1992–1993. Geneva.

97. Ishikawa S, Miyata M (1980) Development of myopia following chronic organophosphate pesticide intoxication: An epidemiological and experimental study. In: *Neurotoxicity of the Visual System*. Merigan WH, Weiss B eds. Raven Press, New York p. 233.

98. Jager KW, Roberts DV, Wilson A (1970) Neuromuscular function in pesticide workers. *Brit J Ind Med* **27**, 273.

99. Jedrzejowska H, Rowinska-Marcinska K, Hoppe B (1980) Neuropathy due to phytosol (agritox). Report of a case. *Acta Neuropathol* **49**, 163.

100. Jeyaratnam J, Maroni M (1994) Organophosphorus compounds. In: *Health Surveillance of Pesticide Workers*. Tordoir WF, Maroni M, He F eds. *Toxicology* **91**, 15.

101. Johnson MK (1975) Organophosphorus esters causing delayed neurotoxic effects: Mechanism of action and structure/activity studies. *Arch Toxicol* **34**, 259.

102. Johnson MK (1975) The delayed neuropathy caused by some organophosphorus esters: Mechanism and challenge. *CRC Crit Rev Toxicol* **3**, 289.

103. Johnson MK (1977) Improved assay of neurotoxic esterase for screening organophosphates for delayed neurotoxicity potential. *Arch Toxicol* **37**, 113.

104. Johnson MK (1982) The target for initiation of delayed neurotoxicity by organophosphorus esters: Biochemical studies and toxicological applications. In: *Reviews in Biochemical Toxicology. Vol 4*. Hodgson E, Bend JR, Philpot RM eds. Elsevier, New York p. 141.

105. Johnson MK (1984) Check your paraoxon and parathion for neurotoxic impurities. In: *Delayed Neurotoxicity Workshop. Proceedings of the Delayed Neurotoxicity Workshop*. Crammer JM, Hixson JE eds. IUTOX Press, Little Rock.

106. Johnson MK (1990) Organophosphates and delayed neuropathy—Is NTE alive and well? *Toxicol Appl Pharmacol* **102**, 385.

107. Johnson MK, Read DJ (1993) Prophylaxis against and promotion of organophosphate-induced delayed neuropathy by phenyl di-*n*-pentylphosphinate. *Chem-Biol Inter* **87**, 449.

108. Johnson MK, Vale JA (1992) Clinical management of acute organophosphate poisoning: An overview. In: *Clinical & Experimental Toxicology of Organophosphates and Carbamates*. Ballantyne B, Marrs TC eds. Butterworth-Heinemann, Oxford p. 528.

109. Johnson MK, Vilanova E, Read DJ (1991) Anomalous biochemical responses in tests of the delayed neuropathic potential of methamidophos (*O,S*-dimethyl phosphothioamidate), its resolved isomers and of some higher *O*-alkyl homologues. *Arch Toxicol* **65**, 618.

110. Jokanovic M, Moretto A, Lotti M (1998) Repeated low doses of *O*-(2-chloro-2,3,3-trifluorocyclobutyl)-*O*-ethyl *S*-propyl phosphorothioate (KBR-2822) do not cause neuropathy in hens. *Arch Toxicol* **72**, 93.

111. Jusic A, Jurenic D, Milic S (1980) Electromyographical neuromuscular synapse testing and neurological findings in workers exposed to organophosphorus pesticides. *Arch Environ Health* **35**, 168.

112. Kaplan JG, Kessler J, Rosenberg N *et al.* (1993) Sensory neuropathy associated with Dursban (chlorpyrifos) exposure. *Neurology* **43**, 2193.

113. Karademir M, Ertuk F, Kocak R (1990) Two cases of organophosphate poisoning with development of intermediate syndrome. *Hum Exp Toxicol* **9**, 187.

114. Koelle GB (1963) *Handbuch der Experimentellen Pharmakologie, Cholinesterases and Anticholinesterase Agents*. Springer-Verlag, Berlin.

115. Korsak RJ, Sato MM (1977) Effects of chronic organophosphate pesticide exposure on the central nervous system. *Clin Toxicol* **11**, 83.

116. Krueger HR, O'Brien RD (1959) Relationship between metabolism and differential toxicity of malathion in insects and mice. *J Econ Entomol* **52**, 1063.

117. LeQuesne PM (1978) Clinical expression of neurotoxic injury and diagnostic use of electromyography. *Environ Health Perspect* **26**, 89.

118. Levi PE, Hodgson E (1992) Metabolism of organophosphorus compounds by the flavin-containing monooxygenase. In: *Organophosphates. Chemistry, Fate, and Effects.* Chambers JE, Levi PE eds. Academic Press, San Diego p. 141.

119. Levin HS, Rodnitzky RL (1976) Behavioural effects of organophosphorus pesticides in man. *Clin Toxicol* 9, 391.

120. Lotti M (1987) Organophosphate-induced delayed polyneuropathy in humans: Perspectives for biomonitoring. *Trends Pharmacol Sci* 8, 175.

121. Lotti M (1991) Treatment of acute organophosphate poisoning. *Med J Australia* 154, 51.

122. Lotti M (1992) The pathogenesis of organophosphate delayed polyneuropathy. *Crit Rev Toxicol* 21, 465.

123. Lotti M (1992) Central neurotoxicity and behavioural effects of anticholinesterases. In: *Clinical & Experimental Toxicology of Organophosphates and Carbamates.* Ballantyne B, Marrs TC eds. Butterworth-Heinemann, London p. 75.

124. Lotti M (1995) Cholinesterase inhibition: Complexities in interpretation. *Clin Chem* 69, 705.

125. Lotti M, Becker CE, Aminoff MJ (1984) Organophosphate polyneuropathy: Pathogenesis and prevention. *Neurology* 34, 658.

126. Lotti M, Becker CE, Aminoff MJ *et al.* (1983) Occupational exposure to the cotton defoliants DEF and Merphos. A rational approach to monitoring organophosphorus-induced delayed neurotoxicity. *J Occup Med* 25, 517.

127. Lotti M, Caroldi S, Capodicasa E, Moretto A (1991) Promotion of organophosphate induced delayed polyneuropathy by phenylmethanesulfonyl fluoride. *Toxicol Appl Pharmacol* 108, 234.

128. Lotti M, Caroldi S, Moretto A *et al.* (1987) Central-peripheral delayed neuropathy caused by diisopropyl phosphorofluoridate (DFP): Segregation of peripheral nerve and spinal cord effects using biochemical, clinical and morphological criteria. *Toxicol Appl Pharmacol* 88, 87.

129. Lotti M, Johnson MK (1978) Neurotoxicity of organophosphorus pesticides: Predictions can be based on in vitro studies with hen and human enzymes. *Arch Toxicol* 41, 215.

130. Lotti M, Johnson MK (1980) Repeated small doses of a neurotoxic organophosphate. Monitoring of neurotoxic esterase in brain and spinal cord. *Arch Toxicol* 45, 263.

131. Lotti M, Moretto A, Bertolazzi M *et al.* (1995) Organophosphate polyneuropathy and neuropathy target esterase: Studies with methamidophos and its resolved optical isomers. *Arch Toxicol* 69, 330.

132. Lotti M, Moretto A, Capodicasa E *et al.* (1993) Interactions between neuropathy target esterase and its inhibitors and the development of polyneuropathy. *Toxicol Appl Pharmacol* 122, 165.

133. Lotti M, Moretto A, Zoppellari R *et al.* (1986) Inhibition of lymphocytic neuropathy target esterase predicts the development of organophosphate-induced delayed polyneuropathy. *Arch Toxicol* 59, 176.

134. Maizlish N, Schenker M, Weisskopf C *et al.* (1987) A behavioral evaluation of pest control workers with short term, low level exposure to the organophosphate Diazinon. *Amer J Ind Med* 12, 153.

135. Marrs TC (1993) Organophosphate poisoning. *Pharmacol Ther* 58, 51.

136. Matsushita T, Aoyama K, Yoshimi K *et al.* (1985) Allergic contact dermatitis from organophosphorus insecticides. *Ind Health* 23, 145.

137. Metcalf DR, Holmes JH (1969) EEG, psychological and neurological alterations in humans with organophosphorus exposure. *Ann N Y Acad Sci* 160, 357.

138. Milatovic D, Johnson MK (1993) Reactivation of phosphorodiamidated acetylcholinesterase and neuropathy target esterase by treatment of inhibited enzyme with potassium fluoride. *Chem-Biol Inter* 87, 425.

139. Moretto A, Bertolazzi M, Capodicasa E *et al.* (1992) Phenylmethanesulfonyl fluoride elicits and intensifies the clinical expression of neuropathic insults. *Arch Toxicol* 66, 67.

140. Moretto A, Bertolazzi M, Lotti M (1994) The phosphorothioic acid-O-(2-chloro-2,3,3-trifluorocyclobutyl)-O-ethyl S-propyl ester promotes organophosphate polyneuropathy without inhibition of neuropathy target esterase. *Toxicol Appl Pharmacol* 129, 133.

141. Moretto A, Capodicasa E, Lotti M (1992) Clinical expression of organophosphate-induced delayed polyneuropathy in rats. *Toxicol Lett* 63, 97.

142. Moretto A, Capodicasa E, Peraica M, Lotti M (1991) Age sensitivity to organophosphate-induced delayed polyneuropathy. Biochemical and toxicological studies in developing chicks. *Biochem Pharmacol* 41, 1497.

143. Moretto A, Capodicasa E, Peraica M, Lotti M (1993) Phenylmethanesulfonyl fluoride delays recovery from crush of peripheral nerves in hens. *Chem-Biol Inter* 87, 457.

144. Moretto A, Lotti M (1998) Poisoning by organophosphorus insecticides and sensory neuropathy. *J Neurol Neurosurg Psych* 64, 463.

145. Moretto A, Lotti M, Sabri MI, Spencer PS (1987) Progressive deficit of retrograde axonal transport is associated with the pathogenesis of di-*n*-butyl dichlorvos axonopathy. *J Neurochem* 49, 1515.

146. Moretto A, Lotti M, Spencer PS (1989) *In vivo* and *in vitro* regional differential sensitivity of neuropathy target esterase to di-*n*-butyl-2,2 dichlorovinyl phosphate. *Arch Toxicol* 63, 469.

147. Morgan DP, Hetzler HL, Slach EF, Lin LI (1977) Urinary excretion of paranitrophenol and alkyl phosphates following ingestion of methyl and ethyl parathion by human subjects. *Arch Environ Contam Toxicol* 6, 159.

148. Morgan JP, Penovich P (1978) Jamaica ginger paralysis. Forty-seven-year follow-up. *Arch Neurol* **35**, 530.

149. Moriya M, Ohata T, Watanabe K *et al.* (1983) Further mutagenicity studies on pesticides in bacterial reversion assay systems. *Mutation Res* **116**, 185.

150. Motoyama N, Dauterman WC (1980) Glutathione S-transferases: Their role in the metabolism of organophosphorus insecticides. In: *Review of Biochemistry and Toxicology. Vol 2.* Hodgson E, Bend JR, Philpot RM eds. Elsevier/North Holland, Amsterdam p. 49.

151. Murphy SD (1966) Liver metabolism and toxicity of thiophosphate insecticides in mammalian, avian and piscine species. *Proc Soc Exp Biol Med* **123**, 392.

152. Murphy SD (1986) Toxic effects of pesticides. In: *Casarett and Doull's Toxicology. The Basic Science of Poisons. 3rd Ed.* Klaassen CD, Amdur MO, Doull J eds. Macmillan, New York p. 519.

153. Murray WJ, Franklin CA (1992) Monitoring for exposure to anticholinesterase-inhibiting organophosphorus and carbamate compounds by urine analysis. In: *Clinical & Experimental Toxicology of Organophosphates and Carbamates.* Ballantyne B, Marrs TC eds. Butterworth-Heinemann, Oxford p. 430.

154. Nakatsugawa T (1992) Hepatic disposition of organophosphorus insecticides: A synthesis of *in vitro, in situ,* and *in vivo* data. In: *Organophosphates. Chemistry, Fate, and Effects.* Chambers JE, Levi PE eds. Academic Press, San Diego p. 201.

155. Namba TL, Nolte CT, Jackrel J, Grob D (1971) Poisoning due to organophosphate insecticides. Acute and chronic manifestations. *Amer J Med* **50**, 475.

156. National Research Council (US) (1993) *Pesticides in the Diets of Infants and Children.* National Academy Press, Washington, DC.

157. Natoff IL (1976) The effects of antidotes in experimental animals intoxicated by carbamate and organophosphorus cholinesterase inhibitors. In: *Medical Protection Against Chemical Warfare Agents.* Stockholm International Peace Research Institute ed. Almquist and Wiskall, Uppsala p. 53.

158. Newcombe DS (1992) Immune surveillance, organophosphorus exposure and lymphomagenesis. *Lancet* **339**, 539.

159. Nordgren I, Bergstrom M, Holmstedt B, Sandoz M (1978) Transformation and action of metrifonate. *Arch Toxicol* **41**, 31.

160. Nordgren I, Holmstedt B, Bengtsson E, Finkel Y (1980) Plasma levels of metrifonate and dichlorvos during treatment of schistosomiasis with Bilarcil. *Amer J Trop Med Hyg* **29**, 426.

161. Padilla S, Veronesi B (1985) The relationship between neurological damage and neurotoxic esterase inhibition in rats acutely exposed to tri-ortho-cresyl phosphate. *Toxicol Appl Pharmacol* **78**, 78.

162. Peraica M, Capodicasa E, Moretto A, Lotti M (1993) Organophosphate polyneuropathy in chicks. *Biochem Pharmacol* **45**, 131.

163. Plestina R, Piukovic-Plestina M (1978) Effect of anticholinesterse pesticides on the eye and on vision. *CRC Crit Rev Toxicol* **6**, 1.

164. Pope CN, Padilla S (1990) Potentiation of organo-phosphorus-induced delayed neurotoxicity by phenylmethylsulfonyl fluoride. *J Toxicol Environ Health* **31**, 261.

165. Prineas J (1969) The pathogenesis of dying-back polyneuropathies. Part I. An ultrastructural study of experimental tri-orthocresyl phosphate intoxication in the cat. *J Neuropathol Exp Neurol* **28**, 571.

166. Reiff B, Lambert SM, Natoff IL (1971) Inhibition of brain cholinesterase by organophosphorus compounds in rats. *Arch Int Pharmacodyn* **192**, 48.

167. Reiner E, Aldridge WN, Hoskin FCG (1989) *Esterases Hydrolysing Organophosphorus Compounds.* Ellis Horwood Ltd, Chichester.

168. Reiner E, Lotti M (guest eds) (1993) Enzymes interacting with organophosphorus compounds. *Chem-Biol Inter* **87**, Special Issue.

169. Reiner E, Plestina R (1979) Regeneration of cholinesterase activity in humans and rats after inhibition by O,O-dimethyl-2,2-dichlorovinyl phosphate. *Toxicol Appl Pharmacol* **49**, 451.

170. Richardson RJ (1992) Interactions of organophosphorus compounds with Neurotoxic Esterase. In: *Organophosphates. Chemistry, Fate, and Effects.* Chambers JE, Levi PE eds. Academic Press, San Diego p. 299.

171. Roberts DV (1976) EMG voltage and motor nerve conduction velocity in organophosphorus pesticide factory workers. *Int Arch Occup Environ Health* **36**, 267.

172. Roberts NL, Fairley C, Phillips C (1983) Screening, acute delayed and subchronic neurotoxicity studies in the hen: Measurements and evaluations of clinical signs following administration of TOCP. *Neurotoxicology* **4**, 263.

173. Robertson DG, Schwab BW, Sills RD *et al.* (1987) Electrophysiologic changes following treatment with organophosphorus-induced delayed neuropathy-producing agents in the adult hen. *Toxicol Appl Pharmacol* **87**, 420.

174. Rodgers KE, Devens BH, Imamura T (1992) Immunotoxic effects of anticholinesterases. In: *Clinical & Experimental Toxicology of Organophosphates and Carbamates.* Ballantyne B, Marrs TC eds. Butterworth-Heinemann, Oxford p. 211.

175. Rodnitzky RL, Levin HS, Mick DL (1975) Occupational exposure to organophosphate pesticides. A neurobehavioural study. *Arch Environ Health* **30**, 98.

176. Rosenstock L, Keifer M, Daniell WE *et al.* (1991) Chronic central nervous system effects of acute organophosphate pesticide poisoning. *Lancet* **338**, 223.

177. Russel RW, Overstreet DH (1987) Mechanisms under-

lying sensitivity to organophosphorus anticholinesterase compounds. *Prog Neurobiol* **28**, 97.

178. Salem H, Olajos EJ (1988) Review of pesticides: Chemistry, uses and toxicology. *Toxicol Ind Health* **4**, 291.

179. Savage EP, Keefe TJ, Mounce LM *et al.* (1988) Chronic neurological sequelae of acute organophosphate pesticide poisoning. *Arch Environ Health* **43**, 38.

180. Senanayake N (1981) Tri-cresyl phosphate neuropathy in Sri Lanka: A clinical and neurophysiological study with a three-year follow up. *J Neurol Neurosurg Psychiat* **44**, 775.

181. Senanayake N, Johnson MK (1982) Acute polyneuropathy after poisoning by a new organophosphate insecticide. *N Engl J Med* **306**, 155.

182. Senanayake N, Karalliedde L (1987) Neurotoxic effects of organophosphorus insecticides: An intermediate syndrome. *N Engl J Med* **316**, 761.

183. Sharma RP, Tomar RS (1992) Immunotoxicology of anticholinesterase agents. In: *Clinical & Experimental Toxicology of Organophosphates and Carbamates.* Ballantyne B, Marrs TC eds. Butterworth-Heinemann, Oxford p. 203.

184. Shaw KP, Aracava C, Akaike A *et al.* (1985) The reversible cholinesterase inhibitor physostigmine has channel-blocking and agonist effects on the acetylcholine receptor-ion channel complex. *Mol Pharmacol* **28**, 527.

185. Sheets LP, Hamilton BF, Sangha GK, Thyssen JH (1997) Subchronic neurotoxicity screening studies with six organophosphate insecticides: An assessment of behavior and morphology relative to cholinesterase inhibition. *Fund Appl Toxicol* **35**, 101.

186. Sivam SP, Hoskins B, Ho IK (1984) An assessment of comparative acute toxicity of diisopropyl-fluorophosphate, tabun, sarin and soman in relation to cholinergic and GABAergic enzyme activities in rats. *Fund Appl Toxicol* **4**, 531.

187. Sivam SP, Norris JC, Kim DK *et al.* (1983) Effect of acute and chronic cholinesterase inhibition with diisopropyl-fluorophosphate on muscarinic, dopamine and GABA receptors of the rat striatum. *J Neurochem* **40**, 1414.

188. Somkuti SG, Lapadula DM, Chapin RE *et al.* (1987) Reproductive tract lesions resulting from subchronic administration (63 days) of tri-o-cresyl phosphate in male rats. *Toxicol Appl Pharmacol* **89**, 49.

189. Stamboulis E, Psimaras A, Vassilopoulos D *et al.* (1991) Neuropathy following acute intoxication with mecarbam (OP ester). *Acta Neurol Scand* **83**, 198.

190. Stavinoha WB, Modak AT, Weintraub ST (1976) Rate of accumulation of acetylcholine in discrete regions of the rat brain after dichlorvos treatment. *J Neurochem* **27**, 1375.

191. Stephens R, Spurgeon A, Beach J *et al.* (1995) An investigation into the possible chronic neurophysiological and neurological effects of occupational exposure to organophosphates in sheep farmers. *HSE Contract Research Report 74/1995,* UK.

192. Stephens R, Spurgeon A, Calvert IA *et al.* (1995) Neurophysiological effects of long-term exposure to organophosphates in sheep-dip. *Lancet* **345**, 1135.

193. Stokes L, Stark A, Marshall E, Narang A (1995) Neurotoxicity among pesticide applicators exposed to organophosphates. *Occup Environ Med* **56**, 648.

194. Sultatos LG (1992) Role of glutathione in the mammalian detoxication of organophosphorus insecticides. In: *Organophosphates. Chemistry, Fate, and Effects.* Chambers JE, Levi PE eds. Academic Press, San Diego p. 155.

195. Sultatos LG, Costa LG, Murphy SD (1982) Factors involved in the differential acute toxicity of the insecticides chlorpyrifos and methyl chlorpyrifos in mice. *Toxicol Appl Pharmacol* **65**, 144.

196. Sussman JL, Harel M, Frolow F *et al.* (1991) Atomic structure of acetylcholinesterase from *Torpedo californica*: A prototypic acetylcholine-binding protein. *Science* **253**, 872.

197. Suzuki T, Morita H, Ono K *et al.* (1995) Sarin poisoning in Tokyo subway. *Lancet* **345**, 980.

198. Tabershaw IR, Cooper WC (1966) Sequelae of acute organic phosphate poisoning. *J Occup Med* **8**, 5.

199. Talcott RE, Denk H, Mallipudi NM (1979) Malathion carboxylesterase activity in human liver and its inactivation by isomalathion. *Toxicol Appl Pharmacol* **49**, 373.

200. Tanaka D Jr, Bursian SJ, Lehning E (1990) Selective axonal and terminal degeneration in the chicken brainstem and cerebellum following exposure to bis(1-methylethyl)phosphorofluoridate (DFP). *Brain Res* **519**, 200.

201. Taylor P (1990) Anticholinesterase agents. In: *Goodman and Gilman's The Pharmacological Basis of Therapeutics. 8th Ed.* Goodman Gilman A, Rall TW, Nies AS, Taylor P eds. Pergamon Press, New York p. 131.

202. Teidt TN, Albuquerque EX, Hudson CS, Rash JE (1978) Neostigmine-induced alterations at the mammalian neuromuscular junction. I. Muscle contraction and electrophysiology. *J Pharmacol Exp Ther* **205**, 326.

203. Tracey JA, Gallagher H (1990) Use of glycopyrrolate and atropine in acute organophosphorus poisoning. *Hum Exp Toxicol* **9**, 99.

204. Umetsu N, Grose FH, Allahyari R *et al.* (1977) Effect of impurities on the mammalian toxicity of technical malathion and acephate. *J Agr Food Chem* **25**, 946.

205. Vasilescu C, Alexianu M, Dan A (1984) Delayed neuropathy after organophosphorus insecticide (Dipterex) poisoning: A clinical, electrophysiological and nerve biopsy study. *J Neurol Neurosurg Psychiat* **47**, 543.

206. Vasilescu C, Florescu A (1980) Clinical and electrophysiological study of neuropathy after organophosphorus compounds poisoning. *Arch Toxicol* **43**, 305.

207. Veronesi B (1984) A rodent model of organophosphorus-induced delayed neuropathy: Distribution of central (spinal cord) and peripheral nerve damage. *Neuropathol Appl Neurobiol* **10**, 357.

208. Veronesi B, Ehrich M (1993) Differential cytotoxic sensi-

tivity in mouse and human cell lines exposed to organophosphate insecticides. *Toxicol Appl Pharmacol* **120**, 240.

209. Veronesi B, Padilla S, Blackmon K, Pope C (1991) Murine susceptibility to organophosphorus-induced delayed neuropathy (OPIDN). *Toxicol Appl Pharmacol* **107**, 311.

210. Wadia RS, Sadagopan C, Amin RB, Sardesai HV (1974) Neurological manifestations of organophosphorus insecticide poisoning. *J Neurol Neurosurg Psychiat* **37**, 841.

211. Wadia RS, Shinde SN, Vaidya S (1985) Delayed neurotoxicity after an episode of poisoning with dichlorvos. *Neurology-India* **33**, 247.

212. Walker CH, Mackness MI (1987) "A" esterases and their role in regulating the toxicity of organophosphates. *Arch Toxicol* **60**, 30.

213. Wallace KB (1992) Species-selective toxicity of organophosphorus insecticides: A pharmacodynamic phenomenon. In: *Organophosphates. Chemistry, Fate, and Effects.* Chambers JE, Levi PE eds. Academic Press, San Diego p. 79.

214. WHO (1986) *Organophosphorus Insecticides: A General Introduction.* Environmental Health Criteria 63, World Health Organization, Geneva.

215. WHO (1989) *Dimethoate.* Environmental Health Criteria 90, World Health Organization, Geneva.

216. WHO (1990) *Principles for the Toxicological Assessment of Pesticide Residues in Food.* Environmental Health Criteria 104, World Health Organization, Geneva.

217. WHO (1993) *Methylparathion.* Environmental Health Criteria 145, World Health Organization, Geneva.

218. WHO/UNEP (1990) *Public Health Impact of Pesticides Used in Agriculture.* World Health Organization, Geneva.

219. Wilson BW, Hooper M, Chow E *et al.* (1984) Antidotes and neuropathic potential of isofenphos. *Bull Environ Contam Toxicol* **33**, 386.

220. Wilson BW, Hooper MJ, Hansen ME, Nieberg PS (1992) Reactivation of organophosphorus inhibited AChE with oximes. In: *Organophosphates. Chemistry, Fate, and Effects.* Chambers JE, Levi PE eds. Academic Press, San Diego p. 107.

221. Worthing CR, Hance RJ (1991) *The Pesticide Manual. 9th Ed.* The British Crop Protection Council, Old Woking, UK.

222. Xintaras C, Burg JR (1980) Screening and prevention of human neurotoxic outbreaks: Issues and problems. In: *Experimental and Clinical Neurotoxicology.* Spencer PS, Schaumburg HH eds. Williams & Wilkins, Baltimore p. 663.

223. Xintaras C, Burg JR, Tanaka S *et al.* (1978) *Occupational Exposure to Leptophos and Other Chemicals.* U.S. Department of Health and Welfare, National Institute of Occupational Safety and Health (NIOSH), Cincinnati, Ohio, US NIOSH Publication No. 78–136.

β-N-Oxalylamino-L-Alanine

Jacques Hugon
Albert C. Ludolph
Peter S. Spencer

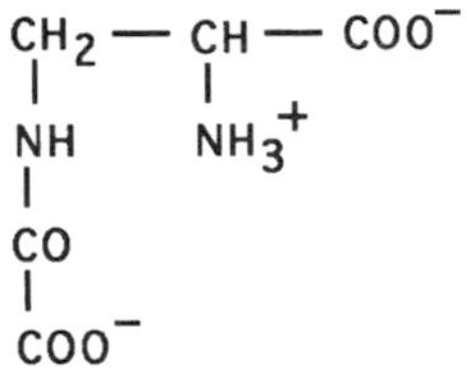

$$CH_2 - CH - COO^-$$
$$| \quad\quad |$$
$$NH \quad NH_3^+$$
$$|$$
$$CO$$
$$|$$
$$COO^-$$

L-BOAA
C₅H₇N₂O₅

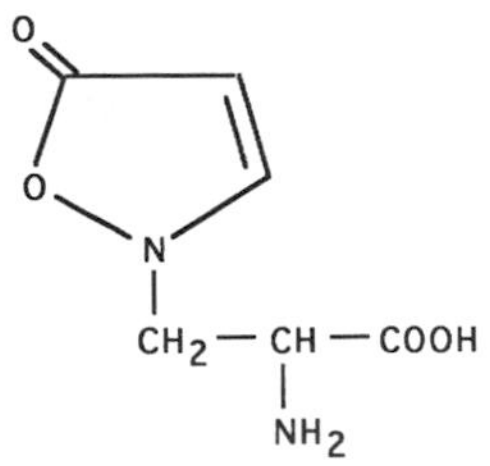

β-(ISOXAZOLIN-5-ON-2YL)ALANINE
C₆H₈N₂O₄

3-N-Oxalyl-2,3-diaminopropanoic acid; β-N-oxalylamino-α,β-diaminopropionic acid; L-3-Oxalylamino-2-aminopropionic acid; OAP; Ox-dapro; ODAP; BOAA

NEUROTOXICITY RATING

Clinical

A   Spastic paraparesis (*Lathyrus sativus*)

Experimental

A   Seizure disorder

A   Central motor-system disorder

β-N-Oxalylamino-L-alanine (L-BOAA) is a stereospecific neurotoxic amino acid present in free form in certain plants used by humans for food and medicine, notably many species of the leguminous genus *Lathyrus*, but also cycads (*Macrozamia* spp.) and ginseng (*Panax* spp.) (7,69,86,95). Clinical and experimental interest in L-BOAA, a glutamate analogue and potent excitatory neurotoxin, is largely based on the fact that the amino acid is held responsible for the motor neuron disease lathyrism (neurolathyrism). This disorder—described since ancient times in humans and animals—is caused by the continuous heavy ingestion of *Lathyrus sativus* (chickling vetch, chickling pea, or grass pea), *L. cicera* (flat-podded vetch), or *L. clymenum* (Spanish vetchling) (124,129). Other compounds have been erroneously linked to the etiopathogenesis of neurolathyrism: (a) β-aminopropionitrile, which induces experimental angio- and osteolathyrism, is not neurotoxic, and (b) β,β'-iminodipropionitrile (IDPN)—once considered an "experimental neurolathyrogen" (122)—is not detected in *Lathyrus* spp. and induces a neurotoxic disorder distinct from lathyrism (*see* β,β'-Iminodipropionitrile, this volume) (46,116).

The ancient Hindus, Hippocrates (460–377 BC), Pliny the Elder (23–79 AD), Pedanius Dioskurides (50 AD), and Galen (130–210 AD) were aware of a causal association between prolonged intake of grass pea and the development of spastic paraplegia in man (24,42,44,99,120,130). Hippocrates described an outbreak of leg weakness in inhabitants of the village of Eno in Thrakia after prolonged consumption of *ervo* (peas) during a time of food shortage (42). In central, east, and southern Europe, *Lathyrus* seeds were often cultivated to feed horses, or the flour was mixed with wheat and used to bake bread for human consumption (120). In Germany in 1671, Duke Georg banned the use of *Lathyrus* flour in the county of Württemberg because of its ability to paralyze the legs ("*wegen seiner lähmenden Wirkung auf die Beine*"); this ban was apparently only partly successful since further action by his successor Leopold followed in 1705 and 1714 (120). The Italian Bernadino Ramazzini described an outbreak of lathyrism in Modena in 1690 (125). Kinlock Kirk discussed the disease in India in 1861 and pointed out that consumption of *Lathyrus dal* is restricted to the poorest villages and families; he concluded that village poverty varied directly with the amount of *Lathyrus* sold in the market place (56, *see also* 2). Repeated epidemics of lathyrism were described in Toscany in the eighteenth century (22). In 1873, Arnoldo Cantani of Naples observed three brothers aged 8, 10, and 20 years old suffering from spastic paraparesis, and used the word "lathyrismus" (*latirismo*) to describe the clinical disease (13,22) in humans; this replaced the older Italian descriptors *Crurum exsolutio*, *Crurum impotentia*, *Crurum imbecillia*, and "*storpio delle gambe*" (13,22,120). Prolonged consumption of *L. sativus* was identified as the causal factor, and exposure to cold was considered an important precipitating factor (13,22). Although Cantani clinically described a typical spastic paraparesis, he actually suspected the presence of a generalized muscle disease since he detected lipid vacuoles in a muscle biopsy (13,22). In his inaugural lecture, Strümpell concluded that the clinical picture of lathyrism resem-

bles the signs and symptoms of "*spastische Spinal paralyse*" (which included hereditary spastic paraparesis and primary lateral sclerosis) (129,136). Later, in the nineteenth century, several outbreaks of lathyrism were described in different parts of the world (*see* 120,124). In 1897, lathyrism patients were described for the first time in Ethiopia (Abyssinia) (35). However, several historical reports, in particular those from North Africa, describe a clinical picture that is possibly partly due to contamination of *Lathyrus* seeds with ergot (120). In the early twentieth century, the disease was seldom seen in Europe (with the exception of Russia [28,32]), but later food shortages led to the reappearance of lathyrism in western Europe. During the late 1930s and early 1940s, an outbreak occurred among peasants in the Spanish Civil War (34,51); this was followed during World War II by an epidemic of lathyrism among prisoners in a German forced-labor camp in the Ukrainian town of Wapniarka (20,21,53). Prisoners-of-war were also affected by the stereotypical paraparesis (27,81). Today, lathyrism is restricted to parts of the world where populations continue to consume *L. sativus* and rely on the hardy legume during periods of flood and drought. Numerous cases are found in parts of India, Bangladesh, Nepal, Pakistan, Ethiopia, China, and Chile (30,33,70,73,124,138,139). Because *L. sativus* remains a valuable food and fodder crop in parts of Asia and the Horn of Africa, an international network of scientists of various disciplines (International Network for the Improvement of *Lathyrus sativus* and Eradication of Lathyrism [INILSEL]) has operated with the goal of developing a nonneurotoxic strain of the grass pea to exploit its valuable nutritional and other properties. Common names for *L. sativus* include *khesari* in India and Bangladesh, *guaya* in Ethiopia, *san li dow* in China, *pois carré* in France, and *las gachas* in Spain (34,55).

General Toxicology

L-BOAA was isolated from the grass pea in 1964 (7,86,104) and, in 1969 and 1975, the compound was synthesized (101,112). β-(Isoxazolin-5-on-2-yl)alanine (BIA) is the biosynthetic precursor of BOAA in *L. sativus* seedlings (48). L-BOAA is a white, crystalline, water-soluble compound with a melting point of 206°C (with decomposition) and specific optical rotation, $(\alpha)^{27}$D − 28.7 (C2, 0.5 N HCl) (116). In mature seed, the concentration of L-BOAA varies from 0.1%–2.5% of its dry weight (54,116); a paucity of zinc and excess iron in the soil serve to increase the content of BOAA in mature seed (66). The biological function of BOAA may be related to uptake and transport of zinc ions (66). L-BOAA exists with its α-isomer in the seed of *L. sativus* in a proportion of 95%:5%, respectively (14,115,116); the proportion of the α-isomer slowly increases in a standing aqueous solution until a 4:6 equilibrium is reached; this isomerization is enhanced by heating (23,54). Both the α-isomer, L-2-oxalylamino-3-aminopropionic acid, and D-BOAA, lack neurotoxic activity (14,87). Methods of chemical synthesis and detection of BOAA are described (23,54,60,101,102,112,116). α- and β-Isomers are separated by high-performance liquid chromatography after precolumn derivitization with phenylisothiocyanate (54). Precolumn derivitization with 9-fluorenylmethyl chloroformate followed by gradient reverse-phase chromatography and fluorescence detection has been used to detect picomolar concentrations of L-BOAA in plant and animal tissues (57).

Absorption and distribution of L-BOAA are largely unstudied. After intraperitoneal (i.p.) administration of radiolabeled L-BOAA to rats, 50%–70% of the radioactivity is excreted in the urine within 24 h (16,17). Intravenous injection of radiolabeled L-BOAA to squirrel monkeys resulted in excretion of about 20% radioactivity within one hour of administration (79). After injection of L-BOAA into rats, a ketoacid derivative is found in liver and kidneys (16,17). Blood levels of L-BOAA are low in monkeys with pyramidal-tract dysfunction produced by prolonged oral administration of L-BOAA (116). How and to what extent L-BOAA crosses the blood-brain barrier during states of adequate nutrition is unknown, although it is clear the amino acid induces neuropharmacological and behavioral responses that provide indirect evidence of its access to CNS neurons (77,80,103,105). The distribution and metabolic fate of L-BOAA in the brain and spinal cord are unstudied, and there is no entirely satisfactory explanation for why central motor-system disease follows prolonged dietary exposure to L-BOAA in humans and nonhuman primates (see also, 125). Young animals are more susceptible than adults to the neurotoxic effects of L-BOAA; however, older animals reportedly become more vulnerable under acidotic conditions (16,105).

Animal Studies

Early Studies

The acute lethal dosage is high; a dosage of 10–12 g L. sativus/100 g body weight is required in rabbits (29). Numerous historical references and some recent reports note the effects of prolonged ingestion of the neurotoxic seed of Lathyrus spp. Reports describe neurological disorders in birds, turtles, ducks, geese, frogs, guinea pigs, hens, rabbits, peacocks, pigs, oxen, sheep, cows, bullocks, horses, macaques, and even elephants (6,8,29,32,51,74,76,83,84,113, 114,120–122,124,130,133,134,137,141). Taken together, these studies show that two different neurological responses can be obtained: an acute response characterized by som-

nolence and death and sometimes accompanied by hindlimb paresis, and a more chronic form that results in hindlimb weakness that is reversible in most cases. Neuropathological studies are comparatively rare; some of the authors describe reversible changes (32,134), others chromatolysis and dendritic atrophy of anterior horn cells and of cells in brain gray matter associated with changes of the lateral pyramidal tract and fasciculus gracilis (84). The majority of authors finds no convincing change; one describes abnormalities in the dorsal horn (see 29).

Horses are exceptionally vulnerable to the neurotoxic effects of Lathyrus spp. (29,67,75,83,120). Days to months of a diet of L. sativus or other neurotoxic Lathyrus spp. is sufficient for horses to develop muscular weakness accompanied by signs of laryngeal nerve palsy ("roaring," "Dampf," "le cornage"); this appears most commonly during exercise, and the animal may die. Hyperacusis, hyperesthesia, tremor, and irritability have been observed later in the course of the disease (29). A thorough description of equine lathyrism is available from an outbreak in 1867 that occurred in Rouen, France: 29 of 45 animals fed a diet containing only up to 20% Lathyrus spp. developed laryngeal and hindlimb paralysis within 6 months ("jarosse" disease) (120). The neuropathology is consistent with the clinical syndrome: degenerative changes were present in the "ganglion cells" of spinal cord gray matter, the lateral columns and the motor roots, in the vagal and accessory nuclei, and the recurrent laryngeal nerves (134). A similar outbreak of equine lathyrism is described in Liverpool, England, during which 31 of 78 animals died (29); only adult male horses (with the exception of a single female horse) were affected by the disease.

Controlled Studies

Rats receiving L-BOAA by i.p. injection (50 mg/kg) or oral intake (100 mg/kg) of an alcoholic extract of grass pea showed a L-BOAA concentration of 100 and 150 μg/g wet weight tissue, respectively (64). Since the animals were not systemically perfused with fluid prior to termination, these estimations include L-BOAA in blood and in neural tissue.

Results of short-term administration of L-BOAA are described in birds, rodents, and primates (79,80,105, 106,111,113). Relative to C57BL/6J (black) mice, Wistar rats and BALB/c mice are relatively resistant to L-BOAA neurotoxicity; they become susceptible to L-BOAA following pretreatment with tyrosine or phenylalanine (123). Seizures and opisthotonus also appear in young mice given a large i.p. (225–1350 mg/kg body weight) or oral (3900 mg/kg) dose of L-BOAA (80). Convulsions and behavioral changes in mice are blocked by intracerebroventricular administration of non–N-methyl-D-aspartate antagonists

(111). Neuropathological changes are found in those areas of the brain unprotected by the blood barrier, *i.e.*, the circumventricular organs such as the area postrema, the subfornical and subcommisural organ, the organum vasculosum of the lamina terminalis, and the arcuate-eminence region of the hypothalamus (88,90). Spinal cord changes are restricted to areas around the central canal. These changes show the morphological hallmarks of excitotoxicity, *i.e.*, postsynaptic vacuolar degeneration of dendrites (88–90). In squirrel monkeys, a similar syndrome with muscle tremors, sedation, opisthotonus, seizures, and death is observed after oral administration of 8.0–8.5 mg/g L-BOAA or 2.0 mg/kg i.p. (78,96). Chronic oral feeding of the same species with a high dosage of L-BOAA (0.6–6.0 mg/g) did not result in any observable neurological deficits (78).

Several attempts have been made to model the human disease by controlled feeding of *L. sativus*. A 1929 review describes the following results (134):

Feeding experiments have frequently been carried out on all kinds of domestic and laboratory animals with very varying results—in many cases the animals have fattened and thriven, while in others weakness or paralysis of the limbs developed or a more generalized paralysis and death.

The underlying reasons for the poorly reproducible results remain unexplained more than 60 years later. Part of the problem undoubtedly lies in the observer's expectation of overt and permanent hind-limb paralysis rather than the subtle spastic paraparesis that characterizes the initial and potentially reversible phase of the human disease. Neurological deficits of unknown relationship to lathyrism are reported in macaques fed L-BOAA–containing materials to animals with uncontrolled nutritional status (131) or vitamin C deficiency (50). Chronic oral administration of a high dosage of L-BOAA (0.6–6.0 mg/g body weight) to squirrel monkeys reportedly did not result in neurological deficits (78).

Modern studies have shown that prolonged treatment of well-nourished macaques with *L. sativus* or L-BOAA induces a reversible motor-system disorder comparable to beginning human lathyrism (126,127,129). Four groups of adult cynomolgus monkeys (*Macaca fasicularis*) fed a carefully constructed nutritious diet were examined neurologically: The first received pellets of enriched flour prepared from *L. sativus* seed plus a daily oral gavage of an alcoholic extract of *L. sativus* seed, with an estimated L-BOAA intake of 1.1–1.5 g/kg body weight/day. After 3–10 months of this regimen, the primates developed stimulus-sensitive myoclonic jerks affecting the legs, and, occasionally, the upper extremities. Later, an abnormal posture and exaggerated deep tendon reflexes of the hindlimbs were observed. A

mild-to-moderate increase in leg-muscle tone resulted in a gait disorder characterized by a stiff, sometimes upright bipedal gait associated with early tiring (126,127). Cessation of *L. sativus* treatment resulted in functional recovery. A second (negative) control group of animals remained neurologically intact while maintained on a closely matched diet prepared from the chick pea, *Cicer arietinum*. A third group of animals on a chick pea diet received by gavage a daily dose of grass pea extract plus synthetic L-BOAA, or L-BOAA alone (300 mg/kg/day increasing by 300 mg/kg/day every 15 days). Within weeks, these animals rapidly developed a pattern of neurological deficit comparable to that seen in animals fed the grass pea diet. These experiments show that L-BOAA is the major or exclusive neurotoxic component of *L. sativus*.

The observed pattern of functional vulnerability to L-BOAA was further defined by examination of corticospinal tract function with noninvasive electric brain (principally motor cortex) stimulation (46) and intradural spinal-cord recording electrodes. The calculated maximum velocity for impulse conduction along the fast descending fibers was 65–70 m/sec, a value consistent with the results of invasive measurements of corticospinal neurons (98). Complementary results were obtained in positive-control animals chronically intoxicated with IDPN which had well-defined multifocal axonal lesions of the corticospinal tract. At cervical and lumbar levels, *L. sativus*– and L-BOAA–treated animals showed a 10%–20% decrease in central motor conduction velocity (60 m/sec) and a greatly decreased amplitude of the descending volley. While this pattern suggested the presence of proximal corticospinal deficits, histopathological examination of Betz cells and corticospinal tracts in well-fixed tissue revealed minor, if any, changes.

Neuronal vacuolation is found in the retina and area postrema of newborn mice after systemic injection of L-BOAA (90). Adult rats given repeated subconvulsive doses of L-BOAA develop a reversible excitatory state associated with changes in glutamate receptor function. Rats treated by gavage daily for 14 days with an alcoholic grass pea extract display down-regulation of low-affinity glutamate receptors in the frontal cortex and cerebellum, but not in the hippocampus. When ^{3}H-glutamate binding is assayed in the presence of excess N-methyl-D-aspartic acid (NMDA), there is a decrease in low-affinity glutamate-binding sites, with an increase in binding affinity in the remaining sites, selectively in the frontal cortex (63,64). A dose- and time-dependent increase of cerebellar cyclic guanosine monophosphate (cGMP) level is observed after intraperitoneal administration of synthetic L-BOAA or *Lathyrus sativus* seed extract; the increase is blocked by administration of kynurenic acid, a nonspecific excitatory amino acid antagonist (63). Wistar rats fed a diet of *L. sativus* seed showed significantly increased open-field activity consistent with a reversible excitable state (65).

Direct application of L-BOAA to the brain or spinal cord of primates and rats has also been used to assess the neurotoxic actions of L-BOAA (14,106). Introduction of α and β-N-oxalyl-L-α,β-diaminopropionic acids into rat cerebrospinal fluid showed that L-BOAA is a potent direct-acting neurotoxin, while its α-isomer lacks neurotoxic activity (14). L-BOAA decreased norepinephrine levels but did not affect levels of dopamine or dopamine metabolites after intranigral injection in rats; neuronal damage and substance P–immunoreactive terminals in the substantia nigra pars reticulata disappeared (68). Direct injection of L-BOAA (50 nmol) or α-amino-3-hydroxy-5-methyl-4-isoxazole 4-propionic acid (AMPA) (1 nmol) into rat dorsal hippocampus produced heavy damage in hippocampal subfields CA1, CA4 and in dentate granule neurons, with minimal damage in CA2 and CA3. Similar patterns are seen with NMDA (25 nmol). Microinjection of L-BOAA (1 μg per animal) or AMPA (0.05 μg per animal) into the ventrolateral periaqueductal gray matter induced immobility, running, grooming, and clonus that were antagonized by pretreatment with the AMPA antagonist 6-cyano-7-nitroquinozaline-2,3-dione (CNQX), but not with the specific NMDA receptor antagonist, 2-amino-5-phosphonovalerate or the weak glutamate metabotropic receptor antagonist L (+)-2-amino-3-phosphonopropionic acid (72). L-BOAA–induced injury was attenuated dose-dependently by focal co-injection or delayed (2 h) injection of the AMPA agonist 2,3-dihydroxy-6-nitro-7-sulfamoyl-benzo(F)quinoxaline, but not by intraperitoneal administration of the NMDA open-channel antagonist MK-801 (145). Damage induced by L-BOAA, but not by AMPA, kainic acid (0.5 nmol), or NMDA (25 nmol) was attenuated dose-dependently by focal co-injection of four potential free-radical scavengers (dimethyl sulfoxide, dimethylthiourea, dimethylformamide, mannitol). These findings suggest that L-BOAA–induced hippocampal damage involves an interaction between AMPA receptors and free radicals (144). Major increases in heat-shock protein 70, c-fos and brain-derived neurotrophic factor mRNAs are seen in rat hippocampus 1 h after intracerebroventricular injection of L-BOAA (4).

In Vitro Studies

There is convincing evidence that L-BOAA neurotoxicity is mediated by the AMPA class of glutamate receptor subtype, as shown by several pharmacological and electrophysiological in vitro studies (3,9,11,59,109,110,143). The affinity of L-BOAA for synaptic membranes from mouse cortex (IC_{50} of L-BOAA to displace ^{3}H-AMPA 0.79 mmol) is larger than for those from hippocampus (3.83 mmol), cerebellum

(5.9 mmol), and spinal cord (90 mmol), a result broadly consistent with the apparent distribution of neuronal involvement in lathyrism.

L-BOAA concentration-dependently reduces transport of ^{3}H-glutamate > transport of ^{3}H-aspartate in rat brain and spinal cord synaptosomes; by contrast, 1 mmol L-BOAA has no effect on high-affinity transport of ^{3}H–γ-aminobutyric acid (GABA), ^{3}H-glycine, or ^{3}H-choline, or the enzyme activity of glutamate decarboxylase (108). L-BOAA reduces high-affinity ^{3}H-norepinephrine uptake in cortical synaptosomes, but striatal ^{3}H-dopamine uptake and cortical high-affinity ^{3}H-5-HT uptake are unaffected (68). L-BOAA (200 μmol) increases basal cytosolic and KCl-stimulated vesicular release of glutamate from guinea-pig hippocampal mossy fibers (31).

Tissue culture studies show that L-BOAA exhibits a time- and concentration-dependent damage of cortical neurons, with an EC_{50} of 20 μmol (143). Neuropathological changes, consisting of postsynaptic dendritic edematous vacuolation and neuronal degeneration, are consistent with an excitotoxic action of L-BOAA, and antagonists to non-NMDA glutamate receptor subtypes attenuate this damage in a concentration-dependent manner (87,111).

L-BOAA induces widespread neuronal injury in cortical cell cultures that is substantially attenuated by addition of 10^{-7}–10^{-6} mole of tetrandrine, a Ca^{2+} antagonist isolated from a traditional Chinese herb (15). L-BOAA is less potent than glutamate in killing cerebellar granule cells in vitro, and the effect is blocked by kynurenic acid. L-BOAA induces hallmarks of both necrotic and apoptotic-like cell death in vitro (132). L-BOAA (0.5–1.0 mmol) induces cell degeneration through an apoptotic mechanism in a ventral spinal-cord motoneuron hybrid cell line in the absence of functional synaptic excitatory amino acid receptors (62,64).

L-BOAA damages chick retina in vitro via a non-NMDA receptor and causes a dose-dependent increase in the release of GABA (146). Treatment of embryonic day-15 chick retina for 5 min with L-BOAA (200 μmol), glutamate (1 mmol), NMDA (100 μmol), kainate (100 μmol), or domoate (20 μmol) increases cyclic guanosine monophosphate; the L-BOAA response is blocked by CNQX, by the nitric oxide synthase inhibitor N-nitro-L-arginine and by hemoglobin, a nitric oxide scavenger (147). L-BOAA inhibits norepinephrine-stimulated phosphoinositide hydrolysis in rat cerebral cortex; this effect is insensitive to excitatory amino acid antagonists (52,91).

Rat cortical astrocytes in culture express a glutamate receptor activated by kainate, quisqualate, and L-BOAA (5). High concentrations of L-BOAA (IC_{50} = 2.1 mmol) are required to induce swelling, vacuolation, and death of astrocytes over a 24-h period (10). Lower concentrations (IC_{50}

= 55 μmol) increase the activity of glutamine synthetase in cortical astrocyte cultures. Increased enzyme activity (up to 155% of that in untreated cells) is enantiomer- and isomer-specific, dose-dependent, blocked by cycloheximide, but not by actinomycin D, suggesting that L-BOAA–induced regulation of glutamine synthetase synthesis occurs at the level of translation (82).

The L-BOAA plant precursor BIA and its higher homologue, α-amino-γ-(isoxazolin-5-on-2-yl) alanine (ACI), have been examined for neurotoxic potential (107). BIA is approximately 100-fold less potent than L-BOAA in vitro (107). BIA (0.5–2.0 mmol) but not ACI (2.0 mmol) produced concentration-dependent neurodegeneration in mouse cortical explants; the action of BIA was blocked by the non-NMDA receptor antagonist CNQX. BIA activates CNQX-sensitive currents that are smaller than those activated by L-BOAA or AMPA in a majority of neurons. In some neurons, BIA (2 mmol) produced currents similar in amplitude to those produced by L-BOAA (50 μmol) (107). BIA is inactive on rat brain NMDA receptors, while L-BOAA inhibits receptor binding with an IC_{50} of 4.7×10^{-5} mole (49).

Three studies have examined the interaction of L-BOAA with human brain tissue in vitro. Inhibition of ^{3}H-AMPA binding in postmortem human hippocampal membranes reveals a rank order of potency as quisqualate = AMPA > L-BOAA > L-glutamate = DNQX = CNQX > kainate > L-aspartate = NMDA. AMPA receptors in human fetal brain tissue show a comparable pharmacology (119). L-BOAA, relative to domoate (see Domoic Acid, this volume), shows very low affinity for kainate-binding sites in CA2/3-equivalent regions and higher affinity in CA1-equivalent regions of the human hippocampus (58). L-BOAA and L-glutamate are equipotent in displacing ^{3}H-AMPA binding in human hippocampus (59). L-BOAA potently inhibits AMPA binding in human cerebral cortex membranes (61).

Human Studies

The best documented evidence of a causal relationship between heavy consumption of grass pea and development of spastic paraparesis is found in the writings of Kessler (53), a victim and observer of an epidemic of lathyrism affecting approximately 800 political prisoners during World War II. On September 16, 1942, some 1200 Roumanian Jews aged 14–25 years were interned in a forced-labor camp in the Ukrainian town of Wapniarka. Inmates received daily food rations consisting of 400 g of grass pea cooked in salt water, plus 200 g of bread made from barley (80%) and chopped straw (20%). Within a couple of months, many developed muscle spasms and weakness in the legs. By the end of December 1942, spastic weakness of the legs was prominent, and some severely affected individuals were bedridden. Kessler recognized the crippling disease as lathyrism and, on January 22, 1943, managed to persuade the camp guards to stop using the neurotoxic legume to feed the prisoners, whereupon no fresh cases of lathyrism appeared. While Kessler explicitly states that dosage is the only risk factor (53), it is noteworthy that disease appeared earlier and was more widespread in those inmates who had been brought from another labor camp relative to those taken from their homes who were, one may assume, in a better state of nourishment. After the War, many victims migrated to Israel, where the clinical course of over 200 has been followed for over 50 years: All surviving patients have varying degrees of spastic paraparesis dominated by marked stiffness, mild weakness, cramps, and pathological reflexes in the legs (20,21). Analysis of the cause of death of 81 of these patients shows that 16 of 40 subjects died of malignancy, an apparently high rate that is unexplained (18).

Lathyrism is presently endemic in several regions of the world including Bangladesh, China, India, and Ethiopia (125). The epidemiology of lathyrism has been extensively studied in drought-prone areas of India and Ethiopia where the environmentally tolerant grass pea is an important and popular crop (26,36,37). In the horn of Africa, lathyrism impacts subsistence farmers who cultivate grass pea to serve as a regular component of the diet as well as an insurance crop (138,139). Production of grass pea is largely restricted to the northwest and central region of Ethiopia; in 1988–1989, the total annual production was estimated as 4100 tons cultivated on a surface of 37,800 hectares. Since L. sativus is usually consumed in spring and summer, more than 80% of cases appear in this timeframe or shortly thereafter. New cases accompany food shortages and unusually heavy reliance on grass pea. The highest prevalence of lathyrism is found in the Gojam region (7.5/1000). Lathyrism is more common among males than females (2.6:1) and is largely restricted to those under the age of 40 years. Comparable epidemiological findings have been obtained in affected areas of India and Bangladesh (26,30,70,73). The estimated prevalence of lathyrism in pockets of the disease in northwest Bangladesh approached 10% in the period 1976–1989 (41).

Lathyrism often commences suddenly but may also develop more slowly. Patients consistently report improvement and stabilization of symptoms after exposure to L. sativus has ceased (20,21,34). Factors associated with disease onset are physical work, coldness, exhaustion, malnutrition and, sometimes, fever. Historical descriptions also emphasize the association between disease onset, environmental factors (rain, wind, and cold), and sometimes the presence of fever. The older clinical descriptions also emphasize the frequent, but transitory, presence of muscle cramps, incontinence, and impotency (120). Symptoms likely referable to the limbic system (*e.g.*, cognitive deficits, mood disturbances, vivid dreams) are occasionally noted (53,59,81).

Seventeen Bangladeshi subjects were given a detailed neurological and neurophysiological examination more than 10 years after the onset of lathyrism during the famines of 1972, 1973–1974, or 1976 when more than 100,000 people were affected by the disease (70). At the time of onset in 1972, cerebrospinal fluid samples were found to be normal but all patients had mild to severe anemia, possibly indicating the presence of malnutrition (73). Typical early symptoms were weakness, heaviness, and stiffness of both legs; six patients described pain and cramps (in particular, calf muscles) of the lower extremities, and fever. Consistent with reports of others (53,81), patients stated they had initially experienced tremulousness and tremor, diffuse pain, falls, unsteadiness, paresthesias, formication and numbness, urgency of micturition, sphincteric spasms, impotency, nocturnal erection, and ejaculation. None complained of myoclonus, increased nocturnal dreaming, or impairment of short-term memory, symptoms occasionally reported by other authors (53,81). More than 10 years after onset, overt malnutrition was absent, and clinical examination revealed the presence of a stereotyped spastic paraplegia.

Lathyrism causes its victims to walk on the balls of their feet with the pelvis tilted; thigh adductor spasticity produces a characteristic scissoring gait. On the Indian subcontinent, the stage of lathyrism is crudely but usefully classified on a four-point scale of increasing physical impairment: no-stick cases (mildly affected), one-stick cases, two-stick cases (severe impairment), and crawler-stage cases, when victims are unable to move the legs and the hands are used to move the body on the rump (2). Pyramidal signs consist of brisk tendon reflexes, extensor plantar reflexes (Babinski's sign), crossed adductor responses, and ankle clonus which, in the more severely affected individuals, are associated with muscle spasms in the thigh adductor and gastrocnemius muscles. Bladder or bowel dysfunction is not present in the chronic stage of the disease. Examination of cranial nerves, the sensory system, and the cerebellum is unremarkable.

Electrophysiological studies were performed in 11 Spanish patients approximately 50 years after onset of lathyrism associated with a period of food shortage during the Spanish Civil War in the late 1930s. Magnetic cortical stimulation was used to obtain motor evoked potentials in patients and in controls (34,45,47). Central conduction times were more prolonged in severely affected individuals compared with mildly affected patients, and a correlation between the degree of motor impairment and central conduction deficits

was obtained. Deficits in pathways supplying the upper extremities were found in only one severely affected patient. These results show that pyramidal dysfunction is a major feature of human lathyrism. In longstanding lathyrism patients from Bangladesh, somatosensory evoked potentials were recorded after median and tibial nerve stimulation (45). Median nerve potentials were normal in all subjects, but cortical latencies after tibial nerve stimulation were abnormal in 3 of 13. Peripheral nerve studies were performed in Israel on former Rumanians who developed lathyrism in a German forced labor camp during World War II (*vide supra*) (19–21,25); sensorimotor neuropathy and late muscle denervation were detected in 7% of the patients. A neuropathy was also seen in a few patients examined in Spain and Bangladesh (45,47). However, there was no direct correlation between the presence of peripheral neuropathy and the degree of clinical or electrophysiological central motor deficit; this suggests that peripheral nerve disease developed independently from the neurotoxic CNS disease and is not a component of lathyrism (128). In addition, Spanish patients with longstanding disease showed neither clinical nor electrophysiological evidence of anterior horn cell involvement, an observation that failed to confirm a suggestion that lathyrism slowly progresses into a clinical picture resembling amyotrophic lateral sclerosis (19,34,45,47). Mild progression of symptomatology decades after onset was reported by 9 of 12 Spanish lathyrism patients, but their description of increased stiffness, shortening of steps, and calf muscle cramps was suggestive of slowly advancing CNS (but not lower-motor-neuron) dysfunction (34).

Neuropathological studies of human lathyrism are rare. A 1926 description reports loss and shrinkage of large pyramidal neurons in the brain (presumably the precentral gyrus) of a patient who developed lathyrism 31 years before death (28). Other studies are limited to description of spinal cord alterations (12,28,30,43,100,118,135). Lesions consist of distal and symmetrical degeneration of lateral and ventral corticospinal tracts accompanied in a number of cases by distal degeneration of spinocerebellar and gracile tracts. In a report of an individual who developed the disease 32 years before death, autopsy showed anterior horn cell changes, the presence of Hirano bodies, and diminished Nissl substance, but no loss of neurons (135). It is not possible to determine from these sparse reports whether the primary lesion is in the cell soma or the distal axon. However, if L-BOAA is the culpable agent in lathyrism, the molecular pathology of the dominant central motor pathway would be expected to be focused at the cell body or dendrites of pyramidal neurons in the motor cortex. This is supported by the observation that Betz cells in the cat are exquisitely sensitive to L-BOAA (142). Primary degeneration of cortical motor neurons supporting the longest nerve fibers in the spinal cord would give rise to a pattern of symmetrical axonal degeneration that is more apparent in caudal regions of the spinal cord.

Diagnosis and Treatment

The clinical features of lathyrism closely resemble those of hereditary spastic paraplegia. Most observers of lathyrism are impressed by the stereotypy of the clinical picture. Diagnosis is based on four criteria (53,125): (a) a history of ingestion of large amounts of a neurotoxic *Lathyrus* spp. during the weeks preceding clinical signs and symptoms; (b) the presence of a clear-cut spastic paraparesis or paraplegia; (c) the absence of other neurological signs and symptoms suggesting the presence of cerebellar, sensory, or cranial nerve dysfunction; (d) absence of clinical progression (improvement is common, especially among children) after cessation of exposure to *L. sativus*; and (e) the absence of any other cause. Minimal nutrition may be evident. Disease is not reported in patients younger than 2 years old, is more common and more severe in males than females, and may show a familial pattern. Cerebrospinal fluid from 50 Bangladeshi patients relative to 12 healthy controls showed alterations in the concentration of glutamate (281%), aspartate (71%), glycine (277%), and taurine (198%), with significant correlation between glycine level and disease duration. Levels of threonine, serine, and alanine were increased and isoleucine decreased (55).

Lathyrism (neurolathyrism) may coexist with osteolathyrism, a collagen disorder associated with ingestion of 2-cyanoethyl-isoxazolin-5-one, a compound in the green parts of *L. sativus* that chemically and metabolically can produce the osteolathyrogen β-aminopropionitrile (39,94,116). Sixty male subjects of 500 Bangladeshi lathyrism patients of both genders complained of bone pain and showed skeletal abnormalities suggestive of osteolathyrism. Two patients aged 30 and 37 years showed radiographic evidence of fusion failure of both vertebral and iliac epiphyses (39).

The differential diagnosis of lathyrism includes hereditary spastic paraplegia and cerebral palsy (Little's disease). The motor deficit of lathyrism is closely similar to that of *konzo* (125), a form of severe spastic paraparesis (with additional visual and auditory deficits) of southern and western African populations with heavy dietary dependence on the roots of *Manihot esculenta*, (see Cassava, this volume) (140). Multiple sclerosis and human T-cell lymphotropic virus type 1 (HTLV-1)-related tropical spastic paraparesis may show some clinical similarities to lathyrism. Only 4 of 415 male and 29 female Bangladeshi patients with lathyrism were seropositive for HTLV-1 (40). HTLV-1 is also uncommon in Ethiopian patients with tropical spastic parapareses that include lathyrism (1).

Treatment with a centrally acting muscle relaxant reduces the degree of spasticity associated with lathyrism (38). Incomplete surgical release of spastic thigh adductor muscles has also been employed in India.

Toxic Mechanisms

L-BOAA interferes with CNS excitatory neurotransmission (11,71,90,97,107,110,111,142). Central excitant actions of L-BOAA are responsible for the initial, reversible phase of lathyrism. Unlike the human disease, which consistently develops in the setting of severe food shortage, well-fed macaques only display the mild, reversible signs of spastic paraparesis. Evidence of a central motor disorder developed in macaques 3–10 months after an estimated daily dosage of L-BOAA 10 to 100-fold greater than the intake of L-BOAA required to induce lathyrism in poorly nourished human subjects consuming a diet of *L. sativus* for 3 months (20,21,53). While differences in L-BOAA toxicodynamics and metabolism may exist between humans and macaques, it is hypothesized that a poor nutritional state substantially modifies susceptibility by increasing transfer of amino acid across the blood-brain barrier or reducing availability of antioxidants. Additional open questions concern the potential etiological role of factors frequently associated with acute onset of human lathyrism, such as physical work, cold, and fever (70). The preferential involvement of young males (70,125) and the latency of 2–3 months consistently observed before disease onset are also unexplained features of the human disease. Widespread L-BOAA excitation of glutamatergic receptors presumably accounts for the reversible neurological manifestations (myoclonus, tremor, global muscle spasm, and involuntary voiding) of the prodromal phase of the disease.

Onset of irreversible weakness probably corresponds with L-BOAA–induced excitotoxic degeneration of those neurons (Betz cells supplying lower limbs?) that are most sensitive to this plant amino acid (125). If L-BOAA is injected systemically into newborn mice, lesions are restricted to regions unprotected by the blood-brain barrier, such as the retina and the area postrema (90). Damage can be prevented by the administration of antagonists to non-NMDA glutamate receptor subtypes (110,111). Electrophysiological recordings confirm these morphological and pharmacological studies (3,11,71,97,107) and further demonstrate that L-BOAA is an agonist at the AMPA glutamate receptor subtype. Binding studies are also consistent, since they show that L-BOAA preferentially binds to AMPA receptors in rat brain (11,109). Based on these studies, the major mechanism of L-BOAA toxicity is likely to be excitotoxicity mediated by AMPA receptors. Overstimulation of these receptors would result in a cellular influx of Na^+ and Cl^- ions, and water; direct Ca^{2+} influx and indirect intracellular Ca^{2+} accumulation by progressive failure of ion pumps would follow and activate a cascade of events that eventuate in cell degeneration. It is presently unknown whether the effects of comparatively large concentrations of L-BOAA on high-affinity glutamate transport (108), glial glutamine synthetase (82), astrocytes (10), kainate receptors (11), and presynaptic glutamate release (31), are of any relevance in the pathogenesis of the human and animal diseases.

Three additional mechanisms of L-BOAA neurotoxicity have been proposed:

1. L-BOAA is reported to inhibit the enzyme activity of NADH dehydrogenase (part of mitochondrial complex I) in mouse brain slices; in mouse brain mitochondria, picomolar concentrations of L-BOAA reportedly inhibit NADH dehydrogenase, a part of mitochondrial complex I (92,93). An attempt to replicate these findings was unsuccessful (117).
2. L-BOAA toxicity in rat hippocampus is partly blocked by scavengers of free radicals (144). Since neuroprotection by scavengers of free radicals is restricted to the action of L-BOAA, with no effect on AMPA neurotoxicity, there must be an additional mechanism of neurotoxicity peculiar to L-BOAA.
3. L-BOAA kills ventral spinal cord motoneuron hybrid cells lacking non-NMDA receptors (62). Cell death develops after 36–48 h and is not influenced by antagonists of non-NMDA glutamate receptor subtypes. Lesioned cell concentration dependently show morphological criteria suggestive of apoptosis, and cysteine (1 mmol) prevents cell death. This is consistent with the observation that L-BOAA is neurotoxic in immature primary cultures and also inhibits the cystine/glutamate antiporter in this system (85). Protection experiments show that tocopherol partially blocks L-BOAA neurotoxicity suggesting that free radicals play a potential role in toxicity (62). In summary, it is suggested that, in these motorneuron hybrid cells, the neurotoxic action of L-BOAA is associated with an apoptotic mechanism that may be mediated by a block of the cystine/glutamate antiporter (62).

Editors' Note: A comparative study of the metabolism of ^{14}C-radiolabeled BOAA species shows that the amino acid undergoes incomplete oxidation leading to the formation of CO_2 and oxalate. After oral administration of 1,2,3-^{14}C-BOAA, radioactivity appeared in expired CO_2 within 8 hours in amounts of 16% (mouse), 3% (rat), and <2% (chick). Since detectable amounts of BOAA do not appear in the urine of humans consuming *Lathyrus sativus* or after oral ingestion of BOAA, the authors suggest a similar but more efficient metabolic pathway may exist in humans (52).

REFERENCES

1. Abebe M, Haimanot RT, Gustafsson A *et al.* (1991) Low HTLV-1 seroprevalence in endemic tropical spastic paraparesis in Ethiopia. *Trans Roy Soc Trop Med Hyg* **85**, 109.
2. Acton WH (1922) An investigation into the causation of lathyrism in man. *Ind Med Gaz* **57**, 241.
3. Allen CN, Ross SM, Spencer PS (1990) Properties of the neurotoxic amino acids β-N-methylamino-L-alanine (BMAA) and β-N-oxalylamino-L-alanine (BOAA). In: *ALS: New Advances in Toxicology and Epidemiology.* Ross FC, Norris FH eds. Smith-Gordon, London p. 49.
4. Andersson H, Lundqvist E, Olson L (1997) Plant-derived amino acids increase hippocampal BDNF, NGF, c-fos and hsp70 mRNAs. *NeuroReport* **8**, 1813.
5. Backus KH, Kettenmann H, Scahchner M (1989) Pharmacological characterization of the glutamate receptor in cultured astrocytes. *J Neurosci Res* **22**, 274.
6. Barrow MV, Simpson CF, Miller EJ (1974) Lathyrism: A review. *Quart Rev Biol* **49**, 101.
7. Bell EA, O'Donovan JP (1966) The isolation of α- and γ-oxalyl derivatives of diamino butyric acid from seeds of *Lathyrus latifolius*, and the detection of the α-oxalyl isomer of the neurotoxic α-amino-β-oxalyl-aminopropionic acid which ocuurs with the neurotoxin in this and other species. *Phytochemistry* **5**, 1211.
8. Bourlier A (1882) Le lathyrisme. *Gaz Med Algerie* **17**, 139.
9. Bridges RJ, Hatalski C, Shim SN, Nunn PB (1991) Gliotoxic properties of the *Lathyrus* excitotoxin β-N-oxalyl-L-α,β-diaminopropionic acid-(β-L-ODAP). *Brain Res* **561**, 262.
10. Bridges RJ, Kadri MM, Monaghan DT *et al.* (1988) Inhibition of ^{3}H-α-amino-3-hydroxy-5-methyl-4-isoxazolepropionic acid binding by the excitotoxin β-N-oxalyl-L-α,β-diaminopropionic acid. *Eur J Pharmacol* **145**, 357.
11. Bridges RJ, Stevens DR, Kahle JS *et al.* (1989) Structure-function studies on N-oxalyl-diamino-dicarboxylic acids and excitatory amino acid receptors: Evidence that L-ODAP is a selective non-NMDA agonist. *J Neurosci* **9**, 2073.
12. Buzzard EF, Greenfield JG (1921) *Pathology of the Nervous System.* Constable, London p. 232.
13. Cantani A (1873) Latirismo (Lathyrismus) illustrata de tre casa clinici. *Il Morgagni* **15**, 745.
14. Chase RA, Pearson SA, Nunn PB, Lantos PL (1985) Comparative toxicities of α- and β-N-oxalyl-L-α,β-diaminopropionic acids to rat spinal cord. *Neurosci Lett* **55**, 89.
15. Che JT, Zhang JT, Qu ZQ (1996) Protective effect of

tetrandrine on neuronal injury in cultured cortical neurons of rats. *Yao Hsueh Hsueh Pao* **31**, 161. [In Chinese]

16. Cheema PS, Malathi K, Padmanaban G, Sarma PS (1969) The neurotoxicity of β-N-oxalyl-α,β-diaminopropionic acid, the neurotoxin from the pulse *Lathyrus sativus*. *Biochem J* **112**, 29.

17. Cheema PS, Padmanaban G, Sarma PS (1971) Transamination of β-N-oxalyl-α,β-diaminopropionic acid, the *Lathyrus sativus* neurotoxin, in tissues of rat. *Ind J Biochem Biophys* **8**, 16.

18. Cohn DF (1994) Does neurolathyrism affect longevity? In: *Nutrition, Neurotoxins, and Lathyrism. The ODAP Challenge.* Abegaz BA, Tekle-Haimanot R, Palmer VS, Spencer PS eds. Third World Medical Research Foundation, New York p. 33.

19. Cohn DF, Streifler M (1977) Das motorische Neuron im chronischen Lathyrismus. *Nervenarzt* **48**, 127.

20. Cohn DF, Streifler M (1981) Human neurolathyrism, a follow-up study of 200 patients. Part I. Clinical investigation. *Schweiz Arch Neurol Neurochir Psychiat* **128**, 151.

21. Cohn DF, Streifler M (1981) Human neurolathyrism, a follow-up study. Part II. *Schweiz Arch Neurol Neurochir Psychiatr* **128**, 157.

22. Czarda (1876) Über Lathyrismus. Nach einem klinischen Vortrage des Prof. Cantani in Neapel. *Prag Med Wochenschr* **23, 24**, 442, 459.

23. De Bruyn A, van Haver D, Lambein F (1993) Chemical properties of the natural neurotoxin of *Lathyrus sativus* 3-N-oxalyl-2,3-diamino-propanoic acid (β-ODAP), its nontoxic 2-N-oxalyl isomer, and its hydrolysis product 2,3-diamino-propanoic acid by (DAPRO) by ^{1}H and ^{13}C-NMR spectroscopy. *Nat Toxins* **1**, 328.

24. Desparanches T (1829) Le lathyrisme. *Bull Sci Med* **18**, 433.

25. Drory VE, Rabey MJ, Cohn DF (1992) Electrophysiological features in patients with chronic neurolathyrism. *Acta Neurol Scand* **85**, 401.

26. Dwivedi MP (1989) Epidemiological aspects of lathyrism in India—a changing scenario. In: *The Grass Pea: Threat and Promise.* Spencer PS ed. Third World Medical Research Foundation, New York p. 1.

27. Faust C (1947) Drei Fälle von Lathyrismus. *Dtsch Med Wochenschr* **12**, 122.

28. Filimonoff IN (1926) Zur pathologisch-anatomischen Charakteristik des Lathyrismus. *Z Ges Neurol Psychiatr* **105**, 76.

29. Fumorala G, Zanelli CF (1914) Anatomisch-experimentelle Forschungen über den Lathyrismus. *Arch Psychiatr* **54**, 489.

30. Ganapathy KT, Dwivedi MP (1961) *Studies on the Clinical Epidemiology of Lathyrism.* Indian Council of Medical Research, Gandhi Memorial Hospital, Lathyrism Enquiry Field Unit, Rewa, MP.

31. Gannon RL, Terrian DM (1989) L-BOAA selectively enhances L-glutamate release from guinea pig hippocampal mossy fiber synaptosomes. *Neurosci Lett* **107**, 289.

32. Gardner AF, Sakiewicz N (1963) A review of neurolathyrism including the Russian and Polish literature. *Exp Med Surg* **21**, 164.

33. Gebre-Ab T, Gabriel ZQ, Maffi M *et al.* (1978) Neurolathyrism: A review and a report of an epidemic. *Ethiop Med J* **16**, 1.

34. Giménez-Roldán S, Ludolph AC, Hugon J *et al.* (1994) Lathyrism in Spain: Progressive central deficits in lathyrism patients more than 45 years after onset. In: *Nutrition, Neurotoxins, and Lathyrism: The ODAP Challenge.* Abegaz BA, Tekle-Haimanot R, Palmer VS, Spencer PS eds. Third World Medical Research Foundation, New York p. 10.

35. Goltzinger H (1897) *Du lathyrisme en Abissinie.* Clinique Neuropathie de St. Pétersbourg.

36. Haimanot RT, Kidane Y, Wuhib E *et al.* (1993) The epidemiology of lathyrism in north and central Ethiopia. *Ethiop Med J* **31**, 15.

37. Haimanot RT, Kidane Y, Wuhib E *et al.* (1993) The epidemiology of lathyrism in Ethiopia. In: *Nutrition, Neurotoxins, and Lathyrism: The ODAP Challenge.* Abegaz BA, Tekle-Haimanot R, Palmer VS, Spencer PS eds. Third World Medical Research Foundation, New York p. 1.

38. Haque A, Hossain M, Khan JK *et al.* (1994) New findings and symptomatic treatment for neurolathyrism, a motor neuron disease occurring in north west Bangladesh. *Paraplegia* **32**, 193.

39. Haque A, Hossain M, Lambein F, Bell EA (1997) Evidence of osteolathyrism among patients suffering from neurolathyrism in Bangladesh. *Nat Toxins* **5**, 43.

40. Haque A, Khan JK, Wouters G *et al.* (1995) Study of HTLV-I antibodies in CSF and serum of neurolathyrism patients in Bangladesh. *Ann Soc Belg Med Trop* **75**, 131.

41. Haque A, Mannan MA (1989) The problem of lathyrism in Bangladesh. In: *The Grass Pea: Threat and Promise.* Spencer PS ed. Third World Medical Research Foundation, New York p. 27.

42. Hippocrates (1846) *On Epidemics, Vol 5. Book 2. Section IV, 3rd Ed.* Littre F ed. Paris p. 126.

43. Hirano A, Llena JJ, Streifler M, Cohn DF (1976) Anterior horn cell changes in a case of neurolathyrism. *Acta Neuropathol* **35**, 277.

44. Huber JC (1886) Historische Notizen über den Lathyrismus. *Friedreich's Blätter für Gerichtliche Medizin* **1**, 34.

45. Hugon J, Ludolph AC, Giménez-Roldán S *et al.* (1990) Electrophysiological evaluation of human lathyrism: Results in Bangladesh and Spain. In: *ALS: New Advances in Toxicology and Epidemiology.* Rose FC, Norris FH eds. Smith-Gordon, London p. 49.

46. Hugon J, Ludolph AC, Roy DN *et al.* (1988) Studies on the etiology and pathogenesis of motor neuron diseases. II. Clinical and electrophysiological features of pyramidal

dysfunction in macaques fed *Lathyrus sativus* and IDPN. *Neurology* **38**, 435.

47. Hugon J, Ludolph AC, Spencer PS *et al.* (1993) Studies on the etiology and pathogenesis of motor neuron diseases. III. Magnetic cortical stimulation in patients with lathyrism. *Acta Neurol Scand* **88**, 412.

48. Ikegami F, Itagaki S, Ishikawa T *et al.* (1991) Biosynthesis of β-(isoxazolin-5-on-2-yl)alanine, the precursor of the neurotoxic amino acid β-N-oxalyl-L-α,β-diaminopropionic acid. *Chem Pharm Bull (Tokyo)* **39**, 3376.

49. Ikegami F, Kusama-Eguchi K, Sugiyama E *et al.* (1995) Interaction of some plant heterocyclic β-substituted alanines with rat brain N-methyl-D-aspartate (NMDA) receptors. *Biol Pharm Bull* **18**, 360.

50. Jahan K, Ahmad K (1993) Studies on neurolathyrism. *Environ Res* **60**, 259.

51. Jiminez Dias C, Roda E, Ortiz de Landaruzi E *et al.* (1942) Investigations sobre el latirismo. II. El cuadro clinco. *Rev Clin Esp* **5**, 168.

52. Jyothi P, Rudra MP, Rao SLN (1998) *In vivo* metabolism of β-N-oxalyl-L-α,β-diaminopropionic acid: the *Lathyrus sativus* neurotoxin in experimental animals. *Nat Toxins* **6**, 189.

53. Kessler A (1947) Lathyrismus. *Monatsschr Psychiatr Neurol* **113**, 345.

54. Khan JK, Kebede N, Kuo Y-H *et al.* (1993) Analysis of neurotoxin β-ODAP and its α-isomer by precolumn derivatization with phenylisothiocyanate. *Anal Biochem* **208**, 237.

55. Khan JK, Kuo YH, Haque A, Lambein F (1995) Inhibitory and excitatory amino acids in cerebrospinal fluid of neurolathyrism patients, a highly prevalent motorneurone disease. *Acta Neurol Scand* **91**, 506.

56. Kirk K (1861) On the injurious effects arising from the use of the leguminous seed, common in India as articles of food. *Ind Ann Med Sci* **7**, 144.

57. Kisby G, Roy DN, Spencer (1989) A sensitive HPLC method for the detection of β-N-oxalylamino-L-alanine in *Lathyrus sativus* and animal tissue. In: *The Grass Pea: Threat and Promise*. Spencer PS ed. Third World Medical Research Foundation, New York p. 133.

58. Künig G, Hartmann J, Krause F *et al.* (1995) Regional differences in the interaction of the excitotoxins domoate and L-β-oxalyl-amino-alanine with ³H-kainate binding sites in human hippocampus. *Neurosci Lett* **187**, 107.

59. Künig G, Hartmann J, Niedermeyer B *et al.* (1994) Excitotoxins L-β-oxalyl-amino-L-alanine (L-BOAA) and 3,4,6-trihydroxyphenylalanin (6-OH-DOPA) inhibit ³H-α-amino-3-hydroxy-5-methyl-4-isoxazole-propionic acid (AMPA) binding in human hippocampus. *Neurosci Lett* **169**, 219.

60. Kuo Y-H, Lambein F (1991) Biosynthesis of the neurotoxin β-N-oxalyl-α,β-diaminopropionic acid in callus tissue of *Lathyrus sativus*. *Phytochemistry* **30**, 3241.

61. Kurumaji A, Ishimaru M, Toru M (1992) α-³H-Amino-3-hydroxy-5-methylisoxazol propionic acid binding in human cerebral cortical membranes: Minimal changes in postmortem brains of chronic schizophrenics. *J Neurochem* **59**, 829.

62. La Bella V, Alexianu ME, Colom LV *et al.* (1996) Apoptosis induced by β-N-oxalylamino-L-alanine on a motoneuron hybrid cell line. *Neuroscience* **70**, 1039.

63. La Bella V, Brighina F, Piccoli F, Guarneri R (1993) Effect of β-N-oxalylamino-L-alanine on cerebellar cGMP level *in vivo*. *Neurochem Res* **18**, 171.

64. La Bella V, Guarneri R, Piccoli F (1993) Effect of chronic oral intake of *Lathyrus sativus* extract containing β-N-oxalyl-amino-L-alanine, on ³H-glutamate binding in different areas of rat brain. *Neurodegeneration* **2**, 253.

65. La Bella V, Rizza ML, Alfano F, Piccoli F (1997) Dietary consumption of *Lathyrus sativus* seeds induces behavioral changes in the rat. *Environ Res* **74**, 61.

66. Lambein F, Haque R, Khan JK *et al.* (1994) From soil to brain: Zinc deficiency increases the neurotoxicity of *Lathyrus sativus* and may affect the susceptibility for the motorneurone disease neurolathyrism. *Toxicon* **32**, 461.

67. Leather J and Sons (1885) *Lathyrus* poisoning in horses. *Vet J Ann Comp Pathol* **20**, 233.

68. Lindstrom H, Luthman J, Mouton P *et al.* (1990) Plant-derived neurotoxic amino acids (β-N-oxalyl-amino-L-alanine and β-N-methylamino-L-alanine): Effects on central monoamine neurons. *J Neurochem* **55**, 941.

69. Long YC, Ye YH, Xing QY (1996) Studies on the neuroexcitotoxin β-N-oxalo-L-α,β-diaminopropionic acid and its isomer α-N-oxalo-L-α,β-diaminopropionic acid from the root of *Panax* species. *Int J Pept Protein Res* **47**, 42.

70. Ludolph AC, Hugon J, Dwivedi MP *et al.* (1987) Studies on the aetiology and pathogenesis of motor neuron diseases. I. Lathyrism: Clinical findings in established cases. *Brain* **110**, 149.

71. MacDonald JF, Morris ME (1984) Lathyrus excitotoxins: Mechanism of neuronal excitation by L-2-oxalylamino-3-amino- and L-3-oxalylamino-2-amino-propionic acid. *Exp Brain Res* **57**, 158.

72. Maione S, Berrino L, Leyva J *et al.* (1995) Behavioral effects induced by microinjection of L-BOAA into the ventrolateral PAG matter of the mouse. *Pharmacol Biochem Behav* **50**, 453.

73. Mannan MA (1985) Lathyrism. *Bangladesh J Neurosci* **1**, 5.

74. Marie P (1883) Des manifestations médullaires de l'Ergotisme et du Lathyrisme. *Le Progrès Médical*. Tom XI, 84.

75. McCall (1886) Notes of two lectures of poisoning of horses by *L. sativus*. *Veterinarian, London* **59**, 789.

76. McCarrisson R, Krishman BG (1934) Lathyrism in the rat. *Ind J Med Res* **22**, 65.

77. Mehta T, Parker AJ, Cusick PK *et al.* (1980) The *Lathyrus sativus* neurotoxin: Evidence of selective retention in monkey tissue. *Toxicol Appl Pharmacol* **52**, 54.

78. Mehta T, Parker AJ, Cusick PK *et al.* (1983) The *Lathyrus sativus* neurotoxin: Resistance of the squirrel monkey to prolonged oral high doses. *Toxicol Appl Pharmacol* **69**, 480.

79. Mehta T, Zarghami NS, Cusick PK *et al.* (1976) Tissue distribution and metabolism of *Lathyrus sativus* neurotoxin, L-3-oxalylamino-2-aminopropionic acid, in the squirrel monkey. *J Neurochem* **27**, 1327.

80. Mehta T, Zarghami NS, Parker AJ *et al.* (1979) Neurotoxicity of orally or intraperitoneally administered L-3-oxalylamino-2-aminopropionic acid in the mouse. *Toxicol Appl Pharmacol* **48**, 1.

81. Mertens HG (1947) Zur Klinik des Lathyrismus. *Nervenarzt* **18**, 493.

82. Miller S, Nunn PB, Bridges RI (1993) Induction of astrocyte glutamine synthetase activity by the *Lathyrus* toxin β-N-oxalyl-L-α,β-diaminopropionic acid (β-L-ODAP). *Glia* **7**, 329.

83. Mingazzini G, Buglioni GB (1896) Studio clinico col anatomico sul laterismo. *Riv Sper Freniatr Med Leg* **XL**, 79.

84. Mirto D (1897) Sulle alterazioni degli elementi nevrosi nel latirismo sperimentale acuto. *Pisani, Palermo* **18**, 109.

85. Murphy TH, Schuarr PL, Coyle JT (1990) Immature cortical neurons are uniquely sensitive to glutamate toxicity by inhibition of cystine uptake. *Fed Amer Soc Exp Biol* **4**, 1624.

86. Murti VVS, Seshadri TR, Venkitasubramanian TA (1964) Neurotoxic compounds of the seeds of *Lathyrus sativus*. *Phytochemistry* **3**, 73.

87. Nunn PB, Seelig M, Zagoren JC, Spencer PS (1987) Stereospecific acute neuronotoxicity of "uncommon" plant amino acids linked to human motor-system diseases. *Brain Res* **410**, 375.

88. Olney JW (1980) Excitotoxic mechanisms of neurotoxicity. In: *Experimental and Clinical Neurotoxicology*. Spencer PS, Schaumburg HH eds. Williams & Wilkins, Baltimore p. 272.

89. Olney JW (1994) Excitotoxins in food. *Neurotoxicology* **3**, 535.

90. Olney JW, Misra CH, Rhee V (1976) Brain and retinal damage from *Lathyrus* excitotoxin, β-N-oxalyl-L-α,β-diaminopropionic acid. *Nature* **264**, 659.

91. Ormandy GC, Jope RS (1990) Inhibition of phosphoinositide hydrolysis by the novel neurotoxin β-N-oxalyl-L-α,β-diaminopropionic acid (L-BOAA). *Brain Res* **510**, 53.

92. Pai KS, Ravindranath V (1993) L-BOAA induces selective inhibition of brain mitochondrial enzyme, NADH-dehydrogenase. *Brain Res* **621**, 215.

93. Pai KS, Shankar SK, Ravindranath V (1993) Billion-fold-difference in the toxic properties of the two excitatory amino acids, L-BOAA and L-BMAA: Biochemical and morphological studies using mouse brain slices. *Neurosci Res* **17**, 241.

94. Paissios CS, Demopoulos T (1962) Human lathyrism. A clinical and skeletal study. *Clin Orthop Relat Res* **23**, 236.

95. Pan M, Mabry TJ, Cao P, Moini M (1997) Identification of nonprotein amino acids from cycad seeds as N-ethyoxycarbonyl ethyl ester derivatives by positive chemical-ionization gas chromatography-mass spectrometry. *J Chromatogr* **787**, 288.

96. Parker AJ, Mehta T, Zarghami NB *et al.* (1979) Acute neurotoxicity of the *Lathyrus sativus* neurotoxin, L-3-oxalyl-2-amino-propionic acid in the squirrel monkey. *Toxicol Appl Pharmacol* **47**, 135.

97. Pearson S, Nunn PB (1981) The neurolathyrogen β-N-oxalyl-L-α,β-diaminopropionic acid is a potent agonist at "glutamate preferring" receptors in the frog spinal cord. *Brain Res* **206**, 178.

98. Philips CG, Porter R (1977) *Corticospinal Neurons: Their Role in Movement*. Academic Press, London.

99. Proust A (1883) Du lathyrisme medullaire spasmodique. *Bull Acad Med* **12**, 829.

100. Puig JS, Devinals RR (1943) Aportacion a la anatomia patologica del latirismo. *Rev Clin Esp* **8**, 107.

101. Rao SLN (1975) Chemical synthesis of β-N-oxalyl-L-α,β-diaminopropionic acid and optical specificity in its neurotoxic action. *Biochem J* **14**, 5218.

102. Rao SLN (1978) A sensitive and specific calorimetric method for the determination of α,β-diaminopropionic acid and the *Lathyrus sativus* neurotoxin. *Anal Biochem* **86**, 386.

103. Rao SLN (1978) Entry of β-N-oxalyl-L-α,β-diaminopropionic acid into the central nervous system of the adult rat, chick, and rhesus monkey. *J Neurochem* **30**, 1467.

104. Rao SLN, Adiga PR, Sarma PS (1964) The isolation and characterization of β-N-α,β-diaminopropionic acid: a neurotoxin from the seeds of *Lathyrus sativus*. *Biochem J* **3**, 432.

105. Rao SLN, Sarma PS (1967) Neurotoxic action of β-N-oxalyl-α,β-diaminopropionic acid. *Biochem Pharmacol* **16**, 218.

106. Rao SLN, Sarma PS, Mani KS *et al.* (1967) Experimental neurolathyrism in monkeys. *Nature* **214**, 610.

107. Riepe M, Spencer PS, Lambein F *et al.* (1995) *In vitro* toxicological investigations of isoxazolinone amino acids of *Lathyrus sativus*. *Nat Toxins* **3**, 58.

108. Ross SM, Roy DN, Spencer PS (1985) β-N-Oxalylamino-L-alanine: Action on high-affinity transport of neurotransmitters in rat brain and spinal cord synaptosomes. *J Neurochem* **44**, 886.

109. Ross SM, Roy DN, Spencer PS (1989) β-N-Oxalylamino-L-alanine: Action on glutamate receptors. *J Neurochem* **53**, 710.

110. Ross SM, Seelig M, Spencer PS (1987) Specific antagonism of excitotoxic action of "uncommon" amino acids assayed in organotypic mouse cortical cultures. *Brain Res* **425**, 120.

111. Ross SM, Spencer PS (1987) Specific antagonism of behavioral action of "uncommon" amino acids linked to motor-system diseases. *Synapse* **1**, 248.

112. Roy DN (1969) Biosynthesis of β-(N)-oxalylaminoalanine: Evidence that serine is not the precursor. *Ind J Biochem* **6**, 147.

113. Roy DN (1973) Effect of oral administration of β-(N)-oxalylamino-L-alanine (BOAA) with or without *Lathyrus sativus* trypsin inhibitor (LS-TI) in chicks. *Environ Physiol Biochem* **3**, 192.

114. Roy DN, Nagarajan V, Gopalan C (1963) Production of neurolathyrism in chicks by the injection of *L. sativus* concentrates. *Curr Sci (India)* **3**, 116.

115. Roy DN, Narasinga Rao BS (1968) Distribution of α- and β-isomers of N-oxalyl-α,β-diaminopropionic acid in some Indian varieties of *Lathyrus sativus*. *Curr Sci (India)* **14**, 395.

116. Roy DN, Spencer PS (1989) Lathyrogens. In: *Toxicants of Plant Origin. Vol III. Proteins and Amino Acids.* Cheeke PR ed. CRC Press, Boca Raton, Florida p. 169.

117. Sabri MI, Lystrup B, Roy DN, Spencer PS (1995) Action of β-N-oxalylamino-L-alanine on mouse brain NADH-dehydrogenase activity. *J Neurochem* **65**, 1842.

118. Sachdev S, Sachdev JC, Puri D, Devinder P (1969) Morphological study in a case of lathyrism. *J Indian Med Assoc* **52**, 320.

119. Sawutz DG, Krafte DS, Oleynek JJ, Ault B (1995) AMPA (amino-3-hydroxy-5-methylisoxazole-4-propionic acid) receptors in human brain tissue. *J Recept Signal Transduct Res* **15**, 829.

120. Schuchardt B (1887) Zur Geschichte und Kasuistik des Lathyrismus. *Dtsch Arch Klin Med* **40**, 312.

121. Selye H (1957) Lathyrism. *Rev Can Biol* **16**, 1.

122. Sharan RK (1973) Experimental neurolathyrism in chicks. *Paraplegia* **10**, 249.

123. Shasi Vardhan K, Pratap Rudra MP, Rao SI (1997) Inhibition of tyrosine aminotransferase by β-N-oxalyl-L-α,β-diaminopropionic acid, the *Lathyrus sativus* neurotoxin. *J Neurochem* **68**, 2477.

124. Spencer PS (1994) Lathyrism. In: *Handbook of Clinical Neurology 65. Intoxications of the Nervous System, Part II.* Vinken PJ, Bruyn GW eds. Elsevier, North Holland p. 1.

125. Spencer PS (1999) Food toxins, AMPA receptors, and motor neuron diseases. *Drug Metab Rev* **31**, 561.

126. Spencer PS, Roy DN, Ludolph A *et al.* (1986) Lathyrism: Evidence for role of the neuroexcitatory amino acid BOAA. *Lancet* **ii**, 1066.

127. Spencer PS, Roy DN, Ludolph AC *et al.* (1988) Primate model of lathyrism: A human pyramidal disorder. In: *Neurodegenerative Disorders: The Role Played by Endotoxins and Xenobiotics.* Nappi G, Hornykiewicz L, Fariello R eds. Raven Press, New York p. 233.

128. Spencer PS, Schaumburg HH (1983) Lathyrism: A neurotoxic disease. *Neurobehav Toxicol Teratol* **5**, 625.

129. Spencer PS, Schaumburg HH, Cohn DF, Seth PK (1984) Lathyrism: A useful model of primary lateral sclerosis. In: *Research Progress in Motor Neurone Disease.* Rose FC ed. Pitman, London p. 312.

130. Spirtoff I (1903) Changes in the spinal cord and brain cells under the influence of poisoning by *Lathyrus*. *Obozr Psichiat Nevrol* **8**, 675.

131. Srinivasa Rao P, Roy DN (1981) Effect of administration of *Lathyrus sativus* extract on lipid composition of nervous tissue of monkey. *Baroda J Nutr* **8**, 36.

132. Staton PC, Bristow DR (1997) The dietary excitotoxins β-N-methylamino-L-alanine and β-N-oxalylamino-L-alanine induce necrotic- and apoptotic-like death of cerebellar granule cells. *J Neurochem* **69**, 1508.

133. Stockman R (1917) Lathyrism. *Edinburgh Med J* **19**, 277.

134. Stockman R (1929) Lathyrism. *J Pharmacol Exp Ther* **37**, 43.

135. Streifler M, Cohn DF, Hirano A, Schujman E (1977) The central nervous system in a case of neurolathyrism. *Neurology* **27**, 1176.

136. Strümpell (1884) Über die Ursachen der Erkrankungen des Nervensystems. Antrittsvorlesung. Leipzig, Vogel p. 13.

137. Sugg RS, Simms BT, Baker KG (1944) Studies of toxicity of winter peas (*Lathyrus hirsatus*) for cattle. *Vet Med* **39**, 308.

138. Tekle-Haimanot R, Kidane Y, Wuhib E *et al.* (1990) Lathyrism in rural northwestern Ethiopia: A highly prevalent neurotoxic disorder. *Int J Epidemiol* **19**, 664.

139. Tekle-Haimanot R, Kidane Y, Wuhib E *et al.* (1993) The epidemiology of lathyrism in North and Central Ethiopia. *J Ethiop Med* **31**, 15.

140. Tyleskär T, Rwiza HT, Banea M *et al.* (1994) Similarities between konzo and lathyrism suggest a common pathogenetic mechanism. In: *Nutrition, Neurotoxins, and Lathyrism: The ODAP Challenge.* Abegaz BA, Tekle-Haimanot R, Palmer VS, Spencer PS eds. Third World Medical Research Foundation, New York p. 26.

141. Visco S (1924) Exclusive and prolonged feeding of rats with *Lathyrus sativus*. *Arch Farmacol Sper* **37**, 269.

142. Watkins JC, Curtis DR, Biscoe TE (1966) Central effects of β-N-oxalyl-α,β-diaminopropionic acid and other *Lathyrus* factors. *Nature* **211**, 637.

143. Weiss JH, Koh JH, Choi DW (1989) Neurotoxicity of β-N-methylamino-L-alanine (BMAA) and β-N-oxalyl-amino-L-alanine (BOAA) on cultured cortical neurons. *Brain Res* **497**, 64.

144. Willis CL, Meldrum BS, Nunn PB *et al.* (1994) Neuroprotective effect of free radical scavengers on β-N-oxalyl-amino-L-alanine (BOAA)-induced neuronal damage in rat hippocampus. *Neurosci Lett* **182**, 159.

145. Willis CL, Meldrum BS, Nunn PB *et al.* (1994) Neuronal damage induced by β-N-oxalylamino-L-alanine, in the rat hippocampus, can be prevented by a non-NMDA antagonist, 2,3-dihydroxy-6-nitro-7-sulfamoyl-benzo(F) quinoxaline. *Brain Res* **627,** 55.
146. Zeevalk GD, Nicklas WJ (1989) Acute excitotoxicity in

chick retina caused by the unusual amino acids BOAA and BMAA: Effects of MK-801 and kynurenate. *Neurosci Lett* **102,** 284.
147. Zeevalk GD, Nicklas WJ (1994) Nitric acid in retina: Relation to excitatory amino acids and excitotoxicity. *Exp Eye Res* **58,** 343.

Oxotremorine

Albert C. Ludolph
Peter S. Spencer

OXOTREMORINE
$C_{12}H_{18}N_2O$

1-[4-(1-Pyrrolidinyl)-2-butynyl]-2-pyrrolidinone

NEUROTOXICITY RATING

Clinical

B   Psychobiological reaction (anxiety, depression)

Experimental

A   CNS muscarinic receptor activation (notably M2)

Oxotremorine is a synthetic, nonselective muscarinic agonist that (a) stimulates G-protein-coupled production of inositol 1,4,5-triphosphate resulting from activation of phospholipase C and (b) inhibits activated adenylate cyclase, resulting in decreased cyclic adenosine monophosphate production. The drug's effects are attenuated in mice with genetic deletion of the M2 muscarinic receptor, which regulates cardiac function and mediates muscarinic-dependent movement, temperature control, and analgesia (2).

Derivatives of oxotremorine have been used to probe muscarinic receptor function (3,5). Slight structural modification reduces affinity for the cholinergic system. For example, phenyl-substituted analogs of oxotremorine are devoid of intrinsic muscarinic activity but behave as competitive muscarinic antagonists (4). They have less or similar affinity for the receptor compared with corresponding methyl-substituted analogs, but display approximately one-tenth the antimuscarinic potency of methyl-substituted compounds (4).

After short-term application of oxotremorine intracerebroventricularly (ED_{50}, 0.03–0.3 μmol/kg) or subcutaneously (ED_{50}, 0.2–1.0 μmol/kg), mice develop tremor and

akinesia (M2-mediated), salivation (*via* M3), and hypothermia (largely *via* M2) within 10–40 min (2,6) . Tremor is likely exclusively caused by activation of central muscarinic receptors, whereas hypothermia and salivation are consequences of both activation of peripheral (parasympathetic) nerves and central cholinergic receptors (6). Subcutaneous treatment of mice with 0.5 mg/kg body weight oxotremorine for 6 days causes loss of muscarinic receptors, development of tolerance, and temporary impairment of spatial learning (7). In an attempt to ameliorate memory loss in Alzheimer's disease with oral oxotremorine (0.25–2.0 mg/kg body weight), five of seven patients developed severe depression and two others (on a lower dose) reported anxiety. The symptoms were so severe that the cognitive status could not be assessed; the study was discontinued (1).

REFERENCES

1. Davis KL, Hollander E, Davidson M *et al.* (1987) Induction of depression with oxotremorine in patients with Alzheimer's disease. *Amer J Psychiat* **144,** 468.
2. Gomeza J, Shannon H, Kostenis E *et al.* (1999) Pronounced pharmacologic deficits in M2 muscarinic acetylcholine receptor knockout mice. *Proc Natl Acad Sci USA* **96,** 1692.
3. Messer WS Jr, Ngur DO, Abuh YF *et al.* (1992) Stereoselective binding and activity of oxotremorine analogs at muscarinic receptors in the brain. *Chirality* **4,** 463.
4. Nilsson BM, Vargas HM, Ringdahl B, Hacksell U (1992) Phenyl-substituted analogues of oxotremorine as muscarinic antagonists. *J Med Chem* **35,** 285.
5. Ringdahl B, Jenden DJ (1983) Pharmacological properties of oxotremorine and its analogs. *Life Sci* **32,** 2401.
6. Sanchez C, Meier E (1993) Central and peripheral mediation of hypothermia, tremor and salivation induced by muscarinic agonists in mice. *Pharmacol Toxicol* **72,** 262.
7. Wehner JM, Upchurch M (1989) The effects of chronic oxotremorine treatment on spatial learning and tolerance development in mice. *Pharmacol Biochem Behav* **32,** 543.

Oxybate

Peter S. Spencer

4-Hydroxybutanoic acid; γ-Hydroxybutyric acid; GHB

NEUROTOXICITY RATING

Clinical

A Acute encephalopathy (sedation)

A Seizure disorder (myoclonus)

Oxybate ($C_4H_8O_3$), a metabolite of the inhibitory neurotransmitter γ-aminobutyric acid (GABA), is present in the brain in about one thousandth of the concentration of GABA (3). Formerly employed as an anesthetic, oxybate (GHB) continues to be used in Europe for treatment of narcolepsy, alcohol dependence, and opiate dependence (8). In the United States, oxybate (GHB) was sold in health food stores and mostly purchased by body builders until 1990 when sale was banned. More recently, it has been used recreationally and for the purpose of intended sexual assault ("date-rape") (1,4,5). GHB is the active metabolite of γ-butyrolactone, a substance found in products that claim to induce sleep, release growth hormone, enhance sexual activity and athletic performance, relieve depression, and prolong life (2).

The street form of GHB ("Liquid E," "Fantasy," "Nature's Quaalude") is said to be a clear liquid with a taste of seawater. Ingestion of GHB with alcohol and other drugs is common and may prove fatal. Toxic effects of GHB include rapid-onset drowsiness, nausea, vomiting, bradycardia, hypothermia, myoclonic seizures, and short-duration coma (2,8). During August 1995–September 1996, poison control centers in New York and Texas received reports of 69 acute poisonings and one death attributed to ingestion of GHB (1). Withdrawal from physical dependence on GHB is associated with insomnia, anxiety and tremor (7).

GHB is behaviorally, biochemically and physiologically distinct from GABA, and it does not consistently effect $GABA_A$ or $GABA_B$ agonist-induced responses (4,6). The central dopamine system is markedly affected by GHB (4); it increases potassium conductance in rat ventral tegmental dopamine neurons (10). GHB is twenty times more active than γ-butyrolactone in depressing evoked synaptic field potentials in the CA1 region of rat hippocampus *in vitro* (9).

REFERENCES

1. *Anon.* (1997) Gamma hydroxy butyrate use: New York and Texas, 1995–1996. *MMWR Morb Mortal Wkly Rep* **46**, 281.
2. *Anon.* (1999) Adverse events associated with ingestion of gamma-butyrolactone: Minnesota, New Mexico, and Texas, 1998–1999. *MMWR Morb Mortal Wkly Rep* **48**, 137.
3. Cash CD (1994) Gamma-hydroxybutyrate: an overview of the pros and cons for it being a neurotransmitter and/or a useful therapeutic agent. *Neurosci Biobehav Rev* **18**, 291.
4. Centers for Disease Control (1991) Multistate outbreak of poisonings associated with illicit use of gamma hydroxy butyrate. *J Amer Med Assoc* **265**, 447.
5. ElSohly MA, Salamone SJ (1999) Prevalence of drugs used in cases of alleged sexual assault. *Anal Toxicol* **23**, 141.
6. Feigenbaum JJ, Howard SG (1996) Gamma hydroxybutyrate is not a GABA agonist. *Prog Neurobiol* **50**, 1.
7. Galloway GP, Frederick SL, Staggers FE Jr *et al.* (1997) Gamma-hydroxybutyrate: an emerging drug of abuse that causes physical dependence. *Addiction* **92**, 89.
8. Kam PC, Yoong FF (1998) Gamma-hydroxybutyric acid: an emerging recreational drug. *Anaesthesia* **53**, 1195.
9. King MA, Thinschmidt JS, Walker DW (1997) Gamma-hydroxybutyrate (GHB) receptor ligand effects on evoked synaptic field potentials in CA1 of the rat hippocampal slice. *J Neural Transm* **104**, 1177.
10. Madden TE, Johnson SW (1998) Gamma-hydroxybutyrate is a $GABA_B$ receptor agonist that increases a potassium conductance in rat ventral tegmental dopamine neurons. *J Pharmacol Exp Ther* **287**, 261.

Palytoxin

Alexander Storch
Albert C. Ludolph

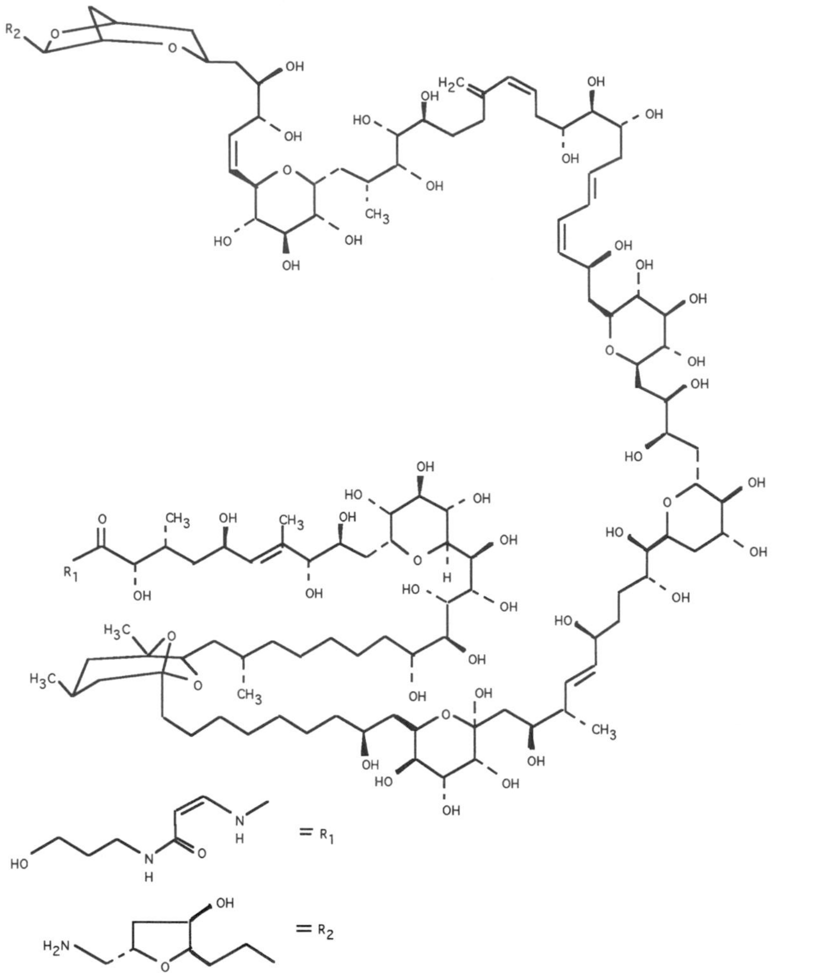

PALYTOXIN
$C_{129}H_{233}N_3O_{54}$

Palytoxin (C51–55 hemiacetal); PTX

NEUROTOXICITY RATING

Clinical

B   Ion channel syndrome

Experimental

A   Ion channel dysfunction

A   Inhibition of Na^+,K^+-ATPase

Palytoxin was isolated from the marine coelenterate *Palythoa toxica* in 1963 (11). The toxin was subsequently found in several other species of the genus *Palythoa*, including *P. vestitus*, *P. mammilosa*, *P. caribaerum*, *P. tuberculosa*, and a Tahitian *Palythoa* spp. (10). On the basis of chromatographic properties and dose–response relationships in ani-

mal models, palytoxin or palytoxin-like toxins were also detected in the trigger fish *Melichthys vidua* (family Balistidae), the file fish *Alutera scripta* (family Monoacanthidae), the parrotfish *Ypsiscarus ovifrons,* the mackarel *Decapterus macrosoma,* and in three species of xanthid crabs (*Demania alcalai et reynaudii, Lophozozymus pictor*) (1,3,5,8,9, 12,17). In some, the toxin was from ingested *Palythoa* spp.; therefore, it is unknown whether these species synthesize the toxin *de novo* (3,5,8).

Palytoxin is a white, amorphous, hygroscopic solid. It is soluble in water, dimethyl sulfoxide, and pyridine; sparingly soluble in methanol and ethanol; and insoluble in chloroform, ether, and acetone (10,11). The ultraviolet absorption spectrum in water shows two intense peaks at 233 nm and

263 nm. The MW of palytoxin is 2678.5 daltons; physical properties are available (10).

Palytoxin is one of the most poisonous low-molecular-weight substances known. It is surpassed only by some bacterial toxins (*e.g.*, botulinum). The LD_{50} of palytoxin in mice has been estimated as 0.15 μg/kg following intravenous injection and 0.4 μg/kg following intraperitoneal injection (11). Intravenous LD_{50}s between 0.25 μg/kg (rabbit) and 0.45 μg/kg (mouse) are reported (15,16). Intragastric or intrarectal applications are relatively nontoxic [LD_{50} >40 μg/kg and 10 μg/kg, respectively (16)]. Toxic potency is not increased by intraventricular injection (7).

Clinical signs noted after intravenous administration of palytoxin vary between species. Rodents become drowsy and inactive. Prostration, dyspnea, and convulsions appear soon after injection and immediately before death. Monkeys become drowsy, weak, and ataxic; this is followed by collapse and death (16). Death from palytoxin is due to intense spasm of vascular smooth muscle of coronary and pulmonary vessels (6,15,16).

Palytoxin promotes development of tumors in a two-stage mouse skin assay without binding to protein kinase C or inducing ornithine decarboxylase (2).

There is one case of a dog poisoned from ingestion of the palytoxin-containing crab *Demania reynaudii* (1); the animal died 1 h after eating three-fourths of a crab.

In vitro studies show that palytoxin both inhibits Na$^+$,K$^+$-adenosine triphosphatase (ATPase) and increases cell permeability for small cations by using the ATPase as its receptor in an agonist-like manner (4). High concentrations ($\geq$100 nmol) are required to affect enzyme acitivity (4). In lower concentrations (picomolar range), palytoxin causes a rapid K$^+$ outflow and Na$^+$ influx into several cell types by increasing plasmalemma ion permeability (4); this leads to depolarization of the cell (4,7). The effects of palytoxin are enhanced by extracellular Ca^{2+} and borate; they are potently inhibited by ouabain. In addition, palytoxin binds to a receptor that is very similar to that for ouabain. Patch-clamp studies and experiments with planar bilayers show that palytoxin affects a 9.0 to 9.5-pS single channel permeable for small cations, probably acting through Na$^+$,K$^+$-ATPase (4). Recent studies demonstrate that palytoxin binds to and forms a channel within Na$^+$,K$^+$-ATPase in a manner that does not require adenosine triphosphate hydrolysis or phosphorylation of the plasmalemmal enzyme (13,14).

In organ preparations, palytoxin has contractile effects on all investigated muscles, including smooth, cardiac, and striated muscles (4,7). Nerve fiber preparations show depolarization in response to low concentrations of palytoxin (4,7).

There are few cases of human poisoning with palytoxin or palytoxin-like toxins (1,8,12,17). Occasional outbreaks of fatal crab poisoning have occurred in the Philippines (1). In some cases, the agent was identified as palytoxin or a palytoxin-like toxin in *Demania alcalai et reynaudii* and *Lophozozymus pictor* (1,17). In other reports, the victims consumed smoked mackerel (*Decapterus macrosoma*) or the parrotfish *Ypsiscarus ovifrons*. Clinical signs, comparable in all, commenced a few minutes to several hours after ingestion of the animal. Victims experienced weakness, excessive sweating, abdominal cramps, nausea, diarrhea, cardiac arrhythmia, renal failure, circumoral paresthesia, parasthesia and numbness of the extremities, dysesthesia, plus severe muscle spasms and tremor (1,8,12,17). A spinal seizure-like syndrome with contraction of all muscle groups was also reported (8). Laboratory findings included abnormally high serum levels of creatine phosphokinase, lactate dehydrogenase, and serum glutamic oxaloacetic transaminase, and myoglobinuria (8,12), reflecting tissue damage. Most died within a few days of the tainted meal, usually from cardiac and renal failure (1,8,12,17).

Diagnosis, usually simple if a history of ingestion is available, can be confirmed by identifying the causative toxin in the remnants of the toxic animal.

Treatment is supportive. Pretreatment with hydrocortisone protected against lethal doses in experimental animals (15). Tests in animals with various vasodilators showed that papaverine and isosorbide dinitrate injected intraventricularly are effective antidotes (15).

All effects of palytoxin can be explained by its action on Na$^+$,K$^+$-ATPase. The fast increase of permeability for small ions (*vide supra*), especially for K$^+$ and Na$^+$, causes depolarization of affected cells. This leads to muscle contraction and neuronal hyperexcitability (4,7).

REFERENCES

1. Alcala AC, Alcala LC, Garth JS *et al.* (1988) Human fatality due to ingestion of the crab *Demania reynaudii* that contained a palytoxin-like toxin. *Toxicon* 26, 105.
2. Fujiki H, Sugimura T (1987) New classes of tumor promotors: Teleocidin, aplysiatoxin, and palytoxin. *Adv Cancer Res* 49, 223.
3. Fukui M, Murata M, Inoue A *et al.* (1987) Occurrence of palytoxin in the trigger fish *Melichtys vidua*. *Toxicon* 25, 1121.
4. Habermann E (1989) Palytoxin acts through Na$^+$,K$^+$-ATPase. *Toxicon* 27, 1171.
5. Hashimoto Y, Fusetani N, Kimura S (1969) Aluterin: A toxin of filefish, *Alutera scripta*, probably originated from a zoantharian, *Palythoa tuberculosa*. *Bull Jpn Soc Sci Fish* 35, 1086.
6. Ito K, Urakawa N, Koike H (1982) Cardiovascular toxicity of palytoxin in anesthetized dogs. *Arch Int Pharmacodyn* 258, 146.

7. Kaul PN (1976) Palytoxin—a new physiological tool. In: *Food and Drugs from the Sea*. Proc U.S. Marine Technol Soc, Washington, DC p. 311.

8. Kodama AM, Hokama Y, Yasumoto T *et al.* (1989) Clinical and laboratory findings implicating palytoxin as cause of ciguatera poisoning due to *Decapterus macrosoma* (mackarel). *Toxicon* 27, 1051.

9. Lau CO, Khoo HE, Yuen R *et al.* (1993) Isolation of a novel fluorescent toxin from the coral reef crab, *Lophozozymus pictor*. *Toxicon* 31, 1341.

10. Moore RE (1985) Structure of palytoxin. *Prog Chem Org Nat Prod* 48, 82.

11. Moore RE, Scheuer PJ (1971) Palytoxin: A new marine toxin from a coelenterate. *Science* 172, 495.

12. Noguchi T, Hwang D, Arakawa O *et al.* (1987) Palytoxin as the causative agent in the parrotfish poisoning. In: *Progress in Venom and Toxin Research*. Gopalakrishna-kone P, Tan CK eds. National University of Singapore, Kent Ridge, Singapore p. 325.

13. Scheiner-Bobis G (1998) Ion-transporting ATPases as ion channels. *Naunyn Schmied Arch Pharmacol* 357, 477.

14. Scheiner-Bobis G, Schneider H (1997) Palytoxin-induced channel formation within the Na^+/K^+-ATPase does not require a catalytically active enzyme. *Eur J Biochem* 248, 717.

15. Vick JA, Wiles JS (1975) The mechanism of action and treatment of palytoxin poisoning. *Toxicol Appl Pharmacol* 34, 214.

16. Wiles JS, Vick JA, Christensen MK (1974) Toxicological evaluation of palytoxin in several animal species. *Toxicon* 12, 427.

17. Yasumoto T, Yasumura D, Ohizumi Y *et al.* (1986) Palytoxin on two species of xanthid grabs from Philippines. *Agr Biol Chem* 50, 163.

Pandinus imperator Toxin

Albert C. Ludolph
Peter S. Spencer

NEUROTOXICITY RATING

Experimental

A   Ion channel dysfunction (potassium channel—nerve)

One component of the venom of the scorpion *Pandinus imperator* blocks voltage-gated K^+ channels (6). Several 35-amino-acid (pandinotoxins) and 38-amino-acid K^+-channel toxins have been isolated and characterized (1,2,4,5,8). The venom irreversibly blocks the delayed-rectifier axonal K^+ channels of bullfrog myelinated nerve fibers (6). The same concentration-dependent effect has been observed in cultured clonal rat anterior pituitary cells (7). Venom slowed channel opening, speeded deactivation, and increased inactivation rates. In these cells, the venom also blocked sodium and calcium currents, possibly secondary to zinc present in *Pandinus* venom (7). The venom of *P. imperator* facilitates evoked acetylcholine release at the neuromuscular junction by blockade of neuronal K^+ currents (1). No effect on Na^+ channels has been detected (3).

Two other peptide toxins from *P. imperator* venom act on ryanodine receptors in skeletal muscle (9,10). "Imperatoxin inhibitor" (estimated MW of 10,500) inhibits and "imperatoxin activator" (estimated MW of 8700), now known as imperatoxin A, stimulates ^{3}H-ryanodine binding to skeletal muscle sarcoplasmic reticulum. They also block and stimulate Ca^{2+}-release channels of skeletal muscle incorporated into planar bilayers in low nanomolar concentrations.

REFERENCES

1. el-Hayek R, Lokuta AJ, Arevalo C, Valdivia HH (1995) Peptide probe of ryanodine receptor function. Imperatoxin A, a peptide from the venom of the scorpion *Pandinus imperator*, selectively activates skeletal-type ryanodine receptor isoforms. *J Biol Chem* 270, 28696.

2. Gomez-Lagunas F, Olamendi-Portugal T, Zamudio FZ, Possani LD (1996) Two novel toxins from the venom of the scorpion *Pandinus imperator* show that the N-terminal amino acid sequence is important for their affinities towards Shaker B K^+ channels. *J Membr Biol* 152, 49.

3. Marshall DL, Harvey AL (1989) Block of potassium channels and facilitation of acetylcholine release at the neuromuscular junction by the venom of the scorpion *Pandinus imperator*. *Toxicon* 27, 493.

4. Olamendi-Portugal T, Gomez-Lagunas F, Gurrola GB, Possani LD (1996) A novel structural class of K^+-channel blocking toxin from the scorpion *Pandinus imperator*. *Biochem J* 315, 977.

5. Olamendi-Portugal T, Gomez-Lagunas F, Gurrola GB, Possani LD (1998) Two similar peptides from the venom of the scorpion *Pandinus imperator*, one highly effective blocker and the other inactive on K^+ channels. *Toxicon* 36, 759.

6. Pappone PA, Cahalan MD (1987) *Pandinus imperator* scorpion venom blocks voltage-gated potassium channels in nerve fibers. *J Neurosci* 7, 3300.

7. Pappone PA, Luccro MT (1988) *Pandinus imperator* scorpion venom blocks voltage-gated potassium channels in GH3 cells. *J Gen Physiol* 91, 817.

8. Rogowski RS, Collins JH, O'Neil TJ *et al.* (1996) Three new toxins from the scorpion *Pandinus imperator* selectively block certain voltage-gated K$^+$ channels. *Mol Pharmacol* **50**, 1167.

9. Valdivia HH, Fuentes O, El Hayek R *et al.* (1991) Activation of the ryanodine receptor Ca^{2+} release channel of sarcoplasmic reticulum by a novel scorpion toxin. *J Biol Chem* **266**, 19135.

10. Valdivia HH, Kirby MS, Lederer W, Coronado R (1992) Scorpion toxins targeted against the sarcoplasmic reticulum Ca^{2+} release channel of skeletal and cardiac muscle. *Proc Nat Acad Sci USA* **89**, 12185.

Paraquat

Herbert H. Schaumburg

PARAQUAT
$$[C_{12}H_{14}N_2]^{2+}$$

1,1'-Dimethyl-4,4'-bipyridinium

NEUROTOXICITY RATING

Clinical

C   Acute encephalopathy

C   Extrapyramidal syndrome (Parkinson's disease)

Experimental

C   Extrapyramidal dysfunction (substantia nigra dysfunction)

Paraquat is a bipyridal herbicide and one of the most specific pulmonary toxicants. Because of its high risk for permanent and fatal pulmonary damage, it is no longer widely used in North America. Pulmonary edema and fibrosis follow ingestion in humans and laboratory animals. The mechanism of pulmonary toxicity is well studied; it includes free radical formation with conversion of the superoxide anion to hydrogen peroxide and resultant alveolar membrane damage.

Paraquat is little metabolized by the body, and the parent compound has limited entry into the brain (8). Systemically administered paraquat may produce CNS dysfunction in immature animals (2) but appears to be without serious neurotoxicity in the adult rodent (6,10). One study describes behavioral effects associated with paraquat deposition in the area postrema (1). Some experimental animal studies describe an effect of paraquat upon hippocampal, basal ganglia or motor function following direct intracerebral injection (7,9,12). Paraquat appears to kill PC12 cells *in vitro* by cellular lipid peroxidation (11).

There have been many instances of human survival from severe paraquat intoxication; most have displayed profound pulmonary dysfunction, none has displayed clinical evidence of CNS disease, and it appears unlikely that paraquat is neurotoxic to humans. Isolated reports of nonspecific CNS changes in fatal cases reflect anoxia and are not convincing evidence of a primary effect of paraquat upon the CNS (3,5).

The structure of paraquat resembles that of methyl phenyl tetrahydropyridine (MPTP), an agent that produces degeneration in the substantia nigra of humans and primates (*see* MPTP and Analogs, this volume). Epidemiological studies of rural and urban populations have failed to demonstrate a robust correlation between historical deployment of paraquat and clusters of Parkinson's disease cases (4).

REFERENCES

1. Edmonds BK, Edwards GL (1996) The area postrema is involved in paraquat-induced conditioned aversion behavior and neuroendocrine activation of the hypothalamic-pituitary-adrenal axis. *Brain Res* **712**, 127.

2. Fredriksson A, Fredriksson M, Eriksson P (1993) Neonatal exposure to paraquat or MPTP induced permanent changes in striatum dopamine and behavior in adult mice. *Toxicol Appl Pharmacol* **122**, 258.

3. Grčevic N, Jadro-Santel D, Jukic S (1977) Cerebral changes in paraquat poisoning. In: *Neurotoxicology*. Roizen L, Shiraki H, Grčevic N eds. Raven Press, New York p. 469.

4. Ho SC, Woo J, Lee CM (1989) Epidemiologic study of Parkinson's disease in Hong Kong. *Neurology* **39**, 1314.

5. Hughes JT (1988) Brain damage due to paraquat poisoning: A fatal case with neuropathological examination of the brain. *Neurotoxicology* **9**, 243.

6. Lin-Shiau SY, Hsu KS (1994) Studies on the neuromuscular blocking action of commercial paraquat in mouse phrenic nerve-diaphragm. *Neurotoxicology* **15**, 379.

7. Liou HH, Chen RC, Tsai YF *et al.* (1996) Effects of paraquat on the substantia nigra of the Wistar rats: Neurochemical, histological, and behavioral studies. *Toxicol App Pharmacol* **137**, 34.

8. Naylor JL, Widdowson PS, Simpson MG *et al.* (1995) Further evidence that the blood/brain barrier impedes paraquat entry into the brain. *Hum Exp Toxicol* **14**, 587.

9. Rispoli V, Rotiroti D, Nistico G (1994) Neurodegeneration produced by intrahippocampal injection of paraquat

is reduced by systemic administration of the 21-aminosteroid U74389F in rats. *Free Radical Res* **21**, 85.

10. Widdowson PS, Farnworth MJ, Upton R, Simpson MG (1996) No changes in behavior, nigro-striatal system neurochemistry or neuronal cell death following toxic multiple oral paraquat administration to rats. *Hum Exp Toxicol* **15**, 583.

11. Yang WL, Sun AY (1998) Paraquat-induced cell death in PC12 cells. *Neurochem Res* **23**, 1387.

12. Yoshimura Y, Watanabe Y, Shibuya T (1993) Inhibitory effects of calcium channel antagonists on motor dysfunction induced by intracerebroventricular administration of paraquat. *Pharmacol Toxicol* **72**, 229.

Parmelia molliuscula

Albert C. Ludolph

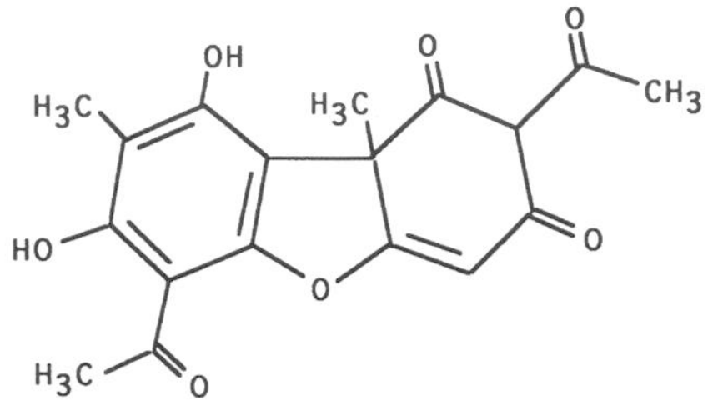

USNIC ACID
$C_{18}H_{16}O_7$

Usnic acid; 2,6-Diacetyl-7,9-dihydroxy-8,9b-dimethyl-1,3(2*H*,9b*H*)-dibenzofurandione; Usninic acid; Usniacin

NEUROTOXICITY RATING

Clinical

B Ataxia (sheep)

Experimental

A Mitochondrial uncoupler

Parmelia molliuscula (ground lichen) is a gray-green leathery plant native to Nebraska and North Dakota in the United States. Its toxic moiety is thought to be usnic acid, a yellow compound with a MW of 344.32. Usnic acid has antimicrobial activity, and low concentrations (1 μM) uncouple mitochondrial oxidative phosphorylation (1,2,4). Intoxication of cattle and sheep with *P. molliuscula* leads to ataxia and paralysis (3); if a dosage of >1%/kg body weight is ingested, animals die within days (3).

REFERENCES

1. Abo-Khatwa AN, al-Robai AA, al-Jawhari DA (1996) Lichen acids as uncouplers of oxidative phosphorylation of mouse-liver mitochondria. *Nat Toxins* **4**, 96.

2. Gonzalez AG, Rodriquez-Perez EM, Barrera JB (1991) Biologically active compounds from the lichen *Ramalina hierrensis*. *Planta Med* **57**, A2.

3. Kingsbury JM (1964) *Poisonous Plants of the United States and Canada*. Prentice Hall, Englewood Cliffs, New Jersey p. 86.

4. Reynolds JEF (1982) *Martindale: The Extra Pharmacopoeia*. 28th Ed. The Pharmaceutical Press, London.

Pelamitoxin

Albert C. Ludolph

NEUROTOXICITY RATING

Clinical

A Neuromuscular transmission syndrome

Experimental

A Neuromuscular transmission dysfunction (postsynaptic)

Pelamitoxins a, b, and c are basic 60-amino-acid proteins from the venom of the sea snake *Pelamis platurus* (yellow-bellied sea snake). The structure of pelamitoxin b differs by a single amino acid from pelamitoxin a (1). *P. platurus* is found in coastal southern California, U.S.A., along the entire coast of Central America, and south to the northern coast of Chile (3).

Similar to other sea snake neurotoxins, pelamitoxin is a postsynaptic (α) neurotoxin that binds to the α-subunit of the acetylcholine receptor. The LD$_{50}$ in mice after intravenous administration is 0.044–0.44 μg/g (3). Treated rabbits show a reduced twitch response to nerve stimulation and develop respiratory paralysis (4).

Sea snake bites are practically unknown along the Pacific coast of the United States (2). Those species that pose potential danger to humans include, in descending order of threat (2): *Enhydrina schistosa, Hydrophis cyanocinctus, Lapemis hardwickii, Hydrophis spiralis, Kerilia jerdoni,* and *P. platurus*. For more general information on sea snake neurotoxins, *see* Hydrophiidae Toxins and also Erabutoxins, this volume—the best characterized group of sea-snake neurotoxins.

REFERENCES

1. Mori N, Ishizaki H, Tu AT (1989) Isolation and characterization of *Pelamis platurus* (yellow-bellied sea snake) postsynaptic isoneurotoxin. *J Pharm Pharmacol* **41**, 331.
2. Reid HA (1975) Epidemiology of sea snake bites. *J Trop Med Hyg* **78**, 106.
3. Tu AT (1988) Sea snakes and their venoms. In: *Handbook of Natural Toxins. Vol 3. Marine Toxins and Venoms*. Tu AT ed. Marcel Dekker, New York p. 424.
4. Tu T, Tu AT, Lin TS (1976) Some pharmacological properties of the venom, venom fractions and pure toxin of the yellow-bellied sea snake *Pelamis platurus*. *Pharm Pharmacol* **28**, 139.

Pemoline

Herbert H. Schaumburg

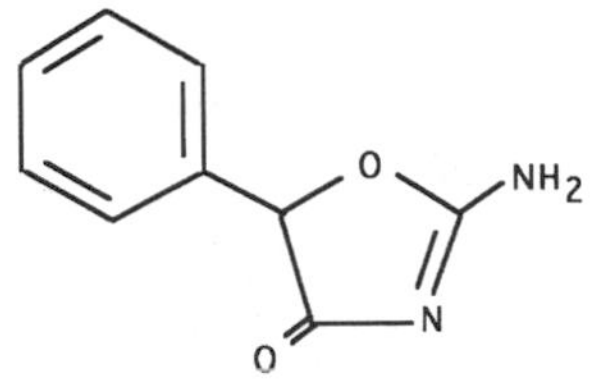

PEMOLINE
$C_9H_8N_2O_2$

2-Amino-5-phenyl-4(5*H*)-oxazolone

NEUROTOXICITY RATING

Clinical

A Acute encephalopathy (agitation, irritability, seizures)

A Extrapyramidal syndrome (chorea)

Experimental

A CNS dopaminergic reaction

A CNS stimulant

Pemoline, an oxazolidine derivative, is a CNS stimulant with a chemical structure dissimilar to the amphetamines or methylphenidate. It is used exclusively, but infrequently, in North America to treat children with attention deficit disorder (ADD); methylphenidate is the first-line CNS stimulant therapy for this condition. Pemoline is pharmacologically classified as an amphetamine-class CNS stimulant; experimental animal studies indicate it has a dopaminergic action that is unaffected by prior administration of reserpine. The drug is rapidly absorbed from the gastrointestinal tract and is widely distributed; its half-life is 12 h, and it takes 2 weeks of daily administration before the desired CNS effect appears. There is a considerable variation in systemic availability of pemoline in hyperactive children; this has made appearance of adverse effects somewhat unpredictable and accounts, in part, for the drug's unpopularity in treating ADD. The principal systemic adverse effects are growth retardation, mild hepatic dysfunction and, rarely, liver failure (1).

Guinea pigs receiving pemoline develop behavioral stereotypy in a dose-related manner (4). This effect is characteristic of amphetamine-induced striatal dopaminergic activity (5).

Pemoline therapy may cause the full spectrum of untoward human effects associated with chronic CNS stimulant therapy, namely, insomnia, agitation, generalized seizures, irritability, extraocular muscle palsies, and hallucinations. Most patients adapt to insomnia, and agitation generally subsides within a few months. Overdose of pemoline has been associated with transient chorea and a Tourette's-like syndrome (2,4). One instance of choreoathetosis following ingestion of 1 g of pemoline was so severe as to cause myoglobinuria (3).

REFERENCES

1. Adcock KG, MacElroy DE, Wolford ET, Farrington EA (1998) Pemoline therapy resulting in liver transplantation. *Ann Pharmacother* **32**, 422.
2. Bonthala CM, West A (1983) Pemoline induced chorea and Gilles de la Tourette's syndrome. *Brit J Psychiat* **143**, 300.
3. Briscoe JG, Curry SC, Gherkin RD, Ruin RR (1988) Pemoline-induced choreoathetosis and rhabdomyolysis. *Med Toxicol* **3**, 72.
4. Nausieda PA, Koller WC, Weiner WJ, Klawans HL (1981) Pemoline-induced chorea. *Neurology* **31**, 356.
5. Randrup A, Munkvard I (1967) Stereotypic activities produced by amphetamines in several animal species and man. *Psychopharmacology* **11**, 300.

Penicillamine

Steven Herskovitz

PENICILLAMINE
$C_5H_{11}NO_2S$

3-Mercapto-D-valine; β,β-Dimethylcysteine

NEUROTOXICITY RATING
Clinical

A   Myasthenia gravis

A   Myopathy (inflammatory)

B   Peripheral neuropathy

B   Optic neuropathy

Experimental

A   Neuromuscular transmission dysfunction (acetylcholine receptor antibody—myesthenia)

A   Myopathy (inflammatory)

Penicillamine is a degradation product of penicillin. Only the D-isomer is used clinically, since the L-isomer and DL-racemate induce pyridoxine deficiency and are toxic. Penicillamine is an effective chelator of copper, zinc, mercury, and lead. Clinical uses include the chelation and elimination of copper in Wilson's disease, the treatment of cystinuria by forming a relatively soluble disulfide compound with cysteine, and the suppression of rheumatoid arthritis, perhaps by reducing the concentration of immunoglobulin M rheumatoid factor (7). It has also been used in the treatment of scleroderma and primary biliary cirrhosis. Neurotoxicity includes the induction of myasthenia gravis and polymyositis/dermatomyositis; isolated clinical reports also suggest peripheral neuropathy, neuromyotonia, fasciculations, and optic neuropathy.

Penicillamine is rapidly absorbed from the gastrointestinal tract (40%–70%), with peak plasma concentrations between 1 and 3 h of ingestion (7,9,21,23). About 80% is protein-bound. There is biphasic plasma clearance; a rapid phase with a half-life of about 1 h is followed by a slower elimination phase with a half-life of about 8 days. Elimination is mainly renal, with disulfide forms representing the main compounds found in the urine.

In animal experiments, long-term administration of penicillamine to guinea pigs produces in muscle an edrophonium-reversible decrement on repetitive stimulation, significant elevations of acetylcholine receptor (AChR) antibody, and nonspecific inflammatory and necrotic changes in muscle (20). Another study in guinea pigs produced polymyositis (15). Long-term administration of penicillamine to certain strains of mice caused no clinical weakness or anti-AChR antibody, but augmented antibody responses to challenge with purified AChR in adjuvant and increases susceptibility to experimental autoimmune myasthenia gravis (3).

Adverse side effects, common with penicillamine treatment, include a variety of skin rashes, gastrointestinal toxicity, reversible elevation of liver enzymes, pancytopenia, and renal toxicity (9,21). Induced autoimmune syndromes include a systemic lupus erythematosus–like illness in as many as 2% of patients, a Goodpasture's-like pulmonary and renal syndrome, pemphigus, hemolytic anemia, thyroiditis, myasthenia gravis, polymyositis, and dermatomyositis. Poor sulfoxidation status is a risk factor for penicillamine toxicity (31).

Penicillamine can induce myasthenia gravis in up to 7% of patients (2). Instances are reported in patients treated for rheumatoid arthritis, scleroderma, and Wilson's disease. Clinical, electrophysiological, and serological features are identical to idiopathic myasthenia gravis, except that most cases resolve within several months of discontinuing the drug (1,6,9,11,17,19,21). Relative to idiopathic myasthenia gravis, there is a higher female/male ratio at presentation. Ocular, bulbar, respiratory, or generalized muscle dysfunction can occur; this may appear after widely varying doses and durations of treatment. Characteristic decremental responses to repetitive stimulation and jitter, and blocking on single-fiber electromyography (EMG), can be demonstrated (1). AChR antibody is present in almost all cases and decreases gradually after withdrawal of penicillamine, concomitant with clinical improvement (6). Many also have antinuclear antibodies and anti–ds-DNA. Antistriational muscle antibodies and even thymic hyperplasia may develop (19). There is a response to edrophonium and pyridostigmine. Occasional severe cases have had to be managed with steroids, plasmapheresis. or thymectomy, in addition to withdrawing penicillamine. There is an association reported with HLA antigens BW35 and DR1.

Penicillamine can induce polymyositis or dermatomyositis in approximately 1% of patients, without a clear relationship to dose or duration of treatment (4,5,10,18,22, 27,32). The clinical, electrophysiological, and pathological features are indistinguishable from the idiopathic variety. They are generally less severe but can be associated with severe weakness, myocarditis, arrhythmia, and fatality. Recovery is usually rapid after withdrawal of penicillamine. Antinuclear antibodies are common, and anti–Jo-1 antibody was detected in one case (10). There is an association reported with HLA antigens B18, B35, and DR4.

Some reports have suggested peripheral nerve dysfunction in association with penicillamine. After 6 months of therapy, a patient with rheumatoid arthritis developed electromyographically confirmed diffuse fasciculations that disappeared after discontinuing the drug and recurred on rechallenge (28). Another individual developed reversible neuromyotonia (30). A severe, symmetrical, sensorimotor polyneuropathy, unlike the types seen in rheumatoid arthritis, progressed over several months in a patient after 10 months of penicillamine therapy (29). Nerve conduction studies and sural nerve biopsy suggested both demyelination and axonal degeneration; the cerebrospinal fluid (CSF) was not examined. A clinical response to pyridoxine and subsequent complete resolution after discontinuing penicillamine suggested that pyridoxine antagonism might be responsible. In another case, a predominantly motor polyneuropathy with a clinical, electrophysiological and CSF picture consistent with Guillain-Barré syndrome occurred simultaneously with the appearance of *pemphigus foliaceus*, and resolved completely within a few weeks of discontinuing the drug; the pyridoxine level was normal (13). Another report describes a skin rash, nephrotic syndrome and reversible proximal muscle weakness without sensory involvement, and normal CSF and normal creatine kinase values; the reported nerve conduction and EMG studies are said to suggest a demyelinating polyradiculopathy, but they are difficult to interpret (25). These reports suggest that penicillamine may induce a demyelinating polyneuropathy.

Initial deterioration of neurological function may occur after starting penicillamine treatment in symptomatic or presymptomatic patients with Wilson's disease (8,24). A few cases of penicillamine-associated optic neuropathy have appeared (12,16).

Penicillamine-induced and naturally occurring myasthenia gravis share the same essential pathophysiological features. Serial studies, including motor point biopsies, in a patient with penicillamine-induced myasthenia gravis, demonstrate the presence of AChR antibody titers correlating with the temporal course of the disease, serum-induced blockade of AChRs, antibody-mediated accelerated degradation of AChRs, and a reduction in available junctional AChRs (14). Clinical and junctional AChR recovery occurred within 8 months of stopping penicillamine. It is likely that penicillamine produces myasthenia gravis not by enhancing pre-existing/ongoing autoimmunity, but rather by initiating a new autoimmune response. That antigenic alteration of the AChR may be the underlying mechanism is suggested by penicillamine's binding to sulfhydryl bands of the AChR; in long-term studies with rabbits, penicillamine can alter the AChR *in vivo*, so that it is perceived as antigenic (26).

REFERENCES

1. Albers JW, Hodach RJ, Kimmel DW, Treacy WL (1980) Penicillamine-associated myasthenia gravis. *Neurology* 30, 1246.
2. Andonopoulos AP, Terzis E, Tsibiri E *et al.* (1994) D-Penicillamine induced myasthenia gravis in rheumatoid arthritis: An unpredictable common occurrence? *Clin Rheumatol* 13, 586.
3. Bever CT, Dretchen KL, Blake GJ *et al.* (1984) Augmented anti-acetylcholine receptor response following long-term penicillamine administration. *Ann Neurol* 16, 9.
4. Carroll GJ, Will RK, Peter JB *et al.* (1987) Penicillamine induced polymyositis and dermatomyositis. *J Rheumatol* 14, 995.
5. Doyle DR, McCurley TL, Sergent JS (1983) Fatal polymyositis in D-penicillamine-treated rheumatoid arthritis. *Ann Intern Med* 98, 327.
6. Drosos AA, Christou L, Galanopoulou V *et al.* (1993) D-Penicillamine-induced myasthenia gravis: Clinical, serological and genetic findings. *Clin Exp Rheumatol* 11, 387.
7. Gilman AG, Rall TR, Nies AS, Taylor P (1990) *The Pharmacological Basis of Therapeutics. 8th Ed.* Pergamon Press, New York p. 1610.
8. Glass JD, Reich SG, DeLong MR (1990) Wilson's disease. Development of neurological disease after beginning penicillamine therapy. *Arch Neurol* 47, 595.
9. Howard-Lock HE, Lock CJL, Mewa A, Kean WF (1986) D-Penicillamine: Chemistry and clinical use in rheumatic disease. *Semin Arthritis Rheum* 15, 261.
10. Jenkins EA, Hull RG, Thomas AL (1993) D-Penicillamine and polymyositis: The significance of the anti-Jo-1 antibody. *Brit J Rheumatol* 32, 1109.
11. Katz LJ, Lesser RL, Merikangas JR, Silverman JP (1989) Ocular myasthenia gravis after D-penicillamine administration. *Brit J Ophthalmol* 73, 1015.
12. Klingele TG, Burde RM (1984) Optic neuropathy associated with penicillamine therapy in a patient with rheumatoid arthritis. *J Clin Neuro-ophthalmol* 4, 75.
13. Knezevic W, Mastaglio FL, Quinter J, Zilko PJ (1984) Guillain-Barré syndrome and pemphigus foliaceus associated with D-penicillamine therapy. *Aust N Z J Med* 14, 50.
14. Kuncl RW, Pestronk A, Drachman DB, Rechthand E (1986) The pathophysiology of penicillamine-induced myasthenia gravis. *Ann Neurol* 20, 740.
15. Lava NS, McVicker J, Ringel SP (1979) D-Penicillamine-induced neuromuscular disease in guinea pigs. *Neurology* 29, 564.
16. Lee AH, Lawton NF (1991) Penicillamine treatment of Wilson's disease and optic neuropathy. *J Neurol Neurosurg Psychiat* 54, 746. [Letter]

17. Liu GT, Bienfang DC (1990) Penicillamine-induced ocular myasthenia gravis in rheumatoid arthritis. *J Clin Neuro-ophthalmol* **10**, 201.

18. Lund HI, Nielson M (1983) Penicillamine-induced dermatomyositis. A case history. *Scand J Rheumatol* **12**, 350.

19. Masters CL, Dawkins RL, Zilko PJ *et al.* (1977) Penicillamine-associated myasthenia gravis, acetylcholine receptor and antistriational antibodies. *Amer J Med* **69**, 689.

20. McVicker JH, Lava NS, Mittag TW, Ringel SP (1982) D-Penicillamine-induced neuromuscular disease in guinea pigs. *Exp Neurol* **76**, 46.

21. Meyboom RHB (1992) Metal antagonists. In: *Meyler's Side Effects of Drugs. 12th Ed.* Dukes MNG ed. Elsevier, Amsterdam p. 537.

22. Morgan GJ, McGuire JL, Ochoa J (1981) Penicillamine-induced myositis in rheumatoid arthritis. *Muscle Nerve* **4**, 137.

23. Netter P, Bannwarth B, Pere P, Nicolas A (1987) Clinical pharmacokinetics of D-penicillamine. *Clin Pharmacokinet* **13**, 317.

24. Pall HS, Williams AC, Blake DR (1989) Deterioration of Wilson's disease following the start of penicillamine therapy. *Arch Neurol* **46**, 359.

25. Pederson PB, Hogenhaven H (1983) Penicillamine-induced neuropathy in rheumatoid arthritis. *Acta Neurol Scand* **81**, 188.

26. Penn AS, Lamme E, Mitelman R (1984) Chronic D-penicillamine administration creates a new antigenic determinant reactive in D-penicillamine myasthenia gravis. *Neurology* **34**, 240.

27. Petersen J, Halberg P, Hjgaard K *et al.* (1978) Penicillamine-induced polymyositis-dermatomyositis. *Scand J Rheumatol* **7**, 113.

28. Pinals RS (1983) Diffuse fasciculations induced by D-penicillamine. *J Rheumatol* **10**, 809.

29. Pool KD, Feit H, Kirkpatrick J (1981) Penicillamine-induced neuropathy in rheumatoid arthritis. *Ann Intern Med* **95**, 457.

30. Reeback J, Benton S, Swash M, Schwartz MS (1979) Penicillamine-induced neuromyotonia. *Brit Med J* **1**, 1465.

31. Seideman P, Ayesh R (1994) Reduced sulphoxidation capacity in D-penicillamine-induced myasthenia gravis. *Clin Rheumatol* **13**, 435.

32. Takahashi K, Ogita T, Okudaira H *et al.* (1986) D-Penicillamine-induced polymyositis in patients with rheumatoid arthritis. *Arthritis Rheum* **29**, 560.

Penicillins

Libor Velísek
Solomon L. Moshé

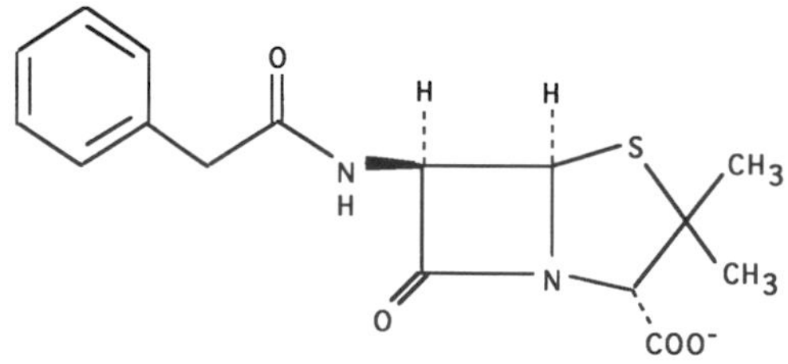

PENICILLIN G
C₁₆H₁₆N₂O₄S

[2S-(2α,5α,6β)]-3,3-Dimethyl-7-oxo-6-[(phenylacetyl)amino]-4-thia-1-azabicyclo[3.2.0]heptane-2-carboxylic acid

NEUROTOXICITY RATING
Clinical

A Seizure disorder

A Headache (intrathecal edema)

Experimental

A GABA receptor blockade

A Seizure disorder (local & systemic administration)

The discovery of penicillin by Sir Alexander Fleming in 1928 opened a new era in the treatment of infections. Penicillins are natural antibiotics produced by the fungi of the *Penicillium* genus. There are also semisynthetic penicillins resulting from chemical modifications of natural *Penicillium* products (Table 54). Penicillins are acids; their sodium salts differ in solubility and stability. The naturally occurring benzylpenicillin is unstable and water-insoluble. In contrast, its sodium and potassium salts are relatively stable and water-soluble. Penicillins inhibit the final step in the synthesis of the bacterial cell wall; the resultant defective cell wall cannot resist the osmotic pressure difference between the inner and outer environment. Penicillins exert bacteriostatic effects especially in fast-growing bacterial populations where there is an immediate need for new cell-wall synthesis. In static bacterial populations, penicillins are much less effective.

There are individual differences in the absorption of penicillins. Natural benzylpenicillin is almost completely decomposed in the acidic environment of the stomach. Par-

TABLE 54. Penicillins

Drug	R-Substituent
Penicillin G	(phenyl)–CH_2–
Penicillin V	(phenyl)–OCH_2–
Ampicillin	(phenyl)–$\underset{NH_2}{\overset{\textstyle |}{CH}}$–

enteral administration of its sodium or potassium salt produces peak plasma concentrations within 15–30 min. Phenoxymethylpenicillin is well absorbed from the gastrointestinal tract. Approximately 50%–65% of the absorbed penicillin is reversibly bound to serum albumins. Penicillins are widely distributed in the body, but there are mild differences in concentration in various tissues and fluids. A portion is metabolized (10%–40%); the rest is excreted unchanged, mostly by the kidneys, either by glomerular filtration (20%) or *via* tubular secretion (80%).

The most serious neurological side effect of penicillin treatment is seizures. The epileptiform activity of penicillin was first reported in 1945 in laboratory animals (19). Administration of 500 U into the motor cortex of monkeys elicited muscular twitching. Cats developed seizures after instillation of 1000–2000 U of penicillin into the motor cortex (19). Since then, the epileptogenic activity of penicillin has been studied in many species (14). The reliability and reproducibility of penicillin-induced epileptiform discharges resulted in a penicillin-induced model of seizures (*i.e.*, penicillin-induced epileptiform activity as a tool in neuroscience and epilepsy research). Because penicillin crosses the blood-brain barrier poorly, most of the penicillin-induced models of epileptiform discharges require local application of penicillin, thus creating an epileptic focus at the site of application. By adjusting the dose of penicillin, the seizure threshold can be determined for the injected site. In a comparative study, epileptogenic potency of different penicillins and their derivatives was determined following local application on the neocortex of rats and cats (10). The order of epileptiform potency of penicillin-like compounds is: benzylpenicillin (threshold concentration ~25 mmol/l) ≥ phenoxymethylpenicillin (~100 mmol/l) > oxacillin (~150 mmol/l) > methicillin (~150 mmol/l) > ampicillin (~175 mmol/l) (10). Similar studies successfully determined

the seizure thresholds of the developing rat sensorimotor neocortex (11). Cats are extremely sensitive to parenterally administered penicillin, and generalized seizures can be induced using the dose of 350,000 U/kg intramuscularly (9), 0.5–1.0 million U/kg intravenously (2), or 1–2 million U/kg intraperitoneally (2). Seizures consist of brief myoclonic jerks followed by generalized tonic convulsions of all limbs and, eventually, *status epilepticus* may occur (2). Myoclonic jerks and seizures are associated with isolated and generalized electroencephalographic (EEG) spike-and-wave discharges, respectively. During generalized seizures, generalized spike-and-wave EEG discharges are present (2,9). Systemic penicillin can also induce seizures in rats and mice; however, substantially higher doses are required. For example, in rats, the penicillin dose of 2.5–5.0 million U/kg intraperitoneally is necessary to provoke behavioral seizures (2); in mice, 2 million U of penicillin/mouse (20 g) is required to induce seizures. The resulting plasma levels of penicillin were between 6 and 7 mg/ml (7). Although there are no long-term studies, one report suggests a potentiation (or kindling effect) after repeated focal applications of penicillin in rats (3). Repeated administration of penicillin therefore may lead to an increased susceptibility of seizures in laboratory animals. There are no such data in primates or humans.

In vitro hippocampal slices are a convenient system to study mechanisms of penicillin-induced epileptogenesis because of the relatively high sensitivity to epileptiform stimuli and simple synaptic arrangement. Penicillin induces interictal as well as ictal discharges in hippocampal slices (13). Ictal activity requires concentrations between 90 and 300 mg/l (8). In contrast, neocortical slices require much larger concentrations for the induction of epileptiform discharges; ictal bursting begins with 600 mg/l of penicillin (4). Thus, ability to evoke seizures by penicillin may be a measure of the epileptogenic potential of the tissue. This paradigm was applied in slices from developing rats; in hippocampal slices from 9- to 19-day-old rats, penicillin induced more frequent and longer discharges than in tissue from older or younger animals (17). This *in vitro* window of increased seizure susceptibility correlates well with *in vivo* data from many seizure models (12,18).

There are numerous reports of acute seizures occurring in patients treated with local and systemic penicillin (16). In adult humans, the threshold for the epileptogenic action of penicillin after intracortical administration appears to be higher (~20,000 U) than the penicillin-induced seizure thresholds in cats or monkeys. The threshold is lower in children (10,000 U) (20). Intrathecal administration of penicillin (from doses as low as 3000–5000 U) may also have convulsant effects that are associated with vomiting, convulsions, and meningeal irritation (16). Higher doses of penicillin administered intrathecally (200,000–500,000 U) or intracisternally (40,000–100,000 U) are associated with muscular twitches and generalized seizures, and rarely with death (16). There is also evidence that high doses of systemically administered penicillin may provoke seizures (1). In one study, 44% of patients who received 180,000 U/kg of penicillin intravenously after heart surgery developed seizures (5). Penicillin concentrations in the cerebrospinal fluid of patients with seizures after intravenous drug administration are in the range 75–220 mg/l, corresponding with the penicillin concentrations necessary to induce *in vitro* epileptiform activity (15). Patients with deteriorated renal function are especially prone to develop seizures after penicillin if dose adjustments are not made. There is also a high risk for penicillin-induced seizures in patients with endocarditis or in patients who receive large doses of penicillin (10–60 million U/day) after heart surgery (*vide supra*). Both conditions result in a decreased cardiac output leading to a deterioration of renal function that further increases plasma concentrations of penicillin. Convulsions have also been reported after administration of other penicillin-related compounds: carbenicillin, oxacillin, cloxacillin, and ampicillin (16). Other side effects of penicillin involve mild to severe pain in toes or legs, bladder hypotonia, paralysis of the legs, radiculitis, and leptomeningeal thickening. These side effects occur after prolonged intrathecal administration of penicillin at doses of 10,000 U/day (16).

The mechanism of convulsant action of penicillin is associated with a blockade of γ-aminobutyric acid (GABA) inhibitory transmission. Penicillin has been shown to block the chloride channel associated with the GABA$_A$ receptor, thereby limiting Cl$^-$ entry through the channel (6). Depending on the membrane resting potential, the Cl$^-$ current either elicits hyperpolarization and/or leads to a large decrease in membrane resistance and shunting of the excitatory currents. Any of these effects results in membrane stability; blockade of the Cl$^-$ channel induced by penicillin therefore results in increased membrane excitability.

REFERENCES

1. Borman JB, Eyal Z (1968) Neurotoxic effects of large doses of penicillin administered intravenously. *Arch Surg* **97**, 662.
2. Chen R-C, Huang Y-H, How S-W (1986) Systemic penicillin as an experimental model of epilepsy. *Exp Neurol* **92**, 533.
3. Collins RC (1978) Kindling of neuroanatomic pathways during recurrent focal penicillin seizures. *Brain Res* **150**, 503.
4. Connors BW, Gutnick MJ (1984) Cellular mechanisms of neocortical epileptogenesis in an acute experimental model. In: *Electrophysiology of Epilepsy*. Schwartzkroin PA, Wheal HV eds. Academic Press, London p. 79.
5. Currie TT, Hayward NJ, Westlake G (1971) Epilepsy in cardiopulmonary bypass patients receiving large intravenous doses of penicillin. *J Thorac Cardiovasc Surg* **62**, 1.
6. DeLorey TM, Olsen RW (1994) GABA and glycine. In: *Basic Neurochemistry*. Siegel GJ, Agranoff BW, Albers RW, Molinoff PB eds. Raven Press, New York p. 389.
7. Eng RHK, Munsif AN, Yangco BG *et al.* (1989) Seizure propensity with imipenem. *Arch Intern Med* **149**, 1881.
8. Esplin B, Theoret Y, Seward E, Capek R (1985) Epileptogenic action of penicillin derivatives: Structure-activity relationship. *Neuropharmacology* **24**, 571.
9. Gloor P, Testa G (1974) Generalized penicillin epilepsy in the cat: Effect of intracarotid and intravertebral pentylenetetrazol and amobarbital injections. *Electroencephalogr Clin Neuro* **36**, 499.
10. Gutnick MJ, Van Duijn H, Citri N (1976) Relative convulsant potencies of structural analogues of penicillin. *Brain Res* **114**, 139.
11. Maré P (1973) Symmetrical epileptogenic foci in cerebral cortex of immature rat. *Epilepsia* **14**, 427.
12. Moshé SL, Albala BJ, Ackermann RF, Engel JJ (1983) Increased seizure susceptibility of the immature brain. *Dev Brain Res* **7**, 81.
13. Schwartzkroin PA, Prince DA (1977) Penicillin-induced epileptiform activity in the hippocampal *in vitro* preparation. *Ann Neurol* **1**, 463.
14. Servít Z (1972) Phylogenetic correlations. In: *Experimental Models of Epilepsy—A Manual for the Laboratory Worker*. Purpura DP, Penry JK, Tower D *et al.* eds. Raven Press, New York p. 509.
15. Smith H, Lerner PI, Weinstein L (1967) Neurotoxicity and "massive" intravenous therapy with penicillin. A study of possible predisposing factors. *Arch Intern Med* **120**, 47.
16. Snavely SR, Hodges GR (1984) The neurotoxicity of antibacterial agents. *Ann Intern Med* **101**, 92.
17. Swann JW, Brady RJ (1984) Penicillin-induced epileptogenesis in immature rat CA3 hippocampal pyramidal cells. *Develop Brain Res* **12**, 243.
18. Velísek L, Kubová H, Pohl M *et al.* (1992) Pentylenetetrazol-induced seizures in rats: An ontogenetic study. *Naunyn-Schmied Arch Pharmacol* **346**, 588.
19. Walker AE, Johnson HC (1945) Convulsive factor in commercial penicillin. *Arch Surg* **50**, 69.
20. Walker AE, Johnson HC, Kollros JJ (1945) Penicillin convulsions: The convulsive effects of penicillin applied to the cerebral cortex of monkey and man. *Surg Gynecol Obstet* **81**, 692.

CASE REPORT

A 44-year-old man had a calcified stenotic mitral valve replaced by a prosthetic device. The procedure required car-

diopulmonary bypass for 4 h. During surgery, the patient received continuous infusion of 5 million U of sodium penicillin G. At the end of the operation, the patient was stuporous. Generalized muscle twitches appeared soon after. Postoperatively, he received 60 million U of sodium penicillin G in a continuous intravenous infusion, 3 g of methicillin sodium every 6 h, and 0.5 g of streptomycin sulfate every 12 h. The next morning, the patient experienced generalized convulsions that intermittently continued for 24 h despite intensive anticonvulsant therapy, including intramuscular barbiturates and rectal chloral hydrate. The penicillin treatment was discontinued. The patient stopped having seizures and was discharged with no physical or mental sequlae. [Adapted according to Albers et al. (1).]

Penitrems and Other Tremorgens

Albert C. Ludolph

Peter S. Spencer

The metabolic products of fungi are best known for their beneficial use as antibiotics. The broad term fungus *toxin* (mycotoxin) includes all toxic metabolites of true fungi (Eumycetes). The targets of mycotoxins include liver (aflatoxin, sporidesmin, phomopsin), renal (ochratoxin, citrinin), and dermal (trichothecenes). Animal and human diseases caused by fungi are referred to as mycotoxicoses. *Neurotoxic* effects of mycotoxins in humans are restricted to (a) ergot toxicity (*see* Ergot Alkaloids, this volume), the first mycotoxicosis recognized to affect man; (b) the known side effects of fungal products used as antibiotics (*see* the respective compounds); (c) the selective striatal necrosis produced by 3-nitropropionic acid—an inhibitor of complex II of the mitochondrial electron transport chain (*see* 3-Nitropropionic Acid and Related Compounds, this volume); and (d) the neurotoxicity of mushrooms (*see* *Amanita* toxins, *Gyromitrin*, and *Psilocybin*, and *Psilocin*, this volume).

Historically, poisoning of animals and humans by moldy food has often been suspected (for references, *see* 85,95,98,105). However, in most cases, a critical review of these accidental poisonings does not reveal convincing evidence for a cause-and-effect relationship. Moreover, fungi have been misidentified in the past, and mycotoxins have been named after fungi that are now known not to produce them (28).

In vertebrate animals, mycotoxins are suspected of producing a number of neurological syndromes (15,56,57,101). In most cases, the precise pathophysiological and biochemical link to the respective etiologically responsible organism is not established. The presence of a sustained or intermittent tremor seems to be a common clinical feature of the majority of these syndromes (hence, the term "tremorgens") and, at higher dosages, seizures occur. Apart from these common aspects, some of the syndromes show some variation and await detailed clinical, biochemical, and neuropathological description.

Accidental human or animal disease caused by mycotoxins has the following characteristics (11):

1. The diseases are not transmissible.
2. Drug and antibiotic treatment have, with few exceptions, little or no effect.
3. Field outbreaks often occur seasonally.
4. An outbreak is usually associated with a specific food or foodstuff.
5. The degree of toxicity is often influenced by age, sex, and nutritional state of the host.
6. Examination of the suspected food or feed reveals signs of fungal activity.

Neurotoxicity is rare, although present knowledge of neurotoxicity of mycotoxins is restricted to acute effects; chronic, slowly accumulating damage is unknown and unexplored. The epidemiology of mycotoxicoses is associated with climate, since growth and metabolism of most fungi are greatly dependent on environmental conditions such as light, humidity, and temperature. In moderate climatic zones, outbreaks are seasonal and occur most frequently after long-term storage of food. The chemical characteristics of the individual neurotoxin determine the amount of decontamination or degradation obtained by washing, cooking, or baking procedures. Visual characteristics of food, taste, or smell usually limit oral intake, but these warning signals may not be present or may be overlooked by animals and humans during times of food shortages. Presently, there is no firm evidence that neurotoxic fungal products are secreted into the milk of lactating animals. Preventive measures for mycotoxin production in stored foodstuffs are diverse, and each of them has advantages and disadvantages; cost and effectiveness must be considered for each foodstuff, and the use of the methods depends on the specific environmental conditions (49).

The first tremorgenic mycotoxin to be discovered was in 1964 (103). Since then, the number of known neurotoxic fungal products has steadily increased. On structural grounds, six groups of compounds exist (93):

1. The penitrems, janthitrems, lolitrems, aflatrem, paxilline, paspaline, paspalicine, paspalinine, and paspalitrems A and B
2. The territrems
3. Verrucosidin
4. Verruculotoxin
5. Verruculogens and fumitremorgins
6. The tryptoquivalines

Other neurotoxic but "nontremorgenic" mycotoxins considered here include citreoviridin, and cyclopiazonic acid. The significance of this group of mycotoxins in human disease is unclear. Interest centers on their relation to some syndromes in veterinary medicine (*see* Chapter 3, this volume) and, more recently, their selective pharmacological properties.

Penitrems

(A) R_1 = Cl, R_2 = OH, R_3 = H; 23α,24α-epoxide
(B) R_1 = R_2 = R_3 = H; 23α,24α-epoxide
(C) R_1 = Cl, R_2 = R_3 = H
(D) R_1 = R_2 = R_3 = H
(E) R_1 = R_3 = H, R_2 = OH; 23α,24α-epoxide
(F) R_1 = Cl, R_2 = R_3 = H; 23α,24α-epoxide

PENITREMS

A: $C_{37}H_{44}ClNO_6$
B: $C_{37}H_{45}NO_5$
C: $C_{37}H_{44}ClNO_4$
D: $C_{37}H_{45}NO_4$
E: $C_{37}H_{45}NO_6$
F: $C_{37}H_{44}ClNO_5$

NEUROTOXICITY RATING

Experimental

A Tremor

A Cerebellar degeneration (penitrem A)

Penitrems are produced by *Penicillium clavigerum*, *P. crustosum*, and *P. glandicola*, less frequently by *P. aurantiogriseum* var. *aurantiogriseum* (28). These toxin-producing fungi can be found on silage, maize, and other agricultural commodities. Penitrem A is a white amorphous solid that chemically resembles penitrems B, C, D, E, and F. Methods of growth for penitrem-producing fungi, separation, and detailed structural considerations have been summarized (93). Penitrems were suspected to play a role in the etiology of migram and ryegrass staggers among cattle (73), and in a condition closely resembling the staggers syndrome observed in England (90). In another epidemic of cattle intoxication, penitrem A was isolated from fungi present on moldy corn associated with the outbreak (23). A causal role for penitrem A and penitrem B in the etiology of "huecu's disease" (a disease of sheep, horses, cattle, and goats) is suspected (86). "Huecu's disease" develops in animals grazing on *Poa huecu* Parodi grass in the Andean mountain range. Mice injected with the identified mycotoxins reportedly developed signs characteristic of tremorgens and similar to those observed in sheep (86). Murine signs (males and females) included motor incoordination, transient ataxia, rough hair, tremors and muscle contractions and, occasionally, blindness. Doses greater than 1.5 g/kg per mouse were lethal (78). A canine intoxication with moldy cream cheese was also attributed to penitrem A toxicosis (14).

The nonpolar compounds cross the blood-brain barrier readily. After intraperitoneal (i.p.) injection of penitrem A into rats, animals develop tremor of the whole body, typically followed by repeated tonic convulsions (104). Glutamic acid enhances this tremor (92). When calves are dosed with mycelia containing penitrem A, animals develop tremor, rigidity, and convulsions (21). Similar observations have been made in dogs (39). The seizures respond to administration of pentobarbital. Tremors also develop in sheep chronically dosed with penitrem A, but consistent CNS morphological changes have not been detected in these animals (76).

Two groups have examined the brain of rats after intracerebroventricular or i.p. administration of penitrem A. These studies revealed neuropathological changes restricted to the cerebellum, with loss of Purkinje cells most prominent in the vermis and para-vermis, and significant vacuolation of the molecular layer (6,9). Treatment is initially associated with transient alteration of the electroencephalogram, increased blood flow to the cerebellar cortex, and tremor (6,9). Tremor may persist for some time, and seizures may develop. Tremor eventually disappears, and animals that have sustained cerebellar damage may have persistent neuromotor changes or return to a largely normal pattern of behavior (6,9). Purkinje cells initially (2h after 3 mg/kg i.p.) exhibit pathological changes in dendrites consisting of cytoplasmic condensation and vacuolation of smooth endoplasmic reticulum accompanied by enlargement of perikaryal mitochondria. With time, some Purkinje cells show intense cytoplasmic condensation (6 h), while others exhibit edema and swelling (12 h). Stellate and basket cells display swollen mitochondria within 30 min of dosing: this condition persists for more than 12 hours without leading to cell death. Astrocytes also swell (0.5 h) and later (6 h) display organelle hypertrophy. These changes are accompanied (from 8 h) by increased permeability of overlying meningeal vessels to horseradish peroxidase. The authors attributed these changes to excitotoxicity associated with the action of penitrem A on high-conductance Ca^{2+}-dependent K^+ channels and γ-aminobutyric acid (GABA) receptors (9). The striking preponderance of pathological change in the cerebellar vermal region is a pattern of brain damage seen in certain other neurotoxic disorders, such as chronic alcoholism. The phenomenon has been discussed in light of the possibility that the vermal region is heavily exposed to substances in cerebrospinal fluid (CSF), and the ability of Purkinje cell dendrites and Bergmann glial procesess to extract materials from the CSF (8).

In vitro studies of penitrem A have utilized bovine aortic smooth-muscle sarcolemmal membranes (42). Here, the compound inhibits binding of ^{125}I-charybdotoxin to high-conductance Ca^{2+}-activated K^+ (maxi K) channels. In electrophysiological experiments, the mycotoxin inhibited maxi-K channels. Penitrem A also increases GABA and aspartate release from cerebrocortical but not from spinal cord or medullary synaptosomes (71). In contrast, even high doses of penitrem A do not influence acetylcholinesterase activity and cerebral catecholamine levels (76,102). Penitrem B concentration-dependently enhances the electrically induced twitch contractions of the guinea pig ileum, but its effects are weaker than those seen after paxilline and verruculogen administration (88). The authors of the foregoing study advance a presynaptic action as causative (88,89), an effect previously discussed by others after studies of the rat phrenic nerve–diaphragm preparation (102). There are no reports on the effects of acute or chronic exposures of humans to tremorgenic mycotoxins of the penitrem group.

Understanding of the mechanisms of penitrem neurotoxicity is largely based on *in vitro* studies. Penitrem A increases the spontaneous release of glutamate, aspartate, and GABA in cerebrocortical synaptosomal preparations from rats and sheep (71,77) and, like paspalitrem A, paspalitrem C, aflatrem and paspaline, and penitrem A, inhibits maxi-K channels. The latter effect is likely to cause the former. However, the nontremorgen paspalicine has the same effect on high-conductance Ca^{2+}-activated K^+ channels, indicating that this mechanism is unrelated to tremor induction (42). As with related compounds, a GABAergic mechanism might be responsible for the induction of tremor (*see* Aflatrem, *vide infra*).

Janthitrems

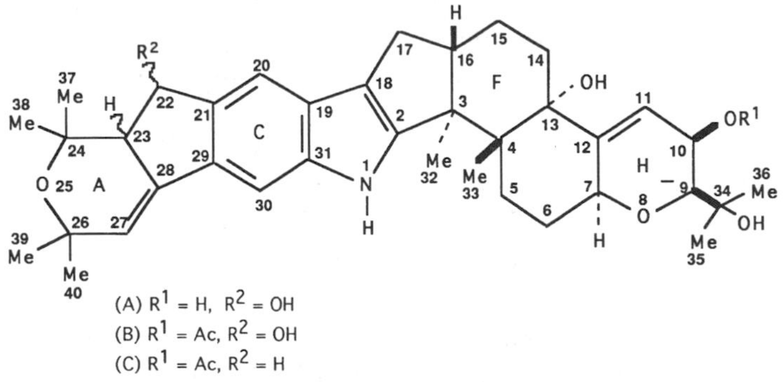

(A) R^1 = H, R^2 = OH
(B) R^1 = Ac, R^2 = OH
(C) R^1 = Ac, R^2 = H

JANTHITREMS

A: $C_{37}H_{47}NO_6$ D: $C_{37}H_{49}NO_6$
B: $C_{37}H_{47}NO_5$ E: $C_{39}H_{51}NO_7$
C: $C_{37}H_{47}NO_4$ F: $C_{39}H_{51}NO_6$

Janthitrems A, B, and C are tremorgenic mycotoxins produced by some isolates of *Penicillium janthinellum* (28). These tremorgenic strains were isolated from ryegrass pastures associated with outbreaks of ryegrass staggers in sheep in New Zealand (33). Janthitrems A, B, and C have a MW of 601, 585, and 569, respectively. Others include

janthitrem D and janthitrems E, F, and G (MW 603, 645, 629, respectively) (22,47). Janthitrems display a purple-blue fluorescence when irradiated with long-wave ultraviolet light. A detailed description of the isolation, analytical procedures, and the structure of janthitrems is available (93). Tremors in mice were induced by injecting 200 μg of janthitrem B in 0.1 ml of propylene glycol i.p. (33); tremor was accompanied by hypersensitivity to touch and sound. There are no reports of accidental exposures of humans to tremorgenic janthitrems.

Lolitrems

LOLITREMS

The lolitrems (A, B, C, and D) are produced by the toxic endophyte *Acremonium* spp., which infects perennial ryegrass (*Lolium perenne*) in countries such as Australia and New Zealand (29,93). Lolitrem B has the chemical formula $C_{42}H_{55}NO_7$ and a MP of 303°–304°C. Structural details have been reported (93). Lolitrems cause perennial ryegrass staggers, a disorder of sheep, cattle, horses, and deer associated with overgrazing of pastures and ingestion of the lowest, most mycotoxic parts of the leaves (46,59). The syndrome of ryegrass staggers in sheep includes fasciculation, tremor, incoordination, and tetanic spasms (79). Additional information on the neurological picture is given in Chapter 3 (page 90). Lolitrem neurotoxicity may reflect an increased concentration of the excitatory amino acids aspartate and glutamate in the cerebral cortex of animals exhibiting tremors (54). It is possible that lolitrems bind to GABA receptors in the CNS (25). In addition, lolitrem B induced prolonged stimulation of smooth muscle of the reticulorumen in conscious sheep; this action was sensitive to

atropine, suggesting the involvement of cholinoceptors. A non-tremorgenic isomer of lolitrem B (31-epilolitrem B) had no effect on the reticulorumen (58).

Aflatrem

AFLATREM
$C_{32}H_{39}NO_4$

Aflatrem was the first tremorgenic mycotoxin to be discovered (103). The MW is 501 and the MP is 233°–235°C.

Detailed structural features have been summarized (93). The compound is produced by *Aspergillus flavus* and *A. clavatoflavus* (17,28); it grows on various foods, such as corn, millet, rice, and potatoes (34,103), and is structurally similar to paspalinine. Its metabolites, aflavinine and dihydroxyaflavanine, are not tremorgenic (93). Mice given aflatrem (0.5–4.0 mg/kg) initially are inactive and immobile, then show an increased response to auditory and tactile stimuli, develop a tremor of the entire body and, finally, display convulsive activity (31,103). There are no reports of accidental exposures of humans. Aflatrem inhibits binding of ^{125}I-charybdotoxin to maxi-K channels in bovine aortic smooth muscle sarcolemmal membranes (42). Aflatrem (like paspalinin, paxillin, and verruculogen) also binds close to the Cl$^-$ channel associated with the inhibitory GABA$_A$ receptor (35) and inhibits GABA-induced ^{36}Cl$^-$ influx. However, at lower concentrations (1:30), aflatrem potentiates GABA-induced chloride currents (110) by acting as an allosteric modulator of the GABA$_A$ channel as expressed in *Xenopus* oocytes. This stimulatory effect on an inhibitory system may cause the early clinical symptomatology of aflatrem intoxication. Higher doses induce a different clinical picture reflecting inhibition of Cl$^-$ influx or release of excitatory neurotransmitters (110).

Paxilline, Paspaline, Paspalicine, Paspalinine, Paspalitrems

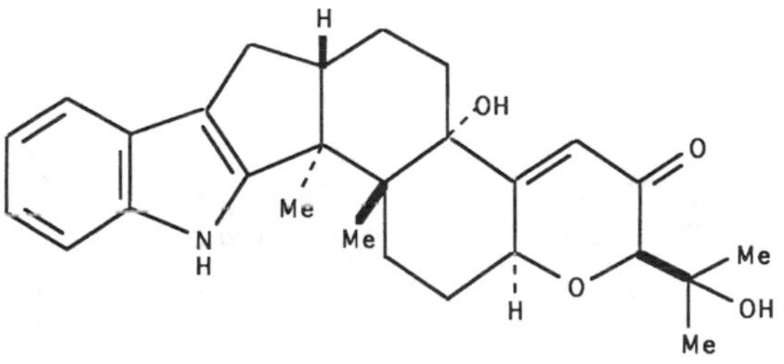

Paxilline was discovered in 1974 (20); it is produced by *Penicillium paxilli*, *Aspergillus clavatoflavus* (28), and by the genus *Emericella* (*E. desertorum*, *E. foveolata*, *E. striata*). *E. striata* additionally produces the related tremorgenic compound, 10-acetylpaxilline (72). The tremorgenic crystal paxilline has a MP of 252°C and a MW of 435.24 (93). Details of the structure of the compound are described (20). Severe tremors were observed in mice and cockerels after a 25-mg/kg injection of paxilline (20). The same effect was seen after injection of 4 mg/kg i.p.; the dioxygenated compound was apparently inactive (55). There are no reports of the effects on humans of exposure to paxilline.

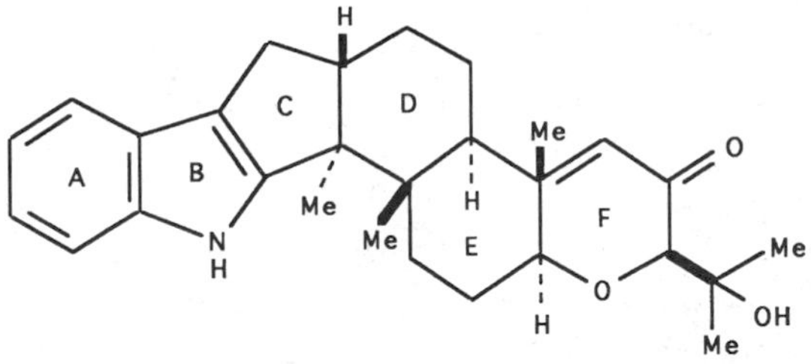

PASPALINE
$C_{28}H_{39}NO_2$

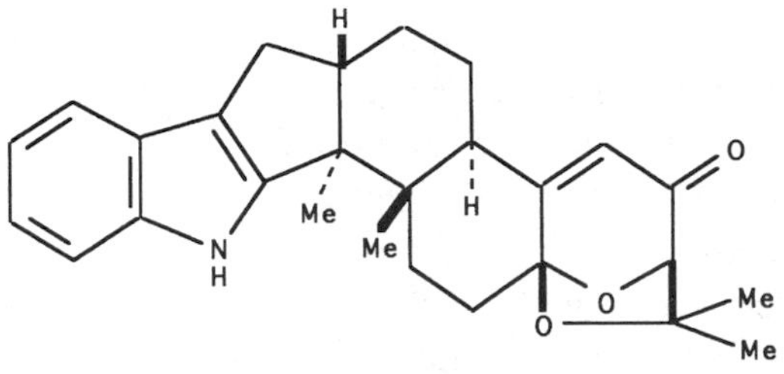

PASPALICINE
$C_{27}H_{31}NO_3$

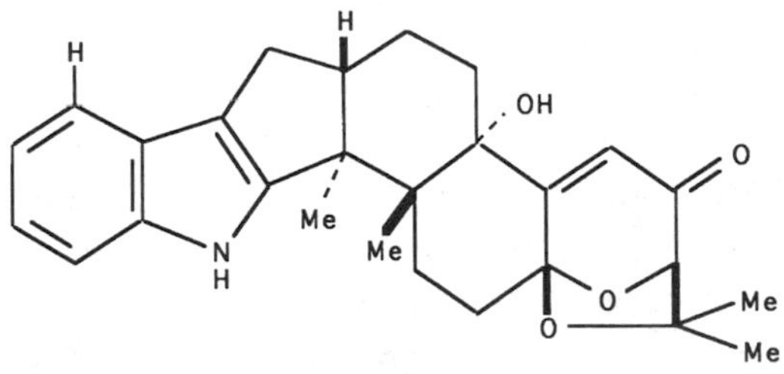

PASPALININE
$C_{27}H_{31}NO_4$

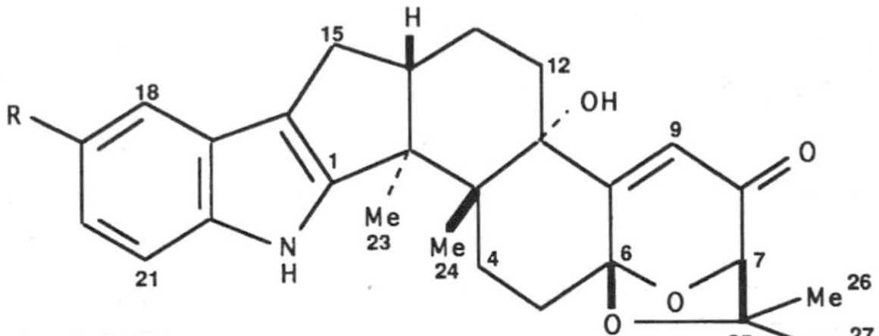

PAXILLINE
$C_{27}H_{33}NO_4$

PASPALITREMS

A: $C_{39}H_{39}NO_4$
B: $C_{32}H_{39}NO_5$

(A) R = Me$_2$C=CHCH$_2$
(B) R = Me$_2$C(OH)CH=CH–CH–

NEUROTOXICITY RATING
Experimental
A Tremor

In vitro, like aflatrem, paxilline inhibits GABA-induced $^{36}Cl^-$ influx into microsacs in rat brain (IC$_{50}$, 39.2 ± 6.9 μmol) and ^{35}S-*t*-butylbicyclophosphorothionate (^{35}S-TBPS) binding to rat brain membranes (IC$_{50}$, 11.2 ± 1.3 μmol). Also, like aflatrem, the mycotoxin binds to a site other than GABA-, benzodiazepine-, or barbiturate-binding sites (35). Like verruculogen and paspalicine, paxilline enhances binding of ^{125}I-charybdotoxin to maxi-K channels in bovine aortic smooth muscle sarcolemmal membranes (42); electrophysiologically, it is a specific, calcium-sensitive inhibitor of these channels in *Xenopus* oocytes and in mammalian cortical neurons and smooth muscle (38,40,83). This explains the finding that paxilline enhances the electrically evoked twitch contractions in the guinea pig ileum likely caused by presynaptic acetylcholine release (88,89).

Paspaline, paspalicine, paspalinine, and paspalitrems A and B are chemically related mycotoxins produced by *Aspergillus* and *Claviceps* spp. Paspalinine is elaborated by *Aspergillus flavus*, *A. leporis*, and *A. clavatoflavus* (28). Paspaline was isolated from *Aspergillus alliaceus* sclerotia (43). The ergot fungus *Claviceps paspali* also produces paspalinine (16,30) and the related compounds paspaline (MP, 254°C), paspalicine (MP, 230°C), and the paspalitrems A and B. Paspaline is a colorless crystal with a MP of 264°C and a MW of 457. The corresponding numbers for paspalicine are 230°C and 485. The MWs of paspalinine and paspalitrem A are 433 and 501, respectively (93). *Claviceps paspali* infects the grass *Paspalum dilatatum* which, when consumed by cattle, induces a disorder known as "paspalum staggers." The syndrome is observed sporadically in the southern parts of the United States and in New Zealand (93) and is caused by ingestion of dallis grass (*Paspalum dilatatum*) or bahia grass (*Bahia oppositifolia*). The syndrome, which resembles perennial ryegrass staggers, affects cattle, sheep, and horses (*see also* Chapter 3, p 91). When injected into mice, the effects of this group of compounds are comparable to those observed after paxilline administration. There are no reports on human exposures to these tremorgenic mycotoxins.

Of this group of compounds, only paspalinine, and paspalitrem A and B are tremorgenic. Paspalicine, which does not induce tremors, does not have a hydroxyl group at C-19, a common feature of all the tremorgenic indole-terpene alkaloids. The mechanism of tremorgenesis is held to be related to competitive inhibition of GABA-induced chloride ion influx (88). Like paxilline, paspalinine inhibits GABA-induced $^{36}Cl^-$ influx into microsacs in rat brain (IC$_{50}$, 78.7 ± 5.4 μmol) and ^{35}S-TBPS binding to rat brain membranes (IC$_{50}$, 3.5 ± 0.9 μmol) (35). Like aflatrem and penitrem A, paspalitrem A, C, and paspalinine inhibit binding of ^{125}I-charybdotoxin to maxi-K channels in bovine aortic smooth

muscle sarcolemmal membranes (42); electrophysiologically—like all the other tremorgenic indole alkaloids—the compounds are specific and potent inhibitors of these channels. Paspalicine—which is not tremorgenic—also blocks maxi-K channels, indicating that this effect on K$^+$ channels is unrelated to the pathogenesis of tremorgenesis.

Territrems

(A) R$_1$ = OMe; R$_2$,R$_3$ = −OCH$_2$O−
(B) R$_1$ = R$_2$ = R$_3$ = OMe
(C) R$_1$ = R$_3$ = OMe; R$_2$ = OH

TERRITREMS

A: $C_{28}H_{30}O_9$
B: $C_{29}H_{34}O_9$
C: $C_{28}H_{32}O_9$

NEUROTOXICITY RATING
Experimental
A   Tremor
A   Seizure disorder

Territrems A and B were first isolated in 1968 (10,96). Eleven isolates of *Aspergillus terreus* found on rice were able to synthesize metabolites that induced tremors and convulsions in mice after i.p. injection (50,51,53). Later, similar compounds, designated territrems C, A', and B', were described. Structurally, territrems differ from other known tremorgenic mycotoxins since they do not contain a nitrogen. The MWs and MPs of these compounds are 510 and 288°–290°C, 526 and 200°–203°C, and 512 and 172.5°–173.5°C, respectively (53,93). Methods of isolation, separation, other physicochemical data, and detailed structures of territrems A, B, and C are described elsewhere (51,93). Acute i.p. injection of territrems A, B, and C into mice induces a sustained whole-body tremor that is followed by convulsions and, in higher dosages, death (50,53). A median "tremulous dose" of 0.31, 0.21, and 0.24 mg/kg body weight was calculated for territrem A, B, and C, respectively. The tremorgenic effect is not seen after injection of territrems A' and B'. No reports exist on human exposures to territrems.

It has been proposed that the body tremor characteristically observed after administration of territrems is due to an effect of the compound on neuromuscular transmission (51). Several modulators of neuromuscular transmission (such as *d*-tubocurarine, magnesium, and calcium) influence the muscle twitching induced by territrem B; territrem B also interacts with presynaptic potassium currents. In the molluscan ganglion, territrem B potentiates acetylcholine-induced currents, but does not interfere with GABA- or glutamate-elicited currents. This suggests that territrems block presynaptic potassium currents and possibly inhibit acetylcholinesterase in the molluscan neuron (51). Incubation of territrem B with rat liver microsomes produces metabolites that act as potent acetylcholinesterase inhibitors (74,75). A recent review of territrem neurotoxicity is available (52).

Verrucosidin

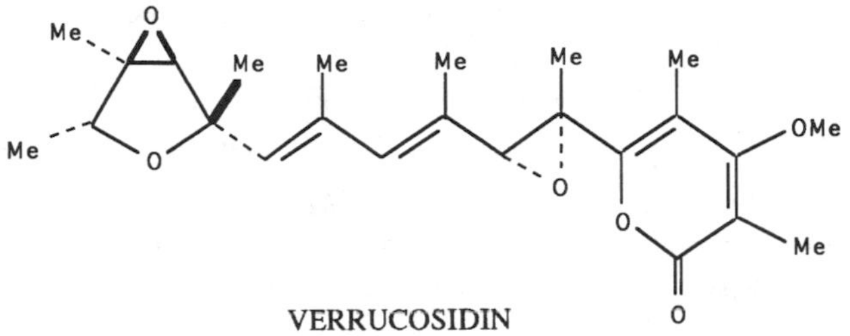

VERRUCOSIDIN
$C_{24}H_{32}O_6$

NEUROTOXICITY RATING

Experimental

A Tremor

Verrucosidin is a crystal with a MP of 90°–91°C; structural data are available (93). Verrucosidin (S-toxin) is a tremorgenic mycotoxin produced by *Penicillium aurantiogriseum* var. *polonicum* (24). Structurally, this mycotoxin resembles citreoviridin and the aurovertins but, in contrast to these compounds, induces tremors in experimental animals. The isolation of verrucosidin was first reported in relation to a disease observed in cattle (101).

Verruculotoxin

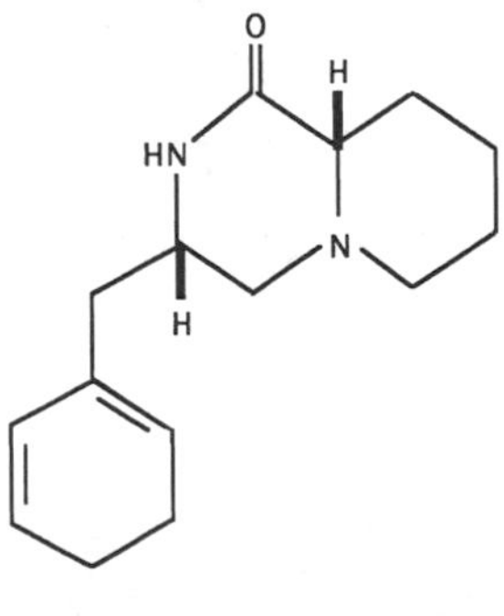

VERRUCULOTOXIN
$C_{15}H_{20}N_2O$

NEUROTOXICITY RATING

Experimental

A Myotoxin

Verruculotoxin, a cyclic dipeptide (19), is the metabolic product of *Penicillium brasilianum* (28); the crystal compound has a MP of 152°C. The fungus grows on green peanuts and wheat. Further information on chemical synthesis, isolation, and structure is available (93). Although sometimes classified as a tremorgen (93), this mycotoxin is nontremorgenic; it does not interact with the $GABA_A$ receptor–associated ion channel, and does not inhibit ^{35}S-TBPS binding to rat brain (35). This indicates that interaction with GABA receptors may be specific for tremorgenic mycotoxins. The LD_{50} of verruculotoxin in mice is 20 mg/kg body weight (19). Effects on the neuromuscular system of mice are likely to be mediated by a direct effect on skeletal muscle since it potentiates twitch tension to 150% of controls (26).

Verruculogens, Fumitremorgens

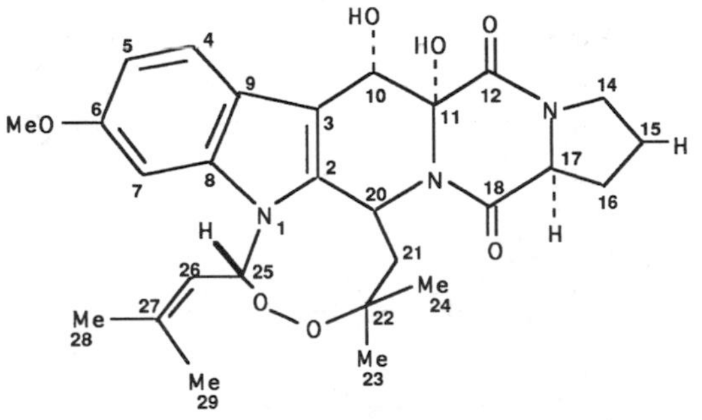

VERRUCULOGENS
$C_{27}H_{33}N_3O_7$

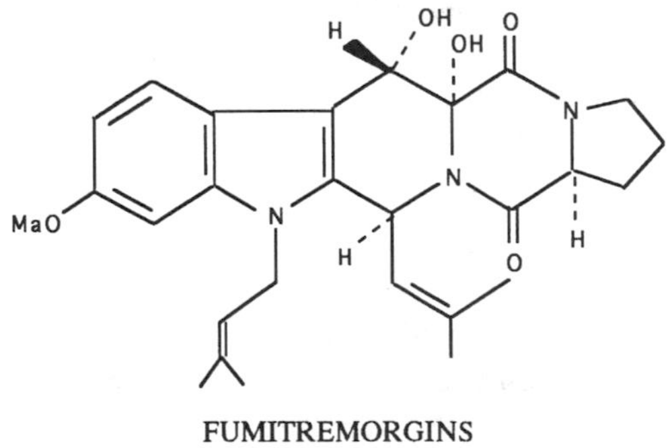

FUMITREMORGINS

A: $C_{32}H_{41}N_3O_7$
B: $C_{27}H_{33}N_3O_5$
C: $C_{32}H_{25}N_3O_3$

NEUROTOXICITY RATING

Experimental

A Seizure disorder, tremor

Verruculogens and fumitremorgens have in common a 5-methoxyindole moiety. The fumitremorgins A, B (synonym, lanosulin), and C were first isolated from *Aspergillus fumigatus* from rice in 1971 (109) and later also detected in cultures of *Aspergillus caespitosus* and *Penicillium lanosum* (3). The growth of fumitremorgens in culture is dependent on the presence of L-tryptophan. The MWs of fumitremorgin A and B are 579 and 479, respectively (93). The MPs of fumitremorgins A and B are 206°–209°C and 211°–212°C (93). The corresponding data for fumitremorgin C are 499 and 125°–130°C. The compounds can be detected by thin-layer chromatography (3). Clinically, they induce tremors and convulsions in animal species such as mice, rats, and rabbits (65,107,108). Their structure and clinical effects are similar to that of verruculogen, which was isolated from *Penicillium verruculosum* in 1972 (18) ("fumitremorgen-verruculogen group"). Fumitremorgin A is the most potent compound of this group (65); fumitremorgins B and C are less potent (61,100,108). Verruculogen was initially isolated from *Penicillium verruculosum* on peanuts (18); later, the compound was also obtained from cultures of *Aspergillus caespitosus*, *A. fumigatus*, *Penicillium paraherquei*, *P. janthinellum*, *P. paxilli*, and *P. piscarium* (15,29,44,84). The latter fungus was detected in ryegrass pastures (32). The MP of verruculogen is 233°–235°C (93). Further information on growth, isolation, and structure of verruculogen is available (93).

The products of heat-resistant molds, fumitremorgin A and C, along with verruculogen, are found in pasteurized and canned fruit and fruit products that have spoiled (95).

In mice, fumitremorgin A induces tremor, a gait disorder, and, at higher dosages, generalized tonic-clonic convulsions (94,108) after parenteral and oral administration. Verruculogen causes a similar syndrome in rats (5). Verruculogen induces severe tremors if administered orally to mice or 1-day-old cockerels (18). Sheep fed verruculogen developed tremors (5). Studies with fumitremorgin A in the rabbit revealed that seizures (dosage, 10–200 μg/kg body weight) were not accompanied by electroencephalographic evidence of hypersynchronized cortical activity and were still present in decorticated or decerebrated animal (65). Studies of the effects of fumitremorgin A on spinal cord and brainstem showed that convulsions could be interrupted by transection of the spinal cord at an upper level (66) and that they were associated with increased excitability of midbrain reticular neurons (67). This suggests that abnormal excitation of the reticulospinal pathway may cause the seizures induced by fumitremorgin A. Convulsions can be antagonized by D,L-2-aminophosphonovalerate, an antagonist at the *N*-methyl-D-aspartate glutamate receptor subtype, indicating that excitatory amino acid transmitters may be part of their pathogenesis. Verruculogen increases cerebral (but not spinal) glutamate and aspartate release in rat and sheep synaptosomal preparations (71); similar results have been obtained *in vivo* (77). In contrast to penitrem A, verruculogen does not increase GABA release (5). In guinea pig ileum, verruculogen increases release of acetylcholine from presynaptic terminals (89). Like a number of other tremorgenic indole alkaloids, verruculogen inhibits smooth-muscle high-conductance Ca^{2+}-activated potassium channels and enhances binding of ^{125}I-charybdotoxin to these channels. Like aflatrem, paspalinine, and paxilline, verruculogen inhibits GABA-induced $^{36}Cl-$ influx and ^{35}S-TBPS binding in rat brain membranes, a result consistent with earlier pharmacological experiments (41). Verruculogens in soil and animal feces were linked to an outbreak of ryegrass staggers in cattle in Australia (13). Another epidemic has been reported (44).

The effect of verruculogen on amino acid release may stem from its primary effect on K^+ channels; however, the effect on K^+ channels does not explain its tremorgenic properties (42). These likely reflect inhibition of GABAergic neurotransmission, in particular, since concentrations used in *in-vitro* experiments are consistent with dosages used *in vivo* (35).

Tryptoquivalines

TRYPTOQUIVALINES

A: $C_{29}H_{30}N_4O_7$
B: $C_{26}H_{24}N_4O_6$

NEUROTOXICITY RATING

Experimental

A   Tremor

The tryptoquivalines A (synonym, tryptoquivaline C) and B (synonyms, tryptoquivalone, nortryptoquivalone) are cyclic tetrapeptides produced by *Aspergillus clavatus* and *A. fumigatus* (28). Both fungi grow on rice. *A. clavatus* toxicosis was implicated in the death of a child in Thailand; however, a cause-and-effect relationship could not be proven (12). Tryptoquivaline was also identified in a bioareosol in a German compost facility (27). A number of compounds other than, but structurally similar to, tryptoquivalines A and B has been described (93,106). Tryptoquivaline A is a crystalline compound with a MP of 155°–157°C; tryptoquivaline B has a MP of 208°–209°C. Further details on growth, synthesis, and structure of the tryptoquivalines and their toxic and nontoxic metabolites are available (93). Intraperitoneal injection of 500 mg of tryptoquivaline and nortryptoquivaline induced fine tremors in weanling rats (36). In contrast, even at higher dosages, the tryptoquivalines C, D, E, F, G, H, I, and J did not provoke changes in mice.

Citreoviridin

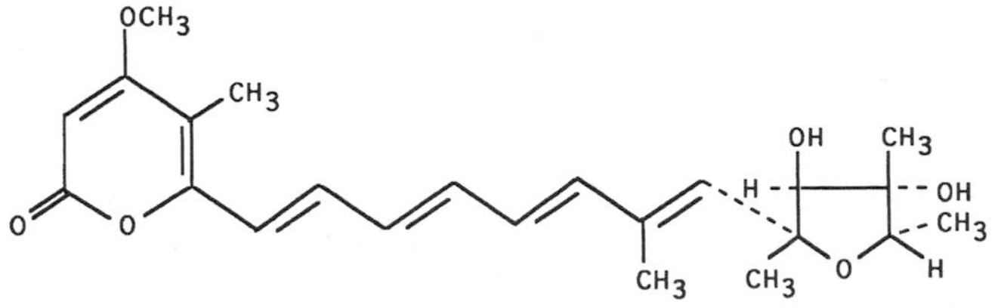

CITREOVIRIDIN
$C_{22}H_{30}O_6$

NEUROTOXICITY RATING

Experimental

A   Seizure disorder

Citreoviridin is produced by *Penicillium citreonigrum*, *P. miczynskii*, *P. manginii*, and *P. corynephorum*; *Eupenicillium ochrasalmoneum*; and *Aspergillus* spp. (28). The yellow compound is usually found on molded rice (81). It was also isolated in throat swabs taken from Czechoslovakian uranium miners (91). The chemical structure of citreoviridim (81,82) resembles that of aurovertin B1, an inhibitor of adenosine triphosphate synthesis and hydrolysis. Citreoviridin appears to inhibit protein synthesis in test systems (99). The toxicity of citreoviridin is abolished by ultraviolet radiation or sunlight (81). Studies of short-term, controlled exposure have been done in experimental mice and rabbits. After oral or parenteral administration of citreoviridin to mice, convulsions, an ascending paralysis (97), hypokinesia, and stereotyped movements were observed (63). In rabbits (63), respiratory failure preceded electrocardiographic and electroencephalographic alterations, indicating that clinical signs of neurotoxicity may be a secondary, rather than the primary effect of the compound.

Cyclopiazonic Acid

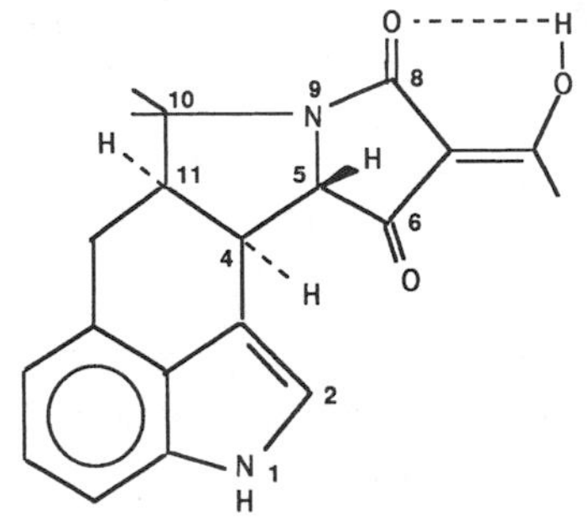

CYCLOPIAZONIC ACID
$C_{20}H_{20}N_2O_3$

NEUROTOXICITY RATING

Experimental

A   Myopathy

B   Acute encephalopathy

Cyclopiazonic acid (CPA) is consistently produced by *Aspergillus flavus*, *A. oryzae* (only some isolates), *A. tamarii*, *A. subolivaceus*, *Penicillium griseofulvum*, *P. camemberti*, and *P. commune* (28). CPA has been detected on cheese, fermented sausages, cereal products, corn, peanuts, and stored grains (45,48,79). A report from India indicates that CPA can be isolated from kodo millet obtained from *Paspalum* grass (80). CPI is eliminated from pigs with a half-life of 24 h (7).

After controlled short-term administration to mice, CPA induces hypokinesia, convulsions, catalepsy, and opisthotonus (62,64,80); changes in brain catecholamines correlate with these behavioral abnormalities, but structural abnormalities have not been found (62,64). Uncontrolled exposure of cattle has been observed in India (2). Oral intake of kodo millet (*Paspalum scrobiculatum*) causes nervousness, lack of muscular coordination, staggering gait, depression, and spasms in these animals; rarely, animals may die (60). Contamination of the millet with CPA-producing fungi is the suspected cause (2,4,80). Possible consequences of human exposure to CPA have also been observed in India. Here, in several regions, *Paspalum scrobiculatum* L. is used as an emergency food. The dehusked grain is cooked like rice or used for bread; poisonings have been repeatedly reported and fungus contamination suspected as the cause

(1). The symptomatology (sleepiness, tremor, and giddiness for 1–3 days) of "kodua poisoning" (or "kodo") may indicate CNS involvement (4). Two samples of millet seeds that caused "giddiness and nausea" after consumption were contaminated with *A. flavus* and *A. tamarii* (80). A toxin was extracted from seed, and mice injected with the toxin developed signs of CPA toxicity.

Although CPA is clearly toxic to muscle in accidentally and experimentally poisoned animals, it is unclear whether the compound disturbs CNS function directly or indirectly. CPA accumulates in striated, smooth, and cardiac muscles, and specifically inhibits Ca^{2+}-ATPase of the sarcoplasmic reticulum (37,69,70,87). Fast Ca^{2+} imaging has demonstrated that CPA reduces action-potential evoked Ca^{2+} transients in rodent hippocampal CA1 pyramidal neurons (83). CPA also enhanced whole-cell membrane currents induced by treatment of human astrocytes *in vitro* with N-methyl-D-aspartate (68).

REFERENCES

1. Agarwal ON, Negi SS, Mahadevan V (1964) Studies on the toxicity and nutritive value of fungus-free *Paspalum scrobiculatum* grains. *Ind Vet J* **41**, 43.
2. Bazlur M (1960) Probable mona grass (*P. commersoni*) poisoning. *Ind Vet J* **37**, 31.
3. Betina V (1984) Indole-derived tremorgenic toxins. In: *Mycotoxins—Production, Isolation, Separation, and Purification.* Betina V ed. Elsevier Science, Amsterdam p. 415.
4. Bhide NK (1962) Pharmacological study and fractionation of *P. scrobiculatum* extract. *Brit J Pharmacol* **18**, 7.
5. Bradford HF, Norris PJ, Smith CC (1990) Changes in transmitter release patterns *in vitro* induced by tremorgenic mycotoxins. *J Environ Pathol Toxicol Oncol* **10**, 17.
6. Breton P, Bizot JC, Buee J, De La Manche I (1998) Brain neurotoxicity of Penitrem A: electrophysiological, behavioral and histopathological study. *Toxicon* **36**, 645.
7. Byrem TM, Pestka JJ, Chu FS, Strasburg GM (1999) Analysis and pharmacokinetics of cyclopiazonic acid in market weight pigs. *J Anim Sci* **77**, 173.
8. Cavanagh JB, Holton JL, Nolan CC (1997) Selective damage to the cerebellar vermis in chronic alcoholism: a contribution from neurotoxicology to an old problem of selective vulnerability. *Neuropathol Appl Neurobiol* **23**, 355.
9. Cavanagh JB, Holton JL, Nolan CC et al. (1998) The effects of the tremorgenic mycotoxin penitrem A on the rat cerebellum. *Vet Pathol* **35**, 53.
10. Chung CH, Ling KH, Tsai SE et al. (1971) Study on fungi of the stored, unhulled rice of Taiwan (2) Aflatoxin B₁ like compounds from the culture of *Aspergillus* genus. *J Formosa Med Assoc* **70**, 258.
11. Ciegler A, Burmeister HR, Vesonder HF (1983) Poisonous fungi: Mycotoxins and mycotoxicosis. In: *Fungi Pathogenic for Humans and Animals.* Howard DH ed. Marcel Dekker, New York p. 413.
12. Clardy J, Springer JP, Büchi G et al. (1975) Tryptoquivaline and tryptoquivalone, two tremorgenic metabolites of *Aspergillus clavatus. J Amer Chem Soc* **97**, 663.
13. Cockrum PA, Culvenor CCJ, Edgar JA, Payne AL (1979) Chemically different tremorgenic mycotoxins in isolates of *Penicillium paxilli* from Australia and North America. *J Nat Prod* **42**, 534.
14. Cole RJ (1981) Fungal tremorgens. *J Food Protect* **9**, 715.
15. Cole RJ, Dorner JW (1985) Role of fungal tremorgens in animal disease. In: *Mycotoxins and Phycotoxins.* Steyn PS, Vleggaar R eds. Elsevier Science Publishers, Amsterdam p. 501.
16. Cole RJ, Dorner WJ, Lamsden JA et al. (1977) Paspalum staggers: Isolation and identification of tremorgenic metabolites from sclerotia of *Claviceps paspali. Agr Food Chem* **25**, 1197.
17. Cole RJ, Kirksey JW, Dorner JW et al. (1977) Mycotoxins produced by *Aspergillus fumigatus* species isolated from molded silage. *J Agr Food Chem* **25**, 826.
18. Cole RJ, Kirksey JW, Moore JH et al. (1972) Tremorgenic toxin from *Penicillium verruculosum. Appl Microbiol* **24**, 248.
19. Cole RJ, Kirksey JW, Morgan-Jones G (1975) Verruculotoxin, a new mycotoxin from *Penicillium verruculosum. Toxicol Appl Pharmacol* **31**, 465.
20. Cole RJ, Kirksey JW, Wells JM (1974) A new tremorgenic metabolite from *Penicillium paxilli. Can J Microbiol* **20**, 1159.
21. Cysewski SJ, Baetz AL, Pier AC (1975) Penitrem A intoxication of calves: Blood chemical and pathologic changes. *Amer J Vet Res* **36**, 53.
22. DeJesus AE, Steyn PS, Van Heerden FR, Vleggaar R (1984) Structure elucidation of the janthitrems: Novel tremorgenic mycotoxins from *Penicillium janthinellum* isolates from ryegrass pastures. *J Chem Soc Perkin Trans* I, 697.
23. Dorner JW, Cole RJ, Hill RA (1984) Tremorgenic mycotoxins produced by *Aspergillus fumigatus* and *Penicillium crustosum* from molded corn implicated in a natural intoxication in cattle. *J Agr Food Chem* **32**, 411.
24. El-Banna AA, Pitt JI, Leistner L (1987) Production of mycotoxins by *Penicillium* species. *Syst Appl Microbiol* **10**, 42.
25. Eldefrawi ME, Gant DB, Eldefrawi AT (1990) The GABA receptor and the action of tremorgenic mycotoxins. In: *Microbial Toxins in Foods and Feeds.* Pohland AE ed. Plenum Press, New York p. 291.
26. Field DJ, Bowen JM, Cole RJ (1978) Verruculotoxin po-

tentiation of twitch tension in skeletal muscle. *Toxicol Appl Pharmacol* **46**, 529.

27. Fischer G, Muller T, Ostrowski R, Dott W (1999) Mycotoxins of *Aspergillus fumigatus* in pure culture and in native bioaerosols from compost facilities. *Chemosphere* **38**, 1745.

28. Frisvad JC (1989) The connection between the *Penicillia* and *Aspergilli* and mycotoxins with special emphasis on misidentified isolates. *Arch Environ Contam Toxicol* **18**, 452.

29. Gallagher RT, Campbell AG, Hawkes AD et al. (1982) Ryegrass staggers: The presence of lolitrem neurotoxins in perennial ryegrass seed. *N Z Vet J* **30**, 183.

30. Gallagher RT, Finer J, Clardy J et al. (1980) Paspalinine, a tremorgenic metabolite from *Claviceps paspali* Stevens et Hall. *Tetrahedron Lett* **21**, 235.

31. Gallagher RT, Hawkes AD (1986) The potent tremorgenic neurotoxins lolitrem B and aflatrem: A comparison of the tremor response in mice. *Experientia* **42**, 823.

32. Gallagher RT, Latch GCM (1977) Production of the tremorgenic mycotoxins verruculogen and fumitremorgin B by *Pencillium piscarium* Westling. *Appl Environ Microbiol* **33**, 730.

33. Gallagher RT, Latch GCM, Keogh RG (1980) The janthitrems: Fluorescent tremorgenic toxins produced by *Penicillium janthinellum* isolates from ryegrass pastures. *Appl Environ Microbiol* **39**, 272.

34. Gallagher RT, Wilson BJ (1978) Aflatrem, the tremorgenic mycotoxin from *Aspergillus flavus*. *Mycopathologia* **66**, 183.

35. Gant DB, Cole RJ, Valdes JJ et al. (1987) Action of tremorgenic mycotoxins on GABA$_A$ receptor. *Life Sci* **41**, 2207.

36. Glinsukon T, Yuan SS, Wightman R et al. (1974) Isolation and purification of cytochalasin E and two tremorgens from *Aspergillus clavatus*. *Plant Foods Man* **1**, 113.

37. Goeger DE, Riley RT, Dorner JW, Cole RJ (1988) Cyclopiazonic acid inhibition of Ca^{2+} ATPase in rat skeletal muscle sarcoplasmic reticulum vesicles. *Biochem Pharmacol* **37**, 978.

38. Gribkoff VK, Lum-Ragan JT, Boissard CG et al. (1996) Effects of channel modulators on cloned large-conductance calcium-activated potassium channels. *Mol Pharmacol* **50**, 206.

39. Hayes AW, Presley DB, Neville JA (1976) Acute toxicity of penitrem A in dogs. *Toxicol Appl Pharmacol* **35**, 311.

40. Holm NR, Christophersen P, Olesen SP, Gammeltoft S (1997) Activation of calcium-dependent potassium channels in mouse [correction of rat] brain neurons by neurotrophin-3 and nerve growth factor. *Proc Natl Acad Sci USA* **94**, 1002.

41. Hotujac L, Muftie RH, Filipovic N (1976) Verruculogen, a new substance for decreasing GABA levels in CNS. *Pharmacology* **14**, 297.

42. Knaus H-G, McManus OB, Lee SH et al. (1994) Tremorgenic indole alkaloids potently inhibit smooth muscle high-conductance calcium-activated potassium channels. *Biochemistry* **33**, 5819.

43. Laakso JA, Narske ED, Gloer JB et al. (1994) Isokotanins A-C: New bicoumarins from the sclerotia of *Aspergillus alliaceus*. *J Nat Prod* **57**, 128.

44. Lanigan GW, Payne AL, Cockrum PA (1979) Production of tremorgenic toxins by *Penicillium janthinellum* Biourge: A possible aetiological factor in ryegrass staggers. *Austr J Exp Biol Med Sci* **57**, 31.

45. Lansden JA, Davidson JL (1983) Presence of cyclopiazonic acid in peanuts. *Appl Environ Microbiol* **45**, 766.

46. Latch GCM (1985) Endophytes and ryegrass staggers. In: *Trichothecenes and Other Mycotoxins*, Lacey J ed. John Wiley, New York p. 135.

47. Lauren DS, Gallagher RT (1982) High-performance liquid chromatography of the janthitrems: Fluorescent tremorgenic mycotoxins produced by *Penicillium janthinellum*. *J Chromatogr* **150**, 248.

48. Le Bars J (1979) Cyclopiazonic acid production by *Penicillium camberti* Thom and natural occurence of this mycotoxin in cheese. *Appl Environ Microbiol* **38**, 1052.

49. Leitao J, de Saint Blanquat G, Bailly JR, Derache R (1990) Preventive measures for microflora and mycotoxin production in foodstuffs. *Arch Environ Contam Toxicol* **19**, 437.

50. Ling KH (1976) Studies on mycotoxins contaminated in food in Taiwan. (2) Tremor inducing compounds from *Aspergillus terreus*. *Proc Nat Sci Council Repub China*, **9**, 121.

51. Ling KH (1994) Territrems, tremorgenic mycotoxins isolated from *Aspergillus terreus*. *J Toxicol-Toxin Rev* **13**, 243.

52. Ling KH (1998) Territrem: neurotoxicity and biotransformation. *J Toxicol Sci* **23** Suppl 2:189.

53. Ling KH, Huang MT (1975) Studies on mycotoxins contaminated in food in Taiwan. (1) Study on pseudoaflatoxin B2 from *Aspergillus terreus*. *Proc Nat Sci Council Repub China* **8**, 65.

54. Mantle PG (1983) Amino acid neurotransmitter release from cerebrocortical synaptosomes of sheep with severe rye grass staggers in New Zealand. *Res Vet Science* **34**, 373.

55. Mantle PG, Burt SJ, MacGeorge KM et al. (1990) Oxidative transformation of paxilline in sheep bile. *Xenobiotica* **20**, 809.

56. Mantle PG, Mortimer PH, White EP (1977) Mycotoxic tremorgens of *Claviceps paspali* and *Penicillium cyclopium*: A comparative study of effects of sheep and cattle in relation to natural staggers syndromes. *Rev Vet Sci* **24**, 49.

57. Mantle PG, Penny HRC (1981) Tremorgenic mycotoxins and neurological disorders—a review. *Vet Annu* **21**, 51.

58. McLeay LM, Smith BL, Munday-Finch SC (1999) Tremorgenic mycotoxins paxilline, penitrem and lolitrem B, the non-tremorgenic 31-epilolitrem B and electromyographic activity of the reticulum and rumen of sheep. *Res Vet Sci* **66**, 119.

59. Mortimer PH (1978) Perennial ryegrass staggers in New Zealand. In: *Effects of Poisonous Plants on Livestock.* Keeler RF, Van Kampen KR, James LF eds. Academic Press, New York p. 353.

60. Nayak NC, Misra DB (1962) Cattle poisoning by *Paspalum scrobiculatum* (kodua poisoning). *Ind Vet J* **39**, 501.

61. Nielsen PV, Beuchat LR, Frisvad JC (1988) Growth of and fumitremorgin production by *Neosartorya fischeri* as affected by temperature, light and water activity. *Appl Environ Microbiol* **54**, 1504.

62. Nishie K, Cole RJ, Dorner JW (1988) Toxicity and neuropharmacology of cyclopiazonic acid. *Food Chem Toxicol* **23**, 831.

63. Nishie K, Cole RJ, Dorner JW (1988) Toxicity of citreoviridin. *Res Commun Chem Pathol Pharmacol* **59**, 31.

64. Nishie K, Porter JK, Cole RJ, Dorner JW (1986) Neurochemical and pharmacological effects of cyclopiazonic acid, chlorpromazine, and reserpine. *Res Commun Psychol Psychiat Behav* **10**, 291.

65. Nishiyama M, Kuga T (1986) Pharmacological effects of the tremorgenic mycotoxin fumitremorgin A. *Jpn J Pharmacol* **40**, 481.

66. Nishiyama M, Kuga T (1989) Central effects of the neurotropic mycotoxin fumitremorgin a in the rabbit. (I). Effects on the spinal cord. *Jpn J Pharmacol* **50**, 167.

67. Nishiyama M, Kuga T (1990) Central effects of the neurotropic mycotoxin fumitremorgin a in the rabbit. (II). Effects on the brain stem. *Jpn J Pharmacol* **52**, 201.

68. Nishizaki T, Matsuoka T, Nomura T et al. (1999) Store Ca^{2+} depletion enhances NMDA responses in cultured human astrocytes. *Biochem Biophys Res Commun* **16**, 661.

69. Norred WP, Morissey RE, Riley RT et al. (1985) Distribution, excretion, and skeletal muscle effects of the mycotoxin (^{14}C) cyclopiazonic acid in rats. *Food Chem Toxicol* **23**, 1069.

70. Norred WP, Porter JK, Dorner JW, Cole RJ (1988) Occurrence of the mycotoxin, cyclopiazonic acid, in meat after oral administration to chickens. *J Agr Food Chem* **36**, 113.

71. Norris PJ, Smitt CCT, De Belleroche J et al. (1980) Actions of tremorgenic fungal toxins on neurotransmitter release. *J Neurochem* **34**, 33.

72. Nozawa K, Horie Y, Udagawa S et al. (1989) Isolation of a new indoloditerpene, 1'-O-acetylpaxilline from *Emericella striata* and distribution of paxilline in *Emericella* spp. *Chem Pharm Bull Tokyo* **37**, 1387.

73. Patterson DSP, Roberts BA, Shreeve BJ et al. (1979) Tremorgenic toxins produced by soil fungi. *Appl Environ Microbiol* **37**, 172.

74. Peng FC (1995) Acetylcholinesterase inhibition by territrem B derivatives. *J Nat Prod* **58**, 857.

75. Peng FC (1997) Structure and anti-acetylcholinesterase activity of 4 α-(hydroxymethyl)-4 α-demethylterritrem B. *Nat Prod* **60**, 842.

76. Penny RHC, O'Sullivan BM, Shaw BI, Mantle PG (1979) Clinical investigation of tremorgenic mycotoxicoses in sheep. *Vet Rec* **104**, 215.

77. Peterson DW, Bradford HF, Mantle PG (1982) Action of tremorgenic mycotoxins on amino acid transmitter release *in vivo*. *Biochem Pharmacol* **31**, 2807.

78. Pomilio AB, Rofi RD, Gambino MP et al. (1989) The lethal principle of *Poa huecu* (coiron blanco): a plant indigenous to Argentina. *Toxicon* **27**, 1251.

79. Porter KJ, Norred WP, Cole RJ, Dorner JW (1988) Neurochemical effects of cyclopiazonic acid in chickens. *Proc Soc Exp Biol Med* **187**, 335.

80. Rao BL, Husain A (1985) Presence of cyclopiazonic acid in kodo millet (*Paspalum scrobiculatum*) causing "kodua" poisoning in man and its production by associated fungi. *Mycopathologia* **89**, 177.

81. Sakabe N, Goto T, Hirata Y (1964) The structure of citreoviridin, a toxic compound produced by *P. citreoviride* molded on rice. *Tetrahedron Lett* **27**, 1825.

82. Sakabe N, Goto T, Hirata Y (1977) The structure of citreoviridin, a mycotoxin produced by *Penicillium citreoviride* molded on rice. *Tetrahedron Lett* **33**, 3077.

83. Sanchez M, McManus OB (1996) Paxilline inhibition of the alpha-subunit of the high-conductance calcium-activated potassium channel. *Neuropharmacology* **35**, 963.

84. Schroeder HW, Cole RJ, Hein H, Kirksey JW (1975) Tremorgenic mycotoxins from *Aspergillus caespitosus*. *Appl Microbiol* **24**, 248.

85. Schuchardt B (1887) Zur Geschichte und Kasuistik des Lathyrismus. *Deut Arch Klin Med* **40**, 312.

86. Scuteri M, Sala de Miguel MA, Blanco Viera J, Planes de Banchero E (1992) Tremorgenic mycotoxins produced by strains of *Penicillium* spp. isolated from toxic *Poa huecu* Parodi. *Mycopathologia* **120**, 177.

87. Seidler NW, Jona I, Vegh M, Martonisi M (1989) Cyclopiazonic acid is a specific inhibitor of the Ca^{2+} ATPase of sarcoplasmic reticulum. *J Biol Chem* **264**, 17816.

88. Selala MI, Daelemans F, Schepens PJ (1989) Fungal tremorgens: The mechanism of action of single nitrogen containing toxins—a hypothesis. *Drug Chem Toxicol* **12**, 237.

89. Selala MI, Laekeman GM, Loenders B et al. (1991) *In vitro* effects of tremorgenic mycotoxins. *J Nat Prod* **54**, 207.

90. Shreeve BJ, Pattersson DSP, Roberts BA, MacDonald SM (1983) Tremorgenic fungal toxins. *Vet Res Commun* 7, 155.

91. Sram RJ, Dobias L, Rossner P *et al.* (1993) Monitoring genotoxic exposure in uranium mines. *Environ Health Perspect* 101 Suppl 3:155.

92. Stern P (1971) Pharmacological analysis of the tremor induced by Cyclopium toxin. *Jugoslav Physiol Pharmacol Acta* 7, 187.

93. Steyn PS, Vleggaar R (1985) Tremorgenic mycotoxins. *Fortschr Chem Org Naturst* 48, 1.

94. Suzuki S, Kikkawa K, Yamazaki M (1984) Abnormal behavioral effects elicited by a neurotropic mycotoxin, fumitremorgin A, in mice. *J Pharmacobiodyn* 7, 935.

95. Tournas V (1994) Heat-resistant fungi of importance to the food and beverage industry. *Crit Rev Microbiol* 20, 243.

96. Tung SS, Ling KH, Tsai SE *et al.* (1971) Study on fungi of the stored, unhulled rice of Taiwan (1) Mycological survey of the stored unhulled rice. *J Formosa Med Assoc* 70, 251.

97. Uraguchi K (1971) Citreoviridin. In: *Microbial Toxins. Vol 6. Fungal Toxins.* Ciegler A, Kadis S, Ajl SJ eds. Academic Press, New York p. 299.

98. Verhaart WJC (1938) Symmetrical degeneration of the neostriatum in Chinese infants. *Arch Dis Child* 13, 225.

99. Vieta I, Savarino A, Papa G *et al.* (1996) *In vitro* inhibitory activity of citreoviridin against HIV-1 and an HIV-associated opportunist: *Candida albicans. Chemother* 8, 351.

100. Weiser M, Fink-Gremmels J (1991) Effects of verrucologen and fumitremorgin B on neurotransmitter release *in vivo. Acta Vet Scand Suppl* 87, 193.

101. Wilson BJ, Byerly CS, Burka LT (1981) Neurological disease of fungal origin in three herds of cattle. *J Amer Vet Med Assn* 179, 480.

102. Wilson BJ, Hoekman T, Dettbarn W-D (1972) Effect of fungus tremorgenic toxin (penitrem A) on transmission in rat phrenic nerve-diaphragm preparations. *Brain Res* 40, 540.

103. Wilson BJ, Wilson CH (1964) Toxin from *Aspergillus flavus:* Production on food materials of a substance causing tremors in mice. *Science* 144, 177.

104. Wilson BJ, Wilson CH, Hayes AW (1968) Tremorgenic toxin from *Penicillium cyclopium* grown on food materials. *Nature* 220, 77.

105. Woods AH, Pendleton L (1925) Fourteen simultaneous cases of an acute degenerative striatal disease. *Arch Neurol Psych* 13, 549.

106. Yamazaki M, Fujimoto H, Okuyama E (1976) Structure determination of six tryptoquivaline-related metabolites from *Aspergillus fumigatus. Tetrahedron Lett* 28, 61.

107. Yamazaki M, Suzuki S (1986) Toxicology of tremorgenic mycotoxins, fumitremorgin A and B. *Develop Toxicol Environ Sci* 12, 273.

108. Yamazaki M, Suzuki S, Kukita K (1979) Neurotoxicological studies on fumitremorgin A, a tremorgenic mycotocin, on mice. *J Pharmacobiodyn* 2, 119.

109. Yamazaki M, Suzuki S, Miyaki K (1971) Tremorgenic toxins from *Aspergillus fumigatus. Fres Chem Pharm Bull (Tokyo)* 19, 1739.

110. Yao Y, Peter AB, Baur R, Sigel E (1989) The tremorogen aflatrem is a positive allosteric modulator of the gamma-aminobutyric acid A receptor channel expressed in expressed in *Xenopus* oocytes. *Mol Pharmacol* 35, 319.

Pennyroyal Oil

Peter S. Spencer

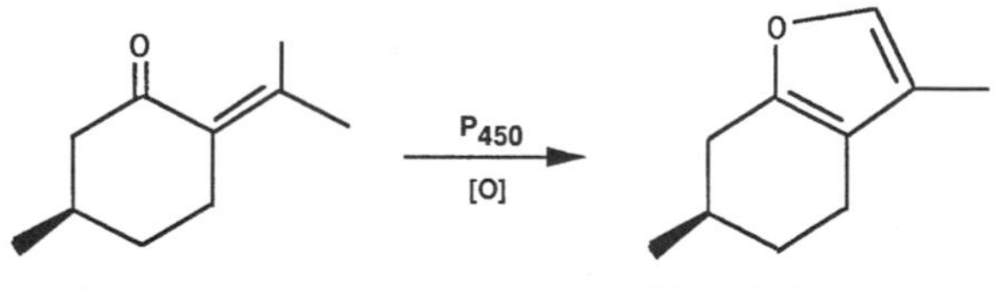

(R)-PULEGONE
$C_9H_{14}O$

(R)-MENTHOFURAN
$C_9H_{12}O$

Squaw mint, mosquito plant

NEUROTOXICITY RATING

Clinical

B   Acute encephalopathy

American pennyroyal, *Hedeoma pulegioides* (Linné) Persoon (Fam. Labiatae), is distributed from Canada to Florida and west to Nebraska (7). Pennyroyal has a long history of folk-medicine use as an aromatic stimulant, a carminative, a diaphoretic, an emmenagogue and, among Native Americans, a treatment for headache (7). The herb and oil of pennyroyal (also known as *Mentha pulegium*) are used in flea collars for cats and dogs (4). The oil contains (−)-methone, (+)-isomethone, and an hepatotoxic monoterpene, R-(+)-pulegone, which depletes plasma and hepatic glutathione. Pulegone is metabolized by human liver cytochrome P-450s to menthofuran (*vide supra*), a proximate hepatotoxic metabolite of pulegone (3,4). Rats treated with pulegone develop severe hepatotoxicity (3,5); the nervous system appears not to have been examined. Ingestion of pennyroyal in herbal teas has resulted in severe and sometimes fatal poisoning (1,2,6); most cases have occurred in adult women who used pennyroyal as an abortifacient (4). Two infants developed hepatic and neurologic illness after ingestion of home-brewed mint tea (2). One infant developed hepatic dysfunction and severe epileptic encephalopathy. Fulminant liver failure with cerebral edema and necrosis developed in the second. Sera from both individuals were positive for pulegone (25 ng/ml) and/or menthofuran (41 ng/ml) (2).

REFERENCES

1. Anderson IB, Mullen WH, Meeker JE et al. (1996) Pennyroyal toxicity: measurement of toxic metabolite levels in two cases and review of the literature. Ann Intern Med 124, 726.

2. Bakerink JA, Gospe SM Jr, Dimand RJ, Eldridge MW (1996) Multiple organ failure after ingestion of pennyroyal oil from herbal tea in two infants. Pediatrics 98, 944.

3. Gordon WP, Huitric AC, Seth CL et al. (1987) The metabolism of the abortifacient terpene, (R)-(+)-pulegone, to a proximate toxin, menthofuran. Drug Metab Dispos 15, 589.

4. Khojasteh-Bakht SC, Chen W, Koenigs LL et al. (1999) Metabolism of (R)-(+)-pulegone and (R)-(+)-menthofuran by human liver cytochrome P-450s: evidence for formation of a furan epoxide. Drug Metab Dispos 27, 574.

5. Mizutani T, Nomura H, Nakanishi K, Fujita S (1987) Effects of drug metabolism modifiers on pulegone-induced hepatotoxicity in mice. Res Commun Chem Pathol Pharmacol 58, 75.

6. Sullivan JB Jr, Rumack BH, Thomas H Jr et al. (1979) Pennyroyal oil poisoning and hepatotoxicity. J Amer Med Assoc 242, 2873.

7. Tyler V, Brady LR, Robbers JE (1981) Pharmacognosy. 8th ed. Lea & Febiger, Philadelphia, p. 492.

Pentaborane

Steven A. Sparr

B_5H_9

Pentaborane (9); Pentaboron nonahydride

NEUROTOXICITY RATING
Clinical
A   Seizure disorder (generalized myoclonic)
A   Acute encephalopathy (lethargy, hallucinations, coma)
B   Myopathy (rhabdomyolysis)
Experimental
A   Seizure disorder

Pentaborane, a member of the boron hydride family, was first synthesized in the 1870s (10). These compounds are highly effective reducing agents (10). During and after World War II, boron hydrides were studied for use as rocket fuels (4). In the 1960s, borane hydrides were used as dopants in the manufacture of semiconductors (10) and as industrial catalysts in synthetic reactions (6). Pentaborane is highly neurotoxic and is capable of causing profound, diffuse CNS damage in humans (1,2,5,6,10) and in laboratory animals (2,4,7,8).

There are three relatively stable boron hydrides: diboranc, a gas at standard atmospheric conditions; pentaborane, a liquid; and decaborane, a solid. The toxicity of the latter two compounds is similar, both produce severe CNS damage; diborane induces severe pulmonary toxicity (10). All of the compounds rapidly oxidize in water to form boric oxide in highly exothermic reactions (10). The high reactivity of pentaborane, boric oxide, or possible intermediates in the reaction (4), cause widespread organ toxicity. Particularly affected are enzymes that have pyridoxal phosphate as a cofactor, including dopa decarboxylase, necessary for the synthesis of dopamine and norepinephrine, and 5-hydroxytryptophan decarboxylase, required for the synthesis of serotonin (4). Although the specific cause of neurotoxicity is unknown, depletion of these biogenic amines is probably a major factor (4).

Pentaborane may enter the body by inhalation, ingestion, or through the skin (3,10). In animal models, toxicity has been produced by intraperitoneal injections (2,4,8) or by inhalation (7,8). As the substance is highly toxic, great care must be taken to avoid exposure in the workplace. The recommended threshold of 0.005 ppm is well below the odor threshold of 0.8 ppm, so that smelling the substance (which has an odor reminiscent of burnt rubber) already implies an exposure beyond that recommended (3,8,10).

Animal studies have confirmed the severe toxicity of pentaborane (2,4,7,8). Rats die immediately after exposure to concentrations of 14 ppm (8). Exposure to 10 ppm causes death after 2 h, and exposure to 3.5 ppm for 5 h daily leads to 100% mortality by 4 days (4). Dogs exposed to toxic sublethal concentrations of pentaborane exhibit hyperactivity, followed by lethargy, increased salivation, muscle spasms, catatonia, myoclonic jerks, and seizures (7,8). After recovering from acute toxic reactions, animals remain lethargic and apprehensive for several days, and have a poor appetite (8). Comparable toxicity with repeated low-dose exposures suggest cumulative effects (8).

Exposure of animals to either pentaborane or decaborane is followed by depletion of brain norepinephrine, serotonin, and dopamine (2,4), although one rat study found a slight increase in brain serotonin associated with a profound decrease of norepinephrine (9). Treatment of mice with pyridoxine prior to exposure attenuates the neurotoxic effect of pentaborane (4), and some reversal of hemodynamic compromise in dogs was achieved by treatment with norepinephrine (7).

The toxicity of pentaborane in humans has been elucidated from the clinical histories of patients exposed to the substance in industrial accidents (1,3,5,6,10). With major exposures, patients develop cardiac depression with hypotension, bradycardia, and severe metabolic acidosis, with arterial pH as low as 6.4. Rhabdomyolysis, with elevated muscle enzymes in the serum and myoglobinuria, has been reported, as has toxic hepatitis, with elevated hepatic parenchymal enzymes, and biopsy-proven necrosis and fatty degeneration (10).

Neurological effects may be evident within minutes of exposure or are delayed up to 40 h (10). Early manifestations include lethargy, anxiety, dizziness, headache, inattentiveness, and personality change (3,6,10). These may be followed by sialorrhea, hypesthesia, myoclonic muscle jerks, opisthotonic spasms, visual hallucinations, generalized seizures, coma, and death (3,6,10). Patients who survive may recover completely or may have permanent neurological sequelae with incoordination, visual abnormalities, and spasticity (10). Residual cognitive deficits, especially in memory and visuospatial processing, and persistent computed tomography (CT) evidence of brain atrophy, have appeared in patients exposed to pentaborane (1,5,6). Many patients had persistent psychiatric symptoms that met DSM III criteria for posttraumatic stress disorder (5,6).

Electroencephalograms of patients with major toxic CNS reactions show bitemporal or diffuse slowing (3,10), tri-phasic waves (10), or convulsive spikes (3). Serial CT scans may disclose cerebral edema followed by progressive diffuse brain atrophy with ventriculomegaly (10).

There is no known antidote for pentaborane toxicity. Treatment with intravenous catecholamines and pyridoxine is recommended for victims of major exposure, although it is unclear if these therapies alter the course (10).

Depletion of CNS catecholamines is thought to have a major role in the production of toxicity; however, reserpine causes even greater depletion but has lower toxic potential (10). Many other enzyme systems are disrupted by pentaborane, such as lactic and malic dehydrogenase, and those involved in oxidative phosphorylation (4), and pentaborane reacts avidly with saturated hydrocarbons and heterocyclic amines (6). Thus, widespread disruption of many biological processes is predictable with exposure.

REFERENCES

1. Hart RP, Silverman JJ, Garrettson LK et al. (1984) Neuropsychological function following mild exposure to pentaborane. Amer J Ind Med 6, 37.
2. Merritt JH, Shultz EJ (1966) The effect of decaborane on the biosynthesis and metabolism of norepinephrine in the rat brain. Life Sci 5, 27.
3. Mindrum G (1964) Pentaborane intoxication. Arch Intern Med 114, 364.
4. Naeger LL, Leibman KC (1972) Mechanism of decaborane toxicity. Toxicol Appl Pharmacol 22, 517.
5. Silverman JJ (1986) Post-traumatic stress disorder. Adv Psychosom Med 16, 115.
6. Silverman JJ, Hart RP, Garrettson LK et al. (1985) Post-traumatic stress disorder from pentaborane intoxication. Neuropsychiatric evaluation and short-term follow-up. J Amer Med Assn 254, 2603.
7. Weir FW, Meyers FH (1966) The similar pharmacologic effects of pentaborane, decaborane and reserpine. Ind Med Surg 35, 696.
8. Weir FW, Seabaugh VM, Mershon MM et al. (1964) Short exposure inhalation toxicity of pentaborane in animals. Toxicol Appl Pharmacol 6, 121.
9. Wykes AA, Landez JH (1965) The effect of decaborane and pentaborane on brain amines as influenced by pargyline hydrochloride and iproniazid phosphate. Fed Proc 24, 194.
10. Yarbrough BE, Garrettson LK, Zolet DI et al. (1985–6) Severe central nervous system damage and profound acidosis in persons exposed to pentaborane. J Toxicol-Clin Toxicol 23, 519.

2,4-Pentanedione

Peter S. Spencer

$$CH_3CCH_2CCH_3$$

with O double bonds above the first and third carbons

2,4-PENTANEDIONE
$C_5H_8O_2$

Acetylacetone; 2,4-PD

NEUROTOXICITY RATING

Experimental

C   Peripheral neuropathy

2,4-Pentanedione (2,4-PD), a colorless or slightly yellow flammable liquid, is miscible with most organic solvents and forms organometallic complexes (*e.g.*, bis[2,4-pentanedionato-O,O']nickel, a catalyst). These are used as additives for gasoline and lubricants, as driers for varnishers' and printers' inks, and as fungicides and insecticides (1). A novel bisubstituted catechol, 3-[3,4-dihydroxybenzylidine]-2,4-pentanedione, is an orally active and highly selective inhibitor of peripheral but not striatal catechol-O-methyltransferase (4).

2,4-PD was fetotoxic (reduced body weight and ossification) when pregnant Fischer 344 rats were exposed to 398 ppm on gestational days 6–15; at 53 ppm, no observable fetal or maternal effects were seen (7).

The rat LC_{50} for 2,4-PD is 1000 ppm (1). Most male and female Fischer 344 rats exposed for 4 h to 1811 ppm died within hours of exposure; 10% died after exposure to 1265 ppm (3). All female animals and one-third of males died after 29 daily 4-h exposures to 650 ppm 2,4-PD. Half of the animals that survived and most of those that died reportedly had light microscopical evidence of malacia and gliosis principally in the caudate-putamen, deep cerebellar nuclei, and vestibular nuclei; some had changes in various regions of the cerebral cortex. No neuropathological changes were seen in animals exposed to 307 ppm or 101 ppm 2,4-PD (2,3).

Ultrastructural examination of peripheral nerves removed from rats treated in the aforementioned study for 14 weeks with 650 ppm failed to disclose pathological changes (2,3). However, in a separate report (5), rats treated subcutaneously with 2,4-PD or 2,5-hexanedione (2,5-HD; an established cause of peripheral neuropathy) 200 mg/kg/day, 5 days/week, exhibited significant slowing of maximum motor nerve conduction velocity (MCV) after 6 and 10 weeks, respectively, and sensory nerve conduction velocity (SCV) was decreased in both groups in the eighth week of treatment. Whereas changes in MCV reportedly were more pronounced than those in SCV in 2,5-HD–treated animals, the reverse pattern was seen in rats treated with 2,4-PD. Amplitudes of the motor nerve action potential (NAP) and muscle action potential (MAP) were significantly decreased after 10 and 12 weeks of 2,5-HD treatment and after 16 and 28 weeks of 2,4-pentanedione treatment. Motor distal latencies were markedly prolonged at an early stage only in rats treated with 2,5-HD (5).

2,4-PD is mildly irritating to skin and mucous membranes (1).

2,4-PD is a symmetrical aliphatic diketone which, in contrast to 2,5-hexanedione, lacks the γ-diketo spacing required for the induction of central-peripheral distal axonopathy of the giant axonal type (6). Reports of CNS and PNS disease in animals repeatedly exposed to 2,4-PD require confirmation. Block of normal thiamine biochemistry has been advanced to explain the CNS pathology associated with subchronic 2,4-PD exposure (3).

REFERENCES

1. Budavari S, O'Neil MJ, Smith A *et al.* (1996) *The Merck Index. An Encyclopedia of Chemicals, Drugs, and Biologicals.* 12th Ed. Merck & Co, Whitehouse Station, New Jersey.
2. Dodd DE, Garman H, Pritts IM *et al.* (1986) 2,4-Pentanedione: 9-day and 14-week vapor inhalation studies in Fischer-344 rats. *Fund Appl Toxicol* 7, 329.
3. Garman RH, Dodd DE, Ballantyne B (1995) Central neurotoxicity induced by subchronic exposure to 2,4-pentanedione vapor. *Hum Exp Toxicol* 14, 662.
4. Mannisto PT, Kaakkola S, Nissinen E *et al.* (1988) Properties of novel effective and highly selective inhibitors of catechol-O-methyltransferase. *Life Sci* 43, 1465.
5. Nagano M, Misumi J, Nomura S (1983) An electrophysiological study on peripheral neurotoxicity of 2,3-butanedione, 2,4-pentanedione and 2,5-hexanedione in rats. *Jpn J Ind Health (Sangyo Igaku)* 25, 471.
6. Spencer PS, Bischoff MC, Schaumburg HH (1978) On the specific molecular configuration of neurotoxic aliphatic compounds causing central-peripheral distal axonopathy. *Toxicol Appl Pharmacol* 44, 17.
7. Tyl RW, Ballantyne B, Pritts IM *et al.* (1990) An evaluation of the developmental toxicity of 2,4-pentanedione in the Fischer 344 rat by vapor exposure. *Toxicol Indust Health* 6, 461.

Pentazocine

Herbert H. Schaumburg

PENTAZOCINE
C₁₉H₂₇NO

(2α,6α,11R*)-1,2,3,4,5,6-Hexahydro-6,11-dimethyl-3-(3-methyl-2-butenyl)-2,6-methano-3-benzazocin-8-ol

NEUROTOXICITY RATING

Clinical

A Acute encephalopathy (seizures, stupor, coma)

B Myopathy (myofibrosis—local administration)

Pentazocine, a synthetic benzomorphan opioid, was designed as a drug that could produce analgesia with little potential for abuse. Initially, pentazocine was not subject to special regulation in North America; however, U.S. Federal Controlled Substances Act regulations were instituted following an epidemic of abuse in the addict subculture of a pentazocine-tripelennamine mixture. The drug is uncommonly used now, mostly for chronic pain syndromes and in individuals considered at risk for abuse.

Pentazocine is rapidly absorbed from the gastrointestinal tract following parenteral administration; first-pass hepatic metabolism is extensive, >50% in most individuals (2). There is considerable variability in rate of metabolism, rendering pentazocine's analgesic effect unpredictable. Aside from nausea, tachycardia, and sweating, there are few systemic adverse effects (3). Repeated subcutaneous or intramuscular injection is associated with severe local dermal and muscle necrosis, and eventually these lesions may become disabling and limit proximal limb function (6). Instances of familial pentazocine or meperidine parenteral abuse have been erroneously labeled as hereditary myopathies (1,4).

Experimental animal studies indicate that pentazocine differs from other opioids in its action at μ, κ, and σ opioid receptors. Most therapeutic opioids are agonists at μ and κ receptors and, in high doses, cause respiratory depression, CNS depression, and meiosis. Pentazocine acts both as an agonist and antagonist at μ receptors, a partial agonist at κ receptors and, unlike other opioids, as an agonist at σ receptors. Large amounts of pentazocine increase the excit-ability of the cerebral cortex and release substantial amounts of dopamine and norepinephrine from brain tissue (5,6). The maximum depletion of brain catecholamines co-incides with stimulation of motor activity (9).

Generalized seizures occasionally occur in human over-doses; they may reflect the catecholamine effect (8). Other phenomena in pentazocine-overdose syndromes can be attributed to the drug's effect on specific opioid receptors, as follows: (a) variable degrees of respiratory depression reflect the balance between agonist and antagonist activity at the μ receptor, (b) stupor/coma and meiosis are consistent with agonism at the σ receptor, and (c) psychomimetic effects (dysphoria, bizarre thoughts, anxiety, visual hallucinations) are secondary to agonism at the σ receptor.

The neurotoxicity of pentazocine is unpredictably enhanced by coconsumption of other sedative-hypnotic drugs or ethyl alcohol. Reports describe coma and severe respiratory depression when pentazocine overdose is combined with ingestion of these substances (7,10).

REFERENCES

1. Alberfeld DC, Bienenstock H, Shapiro MS et al. (1968) Diffuse myopathy related to meperidine addiction in a mother and daughter. Arch Neurol 19, 384.
2. Beckett AH, Taylor JF, Kourounakis P (1970) The absorption, distribution and excretion of pentazocine in man after oral and intravenous administration. J Pharmacol 22, 123.
3. Challoner KR, McCarron MM, Newton E (1990) Pentazocine (Talwin) intoxication: Report of 57 cases. J Emerg Med 8, 67.
4. Choucair AK, Ziter FA (1984) Pentazocine abuse masquerading as familial myopathy. Neurology 34, 524.
5. Holtzman SG, Jewelt RF (1972) Some actions of pentazocine on behavior and brain monamines in the rat. J Pharmacol Exp Ther 181, 346.
6. Oh SJ, Rollins JL, Lewis I (1975) Pentazocine-induced fibrotic myopathy. J Amer Med Assn 231, 271.
7. Poklis A, MacKell M (1982) Toxicological findings in deaths due to ingestion of pentazocine: A report of two cases. Forensic Sci Int 20, 89.
8. Roytblat I, Bear R, Gesztes T (1986) Seizures after pentazocine overdose. Isr J Med Sci 22, 385.
9. Soto-Moyan R, Pacile C, Hernandez A (1980) Increase of cortical excitability induced by pentazocine. J Pharm Pharmacol 32, 599.
10. Stahl SM, Kasser IS (1983) Pentazocine overdose. Ann Emerg Med 12, 28.

Pentenenitrile

Mary Beth Genter
Kevin M. Crofton

$$CH_3—CH_2—CH=CH—CN$$

2-PENTENENITRILE
C_5H_7N

2-Pentenenitrile; *cis*-2-Pentenenitrile; 1-Cyano-1-butene

NEUROTOXICITY RATING

Experimental

A Olfactory neuropathy

A Ototoxicity

Pentenenitrile exists as a series of isomers, of which 2-pentenenitrile (2-PN) is the most commercially visible. 2-PN is used as a feedstock in the manufacture of pyridine and polymer derivatives (2). Although information on industrial usage of 2-PN is limited, it appears to be a part of a by-product stream that also contains 2-methyl-2-butenenitrile and 2-methyl-3-butenenitrile (6). Production quantities and potential for human exposure are unknown. No workplace exposure standard or drinking water standards have been established for the pentenenitrile isomers (1,16).

Little toxicity testing has been conducted on any of the isomers of pentenenitrile. Most data are available for 2-PN, which is a neurotoxicant by various routes of exposure.

Acute oral administration of 2-PN (up to 3.0 mmol/kg, with and without carbon tetrachloride pretreatment) results in a syndrome of neurotoxicity very similar to that seen following β,β'-iminodipropionitrile (IDPN) exposure; both rats and mice exhibit head-bobbing, retropulsion, circling, and hyperactivity (13,15). Hyperactivity, spasms, and incoordination were seen in rats following acute oral administration of 200–1000 mg/kg pentenenitrile (5). Evidence that 2-PN is an olfactory system toxicant is derived from a study in which 2-PN was administered intraperitoneally for 3 consecutive days at doses of 0–200 mg/kg/day (10). The highest dose caused a pattern of olfactory damage characterized by complete sloughing of the epithelium and damage to the Bowman's glands. Evidence of damage to the vestibular system and a profound hearing loss were observed following intraperitoneal administration of 100 mg/kg 2-PN (10). A 4-h inhalation study with high-purity (>98%) 2-PN also demonstrated signs of CNS toxicity including circling, foot splay, and head-bobbing (7,10). In summary, the acute toxicity of 2-PN resembles that of IDPN, with similar olfactory pathology, profound hearing loss, and behavioral evidence of vestibular damage (*see* 4,9,11,12).

There is a paucity of information on the effects of long-term exposure to pentenenitrile. Inhalation exposure to 2-PN at concentrations up to 300 ppm for 4 weeks failed to produce neurotoxicity as assessed by functional-observational-battery and motor-activity measures; however, olfactory epithelial damage occurred at airborne concentrations of 30 ppm and above (3,8). This study actually involved exposure to "stripped" 2-PN, which contained approximately 70% *cis*-2-PN and 20% *cis*-2-methyl-2-butenenitrile, along with a number of other minor contaminants. The contribution of 2-PN to the olfactory toxicity observed in this study is clouded somewhat, as acute 2-methyl-2-butenenitrile exposure also causes olfactory mucosal damage (10).

The molecular basis for the neurotoxicity of 2-PN is unknown. Some studies point to alterations in the metabolism of neurotransmitters such as serotonin and dopamine (14,15). Administration of serotonin or dopamine antagonists reduced signs of 2-PN neurotoxicity, whereas administration of a serotonin releaser enhanced the behavioral effects of 2-PN (13).

Neither 3-pentenenitrile (3-PN) nor 4-pentenenitrile (4-PN) are associated with CNS or olfactory system toxicity, even at lethal dosages (10; K.M. Crofton, unpublished data).

There is no information on human exposures to 2-PN.

REFERENCES

1. ACGIH (1994) American Conference of Governmental Industrial Hygienists, Threshold Limit Values, Cincinnati, Ohio.

2. Anonymous (1978) *Chemical Marketing Reporter*, 08/14/78, p. 4.

3. Bogdaffy M (1993) Olfactory mucosal toxicity, integration of morphological and biochemical data in mechanistic studies: Dibasic esters as an example. CIIT Conference: *Nasal Toxicity and Dosimetry of Inhaled Xenobiotics: Implications for Human Health*. Durham, North Carolina.

4. Crofton KM, Janssen R, Prazma G *et al.* (1994) The ototoxicity of β,β'-iminodipropionitrile: Functional and morphological evidence of cochlear dysfunction. *Hear Res* 80, 129.

5. DuPont (1990) Approximate lethal dose (ALD) of 2-pentenenitrile in rats. *FYI Submission to US Environmental Protection Agency* (FYI-OTS-0990–0790), September 26, 1990.

6. DuPont (1991) *FYI Submission to the US Environmental Protection Agency* (FYI-OTS-1991–0790), January 11, 1991.

7. DuPont (1991) Acute inhalation toxicity study with cis-2-

pentenenitrile in rats. *TSCA 8e Submission to the US Environmental Protection Agency* (8EHQ-0691–1121), June 20, 1991.

8. DuPont (1993) *TSCA 8e Submission to the US Environmental Protection Agency* (8EHQ-0693–1121), June 1, 1993.

9. Genter MB, Llorens J, O'Callaghan JP *et al.* (1992) Olfactory toxicity of β,β'-iminodipropionitrile in the rat. *J Pharmacol Exp Ther* **263**, 1432.

10. Genter MB, Zhao X, Crofton KM (1995) Structure-activity studies on the audio-vestibular and olfactory toxicity of nitriles. *Toxicologist* **15**, abstr #119.

11. Llorens J, Demênes D (1994) Hair cell degeneration resulting from β,β'-iminodipropionitrile toxicity in the rat vestibular epithelia. *Hear Res* **76**, 78.

12. Llorens J, Demênes D, Sans A (1993) The behavioral syndrome caused by β,β'-iminodipropionitrile and related nitriles in the rat is associated with degeneration of the vestibular sensory hair cells. *Toxicol Appl Pharmacol* **123**, 199.

13. Tanii H, Hayshi M, Hashimoto K (1989) Nitrile-induced behavioral abnormalities in mice. *Neurotoxicology* **10**, 157.

14. Tanii H, Hayshi M, Hashimoto K (1990) Effects of neurotropic agents with a selectivity for alpha-adrenoreceptors on nitrile-induced dyskinetic syndrome in mice. *Pharmacol Biochem Behav* **36**,317.

15. Tanii H, Hayshi M, Hashimoto K (1991) Behavioral syndrome induced by allylnitrile, crotononitrile or 2-pentenenitrile in rats. *Neuropharmacology* **30**, 877.

16. US EPA (1995b) *Drinking Water Regulations and Health Advisories*. Office of Water, U.S. Environmental Protection Agency (US EPA) Washington, DC.

Perhexiline Maleate

Steven Herskovitz

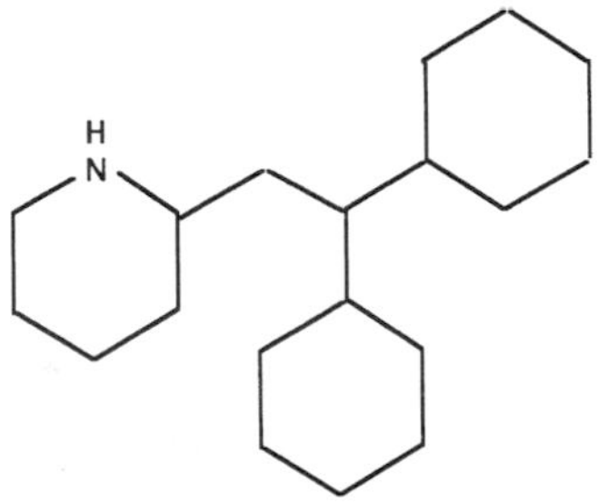

PERHEXILINE
$C_{19}H_{35}N$

2-(2,2-Dicyclohexylethyl)piperidine

NEUROTOXICITY RATING

Clinical

A   Peripheral neuropathy

A   Benign intracranial hypertension

Experimental

A   Peripheral neuropathy (axonal & demyelinating)

Perhexilene maleate (PM) is an orally administered prophylactic agent for treatment of angina pectoris and variant angina (Prinzmetal's) (8,12). Drug actions include coronary vasodilation by a direct effect on vascular smooth muscle and blocking of exercise-induced tachycardia. The principal neurotoxic effect of PM is a peripheral neuropathy. There are additional reports of raised intracranial pressure with papilledema and a proximal myopathy.

PM is absorbed within 6–12 h of ingestion and has a half-life of 3–12 days. It is a lipophilic drug, can be found unchanged along with its metabolites in all tissues examined, and is eliminated in urine and feces after metabolic oxidation in the liver to the more polar mono- and dihydroxylated metabolites (21). Large interindividual variations in plasma half-lives, and thereby risk of toxic drug accumulation, are well described. They may reflect genetically determined differences in rate of metabolism of the drug; poor debrisoquine hydroxylators (poor-metabolizer phenotype) are at greater risk for neuropathy (15–17).

When fed PM orally at 80 mg/kg/day for 4–10 weeks, dark Agouti rats (poor debrisoquine hydroxylators) develop cytoplasmic lipid inclusions similar to those in humans (9). These are most prominent in sensory and autonomic ganglia, but also appear in Schwann cells along with demyelination in spinal roots and mixed demyelination and axonal degeneration in distal nerve segments. The number of inclusions is related to the duration of PM treatment and to tissue and plasma concentrations of PM. There is a prolongation of motor latency in sciatic nerve. Withdrawal of the drug results in decreased numbers of inclusion bodies within 2 weeks, indicating reversibility. Sprague-Dawley rats, which are vigorous hydroxylators, accumulate few inclusion bodies after prolonged treatment. In a study of adult Swiss NMRI strain mice fed PM for 10–18 weeks at 100–200 mg/kg/day, inclusions were present in Schwann and perineurial cells of sciatic nerve as well as in gastrocnemius muscle biopsies (1). In both studies, changes in animal weight, behavior, or nonquantitative measures of neurological function were not noted. Polymorphous inclusions in neurons, satellite cells, Schwann cells, and fibroblasts were noted in mice spinal ganglia treated *in vitro* for 3 days with PM concentrations of 7 and 14 μg/ml (4).

The neuropathy associated with PM therapy appears after treatment for months to years at the commonly used doses of 200–400 mg daily (2,5,6,13,20). The incidence of symptomatic neuropathy may be low (10,14), but subclinical electrophysiological abnormalities occur in up to two-thirds of patients (14,16). It is a symmetrical sensorimotor polyneuropathy, beginning with acral pain and paresthesias, and evolving to both proximal and distal weakness. There may be facial diplegia, perioral numbness or autonomic dysfunction, hyporeflexia or reflexia, and stocking hypesthesia (2,13). After drug withdrawal, recovery evolves gradually over months; it may be incomplete in severe cases.

The protein level in cerebrospinal fluid is typically mildly to moderately elevated—up to several hundred milligrams per deciliter (5,6,13,18,20). There is mild to marked prolongation of distal motor latencies and slowing of motor and sensory conduction velocities to 20 m/sec or even less, consistent with primary demyelination (5,6,13,20).

Examination of human sural nerve biopsies, including teased nerve fibers, shows segmental demyelination along with mild loss of large myelinated fibers. In a study of five patients, segmental demyelination was found in 16%–90% of fibers and axonal degeneration in 3%–20% (13). There is no inflammatory infiltrate (1,13). Numerous polymorphic lysosomal inclusions are present mainly in Schwann cells, but also in endothelial cells, fibroblasts, perineurial cells, phagocytes, and pericytes, as well as in hepatocytes and skin and muscle fibers (1,4,13). Biochemical analysis of biopsy samples in four patients suggested that PM-induced lipid storage consists mainly of gangliosides (11).

PM is occasionally associated with raised intracranial pressure (pseudotumor cerebri) and papilledema, with or without peripheral neuropathy (3,18). Improvement occurs within a few weeks of stopping the drug. A single patient is described with acute proximal weakness, rash, and an electromyogram with myopathic motor units and recruitment pattern; this case is unconvincing as the creatine kinase level was normal and no muscle biopsy was performed (19); resolution occurred within 2 months of drug discontinuation. Systemic effects of PM include weight loss, nausea, dizziness, and hepatotoxicity. Keratopathy is described, including the development of cytoplasmic inclusions in conjunctiva and corneal epithelium (3).

The clinical profile, electrophysiological studies, nerve biopsy data, and experimental animal studies indicate a primary demyelinating polyneuropathy with associated axonal degeneration. The toxic mechanism is likely related to accumulation of lysosomal inclusions in Schwann cells and other tissues. Like amiodarone, PM is a cationic amphophilic drug that can penetrate lysosomes. It is postulated that such compounds form tight but not irreversible complexes with polar lipids leading to impairment of degradation and to intralysosomal accumulation (7). The inclusions resemble those found in patients with inherited lysosomal storage diseases.

REFERENCES

1. Fardeau M, Tomé FMS, Simon P (1979) Muscle and nerve changes induced by perhexilene maleate in man and mice. *Muscle Nerve* 2, 24.
2. Fraser DM, Campbell IW, Miller HC (1977) Peripheral and autonomic neuropathy after treatment with perhexilene maleate. *Brit Med J* 2, 675.
3. Gibson JM, Fielder AR, Garner A, Millac P (1984) Severe ocular side effects of perhexilene maleate: Case report. *Brit J Ophthalmol* 68, 553.
4. Hauw JJ, Mussini JM, Boutry JM *et al.* (1981) Perhexilene maleate induced lipidosis in human peripheral nerve and tissue culture: Ultrastructural and biochemical changes. *Clin Toxicol* 18, 1405.
5. Lhermitte F, Fardeau M, Chedru F, Mallecourt J (1976) Polyneuropathy after perhexilene maleate therapy. *Brit Med J* 1, 1256.
6. Lorentz IT, Shortall M (1983) Perhexilene neuropathy: A report of two cases. *Aust N Z J Med* 13, 517.
7. Lüllmann H, Lüllmann-Rauch R (1978) Perhexilene induces generalized lipidosis in rats. *Klin Wochenschr* 56, 309.
8. Lyon LJ, Nevins MA, Fisch S, Henry S (1971) Perhexilene maleate in treatment of angina pectoris. *Lancet* 1, 1272.
9. Meier C, Wahllaender A, Hess CW, Preisig R (1986) Perhexilene-induced lipidosis in the dark agouti (DA) rat. *Brain* 109, 649.
10. Pilcher J, Chandrasekhar KP, Russell Rees J (1973) Long term assessment of perhexilene maleate in angina pectoris. *Postgrad Med J* 49, 115.
11. Pollet S, Hauw JJ, Escourolle R, Baumann N (1977) Peripheral nerve lipid abnormalities in patients on perhexilene maleate. *Lancet* 1, 1258.
12. Raabe DS Jr (1979) Treatment of variant angina pectoris with perhexilene maleate. *Chest* 75, 152.
13. Said G (1978) Perhexilene neuropathy: A clinicopathological study. *Ann Neurol* 3, 259.
14. Sebille A (1978) Prevalence of latent perhexilene neuropathy. *Brit Med J* 2, 1321.
15. Shah RR, Oates NS, Idle JR *et al.* (1982) Impaired oxidation of debrisoquine in patients with perhexilene neuropathy. *Brit Med J* 1, 295.

16. Shah RR, Oates NS, Idle JR *et al.* (1983) Prediction of subclinical perhexilene neuropathy in a patient with inborn error of debrisoquine hydroxylation. *Amer Heart J* **105**, 159.

17. Singlas E, Goujet MA, Simon P (1978) Pharmacokinetics of perhexilene maleate in anginal patients with and without peripheral neuropathy. *Eur J Clin Pharmacol* **14**, 195.

18. Stephens WP, Eddy JD, Parsons IM, Singh SP (1978) Raised intracranial pressure due to perhexilene maleate. *Brit Med J* **1**, 21.

19. Tomlinson IW, Rosenthal FD (1977) Proximal myopathy after perhexilene maleate treatment. *Brit Med J* **1**, 1319.

20. Wijesekera JC, Critchley EMR, Fahim Y *et al.* (1980) Peripheral neuropathy due to perhexilene maleate. *J Neurol Sci* **46**, 303.

21. Wright GJ, Leeson GA, Zeiger AV, Lang JF (1973) The absorption, excretion and metabolism of perhexilene maleate by the human. *Postgrad Med J* **49**, 8.

Pertussis Vaccine

Neil L. Rosenberg

Diphtheria-pertussis-tetanus vaccine

NEUROTOXICITY RATING

Clinical

A Acute encephalopathy

A Seizure disorder

C Chronic encephalopathy

C Peripheral neuropathy

Neurological complications of triple immunization for diphtheria-pertussis-tetanus (DPT) are secondary to the pertussis component. This triple vaccine consists of diphtheria toxoid (DT), tetanus toxoid, and a whole-cell pertussis preparation.

Natural infection with the pertussis organism produces whooping cough; it primarily affects infants and young children. The most important neurological effect of systemic manifestation is encephalopathy without evidence of inflammation (35,37,51). In cases where some inflammation is evident, it is usually in an older child who developed symptoms subacutely instead of the usual acute illness of infants. One large series of pertussis cases reported an incidence of neurological complications between 1.7%–7.0% (51). The most common neurological sign was seizures; in some cases, permanent encephalopathy developed with residual deficits, including paraplegia, hemiplegia, ataxia, blindness, and deafness (35,37,51).

Mild systemic and local reactions to DPT or pertussis vaccines are frequent (9,10,14,28,31,39–41). The most common local reactions are swelling, redness, and pain at the injection site (10,14,31,39–41). In one study, 96% of DPT recipients, but also 36% of placebo recipients, developed fever, local reactions (pain, tenderness, redness), and adverse behavioral effects (31). In a study comparing DPT

to DT vaccine, severe local redness was seen in 38% and 9%, respectively (40). In a study comparing DPT vaccines with standard and small doses of DT, fewer children developed large local reactions to the modified (smaller dose) vaccine (41). The reactions were uncomfortable but not serious, and were felt to result from the larger amounts of DT in standard vaccines (41).

Mild systemic reactions to pertussis and DPT vaccination include fever, drowsiness, fretfulness, anorexia, and persistent crying (14,31,39). In a study of 538 children (observed from 2–20 months of age) who received 1553 doses of DPT vaccine (either the standard four-dose or modified three-dose schedule), behavioral and local effects occurred maximally in the first 6 h following vaccination, but fever peaked later (31). There was no interrelationship between the occurrence of adverse effects and fever, and age had more effect on the type and severity of adverse effects than did the number of immunizations (31). In a study of 730 children in Mexico (39), 87% had one or more of the following side effects: fever (66%), malaise (37.8%), anorexia (25%), sleep disorder (20.4%), vomiting (7.9%), and continuous crying (7.6%). None of the children in these latter two studies had any serious nervous system complication (31,39).

Prolonged crying has been reported following vaccination (10,14,31); it has primarily been associated with painful local reactions (10) and has not been linked to any serious neurological complication. There is no relationship between DPT immunization and hospitalization for an infectious disease (28).

Though most systemic effects are mild, a case report describes an individual hyperimmunized with pertussis vaccine who developed a diffuse vasculitis and died (9). This case is unusual in that it was an adult who received multiple doses of vaccine.

Neurological complications following pertussis and DPT vaccines have been noted for decades (1,5,6,10–12,14, 15,18,20,23,29,30,32–34,36,47–50). The primary complications are seizures (1,5,6,10,20,23,27,29,30,33,34,36,48), including infantile spasms (5,33,36), febrile seizures (10, 20,23,30), and encephalopathy with resultant permanent brain damage (6,12,14,29,34,47,48). Brachial plexopathy has been implicated, but is not causally related (32,49).

Seizures are commonly reported (1,5,6,10,20,23,27, 29,30,33,34,36,48). Most reports are uncontrolled case series reporting all types of seizures at almost any period of time following immunization (1,5,6,29,34,36). A 1974 report presented data on 36 children evaluated at the Hospital for Sick Children in London, U.K. (29); 32 suffered seizures and 22 were subsequently retarded. Since these complications usually appeared within the first 24 h after pertussis vaccination, a causal association was suggested (29). In a larger uncontrolled series, the first 1000 cases notified to the U.S. National Childhood Encephalopathy Study (NCES) were analyzed (34). Only 35 of the notified children (3.5%) had received pertussis vaccine in the 7-day period before becoming ill; nevertheless, a significant association was reported between serious neurological illness, including seizures, and the vaccine. Subsequently, carefully controlled studies failed to show an association between pertussis or DPT vaccine and development of seizures (20,31,39).

Studies descibe a clear association between DPT vaccination and seizures resembling febrile seizures (10,20,23, 30). These children had the usual risk factors for febrile seizures, including a family history of seizures (23,30). Because of the rare occurrence of neurological events after DPT vaccination and the usually benign outcome of febrile seizures, a history of seizures in siblings or parents is not considered a contraindication to DPT vaccination. Prevention of postvaccination fever may be warranted in children with a family history of seizures. Infantile spasms were formerly attributed to pertussis vaccination (5,33,36). One study concluded the vaccines do not cause infantile spasms but *"may trigger their onset in those children in whom the disorder is destined to develop"* (5). Another stated that, since the introduction of DPT vaccine into Denmark in 1961, there has been no significant change in the age distribution of children with infantile spasms (33).

Severe encephalopathies from pertussis or DPT vaccination have been claimed for decades (6,12,14,29,34,47,48). An early analysis of data collected by questionnaire found that 38 had seizures, two died, and 12 had permanent brain damage (48). A review of the neurological complications of 107 cases of pertussis encephalopathy from 25 different reports (6) noted that 68 were immunized against pertussis alone, 12 against diphtheria-pertussis, and 28 against DPT. Overall, 41 recovered completely, 15 died, 19 developed recurring seizures, 19 had paralysis, and 12 were mentally retarded (6). In a large controlled study from Los Angeles County, California, a high percentage of children developed both local and systemic reactions, but encephalopathy was not reported (14). A United Kingdom study of 36 children with neurological complications from pertussis vaccination noted that two died within 6 months, 22 were mentally retarded and had recurrent seizures, three had seizures only, and four recovered completely (29). This was followed by a retrospective analysis of 197 cases in which brain damage was reported after pertussis vaccination (47).

The NCES report of the first 1000 cases, conducted in response to these two studies, included 35 (3.5%) with severe neurological complications temporally related to pertussis vaccination (34). Thirty-four of the 1955 controls (1.7%) who had neurological events temporally related to pertussis vaccination were matched by age, sex, and area of residence. The relative risk of a child having had pertussis vaccination within the time interval was 2.4 ($p \leq$ 0.001). Of the 35 children, 32 had no prior neurological abnormality. One year later, two had died, nine had developmental retardation, and 21 were normal. There appeared to be a significant association between serious neurological disease and pertussis vaccination, though cases were few and most children recovered completely (34). The estimated risk attributed to pertussis vaccine for the development of neurological disease was 1:310,000.

The neuropathological aspects of pertussis vaccination have been analyzed (15). Literature review and new data on 29 deaths revealed no recurrent pattern of inflammatory or other pathological change attributable to a specific reaction to pertussis immunization. The changes were indistinguishable from those seen in many other encephalopathies of childhood due to hypoxic-ischemic insult (15).

A review of the epidemiological literature in 1991 (50) found that the NCES was the only published case-control study of this issue. Because of the rare association in the NCES study between DPT vaccine and serious illness, the authors suggested that a noncausal relationship (*i.e.,* coincidence and bias) had a role in the results and that the NCES study did not demonstrate that DPT vaccination causes permanent brain damage (50). In a more recent population-based, case-control study of a population of 218,000 children, 1–24 months of age, no statistically significant increased risk of serious acute neurological illness was seen in the 7 days following DPT vaccination (18). The epidemiological data overall do not confirm an association between DPT or pertussis vaccination and serious neurological sequelae.

A relationship between sudden infant death syndrome (SIDS) and DPT vaccination has been suggested (4,7,25,42, 45). A retrospective review of 145 SIDS victims in Los Angeles County, California, revealed that 53 had received a recent DPT vaccination (4). Of these, 27 received the vaccine within 28 days of death, 17 within 1 week, and six within 24 h. However, 46 infants also died following a physician or clinic visit where DPT was not given. The deaths were more than expected, and the data suggest not only a temporal association between DPT vaccination and SIDS, but also a physician visit without DPT vaccination. Another study reported an association between a single lot of DPT vaccine and SIDS (7). However, two controlled studies failed to find an association between DPT vaccination and SIDS (25,42).

In yet another attempt to address this issue, the effects of DPT vaccination on prolonged apnea or bradycardia in siblings of SIDS victims was assessed because of the increased risk of SIDS in this population (45). The results of this study failed to find a link between DPT vaccination and increased frequency or severity of prolonged apnea.

Animal models have been developed to address pertussis encephalopathy (16,38,43,44). In one model, a mouse strain developed a lethal shock-like syndrome following immunization with heat-killed *Bordetella pertussis* and re-challenge with bovine serum albumin (38,43). Diffuse vascular congestion and punctate hemorrhages—both in gray and white matter—resembled the human pathology when death occurs within 48 h of immunization. A follow-up study of the same model revealed that the pertussis toxin itself was the critical constituent of *B. pertussis* responsible for this experimental encephalopathy (44). Another experimental study in mice found that intracerebral pretreatment with pertussis toxin enhanced sensitivity to N-methyl-D-aspartate–induced seizures (16).

Epidemiological studies have absolved pertussis vaccine of serious neurological side effects. However, because of local and other systemic effects, a less reactive vaccine is desirable. The problem of reactivity to whole-cell pertussis vaccines and subsequent side effects has led to the evaluation of less-reactive alternatives (8,19,21,24,26). These have included acellular pertussis vaccines (8,19,24,26) and one with diphtheria and tetanus toxoids for use as the fourth and fifth doses of DPT. Acellular DPT vaccines have been shown to be more immunogenic and less reactive, with fewer and less severe local reactions, fever, and other systemic side effects (8,19,24,26). Another suggested method of reducing adverse reactions to DPT vaccine is to adsorb other noncellular components of the vaccine, such as aluminum compounds, which may also contribute to toxicity (21).

Medical specialty societies and task forces have rendered opinions on the previous controversy surrounding possible neurological reactions to pertussis and DPT vaccines (2,3,11,13,17,22,46). Until more recently, there had been no controlled studies of quantitative data (13). In the United States, the Child Neurology Society (2) and the American Academy of Neurology (3) have stated there is no evidence that DPT vaccine is causally linked to any specific clinical or neuropathological syndrome. Furthermore, there is no means whereby a diagnosis of brain injury due to DPT vaccination can be established in an individual case.

In conclusion, the only neurological complication that seems to be causally linked to pertussis or DPT vaccination is that of febrile seizures, which generally have a benign outcome. Future use of the acellular pertussis component of the DPT vaccine should reduce this risk even further.

REFERENCES

1. Aicardi J, Chevrie JJ (1975) Neurologic manifestations following pertussis vaccination. *Arch Franc Pediat* **32**, 309.
2. Anonymous (1991) Ad Hoc Committee for the Child Neurology Society Consensus Statement on Pertussis Immunization and the Central Nervous System. Pertussis immunization and the central nervous system. *Ann Neurol* **29**, 458.
3. Anonymous (1992) Assessment of DTP vaccination: Report of the therapeutics and technology assessment subcommittee of the American Academy of Neurology. *Neurology* **42**, 471.
4. Baraff LJ, Ablon WJ, Weiss RC (1982) Possible temporal association between diphtheria-tetanus toxoid-pertussis vaccination and sudden infant death syndrome. *Pediat Infect Dis* **2**, 7.
5. Bellman MH, Ross EM, Miller DL (1983) Infantile spasms and pertussis immunization. *Lancet* **1**, 1031.
6. Berg JM (1958) Neurological complications of pertussis immunization. *Brit Med J* **2**, 24.
7. Bernier RH, Frank JA Jr, Dondero TJ Jr *et al.* (1982) Diphtheria-tetanus toxoids-pertussis vaccination and sudden infant deaths in Tennessee. *J Pediat* **101**, 419.
8. Bernstein HH, Rothstein EP, Reisinger KS *et al.* (1994) Comparison of a three-component acellular pertussis vaccine with a whole-cell pertussis vaccine in 15- through 20-month-old infants. *Pediatrics* **93**, 656.
9. Bishop WB, Carlton RF, Sanders LL (1966) Diffuse vasculitis and death after hyperimmunization with pertussis vaccine. Report of a case. *N Engl J Med* **274**, 616.
10. Blumberg DA, Lewis K, Mink CM *et al.* (1993) Severe reactions associated with diphtheria-tetanus-pertussis vaccine: Detailed study of children with seizures, hypotonic-hyporesponsive episodes, high fevers, and persistent crying. *Pediatrics* **91**, 1158.

11. Camfield P (1992) Brain damage from pertussis immunization. A Canadian neurologist's perspective. *Amer J Dis Child* **146**, 327.

12. Cavanagh NP, Brett EM, Marshall WC, Wilson J (1981) The possible adjuvant role of bordetella pertussis and pertussis vaccine in causing severe encephalopathic illness: a presentation of three case histories. *Neuropediatrics* **12**, 374.

13. Cherry JD, Brune PA, Golden GS, Karzon DT (1988) Report of the Task Force on Pertussis and Pertussis Immunization. *Pediatrics* **81**, 939.

14. Cody CL, Baraff RM, Cherry JD *et al.* (1981) Nature and rates of adverse reactions associated with DPT and DT immunizations in infants and children. *Pediatrics* **68**, 650.

15. Corsellis JA, Janota I, Marshall AK (1983) Immunization against whooping cough: A neuropathological review. *Neuropathol Appl Neurobiol* **9**, 261.

16. Durcan MJ, Morgan PF (1991) Intracerebroventricular pertussis toxin enhances sensitivity to N-methyl-D-aspartate-induced seizures in mice. *Eur J Pharmacol* **197**, 209.

17. Fenichel GM (1983) The pertussis vaccine controversy. The danger of case reports. *Arch Neurol* **40**, 193.

18. Gale JL, Thapa PB, Wassilak SG *et al.* (1994) Risk of serious acute neurological illness after immunization with diphtheria-tetanus-pertussis vaccine. A population-based case-control study. *J Amer Med Assn* **271**, 37.

19. Glode M, Joffe L, Reisinger K *et al.* (1992) Safety and immunogenicity of acellular pertussis vaccine combined with diphtheria and tetanus toxoids in 17- to 24-month-old children. *Pediat Infect Dis J* **11**, 530.

20. Griffin MR, Ray WA, Mortimer EA *et al.* (1990) Risk of seizures and encephalopathy after immunization with the diphtheria-tetanus-pertussis vaccine. *J Amer Med Assn* **263**, 1641.

21. Gupta RK, Relyveld EH (1991) Adverse reactions after injection of adsorbed diphtheria-pertussis-tetanus (DPT) vaccine are not due only to pertussis organisms or pertussis components in the vaccine. *Vaccine* **9**, 699.

22. Harding CM (1983) Whooping cough vaccination: A review of the controversy since the 1981 DHSS report. *Child Care Health Dev* **9**, 257.

23. Hirtz DG, Nelson KB, Ellenberg JH (1983) Seizures following childhood immunizations. *J Pediat* **102**, 14.

24. Hodder SL, Mortimer EA (1992) Epidemiology of pertussis and reactions to pertussis vaccine. *Epidemiol Rev* **14**, 243.

25. Hoffman HJ, Hunter JC, Damus K *et al.* (1987) Diphtheria-tetanus-pertussis immunization and sudden infant death: Results of the National Institute of Child Health and Human Development Cooperative Epidemiological Study of Sudden Infant Death Syndrome Risk Factors. *Pediatrics* **79**, 598.

26. Hori H, Afari EA, Akanmori BD *et al.* (1994) A randomized controlled trial of two acellular pertussis-diphtheria-tetanus vaccines in primary immunization in Ghana: Antibody responses and adverse reactions. *Ann Trop Paediat* **14**, 91.

27. Hunt A (1983) Tuberous sclerosis: A survey of 97 cases. I: Seizures, pertussis immunisation and handicap. *Develop Med Child Neurol* **25**, 346.

28. Joffe LS, Glode MP, Gutierrez MK *et al.* (1992) Diphtheria-tetanus toxoids-pertussis vaccination does not increase the risk of hospitalization with an infectious illness. *Pediat Infect Dis J* **11**, 730.

29. Kulenkampff M, Schwartzman JS, Wilson J (1974) Neurological complications of pertussis inoculation. *Arch Dis Child* **49**, 46.

30. Livengood JR, Mullen JR, White JW *et al.* (1989) Family history of convulsions and use of pertussis vaccine. *J Pediat* **115**, 527.

31. Long SS, Deforest A, Smith DG *et al.* (1990) Longitudinal study of adverse reactions following diphtheria-tetanus-pertussis vaccine in infancy. *Pediatrics* **85**, 294.

32. Martin GI, Weintraub MI (1973) Brachial neuritis and seventh nerve palsy—a rare hazard of DPT vaccination. *Clin Pediat* **12**, 506.

33. Melchior JC (1977) Infantile spasms and early immunisation against whooping cough. Danish survey from 1970 to 1975. *Arch Dis Child* **52**, 134.

34. Miller DL, Ross EM, Alderslade R *et al.* (1981) Pertussis immunisation and serious acute neurological illness in children. *Brit Med J Clin Res Ed* **282**, 1595.

35. Miller HG, Stanton JB, Gibbons JL (1955) Parainfectious encephalomyelitis and related syndromes. *Quart J Med* **25**, 427.

36. Millichap JG (1987) Etiology and treatment of infantile spasms: current concepts, including the role of DPT immunisation. *Acta Pediat Jpn* **29**, 54.

37. Olson LC (1975) Pertussis. *Medicine* **54**, 427.

38. Redhead K, Robinson A, Ashworth LA, Melville-Smith M (1987) The activity of purified *Bordetella pertussis* components in murine encephalopathy. *J Biol Standardiz* **15**, 341.

39. Regalado MR, Nieves-Rodriguez B, Ghersy MT *et al.* (1990) Side effects of the vaccine against diphtheria, tetanus and whooping cough. *Bol Med Hosp Infant Mexico* **47**, 295.

40. Scheifele DW, Bjornson G, Halperin SH *et al.* (1994) Role of whole-cell pertussis vaccine in severe local reactions to the preschool (fifth) dose of diphtheria-pertussis-tetanus vaccine. *Can Med Assn J* **150**, 29.

41. Scheifele DW, Meekison W, Grace M *et al* (1991) Adverse reactions to the preschool (fifth) dose of adsorbed diphtheria-pertussis-tetanus vaccine in Canadian children. *Can Med Assn J* **145**, 641.

42. Solberg KJ (1985) DPT immunization, visit to child health center and sudden infant death syndrome (SIDS). Report to the Oslo Health Council, Oslo p. 131.

43. Steinman L, Sriram S, Adelman NE, Zamvil S (1982) Murine model for pertussis vaccine encephalopathy: Linkage to H-2. *Nature* **299**, 738.

44. Steinman L, Weiss A, Adelman N, Lim M (1985) Pertussis toxin is required for pertussis vaccine encephalopathy. *Proc Nat Acad Sci USA* **82**, 8733.

45. Steinschneider A, Freed G, Rhetta-Smith A, Santos VR (1991) Effect of diphtheria-tetanus-pertussis immunization on prolonged apnea or bradycardia in siblings of sudden infant death syndrome victims. *J Pediat* **119**, 411.

46. Stephenson JB (1988) A neurologist looks at neurological disease temporally related to DTP immunization. *Tokai J Exp Clin Med* **13**, 157.

47. Stewart GT (1979) Toxicity of pertussis vaccine: Frequency and probability of reactions. *J Epidemiol Community Health* **33**, 150.

48. Toomey JA (1948) Reactions to pertussis vaccine. *J Amer Med Assn* **139**, 448.

49. Tsairis P, Dyck PJ, Mulder DW (1972) Natural history of brachial plexus neuropathy: Report on 99 patients. *Arch Neurol* **27**, 109.

50. Wentz KR, Marcuse EK (1991) Diphtheria-tetanus-pertussis vaccine and serious neurologic illness: an updated review of the epidemiologic evidence. *Pediatrics* **87**, 287.

51. Zellweger H (1959) Pertussis encephalopathy. *Arch Pediat* **76**, 381.

Pfiesteria piscicida

Edward D. Levin
Howard Glasgow Jr
Donald E. Schmechel
Nora Deamer-Melia
JoAnn Burkholder

NEUROTOXICITY RATING

Clinical

B Chronic encephalopathy (cognitive dysfunction)

Experimental

A Acute and chronic encephalopathy (cognitive dysfunction)

The dinoflagellate *Pfiesteria piscicida* inhabits estuarine waters and is suspected as a cause of mass fish kills in the estuarine environments along the eastern U.S. seaboard, in particular in the states of North Carolina and Maryland. *P. piscicida* is a complex organism with at least 24 distinct life stages (2); the small flagellated zoospores appear to have the most lethal toxic effects (4). Fish appear to be narcotized and show poor fright response after exposure to *P. piscicida* (3). Chemical fractions containing toxins produced by *P. piscicida* have been isolated and structural characterization is in progress. Water-soluble toxins are likely responsible for fish lethality and neurotoxic effects, while lipid-soluble toxins may be responsible for epidermal necrosis.

Experimental exposure of rats to *P. piscicida* caused cognitive dysfunction (6–8). Adult female Sprague-Dawley rats were injected subcutaneously with doses ranging from 35,600 to 961,200 *Pfiesteria* cells/kg of body weight. Starting 2 days after injection, the animals began testing on the win-shift radial-arm maze task, a test of spatial learning and memory. They were tested in 18 sessions over the next 6 weeks. Compared to controls, rats exposed to *Pfiesteria* showed a significant impairment in radial-arm maze learning. With supplemental training, the *Pfiesteria*-treated animals did learn the task and approached control levels of performance. A single exposure to 106,800 *Pfiesteria* cells/kg was sufficient to cause a significant deficit in radial-arm maze acquisition. To differentiate the effects of *Pfiesteria* on learning and memory, rats were pretrained on the radial-arm maze win-shift procedure prior to *Pfiesteria* administration; beginning 2 days after dosing (0, 35,600, or 106,800 cells/kg; n = 12/group), animals were tested for maintenance of working memory choice accuracy. No significant deficits caused by *Pfiesteria* administration were observed on retention of win-shift radial-arm maze choice accuracy. To assess the effects on learning, the rats were switched to the repeated acquisition procedure in the radial-arm maze. A significant deficit was seen in animals receiving the higher dose ($p < 0.05$), but not in the lower dose group, relative to controls. This *Pfiesteria*-induced learning deficit was seen 10 weeks after a single exposure.

No clinical signs of health impairment in rats were noted during the period when cognitive deficits were documented. The Functional Observational Battery failed to detect any consistent behavioral changes other than deficits in habituation of rearing and arousal over repeated test sessions. No *Pfiesteria*-induced effects on blood count and white cell differential or in a standard pathological screening of brain, liver, lungs, kidney, and spleen tissue were seen at 2 months after exposure.

Taken together, the foregoing studies document a selective and persistent learning impairment in otherwise healthy rats that have been exposed to the dinoflagellate *Pfiesteria*. The learning impairment may be related to the cognitive impairments humans have shown after *Pfiesteria* exposure.

Preliminary *in vitro* studies have shown neural cells to be more sensitive than endothelial cells to toxic damage, including lactate dehydrogenase leakage and lower adenosine triphosphate levels (9).

Adverse effects of *Pfiesteria* exposure have been documented in humans. Three medically examined laboratory staff, as well as seven others, reported symptoms after accidental laboratory exposure to *P. piscicida* (5). *Pfiesteria* exposure resulted in a complex syndrome characterized by spatial disorientation, difficulty with memory and concentration, reading impairment, fatigue, excessive mood lability, irritability, dermal lesions, and immunological suppression. These symptoms diminished over a period of weeks to a few months. A similar constellation of symptoms was reported in a small group of people with environmental exposure (10). Individuals exposed to river water containing *Pfiesteria* or *Pfiesteria*-like dinoflagellates reported fatigue, headache, respiratory irritation, diarrhea, weight loss, skin irritation, confusion, difficulty concentrating, and memory impairment. Objective tests of those with heaviest exposure showed deficits in verbal learning and memory, concentration, and response inhibition. Avoidance of ingestion or dermal or inhalation exposure to *Pfiesteria*-containing water is recommended.

Editors' Note: In May 1999, the U.S. Centers for Disease Control and Prevention (CDC) noted that *Pfiesteria piscicida* is an estuarine dinoflagellate that has been associated with fish-kill events in estuaries along the eastern seaboard and possibly with human health effects. CDC, in collaboration with other federal, state, and local government agencies and academic institutions, stated that it was conducting multistate surveillance, epidemiologic studies, and laboratory research for possible estuary-associated syndrome, including possible human illness related to *P. piscicida*.

REFERENCES

1. Anon. (1999) Possible estuary-associated syndrome. *MMWR Morb Mortal Wkly Rep* **48**, 381.
2. Burkholder JM, Glasgow HB Jr (1995) Interactions of a toxic estuarine dinoflagellate with microbial predators and prey. *Arch Protistenkd* **145**, 177.
3. Burkholder JM, Glasgow HB Jr, Noga EJ, Hobbs CW (1993) The role of a new toxic dinoflagellate in finfish and shellfish kills in the Neuse and Pamlico Estuaries. In: *Ablemarle-Pamlico Estuarine Study*. North Carolina Dept Environ Health Natural Resources and EPA Nat Estuarine Prog, Raleigh, North Carolina p. 1.
4. Burkholder JM, Noga EJ, Hobbs CW *et al.* (1992) A new "phantom" dinoflagellate is the causative agent of major estuarine fish kills. *Nature* **358**, 407.
5. Glasgow HB Jr, Burkholder JM, Schmechel DE *et al.* (1995) Insidious effects of a toxic estuarine dinoflagellate on fish survival and human health. *J Toxicol Environ Health* **46**, 501.
6. Levin, ED, Schmechel DE, Burkholder JM *et al.* (1997) Persisting learning deficits in rats after exposure to *Pfiesteria piscicida*. *Environ Health Perspect* **105**, 1320.
7. Levin ED, Schemechel DE, Glasgow HB Jr, Burkholder JM (1997) Cognitive effects seen in rats exposed to the dinoflagellate *Pfiesteria*. *Toxicologist* **36**, 62.
8. Levin ED, Schemechel DE, Glasgow HB Jr *et al.* (1996) *Pfiesteria piscicida* effects on cognitive performance in rats. SE Estuarine Res Soc Meeting, Atlantic Beach, North Carolina.
9. McCellan-Green PD, Noga E, Baden D *et al.* (1997) Cytotoxicity of a putative toxin from the *Pfiesteria piscicida* dinoflagellate. *Toxicologist* **36**, 276.
10. Morris JG, Charache P, Grattan LM *et al.* (1997) Medical evaluation of persons with exposure to water containing *Pfiesteria* or *Pfiesteria*-like dinoflagellates. Interim Report. University of Maryland, Baltimore, MD.

Phalaris Spp.

Alexander Storch
Albert C. Ludolph

N,N-DIMETHYLTRYPTAMINE
$C_{12}H_{16}N_2$

N,N-Dimethyltryptamine; N,N-Dimethyl-1H-indole-3-ethanamine; DMT

NEUROTOXICITY RATING

Clinical

B   Chronic encephalopathy (sheep, cattle—agitation, ataxia, limb
    spasms)

Experimental

B   Serotonin agonist

Phalaris spp. are cool-season annual grasses used in pasture improvement in Australia. Poisoning in sheep and cattle caused by Phalaris spp. has occurred in New Zealand and Australia (P. aquatica; formerly P. tuberosa), California (P. minor and P. tuberosa), Louisiana (P. carolinensis), Scandinavia (P. arundinacea), South America (P. angusta and P. aquatica) and South Africa (5,9,11,13–16). Four chemically related groups of tryptamine alkaloids occur in P. aquatica: N,N-dimethylated indolalkylamines [N,N-dimethyltryptamine (DMT); 5-methoxy-N,N-dimethyl-tryptamine (5-MDMT), and variable amounts of 5-hydroxy-N,N-dimethyltryptamine (5-HDMT)], hordenine, gramine, and 2-methyltetrahydro-β-carboline (4,8,9) (see also Carbolines/Isoquinolines, this volume). The endogenous toxins of Phalaris and other grasses have been reviewed, as has the clinical differentiation of phalaris staggers from other locomotor disorders of sheep (2,7) (see also Chapter 3).

Two syndromes of Phalaris spp. intoxications are described; a hyperactive form and an acute/chronic neurological syndrome. The first is a cardiac disorder, sometimes called "sudden death"; this is characterized by sudden collapse, without previous signs, followed by several minutes of ventricular fibrillation, respiratory disturbances, cyanosis, and death (3,4,11). A polioencephalomalacic disorder has also been implicated as another factor in P. aquatica "sudden death" syndrome (3). The pathogenetic mechanisms are unknown. It has been suggested that tryptamine alkaloids cause the cardiac syndrome (9,11), but field evidence and experimental data implicate other mechanisms (3,4,8), including cyanogenic and/or nitrate compounds or a cardiorespiratory toxin (3).

The (chronic) neurological syndrome, called chronic phalaris toxicosis or "phalaris staggers," varies greatly in time of onset/recovery, and degree of dysfunction. This likely reflects a variable concentration and composition of alkaloids in the plants. Clinical signs appear within days to months and include persistent head nodding, hyperexcitability, ataxia, limb weakness, and muscle twitching. Spasms and extensor rigidity of the legs, chewing, salivation, and tachycardia may appear. Signs are exaggerated by enforced movement or excitement. Animals suffering from the acute form recover quickly and completely following removal from the pasture. In the chronic form, symptoms persist despite removal from the phalaris pasture (death can occur over the ensuing weeks or months), suggesting persistent CNS degenerative lesions (5,6,9,13–16).

Controlled administration of phalaris alkaloids to sheep and laboratory animals, either intravenously (i.v.) or orally (p.o.), induces clinical signs identical to those in grazing domestic animals (4,5,9). The most potent compound is 5-MDMT, followed by 5-HDMT and DMT. After parenteral administration of 5-MDMT to sheep in doses of 0.1–5 mg/kg, clinical signs appeared within 10–15 sec and lasted for 20–90 min. Severity of illness was dose-related. Following ingestion, 5 MDMT was effective in a dose range from 40–85 mg/kg. Some animals died several minutes after the administration of high doses (4,5,9).

Electromyographic studies on sheep injected with N,N-dimethylated tryptamines suggest the convulsive spasms originate in the spinal cord. Lesion experiments indicate that the excessive discharge of motor units is not due to hyperexcitability of the somatosensory or γ-afferent system, nor to direct action of the alkaloids on transmission at either the neuromuscular junction or nerve fibers (10).

Gramine and hordenine, applied intravenously or orally, also induce comparable neurological signs in sheep (lowest effective test dosage were, for gramine, 10 mg/kg i.v. and 500 mg/kg p.o.; and for hordenine, 20 mg/kg i.v. and 800 mg/kg p.o.) (4).

Postmortem examination of sheep that had died of chronic phalaris toxicosis disclosed green-brown pigmented neuronal cytoplasm in multiple nuclei of the thalamus, midbrain, and medulla oblongata. Pigmentation occurred to a lesser degree in neurons of the ventral horn of the spinal cord, deep cerebellar nuclei, and primary olfactory cortex (5,9,12,13). This pigmentation caused a grey greenish discoloration in gross sections of fixed brains (9). Closely related green or brown pigments can be produced *in vitro* from 5-MDMT, DMT, and 5-HDMT by enzymatic degradation (4,6,9). In addition, moderate axonal degeneration and myelin pallor were present diffusely in tracts of the midbrain, the medulla oblongata, and the spinal cord (12,13).

There is no specific therapy for either the sudden death syndrome or the acute form of the nervous syndrome from phalaris toxicity. Dosing with cobalt sulfate or heavy cobalt pellets reduces the incidence of phalaris staggers after an outbreak appears (9,14). The therapeutic or prophylactic mechanisms of this treatment are unknown.

The neurotoxic mechanisms of phalaris poisoning are unknown. It is suggested that the neurological disturbances induced by *Phalaris* spp. result from an influence of phalaris alkaloids on the central serotonergic system *via* a direct action upon serotonergic receptors (5).

The *N,N*-dimethylated tryptamine alkaloids found in *Phalaris* spp. display strong serotonergic activity in the mammalian CNS (1,5). These compounds are agonists and partial antagonists at several central serotonin receptors (5-HT$_1$ and 5-HT$_2$ subtypes; weak action upon 5-HT$_3$) (1,5). Most of the clinical signs can be attributed to serotonergic actions (for details, *see* ref. 5). Furthermore, the neurological symptoms are comparable to those elicited by other serotonergic agonists (5).

In sum, the pharmacological and neuropathological findings implicate an important role of the action of phalaris alkaloids on the central serotonergic system, especially in the brainstem, in generating chronic *Phalaris* toxicosis.

REFERENCES

1. Blackburn TP, Foster GA, Heapy CG, Kemp JD (1980) Unilateral 5,7-dihydroxytryptamine lesions of the dorsal raphe nucleus (DRN) and rat rotational behaviour. *Eur J Pharmacol* 67, 427.
2. Bourke CA (1995) The clinical differentiation of nervous and muscular locomotor disorders of sheep in Australia. *Aust Vet J* 72, 228.
3. Bourke CA, Carrigan MF (1992) Mechanisms underlying *Phalaris aquatica* "sudden death" syndrome in sheep. *Aust Vet J* 69, 165.
4. Bourke CA, Carrigan MF, Dixon RJ (1988) Experimental evidence that tryptamine alkaloids do not cause *Phalaris aquatica* sudden death syndrome in sheep. *Aust Vet J* 65, 218.
5. Bourke CA, Carrigan MF, Dixon RJ (1990) The pathogenesis of the nervous syndrome of *Phalaris aquatica* toxicity in sheep. *Aust Vet J* 67, 356.
6. Bourke CA, Carrigan MF, Seaman JT, Evers JV (1987) Delayed development of clinical signs in sheep affected by *Phalaris aquatica* staggers. *Aust Vet J* 64, 31.
7. Cheeke PR (1995) Endogenous toxins and mycotoxins in forage grasses and their effects on livestock. *Anim Sci* 73, 909.
8. Culvenor CCJ, Dal Bon R, Smith LW (1964) The occurrence of indolealkylamine alkaloids in *Phalaris tuberosa* L. and *P. arundinacea* L. *Aust J Chem* 17, 1301.
9. Gallagher CH, Koch JH, Hoffman H (1966) Diseases of sheep due to ingestion of *Phalaris tuberosa*. *Aust Vet J* 42, 279.
10. Gallagher CH, Koch JH, Hoffman H (1967) Electromyographic studies on sheep injected with the *N,N*-dimethylated tryptamine alkaloids of *Phalaris tuberosa*. *Int J Neuropharmacol* 6, 223.
11. Gallagher CH, Koch JH, Moore RM, Steel JD (1964) Toxicity of *Phalaris tuberosa* for sheep. *Nature* 204, 542.
12. Lean IJ, Anderson M, Kerfoot MG, Marten GC (1989) Tryptamine alkaloid toxicosis in feedlot sheep. *J Amer Vet Med Assn* 195, 768.
13. McDonald IW (1942) A "staggers" syndrome in sheep and cattle associated with grazing on *Phalaris tuberosa*. *Aust Vet J* 18, 182.
14. Nicholson SS (1989) Tremorgenic syndromes in livestock. *Vet Clin N Amer Food Anim Pract* 5, 291.
15. Nicholson SS, Olcott BM, Usenik EA *et al.* (1989) Delayed phalaris grass toxicosis in sheep and cattle. *J Amer Vet Med Assn* 195, 345.
16. Odriozola E, Campero C, Lopez T *et al.* (1991) Neuropathological effects and deaths of cattle and sheep in Argentinia from *Phalaris angusta*. *Vet Hum Toxicol* 33, 465.

Phencyclidine

Daniel C. Javitt

PHENCYCLIDINE
$C_{17}H_{25}N$

1-(1-Phenylcyclohexyl)piperidine

NEUROTOXICITY RATING

Clinical

A Psychobiological reaction (agitation, psychosis, dysphoria)

A Acute encephalopathy (tremor, stupor, nystagmus)

B Psychobiological reaction (schizophreniform psychosis)

Experimental

A Psychobiological reaction (catalepsy, catatonia)

A Neuronal vacuolation and necrosis

A NMDA receptor blockade

Phencyclidine (PCP) is an odorless, white, crystalline substance. Pure PCP has a MW of 243.9, a MP of 234°–236°C, and is highly insoluble in water. The most frequently encountered form of PCP is the hydrochloride salt, which has a MW of 279.9 and is soluble in both water and ethanol. Phencyclidine synthesis involves the use of benzene, piperidine, and p toluene sulfonic acid. Other agents, including ether, cyclohexanone, phenol-MgBr, isopropyl alcohol, hydrochloric acid, ammonium hydroxide, and phenol-lithium, are also used at various stages of its preparation. Failure to remove some of the compounds used in phencyclidine synthesis may also contribute to toxicity associated with street exposure to PCP (17).

In the late 1950s, phencyclidine was developed for use as a nonnarcotic, nonbarbiturate anesthetic agent under the tradename Sernyl. In initial animal and human studies, PCP induced a unique type of anesthesia in which subjects remained awake but were apparently "dissociated" from the environment. Phencyclidine and similarly acting arylcyclohexylamines, such as ketamine, were thus designated "dissociative anesthetics." An advantage of these agents over other available anesthetics was their lack of respiratory depression. In early clinical studies, however, it became clear that a significant percentage of individuals exposed to PCP developed psychotic symptoms upon emergence from anesthesia (7,24,31). These symptoms typically lasted for several hours but, in some cases, persisted for up to 10 days

following treatment. Similar but less severe symptoms were seen in trials in which subanesthetic doses of PCP were used for treatment of chronic pain (40). In 1965, clinical investigation of Sernyl was suspended by the manufacturer. From early 1967 until 1979, phencyclidine was marketed solely for veterinary use under the tradename Sernylan. All legal manufacture of PCP in the United States ceased in 1979. Because of its abuse potential and lack of clinical indication, PCP is now listed as a Schedule II agent by the U.S. Drug Enforcement Agency.

PCP exposure now occurs almost exclusively in the context of drug abuse. In the late 1960s, PCP ("PeaCe Pill") made its first appearance as a street drug in the Haight Ashbury section of San Francisco, California, during the "Summer of Love." Initially, phencyclidine was unpopular due to dysphoria and other negative experiences, as well as its erratic absorption following oral ingestion. In the 1970s, however, phencyclidine abuse increased precipitously because of low cost and ease of synthesis. It was commonly substituted for other drugs, most frequently tetrahydrocannabinol, which is much more difficult to synthesize and degrades rapidly. PCP was frequently added to other drugs to boost potency. The arylcyclohexylamine structure of PCP also proved easy to modify. Until 1986, drug dealers could escape prosecution by synthesizing PCP derivatives instead of PCP itself; this led to the popularization of at least 30 "designer" PCP derivatives, including TCP (thiophene analog), PCE (N-ethyl analog), PHP (phenylcyclohexyl pyrralidine), and PCC (pyridocyclohcxanc-carbonitrilc) (17). In 1979, sales of piperidine were restricted to discourage PCP synthesis.

PCP is available "on the street" in capsule, powder, tablet, leaf mixture, rock crystal, and liquid forms. It is smoked, snorted, or ingested. A typical tablet of "line" of PCP contains approximately 5 mg. PCP-containing "joints" typically contain about 1 mg of drug per 150 mg of leaves, totaling anywhere from 1–10 mg of PCP. Common street names for PCP include "angel dust," animal or elephant tranquilizer, or "hog." "Blunts," which consist of PCP-dipped marijuana cigars, have achieved recent popularity. Ketamine, a PCP-like agent that remains in clinical use as an anesthetic, has also recently emerged as a drug of abuse under the street name "Special K."

General Toxicology

PCP is highly lipid-soluble and well absorbed following oral or parenteral administration. It is a weak base with a pKa of 8.6–9.4. PCP is largely ionized within the stomach; absorption following oral administration occurs primarily in the small intestine. Even when not taken orally, PCP may be actively secreted into the stomach (32). Gastric gavage thus may be effective in the treatment of both oral and parenteral PCP overdose. Because of its high lipophilicity and basic pH, PCP is subject to extensive enterohepatic recirculation; this, in turn, may lead to wide blood-level variability and a fluctuating clinical course. Oral bioavailability of PCP has been estimated at 72% following a 1-mg dose (8). Blood/plasma ratios of PCP are approximately 1.0, and plasma binding of PCP is approximately 65% (8). Because of its basic pKa and high lipophilicity, PCP may be extensively trapped intracellularly. The volume of distribution of phencyclidine, 6.2 l/kg, is therefore high (8,27,58). PCP levels in brain and adipose tissue, moreover, may be significantly higher than those in serum (3,41).

PCP is metabolized in liver to hydroxyl and glucuronide metabolites, which are then excreted by the kidney. In both controlled and overdose settings, the terminal-phase half-lives average 21 ± 3 h (range, 7–46 h) (8,37). PCP can be detected in serum or urine using immunoassay, thin-layer chromatography, gas chromatography (GC), or GC/mass spectrometry. The range of detection of typical clinical assays is approximately 25 ng/ml, although levels as low as 5 ng/ml are measurable using more sensitive methods. PCP can be detected in urine for approximately 7 days following single administration and 2–4 weeks following chronic use. Metabolism of PCP appears to be unaffected by alcohol, although its entry into CNS may be increased (23). In contrast, tetrahydrocannabinol appears to inhibit PCP metabolism, leading to higher serum levels and prolonged serum half-life (23). "Blunts," which contain combined marijuana and PCP, represent a particularly potent combination agent.

A specific brain receptor for PCP was first described in 1979 (48,56,60). The order of potency with which other dissociative anesthetics, including ketamine, bind to brain PCP receptors closely parallels their clinical potency. The behavioral effects of this class of agents is mediated primarily through the PCP receptor. PCP receptors, in turn, have been shown to represent a site located within the ion channel formed by the N-methyl-D-aspartate (NMDA)–type excitatory amino acid receptor, linking NMDA receptors to PCP-induced behavioral toxicity (reviewed in 29,30).

Animal Studies

The behavioral effects of PCP in animals are species-specific (5). In rodents, PCP induces a characteristic syndrome of hyperactivity and stereotypes (4,5,16). These behavioral effects respond partially to treatment with neuroleptics (26); they may also be reversed by agents, such as glycine, that augment NMDA receptor–mediated neurotransmission (55). Rodents typically require doses of PCP higher than those used clinically in humans because the serum half-life of PCP is shorter and the volume of distribution is larger in these animals (46). Sensitization to the behavioral effects of PCP follows daily administration (59). In rodents, PCP may also inhibit social behavior; these effects are poorly reversed by typical or atypical antipsychotic agents (53).

In monkeys, doses of approximately 0.5 mg/kg PCP produce a tranquilization wherein animals appear awake but are unresponsive to the environment (6). At doses of 1.0 mg/kg, PCP induces a cataleptoid state in which animals show waxy flexibility and rigidity closely resembling catatonic schizophrenia. Doses of 2.5 mg/kg lead to stupor; 5 mg/kg, to surgical anesthesia; and 15 mg/kg, to convulsive seizures. PCP also significantly inhibits acquisition of new information in monkeys (42). Ketamine induces behavioral effects similar to those of PCP, albeit with lower potency (42).

In the range of concentrations most associated with behavioral hyperactivity, PCP does not appear to cause significant persistent CNS toxicity. At doses significantly above those used for behavioral studies (e.g., 5–50 mg/kg), however, PCP induces neuronal vacuolization, particularly in neurons in posterior cingulate/retrosplenial cortex (45). Similar vacuolization is observed following administration of MK-801 (dizocilpine) and ketamine, indicating that the effect is probably NMDA receptor–mediated. The effect is initially observed in layers III and IV of the cortex. At lower doses (e.g., 5 mg/kg), the effect is transient, reaching peak levels approximately 12 h after PCP or MK-801 administration and then resolving over 12–18 h. Extremely large doses of drug, however, may lead to neuronal necrosis that is apparent even 48 h after drug administration. Although the posterior cingulate/retrosplenial cortex appears most susceptible to the effects of PCP, other hippocampal and limbic brain regions may be affected at higher dosages. Purkinje cells throughout the cerebellum are also targeted by PCP but not by dizocilpine (43). Along with neuronal vacuolation, administration of high-dose PCP leads to elevation of glucose uptake (13), and expression of heat shock (51) and glial fibrillary acidic proteins (15) in the affected regions. The number of neurons undergoing PCP-induced degeneration in posterior cingulate and retrosplenial cortex is attenuated when animals are pretreated with 1,3-dimethylthiourea; this significantly reduces PCP stimulation of haem oxygenase-1 protein, a heat-shock protein induced by oxidative stress (49). Neuronal vacuolation can also be inhibited by prior administration of antipsychotic, anticholinergic, or γ-aminobutyric acid (GABA)–ergic agents, and is potentiated by pilocarpine. It has been suggested that the pattern of pathological alteration induced by PCP and other noncompetitive antagonists may be relevant to the patho-physiology of schizophrenia and related psychoses (13,44).

Human Studies

PCP was given at doses of 0.25 mg/kg in initial clinical trials (24); this dose permitted the performance of procedures such as skin grafting, orthopedic surgery, and gastrectomy/cholecystectomy. Within a few minutes of intravenous injection, patients lost partial consciousness and became unresponsive to painful and auditory stimuli. They appeared semiconscious, with open eyes, fixed staring flat facies, open mouth, rigid posturing, and waxy flexibility. Nystagmus occurred in all and persisted for 24–36 h. Complete amnesia for the intraoperative period and partial postoperative amnesia were observed. Feelings of numbness frequently persisted for 24 h following exposure. Despite its effectiveness as an anesthetic and analgesic, however, PCP was also found to induce marked confusion, disorientation, psychosis, and excitation. These effects were observed both during induction and, most prominently, during emergence from anesthesia. Patients were described as "noisy and excited" for several hours after anesthesia and experienced vestibular and proprioceptive hallucinations accompanied by distortion of vision. The overall clinical state was described as ranging from "happily drunken" to "violent and aggressive" (31). Subanesthetic doses (0.05–0.1 mg/kg) of PCP induced more subtle cognitive disturbances, including concrete and idiosyncratic proverb interpretation, decreased verbalization, and neuropsychological dysfunction closely resembling those in schizophrenia (50). Effects of a single low dose of PCP typically persisted for 4–6 h, although more prolonged reactions were observed in recompensated chronic schizophrenic subjects treated with a single low dose of PCP (2,10,36).

Similar effects to those induced by PCP have been observed following administration of low doses of ketamine to controls (19,33) and recompensated schizophrenic subjects (34). Like PCP, the central effects of ketamine have been linked to occupancy of brain PCP receptors (25).

PCP became a major drug of abuse in the 1970s and 1980s. Symptoms following clinical overdose with PCP vary considerably and depend on both the dose and the predisposition of the individual user. Presenting symptoms may be predominantly or exclusively psychiatric, without significant alterations in level of consciousness. Behavioral symptoms resemble acute schizophrenic decompensation, with concrete and/or illogical thinking, bizarre behavior, negativism, catatonic posturing, and echolalia. Subjective feelings of "drunkenness" may or may not be present. Prior to the development of serum and urine screening tests for

PCP, PCP psychosis could not be reliably differentiated from acute schizophrenia on the basis of presenting symptomatology (14).

PCP-induced psychosis is associated primarily with serum PCP concentrations that range from undetectable (<5 ng/ml) to 100 ng/ml (35,57). Subjects with blood levels of 100 ng/ml may also present with more minor patterns of behavioral disturbance, including lethargy, or bizarre, violent, agitated, or euphoric behavior. Even at serum PCP concentrations between 25 and 100 ng/ml, however, up to 10% of subjects may be asymptomatic. Concentrations above 100 ng/ml almost always cause gross impairment of consciousness, while concentrations above 250 ng/ml are associated with coma, seizures, and respiratory arrest. The highest recorded serum and cerebrospinal fluid concentrations are in the range of 250–500 ng/ml. Despite these broad outlines, however, particular manifestations are not highly correlated with serum levels. Thus, coma has been observed in patients with undetectable serum PCP levels, while some with serum levels >100 ng/ml may continue to be asymptomatic. The variability may account for the dissociation between serum and brain levels (11), or differences in susceptibility or tissue binding between individuals. Typically, subjects have partial or total amnesia for events that occur during PCP intoxication.

Neurological signs may be observed in subjects with only relatively mild degrees of behavioral disturbance. In one study (38), nystagmus and hypertension occurred in over 50% of subjects who presented with lethargy, bizarre or violent behavior, agitation, or euphoria, while tachycardia was seen in approximately 25%. Coma usually follows a period of confused, violent, or bizarre behavior. In 26 cases of mild coma, each lasting <2 h, the most commonly observed signs and symptoms were nystagmus (69%), hypertension (46%), and tachycardia (31%).

Hypertension resulting from PCP intoxication may be fatal (12,39). Generalized seizures occurred in 11% of subjects, and hyperactive deep tendon reflexes in 8%. Other signs, such as muscular rigidity, tremors, or hypersalivation were not observed. On emergence from mild coma, 54% of subjects continued to display an acute encephalopathy for an additional 2–24 h, and the majority showed some form of continuing behavioral disturbances for hours to days. Only two patients awoke from mild coma to mental clarity. More severe episodes of PCP intoxication, in which coma lasted for several hours to days, were associated with additional neurological signs. Subjects became increasingly unresponsive to deep pain, and there was an increased incidence of localized dystonia or generalized rigidity, loss of deep tendon reflexes, athetosis, facial grimacing, tachypnea, and hypothermia or hyperthermia (38). PCP may induce significant analgesia that predisposes subjects to physical injury which it may then mask. Rhabdomyolysis, commonly seen in PCP psychosis, was observed in 22 of 1000 patients (38); this may be due to a combination of trauma and muscular rigidity or seizures, and can lead to renal failure from myoglobinuria (47).

In addition to its acute effects, which resolve upon drug elimination, PCP intoxication may cause a persistent psychosis in up to 20% of exposed individuals. Such symptoms may manifest on initial presentation following low-dose intoxication, or may emerge as confusion subsides following high-dose intoxication. Symptoms typically persist for up to 2 weeks and then resolve abruptly. In some individuals, however, episodes of PCP psychosis may be the initial manifestation of a prolonged schizophrenic reaction. Individuals with a biological predisposition to schizophrenia may be particularly sensitive to the psychotomimetic effects of PCP. In cases where PCP psychosis fails to resolve within several weeks following intoxication, the syndrome should probably be considered a PCP-precipitated schizophrenic decompensation rather than a prolonged PCP-induced psychosis.

The degree to which PCP-induced behavioral symptoms respond to antipsychotics is unclear. Higher-potency neuroleptics (e.g., haloperidol, pimozide) are superior to lower-potency agents (e.g., chlorpromazine) (22). Furthermore, low-potency neuroleptics, such as chlorpromazine, may be more likely to decrease seizure threshold. However, such agents may also act as effective alpha-blocking agents, and may assist in the management of hypertension. Ascorbic acid has been reported to augment the therapeutic effects of haloperidol (21). Meperidine has also been shown to be effective (20), although its use has not achieved widespread popularity. Benzodiazepines or other sedative-hypnotics are frequently employed for the management of agitation or excitation during acute PCP intoxication (18). Diphenhydramine has been reported to be effective in the management of PCP-induced dystonias but not generalized rigidity (38). Because PCP is frequently taken in combination with other drugs, a toxicological analysis of urine and/or blood for other drugs besides PCP is essential. Urine should also be tested for heme because of the potential complication of myoglobinura. Serum uric acid, creatine phosphokinase, and serum glutamic acid oxaloacetic transferase/serum glutamic acid pyruvate transferase elevations, may also be associated with PCP-induced rhabdomyolysis. Gastric lavage using activated charcoal may be effective in binding PCP and increasing its nonrenal clearance (32). Cathartics, such as sorbitol or magnesium citrate, may also increase gastrointestinal transit time and thus decrease absorption. Because PCP is a weak base, urinary acidification is recommended. Decreasing urinary pH from 7 to 5 and forcing diuresis may increase PCP clearance 100-fold. However, since 90% of PCP is metabolized by the liver, and only 10% is excreted unchanged in urine, the benefits of increased renal clearance may not outweigh the risks (54).

Toxic Mechanisms

PCP induces its behavioral effects primarily by blocking the ion channels associated with NMDA-type glutamate receptors (30). PCP blocks NMDA channels by binding to a specific receptor, termed the PCP receptor, located within the NMDA receptor-associated ion channel. PCP, ketamine, and dizocilpine (MK-801) are thus noncompetitive NMDA antagonists. Similar behavioral effects to those of PCP may be induced by competitive NMDA antagonists (52) that prevent the binding of glutamate or glycine to their recognition sites on the NMDA complex. A number of competitive NMDA antagonists, including D-(−)-4-(3-phosphono-propyl)piperazine-2-carboxylic acid and its unsaturated analogue (D(−)(E)-4-(3-phosphonoprop-2-enyl) piperazine-2-carboxylic acid are under investigation as potential anti-ischemic and antiepileptic medication (54).

At doses approximately tenfold higher than those that block NMDA receptor–mediated neurotransmission, PCP also blocks presynaptic monoamine reuptake and thus directly increases synaptic levels of dopamine and noradrenaline. Levels sufficient to block monoamine reuptake may be achieved during high-dose intoxication and may contribute to the amphetamine-like effects of PCP seen at those doses. Ketamine, even at high dose, does not interact with monoamine transporters; this may explain the rare episodes of extreme agitation and violence following ketamine, but not PCP, intoxication.

PCP blocks neuronal Na^+ and K^+ channels in concentrations associated with high-dose intoxication. Such effects may be relevant to the seizures observed following PCP overdose. PCP also interacts with a variety of other CNS receptors including cholinergic, μ-opiate, and GABA/benzodiazepine receptors. However, the majority of such effects appears at concentration unlikely to be encountered in clinical situations.

A major consequence of PCP-induced NMDA blockade is stimulation of dopaminergic and noradrenergic neurotransmission. In rodents, PCP-induced hyperactivity has been linked to an elevation in presynaptic dopamine release (16,52). NMDA receptors also play a crucial role in initiation of long-term potentiation, which is believed to underlie learning and memory formation (58). NMDA antagonists disrupt long-term potentiation, leading to the amnesia that is commonly observed following PCP intoxication. Furthermore, PCP-induced NMDA-receptor blockade disrupts memory-dependent sensory processing at subcortical and cortical sites (1,28), leading to the sensory distortions seen following PCP administration. Mechanisms underlying experimental high-dose PCP-induced neuronal vacuolization are poorly understood; since vacuolization is significantly potentiated by the cholinergic agonist pilocarpine and inhibited by muscarinic antagonists, NMDA modulation of cholinergic function may be critical (44). PCP is currently less a public health threat than a decade ago. Continued investigation into mechanisms underlying PCP-induced behavioral and neuronal toxicity are useful and may be relevant to the pathophysiology of severe neuropsychiatric illnesses such as schizophrenia (30) or dementia (13).

REFERENCES

1. Bakshi VP, Swerdlow NR, Geyer MA (1994) Clozapine antagonizes phencyclidine-induced deficits in sensorimotor gating of the startle response. *J Pharmacol Exp Ther* **271**, 787.

2. Ban TA, Lohrenz JJ, Lehmann HE (1961) Observations on the action of sernyl—a new psychotropic drug. *Can Psychiat Assn J* **6**, 150.

3. Budd RD, Liu Y (1982) Phencyclidine concentrations in postmortem body fluids and tissues. *J Toxicol-Clin Toxicol* **19**, 843.

4. Carter AJ (1995) Antagonists of the NMDA receptor-channel complex and motor coordination. *Life Sci* **57**, 917.

5. Chen G, Ensor CR, Russell D, Bohner B (1959) The pharmacology of 1-(1-phenylcyclohexyl)piperidine-HCl. *J Pharmacol Exp Ther* **127**, 240.

6. Chen GM, Weston JK (1960) The analgesic and anesthetic effect of 1-(1-phenylcyclohexyl)piperidine-HCl on the monkey. *Anesth Analg* **39**, 132.

7. Collins VJ, Gorospe CA, Rovenstine EA (1960) Intravenous nonbarbiturate, nonnarcotic analgesics: Preliminary studies. I. Cycohexylamines. *Anesth Analg* **39**, 302.

8. Cook CE, Brine DR, Jeffcoat AR et al. (1982) Phencyclidine disposition after intravenous and oral doses. *Clin Pharmacol Ther* **31**, 625.

9. Cotman CW, Monaghan DT, Ganong AH (1988) Excitatory amino acid neurotransmission: NMDA receptors and Hebb-type synaptic plasticity. *Annu Rev Neurosci* **11**, 61.

10. Domino EF, Luby ED (1981) Abnormal mental states induced by phencyclidine as a model for schizophrenia. In: *PCP (Phencyclidine): Historical and Current Perspectives.* Domino EF ed. NPP Books, Ann Arbor, Michigan p. 401.

11. Donaldson JO, Baselt RC (1979) CSF phencyclidine. *Amer J Psychiat* **136**, 10.

12. Eastman JW, Cohen SH (1975) Hypertensive crisis and death associated with phencyclidine poisoning. *J Amer Med Assn* **231**, 1270.

13. Ellison G (1995) The N-methyl-D-aspartate antagonists phencyclidine, ketamine, and dizocilpine as both behavioral and anatomical models of the dementias. *Brain Res Rev* **20**, 250.

14. Erard R, Luisada PV, Peele R (1980) The PCP psychosis: Prolonged intoxication of drug-precipitated functional illness. *J Psychedelic Drugs* **12**, 235.

15. Fix AS (1994) Pathological effects of MK-801 in the rat posterior cingulate/retrosplenial cortex. *Psychopharm Bull* **30**, 577.

16. French ED (1988) Effects of acute and chronic administration of phencyclidine on the A$_{10}$ dopaminergic mesolimbic system: Electrophysiological and behavioral correlates. *Neuropharmacology* **27**, 791.

17. Garey RE (1979) PCP (phencyclidine): An update. *J Psychedelic Drugs* **11**, 265.

18. Garrettson LK, Geller RJ (1990) Acid and alkaline diuresis. When are they of value in the treatment of poisoning? *Drug Safety* **5**, 220.

19. Ghoneim MM, Hindrichs JV, Mewaldt SP, Petersen RC (1985) Ketamine: Behavioral effects of subanesthetic doses. *J Clin Psychopharmacol* **5**, 70.

20. Giannini AJ, Loiselle RH, DiMarzio LR, Giannini MC (1987) Augmentation of haloperidol by ascorbic acid in phencyclidine intoxication. *Amer J Psychiat* **144**, 1207.

21. Giannini AJ, Loiselle RH, Price WA, Giannini MC (1985) Chlorpromazine *vs.* meperidine in the treatment of phencyclidine psychosis. *J Clin Psychiat* **46**, 52.

22. Giannini AJ, Nageotte C, Loiselle RH et al. (1984) Comparison of chlorpromazine, haloperidol and pimozide in the treatment of phencyclidine psychosis: DA-2 receptor specificity. *J Toxicol-Clin Toxicol* **22**, 573.

23. Godley PJ, Moore ES, Woodworth JR, Fineg J (1991) Effects of ethanol and delta 9-tetrahydrocannabinol on phencyclidine disposition in dogs. *Biopharm Drug Disposition* **12**, 189.

24. Greifenstein FE, DeVault M (1958) A study of 1-aryl cyclohexylamine for anesthesia. *Anesth Analg* **37**, 283.

25. Hartvig P, Valtysson J, Lindner K-J et al. (1995) Central nervous system effects of subdissociative doses of (S)-ketamine are related to plasma and brain concentrations measured with positron emission tomography in healthy volunteers. *Clin Pharmacol Ther* **58**, 165.

26. Jackson DM, Johansson C, Lindgren L-M, Bengtsson A (1994) Dopamine receptor antagonists block amphetamine and phencyclidine-induced motor stimulation in rats. *Pharmacol Biochem Behav* **48**, 465.

27. James SH, Schnoll SH (1976) Phencyclidine: Tissue distribution in the rat. *Clin Toxicol* **9**, 573.

28. Javitt DC, Steinschneider M, Schroeder CE, Arezzo JC (1996) Role of cortical N-methyl-D-aspartate receptors in auditory sensory memory and mismatch negativity gen-

eration: Implications for schizophrenia. *Proc Nat Acad Sci USA* **93**, 11962.

29. Javitt DC, Zukin SR (1990) Role of excitatory amino acids in neuropsychiatric illness. *J Neuropsychiat Clin Neurosci* **2**, 44.

30. Javitt DC, Zukin SR (1991) Recent advances in the phencyclidine model of schizophrenia. *Amer J Psychiat* **148**, 1301.

31. Johnstone M, Evans V, Baigel S (1959) Sernyl (Cl-395) in clinical anesthesia. *Brit J Anaesth* **31**, 433.

32. Jones J, McMullen MJ, Dougherty J, Cannon L (1987) Repetitive doses of activated charcoal in the treatment of poisoning. *Amer J Emerg Med* **5**, 305.

33. Krystal JH, Karper LP, Siebyl JP et al. (1994) Subanesthetic effects of the noncompetitive NMDA antagonist, ketamine, in humans. *Arch Gen Psychiat* **51**, 199.

34. Lahti AC, Holcomb HH, Medoff MR, Tamminga CA (1995) Ketamine activates psychosis and alters limbic blood flow in schizophrenia. *Neuroreport* **6**, 869.

35. Liden CB, Lovejoy FH, Costello CE (1975) Phencyclidine: Nine cases of poisoning. *J Amer Med Assn* **234**, 513.

36. Luby ED, Cohen BD, Rosenbaum G et al. (1959) Study of a new schizophrenomimetic drug—Sernyl. *AMA Arch Neuro Psychiat* **81**, 363.

37. Marshman JA, Ramsay MP, Sellers EM (1976) Quantitation of phencyclidine in biological fluids and application to human overdose. *Toxicol Appl Pharmacol* **35**, 129.

38. McCarron MM, Schulze BW, Thompson GA et al. (1981) Acute phencyclidine intoxication: Clinical patterns, complications and treatment. *Ann Emerg Med* **10**, 290.

39. McMahon B, Ambre J, Ellis J (1978) Hypertension during recovery from phencyclidine intoxication. *Clin Toxicol* **12**, 37.

40. Meyer JS, Greifenstein F, Devault M (1959) A new drug causing symptoms of sensory deprivation. *J Nerv Ment Dis* **129**, 54.

41. Misra AL, Pontani RB, Barteolemeo J (1979) Persistence of phencyclidine (PCP) and metabolites in brain and adipose tissue and implications for long-lasting behavioral effects. *Res Commun Chem Pathol Pharmacol* **24**, 3431.

42. Moersbaecher JM, Thompson DM (1980) Effects of phencyclidine, pentobarbital, and d-amphetamine on the acquisition and performance of conditional discriminations in monkeys. *Pharmacol Biochem Behav* **13**, 887.

43. Nakki R, Koistinaho J, Sharp FR, Sagar SM (1995) Cerebellar toxicity of phencyclidine. *Neurosci* **15**, 2097.

44. Olney JW, Farber NB (1995) Glutamate receptor dysfunction and schizophrenia. *Arch Gen Psychiat* **52**, 1015.

45. Olney JW, Labruyere J, Price MT (1989) Pathological changes induced in cerebrocortical neurons by phencyclidine and related drugs. *Science* **244**, 1360.

46. Owens SM, Hardwick WC, Blackall D (1987) Phencyclidine pharmokinetic scaling among species. *J Pharmacol Exp Ther* **242**, 96.

47. Patel R, Connor G (1986) A review of thirty cases of rhabdomyolysis-associated acute renal failure among phencyclidine users. *Clin Toxicol* **23**, 547.

48. Quirion R, Hammer RP, Henkenham M, Pert C (1981) Phencyclidine (angel dust)/sigma "opiate" receptor: Visualization by tritium-sensitive film. *Proc Nat Acad Sci USA* **78**, 5881.

49. Rajdev S, Fix AS, Sharp FR (1998) Acute phencyclidine neurotoxicity in rat forebrain: induction of haem oxygenase-1 and attenuation by the antioxidant dimethylthiourea. *Eur J Neurosci* **10**, 3840.

50. Rosenbaum G, Cohen BD, Luby ED et al. (1959) Comparison of sernyl with other drugs. *AMA Arch Gen Psychiat* **1**, 651.

51. Sharp FR, Butman M, Aardalen K et al. (1994) Neuronal injury produced by NMDA antagonists can be detected using heat shock proteins and can be blocked with antipsychotics. *Psychopharmacol Bull* **30**, 555.

52. Steinpreis RE, Salamone JD (1993) The role of nucleus accumbens dopamine in the neurochemical and behavioral effects of phencyclidine: A microdialysis and behavioral study. *Brain Res* **612**, 263.

53. Steinpreis RE, Sokolowski JD, Papnikolaou A, Salamone JD (1994) The effects of haloperidol and clozapine on PCP- and amphetamine-induced suppression of social behavior in the rat. *Pharmacol Biochem Behav* **47**, 579.

54. Tong TG, Benowitz NL, Becker CE et al. (1975) Phencyclidine poisoning. *J Amer Med Assn* **234**, 512.

55. Toth E, Lajtha E (1986) Antagonism of phencyclidine-induced hyperactivity by glycine in mice. *Neurochem Res* **11**, 393.

56. Vincent JP, Kartalovski B, Geneste P et al. (1979) Interaction of phencyclidine ("angel dust") with a specific receptor in rat brain membranes. *Proc Nat Acad Sci USA* **76**, 4678.

57. Walberg DB, McCarron MM, Schulze BW (1983) Quantitation of phencyclidine in serum by enzyme immunoassay: Results in 405 patients. *J Anal Toxicol* **7**, 106.

58. Woodworth JR, Owens SM, Mayersohn M (1985) Phencyclidine (PCP) disposition kinetics in dogs as a function of dose and route of administration. *J Pharmacol Exp Ther* **234**, 654.

59. Xu X, Domino Ef (1994) Phencyclidine-induced behavioral sensitization. *Pharmacol Biochem Behav* **47**, 603.

60. Zukin Sr, Zukin RS (1979) Specific [^{3}H]phencyclidine binding in rat central nervous system. *Proc Nat Acad Sci USA* **76**, 5372.

Phenelzine and Other Monoamine Oxidase Inhibitors

Arnold E. Merriam

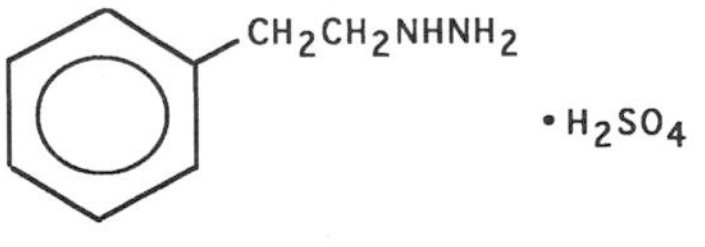

PHENELIZINE SULFATE
$C_8H_{12}N_2 \cdot H_2SO_4$

(2-Phenethyl)hydrazine sulfate

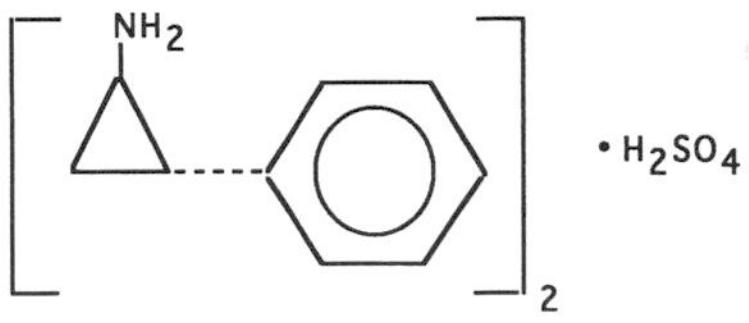

TRANYLCYPROMINE SULFATE
$(C_9H_{11}N)_2 \cdot H_2SO_4$

($\pm$)-*Trans*-2-phenylcyclopropylamine sulfate

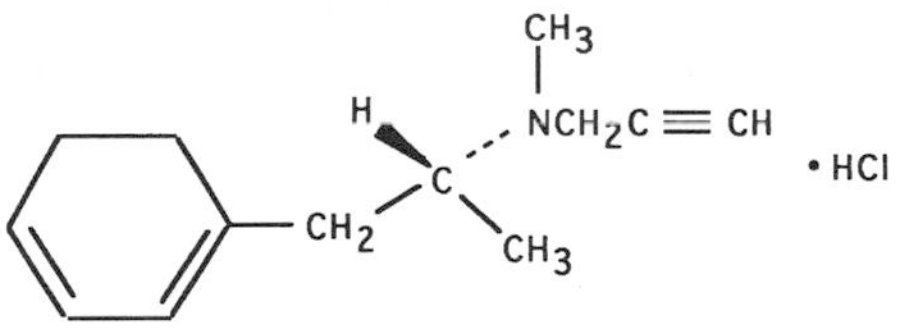

L-DEPRENYL HYDROCHLORIDE
$C_{13}H_{17}N \cdot HCl$

Selegiline hydrochloride; (R)-$(-)$-N,α-Dimethyl-N-2-propynylphenethylamine hydrochloride

NEUROTOXICITY RATING

Clinical

A   Seizure disorder

A   Extrapyramidal syndrome

A   Serotonin syndrome (delirium, mania, autonomic dysfunction, tremor)

Experimental

A   Serotonin dysfunction (rodent)

The monoamine oxidase inhibitors (MAOIs) form the first group of antidepressant compounds to have been discovered; they remain in active use, primarily in the treatment of depression with so-called atypical features (*e.g.*, profound loss of energy, hyperphagia, hypersomnolence); for depression not responsive to medication trials with other agents; and for some cases of anxiety, obsessive-compulsive disorder, and eating disorder. They have a minor place in the management of some cases of vascular headache, par-

ticularly cluster headache. Only phenelzine, a hydrazine derivative, and tranylcypromine, a drug structurally related to amphetamine, remain in use in the United States as psychotropic agents. L-Deprenyl, an agent without a prominent psychiatric role, has been used in the treatment of Parkinson's disease.

The therapeutic efficacy of these agents relates to their potent inhibitory action on the enzyme monoamine oxidase (MAO), key to a principal metabolic pathway by which aminergic neurotransmitters are eliminated from the synaptic space after their release from nerve terminals. MAO inhibition results in an increase in the synaptic concentration of these neurotransmitters; the link between this effect and the alleviation of depression has not been conclusively demonstrated, but clearly depends upon some further physiological alteration, since monoamine concentrations are elevated long before mood symptoms clinically remit.

There are two species of the MAO enzyme: MAO type A preferentially deaminates serotonin and norepinephrine, while MAO type B preferentially deaminates phenethylamine; both types effectively deaminate dopamine and tyramine. The relative proportions of these two enzyme types differ in different species and, within species, the distribution of the two forms differs in the various body tissues: in humans, types A and B are found both in the liver and the brain; type A predominates in the gut, and type B in platelets. Phenelzine and tranylcypromine nonspecifically inhibit both enzyme types, although phenelzine shows a preference for type A substrates and tranylcypromine for type B. L-Deprenyl prefentially inhibits the type-B enzyme at low concentrations; this selectivity is lost at higher dosages.

The MAOIs are readily absorbed after oral administration, are widely distributed, and achieve maximal enzyme inhibition within a few days. Phenelzine and L-deprenyl irreversibly inactivate the MAO enzyme, while the effect of tranylcypromine is reversible. After drug discontinuation, enzyme activity returns to baseline sooner in the case of tranylcypromine (7–10 days) than in the case of phenelzine and L-deprenyl since, in the latter instance, the actual enzyme molecules must be regenerated, a process that takes 2–3 weeks.

The metabolism and excretion of these agents is poorly understood. It was formerly considered that acetylation was a metabolic process prominent in the degradation of phenelzine; it has more recently been discovered that N-acetylation is not a significant pathway in man (7). Free and conjugated aromatic acid forms of this drug are excreted in the urine.

The MAOIs have been confirmed to increase brain monoamine content in the rat (1). A syndrome equivalent to the serotonin syndrome in man (*vide infra*) has been induced in laboratory rodents by the use of MAOIs in conjunction either with various serotonin-reuptake inhibitors or with L-tryptophan: features include tremor, rigidity, hyperreactivity, myoclonus, and seizures (2). The syndrome can be blocked in these animals by pretreatment with serotonin depletors, such as *p*-chlorophenylalanine, or by blocking serotonin receptors. Data from rats and mice indicate that the syndrome is mediated by action at the postsynaptic $5-HT_{1A}$ moiety of serotonin receptor (3,13).

Lethal overdose has been reported in man after ingestion of 375–1500 mg phenelzine, and of 170–650 mg tranylcypromine; toxicity may not become fully manifest until 12 h following ingestion. Manifestations of overdose include confusion, agitation, hyperthermia, tachycardia, and either hypertension or circulatory collapse; in the neurological sphere, symptoms include headache and dizziness, and signs include hyperreflexia, chorea, convulsions, and/or coma. Hemodialysis has been reported to be effective in rapidly reversing poisoning with both tranylcypromine (6) and phenelzine (12); the latter is somewhat surprising given the irreversible nature of its enzyme-inhibiting action.

At therapeutic doses, usually up to 90 mg/day of phenelzine or 60 mg/day of tranylcypromine, the most regularly encountered MAOI-induced neurotoxic effect is the precipitation of myoclonus, often described by patients as "twitchiness." MAOI-induced myoclonus may occur during wakefulness, but is more often seen during rest, sleep onset, and sleep (5). The incidence of MAOI-related myoclonus has not been determined, but it is far from uncommon and appears to be dose-related. Postural tremor is also sometimes encountered but is rarely of clinical significance.

Of the various antidepressants, MAOIs are considered to exert the least effect on seizure threshold, although seizures are often encountered in overdose.

Despite the relatively benign neurological profile of the MAOIs when they are used as solo agents in therapeutic dosage, these compounds have been documented to evoke two different varieties of catastrophic and even lethal reactions in combination with certain foodstuffs and pharmaceuticals: these are the *hypertensive reaction*, and the *serotonin syndrome*. Either type of interaction may occur for a period of up to 3 weeks following MAOI discontinuation, because MAO enzyme levels recover only slowly from their inhibition or depletion.

The MAOI hypertensive crisis is a hyperadrenergic reaction that can occur when tyramine-containing foodstuffs are ingested by patients taking MAOIs. Symptoms include hypertension, headache, diaphoresis, mydriasis, excitation, and cardiac arrhythmia. The syndrome results when tyramine, no longer capable of being deaminated by hepatic MAO after its intestinal absorption, triggers the widespread release of norepinephrine from presynaptic stores. Acute hypertension, which has led to intracerebral hemorrhage or myocardial infarction, is a particularly dangerous aspect of the reaction. Treatment is parallel to that of any acute hypertensive emergency: some have recommended the use of calcium-channel blockers (*e.g.*, nifedipine) for MAOI-induced catastrophic hypertension but have pointed out that the optimal dose and route have yet to be clearly determined (8). Every prescription of MAOI should be accompanied by an explanation of foods to be avoided: these are, principally, aged cheeses, aged meats, concentrated yeast extracts, sauerkraut, broad bean pods, tap beer, and excessive alcohol (9,11).

The other catastrophic MAOI-related reaction is the so-called serotonin syndrome, characterized by restlessness, delirium, incoordination, tremor, myoclonus, shivering, seizures, muscular hypertonia, hyperreflexia, autonomic instability, and hyperpyrexia (10). Other manifestations include diarrhea, hypomania, and disseminated intravascular coagulation. This state may progress to coma and death from cardiovascular collapse, hyperpyrexia, and other systemic complications. While there is some overlap between the manifestations of this syndrome and those of MAOI overdose, the serotonin syndrome has been reported in the context of usual and customary doses of the MAOI when taken in the company of other agents that also perturb serotonergic neurotransmission. The agents recognized to fall into this category include the tricyclic antidepressants (most prominently clomipramine, which of all the tricyclic antidepressant compounds most potently blocks serotonin reuptake); the selective serotonin-reuptake inhibitors (SSRIs); the serotonin precursor L-tryptophan; and the narcotic compounds meperidine and dextromethorphan, both of which inhibit serotonin reuptake. In cases where one of these agents is discontinued and another started, prescribers should be aware of the possiblity of interactions due to persistence of the discontinued agent's lingering effects on the serotonergic system. MAOIs exert prolonged biological effects for a period of up to 3 weeks after drug discontinuation; in the case of phenelzine, replacement enzyme molecules must actually be resynthesized. Among the SSRIs, fluoxetine has the most prolonged action and shows evidence of persistent plasma levels of an active metabolite for up to 5 weeks. Polypharmacy during these periods should be undertaken with the greatest caution.

Treatment of serotonin syndrome would logically consist of serotonin receptor blockade, a strategy that has proven successful in animal models of this disorder (3,13). This approach (in the form of cyproheptadine treatment) was beneficial in a case of serotonin syndrome precipitated by use of a SSRI 11 days after discontinuation of a MAOI (4).

REFERENCES

1. Campbell JC, Robinson DS, Lovenberg W, Murphy DL (1979) The effects of chronic regimens of clorgyline and pargyline on monoamine metabolism in the rat brain. *J Neurochem* **32**, 49.
2. Gerson SC, Baldessarini RJ (1980) Motor effects of serotonin in the central nervous system. *Life Sci* **27**, 1435.
3. Goodwin GM, De Souza RJ, Green AR *et al.* (1987) The pharmacology of the behavioural and hypothermic responses of rats to 8-hydroxy-2-(di-*n*-propylamino)tetralin. (8-OH-DPAT). *Psychopharmacology* **91**, 506.
4. Lappin RI, Auchincloss EL (1994) Treatment of the serotonin syndrome with cyproheptadine. *N Engl J Med* **331**, 1021.
5. Lieberman JA, Kane JM, Reife R (1986) Neuromuscular effects of monoamine oxidase inhibitors. In: *Advances in Neurology. Vol 43. Myoclonus.* Fahn S *et al.* eds. Raven Press, New York p. 231.
6. Matter BJ, Donat PE, Bril ML *et al.* (1965) Tranylcypromine sulfate poisoning. Successful treatment by hemodialysis. *Arch Intern Med* **116**, 18.
7. Robinson DS, Cooper TB, Jindal SP *et al.* (1985) Metabolism and pharmacokinetics of phenelzine: Lack of evidence for acetylation pathway in humans. *J Clin Psychopharmacol* **5**, 333.
8. Shader RI, Greenblat DJ (1992) MAOIs and hypertension. *J Clin Psychopharmacol* **12**, 1.
9. Shulman KI, Walker SE, MacKenzie S, Knowles S (1989) Dietary restriction, tyramine, and the use of monoamine oxidase inhibitors. *J Clin Psychopharmacol* **9**, 397.
10. Sternbach, H. The serotonin syndrome (1991) *Amer J Psychiat* **148**, 705.
11. Tailor SAN, Shulman KI, Walker SE *et al.* (1994) Hypertensive episode associated with phenelzine and tap beer. *J Clin Psychopharmacol* **14**, 5.
12. Versaci AA, Nakamoto S, Kolff WJ (1964) Phenelzine intoxication; report of a case treated by hemodialysis. *Ohio State Med J* **60**, 770.
13. Yamada J, Sugimoto Y, Horisaka K (1988) The behavioural effects of 8-hydroxy-2-(di-*n*-propylamino)tetralin (8-OH-DPAT) in mice. *Eur J Pharmacol* **154**, 299.

Phenol

Herbert H. Schaumburg

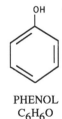

PHENOL
C_6H_6O

Carbolic acid

NEUROTOXICITY RATING
Clinical
A Peripheral neuropathy (local administration)
B Acute encephalopathy (seizures)
Experimental
A Peripheral neuropathy (local administration)

Phenol, carbolic acid, is used both as an industrial and a pharmaceutical agent. In industry, it is a precursor in the synthesis of aromatic substances; it is now rarely associated with serious occupational illness. Phenol has two pharmaceutical uses: one as a topical disinfectant agent for minor skin infections; the other, a locally injected neurolytic agent to treat spasticity. In the late nineteenth century, phenol sprays were deployed in operating rooms during major surgical procedures; hospital personnel were exposed to high levels of airborne phenol with few reported consequences.

Phenol is readily absorbed through the skin, stomach, and respiratory tract. Following absorption, most is oxidized and conjugated with glucuronic and sulfuric acids. Phenol is excreted in the urine as conjugated (63%) and free (37%) forms. Systemic toxicity is directly related to the level of circulating free phenol (7). The effects of high-level oral ingestion (> 1g) or massive dermal exposure (adults falling in a vat of pure phenol, children with massive topical application of calamine lotion) are pallor, cyanosis, slow pulse, respiratory depression, convulsions, and death (2). Many of these manifestations stem from myocardial toxicity. Chronic exposure causes darkened and then depigmented skin, wasting ("phenol marasmus"), and hepatorenal dysfunction.

Acute high-level ingestion or dermal exposure may also cause generalized seizures and episodes of limb rigidity (2). There are no contemporary studies of the neurophysiology of phenol-induced seizures, and the mechanism of this neurotoxic reaction to phenol is unclear. Seizures are not secondary to hypoperfusion, since they almost always antedate evidence of cardiac failure. There are no descriptions of adverse effects on the nervous system in individuals with chronic intoxication, save for muscle pain and fatigue.

Spasticity from human spinal cord lesions has been ameliorated either by local intramuscular injections of aqueous solutions of phenol to motor points (a procedure known as "chemical neurotomy") (4), or by injections of phenol in glycerol solutions into the lumbar subarachnoid space, "chemical rhizotomy" (5). One report additionally describes diminished spasticity without weakness in a lower limb selectively perfused with dilute phenol solution (1). The rationale for these procedures was suggested by experimental animal studies that indicated an ability of local applications of phenol selectively to damage small-diameter myelinated nerve fibers such as the gamma efferents (6). A subsequent experimental and electrophysiological study failed to confirm this notion; it indicated that phenol causes axonal damage to all nerve fibers (8). Considerable local neurotoxicity stemmed from some of these procedures, particularly from the injection of phenol into the lumbar subarachnoid space. Occasional intrathecal injections were followed by multilevel nerve root necrosis and spinal cord infarction from uncontrolled spread of phenol in the subarachnoid space (3). The local proteolytic effect of concentrated phenol produces coagulation necrosis in arteries as well as in peripheral nerves. This risky procedure is now rarely used because there are several effective antispasticity oral medications and safer, surgically implantable pumps that can release less toxic spasmolytic agents into the cerebrospinal fluid. Local limb motor-point muscle injections have had few complications and are still in widespread use. Stellate and celiac ganglion blocks are less safe than limbmuscle blocks because of potential diffusion of phenol into the peritoneal cavity and the fascial planes of the neck (9).

REFERENCES
1. Cooper IS, Hirose T, Matsuoka S et al. (1965) Specific neurotoxic perfusion: A new approach to selected cases of pain and spasticity. *Neurology* **15**, 985.
2. Deichmann WB (1949) Local and systemic effects following skin contact with phenol: A review of the literature. *J Ind Hyg Toxicol* **31**, 146.
3. Hughes JT (1970) Thrombosis of the posterior spinal arteries. *Neurology* **20**, 659.
4. Khalili AA, Betts HB (1967) Peripheral nerve block with phenol in the management of spasticity. *J Amer Med Assn* **200**, 1155.
5. Nathan PW (1959) Intrathecal phenol to relieve spasticity in paraplegia. *Lancet* **2**, 1099.
6. Nathan PW, Sears TA (1961) Effects of phenol on nervous conduction. *J Physiol* **150**, 565.
7. Ruedemann R, Deichmann WB (1953) Blood phenol level after topical application of phenol-containing preparations. *J Amer Med Assn* **152**, 506.
8. Schaumburg HH, Byck R, Weller RO (1970) The effect of phenol on peripheral nerve. *Neuropathol Exp Neurol* **29**, 615.
9. Superville-Sovak B, Rasminsky M, Finlayson MH (1975) Complications of phenol neurolysis. *Arch Neurol* **32**, 226.

Phenytoin

Allison Mann
Mark J. Sinnett
Shlomo Shinnar

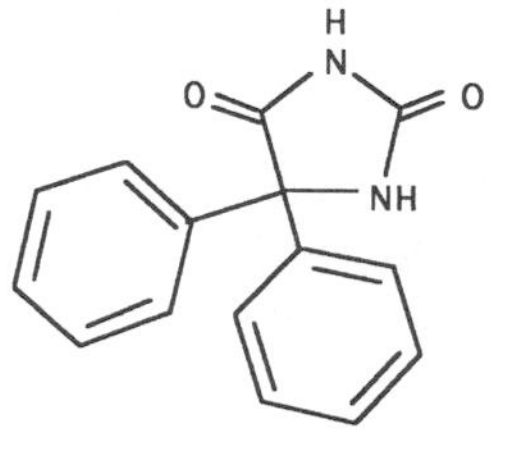

PHENYTOIN
$C_{15}H_{12}N_2O_2$

5,5-Diphenyl-2,4-imidazolidinedione; Diphenylhydantoin

NEUROTOXICITY RATING
Clinical
A Teratogenicity
A Cerebellar syndrome (ataxia, nystagmus)
A Chronic encephalopathy (cognitive dysfunction)
B Extrapyramidal syndrome (chorea, dyskinesia)
B Peripheral neuropathy
Experimental
A Acute encephalopathy (ataxia)
A Teratogenicity

Phenytoin is a prescription antiepileptic drug (AED) derived from hydantoin. Synthesized in 1908, it became available for the treatment of epilepsy in 1938. Although many AEDs have been approved since, phenytoin remains the most widely used anticonvulsant in North America.

Phenytoin is available as either the free acid or the sodium salt. Each 100 mg of phenytoin sodium contains approximately 92 mg of phenytoin. The acid form is utilized in the preparation of a suspension and tablets. Phenytoin sodium is available as both a prompt and extended-release capsule and as a sterile solution for intravenous administration.

Phenytoin, a weak organic acid, is practically insoluble in water, sparingly soluble in alcohol, and soluble in acetone. The drug has a true pKa of 8.06 and is essentially nonionized at pH 5.4 (92). Aqueous phenytoin sodium undergoes hydrolysis to phenytoin, resulting in drug precipitation. Hence, phenytoin for injection is more stable if dissolved in a vehicle containing propylene glycol, ethanol, and sodium hydroxide. Precipitation of phenytoin can occur at pH 11.5 or less.

The mechanism of anticonvulsant action of phenytoin has been studied in both animal and human neurons. Phenytoin affects sodium permeability across the neuronal membrane by binding preferentially to and stabilizing inactivated sodium channels, and thereby slowing the rate of membrane recovery to its resting state. This action reduces the rate of excessive neuronal firing associated with seizure activity (59).

Phenytoin is used primarily in the acute and chronic management of generalized tonic-clonic and partial seizures, and in the prevention and treatment of acute seizures following neurosurgical procedures and head trauma. A typical dose ranges from 200–600 mg/day. Usual therapeutic concentrations for seizure control are between 40 and 80 μM (10–20 μg/ml) for refractory ventricular and atrial arrhythmias, particularly those caused by digitalis intoxication (11). It is also shown to be effective in neurological pain syndromes (99) and, in uncontrolled trials, relieved migraine headache (68) and promoted wound healing (70).

Phenytoin is widely used as an anticonvulsant because of ease of administration in emergencies. It is the only anticonvulsant available that can be given intravenously in a full loading dose without significantly affecting the level of consciousness of the patient. Barbiturates and benzodiazepines decrease consciousness; other anticonvulsants, such as carbamazepine, valproate, gabapentin, and lamotrigine, are not available in an intravenous formulation. These factors and its proven efficacy allows phenytoin to retain its status as the first-line drug for treating seizures in the emergency room (8). It has also remained a first-line drug for chronic therapy because of proven efficacy, low cost, and the availability of a slow-release capsule for once-a-day dosing. There are some disadvantages associated with chronic phenytoin use; these include a variety of side effects and pharmacokinetic issues discussed below. Phenytoin pharmacotherapy can be difficult to manage.

General Toxicology

Phenytoin is completely absorbed from the gastrointestinal tract. It is essentially insoluble at the low pH of the stomach (92). Most phenytoin is absorbed in the duodenum (pH 7.8) although its solubility at pH 7.8 is only 400 μM (100 μg/ml). Peak serum concentrations occur within 4–8 h (75) and are directly proportional to the dose administered (43). It is slowly and erratically absorbed when given intramuscularly.

Phenytoin is about 90% bound to serum albumin in healthy adults; binding decreases in the presence of renal failure and hepatic disease. It is distributed widely in the body and reaches peak brain concentrations within 15 min. Phenytoin brain concentrations are one to three times the plasma concentration. More drug accumulates in white matter than in gray matter (44,74).

Elimination of phenytoin occurs primarily by hepatic biotransformation to several hydroxylated metabolites. Its major route of metabolism is oxidation to the inactive metabolite 5-(p-hydroxy-phenyl-5-phenylhydantoin (Fig. 28). Less than 5% of a phenytoin dose is excreted unchanged in the urine. It is suspected that hepatic enzymes have a limited drug metabolizing capacity. This metabolizing limit is usually well above the metabolic rate of most drugs, but not for phenytoin. Phenytoin exhibits capacity-limited pharmacokinetics in humans. At subtherapeutic phenytoin doses, elimination of phenytoin is linear or directly proportional to serum concentration. However, as serum concentrations reach the therapeutic range, further increases in phenytoin dose cause a disproportionate increase in serum concentration. The half-life of phenytoin is directly proportional to its serum concentration. The mean phenytoin K_m (serum phenytoin concentration at which half the maximum velocity of the enzyme system is attained) is 24.8 μM (6.2 μg/ml) in adults (13).

Potential adverse effects produced by phenytoin are legion. The drug has both acute and chronic effects on several organs, including the gastrointestinal, dermatological, immunological, hematological, cardiovascular, PNS, and CNS. In addition, the 1996 12th edition of *The Merck Index* states phenytoin may reasonably be anticipated to be a carcinogen.

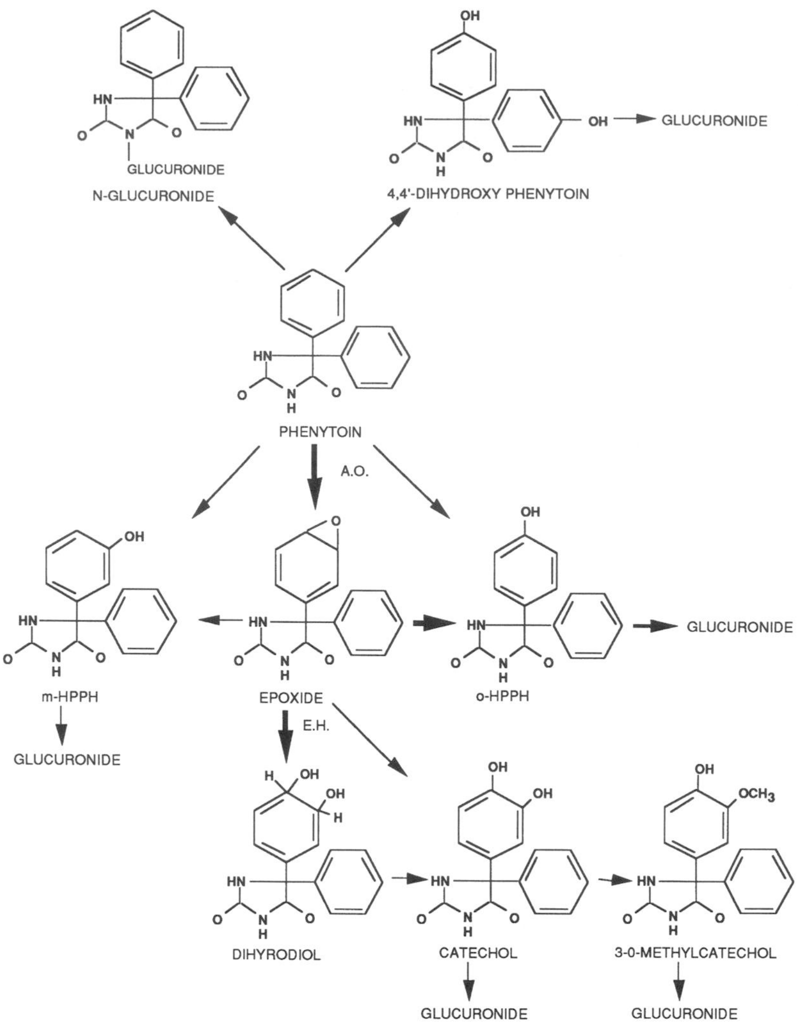

FIGURE 28. Metabolism of phenytoin. Hepatic elimination of phenytoin occurs primarily by oxidation to the inactive metabolite 5-(*p*-hydroxy-phenyl)-5-phenylhydantoin (*p*-HPPH). *p*-HPPH is further metabolized by conjugation with glucuronic acid.

Animal Studies

Neurotoxic effects have been produced in mice, rats, rabbits, pigs, and turkeys. Acute neurotoxicity, as defined by the rotorod procedure (32), was more evident in mice and rats receiving phenytoin than with valproic acid (16,18,101), phenobarbital (18), ethosuximide (18,101), and felbamate (101). Neurological deficits were demonstrated by the inability of the mouse to maintain its equilibrium for 1 min on a rotating rod and in the rat by overt evidence of ataxia, loss of pacing response and muscle tone. Ataxia was produced in rats following a 0.52–1.70 mg/min intravenous phenytoin infusion (85). A correlation between neurotoxic effects and plasma concentrations has been established (62). Phenytoin consistently displayed a higher protective index or safety ratio (median neurotoxic dose/

median dose required to elicit an effect) than most other anticonvulsants. The reversibility of these effects was not evaluated. Phenytoin (50 mg/kg/day) given for 1 week decreased cerebral metabolism in rats (67). Prolonged administration of phenytoin in rats, turkeys, and pigs has not clearly demonstrated its role in cerebellar degeneration (20,73,94); this may have been due to an inadequate study design. Prolonged treatment with high-dose phenytoin (72–88 mg/kg) significantly reduced brain weight, particularly within the cerebral cortex and cerebellum (80). The drug has an oral LD_{50} in mice of 230 mg/kg (18,101).

Experiments with phenytoin in animals have also shown PNS effects (50,61,67). Significant reductions in nerve conduction velocity and muscle action potential were detected in rats within 1 h of phenytoin (250 mg/kg) administration (61). Following 3–4 days of phenytoin administration, guinea pigs exhibited an average 13% decrease in conduction velocity. Phenytoin serum concentrations were found to be >200 μM (50 μg/ml). Effects were reversible upon drug discontinuation (67).

The effect of phenytoin on developing animals has been extensively evaluated. Studies have suggested the drug may decrease protein synthesis in neurons and inhibit neuronal growth. Prolonged exposure of phenytoin (200 mg/kg) administered prenatally in rats during embryonic days 7 through 18 resulted in numerous neuroteratogenic effects that persisted well into adulthood. Phenytoin exhibited fewer effects when given during embryonic days 11 through 14 (109).

In Vitro Studies

In embryonic chick dorsal root ganglia, phenytoin decreased the production of substrate-attached neurite-promoting activity and inhibited process formation in a concentration-dependent manner (31). Long-term exposure of neonatal mouse cerebellar tissue cultures to 36–184 μM (9–46 μg/ml) phenytoin produced cerebellar degeneration, especially of Purkinje cells (12). This effect was not exhibited in mature cerebellar tissue.

Human Studies

The CNS, PNS and tissue of neuroectodermal origin are all potential targets of phenytoin-related neurotoxic effects (86).

Phenytoin can have both acute and chronic dose-dependent effects on the cerebellum and vestibular system. A reversible vestibulo-ocular cerebellar syndrome has been described with acute phenytoin intoxication (86). It is clinically characterized by nystagmus, ataxia, and altered mental status. Nystagmus is the most reliable indicator of acute toxicity (48). A study of 32 phenytoin-treated patients demonstrated a step-wise relationship between phenytoin blood levels and specific signs of toxicity. Nystagmus developed at serum concentrations nearing 80 μM (20 μg/ml); ataxia at levels approaching 120 μM (30 μg/ml); and mental changes at levels >160 μM (40 μg/ml) (48). The severity and specific clinical manifestations of toxicity vary widely among patients with equivalent phenytoin serum levels (47,48,83,86). Diagnosis is based on a history of phenytoin use and determination of serum phenytoin concentrations. In patients with diseases such as uremia or hypoalbuminemia, which impair serum-protein binding of phenytoin, free phenytoin levels are a more accurate indicator of pharmacologically active drug (91). Drug–drug interactions or disease states that elevate phenytoin blood levels may predispose patients to acute intoxication. Such individuals should have their clinical status and serum drug levels monitored carefully (47,81,86).

Abnormalities of eye movement, associated with acute phenytoin intoxication, are varied and may, in part, mimic those resulting from structural brain lesions. Nystagmus is frequently rotational or lateral. Gaze-evoked nystagmus occurs closer to the primary position of gaze with increasing phenytoin serum concentrations (48). Down-beat nystagmus, commonly associated with posterior fossa lesions near the cervicomedullary junction, has been reported with phenytoin intoxication (111). A case of opsoclonus in conjunction with ataxia and dysarthria was reported in a 44-year-old woman loaded with phenytoin and diazepam after a generalized tonic-clonic seizure (24). Case reports have described total external ophthalmoplegia with impairment or complete loss of oculocephalic and cold-caloric test responses in patients with severely depressed levels of consciousness, resulting from oral or intravenous loading of phenytoin to supratherapeutic blood levels, usually >120 μM (30 μg/ml). In contrast to patients with structural brainstem lesions, these individuals maintained pupillary function (78,91,96). All of the described dose-related eye movement abnormalities resolved as phenytoin blood levels dropped to the therapeutic range of 40–80 μM (10–20 μg/ml) (24,78,91,96,111).

Phenytoin use can produce lasting adverse effects on the cerebellum. Irreversible cerebellar atrophy with permanent residual ataxia is most often a long-term, dose-related complication of phenytoin use. Most instances have occurred in patients on long-term phenytoin therapy with chronically elevated phenytoin blood levels. Cerebellar atrophy can occur in all age groups (87). The degree of clinical disability, from ataxia and dysmetria, is loosely correlated with the extent of cerebellar atrophy documented by computed tomography (CT) (10,114). Neuroradiological findings have included enlargement of the fourth ventricle and a decrease in the volume of the cerebellar vermis (10,41). Clinical signs may commence years after the initiation of phenytoin treatment. At the onset of clinical symptoms, reported blood levels have ranged from high therapeutic, 80 μM (20 μg/ml), to toxic, >160 μM (40 μg/ml) (10,41,65,114). Irreversible cerebellar damage has been reported with acute phenytoin intoxication. This is illustrated by the case of a neurologically intact 21-year-old man who developed severe cerebellar atrophy on brain CT and permanent signs of clinical cerebellar dysfunction after ingesting 7 g of phenytoin in a suicide attempt (64). The use of multiple antiepileptic medications and pre-existing brain damage may also predispose patients to this complication (10,41,86).

Unclear is the degree to which cerebellar atrophy is a result of the direct effect of phenytoin or of repeated hypoxia secondary to frequent tonic-clonic seizures (10,21,41,64,65,72,86,114). One study suggests that cerebellar changes in phenytoin-treated patients are primarily the result of the effects of hypoxia. The author reviewed postmortem results of 32 patients with idiopathic *grand mal* epilepsy and found that reduced cerebellar Purkinje cell density correlated better with seizure frequency than with phenytoin dosage (21). It is unclear how these results relate to more recent studies that employ clinical and neuroradiological data to sort out the importance of drug *vs.* seizure effect. A study of 41 chronically institutionalized adults with epilepsy found no association between cerebellar atrophy on brain CT scan and seizure frequency or status epilepticus; there was an association between cerebellar atrophy and peak phenytoin blood levels (114). The role of primarily long-term phenytoin therapy in development of cerebellar atrophy is supported by studies reporting radiologically confirmed cerebellar atrophy in epilepsy patients receiving phenytoin with seizure types and/or frequencies not likely to cause hypoxia (65,72). While it is well established that hypoxia secondary to frequent generalized motor seizures does have an adverse effect on cerebellar function (21,86), the more recent literature strongly suggests that chronic phenytoin therapy is an independent risk factor for the development of cerebellar atrophy (10,65,72,86).

Seizure exacerbation is a possible side effect of any antiepileptic medication. It can be dose-related (51,79,86,97,107) or result from using an inappropriate drug for a given seizure type or epilepsy syndrome (82). One retrospective chart review of patients admitted to the hospital for phenytoin intoxication reported a 10% incidence of phenytoin-activated seizures. In this study, a phenytoin blood level >120 μM (30 μg/ml) correlated with increased risk of seizure exacerbation (97), although higher levels are more commonly cited in the literature (79,107). Atypical neurological findings are sometimes associated with dose-related seizure exacerbation. In one series, two of three patients with phenytoin intoxication and increased seizure frequency developed reversible hemianesthesias and hemipareses (5). A change in the clinical character of the seizures sometimes serves as a clue to the diagnosis. The interictal electroencephalogram (EEG) commonly contains profound background slowing and high-voltage discharges (51).

Seizure exacerbation may also result from prescribing an incorrect antiepileptic medication for a specific seizure type or epileptic syndrome. Not all anticonvulsants are effective against all seizure types. For example, while it is one of the drugs of choice for generalized tonic-clonic seizures, phenytoin, as well as carbamazepine, may aggravate absence seizures. Excessive polytherapy may also have the same effect (82).

An asymptomatic peripheral neuropathy can occur with long-term phenytoin use. Knee and ankle jerks are absent or diminished. Careful examination occasionally will disclose an asymptomatic mild stocking-distribution sensory loss. Distal motor and sensory conduction velocities of the lower leg are minimally reduced, and sensory action potentials may be absent (86). The reported incidence of clinical and electrophysiological signs of neuropathy varies considerably, ranging from 0%–33% and 0%–89%, respectively (93).

A number of variables has been suggested as possible risk factors for phenytoin-related peripheral neuropathy. Phenytoin blood levels >80 μM (20 μg/ml), duration of treatment >10 years, and low serum folate levels have all been implicated (17,33,56,93) or dismissed (100,102) as potential risk factors. There are several explanations for the variability in the reported incidence of neuropathy. Experimental study design and the patient populations examined have differed from study to study. In some studies, patients received multiple antiepileptic medications. Not all studies have distinguished possible acute from chronic effects of phenytoin on nerve physiology. Three findings emerged in a prospective study of 51 adult patients with epilepsy treated 1–5 years with phenytoin, carbamazepine, or barbiturates. First, acute exposure to phenytoin levels >80 μM (20 μg/ml) resulted in a reversible slowing of sensory nerve conduction velocities. Second, of the 32 patients on phenytoin monotherapy with therapeutic drug blood levels at the time of electrophysiological examination, 18% had mild electrophysiological abnormalities. When compared with patients on phenytoin with normal electrophysiology studies, the abnormal group had a greater past history of exposure to high phenytoin blood levels and/or low folate levels. Lastly, of the 19 patients on carbamazepine monotherapy and the six on barbiturate monotherapy, the former group displayed no clinical or electrophysiological evidence of neuropathy, whereas the latter did. This study supports the notion that phenytoin may have both acute and chronic PNS effects (93).

Although uncommon, reversible movement disorders can occur with phenytoin therapy. Choreoathetosis, orofacial dyskinesias, dystonias, ballismus, and asterixis have been described in all age groups (3,15,46,58,86). In some reports, the clinical picture is very similar to that of neuroleptic-induced tardive dyskinesia (15). The onset is usually sudden, occurring soon after the initiation of phenytoin treatment or an increase in drug dosage. Most cases are associated with phenytoin intoxication [*i.e.*, blood levels

≥80 μM (20 μg/ml) (3,15,46,58)], although choreoathetosis has been reported in a patient with therapeutic phenytoin levels (113). Polypharmacy and pre-existing brain damage have been proposed as risk factors for this neurotoxic effect (3,58,86).

Phenytoin can have adverse effects on mental status and cognition. Phenytoin-induced acute encephalopathy is variably characterized by personality changes, psychosis, delirium, obtundation, and even coma (86). Phenytoin blood levels commonly exceed 160 μM (40 μg/ml) but can register in the therapeutic range (5,55,108). The encephalopathy is commonly associated with other signs of phenytoin neurotoxicity, although there is a great deal of variation among patients. Peripheral neuropathy can occur with the encephalopathy (90,108). Unusual neurological features such as dyskinesias have been reported (108). Mental deterioration usually has an acute or subacute onset in cases where long-term toxic dosing has gone unrecognized; it may also be delayed, occurring years after the initiation of phenytoin therapy in the absence of a dose change. The EEG shows some degree of slowing, and cerebrospinal fluid protein is sometimes mildly elevated (86,90). Pre-existing brain damage and polypharmacy predispose to this complication (86,108).

Long-term phenytoin intoxication can produce a nonspecific constellation of neurological abnormalities that suggests diagnosis of a structural brain lesion or neurodegenerative disease (55,86,108). One author described progressive neurological deterioration in four children on phenytoin thought to be due to degenerative disease. Each of these patients had a phenytoin level ≥160 μM (40 μg/ml), and each patient's neurological status improved with a decrease in or discontinuation of phenytoin therapy (55). The reversibility of various neurological deficits may relate to the duration of exposure to toxic phenytoin levels (86). Therefore, phenytoin toxicity should be the first diagnosis investigated in any epilepsy patient with newly appearing neurological symptoms potentially ascribable to the drug.

Phenytoin toxicity can manifest itself as a chronic encephalopathy with deficits in cognition. Changes in memory, concentration, mental speed, and motor speed are also described (4,14,19,26–29,36,57,66,86,95,103–106). Cognitive decline is a dose-dependent phenomenon that has been reported in all age groups. Studies of healthy adult volunteers and epilepsy patients indicate that the severity of cognitive deficits increases with increasing phenytoin blood levels (66,103–106). Polypharmacy is a risk factor for this effect (14,36,66,106), while patient age and duration of therapy are not (19,26,66).

There is a vast literature on the effects of antiepileptic drugs on cognition (4,14,19,26–29,36,57,63,66,95,103–106). When compared with valproic acid and carbamazepine, phenytoin produces neither a unique set of cognitive deficits nor a greater degree of cognitive deficit (26,66). Initial results of a double-blind cross-over study comparing cognitive decline in adults on carbamazepine or phenytoin monotherapy suggested that phenytoin use resulted in greater impairment of memory, visuomotor processing, and attention (27). However, these differential effects disappeared when the data were controlled for antiepileptic blood levels (28). The U.S. Veterans Administration Cooperative Study examined more than 400 patients with new-onset epilepsy and started on monotherapy (carbamazepine, phenytoin, phenobarbital, primidone); at therapeutic levels, cognitive abilities of study patients deteriorated minimally and there were no statistically significant interdrug differences (95). One study examined the intellectual abilities of children with new-onset epilepsy before and 1 year after drug initiation (phenytoin, carbamazepine, or valproate); at therapeutic levels, carbamazepine had some negative effect on memory while valproic acid and phenytoin did not (30). It is widely held that using antiepileptic medication at the lowest possible effective dosage as monotherapy may minimize the risk of cognitive side effects (14,26,57,66,95,103,104).

Any antiepileptic drug taken during the first trimester of pregnancy is a potential teratogen (22,53,86). A constellation of clinical findings dubbed "the fetal hydantoin syndrome" was first described in 1975 (39). The syndrome is characterized by craniofacial defects and the presence of at least two other abnormalities, including prenatal or postnatal growth retardation, limb defects, major malformations, and intellectual impairment (22,38,39,52,86). In one retrospective study, 11% of infants exposed to phenytoin in utero displayed the full-blown syndrome while 33% expressed only limited features of the syndrome (38). However, a more recent prospective study suggests the actual numbers are much lower (22).

Minor and major malformations identified in offspring exposed to antiepileptic medications display variable drug specificity (22,37,53). Craniofacial defects, prenatal and postnatal growth retardation, and developmental delay have been reported in association with phenytoin, barbiturates, carbamazepine, and valproate (22,53). Other defects appear to be more drug specific. Distal digital hypoplasia most commonly, although not exclusively, occurs with phenytoin exposure (37). Major congenital-like heart defects and facial clefts are most frequently described in children exposed to phenytoin or barbiturates. Urogenital defects, especially hypospadia and neural tube defects (primarily spina bifida aperta) occur with valproate and to a lesser extent, carbamazepine exposure (22,53). The risk of spina bifida aperta is about 1%–2% with valproate exposure (77) and 0.5%–1% with carbamazepine (89). Reports of bilateral radial aplasia are specific to valproate (53).

The risk of birth defects in children of mothers with epilepsy is influenced by many factors. The presence of maternal epilepsy, irrespective of antiepileptic drug use, is a risk factor for birth defects. The incidence of birth defects in infants of mothers with epilepsy is two to three times that of infants of mothers without epilepsy (22,53,86). In a prospective study of 121 children born to women with epilepsy, the presence of most infant malformations was correlated with the presence of maternal epilepsy, not exposure to antiepileptic drugs (37). This does not negate the additional teratogenic risk imparted by antiepileptic drug exposure. Several studies have reported an increased incidence of malformations among infants of women with epilepsy exposed to antiepileptic medications when compared to unexposed women with epilepsy. These studies found that the incidence of malformations in the offspring increased with maternal exposure to increasing numbers of antiepileptic medications (52,53,71). The risk of birth defects is also slightly elevated when the mother has active epilepsy during the pregnancy (7,52,71).

Phenytoin's teratogenic potential, as well as other neurotoxic actions of the drug, have been suggested to be linked to an effect on folate metabolism (22,40,86,88). Long-term phenytoin use, like barbiturates, can result in a dose-dependent lowering of serum and red blood cell folate levels (87). Subnormal levels have been reported in 27%–91% of patients on chronic phenytoin therapy (86). It may be of clinical importance in pregnancy because maternal folate deficiency, especially in the early stages of gestation, is associated with adverse pregnancy outcomes (22,53). Folate deficiency has been implicated in neural tube defects (87,88). Yet, there are no reports of neural tube defects in pregnant women on phenytoin monotherapy (88).

Severe deficiency of folate can produce a megaloblastic anemia; some have suggested that a folate deficiency can cause peripheral neuropathy and, in rare cases, subacute combined degeneration (40,86). This controversial notion is somewhat supported by a case report of a patient taking phenytoin (40). Most patients with phenytoin-induced folate deficiency develop only mild reductions in folate levels and a clinically inapparent macrocytosis. Less than 1% of patients develop megaloblastic anemia (86). Peripheral neuropathy is a potential neurotoxic complication of phenytoin independent of folate status (33,56,102). In most cases, there is not a clear causal relationship between neuropathy and folate levels (17,56,86,88,102). Folate deficiency has been implicated in psychiatric disturbances [i.e., depression, psychosis, and dementia (86–88)]. In a review of the literature (86,87), it was emphasized that the etiology of psychological disorders in epilepsy patients is most likely multifactorial and not clearly the result of folate deficiency (87).

Other tissues of neuroectodermal origin are potential targets of phenytoin-related neurotoxicity. Chronic phenytoin therapy is associated with thickening of fibrous subcutaneous tissues. Gingival hyperplasia is the most common of all phenytoin-related side effects; it has been reported in 50% or more of treated patients (6,30,86). It becomes clinically apparent after 2–3 months of phenytoin use and usually regresses, although not necessarily completely, within several months of drug discontinuation (54,86). Children are more often affected than adults (9). The risk of developing gingival hyperplasia has been positively correlated with increasing phenytoin dosage and blood levels (2,54), and poor oral hygiene (6,30).

Long-term chronic phenytoin therapy can also cause the insidious development of craniofacial dysmorphisms, commonly referred to as coarsened facies (86). The changes in facial features have been most frequently described in mentally retarded children who developed epilepsy early in life. They are characterized by enlargement of the lips, broadened nose, and generalized thickening of subcutaneous tissues of the face and scalp (42,49,86). Associated features may include gum hypertrophy, elevated serum alkaline phosphatase blood levels, and calvarial thickening (49,86). Predisposing factors have not been clearly defined (42).

Treatment

The mainstay of treatment for the majority of phenytoin-related neurotoxic effects is a reduction in or discontinuation of phenytoin therapy. The acute vestibulo-ocular-cerebellar syndrome usually resolves fully; so do movement disorders, although they may take weeks to months to remit (58,86). Seizure exacerbation usually remits with a decrease in dosage (51,79,97,107) or a change in medication (82). Not all neurotoxic side effects are reversible. The clinical cerebellar dysfunction associated with long-term, high-dose phenytoin use often improves when phenytoin dosing is reduced or stopped, but residual disability is common. The same can be true of dose-related encephalopathy and peripheral neuropathy (86).

Thickened fibrous connective tissue also recedes with dose reduction or cessation, but may not revert to the normal predrug state (30,42,86). Gingival hyperplasia is treated with good oral hygiene, frequent dental visits and, in severe cases, surgical excision of overgrown gum tissue (30,86). Many patients and families find coarsened facies to be a cosmetically unacceptable side effect. Therefore, the use of phenytoin therapy in patients most likely to experience distress over its possible negative effects on appearance —namely, children and young women, should be carefully considered when an alternative drug treatment is medically equally acceptable.

For epileptic women of childbearing years, preconceptional counseling and close obstetrical follow-up are essential. Patients should be informed of the teratogenic risks posed by both the diagnosis of epilepsy and the anticonvulsant medication(s) they are taking before becoming pregnant. The antiepileptic medications(s) prescribed should be the first-line drug(s) for the patient's seizure type, used as monotherapy, if possible, and administered in the lowest effective dose. Folate supplementation should be initiated prior to conception and continued during the pregnancy. Lastly, the pregnant woman with epilepsy should be offered prenatal diagnosis of birth defect (25).

Toxic Mechanisms

The mechanisms of phenytoin neurotoxicity are unclear. In animal studies, phenytoin has been shown to cause both histological and electrophysiological changes in both the developing and adult cerebellum (12,45,60,76,84). Tissue culture preparations of neonatal mouse cerebellum demonstrated concentration-dependent degeneration of Purkinje cells (12). When compared to controls, mice given 10 mg/kg/day of oral phenytoin on postnatal days 2–14 displayed pyknotic cells in the external granule cell layer, a widening of that cerebellar layer indicating a delay in development and a reduction of cerebellar weight and size in association with abnormal behavioral and motor development (76). In mature mice, high-dose phenytoin produced Purkinje cell axonal swelling in the deep cerebellar nuclei (45). In rats, single toxic (84) and long-term nontoxic (60) administration of phenytoin caused a decrease in the firing rate of cerebellar Purkinje cells.

Experimental studies using a variety of animal models indicate that phenytoin has the capacity to interfere with embryonic development. Facial clefting, hydronephrosis, and skeletal abnormalities have been described (1). Proposed mechanisms of phenytoin-related teratogenicity include a disturbance in folate metabolism (1,23), and the production of a toxic metabolite (an epoxide) of phenytoin able to bind to embryonic nucleic acids[1] (see Fig. 28) (1,34). Low or inadequate levels of epoxide hydroxylase, the en-

---

[1]Oxidation of DNA may be particularly critical, since transgenic mice with +/− or −/− deficiencies in the p53 tumor suppressor gene, which facilitates DNA repair, are more susceptible to phenytoin (110). The apparent importance of antioxidative balance is suggested by the observation that superoxide dismutase promotes while catalase inhibits phenytoin teratogenicity (112) [Note added by the editors].

zyme that detoxifies the oxidative metabolite, may further increase the risk of birth defects (1,34,69). In mice, decreasing fetal exposure to oxidative metabolites with the enzyme inhibitor stiripentol decreased the number of phenytoin-related birth defects (34). In one human study, greater than 30% reduction in amniocyte epoxide hydroxylase activity was predictive of fetal hydantoin syndrome (35,69). Prenatal exposure to phenytoin in fetal mice produced downregulation in the levels of a number of growth and transcription genes, which may relate to teratogenicity (35,98).

Proposed mechanisms for phenytoin-related gum hypertrophy are also numerous; they include gingival changes resulting from direct stimulation of gingival fibroblasts by phenytoin, folate depletion, and alterations in immunological and endocrinological factors (86,99).

REFERENCES

1. Adams J, Vorhees CV, Middaugh LD (1990) Developmental neurotoxicity of anticonvulsants: Humans and animal evidence on phenytoin. *Neurotoxicol Teratol* 12, 203.
2. Addy V, McElnay JC, Campbell N *et al.* (1982) Risk factors in phenytoin-induced gingival hyperplasia. *J Peridontol* 54, 373.
3. Ahmad S, Laidlaw J, Houghton GW, Richens A (1975) Involuntary movements caused by phenytoin intoxication in epileptic patients. *J Neurol Neurosurg Psychiat* 38, 225.
4. Aldenkamp AP, Alpherta MA, Blennow G *et al.* (1993) Withdrawal of antiepileptic medication in children—effects on cognitive function: The multicenter Holmfrid study. *Neurology* 43, 41.
5. Ambrosetto G, Tassinari CA, Baruzzi A, Lugaresi E (1977) Phenytoin encephalopathy as probable idiosyncratic reaction: Case report. *Epilepsia* 18, 405.
6. Angelopoulos AP, Goaz PW (1972) Incidence of diphenylhydantoin gingival hyperplasia. *Oral Surg* 34, 898.
7. Annegers JF, Hauser WA, Elveback LR (1978) Congenital malformations and seizure disorders among offspring of parents with epilepsy. *Int J Epidemiol* 7, 241.
8. Anon (1994) Phenytoin. In: *American Hospital Formulary Service: Drug Information.* McEvoy GK ed. American Society of Hospital Pharmacists, Bethesda, Maryland p. 1359.
9. Babcock JR (1965) Incidence of gingival hyperplasia associated with dilantin therapy in a hospital population. *J Amer Dent Assn* 71, 1447.
10. Baier WK, Kilnge H, Hirsch W (1984) Cerebellar atrophy following diphenylhydantoin intoxication. *Neuropediatrics* 15, 76.
11. Bigger JT, Strauss HC (1972) Digitalis toxicity: Drug interactions promoting toxicity and the management of toxicity. *Semin Drug Treatment* 2, 147.

12. Blank NK, Nishimura RN, Seil FJ (1982) Phenytoin neurotoxicity in developing mouse cerebellum in tissue culture. *J Neurol Sci* 55, 91.

13. Browne TR, Chang T (1989) Phenytoin: Biotransformation. In: *Antiepileptic Drugs. 3rd Ed.* Levey R, Mattson R, Meldrum R *et al.* eds. Raven Press, New York p. 197.

14. Bulmahn A, Wohluter M, Rambeck (1992) Effect of withdrawal of phenytoin of phenytoin on cognitive and psychomotor function in hospitalized epileptic patients in polytherapy. *Acta Neurol Scand* 71, 448.

15. Chadwick D, Reynolds EH, Marsden CD (1976) Anticonvulsant-induced dyskinesias: A comparison with dyskinesias induced by neuroleptics. *J Neurol Neurosurg Psychiat* 39, 1210.

16. Chez MG, Bourgeois BFD, Pippenger CE, Knowles WD (1994) Pharmacodynamic interactions between phenytoin and valproate: Individual and combined antiepileptic and neurotoxic actions in mice. *Clin Neuropharmacol* 17, 32.

17. Chokroverty S, Sayeed ZA (1975) Motor nerve conduction study in patients on diphenylhydantoin therapy. *J Neurol Neurosurg Psychiat* 38, 1235.

18. Clark CR (1988) Comparative anticonvulsant activity and neurotoxicity of 4-amino-N-(2,6-dimethylphenyl)-benzamide and prototype antiepileptic drugs in mice and rats. *Epilepsia* 29, 198.

19. Craig I, Tallis R (1994) Impact of valproate and phenytoin on cognitive function in elderly patients: Results of a single-blind randomized comparative study. *Epilepsia* 35, 381.

20. Dam M (1966) Organic changes in phenytoin-intoxicated pigs. *Acta Neurol Scand* 42, 491.

21. Dam M (1970) Number of Purkinje cells in patients with grand mal epilepsy treated with diphenylhydantoin. *Epilepsia* 11, 313.

22. Dansky LV, Finnel RH (1991) Paternal epilepsy, anticonvulsant drugs, and reproductive outcome: Epidemiologic and experimental findings spanning three decades: 2, human studies. *Reprod Toxicol* 5, 301.

23. Dansky LV, Rosenblatt DS, Anderman E (1992) Mechanisms of teratogenesis: Folic acid and antiepileptic therapy. *Neurology* 42, 32.

24. Dehaene MD, Van Vleymen B (1987) Opsoclonus induced by phenytoin and diazepam. *Ann Neurol* 21, 216.

25. Delgado-Escueta AV, Janz D (1992) Consensus guidelines: Preconception counseling, management and care of pregnant women with epilepsy. *Neurology* 42, 149.

26. Dodrill CB (1992) Problems in the assessment of cognitive effects of antiepileptic drugs. *Epilepsia* 33, S29.

27. Dodrill CB, Troupin AS (1977) Psychotropic effects of carbamazepine in epilepsy: A double-blind comparison with phenytoin. *Neurology* 26, 1023.

28. Dodrill CB, Troupin AS (1991) Neuropsychological effects of carbamazepine and phenytoin, a reanalysis. *Neurology* 41, 141.

29. Dodrill CB, Wilensky AJ (1992) Neuropsychological abilities before and after 5 years of stable antiepileptic drug therapy. *Epilepsia* 33, 327.

30. Dongari A, McDonnell HT, Langlais RP (1993) Drug-induced gingival overgrowth. *Oral Surg Oral Med Oral Path* 76, 543.

31. Dow KE, Riopelle RJ (1988) Differential effects of anticonvulsants on developing neurons in vitro. *Neurotoxicology* 9, 97.

32. Dunham NW, Miya TS (1957) A note on a single apparatus for detecting neurological deficit in rats and mice. *J Amer Pharm Assn* 46, 208.

33. Eisen AA, Woods JF, Sherwin AL (1974) Peripheral nerve function in long-term therapy with diphenylhydantoin. *Neurology* 24, 411.

34. Finnell RH, Dansky LV (1991) Parental epilepsy, anticonvulsant drugs, and reproductive outcome: Epidemiological and experimental findings spanning three decades. 1 Animal studies. *Reprod Toxicol* 5, 281.

35. Finnell RH, Nau H, Yerby MS (1995) General principles: Teratogenicity of antiepileptic drugs. In: *Antiepileptic Drugs.* Levy R, Mattson R, Medlum B *et al.* eds. Raven Press, New York p. 209.

36. Forsythe I, Butler R, Berg I, McGuire (1991) Cognitive impairment in new cases of epilepsy randomly assigned to carbamazepine, phenytoin and sodium valproate. *Develop Med Child Neurol* 33, 524.

37. Gaily E, Granstrom ML, Hiilesmaa V, Bardy A (1988) Minor anomalies in offspring of epileptic mothers. *J Pediat* 112, 520.

38. Hanson JW, Myriantholpoulos NC, Harvey MAS, Smith DW (1976) Risks to the offspring of women treated with hydantoin anticonvulsants, with emphasis on the fetal hydantoin syndrome. *J Pediat* 89, 662.

39. Hanson JW, Smith DW (1975) The fetal hydantoin syndrome. *J Pediat* 87, 285.

40. Hawkins CF, Meynell MJ (1958) Macrocytosis and macrocytic anemia caused by anticonvulsant drugs. *Quart J Med* 27, 45.

41. Iivanainen M, Viukari M, Helle EP (1977) Cerebellar atrophy in phenytoin-treated mentally retarded epileptics. *Epilepsia* 18, 375.

42. Johnson JP (1984) Acquired craniofacial features associated with chronic phenytoin therapy. *Clin Pediat* 23, 671.

43. Jung D, Powell JR, Watson P, Perrier D (1980) Effect of dose on phenytoin absorption. *Clin Pharmacol Ther* 28, 479.

44. Kemp JW, Woodbury DM (1971) Subcellular distribution of 4-^{14}C-diphenylhydantoin in rat brain. *J Pharmacol Exp Ther* 177, 342.

45. Kiefer R, Knoth R, Anagnostopoulos J, Volk B (1989) Cerebellar injury due to phenytoin. Identification and evolution of Purkinje cell axonal swellings in deep cerebellar nuclei of mice. *Acta Neuropathol* 77, 289.

46. Kooiker JC, Sumi SM (1974) Movement disorder as a manifestation of diphenylhydantoin intoxication. *Neurology* 24, 68.

47. Kutt H (1990) Hydantoins. In: *Comprehensive Epileptology*. Dam M, Grun L eds. Raven Press, New York p. 563.

48. Kutt H, Winters W, Kokenge R, McDowell F (1964) Diphenylhydantoin metabolism, blood level and toxicity. *Arch Neurol* 11, 642.

49. Lefebvre EB, Haining RG, Labbe RF (1972) Coarse facies, calavarial thickening and hypophosphatasia associated with long-term anticonvulsant therapy. *N Engl J Med* 286, 1301.

50. Le Quesne PM, Goldberg V, Vajda F (1976) Acute conduction velocity changes in guinea-pigs after administration of diphenylhydantoin. *J Neurol Neurosurg Psychiat* 39, 995.

51. Levy LL, Fenichel GM (1965) Diphenylhydantoin activated seizures. *Neurology* 15, 716.

52. Lindhout D, Hoppener RJEA, Meinardi H (1984) Teratogenicity of antiepileptic drug combinations with special emphasis on epoxidation (of carbamazepine). *Epilepsia* 25, 77.

53. Lindhout D, Omtzigt JGC (1992) Pregnancy and the risk of teratogenicity. *Epilepsia* 33, S41.

54. Little MT, Giris SS, Masotta RE (1975) Diphenylhydantoin-induced gingival hyperplasia: Its response to changes in drug dosage. *Develop Med Child Neurol* 17, 421.

55. Logan WJ, Freeman JM (1969) Pseudodegenerative disease due to diphenylhydantoin intoxication. *Arch Neurol* 21, 631.

56. Lovelace RE, Horowitz SJ (1968) Peripheral neuropathy in long-term diphenylhydantoin therapy. *Arch Neurol* 18, 69.

57. Ludgate J, Keating J, O'Dwyer R, Callaghan N (1985) An improvement in cognitive function following polypharmacy reduction in a group of epileptic patients. *Acta Neurol Scand* 71, 448.

58. Luhdorf K, Lund (1977) Phenytoin-induced hyperkinesia. *Epilepsia* 18, 409.

59. Macdonald RL, Kelly KM (1994) Mechanisms of action of currently prescribed and newly developed antiepileptic drugs. *Epilepsia* 35, S41.

60. Mameli O, Tolu E, Melis F et al. (1984) Correlations between cerebellar activity and chronic nontoxic administration of phenytoin in rats. *Epilepsia* 25, 33.

61. Marcus DJ, Swift TR, McDonald TF (1981) Acute effects of phenytoin on peripheral nerve function in the rat. *Muscle Nerve* 4, 48.

62. Masuda Y, Utsui Y, Shiraishi Y et al. (1979) Relationship between plasma concentrations of diphenylhydantoin, phenobarbital, carbamazepine, and 3-sulfamoylmethyl-1-1,2-benzisoxazole (AD-810), a new anticonvulsant agent, and their anticonvulsant or neurotoxic effects in experimental animals. *Epilepsia* 20, 623.

63. Masur DM, Shinnar S (1992) The neuropsychology of childhood seizure disorders. In: *Handbook of Neuropsychology. Vol 7*. Segalowitz SJ, Rapin I eds. Elsevier, Amsterdam p. 457.

64. Masur H, Elger CE, Ludolph AC, Galanski M (1989) Cerebellar atrophy following intoxication with phenytoin. *Neurology* 39, 432.

65. McLain LW, Martin JT, Allen JH (1980) Cerebellar degeneration due to chronic phenytoin therapy. *Ann Neurol* 7, 18.

66. Meador KJ (1994) Cognitive side effects of antiepileptic drugs. *Can J Neurol Sci* 21, S12.

67. Melisi JW, Dow-Edwards DJ, Hammock MK, Milhorat TH (1988) Effects of chronic diphenylhydantoin on cerebral metabolism in the adult rat. *Exp Neurol* 99, 523.

68. Millichap JG (1978) Recurrent headaches in 100 children: Electroencephalographic abnormalities and response to phenytoin (Dilantin). *Child Brain* 4, 95.

69. Musselman AC, Bennett GD, Greer KA et al. (1994) Preliminary evidence of phenytoin-induced alterations in embryonic gene expression in a mouse model. *Reprod Toxicol* 8, 383.

70. Muthukumarasamy MG, Sivakurmar G, Manoharan G (1991) Topical phenytoin in diabetic foot ulcers. *Diabetes Care* 14, 909.

71. Nakane Y, Okuma T, Takahashi R et al. (1980) Multiinstitutional study on the teratogenicity and fetal toxicity of antiepileptic drugs: A report of a collaborative study group in Japan. *Epilepsia* 21, 663.

72. Ney G, Lantos G, Barr W, Schaul N (1994) Cerebellar atrophy in patients with long-term phenytoin exposure and epilepsy. *Arch Neurol* 51, 767.

73. Nielsen MH, Dam M, Klinken L (1971) The ultrastructure of Purkinje cells in diphenylhydantoin-intoxicated rats. *Exp Brain Res* 12, 447.

74. Noach EL, Woodbury DM, Goodman LS (1958) Studies on absorption, distribution, fate and excretion of 4-^{14}C labeled diphenylhydantoin. *J Pharmacol Exp Ther* 20, 36.

75. O'Doherty DS, O'Malley WE, Denckal MA (1969) Oral absorption of diphenylhydantoin as measured by gas liquid chromatography. *Trans Amer Neurol Assn* 94, 318.

76. Ohmori H, Kobayashi T, Yasuda M (1992) Neurotoxicity of phenytoin administered to newborn mice on developing cerebellum. *Neurotoxicol Teratol* 14, 159.

77. Omtzigt JGC, Los FJ, Grobbee DE et al. (1992) The risk of spina bifida aperta after first trimester valproate exposure in a prenatal cohort. *Neurology* 42, 119.

78. Orth DN, Henderson A, Walsh FB, Honda A (1967) Ophthalmoplegia resulting from diphenylhydantoin and primidone intoxication. *J Amer Med Assn* **201**, 485.

79. Osorio I, Burnstine TH, Remler B *et al.* (1989) Phenytoin-induced seizures: A paradoxical effect at toxic concentrations in epileptic patients. *Epilepsia* **30**, 230.

80. Palm R, Hallmans G, Wahlstrom G (1986) Effects of long-term phenytoin treatment on brain weight and zinc and copper metabolism in rats. *Neurochem Pathol* **5**, 87.

81. Phelps SJ, Baldree LA, Boucher BA, Hogue SL (1993) Neuropsychiatric toxicity of phenytoin. Importance of monitoring phenytoin levels. *Clin Pediatr* **32**, 107.

82. Pinchas L (1986) Seizures induced or aggravated by anticonvulsants. *Epilepsia* **27**, 706.

83. Plaa GL (1975) Acute toxicity of antiepileptic drugs. *Epilepsia* **16**, 183.

84. Puro DG, Woodward DJ (1973) Effects of diphenylhydantoin on activity of rat cerebellar Purkinje cells. *Neuropharmacology* **12**, 433.

85. Ramzam I (1990) Pharmacodynamics of phenytoin-induced ataxia in rats. *Epilepsy Res* **5**, 80.

86. Reynolds EH (1989) Phenytoin toxicity. In: *Antiepileptic Drugs*. Levy R, Mattson R, Medlum B *et al.* eds. Raven Press, New York p. 241.

87. Reynolds EH, Trimble MR (1985) Adverse neuropsychiatric effects of anticonvulsant drugs. *Drugs* **29**, 570.

88. Rivey MP, Schottelius DD, Berg MJ (1984) Phenytoin-folic acid: A review. *Drug Intell Clin Pharm* **18**, 292.

89. Rosa FW (1991) Spina bifida in infants of women treated with carbamazepine during pregnancy. *N Engl J Med* **324**, 674.

90. Roseman E (1961) Dilantin toxicity: A clinical and electroencephalographic study. *Neurology* **11**, 912.

91. Sansyk R (1984) Total external ophthalmoplegia induced by phenytoin. *S Afr Med J* **65**, 141.

92. Schwartz PA, Rhodes CT, Cooper JW (1977) Solubility and ionization characteristics of phenytoin. *J Pharm Sci* **66**, 994.

93. Shorvon SD, Reynolds EH (1982) Anticonvulsant peripheral neuropathy: A clinical and electrophysiological study of patients on single drug treatment with phenytoin, carbamazepine or barbiturates. *J Neurol Neurosurg Psychiat* **45**, 620.

94. Simpson CF, Taylor WJ (1985) Neurotoxic and antihypertensive effects of phenytoin in turkeys. *J Pharmacol Exp Ther* **233**, 853.

95. Smith DB, Mattson RH, Cramer JA *et al.* (1987) Results of a nationwide Veterans Administration Cooperative Study comparing the efficacy and toxicity of carbamazepine, phenobarbital, phenytoin and primidone. *Epilepsia* **28**, S50.

96. Spector RH, Davidoff RA, Schwartzman RJ (1976) Phenytoin-induced ophthalmoplegia. *Neurology* **26**, 1031.

97. Stilman N, Masdeu JC (1985) Incidence of seizures with phenytoin toxicity. *Neurology* **35**, 1769.

98. Strickler SM, Dansky LV, Miller MA *et al.* (1985) Genetic predisposition to phenytoin-induced birth defects. *Lancet* **2**, 746.

99. Swerdlow M, Cundill JG (1981) Anticonvulsant drugs used in the treatment of lancinating pain: A comparison. *Anaesthesia* **36**, 1129.

100. Swift TR, Gross JA, Ward CL, Crout BO (1981) Peripheral neuropathy in epileptic patients. *Neurology* **31**, 826.

101. Swinyard EA, Sofia RD, Kupferberg HJ (1986) Comparative anticonvulsant activity and neurotoxicity of felbamate and four prototype antiepileptic drugs in mice and rats. *Epilepsia* **27**, 27.

102. Taylor JW, Murphy MJ, Rivey MP (1985) Clinical and electrophysiological evaluation of peripheral nerve function in chronic phenytoin therapy. *Epilepsia* **26**, 416.

103. Thompson PJ, Huppert FA, Trimble MR (1981) Phenytoin and cognitive function: Effects on normal volunteers and the implications for epilepsy. *Brit J Clin Psychol* **20**, 150.

104. Thompson PJ, Trimble MR (1982) Anticonvulsant drugs and cognitive function: Relation to serum levels. *J Neurol Neurosurg Psychiat* **46**, 227.

105. Trimble MR, Corbett J, Donaldson D (1980) Folic acid and mental symptoms in children with epilepsy. *J Neurol Neurosurg Psychiat* **43**, 1030.

106. Trimble MR, Thompson PJ (1983) Anticonvulsant drugs, cognitive function and behavior. *Epilepsia* **24**, S55.

107. Troupin AS, Ojemann LM (1975) Paradoxical intoxication—a complication of anticonvulsant administration. *Epilepsia* **16**, 753.

108. Vallarta J, Bell D, Reichert A (1974) Progressive encephalopathy due to chronic hydantoin intoxication. *Amer J Dis Child* **128**, 27.

109. Vorhees CV, Rindler JM, Minck DR (1990) Effects of exposure period and nutrition on the developmental neurotoxicity of anticonvulsants in rats: Short and long-term effects. *Neurotoxicology* **11**, 273.

110. Wells PG, Kim PM, Laposa RR *et al.* (1997) Oxidative damage in chemical teratogenesis. *Mutat Res* **396**, 65.

111. Wheeler SD, Ramsay RE, Weiss J (1982) Drug-induced downbeat nystagmus. *Ann Neurol* **12**, 227.

112. Winn LM, Wells PG (1999) Maternal administration of superoxide dismutase and catalase in phenytoin teratogenicity. *Free Radic Biol Med* **26**, 266.

113. Yoshida M, Yamada S, Oaaki Y, Nakatishi T (1985) Phenytoin-induced orofacial dyskinesias. *J Neurol* **231**, 340.

114. Young GB, Oppenheimer SR, Gordon BA (1994) Ataxia in institutionalized patients with epilepsy. *Can J Neurol Sci* **21**, 252.

Philanthotoxin

Tom Piek

PHILANTHOTOXIN
$C_{23}H_{41}N_5O_3$

Dideaza-PTX-12: $C_{25}H_{43}N_3O_3$

NEUROTOXICITY RATING

Experimental

A   Glutamate antagonist

δ-Philanthotoxin (PTX-4.3.3.) is one of the neuroactive components of the venom of the solitary digger wasp *Philanthus triangulum* (beewolf), a predator of workers of the honey bee, *Apis mellifera*. The notation 4.3.3 refers to the number and succession of CH_2-groups present in the polyamine chain (13). The venom contains the neurotransmitters acetylcholine and glutamate in addition to philanthotoxins. If extracts of the venom are injected into honeybees, they are dose-dependently paralyzed and recover at a dose-dependent rate. The excitatory glutamatergic neuromuscular transmission of insects is antagonized by *P. triangulum* venom and its active toxin component, PTX-4.3.3 (5,10,11).

PTX-4.3.3 modifies the kinetics of open cation channels in the glutamate receptor–ionophore complex present in skeletal muscle fibers of insects (3,7,8,12). Structure–activity studies (2–4,7,8) show that the activity of these polyamines as modifiers of channel kinetics depends on the presence of the aromatic moiety and a certain length of the polyamine chain. Attempts to change the molecule into a more potent antagonist results in increased potency from 10–100 times (6,7). Substitution of two methyl groups for the two internal amino groups of the polyamine chain (dideaza-PTX-12) decreases the potency as a channel blocker in insect muscle by a factor of about 500 (6,7). In contrast, a comparable structure–activity study of the blocking action of philanthotoxin analogues on glutamatergic transmission in the rat hippocampus showed that dideaza-PTX-12 was more potent than all other analogues tested, including the native philanthotoxin (15). In the rat hippocampal slice preparation, philanthotoxins decrease the amplitude of the population spike, the field excitatory postsynaptic potential and the presynaptic volley, as evoked by Schaffer-collateral-commissural inputs to CA_1 pyramidal cells (15). PTX-4.3.3 (the native philanthotoxin) inhibits N-methyl-D-aspartate (NMDA)–induced currents in oocytes expressing these receptors (14). However, in single hippocampal neurons, philanthotoxin selectively blocks Ca^{2+}-permeable α-amino-3-hydroxy-5-methyl-4-isoxazole propionate (AMPA) receptors involved in synaptic transmission of mossy fibers (16). Block is agonist-dependent and is effected either by direct open-channel blockade (1) or by binding to another region of the channel (intrinsic gate) to form a blocking complex that occludes the pore (9).

Dideaza-PTX-12 is a potent antagonist of voltage-dependent Ca^{2+} currents in rat hippocampal CA_1 neurons (6); a concentration of 10 μM dideaza-PTX-12 reduces the Ca^{2+} currents to 40%. Two voltage-dependent potassium currents, the A current and the delayed rectifier, were barely affected by dideaza-PTX-12, indicating a selectivity of this polyamine toxin for Ca^{2+} currents.

REFERENCES

1. Bahring R, Mayer ML (1998) An analysis of philanthotoxin block for recombinant rat GluR6(Q) glutamate receptor channels. *J Physiol* **509**, 635.

2. Benson JA, Kaufmann L, Hue B *et al.* (1993) The physiological analogues of philanthotoxin-4.3.3 at insect nicotinic acetylcholine receptors. *Comp Biochem Physiol* **105**, 303.

3. Benson JA, Schürmann F, Kaufmann L *et al.* (1992) Inhibition of dipteran larval neuromuscular synaptic transmission by analogues of philanthotoxin-4.3.3, a structure-activity study. *Comp Biochem Physiol* **102**, 267.

4. Bruce M, Bukownik R, Eldefrawi AT *et al.* (1990) Structure-activity relationship of analogues of the wasp toxin philanthotoxin: Non-competitive antagonists of quisqualate receptors. *Toxicon* **28**, 1333.

5. Clark RB, Donaldson PL, Gration KA *et al.* (1982) Block of locust muscle glutamate receptors by δ-philanthotoxin occurs after receptor activations. *Brain Res* **241**, 105.

6. Karst H, Joëls M, Wadman W, Piek T (1994) Philanthotoxin inhibits Ca^{2+}-currents in rat hippocampal CA1 neurons. *Eur J Pharmacol* **270**, 357.

7. Karst H, Piek T (1991) Structure-activity relationship of philanthotoxins-II. Effects on the glutamate gated ion channels of the locust muscle fibre membrane. *Comp Biochem Physiol* **98**, 497.

8. Karst H, Piek T, van Marle J *et al.* (1991) Structure-activity relationship of philanthotoxins-I. Pre-and postsynaptic inhibition of the locust neuromuscular transmission. *Comp Biochem Physiol* **98**, 471.

9. Lee JK, John SA, Weiss JN (1999) Novel gating mecha-

nism of polyamine block in the strong inward rectifier K channel Kir2.1. *Gen Physiol* **113**, 555.

10. Nakanishi K, Goodman R, Konno K *et al.* (1990) Philanthotoxin-4.3.3, a non-competitive glutamate receptor inhibitor. *Pure Appl Chem* **62**, 1223.

11. Piek T (1966) Site of action of the venom of the digger wasp *Philanthus triangulum F.* on the fast neuromuscular system of the locust. *Toxicon* **4**, 191.

12. Piek T (1982) Delta-philanthotoxin, a semi-irreversible blocker of ion channels. *Comp Biochem Physiol* **72**, 311.

13. Piek T, Hue B (1989) Philanthotoxins, a new class of neuroactive polyamines, block nicotinic transmission in the insect CNS. *Comp Biochem Physiol* **93**, 403.

14. Ragsdale D, Gant DB, Anis NA *et al.* (1989) Inhibition of rat brain glutamate receptors by philanthotoxin. *J Pharmacol Exp Ther* **251**, 156.

15. Schluter NCM, Piek T, Lopes da Silva F (1992) Philanthotoxins block glutamatergic transmission in rat hippocampus-II. Inhibition of synaptic transmission in the CA₁ region. *Comp Biochem Physiol C* **101**, 41.

16. Toth K, McBain CJ (1998) Afferent-specific innervation of two distinct AMPA receptor subtypes on single hippocampal interneurons. *Nat Neurosci* **1**, 572.

Physalia Toxin

Michael K. Pugsley
Michael J.A. Walker

NEUROTOXICITY RATING

Clinical

B   Ion channel syndrome

Experimental

A   Ion channel dysfunction

Jellyfish are a common source of injury for humans. *Physalia physalis*, more commonly known as the Portuguese man-of-war or blue-bottle, is a coelenterate of the class Hydrozoa and the order Siphonophora (12). *Physalia* spp. are pelagic, colonial organisms composed of a large, gas-containing float or medusa (pneumatophore); located on the underside are polyps modified for processing of food (gastrozooids), reproduction (gonodentra), and prey-capture (dactylozooids) (12). The dactylozooids develop into tentacles; the Atlantic species of jellyfish has eight, the Indo-Pacific species only one. These tentacles, which may be up to 33 m in length (9) and contain batteries of nematocysts (12,16), serve both to capture food and protect the animal. Human contact with the nematocyst-bearing tentacles of many species of jellyfish results in stinging and subsequent injury. Such injury can vary from mild skin irritation to death following cardiovascular and respiratory collapse.

The Physallidae family, of which *P. physalis* was until recently thought to be the only member (10), is distributed across both the Atlantic (as *P. physalis*) and Indo-Pacific (as *P. utriculus*) oceans. Both types of *Physalia* are responsible for a large number of human stings each year along the beaches of both Australia and Florida, United States. Evenomation results in symptoms that range from mild or local stings to severe fatal reactions (3,6).

The toxin complex responsible for the stinging action of the nematocyst is thought to coat the surface of the nematocyst thread (14) which, when extended, penetrates the prey species or others. Stinging organelles, nematocysts, are unique to coelenterates; 17 types have been described. However, of the approximately 10,000 species of marine coelenterates only about 100 are considered to be harmful to man (1). *P. physalis* has only one structural type of nematocyst, classified as holotrichous isorhizus, although its size is bimodally distributed such that large ones are about 23.5 μm in length and the smaller ones about 10.6 μm (3,6,14). Contact of prey or skin with the nematocysts results in rapid contraction and release of the nematocyst thread at a force of approximately 2–5 lb/sq inch (4).

Ultrastructural studies of the nematocyst venom apparatus show that the nematocyst is surrounded by a fibrillar basket that is highly sensitive to both external mechanical or chemical stimuli (9). Each nematocyst basket is composed of a complex microfilamentous tubule system on which there is mounted a trigger-like projection, the cnidocil. The cnidocil is composed of a central flagellum responsive to chemical stimuli and surface stereocilia sensitive to mechanical stimuli. Stimulation of the cnidocil results in contraction of the fibrillar system and a consequent increase in capsular wall pressure together with structural deformation. This deformation dislodges the operculum and, thus, the junction between the capsule and internal venom thread. Thread eversion occurs such that, in a spring-like manner, the thread erupts from the nematocyst to penetrate and affix itself to the victim (14). The tortuous barbed structure of the thread ensures that it achieves penetration and lodges in the victim. The released thread remains attached to the nematocyst keeping the victim in close apposition to the tentacle and thereby increasing the probability of further exposure to nematocyst toxin(s).

Early attempts to purify crude *Physalia* toxin were hampered by the instability of the toxin in solution (15). Lyophilized crude toxin was shown to be heterogeneous, yielding eight to nine fractions when chromatographed. Crude toxin preparations have marked proteolytic actions, with enzyme activity being most prominent in the pH range 7.8–8.0 (3). Such crude preparations contained high levels of inorganic ions such as boron, iron, and aluminum and, when compared to other marine animals, *Physalia* nematocysts contained abnormally high levels of amino acids such as glutamic acid, glycine, proline, and alanine (16).

Many enzymatic components have been isolated from the crude venom of *Physalia* (3). Examination of the lipid content of the toxin shows that extracts can catalyze fatty acid hydrolysis in such a manner as to indicate phospholipase A and B activity. Lipids in the toxin include high levels of free fatty acids that are believed to maintain phospholipases in their inactive states while stored. The lipid components of the crude toxin may also serve to impart biological activity by providing a hydrophobic surface for plasma membrane interaction in victims. In 1981, a high-molecular-weight (250 kDa) protein, physalitoxin, was identified in venom extracts that could account for most of the hemolytic and lethal activity of the toxin (23). This rod-shaped protein is composed of three unequally sized, glycosylated subunits and comprises 28% of the total venom protein. It contains 10.6% carbohydrate by weight, mainly as a major glycoprotein.

Crude toxin administration is lethal to all metazoan animals tested, provided the dose is sufficient. The LD_{50} for mammals apparently does not vary a great deal among species. The intravenous LD_{50} is 50 $\mu g/kg$ in mice and 150 $\mu g/kg$ in dogs (11,13,15). The stages to death are similar for different mammal species; respiratory paralysis is followed by cardiovascular collapse.

The rate of development of cutaneous symptoms following stinging suggests the toxin is easily absorbed from the thread. Perception of a painful stimulus is almost immediate on contact with the tentacle, and systemic symptoms may appear within minutes of a victim being stung (3,4). Apart from this suggestive evidence, no other information is available regarding the pharmacokinetics of the toxin.

Toxin administration produces a wide variety of nonspecific organ effects. Early studies involved injection of crude toxin into the hemolymph of the land crab, *Cardiosoma guanhumi* (15). Immediately upon exposure to the crude toxin, impulse conduction in the crustacean heart stopped.

Mammalian hearts also respond rapidly in a dose-dependent manner to infusion or injection of crude toxin. In rats and dogs, intravenous injection of crude toxin produced marked aberrations in the electrocardiogram including prolongation of the Q-T interval, bifurcation of the QRS complex, and a reduction in the P-R interval followed by loss of the P-wave, bradycardia, and fatal ventricular fibrillation (11,13,15).

Massive hemolysis also occurs in rats and dogs; this is associated with marked increases in serum potassium concentrations (13,15) together with a reduction in serum sodium concentrations. Isotonic KCl administration reverses the electrocardiographic responses and, as a result of this and related observations, it was concluded that the crude toxin interferes with Na^+,K^+-ATPase (13). Both heart rate and blood pressure were reduced by crude toxin, and respiration was also markedly affected (11). The vascular effects of the toxin were examined on dog skeletal muscle and isolated rabbit aortic ring segments (17,18); relaxation occurred in the rings and vasodilation in the vasculature, both of which were inhibited by administration of meclofenamate. From these studies, it was concluded that such effects were due to stimulation of endogenous prostaglandin synthesis.

Biochemical investigations showed that crude toxin reduces mitochondrial calcium uptake and respiration. However, such effects are not due to the lethal component of the crude toxin but to the lipases and proteases that cause cell lysis (3,8). Nuclear cytotoxic actions of the crude venom have been demonstrated in Chinese hamster ovary K1 cells. Upon prolonged exposure to the crude toxin, cells become multinucleated, perhaps due to lectin components in the toxin, and chromatin levels are reduced. The latter may be due to both the protease and lectin components of the crude toxin (21).

In vitro studies suggest that the general muscle contractile effects of the toxin are independent of known membrane receptor systems. Thus rat and guinea pig ileum contract upon exposure to crude toxin; these responses are not inhibited by administration of atropine, chlorpheniramine, hexamethonium, or methysergide (11). These findings prompted study of the action of crude toxin on transmembrane ion fluxes: crude toxin increases frog skin permeability to Na^+, an effect inhibited by ouabain, and blocks frog sciatic nerve conduction due to modification in membrane permeability to ion fluxes (3,15,16). The high-molecular-weight fraction of the toxin reversibly inhibits both the actions of glutamate in snail parietal cells and the amplitudes of excitatory junction potentials in the crayfish neuromuscular junction (19). A purified component of the high-molecular-weight toxin fraction competitively inhibits nicotinic receptors at the frog neuromuscular junction by producing a nonspecific ion-channel block (20). *Physalia* toxin also releases histamine from peritoneal mast cells (3,8,9) and impacts leukocyte, eosinophil, and lymphocyte activity (8).

Studies of the action of crude and purified toxin have been aided by development of monoclonal antibodies (mAb) to the highly antigenic toxic component of the venom (3). Studies confirmed the antigenic nature of the toxin (22) and showed that 56% of patients stung by *P. physalis* had immunoglobulin G (IgG) antibodies, and 13% developed IgE antibodies against the toxin. Interestingly, these patients also developed cross-reacting antibodies directed against the venom of the sea nettle jellyfish (*Chrysaora quinquecirrha*, a Scyphozoan). In view of the existence of this marked antigenic relationship between venoms of diverse jellyfish species, studies were conducted to determine whether a single anti-inflammatory agent could protect against the actions of the toxin on skin permeability. No single antagonist for any of the mediators of increased vascular permeability could be used against all venoms from various jellyfish; thus, treatment should be venom-specific (2). For *Physalia* envenomation, both methysergide and piripost, a leukotriene antagonist, decrease vasopermeability, suggesting the involvement of arachidonic acid metabolites and serotonin in the cutaneous vascular damage produced by the venom (2,3).

A wide variety of local and systemic reactions is induced by *Physalia* envenomation (1,3,4). Acute local reactions, which include pain, urticarial eruptions, and local edema, are most common. Some of these actions may be due to a kinin-like factor in addition to the enzymes, lipases, and toxic component found in the venom (3,4). Cases of both recurrent and delayed lesions have been reported, as have inflammatory eruptions at sites remote from the site of envenomation (3,4). Possible long-term reactions include the appearance of gangrene, keloids, fat atrophy, and scar formation (4). Systemic reactions include malaise, dizziness, weakness, ataxia, and fever; effects can be very severe but are not usually fatal. However, two fatalities have occurred with envenomation from the Atlantic form of *Physalia* (5). Experimental and clinical evidence suggest that such fatal reactions are the result of central respiratory failure, an anaphylactoid reaction (which may be due to histamine release), and hyperkalemia due to shocked-kidney syndrome (3,4).

Treatment for jellyfish stinging includes bathing the area with 4%–6% acetic acid (vinegar) or aluminum sulfate (Stingose). Application of methylated spirits or isopropyl alcohol increases envenomation (1,10). Other remedies reported to be of benefit include rubbing sand, alcohol, antistinger lotion (picric acid, camphor, ethanol and water),

or crystal meat tenderizer (papain); use of calcium antagonists such as verapamil, or topical anesthetics; and immobilization of the sting area; application of ice or cold packs, and a baking soda slurry (1,3–5,7,10). It is also suggested that shaving the area and applying corticosteroids can be of great benefit (1). A 1993 report cites a newly differentiated Indo-Pacific form of the jellyfish that may be as lethal as its Atlantic counterpart (10); stings from this jellyfish may cause severe systemic reactions and application of vinegar may actually cause nematocysts to discharge (1).

REFERENCES

1. Auerbach PS (1991) Marine envenomations. *N Engl J Med* **325**, 486.

2. Burnett JW, Calton GJ (1986) Pharmacological effects of various venoms on cutaneous capillary leakage. *Toxicon* **24**, 614.

3. Burnett JW, Calton GJ (1987) Venomous pelagic coelenterates: Chemistry, toxicology, immunology & treatment of their stings. *Toxicon* **25**, 581.

4. Burnett JW, Calton GJ (1987) Jellyfish envenomation syndromes updated. *Ann Emerg Med* **16**, 1000.

5. Burnett JW, Gable WD (1989) A fatal jellyfish envenomation by the Portugese man-of-war. *Toxicon* **27**, 823.

6. Burnett JW, Ordonez JV, Calton GJ (1986) Differential toxicity of *Physalia physalis* (Portuguese man-of-war) nematocysts separated by flow cytometry. *Toxicon* **24**, 514.

7. Cleland JB, Southcott RV (1965) Injuries from marine invertebrates. In: *Injuries to Man from Marine Invertebrates in the Australian Region.* Lee DJ, Barnes HJ eds. National Health and Medical Research Council Special Series Report No. 12, Canberra, A.C.T.

8. Cormier SM (1984) Exocytotic and cytolytic release of histamine from mast cells treated with Portuguese man-of-war (*Physalia physalis*) venom. *J Exp Zool* **231**, 1.

9. Cormier SM, Hessinger DA (1980) Cellular basis for tentacle adherence in the Portuguese man-of-war (*Physalia physalis*). *Tissue Cell* **12**, 714.

10. Fenner PJ, Williamson JA, Burnett JW, Rifkin J (1993) First aid treatment of jellyfish stings in Australia: Response to a newly differentiated species. *Med J Australia* **158**, 498.

11. Garriott JC, Lane CE (1969) Some autonomic effects of *Physalia* toxin. *Toxicon* **6**, 281.

12. Halstead BW (1978) Invertebrates: Phylum Coelenterata. In: *Poisonous and Venomous Marine Animals of the World.* Halstead LG ed. Darwin Press, Princeton, New Jersey.

13. Hastings SG, Larsen JB, Lane CE (1967) Effects of nematocyst toxin of *Physalia physalis* (Portuguese man-of-war) on the canine cardiovascular system. *Proc Soc Exp Biol Med* **125**, 41.

14. Hulet WH, Belleme JL, Musil G, Lane CE (1974) Ultrastructure of *Physalia* nematocysts. In: *Marine Science: Bioactive Compounds from the Sea*. Humm HJ, Lane CE eds. Marcel Dekker, New York.

15. Lane CE (1967) Pharmacologic action of *Physalia* toxin. *Fed Proc* **26**, 1225.

16. Lane CE (1974) Nematocyst toxins of coelenterates. In: *Marine Science: Bioactive Compounds from the Sea*. Humm HJ, Lane CE eds. Marcel Dekker, New York.

17. Loredo JS, Gonzalez RR, Hessinger DA (1985) Vascular effects of *Physalia physalis* venom in the skeletal muscle of the dog. *J Pharmacol Exp Ther* **232**, 301.

18. Loredo JS, Gonzalez RR, Hessinger DA (1986) Effect of Portuguese man-of-war venom on isolated vascular segments. *J Pharmacol Exp Ther* **236**, 140.

19. Mas R, Memendez R, Garateix A *et al.* (1989) Effects of a high molecular weight toxin from *Physalia physalis* on glutamate responses. *Neuroscience* **33**, 269.

20. Menendez R, Mas R, Garateix A *et al.* (1990) Effects of a high molecular weight polypeptidic toxin from *Physalia physalis* (Portuguese man-of-war) on cholinergic responses. *Comp Biochem Physiol* **95**, 63.

21. Neeman I, Calton GJ, Burnett JW (1980) An ultrastructural study of the cytotoxic effect of the venoms from the sea nettle (*Chrysaora quinquecirrha*) and Portuguese man-of-war (*Physalia physalis*) on cultured Chinese hamster ovary K-1 cells. *Toxicon* **18**, 495.

22. Russo AJ, Calton GJ, Burnett JW (1983) The relationship of the possible allergic response to jellyfish envenomation and serum antibody titers. *Toxicon* **21**, 475.

23. Tamkun MM, Hessinger DA (1981) Isolation and partial characterization of a hemolytic and toxic protein from the nematocyst venom of the Portuguese man-of-war, *Physalia physalis*. *Biochem Biophy Acta* **667**, 87.

Phytolacca Spp.

Albert C. Ludolph

NEUROTOXICITY RATING

Clinical

B   Headache

B   Acute encephalopathy

Consumption of the roots, leaves, or an extract thereof ("poke root tea") of *Phytolacca americana* (pokeweed, pokeberry), a shrub-like plant, causes a gastrointestinal condition that includes nausea, emesis, diarrhea, and tachycardia. The entire plant is toxic. In most cases, complete recovery follows; however, a few fatalities have occurred (2,6). In Africa, the plant was said to be widely used as an instrument of violent death (7). After a severe poisoning incident in 1979, the American state of Wisconsin embargoed all lots of poke roots sold in health-food stores (6).

In a small outbreak in New Jersey in summer 1980, 21 out of 52 subjects (campers and counselors) became ill after consumption of a salad prepared from pokeweed. The leaves of the plant had been boiled and reboiled. Between 30 min and 5.5 h after consumption, 18 of 21 patients developed nausea and stomach cramps, seventeen vomiting, eight burning in the stomach, and six diarrhea. Eleven subjects complained of headache, ten of dizziness. Symptoms resolved within 1–48 h in each patient. Two recovered from continuous vomiting after more than 24 h. Lethargy, stupor, convulsions, weakness, tremor, blurred vision, and vertigo have been reported in the older literature (5); some individuals develop headache (2).

In an experimental study in turkeys, animals were unable to stand or walk (1).

The toxic principle of pokeweed is unknown, although saponins and lectins are suspected (3). In parts of Africa, saponins from *P. dodecandra* are used to control the water snail, *Biomphalaria glabrata*, which transmits schistosomiasis (4,8).

REFERENCES

1. Barnett BD (1975) Toxicity of pokeberries (fruit of *Phytolacca americana*) for turkey poults. *Poultry Sci* **54**, 1215.

2. Callahan R, Piccola F, Gensheimer K *et al.* (1981) Plant poisonings. *N J Morb Mortal Wkly Rep* **30**, 65.

3. Frohne D, Pfänder HJ (1987) *Giftpflanzen*. Wissenschaftliche Verlags-gesellschaft, Stuttgart.

4. Hosttetmann (1985) Saponins and schistosomiasis: Isolation and determination of saponin structure. *Schweiz Apoth Ztg* **123**, 223.

5. Jaeckle K, Freemon FR (1981) Pokeweed (*Phytolacca americana*) poisoning. *Southern Med J* **74**, 639.

6. Lewis W, Smith PR (1979) Poke root herbal tea poisoning. *J Amer Med Assn* **242**, 2759.

7. Mettam RWM (1939) Poisoning by *Phytolacca dodecandra* L'Herit.-family: Phytolacceae. *Vet J* **95**, 135.

8. Webbe G, Lambert JDH (1983) Plants that kill snails and prospects for disease control. *Nature* **302**, 754.

Picrotoxin

Albert C. Ludolph
Peter S. Spencer

PICROTOXININ
$C_{15}H_{16}O_6$

NEUROTOXICITY RATING
Clinical
B   Seizure disorder
Experimental
A   GABA receptor blockade

Picrotoxin is a noncompetitive $GABA_A$ antagonist with a binding site close to the γ-aminobutyric acid (GABA)–activated chloride channel (2,9). It occurs naturally in the seeds of *Anamirta cocculus*; it was formerly used as an insecticide (*cf.* 5). Two to 3 g of the seeds are lethal; generalized seizures occur in humans after ingestion of as little as 10 mg.

Picrotoxin (MW, 602.57) is a polycyclic lactone consisting of two compounds, low-efficiency picrotin and high-efficiency picrotoxinin (4). It is readily soluble in water and ethanol. Even after intravenous application, some latency to onset of effect is observed.

At low dosage (4 mg/kg), female rats are more susceptible to picrotoxin-induced generalized seizures; at high dosage (10 mg/kg), males convulse more readily (11). The LD_{50} in mice is 7.2 mg/kg (1). Cardiac arrythmias appear in rabbits upon intracerebroventricular injection (10). In cats, picrotoxin induces coronary artery spasm (7).

Perinatal exposure to picrotoxin during critical periods of male brain sexual differentiation reportedly has long-term effects on the reproductive physiology and behavior of male rats. Striatal dopamine and homovanillic acid levels were decreased and hypothalamic norepinephrine levels were increased in the offspring of dams treated with picrotoxin (8).

Picrotoxin induces epileptiform discharges in neocortical slices (12). The picrotoxin block of GABA current is use-dependent, suggesting that the toxin-binding site is exposed by the conformational change initiated by the binding of GABA to its receptor (6,14). At the single-channel level, picrotoxinin behaves similarly to dieldrin in decreasing the channel open probability of the $GABA_A$ receptor-channel complex (3). In rodents, treatment with picrotoxin dissolved in drinking water (2 mg/ml) increases the hepatic content of cytochrome P-450 and triples the activity of benzphetamine N-demethylation, indicating that picrotoxin induces liver enzymes (13).

REFERENCES
1. Budavari S (1989) *The Merck Index. 11th Ed.* Merck & Co, New Jersey.
2. Galindo A (1969) GABA-picrotoxin interaction in the mammalian nervous system. *Brain Res* **14**, 763.
3. Ikeda T, Nagata K, Shono T, Narahashi T (1998) Dieldrin and picrotoxinin modulation of GABA(A) receptor single channels. *Neuroreport* **9**, 3189.
4. Jarboe CH, Poerter LA, Buckler RT (1968) Structural aspects of picrotoxin in action. *J Med Chem* **11**, 729.
5. Lummis SCR, Martin IL (1992) Convulsants and gamma-aminobutyric acid receptors. In: *Handbook of Experimental Pharmacology. Vol 102. Selective Neurotoxicity.* Herken H, Hucho F eds. Springer, Berlin p. 507.
6. Newland CF, Cull-Candy SG (1992) On the mechanism of action of picrotoxin on GABA receptor channels in dissociated sympathetic neurones of the rat. *J Physiol-London* **447**, 191.
7. Segal SA, Pearle DL, Gillis RA (1981) Coronary spasm produced by picrotoxin in cats. *Eur J Pharmacol* **76**, 447.
8. Silva MR, Oliveira CA, Felicio LF *et al.* (1998) Perinatal treatment with picrotoxin induces sexual, behavioral, and neuroendocrine changes in male rats. *Pharmacol Biochem Behav* **60**, 203.
9. Simmonds MA (1980) Evidence that bicuculline and picrotoxin act at separate sites to antagonize gamma-aminobutyric acid in the rat cuneate nucleus. *Neuropharmacology* **19**, 39.
10. Sun AY, Li DX (1990) Ventricular arrhythmia evoked by microinjection of picrotoxin into brain areas in rabbits. *Chung Kuo Yao Li Hsueh Pao* **11**, 296.
11. Thomas J (1990) Gender difference in susceptibility to picrotoxin-induced seizures is seizure- and stimulation-dependent. *Brain Res Bull* **24**, 7.
12. Wadman WJ, Gutniock MJ (1993) Non-uniform propagation of epileptiform discharge in brain slices of rat neocortex. *Neuroscience* **52**, 255.
13. Yamada H, Fujisaki H, Kaneko H *et al.* (1993) Picrotoxin as a potent inducer of rat hepatic cytochrome P450, CYP2B1 and CYP2B2. *Biochem Pharmacol* **45**, 1783.
14. Yoon KW, Covey DF, Rothman SM (1993) Multiple mechanisms of picrotoxin block of GABA-induced currents in rat hippocampal. *J Physiol-London* **464**, 423.

Piper methysticum

Albert C. Ludolph

KAVAIN
$C_{14}H_{14}O_3$

Kavain; [R(E)]-5,6-Dihydro-4-methyoxy-6-(2-phenylethenyl)-2H-pyran-2-one

NEUROTOXICITY RATING

Clinical

B   Acute encephalopathy (sedation)

People native to the South Pacific region prepare a beverage from the rootstock of different varieties of the pepper plant *Piper methysticum*, termed *kava*. It is consumed to counteract fatigue, alleviate anxiety, and elicit contentment resulting in a state of well-being (13). Kava is also used as an antianxiety drug in Europe and in the United States. The kava plant is a robust, succulent, well-branched and erect, perennial shrub belonging to the Piperaceae family. It thrives at altitudes of between 150 and 300 m above sea level and grows well in stony ground (13). The cultivated plant is harvested when it is 2.0–2.5 m tall (13). Kava has a bitter taste and has a numbing, astringent effect on the mucuous membranes of the mouth (13). Beverages prepared from fresh roots make stronger drinks (12). The active constituents have anticonvulsive, analgesic, and central muscle-relaxing effects (5,13). The most characteristic CNS effect is a mephenesin-like muscle relaxation (13).

The pharmacologically active components of kava are α-pyrones or substituted 5,6-dihydro-α-pyrones (dihydrokavain, kavain, dihydromethysticin, methysticin, dihydrogynagonin, yangonin) (7,13). Little is known about the pharmacology of the various compounds (11,13). It appears likely that the different constituents act synergistically (13), probably by facilitated penetration into the brain (9). Maximal brain concentration of kavain and dihydrokavain is observed 5 min after intraperitoneal (i.p.) administration (9). A single i.p. injection of 120 mg/kg body weight kava resin into mice results in brain concentrations of the active constituents of about 200 nmol (9). Many of the lipid components are secreted in the urine together with several me-tabolites (3). This method can be used to determine whether subjects have recently consumed kava (3).

Kava decreases human spontaneous activity, produces analgesia, induces muscle relaxation, reduces motor control, has hypnotic and anxiolytic effects, has a slight anti-apomorphine effect, and produces hypothermia (7). The lipid-soluble extract, kava resin, produces a greater range of pharmacological actions than the aqueous extract, and the latter is orally inactive in mice and rats (7). Tolerance develops faster for the aqeuous extract than for the lipid-soluble extract (2). The hypnotic effects of ethanol and kava augment one another (6).

In a study on the physical health of Australian Aborigines, there was a correlation between the extent of kava usage and signs of multiorgan dysfunction including scaly skin rash; increased patellar reflexes; underweight; reduced levels of albumin, plasma protein, urea, and bilirubin; decreased platelet and lymphocyte count; shortness of breath; and pulmonary hypertension (10). A reduced near point of accommodation and convergence, an increased pupillary diameter, and disturbances of oculomotor balance were noted soon after ingestion of the kava drink (4). In one report, kava pyrones caused coma in a patient who consumed kava from a health-food store while on medication with benzodiazepines (1).

One way kavapyrones mediate sedative effects *in vivo* is by affecting the binding of γ-aminobutyric acid (GABA)-ergic substances to the $GABA_A$ receptor in a concentration-dependent manner (8). The EC_{50} for stimulation of muscimol binding is 200–300 μmol/l for different kavapyrones (8). Kavain, a synthetic kavapyrone, quickly and specifically inhibits voltage-dependent sodium (and calcium) channels with an EC_{50} concentration of <100 μmol/l (5,12).

In summary, kava pyrones have anticonvulsive, analgesic, and central muscle-relaxing effects by affecting $GABA_A$ receptors and voltage-dependent sodium channels. While general ill health was correlated with chronic kava intake in a population-based study, the pattern of human toxicity is undefined. Dopamine antagonism is held responsible for the sedative action of kava extract (11). Acute sedative toxicity may be greatly enhanced by simultaneous consumption of other sedative drugs, such as ethanol and benzodiazepines.

REFERENCES

1. Almeida JC, Grimsley EW (1996) Coma from the health food store: Interaction between kava and alprazolam. *Ann Intern Med* **125**, 940.

2. Duffield AM, Jamieson DD, Lidgard RO *et al.* (1989) Identification of some human urinary metabolites of the intoxicating beverage kava. *J Chromatogr* **475**, 273.

3. Duffield PH, Jamieson D (1991) Development of tolerance to kava in mice. *Clin Exp Pharmacol Physiol* **18**, 571.

4. Garner LF, Klinger JD (1985) Some visual effects caused by the beverage kava. *J Ethnopharmacol* **13**, 307.

5. Gleitz J, Beile A, Peters T (1995) (+/−)-Kavain inhibits veratridine-activated voltage-dependent Na⁺-channels in synaptosomes prepared from rat cerebral cortex. *Neuropharmacology* **34**, 1133.

6. Jamieson DD, Duffield PH (1990) Positive interaction of ethanol and kava resin in mice. *Clin Exp Pharmacol Physiol* **17**, 509.

7. Jamieson DD, Duffield PH, Cheng D, Duffield AM (1989) Comparison of the central nervous system activity of the aqueous and lipid extract of Kava (*Piper methysticum*). *Arch Intern Pharmacodyn* **301**, 66.

8. Jussofie A, Schmiz A, Hiemke C (1994) Kavapyrone enriched extract from *Piper methysticum* as modulator of the GABA binding site in different regions of rat brain. *Psychopharmacology* **116**, 469.

9. Keledjian J, Duffield PH, Jamieson DD *et al.* (1988) Uptake into mouse brain of four compounds present in the psychoactive beverage kava. *J Pharm Sci* **77**, 1003.

10. Mathews JD, Riley MD, Fejo L *et al.* (1988) Effects of the heavy usage of kava on the physical health: Summary of a pilot survey in an aboriginal community. *Med J Australia* **148**, 548.

11. Schelosky L, Raffauf C, Jendroska K, Poewe W (1995) Kava and dopamine antagonism. *J Neurol Neurosurg Psychiat* **58**, 639.

12. Schirrmacher K, Busselberg D, Langosch JM *et al.* (1999) Effects of (+/−)-kavain on voltage-activated inward currents of dorsal root ganglion cells from neonatal rats. *Eur Neuropsychopharmacol* **9**, 171.

13. Singh YN (1992) Kava: An overview. *J Ethnopharmacol* **37**, 13.

Piperazine

Steven A. Sparr

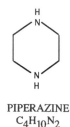

PIPERAZINE
$C_4H_{10}N_2$

Piperazine-1,2,3-propanetricarboxylate (3:2)

NEUROTOXICITY RATING

Clinical

A   Acute encephalopathy (ataxia, confusion, seizures)

Salts of piperazine, a cyclic secondary amine, were introduced into clinical medicine in the 1880s for the treatment of gout and other rheumatic disorders; they were found in the 1950s to have anthelmintic activity (3–5). Piperazine is used for the treatment of intestinal infestation with *Ascaris lumbricoides* (roundworm) and *Enterobius vermicularis* (pinworm) (2,5,6). Although side effects are rare and usually mild, the drug has the potential to cause neurological toxicity that can be severe, especially in children with epilepsy or other brain abnormalities (6). Given these risks and the availability of alternative treatments, piperazine is now rarely used in the United States but continues to be used widely elsewhere (6).

In ascariasis, piperazine is believed to act by hyperpolarizing the worms' muscle membranes, thus blocking the effects of acetylcholine at the neuromuscular junction (2,5). The worms become paralyzed, released into the bowel, and excreted. The mode of action in pinworm infections is not yet defined (2).

Various salts of piperazine are used throughout the world, including the hexahydrate, phosphate, tartrate, adipate, and citrate, but only the citrate salt is available in the United States (2). Piperazine is readily absorbed from the gastrointestinal tract following oral administration and is excreted primarily unchanged in the kidneys; hepatic metabolism plays a minor role in its pharmacology (2). Rate of renal excretion and plasma half-life are highly variable (2).

Adverse effects are rare. Nausea, diarrhea, and abdominal cramping, as well as hypersensitivity reactions, are the most common nonneurological side effects (2). Neurological toxicity is rare but potentially serious, with ataxia, headache, weakness, tremors, hypotonia (so-called *worm wobble*), and seizures reported (2,4). Toxicity is more commonly associated with overdose of the medication or renal failure impairing elimination, but is also seen in patients without these risk factors (4,6). Other risk factors for neurotoxicity include history of epilepsy and concurrent use of psychotropic drugs (3). More soluble piperazine salts, such as the hexahydrate salt, may have a greater incidence of neurotoxicity (3,6).

Potential neurological toxicity has been recognized since the nineteenth century, with descriptions of hypotonia, weakness, ataxia, and confusion in patients treated with piperazine for gout. Similar neurological toxicity in adult and pediatric patients treated for worm infections were described in 1953 (4). Ten pediatric patients treated with piperazine developed ataxia, confusional states, incoordination, myoclonic jerks, and exacerbation of epilepsy. Two developed status epilepticus with seizures lasting hours; one died, an 11-year-boy with anemia and a history of brief "staring spells" who developed confusion and unsteady gait 3 days after the initiation of piperazine for ascariasis. He subsequently developed myoclonic twitches, then generalized seizures that were refractory to anticonvulsants. He became comatose and lost all brainstem reflexes prior to death. Electroencephalography (EEG) initially showed 2–4/sec, high-amplitude slow waves, spikes, and polyspikes. As his condition deteriorated, the EEG showed slow, low-amplitude activity with spike and slow wave abnormalities. An incidence of neurological toxicity was noted in 10 of 19 children with previous CNS disorders, and in 1 of 16 previously normal children.

A consistent pattern of EEG abnormalities has been documented in several cases of piperazine neurotoxicity. These abnormalities consist of diffuse high-amplitude slow-wave activity; bursts of 2- to 4-Hertz rhythmic delta activity; and spike, polyspike, or spike and slow wave activity (1,3,4,6).

EEG studies performed on a group of 11 children routinely treated with a 5-day course of piperazine revealed abnormalities in all but one (1); these abnormalities resolved with cessation of drug treatment. Only one child was reported to be symptomatic with vertigo, tremor, and vomiting. When six of these children were rechallenged with the same dose of piperazine and cotreated with oral prednisone, EEG abnormalities were much less pronounced or absent.

Mechanisms of piperazine neurotoxicity are unknown. Several hypotheses have been proposed ranging from central inhibition of γ-aminobutyric acid pathways (6) to peripheral postsynaptic blockade at the neuromuscular junction (4). Noteworthy is the structural similarity between piperazine and several antipsychotic drugs (fluphenazine, thiothixene) and antitussive agents (zipeprol, eprazinone) known to lower seizure threshold in epileptic patients or to induce seizures in patients no history of prior seizures (6).

REFERENCES

1. Belloni C, Rizzoni G (1967) Neurotoxic side-effects of piperazine. *Lancet* **2**, 369.
2. McEvoy GK (1995) *American Hospital Formulary Service Drug Information*. American Society of Health System Pharmacists, p. 47.
3. Neau JP, Rogez R, Boissonnot L *et al.* (1984) Accidents neurologiques de la piperazine. *Acta Neurol Belg* **84**, 26.
4. Parsons AC (1971) Piperazine neurotoxicity: "Worm Wobble." *Brit Med J* **4**, 792.
5. Tracy JW, Webster LT (1996) Drugs used in the chemotherapy of protozoal infections. In: *The Pharmacologic Basis of Therapeutics. 9th Ed.* Hardman JG, Goodman AG, Limbird LE eds. McGraw-Hill, New York p. 987.
6. Yohai D, Barnett SH (1989) Absence and atonic seizures induced by piperazine. *Pediat Neurol* **5**, 393.

α-*Plectreurys tristis* Toxins

Albert C. Ludolph
Peter S. Spencer

NEUROTOXICITY RATING

Experimental

A Ion channel dysfunction

The venom of the spider *Plectreurys tristis* contains a number of inhibitory and excitatory fractions (1); approximately 50 peptide toxins have been purified (6), and some have been cloned and sequenced (4). The excitatory components have not been purified; the inhibitory activities are named PLTX I–III (1). α-PLTX II is a 44-amino-acid polypeptide that inhibits presynaptic Ca^{2+} channels in *Drosophila* (5); PLTX I and III have not been characterized. α-PLTX II, a small fraction (0.1% of the protein) of the spider venom, has a MW of about 7000 Da and is soluble in organic solvents. α-PLTX II is active at the neuromuscular junction of *Drosophila* (1) but not of the frog. It noncompetitively and allosterically inhibits the binding of (^{125}I-tyrosyl)-ω-conotoxin GVIA to rat brain synaptic plasma membranes (3). Structurally, α-PLTX II is a peptide with an

O-palmitoyl threonine amide residue at the carboxy terminus (2); this may have functional impact, since it might allow the toxin to penetrate membranes and act intracellularly (2).

REFERENCES

1. Branton WD, Kolton L, Jan YN, Jan LY (1987) Neurotoxins from *Plectreurys* spider venom are potent presynaptic blockers in *Drosophila*. *J Neurosci* 7, 4195.
2. Branton WD, Rudnick MS, Zhou Y *et al.* (1993) Fatty acylated toxin structure. *Nature* 365, 496.
3. Feigenbaum P, Garcia ML, Kaczorowski EJ (1988) Evidence for distinct sites coupled to high affinity omega-conotoxin in rat brain synaptic plasma membrane vesicles. *Biochem Biophys Res Commun* 154, 298.
4. Leisy DJ, Mattson JD, Quistad GB *et al.* (1996) Molecular cloning and sequencing of cDNAs encoding insecticidal peptides from the primitive hunting spider, *Plectreurys tristis* (Simon). *Insect Biochem Mol Biol* 26, 411.
5. Leung H-T, Branton WD, Phillips H *et al.* (1989) Spider toxins selectively block calcium currents in *Drosophila*. *Neuron* 3, 767.
6. Quistad GB, Skinner WS (1994) Isolation and sequencing of insecticidal peptides from the primitive hunting spider, *Plectreurys tristis* (Simon). *J Biol Chem* 269, 11098.

Podophyllotoxin and Related Compounds

Fung-Chow Chui

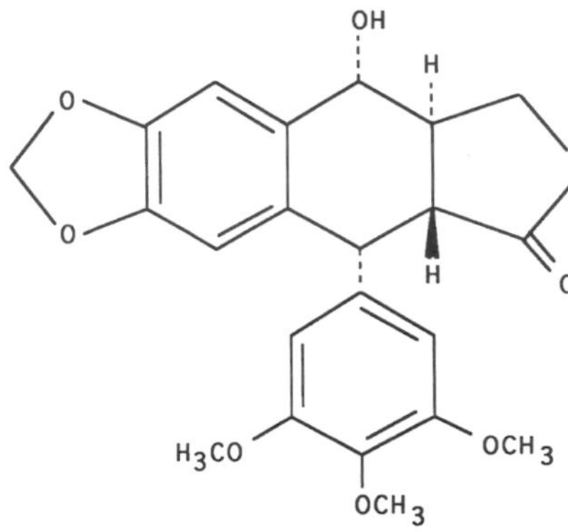

PODOPHYLLOTOXIN
$C_{22}H_{22}O_8$

[5R-(5α,5αβ,8aα,9α)]-5,8,8a,9-Tetrahydro-9-hydroxy-5-(3,4,5-trimethoxyphenyl)furo[3',4':6,7]naphtho[2,3-d]-1,3-dioxol-6(5aH)-one

NEUROTOXICITY RATING

Clinical

A Peripheral neuropathy

B Psychobiological reaction (hallucinations)

Experimental

A Microtubule binding

A Neuronal and axonal pathology

Podophyllotoxin is found in the rhizomes of *Podophyllum peltatum*, known in North America as May apple. It was used as a purgative by Native Americans. There is a cogent review of the early use of podophyllum in the Americas (11); podophyllum, a herbal preparation of podophyllotoxin, *gui jiu*, has been used for centuries in Chinese medicine. *Gui jiu*, extracted from the root of *Dysosma versipellis* (*ba jiao lian*), was described in *The Herbal Catalog* (*ben cao gan mu*) by Li Shih-zheng (1518–1593 AD) who wrote that gui jiu, used at one qian (about 4 g) per dose in an alcoholic extract, was highly effective in aborting still births, in treating snake bites, and in purging intestinal parasites. However, Li cautioned that gui jiu was toxic. The neurotoxicity of gui jiu was noted in early Chinese medical texts, in particular, its ability to induce "madness."

Since 1942, the alcohol-extracted podophyllum resin has been widely used topically to treat genital warts (10). Two semisynthetic derivatives of podophyllotoxin, etoposide and teniposide, have been employed as antineoplastic agents against a broad spectrum of malignancies. Both podophyllotoxin and etoposide have neurotoxic potential, affecting both the CNS and PNS. In addition to the antimitotic lignins, which include podophyllotoxin and its derivatives, the podophyllum resin contains flavonoids, in particular quercetin and kaempherol (8). While these flavonoids are not toxic at low doses, they have anti-inflammatory properties and are powerful modulators of the immune system.

Podophyllin and podophyllotoxin are strong purgatives and can be lethal if taken orally. However, the amount absorbed into the bloodstream is low. Topical application of podophyllin, in a 20% solution, has resulted in several reported cases of toxicity. An ointment containing 0.5% podophyllotoxin has been extensively tested to treat genital warts; it appears to be highly effective, without any negative side effects.

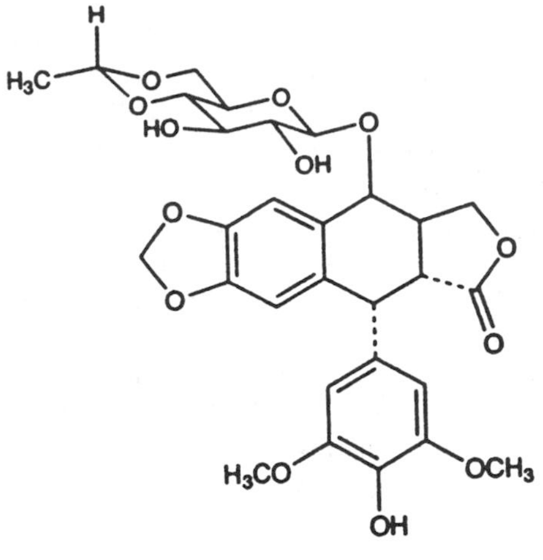

ETOPOSIDE

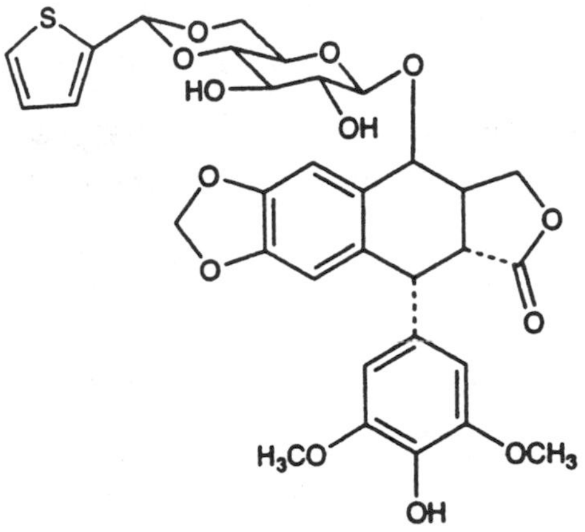

TENIPOSIDE

Intravenously injected podophyllotoxin is metabolized within 1 h in rat with no evidence of retention in liver, kidney, spleen, blood, or tumor tissue (12). In contrast, incubation with tissue homogenates resulted in no significant degradation of podophyllotoxin in 4 h. Injections of low dosages (5–20 mg) into humans caused mimimal intestinal discomfort and no toxic symptoms (11). Etoposide and teniposide are both poorly absorbed in humans. Only 50% of oral etoposide is bioavailable, with no evidence of accumulation in tissue following multiple consecutive doses (4).

Podophyllotoxin, a powerful inhibitor of DNA, RNA, and protein synthesis, is a systemic toxin (1,2,19). It binds strongly but reversibly to microtubules, and it disrupts mitosis. The alcohol-extracted podophyllum resin is extremely caustic to skin, mucous membranes, and eyes. The LD_{50} of subcutaneously injected podophyllotoxin is 22 mg/kg in rats and 24.6 mg/kg in mice. In contrast, oral administration of podophyllotoxin is less toxic; the LD_{50} is 90 mg/kg in mice. Podophyllotoxin is more toxic in weanlings (LD_{50} of 8 mg/kg) than in adult rats (15).

Following parenteral administration of fatal doses of podophyllotoxin, rats become flaccid and display slow, labored respiration (15). This is followed by a period of somnolence and unconsciousness; death occurs within 12–15 h of injection. Histopathological changes include enteritis with chromatolysis of the intestinal mucosa and necrosis of the underlying lymphoid tissue. There is also necrosis in the lymphoid follicles in the spleen. Except for an increase in mitotic figures, there is no apparent change in the mucosal epithelia. Injection of a lethal dose of podophyllin resin results in a period of excitation that eventuates in generalized seizures. Otherwise, the terminal stage of flaccidity and microscopic damage are similar to that induced by podophyllotoxin. Death finally occurs about 15–18 h following injection of podophyllin.

Neuronal changes are observed following a single injection of a sublethal dose (10–15 mg/kg) of podophyllotoxin in rats (1). Motor neurons of the anterior horn in the spinal cord appear swollen. More serious abnormalities are found in the dorsal root ganglion neurons, which become depleted of Nissl substance. Focal axonal swellings appear throughout the PNS and CNS.

Quercetin, a flavonoid that constitutes as much as 10% by weight of the podophyllin resin, is toxic at high dosages. Subcutaneous injection of a lethal dose of quercetin in mice (LD_{50} of 97–98 mg/kg) produced a terminal illness different from that of podophyllotoxin (15). Within 30 min of quercetin injection, mice displayed a rapid swimming motion of the forepaws, followed by forelimb paralysis. Within 1 h of injection, the animals became somnolent, with labored respiration. Thereafter, the animals became flaccid, and death usually occurred within 4 h of injection. Like podophyllotoxin, ingested quercetin is poorly absorbed, with a LD_{50} of about 160 mg/kg.

Podophyllin-induced human neurotoxicity has been reported following oral, topical, and parenteral exposures. Topical application of podophyllin resulted in coma in one instance (14). Another individual became stuporous following oral ingestion of the resin (3). Sensorimotor neuropathy subsequently developed in both instances. A third patient developed hallucinatory psychosis and autonomic disturbances, in addition to sensorimotor neuropathy, after a single topical exposure (5). High doses of etoposide, a derivative of podophyllotoxin used as an antineoplastic agent, have also produced acute neurological dysfunction. Within 9 days of the initiation of high doses of etoposide, six of eight patients suffering from recurrent glioma developed confusion, papilledema, somnolence, exacerbation of weakness, and increases in seizure activity (13). In a recent incident, a 25-year-old male self-injected 5 ml of topical podophyllin resin. Within 3 days, he developed distal paresthesia and weakness, which subsequently progressed to a symmetrical polyneuropathy with profound distal sensory loss and pseudoathetosis. Autonomic dysfunction was detected by laboratory testing (6).

Podophyllotoxin binds reversibly to microtubules and exerts a colchicine-like activity evident in mitotic arrest, depolymerization of mitotic spindles, and disruption of axonal cytoarchitecture (16,17). It competes with colchicine for the same binding site but does not displace bound colchicine (16). Unlike colchicine, stereotaxically-injected podophyllotoxin causes only limited damage to neurons, mostly restricted to the vicinity of the injection site (7). Podophyllotoxin and its derivatives inhibit topoisomerase II, which uncoils DNA, and thus suppress the ability of the cell to synthesize nucleic acids during cell division and transcription (9,19). Several podophyllotoxin derivatives, when complexed with copper, are able to cleave DNA (18).

REFERENCES

1. Chang LW, Yang CM, Chen CF, Deng JF (1992) Experimental podophyllotoxin (bajiaolian) poisoning: I. Effects on the nervous system. *Biomed Environ Sci* 5, 283.
2. Chang LW, Yang CM, Chen CF, Deng JF (1992) Experimental podophyllotoxin (bajiaolian) poisoning: II. Effects on the liver, intestine, kidney, pancreas and testis. *Biomed Environ Sci* 5, 293.
3. Clark ANG, Parsonage MJ (1957) A case of podophyllum poisoning with involvement of the nervous system. *Brit Med J* 2, 1155.
4. Clark PI (1992) Clinical pharmacology and schedule dependency of the podophyllotoxin derivatives. *Semin Oncol* 19, 20.
5. Filley CM, Graff-Radford NR, Lacy JR *et al.* (1982) Neurologic manifestations of podophyllin toxicity. *Neurology* 32, 308.
6. Freeman MC, Weimer LH, Arnaudo E, Brust JCM (1997) Neuropathy and autonomic effects of intramuscular podophyllin. *Ann Neurol* 42, 416.
7. Goldschmidt RB, Steward O (1989) Comparison of the neurotoxic effects of colchicine, the vinca alkaloids, and other microtubule poisons. *Brain Res* 486, 133.
8. Hartwell JL, Schrecker AW (1958) The chemistry of podophyllum. *Fortschr Chem Org Naturst* 15, 98.
9. Kamal A, Atchison K, Daneshtalab M, Micetich RG (1995) Synthesis of podophyllotoxin congeners as potential DNA topoisomerase II inhibitors. *Anti-cancer Drug Design* 10, 545.
10. Kaplan IW (1942) *Condylomata acuminata. New Orleans Med Soc J* 94, 388.
11. Kelly MG, Hartwell JL (1954) The biological effects and the chemical composition of podophyllin. A review. *J Nat Cancer Inst* 14, 967.
12. Kelly MG, Leiter J, Bourke AR, Smith PK (1951) Fate and distribution of podophyllotoxin in animals. *Cancer Res* 11, 263.
13. Leff RS, Thompson JM, Daly MB *et al.* (1988) Acute neurologic dysfunction after high-dose etoposide therapy for malignant glioma. *Cancer* 62, 32.
14. Slater GE, Rumack BH, Peterson RG (1978) Podophyllin poisoning: Systemic toxicity following cutaneous application. *Obstet Gynecol* 52, 94.
15. Sullivan M, Follis RH Jr, Hilgartner M (1951) Toxicology of podophyllin. *Proc Soc Exp Biol Med* 77, 269.
16. Wilson L, Bamburg JR, Mizel SB *et al.* (1974) Interaction of drugs with microtubule proteins. *Fed Proc* 33, 158.
17. Wisniewski H, Shelanski ML, Terry RD (1968) Effects of mitotic spindle inhibitors on neurotubules and neurofilaments in anterior horn cells. *J Cell Biol* 38, 224.
18. Yamashita A, Tawa R, Imakura Y *et al.* (1994) Site-specific DNA cleavage by Cu(II) complexes of podophyllotoxin derivatives. *Biochem Pharmacol* 47, 1920.
19. Yang CM, Deng JF, Chen CF, Chang LW (1994) Experimental podophyllotoxin (bajiaolian) poisoning: III. Biochemical bases for toxic effects. *Biomed Environ Sci* 7, 259.

Polio Virus Vaccine

Neil L. Rosenberg

NEUROTOXICITY RATING

Clinical

A Vaccine-associated paralytic poliomyelitis (VAPP)
C Peripheral neuropathy (Guillain-Barré syndrome)

During the twentieth century, large epidemics of poliomyelitis have occurred in the United States, peaking at 57,879 reported cases of both paralytic and nonparalytic poliomyelitis in 1952 (10). Inactivated poliovirus vaccine (IPV) was introduced by Salk in 1955 and the oral poliovirus vaccine (OPV) by Sabin in 1961; both were effective. OPV became the preferred vaccine because of its ease of administration and effectiveness; IPV has not been as widely used. IPV continues to have an excellent safety record, and the only reported complications are a febrile reaction in 5% of children and restlessness occurring in 15% (30).

The last epidemic of poliomyelitis in the United States was in 1979, and the last sporadic case caused by the wild

TABLE 55. History of Poliomyelitis and VAPP in the United States

Event	Year
Epidemic poliomyelitis appears in United States	Turn of the 20th century
Peak epidemic year: 57,879 cases	1952
IPV introduced	1955
Monovalent OPV introduced	1961
Trivalent OPV introduced	1963
229 cases of VAPP reported	1961–1984
Last epidemic and sporadic case of "wild virus" poliomyelitis	1979
Last "imported" case of paralytic poliomyelitis to United States	1986
eIPV introduced	1987
80 cases of VAPP reported (1 case per 2.5 million doses)	1980–1989

VAPP, vaccine-associated paralytic poliomyelitis; IPV, inactivated poliovirus vaccine; OPV, oral poliovirus vaccine; eIPV, enhanced-potency IPV.

virus occurred in the same year (15); the disease continues to occur in other parts of the world. Currently, if wild poliovirus was imported into the United States, circulation of the virus in the general population would be prevented because of the high levels of immunity due to effective vaccination. There are at-risk populations in the United States that would be more susceptible because of lower rates of vaccination. These populations are found in religious communities opposed to vaccinations: there were outbreaks of poliomyelitis in a Christian Scientist school in 1972 (4) and among the Amish people in 1979 (31). An outline of the history of poliomyelitis and poliovaccines is given in Table 55.

The principal complication is vaccine-associated paralytic poliomyelitis (VAPP) (1,2,6,7,13,17,19,20,23–25,28,32–38). Those at greatest risk for VAPP are vaccinated individuals with immunodeficiencies (1,2,7,13,19,23,25,28,33–38). VAPP has not followed IPV use (24,32). Cases of VAPP are rare, with a range of 1–14 cases reported annually since 1965 (24,34) and an estimated incidence of 1 case per 2.5 million doses of vaccine distributed between 1980 and 1989 (32). Between 1980 and 1989, there were 80 cases of VAPP, no indigenous wild-virus cases, and five imported wild-virus cases reported in the United States (32). Cases of VAPP develop in three at-risk groups: infants receiving their first dose of OPV, immunologically compromised individuals receiving OPV, and unvaccinated or inadequately vaccinated persons in contact with OPV recipients (32). Immunodeficiencies associated with the development of VAPP include hypogammaglobulinemia (7,25,36–38), sex-linked agammaglobulinemia (34), human immunodeficiency virus positivity (13), ataxia-telangiectasia (28), and other less clearly defined immunodeficiencies (1,38).

Although the risk of development of VAPP is small, the development of an enhanced-potency IPV (eIPV) in 1987 (11) led to a re-evaluation of vaccine policy for the United States in 1988 (12,18). A National Academy of Sciences panel recommended consideration of a sequential eIPV/OPV vaccination schedule to reduce the risk of VAPP even further. The rationale for this recommendation was that eIPV, as the first-dose vaccine in infants (when risk of developing VAPP is highest), might confer effective immunity so that subsequent doses of OPV (the most effective vaccine for long-term immunity to poliovirus) would not result in the development of VAPP.

Epidemiological studies have addressed the safety of poliovaccines in pregnancy (8,9,26) and the occurrence of Guillain-Barré syndrome (GBS) (29). Several studies have demonstrated a complete lack of impact on fetal development and perinatal outcome (8,9,26).

A cluster of cases of GBS in southern California following a mass vaccination program using OPV and the experience with swine flu vaccine prompted epidemiological studies that failed to reveal evidence of a causal association (29).

Experimental studies suggest that enhanced neurovirulence in some individuals occurs through genomic modifications (i.e., mutations) that take place in the gastrointestinal tract (3,5,14,16,21,22,27). Viral isolation studies have also demonstrated that the CNS isolate (i.e., that causing VAPP) may not be representative of the virus isolated from stool (5). A wide variety of poliovirus-vaccine genomic structures has been implicated in the etiology of VAPP (5).

In sum, the only neurological complication of poliovirus vaccine (OPV) is VAPP. The risk is low, approximately 1 case per 2.5 million doses distributed, and may become even lower if recommendations utilizing sequential eIPV/OPV administration are enacted (see 34).

REFERENCES

1. Arya SC (1994) Vaccine-associated poliomyelitis. *Lancet* **343**, 610.
2. Davis LE, Bodian D, Price D *et al.* (1977) Chronic progressive poliomyelitis secondary to vaccination of an immunodeficient child. *N Engl J Med* **297**, 241.

3. Evans DHA, Dunn G, Minor PD *et al.* (1985) Increased neurovirulence associated with a single nucleotide change in a noncoding region of the Sabin type 3 poliovaccine genome. *Nature* **314**, 548.

4. Foote FM, Kraus G, Andrews MD, Hart JC (1973) Polio outbreak in a private school. *Conn Med* **37**, 643.

5. Georgescu M-M, Delpeyroux F, Tardy-Panit M *et al.* (1994) High diversity of poliovirus strains isolated from the central nervous system from patients with vaccine-associated paralytic poliomyelitis. *J Virol* **68**, 8089.

6. Gold R, Scheifele D, Fast M *et al.* (1991) Evaluation of poliovirus-related cases occurring in Canada in 1989. *Can Dis Wkly Rep* **17**, 75.

7. Groom SN, Clewley J, Litton PA, Brown DW (1994) Vaccine-associated poliomyelitis. *Lancet* **343**, 609.

8. Harjulehto-Mervaala T, Aro T, Hiilesmaa VK *et al.* (1993) Oral polio vaccination during pregnancy: No increase in the occurrence of congenital malformations. *Amer J Epidemiol* **138**, 407.

9. Harjulehto-Mervaala T, Aro T, Hiilesmaa VK *et al.* (1994) Oral polio vaccination during pregnancy: Lack of impact on fetal development and perinatal outcome. *Clin Infect Dis* **18**, 414.

10. Hinman AR, Koplan JP, Orenstein WA *et al.* (1988) Live or inactivated poliomyelitis vaccine: An analysis of benefits and risks. *Amer J Public Health* **78**, 291.

11. Immunization Practices Advisory Committee. Poliomyelitis prevention: Enhanced-potency inactivated poliomyelitis vaccine-supplementary statement. *Morb Mort Wkly Rep MMWR* **36**, 795.

12. Institute of Medicine. *An Evaluation of Poliomyelitis Vaccine Policy Options.* Washington, DC: National Academy of Sciences. 1988.

13. Ion-Nedelcu N, Dobrescu A, Strebel PM, Sutter RW (1994) Vaccine-associated paralytic poliomyelitis and HIV infection. *Lancet* **343**, 51.

14. Kew OM, Nottay BK, Hatch MH *et al.* (1981) Multiple genetic changes can occur in the oral poliovaccines upon replication in humans. *J Gen Virol* **56**, 337.

15. Kim-Farley RJ, Bart KJ, Schonberger LB *et al.* (1984) Poliomyelitis in the USA: Virtual elimination of disease caused by wild virus. *Lancet* **2**, 1315.

16. Lipskaya GY, Muzychenko AR, Kutitova OK *et al.* (1991) Frequent isolation of intertypic poliovirus recombinants with serotype 2 specificity from vaccine-associated polio cases. *J Med Virol* **35**, 290.

17. Mashikian MV, Stollerman GH (1994) Vaccine-associated polio: A case and its lessons. *Hosp Pract* **29**, 69.

18. McBean AM, Modlin JF (1987) Rationale for the sequential use of inactivated poliovirus vaccine and the live attenuated poliovirus vaccine for routine poliomyelitis immunization in the United States. *Pediat Infect Dis J* **6**, 881.

19. McLaughlin M, Thomas P, Oronato I *et al.* (1988) Live virus vaccines in human immunodeficiency virus-infected children: A retrospective survey. *Pediatrics* **82**, 229.

20. Mermel L, Sanchez de Mora D, Sutter RW, Pallansch MA (1993) Vaccine-associated paralytic poliomyelitis. *N Engl J Med* **329**, 810.

21. Minor PD, Dunn G (1988) The effect of sequences in the 5' non-coding region on the replication of polioviruses in the human gut. *J Gen Virol* **69**, 1091.

22. Minor PD, John A, Ferguson M, Icenogle JP (1986) Antigenic and molecular evolution of the vaccine strain of type 3 poliovirus during the period of excretion by a primary vaccine. *J Gen Virol* **67**, 693.

23. Mok JQ, Giaquinto C, DeRossi A *et al.* (1987) Infants born to mothers seropositive for human immunodeficiency virus: Preliminary findings from a multicentre European study. *Lancet* **1**, 1164.

24. Nkowane BM, Wassilak SGF, Orenstein WA *et al.* (1987) Vaccine-associated poliomyelitis. United States: 1973 through 1984. *J Amer Med Assn* **257**, 1335.

25. Onorato IM, Markowitz LE, Oxtoby MJ (1988) Childhood immunization, vaccine-preventable disease and infection with human immunodeficiency virus. *Pediat Infect Dis J* **7**, 588.

26. Ornoy A, Ben Ishai P (1993) Congenital anomalies after oral poliovirus vaccination during pregnancy. *Lancet* **341**, 1162.

27. Otelea D, Guillot S, Furione M *et al.* (1993) Genomic modifications in naturally occurring neurovirulent revertants of Sabin 1 polioviruses. *Develop Biol Standard* **78**, 33.

28. Pohl KRE, Farley JD, Jan JE, Junker AK (1992) Ataxia-telangiectasia in a child with vaccine-associated paralytic poliomyelitis. *J Pediat* **121**, 405.

29. Rantala H, Cherry JD, Shields WD, Uhari M (1994) Epidemiology of Guillain-Barré syndrome in children: Relationship of oral polio vaccine administration to occurrence. *J Pediat* **124**, 220.

30. Ruuskanen O, Salmi TT, Stenvik M, Lapinleimu K (1980) Inactivated poliovaccine: Adverse reactions and antibody responses. *Acta Paediat Scand* **69**, 397.

31. Schonberger LB, Kaplan J, Kim-Farley R *et al.* (1984) Control of paralytic poliomyelitis in the United States. *Rev Infect Dis* **6**, S424.

32. Strebel PM, Sutter RW, Cochi SL *et al.* (1992) Epidemiology of poliomyelitis in the United States one decade after the last reported case of indigenous wild virus-associated disease. *Clin Infect Dis* **14**, 568.

33. Von Reyn CF, Clements CJ, Mann JM (1987) Human immunodeficiency virus infection and routine childhood immunization. *Lancet* **2**, 669.

34. Willis E, Sherrod JL (1997) Childhood immunizations: position on the enhanced inactivated poliovirus vaccine and live attenuated oral poliovirus vaccine dilemma. *J Natl Med Assn* **89**, 785.

35. Wright PF, Hatch MH, Kasselberg AG *et al.* (1977) Vaccine-associated poliomyelitis in a child with sex-linked agammaglobulinemia. *J Pediat* **91**, 408.

36. Wyatt HV (1973) Poliomyelitis in hypogammaglobulinemics. *J Infect Dis* **128**, 802.

37. Wyatt HV (1975) Risk of live poliovirus in immunodeficient children. *J Pediat* **87**, 152.

38. Wyatt HV (1994) Vaccine-associated poliomyelitis. *Lancet* **343**, 610.

Polychlorinated Biphenyls

Herbert H. Schaumburg

POLYCHLORINATED BIPHENYLS

X = H or Cl

NEUROTOXICITY RATING

Clinical

C   Peripheral neuropathy

Experimental

A   PNS teratogen

There are potentially 209 possible polychlorinated biphenyls (PCBs), depending on the number of chlorine substitutions. Commercial PCBs range from mixtures rich in dichlorobiphenyl to technical-grade decachlorobiphenyl. Most are yellow liquids at room temperature, nonflammable, chemically and heat-stable, water-insoluble, and of high dielectric capacity (13). The production of these synthetic chemicals involves batch chlorination of biphenyl; the degree of chlorination is proportional to the contact time of the reactants (13). Commercial-grade PCBs may contain small amounts of polychlorinated dibenzofurans (PCDFs). Heating PCBs between temperatures of 200° and 600°C increases the concentration of PCDFs and polychlorinated naphthalenes (PCNs). The epidemics of neurotoxicity attributed to ingestion of rice oils contaminated with PCBs, PCNs, PCDFs, and polychloroquaterphenyls probably reflects the effects of these other polychlorinated substances (8), since neurotoxicity has not been detected in workers with high PCB exposure.

First introduced in 1930, PCB use expanded greatly in 1950–1970; 1.3 billion pounds were produced in the United States from inception until 1976, when production ceased. PCBs were widely used as heat-transfer agents, in hydraulic systems, and in transformers and capacitors. These stable chemicals are widespread in the North American environment and the food chain; many humans have persistent, lipid-associated body burdens. "Clean" PCBs (free of heat-generated impurities) have been associated with developmental delay (6,15,20,21) and CNS heterotopes in spinal roots of immature experimental animals (4). "Unclean" PCBs have been associated with peripheral neuropathy and chloracne in adults and developmental delays in their offspring (9,11,14).

PCBs are, in general, well absorbed from the gastrointestinal tract by passive diffusion across lipophilic cell membranes (16). The major structural determinant governing absorption is degree of chlorination; the greater the chlorination, the better the absorption. Dermal absorption is less efficient (15%–34%). Once absorbed, PCBs are bound to circulating lipoprotein and widely distributed, notably to liver and muscle; subsequently, levels in these tissues decline, and levels in skin and adipose tissue increase (16). Two factors primarily determine persistence and rate of metabolism: degree of chlorination (directly proportional to persistence) and orientation of chlorine substitution (diortho substitution favors persistence).

Metabolism of the lowest chlorinated biphenyl, 4-chlorobiphenyl, yields phenol and glucuronide conjugates (16). Metabolism of the higher chlorinated PCBs is less complete and poorly understood; it involves oxidative metabolism and requires both NADPH and the microsomal monooxygenase system. Since some PCBs are eliminated or metabolized more readily than others, the mixture of PCBs in the body is subject to change; in time, it may have little resemblance to the composition of the agent in the original exposure.

Systemic toxicological studies in experimental animals demonstrate considerable species variation for most organ systems; for example, subhuman primates, guinea pigs, and mink are more vulnerable to neoplasia than are dogs, rats, and rabbits (10). Highly chlorinated mixtures of PCBs produce hepatocellular adenomas and carcinomas in rats, and hepatoma in mice. Subhuman primates with prolonged exposure to some PCB mixtures develop chloracne, thickening of the meibomian glands, and characteristic gastrointestinal mucosal papillary excrescences ("simian gastropathy") (1). Avian species have a unique reaction of diffuse interstitial fluid accumulation ("chick edema disease"). Chronic exposure to PCBs or PCDFs causes depression of humoral-mediated immunity in laboratory animals; it is unclear if they affect cell-mediated immunity. Atrophy of thyroid follicles and hepatic necrosis are seen in mice exposed to high levels. Testicular atrophy occurs in several species after near-lethal exposure; it is uncertain if this is a primary effect of PCBs or secondary to weight loss.

Studies of the systemic toxicity of "clean" PCBs in humans have utilized communities of fish eaters and workers in industries with heavy potential exposure (e.g., capacitor and transformer production and maintenance). Initial claims of cardiovascular and immunological dysfunction have not been supported by subsequent studies; it now appears unlikely that such exposures are associated with serious systemic toxicity (7).

Individuals with repeated high-level exposure to PCBs, PCDFs, chlorinated naphthalenes, and dibenzodioxins from two epidemics of consumption of contaminated rice oil, yusho in Japan and yu-cheng in Taiwan, experienced serious systemic toxicity in a syndrome that included chloracne, hyperpigmentation, meibomian gland enlargement, and immune dysfunction (9,14). Distal-extremity sensory loss and slowed sensory nerve conduction velocities are described in some; this is claimed to be evidence of neuropathy (2,3,10). Neuropathy is uncertain since these studies did not feature measures of nerve impulse amplitude or nerve biopsies, and there are poor longitudinal examination data. Children born to severely affected mothers had hyperpigmentation, short stature, delayed development, and intellectual impairment. Although this illness was initially attributed to PCBs, it now appears unlikely that they played a significant role. Based on subsequent body burden and environmental analyses, most consider PCDFs to have been causal (8). Another study of a reversible peripheral neuropathy in workers exposed to PCBs in an industrial fire may also represent an effect of PCDFs, which were identified by analysis of soot (19).

Neurobehavioral effects from exposure to "clean" PCBs are described in rodents and nonhuman primates. Most of these studies focus on developmental neurotoxicity wherein PCBs are administered pre- or perinatally (15). Hyperactivity is a consistent behavioral finding in all species; some studies also report impaired memory function. Two studies of mice, whose mothers were exposed to PCBs during gestation, describe spinning and circling behavior. Especially convincing is a study that utilized a maternal oral daily dose of 32 mg/kg of pure 3,4,3',4'-tetrachlorobiphenyl for 7 days and detailed histopathological examination of tissue from 24 animals and 24 controls (4). Haloperidol administration abolished the spinning, suggesting dopaminergic dysfunction. Histopathological analysis revealed projections of cylindrical bundles of CNS tissue (axons, oligoden-droglia, and astrocytes) into ventral spinal roots and occasional ectopic anterior horn cells. The relationship, if any, between the morphological abnormalities and spinning behavior is unclear. Several perinatal rodent studies and one adult nonhuman primate study also suggest that "clean" PCBs may deplete dopamine levels in the CNS (17,18). The primate study employed lightly chlorinated PCBs and featured multiple postmortem sampling of tissue and an in vitro analysis of dopamine depletion in pheochromocytoma cell cultures.

There is no convincing case report of human neurotoxicity from "clean" PCB exposure; all inferences have been drawn from two neurobehavior-oriented, population studies of children born to women with ambient environmental exposure (15,20). Children with the highest transplacental exposure displayed hypotonia and deficits in visual-memory processing and in short-term memory. It is difficult to judge the significance of these studies because the tests employed have not been widely used to predict behavioral abnormalities in children (7). In addition, there are uncertainties about maternal health, alcohol consumption, degree of exposure, and their relationships to behavioral changes in the children (12).

There are few studies of workers exposed to "clean" PCBs; most studies that claim occupational neurotoxicity were performed on individuals imperiled in fires; these studies are confounded by the presence of PCDFs (vide supra). One study of capacitor workers demonstrated an elevated body burden and depended on a questionnaire concerning symptoms (5). This study is difficult to interpret because no control group utilized this instrument.

REFERENCES

1. Allen JR, Barsotti DA (1976) The effects of transplacental and mammary movement of PCBs on infant rhesus monkeys. Toxicology 6, 331.

2. Chia LG, Chu FL (1984) Neurological studies on polychlorinated biphenyl (PCB)-poisoned patients. Amer J Ind Med 5, 117.

3. Chia LG, Chu FL (1985) A clinical and electrophysiological study of patients with polychlorinated biphenyl poisoning. J Neurol Neurosurg Psychiat 48, 894.

4. Chou SM, Miike T, Payne WM, Davis GJ (1979) Neuropathology of "spinning syndrome" induced by prenatal intoxication with a PCB in mice. Ann N Y Acad Sci 320, 373.

5. Fishbein A, Wolff MS, Lilis R et al. (1979) Clinical findings among PCB-exposed capacitor manufacturing workers. Ann N Y Acad Sci 320, 703.

6. Jacobson JL, Jacobson SW (1996) Intellectual impairment in children exposed to polychlorinated biphenyls in utero. N Engl J Med 335, 783.

7. Kimbrough RD (1995) Polychlorinated biphenyls (PCBs) and human health: An update. *CRC Crit Rev Toxicol* **25**, 133.

8. Kunita N, Hori S, Obana H et al. (1985) Biological effects of PCBs, PCQs, and PCDFs present in the oil causing Yusho and yu-Cheng. *Environ Health Perspect* **59**, 79.

9. Kuratsune M (1989) Yusho, with reference to Yu-Cheng. In: *Halogenated Biphenyls, Terphenyls, Naphthalenes, Dibenzodioxins and Related Products*. Kimbrough RD, Jensen AA eds. Elsevier, New York p. 381.

10. McConnell EF (1989) Acute and chronic toxicity and carcinogenesis in animals. In: *Halogenated Biphenyls, Terphenyls, Naphthalenes, Dibenzodioxins and Related Products*. Kimbrough RD, Jensen AA eds. Elsevier, New York p. 161.

11. Murai Y, Kuroiwa Y (1971) Peripheral neuropathy in chlorobiphenyl poisoning. *Neurology* **21**, 1173.

12. Paneth N (1991) Human reproduction after eating PCB-contaminated fish. *Health Environ Digest* **5**, 4.

13. Rappe C, Buser HE (1989) Chemical and physical properties, analytical methods, sources and environmental levels of halogenated dibenzodioxins and dibenzofurans. In: *Halogenated Biphenyls, Terphenyls, Naphthalenes, Dibenzodioxins and Related Products*. Kimbrough RD, Jensen AA eds. Elsevier, New York p. 71.

14. Rogan WJ (1989) Yu-Cheng. In: *Halogenated Biphenyls, Terphenyls, Naphthalenes, Dibenzodioxins and Related Products*. Kimbrough RD, Jensen AA eds. Elsevier, New York p. 401.

15. Rogan WJ, Gladen BC (1992) Neurotoxicology of PCBs and related compounds. *Neurotoxicology* **13**, 27.

16. Safe S (1989) Polyhalogenated aromatics: Uptake, disposition and metabolism. In: *Halogenated Biphenyls, Terphenyls, Naphthalenes, Dibenzodioxins and Related Products*. Kimbrough RD, Jensen AA eds. Elsevier, New York p. 1131.

17. Seegal RF, Bush B, Brosch KO (1994) Decreases in dopamine concentrations in adult, nonhuman primate brain persist following removal from polychlorinated biphenyls. *Toxicology* **86**, 71.

18. Seegal RF, Bush B, Shain W (1990) Lightly chlorinated ortho-substituted PCB congeners decrease dopamine in nonhuman primate brain and in tissue culture. *Toxicol Appl Pharmacol* **106**, 136.

19. Seppäläinen AM, Vuojolahti, Elo O (1985) Reversible nerve lesions after accidental polychlorinated biphenyl exposure. *Scand J Work Environ Health* **11**, 91.

20. Tilson HA (1990) Polychlorinated biphenyls and the developing nervous system: Cross-species comparisons. *Neurotoxicol Teratol* **12**, 239.

21. Tilson HA, Kodavanti PR (1998) The neurotoxicity of polychlorinated biphenyls. *Neurotoxicology* **19**, 517.

Polymyxin

Herbert H. Schaumburg

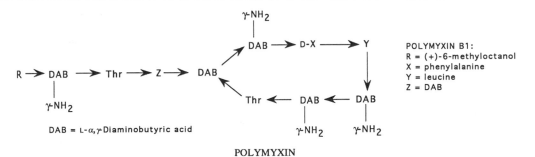

POLYMYXIN

NEUROTOXICITY RATING

Clinical

A   Neuromuscular transmission syndrome

Experimental

A   Neuromuscular transmission dysfunction (postsynaptic neuromuscular blockade)

Polymyxin B and polymyxin E (colistin) are microorganism-derived antibiotics effective against Gram-negative bacteria. Although parenteral administration is accompanied by nephrotoxicity and neurotoxicity, intravenous colistin is effective in treating acute respiratory exacerbations associated with *Pseudomonas aeruginosa* in patients with cystic fibrosis (1). Polymyxins are surface-active, amphipathic agents; they interact strongly with phospholipids. They penetrate into and disrupt the structure of cell membranes.

The polymyxins are not absorbed through mucous membranes and must be administered parenterally for a systemic antibacterial effect. With parenteral administration, polymyxins are largely unmetabolized and excreted intact in the urine. Individuals with renal compromise are especially susceptible to adverse effects. Approximately 20% of persons receiving conventional doses of polymyxin develop renal dysfunction (2). Azotemia or rising creatinine levels are universal in all experiencing nephrotoxicity. In most instances, blood urea nitrogen and creatine levels gradually return to normal if polymyxin is promptly discontinued. Six percent of patients have developed acute tubular necrosis, which may be fatal. Topical polymixin therapy is unaccompanied by serious systemic toxicity.

Transient facial and limb paresthesias of unknown pathogenesis frequently accompany polymyxin therapy (2). There are rare reports of polymyxin-induced acute gait ataxia, with poor position sense in the lower limbs, in patients with pre-existing renal compromise. The ataxia can be incapacitating; it appears within a few days of commencement of conventional therapy and gradually improves following drug withdrawal (5). Ataxia has not been accompanied by signs of cerebellar dysfunction (nystagmus, dysarthria, limb tremor), and it is possible that sensory impairment in the lower limbs has a role in this curious syndrome.

The most serious neurotoxic effect of polymyxin is impaired neuromuscular transmission. Limited experimental animal studies indicate that polymyxin has its most prominent effect on the postsynaptic membrane of the neuromuscular junction (4); this effect is nondepolarizing and noncompetitive. There is also slight presynaptic inhibition of transmitter release that is partially reversible by calcium chloride.

Neuromuscular blockade occurs in 2% of patients receiving polymyxins (2). This effect is more potent than the neuromuscular blockade from the aminoglycoside antibiotics, and polymyxin blockade is not reversed by neostigmine or calcium chloride. The usual clinical manifestation of polymyxin blockade is apnea; this suddenly appears after only 1 or 2 days of conventional therapy. It is more common in older individuals and in patients with pre-existing renal insufficiency; this probably reflects high peak blood concentrations of the drug. Other manifestations of neuromuscular blockade (diplopia, ptosis, and limb fatigue) may accompany respiratory compromise. Polymyxin therapy is absolutely contraindicated in individuals with myasthenia gravis. In one series of 11 patients with polymyxin-induced apnea, all required ventilatory support and then gradually recovered within 5 days of drug withdrawal (3).

REFERENCES
1. Conway SP, Pond MN, Watson A (1997) Intravenous colistin sulphomethate in acute respiratory exacerbations in adult patients with cystic fibrosis. *Thorax* **52**, 987.
2. Koch-Weser J, Sidel VW, Federman EB *et al.* (1970) Adverse effects of sodium colistimethate. Manifestations and specific reaction rates during 317 courses of therapy. *Ann Intern Med* **72**, 857.
3. Linswanith LA, Baines RD Jr, Bigelow DB *et al.* (1968) Reversible respiratory paralysis associated with polymyxin therapy. *Ann Intern Med* **68**, 318.
4. Viswanath DV, Jenkins HJ (1978) Neuromuscular block of the polymyxin group of antibiotics. *J Pharm Sci* **67**, 1275.
5. Wolinsky E, Hines JD (1962) Neurotoxic and nephrotoxic effects of colistin in patients with renal disease. *N Engl J Med* **266**, 759.

Poneratoxin

Tom Piek

```
Phe — Leu — Pro — Leu — Leu

Ile — Leu — Gly — Ser — Leu

Leu — Met — Thr — Pro — Pro

Val — Ile — Gln — Ala — Ile

His — Asp — Ala — Gln — Arg-NH2
```

PONERATOXIN
$C_{129}H_{215}N_{33}O_{31}S_1$

NEUROTOXICITY RATING
Clinical
B   Tremor

Experimental

A   Ion channel dysfunction (sodium ion channel)

Poneratoxin (PoTX) is a potent neurotoxin present in the venom of a ponerine ant, *Paraponera clavata*, a resident of Central and South America (4,3). PoTX is an amidated polypeptide containing 25 amino-acid residues (4,3); the peptide has been synthesized (3). Most ant species that use venoms for defense and killing prey belong to the subfamilies Myrmicinae and Ponerinae, including *Paraponera clavata*. Envenomation by *P. clavata* causes pain and uncontrollable tremor in man; the tremor is not caused by pain alone (7). Used in some local Indian rituals to test manhood, the ants were placed inside woven fiber cylinders into which young marriage-seeking men placed their hands to demonstrate their ability to withstand pain (2).

At concentrations from 10^{-8}–10^{-6} M, synthetic PoTX is a strong agonist for smooth muscles. A dose of twenty-five μg of venom of *P. clavata* dissolved in 25 μl added dropwise to a cascade of mammalian smooth muscle preparations caused these muscles to contract slowly and reversibly. PoTX also blocks synaptic transmission in the insect in a concentration-dependent manner; it depolarizes cockroach giant interneurons (3), and affects electrical activity of isolated cockroach axons, as well as isolated frog and rat skeletal muscle fibers (3). In frog skeletal muscle fibers, PoTX induces a concentration-dependent (10^{-9}– 5×10^{-6} M) prolongation of action potentials and, at saturating concentrations, a slow repetitive activity developing at negative potentials (1).

PoTX specifically acts on voltage-dependent Na^+ channels by decreasing the peak current of normal fast sodium channels (I_{Na}) and by simultaneously inducing a slow I_{Na}, which starts to activate at -85 mV and inactivates very slowly. It is suggested that PoTX affects all Na^+ channels and that fast and slow I_{Na} components originate from a possible PoTX-induced interconversion between a fast and a slow operative mode of Na^+ channels (1).

The mechanism of action of PoTX differs from that of other modifiers of Na^+ channel currents like batrachotoxin, ciguatoxin, and a number of well-known α- and β-scorpion toxins. Therefore, PoTX has a specific mechanism, different from those earlier reported for other natural toxins known to affect Na^+ channel function (1).

While controlled studies of PoTX have yet to be performed, there are data concerning the lethal capacity of the crude venom of the ant *P. clavata*. Crude venom also contains a small amount of kinin (5) and a moderate amount of phospholipase A (6). For mice, the LD_{50} of the venom is 6.0 mg/kg (6). Since the average content of the venom reservoir of *P. clavata* is 180 μg, the lethal capacity (expressed as the number of stings for a LD_{50} dose) predictably will be 0.8 μg for a 25-g mammal and 67 μg for a 2-kg mammal (6). Since the colony size of *P. clavata* is estimated to be several hundred, it is clear that a colony of this ant species would be unable to kill an adult human.

Editors' Note: Actions of *P. clavata* venom on adenosine triphosphatase activity in bovine heart mitochondria are also reported (8).

REFERENCES
1. Duval A, Malécot CO, Pelhate M, Piek T (1992) Poneratoxin, a new toxin from an ant venom, reveals interconversion between two gating modes of the Na channels in frog muscle fibres. *Eur J Physiol* **420**, 239.
2. Lange A (1914) *The Lower Amazon*. Putnam Press, New York.
3. Piek T, Duval A, Hue B *et al.* (1991) Poneratoxin, a novel peptide neurotoxin from the venom of the ant, *Paraponera clavata*. *Comp Biochem Physiol* **99**, 487.
4. Piek T, Hue B, Mantel P *et al.* (1991) Pharmacological characterization and chemical fractionation of the venoms of the ponerine ant *Paraponera clavata* (F). *Comp Biochem Physiol* **99**, 481.
5. Piek T, Schmidt JO, de Jong JM, Mantel P (1989) Kinins in ant venoms—a comparison with venoms of related *Hymenoptera*. *Comp Biochem Physiol* **92**, 117.
6. Schmidt JO, Blum MS, Overal WL (1980) Comparative lethality of venoms from stinging *Hymenoptera*. *Toxicon* **18**, 469.
7. Schmidt JO, Blum MS, Overal WL (1984) Hemolytic activities of stinging insect venoms. *Arch Insect Biochem Physiol* **1**, 155.
8. Zaitseva LG, Zaitsev VG, Feniuk BA (1995) Protein composition of venoms from several species of tropical ants and their effect on mitochondrial H^+-ATPase. *Bioorg Khim* **21**, 563. [Russian]

Praziquantel

Steven A. Sparr

PRAZIQUANTEL
$C_{19}H_{24}N_2O_2$

2-(Cyclohexylcarbonyl)-1,2,3,6,7,11b-hexahydro-4*H*-pyrazino[2,1-*a*]isoquinolin-4-one

NEUROTOXICITY RATING
Clinical

B   Encephalomalacia (neurocysticercosis)

Praziquantel is a pyrazinoisoquinoline derivative with anthelmintic activity for a wide variety of cestodes and trematodes. The compound, a mixture of L- and D-isomers, was initially introduced as a veterinary cesticidal drug and has subsequently been shown to have activity against many human helminth parasites, including trematodes (flukes), including all species of *Schistosoma* (9), liver flukes *Clonorchis sinensis* and *Opisthorchis viverrini*, lung flukes *Paragonimus westermani*, and several intestinal flukes; and cestodes (flatworms) including *Taenia saginata* (beef tapeworm), *Taenia solium* (pork tapeworm), and *Diphyllobothrium latum* (fish tapeworm) (20). The drug is ineffective against nematodes (roundworm) and limited in its effectiveness against *Echinococcus*. It has been widely used for treatment of CNS cysticercosis, which is caused by the larval form of *T. solium*, although its role in treating this disorder has been controversial (4,22); albendazole may be more effective (7,16,18).

The anthelmintic activity of praziquantel is twofold: (a) by inducing muscle contraction with paralysis, the organism releases its attachment to the host, and (b) by causing direct toxic damage (vacuolization of the organism) and a host response. These mechanisms may be mediated by influx of Ca^{2+} and other ions (20).

Praziquantel is usually well tolerated, although transient headache, nausea, vomiting, or abdominal pain are frequent side effects. The primary neurological toxicity is a CNS inflammatory reaction after treatment of brain cysticercosis; this ranges from headache and fever to papilledema, seizures, and focal neurological signs. A single case of vasculitic brain infarction has been reported in a patient receiving praziquantel for cysticercosis (24).

Praziquantel is readily absorbed after oral dosing, with plasma concentration peaking 1–2 h after ingestion. The drug is rapidly metabolized by the liver to inactive metabolites, so that serum half-life is only 1.2 h; metabolites are eliminated in the urine over a 24-h period (20). Bioavailability is decreased by coadministration of steroids (21) or some anticonvulsants (3), and is increased by cimetidine (13,15). Animal studies suggest the L-isomer is the more active component (26).

Dosing for most indications is 25–75 mg/kg/day for 1–2 days, often requiring only a single dose for many helminthic infestations. Prolonged treatment at low dosage (50 mg/kg/day for 15 days) is recommended for CNS cysticercosis (4), although higher doses for shorter periods (100 mg/kg/day for 10 days) may be as effective (2). A regimen of three doses of 25 mg/kg given in a single day has also been proposed (6).

Animal experiments have demonstrated a LD_{50} of approximately 2500 mg/kg for mice, while doses of 120 mg/kg showed no toxic effects (26). There is no animal model of CNS cysticercosis in which toxicity of praziquantel can be studied.

Few neurological side effects have been seen with treatment of helminth infestations outside of the CNS. In a large clinical series performed in Egypt, 3026 patients were treated for schistosomiasis with a single dose of 40 mg/kg praziquantel. Side effects were rare and included dizziness that was short-lived and resolved over 24–48 h (9). About 25% of the patients complained of headache after treatment; this was statistically significant when compared with baseline symptoms prior to treatment. Another study of 204 patients in Egypt treated for schistosomiasis found that when the dose of praziquantel was increased from 40 mg/kg single dose to 20 mg/kg twice daily for 3 days, the incidence of headache rose dramatically from 23% to 61% (10). In a very large Chinese clinical study involving 25,693 patients treated for schistosomiasis with praziquantel ranging from 45–120 mg/kg given over 1–6 days, serious side effects were encountered in <1% of patients: one case of transient ataxia, five cases of psychosis lasting up to 6 months, and eight cases of seizure—all in patients with known seizure disorders (14). Given the large population involved in the study, it is difficult to attribute these disorders to praziquantel treatment; however, another report describes a Spanish patient with epilepsy who had been seizure-free for 7 years and who developed seizures 12 h after receiving praziquantel for schistosomiasis (1).

Major neurological toxicity has been confined to patients treated for CNS cysticercosis. Similar side effects have not been seen in patients treated for CNS schistosomiasis with a single dose of 60 mg/kg (23). A "cerebrospinal fluid reaction" characterized by headache, meningeal signs, focal neurological signs, and seizures is nearly universally seen with praziquantel treatment of CNS cysticercosis (5,17) and may be delayed up to 2 weeks after treatment (5,12,25). Risk of this reaction may be proportional to the burden of cysts present in the brain (8). As the cerebrospinal fluid reaction is likely due to host inflammatory responses to dying organisms, the reaction may be prevented by simultaneous administration of corticosteroids (5,7). However, as steroids may lower the efficacy of praziquantel by lowering its serum level (21), some have suggested reserving steroids for cases with severe intracranial hypertension, while using nonsteroidal anti-inflammatory agents and anticonvulsants for milder reactions (8). Patients treated with praziquantel for other indications may have unrecognized CNS cysticercosis with resultant precipitation of headache or seizures after treatment (11,19).

There is one case report of cerebral infarction concomitant with praziquantel treatment of CNS cysticercosis (24). This patient developed aphasia and right hemiparesis during treatment; a left frontal infarction was evident on serial computed axial tomography. The authors attributed the infarction to inflammatory vasculitis brought on by host responses to cyst destruction.

REFERENCES

1. Bada JL, Trevino B, Carbezos J (1988) Convulsive seizures after treatment with praziquantel. *Brit Med J* **296**, 646.
2. Bittencourt PRM, Gracia CM, Gorz AM *et al.* (1990) High-dose praziquantel for neurocysticercosis: Efficacy and tolerability. *Eur Neurol* **30**, 229.
3. Bittencourt PRM, Gracia CM, Martins R *et al.* (1992) Phenytoin and carbamazepine decrease oral bioavailability of praziquantel. *Neurology* **42**, 492.
4. Carpio A, Santillam F, Leon P *et al.* (1995) Is the course of neurocysticercosis modified by treatment with antihelminthic agents? *Arch Intern Med* **155**, 1982.
5. Ciferri F (1988) Delayed CSF reaction to praziquantel. *Lancet* **1**, 642.
6. Corona C, Lugo R, Medina R, Sotelo J (1996) Single-day praziquantel therapy for neurocysticercosis. *N Engl J Med* **334**, 125.
7. Cruz I, Cruz M, Horton J (1991) Albendazole versus praziquantel in the treatment of cerebral cysticercosis: Clinical evaluation. *Trans Roy Soc Trop Med Hyg* **85**, 244.
8. Del Brutto OH (1988) Delayed CSF reaction to praziquantel. *Lancet* **1**, 341.
9. El-Alamy MA, Habib MA, McNeely DF, Cline BL (1981) Preliminary results of chemotherapy on a large scale in Qalyub bilharziasis project where simultaneous infection with *S. mansoni* and *S. haematobium* exists. *Arzneim-Forsch-Drug Res* **31**, 612.
10. el-Masry NA, Bassily S, Farid Z (1988) A comparison of the efficacy and side effects of various regimens of praziquantel for the treatment of schistosomiasis. *Trans Roy Soc Trop Med Hyg* **82**, 719.
11. Flisser A, Madrazo I, Plancarte A (1993) Neurological symptoms in occult neurocysticercosis after single taeniacidal dose of praziquantel. *Lancet* **342**, 748.
12. Markwalder K, Hess K, Valvanis A, Witassek F (1989) Cerebral cysticercosis: Treatment with praziquantel: Report of 2 cases. *Amer J Trop Med Hyg* **33**, 273.
13. Metwally A, Bennett JL, Botros S, Ebeid F (1995) Effect of cimetidine, bicarbonate and glucose on the bioavailability of different formulations of praziquantel. *Arzneimforsch* **45**, 516.
14. Minggang C, Sui F, Xiangjin H, Huimin W (1983) A prospective survey on side effects of praziquantel among 25,693 cases of *Schistosomiasis japonica*. *SE Asian J Trop Med Publ Health* **14**, 495.
15. Overbosch D (1992) Neurocysticercosis. An introduction with special emphasis on new developments in pharmacotherapy. *Schweiz Med Wochenschr* **122**, 893.
16. Sotelo J, del Brutto OH, Penagos P *et al.* (1990) Comparison of the therapeutic regimen of anticysticercal drugs on parenchymal brain cysticercosis. *J Neurol* **237**, 69.
17. Sotelo J, Escobedo F, Rodriguez-Cabajal J *et al.* (1984) Therapy of parenchymal brain cysticercosis with praziquantel. *N Engl J Med* **310**, 1001.
18. Takayanagui OM, Jardim E (1992) Therapy for neurocysticercosis. Comparison between albendazole and praziquantel. *Arch Neurol* **49**, 290.
19. Torres JR (1989) Use of praziquantel in populations at risk of neurocysticercosis. *Rev Inst Med Trop* **31**, 290.
20. Tracy JW, Webster LT (1996) Drugs used in chemotherapy of helminthiasis, In: *Goodman and Gilman's The Pharmacological Basis of Therapeutics.* 9th Ed. Hardman JG, Limbird LE eds. McGraw-Hill, New York p. 1009.
21. Vasquez ML, Jung H, Sotelo J (1987) Plasma levels of praziquantel decrease when dexamethasone is given simultaneously. *Neurology* **37**, 1561.
22. Vazquez V, Sotelo J (1992) The course of seizures after treatment for cerebral cysticercosis. *N Engl J Med* **327**, 696.
23. Watt G, Long GW, Ranoa CP *et al.* (1986) Praziquantel in treatment of cerebral schistosomiasis. *Lancet* **2**, 529.
24. Woo E, Yu YL, Huang CY (1988) Cerebral infarct precipitated by praziquantel in neurocysticercosis—a cautionary note. *Trop Geograph Med* **40**, 143.
25. Worthington M, Horowitz H (1987) Case 11. *N Engl J Med* **316**, 693.
26. Yue-han L, Qian M, Wang X *et al.* (1993) Levopraziquantel versus praziquantel in experimental and clinical treatment of *Schistosomiasis japonica*. *Chin Med J* **106**, 593.

n-Propanol

Peter S. Spencer

$$CH_3-CH_2-CH_2OH$$

n-PROPANOL

$$C_3H_8O$$

NEUROTOXICITY RATING

Experimental

A   Neuroteratogen

n-Propanol (1-propanol, propyl alcohol) is a colorless solvent with a sweet, alcoholic odor; it has a vapor pressure of 14.5 mm at 20°C. While the substance has a low order of acute toxicity in animals, congenital malformations (including microcephaly) are reported in the offspring of dams treated 7 h/day on days 1 and 19 of gestation with >5000 ppm *n*-propanol, *n*-butanol, or isopropanol (2) (*see also* page 697, this volume). It has been suggested that muscarinic receptor-stimulated phosphoinositide metabolism is a common neurochemical target for the developmental neurotoxicity of short-chain alcohols (1).

REFERENCES

1. Candura SM, Balduini W, Costa LG (1991) Interaction of short chain aliphatic alcohols with muscarinic receptor-stimulated phosphoinositide metabolism in cerebral cortex from neonatal and adult rats. *Neurotoxicology* **12**, 23.
2. Nelson BK, Brightwell WS, Krieg EF Jr (1990) Developmental toxicology of industrial alcohols: a summary of 13 alcohols administered by inhalation to rats. *Toxicol Ind Health* **6**, 373.

Propranolol and Other β-Adrenergic Receptor Antagonists

Steven A. Sparr

PROPRANOLOL
$C_{16}H_{21}NO_2$

1-[(1-Methylethyl)amino]-3-(1-naphthalenyloxy)-2-propanol

NEUROTOXICITY RATING
Clinical

A Tremor (pindolol)

A Acute encephalopathy (headache, fatigue, sleep disturbances)

B Psychological reaction (hallucination, depression)

Propranolol is the prototype of a class of drugs that blocks adrenergic stimulation of β-adrenergic receptors in various organs of the body. The discovery of α- and β-adrenergic receptors in the 1950s was followed by the development of drugs to modulate the activity of the adrenergic system on these receptors (14). The first drug of this class to gain widespread clinical use was propranolol in the 1960s (14). Since then, numerous β-adrenergic blockers ("β-blockers") have been developed; they differ in their relative selectivity for receptor subtypes, partial-agonist properties, lipid solubility, and membrane-stabilizing properties (19). These pharmacological profiles influence both drug efficacy and side effects (14,19).

β-Blockers are used to treat a wide variety of conditions such as ischemic heart disease, hypertension, cardiac arrhythmia, migraine, essential tremor, pheochromocytoma, thyrotoxicosis, and anxiety states (14,21). As a class, β-blockers are usually well tolerated, with incidence of toxicity estimated at 10%–20% (19). Although most toxic reactions are mild, β-blockers can have serious cardiovascular, pulmonary, and neurological side effects that limit their use in some patients. Careful selection of agents and close monitoring of patients are mandatory (19).

Propranolol, the prototype of this class of drug, nonselectively blocks both β₁- and β₂-receptors and has no agonist activity (14). Other drugs in the class, such as atenolol and metaprolol, are more potent β₁-receptor blockers and thus purported to be more "cardioselective" (14). However, in higher doses, the relative specificity for β₁-receptors is lost (19). Other agents, such as pindolol, demonstrate β-agonist properties and cause stimulation of the β-adrenergic system even in the absence of catecholamines (19). Labetalol not only blocks β-receptors but also has α₁-receptor-blocking effects (19). The drugs differ widely in their lipid solubility, an important factor in the ability of the drug to cross the blood-brain barrier and have direct effects on the CNS (20). A recently developed β-blocker, sotalol, has quinidine-like membrane-stabilizing effects useful in the treatment of ventricular arrhythmias (19). Selection of the appropriate β-blocker in clinical practice is further complicated by the fact that theoretical predictions of the effects and toxicities, based on known pharmacological properties of each drug, are often not well correlated with clinical experience (19).

Propranolol can be administered orally and by intravenous injection. Oral doses are well absorbed from the gastrointestinal tract, with peak plasma concentrations occurring within 60–90 min of ingestion (21). Extended-release preparations with prolonged absorption times are also available. There is extensive first-pass metabolism in the liver, so that only ~25% of the ingested drug reaches the systemic circulation (14). The drug is 90% bound to plasma proteins and has wide distribution to body tissues, including the brain (14). Propranolol is metabolized in the liver to metabolites, some of which have β-blocking activity but short half-lives (21). The half-life of the parent drug is approximately 2–3 h after a single dose, and 3–6 h with chronic administration (21).

β-Blockers that are highly lipid-soluble, such as propranolol, exhibit complete gastrointestinal absorption, are metabolized chiefly by the liver, are highly protein-bound in the plasma, and are widely distributed throughout body tissues including to the CNS (20). β-Blockers that are highly water-soluble, such as atenolol and sotalol, have less absorption from the gastrointestinal tract, are excreted unchanged by the kidneys, are less bound by plasma proteins, and penetrate poorly into the CNS (20). Cerebrospinal fluid and plasma concentrations of lipophilic β-blockers are similar, and are much higher in the brain parenchyma (e.g., brain/plasma ratio of 26 for propranolol), whereas spinal fluid and brain concentrations are much lower than plasma levels of hydrophilic agents (e.g., brain/plasma ratio of 0.2 for atenolol) (23).

As β-adrenergic receptors are present in many different body tissues, the clinical effects of β-blockade are complex. In the heart, blocking β-receptors (chiefly β_1, but also β_2) causes slowing of heart rate and negative inotropic effects on cardiac muscle (14). Sinus rate is diminished, and there is slowing of conduction through the atrioventricular node (14). Propranolol may have membrane-stabilizing effects apart from its β-blocking action; this may account for some activity in suppressing ventricular arrhythmia (14). Propranolol blocks catecholamine-induced release of renin from the juxtaglomerular apparatus in the kidneys and may account for some of the drug's antihypertensive effects (14). Propranolol can cause vasoconstriction due to unopposed α-adrenergic activity in arterial smooth muscle; however, with chronic administration, propranolol reduces peripheral vascular resistance by unknown mechanisms. Proposed mechanisms include α-receptor blockade, β-receptor agonist effects, and CNS effects (14). In the bronchial tree, bronchoconstriction results from blockade of β_2-receptors (14). In addition to blocking the effects of cathecholamines on peripheral organs, propranolol may also block release of norepinephrine by acting on β-receptors on presynaptic sympathetic nerve terminals (14). The clinical effects of β-blockade on the brain are poorly understood.

The major nonneurologic side effects of β-blockers are cardiovascular, including hypotension, bradycardia, complete heart block, and congestive heart failure, all readily predictable from the pharmacology of the drug (21). Abrupt cessation of propranolol can precipitate a syndrome of autonomic hyperactivity with anxiety, tachycardia, sweating, and exacerbation of angina (21). Propranolol can precipitate peripheral vascular disease with worsening claudication and even development of gangrene (21), although several studies have found no such correlation (19). Patients may develop Raynaud's symptomatology during treatment with propranolol, and the drug can exacerbate bronchospastic lung disease (21). Other nonneurologic side effects are rare.

Neurological toxicity, usually mild, is common with use of propranolol and other β-blockers, although there are no animal models of direct CNS neurotoxicity.

The most common side effect of propranolol is fatigue, occurring in about 20% of patients (19,20). The mechanism is unclear and may be due to several factors, such as reduced cardiac output, diminished blood supply to skeletal muscles, direct effects on skeletal muscle contractility (especially fast-twitch fibers), and possible CNS effects (19).

A review of the CNS side effects of β-blockers describes depression, dizziness, headache, memory impairment, hallucinations, sleep disturbances, and psychomotor slowing (20). This study considered four drugs: propranolol, pindolol, metoprolol, and atenolol, which vary in their lipid solubility, receptor selectivity, and receptor agonist properties. The goal was to determine if there is a relationship between the degree of lipid solubility of the various β-blockers and their potential for CNS toxicity. In all, 276 published reports and clinical series were reviewed. The incidence of possible CNS toxicity was found to be low, but drugs of high lipid solubility, such as propranolol and pindolol, were more frequently implicated in CNS side effects than those, such as atenolol, which are highly water soluble (20).

The magnitude and nature of direct CNS effects of the β-blockers have been controversial, as is the relationship to lipid solubility. Numerous studies have attempted to elucidate these effects (6). A controlled double-blind study of normal volunteers found similar electroencephalographic changes, including diminution of wakeful α activity, with both propranolol and atenolol (5,24). Another study found impaired performance on a battery of psychomotor and visual tasks in normal volunteers given atenolol (28). These studies suggest that the hydrophilic drug atenolol may have significant CNS effects; however, other reports describe no difference from placebo in performance on 22 items of a neuropsychological battery in volunteers given atenolol or propranolol, with the exception of increased reaction time with propranolol (15,17,25). Since motor-response impairment may be attributed to effects on skeletal muscle, there may be little evidence for CNS toxicity with β-blockers.

A comprehensive review of 55 published studies on the effects of β-blockers on cognitive tests divided neuropsychological tests into four general categories: perceptual/motor, memory, abstraction, and learning (6). Impairment of functioning was documented in 16% of observations, improvement of function in 17%, and no significant effect in the remainder. There was no consistent relationship with drug lipid solubility for any of these measures. Other than subjective feelings of sedation and fatigue, no consistent evidence implicated CNS impairment by β-blockers.

Various forms of sleep disturbance have been reported with β-blockers. Polysomnography testing of 30 volunteers treated with atenolol, metoprolol, propranolol, or pindolol revealed that the lipophilic agents, but not the hydrophilic agents, caused a significant incidence of sleep disturbances (15). These included subjective complaints of restless sleep and an increase in the number of nocturnal awakenings on polysomnography. Only pinolol affected sleep architecture with increased rapid-eye-movement (REM) latency and decreased total time spent in REM sleep. Nightmares were experienced by patients with all β-blockers studied. These effects on sleep were attributed by the authors to possible effects of β-blockers on central adrenergic or serotonergic pathways. Similar effects were described in ten female volunteers treated with atenolol, propranolol, metoprolol, and pindolol: early awakenings, increased dreaming (especially with pindolol), and subjective symptoms of restless sleep (4). Only atenolol did not differ from placebo in these parameters. Hypnopompic and hypnogogic visual hallucinations occurred in 17% of patients treated with propranolol in a hypertension clinic (9). These hallucinations were devoid of color, but vivid in content, and often recurred. Only one study found no increased incidence in symptoms of sleep disturbance or nightmares in 165 hypertensive women taking β-blockers when compared with patients taking other classes of antihypertensive drugs, or compared with the population-at-large (3).

There are several case reports of toxic delerium or psychosis associated with β-blocker therapy (10,12,16,22, 30,32). The patients described in these reports developed confusion, auditory hallucinations, and agitation. In general, symptoms abated within 1–2 days of discontinuing the medication. However, the relationship of the medication to the mental side effects is not clear in several of these reports. Most patients had concurrent illnesses (that may have had effects on the sensorium) such as thyrotoxicosis (32), right hemispheric stroke (22), lymphoma with ill-defined lesion on computed tomography (12), and premorbid schizoid personality (30) although, in some reports (10,16) no such condition was evident. Many of these patients developed symptoms months to years after tolerating therapy with β-blockers, making the relationship between their symptoms and medication tenuous.

Depression has been associated with use of β-blockers (21,27,29,31). In one case, a 35-year-old hypertensive man developed depression and suicidal ideation 2 days after initiating nadalol therapy (27); symptoms abated with cessation of the drug. A review of medications prescribed in one prescription drug plan found a 4.8-fold increase in the use of antidepressant medications in patients treated with β-blockers in general, and even higher incidence in those on propranolol (31). One study reports no significant incidence of depression in a series of 25 patients treated with atenolol and nifedipine in a double-blind crossover trial (29).

Although β-blockers are frequently used as a prophylac-

tic agent for migraine, there are case reports of precipitation of migraine and other forms of headache in patients treated with these agents (1,2,13,26). A review of 10,506 reports to the World Health Organization Collaboration Centre describes possible drug-induced headaches (1). There were approximately 400 cases of headache associated with β-blockers (atenolol, metoprolol, and propranolol) and 20 reports of migraine associated with atenolol. A case report is illustrative: a 70-year-old woman with a history of migraine that had been quiescent for almost 40 years developed headache and photophobia 3 days after beginning propranolol for angina (26). Symptoms resolved with drug discontinuation. When later rechallenged in a placebo-controlled double-blind fashion, her headaches recurred with propranolol but not with placebo.

There are case reports of patients with migraine who had strokes while on β-blocker therapy (2,11), but with widespread use of these agents and an incidence of stroke of 1% in migraineurs, chance association cannot be excluded.

One individual developed diplopia while taking propranolol and oxprenolol due to medication error; this resolved with discontinuation of propranolol (34). Twenty-four instances of diplopia reported to the Committee on Safety of Medications could have been induced by various β-blockers. In four, symptoms recurred with rechallenge; in three, symptoms responded to decreased dosage of the β-blocker; one patient had myasthenia gravis. Another report describes a 55-year-old woman who developed diplopia 45 days after commencing antihypertensive therapy with labetolol (18). Symptoms responded to neostigmine, and neuromuscular blockade was confirmed by repetitive-stimulation electromyography. The patient was found to have thymic hyperplasia. Diplopia abated within 36 h of discontinuing labetalol. These putative side effects of β-blockade were attributed to direct effects of the drugs on the neuromuscular junction where they may have a curare-like effect in inhibiting postsynaptic acetylcholine receptors (18) or some other membrane-stabilizing effect on muscle cells (24).

Other possible neurological side effects of β-blockers are rare and have been described in reports of single cases or of small series. Hand tremors may be caused by pidolol (13). Tremors affect both hands, are fine in amplitude, appear in 1–3 days after initiating treatment, and cease 1–3 days after discontinuing medication. Pindolol differs from other β-blockers in its strong agonist properties, which may precipitate tremors due to sympathetic stimulation.

There is one report of three patients who developed carpal tunnel syndrome after 8–11 years of therapy with propranolol or metoprolol (7). Symptoms were bilateral in one, unilateral in two, and abated 6–10 weeks after cessation of therapy. Given the large number of patients on β-blockers in the population, and the high prevalence of carpal tunnel syndrome, a causal association is unproven.

Myotonia appeared in a 20-year-old woman who developed stiffness in her hands while on propranolol for migraine (33). Symptoms ceased 2 months after discontinuing the medication and recurred with rechallenge. There was insufficient evidence by history of muscle biopsy to make the diagnosis of myotonic dystrophy in this patient, but the authors speculated that propranolol may unmask a clinically silent muscle abnormality.

A 43-year-old man developed hearing loss after switching from propranolol to metoprolol (8). Hearing improved during the months following drug discontinuation. Tinnitus and hearing loss, noted in 36 patients treated with β-blockers, had previously reported to the British Committee on the Safety of Medications. The mechanism underlying drug-induced hearing loss in unknown.

REFERENCES

1. Ashmark H, Lundber P, Olsson S (1989) Drug related headache. *Headache* **29**, 441.
2. Bardwell A, Trott JA (1987) Stroke in migraine as a consequence of propranolol. *Headache* **27**, 381.
3. Bengtsson C, Lennartsson J, Linquist O *et al.* (1980) Sleep disturbance, nightmares and other possible central nervous disturbances in a population sample of women, with special reference to those on antihypertensive drugs. *Eur J Clin Pharmacol* **17**, 173.
4. Betts TA, Alford C (1985) Beta-blockers and sleep: A controlled trial. *Eur J Clin Pharmacol* **28**, Suppl 65–8.
5. Currie D, Lewis RV, McDevitt DG *et al.* (1988) Central effects of β-adrenoceptor antagonists. I. Performance and subjective assessments of mood. *Brit J Clin Pharmacol* **26**, 121.
6. Dimsdale JE, Newton RP, Joist T (1989) Neuropsychological side effects of β-blockers. *Arch Intern Med* **149**, 514.
7. Emara MK, Saadah AM (1988) The carpal tunnel syndrome in hypertensive patients treated with β-blockers. *Postgrad Med J* **64**, 191.
8. Faldt R, Liedholm H, Aursnes J (1984) β Blockers and loss of hearing. *Brit Med J* **289**, 1490.
9. Fleminger R (1978) Visual hallucinations and illusions with propranolol. *Brit Med J* **1**, 1182.
10. Gershon ES, Goldstein RE, Moss AJ, Kammen DP (1979) Psychosis with ordinary doses of propranolol. *Ann Intern Med* **90**, 928.
11. Gilbert GJ (1982) The occurrence of complicated migraine during propranolol therapy. *Headache* **22**, 81.
12. Helson L (1978) Acute brain syndrome after propranolol. *Lancet* **1**, 98.
13. Hod H, Kaplinsky N, Har-Zahav J, Frankl O (1980) Pindolol-induced tremor. *Postgrad Med J* **56**, 346.
14. Hoffman BB, Lefkowitz RJ (1996) Catecholamines, sympathomimetic drugs, and adrenergic receptor antagonists. In: *The Pharmacologic Basis of Therapeutics. 9th Ed.* Hardman JG, Goodman AG, Limbird LE eds. McGraw-Hill, New York p. 199.
15. Kostis JB, Rosen RC (1987) Central nervous system effects of β-adrenergic-blocking drugs: The role of ancillary properties. *Circulation* **75**, 204.
16. Kurland ML (1970) Organic brain syndrome with propranolol. *N Engl J Med* **300**, 366.
17. Landauer AA, Pocock DA, Prott FW (1979) Effects of atenolol and propranolol on human performance and subjective feeling. *Pscyhopharmacology* **60**, 211.
18. Leys D, Pasquier F, Vermersch P *et al.* (1987) Possible revelation of latent myasthenia gravis by labetolol chlorhyrate. *Acta Clin Belg* **42**, 475.
19. MacDonald TM, McDevitt DG (1992) Antianginal and β-adrenoceptor blocking drugs: In: *Meyler's Side Effects of Drugs. 12 Ed.* Dukes MNG ed. Elsevier, Amsterdam BV p. 431.
20. McAinsh J, Cruickshank JM (1990) β-Blockers and central nervous system side effect. *Pharmacol Ther* **46**, 163.
21. McEvoy GK (1995) *American Hospital Formulary Service Drug Information.* American Society of Health System Pharmacists, p. 1123.
22. McGahan DJ, Wojslaw A, Prasad V, Blanjkenship S (1984) Propranolol-induced psychosis. *Drug Intell Clin Pharm* **18**, 601.
23. Neil-Dwyer G, Bartlett J, McAinsh J, Cruickshank JM (1981) β-Adrenoceptor blockers and the blood-brain barrier. *Brit J Clin Pharmacol* **11**, 549.
24. Nicholson AN, Wright NA, Zeitlin MB *et al.* (1988) Central effects of β-adrenoceptor antagonists. II. Electroencephalogram and body sway. *Brit J Clin Pharmacol* **26**, 129.
25. Ogle CW, Turner P, Markomihelakis H (1976) The effects of high doses of oxprenolol and of propranolol on pursuit rotor performance, reaction time and critical flicker fusion. *Psychopharmacologia* **46**, 295.
26. Robson RH (1977) Recurrent migraine after propranolol. *Brit Heart J* **39**, 1157.
27. Russell JW, Schuckit MA (1982) Anxiety and depression in patient on nadolol. *Lancet* **2**, 1286.
28. Salem SA, DcDevitt DG (1983) Central effects of β-adrenoceptor antagonists. *Clin Pharmacol Ther* **33**, 52.
29. Skinner MH, Futterman A, Morrissette D *et al.* (1992) Atenolol compared with nifedipine: Effect on cognitive function and mood in elderly hypertensive patients. *Ann Intern Med* **116**, 615.
30. Steinert J, Pugh CR (1979) Two patients with schizophrenic-like psychosis after treatment with β-adrenergic blockers. *Brit Med J* **1**, 790.
31. Thiessen BQ, Wallace SM, Blackburn JL *et al.* (1990) Increased prescribing of antidepressants subsequent to β-blocker therapy. *Arch Intern Med* **150**, 2286.
32. Topliss D, Bond R (1977) Acute brain syndrome after propranolol treatment. *Lancet* **2**, 1133.
33. Turkewitz LJ, Sahgal VS, Spiro A (1984) Propranolol-induced myotonia. *Mt Sinai J Med* **51**, 207.
34. Weber JCP (1982) β-Adrenoceptor antagonists and diplopia. *Lancet* **2**, 826.

Propylene Glycol

Brent T. Burton

$$CH_3CHCH_2$$
$$|\quad |$$
$$OH\ OH$$

PROPYLENE GLYCOL
$C_3H_8O_2$

1,2-Propanediol

NEUROTOXICITY RATING

Clinical

B   Seizure disorder

B   Acute encephalopathy (sedation, confusion, coma)

Propylene glycol, a clear, colorless, odorless, viscous liquid with a MW of 76.09, is a solvent used in many industrial, cosmetic, and pharmaceutical applications. Numerous injectable medications contain propylene glycol as a preservative (17) and account for many of the reported adverse affects. Propylene glycol has been used as a topical solution in concentrations of 40%–60% for the treatment of ichthyosis (9) and is available in some over-the-counter moisturizing lotions. Industrial uses include incorporation into antifreeze, hydraulic fluids, plasticizers, and resins (6). Propylene glycol is also added to some foods as a moistening agent or preservative (16). Some pet foods contain up to 13% propylene glycol as a source of calories (3). Its daily acceptable intake as a food additive is estimated to be 25 mg/kg (19).

Propylene glycol is rapidly absorbed following oral ingestion and peaks within 1 h of administration (20). The volume of distribution is ~ 0.6 l/kg (20). It is metabolized to pyruvic acid, acetic acid, lactic acid, and propionaldehyde (13). Approximately 12%–45% is excreted as the parent compound into urine, primarily as the glucuronide conjugate (16). The half-life is ~ 2.4–5.2 h in adults (20) but considerably longer, 10.8–30.5 h, in infants (7).

The oral LD_{50} for propylene glycol is ~ 20–30 ml/kg for rats and 20 ml/kg for dogs. Drinking water containing up to 10% propylene glycol produced no demonstrable effects on rats treated for 24 weeks (16). The intravenous LD_{50} for rats is 13 ml/kg (16). An atmosphere saturated with propylene glycol produced no evidence of measurable physiological effects in rats exposed for periods of 12–18 months (15). One study found that daily intraperitoneal injections of 4 ml/kg to rats for 3 days resulted in increased liver microsomal metabolism of aniline and p-nitroanisole and no change in cytochrome P-450 activity (4). "Large doses" of propylene glycol administered to animals resulted in dysequilibrium, depression, analgesia, coma, and death (16).

Acute accidental oral ingestion of propylene glycol by humans is generally considered relatively innocuous. In contrast, rapid injection of medications containing propylene glycol may produce hypotension, bradycardia, hemolysis, and possible cardiac arrest. Patients with underlying renal failure may develop lactic acidosis following topical, oral, or intravenous administration (2,5,10). Patients receiving propylene glycol may develop a hyperosmolality syndrome due to high propylene glycol blood levels. It produces minor skin irritation but has a low potential for sensitization (18).

CNS depression is considered to be the most prominent consequence of propylene glycol overdose and is manifest by effects such as drowsiness, dysarthria, and confusion, similar to those seen with ethanol overdose. Oral doses of 1.5 g/kg used in the treatment of glaucoma have caused dizziness in adults (8). An infant was reported to develop recurrent episodes of CNS depression while receiving daily doses of ascorbic acid suspended in 7.5 ml of propylene glycol. The mechanism of CNS depression was attributed to hypoglycemia that was documented by blood glucose levels of 41 and 42 mg/dl (12). Propylene glycol intoxication has also been suspected in patients receiving oral solutions of phenytoin with propylene glycol. In one investigation, patients were assessed as their own controls in a crossover study while taking phenytoin without propylene glycol during which time CNS depression was reportedly absent (20). However, the dosage of propylene glycol in this study was relatively high, namely at 20.7 g every 8 h or 41.4 g every 12 h.

Generalized seizures have been reported following relatively large doses of propylene glycol. After more than 1 year of taking dihydrotachysterol dissolved in propylene glycol with alcohol for "candidiasis-endocrinopathy syndrome with hypoparathyroidism," an 11-year-old boy was reported to have experienced a generalized seizure (1). Neonates receiving 3 g/day of propylene glycol contained in an intravenous multivitamin solution have been reported to have a higher incidence of seizures than infants receiving 300 mg/day of propylene glycol (11).

Though probably more a direct injury, rather than a primary neurotoxic effect, instillation of propylene glycol into the middle ear of patients with tympanostomy tubes results in cochlear toxicity (14).

REFERENCES

1. Arulanantham K, Genel M 1978) Central nervous system toxicity associated with ingestion of propylene glycol. *J Pediat* 93, 515.

2. Cate JC, Hedrick R (1980) Propylene glycol intoxication and lactic acidosis. *N Engl J Med* **303**, 1237.

3. Christopher MM, Perman V, Eaton JW (1989) Contribution of propylene glycol-induced Heinz body formation to enemia in cats. *J Amer Vet Med Assn* **194**, 1045.

4. Dean ME, Stock BH (1974) Propylene glycol as a drug solvent in the study of hepatic microsomal metabolism in the rat. *Toxicol Appl Pharmacol* **28**, 44.

5. Demey H, Daelemans R, De Broe ME *et al.* (1984) Propylene glycol intoxication due to intravenous nitroglycerin. *Lancet* **1**, 1360.

6. Fisher AA (1978) Propylene glycol dermatitis. *Curtis* **21**, 166.

7. Glasgow AM, Boeckx RL, Miller MK *et al.* (1983) Hyperosmolality in small infants due to propylene glycol. *Pediatrics* **72**, 353.

8. Goldsmith LA (1978) Propylene glycol. *Int J Dermatol* **17**, 703.

9. Goldsmith LA, Baden HP (1972) Propylene glycol with occlusion for treatment of ichthyosis. *J Amer Med Assn* **220**, 579.

10. Kelner MJ, Bailey DN (1985) Propylene glycol as a cause of lactic acidosis. *J Anal Toxicol* **9**, 40.

11. MacDonald MG, Getson PR, Glasgow AM *et al.* (1987) Propylene glycol: Increased incidence of seizures in low birth weight infants. *Pediatrics* **79**, 622.

12. Martin G, Finberg L (1970) Propylene glycol: A potentially toxic vehicle in liquid dosage form. *J Pediat* **77**, 877.

13. Miller DN, Bazzano G (1965) Propanediol metabolism and its relation to lactic acid metabolism. *Ann N Y Acad Sci* **119**, 957.

14. Morizono T, Paparella MM, Juhn SK (1980) Ototoxicity of propylene glycol in experimental animals. *Amer J Otolaryngol* **1**, 393.

15. Robertson OH, Loosli CG, Puck TT *et al.* (1947) Tests for the chronic toxicity of propylene glycol and triethylene glycol on monkeys and rats by vapor inhalation and oral administration. *J Pharmacol Exp Ther* **91**, 52.

16. Ruddick JA (1972) Toxicology, metabolism, and biochemistry of 1,2-propanediol. *Toxicol Appl Pharmacol* **21**, 102.

17. Smolinske SC, Vandenberg SA, Spoerke DG *et al.* (1987) Propylene glycol content of parenteral medications. *Vet Hum Toxicol* **29**, 491. [Abstract]

18. Shmunes E (1990) *Solvents and Plasticizers in Occupational Skin Disease. 2nd Ed.* Adams RM ed. WB Saunders Co, Philadelphia.

19. WHO (1974) Toxicological evaluation of certain food additives with a review of general principles and of specifications. *17th Report of the Joint FAO/WHO Expert Committee on Food Additives, Technical Report Series, No 539.* World Health Organization, Geneva.

20. Yu DK, Elmquist WF, Sawchuk RJ (1985) Pharmacokinetics of propylene glycol in humans during multiple dosing regimens. *J Pharm Sci* **74**, 876.

Pseudomonas Toxins

Albert C. Ludolph

NEUROTOXICITY RATING

Experimental

A   G-protein system

A   Peptide elongation

Pseudomonas toxins are products of the gram-negative bacteria *Pseudomonas aeruginosa* (2). Opportunistic infections produced by these bacteria are difficult to control, since they are resistant to a number of commonly used antibiotics. *P. aeruginosa* produces a large number of compounds (2) that contribute to the pathogenesis of the infection. Exotoxin A is a valuable experimental tool in cellular neurobiology (1).

The heat-labile *P. aeruginosa* exotoxin (MW, 66,853 Da) has a structure similar to those of pertussis toxin (*Bordetella pertussis*), cholera toxin (*Vibrio cholerae*), and the heat-labile toxin of *Escherichia coli* (2,3). It is characterized by a two-component A-B structure with three domains: domain I binds to receptors of the cell surface, domain III carries the enzymatic activity, and domain II presumably translocates domain III to the cytosol. The exotoxin has effects on intracellular signaling pathways, specifically on guanine nucleotide-binding proteins (G proteins), and by its adenosine diphosphate–ribosyltransferase activity. Like diphtheria toxin, the molecule binds to a receptor of the target cell, enters the cell by endocytosis, and is then translocated across the membranes of intracellular organelles. Exotoxin A inhibits synthesis of cellular proteins by blocking polypeptide chain elongation; this results from enzymatic inactivation of elongation factor 2.

After injection into mice, the primary target of the toxin is the liver; under physiological circumstances, pseudomonas toxins will not cross the blood-brain barrier. Like cholera and pertussis toxins, pseudomonas exotoxin A and other toxins produced by these bacteria are not known to have neurotoxic potential.

REFERENCES

1. Gierschik P, Jakobs KH (1992) ADP-ribosylation of signal-transducing guanine nucleotide binding proteins by cholera and pertussis toxin. In: *Handbook of Experimental Pharmacology. Vol 102. Selective Neurotoxicity.* Herken H, Hucho F eds. Springer Verlag, Berlin, Heidelberg, New York p. 808.

2. Iglewski BH (1988) Pseudomonas toxins. In: *Handbook of Natural Neurotoxins. Vol 4. Bacterial Toxins.* Tu AT ed. Marcel Dekker, New York p. 249.

3. Liu PV (1966) The roles of various fractions of *Pseudomonas aeruginosa* in its pathogenesis. III. Identity of the lethal toxin produced *in vitro* and *in vivo. J Infect Dis* 1328, 514.

Psilocybin and Psilocin

John C.M. Brust

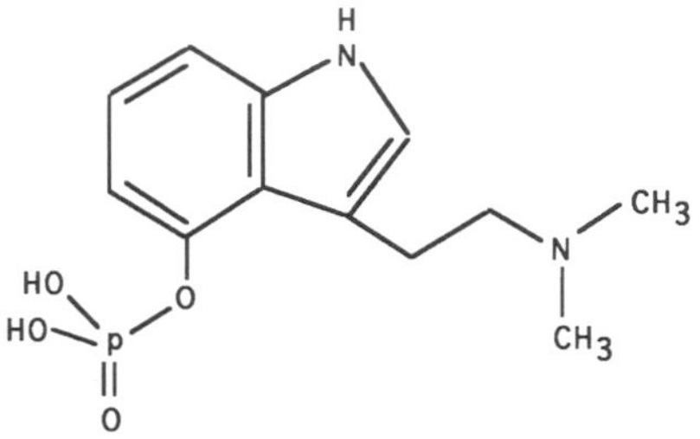

PSILOCYBIN
$C_{12}H_{17}N_2O_4P$

3-[2-(Dimethylamino)ethyl]-1*H*-indol-4-ol dihydrogen phosphate ester

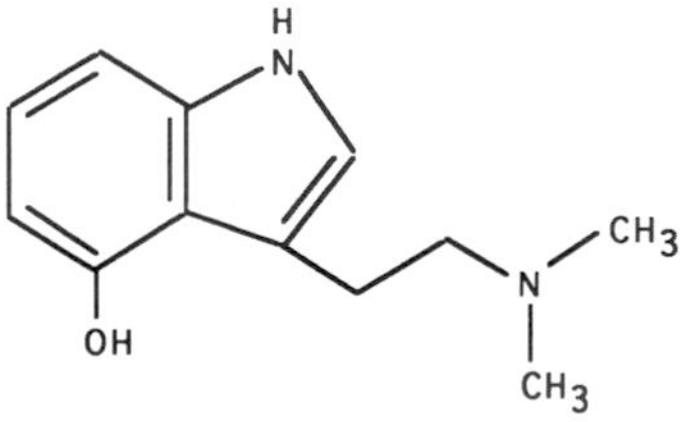

PSILOCIN
$C_{12}H_{16}N_2O$

3-[2-(Dimethylamino)ethyl]-1*H*-indol-4-ol

NEUROTOXICITY RATING

Clinical

A   Acute encephalopathy

A   Psychobiological reaction (anxiety, euphoria, hallucinations, paranoia, seizures)

C   Chronic encephalopathy

Experimental

A   Serotonin receptor blockade

Psilocybin and psilocin are indolealkylamines present in Central American *Psilocybe* species of mushrooms and in *Panaeolus* mushroom species of the United States (3,4). For thousands of years, Mexican Native Americans have eaten *Psilocybe* mushrooms ritualistically for their hallucinatory

and psychedelic ("mind-revealing") properties. In the United States during the 1980s, recreational use of mushrooms became popular among adolescents (1). A survey of American college students revealed that 15% had used mushrooms compared to only 5% who had used D-lysergic acid diethylamide (LSD) (7). A survey in California found that psilocybin-containing mushrooms had been used by 3.4% of seventh graders and 8.8% of eleventh graders (6). Mail-order catalogues directed toward the drug culture advertise spores of various psilocybin- and psilocin-containing species that can be grown at home (3). Both *Psilocybe* and *Panaeolus* species are used to induce hallucinatory effects (1,3,5). Mushrooms are usually dried or frozen; cooking does not destroy the psychoactive compounds.

Psilocybin is classified by the U.S. Food and Drug Administration as a Schedule I drug ("high potential for abuse, no accepted medical use").

Studies with animals and humans show that psilocybin and psilocin produce behavioral and psychic effects indistinguishable from those caused by LSD and mescaline. The mechanism of action of LSD, mescaline, psilocybin, and psilocin is mainly if not exclusively through agonism or partial agonism at serotonin receptors, especially the 5-HT$_2$ and 5-HT$_{1C}$ types. In drug discrimination studies, animals generalize from psilocybin to LSD and mescaline but not to amphetamine. Animals do not self-inject psilocybin. They display cross-tolerance between psilocybin, LSD, and mescaline, and abstinence following prolonged psilocybin exposure does not lead to discernable withdrawal signs.

In most people, two to six mushrooms produce psychic symptoms, but there is much variability. Agitation and hallucinations have followed ten mushrooms, yet gastritis without psychic effect has followed 200. Some users have experienced anticholinergic effects or seizures. Psilocybin is less potent than LSD; 150–200 μg of psilocybin are equivalent to 1 μg of LSD. Its hallucinogenic effects begin sooner after injection—about 30 min for psilocybin compared to

60–90 min for LSD; otherwise, even experienced users cannot tell them apart. Within minutes of ingestion, there are mild somatic symptoms and either euphoria or anxiety; illusions emerge, progressing to unformed and then formed hallucinations; subjective time is slowed, and there is depersonalization, derealization, and a sense of mystical profundity; elation may alternate with paranoia, and panic reactions occur unpredictably. There may be fever, hypertension, tachycardia, piloerection, and mydriasis. Symptoms wane over several hours. Intoxication has resulted in ataxia, seizures, and fatal accidents, but fatal overdose has not been documented. Tolerance develops to the effects of psilocybin, with cross-tolerance to LSD and mescaline. There is no withdrawal syndrome. Reports of prolonged psychosis or subtle cognitive abnormalities after LSD use (8) raise the possibility of lasting neurobehavioral changes in abusers of psilocybin and psilocin; the causal relationship of LSD to such abnormalities remains uncertain, however, and with psilocybin and psilocin it is entirely theoretical.

Pure psilocybin or psilocin has not emerged as a street drug. Intravenous injection of psilocybe mushroom extract produced chills, fever, dyspnea, vomiting, myalgia, weakness, and methemoglobinemia (2).

Psilocybin and psilocin exert striking CNS toxicity by mechanisms similar, if not identical, to LSD and mescaline. Permanent CNS damage has not been documented.

REFERENCES

1. Brust JCM (1993) *Neurological Aspects of Substance Abuse.* Butterworth-Heinemann, Stoneham, Massachusetts p. 149.
2. Curry SC, Rose MC (1985) Intravenous mushroom poisoning. *Ann Emerg Med* 14, 900.
3. Goldfrank LR, Kulberg AG, Bresnitz EA (1990) Mushrooms: Toxic and hallucinogenic. In: *Toxicologic Emergencies. 4th Ed.* Goldfrank LR, Flomenbaum NE, Lewin NA *et al.* eds. Appleton & Lange, Norwalk, Connecticut p. 575.
4. Hatfield GM, Brady LR (1975) Toxins of higher fungi. *Lloydia* 38, 36.
5. Jaffe JH (1990) Drug addiction and drug abuse. In: *The Pharmacological Basis of Therapeutics. 8th Ed.* Gilman AG, Rall TW, Nies AS, Taylor P eds. Pergamon Press, New York p. 522.
6. Schwartz RH, Smith DE (1988) Hallucinogenic mushrooms. *Clin Pediat* 27, 70.
7. Thompson JP, Anglin MD, Emboden W *et al.* (1985) Mushroom use by college students. *J Drug Educ* 25, 111.
8. Vardy MM, Kay SR (1983) LSD psychosis or LSD-induced schizophrenia? *Arch Gen Psychiat* 40, 877.

Pteridium aquilinum

Albert C. Ludolph
Peter S. Spencer

Bracken

NEUROTOXICITY RATING

Clinical

A Tremor (horses)

Experimental

A Polioencephalopathy

Bracken fern (*Pteridium aquilinum*) is a plant (family Polydodiaceae) containing thiaminase I; this enzyme causes thiamine and thiamine diphosphate depletion. Ingestion of the fern by livestock causes significant neurotoxicity, which is dependent on plant part, season, maturity of the plant, and rainfall. Apart from its antithiaminase activity, bracken fern also contains pterosin Z (a smooth muscle relaxant), tannin, quercetin, shikimic acid, prunasin, ptaquiloside, and kaemferol (10,11). Some of these substances are carcinogens (8,10); their human effects are unkown (2,9,12).

Bracken fern neurotoxicity is related to its antithiaminase activity. Thiamine (vitamin B_1) in the form of its diphosphate is a coenzyme of the mitochondrial pyruvate and α-ketoglutarate dehydrogenase enzyme complexes, which decarboxylate the corresponding α-keto acids. Thiamine deficiency leads to an increase of blood pyruvate and lactate. The enzyme transketolase that catalyzes several reactions of the pentose pathway is also thiamine-dependent. In thiamine deficiency, the activity of transketolase is used as a specific test for diagnosis.

Horses fed bracken-fern hay develop signs of poisoning (4); clinical and biochemical responses are typical of thiamine deficiency. Autoclaving the fern prevents the toxic effect, which is characterized by cardiotoxicity and neurotoxicity; the latter includes tremor and seizures. In experimental pigs, cardiotoxicity is prominent. Prior parenteral administration of vitamin B_1 in horses and pigs (5,7) prevents toxicity. The etiology of polioencephalomalacia (cerebrocortical necrosis) in ruminants has also been associated with intake of thiaminase-containing plants, including *P. esculentum* (1,3,5,6). Human neurotoxicity of bracken fern is not described (2,9,12).

REFERENCES

1. Bakker HJ, Dickson, J, Steele P, Nottle MC (1980) Experimental induction of ovine polioencephalomalacia. *Vet Rec* **107**, 464.

2. Caldwell ME, Brewer WR (1980) Possible hazards of eating bracken fern. *N Engl J Med* **303**, 164.

3. Chick BF, Caroll SN, Kennedy C, McCleary BV (1981) Some biochemical features of an outbreak of polioencephalomalacia in sheep. *Aust Vet J* **57**, 251.

4. Evans ETR, Evans WC, Roberts HE (1951) Studies on bracken poisoning in the horse. *Brit Vet J* **107**, 364.

5. Evans WC (1975) Thiaminases and their effects on animals. *Vita Hormone* **33**, 467.

6. Evans WC, Evans IA, Humphreys DJ *et al.* (1975) Induction of thiamine deficiency in sheep, with lesions similar to cerebrocortical necrosis. *J Comp Pathol* **85**, 253.

7. Evans WC, Widdop B, Harding JD (1972) Experimental poisoning by bracken rhizomes in pigs. *Vet Rec* **90**, 471.

8. Hirono I (1986) Human carcinogenic risk in the use of the bracken fern diet. In: *Nutrition and Cancer*. Japan Sci Soc Press, Tokyo p. 139.

9. Hodgson ES (1991) Is bracken a health hazard? *Lancet* **337**, 493.

10. Hopkins NCG (1986) Aetiology of enzootic hematuria. *Vet Rec* **118**, 715.

11. Sheridan H, Frankish N, Farrell R (1999) Smooth muscle relaxant activity of pterosin Z and related compounds. *Planta Med* **65**, 271.

12. Trotter WR (1990) Is bracken a health hazard? *Lancet* **336**, 1563.

Pyrethroids

Henk P.M. Vijverberg

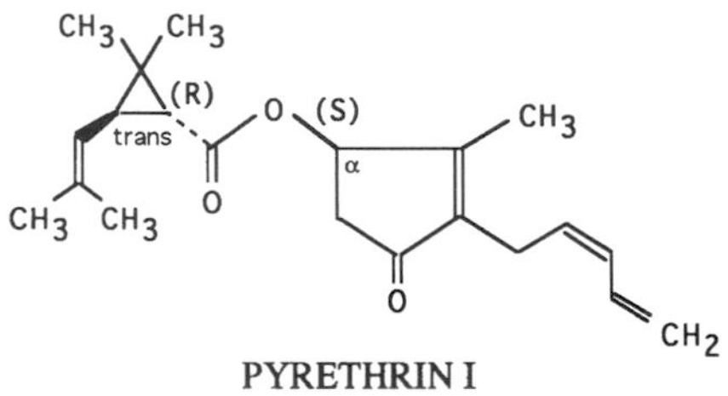

PYRETHRIN I
$C_{21}H_{28}O_3$

[1R-[1α]S*(Z)],3β]]-2,2-Dimethyl-3-(2-methyl-1-propenyl) cyclopropanecarboxylic acid 2-methyl-4-oxo-3-(2,4-pentadienyl)-2-cyclopenten-1-yl ester

NEUROTOXICITY RATING

Clinical

A   Ion channel syndrome (paresthesia)

A   Seizure disorder

Experimental

A   Ion channel dysfunction (sodium channel agent—types I & II)

A   GABA receptor inhibitor (type II)

A   Tremor

A   Extrapyramidal dysfunction (choreoathetosis—type II)

Pyrethroids are derived from the natural pyrethrins, the insecticidal ingredients of pyrethrum flowers (*Chrysanthemum* spp.) (82). Early synthetic pyrethroid insecticides,

[*e.g.*, allethrin (112)], resemble pyrethrin I, a major constituent of the natural pyrethrins. Pyrethrins and most pyrethroids are esters with an acid moiety derived from or sterically resembling chrysanthemic acid, and an aromatic alcohol moiety. However, the structure of some synthetic pyrethroids is only remotely related to that of the natural pyrethrins. Chemical structures of some of the current pyrethroid insecticides are shown in Figure 29. Activity and stability of pyrethroids have been greatly enhanced by the halogenation of the isobutenyl side chain of chrysanthemic acid, and by the introduction of novel alcohol moieties, in particular the 3-phenoxy-benzyl alcohol. Pyrethroids containing an α-cyano-substituted 3-phenoxybenzyl alcohol moiety are commonly referred to as α-cyano or type II pyrethroids. Virtually all pyrethroids are chiral molecules; up to 16 isomers of a single compound may be distinguished. With few exceptions, technical pyrethroids are mixtures of several active and several inactive isomers. Some products are enriched in specific isomer content, and this is generally indicated by a prefix to the common name [*e.g.*, bioallethrin (1R,*trans*,αS-allethrin); β-cyfluthrin, λ-cyhalothrin, α-methrin (1:1 mixtures of active 1R,*cis*,αS and inactive 1S,*cis*,αR enantiomers of cyfluthrin, cyhalothrin, and cypermethrin, respectively); and esfenvalerate (2S,αS fenvalerate)].

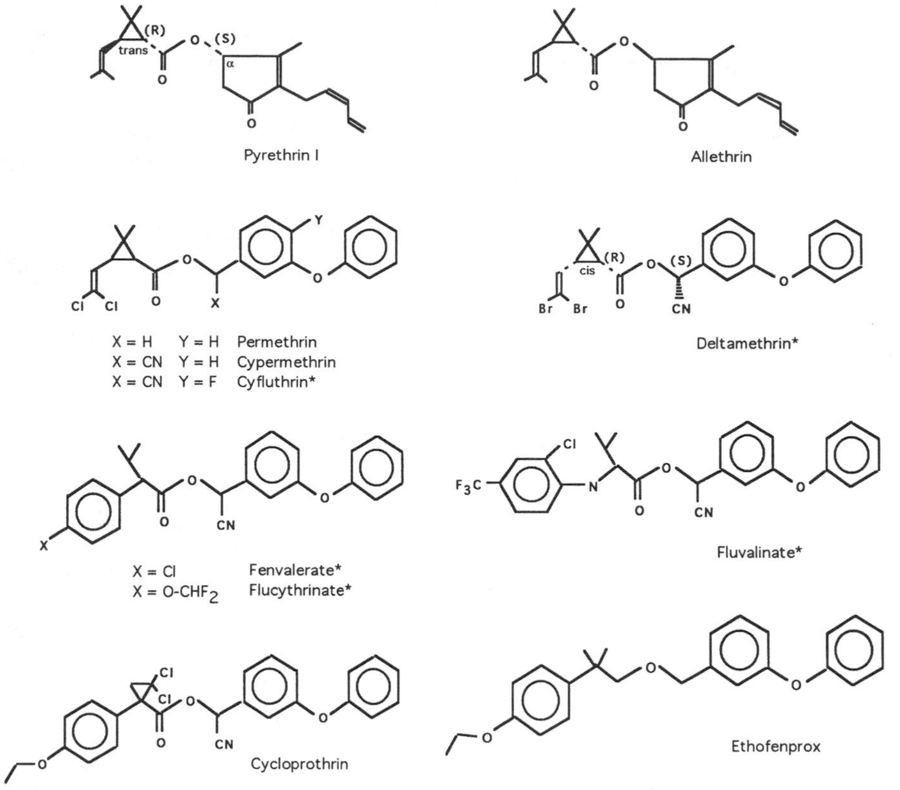

FIGURE 29. Chemical structure of the natural pyrethrin I, allethrin, the first synthetic pyrethroid insecticide, and a number of more recently developed phenoxybenzyl pyrethroids. Pyrethrin I and deltamethrin are synthesized as single enantiomers and ethofenprox is a nonchiral molecule. All other compounds are isomer mixtures. *α-Cyanopyrethroids (type II pyrethroids).

The few dozen pyrethroids that have found widespread use as insecticides comprise several compounds that are among the most potent insecticides known. Despite the high insecticidal potency, the mammalian toxicity of the pyrethroids is generally lower than that of other classes of insecticides (36,87).

Pure pyrethroids are viscous liquids or crystalline solids at room temperature. Pyrethroids are poorly soluble or insoluble in water. Their octanol/water partition coefficients ($\log P_{oct}$ values) range between 4 and 9. Most of the pyrethroids have a low vapor pressure. In the environment, pyrethroids readily adsorb to organic material and soil. The natural pyrethrins and early, nonhalogenated pyrethroids are rapidly inactivated in the environment under the influence of ultraviolet (UV) light and air (87). Halogenated pyrethroids with the phenoxybenzyl alcohol appear more stable, particularly in the indoor environment. After indoor spraying, significant residues of these pyrethroids remain on surfaces and in dust for periods of at least several months (142,152). The half-lives of permethrin and deltamethrin in impregnated mosquito nets are 1 and 2 months, respectively, (153). Commercial formulations of pyrethroid insecticides generally contain a variety of substances, which may include antioxidants, ultraviolet absorbers, dyes, propellants, organic solvents, emulsifiers, inorganic carrier particles, and metabolic inhibitors as synergists (87). Differences in formulation and isomer content of pyrethroids are generally associated with differences in toxic properties (77), and the ingredients added in commercial formulations of pyrethroids may contribute to toxicity (147).

Pyrethroids are widely used as agricultural and household insecticides and, for specific purposes, in animal and human health care. In large-scale field applications, these insecticides are employed to combat a variety of pests in crop protection. In the domestic environment, pyrethroids are applied as insecticides and as insect repellents either by spraying, evaporation (mosquito coils), surface treatment, or impregnation (mosquito nets, clothing, wood preservation). In addition, pyrethrin- and pyrethroid-containing preparations are applied dermally to cure and prevent various ectoparasitical infections in animals and man.

For airborne occupational exposure to pyrethroids, the 8-h Time-Weighted Average Threshold Limit Value (TWA/TLV) as determined by the American Conference of Government Industrial Hygienists in 1987 is 5 mg/m³. The same TWA/TLV value and a maximum limit of 25 mg/m³ have been adopted by the Health and Safety Directorate of the Commission of the European Community. Short-Term (30 min) Exposure Limit values of 10–50 mg/m³ are imposed by several countries. Recommended Acceptable Daily Intake values are 0.01–0.05 mg/kg body weight for the various pyrethroid insecticides (32).

General Toxicology

Intestinal absorption of pyrethroids varies considerably. In rodents, oral doses of some pyrethroids (*e.g.*, bioresmethrin, cismethrin, and terallethrin) are virtually completely absorbed. For various other pyrethroids, a fraction of the oral dose has been reported to remain unchanged on passage through the intestinal tract; for example *cis*-permethrin 3%, *trans*-permethrin 6%, tetramethrin 16%, and various α-cyano pyrethroids, including cypermethrin and fluvalinate, up to 50% (reviewed in 74). Incomplete absorption of oral doses of cypermethrin and fluvalinate, similar to that in the rat, has been reported in man and rhesus monkey, respectively (30,98,149). Estimated half-times of intestinal absorption of permethrin are 0.9 h for a corn oil solution given to rats (9) and 3 h for an Emulphor/ethanol emulsion in water administered to mice (3).

Percutaneous absorption of pyrethroids is less than intestinal absorption but also appears to vary. In the rat, 8%–17% of phenothrin, applied as a dust formulation to the skin, is absorbed over a 24-h period with an estimated half-time of 10 h. When applied as an emulsifiable concentrate, two to three times less phenothrin is absorbed with a half-time of 2–3 h (67). In rats treated dermally with acetone solutions of *trans*- and *cis*-permethrin, 43%–46% of the dose is absorbed within 24 h (116). In mice, anomalous high (39% in 1 h) and rapid (6 min half-time) absorption of permethrin, applied as an acetone solution to the skin, has been reported (114). In rhesus monkeys, percutaneous absorption of *trans*- and *cis*-permethrin, applied as an acetone solution, is less than that in rats and amounts to 5%–12% and 14%–28% within 24 h for the forearm and forehead, respectively (116). In human volunteers, absorption of pyrethrin from a formulation used to treat head lice has been investigated. Within 30 min, 1.9% of the dose is absorbed through the skin on the forearm. Based on known relative percutaneous absorption rates, this value extrapolates to 7.5% for the skin on the scalp (144). Only 1%–2% of cypermethrin, mixed with surfactants and wetting agents and diluted in soy bean oil, is absorbed through the back skin of human volunteers over an 8-h period (149).

Absorbed pyrethroids are rapidly distributed throughout the body. Within 1 min after intravenous administration of a toxic dose to rats, the plasma level of deltamethrin is reduced by a factor of 2, and small amounts of the pyrethroid are present in every tissue examined, including brain, sciatic nerve, liver, kidney, muscle, salivary glands, and fat (52,53). The non–cyano pyrethroids cismethrin and bioresmethrin also rapidly partition into rat tissues (51). Brain levels attain maximum values within the first minutes following injection and subsequently decline with a biphasic time course. Steady-state distribution volumes estimated from the kinetics of tetramethrin (117) and permethrin (9) in rats also indicate extensive partitioning of the pyrethroids in tissues. At late times after dosing, the main residues of pyrethroids are found in fat. In nervous tissue, partitioning into myelin may occur (53).

The pyrethrins and pyrethroids are rapidly metabolized in the mammalian liver (74). The major mechanisms are cleavage of the ester bond, and hydroxylation and oxidation of alkyl and aromatic carbon atoms (Figure 30). Ester cleavage results in effective detoxification (145). Either hydrolytic or oxidative metabolism may predominate; this depends on the structure and stereochemistry of the pyrethroid molecule and on animal species. In rat liver, hydrolysis is the major metabolic process for *trans*-substituted cyclopropane carboxylates, but oxidation occurs as well. The *cis*-isomers as well as pyrethroids with a secondary alcohol moiety (*e.g*, pyrethrin I, allethrin, and α-cyano pyrethroids) are hydrolyzed at much slower rates and are mainly metabolized through oxidation. Hydrolysis of *cis*- and *trans*-permethrin by rat and mouse liver involves several microsomal carboxylesterases with distinct substrate specificity and inhibitor sensitivity (119). It has been suggested that oxidative metabolism also contributes to ester cleavage (23). Cyanide ions are rapidly released from ester cleavage products of α-cyano pyrethroids and are mainly converted into thiocyanate (22,110). Metabolism of pyrethroids lacking the cyclopropane ring (*e.g.*, fenvalerate and fluvalinate) appears to be governed by the same two basic mechanisms that operate at comparable rates as with other pyrethroids (68,99). Data on the mammalian metabolism of pyrethroids lacking the ester bond are not available. Enterohepatic circulation may occur with some pyrethroids [*e.g.*, resmethrin, proparthrin (83), and *trans*-tetramethrin (117)], but significant biliary excretion is not observed with cypermethrin (22). Although some metabolism of pyrethroids may occur in tissue compartments other than liver (*e.g.*, blood, stomach, kidney, and brain), the contribution of metabolism in these tissues to the detoxification of pyrethroids *in vivo* is generally considered to be marginal (47,53,109,110,145).

Hydrolysis of pyrethroids has been demonstrated in all mammalian species tested thus far, but the efficacy and the stereoselectivity of hydrolytic enzymes appears to vary

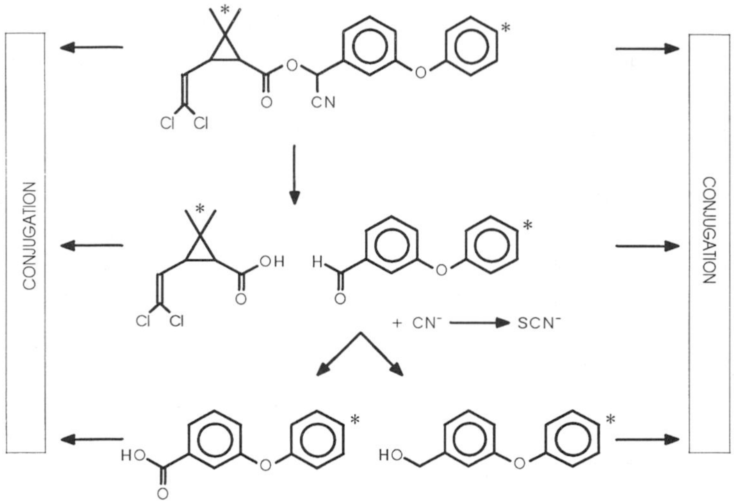

FIGURE 30. Major metabolic pathways of pyrethroid insecticides. Ester cleavage may occur as a result of hydrolysis or oxidation. The α-cyano-phenoxybenzyl-aldehyde rapidly releases a cyanide ion that is converted into thiocyanate, and the remaining aldehyde is further oxidized or reduced. Hydroxylation occurs mainly at one of the methyl groups of the cyclopropane ring, which is hydroxylated in a stereospecific manner, and at the 4' position of the alcohol moiety. These sites are indicated by an asterisk. In addition, some hydroxylation may occur at the 2', 5, and 6 positions of the alcohol metabolites. The sites of hydroxylation and the nature of the subsequently formed conjugates vary with pyrethroid structure and with species [(for a detailed review, *see* Leahey (74)].

(60,74). Human carboxylesterase solubilized from liver microsomes hydrolyzes cypermethrin more rapidly than that from rat liver, and the human esterase appears to hydrolyze the *cis*- and *trans*-isomers at similar rates (62). Preferred sites of hydroxylation and the nature of the subsequently formed conjugates (*e.g.*, with sulfate, glucuronic acid, amino acids, bile acids, and glycerols) also vary between species (60).

In mammals, pyrethroid metabolites are readily excreted. Metabolites of the acid and alcohol moieties are found mainly in urine, whereas intact ester metabolites and their conjugates are excreted in the feces. In the rat, orally administered *cis*- and *trans*-permethrin are virtually completely recovered in feces and urine. Approximately 70% of the dose is excreted after 1 day and 97%–100% after 12 days. Little or no radiolabel is expired (46). The estimated half-time of plasma elimination of a high dose of permethrin is 12.4 h (9). Low oral doses of deltamethrin in the rat are excreted 80%–90% at 1 day, and 98%–99% at 8 days after dosing. The distribution and excretion pattern of the cyano metabolites is very similar to that after cyanide administration. Thiocyanate, the main cyano metabolite, is mainly retained in skin and stomach and is 70%–80% eliminated at 8 days (110). Tissue retention of pyrethroids is generally low. The *cis*-isomers are retained for a somewhat longer period, particularly in fat, which may contain small but significant amounts of mainly unchanged pyrethroids. Elimination of *cis*-isomers of cypermethrin from fat in various rat organs is biphasic, with half-times of 1.6–2.7 days and 17–40 days (61).

Human urinary excretion has been monitored in adult male volunteers after oral doses of 0.25–1.5 mg cypermethrin in corn oil contained in a gelatin capsule (30,31). In the first 24 h after dosing, 43%–49% of the *cis*-isomer dose and 72%–78% of the *trans*-isomer dose were excreted in the urine as free and conjugated acid metabolites. During repeated daily dosing for 5 days, the daily amounts of excreted metabolites remained unchanged. In a similar study, 3.3 mg of 1:1 *cis:trans*-cypermethrin adsorbed to a sugar cube was given orally to male volunteers and urinary metabolites were monitored for up to 120 h. Acid metabolites had a 1:2 *cis:trans* ratio and peaked within the first 4 h, whereas the alcohol metabolites peaked 4–24 h after application. Nearly equal amounts of acid and alcohol metabolites were recovered from the urine after oral dosing. After dermal application of a 31-mg dose of 56:44 *cis:trans* technical cypermethrin to the skin on the back, the pattern of urinary metabolites was quite different. The *cis:trans* ratio of acid metabolites was approximately 1:1, and the amount of acid metabolites was four times smaller than the amount of alcohol metabolites in urine. All metabolites peaked 12–36 h after dermal application (149). Urinary excretion patterns of acid and alcohol metabolites of cypermethrin in eight cotton sprayers were consistent with oral, rather than dermal, absorption (146).

Natural pyrethrins and pyrethroids may cause slight induction of mixed-function oxidases and liver enlargement in the rat (18,121). This condition does not change during prolonged exposure and reverses after cessation of exposure (77). Enzyme induction by phenobarbitone reduces the acute oral toxicity of the α-cyanopyrethroid fenpropathrin in the rat (23). Esterase inhibition by organophosphorus compounds may enhance pyrethroid toxicity (2,45,145); young animals may be more sensitive due to incomplete development of enzymes involved in hydrolysis (17,115).

The nervous system is the target organ of pyrethroids. Gross exposure may cause neuroexcitatory symptoms, which are due to direct modulatory effects of pyrethroids on neuronal activity. Effects of pyrethroids on both the CNS and PNS have been reported. Exposure to low doses of specific formulations of some pyrethroids causes paresthesias and respiratory irritation.

Animal Studies

The doses of pyrethroids that cause acute toxicity in mammals are generally very high compared to the dose required to kill insects (36,87). Studies in rodents have shown that the mammalian toxicity of pyrethroids depends greatly on the route of exposure, on the isomer ratio, and on the vehicle used.

On dermal application, the toxicity of the pyrethroids is generally too low to establish LD_{50} values. However, pyrethroids may cause sensory stimulation at extremely low dermal doses and evoke licking, rubbing, scratching, and biting of the exposed area as demonstrated in guinea pigs. The α-cyano pyrethroids fenvalerate, cypermethrin, deltamethrin, and flucythrinate produce sensory stimulation at threshold doses as low as 10 μg. More intense effects were obtained at 100-fold higher doses; with higher doses, sensory stimulation declined. Effects were maximal approximately 1 h after application and disappeared within 24 h. The non–cyano pyrethroid permethrin was shown to cause little or no sensory stimulation in the guinea pig (16,81).

Oral toxicities of pyrethroids to rodents vary over a wide range. Some pyrethroids are virtually nontoxic when given orally [e.g., phenothrin had no mortality at 5000 mg/kg in mice (83)]. Mouse oral LD_{50} values of the two toxic isomers 1R,cis and 1R,trans-permethrin are approximately 100 mg/kg and >3000 mg/kg, respectively. By comparison, the more toxic 1R,cis,αS enantiomer of deltamethrin has a relatively low acute oral LD_{50} for mice of 20 mg/kg. These LD_{50} values were obtained using lipophilic carriers; toxicity is reduced by a factor of up to 10 when polar carriers are used. Oral toxicity of pyrethroids to rats is generally slightly less than that to mice (87).

Pyrethroid toxicity is higher after intravenous application (136) and is enhanced dramatically by intracerebral administration (53,72). The relation between the route of application and toxicity of pyrethroids (Table 56) is indicative of their neurotoxic mechanism of action.

The systemic symptoms of acute pyrethroid poisoning in rats, as observed following intravenous administration, have been divided into two classes (136). Non–cyano pyrethroids initially cause aggressive sparring behavior and increased sensitivity to external stimuli. This is followed by fine tremors, which gradually intensify until the animal becomes prostrate with coarse whole-body tremor. Most of the α-cyano pyrethroids cause a distinct sequence of symptoms. After initial pawing and burrowing behavior, the rat shows profuse salivation, coarse whole-body tremor, increased startle response, and abnormal locomotion involving the hindlimbs. The coarse tremor progresses into choreoathetosis, which gradually becomes more severe, and seizures may be observed before death. Some α-cyano pyrethroids (e.g., fenpropathrin and 1R,trans-cyphenothrin) cause effects similar to those of the non–cyano pyrethroids or may induce mixed signs. Toxic signs usually appear rapidly after intravenous injection, and surviving animals recover completely within several hours (136,151). A detailed study with deltamethrin in the rat has shown that distinct threshold levels of the parent compound in the nervous system need to be exceeded for the occurrence of the various toxic signs. This finding accounts for the characteristic sequence of onset and reversal of signs with dose and time (101). Although the intensity of specific signs may vary slightly, similar structure-dependent sequences of effects are produced by pyrethroids after intraperitoneal and intracerebral administration in mice (72). In dogs, intravenous infusion of deltamethrin (1 mg/min) induces a sequence of signs similar to that described in the rat. Death occurs at doses >2 mg/kg, and signs induced by doses ≤1 mg/kg reverse gradually and completely after persisting for several hours (130).

Neurobehavioral investigations into the effects of pyrethroids have revealed more subtle effects of these agents at doses that cause little or no overt toxic signs. Permethrin and deltamethrin cause a dose-dependent, reversible decrease in the rate of lever pressing during operant behavior. The size of the effects produced by deltamethrin, cis-permethrin and trans-permethrin is correlated with the toxicity of these pyrethroids (11). In the rat, non–cyano pyrethroids enhance the acoustic startle reflex, but the latency of the startle reflex is unaffected. By contrast, α-cyano pyrethroids variably affect the amplitude and latency of the startle reflex and may cause a direct effect on muscle. A rapid onset and recovery of these effects is generally observed

TABLE 56. Relation Between the Route of Administration of *Cis* and *Trans* Isomers of Non–Cyano Pyrethroid Permethrin and of the α-Cyano Pyrethroid Deltamethrin, and Acute Toxicity to Mice (LD_{50} Values in mg/kg)

	Dermal	Oral	i.p.	i.v.	i.c.v.
1*RS,trans*-permethrin	NT*	3100	>1000	93	1.1
1*RS,cis*-permethrin	NT*	100	1000	20	0.1
1*R,cis,αS* deltamethrin	—	30	10	2.4	0.01

*No LD_{50} at the highest possible dose.

i.p., intraperitoneal; i.v., intravenous; i.c.v., intracerebroventricular.

[Dermal and oral data from Miyamoto (83); oral deltamethrin data from Ruzo and Casida (108); i.p. data from Soderlund and Casida (120); i.v. and i.c.v. data from Staatz *et al.* (122)].

(25,59). In all treated animals, locomotor activity in a set of figure-eight mazes is transiently decreased (25). Conversely, hyperactive spontaneous behavior has been reported 4 months after neonatal exposure of mice for 7 days starting at postnatal day 10 to low oral doses (≤0.7 mg/kg/day) of bioallethrin and deltamethrin. Behavioral changes are not observed at postnatal day 17. Subtle changes in the levels of muscarinic acetylcholine (ACh) receptors in the cerebral cortex are observed both at day 17 and 4 months later, but after 100-fold higher doses of bioallethrin, associated with toxic signs and a depression of spontaneous activity, receptor levels remain constant (4,39).

Electrophysiological studies of short- and long-term effects of pyrethroids in the rat revealed that excitability of the tail nerve was enhanced following supramaximal electrical stimulation. The period of enhanced excitability following the nerve impulse was much longer after deltamethrin than after cismethrin. Deltamethrin at 50–200 ppm in the diet for 7 days produced excitability changes similar to those produced by a single intravenous injection of 0.5–1.5 mg/kg. The chronic effects tended to decrease over a period of 8 weeks. Cumulative effects of feeding deltamethrin were not observed, and nerve responses were back within normal limits 24–48 h after return to a normal diet (96,124). Histopathological investigations of rat and mouse peripheral nerve have reported that repeated as well as single lethal and near-lethal oral doses of pyrethroids may cause sparse axonal damage in peripheral nerves of rats and mice. Even at lethal doses, lesions resembling wallerian degeneration were detected only in a fraction of treated animals (6,92). Prolonged feeding with diets containing various dose levels of fenvalerate, with a maximum of 250 ppm for rats and of 1250 ppm for mice up to 2 years, did not produce compound-related nerve damage (93,94). Oral administration of tefluthrin (5 mg/kg/day, 5 days/week for 8 weeks) to rats caused no functional signs of peripheral neuropathy. Motor and sensory nerve conduction velocities were identical to control values (7). After 6 months of feeding fenvalerate to beagle dogs, with prominent neurological signs observed in

the highest dose groups (500 and 1000 ppm), microscopic examination of brain, spinal cord, and peripheral nerves did not reveal treatment-related neuropathological effects (95). Nerve damage could not be detected in hens, even after massive doses of pyrethroids.

Permethrin, cypermethrin, and deltamethrin, but not resmethrin, cause an increase of the activity of the lysosomal enzymes β-glucuronidase and β-galactosidase in the distal portion of the sciatic/posterior tibial nerves of the rat. Effects were observed 2–3 weeks following 1 week of daily oral doses, which were near to the acute LD_{50}. Although the changes in lysosomal enzyme activity are qualitatively similar to those observed in wallerian degeneration, the effects of pyrethroids were an order of magnitude smaller than those induced by the neurotoxic reference compounds acrylamide and methyl mercury (102). From the minor extent of nerve damage and from its quite different time course, it has been concluded that the neuropathological changes are unrelated to the symptoms of acute pyrethroid poisoning (92,102).

The use of products containing both fenvalerate and the insect repellent Deet (*N,N*-diethyl-*m*-toluamide) to control fleas and ticks on cats and dogs is associated with a relatively high incidence of sublethal and lethal poisoning. Although toxic signs resemble those induced by the α-cyano pyrethroids, the low amount of fenvalerate contained in these products suggests that Deet, or a synergistic effect of Deet and fenvalerate, is the cause of the toxicity (29,85; *see also N,N*-Diethyl-*m*-toluamide and Other Dialkylamides, this volume).

In Vitro Studies

The pronounced excitatory effects of pyrethroids in the invertebrate as well as in the vertebrate nervous system are due to a direct action on excitable membranes. The most readily observed effect of pyrethroids is repetitive activity in afferent nerves of sense organs in the skin (19,133). The duration of repetitive nerve-impulse trains varies with pyre-

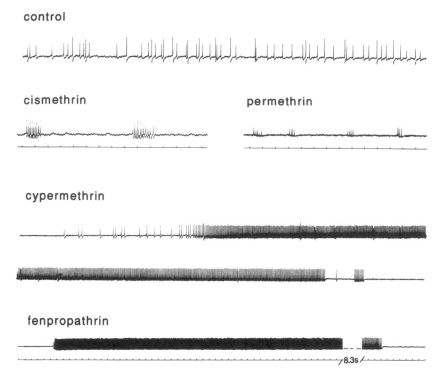

FIGURE 31. Pyrethroid-induced repetitive activity in afferent nerve fibers of the lateral-line sense organ in the skin of the clawed frog, *Xenopus laevis*. Normal activity consists of a stochastic pattern of single nerve impulses. The non-cyano pyrethroids (*e.g.*, cismethrin and permethrin) induce repetitive activity in the form of short nerve impulse trains alternated by silent periods. The α–cyano pyrethroids (*e.g.*, cypermethrin and fenpropathrin) cause long-lasting repetitive discharges. Pyrethroids were applied at the external side of the excised skin at a concentration of 5 μmol and the temperature was 19°C (control) and 13°–17°C (pyrethroids). Time calibrations for the upper traces and for the lower traces are 100 msec/div [Modified from Vijverberg *et al.* (138).]

throid structure, and α-cyano pyrethroids cause particularly prolonged discharges in sense organs (Fig. 31) (138). Intracellular recordings have demonstrated that the pyrethroid-induced repetitive activity is primarily due to enhancement of the inward Na$^+$ current, which results in membrane depolarization. Different degrees of membrane depolarization may variably affect neuronal activity and even cause a block of excitability.

All insecticidally active pyrethroids share the same mechanism of action on voltage-gated Na$^+$ channels. In myelinated nerve fibers of the clawed frog, *Xenopus laevis*, pyrethroids induce a prolonged inward Na$^+$ tail current, which follows the Na$^+$ current evoked by a step depolarization of the membrane (140). The kinetics of Na$^+$ tail current decay vary greatly with pyrethroid structure. The Na$^+$ tail currents induced by α-cyano pyrethroids decay much more slowly than those induced by non–cyano pyrethroids (Fig. 32). For the various pyrethroids, the duration of the tail current relates to the duration of nerve impulse trains during repetitive activity in sense organs (*see* Fig. 31) and both increase at lower temperature (138,141).

In cultured mouse neuroblastoma cells, pyrethroids enhance Na$^+$-current amplitude and slow its kinetics both

during depolarization and after repolarization. The decay of pyrethroid-induced Na$^+$ tail currents in neuroblastoma cells is more rapid than that in frog nerve fibers (106). The recording of Na$^+$-channel opening and closing events in single-channel patch-clamp experiments on mouse neuroblastoma cells and frog spinal ganglion neurons has demonstrated that pyrethroids greatly prolong the open time of individual Na$^+$ channels (Fig. 33) (21,27). In dissociated rat dorsal root ganglion neurons, pyrethroids cause similar but distinct effects on two types of voltage-gated Na$^+$ channels that are sensitive and insensitive to tetrodotoxin (TTX) (50,128). The threshold concentration of tetramethrin to modify TTX-resistant Na$^+$ current is 10 nmol, which is an order of magnitude lower than that required to modify TTX-sensitive Na$^+$ current. At a high concentration of 10 μmol tetramethrin, most of the TTX-resistant and only a small fraction of the TTX-sensitive Na$^+$ channels are modified (128). Pyrethroids also interact with CNS Na$^+$ channels; in rodent brain synaptosomes, as in mouse neuroblastoma cells, pyrethroids enhance TTX-sensitive Na$^+$ influx and stereoselectively modulate the binding of batrachotoxin A 20-α-benzoate, a voltage-gated Na$^+$ channel ligand (15,48,64,79,104). The absence of further interactions

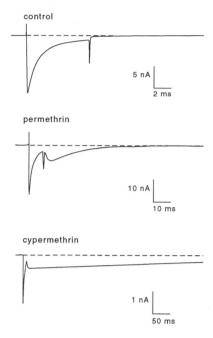

control

5 nA
2 ms

permethrin

10 nA
10 ms

cypermethrin

1 nA
50 ms

FIGURE 32. Voltage-gated Na⁺ current in voltage-clamped myelinated nerve fibers of the clawed frog, *Xenopus laevis*. In the control experiment, membrane depolarization evokes a transient inward current (downward deflection), which rapidly ceases on termination of the depolarizing step after 8 msec. In the presence of permethrin, the Na⁺ current evoked by an identical membrane depolarization is followed by a slowly decaying Na⁺ tail current. Cypermethrin induces a similar Na⁺ tail current, but the cypermethrin-induced tail current decays much more slowly than that induced by the non-cyano analog permethrin. Note the difference in time scale between the three traces. [Modified from Vijverberg *et al.* (141).]

between pyrethroids and toxin binding at different sites of the voltage-gated Na⁺ channel suggests that pyrethroids interact with sites that are distinct from those of other known classes of Na⁺-channel toxins (79). Autoradiography has revealed differences in the regional distributions of pyrethroid-binding sites; that is, the enhancement of labeling with ³H-batrachotoxin A 20-α-benzoate by the α-cyano pyrethroid RU39568, and of ³H-TTX-binding sites in rat brain. These results indicate that pyrethroids interact not only with TTX-sensitive, but also with TTX-insensitive voltage-gated Na⁺ channels in the CNS (79). Although pyrethroids modify voltage-gated Na⁺ current in mammalian, other vertebrate, and invertebrate neurons in a qualitatively similar way, marked species-dependent differences in potency and efficacy of pyrethroids are apparent (71,80,106,128,141).

Inhibitory effects on voltage-gated Na⁺ and K⁺ currents are observed at concentrations of pyrethroids much higher than those required to cause significant prolongation of Na⁺ current (111). Deltamethrin, but not the non-cyano pyrethroid cismethrin, reduces Cl⁻ conductance in rat skel-

etal muscle and vagus nerve; this precedes the prolongation of Na⁺ current (42). Deltamethrin also inhibits large-conductance Cl⁻ channels in mouse N1E-115 neuroblastoma cells (41). Inhibitory effects of pyrethroids on Cl^ins and K⁺ conductance would enhance the tendency of excitable membranes to generate repetitive firing. Tetramethrin blocks low-voltage-activated, transient-type Ca²⁺ channels in cultured mouse neuroblastoma cells (86), in rabbit dissociated sinoatrial node cells (56), and in smooth muscle cells isolated from guinea pig *Taenia coli* (154). Ca²⁺-channel block has not been observed with permethrin and cypermethrin in neuroblastoma cells (105).

Several studies suggest that pyrethroids also affect ligand-gated ion channels. High concentrations of α-cyano pyrethroids cause a stereoselective, partial inhibition of radioligand binding to the picrotoxin site of γ-aminobutyric acid (GABA) receptors in rat brain membranes (73). However, deltamethrin does not affect GABA receptor-gated Cl⁻ current in rat dorsal root ganglion neurons *in vitro* (89). Pyrethroids also inhibit perhydrohistrionicotoxin binding to allosteric channel sites of the end-plate type ACh receptor (1). Inhibitory effects of pyrethroids on the neuronal-type nicotinic ACh receptor-gated ion current in mouse neuroblastoma cells are nonspecific. The effects are equally produced by insecticidally active (1R,*cis*) and inactive (1S,*cis*) isomers of fenfluthrin, and cyphenothrin equally blocks ACh receptor- and serotonin receptor-gated ion currents in these cells (90).

In addition to their effects on ion channels, pyrethroids affect a range of CNS biochemical parameters. In synaptosomes and slices of specific regions of mammalian brain, pyrethroids enhance the release of ACh, GABA, and catecholamine neurotransmitters (14,28,34,88). The smaller efficacy of non–cyano pyrethroids, inhibition of effects by TTX, and the correlation of release with pyrethroid-induced synaptosomal membrane depolarization (33) all suggest that the prolongation of voltage-gated Na⁺ current is the major cause of enhanced neurotransmitter release. Enhanced neuronal activity may result in elevated cytoplasmic Ca²⁺ and Na⁺ concentrations, both of which are involved in the triggering of intracellular processes (5,54). Alterations of cyclic nucleotide contents (13), phosphoinositide turnover (55), protein phosphorylation, and dephosphorylation (37,38,63) occur in the presence of pyrethroids. A photoactivatable arylazide derivative of fenvalerate covalently binds to the β-subunit of G proteins (103). Some of these biochemical changes are also secondary to Na⁺ current prolongation, and some may not originate from within the CNS (13,78). Nonetheless, highly potent effects [*e.g.*, the inhibition of calcineurin by α-cyano pyrethroids (38)] have been observed in isolated enzyme systems *in vi*-

control   cyphenothrin

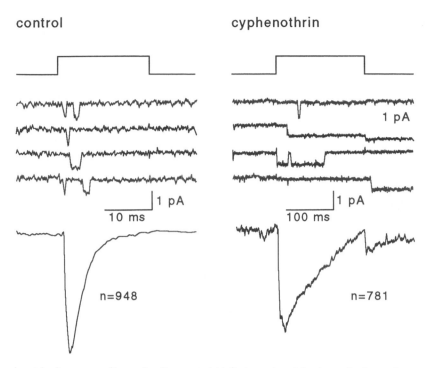

FIGURE 33. Single-channel patch-clamp recordings of voltage-gated Na$^+$-channel activity in excised membrane patches of cultured mouse neuroblastoma cells. In the control experiment, rapid, discrete openings of single Na$^+$ channels (downward deflections) are observed during step depolarizations of the membrane patch. The α-cyano pyrethroid, 1R,cis-cyphenothrin, greatly prolongs the open time of Na$^+$ channels and also causes Na$^+$ channels to (remain) open after termination of the depolarizing step. The summation of large numbers (n) of single channel records (*lower traces*) shows that the unitary events add to a rapid, transient Na$^+$ current in the control experiment and to a prolonged Na$^+$ current followed by a Na$^+$ tail current in the presence of cyphenothrin. [Results from T. Leinders and J.R. de Weille, modified from Vijverberg *et al.* (139).]

tro. The role of most of these effects in the neuroexcitatory symptoms produced by the pyrethroids remains to be resolved.

Human Studies

Cutaneous effects of pyrethroids have been investigated in human volunteers. Fenvalerate dissolved in ethyl alcohol applied to a 4-cm^2 area of one ear lobe at a concentration of 81 mg/cm^2 caused sensations of warmth, numbness, itching, tingling, and burning. These paresthetic effects were virtually absent in the other ear lobe treated with the solvent alone in a double-blind experimental design involving 36 volunteers (69). Of four pyrethroid formulations dissolved in distilled water and applied in a concentration of 130 mg/cm^2 to the ear lobe of six volunteers, flucythrinate caused pronounced paresthesias; fenvalerate and cypermethrin caused intermediate and permethrin only minor effects (40). Application of vitamin E oil, vitamin E acetate, and mineral oil relieved the pyrethroid-induced paresthesias, possibly by a leaching effect (40,132).

Pyrethrin- and permethrin-containing preparations are widely used to treat pediculosis and scabies in humans of all ages. Side effects of pyrethrins are nonneurological and consist of allergic reactions. Allergic reactions, which may be quite severe in specific cases (143), are generally attributed to components of crude pyrethrum extracts other than the natural pyrethrins (125). Clinical trials involving >20,000 patients have been performed with a cream rinse hair conditioner (Nix) containing 1% permethrin with a *trans:cis* ratio of 75:25. In over 95% of the patients, head lice were killed following a single 10-min application to the scalp (126). Minor adverse effects, including pruritus, which is a common feature of the infestation itself, were reported at an incidence of 2.2/1000 on follow-up 7–14 days after permethrin treatment (10).

In the treatment of scabies, a single application of permethrin to the entire human skin is effective. A 1% (w/w) permethrin solution in liquid paraffin was used by 95 patients in Zimbabwe. The amount applied ranged from 3 ml for babies and children to 7 ml for adults. Adverse effects were not reported in this study (129). Studies with 5% permethrin (*trans:cis* = 75:25) in a thixotropic cream base gave >90% cure rates in three separate groups of 23, 10, and 234 patients 1 month following a single whole-body application of the preparation. Amounts of 1.0–1.5 g permethrin, which remained on the skin for up to 14 h, appeared without adverse effects. Mild burning and stinging was experienced during a 1-h period immediately after application in 10% of the cases, but the incidence of this effect was only slightly lower in patients treated with lindane (113,127,135).

Forestry workers exposed to wettable powders of permethrin (*trans:cis* = 75:25) and fenvalerate frequently experience itching and burning sensations, paresthesias, blisters, nasal hypersecretion, sneezing, coughing, dyspnea, and eye irritation. On similar exposure to an organic solvent emulsion of permethrin (*trans:cis* = 60:40), the frequency of symptoms appeared much lower. Burning and tingling skin sensations in the face and hands, experienced after work with fenvalerate, were transient and disappeared overnight (70). Neurological examination of a group of 19 workers exposed to several pyrethroids, who had previously experienced transient sensory symptoms, revealed no abnormalities. Motor and sensory nerve conduction velocities were unaffected as compared to those of a matched control group (75).

In another group of 16 agricultural workers, field exposure to fenvalerate (Pydrin) caused burning and tingling sensations in all and subsequent numbness in four subjects. The symptoms were exacerbated by perspiration, sun, heat, and exposure to water, and generally disappeared overnight. Neither edema nor vesiculation was apparent, indicating the absence of a primary inflammatory reaction (131).

Selective cases of adverse effects following indoor use and abuse of pyrethroids have been reported (43,76,84). Although the causal relation between insecticide application and specific symptoms is often difficult to establish, sensory effects and respiratory irritation are common.

Previously reviewed industrial research data (139) indicate that flowable formulations as well as emulsifiable concentrates and wettable powders of α-cyano pyrethroids may produce skin and respiratory irritation in man. The distinct irritative potential of various insecticidal formulations of permethrin mentioned before, and the virtual absence of skin sensory symptoms with dermatological preparations containing large amounts of permethrin, illustrate the variability in adverse sensory effects.

Examination of 199 workers engaged for 0.5–4.5 months in dividing and packaging emulsions of 20% fenvalerate, 2.5% deltamethrin, and 10% cypermethrin revealed abnormal facial sensations, sneezing, increased nasal secretion, dizziness, and red miliary papules as the main symptoms. No clinical signs of acute pyrethroid poisoning were observed, and functional tests showed no aberrations in blood, heart, lung, liver, kidney, and nervous system. In summer, all symptoms, except sneezing and nasal secretion, were more pronounced, despite the lower air concentrations of the pyrethroids during this season. The sensory symptoms developed with an approximate 30-min latency and generally did not last longer than 24 h (57). A survey of over 3000 persons spraying diluted emulsions of the aforementioned pyrethroids, often mixed with organophosphates, revealed skin sensations, dizziness, headache, fatigue, and nausea as the main symptoms. Due to ignorance of toxicity and of the safe handling of the insecticides, dermal exposure was generally high and 27% of the subjects experienced symptoms related to exposure. Systemic symptoms of acute poisoning developed in 0.3%–0.4% of the spraymen surveyed (20,155).

A simple criterion for diagnosis of pyrethroid poisoning is not available. Apart from frequently reported transient skin and respiratory irritation, which may be caused by low doses of pyrethroids, severe poisoning has always been associated with overt, recent exposure to high doses of pyrethroids. Therefore, diagnosis is based on verified exposure to pyrethroids within 2 days before the onset of toxic signs and on the reasonable exclusion of other diseases (58).

A detailed description of human symptoms has emerged from a large number of cases of occupational and accidental pyrethroid poisoning; illness in these Chinese cases was generally caused by inappropriate handling and ingestion of the pyrethroids deltamethrin (325 cases), fenvalerate (196 cases), and cypermethrin (45 cases) (58). Following ingestion of pyrethroids, initial symptoms develop within 10 min to 1 h and are mainly digestive (*i.e.*, epigastric pain, nausea and vomiting); skin sensations are not significant in these patients. Systemic symptoms include dizziness, headache, nausea, anorexia, and fatigue. In more serious illness, coarse muscular fasciculations, associated with repetitive electromyographic discharges, develop in large muscles of the extremities. In 51 cases, consciousness was disturbed to some degree and some patients, who ingested large amounts (200–500 ml) of emulsifiable-concentrate formulations of pyrethroid, developed coma within 15–20 min. Thirty-five patients suffered convulsive attacks; these lasted 30 sec to 2 min and manifested as flexion of the upper limbs and extension of lower limbs, with opisthotonos and transient loss of consciousness. In two out of three reported cases of moderate to severe acute deltamethrin poisoning, the routine electroencephalogram (EEG) appeared normal and, in the other patient, the EEG showed high-amplitude slow and sharp waves during hyperventilation in the absence of convulsions. Pathological reflexes were not observed. GABA levels in the cerebrospinal fluid were consistently elevated. Convulsive attacks occurred at a frequency up to 10–30/day in the first week after exposure and subsequently decreased gradually to recover completely within 2–3 weeks. Nearly all patients recovered within 1–6 days, though some of the severely affected patients with convulsions were hospitalized for longer periods. In the follow-up of 15 cases, no longstanding or residual symptoms were found. The total number of seven casualties included two cases of acute occupational deltamethrin poisoning, three following fenvalerate ingestion, one acute poisoning with fenvalerate/dimethoate, and one patient misdiagnosed as having acute organophosphate poisoning who died from atropine overdose. Myopia is absent or less pronounced in poisoning with pyrethroids, and inhibition of blood cholinesterase, another indicator of organophosphate poisoning, is not observed with pyrethroids (58).

Despite the lack of specific antidotes (reviewed in 139), the prognosis of pyrethroid poisoning is generally good when adequate symptomatic and supportive treatment is provided. In cases of pyrethroid ingestion, gastric lavage with water or 2%–4% sodium bicarbonate is generally performed. Patients with severe deltamethrin poisoning respond poorly to anticonvulsant therapy, as convulsions are not controlled by diazepam, baclofen, barbiturates, chloral hydrate, chlorpromazine, phenytoin, or hydrocortisone. Low doses of atropine reduce salivation and pulmonary edema in severe cases, but atropine intoxication in patients with pyrethroid poisoning has been reported following injections totalling 12–75 mg (58).

Toxic Mechanisms

Available evidence indicates that the neurotoxic signs of pyrethroids are a consequence of their modification of voltage-gated Na^+ channels in excitable membranes. The distinct syndromes of pyrethroid poisoning in the rat correlate with the efficacy by which pyrethroids prolong the voltage-gated Na^+ current (Table 57) (137). In various vertebrate and invertebrate species, pyrethroids cause similar structure-related, stereoselective effects on voltage-gated Na^+ channels, with analogous manifestations of poisoning (35,44,72,136). Nerve insensitivity in insects, caused by a mutation of the Na^+-channel gene, results in resistance to pyrethroid and dichlorodiphenyltrichloroethane (DDT) insecticides (8,91,97,148). As the mechanism of action by which DDT modifies voltage-gated Na^+ channels is the same as that of the pyrethroids (140), the cross-resistance to DDT also indicates that the voltage-gated Na^+ channel is the primary target of pyrethroids.

Within the nervous system, effects of pyrethroids appear not to be confined to a specific site or region. Effects have been reported on peripheral sensory nerves (134), motor nerve endings (150), skeletal muscle (107,151), spinal neurons (19,118,123), and the brain (100). Studies with spinal rats have demonstrated that pyrethroids can induce their toxic symptoms at the level of the spinal cord (12,53). Despite the pronounced excitatory effects often observed at

TABLE 57. Time Constants of Decay of Prolonged Na^+ Tail Currents Induced *In Vitro* by Various Pyrethroids in Frog Nerve Fibers and in Cultured Mouse Neuroblastoma Cells Compared to *In Vivo* Poisoning Syndromes Reported in Mammals

Compound	Configuration	t_{tail}(ms) Frog*	t_{tail}(ms) Mouse[†]	Syndrome Rat[‡]
Non–cyano pyrethroids				
Phenothrin	(1R),*trans*	6		N
Permethrin	(1R),*trans*	7		N
Phenothrin	(1R),*cis*	13	4	N
Cismethrin	(1R),*cis*	21		T
Permethrin	(1R),*cis*	28		T
Fenfluthrin	(1R),*cis*	105	14–30	
S-5655[§]	(2R,S),(αR,S)	150		T(S)
α-Cyano pyrethroids				
Cyphenothrin	(1R),*trans*,(αS)	290		T
Cyphenothrin	(1R),*cis*,(αS)	385	140	CS
Fenvalerate	(2S),(αS)	600		CS
Cypermethrin	(1R),*cis*,(αS)	1115		CS
Deltamethrin	(1R),*cis*,(αS)	1770	440–800	CS

*Measured in frog myelinated nerve fibers at 15°C.
[†]Measured in mouse neuroblastoma cells at 18°C.
[‡]Intravenous toxicity data from Verschoyle and Aldridge (136).
[§]α-Ethynyl analog of fenvalerate.
N, no symptoms; T, tremor; S, salivation; C, choreoathetosis.
[From Vijverberg *et al.* (137).]

the cellular level, pyrethroids induce CNS excitation as well as inhibition. By enhancing release of the inhibitory neurotransmitter GABA from interneurons, pyrethroids inhibit rat hippocampal activity (49,65,66). On the other hand, release of catecholamines and corticosterone, increased brain glucose utilization, and generalized EEG spiking during choreoathetosis in the rat—all of which are also caused by pyrethroids—are associated with stress and increased nervous system activity (24,26,100).

It can be concluded that the voltage-gated Na^+ channel is the primary cellular target through which pyrethroids cause their acute neurotoxic effects in mammals. In the skin, this results in pronounced repetitive firing of sensory nerve endings and in paresthetic symptoms. The toxic mechanism by which pyrethroids induce manifestation of systemic poisoning is likely to be a combination of excessive afferent activity, direct effects on the neuromuscular system, and disruption of the delicate balance between excitation and inhibition in the CNS, which add to a level beyond the range of physiological compensatory feedback.

REFERENCES

1. Abbassy MA, Eldefrawi ME, Eldefrawi AT (1983) Pyrethroid action on the nicotinic acetylcholine receptor/channel. *Pestic Biochem Physiol* 19, 299.
2. Abernathy CO, Ueda K, Engel JL et al. (1973) Substrate-specificity and toxicological significance of pyrethroid-hydrolyzing esterases of mouse liver microsomes. *Pestic Biochem Physiol* 3, 300.
3. Ahdaya SM, Monroe RJ, Guthrie FE (1981) Absorption and distribution of intubated insecticides in fasted mice. *Pestic Biochem Physiol* 16, 38.
4. Ahlbom J, Fredriksson A, Eriksson P (1994) Neonatal exposure to a type-I pyrethroid (bioallethrin) induces dose-response changes in brain muscarinic receptors and behaviour in neonatal and adult mice. *Brain Res* 645, 318.
5. Ahnert-Hilger G, Habermann E (1981) Increase of cGMP and accumulation of $^{45}Ca^{2+}$ evoked by drugs acting on sodium or potassium channels. *Eur J Pharmacol* 70, 301.
6. Aldridge WN (1980) Mode of action of pyrethroids in mammals: Summary of toxicity and histological, neurophysiological and biochemical studies. In: *Pyrethroid Insecticides; Chemistry and Action.* Table Ronde 37, Casida JE, Elliott M eds. Institut Scientifique Roussel UCLAF, Romainville, France p. 45.
7. Allen SL, Sheldon R (1987) Investigations into the neurotoxicity of 2,5-hexanedione and tefluthrin (a synthetic pyrethroid). *First Meeting of the International Neurotoxicology Association.* Lunteren, The Netherlands p. 172.
8. Amichot M, Castella C, Cuany A et al. (1992) Target modification as a molecular mechanism of pyrethroid resistance in *Drosophila melanogaster. Pestic Biochem Physiol* 44, 183.

9. Anadón A, Martinez-Larrañaga MR, Diaz MJ, Bringas P (1991) Toxicokinetics of permethrin in the rat. *Toxicol Appl Pharmacol* 110, 1.
10. Andrews EB, Joseph MC, Magenheim MJ et al. (1992) Postmarketing surveillance study of permethrin creme rinse. *Amer J Public Health* 82, 857.
11. Bloom AS, Staatz CG, Dieringer T (1983) Pyrethroid effects on operant responding and feeding. *Neurobehav Toxicol Teratol* 5, 321.
12. Bradbury JE, Forshaw PJ, Gray AJ, Ray DE (1983) The action of mephenesin and other agents on the effects produced by two neurotoxic pyrethroids in the intact and spinal rat. *Neuropharmacology* 22, 907.
13. Brodie ME, Aldridge WN (1982) Elevated cerebellar cyclic GMP levels during the deltamethrin-induced motor syndrome. *Neurobehav Toxicol Teratol* 4, 109.
14. Brooks MW, Clark JM (1987) Enhancement of norepinephrine release from rat brain synaptosomes by alpha cyano pyrethroids. *Pestic Biochem Physiol* 28, 127.
15. Brown GB, Gaupp JE, Olsen RW (1988) Pyrethroid insecticides: Stereospecific allosteric interaction with the batrachotoxin-A benzoate binding site of mammalian voltage-sensitive sodium channels. *Mol Pharmacol* 34, 54.
16. Cagen SZ, Malley LA, Parker CM et al. (1984) Pyrethroid-mediated skin sensory stimulation characterized by a new behavioral paradigm. *Toxicol Appl Pharmacol* 76, 270.
17. Cantalamessa F (1993) Acute toxicity of two pyrethroids, permethrin and cypermethrin, in neonatal and adult rats. *Arch Toxicol* 67, 510.
18. Carlson GP, Schoenig GP (1980) Induction of liver microsomal NADPH cytochrome *c* reductase and cytochrome P-450 by some new synthetic pyrethroids. *Toxicol Appl Pharmacol* 52, 507.
19. Carlton M (1977) Some effects of cismethrin on the rabbit nervous system. *Pestic Sci* 8, 700.
20. Chen SY, Zhang ZW, He FS et al. (1991) An epidemiological study on occupational acute pyrethroid poisoning in cotton farmers. *Brit J Ind Med* 48, 77.
21. Chinn K, Narahashi T (1986) Stabilization of sodium channel states by deltamethrin in mouse neuroblastoma cells. *J Physiol-London* 380, 191.
22. Crawford MJ, Croucher A, Hutson DH (1981) Metabolism of *cis*- and *trans*-cypermethrin in rats. Balance and tissue retention study. *J Agr Food Chem* 29, 130.
23. Crawford MJ, Hutson DH (1977) The metabolism of the pyrethroid insecticide (±)-α-cyano-3-phenoxybenzyl 2,2,3,3-tetramethyl-cyclopropanecarboxylate, WL 41706, in the rat. *Pestic Sci* 8, 579.
24. Cremer JE, Cunningham VJ, Ray DE, Sarna GS (1980) Regional changes in brain glucose utilization in rats given a pyrethroid insecticide. *Brain Res* 194, 278.
25. Crofton KM, Reiter LW (1988) The effects of type I and

II pyrethroids on motor activity and the acoustic startle response in the rat. *Fund Appl Toxicol* **10**, 624.

26. De Boer SF, van der Gugten J, Slangen JF, Hijzen TH (1988) Changes in plasma corticosterone and catecholamine contents induced by low doses of deltamethrin in rats. *Toxicology* **49**, 263.

27. De Weille JR, Leinders T (1989) The action of pyrethroids on sodium channels in myelinated nerve fibres and spinal ganglion cells of the frog. *Brain Res* **482**, 324.

28. Doherty JD, Lauter CJ, Salem N (1986) Synaptic effects of the synthetic pyrethroid resmethrin in rat brain *in vitro*. *Comp Biochem Physiol C* **84**, 373.

29. Dorman DC, Buck WB, Trammel HL *et al.* (1990) Fenvalerate/*N,N*-diethyl-*m*-toluamide (Deet) toxicosis in two cats. *J Amer Vet Med Assn* **196**, 100.

30. Eadsforth CV, Baldwin MK (1983) Human dose-excretion studies with the pyrethroid insecticide cypermethrin. *Xenobiotica* **13**, 67.

31. Eadsforth CV, Bragt PC, van Sittert NJ (1988) Human dose-excretion studies with pyrethroid insecticides cypermethrin and alphacypermethrin: Relevance for biological monitoring. *Xenobiotica* **18**, 603.

32. ECDIN (1993) *Environmental Chemicals Data and Information Network* (CDROM). Joint Research Centre of the European Communities Environment Institute, Springer Verlag, Heidelberg.

33. Eells JT, Bandettini PA, Holman PA, Propp JM (1992) Pyrethroid insecticide-induced alterations in mammalian synaptic membrane potential. *J Pharmacol Exp Ther* **262**, 1173.

34. Eells JT, Dubocovich ML (1988) Pyrethroid insecticides evoke neurotransmitter release from rabbit striatal slices. *J Pharmacol Exp Ther* **246**, 514.

35. Eells JT, Rasmussen JL, Bandettini PA, Propp JM (1993) Differences in the neuroexcitatory actions of pyrethroid insecticides and sodium channel-specific neurotoxins in rat and trout brain synaptosomes. *Toxicol Appl Pharmacol* **123**, 107.

36. Elliott M, Janes NF (1978) Synthetic pyrethroids—a new class of insecticide. *Chem Soc Rev* **7**, 473.

37. Enan E, Matsumura F (1992) Specific inhibition of calcineurin by type-II synthetic pyrethroid insecticides. *Biochem Pharmacol* **43**, 1777.

38. Enan E, Matsumura F (1993) Activation of phosphoinositide/protein kinase-C pathway in rat brain tissue by pyrethroids. *Biochem Pharmacol* **45**, 703.

39. Eriksson P, Nordberg A (1990) Effects of two pyrethroids, bioallethrin and deltamethrin, on subpopulations of muscarinic and nicotinic receptors in the neonatal mouse brain. *Toxicol Appl Pharmacol* **102**, 456.

40. Flannigan SA, Tucker SB (1985) Variation in cutaneous sensation between synthetic pyrethroid insecticides. *Contact Dermatitis* **13**, 140.

41. Forshaw PJ, Lister T, Ray DE (1993) Inhibition of a neuronal voltage-dependent chloride channel by the type II pyrethroid, deltamethrin. *Neuropharmacology* **32**, 105.

42. Forshaw PJ, Ray DE (1990) A novel action of deltamethrin on membrane resistance in mammalian skeletal muscle and non-myelinated nerve fibres. *Neuropharmacology* **29**, 75.

43. Fromme H (1991) Anwendung von Pestiziden in Innenräumen unter besonderer Berücksichtigung der Pyrethroide. Problemdarstellung und Lösungsansatze aus der Sicht des ökologischen Gesundheitsschutzes, Teil 1. *Off Gesundh Wes* **53**, 132.

44. Gammon DW, Brown MA, Casida JE (1981) Two classes of pyrethroid action in the cockroach. *Pestic Biochem Physiol* **15**, 181.

45. Gaughan LC, Engel JL, Casida JE (1980) Pesticide interactions: Effects of organophosphorus pesticides on the metabolism, toxicity, and persistence of selected pyrethroid insecticides. *Pestic Biochem Physiol* **14**, 81.

46. Gaughan LC, Unai T, Casida JE (1977) Permethrin metabolism in rats. *J Agr Food Chem* **25**, 9.

47. Ghiasuddin SM, Soderlund DM (1984) Hydrolysis of pyrethroid insecticides by soluble mouse brain esterases. *Toxicol Appl Pharmacol* **74**, 390.

48. Ghiasuddin SM, Soderlund DM (1985) Pyrethroid insecticides are potent stereospecific enhancers of mouse brain sodium channel activation. *Pestic Biochem Physiol* **24**, 200.

49. Gilbert ME, Mack CM, Crofton KM (1989) Pyrethroids and enhanced inhibition in the hippocampus of the rat. *Brain Res* **477**, 314.

50. Ginsburg KS, Narahashi T (1993) Differential sensitivity of tetrodotoxin-sensitive and tetrodotoxin-resistant sodium channels to the insecticide allethrin in rat dorsal root ganglion neurons. *Brain Res* **627**, 239.

51. Gray AJ, Connors TA, Hoellinger H, Nguyen-Hoang-Nam (1980) The relationship between the pharmacokinetics of intravenous cismethrin and bioresmethrin and their mammalian toxicity. *Pestic Biochem Physiol* **13**, 281.

52. Gray AJ, Rickard J (1981) Distribution of radiolabel in rats after intravenous injection of a toxic dose of ^{14}C-acid, -alcohol or -cyano labelled deltamethrin. *Pestic Biochem Physiol* **16**, 79.

53. Gray AJ, Rickard J (1982) Toxicity of pyrethroids to rats after direct injection into the central nervous system. *Neurotoxicology* **3**, 25.

54. Gusovsky F, Daly JW (1988) Formation of second messengers in response to activation of ion channels in excitable cells. *Cell Mol Neurobiol* **8**, 157.

55. Gusovsky F, Secunda SI, Daly JW (1989) Pyrethroids: Involvement of sodium channels in effects on inositol phosphate formation in guinea pig synaptoneurosomes. *Brain Res* **492**, 72.

56. Hagiwara N, Irisawa H, Kameyama M (1988) Contri-

bution of two types of calcium currents to the pacemaker potentials of rabbit sino-atrial node cells. *J Physiol-London* **395**, 233.

57. He F, Sun H, Han K *et al.* (1988) Effects of pyrethroid insecticides on subjects engaged in packaging pyrethroids. *Brit J Ind Med* **45**, 548.

58. He F, Wang S, Liu L *et al.* (1989) Clinical manifestations and diagnosis of acute pyrethroid poisoning. *Arch Toxicol* **63**, 54.

59. Hijzen TH, Slangen JL (1988) Effects of type I and type II pyrethroids on the startle response in rats. *Toxicol Lett* **40**, 141.

60. Hutson DH (1979) The metabolic fate of synthetic pyrethroid insecticides in mammals. In: *Progress in Drug Metabolism. Vol 3.* Bridges JW, Chasseaud IF eds. John Wiley, Chichester p. 215.

61. Hutson DH, Logan CJ (1986) The metabolic fate in rats of the pyrethroid insecticide WL85871, a mixture of two isomers of cypermethrin. *Pestic Sci* **17**, 548.

62. Hutson DH, Millburn P (1991) Enzyme-mediated selective toxicity of an organophosphate and a pyrethroid: Some examples from a range of animals. *Biochem Soc Trans* **19**, 737.

63. Ishikawa Y, Charalambous P, Matsumura F (1989) Modification by pyrethroids and DDT of phosphorylation activities of rat brain sodium channel. *Biochem Pharmacol* **38**, 2449.

64. Jacques Y, Romey G, Cavey MT *et al.* (1980) Interaction of pyrethroids with the Na^+ channel in mammalian neuronal cells in culture. *Biochim Biophys Acta* **600**, 882.

65. Joy RM, Albertson TE, Ray DE (1989) Type I and type II pyrethroids increase inhibition in the hippocampal dentate gyrus of the rat. *Toxicol Appl Pharmacol* **98**, 398.

66. Joy RM, Lister T, Ray DE, Seville MP (1990) Characteristics of the prolonged inhibition produced by a range of pyrethroids in the rat hippocampus. *Toxicol Appl Pharmacol* **103**, 528.

67. Kaneko H, Ohkawa H, Miyamoto J (1981) Absorption and metabolism of dermally applied phenothrin in rats. *J Pestic Sci* **6**, 169.

68. Kaneko H, Ohkawa H, Miyamoto J (1981) Comparative metabolism of fenvalerate and the 2S,aS-isomer in rats and mice. *J Pestic Sci* **6**, 317.

69. Knox JM, Tucker SB, Flannigan SA (1984) Paresthesia from cutaneous exposure to a synthetic pyrethroid insecticide. *Arch Dermatol* **120**, 744.

70. Kolmodin-Hedman B, Swensson Å, Åkerblom M (1982) Occupational exposure to some synthetic pyrethroids (permethrin and fenvalerate). *Arch Toxicol* **50**, 27.

71. Laufer J, Roche M, Pelhate M *et al.* (1984) Pyrethroid insecticides: Actions of deltamethrin and related compounds on insect axonal sodium channels. *J Insect Physiol* **30**, 341.

72. Lawrence LJ, Casida JE (1982) Pyrethroid toxicology: Mouse intracerebral structure-toxicity relationships. *Pestic Biochem Physiol* **18**, 9.

73. Lawrence LJ, Casida JE (1983) Stereospecific action of pyrethroid insecticides on the γ-aminobutyric acid receptor-ionophore complex. *Science* **221**, 1399.

74. Leahey JP (1985) Metabolism and environmental degradation. In: *Pyrethroid Insecticides.* Leahey JP ed. Taylor and Francis, London p. 263.

75. LeQuesne PM, Maxwell IC, Butterworth STG (1980) Transient facial sensory symptoms following exposure to synthetic pyrethroids: A clinical and electrophysiological assessment. *Neurotoxicology* **2**, 1.

76. Lessenger JE (1992) Five office workers inadvertently exposed to cypermethrin. *J Toxicol Environ Health* **35**, 261.

77. Litchfield MH (1985) Toxicity to mammals. In: *Pyrethroid Insecticides.* Leahey JP ed. Taylor and Francis, London p. 99.

78. Lock EA, Berry PN (1981) Biochemical changes in the rat cerebellum following cypermethrin administration. *Toxicol Appl Pharmacol* **59**, 508.

79. Lombet A, Mourre C, Lazdunski M (1988) Interaction of insecticides of the pyrethroid family with specific binding sites on the voltage-dependent sodium channel from mammalian brain. *Brain Res* **459**, 44.

80. Lund AE, Narahashi T (1983) Kinetics of sodium channel modification as the basis for the variation in the nerve membrane effects of pyrethroids and DDT analogs. *Pestic Biochem Physiol* **20**, 203.

81. McKillop CM, Brock JAC, Oliver GJA, Rhodes C (1987) A quantitative assessment of pyrethroid-induced paraesthesia in the guinea pig flank model. *Toxicol Lett* **36**, 1.

82. McLaughlin GA (1973) History of pyrethrum. In: *Pyrethrum, the Natural Insecticide.* Casida JE ed. Academic Press, New York p. 3.

83. Miyamoto J (1976) Degradation, metabolism and toxicity of synthetic pyrethroids. *Environ Health Perspect* **14**, 15.

84. Moretto A (1991) Indoor spraying with the pyrethroid lambda-cyhalothrin: Effects on spraymen and inhabitants of sprayed houses. *Bull WHO* **69**, 591.

85. Mount ME, Moller G, Cook J *et al.* (1991) Clinical illness associated with a commercial tick and flea product in dogs and cats. *Vet Hum Toxicol* **33**, 19.

86. Narahashi T, Tsunoo A, Yoshii M (1987) Characterization of two types of calcium channels in mouse neuroblastoma cells. *J Physiol-London* **383**, 231.

87. Naumann K (1990) Synthetic pyrethroids insecticides. In: *Chemistry of Plant Protection. Vol 4.* Bowerse WS, Ebing W, Martin D, Wegler R eds. Springer-Verlag, Berlin.

88. Nicholson RA, Wilson RG, Potter C, Black MH (1983) Pyrethroid- and DDT-evoked release of GABA from the nervous system *in vitro*. In: *Pesticide Chemistry, Human Welfare and the Environment, Mode of Action, Metab-*

olism and Toxicology. Vol 3. Miyamoto J, Kearney PC eds. Pergamon Press, Oxford p. 75.

89. Ogata N, Vogel SM, Narahashi T (1988) Lindane but not deltamethrin blocks a component of GABA-activated chloride channels. *FASEB J* **2**, 2895.

90. Oortgiesen M, van Kleef RGDM, Vijverberg HPM (1989) Effects of pyrethroids on neurotransmitter-operated ion channels in cultured mouse neuroblastoma cells. *Pestic Biochem Physiol* **34**, 164.

91. Osborne MP, Hart RJ (1979) Neurophysiological studies of the effects of permethrin upon pyrethroid resistant (kdr) and susceptible strains of dipteran larvae. *Pestic Sci* **10**, 407.

92. Parker CM, Albert JR, van Gelder GA *et al.* (1985) Neuropharmacologic and neuropathologic effect of fenvalerate in mice and rats. *Fund Appl Toxicol* **5**, 278.

93. Parker CM, McCullough CB, Gellatly JBM, Johnston CD (1983) Toxicologic and carcinogenic evaluation of fenvalerate in the B6C3F1 mouse. *Fund Appl Toxicol* **3**, 114.

94. Parker CM, Patterson DR, van Gelder GA *et al.* (1984) Chronic toxicity and carcinogenicity evaluation of fenvalerate in rats. *J Toxicol Environ Health* **13**, 83.

95. Parker CM, Piccirillo VJ, Kurtz SL *et al.* (1984) Six-month feeding study of fenvalerate in dogs. *Fund Appl Toxicol* **4**, 577.

96. Parkin PJ, LeQuesne PM (1982) Effect of a synthetic pyrethroid deltamethrin on excitability changes following a nerve impulse. *J Neurol Neurosurg Psychiat* **45**, 337.

97. Pauron D, Barhanin J, Amichot M *et al.* (1989) Pyrethroid receptor in the insect Na⁺ channel: Alteration of its properties in pyrethroid-resistant flies. *Biochemistry* **28**, 1673.

98. Quistad GB, Selim S (1983) Fluvalinate metabolism by rhesus monkeys. *J Agr Food Chem* **31**, 596.

99. Quistad GB, Staiger LE, Jamieson GC, Schooley DA (1983) Fluvalinate metabolism by rats. *J Agr Food Chem* **31**, 589.

100. Ray DE (1980) An EEG investigation of decamethrin-induced choreoathetosis in the rat. *Exp Brain Res* **38**, 221.

101. Rickard J, Brodie ME (1985) Correlation of blood and brain levels of the neurotoxic pyrethroid deltamethrin with the onset of symptoms in rats. *Pestic Biochem Physiol* **23**, 143.

102. Rose GP, Dewar AJ (1983) Intoxication with four synthetic pyrethroids fails to show any correlation between neuromuscular dysfunction and neurobiochemical abnormalities in rats. *Arch Toxicol* **53**, 297.

103. Rossignol DP (1991) Binding of a photoreactive pyrethroid to β subunit of GTP-binding proteins. *Pestic Biochem Physiol* **41**, 121.

104. Rubin JG, Payne GT, Soderlund DM (1993) Structure activity relationships for pyrethroids and DDT analogs as modifiers of ³H-batrachotoxinin-A 20-α-benzoate binding to mouse brain sodium channels. *Pestic Biochem Physiol* **45**, 130.

105. Ruigt GSF (1984) *An Electrophysiological Investigation into the Mode of Action of Pyrethroid Insecticides.* Dissertation, Utrecht University, The Netherlands.

106. Ruigt GSF, Neyt HC, van der Zalm JM, van den Bercken J (1987) Increase of sodium current after pyrethroid insecticides in mouse neuroblastoma cells. *Brain Res* **437**, 309.

107. Ruigt GSF, van den Bercken J (1986) Action of pyrethroids on a nerve-muscle preparation of the clawed frog, *Xenopus laevis. Pestic Biochem Physiol* **25**, 176.

108. Ruzo LO, Casida JE (1977) Metabolism and toxicology of pyrethroids with dihalovinyl substituents. *Environ Health Perspect* **21**, 285.

109. Ruzo LO, Engel JL, Casida JE (1979) Decamethrin metabolites from oxidative, hydrolytic, and conjugative reactions in mice. *J Agr Food Chem* **27**, 725.

110. Ruzo LO, Unai T, Casida JE (1978) Decamethrin metabolism in rats. *J Agr Food Chem* **26**, 918.

111. Salgado VL, Herman MD, Narahasi T (1989) Interactions of the pyrethroid fenvalerate with nerve membrane sodium channels: Temperature dependence and mechanism of depolarization. *Neurotoxicology* **10**, 1.

112. Schechter MS, Green N, LaForge FB (1949) Constituents of pyrethrum flowers. XXIII. Cinerolone and the synthesis of related cyclopentenolones. *J Amer Chem Soc* **71**, 3165.

113. Schultz MW, Gomez M, Hansen RC *et al.* (1990) Comparative study of 5% permethrin cream and 1% lindane lotion for the treatment of scabies. *Arch Dermatol* **126**, 167.

114. Shah PV, Monroe RJ, Guthrie FE (1981) Comparative rates of dermal penetration of insecticides in mice. *Toxicol Appl Pharmacol* **59**, 414.

115. Sheets LP, Doherty JD, Law MW *et al.* (1994) Age-dependent differences in the susceptibility of rats to deltamethrin. *Toxicol Appl Pharmacol* **126**, 186.

116. Sidon EW, Moody RP, Franklin CA (1988) Percutaneous absorption of *cis*- and *trans*-permethrin in rhesus monkeys and rats: Anatomic site and interspecies variation. *J Toxicol Environ Health* **23**, 207.

117. Silver IS, Dauterman WC (1989) The pharmacokinetics and metabolism of (1*R,cis*)- and (1*R,trans*)-tetramethrin in rats. *Xenobiotica* **19**, 301.

118. Smith PR (1980) The effect of cismethrin on the rat dorsal root potentials. *Eur J Pharmacol* **66**, 125.

119. Soderlund DM, Abdel-Aal YAI, Helmuth DW (1982) Selective inhibition of separate esterases in rat and mouse liver microsomes hydrolyzing malathion, *trans*-permethrin and *cis*-permethrin. *Pestic Biochem Physiol* **17**, 162.

120. Soderlund DM, Casida JE (1977) Effects of pyrethroid structure on rates of hydrolysis and oxidation by mouse

liver microsomal enzymes. *Pestic Biochem Physiol* 7, 391.

121. Springfield AC, Carlson GP, DeFeo JJ (1973) Liver enlargement and modification of hepatic microsomal drug metabolism in rats by pyrethrum. *Toxicol Appl Pharmacol* 24, 298.

122. Staatz CG, Bloom AS, Lech JJ (1982) A pharmacological study of pyrethroid neurotoxicity in mice. *Pestic Biochem Physiol* 17, 287.

123. Staatz-Benson CG, Hosko MJ (1986) Interaction of pyrethroids with mammalian spinal neurons. *Pestic Biochem Physiol* 25, 19.

124. Takahashi M, LeQuesne PM (1982) The effects of the pyrethroids deltamethrin and cismethrin on nerve excitability in rats. *J Neurol Neurosurg Psychiat* 45, 1005.

125. Taplin D, Meinking TL (1987) Pyrethrins and pyrethroids for the treatment of scabies and pediculosis. *Semin Dermatol* 6, 125.

126. Taplin D, Meinking TL (1990) Pyrethrins and pyrethroids in dermatology. *Arch Dermatol* 126, 213.

127. Taplin D, Meinking TL, Porcelain SL *et al.* (1986) Permethrin 5% dermal cream: A new treatment for scabies. *J Amer Acad Dermatol* 15, 995.

128. Tatebayashi H, Narahashi T (1994) Differential mechanism of action of the pyrethroid tetramethrin on tetrodotoxin-sensitive and tetrodotoxin-resistant sodium channels. *J Pharmacol Exp Ther* 270, 595.

129. Taylor P (1979) Scabies in Zimbabwe Rhodesia: Distribution on the human body and the efficacy of lindane and permethrin as scabicides. *Cent Afr J Med* 8, 165.

130. Thiebault JJ, Bost J, Foulhoux P (1985) Intoxication expérimentale par la deltaméthrine chez le chien et son traitement. *J Toxicol Clin Exp* 5, 47.

131. Tucker SB, Flannigan SA (1983) Cutaneous effects from occupational exposure to fenvalerate. *Arch Toxicol* 54, 195.

132. Tucker SB, Flannigan SA, Ross CE (1984) Inhibition of cutaneous paresthesia resulting from synthetic pyrethroid exposure. *Int J Dermatol* 10, 686.

133. Van den Bercken J (1977) The action of allethrin on the peripheral nervous system of the frog. *Pestic Sci* 8, 692.

134. Van den Bercken J, Kroese ABA, Akkermans LMA (1979) Effects of insecticides on the sensory nervous system. In: *Neurotoxicology of Insecticides and Pheromones.* Narahashi T ed. Plenum Press, New York p. 183.

135. Van der Rhee HJ, Farquhar JA, Vermeulen NPE (1989) Efficacy and transdermal absorption of permethrin in scabies patients. *Acta Dermato-Venereol* 69, 170.

136. Verschoyle RD, Aldridge WN (1980) Structure-activity relationships of some pyrethroids in rats. *Arch Toxicol* 45, 325.

137. Vijverberg HPM, de Weille JR, Ruigt GSF, van den Bercken J (1986) The effect of pyrethroid structure on the interaction with the sodium channel in the nerve membrane. In: *Neuropharmacology and Pesticide Action.* Ford MG, Lunt GG, Reay RC, Usherwood PNR eds. Ellis Horwood, Chichester, England p. 267.

138. Vijverberg HPM, Ruigt GSF, van den Bercken J (1982) Structure related effects of pyrethroid insecticides on the lateral-line sense organ and on peripheral nerves of the clawed frog, *Xenopus laevis. Pestic Biochem Physiol* 18, 315.

139. Vijverberg HPM, van den Bercken J (1990) Neurotoxicological effects and the mode of action of pyrethroid insecticides. *CRC Crit Rev Toxicol* 21, 105.

140. Vijverberg HPM, van der Zalm JM, van den Bercken J (1982) Similar mode of action of pyrethroids and DDT on sodium channel gating in myelinated nerves. *Nature* 295, 601.

141. Vijverberg HPM, van der Zalm JM, van Kleef RGDM, van den Bercken J (1983) Temperature- and structure-dependent interaction of pyrethroids with the sodium channels in frog node of Ranvier. *Biochim Biophys Acta* 728, 73.

142. Walker G, Keller R, Beckert J, Butte W (1994) Anreicherung von Bioziden in Innenräumen am Beispiel der Pyrethroide. *Zbl Hyg Umweltmed* 195, 450.

143. Wax PM, Hoffman RS (1994) Fatality associated with inhalation of a pyrethrin shampoo. *J Toxicol-Clin Toxicol* 32, 457.

144. Wester RC, Bucks DAW, Maibach HI (1994) Human *in vivo* percutaneous absorption of pyrethrin and piperonyl butoxide. *Food Chem Toxicol* 32, 51.

145. White INH, Verschoyle RD, Moradian MH, Barnes JM (1976) The relationship between brain levels of cismethrin and bioresmethrin in female rats and neurotoxic effects. *Pestic Biochem Physiol* 6, 491.

146. Wilkes MF, Woollen BH, Marsh JR *et al.* (1993) Biological monitoring for pesticide exposure—the role of human volunteer studies. *Int Arch Occup Environ Health* 65, S189.

147. Williamson EG, Long SF, Kallman MJ, Wilson MC (1989) A comparative analysis of the acute toxicity of technical grade pyrethroid insecticides and their commercial formulations. *Ecotoxicol Environ Safety* 18, 27.

148. Williamson MS, Denholm I, Bell CA, Devonshire AL (1993) Knockdown resistance (*kdr*) to DDT and pyrethroid insecticides maps to a sodium channel gene locus in the housefly (*Musca domestica*). *Mol Gen Genet* 240, 17.

149. Woollen BH, Marsh JR, Laird WJD, Lesser JE (1992) The metabolism of cypermethrin in man: Differences in urinary metabolite profiles following oral and dermal administration. *Xenobiotica* 22, 983.

150. Wouters W, van den Bercken J, van Ginneken A (1977) Presynaptic action of the pyrethroid insecticide allethrin in the frog motor end plate. *Eur J Pharmacol* 43, 163.

151. Wright CDP, Forshaw PJ, Ray DE (1988) Classification

of the actions of ten pyrethroid insecticides in the rat, using the trigeminal reflex and skeletal muscle as test systems. *Pestic Biochem Physiol* **30**, 79.

152. Wright CG, Leidy RB, Dupree HE (1993) Cypermethrin in the ambient air and on surfaces of rooms treated for cockroaches. *Bull Environ Contam Toxicol* **51**, 356.

153. Wu N, Xiao Y, Chen DZ, Huang FM (1991) Laboratory evaluation of efficacy of bednets impregnated with pyrethroids. *J Amer Mosquito Contr Assn* **7**, 294.

154. Yabu H, Yoshino M, Someya T, Totsuka M (1989) Two types of Ca channels in smooth muscle cells isolated from guinea pig *Taenia coli*. *Adv Exp Med Biol* **255**, 129.

155. Zhang ZW, Sun JX, Chen SY *et al.* (1991) Levels of exposure and biological monitoring of pyrethroids in spraymen. *Brit J Ind Med* **48**, 82.

Pyridoxine/Vitamin B$_6$

Herbert H. Schaumburg

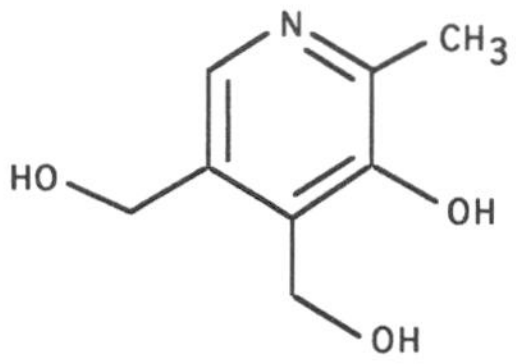

PYRIDOXINE
C$_8$H$_{12}$ClNO$_3$

5-Hydroxy-6-methyl-3,4-pyridinemethanol

NEUROTOXICITY RATING

Clinical

A Peripheral neuropathy (sensory)

A Sensory neuronopathy

Experimental

A Peripheral neuropathy (sensory)

A Sensory neuronopathy

Six substances (vitamers) are collectively designated as vitamin B$_6$: pyridoxine (PN), pyridoxal (PL), pyridoxamine (PM), pyridoxine 5'-phosphate (PNP), pyridoxal 5'-phosphate (PLP), and pyridoxamine 5'-phosphate (PMP) (5). Three vitamers are present in the diet: grain cereals contain PN; and meat and milk, PLP and PMP. The recommended daily requirement of vitamin B$_6$ is 2–4 mg/100 g of dietary protein.

Vitamin B$_6$ is available as the hydrochloride salt of pyridoxine in both tablet and parenteral forms. Pyridoxine hydrochloride, a component of many commercial multivitamin preparations, also appears in nutritional food supplements, fortified foods, and animal feeds. It is a white, odorless, crystalline powder at room temperature and is soluble in water.

The recommended daily requirement is readily available in the North American diet. Pyridoxine supplements are routinely administered to certain individuals, alcoholics and food faddists, considered at risk for vitamin deficiency. Other legitimate uses of pyridoxine supplements (usually 100 mg daily) include treatment of individuals receiving hydralazine, oral contraceptives, or isoniazid therapy (13). Short-term, intravenous, megadose therapy (10 g in 3 h) is used for acute hydrazine poisoning (9). Persons with genetically determined pyridoxine dependency such as pyridoxine-responsive anemia, pyridoxine-dependent seizures of infancy, and xanthurenic aciduria clearly require long-term therapy (3). Pyridoxine is advocated, with less justification, for a variety of conditions such as schizophrenia (15), premenstrual syndrome (1), mushroom (*Gyromytra esculenta*) poisoning (18), and the carpal tunnel syndrome (17).

Pyridoxine is generally regarded as safe (GRAS) and is not regulated. Reports of self-induced nervous system damage from ingestion of megadoses of pyridoxine have led to discontinuance of the 1-g tablets.

General Toxicology

PN is rapidly absorbed from the intestine by nonsaturable diffusion. Low concentrations of dietary PLP and PMP are hydrolyzed to PL or PM by intestinal mucosal cells. High dietary levels of PLP and PMP are absorbed unchanged (12).

Figure 34 outlines the principal metabolic pathways of the six vitamers. Only PLP and PMP, the principal B$_6$ vitamers in mammalian tissues, can function as coenzymes. Pyridoxic acid is the terminal catabolite and urinary excretory product of B$_6$ metabolism.

The liver converts the bulk of absorbed PN to PNP or PL, the major plasma transport vitamers. PNP is converted to PL before utilization by target issues. Plasma PNP values of 62 ± 11 nmol/ml are normal for a 70-kg male on a regular diet. Measurement of tryptophan metabolites is

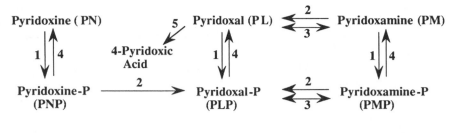

1 - Pyridoxal kinase

2 - Pyridoxamine-P (pyridoxine-P) oxidase

3 - Aminotransferase

4 - Alkaline phosphatase

5 - Aldehyde oxidase and dehydrogenase

FIGURE 34. Principal metabolic pathways of the vitamin B$_6$ vitamers.

used in the diagnosis of B$_6$ deficiency; specifically, urinary xanthurenic acid is elevated following a tryptophan load. The normal plasma level of pyridoxal 5-phosphate is 3.6–18 ng/ml.

Several biochemical interactions with drugs of B$_6$ are clinically relevant. Isoniazid inhibits the formation of the coenzyme form of B$_6$; hydralazine and cycloserine also cause B$_6$ deficiency. B$_6$ enhances dopa decarboxylation and can reduce the effects of L-dopa in Parkinson's disease (13).

Animal Studies

Huge oral doses (2–6 g/kg) cause seizures and death in rats and mice. Rats dosed at 600 mg/kg/day and dogs at 1 g/kg/day develop an unsteady gait within a few days (10,11). Histopathological examination demonstrates vacuolar changes in the axon hillocks of dorsal root ganglion cells, with acute somal chromatolytic reaction. Many sensory axons of peripheral nerves appear to be "transected" near their junction with dorsal root ganglion cells. The dorsal columns of the spinal cord and the descending fibers of the trigeminal tract in the brainstem also display severe axonal destruction. A detailed description is available of the spatiotemporal sequence of CNS and PNS pathology in rats treated by intraperitoneal injection with 1200 mg/kg/day pyridoxine hydrochloride (23). Initial lesions (day 2) consisted of eccentricity and crenation of the nucleus and vacuole formation in the cytoplasm of large lumbar dorsal root ganglion neurons. These lesions were followed by segregation of the nucleolus, axon reaction-like changes in the cytoplasm, and axonal degeneration of both peripheral axons in the sural nerve and central axons in the fasciculus gracilis (more pronounced in the third than the fifth cervical segment). Accumulation of mitochondria, vesicles, multilamellar and dense bodies was found in the nodal and distal paranodal axons of myelinated fibers in the L6 dorsal root

ganglion on the 2nd day; this preceded degeneration of both peripheral and central axons. It is suggested that the accumulation of vesicular structures reflects a blockade of fast axonal transport in the proximal axon and cell body of the primary sensory neuron that causes the degeneration of its peripheral and central axons (23).

Moderately high levels (200 mg/kg/day in the rat) of parenteral intoxication produce, after about 6 weeks, an unsteady gait progressing to an inability to walk; recovery commences after pyridoxine is discontinued (19,21). Histological analysis of peripheral nerves and dorsal root ganglion cells from these animals shows severe axonal destruction in sensory nerves. Dorsal root ganglion cells show only minimal vacuolar changes; motor roots are normal. Guinea pigs appear approximately equally susceptible at this level of intoxication. One study failed to produce neuropathy in mice treated with 300 mg/kg/day for 12 weeks, suggesting variable intermurine species susceptibility (22).

In sum, extremely high doses of pyridoxine produce a toxic sensory neuronopathy syndrome with rapid destruction of either dorsal root ganglion cells or their axon hillocks, while lower doses spare the cells but damage axons.

In Vitro Studies

Tissue culture study of pyridoxine analogs, PN, PL, and PM, indicates that each equally impairs sensory neurite outgrowth (20). Neither PMP, which cannot enter cells, nor pyridoxic acid, the metabolite of pyridoxine, is toxic.

Human Studies

It is claimed that daily injection of 200 mg pyridoxine causes a dependency syndrome and withdrawal symptoms following cessation of the drug (5); however, a study of women consuming 50–300 mg daily for over 1 year discerned no symptoms or signs of dependency upon withdrawal (6).

Pyridoxine excess causes either a reversible sensory neuropathy, following high doses, or an irreversible sensory neuronopathy following extremely high doses. A prospective clinical study of five volunteers taking either 1 or 3 g daily disclosed that (a) there is a clear dose–effect relationship for pyridoxine-induced peripheral neuropathy, (b) quantitative sensory testing (QST) is a sensitive measurement for detecting early neuropathy—QST abnormalities may precede changes in nerve conduction studies, (c) coasting (worsening of symptoms for 2–6 weeks before recovery commences) appears unrelated to persistently elevated blood levels of the toxin, and (d) a dose-dependent vulnerability may exist among nerve fibers of different caliber when exposed to an axonal toxin, such as pyridoxine (4).

Humans who daily ingest high doses of pyridoxine (200 mg to 10 g), usually as part of a self-administered regimen for the premenstrual syndrome or for body building, develop sensory distal axonopathy that is largely reversible (14). Authors of one uncritical study claimed that 2 years of consumption of an average of 117 mg/kg daily is associated with sensory symptoms (7); it has also been alleged that fetal phocomelia is associated with maternal abuse of pyridoxine (8).

The sensory axonopathy is remarkably stereotyped; its intensity correlates with dosage levels (16). Individuals taking 500 mg/d are asymptomatic for several years, while those taking 7–10 g generally experience symptoms within 2 months. All develop distal symmetrical sensory neuropathy. The initial symptoms are unsteady gait and numb feet; sensory loss and clumsiness of the hands follows, frequently heralded by Lhermitte's sign. Neurological examination reveals depressed or absent tendon reflexes and a stocking-and-glove distribution of sensory loss. Cerebrospinal fluid is unremarkable. Sural nerve biopsy reveals widespread nonspecific axonal degeneration. Sensory nerve conduction studies of distal nerve segments show diminished sensory potential amplitudes and slowed conduction. Motor nerve conduction remains normal or is only slightly slowed. Following withdrawal, coasting is frequent before improvement commences. Most make a satisfactory recovery.

Individuals receiving 180 g of pyridoxine intravenously over a 2-day period develop a diffuse sensory neuronopathy syndrome that includes clumsiness of all limbs, inability to swallow, autonomic disturbances (postural hypotension), loss of sensation over the entire body, absent tendon reflexes, and only slight weakness (2). Recovery is poor. It appears that massive parenteral doses of pyridoxine in humans elicits a syndrome that closely mimics that produced in animals, reflecting irreversible destruction of dorsal root ganglion cells.

The diagnosis is established by eliciting a history of pyridoxine consumption in amount and duration sufficient to produce this stereotypical syndrome, and observing improvement following withdrawal. Diagnosis does not depend upon body-burden analysis. The early stage of pyridoxine neuropathy in young women is sometimes erroneously diagnosed as multiple sclerosis.

There is no specific therapy. Most patients recover satisfactorily within a year after withdrawal.

Toxic Mechanisms

The pathogenesis and biochemical basis of pyridoxine neurotoxicity are unknown. It is widely held that the toxic peripheral sensory neuronopathy (high dose) and axonopathy (low dose) syndromes reflect the vulnerability of dorsal root ganglion neurons to circulating toxins, probably due to local vascular permeability, *viz*, the absence of a blood-nerve barrier. The sensory syndromes produced by megadoses of pyridoxine may also reflect the anatomical vulnerability of dorsal root ganglion cells, since vitamin B$_6$ is transported into the CNS by means of a saturable transport mechanism (19), and since central neurons may be shielded from excessive levels of circulating pyridoxine. Tissue-culture study suggests that the neurotoxicity of pyridoxine is a specific effect, is related to its coenzyme activity, and is not due to impurities in commercial preparations (20).

REFERENCES

1. Abraham GE, Hargrove JT (1980) Effects of vitamin B$_6$ on premenstrual symptomatology in women with premenstrual tension syndrome: A double-blind crossover study. *Infertility* 3, 155.
2. Albin RL, Greenberg HS, Townsend JB *et al.* (1986) Acute sensory neuropathy from pyridoxine overdose. *Neurology* 36, 175.
3. Bankier A, Turner M, Hopkins JJ (1983) Pyridoxine dependent seizures—a wider clinical spectrum. *Arch Dis Child* 58, 415.
4. Berger AB, Schaumburg HH, Schroeder C *et al.* (1992) Dose response, coasting, and differential fiber vulnerability in human toxic neuropathy: A prospective study of pyridoxine neurotoxicity. *Neurology* 42, 1367.
5. Canham JT, Nunes WT, Eberlin EW (1964) Electroencephalographic and central nervous system manifestations of B$_6$ dependency in normal human adults. In: *Proceedings of the Sixth International Congress on Nutrition.* E and S Livingston Ltd, Edinburgh p. 337.
6. Dalton K (1985) Pyridoxine overdose in premenstrual syndrome. *Lancet* 1, 1398.
7. Dalton K, Dalton MJT (1987) Characteristics of pyridoxine overdose syndrome. *Acta Neurol Scand* 76, 8.
8. Gardner LI, Welsh-Sloam J, Cady R (1985) Phocomelia in an infant whose mother took large doses of pyridoxine during pregnancy. *Lancet* 1, 636.

9. Harati Y, Niakan E (1986) Hydrazine toxicity, pyridoxine therapy, and peripheral neuropathy. *Ann Intern Med* **104**, 728.

10. Krinke G, Naylor DD, Skorpil V (1985) Pyridoxine megavitaminosis: An analysis of the early changes induced with massive doses by vitamin B$_6$ in rat primary sensory neurons. *J Neuropathol Exp Neurol* **44**, 117.

11. Krinke G, Schaumburg HH, Spencer PS (1980) Pyridoxine megavitaminosis produces degeneration of peripheral sensory neurons (sensory neuropathy) in the dog. *Neurotoxicology* **2**, 13.

12. Lumeng L, Li TK, Lui A (1985) The inter-organ transport and metabolism of vitamin B$_6$. In: *Vitamin B-6: Its Role in Health and Disease.* Reynolds RD, Leklem JE eds. Alan R Liss, New York p. 35.

13. Marcus R, Coulston AM (1985) The vitamins. In: *The Pharmacological Basis of Therapeutics. 7th Ed.* Gilman AG, Goodman LS, Rall TW, Murad F eds. Macmillan, New York p. 1559.

14. Parry GJ, Bredsen DE (1985) Neuropathy due to pyridoxine intoxication. *Neurology* **35**, 1466.

15. Pauling L, Robinson AB, Oxley SS (1973) Results of a loading test of ascorbic acid, niacinamide and pyridoxine in schizophrenic subjects and controls. In: *Orthomolecular Psychiatry: Treatment of Schizophrenia.* Hawkins D, Pauling L eds. WH Freeman, San Francisco p. 18.

16. Schaumburg HH, Kaplan J, Windebank A *et al.* (1983) Sensory neuropathy from pyridoxine abuse. *N Engl J Med* **309**, 445.

17. Smith GP, Rudge JJ, Peters TJ (1984) Biochemical studies of pyridoxal and pyridoxal phosphate and therapeutic trial of pyridoxine in patients with carpal tunnel syndrome. *Ann Neurol* **15**, 104.

18. Southgate MT (1984) Mushroom poisoning. *J Amer Med Assn* **251**, 1057.

19. Spector R (1978) Vitamin B$_6$ transport in the central nervous system: *in vivo* studies. *J Neurochem* **30**, 881.

20. Windebank AJ (1985) Neurotoxicity of pyridoxine analogs is related to coenzyme structure. *Neurochem Pathol* **3**, 159.

21. Windebank AJ, Low PA, Blexrud MD (1985) Pyridoxine neuropathy in rats: Degeneration of sensory axons. *Neurology* **35**, 1617.

22. Xu Y, Sladky JT, Brown MB (1989) Dose-dependent expression of neuronopathy after experimental pyridoxine intoxication. *Neurology* **39**, 1077.

23. Yamamoto T (1991) Pathologic processes of lumbar primary sensory neurons produced by high doses of pyridoxine in rats—morphometric and electron microscopic studies. *Sangyo Ika Daigaku Zasshi* **13**, 109. [Japanese]

CASE REPORT

A 27-year-old woman sought medical attention because of increased difficulty in walking. Approximately 2 years previously, she had been told that vitamin B$_6$ provided a natural way to get rid of body water, and she began to take 500 mg/day for premenstrual edema. One year before presentation, she had started to increase her intake, until she reached a daily intake of 5 g/day. During this period of increase in dosage, she initially noticed that neck flexion produced a tingling sensation down the neck and into her legs and soles of her feet (Lhermitte's sign). In the 4 months before neurological evaluation, she became progressively unsteady when walking, particularly in the dark, and noticed difficulty handling small objects. She also noticed some change in feeling in her lips and tongue, but she had no other positive sensory symptoms and was not aware of any limb weakness.

Examination showed that she could walk only with the assistance of a cane. Her gait was broad-based and stamping, and she was unable to walk at all with her eyes closed. She had marked pseudoathetosis (writhing motions) of the outstretched arms; strength was normal. All limb reflexes were absent. Babinski's signs were absent. The sensations of touch, temperature, pinprick, vibration, and joint position were severely impaired in both upper and lower limbs. There was mild subjective alteration of touch-pressure and pinprick sensation over the cheeks and lips but not over the forehead. Electrophysiological studies determined that no sensory nerve action potentials could be elicited, while motor nerve conduction velocities and electromyogram were normal.

Approximately 2 months after withdrawal from pyridoxine supplementation, she reported the beginning of improvement in gait and sensation. Seven months after withdrawal, she felt much improved; she could walk steadily without a cane, could stand with her eyes closed, and had returned to work. Neurological examination disclosed that her strength was still normal and that tendon reflexes remained absent throughout. Her feet still had a severe loss of vibration sensation, but definite improvement was evident in the sense of joint position, touch, temperature, and pinprick. In the upper limbs, there was only a mild impairment of vibration sensation, and joint-position sense was normal.

Comment

This clinical presentation is a stereotyped sensory distal axonopathy with initial dysfunction in long large-diameter fibers of the lower limb. Prolonged, high-level consumption eventually caused symptoms to appear in the hands and face, structures supplied by shorter nerve fibers. Lhermitte's sign reflects early dysfunction in dorsal column axons from the lumbar sensory ganglion cells.

Pyrimethamine

Herbert H. Schaumburg

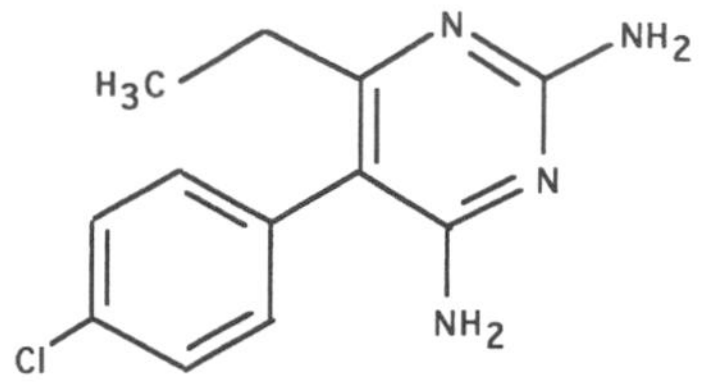

PYRIMETHAMINE
$C_{12}H_{13}ClN_4$

5-(4-Chlorophenyl)-6-ethyl-2,4-pyrimidinediamine

NEUROTOXICITY RATING

Clinical

B Seizure disorder

Experimental

A Seizure disorder

Pyrimethamine, an amyl analog of 2,4-diaminopyrimidine, is used in treatment and prophylaxis of toxoplasmosis and malaria; it is usually employed in combination with sulfonamides or sulfones. Pyrimethamine inhibits difolate reductase of microorganisms and prevents nuclear division during mitosis; this inhibition occurs at concentrations far lower than levels that affect corresponding mammalian enzymes. Absorption from the gastrointestinal tract is slow but complete; the plasma half-life is 80–95 h. Save for skin rash and mild depression of hematopoiesis, little systemic toxicity accompanies conventional (25 mg weekly) pyrimethamine therapy. Chronic high-level therapy may cause folate-deficiency megaloblastic anemia.

Pyrimethamine, in massive doses of 5 mg/kg, causes generalized seizures in experimental animals; similar effects are seen in children following accidental ingestion of the drug (1,2,4). It is alleged that persons with well-controlled epilepsy may experience seizures with conventional doses of pyrimethamine (3,4).

REFERENCES

1. Akinyanju O, Goddell JC, Ahmed I (1973) Pyrimethamine poisoning. *Brit Med J* 4, 147.
2. Duveau E, Chomienne F, Seguin G (1996) Convulsions associated with pyrimethamine overdose. *Arch Pediatr* 3, 286.
3. Fish DR, Espir MLE (1988) Convulsions associated with prophylactic antimalarial drugs: Implications for people with epilepsy. *Brit Med J* 299, 1524.
4. Grisham RSC (1962) Central nervous system toxicity of pyrimethamine (Daraprim) in man. *Amer J Ophthalmol* 54, 1119.

Pyriminil

Albert C. Ludolph
Peter S. Spencer

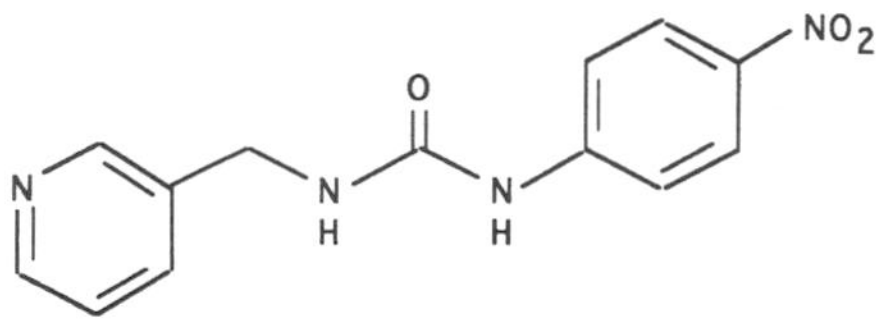

PYRIMINIL
$C_{13}H_{12}N_4O_3$

N-3-Pyridylmethyl-N'-p-nitrophenylurea; Vacor

NEUROTOXICITY RATING

Clinical

A Peripheral neuropathy

A Acute encephalopathy (hallucinations, coma)

B Extrapyramidal syndrome (chorea)

B Cerebellar syndrome

Experimental

A Peripheral neuropathy (axonal neuropathy; axonal transport dysfunction)

A Retinopathy

Pyriminil, a structural analogue of nicotinamide used as a rat poison in the late 1970s, is a powder soluble in dimethylsulfoxide (DMSO) that can be suspended in glycerol (6–11). The principal acute clinical effect of pyriminil poisoning is the induction of diabetes mellitus and orthostatic hypotension, but peripheral nerve damage and encephalopathy are also part of the picture. Neurological deficits, characterized by distal limb weakness, sensory loss, and autonomic disturbances, develop within hours or days of ingestion. Large doses are associated with more generalized weakness, loss of postural reflexes, cranial nerve involvement, and urinary retention. Hyperglycemia, ketosis, orthostatic hypotension, hypothermia, and gastrointestinal hypomotility, including dysphagia, are common features of the syndrome. Much rarer and after higher dosages, blurred vision and acute encephalopathies (coma, hallucinatory states, slurred speech, impaired short-term recall) are observed (8,10). Choreiform movements, myoclonic jerks, nystagmus, and other signs of cerebellar dysfunction are occasionally reported (8). Ocular toxicity has also been seen in a few patients (9). Some of the toxic effects, in particular diabetes mellitus and orthostatic hypotension, frequently persist but neuropathy greatly improves. Additional and apparently unusual features of a well-documented intoxication of a 25-month-old child were nausea and vomiting, motor seizures with multifocal spiking in the electroencephalogram, lethargy, a Babinski's sign, and brisk symmetrical tendon reflexes associated with dysesthesias (6). Neuropathological studies did not reveal further clues.

The therapeutic use of parenteral niacinamide has been suggested (6,8) and early gastric lavage may also be useful. Cardiac arrhythmias are considered life-threatening, and hypoglycemia was seen in some patients (6–8). Morphological studies of the pancreas showed selective β-cell destruction, although α-cells were also affected to some extent (7).

The neuropathy can be modeled in experimental rats (13). The morphological picture in rodents is characterized by degeneration of distal nerve terminals accompanied by selective impairment of fast anterograde axonal transport. Changes in axon terminals of interosseous muscles in the hindfeet of rats appear 3 days after a single oral dose of 80 mg/kg pyriminil. There is swelling of endoplasmic reticulum and reduction of synaptic vesicles followed by focal disruption of the plasma membrane, with subsequent flattening of postsynaptic folds (1). A model for the retinopathy was established in adult Dutch belted rabbits (9); in these animals, oral pyriminil reportedly induced a loss of the rod portion of the b wave of the electroretinogram, and electron microscopy revealed degeneration of the retinal pigment epithelium.

Since pyriminil is a structural analogue of nicotinamide and, if given early, nicotinamide protects against its neurotoxic effects, it has been suggested that pyriminil inhibits carbohydrate and fat utilization (3,7,13). Pyriminil neuropathy may be an instructive example of the strong pathophysiological and biochemical relation between impairment of energy metabolism, decreased nucleotide supply to the nerve, functional impairment of axonal transport, and the resulting morphological picture of a distal axonopathy (12). However, pyriminil also has other toxic effects, such as inhibition of superoxide dismutase (2,5,14) and serum cholinesterase (4), which might also contribute to its toxicity.

REFERENCES

1. Ahn JS, Lee TH, Lee MC (1998) Ultrastructure of neuromuscular junction in vacor-induced diabetic rats. *Korean J Intern Med* **13**, 47.

2. Crouch RK, Gandy SE, Kimsey G *et al.* (1981) The inhibition of islet superoxide dismutase by diabetogenic drugs. *Diabetes* **30**, 235.

3. Deckert FW, Moss JN, Sambuca AS *et al.* (1977) Nutritional and drug interactions with Vacor™ rodenticide in rats. *Fed Proc* **36**, 990.

4. Devi SVU, Krishnamoorthy RV (1979) Non-competitive inhibition of serum acetylcholinesterase (E.C. 3.1.1.7) by Vacor (N-3-pyridyl methyl-N'-p-nitrophenyl urea) in bandicoot rats. *Indian J Physiol Pharmacol* **23**, 285.

5. Gandy SE, Buse MG, Crouch RK (1982) Protective role of superoxide dismutase against diabetogenic drugs. *J Clin Invest* **70**, 650.

6. Johnson D (1980) Accidental ingestion of Vacor rodenticide. The symptoms and sequela in 25-month-old child. *Amer J Dis Child* **134**, 161.

7. Kenney RM, Michaels IAL, Flomenbaum NE, Yu GSM (1981) Poisoning with N-3-pyridylmethyl-N'-p-nitrophenylurea (Vacor). Immunoperoxidase demonstration of β-cell destruction. *Arch Pathol Lab Med* **105**, 367.

8. LeWitt P (1980) The neurotoxicity of the rat poison Vacor. *N Engl J Med* **302**, 73.

9. Mindel JS, Kharlamb AB, Friedman AH *et al.* (1988) N-3-Pyridylmethyl-N'-p-nitrophenylurea ocular toxicity in man and rabbits. *Brit J Ophthalmol* **72**, 584.

10. Osterman J, Zmyslinski RW, Hopkins CB *et al.* (1981) Full recovery from severe orthostatic hypotension after Vacor rodenticide ingestion. *Arch Intern Med* **141**, 1505.

11. Pont A, Rubino JM, Bishop D *et al.* (1979) Diabetes mellitus and neuropathy following Vacor ingestion in man. *Arch Intern Med* **139**, 185.

12. Spencer PS, Miller MS, Ross SM *et al.* (1985) Biochemical mechanisms underlying primary degeneration of axons. In: *Handbook of Neurochemistry. 2nd Ed. Vol 9, Alterations of Metabolites in the Nervous System.* Lajtha A ed. Plenum Press, New York p. 31.

13. Watson DF, Griffin JW (1987) Vacor neuropathy: Ultrastructural and axonal transport studies. *J Neuropathol Exp Neurol* **46**, 96.

14. Wilson GL, Gaines KL (1983) Effects of the rodenticide Vacor on cultured rat pancreatic cells. *Toxicol Appl Pharmacol* **68**, 375.

Pyrithione

Zarife Sahenk

Jerry R. Mendell

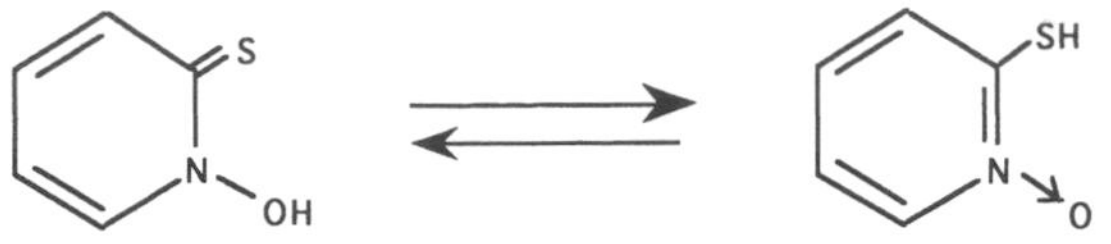

1-HYDROXY-2-PYRIDINETHIONE
C_5H_5NOS

2-PYRIDINETHIOL-1-OXIDE
C_5H_5NOS

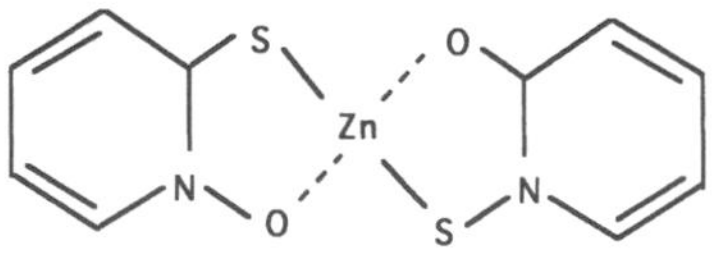

ZINC PYRIDINETHIONE
$C_{10}H_8N_2O_2S_2Zn$

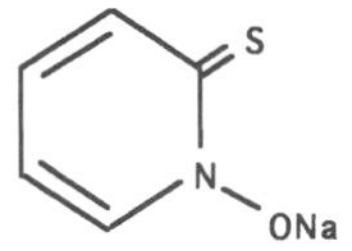

SODIUM PYRIDINETHIONE
C_5H_4NNaOS

1-Hydroxy-2(H1)-pyridinethione; 2-Pyridinethiol 1-oxide

NEUROTOXICITY RATING

Experimental

A   Peripheral neuropathy

A   Retinopathy (Zn chelation)

1-Hydroxy-2-pyridinethione (HPT) and its tautomeric form, 2-pyridinethiol-1-oxide, combine with metal ions to form complexes known as pyridinethiones. Many of the heavy metal salts of HPT have no net charge and exist in the form of lipophilic complexes (24). The water-insoluble zinc salt of HPT, zinc pyridinethione (ZPT), exists as a single dimer in the solid state (4). Both ZPT and the water-soluble sodium salt of HPT (NaPT) are used as antiseborrheic agents in shampoos and as cosmetic and industrial preservatives (7). Pyridinethiones are also used to control various plant diseases (20,26). Some pyridinethione complexes can be extracted into organic solvents and this property has found applications in metal ion determination (14–16).

Since the late 1950s, the toxic effects of pyridinethiones have been extensively studied, leading to the recognition of two significant reproducible complications. Feeding ZPT (10,45) or HPT (13) to animals that have a tapetum lucidum (42) produces ocular lesions causing blindness. Oral administration of ZPT to rodents or percutaneous absorption of NaPT in rabbits causes progressive hindlimb paralysis (11,44,45,50) resulting from a distal axonopathy characterized by accumulation of tubulovesicular membranous organelles in the motor nerve terminals (40). The toxicity of ZPT appears to be independent of zinc, since hindlimb paralysis and tapetal degeneration follow the administration of NaPT (11,50).

The widespread usage of ZPT as an active ingredient in antidandruff shampoos and hair dressings raises the concern for potential hazards. Absorption studies performed with a variety of species, using different methods of application, reportedly indicate that the currently used 1%–2% level of ZPT in shampoo formulations provides an adequate margin of safety for subjects with intact skin (45).

Other than accidental ingestion, scalp and hand contact with commercial shampoos or hair-dressing creams is the major potential source of exposure for humans. Although it has been established that pyridinethiones can cause hindlimb paralysis in experimental animals when absorbed in sufficient amounts through the skin, it is not known whether humans are susceptible to this toxic effect when exposed to high levels. The syndrome has not been observed in primates (10,45).

General Toxicology

Studies of skin retention and absorption using radiolabeled pyridinethiones have been done by several investigators (22,23,33,45). Following the application of shampoo containing 2%–20% ^{35}S-ZPT on the forearm up to 5 min, the maximum amount of ZPT retained on the skin was approximately 2 $\mu g/cm^2$ or about 2% (45). A 1% solution of ^{35}S-NaPT applied to the skin of rats and monkeys for 15 min and 1 h, respectively, was retained locally on the skin and very little was recovered in the urine (33). Using autoradiography, another study with guinea pig skin treated with ^{35}S-ZPT in a 1.7% (w/v) shampoo base showed entry of ^{35}S-ZPT into the hair follicles, but not the sebaceous glands of the dermis (34,37).

Excretion of NaPT following topical application to the nails of monkeys was 10% of the applied topical dose (1). Repeated applications at hourly intervals on the same day increased excretion. Application of NaPT to traumatized skin, or pretreatment of skin with a surfactant that removes sebaceous secretions, enhances skin permeability, resulting in increased absorption and urinary excretion.

Salts of pyridinethione undergo extensive alteration when administered to animals, and the metabolic products from the compounds are excreted mainly in the urine (1,22,23,47). Urinary excretion takes precedence over tissue concentration. There appears to be a two-compartment model for distribution of metabolites (1). The half-life of the initial phase of plasma clearance for both compounds is approximately 3 h. Plasma clearance for the slower secondary phase is 26–36 h, reflecting strongly bound tissue- or plasma-storage compartments. The liver accumulates the highest concentrations over a 24-h period. A study examining tissue distribution of ^{35}S-NaPT (110 mg/kg) following dermal application at 4 h showed a liver concentration of 0.10 mg/kg compared to 0.49 mg/kg for urine (23). All other tissue concentrations were less than those in the liver. At 24 h, there was a threefold increase in liver, kidney, and lung concentrations but, at the same time, urinary excretion increased about 14-fold. Concentrations in the brain were quite low at 4 h, increasing nearly tenfold to 0.0142 mg/kg at 24 h. Although still small, this increase might have implications in a prolonged exposure (34,40,45).

Zinc and the pyridinethione portions of the molecule are metabolized separately (27). Oral administration of double-labeled ^{35}S- and ^{65}Zn-ZPT resulted in a wide tissue distribution and subsequent urinary excretion of ^{35}S. Zinc was excreted in the feces, suggesting that ZPT was decomposed in the gastrointestinal tract (31).

Glucuronide conjugation is a primary feature in ZPT metabolism, especially during the first 24 h following oral administration in rats, rabbits, monkeys, and dogs (25). The biotransformation is similar in all species; the major urinary metabolites are 2-pyridenthiol-1-oxide-S-glucoside, 2-pyridinethiol-S-glucuronide, and 2-pyridinethiol-1-oxide-S-glucuronide, the last being the most abundant (25). In each species tested, 2-methyl sulfonylpyridone has been identified as the terminal plasma pyridinethione metabolite (17). The same metabolite was detected in the systemic circulation of humans involved in the chemical manufacturing process, confirming that the terminal pyridinethione metabolite is identical across species (28).

NaPT has been shown to induce marked effects on the uptake and distribution of nickel, cadmium, and zinc in mice (24). Oral administration of NaPT, together with radiolabeled nickel, cadmium, and zinc, resulted in increased levels of these metals in several tissues when compared to animals given the metals alone. All three metals formed lipophilic complexes with pyridinethiones. This likely facilitates penetration of the complex metals through cellular membranes.

The microbial activities of pyridinethiones are closely linked to the metal-chelating property and are only exhibited in the presence of a metal ion (2,3). A series of in vitro studies has shown that ZPT is primarily cytotoxic, rather than cytostatic (18).

Percutaneous application of 2% ZPT in a shampoo base, conducted with rabbits (30) and Yorkshire pigs (47,48) to assess teratogenicity and embryotoxicity, had no adverse effects on fetal development. The mitogenic potential of ZPT has been evaluated using in vitro gene mutation assays. Using the mouse micronucleus test in vivo, ZPT, at the maximal tolerated dose, did not induce increased frequencies of micronuclei in bone marrow cells (42).

Because of the potential for eye and skin irritation by ZPT in shampoos, the local effects on these tissues have been examined in both animals and humans (11,28,32,35). Repeated-insult close-patch test studies on human volunteers using active solutions of shampoo containing 2% (46) and 0.5% (32) ZPT failed to produce sensitization or undue irritation of the skin. Topical application of ZPT in a 20% suspension was not an overt irritant to mice or rabbits, but induced a marginal hyperplasia and increased epidermal hair growth in these species (28). Two concentrations (0.02% and 0.002%) of ZPT in water, applied to the normal forearms of human volunteers, showed no effects on epidermal renewal in normal skin (42).

The effect of ZPT on epidermal renewal has been investigated with rat skin. Autoradiography was used to determine the percentage of epidermal cells radiolabeled with thymidine. ZPT, at 1% in shampoo base, caused a slight increase in the labeling index in normal skin, similar to the effects of shampoo base alone (19). Although no significant toxic disorder has been conclusively linked to ZPT in humans, occupational contact dermatitis due to NaPT has been reported (46).

Animal Studies

The ocular toxicity of pyridinethiones is clearly established (10,13,29,45). Oral administration of ZPT to dogs and cats at doses of 12.5–25.0 mg/kg produced ocular lesions in 6–14 days. Ophthalmological changes in cats include loss of normal tapedal coloration, intraretinal hemorrhage, subretinal edema and inflammation, and retinal detachment; eventually, severe exudative chorioretinitis and blindness occur. No ocular effects occur in the atapetal beagle dog and rhesus monkey. This suggests that the pyridinethione-induced ocular toxicity is related to zinc chelation in the tapetum lucidum which, in some carnivores, has a high zinc content (49). Other chelating compounds also cause ocular lesions in animals with a tapetum lucidum (8,21).

The effects of intravenous administration of NaPT (50 mg/kg) and ZPT (5 mg/kg) have been studied in guinea pigs. Intravenous ZPT at higher doses (25 mg/kg) in dogs, monkeys, and rabbits resulted in death within 24 h (6). Acute toxic effects included salivation, vasodilation, urination, defecation, and emesis, in addition to muscle fasciculation, ataxia, and muscle weakness. These effects were attributed to cholinergic stimulation of both muscarinic and nicotinic receptors lasting 30–60 min. Acute hindlimb weakness observed following intravenous ZPT (10 mg/kg) and NaPT (200–300 mg/kg) in rabbits was described as being "curare-like" (50), and showed no response to edrophonium or eserine (11).

Progressive hindlimb paralysis and muscle atrophy appear in rats and rabbits fed a diet containing ZPT. These effects occur in the rat at diets above 50 ppm ZPT and in the rabbit at a dose of 17.5 mg/kg for 2 weeks. Sequential morphological studies in rats fed a diet containing 166 ppm ZPT show that the hindlimb paralysis is caused by a central-peripheral distal axonopathy (40) (see Chapter 1). The earliest observable morphological changes, present at 7–10 days of ZPT feeding, occur at the motor nerve terminals in distal hindlimb muscles. Axon terminals show accumulation of tubulovesicular membranous structures and occasional branched membranous arrays, measuring 25–40 nm in diameter. Subsequently, nerve-terminal swelling with autophagic vacuoles and degeneration takes place. Continued exposure results in a centripetal spread of abnormalities to intramuscular nerves and later to peroneal and posterior tibial nerves. CNS axons in long descending tracts of the spinal cord and in the cerebellar vermis show similar, but quantitatively fewer, axonal changes, compared to the peripheral nerves after approximately 4 weeks of ZPT exposure.

Correlative electromyographic studies of rats fed a diet of 166 ppm show trains of positive waves and fibrillation potentials recorded on the fifth day becoming more prominent at 10–14 days. Diminution of evoked muscle potentials recorded from the distal tail muscles occurs on the sixth day. Subsequently, a decrementing response of the evoked potential is observed correlating with the morphological changes preferentially affecting the distal nerve terminal. Electrophysiological abnormalities preceed functional signs (36).

Human Studies

Of the two known serious ZPT-induced toxic conditions in animals, ocular lesions and central-peripheral distal axonopathy, the former probably need not be considered as a potential human disorder. The human retina does not have a tapetum lucidum and the animals lacking this choroidal structure escaped from the adverse ocular effects following oral administration of ZPT (42).

Central-peripheral distal axonopathy has not been observed in primates after thorough studies (10,45). Although a brief report of a case of "mononeuritis multiplex," presenting as left footdrop and weak hand grip, has been linked to ZPT (5), it is more likely that this form of neuropathy was caused by another factor(s). Only symmetrical distal axonopathy, not multiple mononeuropathies, have been secondary to ZPT in experimental paradigms.

Toxic Mechanisms

The biological activity of pyridinethione in vertebrates is not known but could be related to inactivation of enzymes through the ability to chelate metal cofactors (12) or by reducing thiol groups (9). Extensive studies of bidirectional transport in ZPT-induced neuropathy strongly suggest an abnormality in the "turnaround" of fast transported material reaching the nerve terminal correlating with the site of accumulation of tubulovesicular membranous structures (41).

The distal turnaround process can also be impaired by inhibitors of thiol proteases (39). Using the nascent axon-tip model, it has been demonstrated that E-64, a specific inhibitor of thiol proteases, effectively inhibits this process; electron microscopy of the axon tips reveals numerous densely packed membranous tubules similar to those observed in the presence of pyridinethione (38,39). There is a novel protein involved in the membrane-fusion events that is sensitive to N-ethylmaleimide, a sulfhydryl reagent that effectively blocks -SH groups by forming covalent bonds (43). The hallmark of distal axonopathy induced by pyridinethione, the accumulation of tubulovesicular membranous structures at distal nerve terminals, might reflect impairment of fusion events essential for membrane recycling.

REFERENCES
1. Adams MD, Wedig JH, Jordan RL *et al.* (1976) Urinary excretion and metabolism of salts of 2-pyridinethiol-1-oxide following intravenous administration to female Yorkshire pigs. *Toxicol Appl Pharmacol* **36**, 523.
2. Albert A (1973) Metal binding substances. In: *Selective*

Toxicity. 5th Ed. Albert A ed. Chapman & Hall, London p. 334.

3. Albert A, Rees CW, Tomlinson AJH (1956) Why are some metal binding substances antibacterial? *Chem Abstr* **50**, 16975.

4. Barnett BL, Kretschmar HC, Hartman FA (1977) Structural characterization of bis(*N*-oxopyridine-2-thionato)-zinc (II). *Inorg Chem* **16**, 1834.

5. Beck JE (1978) Zinc pyridinethione and peripheral neuritis. *Lancet* **1**, 444.

6. Bernstein J, Losee KA (1958) Heavy metal derivatives of 1-hydroxy-2-pyridinethiones. *Chem Abstr* **52**, 2932.

7. Black JG, Howes D (1979) Toxicity of pyrithiones. *Toxicol Ann* **3**, 1.

8. Budinger JM (1961) Diphenylthiocarbazone blindness in dogs. *Arch Pathol* **71**, 304.

9. Chandler CJ, Segel IH (1978) Mechanism of the antimicrobial action of pyrithione: Effects on membrane transport, ATP levels and protein synthesis. *Antimicrob Agents Chemother* **14**, 60.

10. Cloyd GG, Wyman M, Shadduck JA *et al.* (1978) Toxicity studies with zinc pyridinethione. *Toxicol Appl Pharmacol* **45**, 771.

11. Collum WD, Winek CL (1967) Percutaneous toxicity of pyridinethiones in a dimethylsulfoxide vehicle. *J Pharm Sci* **56**, 1673.

12. Cotton JE (1964) Some cytological and biochemical effects of 2-pyridinethiol-1-oxide. *Dissertation Abstr* **24**, 2673.

13. Delahunt CS, Stebbins RB, Anderson J, Bailey J (1962) The cause of blindness in dogs given hydroxypyridinethione. *Toxicol Appl Pharmacol* **4**, 286.

14. Edrissi M, Massoumi A (1971) 2-Mercaptopyridine-1-oxide (sodium salt) as a selective absorptiometric reagent for determination of palladium (II). *Microchem J* **16**, 177.

15. Edrissi M, Massoumi A (1971) Selective determination of iron as tris(2-thio-4-methyl-pyridine-1-oxide)-iron (III) and the application of this substance for the analysis of mercury (II). *Microchem J* **16**, 353.

16. Edrissi M, Massoumi A, Dalziel JAW (1970) A selective differential spectrophotometric method for the determination of mercury (II) using tris(2-thio-pyridine-1-oxide) iron (III) a reagent. *Microchem J* **15**, 579.

17. Gibson B, Jeffcoat AR, Rodriguez D *et al.* (1982) Zinc pyridinethione: Serum metabolites of zinc pyridinethione in rabbits, rats, monkeys and dogs after oral dosing. *Toxicol Appl Pharmacol* **62**, 237.

18. Gibson WT, Chamberlain M, Parsons JF *et al.* (1985) The effect and muscle action of zinc pyrithione in cell growth. *Food Chem Toxicol* **23**, 93.

19. Gibson WT, Hardy WS, Groom MH (1985) The effect and mode of action of zinc pyrithione on cell growth. II. *In vivo* studies. *Food Chem Toxicol* **23**, 103.

20. Hamilton JM, Szkolnik M (1957) Performance of omodine, AC 5223 and other promising fungicides in the control of apple scab and cedar-apple rust. *Plant Dis Rep* **41**, 293.

21. Howell JM, Ishmael J, Ewbank R, Blake-More WB (1970) Changes in the central nervous system of lambs following administration of sodium diethyldithiocarbamate. *Acta Neuropathol* **15**, 1970.

22. Howes D, Black JG (1975) Comparative percutaneous absorption of pyrithiones. *Toxicology* **5**, 209.

23. Howlett HCS, Van Abbe NJ (1975) The action and fate of sodium pyridinethione when applied topically to the rabbit. *J Soc Cosmet Chem* **26**, 3.

24. Jasim S, Tjälve H (1986) Effects of sodium pyridinethione on the uptake and distribution of nickel, cadmium and zinc in pregnant and non-pregnant mice. *Toxicology* **38**, 327.

25. Jeffcoat AR, Gibson WB, Rodriguez PA *et al.* (1980) Zinc pyridinethione: Urinary metabolites of zinc pyridinethione in rabbits, rats, monkeys and dogs after oral dosing. *Toxicol Appl Pharmacol* **56**, 141.

26. Kenaga CB, Kiesling RL (1975) Control of three foliar diseases by several fungicides in greenhouse tests. *Plant Dis Rep* **41**, 303.

27. Klaassen CD (1976) Absorption, distribution and excretion of zinc pyridinethione in rabbits. *Toxicol Appl Pharmacol* **35**, 581.

28. Landsdown AB (1991) Interspecies variations in response to topical application of selected zinc compounds. *Food Chem Toxicol* **29**, 57.

29. Moe RA, Kirpan K, Linegar CR (1960) Toxicology of hydroxypyridinethione. *Toxicol Appl Pharmacol* **2**, 156.

30. Nolen GA, Patrick LF, Dierckman TA (1975) A percutaneous teratology study of zinc pyrithione in rabbits. *Toxicol Appl Pharmacol* **31**, 430.

31. Okamoto K, Ito T, Hasegawa A, Urakubo G (1967) Percutaneous absorption and residual amount on skin surface of zinc bis(2-pyridylthio)-1,1-dioxide. *Eisei Kagaku* **13**, 323.

32. Opdyke DL, Burnett CM, Brauer EW (1967) Antiseborrheic qualities of zinc pyrithione in a cream vehicle; II. Safety evaluation. *Food Cosmet Toxicol* **5**, 321.

33. Parekh C, Min BH, Goldberg L (1970) Experimental studies of sodium pyridinethione. I. Percutaneous absorption in laboratory animals. *Food Cosmet Toxicol* **8**, 147.

34. Parran JJ (1965) Deposition on the skin of particles of agents from detergent bases. *J Invest Dermatol* **45**, 86.

35. Pearse AD, Walker AP, Marks R (1985) Effect of zinc pyrithione on mitotic activity of normal human skin. *Arch Dermatol Res* **227**, 118.

36. Ross JF, Lawhorn GT (1990) ZPT-related distal axonopathy: Behavioral and electrophysiologic correlates in rats. *Neurotoxicol Teratol* **12**, 153.

37. Rutherford T, Black JG (1969) The use of autoradiography to study the localization of germicides in skin. *Brit J Dermatol* **81**, 75.

38. Sahenk Z, Brown A (1991) Weak-base amines inhibit the anterograde-to-retrograde conversion of axonally transported resides in nerve terminals. *J Neurocytol* **20**, 365.

39. Sahenk Z, Lasek RJ (1988) Inhibition of proteolysis blocks anterograde-to-retrograde conversion of axonally transported vesicles. *Brain Res* **460**, 199.

40. Sahenk Z, Mendell JR (1979) Ultrastructural study of zinc pyridinethione-induced peripheral neuropathy. *J Neuropathol Exp Neurol* **38**, 532.

41. Sahenk Z, Mendell JR (1980) Axoplasmic transport in zinc pyridinethione neuropathy: Evidence for an abnormality in distal turn-around. *Brain Res* **186**, 343.

42. Skoulis NP, Barbee SJ, Jacobson-Kram D *et al.* (1993) Evaluation of the genetic potential of zinc pyrithione in the salmonella mutagenicity (Ames) assay, CHO/HGPRT gene mutation assay and mouse micronucleus assay. *J Appl Toxicol* **13**, 283.

43. Söllner T, Rothman JE (1994) Neurotransmission: Harnessing fusion machinery at the synapse. *Trends Neurosci* **17**, 344.

44. Snyder DR, Gralla EJ, Coleman GL, Wedig JH (1977) Preliminary neurological evaluation of generalized weakness in zinc pyrithione-treated rats. *Food Cosmet Toxicol* **15**, 43.

45. Snyder FH, Buehler EV, Winek CL (1965) Safety evaluation of zinc 2-pyridinethiol-1-oxide in a shampoo formulation. *Toxicol Appl Pharmacol* **7**, 425.

46. Tosti A, Piraccini B, Brasile GP (1990) Occupational contact dermatitis due to sodium pyrithione. *Contact Dermatitis* **22**, 118.

47. Wedig JH, Goldhamer R, Henderson R (1974) Percutaneous absorption, distribution, and excretion of three 2,6-^{14}C pyridinethiones in female Yorkshire pigs. *Pharmacologist* **16a**, 252.

48. Wedig JH, Kennedy GI, Jenkins DH *et al.* (1975) Teratologic evaluation of zinc omadine when applied dermally on Yorkshire pigs. *Toxicol Appl Pharmacol* **33**, 123.

49. Weitzel G, Strecker FJ, Rouster U *et al.* (1954) Zinc in tapetum lucidum. *Hoppe-Seyler's Z Physiol Chem* **296**, 19.

50. Winek CL, Buehler EV (1966) Intravenous toxicity of zinc pyridinethione and several zinc salts. *Toxicol Appl Pharmacol* **9**, 269.

Quinacrine

Byron A. Kakulas

QUINACRINE
$C_{23}H_{30}ClN_3O$

N^4-(6-Chloro-2-methoxy-9-acridinyl)-N^1,N^1-diethyl-1,4-pentanediamine

NEUROTOXICITY RATING

Clinical

A   Seizure disorder

A   Acute encephalopathy

A   Psychobiological reaction (confusion, mania)

Quinacrine is an acridone derivative used as an intestinal anthelmintic and as an antimalarial; it is also frequently utilized for treatment of giardiasis, and its suitability as a female sterilization agent has been suggested. Veterinary uses include antiprotozoal and taeniacide treatment (9). The drug is no longer available in North America. Its mode of action is believed to be due to the inhibition of arachidonic acid derivatives, including the prostagladins. Prostaglandin E_2 inhibits the transport of norepinephrine from the sympathetic nerve endings. A reduction in the production of prostaglandin E_2 amplifies the effects of norepinephrine release (12).

Crystalline quinacrine forms bitter, bright-yellow crystals. The moderate solubility of the crystals (1 g dissolves in about 35 ml water) increases in hot water. It is slightly soluble in ethanol and somewhat more soluble in methanol. Quinacrine is insoluble in ether, benzene, and acetone. The pH of a 1% aqueous solution is about 4.5. The yellow aqueous solution of quinacrine exhibits a vivid fluorescence under ultraviolet light and is detectable at a dilution of 1: 5,000,000 (9).

The usual doses of quinacrine in the treatment of giardiasis in adults are 100 mg t.i.d. for 5–7 days. In children, effective doses are 7 mg/kg/day in three divided doses for 5 days, with a maximum dose of 300 mg daily (4).

Quinacrine is well absorbed, producing peak plasma levels in 1–3 h. The drug is well metabolized, with approximately 10% of each dose being excreted unchanged in the urine. The elimination half-life of quinacrine is approximately 5 days. The oral LD_{50} in roosters is 714 mg/kg (4,9).

Administration of large doses of quinacrine for the treatment of cestodiasis can produce headache, nausea and vomiting, abdominal cramps, and diarrhea. Doses prescribed for antimalarial activity may cause mild and transient headache; dizziness; and gastrointestinal disorders such as diarrhea, anorexia, nausea, and abdominal cramps. Small numbers of drug-treated patients report nightmares, irritability, and nervousness (15,16).

The development of toxic psychosis is a common dose-related effect of quinacrine-based treatment; several hundred cases are reported (6–8,10,13,14). Incidence of quinacrine-induced psychosis at normal doses is low, ranging from 1–4 per 1000 (5,7). The psychosis may occur as early as day 3 or 4 of the treatment or up to 12 days following the last dose (8). The psychosis may last 8–25 days following withdrawal of the drug (5).

A 33-year-old woman with no previous history developed mania following a 5-day course of quinacrine (250 mg orally, *t.i.d.*) for giardiasis. Her manic symptoms disappeared within 3 days after treatment with thiothixene and lithium (11).

Seizures have also been noted in patients following administration of quinacrine. The cerebral cortical stimulating effect of the drug may be responsible (2). Quinacrine should be administered cautiously to patients with epilepsy. Electroencephalographic studies confirm the stimulatory action of quinacrine, which is similar to high doses of amphetamines (3). Chloroquine, a closely related drug, causes both skeletal and cardiac myopathy (1).

REFERENCES

1. Aguayo AJ, Hudgson P (1970) Observations on the short-term effects of chloroquine on skeletal muscle. An experimental study in the rabbit. *J Neurol Sci* 11, 301.

2. Borda I, Krant M (1967) Convulsions following intrapleural administration of quinacrine hydrochloride. *J Amer Med Assn* 201, 899.

3. Engel GL, Romano J, Ferris FB (1947) Effect of quinacrine on the central nervous system. *Arch Neurol Psychiat* 58, 337.

4. DRUGDEX Editorial Staff (1995) Quinacrine. DRUGDEX Microdex Inc. Denver, CO.

5. Gaskill HS, Fitz-Hugh T (1945) Toxic psychosis following Atabrine®. *Bull U S Army Med Dept* 86, 63.

6. Good MI, Shader RL (1977) Behavioral toxicity and

equivocal suicide associated with chloroquine and its derivative. *Deliv Syst* **5**, 131.

7. Lidz T, Kahn RL (1946) Toxicity of quinacrine (Atabrine®) for the central nervous system. *Arch Neurol Psychiat* **56**, 284.

8. Lindemayer JP, Vargus P (1981) Toxic psychosis following use of quinacrine. *J Clin Psychiat* **42**, 162.

9. *Merck Index* (1983) Merck & Co, Rahway, New Jersey p. 1161.

10. Miller LG, Kraft IA (1991) Quinacrine-induced psychosis in a pediatric patient. *J Fam Pract* **32**, 526.

11. Moreno TJ, Green J (1989) Quinacrine associated mania. *Mayo Clin Proc* **64**, 129.

12. Robertson RP (1991) Eicosanoids and human disease In: *Harrison's Principles of Internal Medicine. 12th Ed.* Wilson JD, Braunwald E, Isselbacher KJ *et al.* eds. McGraw-Hill, New York p. 397.

13. Rockwell DA (1968) Psychiatric complications with chloroquine and quinacrine. *Amer J Psychiat* **124**, 1257.

14. Weisholtz SJ, McBride PA, Murray HW, Shear MK (1982) Quinacrine-induced psychiatric disturbances. *South Med J* **75**, 359.

15. Winthrop-Breon (1990) Product information: Atabrine®, quinacrine hydrochloride. Winthrop-Breon, New York.

16. Zipper JA, Stachetti E, Medel M (1970) Human fertility control by transvaginal application of quinacrine on the fallopian tube. *Fert Steril* **21**, 581.

Quinidine

Herbert H. Schaumburg

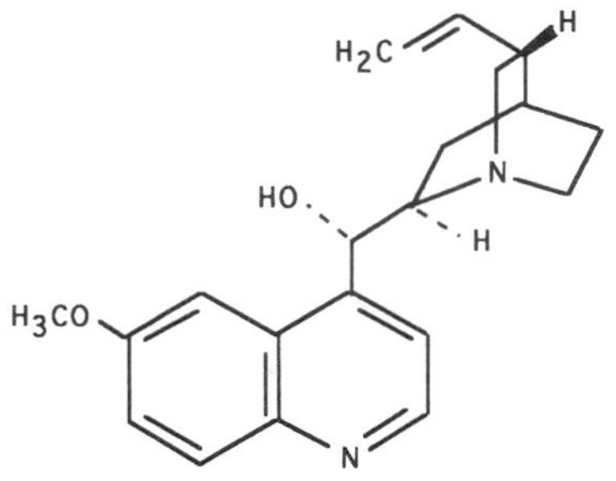

QUINIDINE
$C_{20}H_{24}N_2O_2$

(9S)-6'-Methoxycinchonan-9-ol

NEUROTOXICITY RATING

Clinical

A   Ototoxicity (tinnitus, hearing loss)

B   Chronic encephalopathy (cognitive dysfunction)

Quinidine is a chincona alkaloid widely used in the treatment of cardiac ventricular and atrial arrhythmias. Systemic adverse effects may occur at therapeutic doses, and patients must be monitored closely. Myocardial toxicity with slowed conduction in the Purkinje fibers is a major concern, as are hypotension, arterial embolization (following conversion of atrial fibrillation to normal sinus rhythm), and gastroenteritis.

Prolonged therapy with quinidine at conventional doses may cause a mild, limited form of cinchonism (*see* Quinine, this volume). The symptoms are tinnitus, hearing loss, and vertigo; presumably the auditory phenomena reflect a quinine-like dysfunction in the cochlear outer hair cells (3). Visual symptoms associated with chincona alkaloid toxicity are not convincingly described with quinidine therapy.

Three case reports depict chronic cognitive decline or psychosis in elderly individuals receiving conventional antiarrhythmic maintenance therapy with quinidine; all recovered following drug withdrawal (1,2).

Quinidine decreases the myocardial Purkinje fiber firing rate by a direct action; the molecular mechanism of the antiarrhythmic action is unknown. Quinidine has multiple effects on the autonomic nervous system: it blocks the effect of vagal stimulation by an anticholinergic atropine-like action and also has an α-adrenergic blocking action.

REFERENCES

1. Akinyanju O, Goddell JC, Ahmed I (1973) Pyrimethamine poisoning. *Brit Med J* **20**, 147.

2. Fish DR, Espir MLE (1989) Convulsions associated with prophylactic antimalarial drugs: Implications for people with epilepsy. *Brit Med J* **299**, 1524.

3. Rhuedi L, Furrer W, Luthy F *et al.* (1952) Further observation concerning the toxic effects of streptomycin and quinine on the auditory organ of guinea pigs. *Laryngoscope* **62**, 333.

Quinine

Steven Herskovitz

QUININE
$C_{20}H_{24}N_2O_2$

(8α,9R)-6'-Methoxycinchonan-9-ol

NEUROTOXICITY RATING

Clinical

A Ototoxicity

A Neuromuscular transmission syndrome

A Retinopathy

B Acute encephalopathy (seizures, sedation, coma)

Experimental

A Retinopathy

Quinine, a stereoisomer of quinidine, is the primary alkaloid derived from the bark of the cinchona tree. Historical records suggest that its use dates from the seventeenth century. Uses include the treatment of chloroquine-resistant malaria, nocturnal leg cramps, and the symptoms of myotonia congenita. It is an ingredient in tonic water, may be found as an adulterant in illicit heroin, and was used in the past as an abortifacient. Toxicity results in a constellation of features known as cinchonism, including CNS, ocular, auditory, gastrointestinal, and cardiac abnormalities. It may cause deterioration in patients with myasthenia gravis.

Oral quinine is readily and almost completely absorbed, mainly from the upper small intestine (8,11). Peak plasma concentrations occur within 1–3 h. It is widely distributed to body tissues. Drug concentration in cerebrospinal fluid is only about 2%–5% of that in plasma. About 70%–90% is bound to plasma proteins. The elimination half-life is about 11 h. Metabolism occurs in the liver by hydroxylation; <25% is excreted unchanged in the urine. The pharmacokinetics may be altered in patients with malaria.

Animal toxicity studies are limited. Long-term oral dosing in rats showed some hepatic and renal toxicity, but did not cause any permanent ototoxicity or ophthalmic toxicity in dosages up to 200 mg/kg/day (6). In cats given sublethal doses, anatomical changes in the eye include pyknosis followed by generalized loss of retinal ganglion cells (8).

Quinine toxicity in humans is related to plasma drug concentration; levels >10 mg/l are associated with an increasing risk of toxicity (3,4). Low-level repeated dosing in healthy volunteers is without adverse physiological, ophthalmic, or audiometric effects at daily consumption of up to 80 mg for 21 days (7). The average fatal single dose is about 8 g, but the range is wide (11). Most clinical toxicity results from intentional overdose in suicide attempts or accidental exposure to adulterated street drugs. There are no known effective elimination techniques for the treatment of quinine overdosage (3,4).

The symptoms of cinchonism begin an average of 3.5 h after acute ingestion and are similar in cases of chronic drug accumulation during therapy for malaria (4,11). They include nausea, vomiting, abdominal pain, diarrhea, flushing, diaphoresis, headache, tinnitus, and hearing loss. The auditory symptoms nearly always resolve. As plasma quinine concentrations rise further, increasingly severe visual, cardiac, and neurological features occur (4,11).

Though less potent than quinidine, quinine is also a class 1 antiarrhythmic. Oculotoxicity, associated with concentrations >10 mg/l, typically appears several hours after initial presentation, beginning with visual blurring and disturbance of color perception. Severe cases can progress to constriction of visual fields, decreased central acuity, and blindness. Pupils may be fixed and dilated for some time before light perception is lost. Partial recovery is usual and may be complete, but residua can be severe. A chronic, low-grade quinine maculopathy has been suggested in a study of heroin users (10).

CNS effects include ataxia, headache, vertigo, syncope, and encephalopathy; in severe poisoning, seizures, coma, and respiratory depression are seen (4,11). A single case is reported of so-called myelo-optico-neuropathy after quinine poisoning, but other factors are possible explanations for the clinical features in this alcoholic patient (2). Quinine may interfere with neuromuscular transmission in a complex fashion and cause deterioration in patients with myasthenia gravis (8,9).

The mechanism for the CNS effects of quinine is not well described. It decreases the excitability of the motor endplate region; this may be the basis for its effect in the symptomatic relief of myotonia congenita and in its use for nocturnal leg cramps (8). Oculotoxicity is likely related to a direct toxic effect on cellular elements of the retina, although the exact mechanism is unknown (1,4). The frequently observed retinal vascular changes are probably secondary. Quinine is postulated to block cholinergic neurotransmission in the inner synaptic layer of the retina (5).

REFERENCES

1. Bacon P, Spalton DJ, Smith SE (1988) Blindness from quinine toxicity. *Brit J Ophthalmol* **72**, 219.

2. Banerji NK, Martin VAF (1974) Myelo-optico-neuropathy following quinine poisoning. *J Irish Med Assn* **67**, 46.

3. Bateman DN, Blain PG, Woodhouse KW *et al.* (1985) Pharmacokinetics and clinical toxicity of quinine overdosage: Lack of efficacy of techniques intended to enhance elimination. *Quart J Med* **54**, 125.

4. Bateman DN, Dyson EH (1986) Quinine toxicity. *Adverse Drug React Ac Pois Rev* **4**, 215.

5. Canning CR, Hague S (1988) Ocular quinine toxicity. *Brit J Ophthalmol* **72**, 23.

6. Colley JC, Edwards JA, Heywood R, Purser D (1989) Toxicity studies with quinine hydrochloride. *Toxicology* **54**, 219.

7. Drewitt PN, Butterworth KR, Springall CD (1993) Toxicity threshold of quinine hydrochloride following low-level repeated dosing in healthy volunteers. *Food Chem Toxicol* **31**, 235.

8. Gilman AG, Rall TR, Nies AS, Taylor P (1990) *The Pharmacological Basis of Therapeutics. 8th Ed.* Pergamon Press, New York p. 991.

9. Layzer RB (1985) *Neuromuscular Manifestations of Systemic Disease.* FA Davis, Philadelphia p. 383.

10. Maltzman B, Sutula F, Cinotti AA (1975) Toxic maculopathy, part 1. A result of quinine usage. *Ann Ophthalmol* **7**, 1321.

11. Wolf LR, Otten EJ, Spadafora MP (1992) Cinchonism: Two case reports and review of acute quinine toxicity and treatment. *J Emerg Med* **10**, 295.

3-Quinuclidinyl Benzilate

Peter S. Spencer

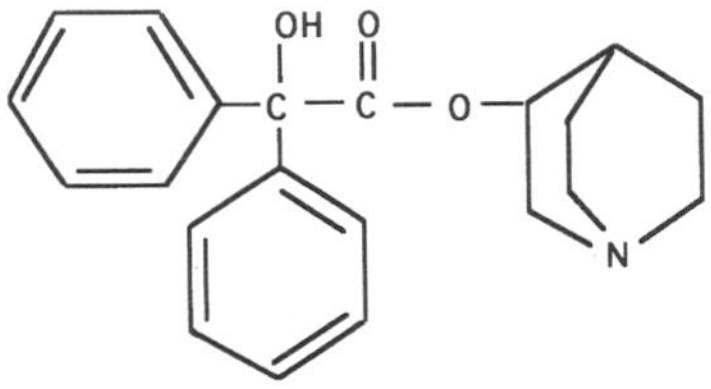

3-QUINUCLIDINYL BENZILATE
$C_{21}H_{23}NO_3$

3-Hydroxyquinuclidine benzilate; QNB; BZ

NEUROTOXICITY RATING

Experimental

A Anticholinergic

3-Quinuclidinyl benzilate (QNB) is a potent, atropine-like glycolic acid ester that blocks acetylcholine muscarinic neurotransmission in the CNS and PNS (6). Halogenated derivatives of QNB are under development as clinical tools to quantify the regional brain distribution of cell-surface muscarinic receptors by single photon emission computed tomography (SPECT) or positron emission tomography (PET) (8,11,16,22,35,45).

From the 1950s onward, QNB was explored by the United States and the former Soviet Union as a potential antidote for potent anticholinesterase nerve agents (38,41,43). The marked hallucinogenic actions of low doses of QNB subsequently led the U.S. Army to adopt the compound (known as *BZ*) as an incapacitating psychochemical (43). The U.S. Army facility at Pine Bluff Arsenal, Arkansas, produced and stockpiled approximately 10 tons of BZ in bulk and weaponized form (6,38). Destruction of the U.S. stockpile of BZ held at Pine Bluff Arsenal began in the 1980s (36) and was complete by 1987. Iraq began investigating esters of glycolic esters before 1985 and, by 1991, may have had large quantities of an incapacitant (known as *Agent 15*) consisting of BZ or a derivative thereof (26). Extensive reviews on the physicochemical, analytical, biological, and toxicological properties of BZ (QNB) are available (27,31,43).

QNB, the benzilate ester of 3-quinuclidinol, has two asymmetric centers on the quinuclidinyl and benzilic acid centers and therefore exists in four different diasteromeric forms (45). Pure QNB is a crystalline solid with a MW of 337.4, a BP of 412°C, and a MP of 167.5°C. It is 11.6 times heavier than air. Volatility at 15°C is insignificant. At 25°C, QNB hydrolyzes rapidly (1.8 min) at pH 13, over 16 days at pH 9.8, and slowly (4 weeks) at pH 7.0; hydrolysis products are 3-quinuclidinol and hydrochloric acid (6). QNB is blended in U.S. weapons with an energetic pyrotechnic mixture (50% BZ, 23% $KClO_3$, 9% S, and 18% $NaHCO_3$) which, after detonation, produces an aerosol cloud of BZ (40).

General Toxicology

QNB and the 3-quinuclidinyl esters of various phenyl-thienyl- and dithienyl-glycolic acids are potent members of a group of glycolate esters that have atropine-like actions on the CNS and PNS (37,38).

QNB is rapidly removed from rat liver perfusates. The brain is the only organ containing radioactivity 48 h after intraperitoneal injection of ^{3}H-QNB to mice (14). Binding of radiolabel to rat brain is strongly inhibited by both muscarinic anticholinergic agonist drugs (scopolamine, isopropamide, atropine) and muscarinic agonists (oxotremorine, acetylcholine, methacholine), but not by nicotinic anticholinergic drugs (hexamethonium, D-tubocurarine) (43). Monkey brain homogenates incubated with ^{3}H-QNB show the following decreasing order of radioligand uptake: putamen, caudate nucleus, occipital cortex, cingulate gyrus, postcentral gyrus, hippocampus, amygdala, precentral gyrus, pyriform cortex, frontal cortex, superior colliculi, thalamus, and inferior colliculi (44). Brain uptake of radiolabel from ^{3}H-QNB shows some correlation with choline uptake and choline acetylase activity, but not with acetylcholinesterase activity (44). QNB decreases brain acetylcholine concentration in a linear relationship with the dose of QNB (9).

The two major urinary metabolites of QNB are 3-quinuclidinol and benzilic acid; trimethylsilyl derivatives thereof are used to analyze the compounds by gas chromatography–mass spectrometry (3). Detection limits for these compounds exceed 0.5 ng/ml and 5 ng/ml, respectively (4).

After intravenous (i.v.) administration of ^{3}H-QNB to the cat, regions retaining radiolabel are motor cortex > sensory cortex > caudate nucleus > lateral geniculate nucleus. Smaller amounts are found in other CNS areas in the following decreasing concentration: thalamus > hippocampus > hypothalamus > medulla oblongata > colliculi > cerebellar cortex > medullary pyramids > cerebral white matter > and cerebellar white matter (1). Intramuscular (i.m.) injection of atropine 30 min before i.v. administration of ^{3}H-QNB decreases regional binding in proportion to QNB uptake and in the following decreasing order: corpus striatum > cerebral cortex > hippocampus > hypothalamus > pons-medulla oblongata > cerebellum. There is therefore agreement in the rank order for QNB binding and that for the reduction by atropine of benzilate binding (43).

Animal Studies

The mouse LD$_{50}$s for QNB are: intravenous, 18–25 mg/kg body weight (vs. 74 mg/kg for atropine); intraperitoneal, 110 mg/kg (vs. 119 mg/kg for scopalamine); subcutaneous, 215 mg/kg; and per os, 290 mg/kg. Intravenous LD$_{50}$s for other species are established for the guinea pig (14 mg/kg), rabbit (10 mg/kg), cat (12 mg/kg), pig (5 mg/kg), and goat (7 mg/kg) (43).

QNB is absorbed percutaneously (p.c.) when the agent is applied in a mixture of alcohol and cresol to the shaven skin of animals (25). Doses up to 500 mg/kg elicit ataxia in cats and dogs after 30 min and 55 min, respectively; lower doses produce ocular effects that persisted for at least 2 days in a single monkey treated p.c. with 250 mg/kg QNB (25). Other reported effects in rats, dogs, and monkeys exposed to clouds of QNB include ataxia, dyspnea, mydriasis, tachycardia, sedation, and hyperactivity (15).

Administration of 0.01, 0.1, or 1.0 mg/kg/day QNB i.v. to male albino rats over a 4-week period results in a consistent daily pattern of mydriasis; this suggests metabolic inactivation of the agent within a 24-h period and an absence of tolerance for this effect. The progressive development of tolerance or decreased responsiveness to QNB is noted at high doses for pharmacotoxic signs other than mydriasis (27). Male and female mongrel dogs given repeated i.v. doses of 0.1 or 1.0 mg/kg/day exhibited mydriasis, ptosis, decreased activity, ataxia and weakness of limbs. A dose of 10 mg/kg induced bradycardia in five of five dogs and death in two of five due to cardiac arrest. Dogs given daily i.v. doses of 100 μg/kg showed an interval to onset of ataxia that increased from 4 min to 14 min over a 14-day treatment period (25). Male and female monkeys treated i.v. with 0.01, 0.1, or 1.0 mg/kg/day showed mydriasis at all dosage levels and decreased activity and ataxia at the two higher dosages (14).

QNB has a biphasic effect on spontaneous rat motor activity: low doses (0.1 mg/kg) depress activity, while higher doses (0.3–10 mg/kg) increase activity in a dose-related manner (23). Physostigmine, amobarbital, or chlorpromazine block the effect (13). ^{3}H-QNB binding in caudate-putamen, cerebral cortex, and hippocampus does not change as a result of forced swimming (5). Doses of 0.5, 1.0, and 2.0 mg/kg of QNB hasten learning of a conditioned response in rats; however, performance of some animals worsened after a dose of 1.0 mg/kg.

Human Studies

Effective doses of anticholinergic glycolates can be delivered by inhalation (fast) or via skin (slow); in dimethyl sulfoxide, percutaneous transfer of QNB increases 25-fold (14,15,39). For aerosol inhalation, the ED$_{50}$ is about 60 mg.min/m^3 for a man with a body weight of 75 kg and minute volume of respiration of 15 liters (15). The estimated 50% concentration (C) X time (t) human incapacitation dose (I(C$_t$)$_{50}$) is 110–170 mg/min/m^3 (20,43). The 7-day standards for daily consumption of 5 liters and 15 liters of potable water are 7 μg/l and 2.33 μg/l QNB, respectively (29).

Experimental trials to determine the effects of QNB on human performance ($n = 354$) were undertaken by the U.S. Army in 1964 and 1969 (25). Effects of QNB decrease in the following order of administration: i.v., i.m., inhalation, oral, dermal (14).

Intramuscular injection of 2 μg/kg body weight results in decrements in task performance, increased heart rate, decreased systolic, and increased diastolic blood pressure (10,17,18). Dizziness, drowsiness, mydriasis, and difficulty in visual accommodation to near objects follow intramuscular injection of 4 mg/kg QNB (vide infra). Performance on the Number Facility Test of the Minnesota Multiphasic Personality Inventory drops as a function of i.m. dose of QNB (19). An i.m. injection of 1.5–1.7 μg/kg VX, S-(2-diisopropylaminoethyl)-ethylmethylphosphonothioate (see Sarin, Other "Nerve Agents," and Their Antidotes, this volume), rapidly improved performance on the Number Facility Test of three volunteers previously given 6 mg/kg QNB (34). Dramatic improvement in performance on this test was seen in four volunteers given 7 mg/kg QNB i.m. after an i.m. injection of 7 or 11 mg of physostigmine salicylate followed by oral administration of 24 or 12 mg, respectively, of the same drug during total periods of treatment of 43 and 42 h, respectively (33).

Clinical manifestations of inhalation exposure to a BZ aerosol appear within 30 min, peak in 4–8 h, and may persist for days. Effects have been graphically described as follows:

> During the first 4 hours, the victim's nose, mouth and throat become parched, and his skin dry and flushed. He may vomit, and his head may ache. His vision blurs, and he becomes dizzy, confused and sedated to the point of stupor. He may stagger and stumble about, talking in a slurred voice or mumbling nonsensically, failing to respond appropriately when spoken to. During the next 4 hours, when he will be feeling highly disoriented, experiencing visual and auditory hallucinations, he may be unable to move about or react effectively to his surroundings. His memory may fade. Later, his activity returns, but for the next day or two his behaviour may remain random and unpredictable, even maniacal, only gradually returning to normal. (32,33)

Aerosolized QNB has about 20 times the potency of atropine in altering CNS functions, and effects last about six times longer (32). Low doses of aerosolized QNB result in dry mouth, decreased gastric motility, inhibition of sweating, increased heart rate, pupillary dilatation and loss of accommodation, mild sedation, and mental slowing. There is decline in motor coordination, attentiveness, and control of thought and learning processes. Other effects include confusion, restlessness, impairment in perception, interpretation, and memory span, poor judgment, and deficient insight. True hallucinations are present. High doses may result in stupor or coma lasting several hours (32).

Six patients given 0.1 mg QNB t.i.d. as a treatment for parkinsonism experienced nocturnal confusion (27).

Treatment

Children are generally more sensitive than adults to antimuscarinic drugs with actions comparable to those of QNB (30). QNB has two potentially life-threatening effects. First, suppression of the ability to sweat may lead to fatal hyperthermia; this is a major health hazard for individuals engaging in strenuous activity in hot weather and/or while wearing chemical protective suits. Second, actions of QNB on the heart may give rise to serious arrhythmias, including ventricular fibrillation (43). The CNS actions of QNB, which may be present for days after exposure, are mediated by actions on acetylcholine muscarinic receptors that are considered to be fully reversible. Both cholinergic and anticholinesterase drugs antagonize the clinical effects of QNB (43).

The following regimen is recommended in U.S. Army technical manuals for treatment of QNB intoxication (7,42): 3 mg physostigmine salicylate i.m., a second equivalent dose 40 min later if required, and oral maintenance doses of 2–5 mg every 1–2 h, with reduction in dosing as the mental state improves. Adequacy of therapy is indicated by a heart rate of 70–80 bpm, with reductions in the frequency and/or magnitude of the dose if the heart rate falls below 70 bpm. Peripheral effects of physostigmine overdose (sweating, vomiting, muscle twitching, tremor, weakness) may be antagonized by small doses of methylatropinium or, if unavailable, atropine.

Healthy male volunteers in their mid twenties showed the following temporal sequence of clinical manifestations following a single intramuscular dose of QNB, 5.0–6.4 μg/kg body weight, followed by treatment at various times with cholinomimetics such as physostigmine or tetrahydroaminoacridine:

10 min—lightheadedness and giggling

30 min—dry mouth, blurred vision, nausea, chilly sensations, and twitching

1 h—flushed skin, incoordination, fatigue, unsteadiness, sleepiness, and quivering legs

2 h—many of the above, plus poor concentration, restlessness, hallucinations, slurred speech, and muscle fasciculation

3 h—as above, plus tremors

4 h—as above, plus belligerence accompanied by difficulty in handling the subject; pulse, 136

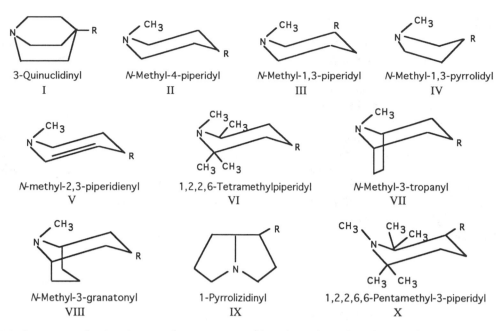

FIGURE 35. Chemical structures of various heterocyclic amino esters of benzilic acid. **R** = benzilate. Psychomimetic potency decreases from I to X. [From National Research Council (27).]

8 h—as above, plus delirium and hallucinations

24 h—persistent delirium, hallucinations, restlessness, unsteadiness, and increased pulse in some

48 h—persistent impairment of function in some and return to an apparently normal state in others, depending on vigor of antidotal treatment (27)

Toxic Mechanisms

QNB binds reversibly to acetylcholine receptors. Diasteromers of quinuclinyl-4^{18}F-fluoromethyl-benzilate (FMeQNB) are high-affinity ligands for muscarinic (m) acetylcholine receptors (16). The nonradioactive (R,R) diasteromer has an eightfold selectivity for m1 over m2 receptors, while the nonradioactive (R,S) diasteromer has a 7-fold selectivity for m2 over m1 receptors *in vitro* (16). Uptake of (R,S)-^{18}F-FMeQNB may be specific for m2 receptors in rat brain *in vivo*, while (R,R)-^{18}F-FeQNB may be m1-selective *in vivo* (2,16,21).

QNB and related anticholinergic drugs inhibit the actions of acetylcholine (a) on autonomic effectors innervated by postganglionic cholinergic nerves, and (b) on smooth muscles that lack cholinergic innervation. Small doses of atropinic agents inhibit salivary and bronchial secretion and sweating; larger doses cause pupillary dilatation and block vagal restraint of heart rate. Still larger doses inhibit the parasympathetic control of bladder and gastrointestinal tract, with inhibition of micturition and decreased intestinal tone and mobility. Very large doses of atropine-like drugs are required to exert effects at nicotinic receptors in auto-nomic ganglia and neuromuscular junctions. CNS acetylcholine postsynaptic receptors are predominately nicotinic in the spinal cord (very low QNB binding) and muscarinic and nicotinic in the brain (high QNB binding regionally) (27). Antimuscarinic drugs like QNB also increase release and turnover of acetylcholine in the CNS; this may result in activation of both muscarinic and nicotinic receptors and contribute to their central effects (27). The psychomimetic effects of QNB in relation to those of structural relatives is shown in Figure 35.

QNB also binds to rat brain mitochondrial fractions with an avidity 2.6–3.3 times greater than that of atropine (46). QNB decreases oxygen consumption in rats and rat brain slices (12). A related compound, ditran (3:7 mixture of the phenylcyclopentyl glycolates of N-ethyl-3-piperidinol and N-ethyl-3-pyrrolidylmethanol), interferes with production of adenosine triphosphate (24). The possibility of a presynaptic (as well as the postsynaptic) action of QNB on calcium metabolism has been raised (28).

REFERENCES

1. Becker MJ (1964) *Biochemical Studies of BZ and EA 3443*. Final Report. Contract No DA-18-104-CML-6631. [Cited in ref. 27]

2. Boulay SF, Sood VK, Rayeq MR *et al.* (1996) Autoradiographic evidence that 3-quinuclidinyl-4-fluorobenzilate (FQNB) displays *in vivo* selectivity for the m2 subtype. *Neuroimage* **3**, 35.

3. Byrd GD, Paul RC, Sander LC *et al.* (1992) *Determination of 3-Quinuclidinyl Benzilate (Qnb) and Its Major Metab-*

olites in Urine by Isotope Dilution Gas Chromatography Mass Spectrometry. Final Report. US Natl Inst of Standards and Technology (NML), Gaithersburg, Maryland.

4. Byrd GD, Sniegoski LT, White E (1987) *Development of a Confirmatory Chemical Test for Exposure to 3-Quinuclidinyl Benzilate (BZ)*. Final Report. U.S. Natl Bureau of Standards (NML), Washington, DC.

5. Carrizo E, Cano G, Suarez-Roca H, Bonilla E (1997) Motor activity and quantitative autoradiographic analysis of muscarinic receptors in the brain of rats subject to the forced swimming test. *Brain Res Bull* **42**, 133.

6. Compton JAF (1987) *Military Chemical and Biological Agents. Chemical and Toxicological Properties*. Telford Press, Caldwell, New Jersey.

7. Directorate of Medical Research (1965) *Guide to the Management of BZ Casualties*. U.S. Dept of Army, Edgewood Arsenal, Maryland.

8. Eckleman WC (1995) Designing a molecular probe for muscarinic acetylcholine receptor (mAChR) imaging. *J Nucl Med* **36**, 5S.

9. Frances H, Jacob J (1971) Comparison des effets de substances cholinergiques et anticholinergiques sur les taux cerebraux d'acetylcholine et sur la motilité chez la souris. *Psychopharmacology* **21**, 338.

10. Freedman T (1962) *Effects of BZ on Pilot Performance*. Final Report, Contract No. DA-18-108-CML-6644. [Cited in ref. 27]

11. Gibson RE, Schneidau TA, Gitler M *et al.* (1994) Muscarinic receptor selectivities of 3-quinuclidinyl 8-xanthenecarboxylate (QNX) in rat brain. *Life Sci* **54**, 1757.

12. Jovic RC, Zupanc S (1973) Inhibition of stimulated cerebral respiration *in vitro* and oxygen consumption *in vivo* in rats treated by cholinolytic drugs. *Biochem Pharmacol* **22**, 1189.

13. Kabes J, Fusek J, Fink Z (1972) Effects of 3-quinuclidinyl-benzilate on spontaneous motor activity in rats and management of the anticholinergic syndrome by some psychotropic drugs. *Activ Nerv Suppl* **14**, 163.

14. Ketchum J (1963) *The Human Assessment of BZ*. U.S. Army Chemical Research and Development Lab Technical Memo 20-29.

15. Ketchum JS, Tharp BR, Crowell EB *et al.* (1967) *The Human Assessment of BZ Disseminated Under Field Conditions*. Technical Report 4140, U.S. Dept of Army, Edgewood Arsenal, Maryland.

16. Kiesewetter DO, Carson RE, Jagoda EM (1997) *In vivo* muscarinic binding selectivity of (*R,S*)- and (*R,R*)-[^18F]-fluoromethyl QNB. *Bioorg Med Chem* **5**, 1555.

17. Kitzes DL, Ketchum JS, Crowell EB Jr, Balter L (1966) *Factors Contributing to Individual Differences in Response to Incapacitating Agents. l. The Contribution to Difference in Body Weight and Performance Agility to Response Variance*. Technical Memo 114-3, U.S. Dept of Army, Edgewood Arsenal, Maryland.

18. Kitzes DL, Vancil ME (1965) *Estimate of Minimal Effective Doses of BZ by the Intramuscular Route in Man*. U.S. Army Chem Res Develop Labs Technical Memo 2-30.

19. Klapper JA, McColloch MA, Kysor KP, Sim VP (1972) *Personality Correlates of Response to Atropine, Scopalamine, and Glycolate Compounds*. Technical Report 4616, U.S. Dept of Army, Edgewood Arsenal, Maryland.

20. Klose K (1968) Psychogifte. *Militärtechnik* **11**, 493.

21. Lee J, Paik CH, Kiesewetter DO *et al.* (1995) Evaluation of stereoisomers of 4-fluoroalkyl analogues of 3-quinuclidinyl benzilate in *in vivo* competition studies for the M1, M2, and M3 muscarinic receptor subtypes in brain. *Nucl Med Biol* **22**, 773.

22. Lee KS, He XS, Jones DW (1996) An improved method for rapid and efficient radioiodination of iodine-123-IQNB. *J Nucl Med* **37**, 2021.

23. Liu WF, Hu NW, Beaton JM (1984) Biphasic effects of 3-quinuclidinyl benzilate on spontaneous motor activity in mice. *Psychopharmacology* **84**, 486.

24. Lowy K, Abood LG, Raines H (1976) Behavioral effects and binding affinities of two stereoisomeric psychotomimetic glycolates. *J Neurosci Res* **2**, 157.

25. McNamara BP (1960) *Research in Toxicology Division on Effects of CS 4030 in Animals*. U.S. Chemical Warfare Laboratories Special Publ 2-28. [Cited in ref. 27]

26. Ministry of Defence (1998) *Iraqi Capability During the Gulf War*. Brit Min Defence Home Page, February 9.

27. National Research Council (1982) *Possible Long-Term Health Effects of Short-Term Exposure to Chemical Agents. Vol 1. Anticholinesterases and Anticholinergics*. National Academy Press, Washington, DC.

28. O'Neill JO (1992) Biochemical aspects of anticholinergic chemicals. In: National Research Council (1982) *Possible Long-Term Health Effects of Short-Term Exposure to Chemical Agents. Vol 1. Anticholinesterases and Anticholinergics*. National Academy Press, Washington, DC p. K1.

29. Palmer WG (1990) *Field-Water Quality Standards for BZ*. Technical Report. U.S. Army Biomed Res Dev Lab, Fort Detrick, Maryland.

30. Pfeiffer CC, Murphee HB, Jenney EH *et al.* (1959) Hallucinatory effect in man of acetylcholine inhibitors. *Neurology* **9**, 249.

31. Rosenblatt DH, Dacre JC, Shiotsuka RN, Rowlett CD (1985) *Problem Definition Studies of Potential Environmental Pollutants. VIII. Chemistry and Toxicology of BZ (3-Quinuclidinyl Benzilate)*. Technical Report. April-August. U.S. Army Med Bioeng Res Dev Lab, Fort Detrick, Maryland.

32. Sidell FR (undated) *A Summary of Investigations in Man with BZ Conducted by the U.S. Army, 1960–1969*. CSL 000-137. [Cited in ref. 27]

33. Sidell FR (1976) *Use of Physostigmine by the Intravenous, Intramuscular, and Oral Routes in the Therapy of Anti-*

cholinergic Drug Intoxication. Technical Report 76012. U.S. Dept of Army, Edgewood Arsenal, Maryland.

34. Sidell FR, Aghajanian GK, Groff WA (1973) The reversal of anticholinergic intoxication in man with cholinesterase inhibitor VX. *Proc Soc Exp Biol Med* **144**, 725.

35. Sood VK, Lee KS, Boulay SF *et al.* (1997) *In vivo* autoradiography of radioiodinated (R)-3-quinuclidinyl (S)-4-iodobenzilate [(R,S)-IQNB] and (R)-3-quinuclidinyl (R)-4-iodobenzilate [(R,R)-IQNB]. Comparison of the radiolabelled products of a novel tributylstannyl precursor with those of the established triazene and exchange methods. *Appl Radiat Isotop* **48**, 27.

36. Spurgeon WE, Roux RG, Meseke EL *et al.* (1985) *M55 Rocket Disposal Program Study M55-CD-07: Concept Plan, Demilitarization of M55 Rockets at Pine Bluff Arsenal (PBA).* Final Report. U.S. Army Toxic and Hazardous Materials Agency, Aberdeen Proving Ground, Maryland.

37. Sternbach LH, Kaiser S (1952) Antispasmotics. II. Esters of basic bicyclic alcohols. *J Amer Chem Soc* **74**, 2219.

38. Stockholm International Peace Research Institute (1971) *The Problem of Chemical and Biological Warfare: A Study of the Historical, Technical, Military, Legal, and Political Aspects of Chemical and Biological Warfare and Possible Disarmament Measures. Vol 1. The Rise of Chemical and Biological Weapons.* Almqvist & Wiksell, Stockholm.

39. Stoughton RB, Fritsch W (1964) Influence of DMSO on human percutaneous absorption. *Arch Dermatol* **90**, 512.

40. Trott BD, Stuart JC (1982) *Minutes of the Explosives Safety Seminar (20th).* Norfolk, Virginia, 24–26 August, Vol. 1. AD-A124 400, Batelle Columbus Laboratories, Ohio.

41. US Department of Army (1967) *Military Chemistry and Chemical Agents.* Technical Manual 3-215/C-2.

42. US Department of Army (1968) *Treatment of Chemical Agent Casualties.* Technical Manual TM 8-285.

43. Wills JH (1982) Digest report: Anticholinergic chemicals. In: National Research Council, *Possible Long-Term Health Effects of Short-Term Exposure to Chemical Agents. Vol 1. Anticholinesterases and Anticholinergics.* National Academy Press, Washington, DC p. I 1.

44. Yamamura HI, Kuhar MJ, Greenberg D, Snyder SH (1974) Muscarinic cholinergic receptor binding: Regional distribution in monkey brain. *Brain Res* **66**, 541.

45. Zeeberg BR, Boulay SF, Gitler MS *et al.* (1997) Correction of the stereochemical assignment of the benzilic acid center in (R)-(−)-3-quinuclidinyl (S)-(+)-4-iodobenzilate [R,S]-4-IQNB]. *Appl Radiat Isot* **48**, 463.

46. Zvirblis P, Kondritzer AA (1966) *Adsorption of H³-BZ and C¹⁴-Atropine to the Mitochondrial Fractions of the Rat Brain.* Technical Report 4042, U.S. Dept of Army, Edgewood Arsenal, Maryland.

CASE REPORT

A male chemist ingested about 0.5 mg QNB. Acute symptoms included dryness of the mouth, mydriasis, and a sensation of weakness in the knees. Several subcutaneous doses of neostigmine were administered as therapy. He slept fitfully that night and spoke incoherently during waking periods. Next morning, he was still unsteady on his feet, and his pupils were dilated. On the second morning, all symptoms except those due to persistent mydriasis had disappeared. He stated that he felt confused and that time had seemed to pass very slowly (33).

Rabies Vaccine

Neil L. Rosenberg

NEUROTOXICITY RATING
Clinical

Neural tissue–derived	Duck embryo–derived	Human diploid cell–derived	
A	A	C	Postvaccinial encephalomyelitis
A	C	B	Peripheral neuropathy (Guillain-Barré syndrome)
A	C	C	Aseptic meningitis

Many neurological complications of rabies vaccine have occurred, most notably postvaccinial encephalomyelitis (PVE), since its initial administration in 1885 (29). PVE and other neurological complications have varied considerably with the type of vaccine.

Human rabies has decreased markedly in North America as a result of widespread dog vaccination and stray-animal control programs (1). Between 1960 and 1979, only 38 cases occurred in the United States and its territories, and the source had shifted from stray dogs and cats to wild carnivores and bats (11 of 27 cases with known exposures) (1).

Each year, approximately 25,000 persons in North America receive rabies prophylaxis (3,5). When appropriately used, postexposure prophylaxis combining local wound treatment, some type of rabies vaccine, and rabies immune globulin, are effective in preventing clinical rabies. Postexposure rabies treatment includes administration of both antibody [either the more preferable human rabies immune globulin (HRIG) or equine antirabies serum] and vaccine (5). Vaccine *only* should be administered in individuals previously immunized with the recommended pre-exposure or postexposure regimens with human diploid cell vaccine (HDCV) or those who have been immunized with other vaccines and have a demonstrably adequate rabies antibody titer. Different vaccines are currently in use around the world; in the United States, only the HDCV is currently available. A single dose of HRIG and five doses of HDCV are safe and effective in preventing development of rabies (5). Rabies prophylaxis varies with the origin of the bite. Individuals bitten by domestic animals can usually be observed for a period of time if the animal is not believed to be rabid; however, bites from wild animals are usually treated on the presumption the animals are rabid, since they are rarely available for observation. Efforts have been made to vaccinate populations of wild animals that pose a risk of transmitting rabies to humans (21).

Despite the successes of rabies postexposure prophylaxis,

some failures have occurred (6,10). Reports of two individuals who received appropriate HDCV and HRIG administration within 24 h of exposure, but nevertheless died from rabies encephalitis, suggested that injection into the buttock (rather than the recommended deltoid) was the chief factor in the vaccine failure (6,10). These failures are rare, and numerous studies have demonstrated the safety, immunogenicity, and efficacy of HDCV (7,11,12,26,36), purified Vero-cell rabies vaccine (PVCV) (17,30), and suckling mouse brain rabies vaccine (22).

Side effects of the various vaccines vary depending on how the vaccine is produced. In general, HDCV is the safest. By contrast, vaccines derived from neural tissues have the greatest number of neurological complications.

Neural Tissue–Derived Vaccines

Early rabies vaccines were crude preparations of rabbit, sheep, or goat CNS tissue infected with the rabies virus (23). The most widely used was the Semple vaccine, which employed phenol to inactivate the virus. Neurological complications were frequently reported with the use of these vaccines (8,9,15,23,32,33,35). Adverse effects included neuroparalytic events of several types (23,32,33) and systemic signs such as fever, headache, and myalgias (23,32). In addition, spongiform encephalopathies apparently have been occasionally transmitted with these vaccines (8,9).

The immune mechanism responsible for the neuroparalytic events is not known, but recent studies have demonstrated the presence of both antibodies to peptides of human myelin basic protein (35) and cardiolipin (15) in serum and cerebrospinal fluid of patients with neurological complications from the Semple vaccine.

Duck Embryo–Derived Vaccines

Duck embryo–derived vaccine was developed in 1955 (27,28). Neurological complications from this type of vaccine have been rare. Its use has been limited, since many individuals have hypersensitivity to egg products. Between 1958 and 1971, approximately 424,000 individuals received duck embryo–derived vaccine (27). A retrospective analysis of voluntary reporting of complications revealed 22 reports of anaphylaxis, 11 of abdominal pain with nausea and vomiting, and 13 cases with neurological complications (27): transverse myelitis (four cases), focal peripheral or cranial neuropathies (five cases), and PVE (four cases, two of which were fatal). Two additional cases with neurological complications were reported from Germany; one case of transverse myelitis and one possible case of Guillain-Barré syndrome (28).

Verocell Rabies Vaccine

PVCV is used extensively in other countries, primarily for its safety, effectiveness, and low cost (16,30). It is currently administered intramuscularly at two sites on day 0 (day of exposure), and at one site on days 7 and 21 (the 2-1-1 dosing regimen). In a study from Thailand (16), 100 individuals who were "severely" exposed to rabies were given PVCV in a 2-1-1 schedule and followed for 1 year. All survived, adverse reactions were mild, and there were no reports of neuroparalytic events. In a study from India (30), 55 individuals bitten by rabid animals were given a total of 327 inoculations of PVCV. All developed protective antibody titers of rabies virus that persisted for 15 months (the duration of follow-up). Adverse local or mild systemic reactions were observed after 10.6% of inoculations.

Chick Embryo Culture Vaccine

Chick embryo culture vaccine has been studied in normal volunteers (31) and to assess its potential for pre-exposure prophylaxis in normal individuals at risk for exposure to rabies (19). These studies have shown this vaccine to be effective and safe; no neuroparalytic complications have been reported.

Human Diploid Cell Vaccine

Systemic complications of HDCV occur infrequently and are generally mild (2,4,13,14,18–20,24–26,34). HDCV rapidly replaced the duck embryo–derived vaccines because of greater antibody production and fewer adverse reactions (2). With the first 25,200 doses of HDCV administered, severe systemic reactions were reported in only eight patients, and there were no reports of deaths or neuroparalytic events (2). After almost 4 years of use and approximately 400,000 doses administered to an estimated 100,000 per-

sons in the United States, there were no deaths secondary to the systemic allergic reactions (4), which are likely related to an immune-complex disease; all have recovered without sequelae (18). These side effects are related to the subsequent booster vaccinations rather than the primary vaccination (20).

Only four cases of possible neurological complications have been reported with HDCV (13,14,25,34). Three cases have been diagnosed as Guillain-Barré syndrome (14,25) or as having a Guillain-Barré-like illness (13). One individual developed a CNS demyelinating illness 8 days following the second dose of HDCV (34). There was right hemiparesis, and the cerebrospinal fluid revealed four oligoclonal bands. Magnetic resonance imaging revealed increased signal intensity bilaterally in the periventricular regions. This may represent coincidental multiple sclerosis, but since it was an initial event, and there has been no published follow-up, one cannot exclude the possibility that HDCV can be associated with neurological complications.

Albumin-Free HDCV

In an attempt to reduce even further the risk of systemic reactions to HDCV, albumin-free vaccine was recently tested and was without significant side effects (36).

REFERENCES

1. Anderson LJ, Nicholson KG, Tauxe RV, Winkler WG (1984) Human rabies in the United States, 1960 to 1979: Epidemiology, diagnosis, and prevention. *Ann Intern Med* 100, 728.
2. *Anon.* (1980) Adverse reactions to human diploid cell rabies vaccine. *Morb Mortal Wkly Rep* 29, 609.
3. *Anon.* (1983) General recommendations on immunization. *Morb Mortal Wkly Rep* 32, 1.
4. *Anon.* (1984) Systemic allergic reactions following immunization with human diploid cell rabies vaccine. *Morb Mortal Wkly Rep* 33, 185.
5. *Anon.* (1984) Rabies prevention—United States, 1984. *Morb Mortal Wkly Rep* 33, 393.
6. *Anon.* (1987) Human rabies despite treatment with rabies immune globulin and human diploid cell rabies vaccine—Thailand. *Morb Mortal Wkly Rep* 36, 759.
7. Aoki FY, Tyrrell DA, Hill LE (1975) Immunogenicity and acceptability of a human diploid-cell culture rabies vaccine in volunteers. *Lancet* 1, 660.
8. Arya SC (1991) Acquisition of spongiform encephalopathies in India through sheep-brain rabies vaccination. *Indian J Pediat* 58, 563.
9. Arya SC (1991) Spread of "unconventional viruses" through sheep-brain rabies vaccines. *Vaccine* 9, 70.
10. Baer GM, Fishbein DB (1987) Rabies post-exposure prophylaxis. *N Engl J Med* 316, 1270.

11. Bahmanyer M, Fayaz A, Nour-Salehi S et al. (1976) Successful protection of humans exposed to rabies infection: Postexposure treatment with the new human diploid cell rabies vaccine and antirabies serum. *J Amer Med Assn* **236**, 2751.

12. Bernard KW, Roberts MA, Sumner S et al. (1982) Human diploid cell rabies vaccine: Effectiveness of immunization with small intradermal or subcutaneous doses. *J Amer Med Assn* **247**, 1138.

13. Bernard KW, Smith PW, Kader FJ, Moran MJ (1982) Neuroparalytic illness and human diploid cell rabies vaccine. *J Amer Med Assn* **248**, 3136.

14. Boe E, Nyland H (1980) Guillain-Barre syndrome after vaccination with human diploid cell rabies vaccine. *Scand J Infect Dis* **12**, 231.

15. Chaleomchan W, Hemachudha T, Sakulramrung R, Deesomchok U (1990) Anticardiolipin antibodies in patients with rabies vaccination induced neurological complications and other neurological diseases. *J Neurol Sci* **96**, 143.

16. Chutivongse S, Wilde H, Fishbein DB et al. (1991) One-year study of the 2-1-1 intramuscular postexposure rabies vaccine regimen in 100 severely exposed Thai patients using rabies immune globulin and vero cell rabies vaccine. *Vaccine* **9**, 573.

17. Chutivongse S, Wilde H, Supich C et al. (1990) Postexposure prophylaxis for rabies with antiserum and intradermal vaccination. *Lancet* **335**, 896.

18. Dreesen DW, Bernard KW, Parker RA et al. (1986) Immune complex-like disease in 23 persons following a booster dose of rabies human diploid cell vaccine. *Vaccine* **4**, 45.

19. Dreesen DW, Fishbein DB, Kemp DT, Brown J (1989) Two-year comparative trial on the immunogenicity and adverse effects of purified chick embryo cell rabies vaccine for pre-exposure immunization. *Vaccine* **7**, 397.

20. Fishbein DB, Yenne KM, Dreesen DW et al. (1993) Risk factors for systemic hypersensitivity reactions after booster vaccinations with human diploid cell rabies vaccine: a nationwide prospective study. *Vaccine* **11**, 1390.

21. Hanlon CA, Ziemer EL, Hamir AN, Rupprecht CE (1989) Cerebrospinal fluid analysis of rabid and vaccinia-rabies glycoprotein recombinant, orally vaccinated raccoons (*Procyon lotor*). *Amer J Vet Res* **50**, 364.

22. Harry TO, Nasidi A, Fritzell B et al. (1989) Trial of economical regimens of suckling mouse brain rabies vaccine for postexposure prophylaxis in Lagos, Nigeria. *Vaccine* **7**, 329.

23. Hemachuda T, Phanuphak P, Johnson RT et al. (1987) Neurologic complications of Semple-type rabies vaccine: Clinical and immunologic studies. *Neurology* **37**, 550.

24. Kagawa KJ, Chomel BB, Lery L (1992) Rabies and brucellosis immunization status and adverse reactions to rabies vaccines in veterinary students. *Comp Immunol Microbiol Infect Dis* **15**, 79.

25. Knittel T, Ramadori G, Mayet W-J et al. (1989) Guillain-Barré syndrome and human diploid cell rabies vaccine. *Lancet* **1**, 1334.

26. Majchrowicz H (1989) Post-vaccination reactions to diploid rabies vaccine. *Przegl Epidemiol* **43**, 259.

27. Rubin RH, Hattwick MAW, Jones S et al. (1973) Adverse reactions to duck embryo rabies vaccine. *Ann Intern Med* **78**, 643.

28. Schlenska GK (1976) Neurological complications following rabies duck embryo vaccination. *J Neurol* **214**, 71.

29. Scott TF (1967) Postinfectious and vaccinal encephalitis. *Med Clin N Amer* **51**, 701.

30. Sehgal S, Bhattacharya D, Bhardwaj M (1994) Clinical evaluation of purified vero-cell rabies vaccine in patients bitten by rabid animals in India. *J Commun Dis* **26**, 139.

31. Suntharasamai P, Chaiprasithikul P, Wasi C et al. (1994) A simplified and economical intradermal regimen of purified chick embryo cell rabies vaccine for postexposure prophylaxis. *Vaccine* **12**, 508.

32. Swamy HS, Anisya V, Nandi SS, Kaliaperumal VG (1991) Neurological complications due to Semple-type antirabies vaccine. Clinical and therapeutic aspects. *J Assn Physician India* **39**, 667.

33. Swamy HS, Vasanth A, Sasikumar (1992) Brown-Sequard syndrome due to Semple antirabies vaccine: Case report. *Paraplegia* **30**, 181.

34. Tornatore CS, Richert JR (1990) CNS demyelination associated with diploid cell rabies vaccine. *Lancet* **335**, 1346.

35. Ubol S, Hemachudha T, Whitaker JN, Griffin DE (1990) Antibody to peptides of human myelin basic protein in post-rabies vaccine encephalomyelitis sera. *J Neuroimmunol* **26**, 107.

36. Wilde H, Glueck R, Khawplod P et al. (1995) Efficacy study of a new albumin-free human diploid cell rabies vaccine (Lyssavac-HDC, Berna) in 100 severely rabies-exposed Thai patients. *Vaccine* **13**, 593.

Reserpine

John D. Rogers

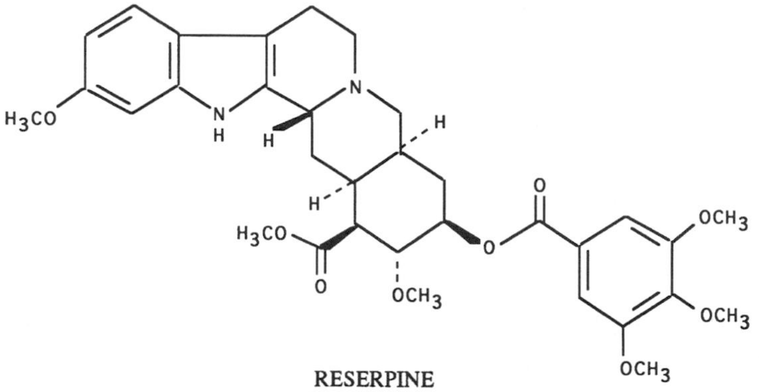

RESERPINE
$C_{33}H_{40}N_2O_9$

$(3\beta,16\beta,17\alpha,18\beta,20\alpha)$-11,17-Dimethoxy-18-[(3,4,5-trimethoxybenzoyl)oxy]yohimban-16-carboxylic acid methyl ester

NEUROTOXICITY RATING

Clinical

A   Extrapyramidal syndrome (parkinsonism)

A   Acute encephalopathy (sedation, cognitive dysfunction)

A   Psychobiological reaction (depression)

Experimental

A   Inhibition of dopamine synthesis

A   Extrapyramidal dysfunction

Reserpine is a naturally occurring substance derived from the shrub *Rauwolfia serpentina*. Introduced in the 1950s for the treatment of hypertension, reserpine has been replaced by agents with greater efficacy and fewer side effects. As an inhibitor of dopamine synthesis, reserpine is occasionally used to treat chorea, tics, tardive dystonia, and myoclonus.

Reserpine is of considerable historical interest because the agent was formerly used to create experimental animal models of reversible parkinsonism from dopamine depletion. Its experimental use led to the initial realization that dopamine was the neurotransmitter involved in this disorder. The term *neuroleptic*, which means the ability of a drug to cause parkinsonism, was initially coined for reserpine.

Reserpine depletes norepinephrine from postganglionic adrenergic neurons and monoamines (serotonin and catecholamines) from CNS neurons. Reserpine irreversibly binds to storage vesicles of adrenergic neurons; the vesicles are unable to concentrate and store norepinephrine, dopamine, and 5-hydroxytryptamine. Residual catecholamines are also subject to catabolism by intraneuronal monoamine oxidase, thus depleting biogenic amines (3). Recovery of sympathetic adrenergic function requires synthesis of new storage vesicles, which can take days to weeks after cessation of reserpine treatment.

Dose-dependent side effects include orthostatic hypotension, cognitive dysfunction, depression, and pronounced sedation. Depression develops insidiously, may be severe with suicidal ideation, and persists for months following drug withdrawal. Reserpine has been listed as a carcinogen by the U.S. Environmental Protection Agency (4), but a more recent review challenged this designation (2).

Editors' Note: Acute and chronic administration of reserpine to rats produces persistent oral dyskinesia accompanied by severe dopamine depletion in the caudate-putamen (1,6). The role of the dopaminergic nigrostriatal dopaminergic system in this model of tardive dyskinesia is unresolved (1,5–7).

REFERENCES

1. Bergamo M, Abilio VC, Queiroz CM et al. (1997) Effects of age on a new animal model of tardive dyskinesia. *Neurobiol Aging* **18**, 623.

2. Feinstein AR (1988) Scientific standards in epidemiologic studies of the menace of daily life. *Science* **242**, 1257.

3. Giachetti A, Shore PA (1978) The reserpine receptor. *Life Sci* **23**, 89.

4. National Toxicology Program 81-43 (1981) *Second Annual Report on Carcinogens*. p. 214.

5. Neisewander JL, Castaneda E, Davis DA et al. (1996) Effects of amphetamine and 6-hydroxydopamine lesions on reserpine-induced oral dyskinesia. *Eur J Pharmacol* **305**, 13.

6. Queiroz CM, Piovezan RD, Frussa-Filho R (1998) Reserpine does not induce orofacial dyskinesia in spontaneously hypertensive rats. *Eur J Pharmacol* **356**, 105.

7. Sussman AN, Tran-Nguyen LT, Neisewander JL (1997) Acute reserpine administration elicits long-term spontaneous oral dyskinesia. *Eur J Pharmacol* **337**, 157.

Rhodactis howesii

Albert C. Ludolph

NEUROTOXICITY RATING

Clinical

B   Acute encephalopathy (stupor, coma)

Human neurotoxicity of the toxic sea anemone *Rhodactis howesii* was initially reported in three cases in 1960 (2). *R. howesii* (locally in American Samoa, *matamalu*) lives on reefs in the Pacific Ocean, where it is consumed after cooking (2). Oral ingestion of uncooked sea anemone induces an unconcious, stuporous state for 8–36 h (1,3). During this time, tendon reflexes are absent and pupillary light reflexes disappear. Shock and pulmonary edema contribute to a fatal outcome. A bioassay in the toad *Bufo marinus* demonstrated that the putative toxin was heat-labile and non-dialyzable (2,3). The culpable chemical agent is unknown (3).

REFERENCES

1. Farber L, Lerke P (1963) Studies on the toxicity of *Rhodactis howesii* (matamulu). In: *Venomous Animals and Noxious Plants of the Pacific Region*. Keegan HL, MacFarlane WV eds. Pergamon Press, Oxford p. 67.
2. Martin EJ (1960) Observations on the toxic sea anemone, *Rhodactis howesii* (Coelenterata). *Pacific Sci* **14**, 403.
3. Southcott RV (1979) Marine Toxins. In: *Handbook of Clinical Neurology. Vol 36. Intoxications of the Nervous System. Part I*. Vinken PJ, Bruyn GW, eds. North-Holland, Amsterdam p. 54.

Ricin

Herbert H. Schaumburg
Peter S. Spencer

NEUROTOXICITY RATING

Experimental

A   Neuronopathy (suicide transport)

A   Neuronal immunotoxin

Ricin is a highly cytotoxic lectin derived from the seed of the castor bean, *Ricinis communis* (Euphorbiaceae). Aqueous extracts of the bean contain two different lectins: the cytotoxic RCA$_{II}$ (ricin) and a hemagglutinin RCA$_I$. The entire plant of the castor bean is toxic: in addition to the lectins, there is a powerful allergen in the leaf and seeds, and the seeds are also rich in a purgative oil (ricinoleic triglyceride) and contain the cyanogenic compound, ricinine.

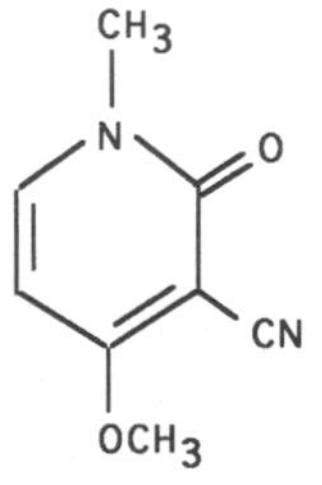

RICININE

The colorful seed is used in ornamental necklaces; wearing these necklaces may cause contact allergy. Ingestion of seed may cause gastroenteritis.

Ricin is a dimeric glycoprotein composed of two different peptide chains, A and B, linked by a disulfide bridge. The molecular mechanisms of ricin toxicity have been well elucidated and are the subject of a comprehensive review (15). The initial step in cellular toxicity is binding by the B chain to cell-surface receptors containing terminal galactoside residues; this facilitates endocytosis of the highly toxic A chain. The A chain is an enzyme (an endoglycosidase) that rapidly inactivates ribosomal protein synthesis and precipitates cell death. The A chain is among the most potent natural toxins: weight for weight, it is twice as potent as cobra venom, and a single molecule in the cytosol is sufficient to kill a cell (15). Oral ingestion by humans and domestic animals is accompanied by severe focal necrosis in the gastrointestinal tract with diarrhea and dehydration. Ingestion rarely causes systemic toxicity or is fatal because the peptide has a pronounced local necrotizing action and any excess is largely destroyed in the intestine (7). Inhalation of ricin in an aerosol causes fulminate fatal pulmonary edema and tracheobronchitis in experimental animals. Systemic administration to experimental animals and humans causes an acute febrile reaction followed by progressive hypotension and shock that are unresponsive to pharmacotherapy; most die within 2 days. The minimum lethal dose for a rabbit is 0.22 μg/kg, and a parenteral dose embedded in a small pellet was the cause of an adult homicide (5,9). The exact mechanism of the hypotensive crisis is unclear; it is likely related to a local vascular effect of ricin. This effect includes both profound peripheral vasodilation stemming from decreased vascular contraction in response to norepinephrine, and increased endothelial-dependent vascular relaxation (4,5). Neither ingested nor systemically administered ricin appears neurotoxic to humans or experimental animals (15).

Experimental animal studies have exploited the retrograde "suicide" transport of ricin injected into peripheral nerve to destroy the corresponding dorsal root ganglion cells and anterior horn cells (14). Such anatomically selective studies have used ricin and related cytotoxic peptides including monensin and volkensin. Ricin is solely transported by peripheral axons; injection into the CNS produces local necrosis and hydrocephalus (8), but not anatomically specific transport to the corresponding CNS neurons (3,10). Volkensin has proven reliable in studies of retrograde transport in the CNS (3). Since systemic toxicity may accompany even minute misapplications of ricin in experiments, preoperative administration of subcutaneous antiricin antibodies has been used to ensure that retrograde axonal transport of ricin proceeds in the absence of fluctuating blood pressure (13).

Ricin bound to monoclonal antibodies ("ricin immunotoxins") has been exploited as a means of ablating specific neuropeptide-containing CNS neurons and determining the physiological consequences (2). Saporin conjugates have also been used in specific immunolesioning experiments (16).

Ricin immunotoxin therapy has been used with modest success in an experimental model of carcinomatous meningitis (12), and has been employed in preliminary clinical trials as a human anticancer agent (11). A dose-limiting side effect of human ricin immunotherapy is hypoalbuminemia resulting from a vascular leak syndrome attributed to dysfunction in ricin-damaged endothelial cells (11).

Ricin has been evaluated as a biological warfare agent and is likely to be effective by most routes of exposure (1); however, it is several hundred times more toxic when administered parenterally than by ingestion (6). Direct injection has been used as an instrument of homicide (8). Aerosol exposure would be expected to have local pulmonary and systemic effects (1). Prophylaxis and specific therapy are unavailable, although it is known that ricin can be neutralized by a specific antibody. Hemodialysis and forced diuresis are not indicated because ricin is not dialyzable and little is excreted in the urine (6). Patient isolation is not required (1).

REFERENCES

1. Bunner DL (1992) Biological warfare agents: An overview. In Somani SM, ed, *Chemical Warfare Agents*, Academic Press, San Diego p. 387.

2. Burlet A, Grouzmann E, Musse N *et al.* (1995) The immunological impairment of arcuate neuropeptide Y neurons by ricin A chain produces persistent decrease of food intake and body weight. *Neuroscience* **66**, 151.

3. Cevolani D, Strocchi P, Bentivoglio M, Stirpe F (1995) Suicide retrograde transport of volkensin in cerebellar afferents: Direct evidence, neuronal lesions and comparison with ricin. *Brain Res* **689**, 163.

4. Christiansen VJ, Hsu CH, Robinson CP (1994) The effects of ricin on the sympathetic vascular neuroeffector system of the rabbit. *J Biochem Toxicol* **9**, 219.

5. Christiansen VJ, Hsu CH, Zhang L, Robinson CP (1995) Effects of ricin on the ability of arteries to contract and relax. *J Appl Toxicol* **15**, 37.

6. Ellenhorn MJ (1997) *Ellenhorn's Medical Toxicology. Diagnosis and Treatment of Poisoning.* 2nd ed. Williams & Wilkins, Baltimore, p. 1847.

7. Fodstad O, Olsnes S, Pihl A (1976) Toxicity, distribution and elimination of the cancerostatic lectins abrin and ricin after parenteral injection into mice. *Brit J Cancer* **34**, 418.

8. Kaur C, Ling EA (1993) Induced hydrocephalus in postnatal rats following an intracerebral injection of ricin. *J Hirnforschung* **34**, 493.

9. Knight B (1979) Ricin—a potent homicidal poison. *Brit Med J* **1**, 350.

10. Roberts RC, Harrison MB, Francis SM, Wiley RG (1993) Differential effects of suicide transport lesions of the striatonigral or striatopallidal pathways on subsets of striatal neurons. *Exp Neurol* **124**, 242.

11. Soler-Rodriguez AM, Ghetie MA, Oppenheimer-Marks N *et al.* (1993) Ricin A-chain and ricin A-chain immunotoxins rapidly damage human endothelial cells: Implications for vascular leak syndrome. *Exp Cell Res* **206**, 227.

12. Walbridge S, Rybak SM (1994) Immunotoxin therapy of leptomeningeal neoplasia. *J Neuro-oncol* **20**, 59.

13. Wiley RG, Oeltmann TN (1989) Anti-ricin antibody protects against systemic toxicity without affecting suicide transport. *J Neurosci Meth* **27**, 203.

14. Wiley RG, Oeltmann TN (1986) Anatomically selective peripheral nerve ablation using intraneural ricin injection. *J Neurosci Meth* **17**, 43.

15. Wiley RG, Oeltmann TN (1991) Ricin and related plant toxins: Mechanism of action and neurobiological applications. In: *Toxicology of Plant and Fungal Compounds.* Keeler RF, Tu AT eds. Marcel Dekker, New York p. 243.

16. Wiley RG, Oeltmann TN, Lappi DA (1991) Immunolesioning: Selective destruction of neurons using immunotoxin to rat NGF receptor. *Brain Res* **562**, 149.

Rotenone

Matthias Riepe

ROTENONE
$C_{23}H_{22}O_6$

[2R-(2α,6aα,12aα)]-1,2,12,12a-Tetrahydro-8,9-dimethoxy-2-
(1-methylethyl)-[1]benzopyrano[3,4-b]furo
[2,3-h][1]benzopyran-6(6aH)-one

NEUROTOXICITY RATING

Clinical

B Seizure disorder

Rotenone and rotenoids, which are found in several strains
of the *Derris* (e.g., *Derris elliptica*) and *Lonchocarpus* (e.g.,
Lonchocarpus utilis, *L. urucu*, *L. nicou*) genera (9), have
been used by native people as a fish poison. In recent times,
rotenone has been employed extensively as an agricultural
and household insecticide and pesticide. Humans are widely
exposed to this substance (7) but exposure is low, since
rotenone is unstable in air and light, and poorly soluble in
water (9).

Rotenone forms orthorhombic six-sided plates when prepared from trichloroethylene. An analytical procedure using
high-performance liquid chromatography is described with
limits of detection of 0.025 μg/g for sediments and 0.005
μg/g for tissue samples (3). Rotenone decays upon exposure
to light and air (9).

Uptake of rotenone from the gastrointestinal tract is
probably low; inhalation seems more hazardous than ingestion (16). Acute intoxication of rotenone in mammals
induces hypotension, bradycardia, and respiratory arrest of
central origin. Ectopic foci, membrane depolarization, contractures, and neuromuscular block are not observed (17).
The LD_{50} in rats has been reported to be from 60–132 mg/
kg orally, 1.6 mg/kg intraperitoneally, and 0.2 mg/kg intravenously (9). At a dose of 10 mg/kg, a 10-day exposure to
rotenone increases the number of nonpregnant rats and re-
sorptions (10). Also reported at doses of 5 and 10 mg/kg

are reductions in maternal body weight gain, fetal weight,
and skeletal ossification, and increased incidence of extra
rib (10).

The reported carcinogenic effect of rotenone after
chronic treatment of rats with 2.0–2.5 ppm (7) could not
be reproduced in other studies. Rotenone added to the diet
of rats in concentrations up to 75 ppm for F344/N rats and
1200 ppm for B6C3F1 mice for up to 103 weeks did increase parathyroid adenomas; no effect was seen on survival of rats of either sex, and a reduced incidence of hepatocellular carcinomas was observed (1,8).

In cultured Chinese hamster cells, rotenone induced
aneuploidy, polyploidy, and endoreduplication, but not
structural chromosome aberrations (15). Some *in vitro* experiments suggest that some rotenoids might be valuable
antitumor agents (11). In isolated hearts, a negative inotropic effect of rotenone has been observed (13).

A case of acute fatal rotenone intoxication upon ingestion of an unknown amount has been reported in a 3½-
year-old girl (5). Systemic exposure to rotenone causes
numbness, nausea, vomiting, tremors, convulsions and,
eventually, respiratory arrest (9). Toxic effects after local
exposure include dermatitis, conjunctivitis, and rhinitis.

Rotenone is a potent inhibitor of nicotinamide adenine
dinucleotide dehydrogenase oxidation to nicotinamide adenine dinucleotide (NAD^+) in mitochondria (complex I),
thereby blocking the oxidation of substrates such as glutamate, α-ketoglutarate, and pyruvate by NAD^+. In higher
concentrations, it binds to more than one region of the respiratory chain (9), in particular to complex III (4), as does
resveratrol (18). Rotenone decreases the electrochemical
proton potential under active state conditions (6) and
thereby causes lactate production to increase severalfold
(2). Cells at all stages of cell cycle are affected by rotenone;
vulnerability is greatest as soon as the acute block at mitosis
is abolished and cells re-enter the cycle (12). Rotenone, like
other uncouplers and respiratory inhibitors, causes the appearance of ring-like and dumbell-like mitochondria; this
effect does not correlate with decreased adenosine triphosphate concentration, changes in oxygen consumption, or
condensation of the mitochondrial matrix (14).

Acute intoxication might be fatal due to respiratory arrest of central origin. Chronic toxicity in humans has not
been reported. Carcinogenicity data are ambiguous.

REFERENCES

1. Abdo KM, Eustis SL, Haseman J *et al.* (1988) Toxicity
   and carcinogenicity of rotenone given in the feed to F344/

N rats and B6C3F1 mice for up to two years. *Drug Chem Toxicol* **11**, 225.

2. Dagani F, Ferrari R, Tosca P, Canevari L (1992) Effects of calcium antagonists on glycolysis of rat brain synaptosomes. *Biochem Pharmacol* **43**, 371.

3. Dawson VK, Allen JL (1988) Liquid chromatographic determination of rotenone in fish, crayfish, mussels, and sediments. *J Assn Off Anal Chem* **71**, 1094.

4. Degli EM, Ghelli A, Crimi M *et al.* (1993) Complex I and complex III of mitochondria have common inhibitors acting as ubiquinone antagonists. *Biochem Biophys Res Commun* **190**, 1090.

5. DeWilde AR, Heyndrickx A, Carton D (1986) A case of fatal rotenone poisoning in a child. *J Forensic Sci* **31**, 1492.

6. Duszynski J, Bogucka K, Wojtczak L (1984) Homeostasis of the protonmotive force in phosphorylating mitochondria. *Biochim Biophys Acta* **767**, 540.

7. Gosalvez M (1983) Carcinogenesis with the insecticide rotenone. *Life Sci* **32**, 809.

8. Greenman DL, Allaben WT, Burger GT, Kodell RL (1993) Bioassay for carcinogenicity of rotenone in female Wistar rats. *Fund Appl Toxicol* **20**, 383.

9. Haley TJ (1978) A review of the literature on rotenone, 1,2,12,12a-tetrahydro-8,9-dimethoxy-2-(1-methylethenyl)-1-benzopyrano(3,4-b)furo(2,3-h)(1)benzopyran-6(6aH)-one. *J Environ Pathol Toxicol* **1**, 315.

10. Khera KS, Whalen C, Angers G (1982) Teratogenicity study on pyrethrum and rotenone (natural origin) and ronnel in pregnant rats. *J Toxicol Environ Health* **10**, 111.

11. Konoshima T, Terada H, Kokumai M *et al.* (1993) Studies on inhibitors of skin tumor promotion, XII. Rotenoids from *Amorpha fruticosa*. *J Nat Prod* **56**, 843.

12. Loffer M, Schneider F (1982) Further characterization of the growth inhibitory effect of rotenone on *in vitro* cultured Ehrlich ascites tumour cells. *Mol Cell Biochem* **48**, 77.

13. Lynch JJ, Rahwan RG (1983) Comparison of the characteristics of the negative inotropic actions of dinitrophenol, rotenone, antimycin A and the intracellular calcium antagonist, propyl-methylenedioxyindene. *Gen Pharmacol* **14**, 437.

14. Markova OV, Mokhova EN, Tarakanova AN (1990) The abnormal-shaped mitochondria in thymus lymphocytes treated with inhibitors of mitochondrial energetics. *J Bioenerg Biomembrane* **22**, 51.

15. Matsumoto K, Ohta T (1991) Rotenone induces aneuploidy, polyploidy and endoreduplication in cultured Chinese hamster cells. *Mutat Res* **263**, 173.

16. Taylor JR, Calabrese VP, Blanke RV (1979) Organochlorine and other insecticides. In: *Handbook of Neurology. Vol 36.* Vinken PJ, Bruyn GW eds. North-Holland, Amsterdam p. 391.

17. Teixeira JR, Lapa AJ, Souccar C, Valle JR (1984) Timbos: Ichthyotoxic plants used by Brazilian Indians. *J Ethnopharmacol* **10**, 311.

18. Zini R, Morin C, Bertelli A *et al.* (1999) Effects of resveratrol on the rat brain respiratory chain. *Drugs Exp Clin Res* **25**, 87.

Rubella Vaccine

Neil L. Rosenberg

NEUROTOXICITY RATING

Clinical

B Peripheral neuropathy

C Myelopathy

Rubella vaccines are derived from human diploid cells (3). Minor and self-limiting side effects commonly follow rubella vaccination (4); the most common is arthralgia (3). There have been cases of a chronic arthritis or arthropathy associated with rubella vaccine (7,11,15–17); these were associated with RA 27/3 rubella immunization (7,15–17). In an 18-month follow-up study, it was found that wild rubella infections in adult populations were associated with a higher incidence, increased severity, and more prolonged duration of joint manifestations than after RA 27/3 rubella immunization (15). It has been suggested the RA 27/3 vaccine is associated with chronic fatigue syndrome (1). There is no later risk of developing cancer in individuals receiving rubella vaccine (10).

Rubella vaccine crosses the placenta and there is potential risk of congenital rubella syndrome in the fetus (12,18); however, two studies have failed to detect postrubella-vaccine congenital rubella syndrome (12,18). The risk of giving inadvertent rubella vaccination during pregnancy appears negligible and should not lead to termination of the pregnancy.

Unconvincing reports of neurological dysfunction include transitory arthralgias and paresthesias beginning 7–21 days after immunization (3,8). Some are alleged to have developed idiopathic polyneuropathy (13), carpal tunnel syndrome (16), or pain and paresthesias without an identifiable polyneuropathy (8,16). Isolated reports of rubella vaccination associated with vasculitis and myositis (5), optic neuritis or recurrent blurred vision (9,16), and myelitis (6,9), appear to be chance associations.

Editors' Note: A recent report describes a mild, distal demyelinating neuropathy associated with antimyelin basic protein antibodies that developed in a 23-year-old woman after immunization with the live attenuated RA 27/3 rubella strain (2). A recent epidemiological study of 293 cases of confirmed autism among children born since 1979 found no evidence to support a causal association between autism and prior immunization with measles, mumps, and rubella vaccine (14).

REFERENCES

1. Allen AD (1988) Is RA27/3 rubella immunization a cause of chronic fatigue? *Med Hypotheses* **27**, 217.
2. Cusi MG, Bianchi S, Santini L *et al.* (1999) Peripheral neuropathy associated with anti-myelin basic protein antibodies in a woman vaccinated with rubella virus vaccine. *Neurovirol* **5**, 209.
3. Fenichel GM (1982) Neurological complications of immunization. *Ann Neurol* **12**, 119.
4. Griffin GV, Byrett KA (1986) Rubella vaccine-how "reactogenic" is it? *J Int Med Res* **14**, 316.
5. Hanissian AS, Martinez AJ, Jabbour JT, Duenas DA (1973) Vasculitis and myositis secondary to rubella vaccination. *Arch Neurol* **28**, 202.
6. Holt S, Hudgins D, Krishnan KR, Critchley EM (1976) Diffuse myelitis associated with rubella vaccination. *Brit Med J* **2**, 1037.
7. Howson CP, Katz M, Johnston RB, Fineberg HV (1992) Chronic arthritis after rubella vaccination. *Clin Infect Dis* **15**, 307.
8. Kilroy AW, Schaffner W, Fleet WF *et al.* (1970) Two syndromes following rubella immunization: Clinical observations and epidemiological studies. *J Amer Med Assn* **214**, 2287.
9. Kline LB, Margulies SL, Oh SJ (1982) Optic neuritis and myelitis following rubella vaccination. *Arch Neurol* **39**, 443.
10. Mellor JA, Langford DT, Zealley H *et al.* (1983) A survey of cancer morbidity and mortality in vaccines seven to 12 years after the administration of live vaccine propagated in human diploid cells. *J Biol Scand* **11**, 221.
11. Mitchell LA, Tingle AJ, Shukin R *et al.* (1993) Chronic rubella vaccine-associated arthropathy. *Arch Intern Med* **153**, 2268.
12. Preblud SR, Williams NM (1985) Fetal risk associated with rubella vaccine: Implications for vaccination of susceptible women. *Obstet Gynecol* **66**, 121.
13. Schaffner W, Fleet WF, Kilroy AW *et al.* (1974) Polyneuropathy following rubella immunization. A follow-up study and review of the problem. *Amer J Dis Child* **127**, 684.
14. Taylor B, Miller E, Farrington CP *et al.* (1999) Autism and measles, mumps, and rubella vaccine: no epidemiological evidence for a causal association. *Lancet* **353**, 2026.
15. Tingle AJ, Allen M, Petty RE *et al.* (1986) Rubella-associated arthritis. I. Comparative study of joint manifestations associated with natural rubella infection and RA 27/3 rubella immunisation. *Ann Rheum Dis* **45**, 110.
16. Tingle AJ, Chantler JK, Pot KH *et al.* (1985) Postpartum rubella immunization: Association with development of prolonged arthritis, neurological sequelae, and chronic rubella viremia. *J Infect Dis* **152**, 606.
17. Tingle AJ, Pot KH, Yong FP *et al.* (1989) Kinetics of isotype-specific humoral immunity in rubella vaccine-associated arthropathy. *Clin Immunol Immunopathol* **53**, S99.
18. Tookey PA, Jones G, Miller BH, Peckham CS (1991) Rubella vaccination in pregnancy. *CDR (Lond Engl Rev)* **1**, R86.

Sarin, Other "Nerve Agents," and their Antidotes

Peter S. Spencer
Barry W. Wilson
Edson X. Albuquerque

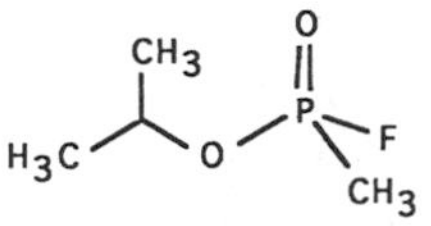

SARIN
$C_4H_{10}FO_2P$

Isopropyl methylphosphonofluoridate; GB; Sarin; Zarin

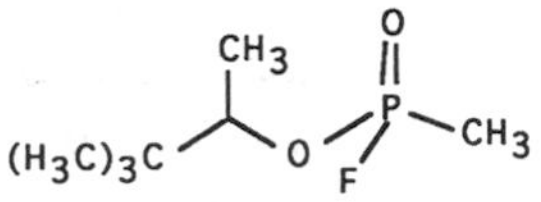

SOMAN
$C_7H_{16}FO_2P$

Methylphosphonofluoridic acid 1,2,2-trimethylpropyl ester;
Pinacolyl methylphosphonofluoridate; GD; Soman; Zoman

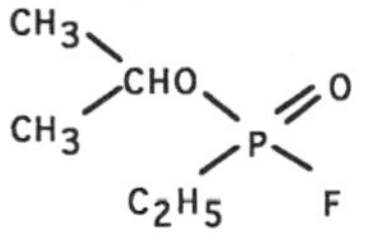

GE
$C_5H_{12}FO_2P$

Isopropyl ethylphosphonofluoridate; GE

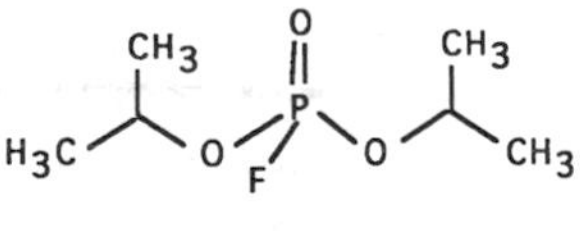

DFP
$C_6H_{14}FO_3P$

Diisopropylphosphorofluoridate; DFP

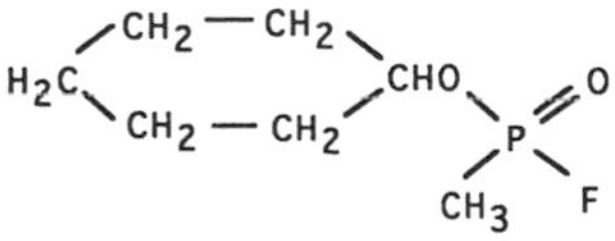

GF
$C_7H_{14}FO_2P$

Cyclohexyl methylphosphonofluoridate; GF

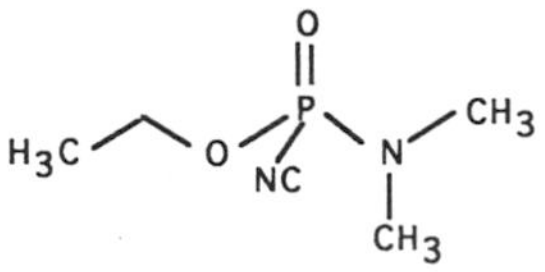

TABUN
$C_5H_{11}N_2O_2P$

Ethyl N-dimethylphosphoramidocyanidate; GA; Tabun;
Taboon A; Trilon 83; Gelan I

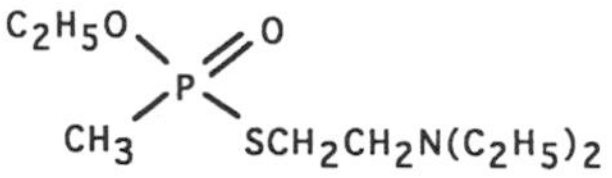

VM
$C_9H_{22}NO_2PS$

O-Ethyl S-[2-(diethylamino)ethyl] methylphosphonothiolate;
VM

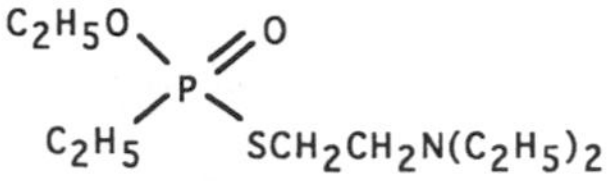

VE
$C_{10}H_{14}NO_2PS$

O-Ethyl-S-[2-(diethylamino)ethyl] ethylphosphonothiolate;
VE

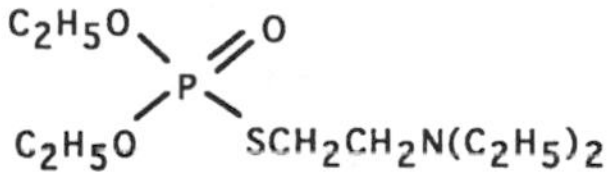

VG
$C_{10}H_{24}NO_3PS$

O,O-Diethyl S-[2-(diethylamino)ethyl] phosphorothiolate;
VG

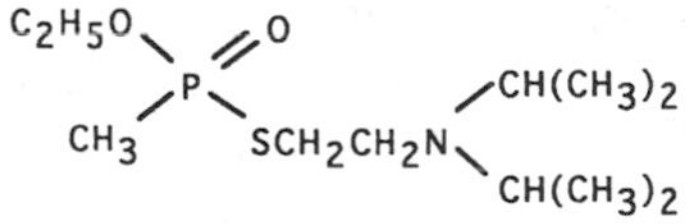

VX
$C_{11}H_{25}NO_2PS$

O-Ethyl S-[2-(diisopropylamino)ethyl]
methylphosphonothiolate; VX

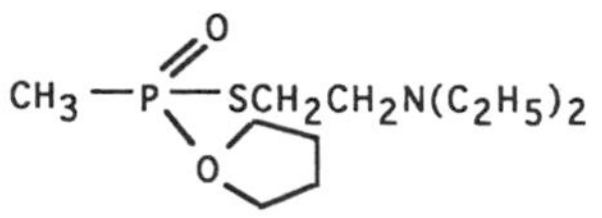

EA3148
$C_{12}H_{26}NO_2PS$

Cyclopentyl S-[2-(diethylamino)ethyl]
methylphosphonothiolate; EA3148

NEUROTOXICITY RATING
Clinical

A   Seizure disorder
B   Peripheral neuropathy

Experimental

A Cholinergic crisis

A Seizures

A Peripheral neuropathy (if protected from supra LD_{50} doses)

Sarin and other anticholinesterase nerve agents are organophosphorus compounds of exceptionally high toxic potency that were developed in a search for contact pesticides. Sarin and tabun were synthesized in Germany in 1937 and soman in 1944, and VX by Great Britain in 1952 (45,70,103,176). Research on nerve agents ceased in Britain in 1959 and, in the United States, in 1969; however, the United States began again in 1981 to produce components for binary weapons in which precursors of nerve agents are stored in separate warhead chambers and mixed on firing to form the lethal compounds (110). Tabun was probably used offensively by Iraq during the Iran-Iraq war in the 1980s. In late January and February 1991, Coalition forces amassed against Iraq conducted aerial bombing that damaged chemical munitions at two sites in the central part of the country where 2.9 and 16.8 metric tons of sarin and cyclosarin, respectively, were stored (133). A large release of sarin and cyclosarin occurred in association with the post–Gulf War destruction of a major Iraqi chemical storage depot housed in Bunker 73 at Khamisiyah, Coalition-Occupied Iraq. While very low-level exposure to Coalition troops is presumed to have occurred, no acute illness is known to have been reported (133). In June 1994 and March 1995, terrorists deployed agents thought to be sarin against civilian populations in the Japanese cities of Matsumoto and Tokyo. During and following the Cold War, the United States stockpiled tens of thousands of tons of sarin and VX loaded in unitary weapons; the former Soviet Union held reserves of tabun, soman, and a substance code-named *VR-55* (*structure not shown*) (162). The U.S. Department of Army is currently engaged in the destruction of aging (30 to 48-year-old) stockpiles of weapons containing sarin, VX, or mustard agents; this program of carefully controlled incineration began in 1990 and will continue into the opening decade of the next millennium. Peripheral neuropathy and electroencephalographic (EEG) changes (*vide infra*), together with birth defects and keratitis, have been cited by the U.S. Centers for Disease Control and Prevention as potential hazards associated with mishaps during stockpile destruction (45).

Physical and Chemical Properties

The principal organophosphorus nerve agents are the fluorine- and cyanide-containing G agents (sarin, tabun, soman) and the somewhat more potent sulfur-containing V agents (*e.g.*, VX). All four organophosphates contain a chiral phosphorus atom and therefore exist in the form of stereoisomers (166). Sarin has two stereoisomers: P(−)-sarin has greater acute toxicity than P(+)-sarin (20). Soman has four enantiomers: C(−)P(−)-soman and (C+)P(−)-soman are one to two orders of magnitude more acutely toxic to rodents than C(+)P(+)-soman or C(−)P(+)-soman (18,91). The *SP* enantiomer of VX has greater anticholinesterase activity than its *RP* counterpart (2).

Physicochemical properties of the nerve agents are shown in Table 58. All are viscous liquids of high (G agents) or low (VX) volatility; they may be deployed as vapor, liquid, or in an artificially thickened state (103). G agents pose a vapor as well as a liquid hazard and spread rapidly on skin surfaces. Under temperate conditions, the volatility and inhalation hazard for VX are low, and spread of the agent on skin is less rapid (45,103). Liquid nerve agents rapidly traverse unbroken skin and mucous membranes, and vapor is readily absorbed by the cornea where it rapidly produces

TABLE 58. Physicochemical Properties of G-Agents and VX

	Tabun	Sarin	Soman	VX
Color	Colorless–straw	Colorless	Colorless	Colorless–brown
Consistency, 25°C	Liquid	Liquid	Liquid	Oily
Odor	Fishy	Fruity	Camphor	Rotten fish
Molecular weight	162.3	140.1	182.2	267.4
Vapor density	5.6	4.8	6.3	9.2
Liquid density, g/ml, 25°C	1.08	1.09	1.02	1.0083
Vapor pressure, mmHg, 20°–25°C	0.07	1.48–2.9	0.5	0.0007
Vapor concentration, mg/m³, 25°C	576–610	16,400–22,000	3060	3–30
Solubility, 100 g water, 25°C	9.8	miscible	2.1 (20°C)	3.0
Half-life in water, hours, pH >8–9	2–3	24 (25°C)		
Half-life in water, hours, pH >6.5		8300 (0°C)	10 (30°C)	400–1000 (50%)
Life in soil, days	1–1.5 (50%)	5 (90%)	hydrolyzes	15 (90%)

Adapted largely from Health Risk Assessment for RfDs, Subcommittee on Chronic Reference Doses (RfDs) for Selected Chemical Warfare Agents, Committee on Toxicology, U.S. National Research Council, prepared by Oak Ridge National Laboratory, Oak Ridge, Tennessee, 1996.

a characteristic local neurotoxic effects (miosis). Lungs rapidly absorb more than 80% of inhaled nerve agent vapor; the amount absorbed per unit time varies directly with the rate of ventilation (102). The $L(C_t)_{50}$ (*vide infra*) for VX is 250–500 times lower than that for the highly toxic gas hydrogen cyanide! (155).

Metabolic detoxification of nerve agents varies by species and route of administration (166). Diisofluorophosphate (DFP), sarin, soman, and tabun are metabolized by an organophosphate hydrolase (95). Metabolites of sarin, soman, and VX include isopropylphosphonic acid, pinacolyl methylphosphonic acid, ethyl methylphosphonic acid, and methylphosphonic acid (80,120). Sarin is more rapidly hydrolyzed by the mouse (0.064 μg/kg/min) than the guinea pig (0.009 μg/kg/min), a distinction that parallels the sevenfold difference in acute LD_{50} values for these species (48). Intraperitoneal soman is largely hydrolyzed by the liver, but subcutaneous soman is mostly sequestered by blood and tissue aliesterases (*vide infra*) (48). In humans, organophosphate detoxification involves a high-density lipoprotein-associated polymorphic enzyme known as paraoxonase (137,184,186). The Arg192 isoform of paraoxonase, which is more common among Japanese (allele frequency: 0.66) relative to other human races (0.24–0.31), hydrolyzes sarin and soman less rapidly than the Gln192 isoform (203).

Occupational and population exposure limits have been recommended by the U.S. Army and endorsed by the U.S. Centers for Disease Control and Prevention. They are based on the lowest doses of sarin that cause miosis and cholinesterase depression in human volunteers; they do not consider performance decrements in primates that may be present without signs of acute toxicity such as miosis (*vide infra*) (65). Even long-term exposure to levels up to the recommended limits are not expected to produce an adverse health effect in the short- or long-term. The recommended inhalation exposure limit for tabun and sarin for workers without respiratory protection is 1×10^{-4} mg/m^3 averaged over 8 h; the general population limit for sarin is 3×10^{-6} mg/m^3 averaged over 72 h. A person exposed to sarin for 8 h at the occupational limit would sustain a calculated cumulative dose over time of 0.048 mg/min/m^3. The corresponding occupational and population control limits for VX are 1×10^{-5} and 3×10^{-6} mg/m^3, respectively.

Description of the large number of methods available to detect nerve agents is beyond the scope of this summary. The U.S. Armed Services is currently seeking a sensitive system capable of detecting, identifying, and quantifying nerve (GA, GB, GD, VX), mustard (*see* Mustard Warfare Agents and Related Substances, this volume), and blood agents both to provide rapid indication of a chemical attack and to monitor airborne levels of agents. Parts per trillion of sarin, tabun, soman, VX, and DFP are presently detectable in freshly prepared water samples (38).

General Toxicology

OP anhydride nerve agents are rapid and stoichometric inhibitors of serine hydrolases (113) that bind in particular to the active site of neural (synaptic) acetylcholinesterase (AChE) [E.C.3.1.1.7]. The enzyme activity of a major rat brain AChE isoform with low mobility (when electrophoresed on polyacrylamide gels) reportedly is most sensitive to the effects of sarin, soman, and VX; a high-mobility form is less sensitive (14). Cholinesterases in plasma (notably the glycoprotein butyrylcholinesterase, BuChE [E.C. 3.1.1.8] and AChE on the surface of red blood cells bind (scavenge) and temporally sequester organophosphates, and may minimize agent access to the nervous system (115). Organophosphate esters differentially inhibit blood cholinesterases in humans; whereas sarin and VX preferentially inhibit the erythrocytic AChE form, DFP has a much greater inhibitory effect on the plasma enzyme (60,82,156,159). Exposure to high levels of nerve agents abolishes the enzyme activities of both cellular and plasma enzymes (154). In dogs, tabun similarly inhibits cellular and plasma enzyme activities (69). Rodents have an additional blood and tissue enzyme group (aliesterases) that may act as a sink for organophosphates such as soman (48,108). In rats, marmosets, and guinea pigs, soman may bind reversibly to aliesterases and to other, unknown sites in lung and muscle, with apparent slow releases of agent into the circulatory system and reappearance of toxic signs (166,183,197). Soman binds to chymotrypsin, trypsin, and other serine-containing hydrolase enzymes (166), as do other nerve agents (*e.g.*, DFP) when present in high concentration.

Administration of exogenous AChE to mice confers protection from soman and VX poisoning (101,196). Single doses of AChE derived from fetal bovine serum (FBS) reportedly protect animals against the acute neurotoxic actions of the potent quaternary organophosphate 7-(methylethoxyphosphinyloxy)-1-methyl-quinolinium iodide (136). Moreover, prophylaxis with human BuChE or FBS AChE protects animals against soman poisoning (12). Human BuChE administered to mice and rats (half-life, 21 h and 46 h, respectively) prior to multiple median lethal doses of a wide range of potent organophosphates alleviates symptoms and obviates the need for postexposure therapy (137). A protein-engineered form of BuChE (termed G117H/E197Q), which features the properties of both spontaneous dephosphonylation and slow dealkylation ("aging", *vide infra*), catalyzes soman hydrolysis and accepts all four soman isomers, sarin, and VX as substrates (113). Under experimental conditions with animal tissues, high-affinity and monoclonal anti-VX antibodies block the effects of VX *in vitro* and *in vivo*, respectively (30,61).

Erythrocyte AChE and plasma BuChE are often used to monitor for exposure to organophosphate pesticides and chemical warfare agents. The steep slope of the dose–response curve for chemical warfare agents makes such biochemical markers especially important even though physiological effects may occur at levels lower than those that cause a detectable inhibition of blood cholinesterases (*vide infra*). There may be some temporal variation in erythrocyte AChE; enzyme activity over the course of 1 year varied by 11% in male and 16% in female subjects (158). Enzyme activity is depressed in certain hematological disorders such as pernicious anemia (67). The smallest measureable decrease in erythrocyte AChE with one pre-exposure measure is estimated to be about 15% (23). Recovery of enzyme activity depends on replacement of blood cells (approximately 1% per day in *Homo sapiens*) (155). While blood AChE estimation provides a valuable diagnostic tool, there may be a poor correlation between enzyme activity and clinical manifestations of acute cholinergic neurotoxicity (69,205). Moreover, although the degree of *in vitro* inhibition of human erythrocyte AChE and brain AChE is the same for tabun (1.5×10^{-8} mol/l) and similar for sarin (3.0 and 3.3×10^{-9} mol/l, respectively) (59), rats treated with acutely toxic concentrations of soman may show a poor correlation between the inhibition of blood and brain AChE activities (77). Other rodent studies with soman suggest that while changes in erythrocyte AChE activity may serve as a useful marker of soman-induced CNS AChE inhibition, those in serum cholinesterase do not (65). There is also evidence that prolonged, low-level exposure to organophosphate pesticides may result in tolerance to their potential effects, and individuals with markedly depressed erythrocyte AChE activity may lack symptoms or signs of toxicity (16,43,72,169). There was no evidence of tolerance of rodent CNS AChE to repeated systemic injection of soman (65).

BuChE (plasma cholinesterase, pseudocholinesterase), so-called because of its high affinity for butyrocholine, is synthesized by the liver and has a replacement time in humans of approximately 50 days (155); however, rodent plasma cholinesterase showed a very fast recovery (within 24–48 h) after the last of a series of daily soman injections (65). Enzyme activity of BuChE is higher in men than women, fluctuates widely over a year, and is lower in those with liver disease and among women taking oral contraceptives (67,140,157,189). Some 26 variants of plasma BuChE are described (27), one of which is a point mutation at the anionic active site that changes aspartate to glycine (107).

While homozygotes for this genetic polymorphism are rare (1:2500), heterozygotes make up 4%–5% of the general population (188). Subjects with BuChE variants may have reduced binding capacity for, and increased susceptibility to, anticholinesterase agents such as succinylcholine, a drug used as a muscle relaxant during surgery which, in genetically susceptible individuals, may elicit apneic periods (76). Pyridostigmine bromide, a carbamate anticholinesterase, triggered a cholinergic crisis in an Israeli soldier found to be homozygous for the aforementioned BuChE genotype (96). Organophosphate-inhibited BuChE can be reactivated by fluoride ions at pH 4 and the resulting phosphofluoridate used to estimate the nerve agent both qualitatively and quantitatively. Since the plasma enzyme represents the bulk of blood cholinesterase, it may be possible to use this method retrospectively to estimate nerve agent dose (132).

While organophosphates inhibit a variety of tissue enzymes and have effects on noncholinergic pathways and neuroendocrine systems, it is generally true that most of the acute neurotoxic responses to these agents result principally from perturbation of neurotransmission *via* inhibition of neural (synaptic) AChE (166). This enzyme normally hydrolyzes the neurotransmitter acetylcholine (ACh) and thereby terminates signal transfer at CNS and PNS cholinergic synapses. The tertiary structure and amino acid sequences of several AChEs and BuChEs has been determined (178,179), and relationships among their structures and the mechanisms of their action and inhibition by chemical agents are under intensive study (47,50). A notable feature of the active site of AChE is a gorge lined with aromatic residues that is about 20 Å deep; the active-site gorge contains two sites of ligand binding, an acylation site near the base of the gorge with a catalytic triad characteristic of serine hydrolases (inhibited by organophosphates and carbamates), and a peripheral site at the mouth of the gorge 10–20 Å from the acylation site (47,150,171,173) (*see* Fig. 27, p. 915). The action of AChE on its substrate ACh is a multistep process initiated by the formation of a reversible enzyme substrate complex (EAX); the serine catalytic site (EA) on the enzyme is acetylated, followed by hydrolysis of the enzyme-substrate complex to yield acetic acid, choline, and the regenerated enzyme (E + A).

$$E + AX \underset{k-1}{\overset{k+1}{\longleftrightarrow}} EAX \overset{k2}{\longleftrightarrow} EA \overset{k3}{\longrightarrow} > E + A$$

Organophosphate chemical warfare agents phosphorylate the serine catalytic site and prevent it from hydrolyzing ACh. The organophosphate-inhibited enzyme can be reactivated by dephosphorylation, but this occurs at a rate that is slower than the rate of reactivation of ACh (deactivated by AChE); consequently, there is depletion of active AChE and a build-up of ACh. The third step, known as *aging*, is thought to involve loss of an alkyl or alkoxy group from the nerve agent moiety of the inhibited enzyme, which leaves a stable enzyme-modified nerve agent complex resistant to dephosphorylation (100). The rate of chemical aging varies with the nerve agent; measured half-lives for aging of nerve agents bound to bovine erythrocyte AChE include tabun (46 h), sarin (12 h), soman (4 min), and VX (>12 days) (103). Rates of chemical aging of the enzyme-agent complex at synaptic junctions have relevance for therapeutic enzyme reactivation with oximes (*vide infra*). The common end result is synaptic accumulation of ACh and consequent abnormal persistence of neurotransmission (84). Recovery of normal neurotransmission depends on the slow process of AChase synthesis (57). Correlation between the enzyme inhibition of erythrocyte and neural AChE inhibition is poor, perhaps because of differences in agent concentration and the sensitivity and inhibition kinetics of enzymes in different locations (77).

Organophosphates also have direct effects on synaptic function in addition to those resulting from the buildup of ACh (3–5,15,74,135). Many of these direct actions have been observed in regions other than the neuromuscular junction and are now known to take place pre- and postsynaptically in CNS neurons. Some of these effects entail direct interactions with cholinergic and noncholinergic receptors (*e.g.*, glutamatergic receptors) and with voltage-gated channels. Evidence has been provided that muscarinic receptors with high affinity for ^{3}H-*cis*-methyldioxalane are directly impacted by nanomolar concentrations of soman or VX (29), and that at higher (micromolar) concentrations these compounds can act as open-channel blockers at muscle nicotinic ACh receptors (6,15,139). Activation of muscarinic receptors by excess ACh is a possible method to activate an uncontrolled excitatory wave that spreads to involve other neural pathways, including those that employ glutamate as neurotransmitter (10,167).

Studies of the effects of soman and tabun on neurotransmitter release from synaptosomes prepared from the cortex of guinea pig indicate that only at micromolar concentrations would these nerve agents affect the basal release of γ-aminobutyric acid (GABA) and glutamate, and that only soman affects the evoked release of these amino acids (174). These findings have been corroborated by the demonstration that, even at micromolar concentrations, soman does not affect synaptic transmission in hippocampal neurons (144). Although it is possible that convulsions induced by soman and tabun are not due to changes in the release of glutamate and GABA (99), the latest available electrophysiological studies of mammalian CNS neurons indicate that VX at low nanomolar concentrations can increase the spontaneous and evoked release of GABA and glutamate as evidenced by the ability of this organophosphate to enhance, respectively, the frequency of GABA- and glutamate-mediated miniature postsynaptic currents and the amplitude of GABA- and glutamate-mediated postsynaptic currents evoked by electric stimulation of presynaptic neurons (142,143,145). Sarin has also been shown to facilitate transmitter release from hippocampal neurons (141). Of greater potential importance, however is the finding that a concentration as low as 100 pmol of VX—approximately 200-fold lower than the IC_{50} for AChE inhibition—increases neuronal excitability apparently by affecting the inactivation of voltage-gated Na^+ channels, and consequently increasing Na^+ conductance (142,145). It is therefore conceivable that by acting on voltage-gated Na^+ channels, VX increases the release of a wide range of CNS neurotransmitters, including glutamate, a mechanism that might contribute to the induction of seizures and neuronal damage. Another clue regarding the toxicology of nerve agents has come from the recent demonstration in rat hippocampal slice experiments that choline, a by-product of ACh hydrolysis, serves as a selective full agonist at CNS nicotinic receptors made up of the α7 subunit (7,9). The finding, coupled with the discovery that these receptors have a critical role in controlling GABA release from interneurons of the CA1 field of the hippocampus (8,9), and glutamate release from pyramidal neurons of the CA3 field of the hippocampus (58), suggests that the neurotoxic effects of some AChE inhibitors might be associated with their ability to alter choline levels in the CNS (142,145). Earlier studies suggested that neither soman, sarin, tabun, nor VX appears to induce convulsions by modulating uptake or release of GABA or glutamate in guinea-pig cerebral cortical synaptosomes (174), and they have no effect on chloride-generated chloride channels (51). VX (>10 nmol/l), but not soman, sarin, or tabun, inhibits binding of ^{125}I-α-cobratoxin to the nicotinic receptor (28). GABA levels and the activity of glutamate decarboxylase and GABA transaminase are unaffected at the onset of soman-induced convulsions (99).

Animal Studies

The rat subcutaneous LD_{50}s are 193 μg/kg body weight (tabun), 103 μg/kg (sarin), 75 μg/kg (soman), and 12 μg/kg (VX); the mouse inhalation G-agent $L(C_t)_{50}$s are 15 (tabun), 5 (sarin), and 1 (soman) mg.m^{-3}/30 min (103). Relative to the mouse intravenous LD_{50} values for tabun, sarin, and soman, the ED_{50} values for inhibition of whole mouse brain AChE are 66%, 38%, and 69%, respectively (181). Rat brain AChE is dose-dependently inhibited in whole brain and in brain regions (cerebral cortex > hippocampus >

midbrain > cerebellum > striatum = brainstem) (21,114,153). Acute neurotoxic effects of soman on rats increase when animals are stressed by exposure to cold or hot environments (187). Blood flow is the single most important determinant of soman-induced cholinesterase inhibition in various rat tissues, including the brain (102). Recovery of mouse brain AChE following systemic exposure to sublethal concentrations of nerve agents is measured in weeks (181).

Seizures followed by cessation of respiration are important components of the acute neurotoxic response to organophosphorus nerve agents. Neuronal damage is proposed to occur by way of a glutamate-mediated excitotoxic mechanism: nerve cells targeted by glutamatergic neurons experience unrelenting stimulation that results in failure of their homeostatic mechanisms, cytoplasmic changes, and cell death (165). This explains why pretreatment with muscarinic receptor antagonists blocks initiation of seizure activity (105,106), but once seizures are fully developed, they become refractory to these agents and only glutamate- (specifically, N-methyl-D-aspartate [NMDA])-receptor antagonists are effective in controlling convulsions (10,167). Microdialysis and receptor-binding studies support this thesis by demonstrating that extracellular levels of glutamate rise in soman intoxication (86,87). Continued release of synaptic glutamate causes an influx of Na^+ ions through NMDA receptor channels in the plasmalemma of targeted neurons; this is followed by movement of water down the osmotic gradient into the nerve cell, with consequent edematous swelling of postsynaptic regions of dendrites and neuronal perikarya. These events are followed by a delayed intracellular influx of Ca^{2+}, which activates a number of intracellular processes that culminate in cell death. Given that NMDA-mediated glutamate excitotoxicity is also activated by reducing oxygen-generated energy available to sustain membrane ion pumps, it seems likely that the indirect glutamatergic effects of organophosphates are exacerbated by their actions on the central respiratory center and on peripheral neuromuscular sites (in intercostal muscles and diaphragm) involved in breathing. Additionally, brain mitochondrial respiration would also be interrupted by hypoxic and anoxic states associated with organophosphate-induced convulsions, and excessive bronchial secretions may interrupt air flow and contribute to cyanosis.

A recent study of the effects of soman on primates illustrates these principles (88). Cynomolgus monkeys pretreated with the carbamate pyridostigmine bromide (producing 30–40% erythrocyte AChE inhibition) received a single intramuscular (i.m.) injection of soman (equivalent to 8 times the LD_{50} dosage); they were rescued 1 min later by i.m. administration of a combination of atropine sulfate and pralidoxime plus diazepam (vide infra). All an-

imals developed muscle fasciculation and tremor within 1–2 min of soman exposure and then exhibited tonic-clonic convulsions associated with opisthotonus and cyanosis. Within 5–8 min and for a continuing period of approximately 30 min, animals were comatose, had copious bronchial secretions, and displayed dyspneic movements. Severe respiratory disturbances and tremor persisted. Forty-five min after soman administration, some animals received an intravenous injection of the glutamate receptor antagonist gacyclidine (GK-11) (89). Treatment with GK-11 stopped convulsions and respiratory disturbances within 5–10 min of drug administration. Treated monkeys recovered biting and grasping reflexes and visual tracking 2–2.5 h after poisoning and survived until the animals were terminated at 3 weeks. Frontal cortex, entorhinal cortex, amygdala, caudate, hippocampus, thalamus, midbrain, pons, medulla oblongata, and cerebellum lacked neuropathological changes when formalin-fixed tissue was examined by light microscopy. By contrast, a single animal that had survived for 3 weeks without GK-11 treatment showed "neuronal rarefaction in the frontoparietal cortex," "neuronal depopulation in the CA1 hippocampal pyramidal layer," and "severe alterations of the dentate gyrus." While these neuropathological descriptions lack the definition that would have been afforded by examination of glutaraldehyde-perfused tissues with optimal preservation of cytological ultrastructure, they are consistent with the results of in-life EEG recordings in these animals. EEG analysis within the classical frequency bands (beta, theta, alpha, delta) showed that GK-11 treatment alone restored normal brain electrical activity (88). Others have shown previously that rhesus monkeys with convulsions induced by soman display neuronal necrosis and astrocytic gliosis in the hippocampus, cerebral cortex, amygdaloid complex, caudate nucleus, and dorsal thalamic nuclei (129–131,185). A neuropathological study of rats repeatedly treated with soman in doses sufficient to induce prostration showed that piriform cortex was most sensitive, while hypothalamus and neocortex were least sensitive, to the nerve agent (65). Animals that displayed seizures showed extensive neuropathological changes in limbic structures (septum, amygdala, hippocampus), with associated effects on animal behaviors utilizing limbic pathways (65). Intense glial fibrillary protein mRNA expression, reportedly related to excessive neuronal activity rather than to cell death, was evident in the molecular layer of the dentate gyrus within 5 h of soman administration to rats, with lower expression levels in other dentate areas and hippocampal subfields CA1, CA3, and CA4 (13). Direct microinjection of soman or VX into the amygdala produced limbic convulsions and associated neuropathological changes (105).

Organophosphate nerve agents (DFP, tabun, sarin, soman) and carbamate cholinesterase inhibitors (physostigmine, pyridostigmine bromide) also have the potential to induce localized pathological changes at the neuromuscular junction; this seems primarily to involve the muscle fiber and only secondarily affects the motor terminal (46,53). Experimental studies suggest this junctional myopathy is initiated by sustained accumulation of ACh at the motor endplate; this causes an increase in sarcoplasmic reticulum Ca^{2+} that triggers events to leading to local muscle fiber necrosis (35–37,40,93,111,128,164). Neuromuscular junctions in the diaphragm are among the most severely affected in organophosphorus-treated animals (186), and pathological changes are also prominent in soleus, gastrocnemius, and quadriceps muscles. Ultrastructural changes appear within hours of anticholinesterase drug administration, progress over a few days, and resolve within a couple of weeks (40). These pathological changes correlate with the appearance of decreased contractile strength a few days after DFP administration and then a return to near-normal strength after several more days (97). Development of junctional myopathy seems to depend on the degree and duration of AChE inhibition; induction of muscle pathology is blocked by curare or pralidoxime (186). Muscle fiber necrosis in rats is more frequent with DFP than with an equivalent dose of soman (62,63). Studies with denervated muscles show that soman produces mainly centrally generated motor unit activity (leading to tremor and complex posturing), while DFP more profoundly inhibits muscle AChE, and elicits more peripherally generated neuromuscular activity coupled with pronounced fasciculation of trunk and extremity muscles (114).

Motor nerve terminals show varying degrees of subcellular change within 30 min to 2 h after injection of soman. Pathological changes include the appearance of intraaxonal myelin figures, membrane enclosures, and an increased number of large-coated vesicles. Three days after DFP injection, motor terminals in soleus muscle are reduced in number and naked endplates are common. Subjacent muscle displays swollen mitochondria, myelin figures, enlarged nucleoli, dilatation of sarcoplasmic reticulum, loss of myofibrillar striae and, later, myofilament loss and fragmentation of Z bands (92).

Junctional myopathy is likely to underly a life-threatening but spontaneously reversible syndrome of proximal limb and intercostal muscle weakness that follows within days or longer after successful treatment and resolution of a severe organophosphate-induced cholinergic crisis (152). This phenomenon is termed the "intermediate syndrome" because it follows a severe cholinergic crisis and precedes the appearance of peripheral neuropathy—in the event the offending organophosphate has the potential to age-inhibit both AChE and another neural enzyme, neuropathy target esterase (NTE) (*vide infra*). The intermediate syndrome has not been described in humans exposed to nerve agents but, *a priori*, is likely to occur in subjects who survive prominent neuromuscular effects in the acute phase of organophosphate intoxication.

Peripheral neuropathy follows single or repeated systemic exposure to organophosphates that age-inhibit NTE, a poorly characterized neuronal enzyme of unknown function. As discussed by Lotti (*see* Organophosphorus Compounds, this volume), a high degree of NTE inhibition in the nervous system of susceptible species (measured within hours of dosing) correlates with the onset 10–20 days later of clinical signs (flaccid limb paralysis) of a symmetrical distal polyneuropathy. Inhibited NTE undergoes irreversible inactivation (aging) through dealkylation of the bonded organophosphate or amide (75,78). There is *no* association between the propensity for an organophosphate to age-inhibit the enzyme activity of NTE and its ability to age-inhibit AChE. An organophosphorus compound such as tri-ortho-cresyl phosphate (TOCP) has weak anticholinesterase activity but single high doses have the potential to induce severe peripheral neuropathy in humans, mammals, and birds within 1–3 weeks of exposure (55). Conversely, nerve agents are potent anticholinesterase chemicals but have modest effects on the enzyme activity of NTE (32,190).

While soman and tabun reportedly have the potential to induce peripheral neuropathy in laboratory species (56), it is necessary to administer doses that greatly exceed the lethal concentration and to protect organophosphorus-treated animals from the anticholinesterase effects of these agents. Studies with fowl indicate that sarin will produce polyneuropathy in protected animals receiving dosages exceeding the $LD_{50}s$ values by 1–2 orders of magnitude (33,55,73,194). For soman, sarin, and tabun, the 50% incapacitation concentration for NTE inhibition corresponds to 0.1 μM, 0.33 μM and 3.6 μM, respectively, or 10–100 times the lethal concentration (191). Approximately 70% inhibition of brain NTE activity 24–48 h after organophosphate exposure correlates with the subsequent appearance of peripheral neuropathy; this level is reached by the oral administration of 200 $\mu g/kg$ body weight of sarin and 3 $\mu g/kg$ of tabun (32,191). However, atropinized hens treated with the highest tolerated i.m. doses of tabun failed to develop behavioral or histological evidence of peripheral neuropathy (68). Chickens protected with atropine and 2-pralidoxamine given single i.m. injections of VX as high as 150 $\mu g/kg$ (5 times LD_{50}) failed to develop the locomotor signs or histological evidence of peripheral neuropathy displayed by animals given a single injection of 400 mg/kg of

TOCP (193). There was no evidence of peripheral neuropathy in hens given repeated doses of VX at or above the LD$_{50}$ (194). Evidence of peripheral neuropathy was also lacking in ewes dosed orally with 30 μg VX/day for 4 weeks (138).

While G agents are considered unlikely to cause peripheral neuropathy in humans, this proposition is essentially based on the results of the foregoing animal studies. Conceivably, individuals who are rescued from the otherwise supralethal effects of a G agent such as sarin, or who are exposed to low levels of these substances for prolonged periods, might be at risk for mild polyneuropathy. Noteworthy is a poorly documented report of electromyographic changes—interpreted as subclinical neuropathy—weeks after exposure to inhalation of an anticholinesterase agent believed to be sarin (119). Concern also arises from a report of significant sarin-induced inhibition of NTE activity in the brain and spinal cord of mice which developed delayed-onset limb weakness and spinal cord damage (73). Additionally, cats were found to have reduced numbers of mechanoreceptors and decreased conduction velocities of muscle spindle and mechanoreceptor afferents after repeated sublethal doses of sarin or soman (54). Nerve agent exposures in the feline and murine studies were both insufficient to induce signs of an acute cholinergic crisis (54,73).

While the clinical picture in organophosphate polyneuropathy is largely referrable to the peripheral somatic and autonomic nervous system, and characterized by a stocking-and-glove distribution of deficits that are dominated by motor signs, the underlying pathological picture is one of retrograde axonal degeneration of elongate CNS as well as PNS nerve fibers. This type of *central-peripheral distal axonopathy* is a pattern of neuropathology common to a number of toxic, metabolic, and certain inherited polyneuropathies (168). Nerve fiber vulnerability is related to their length and size, such that long and large-diameter myelinated fibers undergo retrograde degeneration prior to those that are shorter and thinner. Characteristically, therefore, distal regions of nerves supplying the extremities and the terminal regions of the longest descending (corticospinal to lumbar regions) and ascending (gracile and lumbosacral spinocerebellar) spinal tracts undergo degeneration contemporaneously. With time, pathological changes ascend these pathways (a phenomenon known as "dying-back"), and shorter and thinner nerve fibers also become involved in the dying-back process. Studies of domestic fowl treated with 500 mg TOCP per kg body weight reveal the extent of CNS damage in organophosphate polyneuropathy: nerve fiber degeneration was found in the lateral vestibular, gracile, external cuneate, and lateral cervical nuclei at the level of the medulla oblongata; the lumbar part of the medial pontine spinal tract; in lamina VII of the lumbar ventral horn; and in cranial regions of the dorsal and ventral spinocerebellar tracts and mossy fiber terminals of the cerebellum. Affected to a lesser extent were the solitary, inferior olivary, and raphae nuclei; the medial, descending, and lateral vestibular nuclei; and the lateral paragigantocellular, gigantocellular, and lateral reticular nuclei (177). Since recovery from CNS damage in organophosphate neuropathy may be incomplete, mild spasticity and ataxia may persist as a reflection of permanently damaged motor and sensory spinal pathways.

Exposure of rodents and primates to levels of nerve agents lower than those required to induce signs of acute toxicity are reportedly associated with changes in behavior. In rat studies, tabun produced flavor aversion (146), soman suppressed rates on schedule-controlled behavior (21), and sarin produced alterations in motor coordination (163). Some studies have reported adverse effects of soman on learning ability (52,116); others have not (65). Performance decrements on an equilibrium platform were found in rhesus monkeys given soman in single (2–3 μg/kg body weight) or repeated doses ($\sim$ 1 μg/kg/day) that produced increasing inhibition of serum cholinesterase (up to 80% over 5 days) (65). Large subject-to-subject variation was noted in the responses of primates to low-levels of soman, especially in the presence of carbamate (65). Neither pyridostigmine bromide nor physostigmine—drugs that are effective against high-level acute exposures to soman—protect primates against the appearance of performance decrements induced by low-level exposure to nerve agents. Primate performance decrements induced by low-level exposure to nerve agents generally are not associated with extensive physical signs (*e.g.*, miosis, salivation, fasciculation), and they reverse within 24 h of treatment with soman (19). However, repeated low-level exposure of a monkey for 8 days resulted in unspecified neurological signs that gradually abated over 2–3 weeks, an observation that prompted the suggestion that subtle performance deficits may be an indicator of incipient neuronal damage (65).

Human Studies

Controlled studies of the acute effects of relatively low doses of organophosphate nerve agents have been performed in a sizeable number of healthy humans. Single oral doses of 2.0–4.5 μg VX produced gastrointestinal symptoms in 5 of 32 subjects (156). A single oral dose of 2 μg sarin/kg body weight caused excessive dreaming and talking during sleep, while 22 μg sarin/kg body weight precipitated anorexia, nausea, heartburn, tightness of the chest and stomach, increased fatigue, nervous tension, anxiety, insomnia, and excessive dreaming (59,180). Multiple exposures to sarin had cumulative toxic effects (59). No signs of toxicity were seen in volunteers given 1.43 μg VX/kg/day for 7 days orally in drinking water, although average erythrocyte AChE was reduced to 40% of baseline values (160). Headache, tiredness, and irritability were reported by an adult volunteer who had received an intravenous (i.v.) injection of 0.04 μg VX/kg (83). Administration of 1.5 μg VX/kg i.v. to each of 18 volunteers resulted in dizziness, nausea, and vomiting in 11, 4, and 6 subjects, respectively (156). Performance of volunteers on a number-facility test declined significantly within 1 h of receiving 1.5 μg VX/kg i.v. (156). The calculated no-effect dose for VX-induced tremor in humans is 0.34 μg/kg (109).

The acute manifestations of low-level nerve agent vapor exposure are considered to result from inhibition of synaptic AChE at peripheral muscarinic sites. Local effects are evident within seconds to minutes of exposure and disappear in hours (low dose) to days (moderate dose). Direct contact between the organophosphate and mucous membranes of the eye results in pupillary constriction (miosis), with the nasal passages (rhinorrhea) and with the bronchial tree (bronchoconstriction, increased secretions, and cough). Local exposure of the ciliary body may cause blurring of vision, eye pain, and frontal headache. Dermal exposure to small amounts of nerve agent elicits locally increased sweating (muscarinic effect) and localized muscular fasciculation (nicotinic effect). With increased dermal exposure and systemic distribution, subjects experience nausea, increased salivation, and vomiting. Other muscarinic actions result in bradycardia, enhanced lacrimation, and increased urinary frequency. Pallor and changes in blood pressure (hypertension followed by hypotension) are associated with actions on sympathetic ganglia. These effects may appear within minutes to hours and persist for several days. Absorption of larger amounts of nerve agent *via* the lungs (vapor) or skin (liquid) produces additional acute toxic manifestations attributable to agent actions in both the PNS and CNS: depression of central respiratory and circulatory centers, coupled with flaccid paralysis of respiratory muscles, precipitates dyspnea/apnea, cyanosis, and hypotension; convulsions and loss of consciousness may appear; generalized muscle fasciculation, cramps, and weakness reflect involvement of peripheral neuromuscular function, and involuntary micturition and defecation are mediated by actions at muscarinic sites associated with the urinary bladder and gut (155). Death may supervene within 5 min of exposure to lethal concentrations. The estimated inhalation lethal toxicity values for humans, expressed as the concentration of nerve agent in the air multiplied by the duration of inhalation [L(C$_t$)$_{50}$], in mg.min/m^{-3}, correspond to 400 (tabun),

100 (sarin), 50 (soman), and 10 (VX) (155). Estimated i.v. LD$_{50}$ values for nerve agents are: 0.08 (tabun), 0.01 (sarin), 0.025 (soman) and 0.007 (VX) mg/kg. The estimated percutaneous LD$_{50}$ for VX is 0.142 mg/kg. For survivors, delayed effects of nerve agent exposure include sensations of giddiness, tension, anxiety, jitteriness, restlessness, emotional lability, excessive dreaming, insomnia, nightmares, headaches, tremor, withdrawal and depression, difficulty concentrating, slowness of recall, confusion, slurred speech, and ataxia (45).

Four terrorist incidents in 1994 and 1995 resulted in exposures of Japanese civilians to nerve agents believed to be impure sarin (45). A fifth was thought to be related to VX (125). Two sarin-associated events occurred in the city of Matsumoto; the largest, in June 1994, was a presumed terrorist attack on a residential area in which 600 residents and rescuers were exposed, 58 were admitted to hospital and 7 died (117). Eleven Japanese passengers traveling in the Yokohama city subway were hospitalized with complaints of dizziness and eye pain. Approximately 1000 were affected and 12 died as a result of exposure in the Tokyo subway system in March 1995 to an organophosphate thought to be sarin (132,198). Patients with mild poisoning showed marked miosis and complained of headaches, dizziness, nausea, chest discomfort, and abdominal cramps (172). Patients with severe poisoning showed greatly reduced levels of consciousness, miosis, skin flushing, tachycardia, raised blood pressure, respiratory distress, marked muscle fasciculation, and flaccid paralysis (172). Some had illness reportedly in the absence of evidence of erythrocyte AChE inhibition (205). Nicotinic effects on cardiovascular function (tachycardia, increased blood pressure) and striated muscle dominated the clinical picture in severely affected patients (124,172). Creatine kinase was elevated and hypocalcemia was evident in a small proportion of sarin-exposed patients (117,205). Miosis persisted beyond 2 weeks in some subjects.

Three weeks after exposure to sarin in the city of Matsumoto, severely poisoned patients showed decreased activities of plasma cholinesterase and erythrocyte AChE; reduced serum triglyceride, serum potassium, and chloride; and increased serum creatine kinase, leukocytes, and urinary ketones. Some had gait disturbance. At 30 days, some subjects showed polyphasic, high-amplitude potentials on electromyography (suggestive of subclinical motor neuropathy), epileptiform discharges by EEG, and residual miosis (117). All subjects had recovered at 6 months, except one with anoxic encephalopathy (117). Sarin-exposed individuals who exhibited seizures and/or loss of consciousness experienced anoxic-like persistent retrograde and anterograde amnesia for up to 6 months and beyond (66,117,126). Another group of nine women and nine men (mean age 31, 19–58) with mild-to-moderate manifestations of acute sarin toxicity were compared to a sex- and age-matched group 6 months after exposure when obvious clinical abnormalities were absent: group means for event-related P_{300} potentials and visual evoked potentials, but not brainstem auditory evoked potentials, showed slight but significant prolongation (119). Four of seven subjects severely poisoned with sarin showed epileptic discharges when subjected to electroencephalography 1 and 2 years following sarin exposure. One subject reportedly developed sensory polyneuropathy 7 months after exposure, and another still had visual field deficits 1 year after exposure; these had resolved by 17 months (151).

Unresolved is the question of long-term sequelae from exposure to low levels of potent organophosphate chemicals unassociated with acute hypoxic or anoxic episodes. Even more controversial is whether clinical sequelae may occur in the absence of evidence of erythrocyte AChE inhibition, as claimed by one Japanese group (see 205). Minor disorders of affect, emotion, and memory were reported in 38% of 114 subjects after acute organophosphate poisoning (175). Exacerbation of psychiatric conditions was found in a clinical drug trial in which patients with mental illness were treated therapeutically with DFP (148). Others have claimed that symptomatic organophosphate exposure leads to persistent changes in the EEG and in behavior (112,149). The most provocative study relates to unconfirmed persistent effects reported in civilians with one or more documented symptomatic exposures to sarin (41): Subjects reported increased dreaming, decreased libido, memory loss, irritability, and trouble concentrating. Spectral EEG analysis revealed persistent increases in beta activity in the temporal lobes of sarin-exposed individuals (eyes closed and drowsy), as well as the sarin-exposed group ($n = 77$) relative to controls ($n = 38$). Similar changes were observed in rhesus monkeys 1 year after administration of single (5 μg/kg, intramuscular) or repeated weekly doses of sarin (1 μg/kg, intramuscular) sufficient to induce EEG desynchronization and spike-wave discharges consistent with seizure activity (22). Anoxia was precluded by pretreating animals with gallamine triethiodide and providing artificial respiration. The EEG of sarin-exposed civilians vs. controls also revealed increased delta and theta slowing, decreased alpha activity, and increased rapid-eye-movement sleep (42). While confirmatory studies are needed, these findings suggest that single symptomatic exposure, or a series of subclinical exposures, can alter the frequency of the spontaneous EEG for periods of at least 1 year (41).

An epidemiological study that employed a simple questionnaire to assess current state of health suggests that controlled exposures to measured doses of purified nerve agents and other anticholinesterase chemicals sufficient to generate acute cholinergic manifestations does not produce major neurological or psychiatric compromise in the long term. Between 1958 and 1975, the U.S. Army undertook a human volunteer study to investigate the immediate and short-term effects on performance of chemicals with warfare potential (122,123). As a group, the volunteer population ($n = 6720$) was above average in physical and mental qualifications, with a mean Intelligence Quotient of approximately 110, good behavior records, and "normal" neuropsychological (Minnesota Multiphasic Personality Inventory) profiles generally two standard deviations above the population mean on all scales. Subjects ($n = 4826$) received one or more of 254 chemicals in five classes: psychochemicals, sulfur mustard and various other irritants and vesicants, anticholinergics, cholinesterase reactivators (vide infra), and anticholinesterases (notably organophosphate nerve agents and carbamates). In the early 1960s, 1406 healthy U.S. soldier volunteers, mostly 20–25 years of age, were tested with single or multiple doses of one or more of 16 anticholinesterase chemicals: seven organophosphate esters, including sarin ($n = 246$), tabun ($n = 26$), soman ($n = 83$), GF ($n = 21$), VX ($n = 740$), DFP ($n = 11$), or EA3148 ($n = 32$). Some organophosphate-treated subjects were given the antidotal chemicals atropine and/or pralidoxime chloride (2-PAM-Cl). [Other anticholinesterase agents administered included the organophosphate malathion ($n = 10$); three carbamates, including physostigmine ($n = 138$), neostigmine ($n = 22$), and pyridostgmine ($n = 27$); a quaternary ammonium inhibitor, hexafluorenium ($n = 11$); two cholinergic agonists, methacholine and urecholine ($n = 15$); and an acridine, tetrahydroacridine ($n = 15$).] Total anticholinesterase exposures equaled 1820. Routes of administration included i.v., i.m., percutaneous, oral, and whole-body exposure. Doses given i.v. and i.m. rarely exceeded an incapacitating exposure.

Subjects experienced the following acute signs and symptoms: none reported, headache, nausea, nervousness, leg muscle twitching, sweating of the hands and feet, sensation of heaviness of the eyes, dizziness, weakness, shakiness, persistent nausea, vomiting. Erythrocyte AChE levels were normal or depressed after agent treatment. Subjects treated percutaneously with soman, 8.5 μg/kg body weight, remained asymptomatic and showed no decrease in erythrocyte AChE levels over a 2-week period. By contrast, multiple oral doses of VX (probably 3.5 μg/kg) reduced erythrocyte AChE to less than 20% in 2 of 29 subjects reviewed, with return to normal levels within 6–7 days following exposure. Another subject treated i.v. with VX developed leg muscle fasciculation and perspiration of palms and soles 15 min after injection when erythrocyte AChE was 87% of normal; hands and feet felt cold and heavy at 30 min, and AChE levels at 1 h were 17%. Another subject, treated i.m. with VX, 3.2 μg/kg body weight, was dizzy, nauseated, and very drowsy after 2 h; he lacked concentration and stared vacantly into space for the next 10 h and, at 26 h after exposure, when he was treated with the oxime drug 2-PAM-Cl (*vide infra*), complained of slight dizziness and blurred vision, after which he recovered. Two of six subjects treated intravenously with 1–2 μg/kg of soman, plus oxime and/or atropine, experienced "the usual physiological responses, weakness and muscle contraction, persistent nausea," and vomiting to the point of dehydration. One was referred for psychiatric observation; diagnosed for anxiety reaction, acute agitation, and hysterical reaction; and later released for duty.

In 1984, the National Research Council (a nongovernmental organization based in Washington, DC), undertook a study to determine the possibility of pronounced long-term adverse health effects arising from exposure to anticholinesterase agents administered in the U.S. Army's human research program (122,123). Mailed survey questionnaires were returned by 64% of the overall population of soldiers who participated in the program and who were believed to be living at the time of the survey. Greater than half of the respondents had been earlier exposed to multiple chemical groups. Twenty-seven outcome variables relating to health, social adjustment, and reproductive experience of the participants were examined in volunteers who had been assigned to each of the seven classes of chemicals tested. Two comparison groups were used: subjects who received no test chemicals and subjects who received one or more chemicals other than the one under scrutiny in the test. Mean age of all respondents was 42.4 years and, for the anticholinesterase group, the range was 35–54 years. Self-assessment of current health status was similar across and between groups. There were no differences in reported smoking experience, reported alcohol consumption, or reported use of selected substances of abuse. There was no increase in reports of subjects seeking medical care in the 5-year period preceding the survey date. Admission of test subjects to hospitals run by the U.S. Army or U.S. Department of Veterans Affairs for mental disorders (ICD-8, codes 290-315) or diseases of the nervous system or sense organs (ICD-8, codes 320-389), did not appear to be significantly increased, either during the years immediately after testing or thereafter (up to the early 1980s). Relative to controls, there was no evidence of increased mortality rates among participants in the entire program, in the anticholinesterase subprogram, or in subjects treated only with sarin or with VX. While no adverse effects referrable to the nervous system were detected, the study was known to be of low power and had other limitations (123). Funding was insufficient to undertake clinical examination of the subjects as recommended by the NRC Committee. However, in 1999, planning for clinical studies was set to proceed.

Decontamination and Treatment

The first priority in the event of a civilian or military nerve agent release is to protect rescuers and medical personnel from exposure (71, *cf.* 121) and then to decontaminate the casualties (71). Decontamination and aggressive airway maintenance of casualties are followed by the administration of cholinolytics (atropine), AChase reactivators (oximes) and, if indicated, anticonvulsants (benzodiazepines) (71). Blood samples should be obtained to determine erythrocyte and plasma cholinesterase levels and to confirm the presence of nerve agent and its metabolites (80,120). "Hemodiafiltration" and hemoperfusion reportedly have been employed successfully in a sarin-exposed subject for whom treatment with atropine and 2-PAM-Cl failed to provide clinical improvement (204).

Detailed description of decontamination procedures and treatment are available elsewhere (45). An adequately protected responder should remove the casualty's clothing and monitor the subject for evidence of contamination. Assisted ventilation, oxygen, and frequent suctioning may be needed because of copious secretions and respiratory failure. Atropine is administered because it competes with ACh for occupancy of muscarinic receptors; atropinization reverses most muscarinic signs, but not the CNS or peripheral nicotinic effects of organophosphates. Atropine citrate is administered i.v. or i.m. in aliquots of 2 mg as often as every 5 min until secretions are minimal, respiration is adequate, and heart rate is above 90 beats per minute. A 10- to 20-mg cumulative dose of atropine in the first 2–3 h is usually adequate; however, in severe nerve agent poisoning, up to 50 mg of atropine may be required in a 24-h period. Atropine or oxime eye drops are used to relieve eye pain. While atropine possesses anticonvulsant properties, it also enhances the efficacy of anticonvulsants. The GABA agonist diazepam, which blocks convulsions and incapacitation in monkeys treated with soman (25,44), is administered in an i.m. dose of 10 mg given with the third dose of atropine (45). While subjects with nerve-agent exposure have an increased tolerance for atropine, anticholinergic side effects may be associated with excessive atropinization.

Atropine treatment is supplemented by concurrent treatment with an oxime (Fig. 36). The oxime exerts a nucleophilic attack on the phosphorus; the oxime-phosphonate then splits off, dissociates the nerve agent moiety from the

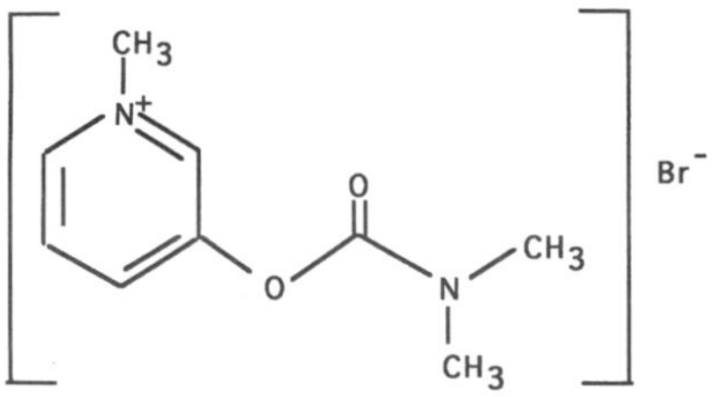

PYRIDOSTIGMINE BROMIDE

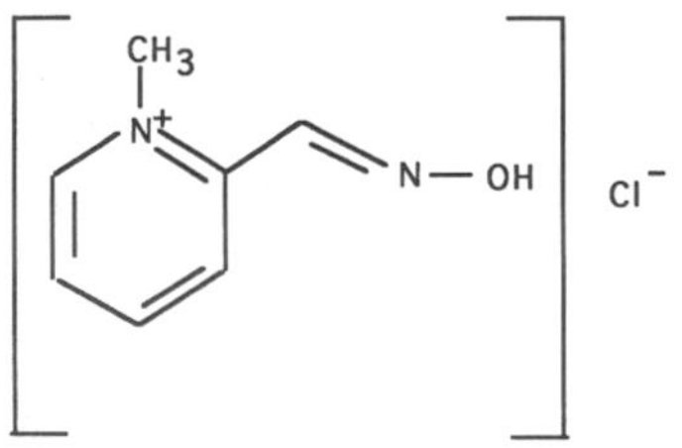

PRALIDOXIME CHLORIDE

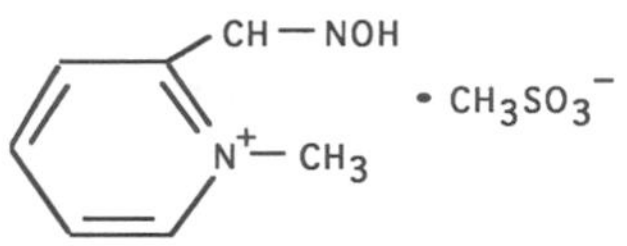

PRALIDOXIMINE METHANESULPHONATE;
N-METHYLPYRIDINIUM-2-ALDOXIME METHANESULFONATE; (P2S)

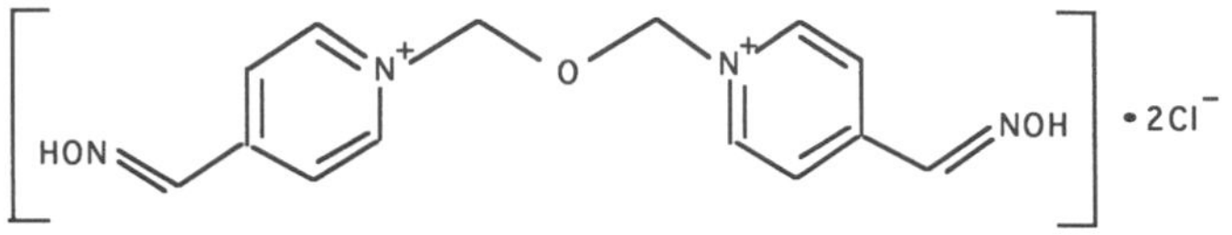

OBIDOXIME; TOXOGONINE DICHLORIDE

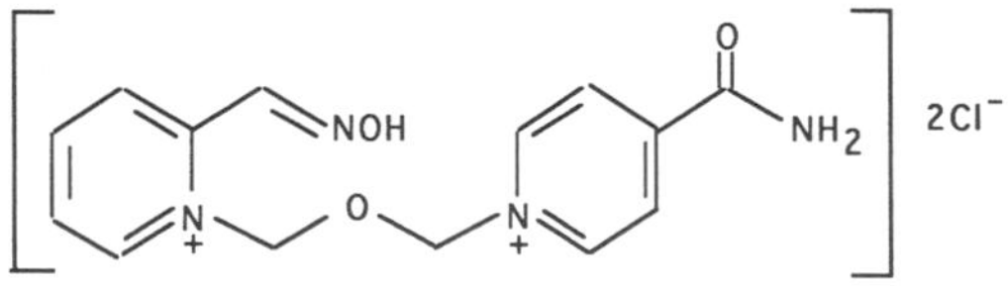

1-[[[4-(AMINO-CARBONYL)PYRIDINIO]METHOXY]METHYL]-2 [HYDROXYIMINO)METHYL]-
PYRIDINIUM DICHLORIDE; ASOXIME CHLORIDE; HI-6

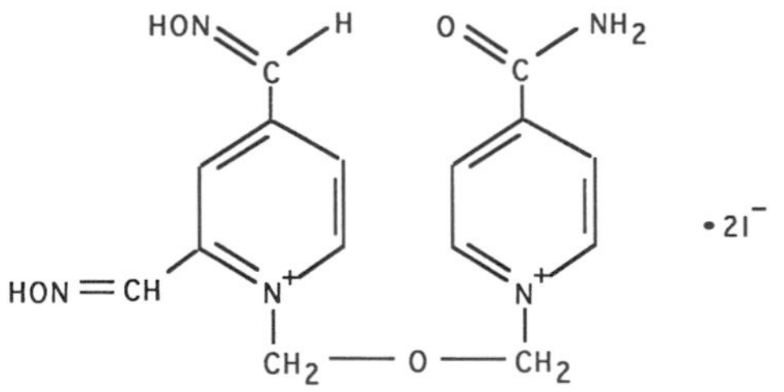

PYRIMIDOXIME DIODIDE; Hlo7

FIGURE 36. Structures of oximes and the carbamate pyridostigmine bromide [From Maynard (103)].

AChE molecule, and thereby reactivates functional enzyme and restores normal synaptic function (34,195). The therapeutic use of oximes evolved from a single cat study demonstrating that i.m. administration of N-methylpyridinium-2-aldoxime methanesulfonate (P2S), resulting in plasma drug levels of >4 mg/ml, succeeded in reversing the anticholinesterase effects (bradycardia, hypotension, respiratory compromise) of intravenous methylisopropoxyphosphoryl thiocholine. Oxime development led to the approval by the U.S. Food and Drug Administration of pralidoximine chloride (2-PAM-Cl) to be used as an adjunct to atropine for organophosphate insecticide poisoning irrespective of the route of exposure (45). An i.v. or i.m. injection of 30 mg/kg body weight 2-PAM-Cl or P2S over a 30-min period

every 4 h is recommended for organophosphorus nerve agents; this is continued until the agent and any active metabolites are fully excreted. P2S overcomes the neuromuscular block produced by sarin but is less effective against tabun (170). Another approach is to administer N,N'-dimethyleneoxide bis(pyridinium-4-aldoxime) dichloride (obidoxime, toxogonine); ambulatory patients receive 250 mg every 2 h (up to 750 mg), while moderately and severely affected patients are given slow intravenous injection of 250 mg every 2 h (up to eight identical doses) (45). Possible side effects of therapeutic doses of pralidoximine may include nausea, vomiting, diarrhea, headache, dizziness, rise in blood pressure, malaise, and blurred vision. Those associated with obidoxime therapy include a menthol taste; a sensation of heat in the upper torso, face, and throat; and perverse circumoral sensations (numbness, tightness).

Tabun, sarin, and soman react with oximes with decreasing reaction velocity (17). Tabun reacts most rapidly with the bispyridinium oxide HI-6 (Fig. 36), sarin with 2-PAM-Cl, and soman with obidoxime (17), but HI-6 is superior to obidoxime in reacting with human erythrocyte AChE *in vitro* (199). Oxime therapy theoretically is not effective against soman poisoning because the agent–enzyme complex rapidly undergoes aging. However, data derived from nonhuman primates lethally intoxicated with soman or tabun suggest that HI-6 may promote recovery of brain respiratory center function and diaphragmatic neuromuscular transmission by a mechanism unrelated to reactivation of inhibited AChE (182). HI-6 was a more effective treatment than either tetroxime or obidoxime in mice administered a median lethal dose of soman (79). HI-6 was superior to 2-PAM-Cl when atropinesterase-free rabbits were intoxicated with soman, tabun, sarin, or VX and given the AChE reactivator 2 min later at onset of signs of toxicity (85,134). Another study showed that HI-6 was therapeutically effective against soman and HLo-7 against tabun and GF (98). Soman intoxication significantly decreased uptake of HI-6 into the rat brain (24). HI-6 significantly reactivated erythrocyte AChE activity in rats given soman with or without pyridostigmine pretreatment; however, pyridostigmine decreased overall recovery of inhibited AChE in VX-challenged rats given HI-6 (11).

Pretreatment with a soman-antidote enhancer, notably the carbamate pyridostigmine bromide (PB), with subsequent administration of atropine and an oxime in the event of soman exposure, provides protection against the acute toxic effects (but not the performance decrements) of this agent (65,202), but not against those of sarin or VX. PB "reversibly"* inhibits a percentage of peripheral cholinesterases and prevents access of soman to the inhibited (protected) enzyme, which subsequently decarbamylates to yield active enzyme (50,56). Acute effects of overdose are attributable to the peripheral anticholinesterase actions of the pyridostigmine moiety, a quaternary carbamate molecule that does not readily traverse the blood-brain barrier; chronic treatment with high dosages of PB may also induce effects associated with the bromine moiety (which readily traverses the blood-brain barrier), namely the neurological and dermatological effects of beginning bromism (*see* Bro-

mide, this volume) (147). It has also been suggested that PB may occupy BuChE sites that would otherwise scavenge and sequester nerve agent (64), thereby making a large amount of an organophosphate, such as sarin, available to the nervous system of PB-treated subjects (64). Hen studies show that repeated oral dosing with PB markedly inhibits BuChE. Fowl given 5 mg PB/kg/day plus 10 mg/kg/day of chlorpyrifos (an organophosphate) reportedly showed an increased neurotoxic response relative to birds treated with either agent alone (1) (*see also* N,N′-Diethyl-*m*-toluamide, this volume). The daily oral dose of PB used in this study appeared to be equivalent to a 13-week no-observed-toxicity level in mice; animals treated by gavage with 15–60 mg/kg/day demonstrated erythrocyte AChE inhibition, exaggerated cholinergic stimulation and tremors (94).

Pyridostigmine bromide (recommended dose: 30 mg once every 8 h) was widely used by U.S. troops serving in southwest Asia during the 1991 Persian Gulf War. Clinical experience with larger doses of PB for the long-term treatment of myesthenia gravis did not predict the large percentage of soldiers who reported drug side effects during wartime use. A study of 41,650 American soldiers (6.5% female), 34,000 of whom had taken PB tablets for 6–7 days at the onset of hostilities, revealed that symptoms (increased flatus, abdominal cramps, soft stools, urinary urgency, headaches, rhinorrhea, diaphoresis, and extremity tingling) were reported in about half of this population (81). Approximately 1% of soldiers believed medical attention had been warranted for their experience with the side effects of PB treatment; most commonly these included severe gastrointestinal disturbance, urinary frequency, and urinary urgency, effects likely attributable to the anticholinesterase action of the pyridostigmine moiety of PB. Some subjects experienced a number of reportedly unexpected responses to the drug, notably bad dreams, vertigo, slurred speech, rashes, edema, and urticaria, and spiking hypertension with epistaxis. By contrast, only minor drug effects were reported in a 2-week, double-blind, placebo-controlled crossover study of seven 18- to 24-year-old healthy males subjected to heat stress while receiving PB 30 mg orally *t.i.d.* for 7 consecutive days (31). This experience may differ from that of Gulf War participants, many of whom were subjected to long periods of heat stress and potential dehydration with water replacement but no salt tablet supplementation. A low-salt diet greatly increases the half-life of bromine and provides the optimum setting for bromide intoxication (127), a likely explanation for the presence of rashes in some Gulf War veterans who ingested PB tablets (81). Headache, bad dreams, and slurred speech are also consistent with the early (and widely forgotten) manifestations of bromism (118). Other factors that might have modulated the effect

---

*It is not appropriate to describe the inhibition of cholinesterase enzyme activity by carbamates as "reversible" and by organophosphates as "irreversible." Some organophosphate-cholinesterase complexes (other than those caused by chemical warfare agents) may reactivate within hours to days, and carbamate-cholinesterase complexes may reactivate in minutes to hours (192).

of PB in Gulf War veterans include concurrent exposure to organophosphorus pesticides and other anticholinesterase agents, and the effects of physical stress. Studies with mice demonstrate that stressful physical activity (forced swimming) apparently increases access of PB to the brain: Less than 1/100th of the dose required in unstressed mice was needed to inhibit brain AChE by 50% in swim-stressed animals (49). Another mouse study showed that PB lethality is increased by exposure to a β-adrenoceptor agonist (isoproterenol), selective β_2-adrenoceptors agonists (salbutamol, terbutaline), α_1- and α_2-adrenoceptor agonists (yohimbine, phentolamine, prazosin), and caffeine (26).

Based on the aforementioned human and animal experience with the delayed effects of severe organophosphate poisoning, subjects successfully treated for acute nerve agent toxicity should be monitored for: (a) potential recurrence of fatal acute toxicity associated with release of agent from unknown sites of sequestration; (b) delayed-onset (days-week), life-threatening but rapidly (days-week) reversible intermediate syndrome characterized by weakness of neck flexors, proximal limb muscles, intercostal muscles and diaphragm, and muscles innervated by certain cranial nerves; (c) insidious onset (weeks/months) distal, mild symmetrical motorsensory polyneuropathy that reverses slowly (months); (d) persistent (months) visual deficits; (e) abnormal subconvulsive brain electrical activity (years); and (f) indices of the post-traumatic stress syndrome (119). Prolongation of the heart rate–adjusted Q-T interval, which contributes to cadiovascular risk, has been reported in acute sarin poisoning (119), and rats recovering from acute sarin or soman intoxication display a cardiomyopathy that is attenuated by anticholinergic drugs administered before the nerve agent (104,161). Studies with guinea pigs suggest that atropine-containing antidote combinations may induce lethal arrhythmias in subjects poisoned with nerve agent (notably tabun and soman at 10 times LD_{50} doses) (200,201).

Although there is no doubt that organophosphate-induced AChE inhibition contributes to the toxicity of nerve agents, there are other important actions of organophosphates that may outweigh the AChE-inhibiting effect in some systems. The limited success in development of antidotes to treat and/or prevent organophosphate intoxication may in part be attributable to a persistent focus on the cholinesterase-inhibiting actions of the organophosphates. Techniques for investigating the interactions of organophosphates with ligand- and voltage-gated ion channels are now prime for molecular studies of the CNS actions of nerve agents. Experimental studies with rats have shown that NMDA receptor antagonists that cross the blood-brain barrier reduce convulsions and protect animals against the lethal effects of soman (39,88,90): they may therefore have

a role in the treatment of human organophosphate neurotoxicity; however, in the absence of muscarinic receptor antagonists, NMDA receptor antagonists may have lethal interactive effects on respiratory function during soman intoxication (165).

REFERENCES

1. Abou-Donia MB, Wilmarth KR, Abdel-Rahman *et al.* (1996) Increased neurotoxicity following exposure to pyridostigmine bromide, DEET, and chlorpyrifos. *Fund Appl Toxicol* **34**, 201.

2. Albaret C, Lacoutiere S, Ashman WP *et al.* (1997) Molecular mechanic study of nerve agent O-ethyl S-[2-(diisopropylamino)ethyl]methylphosphonothioate bound to the active site of *Torpedo californica* acetylcholinesterase. *Proteins* **28**, 543.

3. Albuquerque EX, Aracava Y Cintra WM *et al.* (1988) Structure-activity relationship of reversible cholinesterase inhibitors: Activation, channel blockade and stereospecificity of the nicotinic acetylcholine receptor-ion channel complex. *Braz J Med Biol Res* **21**, 1173.

4. Albuquerque EX, Idriss M, Deshpande SS (1985) Reversible and irreversible anticholinesterase inhibitors interact with the glutamatergic synapse. *Proc 1985 Sci Conf Chem Defense Res, Appendix C* p. 983.

5. Albuquerque EX, Swanson KL, Deshpande SS *et al.* (1987) The direct interaction of cholinesterase inhibitors with the acetylcholine receptor and their involvement with cholinergic autoregulatory mechanisms. In: *Sixth Medical Chemical Defense Bioscience Review.* U.S. Army Medical Research Institute, Maryland p. 27.

6. Albuquerque EX, Swanson KL, Monies JG, Aracava Y (1994) *Molecular Targets and Synaptic Effects of Carbamates, Organophosphates, Oximes and Pyridiniums: Implications for Prophylaxis and Therapy of Organophosphate Toxicity.* U.S. Army Medical Research and Development Command: Final Report of Contract DAMD17-88-C-9119, 300 pp.

7. Alkondon M, Pereira EFR, Albuquerque EX (1997) Choline is a selective agonist of $\alpha 7$ nicotinic acetylcholine receptors in rat hippocampal neurons. *Eur J Neurosci* **9**, 2734.

8. Alkondon M, Pereira EFR, Albuquerque EX (1998) Choline and selective antagonists identify multiple subtypes of nicotinic acetylcholine receptors that modulate γ-aminobutyric acid release from CA1 interneurons in rat hippocampal slices. *J Neurosci* **19**, 2693.

9. Alkondon M, Pereira EFR, Barbosa CTF, Albuquerque EX (1997) Neuronal nicotinic acetylcholine receptor activation modulates GABA release from CA1 neurons of rat hippocampal slices. *J Pharmacol Exp Ther* **283**, 1396.

10. Anderson DR, Harris LW, Woodard CL, Lennox WJ (1992) The effect of pyridostigmine pretreatment on ox-

ime efficacy against intoxication by soman or VX in rats. *Drug Chem Toxicol* **15**, 285.

11. Anderson JJ, Kuo S, Chase TN (1994) Endogenous excitatory amino acids tonically stimulate striatal acetylcholine release through NMDA but not AMPA receptors. *Neurosci Lett* **176**, 264.

12. Ashani Y, Shapira S, Doctor BP *et al.* (1989) *In vivo* stoichiometry of cholinesterase prophylaxis against organophosphate poisoning. *Proc 3rd Int Symp Protection Against Chemical Warfare Agents*, Umeå, Sweden p. 227 [cited by Somani *et al.* 1992].

13. Baille-Le Crom V, Collombet JM, Carpentier P *et al.* (1995) Early regional changes of GFAP mRNA in rat hippocampus and dentate gyrus during soman-induced seizures. *Neuroreport* **7**, 365.

14. Bajgar J (1997) Differential inhibition of the brain acetylcholinesterase molecular forms following sarin, soman and VX intoxication in laboratory rats. *Acta Medica* **40**, 89.

15. Bakry NM, el-Rashidy AH, Eldefrawi AT, Eldefrawi ME (1988) Direct actions of organophosphate anticholinesterases on nicotinic and muscarinic acetylcholine receptors. *J Biochem Toxicol* **3**, 235.

16. Barnes JM (1954) Organo-phosphorus insecticides. The toxic action of organophosphorus insecticides in mammals. *Chem Ind* Jan 2, p. 478.

17. Becker G, Kawan A, Szinicz L (1997) Direct reaction of oximes with sarin, soman or tabun *in vitro*. *Arch Toxicol* **71**, 714.

18. Benschop HP, Konings CAG, van Genderen J, De Jong LPA (1984) Isolation, anticholinesterase properties and acute toxicity in mice of the four stereoisomers of the nerve agent soman. *Toxicol Appl Pharmacol* **72**, 61.

19. Blick DW, Murphy MR, Brown GC *et al.* (1987) Effects of carbamate pretreatment and oxime therapy on soman-induced performance decrements and blood cholinesterase activity in primates. *Soc Neurosci Abst* **13**, 1716.

20. Boter HL, Ooms AJ, Van Den Berg GR, Van Dijk C (1966) The synthesis of optically active isopropyl methylphonofluoridate (sarin). *Rec Trav Chim Phys-Bas* **85**, 147.

21. Brezenoff HE, McGee J, Hymowitz N (1985) Effect of soman on schedule-controlled behavior and brain acetylcholinesterase in rats. *Life Sci* **37**, 2421.

22. Burchfiel JL, Duffy FH, Sim VM (1976) Persistent effects of sarin and dieldrin upon the primate electroencephalogram. *Toxicol Appl Pharmacol* **35**, 365.

23. Callaway S, Davies DR, Rutland JP (1951) Blood cholinesterase levels and range of personal variation in a healthy adult population. *Brit Med J* **2**, 812.

24. Cassel G, Karlsson L, Waara L *et al.* (1997) Pharmacokinetics and effects of HI 6 in blood and brain of soman-intoxicated rats: A microdialysis study. *Eur J Pharmacol* **332**, 43.

25. Castro CA, Larsen T, Finger AV *et al.* (1992) Behavioral efficacy of diazepam against nerve agent exposure in rhesus monkeys. *Pharmacol Biochem Behav* **41**, 159.

26. Chaney LA, Rockhold RW, Mozingo JR *et al.* (1997) Potentiation of pyridostigmine bromide toxicity by selected adrenergic agents and caffeine. *Vet Human Toxicol* **39**, 214.

27. Chatonnet A, Lockridge O (1989) Comparison of butyrylcholinesterase and acetylcholinesterase. *Biochem J* **260**, 625.

28. Chi M, Sun M (1995) Action of organophosphate anticholinesterases on the three conformation states of nicotinic receptor. *Adv Exp Med Biol* **363**, 65.

29. Churchill L, Pazdernik TL, Jackson JL *et al.* (1985) Soman-induced brain lesions demonstrated by muscarinic receptor autoradiography. *Neurotoxicology* **6**, 81.

30. Ci YX, Zhou YX, Guo ZQ *et al.* (1995) Production, characterization and application of monoclonal antibodies against the organophosphorus nerve agent VX. *Arch Toxicol* **69**, 565.

31. Cook JE, Kolka MA (1992) Chronic pyridostigmine bromide administration: Side effects among soldiers working in a desert environment. *Mil Med* **5**, 250.

32. Crowell JA, Parker RM, Bucci TJ, Dacre JC (1989) Neuropathy target esterase in hens after sarin and soman. *J Biochem Toxicol* **4**, 15.

33. Davies DR, Holland P, Rumens MJ (1960) The relationship between the chemical structure and neurotoxicity of alkyl organophosphorus compounds. *Brit J Pharmacol* **15**, 271.

34. Dawson RM (1994) Review of oximes available for treatment of nerve agent poisoning. *J Appl Toxicol* **14**, 317.

35. De Bleeker J, De Reuck JL, Willems JL (1992) Neurological aspects of organophosphate poisoning. *Clin Neurol Surg* **94**, 93.

36. De Bleeker J, Lison D, Van Den Abeele K *et al.* (1994) Acute and subacute organophosphate poisoning in the rat. *Neurotoxicology* **S15**, 341.

37. De Bleeker J, Willems J, De Reuck J *et al.* (1991) Histological and histochemical study of paraoxon myopathy in the rat. *Acta Neurol Belg* **91**, 255.

38. Degenhardt-Langelaan CE, Kientz CE (1996) Capillary gas chromatographic analysis of nerve agents using large volume injections. *J Chromatogr A* **723**, 210.

39. Deshpande SS, Smith CD, Filbert MG (1995) Assessment of primary neuronal culture as a model for soman-induced neurotoxicity and effectiveness of memantine as a neuroprotective drug. *Arch Toxicol* **69**, 384.

40. Dettbarn WD (1984) Pesticide-induced muscle necrosis: Mechanisms and prevention. *Fund Appl Toxicol* **4**, S18.

41. Duffy FA, Burchfiel JL (1980) Long term effects of the organophosphate sarin on the EEG in monkeys and humans. *Neurotoxicology* **1**, 667.

42. Duffy FA, Burchfiel JL, Bartels PH *et al.* (1979) Long-term effects of an organophosphate upon the human electroencephalogram. *Toxicol Appl Pharmacol* **47**, 161.

43. Dulaney MD, Hoskins B, Ho IK (1985) Studies on low dose sub-acute administration of soman, sarin, and tabun in the rat. *Acta Pharmacol Toxicol* **57**, 234.

44. Dunn MA, Sidell FR (1989) Progress in medical defense against nerve agents. *J Amer Med Assn* **262**, 649.

45. Ellenhorn MJ (1997) *Ellenhorn's Medical Toxicology: Diagnosis and Treatment of Human Poisoning. 2nd Ed.* Williams & Wilkins, Baltimore p. 1267.

46. Engle AG, Lambert FH, Santa T (1973) Study of long-term anticholinesterase therapy: Effects on neuromuscular transmission and on motor end-plate structure. *Neurology* **23**, 1273.

47. Faerman C, Ripoll D, Bon S *et al.* (1996) Site-directed mutants designed to test back-door hypotheses of acetylcholinesterase function. *FEBS Lett* **386**, 85.

48. Fonnum F, Sterri S (1981) Factors modifying the toxicity of organophosphorus compounds including soman and sarin. *Fund Appl Toxicol* **1**, 143.

49. Friedman A, Kaufer D, Shemer J *et al.* (1997) Pyridostigmine brain penetration under stress enhances neuronal excitability and induces early immediate transcriptional response. *Nature Med* **2**, 1382.

50. Gall D (1981) The use of therapeutic mixtures in the treatment of cholinesterase inhibition. *Fund Appl Pharmacol* **1**, 214.

51. Gant DB, Eldefrawi ME, Eldefrawi T (1987) Action of organophosphates on GABA receptor and voltage-dependent chloride channels. *Fund Appl Toxicol* **9**, 698.

52. Geller I, Hartmann RJ Jr, Gause EM (1985) Effects of subchronic administration of soman on acquisition of avoidance-escape behavior by laboratory rats. *Pharmacol Biochem Behav* **23**, 225.

53. Glazer EJ, Baker T, Riker WF Jr (1978) The neuropathology of DFP at cat soleus neuromuscular junction. *J Neurocytol* **7**, 741.

54. Goldstein BD, Fincher DR, Searle JR (1987) Electrophysiological changes in the primary sensory neuron following subchronic soman and sarin: Alterations in sensory receptor function. *Toxicol Appl Pharmacol* **91**, 55.

55. Gordon JJ, Inns RH, Johnson MK *et al.* (1983) The delayed effects of nerve agents and some other organophosphorus compounds. *Arch Toxicol* **52**, 71.

56. Gordon JJ, Leadbeater L, Maidment MP (1978) The protection of animals against organophosphorus poisoning by pretreatment with a carbamate. *Toxicol Appl Pharmacol* **43**, 207.

57. Gray AP (1984) Design and structure-activity relationships of antidotes to organophosphorus anticholinesterase agents. *Drug Metab Rev* **15**, 557.

58. Gray R, Rajan AS, Radcliffe KA *et al.* (1996) Hippocampal synaptic transmission enhanced by low concentrations of nicotine. *Nature* **383**, 713.

59. Grob D, Harvey JC (1958) Effects in man of the anticholinesterase compound sarin (isopropyl methyl phosphonofluoridate). *J Clin Invest* **37**, 350.

60. Grob D, Lilienthal JL Jr, Harvey AM, Jones BF (1947) The administration of diisopropylfluorophosphate (DFP) to man. *Bull Johns Hopkins Hosp* **81**, 217.

61. Grognet JM, Ardouin T, Istin M *et al.* (1993) Production and characterization of antibodies directed against organophosphorus nerve agent VX. *Arch Toxicol* **67**, 66.

62. Gupta RC, Patterson GT, Dettbarn WD (1985) Mechanisms of toxicity and tolerance to diisopropylphosphorofluoridate at the neuromuscular junction. *Toxicol Appl Pharmacol* **84**, 541.

63. Gupta RC, Patterson GT, Dettbarn WD (1987) Biochemical and histochemical alterations following acute soman intoxication in the rat. *Toxicol Appl Pharmacol* **87**, 393.

64. Haley RW, Kurt TL (1997) Self-reported exposure to neurotoxic chemical combinations in the Gulf War. A cross-sectional epidemiologic study. *J Amer Med Assn* **15**, 231.

65. Hartgraves SL, Murphy MR (1992) Behavioral effects of low-dose nerve agents. In: *Chemical Warfare Agents.* Somani SM ed. Academic Press, San Diego p. 125.

66. Hatta K, Miura Y, Asukai N, Hamabe Y (1996) Amnesia from sarin poisoning. *Lancet* **347**, 1343.

67. Hayes W (1982) *Pesticides Studied in Man.* Williams & Wilkins, Baltimore.

68. Henderson JD, Higgins RJ, Dacre JC, Wilson BW (1992) Neurotoxicity of acute and repeated treatments of tabun, paraoxon, diisopropyl fluorophosphate and isofenphos to the hen. *Toxicology* **72**, 117.

69. Holmstedt B (1959) Pharmacology of organophosphorus cholinesterase inhibitors. *Pharmacol Rev* **11**, 567.

70. Holmstedt B (1963) Structure-activity relationships of the organophosphorus anticholinesterase agents. In: *Cholinesterases and Anticholinesterase Agents.* Koelle GB sub-ed. *Handbuch der Exp Pharmacol* Eichler O, Farah A eds. **15**, 428.

71. Holstege CP, Kirk M, Sidell FR (1997) Chemical warfare. Nerve agent poisoning. *Crit Care Clin* **13**, 923.

72. Hoskins B, Ho IK (1992) Tolerance of organophosphate inhibitors. In: *Organophosphates: Chemistry, Fate and Effects.* Chambers JE, Lei PE eds. Academic Press, New York p. 285.

73. Husain K, Vijayaraghavan R, Pant SC *et al.* (1993) Delayed neurotoxic effect of sarin in mice after repeated inhalation exposure. *J Appl Toxicol* **13**, 143.

74. Idriss MK, Aguayo LG, Rickett D, Albuquerque EX (1986) Organophosphate and carbamate compounds have pre- and postjunctional effects at the insect glutamertergic synapse. *J Pharmacol Exp Therap* **239**, 279.

75. Jakanovic M, Johnson MK (1993) Interactions *in vitro* of some organophosphoramidates with neuropathy target esterase and acetylcholinesterase of hen brain. *J Biochem Toxicol* 8, 19.

76. Jensen FS, Viby-Mogensen J (1995) Plasma cholinesterase and abnormal reaction to succinylcholine: Twenty years' experience with the Danish cholinesterase research unit. *Acta Anesthiol Scand* 39, 150.

77. Jimmerson VR, Shih T-M, Mailman RB (1989) Variability in soman toxicity in the rat: Correlation with biochemical and behavioral measures. *Toxicology* 57, 241.

78. Johnson MK (1975) Organophosphorus esters causing delayed neurotoxic effects. *Arch Toxicol* 34, 259.

79. Kassa J (1995) Comparison of the effect of selected cholinesterase reactivators combined with atropine on soman and fosdrin toxicity in mice. *Sb Ved Lek Fak Karlovy Univ Hradci Kralove Suppl* 38, 63. [Czech]

80. Katagi M, Nishikawa M, Tatsuno M, Tsuchihashi H (1997) Determination of the main hydrolysis products of organophosphorus nerve agents, methylphosphonic acids, in human serum by indirect photometric detection ion chromatography. *J Chromatogr B Biomed Sci Appl* 698, 81.

81. Keeler JR, Hurst CG, Dunn MA (1991) Pyridostigmine used as nerve agent pretreatment under wartime conditions. *J Amer Med Assn* 266, 693.

82. Ketchum JS, Sidell FR, Drowell EB *et al.* (1973) Atropine, scopalamine, and ditran: Comparative pharmacology and antagonists in man. *Psychopharmacologia* 28, 121.

83. Kimura KK, McNamara BP, Sim VM (1960) *Intravenous Administration of VX in Man.* Technical Report CRDLR 3017. U.S. Army Chemical Corp Res Develop Comm, Chem Res Develop Labs, Army Chem Center, Maryland.

84. Koelle GB (1992) Pharmacology and toxicology of organophosphates. In: *Clinical and Experimental Toxicology of Organophosphates and Carbamates.* Ballantyne B, Marrs TC eds. Butterworth-Heinemann, Oxford p. 33.

85. Koplovitz I, Stewart JR (1994) A comparison of the efficacy of HI6 and 2-PAM against soman, tabun, sarin, and VX in the rabbit. *Toxicol Lett* 70, 269.

86. Lallement G, Carpentier P, Pernot-Marino I *et al.* (1991) Effects of soman-induced seizures on different extracellular amino acid levels and on glutamate uptake in rat hippocampus. *Brain Res* 563, 234.

87. Lallement G, Carpentier P, Pernot-Marino I *et al.* (1991) Involvement of the different rat hippocampal glutamatergic receptors in development of seizures induced by soman. *Neurotoxicology* 4, 655.

88. Lallement G, Clarencon D, Maswueliez C *et al.* (1998) Nerve agent poisoning in primates: Antilethal, antiepileptic and neuroprotective effects of GK-11. *Arch Toxicol* 72, 84.

89. Lallement G, Mestries JC, Privat A (1997) GK ll: Promising additional neuroprotective therapy for organophosphate poisoning. *Neurotoxicology* 18, 851.

90. Lallement G, Veyret J, Masqueliez C *et al.* (1997) Efficacy of huperisine in preventing soman-induced seizures, neuropathological changes and lethality. *Fund Clin Pharmacol* 11, 387.

91. Langenberg JP, Van Dijk C, Sweeney RE *et al.* (1997) Development of a physiologically based model for toxicokinetics of C(+/−)P(+/−)-soman in the atropinized guinea pig. *Arch Toxicol* 71, 320.

92. Laskowski MB, Olsom WH, Dettbarn WF (1975) Ultrastructural changes at the motor end-plate produced by an irreversible cholinesterase inhibitor. *Exp Neurol* 47, 190.

93. Leonard JP, Salpeter MM (1979) Agonist-induced myopathy at the neuromuscular junction is mediated by calcium. *J Cell Biol* 82, 811.

94. Levine BS, Long R, Chung H (1991) Subchronic oral toxicity of pyridostigmine bromide in rats. *Biomed Environ Sci* 4, 283.

95. Little JS, Broomfield CA, Fox-Talbot MK *et al.* (1989) Partial characterization of an enzyme that hydrolyzes sarin, soman, tabun and diisopropyl phosphonofluoridate (DFP). *Biochem Pharmacol* 38, 23.

96. Loewenstein-Lichtenstein Y, Schwarz M, Glick D *et al.* (1995) Genetic predisposition to adverse consequences of anti-cholinesterases in "atypical" BuChE carriers. *Nature Med* 1, 1082.

97. Lowndes HE, Baker T, Riker WF Jr (1974) Motor nerve dysfunction in delayed DFP neuropathy. *Eur J Pharmacol* 29, 66.

98. Lundy PM, Hansen AS, Hand BT, Boulet CA (1992) Comparison of several oximes against poisoning by soman, tabun and GF. *Toxicology* 72, 99.

99. Lundy PM, Magor G, Shaw RK (1978) Gamma aminobutyric acid metabolism in different areas of rat brain at the onset of soman-induced convulsions. *Arch Int Pharmacodyn* 234, 64.

100. Marrs TC (1991) Toxicology of oximes used in treatment of organophosphate poisoning. *Adverse Drug React Toxicol Rev* 10, 61.

101. Maxwell DM, Doctor BP (1992) Use of enzyme as pretreatment for organophosphate toxicity. In: *Chemical Warfare Agents.* Somani SM ed. Academic Press, San Diego p. 67.

102. Maxwell DM, Lenz DE, Grof WA *et al.* (1987) The effects of blood flow on detoxification on *in vivo* cholinesterase inhibition by soman in rats. *Toxicol Appl Pharmacol* 88, 66.

103. Maynard RL (1993) Toxicology of chemical warfare agents. In: *General and Applied Toxicology.* Ballantyne B, Marrs T, Turner P eds. Stockton Press, New York p. 1253.

104. McDonough JH Jr, Dochterman LW, Smith CD, Shih TM (1995) Protection against nerve agent-induced neuropathology, but not cardiac pathology, is associated with the anticonvulsant action of drug treatment. *Neurotoxicology* 16, 123.

105. McDunough JH Jr, Jaax NK, Crowley RA *et al.* (1989) Atropine and/or diazepam therapy protects against soman-induced neural and cardiac pathology. *Fund Appl Toxicol* 13, 256.

106. McDunough JH Jr, McLeod CG Jr, Nipwoda MT (1987) Direct microinjection of soman or VX into the amygdala produces limbic convulsions and neuropathology. *Brain Res* 435, 123.

107. McGuire MC, Nogueira CP, Bartels CF *et al.* (1989) Identification of the structural mutation reponsible for the dibucaine-resistance (atypical) variant form of human serum cholinesterase. *Proc Nat Acad Sci USA* 86, 953.

108. McNamara BP, Leitnaker F (1971) *Toxicological Basis for Controlling Emission of GB into the Environment.* EASP 100-98. AD 91427lL. U.S. Army Med Res Lab, Edgewood Arsenal, Aberdeen Proving Ground, Maryland.

109. McNamara BP, Leitnaker F, Vocci FJ (1973) *Proposed Limits for Human Exposure to VX Vapor in Nonmilitary Operations.* EASP 1100-1 (R-1). AD 770434/9. U.S. Army Med Res Lab, Edgewood Arsenal, Aberdeen Proving Ground, Maryland.

110. Meselson M, Perry Robinson J (1980) Chemical warfare and chemical disarmament. *Sci Amer* 242, 34.

111. Meshul CK (1989) Calcium channel blocker reverses anticholinesterase-induced myopathy. *Brain Res* 497, 142.

112. Metcalfe DR, Holmes JH (1969) EEG, psychological and neurological alterations in humans with organophosphate exposure. *Ann N Y Acad Sci* 160, 357.

113. Millard CB, Lockridge O, Broomfield CA (1998) Organophosphorus acid anhydride hydrolase activity in human butyrylcholinesterase: Synergy results in a somanase. *Biochemistry* 37, 237.

114. Misulis KE, Clinton ME, Dettbarn WD, Gupta RC (1987) Differences in central and peripheral neural actions between soman and diisopropyl fluorophosphate, organophosphorus inhibitors of acetylcholinesterase. *Toxicol Appl Pharmacol* 89, 391.

115. Misulis KE, Sussman J, Bon S, Silman I (1993) Structure and functions of acetylcholinesterase and butyrylcholinesterase. *Prog Brain Res* 98, 139.

116. Modrow HE, Jaax NK (1989) Effect of soman exposure on the acquisition of an operant alternative task. *Pharmacol Biochem Behav* 32, 49.

117. Morita H, Yanagisawa N, Nakajima T *et al.* (1995) Sarin poisoning in Matsumoto, Japan. *Lancet* 29, 346.

118. Moses H, Klawans HL (1979) Bromide intoxication. In: *Handbook of Clinical Neurology. Vol 36. Intoxications of the Nervous System. Pt 1.* Vinken PJ, Bruyn GW eds. North-Holland, Amsterdam p. 291.

119. Murata K, Araki S, Yokoyama K *et al.* (1997) Asymptomatic sequelae to acute sarin poisoning in the central and autonomic nervous system, 6 months after the Tokyo subway attack. *J Neurol* 244, 601.

120. Nagao M, Takatori T, Matsuda Y *et al.* (1997) Detection of sarin hydrolysis products from sarin-like organophosphorus agent-exposed human erythrocytes. *J Chromatogr B Biomed Sci Appl* 701, 9.

121. Nakajima T, Saro S, Morita H, Yanagisawa N (1997) Sarin poisoning of a rescue team in the Matsumoto sarin incident in Japan. *Occup Environ Med* 54, 697.

122. National Research Council (1982) *Possible Long-Term Health Effects of Short-Term Exposure to Chemical Agents. Vol 1. Anticholinesterases and Anticholinergics.* National Academy Press, Washington, DC.

123. National Research Council (1985) *Possible Long-Term Health Effects of Short-Term Exposure to Chemical Agents. Vol 3. Current Health Status of Test Subjects.* National Academy Press, Washington, DC.

124. Nozaki H, Aikawa N (1995) Sarin poisoning in Tokyo subway. *Lancet* 345, 1446.

125. Nozaki H, Aikawa N, Fujishima S *et al.* (1995) A case of VX poisoning and the difference from sarin. *Lancet* 346, 698.

126. Nozaki H, Aikawa N, Shinozawa Y *et al.* (1995) Sarin poisoning in Tokyo subway. *Lancet* 345, 980.

127. Palmer JW, Clark HT (1933) The elimination of bromines from the blood stream. *J Biol Chem* 99, 435.

128. Patterson GT, Gupta RC, Misulis KE, Dettbarn WD (1988) Prevention of diisopropylphosphorofluoridate (DFP)-induced skeletal muscle fiber lesions in the rat. *Toxicology* 48, 237.

129. Petras JM (1981) Soman neurotoxicity. *Fund Appl Toxicol* 1, 242.

130. Petras JM (1984) Brain pathology induced by organophosphate poisoning with the nerve agent soman. *U.S. Army Med Res Develop Command Proc 4th Ann Chem Def Biosci Rev* p. 41.

131. Petras JM (1984) Neurology and neuropathology of Soman-induced brain injury: An overview. *J Exp Anal Behav* 61, 319.

132. Polhuijs M, Langenberg JP, Benschop HP (1997) New method for retrospective detection of exposure to organophosphorus anticholinesterases: Application to alleged sarin victims of Japanese terrorists. *Toxicol Appl Pharmacol* 146, 156.

133. Presidential Advisory Committee on Gulf War Veterans' Illnesses (1996) *Final Report.* U.S. Government Printing Office, Washington, DC.

134. Puu G, Artursson E, Bucht G (1986) Reactivation of nerve agent inhibited human acetylcholinesterases by HI-6 and obidoxime. *Biochem Pharmacol* 35, 1909.

135. Rao KS, Aracava Y, Rickett DL, Albuquerque EX (1987) Noncompetitive blockade of the nicotinic acetylcholine receptor-ion channel complex by an irreversible cholinesterase inhibitor. *J Pharmacol Exp Ther* 240, 337.

136. Raveh L, Ashani Y, Levy D *et al.* (1989) Acetylcholinesterase prophylaxis against organophosphate poisoning. Quantitative correlation between protection and blood-enzyme level in mice. *Biochem Pharmacol* 38, 529.

137. Raveh L, Grunwald J, Marcus D *et al.* (1993) Human butyrylcholinesterase as a general prophylactic antidote for nerve agent toxicity. *In vitro* and *in vivo* quantitative characterization. *Biochem Pharmacol* 45, 2465.

138. Rice GB, Lambert TW, Haas B, Wallace V (1971) *Effects of Chronic Ingestion of VX on Ovine Blood Cholinesterase.* Technical Report DTC 71-512. Desert Test Center, Dugway Providing Ground, Dugway, Utah.

139. Rickett DJ, Glenn JF, Houston WE (1987) Medical defense against nerve agents: New directions. *Mil Med* 152, 35.

140. Robertson GS (1967) Serum protein and cholinesterase changes in association with contraceptive pills. *Lancet* i, 232.

141. Rocha ES, Albuquerque EX (1997) Presynaptic potentiation by sarin of glutamatergic transmission: Non-cholinesterase effects. *Soc Neurosci Abst* 23, 2275.

142. Rocha ES, Alkondon M, Pereira EFR, Albuquerque EX (1998) Choline, a by-product of acetylcholine hydrolysis, is a selective agonist of α7 nicotinic receptors: Relevance for the understanding of the mechanisms underlying the effects of cholinesterase inhibitors on the brain. *U.S. Army Medical Defense Bioscience Review*, Hunt Valley, Maryland p. 203.

143. Rocha ES, Alkondon M, Swanson KL, Albuquerque EX (1996) Stimulatory effects of VX on excitatory synapses of cultured hippocampal neurons. *Soc Neurosci Abst* 22, 1740.

144. Rocha ES, Aracava Y, Albuquerque EX (1992) VX enhances transmitter release in cultured hippocampal neurons. *Soc Neurosci Abst* 18, 634.

145. Rocha ES, Santos MD, Chebabo SR *et al.* (1999) Low concentrations of the organophosphate VX affect spontaneous and evoked transmitter release from hippocampal neurons: Toxicological relevance of cholinesterase-independent actions. *Toxicol Appl Pharmacol* 159, 31.

146. Romano JA, Landauer MR (1986) Effects of the organophosphorus compound, O-ethyl-N-dimethyl-phosphoramidocyanate (tabun), on flavour aversions, locomotor activity, and rotarod performance in rats. *Fund Appl Toxicol* 6, 62.

147. Rothenberg DM, Berns AS, Barkin R, Glantz RH (1990) Bromide intoxication secondary to pyridostgmine bromide therapy. *J Amer Med Assn* 263, 1121.

148. Rowntree DW, Nevin S, Wilson A (1950) The effects of diisopropylfluorophosphonate in schizophrenia and manic depressive psychosis. *J Neurol Neurosurg Psychiat* 13, 47.

149. Savage EP, Keefe TJ, Mounce LM *et al.* (1988) Chronic neurological sequelae of acute organophosphate pesticide poisoning. *Arch Environ Health* 43, 38.

150. Saxena A, Redman AM, Jiang X *et al.* (1997) Differences in active site gorge dimensions of cholinesterases revealed by binding of inhibitors to human butyrylcholinesterase. *Biochemistry* 36, 14642.

151. Sekijima Y, Morita J, Yanagisawa N (1997) Follow-up of sarin poisoning in Matsumoto. *Ann Intern Med* 127, 1042.

152. Senanayake N, Karalliede I (1987) Neurotoxic effects of organophosphorus insecticides: An intermediate syndrome. *N Engl J Med* 316, 761.

153. Shih T-M (1982) Time course effects of soman on acetylcholine and choline levels in six discrete areas of the rat brain. *Psychopharmacology* 78, 170.

154. Sidell FR (1974) Soman and sarin: Clinical manifestations and treatment of accidental poisoning by organophosphates. *Clin Toxicol* 7, 1.

155. Sidell FR (1992) Clinical considerations in nerve agent intoxication. In: *Chemical Warfare Agents.* Somani SM ed. Academic Press, San Diego p. 155.

156. Sidell FR, Groff WA (1974) The reactivatibility of cholinesterase inhibited by VX and sarin in man. *Toxicol Appl Pharmacol* 27, 241.

157. Sidell FR, Kaminskis A (1975) Influence of age, sex, and oral contraceptives on human blood cholinesterase activity. *Clin Chem* 21, 1393.

158. Sidell FR, Kaminskis A (1975) Temporal intrapersonal physiological variability of cholinesterase activity in human plasma and erythrocytes. *Clin Chem* 21, 1961.

159. Sim VM (1962) *Variability of Different Intact Human Skin Sites to the Penetration of VX.* CRDL Report 3122. AD 271163. Edgewood Arsenal, Maryland. [cited by Sidell, 1992]

160. Sim VM, McClure Jr, Vocci FJ *et al.* (1964) *Tolerance of Man to VX-Contaminated Water.* Technical Report CRDLR 3231. USACRDL, Edgewood Arsenal, Maryland.

161. Singer AW, Jaaz NK, Graham JS, Mcleod CG Jr (1987) Cardiomyopathy in soman and sarin intoxicated rats. *Toxicol Lett* 36, 243.

162. SIPRI (1973) *The Problem of Chemical and Biological Warfare. Vol 11. CB Weapons Today.* Stockholm International Peace Research Institute (SIPRI), Almqvist & Wiksell, Stockholm.

163. Sirkka U, Nieminen SA, Ylitalo P (1990) Neurobehavioral toxicity with low doses of sarin and soman. *Meth Find Exp Clin Pharmacol* 12, 245.

164. Sket D, Dettbarn WD, Clinton ME *et al.* (1991) Prevention of diisopropylphosphofluoridate-induced myopathy by botulinum toxin type A blockage of quantal release of acetylcholine. *Acta Neuropathol* **82**, 134.

165. Solberg Y, Belkin M (1997) The role of excitotoxicity in organophosphorus nerve agents central poisoning. *Trends Pharmacol Sci* **18**, 183.

166. Somani SM, Solana RP, Dube SN (1992) Toxicodynamics of nerve agents. In: *Chemical Warfare Agents.* Somani SM ed. Academic Press, San Diego p. 67.

167. Sparenborg S, Brennecke LH, Jaax NK, Braitman DJ (1992) Dizocilpine (MK-801) arrests status epilepticus and prevents brain damage induced by soman. *Neuropharmacology* **31**, 357.

168. Spencer PS, Schaumburg HH (1976) Central-peripheral distal axonopathy—the pathology of dying-back polyneuropathies. In: *Progess in Neuropathology. Vol III.* Zimmerman HM ed. Grune & Stratton, New York.

169. Sumerford WT, Hayes WJ, Johnston JM *et al.* (1953) Cholinesterase response and symptomatology from exposure to organic phosphorus insecticides. *Arch Ind Hyg Occup Med* **7**, 383.

170. Sundwall A (1961) Maximum concentrations of N-methylpyridinium-2-aldoximine methane sulphonate (P2S) which reverse neuromuscular block. *Biochem Pharmacol* **8**, 413.

171. Sussman JL, Harel M, Frolow F *et al.* (1991) Atomic structure of acetylcholinesterase from *Torpedo californica*: A prototype acetylcholine-binding protein. *Science* **253**, 872.

172. Suzuki T, Morita H, Ono K *et al.* (1995) Sarin poisoning in Tokyo subway. *Lancet* **345**, 980.

173. Szegletes T, Mallender WD, Rosenberry TL (1998) Nonequilibrium analysis alters the mechanistic interpretation of inhibition of acetylcholinesterase by peripheral site ligands. *Biochemistry* **37**, 4206.

174. Szilagyi M, Gray PJ, Dawson RM (1993) Effects of the nerve agents soman and tabun on the uptake and release of GABA and glutamate in synaptosomes in guinea pig cerebral cortex. *Gen Pharmacol* **24**, 663.

175. Tabershaw IR, Cooper WC (1966) Sequelae of acute organic phosphate poisoning. *J Occup Med* **8**, 5.

176. Tammelin LE (1957) Dialkoxy-phosphorylcholines, alkoxy-methyl-phosphorothiocholines and analagous choline esters. *Acta Chem Scand* **11**, 1340.

177. Tanaka D Jr, Bursian SJ (1989) Degeneration patterns in the chicken central nervous system induced by ingestion of the organophosphorus delayed neurotoxin tri-*ortho*-tolyl phosphate. A silver impregnation study. *Brain Res* **484**, 240.

178. Taylor P (1994) The cholinesterases: From genes to proteins. *Annu Rev Pharmacol Toxicol* **34**, 281.

179. Taylor P (1996) Cholinesterase agents. In: *Goodman and Gilman's The Pharmacological Basis of Therapeutics. 9th Ed.* Hardman JG, Gilman AG, Limbird LE eds. McGraw-Hill, New York p. 161.

180. Thienes CH Haley TJ (1972) *Clinical Toxicology.* Lea & Febiger, Philadelphia.

181. Tripathi HL, Dewey WL (1989) Comparison of the effects of diisopropylfluorophosphate, sarin, soman, and tabun on toxicity and brain acetylcholinesterase activity in mice. *J Toxicol Environ Health* **26**, 437.

182. Van Helden HPM, Busker RW, Melchers BP, Bruijnzeel PL (1996) Pharmacological effects of oximes: How relevant are they? *Arch Toxicol* **70**, 779.

183. Van Helden HPM, Van der Wiel HJ, Wolthuis OL (1987) Retention of soman in rats, guinea pigs and marmosets: Species-dependent effects of the soman simulator, pinacolyl dimethylphosphate (PDP). *J Pharm Pharmacol* **40**, 35.

184. Walker CH (1993) The classification of esterases which hydrolyse organophosphates: Recent developments. *Chem Biol Interact* **87**, 17.

185. Wall HG, Jaax NK, Hayward IJ (1987) Brain lesions in rhesus monkeys after acute soman intoxication. In: *Sixth Ann Chem Def Biosci Rev.* U.S. Army Medical Research Institute, Maryland p. 155.

186. Wecker L, Dettbarn WD (1976) Paraoxon-induced myopathy: Muscle specificity and acetylcholine involvement. *Exp Neurol* **51**, 281.

187. Wheeler TG (1989) Soman toxicity during and after exposure to different environmental temperatures. *J Toxicol Environ Health* **26**, 349.

188. Whittaker M (1986) Cholinesterase. *Monogr Hum Genet* **2**, 1.

189. Whittaker M, Charlier AR, Ramaswamy S (1971) Changes in plasma cholinesterase isoenzyme due to oral contraceptives. *J Reprod Fertil* **26**, 373.

190. Willems JL, Nicaise M, De Bisschop HC (1984) Delayed neuropathy by the organophosphorus nerve agents soman and tabun. *Arch Toxicol* **55**, 76.

191. Willems JL, Palate BM, Vranken MA, De Bisschop HC (1984) Delayed neuropathy by organophosphorus nerve agents. *Proc Int Symp Protection Against Chemical Warfare Agents*, Stockholm, p. 95.

192. Wilson BW, Henderson JD (1992) Blood esterase determinations as markers of exposure. *Rev Environ Contam Toxicol* **128**, 55.

193. Wilson BW, Henderson JD, Chow E *et al.* (1988) Toxicity of an acute dose of agent VX and other organophosphate esters in the chicken. *J Toxicol Environ Health* **23**, 103.

194. Wilson BW, Henderson JD, Kellner TP *et al.* (1988) Toxicity of repeated doses of organophosphate esters in the chicken. *J Toxicol Environ Health* **23**, 115.

195. Wilson IB (1959) Molecular complementarity and antidotes for alkyl phosphate poisoning. *Fed Proc* **18**, 752.

196. Wolfe AD, Rush RS, Doctor BP *et al.* (1987) Acetylcholinesterase prophylaxis against organophosphate toxicity. *Fund Appl Toxicol* **9**, 266.

197. Wolthuis OL, Benschop HP, Berends F (1981) Persistance of the anticholinesterase soman in rats; antagonism with a non-toxic simulator of this organophosphate. *Eur J Pharmacol* **69**, 379.

198. Woodall J (1997) Tokyo subway gas attack. *Lancet* **350**, 296.

199. Worek F, Backer M, Thiermann H *et al.* (1997) Reappraisal of indications and limitations of oxime therapy in organophosphate poisoning. *Hum Exp Toxicol* **16**, 266.

200. Worek F, Kleine A, Flke K, Szinicz L (1995) Arrhythmias in organophosphate poisoning: Effect of atropine and bispyridinium oximes. *Arch Int Pharmacodyn Ther* **329**, 418.

201. Worek F, Kleine A, Szinicz L (1995) Effect of pyridostigmine pretreatment on cardiorespiratory function in tabun poisoning. *Hum Exp Toxicol* **14**, 634.

202. Xia DY, Wang LX, Pei SQ (1981) The inhibition and protection of cholinesterase by physostigmine and pyridostigmine against soman poisoning *in vivo*. *Fund Appl Toxicol* **1**, 217.

203. Yamasaki Y, Sakamoto K, Watada H *et al.* (1997) The Arg192 isoform of paraoxonase with low sarinhydrolyzing activity is dominant in the Japanese. *Hum Genet* **101**, 67.

204. Yokoyama K, Ogura Y, Kishimoto M *et al.* (1995) Blood purification for severe sarin poisoning after the Tokyo subway attack. *J Amer Med Assn* **274**, 379.

205. Yokoyama K, Yamada A, Mimura A (1996) Clinical profiles of patients with sarin poisoning after the Tokyo subway attack. *Amer J Med* **100**, 586.

CASE REPORT

A healthy American male soldier in his twenties was given EA3148, 1.15 µg/kg i.v. Erythrocyte AChE values dropped precipitously to 22% of normal within 15 min of dosing and to 0% at 48 h; the value recovered to 88% of normal at 72 days post-exposure. Signs of toxicity were evident within 5–8 min of treatment in two comparably dosed subjects who felt dizzy, weak, tired, sweaty, and had hands and feet that were moist. Within 2 h post-exposure, these subjects reportedly were resting, eating, and feeling fine. A U.S. Army report summarizing experience with EA3148 noted anorexia, fatigue, poor sleep, unusual dreams, dizziness, euphoria, blurred vision, increased salivation, restlessness; decrements in a test of numerical facility in four individuals and exaggeration of a schizoid personality in one (139).

Saxitoxin

Richard G. Pellegrino

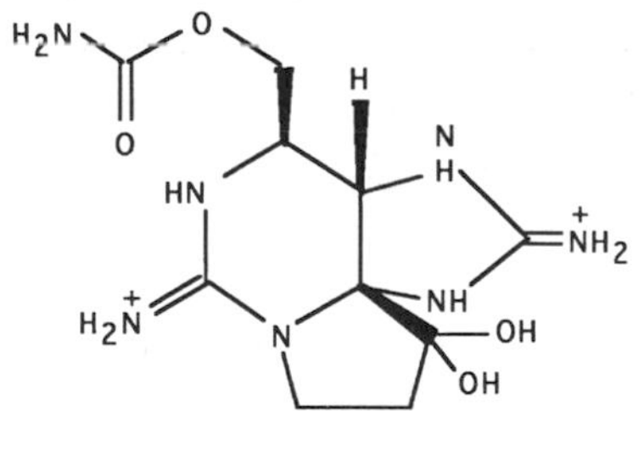

SAXITOXIN
$[C_{10}H_{17}N_7O_4]^{2+}$

STX; Paralytic shellfish poison

NEUROTOXICITY RATING
Clinical
A   Ion channel syndrome
Experimental
A   Ion channel dysfunction (sodium channel agent)

Saxitoxin (STX), a heat-stable neurotoxin produced by some marine dinoflagellates, binds specifically to voltage-sensitive sodium channels. The organisms that produce this molecule are thought to be responsible for the so-called red tides observed since antiquity. The first record of such an event appeared in Exodus 7:20-21:

And all the waters that were in the river were turned to blood. And the fish that were in the river died; and the river stank and the Egyptians could not drink the water of the river.

Although many theories were proposed for the occurrence of poisonous shellfish throughout the eighteenth and nineteenth centuries, the actual cause was not known until 1927, when outbreaks of mussel poisoning occurred along the central California coast. At that time, a connection between red tides and poisonous shellfish was proposed (25). It was suspected that dinoflagellates, upon which the mussels were feeding, might be poisonous. Acidic water extracts of the dinoflagellates in the mussels killed mice in exactly the same manner. The dinoflagellate was identified as *Gonyaulax catanella* (24,25).

The major neurotoxin found in extracts of *G. catanella* was named saxitoxin after the Alaskan butter clam *saxidomus* from which the compound was originally extracted. Several other toxins are present in red tides, and their relative contributions remain to be established.

Tanino and associates (26) reported the first stereospecific total synthesis of racemic STX. STX is a heterocyclic guanidine with a MW of 379; it is water-soluble but insoluble in lipid solvents (3,20). Its diffusion coefficient is 4.9×10^{-6}. The specific optical rotation is 128 degrees and it has a pKa of 8.3 and 11.5 (8). STX is heat-stable; steaming and cooking does not destroy its activity (24).

STX was first tritiated in 1977 (21); since that time, it has been used extensively to characterize STX-binding protein components of the voltage-sensitive Na^+ channel (12). Tritiated STX has enabled the purification of voltage-gated Na^+ channels from electric eel electroplaques (1), rat brain (15), rat and rabbit skeletal muscle (4), and cardiac tissue (18). STX has no medical uses at present; the agent's easily reversible binding has hampered its development as a local anesthetic.

STX's exquisite toxicity has been noted by regulatory agencies around the world. The earliest attempt to establish a public quarantine for paralytic shellfish poisoning is found among the Native Americans on the U.S. Pacific west coast. They were well aware of shellfish poisoning and, during periods of danger, posted sentries to warn the unwary not to consume mussels and clams (20). The processing of clams and mussels is now strictly monitored by both Canadian and U.S. national health agencies. Those interested in details for North America should consult the shellfish sanitation branch of the U.S. Public Health Service, Washington, D.C. An excellent review of the monitoring process is available (14).

Within the European community, directive 91/492/EEC lays down the health conditions for production and marketing of live bivalve mussels. The paralytic shellfish poisoning content of those mussels intended for immediate human consumption is strictly regulated. In spite of this regulation, many cases of paralytic shellfish poisoning continue to be reported (27).

STX acts directly on voltage-gated sodium channels; this action is responsible for the observed toxic effect. STX is readily but incompletely absorbed from the gastrointestinal tract. Pure STX is 130 times more toxic if injected intravenously than if administered orally to mice (7). STX appears to have both CNS and PNS effects; it moves easily and rapidly between the blood and brain along its concentration gradient (5,6).

Studies with tritiated reduced saxitoxin (saxitoxinol) suggest the agent is rapidly excreted primarily in urine (16).

Saxitoxinol was injected into the penile vein of each of six male rats. By 4 h following injection, 60% of the injected radioactivity was excreted in urine. This slowed by 48 h and negligible additional radioactivity was excreted throughout the remainder of the experiment, which was terminated at 144 h. No radioactivity was detectable in the feces at any time. Analysis indicated that excreted toxin was not metabolized, although 28% of the injected radioactivity was not recovered (16).

Animals show a prompt hypotensive response to a subparalytic dose of STX infused into the cranial artery that results in a depressive action on the brainstem vasomotor center. However, with other modes of intoxication, the peripheral effect is dominant over the central effect (5). Other studies have also noted a central effect on the medullary respiratory center (7).

There have been many uncontrolled animal exposures to STX, most of which last a few weeks. The fish kills that accompany red tides have been described since antiquity, but there is mounting evidence that this toxin can travel up the food chain, even to the point of eventually killing mammalian aquatic species. In 1987, during a 5-week period, 14 humpback whales died in Cape Cod Bay, Massachusetts, U.S.A. These whales died at sea, some rapidly, and then washed ashore. Postmortem examination showed the whales had been well immediately before their deaths, many of them had abundant blubber, and fish were present in their stomachs—evidence of a recent feeding. Ingestion of STX-contaminated fish was blamed for the episode (2).

There are no reports of controlled human exposure to STX, but many reports of uncontrolled exposure (14,17). The first detailed description of a case of paralytic shellfish poisoning (PSP) can be found in an account of poisoning in a young woman in 1689 (10). In addition, approximately 200 years ago, Captain Cook and Captain Vancouver described the manifestations of PSP in some of their crew members during their expedition to the coast of the U.S. Pacific Northwest (13).

There is a report of a 53-year-old housewife who became ill following a U.S. Labor Day picnic. She had eaten clams from a supplier from the State of Maine. Her neurological deficits resolved over 5 days. Electrophysiological data were obtained serially on the first, fourth, and sixth hospital days. Nerve conduction studies on the day of admission revealed marked prolongation of distal motor and sensory latencies with a less dramatic but significant decrease in conduction velocities and moderately diminished motor and sensory amplitudes. Needle exam on the fourth hospital day showed a mild decrease in the numbers of voluntary motor units and abnormal variability in the motor unit configuration. No spontaneous activity was noted. This normalized by the sixth hospital day. Conduction deficits were thought to be secondary to complete failure of conduction in some axons, with a graded deficit producing inactivation or blockage of only a portion of the sodium channels in other axons (19).

The reported mortality of PSP ranges from 8.5%–23.2% (20). During red tides, mussels may accumulate 50,000 mouse units per animal. Cell counts of dinoflagellates may approximate 20,000/ml. Mussels may be too hazardous for use as food when seawater dinoflagellate counts are as few as 200/ml (23).

Symptoms of STX poisoning are characterized initially by a tingling and burning sensation of the lips, gums, tongue, and face. The neck, arms, fingertips, legs, and toes gradually become involved, and paresthesias turn to numbness. Gastrointestinal symptoms, such as nausea, vomiting, diarrhea, and epigastric pain, may or may not be present. In the terminal stages, weakness and muscle paralysis supervene, and death occurs as a result of respiratory paralysis within a period of 6–24 h. If the patient survives the acute period, recovery is good (9,14).

There has been a single report of four cases of elevated creatine kinase-MB isoenzyme levels in patients suffering from PSP. Five of these patients presented to a Japanese hospital following an outbreak of PSP that affected 116 people. Electrocardiograms were normal in all patients. The possibility that cardiac damage occurs directly needs to be further substantiated (11).

Treatment of PSP is largely symptomatic; there is no specific antidote. Emetics may help remove poison from the stomach, but the main treatment is maintenance of adequate respiration, by artificial means if necessary (10,14).

STX selectively abolishes sodium currents that are essential for the propagation of impulses in excitable membranes. In the presence of STX, the early current of the action potential that is carried by sodium ions is abolished, while the late current carried by potassium ions remains unaffected. The effect is rapidly reversed after removal of the toxin (22).

REFERENCES

1. Agnew WS, Levinson SR, Brabson JS, Raftery MA (1978) Purification of the tetrodotoxin-binding component associated with the voltage-sensitive sodium channel from *Electrophorus electricus* membranes. *Proc Natl Acad Sci USA* **75**, 2606.
2. Anderson DM (1994) Red tides. *Sci Amer* **271**, 62.
3. Baden DG (1983) Marine food-born dinoflagellate toxins. *Int Rev Cytol* **82**, 99.
4. Barchi RL (1983) Protein components of the purified sodium channel from rat skeletal muscle sarcolemma. *J Neurochem* **40**, 1337.
5. Borison HL, Culp WJ, Gonsalves SF, McCarthy LE (1980) Central respiratory and circulatory depression caused by intravascular saxitoxin. *Brit J Pharmacol* **68**, 301.
6. Borison HL, McCarthy LE (1977) Respiratory and circulatory effects of saxitoxin in the cerebrospinal fluid. *Brit J Pharmacol* **61**, 679.
7. Bower DJ, Hart RJ, Matthews PA, Howden MH (1981) Nonprotein neurotoxins. *Clin Toxicol* **18**, 813.
8. Boyer GJ, Schantz EJ, Schnoes HK (1978) Characterization of 11-hydroxysaxitoxin sulfate, a major toxin in scallops exposed to blooms of the poisonous dinoflagellate, *Gonyaulax tamarensis*. *J Chem Soc Chem Commun* 889.
9. Centers for Disease Control (1976) Paralytic shell fish poisoning—Alaska. *Morbid Mortal Wkly Rep* **25**, 383.
10. Centers for Disease Control (1976) Paralytic shell fish poisoning—New Brunswick, Canada. *Morbid Mortal Wkly Rep* **25**, 347.
11. Cheng HS, Chua SO, Hung JS, Yip KK (1991) Creatine kinase MB elevation in paralytic shellfish poisoning. *Chest* **99**, 1032.
12. Corbett AM, Krueger BK (1990) Isolation of two saxitoxin-sensitive sodium channel subtypes from rat brain with distinct biochemical and functional properties. *J Membrane Biol* **117**, 163.
13. Fortuine R (1975) Paralytic shellfish poisoning in the North Pacific: two historical accounts and implications for today. *Alaska Med* **15**, 71.
14. Halstead BW (1978) *Poisonous and Venomous Marine Animals of the World*. Darwin Press, Princeton, New Jersey.
15. Hartshorne RP, Catterall WA (1984) The sodium channel from rat brain. Purification and subunit composition. *J Biol Chem* **259**, 1667.
16. Hines HB, Naseem SM, Wannemacher RW Jr (1993) Tritiated saxitoxinol metabolism in elimination in the rat. *Toxicon* **31**, 905.
17. Kao CY (1966) Tetrodotoxin, saxitoxin and their significance in the study of excitation phenomena. *Pharmacol Rev* **18**, 997.
18. Lombet A, Lazdunski M (1984) Characterization, solubilization, affinity labeling, and purification of the cardiac sodium channel using *Tityus* toxin gamma. *Eur J Biochem* **141**, 651.
19. Long RR, Sargent JC, Hammer K (1990) Paralytic shellfish poisoning: A case report and serial electrophysiologic observations. *Neurology* **40**, 1310.
20. Morse EV (1977) Paralytic shellfish poisoning: A review. *J Amer Med Assn* **171**, 1178.
21. Ritchie JM, Rogart RB (1977) Characterization of exchange-labelled saxitoxin and the origin of linear uptake by excitable tissue. *Mol Pharmacol* **13**, 1136.
22. Ritchie JM, Rogart RB (1977) The binding of saxitoxin and tetrodotoxin to excitable tissue. *Rev Physiol Biochem Pharmacol* **79**, 1.

23. Schantz EJ (1975) Poisonous red tide organisms. *Environ Lett* **9**, 225.
24. Sommer H, Meyer KF (1937) Paralytic shellfish poisoning. *AMA Arch Pathol* **24**, 560.
25. Sommer H, Whedon WF, Kofoid CA, Stohler R (1937) Relation of paralytic shellfish poison to certain plankton organisms of the genus *Gonyaulax*. *AMA Arch Pathol* **24**, 537.
26. Tanino H, Naketa T, Kaneko T, Kishi Y (1977) Stereospecific total synthesis of D,L saxitoxin. *J M Chem Soc* **99**, 2818.
27. Van Egmond HP, VanDenTop JH, Paulsch WE *et al.* (1994) Paralytic shellfish poison reference materials: An intercomparison of methods for the determination of saxitoxin. *Food Addit Contam* **1**, 39.

Scombroid Fish (Histamine)

Albert C. Ludolph
Peter S. Spencer

NEUROTOXICITY RATING

Clinical

A   Headache

B   Encephalomalacia (hypotension)

Experimental

A   Histamine release

Scombroid fish poisoning (scombrotoxism) is a food-borne disease induced by bacteria contaminating pelagic fish of the tuna, mackerel and other families. In unrefrigerated fish, these bacteria produce large amounts of histamine, which likely accounts for induction of clinical symptoms in the consumer (5). The U.S. Centers for Disease Control and Prevention report that scombroid poisoning is one of the most frequent causes of food-borne illnesses in the United States (3); most hold that the real incidence of scombroid poisoning is underestimated, since many mild cases and outbreaks go unreported. Scombroid fish poisoning occurs worldwide (2–4) and is most frequently caused by fish of the families Scombridae and Scomberesocidae (tuna, mackerel, bonito, and saury) (7), although nonscombroid fish such as mahi-mahi, bluefish, and Clupeidae (sardine, herring, and anchovy) also rarely cause the syndrome (7). Raw, cooked, and canned fish all cause outbreaks (6,7).

Histamine (which is heat-stable) formed by decarboxylation of histidine-rich muscles is considered the major pathogenetic factor in scombroid poisoning. This decarboxylation reaction is catalyzed by bacteria, such as Enterobacteriaceae, *Clostridium*, and *Lactobacillus*, that produce the enzyme histidine decarboxylase, (7). However, attempts to reproduce the clinical picture in human volunteers have met with variable success, and some have challenged the histamine hypothesis (1,3,7).

Clinical signs and symptoms of vasodilation appear after the fish meal within minutes to a few hours. Severe headache is the first symptom; this is followed by a red flushed skin, sweating, and unusual oral sensations. Abdominal pain, nausea, vomiting, diarrhea, tachycardia, and dizziness may accompany the picture. The disorder reverses within hours without sequelae. Elderly patients may experience hypotension and cerebral ischemia. Analytical methods for histamine in fish include fluorometric detection of histamine with o-phthalaldehyde or by thin-layer chromatography (7).

Treatment of scombrotoxism includes administration of antihistaminics if symptoms are severe; a combination of H_1- or H_2-receptor antagonists is preferred (5). Prevention of disease requires the rapid refrigeration of fish (histamine formation is negligible at 0°C).

REFERENCES

1. Clifford MN, Walker R, Wright J *et al.* (1991) Scombroid fish poisoning. *N Engl J Med* **325**, 515.
2. Gellert GA, Ralls J, Brown C *et al.* (1992) Scombroid fish poisoning. Underreporting and prevention among noncommercial recreational fishers. *West J Med* **157**, 645.
3. Hughes JM, Potter ME (1991) Scombroid fish poisoning. From pathogenesis to prevention. *N Engl J Med* **324**, 766.
4. Maire R, Dreiding K, Wyss PA (1992) Incidence and clinical aspects of scombroid fish poisoning. *Schweiz Med Wochenschr* **122**, 1933.
5. Morrow JD, Margolies GR, Rowland J, Roberts LJ II (1991) Evidence that histamine is the causative toxin of scombroid-fish poisoning. *N Engl J Med* **324**, 716.
6. Murray CK, Hobbes G, Gilbert RJ (1982) Scombrotoxin and scombrotoxin-like poisoning from canned fish. *J Hyg* **88**, 215.
7. Taylor SL, Bush RK (1988) Allergy by ingestion of seafoods. In: *Handbook of Natural Toxins. Vol 3. Marine Toxins.* Tu AT ed. Marcel Dekker, New York p. 150.

Scorpion Toxins (α and β)

Albert C. Ludolph
Peter S. Spencer

NEUROTOXICITY RATING
Clinical
A Ion channel syndrome (atypical)
B Seizure disorder
Experimental
A Seizure disorder
A Ion channel dysfunction (sodium channel toxins)

Venom of the scorpion family Buthidae contains neurotoxic compounds[1] that are of major significance for the experimental neurobiologist and of importance for the clinical neurotoxicologist. The selectivity of these compounds is employed experimentally as a tool to localize ion channels in nerve, muscle, neuromuscular junctions, and other structures. Scorpion venoms contain a mixture of compounds including mucopolysaccharides, hyaluronidase and phospholipase, serotonin, histamine, and protease inhibitors. The α- and β-scorpion toxins are exclusively responsible for the clinical neurotoxicity of the venom. α-Scorpion toxins (α-ScTx) are peptides present in the venom of *Androctonus australis* Hector (toxin I), *A. mauretanicus mauretanicus*, *Buthus eupeus* (toxins M7 and 2000), *B. occitanus tunetanus* (toxin I), *Leiurus quinquestriatus* (neurotoxins IV and V), and *Tityus serrulatus* (12) whereas β-scorpion toxins (β-ScTx) can be found in the venom of *Centruroides sculpturatus*, *C. suffusus suffusus*, and *Tityus serrulatus* (*see also* Tityustoxin, this volume) (12). α-ScTx and β-ScTx bind to sites 3 and 4, respectively, of the 6 neurotoxin-binding sites of the voltage-sensitive Na⁺ channel. Detailed reviews on structure–function relationships of scorpion toxins are available (9,12,17).

α-ScTxs and β-ScTxs are basic proteins of about 64 amino acids, four intramolecular disulfide bridges, and a MW of 7000 Da (22). After subcutaneous injection into rodents, they induce similar manifestations of intoxication: hyperexcitability, repetitive firing of motor units, restlessness, jumping, accelerated respiration, trembling associated with convulsions, muscle twitching, and increased muscle tone, especially of hindlimbs. Eventually, respiratory failure occurs. Hyperexcitation may be less extensive after administration of β-ScTxs; respiration is usually heavier and tremor more pronounced.

In contrast to the K⁺ channel toxins, the sodium-channel neurotoxins in scorpion venoms cause toxic disorders and, in severe cases, fatalities in humans. In parts of Tunisia, more than 20 deaths following scorpion stings have been observed per year (4); in Algeria, more than 100 patients died from scorpion stings during the same period of time (1). In Mexico, more than 100,000 *Centruroides* stings, of which about 800 are lethal, are reported in a single year (5,19). The sting of *Leiurus quinquestratus* may be fatal in children (15). Most frequently, scorpion bites occur by accidental contact with an animal residing in clothing, shoes, or bedding.

The local symptomatology of a scorpion sting consists of pain, edema, paresthesia, and numbness. Intoxication with these Na⁺-channel toxins is not associated with a typical axon-channel-toxin syndrome (*see* Chapter 2, this volume) but their clinical effect is rather characterized by the systemic consequences of neurotransmitter release. A catecholaminergic reaction with tachycardia, increased blood pressure, restlessness, and hyperactivity dominates the clinical picture (19). Muscle cramps and fasciculations are observed, and reflexes are often diminished (19). Less frequent are vomiting, abdominal cramps, diarrhea, lacrimation, salivation, dysphagia, dyspnea, nystagmus, and tachypnea (16). Hyperglycemia, hyperkalemia, and hyponatremia often complicate the situation. Patients, in particular children, may die from a number of secondary complications, most commonly shock and pulmonary edema. Convulsions, brain edema, muscular weakness, and paralysis have also been described in severely affected children (4,16). Treatment consists of clinical observation of patients at risk (elderly persons, children), the possible administration of analgesics, and correction of metabolic imbalances. Surgical measures are considered useless. In severe intoxication, early intravenous administration of the (regionally specific) antiserum may be indicated; however, anaphylactic reactions must be anticipated. Antisera are not helpful in the late phase of the intoxication and should not be used (6,8,20, *see also* Editors' Note, *vide infra*).

The *in vivo* effects of scorpion toxins are the consequence of toxin-induced release of presynaptic neurotransmitters (10,14,18). α-Neurotoxins voltage-dependently bind to site 3 at the Na⁺ channel, do not have an effect on channel activation, but slow down or block channel inactivation and stabilize the channel in its open state. In addition, α-ScTxs allosterically enhance persistent activation by toxins, such as batrachotoxin binding to site 2. In contrast, β-

---

[1]These include a large variety of polypeptide toxins that bind to ion channels and modulate ion-channel conductance in excitable tissues. Major toxin classes include "long" toxins that bind to Na⁺ channels (α-type, depressant and excitatory) and "short" toxins that affect K⁺ and Cl⁻ channels (7).

neurotoxins bind to receptor site 4, do not modify channel inactivation, and induce a shift of voltage dependence of activation in the positive direction; after conditioning depolarizing pulses, these toxins shift activation to more negative membrane potentials (13). The same effect is caused by a toxin from *Buthus martensii*, but the shift does not require conditioning (2). Another toxin from *Androctonus australis* shows physiological effects on both the α and β sites of the mammalian Na$^+$ channel (11).

Editors' Note: Two reports address the efficacy of antivenom therapy in the treatment of scorpion envenomation. One study compared the clinical course and outcome of scorpion envenomation in 104 children treated in an Israeli pediatric intensive care unit; 52 who had received specific scorpion antivenom were compared with an historical control group of 52 who had not received antivenom. Demographic, clinical, and laboratory features at presentation were similar, as were lengths of stay in pediatric intensive care and pediatric wards. No difference in outcome between the two groups was found (21). More recently, a matched-pair study of 135 individuals with scorpion envenomation in Tunisia found that systemic administration of scorpion antivenin irrespective of clinical severity did not alter the clinical course (3).

REFERENCES

1. Alamir R, Merad R, Aissa LH et al. (1992) Scorpionic envenoming in Algeria. *Toxicon* 30, 487.
2. Bauer CK, Krylov B, Zhou PA, Schwarz JR (1992) Effects of *Buthus martensii* (Karch) scorpion venom on sodium currents in rat anterior pituitary (CH3/B6) cells. *Toxicon* 30, 581.
3. Belghith M, Boussarsar M, Haguiga H et al. (1999) Efficacy of serotherapy in scorpion sting: a matched-pair study. *Toxicol Clin Toxicol* 37, 51.
4. Champetier de Ribes G (1985) Envenimation scorpionique chez l'enfant. *Ann Pediat* 32, 399.
5. Dahesa-Davila M, Cervantes AF, Velasca DE, Castillo PJ (1990) Clinical and metabolic profile of scorpion sting. *Toxicon* 28, 607.
6. Freire-Maia L, Campos JA (1989) Pathophysiology and treatment of scorpion poisoning. In: *Natural Toxins*. Ownby CL, Odell GV eds. Pergamon Press, Oxford p. 139.
7. Froy O, Sagiv T, Poreh M et al. (1999) Dynamic diversification from a putative common ancestor of scorpion toxins affecting sodium, potassium, and chloride channels. *Mol Evol* 48, 187.
8. Gueron M, Sofer S (1990) Vasodilators and calcium blocking agents as treatment of cardiovascular manifestations of human scorpion envenomation. *Toxicon* 28, 127.
9. Kharrat R, Darbon H, Granier C, Rochat H (1990) Structure-activity relationships of scorpion alpha-neurotoxins: Contribution of arginine residues. *Toxicon* 28, 509.
10. Lin S, Tseng W, Lee CY (1975) Pharmacology of scorpion toxin II in the skeletal muscle. *Naunyn-Schmied Arch Pharmacol* 289, 359.
11. Loret EP, Martin-Euaclare M-F, Mansuelle P et al. (1991) An anti-insect toxin purified from the scorpion *Androctonus australis* Hector also acts on the α- and β-sites of the mammalian sodium channel: Sequence and circular dichroism study. *Biochemistry* 30, 633.
12. Martin-Eauclaire MF, Couraud F (1994) Scorpion neurotoxins: Effects and mechanisms. In: *Handbook of Neurotoxicology*. Chang LW, Dyer RS eds. Marcel Dekker, New York p. 683.
13. Meves H, Simars JM, Watt DD (1986) Interactions of scorpion toxins with the sodium channel. *Ann N Y Acad Sci* 479, 113.
14. Moss J, Colburn RW, Kopin IJ (1984) Scorpion toxin induced catecholamine release from synaptosomes. *J Neurochem* 22, 217.
15. Osman EL, Alamin E (1992) Issues of management of scorpion stings in children. *Toxicon* 30, 111.
16. Piek T, Leeuwin RS (1995) Neurotoxic arthropod venoms. In: *Handbook of Clinical Neurology. Vol 21 (65): Intoxications of the Nervous System. Part II*. Vinken PJ, Bruyn GW eds. Elsevier, Amsterdam, p. 193.
17. Possani LD (1984) Structure of scorpion toxins. In: *Insect, Poisons, Allergens, and Other Invertebrate Venoms. Handbook of Natural Toxins*. Tu AT ed. Marcel Dekker, New York p. 513.
18. Romey G, Chicheportiche R, Lazdunski M et al. (1975) Scorpion neurotoxin—a presynaptic toxin which affects both Na$^+$ and K$^+$ channels in axons. *Biochem Biophys Res Commun* 64, 115.
19. Simard JM, Watt DD (1990) Venoms and toxins. In: *The Biology of Scorpions*. Polis GA ed. Stanford University Press, Stanford, California p. 414.
20. Sofer S, Gueron M (1988) Respiratory failure in children following envenomation by the scorpion *Leiurus quinquestriatus*—hemodynamic and neurological aspects. *Toxicon* 26, 931.
21. Sofer S, Shahak E, Gueron M (1994) Scorpion envenomation and antivenom therapy. *Pediatr* 124, 973.
22. Zlotkin E, Miranda F, Rochat H (1978) Chemistry and pharmacology of *Buthinae* venoms. In: *Arthropod Venoms*. Bettini S ed. Springer-Verlag, Berlin p. 317.

Sea Anemone Toxins

Albert C. Ludolph

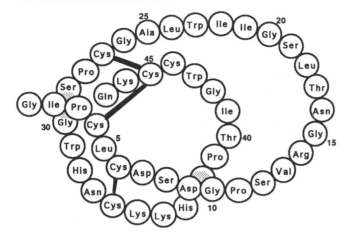

SEA ANEMONE TOXIN

NEUROTOXICITY RATING

Experimental

A   Ion channel dysfunction

Naturally occurring neurotoxins produced by sea anemones play a significant role in experimental neurobiology and pharmacology (4,7,8), but they are of minor importance in clinical neurotoxicology. Sea anemone species with neurotoxic potential are *Stichodactyla* spp. (*see Stichodactyla* spp., this volume), *Anemonia sulcata* , *Anthopleura elegantissima* and *A. xanthogrammatica*, *Bunodosoma caissarum*, *Calliactis parasitica*, *Condylactis gigantea*, *Heteractis macrodactylus*, *Parasicyonis actinostoloides*, *Phyllactis flosculifera*, and *Radianthus paumotensis* (1,6,11,16). Each of these species exclusively produces Na$^+$-channel toxins; *Stichodactyla* spp., *Bunodosoma granulifera* and *Actinia equina* also synthesize K$^+$-channel toxins (4,5,12). A review on chemistry and structure–function relationships of Na$^+$-channel toxins produced by sea anemone is available (16). The polypeptide toxins consist of 27–49 amino acids that are cross-linked by 2–3 disulphide bonds. Toxins I, II, III, and IV (ATX I, II, III, and IV) from *Anemonia sulcata* possess a binding site overlapping with site 3 of the Na$^+$ channel and slow down inactivation of the channel (15,17). This effect is not restricted to neurons; it is also seen in striated and cardiac muscle, and in nonexcitable cells such as glial cells and fibroblasts. ATX II consists of 47-amino-acid residues; ATX III and ATX IV are smaller with 27 residues. Depolarization induced by ATX II releases neurotransmitters from synaptosomal preparations (17) and increases the frequency of miniature end-plate potentials at vertebrate neuromuscular junctions (13). Loss of Na$^+$-channel activation induced by ATX II closely mimics the electrical and mechanical features of myotonia (2). Similar to ATX, the 49-amino-acid peptides anthopleurin A and B from *Anthopleura xanthogrammatica* bind to site 3 of the voltage-dependent Na$^+$ channel and slow channel inactivation; this results in membrane depolarization and prolongation of the nerve action potential (3,14).

The species most vulnerable to sea anemone toxins is *Carcinus maenas*. By contrast, sea anemone channel toxins are less potent in mammals; the LD$_{50}$ of the sodium channel toxin from *Anemona sulcata* is 0.3–20 mg/kg. Present knowledge indicates that the channel toxins of sea anemone are responsible for neither the local reaction occurring after accidental contact nor a systemic reaction in the form of an axon-channel syndrome. Contacts with *Anemonia sulcata* in the Adriatic Sea have resulted in painful local reactions (10).

REFERENCES

1. Alsen C (1983) Biological significance of peptides from *Anemonia sulcata*. *Fed Proc* **42**, 101.
2. Cannon SC, Corey DP (1993) Loss of Na$^+$ channel inactivation by anemone toxin (ATX III) mimics the myotonic state in hyperkalaemic periodic paralysis. *J Physiol London* **466**, 501.
3. Gallagher MJ, Blumenthal KM (1992) Cloning and expression of wild-type and mutant forms of the cardiotonic polypeptide anthopleurin B. *J Biol Chem* **267**, 13958.
4. Karlsson E, Aneiros A, Castaneda O *et al.* (1992) Potassium channel toxins from sea anemone. In: *Recent Advances in Toxinology Research*. Vol 2. Gopalakrishnakone P, Tan CK eds. Venom and Toxin Research Group, National University of Singapore, Singapore p. 378.
5. Kelso GJ, Blumenthal KM (1998) Identification and characterization of novel sodium channel toxins from the sea anemone *Anthopleura xanthogrammatica*. *Toxicon* **36**, 41.
6. Kem WR, Pennington MW, Dunn BM (1990) Sea anemone polypeptide toxins affecting sodium channels. In: *Marine Toxins: Origin, Structure, and Molecular Pharmacology*. Hall S, Strichartz G eds. American Chemical Society, Washington, DC p. 279.
7. Lazdunski M, Barhanin J, Fosset M *et al.* (1987) Polypeptide toxins as tools to study Na$^+$ channels and Ca^{2+}-activated K$^+$ channels. In: *Neurotoxins and Their Pharmacological Implications*. Jenner P ed. Raven Press, New York p. 65.
8. Lazdunski M, Frelin C, Barhanin J *et al.* (1986) Polypeptide toxins as tools to study voltage-sensitive Na$^+$ channels. *Ann N Y Acad Sci* **479**, 204.

9. Malpezzi ELA, Freitas JC (1992) Potassium channel toxins from sea anemone. In: *Recent Advances in Toxinology Research. Vol 2.* Gopalakrishnakone P, Tan CK eds. Venom and Toxin Research Group, National University of Singapore, Singapore p. 408.

10. Maretic C, Russell FE (1983) Stings by the sea anemone *Anemonia sulcata* in the Adriatic sea. *Amer J Trop Med Hyg* **32**, 891.

11. Mebs D, Hucho F (1990) Toxins acting on ion channels and synapses. In: *Handbook of Toxinology.* Shier T, Mebs D eds. Marcel Dekker, New York p. 493.

12. Minagawa S, Ishida M, Nagashima Y, Shiomi K (1998) Primary structure of a potassium channel toxin from the sea anemone *Actinia equina*. *FEBS Lett* **427**, 149.

13. Molgo J, Mallart A (1985) Effects of *Anemonia sulcata* toxin II on presynaptic currents and evoked transmitter release at neuromuscular junctions of the mouse. *Pflugers Arch* **405**, 349.

14. Muramatsu I, Saito K, Ohmura T *et al.* (1991) Supersensitivity to tetrodotoxin and lidocaine of anthopleurin-A-treated Na⁺ channels in crayfish giant axon. *Eur J Pharmacol* **186**, 41.

15. Nishio M, Ohmura T, Kigoshi S, Muramatsu I (1991) Supersensitivity to tetrodotoxin and lignocaine of sea anemone toxin II-treated sodium channel in guinea pig ventricular muscle. *Brit J Pharmacol* **104**, 504.

16. Norton RS (1991) Structure and structure-function relationships of sea anemone proteins that interact with the sodium channels. *Toxicon* **29**, 1051.

17. Romey G, Abita JP, Schweitz H *et al.* (1976) Sea anemone toxin: A tool to study molecular mechanisms of nerve conduction and excitation-secretion coupling. *Proc Nat Acad Sci USA* **73**, 4055.

18. Strichartz G, Rondo T, Wang GK (1987) An integrated view of the molecular toxinology of sodium channel gating in excitable cells. *Annu Rev Neurosci* **10**, 237.

Selenium

Dennis J. Blodgett
Bernard S. Jortner

Sodium selenite Na₂SeO₃
Sodium selenate Na₂SeO₄

NEUROTOXICITY RATING

Clinical

B   Acute encephalopathy (headache, confusion, seizures)

Experimental

A   Multifocal necrotizing encephalomyelopathy

Selenium (Se) and sulfur are both members of group VI elements and they share many similar chemical properties (3). Se occurs in soils and is absorbed by plants. Whereas some geographic areas have highly seleniferous soils, Se is deficient in others. Seleniferous areas in the United States are primarily located in the Great Plains. Other such regions have been identified in Australia, Canada, Israel, Ireland, Colombia, and China.

Elemental Se has several allotropic forms: (a) amorphous; (b) crystalline (red); or (c) metallic (gray). Possible valence states are 2- (selenide), 0 (elemental), 2+, 4+ (selenite), and 6+ (selenate) (3). Many metals react with the selenide form. Se is used as a feed ingredient for animals; a dietary supplement for humans; an ingredient in electronic and photocopier components; a pigment for ceramics, paints, and plastics; and an additive in glass manufacture and in metallurgy. Other forms of Se are being investigated for various therapeutic purposes. The U.S. Food and Drug Administration regulates the amount of Se in animal diets at 0.3 ppm. The Time-Weighted Average Threshold-Limit Value for Se in air is 0.2 mg/m³.

Inorganic and organic forms of Se have different disposition characteristics in the body. Inorganic salt forms are readily absorbed with no homeostatic mechanism regulating absorption (3). However, absorption of inorganic forms is decreased by interactions with other elements and reducing conditions of the intestinal tract (3,10). Organic forms are more bioavailable for animals. Selenomethionine is the

$$CH_3 - Se - CH_2 - CH_2 - \underset{\underset{NH_3^+}{|}}{\overset{\overset{H}{|}}{C}} - COO^-$$

SELENOMETHIONINE

most common organic form, which is believed to be absorbed by methionine-type mechanisms (10). Distribution in the body also depends on the form of Se. Relative orders of magnitude for Se concentrations in tissues are kidney > liver > heart > brain, spinal cord > muscle > fat (3,10). In some short-term Se toxicoses, Se concentration in the liver may exceed that in the kidneys (3). In the CNS of rats, Se in an inorganic or organic form concentrates more in the cerebellum than in the cerebrum or spinal cord (5). Selenomethionine is probably deposited as both a selenoenzyme and as a methionine substitute in various peptides and proteins (5). Metabolism of the inorganic forms occurs by reduction with the aid of glutathione (GSH) (3,8,10). In the process, GSH is oxidized to GSSG, which must be reduced to be reactivated; Se becomes a selenotrisulfide, which is then methylated in the body. Huge doses of Se will be in part exhaled as dimethylselenide, which has a characteristic garlic odor. Most Se is excreted as a trimethylselenonium ion in the urine. Some biliary excretion of Se does occur. Target organs of Se excess are route-, dose-, and species-dependent. Large oral and parenteral doses in most species are primarily cardiotoxic and myotoxic (1,3,10). Lower, but more prolonged oral doses, affect the spinal cord and integument in swine (2,6,18–20). Prolonged oral doses in other animals and humans primarily affect the integument (3,10).

The role of Se in the body as an essential trace element is primarily as a component of two different selenoenzymes (15), both of which contain Se in the form of selenocysteine. Glutathione peroxidase is located in the cytosol of most cells; each mole of enzyme contains 4 g-atoms of Se as selenocysteine. The other selenoenzyme, phospholipid hydroperoxide glutathione peroxidase, is membrane bound and contains one Se atom per molecule. Both selenoenzymes require GSH as a cofactor. These selenoenzymes destroy hydrogen peroxide and lipid peroxides formed by normal oxidative metabolism in the body. The nontoxic by-products are water or lipid alcohols. Peroxides are capable of forming free radicals, which damage various membranes in the body. In addition to the selenoenzymes, vitamin E also provides a line of defense in ridding the body of some of the excess free radicals. At least two types of glutathione peroxidase are found in the brain, one of which is membrane bound (7). The declining order of glutathione peroxidase activity in brain fractions is mitochondria > microsomes > synaptic vesicles > myelin > synaptosomes.

Controlled short-term dosing of animals usually results in cardiac and skeletal muscle necrosis and dystrophic calcification (1,3,10). The lungs may be edematous, and mild perivascular edema in the CNS is suggested (11). Sodium selenite given intracerebrally in mice produces convulsions, whereas the same dose and drug given subcutaneously produces a cardiomyopathy (1).

Prolonged, controlled oral dosing of sodium selenite, sodium selenate, or organic plant forms of Se in swine produces focal symmetrical necrosis in the spinal cord, hair loss, and feet problems (2,6,18,19). Dietary concentrations of Se between 19 and 52 ppm have produced such effects when used for several weeks. Daily oral Se doses of 0.6–1.9 mg/kg body weight as sodium selenite have also reproduced this porcine syndrome. Lesions of poliomyelomalacia in pigs consist of microcavitation of the neuropil, gliosis,

and neuronal degeneration progressing to necrosis. These are best seen in ventral horns of the lumbar and cervical enlargements of the spinal cord, but brainstem nuclei including pontine, olivary, facial, reticular, and trigeminal are also affected.

Uncontrolled exposures in animals result in either short-term problems from iatrogenic administration of too much injectable sodium selenite or long-term exposure from misformulated diets or consumption of plants high in Se content. Prolonged exposures in swine are from misformulation of Se salts in the diet, usually in the form of sodium selenite (6,20). Instead of the recommended amount of 0.3 ppm in the diet, toxic exposures are usually in the range of 12–52 ppm. Clinical signs usually begin within several weeks and consist of emaciation, alopecia, hoof lesions, ataxia, and rear leg paresis progressing to paralysis. Prolonged exposure in cattle and horses from added selenite or organic plant sources produces a syndrome called alkali disease (3,14). These animals also have alopecia and hoof problems in addition to decreased vitality and rough hair coats. Lesions of the CNS have not been noted with alkali disease.

Another disease in sheep and cattle, historically associated with prolonged consumption of Se-containing plants, is "blind staggers" (3,14,16). As the name would imply, the syndrome involves the CNS. Major clinical signs consist of anorexia, impaired vision, circling, ataxia, and paresis (3). Blind staggers has often been reported in animals consuming *Astragalus bisulcatus*, a plant with elevated Se concentrations plus the alkaloid and systemic poison swainsonine. Animals fed this plant have signs and lesions that mimic locoweed swainsonine poisoning (16) (*see* Swainsonine, this volume). Some previous reported cases of blind staggers could have been caused by swainsonine and not Se. The theory is attractive because, unlike alkali disease, blind staggers has not been reproduced experimentally by administration of Se salts (3,14,16). Another etiological theory concerning blind staggers relates to the correlation between seleniferous regions and areas that have high concentrations of sulfates in their plant and water sources (14). Sulfates are capable of inducing thiamine deficiency in ruminants and, thus, producing the bilateral cerebral necrosis of gray matter termed polioencephalomalacia. The clinical signs of polioencephalomalacia are very similar to those found in the blind staggers syndrome.

Clinical manifestations of human selenosis with prolonged exposure usually relate to skin or neurological alterations. The latter include peripheral paresthesias, headache, vertigo, fatigue, and convulsions (4,17). An association between excess Se and human motor neuron disease has been reported. A relatively high incidence (four cases over a 10-year period) of amyotrophic lateral sclerosis was noted in male farmers from a small region of South Dakota where Se toxicosis was endemic in farm animals (9). One of these individuals had a high urinary concentration of Se. Similarly, cervical (but not thoracic or lumbar) spinal cord, liver, and bone concentrations of Se were increased in postmortem studies in a series of adult patients dying with motor neuron disease (12). Among a variety of other trace elements, only manganese also showed spinal cord (cervical and thoracic) tissue elevations in these patients. This association of increased Se exposure and motor neuron disease could not be corroborated by measuring urinary Se (a common method for determining body burden) in 200 patients with amyotrophic lateral sclerosis (4). Similarly, blood Se concentrations were not increased in patients with childhood spinal muscular atrophy and in heterozygote carriers of the gene for this abnormality (13). On balance, Se does not appear to be a primary causative agent of motor neuron disease in humans. However, increased tissue concentrations of Se may occur in a coincidental fashion with small numbers of these conditions where dietary intake of Se is above normal.

The mechanism of Se toxicity is unknown (3). Early investigators assumed Se inhibited enzymes with free sulfhydryl groups. A more recent hypothesis is that, during the metabolism of Se, much of the supply of reduced GSH in the body is oxidized and that in conditions of Se excess, some tissues become deprived of the reduced GSH needed to rid the body of free radicals and other toxic chemicals. This is an attractive hypothesis, since the same myocardial target exists in both Se deficiency and toxicosis. Adequate glutathione peroxidase is missing with Se deficiency; whereas adequate reduced GSH, the cofactor for glutathione peroxidase, is thought to be diminished in Se toxicosis. Another potential mechanism of Se toxicity is the ability of the selenotrisulfide metabolite to inhibit various enzymes in the body (8). Selenotrisulfide is believed to be the molecule active in blocking RNA polymerase in carcinogenic cells. Selenium also inhibits prostaglandin D_2 synthase in the brain of mice and affects sleep (8). Some consideration has been given to a dietary interaction of Se and niacin in porcine poliomyelomalacia (18). Both nutrients share similar metabolic enzymes and deficiency of niacin produces similar lesions to Se excess. However, supplementation of niacin while dosing toxic amounts of Se had only subtle ameliorative effects on the development of selenosis in swine.

REFERENCES

1. Ammar EM, Couri D (1981) Acute toxicity of sodium selenite and selenomethionine in mice after ICV or IV administration. *Neurotoxicology* **2**, 383.
2. Baker DC, James LF, Hartley WJ *et al.* (1989) Toxicosis in pigs fed selenium-accumulating *Astragalus* plant species or sodium selenate. *Amer J Vet Res* **50**, 1396.
3. Burk RF, Diplock AI, Gopalan HNB *et al.* (1987) *Environmental Health Criteria 58: Selenium*. World Health Organization, New York.
4. Conradi S, Ronnevi L-O, Norris F (1982) Motor neuron disease and toxic metals. In: *Human Motor Neuron Diseases*. Rowland LP ed. Rowen Press, New York p. 201.
5. Grønbaek H, Thorlacius-Ussing O (1992) Selenium in the central nervous system of rats exposed to 75-Se L-selenomethionine and sodium selenite. *Biol Tr Elem Res* **35**, 119.
6. Harrison LH, Colvin BM, Stuart BP *et al.* (1983) Paralysis in swine due to focal symmetrical poliomalacia: Possible selenium toxicosis. *Vet Pathol* **20**, 265.
7. Huang K, Lauridsen E, Clausen J (1994) Localization of new glutathione peroxidases in the rat brain. *Biol Tr Elem Res* **46**, 91.
8. Islam F, Watanabe Y, Morii H, Hayaishi O (1991) Inhibition of rat brain prostaglandin D synthase by inorganic selenocompounds. *Arch Biochem Biophys* **289**, 161.
9. Kilness AW, Hochberg FH (1977) Amyotrophic lateral sclerosis in a high selenium environment. *J Amer Med Assn* **237**, 2843.
10. Lo M-T, Sandi E (1980) Selenium: Occurrence in foods and its toxicological significance—a review. *J Environ Pathol Toxicol* **4**, 193.
11. MacDonald DW, Christian RG, Strausz KI, Roff J (1981) Acute selenium toxicity in neonatal calves. *Can Vet J* **22**, 279.
12. Mitchell JD, East BW, Harris IA, Pentland B (1991) Manganese, selenium and other trace elements in spinal cord, liver and bone in motor neuron disease. *Eur Neurol* **31**, 7.
13. Pearn J, McCray CWR (1979) Blood selenium in chronic spinal muscular atrophy. *J Neurol Sci* **42**, 199.
14. Raisbeck MF, Dahl ER, Sanchez DA *et al.* (1993) Naturally occurring selenosis in Wyoming. *J Vet Diagn Invest* **5**, 84.
15. Ursini F, Bindoli A (1987) The role of selenium peroxidases in the protection against oxidative damage of membranes. *Chem Physics Lipids* **44**, 255.
16. Van Kampen KR, James LF (1978) Manifestations of intoxication by selenium-accumulating plants. In: *Effects of Poisonous Plants on Livestock*. Keeler RF, Van Kampen KR, James LF eds. Academic Press, New York p. 135.
17. Van Vleet JF, Ferrans VJ (1992) Etiologic factors and pathologic alterations in selenium-vitamin E deficiency and excess in animals and humans. *Biol Tr Elem Res* **33**, 1.
18. Wilson TM, Cramer PG, Owen RL *et al.* (1989) Porcine focal symmetrical poliomyelomalacia: Test for an interaction between dietary selenium and niacin. *Can J Vet Res* **53**, 454.

19. Wilson TM, Hammerstedt RH, Palmer IS, deLahunta A (1988) Porcine focal symmetrical poliomyelomalacia: Experimental reproduction with oral doses of encapsulated sodium selenite. *Can J Vet Res* **52**, 83.

20. Wilson TM, Scholz RW, Drake TR (1983) Selenium toxicity and porcine focal symmetrical poliomyelomalacia: Description of a field outbreak and experimental reproduction. *Can J Comp Med* **47**, 412.

Shiga Toxin

Albert C. Ludolph
Peter S. Spencer

NEUROTOXICITY RATING

Clinical

B   Acute encephalopathy

Shigellosis in children (rarely in adults) is often associated with lethargy, seizures, and headache; shiga toxin, produced by strains of *Shigella dysenteriae* type 1, has been considered responsible for these effects (1).

Shiga toxin is a representative of a larger family of toxins (verotoxins) produced by *Shigella* spp. and *Escherichia coli*; they share sequence homology with shiga toxin, bind to the same receptor, and have similar biological effects (6,9). Shiga toxin consists of two polypeptide chains with a MW of 32,225 (chain A) and 7691 (chain B). The holotoxin is formed by five B subunits and a single A subunit; the latter consists of two fragments, A_1 and A_2. A_1 is responsible for the catalytic effects, A_2 links the A chain to the B subunit, and the 69-amino-acid B subunit mediates toxin binding to cell-surface glycolipid receptors (4). The A chain has major similarities to the A chain of the plant toxin, ricin. Shiga toxin acts as a specific *N*-glycosidase and cleaves an adenine residue from near the 3' end of the 28S rRNA component of the ribosomal complex, thereby inhibiting the binding of elongation factor 2 to ribosomes (7).

The incidence of neurological complications of shigellosis in humans is high (1,2), but whether they result from a direct action of shiga toxin (verotoxin) on the nervous system has been questioned (1). Intravenous administration of extracts of *Shigella* spp. to rabbits causes paralysis without evidence of CNS histopathological change (1,3). However, recent studies show that verotoxin receptors are present in ependymal cells, myelin sheaths and small dorsal root ganglion cells, as well as capillary endothelial cells (5,8). Rabbits given intravenous verotoxin 2 (VT2) develop hemorrhagic diarrhea, flaccid limb paresis, ataxic gait, opisthotonic posture, and convulsions. Toxin appears to enter cerebrospinal fluid *via* the choroid plexus in these animals (5,6). Magnetic resonance images suggest that lesions initially occur around the third ventricle and later involve the cerebellum and brainstem, with death resulting from involvement of the cardiovascular center (10). Rabbits survive if they are given an intrathecal injection of rabbit anti-VT2 antibody before the intravenous injection of VT2 (6).

REFERENCES

1. Ashkenazi S, Cleary KR, Pickering LK *et al.* (1990) The association of shiga toxin and other cytotoxins with the neurologic manifestations of shigellosis. *J Infect Dis* **161**, 961.

2. Avital A, Maayan C, Goitein KJ (1982) Incidence of convulsions and encephalopathy in childhood *Shigella* infections. *Clin Pediat* **21**, 645.

3. Cavanagh JB, Howard JG, Witby JL (1956) The neurotoxin of *Shigella shigae*. A comparative study of the effects produced in various laboratory animals. *Brit J Exp Pathol* **37**, 272.

4. Donohue-Rolfe A, Acheson DW, Keusch GT (1991) Shiga toxin: Purification, structure, and function. *Rev Infect Dis* **13**, S293.

5. Fujii J, Kinoshita Y, Kita T *et al.* (1996) Magnetic resonance imaging and histopathological study of brain lesions in rabbits given intravenous verotoxin 2. *Infect Immun* **64**, 5053.

6. Fujii J, Kinoshita Y, Yamada Y *et al.* (1998) Neurotoxicity of intrathecal Shiga toxin 2 and protection by intrathecal injection of anti-Shiga toxin 2 antiserum in rabbits. *Microb Pathog* **25**, 139.

7. O'Brien AD, Tesh VL, Donohue-Rolfe A *et al.* (1992) Shiga toxin: Biochemistry, genetics, mode of action, and role in pathogenesis. *Curr Top Microbiol Immunol* **180**, 65.

8. Ren J, Utsunomiya I, Taguchi K *et al.* (1999) Localization of verotoxin receptors in nervous system. *Brain Res* **825**, 183.

9. Tesh VL, O'Brien AD (1991) The pathogenetic mechanisms of Shiga toxin and the Shiga-like toxins. *Mol Microbiol* **5**, 1817.

10. Yamada Y, Fujii J, Murasato Y *et al.* (1999) Brainstem mechanisms of autonomic dysfunction in encephalopathy-associated Shiga toxin 2 intoxication. *Ann Neurol* **45**, 716.

Silicone

Neil L. Rosenberg

$$(H_3C)_3Si - O \left[\begin{matrix} CH_3 \\ | \\ Si - O \\ | \\ CH_3 \end{matrix} \right]_n Si(CH_3)_3$$

POLYDIMETHYLSILOXANE

$$[Si(CH_3)_2O]_n$$

Polydimethylsiloxane, Dimethicone

NEUROTOXICITY RATING

Clinical

C   Peripheral neuropathy

C   Acute encephalopathy

Silicones are synthetic polymers containing a repeating silicon–oxygen (Si-O) backbone, with organic groups attached to the silicon *via* a silicon–carbon bond. The most common of the silicones used medically is polydimethylsiloxane (PDMS) (12). Because of their properties of thermal and oxidative stability, they have numerous uses (*e.g.*, as components of fluids and rubbers). The length of the polymer chain and degree of cross-linking determine the characteristics of the silicone and its uses. Silicone gels, lightly cross-linked PDMS, have been implicated in the development of disorders in women who have received breast implants containing the gel (4,21,24). Though different breast-implant manufacturers may have different silicone gels in their respective implants, the claimed adverse health effects have not varied from manufacturer to manufacturer. Although silicone is contained in a large number of medical devices, interest and discussion have focused on the 1–2 million American women who have undergone breast augmentation or reconstruction procedures with silicone gel–filled elastomer envelope breast prostheses, procedures that have been performed during the past three decades.

The first report of a rheumatological disease associated with silicone breast implants (SBIs) occurred in 1982 (23). Since then, several publications in the form of case reports and small case series have suggested that women with SBIs may develop certain rheumatological disorders (primarily scleroderma) or symptoms of rheumatic disease (4,21,24). Epidemiological studies, however, have failed to find an association between SBIs and rheumatological disease (7,11,18,22).

Studies have suggested that certain neurological disorders, including motor neuron disease (15), multiple sclerosis (14), peripheral neuropathies (13,16), "multiple sclerosis-like" syndrome (14), and memory impairment (16) occur as the result of problems related to SBIs. In addition, a condition termed the "atypical neurological disease syndrome" (ANDS) has been attributed to SBIs (16). There have been no epidemiological studies specifically designed to address the neurological issues. All the case series suggesting that SBIs are associated with certain neurological conditions were reported from only one group (13–16).

This same group published a series of 100 cases of what the authors called "adjuvant breast disease" (16). Numerous studies were performed on these patients, but complete analysis was not performed on all individuals. In addition, no control data were presented, and no specific neurological diagnoses were reported, although the authors offered the diagnosis of "adjuvant breast disease" (ABD) in all patients. Based on this report, ABD is a heterogeneous collection of symptoms and findings (both clinical and laboratory) in patients with silicone breast implants. The only aspect of ABD that discriminates the entity from numerous other similar nonspecific "syndromes" is the presence of silicone implants (or having had silicone injections).

Peripheral nerve disease was described as a cardinal finding in this study. Symptoms that may indicate peripheral nerve disease included "numbness" (77%), "tingling" (72%), and "weakness" (95%). Many patients also had complaints of "fatigue" (95%) and "muscle aches and pain" (91%). Most of these complaints are seen in high frequency in other common disorders, including fibromyalgia, chronic fatigue syndrome, and certain psychiatric disorders, which are also common diagnoses in this patient population. Neurological findings included "weakness" (94%), "loss of vibration" (78%), "loss of pin-prick" (72%), "increased deep tendon reflexes (DTR)" (14%), "decreased DTR" (11%), "facial weakness" (19%), and "muscle atrophy" (4%). Ninety-three individuals underwent electromyography/nerve conduction velocity (EMG/NCV) studies. Of these, 44 (47%) were entirely normal; 24 had "myopathic potentials" (although the distribution of the potentials was not described); 23 had "polyphasia, giant motor units, fibrillations, or decreased recruitment" (again, the distribution was not described); 11 had findings of carpal tunnel syndrome; four had "findings of an axonal neuropathy"; and two patients had myasthenia gravis (with no description on how the diagnosis was made). No details of these EMG/NCV studies were given, nor were any specific diagnoses made based on these studies.

Sural nerve biopsies were performed on 65 patients. The nerve specimens were frozen and prepared for light microscopy; 80% of the biopsies were reportedly abnormal, namely, a "moderate loss" (estimated at "35%–45%" loss) of myelinated fibers (79%). How this estimated loss was determined is not clear. There was no attempt to correlate the symptoms, signs, and other laboratory findings with the nerve or muscle biopsy findings, and whether any individuals had a specific diagnosis of peripheral neuropathy.

An analysis of 131 cases of women with SBIs who were considered to have neurological disease related to SBIs failed to find evidence of neurologic *disease* (including peripheral neuropathy) in the population of women with silicone breast implants (17). It also suggested that other authors failed to follow accepted standards in making neurological diagnoses (17). This was most evident in the diagnosis of chronic inflammatory demyelinating polyneuropathy (CIDP), where not a single criterion necessary to make the diagnosis of CIDP was seen in any of the cases so diagnosed (1). In most cases (82%), patients had numerous symptoms but no objective evidence of a neurological disorder. The remainder of the cases generally had pre-existing physical or psychological disorders that would explain their symtomatology.

There are two other clinical reports relating silicone to neurological dysfunction (8,20). One deals with silicone-coated Dacron dural grafts; grafts were associated with cervical cord compression in two individuals (8). In both cases, extensive scar tissue formation was seen at the site of compression, and two factors were felt possibly to play a role in the formation of the scar tissue: the introduction of the grafts and repeated motion at the graft site. The second report describes a woman who developed compression neuropathies related to silicone gel that had migrated along fascial planes from a ruptured breast implant into the right arm (20). Migration down the arm was demonstrated radiographically; pathologically, patchy areas of inflammation and fibrosis were seen along the course of the median nerve as well as within certain muscle groups. There was no evidence of a generalized disorder of peripheral nerves.

Several epidemiological studies have addressed the association between human disease and silicone breast implants (7,9,18,21). These studies all focused on rheumatological diseases and did not address neurological diagnoses. In the first of these studies (7), 749 women who had received breast implants were compared to 1498 community controls. No association was found between breast implants and connective tissue diseases (scleroderma, systemic lupus erythematosus, rheumatoid arthritis, polymyositis, dermatomyositis, Sjögren's syndrome, Hashimoto's thyroiditis, keratoconjunctivitis sicca), lymphoproliferative disorders, cancer (other than breast cancer), primary biliary cirrhosis, and other symptoms and signs. Other epidemiological studies have failed to find a link between SBIs and rheumatological diseases (18,22). One study (13) included a retro-spective cohort study of 395,543 female health professionals. In this group 10,830 had SBIs and 11,805 reported connective-tissue diseases. A very slight increase in "self-report" of diagnosis of connective tissue diseases was noted [relative risk (RR) of 1.24], but no association with duration of implants was seen. Verification of these diagnoses was not made, and considering the widespread publicity and active litigation associated with SBIs, it is surprising that the RR was not significantly higher. Other epidemiological studies have also failed to find an association between SBIs and breast cancer (2,3) and breast sarcomas (5).

A single experimental study has addressed the possible effects of silicone gel on peripheral nerve (19). In this study, silicone gel was placed either extraneurally adjacent to or injected directly into rat sciatic nerve. The neuropathological changes were assessed every 2 weeks during a 20-week period. Placed extraneurally, the silicone gel elicited an intense inflammatory response that peaked at about 4 weeks; subsequently, collagen deposition increased and inflammation decreased. Perineural fibrosis was marked by 20 weeks, but there was no penetration of the epineurium by the gel. Silicone gel that was injected intraneurally caused a similar response. The intraneural gel did not migrate. There was neither direct toxicity to peripheral nerve nor a generalized disorder of the peripheral nerves.

In a second experimental study, dimethylpolysiloxane fluid, not gel, was injected into rats, rabbits, and monkeys (10). There was no evidence of any neurological effect clinically or pathologically when the compound was injected into the cisterna magna of rats or the spinal canal of rabbits or monkeys.

The American Academy of Neurology found there was no evidence that SBIs or other silicone-containing products are associated with any neurological disorder (6). There may be rare situations where focal fibrosis caused by silicone gel or elastomer may result in constriction around certain neural structures resulting in local symptomatology.

Editors' Note: A committee of the Institute of Medicine (IOM), a non-governmental American organization, noted that a review of 17 epidemiological reports of connective tissue disease in women with breast implants was remarkable for the consistency of finding no elevated relative risk or odds ratio for an association between implants and systemic disease. A review of the toxicology studies of silicones and other substances known to be in breast implants did not provide a basis for health concerns [Bondurant S, Ernster V, Herdman R, eds (1999) *Safety of Silicone Breast Implants*, IOM, Washington D.C.].

REFERENCES

1. American Academy of Neurology (1991) Criteria for diagnosis of chronic inflammatory demyelinating polyneuropathy. *Neurology* **41**, 617.

2. Berkel H, Birdsell DC, Jenkins H (1992) Breast augmentation: A risk factor for breast cancer? *N Engl J Med* **326**, 1649.

3. Deapen DM, Brody GS (1995) Augmentation mammoplasty and breast cancer: A five year update of the Los Angeles study. *J Clin Epidemiol* **48**, 551.

4. Endo LP, Edwards NL, Longley S *et al.* (1987) Silicone and rheumatic diseases. *Semin Arthritis Rheum* **17**, 112.

5. Engel A, Lamm SH, Lai SH (1995) Human breast sarcoma and human breast implantation: A time trend analysis based on SEER data (1973–1990). *J Clin Epidemiol* **48**, 539.

6. Ferguson JH (1997) Silicon breast implants and neurologic disorders. *Neurology* **48**, 1504.

7. Gabriel SE, O'Fallon WM, Kurland LT *et al.* (1994) Risk of connective-tissue diseases and other disorders after breast implantation. *N Engl J Med* **330**, 1697.

8. Gomez H, Little JR (1989) Spinal cord compression: A complication of silicone-coated Dacron dural grafts. Report of two cases. *Neurosurgery* **24**, 115.

9. Hennekens CH, Lee I-M, Cook NR *et al.* (1996) Self-report breast implants and connective-tissue diseases in female health professionals: A retrospective cohort study. *J Amer Med Assn* **275**, 616.

10. Hine CH, Elliott HW, Wright RR *et al.* (1969) Evaluation of a silicone lubricant injected spinally. *Toxicol Appl Pharmacol* **15**, 566.

11. Hochberg MC, Miller R, Wigley FM (1995) Frequency of augmentation mammoplasty in patients with systemic sclerosis: Data from the Johns Hopkins-University of Maryland scleroderma center. *J Clin Epidemiol* **48**, 565.

12. LeVier RR, Harrison MC, Cook RR, Lane TH (1993) What is silicone? *Plastic Reconstr Surg* **92**, 163.

13. Ostermeyer-Shoaib B, Patten BM (1992) Silicone adjuvant breast disease: More neurological cases. *Ann Neurol* **32**, 254.

14. Ostermeyer-Shoaib B, Patten BM (1994) A multiple sclerosis-like syndrome in women with breast implants or silicone fluid injections into breasts. *Neurology* **44**, A158.

15. Ostermeyer-Shoaib B, Patten BM, Ashizawa T (1992) Motor neuron disease after silicone breast implants and silicone injections into the face. *Ann Neurol* **32**, 254.

16. Ostermeyer-Shoaib B, Patten BM, Calkins DS (1994) Adjuvant breast disease: An evaluation of 100 symptomatic women with breast implants or silicone fluid injections. *Keio J Med* **43**, 79.

17. Rosenberg NL (1996) The neuromythology of silicone breast implants. *Neurology* **46**, 308.

18. Sanchez-Guerrero J, Karlson EW, Colditz GA *et al.* (1994) Silicone breast implants (SBI) and connective tissue disease (CTD). *Arthritis Rheum* **37**, S282.

19. Sanger JR, Kolachalam R, Komorowski RA *et al.* (1992) Short-term effect of silicone gel on peripheral nerves: A histologic study. *Plastic Reconstr Surg* **89**, 931.

20. Sanger JR, Matloub HS, Yousif NJ, Komorowski R (1992) Silicone gel infiltration of a peripheral nerve and constrictive neuropathy following rupture of a breast prosthesis. *Plastic Reconstr Surg* **89**, 949.

21. Spierra H (1988) Scleroderma after silicone augmentation mammoplasty. *J Amer Med Assn* **260**, 236.

22. Strom BL, Reidenberg MM, Freundlich B, Schinnar R (1994) Breast silicone implants and risk of systemic lupus erythematosus. *J Clin Epidemiol* **47**, 1211.

23. Van Nunen SA, Gatenby PA, Basten A (1982) Post-mammoplasty connective tissue disease. *Arthritis Rheum* **6**, 694.

24. Varga J, Schumacher HR, Jimenez SA (1989) Systemic sclerosis after augmentation mammoplasty with silicone implants. *Ann Intern Med* **111**, 377.

Smallpox Vaccine

Neil L. Rosenberg

NEUROTOXICITY RATING

Clinical

A   Postvaccinial encephalomyelitis

C   Peripheral neuropathy (Guillain-Barré syndrome)

The eradication of smallpox in 1980 and elimination of the need for vaccination have made postvaccinial neurological complications primarily of historical interest (2,6).

The neurological complications of vaccination against smallpox were the first instances of complications following prophylactic immunization (5,7). The first detailed pathological description of postvaccinial encephalomyelitis (PVE) from smallpox vaccine in seven individuals was published in 1926 (7). A detailed account of the neurological complications followed a smallpox epidemic in South Wales in 1962 (5). Among 39 cases of neurological illness, there were 11 cases of PVE, three cases of an encephalopathy (clinically and pathologically distinct from PVE), six cases with focal lesions of the brain and spinal cord, five peripheral neuropathies, two cases of brachial neuritis, and two cases of myasthenia gravis (5). Other reports suggest a link between smallpox vaccination and other neurological disorders, including multiple sclerosis (3), Guillain-Barré syndrome (1), and transverse myelitis (1).

Neurological complications from smallpox vaccination were more likely to be associated with primary vaccination rather than with revaccination (1,5). While a visible cutaneous reaction (the jennerian vesicle) usually develops, PVE (and presumably other complications) may occur without the appearance of this skin reaction (4).

The frequency of neurological complications from smallpox vaccination was low (1). Of 938 adverse reactions to smallpox vaccination in Australia between 1960 and 1976 (an estimated 5 million vaccinations), only nine were neurological in nature (1). Among these were five cases of PVE, two cases of transverse myelitis, and one case of Guillain-Barré syndrome. With such a low frequency of neurological reactions (only 1% of total complications and <0.0002% of the total vaccinated population), it is difficult to distinguish between causal associations and coincidence.

While there is convincing evidence that PVE occurred as the result of smallpox vaccination, etiological association with other reported complications is unconvincing.

REFERENCES
1. Feery BJ (1977) Adverse reactions after smallpox vaccination. *Med J Australia* 2, 180.
2. Mahy BW, Almond JW, Berns KI *et al.* (1993) The remaining stocks of smallpox virus should be destroyed. *Science* 262, 1223.
3. Ono F (1986) Possible relation of small pox vaccination to multiple sclerosis-like disease. A personal note. *Med Hypotheses* 20, 339.
4. Rockoff A, Spigland I, Lorenstein B, Rose AL (1978) Postvaccinial encephalomyelitis without cutaneous vaccination reaction. *Ann Neurol* 5, 99.
5. Spillane JD, Wells CEC (1964) The neurology of Jennerian vaccination: A clinical account of the neurological complications which occurred during the smallpox epidemic in South Wales in 1962. *Brain* 87, 1.
6. Stuart-Harris C (1984) Prospects for the eradication of infectious diseases. *Rev Infect Dis* 6, 405.
7. Turnbull HM, McIntosh J (1926) Encephalomyelitis following vaccination. *Brit J Exp Pathol* 7, 181.

Sodium Azide

Mohammad I. Sabri

$$NaN_3$$

NEUROTOXICITY RATING

Experimental

A Seizure disorder

A Inhibition of cytochrome c oxidase

Sodium azide (NaN_3) is a highly toxic, colorless, neutral salt of hydrazoic acid (HN_3). In aqueous solutions, NaN_3 is rapidly converted to volatile HN_3, which may be the ultimate toxic metabolite (27). NaN_3 is used commercially as an antibacterial agent, herbicide, fungicide, insecticide; for inflating automobile "air bags"; and in aircraft in inflatable emergency-escape chutes (6,34).

Azide belongs to the class of pseudohalides, such as cyanide, cyanate, and thiocyanate (12). It combines with nonmetals and forms explosively unstable compounds. The azide ion can be oxidized to the azidyl radical (N_3^-) by reacting with hydroxyl radical (30,45). Azide forms well-characterized complexes with the Fe(III) of oxidized heme-containing proteins (9,30) and reversibly inhibits metalloenzymes. Azide is rapidly biotransformed in laboratory animals (14); liver injury does not affect azide toxicity in mice (37). Azide combines with most heme-containing proteins and enzymes to form azide methmyoglobin and azide methemoglobin; the latter has been exploited as a method in the determination of total hemoglobin. Sodium azide is a potent mutagen in bacteria and plants (11), but a weak mutagen in animals (38). Sodium azide is not a carcinogen (28). Experimental studies in Syrian golden hamsters have shown that NaN_3 is embryotoxic but not teratogenic (33). Sodium azide can produce sterility in the common housefly; males are more sensitive than females (41).

Sodium azide (0.1–10 μM) inhibits platelet aggregation, presumably *via* conversion to nitric oxide (NO) (39,40). Azide binds to catalase to form nitrosylcatalase; this complex transfers NO and activates guanylate cyclase (and vasodilation) by transferring NO to the heme-containing enzyme guanylate cyclase (7,29). Azide also competitively binds to ubiquitous heme-containing cytochrome P-450 (39). Azide inhibits catalase activity and reduces glutathione (GSH) in the intact erythrocyte (24). It prevents ethanol oxidation in blood, perhaps by inhibiting catalase activity (35). Azide is a competitive inhibitor of superoxide dismutase (SOD) enzymes containing copper and zinc, iron, or manganese (25).

Unlike cyanide, azide has cumulative effects; animals that have completely recovered from a single dose of azide react much more severely to a second, smaller dose of azide (18). The LD_{50} values for sodium azide in albino mice are 28–34 mg/kg intraperitoneally (i.p.) (1,14), 19 mg/kg intravenously (i.v.), and 27 mg/kg orally. In albino rats, the subcutaneous and intrathecal LD_{50} values are 45 and 48 mg/kg, respectively (14).

Sodium azide (0.5–500 μg/kg) given i.v. causes a sharp, transient fall in blood pressure (19). The hypotensive response to azide may reflect a direct effect on the vascular system. At larger repetitive doses (10–20 mg/kg), azide often produces a rise in blood pressure (14). In the isolated cat heart, azide up to 1 mg had a positive inotropic effect without affecting the rate of contraction (14). In animals, i.v. doses of 10–100 mg/kg produce a temporary bradycardia with a positive inotropic effect. At low doses of azide, an increase in the rate and depth of breathing is reported. Toxic i.v. doses of azide (10–40 mg/kg) cause hypertension, tachycardia, arrhythmia, depressed respiration, seizures, and death (40).

Sodium azide stimulates resting oxygen consumption in frog skeletal muscle; this is followed by an inhibition of oxygen uptake (40). Respiration in rat skeletal muscle and brain cortex decreases with increasing azide concentration (16). Sodium azide increases cyclic guanosine monophosphate (cGMP) levels in guinea pig heart muscle, rat liver, and cerebral cortex without affecting cyclic adenosine monophosphate (20). Since NO also increases tissue levels of cGMP, it was proposed that azide produces these effects by its conversion to NO (8). Azide stimulates catecholamine release from the canine adrenal cortex, perhaps by increasing calcium entry into chromaffin cells (43). It inhibits the sodium ion pump in sympathetic nerves of the rabbit, squid axons and in motor nerve terminals (43).

Azide is a well-known inhibitor of cytochrome-c oxidase (Cox), the terminal enzyme in the mitochondrial electron transport chain (36). Azide inhibits Cox activity in brain tissue both *in vitro* and *in vivo* (42); this can lead to increased azidyl and hydroxyl radical production (30).

Mice injected i.p. with single doses of sodium azide show neurobehavioral changes within minutes of the toxin administration. Animals treated with 9.2 mg/kg display no apparent signs of NaN_3 toxicity; those treated with 19.6 and 28 mg/kg showed dose-related acute neurobehavioral changes. Lethargy, recumbency, arched-back, raised hair coat, and circling movements are some of the typical signs of NaN_3 toxicity. Animals dosed with 28 mg/kg sodium azide became restless and had increased respiration, circling movements and lethargy prior to death. Animals treated with 19.6 mg/kg NaN_3 showed reduced Cox activity in brain mitochondria isolated 24 h after toxin injection (42).

Systemic or local administration of sodium azide causes energy deficits in the brain and damages nerve cells by an excitotoxic mechanism (5). Repeated administration of sodium azide to monkeys produces demyelination, and severe necrosis of the optic nerves, caudate nucleus, and putamen (13,15,18). Electron microscopy shows changes in cortical and subcortical regions of the rat brain (38). The most prominent changes are in cerebellum, cerebral cortex, and basal ganglia (22,23,26). When treated with eight to ten daily doses of 5 mg/kg, monkeys display dyskinesia and choreoathetoid movements associated with mitochondrial and other changes in the striatum (21). Chronic and continuous administration of sodium azide selectively inhibits rat brain Cox activity, impairs learning, and produces a memory deficit (3,4). Mice given sodium azide i.p. (40 mg/kg) develop convulsions and die. An intracerebroventricular dose of 0.4–1.5 mg/kg produced neurobehavioral signs ranging from agitation and tremors to clonic convulsions in unanesthetized, unrestrained rats (39). Pentobarbital-anesthetized cats were, however, refractory to azide at these doses, suggesting that pentobarbital antagonizes the neurotoxic effects of azide. A number of aliphatic azides (*e.g.*, *n*-hexylazide and amylazide) also produced a long-lasting hypotensive response, but these substances were not as neurotoxic as sodium azide (40).

Chronic adminstration of sodium azide to rats, guinea pigs, and hamsters results in behavioral neurotoxicity (3,4,18,34,40,44). Adult rats continuously dosed with 0.2 $\times$ 10^{-2} mM/kg/h NaN_3 showed impairment in the Morris water maze task without motor impairment (4).

Several cases of human poisoning have been documented following accidental ingestion, inhalation, or skin/eye contact with sodium azide (2,10,17,31,32,40,44). Humans died within 1 h to days from cardiac failure (40). No effective antidote is known for acute NaN_3 poisoning.

REFERENCES

1. Abbanat RA, Smith RP (1964) The influence of methemoglobinemia on the lethality of some toxic anions. I. Azide. *Toxicol Appl Pharmacol* 6, 576.
2. Albertson TE, Reed S, Siefkin A (1986) A case of fatal sodium azide ingestion. *J Toxicol Clin Toxicol* 24, 339.
3. Bennet MC, Diamond DM, Stryker SL *et al.* (1992) Cytochrome oxidase inhibition: A novel animal model of Alzheimer's disease. *J Geriatr Psychiatr Neurol* 5, 93.
4. Bennet MC, Rose GM (1992) Chronic sodium azide treatment impairs learning of the Morris water maze task. *Behav Neur Biol* 58, 72.
5. Brouillet E, Hyman BG, Jenkins BG *et al.* (1994) Systemic or local administration of azide produces striatal lesions by an energy impairment-induced excitotoxic mechanism. *Exp Neurol* 129, 175.
6. Budavari S (1989) *The Merck Index. 11th Ed.* Merck & Co, Rahway, New Jersey.

7. Craven PA, DeRubertis FR, Pratt DW (1979) Electron spin resonance study of the role of NO.catalase in the activation of guanylate cyclase by NaN₃ and NH₂OH. Modulation of enzyme responses by heme proteins and their nitrosyl derivatives. *J Biol Chem* **254**, 8213.

8. Dohi T, Morita K, Tsujimoto A (1983) Effect of sodium azide on catecholamine release from isolated adrenal gland and on guanylate cyclase. *Eur J Pharmacol* **94**, 331.

9. Dori Z, Ziolo RF (1973) The chemistry of coordinated azides. *Chem Rev* **73**, 247.

10. Edmonds OP, Bourne MS (1982) Sodium azide poisoning in five laboratory technicians. *Brit J Ind Med* **39**, 308.

11. Frederick KA, Babish JG (1982) Evaluation of mutagenicity and other adverse effects of occupational exposure to sodium azide. *Regul Toxicol Pharmacol* **2**, 308.

12. Golub AM, Kohler K, Skopenko VV (1986) *Chemistry of Pseudohalides*. Elsevier, Amsterdam.

13. Gosselin RE, Smith RP, Hodge HC (1984) *Clinical Toxicology of Commercial Products. Part III-126. 5th Ed.* Williams & Wilkins, Baltimore.

14. Graham JDP (1949) Actions of sodium azide. *Brit J Pharmacol* **4**, 1.

15. Hicks SP (1950) Brain metabolism *in vivo*. II. The distribution of lesions caused by azide, malononitrile, plasmocid and dinitrophenol poisoning in rats. *Arch Pathol* **50**, 545.

16. Hollinger N, Fuhrman FA, Lewis JJ, Field J II (1949) The effect of sodium azide on respiration of rat skeletal muscle and brain cortex *in vitro*. *J Cell Comp Physiol* **33**, 223.

17. Howard JD, Skogerboe KJ, Case GA *et al.* (1990) Death following accidental sodium azide ingestion. *J Forensic Sci* **35**, 193.

18. Hurst EW (1942) Experimental demyelination of the central nervous system. III. Poisoning with potassium cyanide, sodium azide, hydroxylamine, narcotics, carbon monoxide, *etc.*, with some considerations of bilateral necrosis occuring in the basal nuclei. *Aust J Exp Biol Med Sci* **20**, 297.

19. Kaplita PV, Barison HL, McCarthy LE, Smith RP (1984) Peripheral and central actions of sodium azide on circulatory and respiratory homeostasis in anesthetized cats. *J Pharmacol Exp Ther* **231**, 189.

20. Katsuki S, Arnold WP, Murad F (1977) Effects of sodium nitroprusside, nitroglycerin and sodium azide on levels of cyclic nucleotides and mechanical activity of various tissues. *J Cyclic Nucleotide Res* **3**, 239.

21. Mettler FA (1972) Choreoathetosis and striopallidonigral necrosis due to sodium azide. *Exp Neurol* **34**, 291.

22. Mettler FA (1972) Neuropathological effects of sodium azide administration in primates. *Fed Proc* **31**, 1504.

23. Mettler FA, Sax DA (1972) Cerebellar cortical degeneration due to acute azide poisoning. *Brain* **95**, 505.

24. Mills GC, Randall HP (1958) Hemoglobin catabolism. II. The protection of hemoglobin from oxidative breakdown in the intact erythrocyte. *J Biol Chem* **232**, 589.

25. Misra HP, Fridovich I (1978) Inhibition of superoxide dismutases by azide. *Arch Biochem Biophys* **189**, 317.

26. Miyoshi K (1967) Experimental striatal necrosis induced by sodium azide, a contribution to the problem of selective vulnerability and histochemical studies of enzymatic activity. *Acta Neuropathol* **9**, 199.

27. National Research Council, Committee on Hazardous Substances in the Laboratory (1981) *Prudent Practices for Handling Hazardous Chemicals in Laboratories*. National Academy Press, Washington, DC.

28. National Toxicology Program (1991) *Toxicology and Carcinogenesis Studies of Sodium Azide (CAS No. 26628-22-8) in F3441N Rats (Gavage Studies)*. National Toxicology Program, Tech Rep No 389, PB92-13561590, U.S. National Institutes of Public Health, No **91**, 2844.

29. Nicholls P (1964) The reactions of azide with catalase and their significance. *Biochem J* **90**, 331.

30. Partridge RS, Monroe SM, Parks JK *et al.* (1994) Spin trapping of azidyl and hydroxyl radicals in azide-inhibited rat brain submitochondrial particles. *Arch Biochem Biophy* **310**, 210.

31. Richardson SGN, Giles C, Swan CHJ (1975) Two cases of sodium azide poisoning by accidental ingestion of Isoton. *J Clin Pathol* **28**, 350.

32. Roberts RJ, Simmons A, Barrett DAH (1974) Accidental exposure to sodium azide. *J Clin Pathol* **61**, 879.

33. Sana TR, Ferm VH, Smith RP *et al.* (1990) Embryotoxic effects of sodium azide infusions in the Syrian hamster. *Fund Appl Toxicol* **14**, 754.

34. Schmidt EW, Day DJ (1979) *Use of Sodium Azide in Gas Generants for Inflatable Restraint System Inflators*. Rep. No. AOPA 79-1001 Rev. A. prepared for Automotive Occupant Protection Association, Arlington, Virginia August 22.

35. Smalldon KW (1973) Ethanol oxidation by human erythrocytes. *Nature* **254**, 266.

36. Smith L, Kruszyna H, Smith RP (1977) The effect of methemoglobin on the inhibition of cytochrome *c* oxidase by cyanide, sulfide or azide. *Biochem Pharmacol* **26**, 2247.

37. Smith RP, Louis CA, Kruszyna R, Kruszyna H (1991) Acute neurotoxicity of sodium azide and nitric oxide. *Fund Appl Toxicol* **17**, 120.

38. Smith RP, Wilcox DE (1994) Toxicology of selected nitric oxide-donating xenobiotics, with particular reference to azide. *Crit Rev Toxicol* **24**, 355.

39. Sono M, Dawson JH (1982) Formation of low spin complexes of ferric cytochrome P-450-CAM with anionic ligands. *J Biol Chem* **257**, 5496.

40. Stibbe J, Holmsen H (1977) Effects of sodium azide on platelet function. *Thromb Haemost* **38**, 1042.

41. Thakur JN, Mann SK (1981) Infecundity and dominant lethal mutations induced in *Musca domestica* L. by sodium azide (NaN₃). *Experientia* **37**, 824.

42. Tor-Agbidye J, Agoston T, Lystrup B *et al.* (1995) Neurobehavioral changes and *in vitro* and *in vivo* inhibition

of brain mitochondrial cytochrome *c* oxidase by sodium azide. *Toxicologist* **15**, 144.

43. Török TL, Pauló T, Tóth PT *et al.* (1989) Sodium azide evoked noradrenaline and catecholamine release from peripheral sympathetic nerves and chromaffin cells. *Gen Pharmacol* **20**, 143.

44. Vitello W, Kim M, Johnson RM, Miller S (1999) Full-thickness burn to the hand from an automobile airbag. *J Burn Care Rehabil* **20**, 212.

45. Walter TH, Bancroft EE, McIntire GL *et al.* (1982) Spin trapping in heterogenous electron transfer processes. *Can J Chem* **60**, 1621.

Spirogermanium

Herbert H. Schaumburg

SPIROGERMANIUM
$C_{17}H_{36}GeN_2$

8,8-Diethyl-*N*,*N*-dimethyl-2-aza-8-germaspiro[4,5]decane-2-propanamine

NEUROTOXICITY RATING

Clinical

A   Seizure disorder

A   Acute encephalopathy (lethargy, confusion)

Experimental

A   Seizure disorder

Spirogermanium is an organogermanium anticancer agent with a novel chemical structure; it is a member of a class of azaspirene compounds that contain a nitrogen linked to a dimethyl aminopropyl substituent (4,6). Spirogermanium inhibits synthesis of DNA, RNA, and protein in tissue culture. The drug was tried in phase I and II chemotherapy trials against solid tumors of lung and bowel and also against lymphoma; it has now been abandoned as ineffective (7,9). Considerable acute neurotoxicity accompanied its use; in contrast to germanium dioxide and other organogermanium compounds, renal dysfunction is not described following treatment with spirogermanium (6).

In experimental mice and dogs, generalized seizures accompany lethal intramuscular injections and follow nonlethal intravenous infusions (2). Possible malformations have been reported after administration of dimethyl germanium oxide to pregnant animals (1).

In tissue culture, spirogermanium concentrations cytotoxic to tumor cells also lyse rat neurons (4). There is considerable variability in the dose threshold for human neurotoxic reactions. Most patients experience acute and transient (<72 h) signs of CNS dysfunction (7,9).

Permanent sequelae are not described. The most common reactions are lethargy, light-headedness, and visual distortion. Several also experience confusion, lateral gaze nystagmus, and gait ataxia.

Electroencephalograms during the acute encephalopathy stage are unremarkable. In contrast to experimental animals, only one patient experienced generalized seizures, and that followed the accidental administration of ten times the usual dosage (7). In sum, massive doses appear to cause CNS excitation; lower doses induce a widespread, multifocal mixture of CNS depression and excitation.

The neurotoxicity of spirogermanium differs from that of inorganic germanium; germanium dioxide is associated with myopathy and peripheral sensory dysfunction (3,5,8) (*see* Germanium Dioxide, this volume).

REFERENCES

1. Gerber GB, Leonard A (1997) Mutagenicity, carcinogenicity and teratogenicity of germanium compounds. *Mutat Res* **387**, 141.

2. Henry MC, Rosen CD, Levine BS (1980) Toxicity of spirogermanium in mice and dogs after iv or im administration. *Cancer Treatment Rep* **64**, 1204.

3. Higuchi I, Izumo S, Suchara M *et al.* (1989) Germanium myopathy: Clinical and experimental pathological studies. *Acta Neuropathol* **79**, 300.

4. Hill BT, Whatley SA, Bellamy AS *et al.* (1982) Cytotoxic effects and biologic activity of 2-aza-8-germaniumspiro [4,5]-decane-2-propanamin-8,8-diethyl-*N*,*N*-dimethyl dichloride (spirogermanium) *in vitro*. *Cancer Res* **42**, 2852.

5. Kamijo M, Yagihashi S, Kida S *et al.* (1991) An autopsy case of chronic germanium intoxication presenting with peripheral neuropathy, spinal ataxia, and chronic renal failure. *Clin Neurol* **31**, 191.

6. Schauss AG (1991) Nephrotoxicity and neurotoxicity in humans from organogermanium and germanium dioxide. *Biol Tr Elem Res* **29**, 26.

7. Schein PS, Slavik M, Smythe T *et al.* (1980) Phase 1 clinical trial of spirogermanium. *Cancer Treatment Rep* **64**, 1051.

8. Van der Spoel JI, Stricker BHCH, Esseveld MR, Schipper MEI (1990) Dangers of dietary germanium supplements. *Lancet* **ii**, 117.

9. Vogelzang NJ, Gesme DH, Kennedy BJ (1985) A phase II study of spirogermanium in advanced human malignancy. *Amer J Clin Oncol* **8**, 341.

Stichodactyla Spp.

Albert C. Ludolph
Peter S. Spencer

NEUROTOXICITY RATING

Experimental

A   Ion channel dysfunction (sodium & potassium channels)

Naturally occurring neurotoxins produced by the Caribbean sea anemone *Stichodactyla* (formerly *Stoichactis*) *giganteum* and *S. helianthus* serve as experimental tools to interfere with sodium and potassium channel function. The effects of sea anemone toxins are not restricted to the nervous system (3).

S. helianthus produces the 48-amino-acid ("long") polypeptide neurotoxin I (ShI), a compound that prolongs crayfish giant action potentials by slowing Na^+-channel inactivation selectively (10). ShI binds to voltage-gated sodium channels (5), is lethal to crutaceans, but is only moderately toxic to insects and nontoxic to mammals (10). Neurotoxin I has been synthesized (8) and several synthetic analogs have been produced (7). Anionic regions of Asp-6, Asp-7, and Glu-8 are largely responsible for neurotoxicity and binding to neuronal membrancs of crabs (7). The high-resolution structure of ShI has been determined in solution (12), and studies of structure–function relationships by limited proteolysis have shown the importance for biological activity of the protein surface near Asp-6, Asp-7, and Glu-8 (4).

Two K^+-channel toxins have been isolated from *S. helianthus*, the 35-amino-acid polypeptides ShKα (MW, 4069) and ShKβ (MW, 4054) (1,2). ShKα and ShKβ seem to block voltage-dependent K^+ channels in mammals, since they displace ^{125}I-dendrotoxin from rat brain synaptosomal membranes, partially suppress K^+ currents in cultured dorsal root ganglion cells from neonatal rats, and facilitate acetylcholine release at the chick neuromuscular junction (1). Several ShK analogs have been synthesized and their physico-chemical properties studied: these have been used to show that residue Lys22 is essential for ShK binding to rat brain K^+ channels of the Kv1.2 type (6,9,11).

The toxins described are detected in low concentrations in sea anemones and are unlikely to pose a risk for humans.

REFERENCES

1. Karlsson E, Aneiros A, Castaneda O *et al.* (1992) Potassium channel toxins from sea anemone. In: *Recent Advances in Toxinology Research. Vol. 2.* Gopalakrishnakone P, Tan CK eds. Venom and Toxin Research Group, National University of Singapore, Singapore, p. 378.

2. Kem WR, Parten B, Pennington MW *et al.* (1989) Isolation, characterization, and amino acid sequence of a polypeptide neurotoxin occurring in the sea anemone *Stichodactyla helianthus. Biochemistry* **28**, 3483.

3. Lazdunski M, Barhanin J, Fosset M *et al.* (1987) Polypeptide toxins as tools to study Na^+ channels and Ca^{2+} activated K^+ channels. In: *Neurotoxins and Their Pharmacological Implications.* Jenner P ed. Raven Press, New York p. 65.

4. Monks SA, Gould AR, Lumley PE *et al.* (1994) Limited proteolysis study of structure-function relationships in ShI, a polypeptide neurotoxin from a sea anemone. *Biochim Biophys Acta* **1207**, 93.

5. Norton RS (1991) Structure and structure-function relationships of sea anemone proteins that interact with the sodium channel. *Toxicon* **29**, 1051.

6. Pennington MW, Byrnes ME, Zaydenberg I *et al.* (1995) Chemical synthesis and characterization of ShK toxin: a potent potassium channel inhibitor from a sea anemone. *Int J Pept Protein Res* **46**, 354.

7. Pennington MW, Kem WR, Dunn BM (1990) Synthesis and biological activity of six monosubstituted analogs of a sea anemone polypeptide neurotoxin. *Polypep Res* **3**, 228.

8. Pennington MW, Kem WR, Norton RS, Dunn BM (1990) Chemical synthesis of a neurotoxic polypeptide from the sea anemone *Stichodactyla helianthus. J Pep Protein Res* **36**, 335.

9. Pennington MW, Mahnir VM, Krafte DS (1996) Identification of three separate binding sites on SHK toxin, a potent inhibitor of voltage-dependent potassium channels in human T-lymphocytes and rat brain. *Biochem Biophys Res Commun* **219**, 696.

10. Salgado VL, Kem WR (1992) Actions of three structurally distinct sea anemone toxins on crustacean and insect sodium channels. *Toxicon* **30**, 1365.

11. Tudor JE, Pennington MW, Norton RS (1998) Ionisation behaviour and solution properties of the potassium-channel blocker ShK toxin. *Eur J Biochem* **251**, 133.

12. Wilcox GR, Fogh RH, Norton RS (1993) Refined structure in solution of the sea anemone neurotoxin Sh I. *J Biol Chem* **268**, 24707.

Stipa robusta

Frank Bretschneider
Albert C. Ludolph

Sleepygrass

NEUROTOXICITY RATING

Clinical

B   Acute encephalopathy (horses) (stupor)

Stipa robusta (*Stipa vaseyi*, sleepygrass) produces a somnolent or stuporous condition in horses lasting up to several days. When fully recovered, no serious aftereffects have been observed; once poisoned, horses avoid eating the plant (1,4,5).

Sleepygrass is a perennial grass forming stout, erect clumps, 2–6 ft high, in dry plains, hills, and open woods from Colorado to Texas, Arizona, and Mexico, U.S.A. (4). It is consistently infected with a fungus that resembles *Acremonium chisosum* (6,9). The endophyte infection is known to increase productivity and stand persistence of grasses (3). Sleepygrass contains about 20 $\mu g/g$ lysergic acid amide in (dry weight), 8 $\mu g/g$ isolysergic amide, 0.3 $\mu g/g$ 8-hydroxylysergic acid amide, 7 $\mu g/g$ ergonovine, 15 $\mu g/g$ chanoclavine, and 18 $\mu g/g$ N-formylloline (6).

The consistent presence of an *Acremonium* endophyte on *Stipa robusta* suggests that the narcotic effects attributed to this species may be due to alkaloids produced by the fungus (2). The association between endophyte infection and toxicity in other *Stipa* species also supports a causal link in sleepygrass poisoning (9). It is estimated that a horse grazing on sleepygrass for a day (5 kg of fresh plant material) ingests about 47 mg of lysergic acid amide plus isolysergic amide, the dominant alkaloid constituents (6). The narcotic effects of endophyte-infected sleepygrass differ markedly from the effects produced by endophyte-infected tall fescue (*Festuca arundinacea*) (7,8,10), where concentrations of lysergic acid and isolysergic acid amides are much lower (approximately one-tenth those of sleepygrass) (7).

REFERENCES

1. Bailey V (1903) Sleepygrass and its effect on horses. *Science* 17, 392.
2. Clay K (1988) Fungal endophytes of grasses. A defensive mutualism between plants and fungi. *Ecology* 69, 10.
3. Joost RE (1995) *Acremonium* in fescue and ryegrass: Boon or bane? A review. *J Anim Sci* 73, 881.
4. Kingsbury JM (1964) *Poisonous Plants of the United States and Canada*. Prentice-Hall, New Jersey.
5. Marsh CD, Clawson AB (1929) Sleepygrass (*Stipa vaseyi*) as a stock-poisoning plant. *U.S. Dept Agricult Tech Bull* 114, 1.
6. Petroski RJ, Powell RG, Clay K (1992) Alkaloids of *Stipa robusta* (sleepygrass) infected with an *Acremonium* endophyte. *Nat Toxins* 1, 84.
7. Petroski RJ, Powell RG, Hedin PA (1991) Naturally occuring pest bioregulators. Symposium Series 449, *Amer Chem Soc* 426.
8. Petroski RJ, Yates SG, Weisleder D, Powell RG (1989) Isolation, semi-synthesis, and NMR spectral studies of loline alkaloids. *J Nat Prod* 52, 810.
9. White JF, Morgan-Jones G (1987) Endophyte-host associations in forage grasses. VII. *Acremonium chisosum*, a new species isolated from *Stipa eminens* in Texas. *Mycotaxon* 28, 179.
10. Yates SG, Powell RG (1988) Analysis of ergopeptine alkaloids in endophyte-infected tall fescue. *J Agr Food Chem* 36, 337.

Stonefish Venom

Albert C. Ludolph
Peter S. Spencer

NEUROTOXICITY RATING

Experimental

A   Neuromuscular transmission dysfunction (presynaptic neuromuscular blockade)

A   Myopathy (necrotizing)

The venom of the stonefish *Synanceja horrida* contains a toxic compound that targets the neuromuscular junction and, in higher concentrations, muscle. Species carrying the toxin, *Synanceja verrucosa*, *S. trachynis* and *S. horrida* (stonefish), inhabit the Indo-Pacific oceans and the Red Sea (4). Stonefish preferentially live in shallow waters near coral reefs where their colors provide camouflage. These venomous fish often lie buried in the sand and are easily stepped on (4). In comparison to the zebra fish (*Pterois* spp.), the number and disposition of venomous stings are similar, but the 13 dorsal spines of the stonefish are more robust and its integument is thicker (4). The genus *Inimicus* (*I. japonicus* and *I. cirrhosus*) causes similar, but less severe neurotoxic effects.

The venom of the stonefish is a colorless, clear, weakly acid fluid; its lethal fraction is nondialyzable and it loses toxicity at 4°C after 4–5 days (10). The intraperitoneal LD$_{50}$ for mice is reportedly 1.3–2.0 mg/kg body weight (9). Signs in mice include muscular incoordination, tremors, hindlimb paralysis, and respiratory distress (9). The venom remains potent up to 48 h after the death of the animal.

Stonustoxin (SNTx) is a lethal protein isolated from *S. horrida* venom; it also promotes the formation of membrane pores and causes hemolysis (2,3,7). The complete protein sequence of stonustoxin is known; it comprises two subunits, termed alpha and beta, that have molecular masses of 71 and 79 kDa, respectively (1,2,5). The LD$_{50}$ of SNTx in mice reportedly is 0.017 μg/g after intravenous (i.v.) administration (12). Animal studies using the fish venom show that it induces neuromuscular blockade and depolarization of cardiac, skeletal, and smooth muscle cells (11). Electrophysiological studies of murine and frog neuromuscular junction demonstrate that low concentrations (2.5–10 μg/ml) of the venom induce massive neurotransmitter release and presynaptic depletion of acetylcholine (10); this action requires the presence of Ca^{2+} or Mg^{2+} ions, but is independent of Na$^+$—similar to the effect of α-latrotoxin (10). At higher concentrations (100–300 μg/ml), stonefish venom reduces the resting membrane potential of muscle and also induces muscle damage; ultrastructurally, myofibrillar degeneration and mitochondrial damage become a prominent feature (10). In rat brain synaptosomes, stonefish venom also stimulates acetylcholine release and inhibits choline uptake (8). Other components and pharmacological properties of stonefish venom have been reviewed (6,13).

Stonefish stings are extremely painful. Shortly after envenomation, burning pain associated with local edema develops; the latter may affect the entire extremity and result in necrosis and ulceration. The intense pain reaches its peak within 1–2 h and may last a day. Secondary infections may occur. Systemic effects include diarrhea, nausea, vomiting, profuse sweating, local and generalized weakness, difficulty breathing, cardiac arrhythmia, hypotension, and syncope. Stonefish stings are rarely lethal; fatal outcomes in a few cases have been attributed to cardiotoxicity.

Treatment includes induction of local analgesia by lidocaine administration. Hot-water therapy (to inactivate the heat-labile toxin locally) is advocated by some. If necessary, antivenom should be diluted and administered slowly by an i.v. route. The decision to use antivenom depends upon the age of the patient (the younger, the earlier) and the number of stings. The effect is reportedly rapid, although there is no systematic evaluation of the efficacy of the antivenom.

REFERENCES

1. Cheah LS, Gwee MCE, Yuen R *et al.* (1992) Stonustoxin contracts the anococcygeus muscle and then inhibits adrenergic transmission prejunctionally. In: *Recent Advances in Toxinology Research. Vol. 2.* Gopalakrishnakone P, Tan CK eds. Venom and Toxin Research Group, National University of Singapore, Singapore p. 272.

2. Chen D, Kini RM, Yuen R, Khoo HE (1997) Haemolytic activity of stonustoxin from stonefish (*Synanceja horrida*) venom: pore formation and the role of cationic amino acid residues. *Biochem J* **325**, 685.

3. Ghadessy FJ, Chen D, Kini RM *et al.* (1996) Stonustoxin is a novel lethal factor from stonefish (*Synanceja horrida*) venom. cDNA cloning and characterization. *J Biol Chem* **271**, 25575.

4. Halstead BW (1970) *Poisonous and Venomous Marine Animals of the World. Vol. 3.* U.S. Government Printing Office, Washington, DC.

5. Hodgson WC (1997) Pharmacological action of Australian animal venoms. *Clin Exp Pharmacol Physiol* **24**, 10.

6. Hopkins BJ, Hodgson WC, Sutherland SK (1994) Pharmacological studies of stonefish (*Synanceja trachynis*) venom. *Toxicon* **32**, 1197.

7. Kechil AA, Gwee MCE, Low KSY *et al.* (1992) Modification of electric properties of identified central neurones of *Lymnaea* by stonustoxin. In: *Recent Advances in Toxinology Research. Vol 2.* Gopalakrishnakone P, Tan CK eds. Venom and Toxin Research Group, National University of Singapore, Singapore p. 279.

8. Khoo HE, Yuen R, Poh CH, Tan CH (1992) Biological activities of *Synanceja horrida* (stonefish) venom. *Nat Toxins* **1**, 54.

9. Kreger AS (1991) Detection of a cytolytic toxin in the venom of the stonefish (*Synanceia trachynis*). *Toxicon* **29**, 733.

10. Kreger AS, Molgo J, Comellea JX *et al.* (1993) Effects of stonefish (*Synanceia trachynis*) venom on murine and frog neuromuscular junctions. *Toxicon* **31**, 307.

11. Low K, Gwee SY, Yuen R (1990) Neuromuscular effects of the venom of the stonefish *Synanceja horrida*. *Eur J Pharmacol* **183**, 574.

12. Poh CH, Yuen R, Khoo HE *et al.* (1991) Purification and partial characterization of stonustoxin (lethal factor) from *Synanceja horrida* venom. *Comp Biochem Physiol* **99**, 793.

13. Sugahara K, Yamada S, Sugiura M *et al.* (1992) Identification of the reaction products of the purified hyaluronidase from stonefish (*Synanceja horrida*) venom. *Biochem J* **283**, 99.

Strychnine

Charles N. Allen

STRYCHNINE
$C_{21}H_{22}N_2O_2$

Strychnidin-10-one

NEUROTOXICITY RATING

Clinical

A   Seizure disorder (status epilepticus)

A   Muscle contraction (sustained)

Experimental

A   Inhibition of glycine receptor activity

A   Seizure disorder

A   Muscle contraction (sustained)

Strychnine, a naturally occurring toxic alkaloid first isolated from *Strychnos ignatti*, has been used as a poison for the control of vermin since the sixteenth century. Historically, strychnine was used as a stimulant in digestive and circulatory disorders (9). More recently, it has been used for the treatment of children with nonketotic hyperglycinemia (1,8). In the laboratory, strychnine has been used as an experimental tool to study glycine receptors in the brain and spinal cord and as a convulsant agent to model epileptiform activity (2,5,25,26). Strychnine is prepared commercially from *Strychnos nux-vomica* seeds, although a successful synthesis using tryptophan and phenylalanine as starting materials has been described (24).

Strychnine is readily absorbed from the stomach and from subcutaneous or intramuscular injection sites (14,17,23). After ingestion, strychnine appears very rapidly in the blood, is not bound to plasma proteins, and is rapidly cleared from the blood even following a massive oral dose (17). Although the CNS is the primary site of strychnine's toxicity, the liver (where the toxin may be stored) shows the highest concentration (15).

Strychnine is metabolized in the liver by cytochrome P-450 enzymes, in particular, CYP2B (7,19). The primary metabolites are 2-hydroxystrychnine, strychnine-21,22-epoxide, strychnine N-oxide, 11,12-dehydrostrychnine, and $21\alpha,22\alpha$-dihydroxy-22-hydrostrychnine (13). Induction of cytochrome P-450s by pentobarbital makes rats more tolerant to strychnine intoxication (11). Strychnine is also a potent inducer of CYP2B1 and 2B2 isoforms of cytochrome P-450s (7).

Approximately 10%–20% of a strychnine dose is excreted in the urine; the exact amount varies widely and depends on dosage (23).

Human intoxication with strychnine is primarily limited to accidental or self-induced ingestion of rodenticide compounds; use in an attempted homicide has also been reported (9,15–18,20). Strychnine is used in the manufacture of illegal drugs, and accidental poisoning has been linked with their usage (3,14). The lethal strychnine dose is between 50 and 100 mg, although deaths with 5–30 mg occur (15,18). Conversely, some have survived doses as high as 3.7 g (15,18).

Strychnine intoxication manifests initially with muscle spasms, particularly of the head and neck, and anxiety and restlessness (10,14,16,18,20). Subjects become hyperreflexic; and convulsions, triggered by loud noises or sudden movements, develop within 30 min (3,10,18). The number, duration, and severity of convulsions are the primary indicators of outcome; most do not survive more than five convulsions (18). Respiratory paralysis caused by contracture of the respiratory muscles is the usual cause of death (3,18).

The most urgent clinical goals are the maintenance of breathing and the prevention of convulsions. Gastric lavage with activated charcoal has been used to reduce toxin absorption (10,20). Intravenous diazepam, pentobarbital, or phenobarbital have been used to control convulsions (3,10,14). Neuromuscular blockade and artificial ventilation may be required when convulsions are uncontrollable (17,18). Treatment in a dark, quiet room reduces external stimuli that trigger seizure activity (14). Once convulsions are under control, treatment is focused on the severe lactic acidosis, rhabdomyolysis, and hyperthermia that are secondary to the convulsions (3). Patients recover from strychnine intoxication without apparent long-term sequelae.

Mechanisms underlying the toxicity of strychnine are well understood at both molecular and physiological levels. Neuronal excitation is elicited by blockade of inhibitory neurotransmission. Glycine acts as an inhibitory neurotransmitter in the CNS by binding to a high-affinity receptor that activates an integral chloride channel. Activation of this chloride channel tends to hyperpolarize neurons, reducing excitation. This has been most carefully studied in the spinal cord where Renshaw cells provide a glycine-mediated recurrent inhibition of spinal motor neurons (2,6).

Strychnine potently blocks this recurrent inhibition by antagonizing glycine-mediated activation of the chloride channel (4,5).

Strychnine is a competitive inhibitor of glycine receptor binding (25,26). However, strychnine and glycine bind to independent but overlapping sites on the receptor (21,22). Glycine receptors have been cloned and are members of a receptor superfamily that consists of γ-aminobutyric acid and nicotinic acetylcholine receptors. The glycine receptor is a multimer consisting of multiple copies of α- and β-subunits, which form a pentameric structure (12). Strychnine binds to the α-subunit at a site consisting of a lysine at position 200 and a tyrosine located at position 202 (22). The glycine binds to a threonine residue located at position 204 (22). The close physical apposition of these binding sites allows bound strychnine to block the glycine binding site by steric hindrance (22).

REFERENCES

1. Arneson D, Chien LT, Chance P, Wilroy RS (1979) Strychnine therapy in nonketotic hyperglycinemia. *Pediatrics* **63**, 369.

2. Belcher G, Davies J, Ryall RW (1976) Glycine-mediated inhibitory transmission of group 1A-excited inhibitory interneurones by Renshaw cells. *J Physiol-London* **256**, 651.

3. Boyd RE, Brennan PT, Deng J-F et al. (1983) Strychnine poisoning. Recovery from profound acidosis, hyperthermia, and rhabdomyolysis. *Amer J Med* **74**, 507.

4. Curtis DR, Duggan AW, Johnston GAR (1971) The specificity of strychnine as a glycine antagonist in the mammalian spinal cord. *Exp Brain Res* **12**, 547.

5. Curtis DR, Game CJA, Lodge D, McCulloch RM (1976) A pharmacological study of Renshaw cell inhibition. *J Physiol-London* **258**, 227.

6. Curtis DR, Hosli L, Johnston GAR, Johnston IH (1968) The hyperpolarization of spinal motoneurones by glycine and related amino acids. *Exp Brain Res* **5**, 235.

7. Fujisaki H, Mise M, Ishii Y et al. (1994) Strychnine and brucine as the potent inducers of drug metabolizing enzymes in rat liver: Different profiles from phenobarbital on the induction of cytochrome P450 and UDP-glucuronosyltransferase. *J Pharmacol Exp Ther* **268**, 1024.

8. Gitzelmann R, Steinmann B, Otten A et al. (1977) Nonketotic hyperglycinemia treated with strychnine, a glycine receptor antagonist. *Helv Paediat Acta* **32**, 517.

9. Jackson G, Diggle G (1973) Strychnine-containing tonics. *Brit Med J* **2**, 176.

10. Jackson G, Ng SH, Diggle GE, Bourke IG (1971) Strychnine poisoning treated successfully with diazepam. *Brit Med J* **3**, 519.

11. Kato R, Chiesara E, Vassanelli P (1962) Increased activity of microsomal strychnine-metabolizing enzyme induced by phenobarbital and other drugs. *Biochem Pharmacol* **11**, 913.

12. Langosch D, Becker C-M, Betz H (1990) The inhibitory glycine receptor: A ligand-gated chloride channel of the central nervous system. *Eur J Biochem* **194**, 1.

13. Mishima M, Tanimoto Y, Oguri K, Yoshimura H (1985) Metabolism of strychnine in vitro. *Drug Metab Disposition* **13**, 716.

14. O'Callaghan WG, Joyce N, Counihan HE et al. (1982) Unusual strychnine poisoning and its treatment: Report of eight cases. *Brit Med J* **285**, 478.

15. Perper JA (1985) Fatal strychnine poisoning—a case report and review of the literature. *J Forensic Sci* **30**, 1248.

16. Reardon M, Duane A, Cotter P (1993) Attempted homicide in hospital. *Irish J Med Sci* **162**, 315.

17. Sgaragli GP, Mannaioni PF (1973) Pharmacokinetic observations on a case of massive strychnine poisoning. *Clin Toxicol* **6**, 533.

18. Smith BA (1990) Strychnine poisoning. *J Emerg Med* **8**, 321.

19. Tanimoto Y, Kaneko H, Ohkuma T et al. (1991) Site-selective oxidation of strychnine by phenobarbital inducible cytochrome P-450. *J Pharmacobio-Dyn* **14**, 161.

20. Teitelbaum DT, Ott JE (1970) Acute strychnine intoxication. *Clin Toxicol* **3**, 267.

21. Vandenberg RJ, French CR, Barry PH et al. (1992) Antagonism of ligand-gated ion channel receptors: Two domains of the glycine receptor α subunit form the strychnine-binding site. *Proc Nat Acad Sci USA* **89**, 1765.

22. Vandenberg RJ, Handford CA, Schofield PR (1992) Distinct agonist- and antagonist-binding sites on the glycine receptor. *Neuron* **9**, 491.

23. Weiss S, Hatcher RA (1922) Studies on strychnine. *J Pharmacol Exp Ther* **6**, 419.

24. Woodward RB (1955) The total synthesis of strychnine. *Experientia* Suppl II, 213.

25. Young AB, Snyder SH (1973) Strychnine binding associated with glycine receptors of the central nervous system. *Proc Nat Acad Sci USA* **70**, 2832.

26. Young AB, Snyder SH (1974) Strychnine binding in rat spinal cord membranes associated with the synaptic glycine receptor: Cooperativity of glycine interactions. *Mol Pharmacol* **10**, 790.

Styrene

John L. O'Donoghue

STYRENE
C$_8$H$_8$

Ethenylbenzene; Vinylbenzene; Cinnamene; Cinnamol; Styrol; Styrolene; Styropol; Phenylethylene; Phenylethene

NEUROTOXICITY RATING

Clinical

A   Acute encephalopathy (CNS depression)

Experimental

A   Acute encephalopathy (CNS depression)

A   Ototoxicity (hair cell degeneration)

A   Olfactory toxicity (mucosal degeneration)

Styrene is a colorless to slightly yellow, oily liquid that spontaneously polymerizes unless inhibited. At low concentrations, it has a sweet odor; at concentrations above 100 ppm, it is objectionable. Styrene is widely used to make polystyrene, copolymers with acrylonitrile and butadiene, styrene polyesters, and other resins used for surface coatings. It is also used as a chemical intermediate. Styrene-containing polymers are used to make tires, boat hulls, shower stalls, bath tubs, dental restorative plastics, and many other plastic products. Styrene can be synthesized from benzene with ethylene, cumene, or 1-phenylethanol, but is also found naturally in storax, a gum derived from styracaceous trees. The primary exposures to styrene occur during its manufacture and polymerization, particularly in situations where open polymerization processes are used, for example in boat building or shower-stall manufacturing. Styrene is present in tobacco smoke and has been detected in ambient urban air samples.

Styrene has a low vapor pressure and is soluble in organic solvents, but only slightly soluble in water. While styrene is absorbed after oral, inhalation, or dermal exposure, the primary route of human exposure is *via* the lungs. Employees in jobs involving manual application of styrene to fiberglass-reinforced fabric may experience significant dermal exposure to liquid styrene while inhaling styrene vapor. The average retention of styrene in the respiratory tract following inhalation of 4.6–46 ppm was 71% for humans (47). Once absorbed, styrene is widely distributed in the body. Concentrations of styrene in the brain and liver of rats were similar (25 *vs.* 20 mg/dl extract) following exposure to ~2500 ppm (4-h LC$_{50}$) styrene vapor by inhalation (40).

The high lipid solubility of styrene leads to relatively rapid skin penetration and its sequestration in lipid-rich tissues (26).

The metabolism of styrene includes, as an initial step, oxidation of styrene by cytochrome P-450 enzymes to form styrene oxide or styrene-7,8-epoxide, which may be responsible for some of the toxic effects observed following styrene exposure. The major metabolic and detoxication pathway involving styrene oxide results in the formation of styrene glycol, followed by mandelic acid and phenylglycolic acid, which are often used as biological exposure indices. These latter two metabolites account for 85% and 10%, respectively, of the retained dose of styrene in humans (26). A minor detoxication pathway (~1% of dose), quantified in humans exposed to styrene *via* inhalation, involves conjugation of styrene oxide with glutathione *via* cytosolic glutathione-*S*-transferase followed by further transformation to mercapturic acid conjugates, which are excreted in the urine (14). 4-Vinyl phenol, which may be formed through a reactive arene oxide intermediate, is found as a minor (<0.3% of the amount of mandelic acid excreted) metabolite in human urine (33). Metabolism of styrene to 1-phenylethanol and 2-phenylethanol, and excretion of glucuronide conjugates of phenylaceturic acid in the urine, is reported in rats. Major detoxication pathways for styrene in this species include hippuric acid and glutathione metabolites. Styrene metabolism becomes saturated for humans and rodents at ~200 ppm (35).

Due to its relatively high lipid solubility, styrene may be retained in human fat for up to 5 weeks following exposure (11). The half-life of styrene in fat is 2.2–4 days for men exposed to 50 ppm styrene for 1 h (30 min rest plus 30 min exercise) (11).

In rats, the LC$_{50}$ after a 4-h exposure is ~2500–2700 ppm (20,42); a 2-h LC$_{50}$ of ~4900 ppm is reported for mice (40). Rats and guinea pigs exposed to a ~2500 ppm styrene vapor became weak and uncoordinated, and then developed tremors and coma after 10–12 h of exposure (41). At 5000 ppm, animals were weak and unsteady immediately upon exposure to the vapor, and often had seizures (41).

Subchronic and chronic experimental studies with styrene have not clearly identified neurotoxic effects in animals beyond those effects that can be attributed to CNS depression (1,2,7,30,41). Exposure of rats to 100 or 200 mg/kg/day styrene by oral gavage for 14 days did not alter spontaneous locomotor activity, learning ability, or brain concentrations of dopamine or noradrenalin (19). Improved learning (increased conditioned avoidance response) was correlated with increased serotonin levels (200 mg/kg group) in the hypothalamus, hippocampus, and midbrain of rats given 200 mg/kg styrene (19). The effects of styrene on spontaneous motor activity in the rat were examined (16); 8 h following an 8-h exposure to 325 ppm styrene vapor, spontaneous motor activity was reduced. At 349 ppm for 8 h, a reduction in motor activity was also seen 8 h following exposure, but the animals appeared to adapt to the exposure and, on repeated exposures, 985 ppm was required to decrease activity levels. The reduced activity levels may have been due to increased grooming, which interrupted the animals' normal motor activity levels, rather than a CNS effect.

Subchronic neurotoxicity was studied at multiple time points in rats exposed to 0, 350, 700, or 1400 ppm styrene vapor for 16 h/day, 5 days/week for 18 months and following a 6-week postexposure period (25). No effects were observed on coordinated limb movements or tail-nerve conduction velocity. While slight differences were observed for hindlimb grip strength, no consistent or long-lasting effect was detected. During the earlier part of the 18-week exposure period, spontaneous activity was increased for the lower exposure concentration and decreased for the 1400 ppm group, but these effects were not observed during the last week of the study or during the postexposure period. Performance (speed and accuracy) on a visual discrimination task was reduced during the early portion of the exposure period, but not during later time periods, suggesting development of tolerance. No significant subchronic neurotoxic effects were observed.

Rats exposed to 300 ppm styrene for 6 h/day, 5 days/week were reported to have a decrease in tail nerve motor conduction velocity after 6 weeks of exposure, but not after 8 or 11 weeks of exposure (38). Rats and mice exposed to 200–1500 ppm or 50–200 ppm, respectively, of styrene vapor 6 h/day, 5 days/week for 13 weeks did not show microscopic lesions in the sciatic nerve or brain (10). Degeneration of the olfactory mucosa was present at all exposure concentrations in mice and in rats exposed to 500–1500 ppm. Mice were more affected than rats, not only because olfactory changes were observed at lower concentration levels, but because mortality, liver toxicity, and lung toxicity were also observed. While the olfactory epithelium was differentially affected as compared to the respiratory epithelium in the nasal mucosa, it is unclear whether this is due to a specific neurotoxic effect or due to the configuration of the nasal cavity and air flow through the nasal cavity. Styrene vapor at the concentration used in these studies was irritating to the eyes and respiratory system.

Ototoxicity as measured by auditory brainstem and conditioned avoidance responses has been reported in weanling rats exposed to 800, 1000, or 1200 ppm styrene vapor for 14 h/day, 7 days/week for 3 weeks (34). The functional changes occurring at 800 ppm under this exposure paradigm have been correlated with morphological changes, including missing outer hair cells in the basal and lower middle turns of the organ of Corti (48). Ototoxicity has also been observed in rats exposed to 800 ppm, 6 h/day for 13 weeks; ototoxicity was not observed at 50 or 200 ppm exposure levels (1).

Glial fibrillary acidic protein (GFAP) levels were increased in the hippocampus and sensory motor cortex of rats exposed to 320 ppm styrene vapor continuously for 3 months followed by a 4-month waiting period (37). GFAP levels in several other areas of the brain were not affected by this exposure. S-100 protein levels in the brain, brain weight, and regional brain weight were not affected by the exposure. No GFAP effects were observed at 90 ppm styrene.

The effects of styrene on postnatal development in protein-deficient and normal-diet-fed female rats were studied by dosing orally with 250 mg/kg from postnatal day 21 to day 51 (22). Styrene when given alone did not affect amphetamine-induced motor activity levels, but when combined with the low-protein diet, activity levels were increased. Foot-shock-induced aggressive behavior was slight, but not significantly higher in styrene-exposed rats, but protein deficiency especially when combined with styrene significantly increased aggressive behavior in the rats. Styrene-exposed rats also had reduced dopamine levels in the brain; binding to dopamine receptors in the corpus striatum and serotonin levels in the frontal cortex were unchanged. Dopamine, serotonin, and norepinephrine levels in the brain were reduced in styrene-exposed, protein-deficient rats. Binding to dopamine receptors in the corpus striatum and serotonin receptors in the frontal cortex was increased in styrene-exposed, protein-deficient rats. Because styrene exposure to protein-deficient rats, but not to normal-diet rats, reduced body weight more than protein deficiency alone, it is unclear whether the effects observed are a consequence of styrene exposure or the additional reduction in body-weight increase observed in styrene-exposed rats.

Reduced levels of serotonin, 5-hydroxyindolacetic acid, and homovanillic acid were measured in the cerebellum of day-old rat pups exposed in utero during days 7–21 of gestation to 300 ppm (6 h) styrene (24). Similar effects were not observed when the exposure concentration was reduced to 50 ppm. The protein levels in pup brain, pup and maternal brain weights, and pup and maternal histology were not altered at 50 or 300 ppm styrene. Preliminary neurobehavioral tests indicated that at 300 ppm, postnatal open-field behavior was altered, motor activity was increased, and neurobehavioral development was delayed, but learning was not impaired (23). At 50 ppm, disturbances in coordination were observed as well as delays in reflex development (23). By postnatal day 120, no significant differences were present.

The acute effects of styrene on human volunteers (31) are consistent with the acute effects observed in animals. At <10 ppm, its odor is not detected. Between 50 and 100 ppm, styrene has a strong odor that is not objectionable. At 100 ppm, transient eye irritation may be observed, but tests of coordination and dexterity are unaffected. Reaction time is impaired at exposures of 350 ppm for 30 min, but perceptual speed and manual dexterity are unaffected. At 376 ppm for 25 min, performance on the Romberg test is impaired. At 800 ppm for a few hours, styrene is reported to cause listlessness, drowsiness, and impaired balance that lasts beyond the exposure period. Workplace exposures at >100 ppm styrene have resulted in the observation of similar acute effects (43).

Reports of clinically evident neurological disease among styrene workers are uncommon (3,15,30). In general, the neurotoxicology literature for styrene consists of reports of subclinical effects among boat builders. The effects include changes in self-reported symptoms, psychomotor function, color vision, vestibular function, somatosensory evoked potentials, and nerve conduction velocity (2,4–6,8,12,13,17, 21,27,28,32,39,42,44,45,49). The absence of clinical and neurobehavioral effects and nerve conduction changes following chronic workplace exposures has also been reported (43,44). The clinical literature, while fairly voluminous, does not allow conclusions about chronic neurotoxicity, particularly at levels recommended for workplace exposure, which are generally in the range of 20–50 ppm (1,36). Workplace studies have not taken into account the pharmacokinetics of styrene; at most, the delay between the time workers were tested and their last workplace exposure to styrene is a weekend. As the half-life of styrene in body fat is 2–4 days, many of the studies do not provide data that can distinguish between the acute and chronic effects of styrene. Many of the studies use urinary metabolites of styrene as an index of exposure; however, in doing so, they ignore the typical exposure conditions in working with reinforced plastics that can result in peak exposures that are considerably higher than the average exposure level. The groups examined included individuals who worked in many different small-boat-building shops where exposure to relatively high styrene levels and concurrent inhalation and dermal exposures are likely to have occurred. Workplace exposure conditions, including the level of styrene exposure and the presence of other chemicals, is typically not available. This is particularly important because boat building can involve the use of many different materials including paints, solvents, and adhesives. The clean-up procedures to remove excess styrene from equipment and body surfaces, if protective equipment is not worn, may include neurotoxic solvents such as n-hexane and gasoline. Many of the styrene workplace studies are hypothesis-generating studies with different statistical end points; such analytical processes are expected to generate a significant number of false-positive results unless steps are taken to control for statistical errors. Thus, the present database for styrene is inadequate to conclude that chronic low-level exposure to styrene provides a significant neurotoxic risk.

One report identifies two cases of CNS defects (single cases of hydrocephalus and anencephaly) among children of women who had worked in the reinforced plastics industry (18). A second case of anencephaly, whose mother had exposure to plastic resins in her home, was also noted. None of these cases provides a causal link between styrene exposure and birth defects; no similar cases have been described in the 20 years since publication of the original cases.

Cancer bioassays and epidemiology studies have been conducted with styrene (1,9). None of these studies has identified the nervous system as a target tissue; if there is a cancer risk associated with styrene exposure, it is quite small (9). An international cohort study using historical data collected for a cancer mortality study found that in a population of 35,443 employees compared to a World Health Organization mortality databank, mortality was lower in styrene-exposed workers primarily due to deficits in deaths due to cancer, respiratory disease, and cardiovascular disease (46). Deaths due to PNS and CNS diseases were lower than expected; deaths due to mental disorders were as expected. While the authors concluded that styrene exposure may contribute to chronic disease of the nervous system based on trends toward increased mortality to CNS disease (especially epilepsy), with increased exposure levels, the actual number of deaths involved and the differences in incidence rates were small and unimpressive.

In both animals and humans, styrene exposure at sufficiently high levels produces CNS depression. Animal studies also indicate that styrene may alter brain neurochemistry, although the pattern of effects is not well understood. The only long-lasting reproducible effect observed in animal studies is ototoxicity; similar effects have not been clearly demonstrated for humans (5,29). Exposures to styrene at ambient levels in the environment and industrial situations other than the reinforced plastics industry, particularly boat-building shops, have not been associated with long-lasting effects in humans. In spite of the large number of studies of workers in the boat-building industry, it is not clear that the effects reported are more than acute effects. The American Conference of Governmental Industrial Hygienists has recommended a Time-Weighted Threshold-Limit Value of 50 ppm with a Short-Term Exposure Limit of 100 ppm based on the reports of human CNS and PNS changes in the boat-building industry (1). Occupational exposure limits of 20 ppm with short-term excursion limits of 40 ppm and 50 ppm have been set for Germany and Sweden, respectively (1).

The mechanism(s) of styrene's effects on the nervous system is not known. It is likely that the effects of high-level, acute exposure are due to styrene itself, as they appear shortly after exposure and prior to significant metabolism of the parent compound. However, it is unclear if the parent compound or metabolites are neurotoxic at lower exposure levels. Due to its potential reactivity, styrene oxide is an obvious candidate metabolite for concern; its potential reactivity has implications for genotoxicity and carcinogenicity for styrene, although neither animal studies nor human epidemiology studies have validated these concerns to date (1,9).

REFERENCES

1. American Conference of Governmental Industrial Hygienists (1992). Styrene, Monomer. In: *Documentation of the Threshold Limit Values Vol III*. Ed 6. Cincinnati, Ohio p. 1436.
2. Arlien-Søborg P (1992) Styrene In: *Solvent Neurotoxicity*. CRC Press, Boca Raton, Florida p. 129.
3. Behari M, Choudhary C, Roy S *et al.* (1986) Styrene-induce peripheral neuropathy. *Eur Neurol* 25, 424.
4. Bergamaschi E, Smargiassi A, Mutti A *et al.* (1997) Peripheral markers of catecholaminergic dysfunction and symptoms of neurotoxicity among styrene-exposed workers. *Int Arch Occup Environ Health* 69, 209.
5. Calabrese G, Martini A, Sessa G *et al.* (1996) Otoneurological study in workers exposed to styrene in the fiberglass industry. *Int Arch Occup Environ Health* 68, 219.
6. Campagna D, Gobba F, Mergler D *et al.* (1996) Color vision loss among styrene-exposed workers neurotoxicological threshold assessment. *NeuroToxicology* 17, 362.
7. Cavender F (1994) Aromatic hydrocarbons. In: *Patty's Industrial Hygiene and Toxicology. Vol II. Part B. 4th Ed.* Clayton GD, Clayton FE eds. John Wiley, New York p. 1301.
8. Cherry N, Gautrin D (1990) Neurotoxic effects of styrene: further evidence. *Brit J Ind Med* 47, 29.
9. Coggon D (1994) Epidemiological studies of styrene-exposed population. *Crit Rev Toxicol* 24, S107.
10. Cruzan G, Cushman JR *et al.* (1997) Subchronic inhalation studies of styrene in CD rats and CD-1 mice. *Fund Appl Toxicol* 35, 152.
11. Engstrom J (1978) Styrene in subcutaneous adipose tissue after experimental and industrial exposure. *Scand J Work Environ Health* 4, 119.
12. Edling C, Anundi H, Johanson G, Nilsson K (1993) Increase in neuropsychiatric symptoms after occupational exposure to low levels of styrene. *Brit J Ind Med* 50, 843.
13. Fallas C, Fallas J, Maslard P, Dally S (1992) Subclinical impairment of colour vision among workers exposed to styrene. *Brit J Ind Med* 49, 679.
14. Ghittori S, Maestri L, Imbriani M *et al.* (1997) Urinary excretion of specific mercapturic acids in workers exposed to styrene. *Amer J Ind Med* 31, 636.
15. Gobba F, Cavalleri F, Bontadi D *et al.* (1995) Peripheral neuropathy in styrene-exposed workers. *Scand J Work Environ Health* 21, 517.
16. Gut I (1968) Some effects of styrene on the rat. *Cesk Hyg* 13, 27.
17. Härkönen H, Lindström K, Seppäläinen AM *et al.* (1978) Exposure-response relationship between styrene exposure and central nervous functions. *Scand J Work Environ Health* 4, 53.
18. Holmberg PC (1977) Central nervous defects in two children of mothers exposed to chemicals in the reinforced plastics industry. *Scand J Work Environ Health* 3, 212.
19. Husain R, Srivastava SP, Seth PK (1985) Some behavioral effects of early styrene intoxication in experimental animals. *Arch Toxicol* 57, 53.
20. Jaeger RJ, Conolley RB, Murphy SD (1974) Toxicity and biochemical changes in rats after inhalation exposure to 1,1-dichloroethylene, bromobenzene, styrene, acrylonitrile, or 2-chlorobutadiene. *Toxicol Appl Pharmacol* 29, 81.
21. Jégaden D, Amann D, Simon JF *et al.* (1993) Study of the neurobehavioural toxicity of styrene at low levels of exposure. *Int Arch Occup Environ Health* 64, 527.
22. Khanna VK, Husain R, Seth PK (1994) Effect of protein malnutrition on the neurobehavioural toxicity of styrene in young rats. *J Appl Toxicol* 14, 351.
23. Kishi R, Chen BQ, Katakura Y, *et al.* (1995) Effects of prenatal exposure to styrene on the neurobehavioral development, activity, motor coordination, and learning behavior of rats. *Neurotoxicol Teratol* 17, 121.
24. Kishi R, Katakura Y, Ikeda T *et al.* (1992) Neurochemical effects in rats following gestational exposure to styrene. *Toxicol Lett* 63, 141.
25. Kulig BM (1988) The neurobehavioral effects of chronic styrene exposure in the rat. *Neurotoxicol Teratol* 10, 511.
26. Leibman KC (1975) Metabolism and toxicity of styrene. *Environ Health Perspect* 11, 115.
27. Lindström K, Härkönen H, Hernberg S (1976) Disturbances in psychological functions of workers occupationally exposed to styrene. *Scand J Work Environ Health* 2, 129.
28. Matikainen E, Forsman-Grönholm L, Pfäffli P, Juntunen J (1993) Nervous system effects of occupational exposure

to styrene: A clinical and neurophysiological study. *Environ Res* **61**, 84.

29. Muijser H, Hoogendijk EMG, Hoosima J (1988) The effects of occupational exposure to styrene on high-frequency hearing thresholds. *Toxicology* **49**, 331.

30. NIOSH (1983) *Criteria for a Recommended Standard: Occupational Exposure to Styrene*. Dept Health Hum Serv, U.S. Natl Inst Occup Safety Health Publication No. 83-119.

31. O'Donoghue JL (1985) Aromatic Hydrocarbons. In: *Neurotoxicity of Industrial and Commercial Chemicals. Vol II*. O'Donoghue JL ed. CRC Press, Boca Raton, Florida p. 127.

32. Pahwa R, Kalra J (1993) A critical review of the neurotoxicity of styrene in humans. *Vet Human Toxicol* **35**, 516.

33. Pfaffli P, Hesso A, Vaino H et al. (1981) 4-Vinylphenol excretion suggestive of arene oxide formation in workers occupationally exposed to styrene. *Toxicol Appl Pharmacol* **60**, 85.

34. Pryor GT, Rebert CD, Howd RA (1987) Hearing loss in rats caused by inhalation of mixed xylenes and styrene. *J Appl Toxicol* **7**, 55.

35. Ramsey JC, Andersen ME (1984) A physiologically based description of the inhalation pharmacokinetics of styrene in rats and humans. *Toxicol Appl Pharmacol* **73**, 159.

36. Rebert CS, Hall TA (1994) The neuroepidemiology of styrene: A critical review of representative literature. *Crit Rev Toxicol* **24**, S57.

37. Rosengren LE, Haglid KG (1989) Long term neurotoxicity of styrene. A quantitative study of glial fibrillary acidic protein (GFA) and S-100. *Brit J Ind Med* **46**, 316.

38. Seppäläinen AM (1978) Neurotoxicity of styrene in occupational and experimental exposure. *Scand J Work Environ Health* **4**, 181.

39. Seppäläinen AM, Härkönen H (1976) Neurophysiological findings among workers occupationally exposed to styrene. *Scand J Work Environ Health* **2**, 140.

40. Shugaev BB (1969) Concentrations of hydrocarbons in tissues as a measure of toxicity. *Arch Environ Health* **18**, 878.

41. Spencer HC, Irish DD, Adams EM et al. (1942) The response of animals to monomeric styrene. *J Ind Hyg Toxicol* **24**, 295.

42. Stetkároá I, Urban P, Procházka B, Lukás E (1993) Somatosensory evoked potentials in workers exposed to toluene and styrene. *Brit J Ind Med* **50**, 520.

43. Triebig G, Lehrl S, Weltle D et al. (1989) Clinical and neurobehavioral study of the acute and chronic neurotoxicity of styrene. *Brit J Ind Med* **46**, 799.

44. Triebig G, Schaller KH, Valentin H (1985) Investigations on neurotoxicity of chemical substances at the workplace —VII. Longitudinal study with determination of nerve conduction velocities in persons occupationally exposed to styrene. *Int Arch Occup Environ Health* **56**, 239.

45. Tsai S-Y, Chen JD (1996) Neurobehavioral effects of occupational exposure to low level styrene. *Neurotoxicol Teratol* **18**, 463.

46. Welp E, Kogevinas M, Andersen A et al. (1996) Exposure to styrene and mortality from nervous system diseases and mental disorders. *Amer J Epidemiol* **144**, 623.

47. Wieczorek H, Piotrowski J (1985) Evaluation of low exposure to styrene. I. Absorption of styrene vapors by inhalation under experimental conditions. *Int Arch Occup Environ Health* **57**, 57.

48. Yano BL, Dittenber DA, Albee RR, Mattsson JL (1992) Abnormal auditory brainstem responses and cochlear pathology in rats induced by an exaggerated styrene exposure regimen. *Toxicol Pathol* **20**, 1.

49. Yuasa J, Kishi R, Eguchi T et al. (1996) Study of urinary mandelic acid concentration and peripheral nerve conduction among styrene workers. *Amer J Ind Med* **30**, 41.

Succinylcholine

Phyllis L. Bieri

$$[(H_3C)_3{}^+N-CH_2CH_2-O-CO-CH_2CH_2-CO-O-CH_2CH_2-N^+(CH_3)_3] \; 2Cl^-$$

SUCCINYLCHOLINE CHLORIDE
$C_{14}H_{30}Cl_2N_2O_4$

Suxamethonium chloride

NEUROTOXICITY RATING

Clinical

A Neuromuscular transmission syndrome

Experimental

A Neuromuscular transmission dysfunction (postsynaptic
depolarizing neuromuscular blockade)

Succinylcholine is a primary example of a neuromuscular blocking agent that exerts its effects by depolarizing the postsynaptic membrane. It is widely used in general anesthesia, providing rapid muscular paralysis that is readily reversible. The advantages of neuromuscular blockade in general anesthesia have been known since the 1940s, when it became clear that lower doses of generalized anesthetic could be employed if concomitant muscle relaxation was achieved. Similarly, postanesthetic recovery periods are shorter when adjuvant neuromuscular blockade is used.

The depolarizing neuromuscular blocking agents include succinylcholine and decamethonium. They belong to the chemical class of dicholine esters and are characterized by a flexible chain structure that enables variable distances between quaternary groups (12). Of the two compounds, succinylcholine remains the most commonly used in general anesthesia.

Succinylcholine produces muscle paralysis with a very short time of onset as well as duration of action. Mean time of onset is 1.0–1.5 min, with a duration of action of 6–8 min. Drug clearance occurs with rapid hydrolysis by butyrylcholinesterase of the liver and plasma; therefore, therapeutic doses are generally given *via* continuous intravenous infusion.

Succinylcholine initially depolarizes the postjunctional membrane by opening membrane ion channels similarly to acetylcholine. However, the depolarization lasts longer because succinylcholine is resistant to acetylcholinesterase. This initially prolonged period of depolarization is associated with transient muscle fasciculations. The second phase of action is accompanied by flaccid neuromuscular paralysis and is potentiated by anticholinesterase agents. In contrast to the stabilizing neuromuscular blockers of the curare class, depolarizing neuromuscular blockade causes persistent depolarization of both the end plate and the immediately adjacent area of sarcoplasmic reticulum (2).

The depolarizing agents initially function as partial agonists at the end plate, as the probability of channel opening from drug-receptor binding is less than that with acetylcholine (5). Once higher drug concentrations are achieved, the membrane channels are blocked directly, thus impairing ion permeability (1).

Prolonged depolarization of muscle cells can cause extensive K^+ efflux, with Na^+, Cl^-, and Ca^{2+} influx. The degree of K^+ loss can be life threatening in patients with extensive soft tissue injuries. Patients at risk include those with burns, rhadomyolysis, spinal cord injuries, and muscular dystrophies. Those with genetic polymorphisms of plasma cholinesterase experience prolonged neuromuscular blockade due to reduced rates of succinylcholine destruction. Occasionally cardiovascular effects occur. These are most likely due to stimulation of vagal ganglia, causing bradycardia, and sympathetic ganglia, which causes hypertension and tachycardia (12).

In rats, neuromuscular blockade induced by depolarizing agents is potentiated by the histamine H_2 receptor antagonists, including ranitidine (8). Similarly, the duration of neuromuscular block is increased when anticholinesterase agents are administered following succinylcholine (13). The transient jaw muscle contractures observed after succinylcholine administration is dependent on body temperature; they increase with increasing temperature of the jaw area in rats simultaneously given inhalation anesthetics (10).

Drug-induced muscle depolarization is associated with transient muscle fasciculations, particularly over the chest and abdomen. The duration and severity of muscle fasciculations can be attenuated by pretreatment with alfentanil. In the second phase of drug action, paralysis progresses from the neck to the arms and legs, sparing bulbar musculature initially. After a single intravenous bolus, muscle paralysis becomes maximal within 2 min and disappears within 5 min. The degree and duration of muscle relaxation can therefore by adjusted by changing the concentration and rate of continuous intravenous infusion.

Postoperative myalgias can be clinically significant following succinylcholine use. Pretreatment with phenytoin significantly reduced myalgias, as well as the duration and mean intensity of fasciculations (3). Other agents that have been found successful in treating the myalgias include propofol, diclofenac, and atracurium (4,6,7).

A rare cause of death from anesthesia is malignant hyperthermia, which can be triggered by depolarizing neuromuscular blockers and by inhalation anesthetics. Malignant hyperthermia results from excessive release of Ca^{2+} from the sarcoplasmic reticulum; it appears to be associated with mutations in the Ca^{2+}-release channel, known as the ryanodine receptor (9). Clinical features of malignant hyperthermia include tachycardia, hyperthermia, metabolic acidosis, and widespread muscle rigidity. Patients with central core disease are also at risk for malignant hyperthermia, possibly due to allelic variations in the ryanodine receptor gene in both conditions (14). Malignant hyperthermia is treated with rapid cooling and dantroline infusion, which blocks Ca^{2+} release from the sarcoplasmic reticulum, thereby reducing heat production and muscle tone (11). Metabolic acidosis must also be controlled and treated.

REFERENCES

1. Adams PR, Sakmann B (1978) Decamethonium both opens and blocks endplate channels. *Proc Nat Acad Sci USA* 75, 2994.
2. Burns BD, Paton WDM (1951) Depolarization of the motor end-plate by decamethonium and acetylcholine. *J Physiol-London* 115, 41.
3. Hatta V, Saxena A, Kaul HL (1992) Phenytoin reduces suxamethonium-induced myalgia. *Anaesthesiology* 47, 664.
4. Kahraman S, Ercan S, Aypar U, Erdem K (1993) Effect of preoperative i.m. administration of diclofenac on suxamethonium-induced myalgia. *Brit J Anaesth* 71, 238.
5. Katz B, Miledi R (1978) A re-examination of curare action at the motor end plate. *Proc Roy Soc London* 203, 119.
6. Leeson-Payne CG, Nicoll JM, Hobbs GJ (1994) Use of ketorolac in the prevention of suxamethonium myalgia. *Brit J Anaesth* 73, 788.
7. McClymont C (1994) A comparison of the effect of propofol or thiopentone on the incidence and severity of suxamethonium-induced myalgia. *Anaesth Intensive Care* 22, 147.
8. Mishra Y, Ramzan I (1993) Interaction between succinylcholine and ranitidine in rats. *Can J Anaesth* 41, 32.
9. Otsu K, Nishida K, Kimura Y *et al.* (1994) The point mutation Arg615-Cys in the Ca^{2+} release channel of skeletal sarcoplasmic reticulum is responsible for hypersensitivity to caffeine and halothane in malignant hyperthermia. *J Biol Chem* 269, 9413.
10. Shi Y, Keykhah MM, Storella RJ, Rosenberg H (1995) Effect of different volatile anaesthetics on suxamethonium-induced jaw muscle contracture in rats. *Brit J Anaesth* 74, 712.
11. Strazis KP, Fox AW (1993) Malignant hyperthermia: A review of published cases. *Anesth Analg* 77, 297.
12. Taylor P (1996) Agents acting at the neuromuscular junction and autonomic ganglia. In: *The Pharmacological Basis of Therapeutics. 9th Ed.* Hardman JG, Limbird LE, Gilman AG eds. McGraw-Hill, New York p. 177.
13. Valdrighi JB, Fleming NW, Smith BK *et al.* (1994) Effects of cholinesterase inhibitors on the neuromuscular blocking action of suxamethonium. *Brit J Anaesth* 72, 237.
14. Zang Y, Chen HS, Khanna VK *et al.* (1993) A mutation in the human ryanodine receptor gene associated with central core disease. *Nat Genet* 5, 46.

Sulfasalazine

Herbert H. Schaumburg

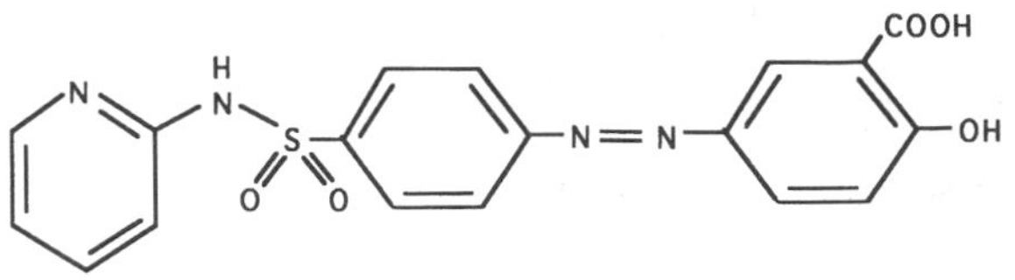

SULFASALAZINE
$C_{18}H_{14}N_4O_5S$

2-Hydroxy-5-[[4-[(2-pyridinylamino)sulfonyl] phenyl]azo]benzoic acid

NEUROTOXICITY RATING
Clinical
B   Peripheral neuropathy

Sulfasalazine (salicylazosulfapyridine) represents the combination of two distinctly different drugs, sulfapyridine and 5-aminosulfasalicylic acid, that are linked by a covalent bond. Sulfasalazine has been widely used for decades for the amelioration of inflammatory bowel diseases; it is also used in the treatment of rheumatoid arthritis. Orally administered sulfasalazine is rapidly cleaved by intestinal bacteria into the two component drugs. The 5-aminosalicylic acid component remains in the bowel and is locally active as an anti-inflammatory agent at the superficial ulcerated lesions. The sulfapyridine component is absorbed into the blood; it has two potential immunosuppressive actions that may account for its effects on rheumatoid arthritis: impairment of lymphocyte transformation and suppression of the activity of natural killer cells.

The sulfapyridine component is responsible for most of the systemic toxic effects of sulfasalazine. These reactions occur most commonly in individuals with a slow-acetylator phenotype who have higher serum concentrations of sulfapyridine. Dose-related, reversible side effects include gastrointestinal intolerance, headache, malaise, arthralgia, drug fever, male infertility, and Heinz-body anemia. Idiosyncratic, presumably hypersensitivity-mediated, reactions are also ascribed to sulfapyridine, including skin rashes, hepatotoxicity, pulmonary fibrosis, agranulocytosis, and a lupus-like syndrome.

Two preliminary reports described sulfasalazine-induced suppression of canine experimental encephalomyelitis and suggested a potential therapeutic use in multiple sclerosis (6,7). This interest was subsequently tempered by the development of multiple sclerosis in a patient receiving sulfasalazine therapy (2) and a recent study that demonstrated enhancement of experimental autoimmune encephalomyelitis in the Lewis rat (1).

Reports of human neurotoxicity associated with sulfasalazine use have depicted multifocal CNS disease (scattered lesions in meninges, cortex, subcortical white matter, and spinal cord) occurring in concert with hypersensitivity dermatitis and hepatitis (3–5,8,9,10). These instances likely reflect a diffuse, CNS hypersensitivity angiitis-type reaction to sulfapyridine. Most have recovered following drug withdrawal and corticosteroid therapy.

There is one report of reversible peripheral neuropathy in a patient treated with sulfasalazine (5) and another in an individual receiving the 5-aminosalicylic acid (mesalamine) component of sulfasalazine (11). Neither instance is documented with thorough electrophysiological examination, and histopathological studies are not described. It is suggested that both reflect toxicity from 5-aminosulfasalicylic acid (11).

REFERENCES

1. Correale J, Olsson T, Bjork J et al. (1991) Sulfasalazine aggravates experimental autoimmune encephalomyelitis and causes an increase in the number of autoreactive T cells. *J Neuroimmunol* **34**, 109.
2. Gold R, Kappa L, Becker T (1990) Development of multiple sclerosis in a patient on long-term sulfasalazine. *Lancet* **335**, 409.
3. Merrin P, Williams IA (1991) Meningitis associated with sulfasalazine in a patient with Sjögren's syndrome and polyarthritis. *Ann Rheumatol Dis* **50**, 645.
4. Olenginski TP, Harrington TM, Carlson JP (1991) Transverse myelitis secondary to sulfasalazine. *J Rheumatol* **18**, 304.
5. Price TR (1985) Sensorimotor neuropathy with sulfasalazine. *Postgrad Med J* **61**, 147.
6. Prosiegel M, Neu I, Mallinger J et al. (1989) Suppression of experimental autoimmune encephalomyelitis by dual cyclooxygenase and 5-lipoxygenase inhibition. *Acta Neurol Scand* **79**, 223.
7. Prosiegel M, Neu I, Rutherstoth-Bauer G et al. (1989) Suppression of experimental autoimmune encephalomyelitis by sulfasalazine. *N Engl J Med* **321**, 545.
8. Schoonjans R, Mast A, Van Den G et al. (1993) Sulfasalazine-associated encephalopathy in a patient with Crohn's disease. *Amer J Gastroenterol* **88**, 1416.
9. Smith MD, Gibson GE, Rowland R (1982) Combined hepatotoxicity and neurotoxicity following sulfasalazine administration. *Austr N Z J Med* **12**, 80.
10. Wallace IW (1970) Neurotoxicity associated with a reaction to sulfasalazine. *Practitioner* **204**, 850.
11. Woodward DK (1989) Peripheral neuropathy and mesalazine. *Brit Med J* **299**, 1224.

Sulfonamides

Steven Herskovitz

SULFANILAMIDE
$C_6H_8N_2O_2S$

4-Aminobenzenesulfonamide; Sulfanilamide

NEUROTOXICITY RATING

Clinical

B   Peripheral neuropathy

B   Acute encephalopathy (hallucinations, delirium)

B   Aseptic meningitis

Experimental

B   Peripheral neuropathy

The sulfonamides, derivatives of 4-aminobenzenesulfonamide, were the first effective antimicrobial agents to be employed systemically for the treatment of human bacterial infections (5). They have a wide range of activity against Gram-positive and Gram-negative bacteria. Their mechanism of action is based on structural analogs and competitive antagonism of *p*-aminobenzoic acid. The earliest preparations included sulfapyridine, sulfadiazine, sulfathiazole, and sulfanilamide; aside from sulfadiazine, they are no longer in general use. Newer compounds, including sulfisoxazole, sulfamethoxazole, sulfametrol, sulfacytine, and sulfamethizole, are more soluble, less toxic, and probably less allergenic. They are often used in combination, as in trimethoprim, with sulfamethoxazole. Long-acting sulfonamides, such as sulfadoxine, are combined with pyrimethamine for malaria prophylaxis. Poorly absorbed agents such as sulfasalazine are used to treat Crohn's disease, ulcerative colitis, and rheumatoid arthritis (*see* Sulfasalazine, this volume). Topical use includes sulfacetamide for ophthalmic infections and silver sulfadiazine for burns.

Most reports of neurotoxicity refer to the use of the earlier compounds; they include case reports of encephalopathy, peripheral neuropathy, ataxia, optic neuritis, transient myopia, and aseptic meningitis.

Sulfonamides are rapidly absorbed from the gastrointestinal tract, variably protein-bound, and widely distributed in tissues, including the cerebrospinal fluid (CSF) (5). They are metabolized primarily by acetylation in the liver and eliminated mostly in the urine, partly as unchanged drug and partly as metabolic products.

Short-term, large doses of sulfanilamide produced in mice what was described as rapidly reversible vestibular dysfunction and spastic paralysis (13). Repeated doses of sulfanilamide in rabbits and chickens produced clinical features suggesting peripheral neuropathy, along with supportive histological abnormalities in some (11).

Human CNS toxicity, reported mostly with the use of some early sulfonamide preparations, includes reversible delirium and psychosis, along with visual and auditory hallucinations (10,11,16,17). Occasionally, more focal symptoms occur such as aphasia, agraphia, and stammering (11). Two cases are described with acute gait and limb ataxia following intravenous trimethoprim-sulfamethoxazole, resolving within 3 days of discontinuing the drug (12). No signs of encephalopathy were detected in a controlled study of normal subjects receiving standard courses of sulfathiazole or sulfadiazine (15).

Aseptic meningitis may complicate the use of sulfonamides; the entity has been most frequently reported with trimethoprim-sulfamethoxazole (1,6,7,9). There may be fever, headache, meningismus and, occasionally, associated encephalopathy and seizures. The CSF usually shows a predominantly polymorphonuclear pleocytosis, elevated protein, and normal glucose.

A single case of reversible toxic "optic neuritis" is reported with the use of sulfanilamide (3). Transient myopia may be induced by sulfonamide therapy, perhaps related to swelling of the ciliary body with narrowing of the anterior chamber (2).

Peripheral neuropathy is rare; it occurred mostly with the use of methylated compounds (10,11,14,16). Descriptions are scanty and difficult to interpret, but include pain, paresthesias, weakness with little or no sensory loss, and depressed tendon reflexes. Gradual and complete recovery is the rule. There are no useful pathological or electrophysiological descriptions. Acetazolamide, a sulfonamide derivative, is associated with transient acral paresthesias (4,18). No cases of neuropathy were recorded in hospitalized patients during 2118 courses of therapy with sulfosoxazole or sulfamethoxazole (8).

The mechanism of sulfonamide-induced neurotoxicity is unknown.

REFERENCES

1. Biosca M, de la Figuera M, Garcia-Bragado F *et al.* (1986) Aseptic meningitis due to trimethoprim-sulfamethoxazole. *J Neurol Neurosurg Psychiat* 49, 332.

2. Bovino JA, Marcus DF (1982) The mechanism of transient

myopia induced by sulfonamide therapy. *Amer J Ophthalmol* **94**, 99.

3. Bucy PC (1937) Toxic optic neuritis resulting from sulfanilamide. *J Amer Med Assn* **109**, 1007.

4. Erdei A, Gyori I, Gedeon A, Szabo I (1990) Successful treatment of intractable gastric ulcers with acetazolamide. *Acta Med Hung* **47**, 171.

5. Gilman AG, Rall TR, Nies AS, Taylor P (1990) *The Pharmacological Basis of Therapeutics. 8th Ed.* Pergamon Press, New York p. 1047.

6. Haas EJ (1984) Trimethoprim-sulfamethoxazole: Another cause of recurrent meningitis. *J Amer Med Assn* **252**, 346.

7. Joffe AM, Farley JD, Linden D, Goldsand G (1989) Trimethoprim-sulfamethoxazole-associated aseptic meningitis: Case reports and review of the literature. *Amer J Med* **87**, 332.

8. Koch-Weser J, Sidel VW, Dexter M *et al.* (1971) Adverse reactions to sulfosoxazole, sulfamethoxazole, and nitrofurantoin: Manifestations and specific reaction rates during 2,118 courses of therapy. *Arch Intern Med* **128**, 399.

9. Kremer I, Ritz R, Brunner F (1983) Aseptic meningitis as an adverse effect of co-trimoxazole. *N Engl J Med* **308**, 1481.

10. Lehr D (1957) Clinical toxicity of the sulfonamides. *Ann N Y Acad Sci* **69**, 417.

11. Little SC (1942) Nervous and mental effects of the sulfonamides. *J Amer Med Assn* **119**, 467.

12. Liu LX, Seward SJ, Crumpacker CS (1986) Intravenous trimethoprim-sulfamethoxazole and ataxia. *Ann Intern Med* **104**, 448.

13. Long PH, Bliss EA (1937) Para-aminobenzenesulfonamide and its derivatives. *J Amer Med Assn* **108**, 32.

14. Ornsteen AM, Furst W (1938) Peripheral neuritis due to sulfanilamide. *J Amer Med Assn* **111**, 2103.

15. Reynolds FW, Shaffer GW (1943) Chemotherapeutic prophylaxis with sulfonamide drugs. *Amer J Syph Gonorrhea Vener Dis* **27**, 563.

16. Snavely SR, Hodges GR (1984) The neurotoxicity of antibacterial agents. *Ann Intern Med* **101**, 92.

17. Stuart MM, Collen MF (1944) Psychoses associated with sulfadiazine therapy. *Perm Found Med Bull* **2**, 153.

18. Theeuwes F, Bayne W, McGuire J (1978) Gastrointestinal therapeutic system for acetazolamide. Efficacy and side effects. *Arch Ophthalmol* **96**, 2219.

Suramin Sodium

Herbert H. Schaumburg

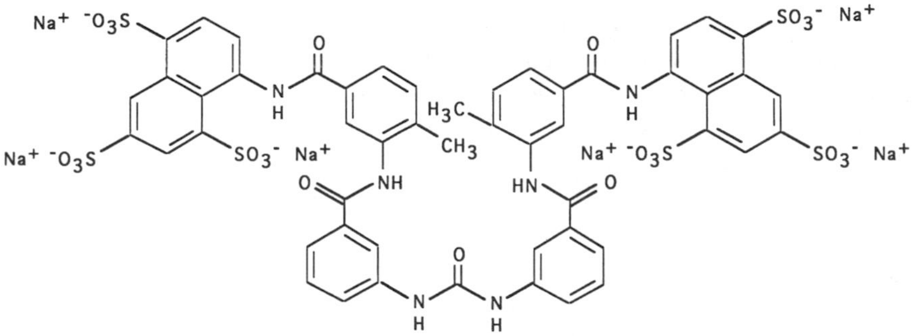

SURAMIN SODIUM
$C_{51}H_{34}N_6Na_6O_{23}S_6$

8,8′-[Carbonylbis[imino-3,1-phenylenecarbonylimino(4-methyl-3,1-phenylene)carbonylimino]] bis-1,3,5-naphthalenetrisulfonic acid hexasodium salt

NEUROTOXICITY RATING

Clinical

A   Peripheral neuropathy

Experimental

A   Peripheral neuropathy (dorsal root ganglion dysfunction—*in vitro*)

Suramin, a polysulfonated naphthylurea used for decades in the treatment and prophylaxis of African trypanosomiasis and onchocerciasis (1), has more recently been tried as a cancer chemotherapy agent for refractory neoplasms. It appears to have therapeutic potential in hormone-unresponsive metastatic prostate cancer and relapsed nodular lymphoma (6). Suramin's antitrypanosome effect is held to reflect inhibition of protozoal glycerol phosphate oxidase. The antineoplastic activity may stem from the demonstrated ability of suramin *in vitro* to inhibit DNA polymerase and several growth factors, including basic fibroblast growth factor, epidermal growth factor, insulin-like growth factor-1, and transforming growth factors α and β (3,5,8). It is suggested that inhibition of nerve growth factor (NGF) is the cause of suramin-associated sensorimotor neuropathy, the principal dose-limiting toxicity of this agent (7,12).

Suramin is administered intravenously (i.v.) and is persistently bound to plasma protein; this accounts for its half-life of 40–50 days. The persistence of suramin in the circulation explains the drug's efficacy in prophylaxis for protozoal diseases. It is not metabolized to any extent and is excreted unchanged by the kidneys. The circulating molecule is a large polar anion that does not enter cells readily; tissue concentrations are uniformly lower than those found in plasma, and the drug has little penetration into the cerebrospinal fluid. Drug dosage for protozoal disease is 1 g/ week for up to 6 weeks; the antineoplastic regimens employ considerably higher dosages (350 mg/m²/day for 3–7 weeks). Plasma levels of 250 µg/ml are necessary for anti-tumor activity. Peak plasma levels in cancer patients are variable, and concentrations between 350 and 400 µg/ml can occur in the course of treatment; these levels have been associated with serious neurotoxicity. This phenomenon probably will restrict the use of suramin to centers with strong pharmacological-monitoring capabilities.

Suramin therapy can cause a variety of systemic adverse reactions; they are more severe in debilitated individuals and in those receiving high-dose (antineoplastic) regimens. Nephrotoxicity with albuminuria is common, since the kidneys retain more of the drug than any other organ; individuals with renal insufficiency must be monitored closely and may be precluded from therapy. Other reactions include headache, upper gastrointestinal distress, leukopenia, adrenal insufficiency, and thrombocytopenia.

The effect of suramin and NGF on the rate of neurite outgrowth of rat dorsal root ganglion cells in culture has been examined (11). These experiments demonstrated that increasing doses of suramin inhibit NGF-specific binding in a concentration-dependent manner, and that high concentrations of NGF can ameliorate suramin-induced damage to dorsal root ganglion. The authors of this study propose that competition between suramin and endogenous NGF for the NGF high-affinity binding sites has a role in the pathogenesis of human suramin-induced sensorimotor neuropathy. Experimental animal studies show that intracerebral injections of suramin cause accumulations of membranous inclusion bodies in the cytoplasm of rodent neurons and oligodendrocytes (9). The inclusion bodies contain arrays of closely packed membranes arrayed concentrically and in layers. A single i.v. dose of 500 mg/kg produced similar changes, suggesting that the blood-brain barrier is not impervious to massive doses. The inclusion bodies probably reflect the ability of suramin to inhibit lysosomal enzymes (including idurodate sulfatase and the acid hydrolase β-hexosiminidase), thus impairing the breakdown of aminoglycans and gangliosides, and causing their intracellular and extracellular accumulation (4). Another set of experiments demonstrated similar lamellar inclusions in dorsal root ganglion neurons of rats given a single intraperitoneal dose of 500 mg/kg. These animals displayed peak serum suramin concentrations of 350–650 µg/ml and peripheral electrodiagnostic changes consistent with axonal polyneuropathy (10).

Persons undergoing suramin treatment for protozoal prophylaxis may experience burning paresthesias of the soles and hands during the initial week of therapy; none of these individuals has undergone careful neurological or neurophysiological evaluation, and the significance of these symptoms is unclear (1). Severe, disabling sensorimotor polyneuropathy may appear in individuals receiving high-dose (antineoplastic) suramin therapy. In a series of 38 patients receiving suramin for various malignancies, four developed neuropathy; in two, neuropathy relentlessly progressed to flaccid quadriplegia with paralysis of respiratory muscles (7). All improved following drug withdrawal; however, the two most affected were left with significant residual disability. Several features suggested a demyelinating component of the neuropathy, including rapid onset, severity of proximal limb weakness, elevated cerebrospinal protein levels, and conduction block on neurophysiological evaluation. The development of polyneuropathy correlated with the maximum plasma suramin level, with an estimated 40% of individuals who experienced plasma levels in excess of 350 µg/ml developing neuropathy. There was no correlation with total dosage or duration of therapy (2).

REFERENCES

1. Burch T, Ashburn L (1951) Experimental therapy of onchocercosis with suramin and hetrazan: Results of a three year study. *Amer J Trop Med Hyg* **31**, 617.
2. Chaudhry V, Eisenberger M, Cornblath DR (1995) Suramin-induced demyelinating neuropathy. *Muscle Nerve* **18**, 1056.
3. Coffey RJ Jr, Leof EB, Shipley GD, Moses HL (1987) Suramin inhibition of growth factor receptor binding and mitogenicity in AKR-2B cells. *J Cell Physiol* **132**, 143.
4. Constantopoulos G, Rees S, Cragg BG *et al.* (1981) Effect of suramin on the activities of degradative enzymes of sphingolipids in rats. *Res Commun Chem Pathol Pharmacol* **32**, 87.
5. Hosang M (1985) Suramin binds to platelet-derived

growth factor and inhibits its biological activity. *J Cell Biochem* **29**, 265.

6. Kim JH, Sherwood ER, Sutkowski DM *et al.* (1991) Inhibition of prostatic tumor cell proliferation by suramin: Alterations in TGF alpha-mediated autocrine growth regulation and cell cycle distribution. *J Urol* **146**, 171.

7. LaRocca RV, Meer J, Gilliatt RW *et al.* (1990) Suramin-induced polyneuropathy. *Neurology* **40**, 954.

8. Pollak M, Richard M (1990) Suramin blockade of insulin like growth factor I-stimulated proliferation of human osteosarcoma cells. *J Nat Cancer Inst* **82**, 1349.

9. Rees S (1978) Membranous neuronal and neuroglial in-
culsions produced by intracerebral injection of suramin. *J Neurol Sci* **36**, 97.

10. Russell JW, Windebank AJ (1993) Electrophysiological and pathological characteristics of suramin-induced neuropathy. *Neurology* **43**, A174.

11. Russell JW, Windebank AJ, Podratz JL (1994) Role of nerve growth factor in suramin neurotoxicity studied *in vitro*. *Ann Neurol* **36**, 221.

12. Soliven B, Dhand UK, Kobayashi K *et al.* (1997) Evaluation of neuropathy in patients on suramin treatment. *Muscle Nerve* **20**, 83.

Swainsonine

Steven U. Walkley

SWAINSONINE
$C_8H_{15}NO_3$

$8\alpha,\beta$-Indolizidine-$1\alpha,2\alpha,8\beta$-triol

NEUROTOXICITY RATING

Clinical

A Neuronal storage disease (α-mannosidosis—livestock)

A Chronic encephalopathy (ataxia, behavioral changes—cattle)

Experimental

A Neuronal storage disease (α-mannosidosis)

A Lysosomal enzyme inhibition (α-mannosidosis)

Swainsonine is an indolizidine alkaloid best known for its occurrence in certain leguminous plants of Australia and the western United States (4). The offending plants are often grazed by livestock, and chronic ingestion has been linked to induction of neurological disease. In Australia, the culpable plant is the darling pea (*Swainsona cancescens*); affected animals are referred to as being "pea-struck." In the United States, the plants are in the locoweed family (*Astragalus* and *Oxytropis* spp.); affected animals are "locoed." More recently, swainsonine has been identified in another Australian plant, the Weir vine (*Ipomoea* spp.), ingestion of which also causes neurological disease (17). Swainsonine has been identified as a mycotoxin produced by *Rhizoctonia leguminicola* when it parasitizes red clover, and ingestion of contaminated feed grain has been linked to generation of neurological disease. Another mold, *Metarhizium anisopliae*, also contains swainsonine and, like *Rhizoctonia*, has been used commercially to produce large quantities of the alkaloid for experimental purposes (4).

The occurrence of a neurological disease in free-ranging herbivores that have plants containing swainsonine is widely known in veterinary medicine. Locoweed poisoning of livestock in the western United States has been characterized as one of the most destructive of all plant intoxications (4,13). Sheep, cattle, and horses are most commonly affected, and reports dating to the early part of the twentieth century document the dramatic clinical disease. Early signs of disease involve loss of condition and appear only after animals have grazed the plants for an extended period of time (several weeks). This rapidly progresses to include evidence of neurological involvement, with affected animals exhibiting dull, depressed behavior and a progressively abnormal gait. Difficulty in eating and drinking, and in rising from a recumbent position, are other common features of the disease. When stressed, animals often show hyperexcitability. Apparent recovery, with return to normal conditioning, is possible if access to the locoweed is eliminated. However, even recovered animals when stressed often demonstrate an impaired gait and abnormal behavior. Disease in humans secondary to ingestion of swainsonine-containing plants has not been reported.

Prolonged oral ingestion of *Swainsona* or locoweed plants has been documented to cause widespread cytoplasmic vacuolation in cells of essentially all tissues, including the brain (10,11). These cytopathological changes (*e.g.*, in cattle with locoweed poisoning) were found closely to resemble the microscopic lesions in a genetic deficiency of lysosomal α-mannosidase (α-mannosidosis) reported in Angus cattle (14). This similarity, and the discovery that animals intoxicated with extracts of *Swainsona* also exhibited tissue accumulation of mannose-rich oligosaccharides in a manner similar to the genetic bovine disease (6), further suggested that the toxic agent might be an inhibitor of a lysosomal enzyme such as α-mannosidase. This was later confirmed through application of extracts from *S. canescens* to various lysosomal enzymes, with the discovery that α-mannosidase was selectively inhibited (5). The enzyme inhibitor in the plant extracts was subsequently isolated, purified to white crystalline needles, and shown by spectroscopic techniques to be an indolizidinetriol (2). It was given the name *swainsonine*. It was later determined that *Astragalus* plants also contained an inhibitor specific for lysosomal α-mannosidase (20), and that this inhibitor was structurally identical to swainsonine in various locoweed species (15) and in the molds (4) as described above. Given its greatest concentration in seed coats of the locoweeds, it may serve as a naturally occurring insecticide (16).

Purified or partially purified preparations of swainsonine have been administered to a variety of experimental animals, including cats, rats, mice, and guinea pigs. The primary goal of these studies has been to compare the pathogenesis of the induced disease state with genetic α-mannosidosis. Some species differences in disease susceptibility have been detected, particularly that rodents appear less likely to develop neurological disease than other animals, possibly due to differences in the blood-brain barrier (*see* 4). Overall, however, these experimental studies have revealed that swainsonine-induced α-mannosidosis is a close phenocopy of the genetic condition. Most notable in this regard are studies in cats, as a genetic model of α-mannosidosis is available for direct comparative study (27). Inherited feline α-mannosidosis, like the gangliosidoses and some other genetic neuronal storage diseases, exhibits remarkable changes in neurons secondary to the metabolic disease. These include growth of ectopic dendrites and formation of new synaptic contacts on otherwise mature pyramidal neurons of the cerebral cortex (22,23,27,29). This so-called phenomenon of "ectopic dendritogenesis" is unique to storage diseases and represents the only circumstance, other than during early brain development, when these neurons generate primary dendrites (21). Elevated expression of a single metabolic product, GM$_2$ ganglioside, has been correlated with dendritic initiation in both the disease states and during development (28). Swainsonine-

induced α-mannosidosis has been shown to be characterized by elevated levels of GM$_2$ ganglioside in brain and by the presence of ectopic dendrites on cortical neurons (8,19,26). Thus, swainsonine represents the only known agent which, after oral ingestion in animals, has the capacity to cause mature cortical pyramidal neurons to sprout new dendrites.

Swainsonine-induced α-mannosidosis, like many genetic lysosomal diseases involving brain, is also characterized by severe neuroaxonal dystrophy (axonal spheroid formation) predominately affecting inhibitory neurons that use γ-aminobutyric acid (GABA) as a neurotransmitter (22,24). In both genetic and induced forms of α-mannosidosis, GABAergic Purkinje cells of the cerebellum are severely affected by this type of axonopathy. This change, and the subsequent loss of Purkinje cells over time, closely correlates with the ataxia characteristic of this disease.

Swainsonine-induced α-mannosidosis has been used to determine the importance of age of disease onset on clinical sequelae, and thus to model, for example, the pathogenesis of infantile *vs.* adult-onset storage disease (29). Additionally, given that swainsonine-induced disease is reversible upon cessation of ingestion of the alkaloid, this model has also been used to evaluate the reversibility of brain lesions and clinical disease after "treatment" to determine what might happen if genetic α-mannosidosis could be treated (12,22,30). Results of these studies show persistence of both ectopic dendrites and axonal spheroids, as well as death of GABAergic neurons. Such residual effects, particularly in the ubiquitous GABAergic system, may account for the re-emergence of clinical disease in animals under stress long after removal from the source of the swainsonine.

Swainsonine has been reported to be strongly lysosomotropic, and an obvious feature of swainsonine intoxication is lysosomal vacuolation (4). However, experimental studies of swainsonine have shown that its effects are not limited to inhibition of this one enzyme. Golgi membrane-associated α-mannosidase II has also been found to be inhibited, but Golgi α-mannosidases type Ia and Ib are not (1,7). Golgi α-mannosidase II is responsible for removal of mannose residues during N-linked oligosaccharide maturation. Swainsonine's ability to modify the processing of aspariginine-linked glycoproteins has been exploited experimentally in a wide variety of studies. Swainsonine-induced alterations in cell-surface oligosaccharides is believed responsible for its capacity to act as an immunomodulator, and swainsonine has been reported to enhance natural killer (NK) cell activity through stimulation of lymphocyte proliferation and lymphokine production (31). The finding that swainsonine inhibited experimental metastasis of B16-F10 murine melanoma cells following injection into mice was believed to be due to its effects on cell-surface oligosaccharide moieties (18). An alternative explanation is that swainsonine directly affects macrophage tumoricidal activity (3). Demonstration of swainsonine's positive effects on tumor growth and metastasis in mouse tumor models led to phase I trials in Canada on its effectiveness in human subjects with advanced malignancies (9). The impact of intravenous injections of swainsonine on lysosomal α-mannosidase and on lysosomal pathology, particularly in brain, was not immediately apparent in these studies, apart from urinary secretion of oligomannosides consistent with lysosomal α-mannosidase inhibition.

REFERENCES

1. Abraham DJ, Sidebothom R, Winchester BG et al. (1983) Swainsonine affects the processing of glycoproteins in vivo. FEBS Lett **163**, 110.

2. Colegate SM, Dorling PR, Huxtable CR (1979) A spectroscopic investigation of swainsonine: An α-mannosidase inhibitor isolated from Swainsona canescens. Aust J Chem **32**, 2257.

3. Das PC, Roberts JD, White SL, Olden K (1995) Activation of resident tissue-specific macrophages by swainsonine. Oncol Res **7**, 425.

4. Dorling PR, Colegate SM, Huxtable CR (1989) Swainsonine: A toxic indolizidine alkaloid. In: Toxicants of Plant Origin. Vol 1. Alkaloids. Cheeke PR ed. CRC Press, Boca Raton, Florida p. 237.

5. Dorling PR, Huxtable CR, Colegate SM (1980) Inhibition of lysosomal α-mannosidase by swainsonine, an indolizidine alkaloid isolated from Swainsona canescens. Biochem J **191**, 649.

6. Dorling PR, Huxtable CR, Vogel P (1978) Lysosomal storage in Swainsona spp. toxicosis: An induced mannosidosis. Neuropathol Appl Neurobiol **4**, 285.

7. Elbein AD, Solf R, Dorling PR, Vosbeck K (1981) Swainsonine: An inhibitor of glycoprotein processing. Proc Nat Acad Sci USA **78**, 7393.

8. Goodman LA, Livingston PO, Walkley SU (1991) Ectopic dendrites occur only on cortical pyramidal neurons containing elevated GM$_2$ ganglioside in α-mannosidosis. Proc Nat Acad Sci USA **88**, 11330.

9. Goss PE, Baptiste J, Fernandes B et al. (1994) A phase I study of swainsonine in patients with advanced malignancies. Cancer Res **54**, 1450.

10. Hartley WJ (1971) Some observations on the pathology of Swainsona spp. poisoning in farm livestock in eastern Australia. Acta Neuropathol **18**, 342.

11. Hartley WJ, Baker DC, James LF (1989) Comparative pathological aspects of locoweed and Swainsona poisoning in livestock. In: Swainsonine and Related Glycosidase Inhibitors. James LF, Elbein AD, Molyneux RJ, Warren CD eds. Iowa State University Press, Ames, Iowa p. 50.

12. Huxtable CR, Dorling PR, Walkley SU (1982) Onset and regression of neuroaxonal lesions in sheep with mannosidosis induced experimentally with swainsonine. Acta Neuropathol **58**, 27.

13. James LF, Panter KE (1989) Locoweed poisoning in livestock. In: Swainsonine and Related Glycosidase Inhibitors. James LF, Elbein AD, Molyneux RJ, Warren CD eds. Iowa State University Press, Ames, Iowa p. 23.

14. Jolly RD, Thompson KG, van de Water NS et al. (1989) Bovine α-mannosidosis. In: Swainsonine and Related Glycosidase Inhibitors. James LF, Elbein AD, Molyneux RJ, Warren CD eds. Iowa State University Press, Ames, Iowa p. 291.

15. Molyneux RJ, James LF (1982) Loco intoxication: Indolizidine alkaloids of spotted locoweed (Astragalus lentiginosus). Science **216**, 190.

16. Molyneux RJ, James LF, Panter KE, Ralphs MH (1989) The occurrence and detection of swainsonine in locoweeds. In: Swainsonine and Related Glycosidase Inhibitors. James LF, Elbein AD, Molyneux RJ, Warren CD eds. Iowa State University Press, Ames, Iowa p. 100.

17. Molyneux RJ, McKenzie RA, O'Sullivan BM, Elbein AD (1995) Identification of the glycosidase inhibitors swainsonine and calystegine B2 in Weir vine (Ipomoea sp. Q6 [aff. calobra]) and correlation with toxicity. J Nat Prod **58**, 878.

18. Olden K, White SL, Matsumoto K, Humphries MJ (1989) Investigation of the possible involvement of glycoprotein glycans in experimental metastasis of B16-F10 murine melanoma cells. In: Swainsonine and Related Glycosidase Inhibitors. James LF, Elbein AD, Molyneux RJ, Warren CD eds. Iowa State University Press, Ames, Iowa p. 445.

19. Siegel DA, Walkley SU (1995) Growth of ectopic dendrites on cortical pyramidal neurons in neuronal storage diseases correlates with abnormal accumulation of GM$_2$ ganglioside. J Neurochem **62**, 1852.

20. Siegel DA, Walkley SU, Suzuki K (1982) Characterization of a specific α-mannosidase inhibitor from "locoweed." Trans Amer Soc Neurochem **13**, 159.

21. Walkley SU (1988) Pathobiology of neuronal storage disease. Int Rev Neurobiol **29**, 191.

22. Walkley SU (1998) Cellular pathology of lysosomal storage disorders. Brain Pathol **8**, 175.

23. Walkley SU, Wurzelmann S (1995) Alterations in synaptic connectivity in cerebral cortex in neuronal storage disease. Mental Retard Dev Disabil Res **1**, 183.

24. Walkley SU, Baker HJ, Rattazzi MC et al. (1991) Neuroaxonal dystrophy in neuronal storage disorders: Evidence for major GABAergic neuron involvement. J Neurol Sci **104**, 1.

25. Walkley SU, Blakemore WF, Purpura DP (1981) Altera-
    tions in neuron morphology in feline mannosidosis: A
    Golgi study. *Acta Neuropathol* **53**, 75.

26. Walkley SU, Siegel DA (1985) Ectopic dendritogenesis oc-
    curs on cortical pyramidal neurons in swainsonine-
    induced feline α-mannosidosis. *Develop Brain Res* **20**,
    143.

27. Walkley SU, Siegel DA (1989) Comparative studies of the
    CNS in swainsonine-induced and inherited feline α-
    mannosidosis. In: *Swainsonine and Related Glycosidase
    Inhibitors*. James LF, Elbein AD, Molyneux RJ, Warren
    CD eds. Iowa State University Press, Ames, Iowa p. 57.

28. Walkley SU, Siegel DA, Dobrenis K (1995) GM₂ ganglio-
    side and pyramidal neuron dendritogenesis. *Neurochem
    Res* **20**, 1287.

29. Walkley SU, Siegel DA, Wurzelmann S (1988) Ectopic
    dendritogenesis and associated synapse formation in
    swainsonine-induced neuronal storage disease. *J Neurosci*
    8, 445.

30. Walkley SU, Wurzelmann S, Siegel DA (1987) Ectopic
    axon hillock-associated neurite growth is maintained in
    metabolically reversed swainsonine-induced neuronal stor-
    age disease. *Brain Res* **410**, 89.

31. White SL, Humphries MJ, Molyneux RJ, Olden K (1989)
    Swainsonine: A new immunomodulator which enhances
    murine lymphoproliferation and natural killer activity. In:
    Swainsonine and Related Glycosidase Inhibitors. James
    LF, Elbein AD, Molyneux RJ, Warren CD eds. Iowa State
    University Press, Ames, Iowa p. 425.

Tacrolimus

Herbert H. Schaumburg
Albert C. Ludolph
Bruce G. Gold

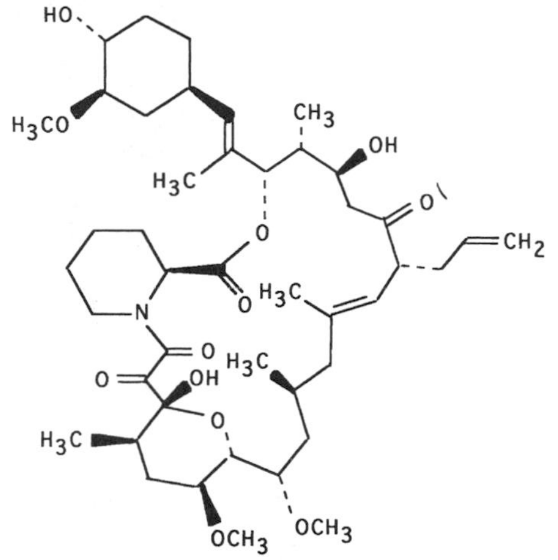

TACROLIMUS
$C_{44}H_{69}NO_{12}$

FK-506; [3S-[3R*[E(1S*,3S*,4S*)]],4S*,5R*,8S*,9E,12R*,
14R*,15S*,16R*,18S*,19S*,26aR*]]-5,6,8,11,12,13,14,15,
16,17,18,19,24,25,26,26a-Hexadecahydro-5,19-dihydroxy-
3-[2-(4-hydroxy-3-methoxycyclohexyl)-1-methylethenyl]-
14,16-dimethoxy-4,10,12,18-tetramethyl-8-(2-propenyl)-
15,19-epoxy-3H-pyrido[2,1-c][1,4]oxaazacyclotricosine-
1,7,20,21(4H,23H)-tetrone

NEUROTOXICITY RATING

Clinical

A   Peripheral neuropathy

A   Leukoencephalopathy

A   Seizure disorder

Tacrolimus (FK-506) is a novel immunosuppressive drug. It was initially used for patients undergoing liver transplantation and has now largely replaced use of cyclosporin A in renal, pancreatic, and cardiac transplantation (17). Tacrolimus is a macrolide antibiotic extracted from the soil microorganism *Streptomyces tsukubaensis*; it suppresses both cell-mediated and humoral immune responses. Tacrolimus therapy is associated with serious neurotoxic side effects. While the tendency to overdose with tacrolimus may contribute to the reported higher incidence of neurotoxicity compared to cyclosporin A (6), it is presently unclear whether its neurotoxic potency exceeds that of cyclosporin A (3,4,22,23).

Tacrolimus is administered intravenously or orally. The elimination half-life is 11.7 ± 3.9 h in liver-transplant patients and in healthy volunteers 21.2 ± 8.5 h (12). Oral bioavailability differs widely, ranging from 6%–56% (25). The compound is metabolized in the liver. FK-506 plasma concentrations are determined by an enzyme-linked immunosorbent assay (ELISA) with a monoclonal antibody (21). There are no animal studies that document neurotoxicity.

Human neurotoxic effects of tacrolimus are common, particularly during the early phase of treatment (3,4,22,25). In a study of 263 patients under immunosuppressive treatment after liver transplantation, the incidence of headache was 25%, tremor 20%, and dysesthesia 15% (21). In another study of tacrolimus neurotoxicity, 14 of 44 patients (32%) developed neurotoxic effects after liver transplantation (24). Akinetic mutism may be an early side effect (3,25); it is reversible after dose reduction and is associated with risk factors such as high plasma levels, pre-existing severe hepatic dysfunction, or disorders of the nervous system such as multiple sclerosis (3). A reversible acute encephalopathy may also develop after administration of tacrolimus; particularly high plasma levels are found (3,25). Clouding of consciousness may range from somnolence to coma. Isolated seizures may appear; they may be generalized, focal motor, or partial complex (3,5,25). Less frequent effects include dysarthria and aphasia, hemiplegia, cortical blindness, and acute psychosis (3,5,15,25).

Sleep disturbances and tremulousness are frequently reported shortly after transplantation and were not associated with high plasma levels (3,25). Other common side effects are visual symptoms, headache (often occipital), tremors, dysesthesia, apraxia of speech, and mood changes (3,25). Patients with migraine reportedly may experience exacerbation of attacks during tacrolimus treatment (4).

In three patients, a severe multifocal demyelinating sensorimotor neuropathy has appeared; it slowly improved after intravenous administration of immunoglobulins or plasma exchange (26). The neuropathy developed 2–10 weeks after initiation of therapy. Cerebrospinal fluid protein was moderately increased in each case. Another report describes a reversible generalized motor axonal neuropathy (1): the pattern of conduction deficits in these patients did not exclude secondary axonal damage from proximal demyelination; therefore, it is unclear presently whether these reports represent two different mechanisms of neuropathy. Experimental studies show a positive dose-dependent effect of tacrolimus on axonal regeneration (7,8,24) after focal nerve injury; this arises from a mechanism distinct from that producing immunosuppression (10,18,19).

Reversible leukoencephalopathy with a parieto-occipital predilection is clearly associated with tacrolimus therapy (3,5,11,15,16,25). Lesions can be seen on both T2-weighted and proton density–weighted magnetic resonance images (MRI) (16). In one report, neuroimaging findings correlated with brain biopsy findings of nonspecific demyelination (16). In a patient with cortical blindness after therapy, MRI also showed diffuse, bilateral, white matter lesions with a posterior predilection (15); these completely disappeared after withdrawal of the drug. One study that monitored lesions induced by cyclosporin A and tacrolimus described infarcts, astrocytosis, and CNS phlebitis (13). In one instance, a brain biopsy revealed the presence of a necrotizing angiopathy (4).

The neurotoxic mechanism of tacrolimus is unknown. The compound binds to a 12-kDa cytosolic protein [FK-506 (tacrolimus)-binding protein, FKBP-12] that associates with and, like cyclosporin A, inhibits calcineurin catalytic activity. Inhibition of calcineurin activity prevents the nuclear translocation of NF-AT (nuclear factor of activated T-cells) leading to a decrease in interleukin-2 synthesis and secretion and, consequently, a reduction in T-cell proliferation. Neurotoxicity is also associated with calcineurin inhibition (2); in contrast, the axon regenerative property of FK-506 appears to be mediated *via* a different FKBP, FKBP-52 (9), a component of the steroid receptor complex. The availability of nonimmunosuppressant (noncalcineurin inhibiting) derivatives of tacrolimus (10,18,19) should help to decipher the role of calcineurin in tacrolimus neurotoxicity. Metabolically, the compound induces hypomagnesemia, hyperkalemia, and hyperglycemia; neurotoxicity was not related to magnesium levels (3). In practice, the neurotoxic effects may be difficult to distinguish from the neurological complications of organ transplantation (14). Elimination of the drug or reduction of the dose leads to rapid resolution of neurotoxicity and helps in differential diagnosis. Effects of drug combinations must also be considered, especially the coadministration of tacrolimus and cyclosporin A (20).

REFERENCES

 1. Ayres RCS, Dousset B, Wixon S *et al.* (1994) Peripheral neurotoxicity with tacrolimus. *Lancet* **343**, 862.
 2. Dumont FJ, Staruch MJ, Koprach SL *et al.* (1992) The immunosuppressant and toxic effects of FK-506 are mechanistically related: Pharmacology of a novel antagonist of FK-506. *J Exp Med* **176**, 751.
 3. Eidelman BH, Abu-Elmagd K, Wilson J *et al.* (1991) Neurologic complications of FK-506. *Transplant Proc* **23**, 3175.
 4. Frank B, Perdrizet GA, White HM *et al.* (1993) Neurotoxicity of FK-506 in liver transplant recipients. *Transplant Proc* **25**, 1887.
 5. Freise CE, Rowley H, Lake J *et al.* (1991) Similar clinical presentation of neurotoxicity following FK-506 and cyclosporine in a liver transplant recipient. *Transplant Proc* **23**, 3173.
 6. Fung JJ, Eliasziw M, Todo S *et al.* (1996) The Pittsburgh randomized trial of tacrolimus compared to cyclosporine for hepatic transplantation. *J Amer Coll Surg* **183**, 117.
 7. Gold BG, Katoh K, Storm-Dickerson T (1995) The immunosuppressant FK-506 increases the rate of axonal regeneration in rat sciatic nerve. *J Neurosci* **15**, 7505.
 8. Gold BG, Storm-Dickerson T, Austin DR (1994) The immunosuppressant FK-506 increases functional recovery and nerve regeneration following peripheral nerve injury. *Restor Neurol Neurosci* **6**, 287.
 9. Gold BG, Yew JY, Zeleny-Pooley M (1998) The immunosuppressant FK506 increases GAP-43 mRNA levels in axotomized sensory neurons. *Neurosci Lett* **241**, 25.
10. Gold BG, Zeleny-Pooley BS, Wang M-S *et al.* (1997) A non-immunosuppressant FKBP-12 ligand increases nerve regeneration. *Exp Neurol* **147**, 267.
11. Hinchey J, Chaves C, Appignani B *et al.* (1996) A reversible posterior leukoencephalopathy syndrome. *N Engl J Med* **334**, 494.
12. Hooks MA (1994) Tacrolimus, a new immunosuppressant —a review of the literature. *Ann Pharmacother* **28**, 501.
13. Lopez OL, Martinez AJ, Torre-Cisneros J (1991) Neuropathologic findings in liver transplantation: A comparative study of cyclosporine and FK-506. *Transplant Proc* **23**, 3181.
14. Patchell RA (1994) Neurological complications of organ transplantation. *Ann Neurol* **36**, 688.
15. Shutter LA, Green JP, Newman NJ *et al.* (1993) Cortical blindness and white matter lesions in a patient receiving FK-506 after liver transplantation. *Neurology* **43**, 2417.
16. Small SL, Fukui MB, Bramblett GT, Eidelman BH (1996) Immunosuppression-induced leukoencephalopathy under tacrolimus (FK-506). *Ann Neurol* **40**, 575.
17. Snyder SH, Sabatini DM (1995) Immunophilins and the nervous system. *Nat Med* **1**, 32.
18. Steiner JP, Connolly MA, Valentine HL *et al.* (1997) Neurotrophic actions of nonimmunosuppressive ligands of immunophilins. *Nat Med* **3**, 1.
19. Steiner JP, Hamilton GS, Ross DT *et al.* (1997) Neurotrophic immunophilin ligands stimulate structural and functional recovery in neurodegenerative animal models. *Proc Nat Acad Sci USA* **94**, 2019.
20. Starzl TE, Todo S, Fung J *et al.* (1989) FK-506 for liver, kidney and pancreas transplantation. *Lancet* **ii**, 1000.
21. Tamura K, Kobayashi M, Hashimoto K *et al.* (1987) A

highly sensitive method to assay FK-506 levels in plasma. *Transplant Proc* **19**, 23.

22. The U.S. Multicenter FK-506 Liver Study Group (1994) A comparison of tacrolimus (FK-506) and cyclosporine for immunosuppression in liver transplantation. *N Engl J Med* **331**, 1110.

23. Venkataramanan R, Jain A, Warty VW *et al.* (1991) Pharmacokinetics of FK-506 following oral administration: A comparison of FK-506 and cyclosporine A. *Transplant Proc* **23**, 931.

24. Wang MS, Zeleny-Pooley M, Gold BG (1997) Comparative dose-dependence study of FK-506 and cyclosporine A on the rate of axonal regeneration in rat sciatic nerve. *J Pharmacol Exp Ther* **282**, 1084.

25. Wijdicks EF, Wiesner RH, Dahlke EJ, Krom RAF (1994) FK-506-induced neurotoxicity in liver transplantation. *Ann Neurol* **35**, 498.

26. Wilson JR, Conwit RA, Eidelman BH *et al.* (1994) Sensorimotor neuropathy resembling CIDP in patients receiving FK-506. *Muscle Nerve* **17**, 528.

Taicatoxin

Albert C. Ludolph
Peter S. Spencer

NEUROTOXICITY RATING

Experimental

A Ion channel syndrome (calcium channels)

A Seizure disorder

Taicatoxin (*Tai*pan and *ca*lcium—*taica*toxin, TCX), an oligomeric toxin isolated from the venom of the Australian taipan snake (*Oxyuranus s. scutellatus*), has a MW of 31,000; it is distinct from taipoxin, a typical presynaptic neurotoxin in the same venom (4; *see* Taipoxin, this volume). TCX consists of three distinct, noncovalently linked components: an α-neurotoxin–like peptide (MW, 8000), a neurotoxic phospholipase (MW, 16,000), and a serine protease inhibitor (MW, 7000) (5). The oligomere is the most potent toxin, although the α-neurotoxin-like peptide and phospholipase are toxic by themselves. In cardiomyocyte cultures, TCX exhibits phospholipase A2 activity leading to the release of lysophospholipids, and acyl CoA and acyl carnitine, which have detrimental effects on cellular integrity and function (3).

In nanomolar concentrations, the basic highly charged toxin produced a voltage-dependent, reversible, and selective blockade of high-threshold (L-type) Ca^{2+} channels in a skeletal muscle cell line (BH_3H_1), in mammalian smooth muscle, and in neurosecretory cells (1,5). TCX does not block low-threshold channel currents and does not affect single-channel conductance; it changes channel gating and has a high affinity for inactivated channels (5). *In vivo*, a fraction of the toxin that displayed Ca^{2+} channel–blocking activity was toxic to mice; signs of intoxication included reduced movement of hindlimbs, "sporadic jumping," and seizures (5). Whole-cell patch-clamp studies of guinea pig ventricular cells revealed that TCX binds to the external but not the internal mouth of the channel; its large charge prevents TCX from penetrating membranes. In isolated cardiac membranes, the compound inhibits binding to dihydropyridine receptors linked to L-type channels (1). The effect on calcium channels is selective; no effect on K^+ or Na^+ channels is observed (1,5).

The foregoing dogma has been questioned by a recent finding that TCX also interacts with apamin-sensitive, small-conductance, Ca^{2+}-activated K^+ channels in rat synaptosomal membranes and specifically blocks affinity-labeling of a 33-kDa ^{125}I-apamin-binding polypeptide on rat brain membranes. In view of these findings, the authors propose that use of TCX as a specific ligand for Ca^{2+} channels should be reconsidered (2).

REFERENCES

1. Brown AM, Yatani A, Lacerda AE *et al.* (1987) Neurotoxins that act selectively on voltage-dependent cardiac calcium channels. *Circ Res* **61**, 6.
2. Doorty KB, Bevan S, Wadsworth JD, Strong PN (1997) A novel small conductance Ca^{2+}-activated K^+ channel blocker from *Oxyuranus scutellatus* taipan venom. Re-evaluation of taicatoxin as a selective Ca^{2+} channel probe. *J Biol Chem* **272**, 19925.
3. Fantini E, Athias P, Tirosh R, Pinson A (1996) Effect of TaiCatoxin (TCX) on the electrophysiological, mechanical and biochemical characteristics of spontaneously beating ventricular cardiomyocytes. *Mol Cell Biochem* **160**, 61.
4. Fohlman J, Eaker D, Karlsson E, Thesleff S (1976) Taipoxin, an extremely potent presynaptic neurotoxin from the venom of the Australian snake taipan (*Oxyuranus s. scutellatus*). *Eur J Biochem* **68**, 457.
5. Possani LD, Martin BM, Yatani A *et al.* (1992) Isolation and physiological characterization of taicatoxin, a complex toxin with specific effects on calcium channels. *Toxicon* **30**, 1343.

Taipoxin

Albert C. Ludolph

NEUROTOXICITY RATING

Clinical

A   Neuromuscular transmission syndrome

A   Myopathy (necrotizing)

Experimental

A   Neuromuscular transmission dysfunction (presynaptic
      neuromuscular blockade)

A   Myopathy (necrotizing)

Taipoxin, a presynaptic neurotoxin, is purified from the potent venom of the southern Papua New Guinean and Australian taipan snake (*Oxyuranus s. scutellatus*). The compound accounts for 16% of the dry weight of the venom and the major part of its neurotoxic property. Taipoxin is an acidic sialoglycoprotein with a MW of 45,600; it consists of a ternary complex of three noncovalently-linked subunits (α, β, and γ). The α-subunit is strongly basic, the β-subunit is neutral, and the γ-subunit is a strongly acidic molecule (6,8,9); α and β components (120 amino acids) are cross-linked by seven disulfide bridges; the γ component consists of 135 subunits and has eight disulfide bridges.

The LD_{50} of crude venom is 12 μg/kg in mice (5); the LD_{50} of taipoxin is 2 mg/kg body weight after intravenous application (5). Mice initially develop paralysis of the hindlimbs (2 h after 2 mg/kg); this spreads within 10–15 h to other muscles and finally affects the respiratory muscles and causes asphyxia. The toxicity of the β- and γ-subunits is low in the mouse (LD_{50} >2000 μg/kg); the α-subunit has a higher potency (LD_{50} of 300 μg/kg). Only the α-subunit displays neuromuscular-blocking activity in physiological experiments (5). Dexamethasone partly reduced lethality of venom-injected mice; diltiazem, nicergoline, nifedipine, piracetam, primaquine, reserpin, verapamil, and vesamicol were not protective (1).

Taipoxin not only affects neuromuscular transmission but—in apparent contrast to some other phospholipase A_2 toxins such as β-bungarotoxin—is also directly myotoxic (7,10). Injection of the venom or the toxin into muscle results, within hours, in muscle necrosis and degeneration, followed by phagocyte infiltration and edema (7). Regeneration is complete after 6 months (10). Ultrastructural changes include lysis of the plasma membrane, hypercontraction of densely clumped myofibrils, and swollen and disrupted mitochondria (7,10). The basal lamina remained intact (7,10). The mechanism of muscle damage is unclear (10) but may include early damage to the plasma membrane followed by calcium influx. Only the α-subunit of taipoxin causes muscle necrosis; injection of γ- and β-subunits did not induce myotoxicity (7). After injection of higher doses of phospholipase A_2, myoglobinuria and renal failure occur and may be fatal (11).

The bite of the taipan snake is almost invariably fatal for humans if therapeutic measures are not readily available. Paralysis of bulbar, extraocular, limb and, finally, respiratory muscles occurs. Symptoms are reversible if the victim receives adequate ventilatory support. Elevations of serum creatine kinase and myoglobinuria—which potentially results in life-threatening renal failure—may accompany this picture. In an analysis of 149 taipan bites in Papua New Guinea, the vast majority of patients (>80%) had prominent signs of neurotoxicity. Coagulopathy was present in >60% of the patients (2); 36% of the patients with signs of neurotoxicity received ventilatory support and all deaths were attributed to neurotoxicity. In some, the myasthenia-like syndrome progressed in spite of antivenom therapy (2).

Taipoxin is an extremely potent compound which—like dendrotoxin, β-bungarotoxin, and crotoxin—irreversibly blocks neuromuscular transmission by interrupting evoked and spontaneous presynaptic acetylcholine release in a triphasic response (4,13–15). In neurons, it has been demonstrated that taipoxin binds with high affinity to a novel 47-kDa protein named pentraxin (NP). The function of NP is not entirely clear but it may be released synaptically and has homology to acute-phase proteins of the immune system and compounds involved in uptake of synaptic macromolecules (12). The concentrations of taipoxin that are gliotoxic are greatly lowered by NP, suggesting that NP mediates the uptake of taipoxin and serves as its receptor (3). Studies performed with antibodies to NP revealed a striking contrast between high message levels and low levels of protein expression (12), possibly indicating the presence of a high turnover of NP. A second protein [taipoxin-associated calcium-binding protein (TCBP-49)] may mediate the activation of internalized taipoxin (3).

REFERENCES

1. Crosland RD (1991) Effect of drugs on the lethality in mice of the venoms and neurotoxins from sundry snakes. *Toxicon* 29, 613.

2. Currie BJ, Theakston RDJ, Warrell DA (1992) Envenoming from the Papuan taipan (*Oxyuranus scutellatus canni*). In: *Recent Advances in Toxinology Research*. Gopalakrishnakone P, Tan CK eds. National University of Singapore, Singapore p. 308.

3. Dodds DC, Omeis IA, Cushman SJ et al. (1997) Neuronal pentraxin receptor, a novel putative integral membrane

pentraxin that interacts with neuronal pentraxin 1 and 2 and taipoxin-associated calcium-binding protein 49. *J Biol Chem* **272**, 21488.

4. Dreyer F, Penner R (1987) The actions of presynaptic snake toxins on membrane currents of mouse motor nerve terminals. *J Physiol* **386**, 455.

5. Fohlman J, Eaker D, Karlsson E, Thesleff S (1976) Taipoxin, an extremely potent presynapic neurotoxin from the venom of the Australian snake taipan (*Oxyuranus s. scutellatus*). *Eur J Biochem* **68**, 457.

6. Fohlman J, Lind P, Eaker D (1977) Snake venom neurotoxin. Elucidation of the primary structure of the acidic carbohydrate-containing taipoxin subunit, a phospholipase analog. *FEBS Lett* **84**, 367.

7. Harris JB, Maltin CA (1982) Myotoxic activity of the crude venom and the principal neurotoxin, taipoxin, of the Australian taipan, *Oxyuranus scutellatus*. *Brit J Pharmacol* **76**, 61.

8. Lind P (1982) Amino acid sequence of the β1 isosubunit of taipoxin, an extremely potent presynaptic neurotoxin from the venom of the Australian snake taipan (*Oxyuranus s. scutellatus*). *Eur J Biochem* **128**, 71.

9. Lind P, Eaker D (1982) Amino acid sequence of the α-subunit of taipoxin, an extremely potent presynaptic neurotoxin from the venom of the Australian snake taipan (*Oxyuranus s. scutellatus*). *Eur J Biochem* **124**, 441.

10. Mebs D, Ownby CL (1990) Myotoxic components of snake venoms: Their biochemical and biological activities. *Pharmacol Ther* **48**, 223.

11. Mebs D, Samejima A (1980) Purification, from Australian elapid venoms, and properties of phospholipases A₂ which cause myoglobinuria in mice. *Toxicon* **18**, 443.

12. Schlimgen AK, Helms JA, Vogel H, Perin MS (1995) Neuronal pentraxin, a secreted protein with homology to acute phase proteins of the immune system. *Neuron* **14**, 519.

13. Simpson LL, Lautenslager GT, Kaiser II, Middlebrook JL (1993) Identification of the site at which phospholipase A2 neurotoxins localize to produce their neuromuscular blocking effects. *Toxicon* **31**, 13.

14. Strong PN (1987) Presynaptic phospholipase A neurotoxins: Relationship between biochemical and electrophysiological approaches to the mechanism of toxin action. In: *Cellular and Molecular Basis of Cholinergic Function*. Dowdall MJ, Hawthorne JN eds. Ellis Horwood, Chichester p. 534.

15. Su MJ, Chang CC (1984) Presynaptic effects of snake venom toxins which have phospholipase A activity (beta-bungarotoxin, taipoxin, crotoxin). *Toxicon* **22**, 631.

Taxoids

Stuart C. Apfel

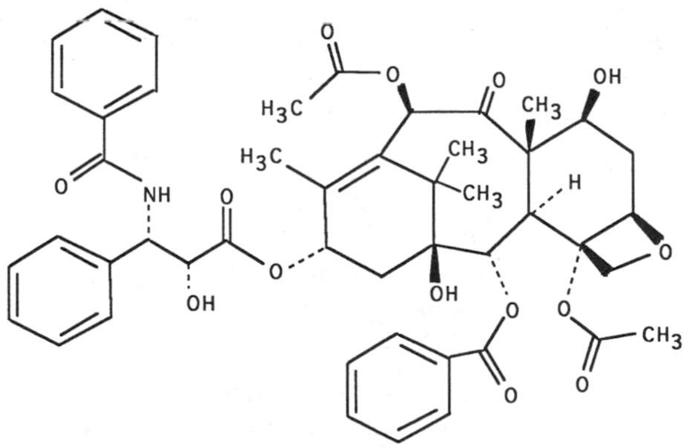

PACLITAXEL
C₄₇H₅₁NO₁₄

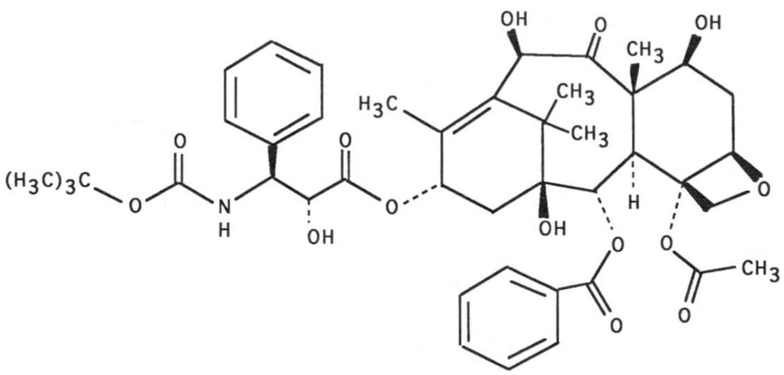

5β,20-Epoxy-1,2α,4,7β,10β,13α-hexahydroxytax-11-en-9-one 4,10-diacetate 2-benzoate 13-ester with (2R,3S)-N-benzoyl-3-phenylisoserine; Taxol A

DOCETAXEL
C₄₇H₅₃NO₁₄

4-Acetoxy-2α-benzoyloxy-5β,20-epoxy-1,7β,10-trihydroxy-9-oxotax-11-ene-13α-yl-(2R,3S)-3-tert-butoxycarbonylamino-2-hydroxy-3-phenylproprionate

NEUROTOXICITY RATING

Clinical

A   Peripheral neuropathy

Experimental

A   Microtubule aggregation

B   Peripheral neuropathy

Paclitaxel and docetaxel are diterpene alkaloids (taxoids) isolated from the Pacific yew tree, *Taxus brevifolia*. Paclitaxel (Taxol) was originally isolated from the bark of the tree during a screening program looking for natural antitumor agents sponsored by the U.S. National Cancer Institute in 1971 (41). Docetaxel was developed by chemically modifying a precursor isolated from needles of *T. baccata* (a different species of yew tree), which resulted in an antitumor agent that was possibly more potent than paclitaxel (3). Paclitaxel had been in short supply, since it is found exclusively in bark extract from the *T. brevifolia* tree; to harvest the drug meant killing the tree, which is found within a limited range. Shortage of the drug abated in the 1990s because of advances in extracting paclitaxel from the needles and other portions of the tree (28), as well as success with semisynthetic methods of manufacturing the drug (8). Availability has been less of an issue with docetaxel since, from its inception, it has been produced semisynthetically from needles of *T. baccata*.

Both drugs are white, odorless crystalline powders that are insoluble in water. Paclitaxel is soluble in Cremophor EL (polyoxyethylated castor oil), polyethylene glycols, ethanol, chloroform, acetone, and methanol (28). It is available clinically as a viscous, colorless fluid that is administered intravenously. Docetaxel is soluble in hydrochloric acid, chloroform, dimethylformamide, ethanol, sodium hydroxide, and methanol (28); it is available only as part of an investigational protocol.

Paclitaxel has been approved for use as chemotherapy for the treatment of metastatic ovarian carcinoma following the failure of first-line therapy, and for the treatment of metastatic breast cancer after the failure of combination chemotherapy or relapse within 6 months of adjuvant chemotherapy (9,26). Paclitaxel has also shown promise in phase II clinical trials testing its efficacy in treating advanced non–small-cell lung cancer (10), advanced small-cell lung carcinoma (10), and advanced head-and-neck cancer (11). Paclitaxel is usually administered intravenously by a 3- to 24-h infusion, at a dose of 200–250 mg/m^2, in courses given at 3-week intervals.

Paclitaxel is considered to be contraindicated in patients with known hypersensitivity reactions to drugs formulated in Cremophor EL, and in patients with a baseline neutropenia of <1500 cells/mm^3. Patients receiving paclitaxel should be pretreated with corticosteroids, diphenhydramine, and H$_2$ antagonists to prevent hypersensitivity reactions; these are common (2%) and potentially life threatening. Paclitaxel should only be administered by a physician experienced with the use of chemotherapeutic neoplastic agents.

Docetaxel has shown considerable promise in phase II trials testing its efficacy in the therapy of a variety of neoplasms. Potential applications include ovarian carcinoma (30), breast cancer (12), and non–small-cell bronchial carcinoma (31). Most phase II clinical trials have used a dose of 100 mg/m^2 given intravenously over 1 h at 3-week intervals. Docetaxel is restricted to investigative use only.

General Toxicology

Pharmacokinetic evaluation for paclitaxel has been limited by lack of adequate biochemical assays owing to its nearly complete lack of aqueous solubility. Paclitaxel is between 89%–92% bound to serum proteins; it is rapidly cleared from the plasma, but its route of elimination is not fully understood (28). Paclitaxel is not significantly cleared by the kidneys. About 20%–40% is found in the bile (22); the balance may be removed by tissue binding or metabolism (28).

More is known about the pharmacokinetics of docetaxel. The drug has a terminal half-life of 11–18 h, and a plasma clearance of 16–21 l/h/m^2 (28). More than 90% is protein-bound in the serum. Like paclitaxel, little is found in urine, but 80% is excreted in the feces (40). Docetaxel has been found to be widely distributed throughout systemic tissues following administration, but it does not gain access to the CNS (36).

Little is known about possible drug interactions with either taxoid. Some of the systemic toxicity associated with paclitaxel is reported to be exacerbated if the patient had previously been treated with cisplatin (36). *In vitro* data also suggest that ketoconazole may inhibit the metabolism of paclitaxel (9); it is therefore recommended that the two drugs are not used together.

Apart from its neurotoxicity, paclitaxel has also been reported to have a variety of systemic toxicities. The most important, and possibly dose-limiting toxicity, is myelosuppression with severe neutropenia (35). This toxicity is diminished by altering infusion schedules (35), and by administration of granulocyte colony-stimulating factor (39). If myelosuppression can be prevented, then neuropathy is usually reported as the dose-limiting toxicity. Other systemic toxicities include hypersensitivity reactions, cardiac arrhythmias, nausea, diarrhea, mucositis, alopecia, and chronic venous changes (35). The spectrum of systemic toxicity seen with docetaxel administration is very similar to that of paclitaxel, but with perhaps a higher incidence of sensitivity reactions and skin lesions (28).

Animal Studies

The earliest animal studies to examine the effects of paclitaxel administration on the nervous system made use of local injections directly into the rat sciatic nerve (37,38) or facial nerve (23). Injection into the sciatic nerve resulted in myelin degeneration, perivascular inflammation, and early wallerian degeneration by the end of the first week. These changes were noted to extend at least 3 weeks following injection. Ultrastructurally, axons were swollen with increased numbers of microtubules. Microtubules were also found to accumulate in Schwann cells as early as 1 day following injection. In addition, arrested mitoses were occasionally seen in Schwann cells, providing a possible explanation for the fact that no attempt at remyelination was seen (39). Similar histological observations were noted when paclitaxel was injected into the facial nerve, but in this study paclitaxel was also found to impair retrograde axonal transport (23).

Systemic administration of paclitaxel to mice and rats has been shown to cause changes in several measures of nerve function. In mice, paclitaxel administration results in an elevation of tail-flick threshold (which tests the sensitivity of the mouse to thermal noxious stimuli), reduction of substance P levels in the dorsal root ganglia, and a reduction in action potential amplitude as recorded from the caudal nerve (2). Conduction velocity was not significantly reduced. These findings are suggestive of a predominantly small-fiber sensory dysfunction. In a rat model of systemic administration, however, the predominant finding was a decrease in conduction velocity, suggestive of large-fiber dysfunction (13). A recent study that utilized two intravenous injections of 12–18 mg/kg paclitaxel to mature rats caused a large-fiber sensory neuropathy without a detrimental effect on general health, a serious limitation in earlier investigations (6). Electrophysiological findings in these animals included reduction in amplitude of H waves in the hindlimbs and in the sensory action potentials in caudal nerves; motor amplitudes were unaffected. Limited histopathological studies disclosed axonal degeneration in the fourth lumbar dorsal spinal root; the corresponding ventral root appeared normal (6). Coadministration of neurotrophic factors was reported to prevent manifestations of paclitaxel neurotoxicity: nerve growth factor (NGF) was reportedly successful in the mouse model (1), and the adrenocorticotropic hormone analog ORG 2766 appeared effective in a rat model (13). Insulin-like growth factor I has also been claimed to prevent neurotoxicity in the mouse model (7,18).

Evidence of docetaxel-induced neuropathy was seen in mice treated for 5 consecutive days at different doses (3). At the lower doses, mice displayed impaired motor activity, with pathological indications of axonal and myelin degeneration. At higher doses, mice developed weakness of the limbs and axonal degeneration in the sciatic nerve.

In Vitro Studies

In spinal cord–dorsal root ganglia explant cultures, paclitaxel has been found to have similar morphological effects to those observed in the aforementioned animal studies (18, 20,21). Microtubules aggregate into bundles and neurite outgrowth is reduced (18). In one study, paclitaxel administration decreased the survival of spinal cord–dorsal root ganglion explant culture neurons, but the effect was prevented by addition of NGF (29). Similarly, paclitaxel-induced decreased neurite outgrowth in sensory ganglion (17) and sympathetic ganglion (14) explant cultures was prevented by NGF. Paclitaxel also induced prominent changes in glial cells in vitro (21).

Human Studies

The most common neurotoxicity associated with paclitaxel administration in clinical trials has been a predominantly sensory peripheral neuropathy. This dose-related complication occurs most commonly at doses of 250 mg/m² or more administered over 6- and 24-h infusions (19,32,33, 35,42,43). Neuropathy also occurs frequently at lower dosage, though it is rarely clinically significant at doses below 200 mg/m² (33). Sensory neuropathy was found to be the dose-limiting toxicity in several phase I trials (42,43) though not in most. It was the major dose-limiting toxicity in trials of paclitaxel combined with granulocyte colony-stimulating factor (a hematopoietic growth factor, given to prevent neutropenia) (34,39). Patients with pre-existing conditions that would predispose to neuropathy, such as diabetes mellitus, kidney disease, or prior exposure to neurotoxic chemotherapy, have a greater risk of developing neuropathy from treatment with paclitaxel. Nerve fiber loss was evident in a sural nerve biopsy from a patient treated with paclitaxel for more than a year (25).

The sensory neuropathy may begin rapidly (within 3 days) after a single high dose, and symptoms may progress after each succeeding treatment (19,33). The most common symptoms include burning dysesthesias, numbness, tingling, and shooting pains. Most often, symptoms appear asymmetrically in the distal lower extremities, but commonly they occur simultaneously in the hands or even the face. Less commonly, symptoms begin in the hands or face before occurring in the feet (19). This pattern is suggestive of a neuronopathy (affecting the neuronal cell body) rather than an axonopathy; however, the symptoms often progress to a stocking-and-glove symmetrical pattern typical of distal axonopathies.

The most common findings on neurological examination are decreased or absent deep tendon reflexes, along with diminished pain, temperature, vibratory and/or propriocep-tive sensation, usually in a stocking-and-glove distribution. Electrophysiologically, patients most often have absent or reduced sensory nerve action potentials, particularly when recorded from the sural nerve (19,33).

Symptoms of sensory neuropathy usually improve with dose reduction or with discontinuation of the chemothera-peutic agent. There is, however, a report that paclitaxel-induced large-fiber dysfunction may be persistent (16). Since severe symptoms are usually seen only at high doses, it is unusual to have to discontinue therapy on the basis of the sensory neuropathy (27). Preclinical studies (2) suggest that nerve growth factor might be useful in the prevention or treatment of paclitaxel-induced sensory neuropathy.

Motor neuropathy is much less commonly seen but has been described in patients receiving the higher doses. Weak-ness is usually mild, affecting the distal extremities, and progressive with continued administration of the drug (19,33). Electrophysiological abnormalities of motor nerves are unusual, but absent or reduced peroneal evoked ampli-tudes have been reported (19,36). It has been suggested that mild distal motor neuropathy might be more common than is usually appreciated, since it rarely affects function signif-icantly (33).

Signs of autonomic dysfunction have also been reported with paclitaxel administration, but clearly defined auto-nomic neuropathy is not as well demonstrated as sensory neuropathy. Possible autonomic abnormalities have in-cluded orthostatic hypotension, gastrointestinal distur-bances, and cardiac arrhythmias. Most studies, however, have not differentiated true autonomic neuropathy from potential systemic causes such as hypovolemia, direct gas-trointestinal toxicity, or cardiac toxicity. One exception is a case report describing the results of formal autonomic testing in two patients with symptomatic orthostatic hy-potension following paclitaxel administration (15).

Muscle may also be affected by paclitaxel administration. There have been isolated reports of probable myopathy in patients receiving very high drug doses. The patients pre-sented with proximal muscle weakness that progressed with continued dosing; electromyography revealed myopathic motor unit potentials (19,33). Myalgias have been fre-quently reported, especially at higher dose levels, but are usually transient and resolve within a few days of dosing.

Paclitaxel does not appear to penetrate into the CNS (33). There have been a few isolated reports of seizures following paclitaxel administration, but in most (though not all) of those cases other explanations for the seizures were likely (33). There is one report that paclitaxel may damage the optic nerve (4): nine of 47 patients receiving high-dose paclitaxel reported experiencing transient scoto-mata soon after completing a paclitaxel infusion. Three also complained of visual loss and were found to have abnormal visual evoked potentials consistent with optic nerve dys-function. Finally, there is one report of a cerebrovascular event 36 h after paclitaxel administration (5); a relationship between these two events is uncertain.

Docetaxel-induced neuropathy has not been studied as well as that of paclitaxel, although reports suggest their neurotoxic effects are similar (1). Most patients have pre-sented with mild to moderate sensory symptoms, such as numbness and paresthesias, but several have developed proximal weakness as well (24,28). Neuropathic symptoms have been reported over a wide dose range. Like paclitaxel, most of the symptoms associated with neurotoxicity appear to be reversible with discontinuation of the drug, though this is rarely necessary since the symptoms are not severe. Neurotoxicity does not appear to be a dose-limiting side effect of docetaxel.

Toxic Mechanisms

The mechanisms responsible for taxoid neurotoxicity are unknown. It is not yet clear whether the neurotoxicity pri-marily affects the nerve cell body (neuronopathy), the axon (axonopathy), or the Schwann cells (demyelinating neurop-athy). Most likely, taxoid neurotoxicity involves all three sites, with some variability among individual patients. One mechanism by which the taxoids may be neurotoxic in-volves their ability to promote the assembly of large arrays of disordered microtubules. This would conceivably inter-fere with axonal transport as well as interactions with other cytoskeletal structures. There is no direct evidence that this mechanism underlies neurotoxicity.

REFERENCES

1. Apfel SC (1996) Docetaxel neuropathy. *Neurology* 46, 2.
2. Apfel SC, Lipton RB, Arezzo JC, Kessler JA (1990) Nerve growth factor prevents toxic neuropathy in mice. *Ann Neurol* 29, 87.
3. Bissery MC, Guenard D, Gueritte-Voegelein F, Lavelle F (1991) Experimental antitumor activity of Taxotere (RP

56976, NSC 628503), a Taxol analogue. *Cancer Res* **51**, 4845.

4. Capri G, Munzone E, Tarenzi E *et al.* (1994) Optic nerve disturbances: A new form of paclitaxel neurotoxicity. *J Nat Cancer Inst* **86**, 1099.

5. Chan AT, Leung WT, Johnson PJ (1994) Cerebrovascular event following taxol infusion. *Clin Oncol* **6**, 202.

6. Cliffer KD, Siuciak JA, Carson ST *et al.* (1998) Physiological characterization of taxol-induced large fiber sensory neuropathy in the rat. *Ann Neurol* **43**, 46.

7. Contreras PC, Steffler C, Gruner JA *et al.* (1995) Insulin like growth factor-I (RHIGF-I) prevents the peripheral neuropathy induced by paclitaxel, cisplatin and vincristine. *Ann Neurol* **38**, 315. [Abstract]

8. Denis JN, Greene AE, Guenard D *et al.* (1988) A highly efficient, practical approach to natural taxol. *J Amer Chem Soc* **110**, 5917.

9. Denniston PL (1995) *Physicians Gen Rx 1995*. Mosby Year Book Inc, St Louis, Missouri.

10. Ettinger DS, Finkelstein DM, Sarma R, Johnson DH (1993) Phase II study of taxol in patients with extensive stage small-cell lung cancer. An Eastern Cooperative Oncology Group Study. *Proc ASCO* **12**, 329.

11. Forastiere AA, Neuberg D, Taylor SG *et al.* (1993) Phase II evaluation of taxol in head and neck cancer. An Eastern Cooperative Oncology Group Trial. *Proc ASCO* **12**, 277.

12. Fumoleau P, Chevallier B, Kerbrat P *et al.* (1993) First line chemotherapy with Taxotere in advanced breast cancer: A phase II study of the EORTC clinical screening group. *Proc ASCO* **12**, 56.

13. Hamers FP, Pette C, Neijt JP, Gispen WH (1993) The ACTH-(4-9) analog, ORG 2766, prevents taxol induced neuropathy in rats. *Eur J Pharmacol* **233**, 177.

14. Hayakawa K, Sobue G, Itoh T, Mitsuma T (1994) Nerve growth factor prevents neurotoxic effects of cisplatin, vincristine and taxol on adult rat sympathetic explants *in-vitro*. *Life Sci* **55**, 519.

15. Jerian SM, Sarosy GA, Link CJ *et al.* (1993) Incapacitating autonomic neuropathy precipitated by taxol. *Gynecol Oncol* **51**, 277.

16. Kaplan JG, Einzig AI, Schaumburg HH (1993) Taxol causes permanent large fiber peripheral nerve dysfunction: A lesson for preventive strategies. *J Neuro-oncol* **16**, 105.

17. Konings PNM, Makkink WK, van Delft AML, Ruigt GSF (1994) Reversal by NGF of cytostatic drug reduction of neurite outgrowth in rat dorsal root ganglia in-vitro. *Brain Res* **640**, 195.

18. Letourneau PC, Ressler AH (1984) Inhibition of neurite initiation and growth by taxol. *J Cell Biol* **98**, 1355.

19. Lipton RB, Apfel SC, Dutcher JP *et al.* (1989) Taxol produces a predominantly sensory neuropathy. *Neurology* **39**, 368.

20. Masurovsky EB, Peterson ER, Crain SM *et al.* (1981) Microtubule arrays in taxol treated mouse dorsal root ganglion–spinal cord cultures. *Brain Res* **217**, 392.

21. Masurovsky EB, Peterson ER, Crain SM *et al.* (1983) Morphological alterations in dorsal root ganglion neurons and supporting cells of organotypic mouse spinal cord-ganglion cultures exposed to taxol. *Neuroscience* **10**, 491.

22. Monsarrat B, Mariel E, Crois S *et al.* (1990) Taxol metabolism. Isolation and identification of three major metabolites of taxol in rat bile. *Drug Metab Disposition* **18**, 895.

23. Nennesmo I, Reinholt FP (1988) Effects of intraneural injection of taxol on retrograde axonal transport and morphology of corresponding nerve cell bodies. *Virchows Arch B Cell Pathol* **55**, 241.

24. New P (1993) Neurotoxicity of Taxotere. *Proc Amer Assn Cancer Res* **34**, 233.

25. New P, Barohn R, Gales T *et al.* (1991) Taxol neuropathy after long term administration. *Proc Amer Assn Cancer Res* **32**, 205.

26. Olin BR (1995) *Drug Facts and Comparisons. 1995 Edition*. Facts and Comparisons, St Louis, Missouri.

27. Onetto N, Canetta R, Winograd B *et al.* (1993) Overview of taxol safety. *Monogr Natl Cancer Inst* **15**, 131.

28. Pazdur R, Kudelka AP, Kavanagh JJ *et al.* (1993) The taxoids: Paclitaxel (Taxol®) and docetaxel (Taxotere®). *Cancer Treatmen Rev* **19**, 351.

29. Peterson ER, Crain SM (1982) Nerve growth factor attenuates neurotoxic effects of taxol on spinal cord–ganglion explants from fetal mice. *Science* **217**, 377.

30. Piccart MJ, Gore M, Ten Bokkel Huinink W *et al.* (1993) Taxotere: An active new drug for the treatment of advanced ovarian carcinoma. *Proc ASCO* **12**, 258.

31. Rigas JR, Francis PA, Kris MG *et al.* (1993) Phase II trial of Taxotere in non-small cell lung cancer. *Proc ASCO* **12**, 336.

32. Rowinsky EK, Burke PJ, Karp JE *et al.* (1989) Phase I and pharmacodynamic study of taxol in refractory acute leukemias. *Cancer Res* **49**, 4640.

33. Rowinsky EK, Chaudhry V, Cornblath DR, Donehower RC (1993) Neurotoxicity of Taxol. *Monogr Natl Cancer Inst* **15**, 107.

34. Rowinsky EK, Chaudhry V, Forastiere AA *et al.* (1993) Phase I and pharmacologic study of paclitaxel and cisplatin with granulocyte colony stimulating factor: Neuromuscular toxicity is dose limiting. *J Clin Oncol* **11**, 2010.

35. Rowinsky EK, Eisenhauer EA, Chaudhry V *et al.* (1993) Clinical toxicities encountered with paclitaxel (Taxol). *Semin Oncol* **20**, 1.

36. Rowinsky EK, Gilbert MR, McGuire WP *et al.* (1991) Sequences of taxol and cisplatin: A phase I and pharmacologic study. *J Clin Oncol* **9**, 1692.

37. Roytta M, Horwitz SB, Raine CS (1984) Taxol induced neuropathy: Short term effects of local injection. *J Neurocytol* **13**, 685.

38. Roytta M, Raine CS (1985) Taxol induced neuropathy: Further ultrastructural studies of nerve fiber changes in situ. *J Neurocytol* **14**, 157.

39. Sarosy G, Kohn E, Stone DA *et al.* (1992) Phase I study of Taxol and granulocyte colony stimulating factor in patients with refractory ovarian cancer. *J Clin Oncol* **10**, 1165.

40. deValeriola D, Brassinne C, Gaillard C *et al.* (1993) Study of excretion balance, metabolism and protein binding of C^{14} radiolabelled Taxotere (RP56976, NSC 628503) in cancer patients. *Proc Amer Assn Cancer Res* **34**, 373.

41. Wani MC, Taylor HL, Wall ME *et al.* (1971) Plant antitumor agents, VI: The isolation and structure of taxol, a novel antileukemic and antitumor agent from *Taxus brevifolia*. *J Amer Chem Soc* **93**, 2325.

42. Wiernik PH, Schwartz EL, Einzig A *et al.* (1987) Phase I trial of taxol given as a 24 hour infusion every 21 days: responses observed in metastatic melanoma. *J Clin Oncol* **5**, 1232.

43. Wiernik PH, Schwartz EL, Strauman JJ *et al.* (1987) Phase I clinical and pharmacokinetic study of taxol. *Cancer Res* **47**, 2486.

CASE REPORT

A 70-year-old man was discovered to have melanoma of the right fifth toe. Following toe amputation, he was started on paclitaxel (250 mg/m²) every 3 weeks, as part of a phase II clinical trial. He received 16 courses with clinical and radiographic disappearance of adenopathy. A few days after each dose, he noted tingling of his feet lasting 2–3 days. He gradually developed constant numbness in his legs up to the thighs, with continuous tingling and burning of his feet. These symptoms improved somewhat with amitryptyline, 50 mg daily. Because of these symptoms, the dose of paclitaxel was reduced to 175 mg/m² and the interval increased to every 4 weeks starting with the 17th course.

Fifteen months later, he was referred for neurological evaluation (after 19 courses of paclitaxel), complaining of diminished agility on the tennis courts and frequent falls. Neurological examination revealed moderate distal weakness of the legs and milder intrinsic hand weakness. Deep tendon reflexes were absent throughout. He was unable to stand on toes or heels. There was a glove-and-stocking sensory deficit in the legs up to the knees and in the hands up to the wrists affecting pin and vibration senses equally. Romberg's sign was present. There was no evidence of diabetes mellitus, renal insufficiency, or vitamin B₁₂ or folate deficiency. Nerve conduction velocities and needle electromyography demonstrated severe generalized peripheral neuropathy, predominantly affecting axons.

Following the reduction of the paclitaxel dose, the neuropathy remained clinically stable, and he was able to continue playing tennis daily.

Tellurium

Kenneth R. Reuhl
Marianne A. Polunas

NEUROTOXICITY RATING

Clinical

B Headache

Experimental

A Fetal neurotoxicity (hydrocephalus)

A Peripheral neuropathy (demyelinating)

The name for element 52, tellurium (Te), is derived from the Latin *tellus*, or earth. Tellurium occurs in the earth's crust at concentrations of 0.002–0.01 ppm (19). Te is a group-16 (formerly group VIB) element: AW, 127.6; MP, 449.5°C; and BP, 989.8°C. The pure crystalline form is silvery white with a metallic luster; amorphous Te is a fine black powder. The chemistry resembles that of selenium and sulfur; it forms compounds in oxidation states -2, $+2$, $+4$, and $+6$. Of greatest neurotoxicological interest are the colorless gases, hydrogen telluride and tellurium hexafluoride, the water-soluble tellurites, and the sparingly soluble tellurium dioxide. Elemental Te is relatively nontoxic.

Industrial emissions and coal combustion are the primary sources of Te in ambient air, with an estimated release of 40 tons Te in fly ash yearly in the United States (12). Estimates of annual world production range from 65–200 tons (12). Te has not been detectable in municipal tap water, nor is it found in principal U.S. rivers. Commercially, Te is utilized in the semiconductor industry and in metal alloys to improve strength and machinability. It has been used as an accelerator in the vulcanization of rubber, a catalyst in the chemical industry, a coloring agent in glass, and in nuclear reactors to produce [131]I. Historically, Te has been used in the treatment of syphilis, leprosy, trypanosomiasis, seborrheic dermatitis, and in pulmonary tuberculosis to decrease sweating.

The U.S. Threshold Limit Value (TLV) for Te in ambient air is 0.1 mg/m^3 (1992), a level that still gives rise to a characteristic garlic odor breath from dimethyl telluride exhalation. A TLV of 0.01 mg/m^3 would eliminate this problem in most workers (19).

Tellurites are approximately 10%–25% absorbed from the gastrointestinal tract; elemental Te and tellurium dioxide are absorbed to a much lesser extent. No quantitative data on respiratory absorption of Te compounds have been reported. Organic esters of Te may be absorbed through intact skin. Te salts are readily transported across both the blood-brain-barrier and the placenta. The estimated half-life in rats varies from 19 h to 15 days; in humans, the half-life is approximately 3 weeks. Inhaled or intravenous Te is excreted in the urine, while ingested Te is mainly excreted in the feces. Small amounts of Te may be exhaled as dimethyl telluride. After short-term exposure, Te accumulates primarily in the kidney, heart, lungs, spleen, blood, and liver. Over the long term, bone becomes the reservoir of about 90% of the total body burden, with an average concentration of 0.12 ppm (16).

The specific manifestation of neurotoxicity depends upon age at the time of exposure; effects are more severe in very young animals and slight in adults. Species/strain differences in toxic response have also been reported.

Dietary administration of Te (500–3500 ppm) to pregnant rats results in a dose-dependent incidence of nonobstructive hydrocephalus in the offspring (8,11). Hydrocephalus is present at birth and is usually fatal within the first month of postnatal life. Pups surviving the first week may develop signs of progressive cerebrospinal fluid obstruction, with stenosis of the cerebral aqueduct, elevated intracranial pressure, neuronal and ependymal degeneration, marked thinning of the cerebral cortices; in some animals, ventriculostomy may form by rupture of the occipital cortex (8). Te-induced hydrocephalus is readily produced by congenital exposure to the element between gestational days 10 and 16; exposure outside this developmental window does not cause the hydrocephalus.

Weanling rats administered Te (1.25% in diet) between postnatal days 15 and 35 manifest a rapidly developing, reversible primary demyelination of peripheral nerve fibers accompanied by transient hindlimb paralysis. The earliest evidence of Schwann cell injury is an accumulation of lipid droplets in the cytoplasm within 12 h of initiating treatment (4,13); this is followed within 36–48 h by development of segmental demyelination, which preferentially involves larger-diameter fibers of the sciatic nerve and spinal roots (5,9). Schwann cells myelinating the longest internodal regions are particularly vulnerable. The myelin sheath undergoes a sequence of nonspecific changes, including splitting at the intraperiod line, vesiculation, and fragmentation of the myelin lamellae. Remyelination is well established within 7–14 days of beginning exposure, even with continued Te administration.

The blood-nerve barrier (BNB) is also affected by Te exposure during the neonatal period, resulting in vasogenic endoneurial edema. Changes in the BNB appear to follow the early changes in Schwann cells and are not believed responsible for the initial Schwann-cell injury. However, a synergistic role for BNB dysfunction in the pathogenesis of Te-induced demyelination has been proposed (4).

Te poisoning in the adult animal is associated with a characteristic garlic odor and variable degrees of growth retardation. A pronounced darkening of the brain is frequently observed at necropsy. This discoloration is the result of cerebral lipofuscinosis, with accumulation of needle-like crystals and black granules within lysosomes (and possibly mitochondria) of large cortical neurons, particularly pyramidal neurons, cerebellar Purkinje cells, and motor neurons of the spinal cord. The presence of Te in these organelles has been confirmed by electron microprobe analysis (10). Despite extensive accumulation of these structures, adverse effects on neuronal functioning have not been identified.

The peripheral nerve of the adult rat is significantly more resistant to Te than that of the developing animal. Dietary consumption of Te for 30 days induces signs of peripheral neuropathy and weakness but no paralysis. Myelin blebbing, edema, segmental demyelination, and remyelination have been noted in spinal roots, sciatic nerve, and brachial plexus (18).

Voluntary ingestion and therapeutic application are the primary means of controlled human exposure to Te. Hansen (1853, cited in 7) deliberately ingested 0.40–0.88 g/day potassium tellurite for 1 week. He reported anorexia, nausea, drowsiness, and cardiac alterations; a strong garlic breath odor developed rapidly and lasted 7 weeks. In the early 1900s, suspensions of elemental Te or tellurium iodide were administered intramuscularly for the treatment of syphilis. Primary side effects of this treatment included garlic breath and a persistent metallic taste. A blue tinge, presumably from systemic distribution, frequently appeared on the face and hands.

Accidental exposure to Te occurs most frequently by inhalation in occupational settings and by ingestion of contaminated food in the general population (6). However, reports of either occupational or dietary Te poisoning are extremely rare. Most patients present with nonspecific neurological complaints such as headache and malaise. A distinct neurological syndrome is lacking, presumably because of insufficient exposure and the relative insensitivity of the adult nervous system. One report describes three workers exposed to Te vapor for approximately 10 min during the production of a tellurium-copper alloy (1). Within 24 h, the men sought medical attention with complaints of transient headache, gastric distress, metallic taste, and heavy garlic odor. Urinary Te concentrations were 0.008–0.016 mg/l 48 h after the incident. Recovery ensued without further manifestations. Two chemists accidentally inhaled tellurium hexaflouride gas (3). The only symptoms reported were tiredness and strong garlic odor. One patient manifested signs of Te skin absorption, with bluish black pigmentation beneath the skin on the webs of the fingers and fainter streaks on his face and neck. Several weeks passed before these Te deposits faded.

Two reports of long-term exposure in humans are available. One describes examination of 13 workers exposed to hydrogen telluride and tellurium dioxide dust at a lead refinery (20). Garlic odor of breath, sweat, and urine, and metallic taste and dryness of mouth were experienced by seven of the workers; five had considerable suppression of sweating, itchy skin, anorexia, nausea and vomiting, depression, and somnolence. Another report described garlic breath in 62 iron-foundry workers exposed to Te fumes at levels of 0.01– 0.1 mg/m³ over a 22-month period (21). Common complaints included garlic odor, dryness and metallic taste in the mouth, somnolence, and occasional nausea.

Reports of nonoccupational accidental exposure are rare. In one incident, sodium tellurite was accidentally substituted for sodium iodide in three patients undergoing retrograde pyelography. Two of the patients received a dose of about 2 g, or 30 mg/kg; they experienced vomiting, renal pain, stupor, loss of consciousness, irregular breathing and cyanosis, followed by death within 6 h of administration. Deposition of black Te pigment was found in the mucosa of the bladder and ureter, and congestion of the lungs, liver, spleen, and kidneys, and fatty change of the liver were noted at autopsy. All tissues smelled of garlic (15).

Diagnostic features of Te poisoning include garlic odor of breath, sweat, or urine; since other compounds (selenium, sulfur) may cause similar signs, identification of Te in blood and urine is important. There is no specific treatment for Te exposure. Eyes or skin should be immediately flushed with water following direct exposure. Treatment of serious acute poisoning is mainly supportive. Evidence that the chelating agent British antilewisite (BAL; dimercaprol) is beneficial in treating Te poisoning is lacking. In fact, it has been proposed to enhance the toxicity of Te (in guinea pigs), and its use is therefore not recommended (2). The obnoxious methyl telluride odor may be reduced by administration of ascorbic acid but reappears when treatment is discontinued.

Altered cholesterol metabolism appears to underlie Te-induced peripheral neuropathy. The period of Schwann cell vulnerability coincides with the period of maximal myelinogenesis in the rat PNS. Dietary exposure of weanling rats to Te causes a 50% decrease in the overall incorporation of [^{14}C]acetate into nerve lipids, but a major concomitant increase in levels of squalene, an intermediate in cholesterol biosynthesis (14). Subsequent studies identified a rapid (within 12 h of treatment), specific inhibitory action of Te (as tellurite) on squalene epoxidase, a microsomal monooxygenase (22). Concentrations of Te as tellurite as low as 5 μM cause 50% reduction of the enzyme, possibly by binding with susceptible sulfhydryl groups on the enzyme. Failure to convert squalene to 2,3-epoxysqualene results in the rapid accumulation of squalene as lipid droplets within Schwann cell cytoplasm. The developing peripheral nerve, with its greater rate of myelin accumulation and high demand for cholesterol, is highly sensitive to disturbances in cholesterol biosynthesis during the first 6 weeks of postnatal life. However, the exact mechanisms leading from the inhibition of the enzyme to primary demyelination are unclear.

REFERENCES

1. Amdur ML (1947) Tellurium. Accidental exposure and treatment with BAL in oil. *Occup Med* **3**, 386.
2. Amdur ML (1958) Tellurium oxide. An animal study in acute toxicity. *Arch Ind Health* **17**, 665.
3. Blackadder ES, Manderson WG (1975) Occupational absorption of tellurium: A report of two cases. *Brit J Ind Med* **32**, 59.
4. Bouldin TW, Earnhardt T, Goines ND, Goodrum J (1989) Temporal relationship of blood-nerve barrier breakdown to the metabolic and morphologic alterations of tellurium neuropathy. *Neurotoxicology* **10**, 79.
5. Bouldin TW, Samsa G, Earnhardt T, Krigman MR (1988) Schwann cell vulnerability to demyelination is associated with internodal length in tellurium neuropathy. *J Neuropathol Exper Neurol* **47**, 41.
6. Braheny SL, Lampert PW (1980) Tellurium. In: *Experimental and Clinical Neurotoxicology*. Spencer PS, Schaumburg HH eds. Williams & Wilkins, Baltimore p. 558.
7. Carson B, Ellis HV III, McCann JL (1986) Tellurium. In: *Toxicology and Biological Monitoring of Metals in Humans*. Lewis Publishing, Inc, Chelsea, Michigan, p. 240.
8. Duckett S (1971) The morphology of tellurium-induced hydrocephalus. *Exp Neurol* **31**, 1.

9. Duckett S, Said G, Streletz L *et al.* (1979) Tellurium-induced neuropathy: correlative physiological, morphological and electron microprobe studies. *Neuropathol Appl Neurobiol* **5**, 265.

10. Duckett S, White R (1974) Cerebral lipofucsinosis induced with tellurium: Electron dispersive X-ray spectrophotometry analysis. *Brain Res* **73**, 205.

11. Garro F, Pentschew A (1964) Neonatal hydrocephalus in the offspring of rats fed during pregnancy non-toxic amounts of tellurium. *Arch Psychiat Z Neurol* **206**, 272.

12. Gerhardsson L, Glover JR, Nordberg GF, Vouk VB (1986) Tellurium. In: *Handbook on the Toxicology of Metals. Vol II. 2nd Ed.* Friberg L, Nordberg GF, Vouk VB eds. Elsevier, New York p. 552.

13. Goodrum JF, Earnhardt TS, Goines ND, Bouldin TW (1990) Lipid droplets in Schwann cells during tellurium neuropathy are derived from newly synthesized lipid. *J Neurochem* **55**, 1928.

14. Harry GJ, Goodrum JF, Bouldin TW *et al.* (1989) Tellurium-induced neuropathy: Metabolic alterations associated with demyelination and remyelination in rat sciatic nerve. *J Neurochem* **52**, 938.

15. Keall JHH, Martin NH, Tunbridge RE (1946) Three cases of accidental poisoning by sodium tellurite. *Brit J Ind Med* **3**, 175.

16. Kobayashi R (1994) Tellurium. In: *Handbook on Metals in Clinical and Analytical Chemistry.* Seiler HG, Sigel A, Sigel H eds. Marcel Dekker, Inc, New York p. 593.

17. Muller R, Zschiesche W, Steffen HM, Schaller KH (1989) Case reports. Tellurium-intoxication. *Klin Wochenschr* **67**, 1152.

18. Said G, Duckett S (1981) Tellurium-induced myelinopathy in adult rats. *Muscle Nerve* **4**, 319.

19. Scansetti G (1992) Exposure to metals that have recently come into use. *Sci Total Environ* **120**, 85.

20. Shie MD, Deeds FE (1920) The importance of tellurium as a health hazard in industry—a preliminary report. *Public Health Rep* **35**, 939.

21. Steinberg HH, Massari SC, Miner AC, Rink R (1942) Industrial exposure to tellurium: Atmospheric studies and clinical evaluation. *J Ind Hyg Toxicol* **24**, 183.

22. Wagner M, Toews AD, Morell P (1995) Tellurite specifically affects squalene epoxidase: Investigations examining the mechanism of tellurium-induced neuropathy. *J Neurochem* **64**, 2169.

CASE REPORT

Te intoxication was reported in a 37-year-old woman with no history of industrial exposure (17). The woman had experienced acute nausea, vomiting, metallic taste, and strong garlic odor of the breath, sweat, and urine a few hours after tasting a piece of meat containing a Te level of 800–1000 μg/kg. Fever developed the following day and spontaneously resolved after 5 days. Hair loss was observed 2 weeks following the onset of symptoms. Upon hospital admission 2 weeks later, clinical findings were unremarkable except for the strong garlic odor. Concentrations in serum and urine were 27.6 and 3.2 μg/l, respectively. The upper normal limit of occupationally nonexposed persons is 1.0 μg/l for both serum and urine (17). The patient was given 200 mg ascorbic acid per day and discharged. Eight weeks after Te exposure, new hair grew in; the garlic odor became less obvious but persisted for 8 months. No further health problems developed, although the patient noticed the garlic odor intensified after alcohol intake.

Tetanospasmin

John W. Griffin
George Oyler

NEUROTOXICITY RATING

Clinical

A Tetanus

A Seizure disorder

Experimental

A Glycinergic inhibition (spinal cord)

A Tetanus

A Seizure disorder

The clinical syndrome of tetanus occurs as a result of the action of the protein neurotoxin *tetanospasmin* on the CNS. The toxin is a 150-kDa protein produced within contaminated wounds by *Clostridium tetani* (3). The spores of this organism are widespread, particularly in the soil, where they are protected from direct sunlight. Any penetrating wound can be considered a potential inoculum. A study in 1938 of samples of dust from the streets of Baltimore documented *Clostridium tetani* in 17% of samples (8). This high incidence may reflect in part the number of horses in use in the city at that time, but a significant incidence of positive cultures would undoubtedly be found today. Within the body, the spores are converted to toxin-producing vegetative forms whose toxin production is favored by anaerobic conditions. Since the toxin is extremely potent, minute wounds can be responsible for fatal tetanus.

Given the ubiquitous distribution of the organism, it is not surprising that tetanus is a major worldwide public health problem with at least 100,000 adult cases annually (31). In unvaccinated populations, young working males are at greatest risk for tetanus, presumably because of their increased incidence of minor wounds that may implant infective material. In North America, the annual incidence of tetanus declined rapidly from 560 cases in 1947 to 36 in 1993 following the availablity of tetanus toxoid inoculations. Childhood inoculation is followed by booster inoculation every 10 years. Nearly all current cases are due to inadequate immunization or failure to obtain postexposure prophylaxis. Historically, large outbreaks of tetanus have been associated with the penetrating wounds produced in wars (11).

Tetanus neonatorum is a special problem; it results from infection of the umbilical stump. In developing countries, the annual toll from neonatal tetanus is estimated to be in excess of 1 million. In the United States, the elderly forms a high-risk population. In addition, urban tetanus—tetanus in unvaccinated drug addicts, which develops after skin penetration with contaminated needles—is an important medical problem (4,13).

Animal Studies
Biochemistry

In vivo study of the clostridial neurotoxins, particularly tetanus toxin, has been central to elucidating the mechanisms of synaptic vesicle release. Tetanus neurotoxin was the first clostridial neurotoxin for which the mechanism of action was identified. Tetanus toxin shares common structural characteristics with the family of clostridial neurotoxins. The toxin is synthesized as a 150-kDa holotoxin by the bacterial host. During or soon after secretion of the toxin, the 150-kDa holotoxin is proteolytically processed to yield a carboxyl-terminal 100-kDa heavy chain and an amino 50-kDa light chain. The toxin heavy and light chains are covalently attached by disulfide bonds and by high-affinity noncovalent interchain binding as well (22).

Intoxication of the presynaptic terminal by clostridial neurotoxins proceeds in four general steps:

1. Heavy chain binding of the toxin complex to the presynaptic membrane.
2. Internalization of the toxin complex by the heavy chain into the presynaptic terminal endosomal compartment.
3. Translocation of the catalytic light chain into the cytosol of the presynaptic terminal.
4. Proteolytic cleavage of a component of the synaptic-vesicle fusion apparatus by the light-chain zinc protease to inhibit neurotransmitter release.

The toxin can undergo retrograde transport from the nerve terminal to the neuronal perikaryon (9,10,19,28). This sequence of events is shared with botulinum toxins, but unlike botulinum toxin, the tetanus heavy chain undergoes a much more extensive transcytosis into glycinergic inhibitory neurons in the spinal cord.

There are eight known forms of clostridial neurotoxins, seven forms of botulinum neurotoxins, designated A–G produced by separate serotype or strains of *Clostridia botulinum*, and tetanus toxin produced by *C. tetani* (12). These are closely related proteins that all share the same general dipeptide 100-kDa heavy-chain and 50-kDa light-chain structure. They also share the molecular functions of the heavy chain in neuronal binding and translocation and light chain zinc-dependent protease activity. The various toxins do differ in the amino acid sequence, sharing approximately 50% identity, indicating a likely common ancestral toxin (15). Curiously, despite the structural and mechanistic similarities of the clostridial neurotoxins, the toxins differ in the substrate specificity for components of the synaptic-vesicle fusion apparatus.

The light chain of the clostridial neurotoxins, including tetanus, contains a histidine zinc-binding motif shared by many zinc proteases (20). The zinc-binding residues of the clostridial neurotoxins have been shown to be invariant. Zinc binding by the clostridial neurotoxin light chains was demonstrated (22,24,25). Based on the shared structural motif of tetanus toxin with zinc proteases, the invariant conservation of zinc coordinate binding residues of the clostridial neurotoxins and the biochemical evidence of zinc binding to tetanus light chain, there existed considerable evidence that the molecular mechanism of tetanus inhibition of neurotransmitter release may be light-chain proteolytic activity. In 1993, the synaptic vesicle protein, synaptobrevin, also referred to as VAMP (*v*esicle *m*embrane *a*ssociated *m*embrane *p*rotein), was proteolyticly cleaved by tetanus toxin light chain (21). Rapidly, a number of researchers demonstrated that the botulinum neurotoxin light chains specifically cleaved one of three proteins associated with either the presynaptic terminal inner membrane, SNAP-25 (*s*ynaptosomal *a*ssociated *p*rotein of 25 kDa) and syntaxin or synaptobrevin associated with the synaptic vesicle (23,30).

Pathophysiology

The discovery of the presynaptic protein substrates of the clostridial neurotoxins converged with advancements in identification of the components of the synaptic-vesicle fusion apparatus by biochemical means and the analysis of the mammalian analogues of yeast secretory protein mutants. A model for the steps involved in synaptic vesicle docking and fusion emerged from these various lines of investigation. The docking and calcium-triggered fusion of synaptic vesicles is a specialized example of the targeting and fusion of transport vesicles of intracellular organelles in general and, as a result, the synaptic vesicles and intracellular transport vesicles utilizes similar molecular machinery. Vesicle targeting and fusion events employ a common docking complex, the NSF particle. The NSF particle is formed by a homotetramer of the NSF protein (*N*-methylmaleimide *s*ensitive *f*actor) with α, β, or γ SNAPS (*s*oluble *NSF a*ssociated *p*roteins) (5). The NSF particle facilitates the docking and fusion of a vesicle to the target membrane (the presynaptic membrane in the case of the synaptic vesicles). Much of the specificity of the targeting of a vesicle to a membrane is the result of a receptor protein on the vesicle (v-SNARE) and a complementary receptor on the target membrane (t-SNARE). In the case of synaptic vesicle docking and fusion with the presynaptic membrane, the v-SNARE is synaptobrevin and the t-SNARES are formed by a complex of SNAP-25 and syntaxin (27). Thus, remarkably, the highly specific proteolytic targets of all the clostridial neurotoxin light chains are one of the v- or t-SNARES (30). By cleaving the v-SNARE, synaptobrevin, tetanus toxin interferes with the ability of the synaptic vesicle to dock and fuse with the presynaptic membrane, thereby preventing neurotransmitter release.

An interesting experiment of evolutionary biology provides further support for this mechanism of vesicle-release inhibition by tetanus toxin. There are at least two isoforms of synaptobrevin associated with synaptic vesicles, both of which appear to be capable of supporting synaptic vesicle fusion (6). In humans, the amino acid sequence at the tetanus toxin light chain cleavage site is conserved between both isoforms (Q_{76}–F_{77}), and both isoforms are cleaved by tetanus toxin. In rats, however, the amino acid sequence differs between the two isoforms as a result of a substitution of valine for glutamine at residue 76 in rat synaptobrevin-1. This amino acid substitution renders the synaptobrevin resistant to tetanus toxin cleavage and rats resistant to tetanus intoxication (25).

Recently, an additional mechanism for tetanus toxin and botulinum toxin B activity has been identified. Independent of the proteolysis of synaptobrevin, tetanus and botulinum B toxins possess transglutaminase activity (2,7). The role that transglutaminase covalent cross-linking of presynaptic proteins may play in inhibiting neurotransmitter release is under investigation. The contribution of transglutaminase activation may in part account for possible preferential inhibition of inhibitory neurotransmitter release.

Tetanus toxin binds with considerable specificity to two gangliosides, GT_1b and GD_1b, which represent the receptors on the neuronal cell membranes (3). *In vivo*, the toxin appears to be bound and taken up by sensory, motor, and autonomic nerve terminals (28). The historically attractive idea that the toxin might directly produce excitation at the level of the motor neuron has proved to be incorrect. In fact, tetanus toxin can produce an opposite effect. For example, at the neuromuscular junction, high concentrations of the toxin prevent the release of acetylcholine, thereby producing a flaccid paralysis similar to that of botulinum toxin (28). The classical manifestations of tetanus result from the action of tetanospasmin within the spinal cord and brainstem. The toxin prevents the release of neurotransmitters, including γ-aminobutyric acid (GABA) and glycine from the presynaptic terminals that surround motor neurons. Glycine is the neurotransmitter used by group 1A inhibitory fibers on motor neurons. Abolition of these inhibitory influences on the motor neuron produces an unrestrained firing that results in sustained muscular contraction. This response can be elicited from a local intraspinal injection of either strychnine—a drug that produces postsynaptic blockade of glycinergic function, or tetanus toxin itself, which produces blockade of glycinergic function presynaptically. In addition, the unopposed excitation of motor neurons produced by tetanus is abolished by iontophoresis of glycine into the spinal cord. Thus, it is clear that clinical tetanus depends entirely on the presence of toxin within the central nervous system.

The means by which tetanospasmin enters the CNS has been the subject of recurrent, often acrimonious debate since the turn of the century, and the phenomenon of local tetanus has been a central element in these arguments. Before 1900, it was suggested by Marie and Morax and others in Europe that local tetanus was best explained by ascent of the toxin from the site of production in wounded extremities to the innervating segments of the spinal cord or brainstem (17). This theory generated a good deal of experimentation, but suffered from two major difficulties: it suggested that a different route, hematogenous spread, must be invoked to explain generalized tetanus; it also depended on the then-unknown mechanisms of translocation of macromolecules within axons. The case against intra-axonal spread was summarized succinctly in *The Bulletin of the Johns Hopkins Hospital* in 1938 by John Jacob Abel and co-workers, who argued (1):

No satisfactory hypothesis has ever been offered to explain how a water-soluble substance of so large a molecular weight as that of tetanus toxin, once it has been absorbed by functional motor end-organs, by naked telodendria, or by the muscle fibers of higher vertebrates, can be transported to central neurons in axis cylinders. The axis cylinder carriage theory assumes the toxins are not bound by the motor end-organs or the cylinders, that they do not immobilize it, that it can move from point to point in its natural unaltered state, and that the axis cylinders serve merely as nature's conduit for its centripetal transportation.

Although this sequence of events was offered as exceedingly unlikely at the time, subsequent developments proved this mechanism to be correct. The recent recognition of the magnitude of bidirectional intra-axonal transport of materials, which normally occurs within nerve fibers, accounts for much of the change in viewpoint.

In the mid-1970s, studies using labeled tetanus toxin demonstrated that the toxin injected into muscle is taken up by motor nerve terminals and carried intra-axonally within membrane-bound vesicles to spinal motor neurons. The maximum rate of transport appeared to be approximately 250 mm/day. Both electrophoretic and immunocytochemical studies have indicated that tetanospasmin remains intact while being transported (10,19,28). This retrograde transport of tetanus toxin can be interrupted by nerve crush, nerve ligation, or by the application of pharmacological agents that focally block axon transport (10,14). When toxin reaches the perikaryon of motor neurons, it appears to pass transsynaptically to the surrounding presynaptic terminals, presumably including those of afferent fibers and the glycinergic inhibitory system (18,26).

The mechanism thus described provides a satisfying explanation for the phenomenon of local tetanus. It seems likely that generalized tetanus also results from retrograde transport of toxin. Generalized tetanus may result from escape of circulating toxin from the vasculature into the extracellular fluid within the muscle, and subsequent uptake and retrograde transport from motor nerve terminals to the spinal cord and brainstem (16). Entry into the CNS by the mechanism of retrograde intra-axonal transport may explain the unusual distribution of affected muscles. The bulbar muscles and the paraspinous muscles may be involved earliest because they are innervated by the shortest axons, and are the first to receive retrogradely transported materials.

Human Studies

The term "tetanus" usually evokes the image of a dramatic neurological syndrome, characterized by lockjaw, opisthotonus, painful spasms and convulsions, and a protracted recovery or death. However, less common but equally striking manifestations are the result of local tetanus.

Local Tetanus

Local tetanus is defined as tetanus predominantly affecting the extremity bearing a contaminated wound. This syndrome has been described since antiquity but has always been uncommon (11,31). In its most severe form, local tetanus includes intense painful spasms developing in the wounded extremity, a presentation that was early recognized to herald the development of generalized tetanus in a high proportion of cases (11). The progression of local tetanus to generalized musculoskeletal involvement early suggested that the active factor might ascend to the CNS through the peripheral nerves. Thus, many nineteenth century physicians advocated neurotomy or amputation of the involved extremity in the hope of preventing more generalized disease.

Detailed neurological descriptions of local tetanus are relatively few in the English literature. The available reports document two features: first, manifestations of local tetanus can be both mild and variable (29). Second, the duration of local tetanus can be prolonged. For example, a report described a 60-year-old man who sustained a minor hand wound with a porcupine quill (29). Following the apparent healing of that wound, he developed pain and tightness in the forearm, which increased in severity over 2 weeks. He showed no loss of hand muscle power, although he was unable to use the hand functionally because of "stiffness." By the end of the second week, he had difficulty in opening his mouth. Spasms that developed in the involved arm and trunk were exacerbated by voluntary movements of the arm. The correct diagnosis of local tetanus was arrived at 3 months after the initial injury and his symptoms gradually subsided over a subsequent 5-month period following treatment of the wound. During the course of his illness, diagnoses of rheumatological disease, dental problems, and parkinsonism were entertained. This individual's clinical course is representative of other previously reported cases of local tetanus.

A striking form of local tetanus follows wounds of the face or head ("cephalic tetanus"). The incubation period is 1 or 2 days followed by partial paralysis and spasms of ocular, facial, and pharyngeal muscles.

Generalized Tetanus

The mild, slowly evolving disease described above contrasts sharply with the dramatic manifestations of generalized tetanus. Recognized in the Hippocratic writings by the triad of wounding, lockjaw, and death, generalized tetanus may follow local tetanus. Trismus, difficulty in swallowing, and the grimace-like contraction of facial muscles termed *risus sardonicus*, are often initial manifestations of generalized tetanus (11,31). Painful spasms begin in the axial musculature and include the neck extensors and paraspinous muscles. These spasms may progress to waves of opisthotonic posturing that are so characteristic of the disease. Respiratory embarrassment due to persistent muscle contraction may occur during the spasms. As the disease progresses, all of the extremities may participate in these episodes of rigidity and spasm, which become increasingly painful. Spasms and generalized convulsions are often elicited by aural or tactile stimuli, although they may occur spontaneously as well. All manipulations should be kept to a minimum and the patient sedated beforehand. Autonomic instability is a particularly ominous manifestation that may result in life-threatening arrhythmias and fluctuations in blood pressure (11,31). Profound diaphoresis and hyperthermia complicate fluid management. Rhabdomyolysis may occur, producing myoglobinuria and acute renal failure.

Treatment of full-blown tetanus is a complex and multifaceted endeavor that includes an attack on the organism and relief of neurological dysfunction. Débridement of a local wound, 10 days of systemic antibiotics (usually penicillin), and administration of a single dose of antitoxin are measures directed at the infection. Muscle spasm may be relieved by chlorpromazine or diazepam. Severe muscle spasms occasionally require neuromuscular blockade and ventilatory support. Tracheostomy is necessary in all patients with generalized spasms; it should not be delayed.

General supportive care may be demanding; airway maintenance is especially vexing and pulmonary complications are common. Involvement of the autonomic nervous system can cause cardiac arrhythmias and hypotension. The mortality rate is 25% despite the advent of intensive care units. Severe cases who survive usually require 4–8 weeks of intensive care; however, recovery is usually complete.

Diagnosis is established from the clinical features; there is no definitive laboratory test. The task is easier if there is a clear history of a previous injury and classic physical findings are prominent. Unfortunately, the injury may have been trivial or forgotten and the organisms may be difficult to culture from the wound by the time the patient encounters the physician. Although the full-blown generalized tetanus syndrome is dramatic and has few imitators, the early phases of the disease are often confusing and accurate diagnosis is delayed by medical personnel in North America who currently rarely encounter tetanus. Differential diagnosis in the early stages includes dystonic spasms from neuroleptic drugs, hysterical spasms, trismus from painful conditions around the mouth, seizures, hypocalcemic tetany, alcohol withdrawal, and strychnine intoxication.

REFERENCES

1. Abel JJ, Firor WM, Chalian W (1938) Researches on tetanus toxin. IX. Further evidence to show that tetanus toxin is not carried to central neurons by way of the axis cylinders in motor nerves. *Bull Johns Hopkins Hosp* **63**, 373.

2. Ashton AC, Li Y, Doussau F, Weller U *et al.* (1995) Tetanus toxin inhibits neuroexocytosis even when its Zn^{2+}-dependent protease activity is removed. *J Biol Chem* **270**, 31386.

3. Bizzini B (1979) Tetanus toxin. *Microbiol Rev* **43**, 224.

4. Cherubin CE (1967) Investigations of tetanus in narcotic addicts in New York City. *Int J Addict* **2**, 253.

5. Clary DO, Griff IC, Rothman JF (1990) SNAPs, a family of NSF attachment proteins involved in intracellular membrane fusion in animals and yeast. *Cell* **61**, 709.

6. Elferink LA, Trimble WS, Scheller RH (1989) Two vesicle-associated membrane protein genes are differentially expressed in the rat central nervous system. *J Biol Chem* **264**, 11061.

7. Facchiano FF, Benfenati F, Valtorta A (1993) Covalent modifications of synapsin I by a tetanus toxin-activated transglutaminase. *J Biol Chem* **268**, 4588.

8. Gilles EC (1938) The isolation of tetanus bacilli from street dust. *J Amer Med Assn* **109**, 484.

9. Glass JD, Brushart TM, George EB, Griffin JW (1993) Prolonged survival of transected nerve fibres in C57BL/Ola mice is an intrinsic characteristic of the axon. *J Neurocytol* **22**, 311.

10. Griffin JW, Price DL, Engel WK, Drachman DB (1977) The pathogenesis of reactive axonal swellings: Role of axonal transport. *J Neuropathol Exp Neurol* **36**, 214.

11. Haberman E (1978) Tetanus. In: *Handbook of Clinical Neurology*. Vinken PJ, Bruyn GW eds. North-Holland Publishing Co, Amsterdam p. 491.

12. Hatheway CL (1989) Bacterial sources of clostridial neurotoxins. In: *Botulinum Neurotoxin and Tetanus Toxin*. Simpson LL ed. Academic Press, San Diego, California.

13. Heurich AG (1973) Management of urban tetanus. *Med Clin N Amer* **57**, 1373.

14. Mellick R, Cavanagh JB (1967) Longitudinal movement of radioiodinated albumin within extravascular spaces of peripheral nerves following three systems of experimental trauma. *J Neurol Neurosurg Psychiat* **30**, 458.

15. Neimann H (1991) *A Sourcebook of Bacterial Protein Toxins*. Alouf JE, Freer JH eds. Academic Press, New York p. 303.

16. Price DL, Griffin JW (1977) Tetanus toxin: Retrograde axonal transport of systemically administered toxin. *Neurosci Lett* **4**, 61.

17. Price DL, Griffin JW (1980) Neurons and ensheathing cells as targets of disease processes. In: *Experimental and Clinical Neurotoxicology*. Spencer PS, Schaumburg HH eds. Williams & Wilkins, Baltimore p. 2.

18. Price DL, Griffin JW (1981) Immunocytochemical localization of tetanus toxin to synapses of spinal cord. *Neurosci Lett* **23**, 149.

19. Price DL, Griffin JW, Young A *et al.* (1975) Tetanus toxin: Direct evidence for retrograde intraaxonal transport. *Science* **188**, 945.

20. Sanders D, Habermann F (1992) Evidence for a link between specific proteolysis and inhibition of noradrenaline release by the light chain of tetanus toxin. *Naunyn-Schmied Arch Pharmacol* **346**, 358.

21. Schiavo G, Benfenati F, Poulain B *et al.* (1992) Tetanus and botulinum-B neurotoxins block neurotransmitter release by proteolytic cleavage of synaptobrevin. *Nature* **359**, 832.

22. Schiavo G, Poulain B, Rossetto F *et al.* (1992) Tetanus toxin is a zinc protein and its inhibition of neurotransmitter release and protease activity depends on zinc. *EMBO J* **11**, 3577.

23. Schiavo G, Rossetto O, Benfenati F *et al.* (1994) Tetanus and botulinum neurotoxins are zinc proteases specific for components of the neuroexocytosis apparatus. *Ann N Y Acad Sci* **710**, 65.

24. Schiavo G, Rossetto O, Santucci A *et al.* (1992) Botulinum neurotoxins are zinc proteins. *J Biol Chem* **267**, 23479.

25. Schiavo GC, Shone O, Rossetto FCG *et al.* (1993) Neurotoxin serotype F is a zinc endopeptidase specific for VAMP/synaptobrevin. *J Biol Chem* **268**, 11516.

26. Schwab ME, Suda K, Thoenen H (1979) Selective retrograde transsynaptic transfer of a protein tetanus toxin subsequent to its retrograde axonal transport. *J Cell Biol* **82**, 798.

27. Sollner T, Whiteheart SW, Brunner M *et al.* (1993) SNAP receptors implicated in vesicle targeting and fusion. *Nature* **362**, 318.

28. Stöckel K, Schwab M, Thoenen H (1975) Comparison between the retrograde transport of nerve growth factor and tetanus toxin in motor, sensory, and adrenergic neurons. *Brain Res* **99**, 1.

29. Struppler A, Struppler E, Adams RD (1963) Local tetanus in man. *Arch Neurol* **8**, 162.

30. Sudhof TC, DeCamilli P, Niemann H, Jahn R (1993) Membrane fusion machinery: Insights from synaptic proteins. *Cell* **75**, 1.

31. Weinstein L (1973) Tetanus. *N Engl J Med* **289**, 1293.

Tetrachlorodibenzodioxin

Marie Haring Sweeney
David A. Dankovic

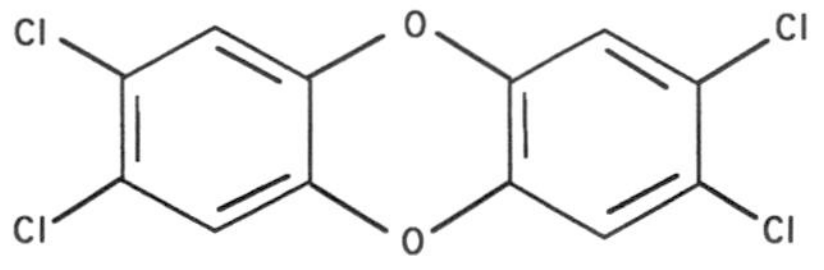

TETRACHLORODIBENZODIOXIN
$C_{12}H_4Cl_4O_2$

2,3,7,8-Tetrachlorodibenzo-*p*-dioxin; TCDD

NEUROTOXOCITY RATING

Clinical

C   Chronic encephalopathy

2,3,7,8-Tetrachlorodibenzo-*p*-dioxin (2,3,7,8-TCDD) is generally produced as an unwanted by-product in several industries; for example, in the production of sodium trichlorophenate, during waste incineration, or by other combustion processes. Occupational exposures to 2,3,7,8-TCDD have occurred during the production of trichlorophenate and related chemicals, such as 2,4,5-trichlorophenoxyacetic acid; as a result of industrial accidents involving trichlorophenol reactors; and during the clean-up of 2,3,7,8-TCDD–contaminated wastes. The general population may be exposed *via* the food chain or through exposures such as incinerator effluents (19,20). 2,3,7,8-TCDD is resistant to chemical oxidation, hydrolysis, and biodegradation. It is also lipophilic, and tends to bioaccumulate (33).

The absorption, distribution, and metabolism of 2,3,7,8-TCDD have recently been reviewed (33). 2,3,7,8-TCDD in oil or feed is 50%–90% absorbed from the gastrointestinal tract in several animal species, and absorption was >86% in a single human subject. The uptake of 2,3,7,8-TCDD from contaminated soil ranges from 2%–43% in rats, depending on soil characteristics. Dermal absorption in rats can be as high as 41%, and is age-, time-, and vehicle-dependent. Transpulmonary absorption was found to be 92% in rats dosed intratracheally (7), which suggests that 2,3,7,8-TCDD should be well absorbed from respirable dust.

Liver and adipose tissue are the major storage sites for 2,3,7,8-TCDD in the rat; skin, intestines, and adrenals also have high concentrations. Approximately 90% of the 2,3,7,8-TCDD body burden of a human subject was sequestered in adipose tissue (33). The concentration of 2,3,7,8-TCDD in serum lipids is essentially equal to the concentration in adipose tissue lipids, allowing human body burdens of 2,3,7,8-TCDD to be estimated from measurements in serum (22). In studies in several countries, the mean concentration of 2,3,7,8-TCDD in the lipid fraction of human blood has ranged from <2.4 to 12 pg/g (parts per trillion, p.p.t.) in the unexposed general population (28). Workers previously employed in the production of 2,4,5-TCP are considered to have levels of 2,3,7,8-TCDD exposure several orders of magnitude higher than that of the general population. In one worker population, lipid-adjusted serum 2,3,7,8-TCDD levels ranged up to 3400 pg/g in workers whose last exposure was 15 years prior to the 2,3,7,8-TCDD measurement (32). Levels up to 50,000 pg/g were measured in community residents of Seveso, Italy, 1 year after a single environmental exposure to 2,3,7,8-TCDD–contaminated industrial effluent (17). These two cohorts have the highest measured serum 2,3,7,8-TCDD levels. In U.S. Air Force Ranch Hand personnel assigned to aerial spraying over Vietnam, the median serum 2,3,7,8-TCDD level adjusted for lipids was 12.8 pg/g, ranging to 618 pg/g (27).

Metabolites of 2,3,7,8-TCDD are excreted primarily in the feces, and to a lesser extent in urine, largely in the form of glucuronides. 2,3,7,8-TCDD is also eliminated *via* lactation. The elimination half-life has been estimated as 12 to 31 days in rats, and 9 to 24 days in several strains of mice. Human elimination of 2,3,7,8-TCDD is slow; the elimination half-life has been estimated as 5.8 years in a volunteer human subject (33), and as 7.1 and 11.3 years in two studies of Air Force veterans (23,35).

In single-dose studies, the acute lethality of 2,3,7,8-TCDD varies over a 5000-fold range across species, with LD_{50} values ranging from 1 μg/kg in the guinea pig to 5000 μg/kg in the hamster. Certain responses to acute 2,3,7,8-TCDD exposure are seen in virtually all animal species studied: weight loss ("wasting syndrome"); thymic atrophy and loss of lymphoid tissue; and hepatotoxicity marked by hyperplasia, hypertrophy, and proliferation of smooth endoplasmic reticulum. Chloracne is a common response in humans, and chloracne-like effects are seen in rhesus monkeys, hairless mice, and rabbits (25).

Prolonged exposure to 2,3,7,8-TCDD produces cancer in rats (14), mice (18), and hamsters (26). The dose of 2,3,7,8-TCDD required to produce an increased incidence of hepatic tumors in female rats is remarkably low: 10 ng/kg/day (14).

Animal studies have examined the relationship between CNS dysfunction and 2,3,7,8-TCDD exposure: Anomalous CNS function appeared in some rats exposed to a single dose of 2,3,7,8-TCDD, and irritability, restlessness, and increased aggression is described in rats administered 2,3,7,8-TCDD (6,8,29). No animal studies have specifically evaluated peripheral or autonomic functions related to 2,3,7,8-TCDD exposure.

Although there are few studies reporting definitive neurological abnormalities related to 2,3,7,8-TCDD exposure in adult animal models, human studies claim a wide spectrum of effects due to 2,3,7,8-TCDD (32). Previous case reports and studies found neurological symptoms shortly after exposure in chemical workers (2,4,5,10,12,21,24) and residents of Seveso, Italy (9); in some cases, effects persisted several years. Symptoms include fatigue, nervousness, anxiety, and decreased libido (2,5,11,12,13,21,30). One case report of exposed workers found mania/hypomania on the Minnesota Multiphasic Personality Inventory (25); another study of chemical workers reported neurasthenia with signs of dementia 10 or more years following exposure (11).

Depression was assessed in a cross-sectional study of 281 production workers and 260 unexposed community-based referents, 15–30 years after exposure to 2,3,7,8-TCDD contaminated chemicals had ceased (1). Exposure durations were up to 18 years in this group of workers. Although the mean serum 2,3,7,8-TCDD levels in the workers was 220 pg/g of lipid and 6 pg/g of lipid in the unexposed referents, no relationship was noted between depressive symptoms and serum 2,3,7,8-TCDD levels.

A cross-sectional study of 1200 U.S. Air Force Ranch Hand personnel assigned to aerial spraying over Vietnam was unable to demonstrate an increased incidence of cognitive or other functional CNS deficits in the exposed Ranch Hand personnel compared to matched, unexposed controls (15,16). An analysis of the cohort using serum 2,3,7,8-TCDD as a measure of exposure found no differences between the highest (>33.3 pg/g lipid) and lowest exposure group (15 to ≤33.3 pg/g lipid).

Overall neurological status of workers (31,32), community residents (3,34), and Vietnam veterans (15,16) exposed to 2,3,7,8-TCDD and evaluated from 5–37 years after last exposure appears to be normal. These studies suggest that, although exposure to 2,3,7,8-TCDD may have been extensive as in exposed workers, Ranch Hand personnel, and Seveso residents, the effects as described in early studies are likely transient. In conclusion, the data suggest that, in adults, no long-term neurological effects are caused by even high exposure to 2,3,7,8-TCDD-contaminated materials.

There is little information on the effects of 2,3,7,8-TCDD exposure on the developing human nervous system.

REFERENCES

1. Alderfer R, Sweeney M, Fingerhut M et al. (1992) Measures of depressed mood in workers exposed to 2,3,7,8-tetrachlorodibenzo-p-dioxin. Chemosphere 25, 247.

2. Ashe WF, Suskind, RR (1950) Reports on Chloracne Cases. Monsanto Chemical Co. Nitro, West Virginia, October 1949 and April 1950. Cincinnati, OH: Department of Environmental Health, College of Medicine, University of Cincinnati (unpublished).

3. Assennato G, Cervino D, Emmet E et al. (1989) Follow-up on subjects who developed chloracne following TCDD exposure of Seveso. Amer J Ind Med 16, 119.

4. Baader EW, Bauer HJ (1951) Industrial intoxication due to pentachlorophenol. Ind Med Surg 20, 286.

5. Bauer H, Schulz K, Spiegelburg W (1961) Industrial poisoning in the manufacture of chlorophenol compounds. Arch Gewerbepath Gewerbehyg 18, 538.

6. Creso E, DeMarino V, Donatelli L, Pagini G (1978) Effette neuropsicofarmacologici deila TCDD. Boll Soc It Sper 54, 1592.

7. Diliberto JJ, Jackson JA, Birnbaum LS (1992) Disposition and absorption of intratracheal, oral, and intravenous ^{3}H-TCDD in male Fischer rats. Toxicologist 12, 79.

8. Elovaara E, Savolainen H, Parkki MG et al. (1977) Neurochemical effects of 2,3,7,8-tetrachlorodibenzo-p-dioxin in Wistar and Gunn rats. Res Commun Chem Pathol Pharmacol 18, 487.

9. Filippini G, Bordo B, Crenna P et al. (1981) Relationship between clinical and electrophysiological findings and indicators of heavy exposure to 2,3,7,8-tetrachlorodibenzodioxin. Scand J Work Environ Health 7, 257.

10. Goldman PJ (1972) Critically acute chloracne caused by trichlorophenol decomposition products. Arbeitsmed Sozialmed Arbeitshygiene 7, 12.

11. Jirasek L, Kalensky K, Kubec K et al. (1974) Chronic poisoning by 2,3,7,8-tetrachlorodibenzo-p-dioxin. Cesk Dermatol 49, 145.

12. Kimmig J, Schulz KH (1957) Chlorinated aromatic cyclic ethers as the cause of so-called chloracne. Naturwissenshaften 44, 337.

13. Kimmig J, Schulz KH (1957) Occupational chloracne caused by aromatic cyclic ethers. Dermatologica 115, 5406.

14. Kociba RJ, Keyes DG, Beyer JE et al. (1978). Results of a two-year chronic toxicity and oncogenicity study of 2,3,7,8-tetrachlorodibenzo-p-dioxin in rats. Toxicol Appl Pharmacol 46, 279.

15. Lathrop GD, Wolfe WH, Albanese RA, Moynihan PM (1984) An Epidemiologic Investigation of Health Effects in Air Force Personnel Following Exposure to Herbicides. Baseline Morbidity Study Results. Brooks Air Force Base, TX: U.S. Air Force School of Aerospace Medicine, Aerospace Medical Division (unpublished).

16. Lathrop GD, Wolfe WH, Michalek JE et al. (1987) An Epidemiologic Investigation of Health Effects in Air Force Personnel Following Exposure to Herbicides. First Follow-up Examination Results, January 1985–September 1987. Brooks Air Force Base, TX: U.S. Air Force School of Aerospace Medicine, Aerospace Medical Division (unpublished).

17. Mocarelli P, Needham LL, Marocchi A et al. (1991) Serum concentrations of 2,3,7,8-tetrachlorodibenzo-p-dioxin and test results from selected residents of Seveso, Italy. J Toxicol Environ Health 32, 357.

18. National Toxicology Program (1982) Bioassay of 2,3,7,8-tetrachlorodibenzo-p-dioxin for possible carcinogenicity (gavage study). U.S. DHHS, PHS. Technical Report Series No. 201. Research Triangle Park, North Carolina.

19. North Atlantic Treaty Organization (NATO) (1988) Pilot study on international information exchange on dioxins and related compounds. Emissions of dioxins and related compounds from combustion and incineration sources. NATO Report No. 172.

20. North Atlantic Treaty Organization (NATO) (1988) Pilot study on international information exchange on dioxins and related compounds. Formation of dioxins and related compounds in industrial processes. NATO Report No. 173.

21. Oliver RM (1975) Toxic effects of 2,3,7,8-tetrachlorodibenzo 1,4 dioxin in laboratory workers. Brit J Ind Med 32, 49.

22. Patterson DG Jr, Needham LL, Pirkle JL et al. (1988) Correlation between serum and adipose tissue levels of 2,3,7,8-tetrachlorodibenzo-p-dioxin in 50 persons from Missouri. Arch Environ Contam Toxicol 17, 139.

23. Pirkle JL, Wolfe WH, Patterson DG (1989). Estimates of the half-life of 2,3,7,8-tetrachlorodibenzo-p-dioxin in Vietnam veterans of operation Ranch Hand. J Toxicol Environ Health 27, 165.

24. Pocchiari F, Silvano V, Zampieri A, Zampieri A (1979) Human health effects from accidental release of tetrachlorodibenzo-p-dioxin (TCDD) at Seveso, Italy. Ann N Y Acad Sci 77, 311.

25. Poland A, Knutson JC (1982) 2,3,7,8-Tetrachlorodibenzo-p-dioxin and related halogenated aromatic compounds: Examination of the mechanism of toxicity. Annu Rev Pharmacol Toxicol 22, 517.

26. Rao MS, Subbarao V, Prasad JD, Scarpelli DC (1988) Carcinogenicity of 2,3,7,8-tetrachlorodibenzo-p-dioxin in the Syrian golden hamster. Carcinogenesis 9, 1677.

27. Roegner RH, Grubbs WD, Lustik MB et al. (1994). Air Force Health Study: An epidemiologic investigation of health effects in Air Force personnel following exposure to herbicides. Serum dioxin analysis of 1987 examination results. NTIS # AD A-237-516 through AD A-237-524.

28. Schecter A, Fürst P, Fürst C *et al.* (1994) Chlorinated dioxins and dibenzofurans in human tissues from general populations: A selective review. *Environ Health Perspect* **102**, 159.

29. Singer R, Moses M, Valciukas J *et al.* (1982) Nerve conduction velocity studies of workers employed in the manufacture of phenoxy herbicides. *Environ Res* **29**, 297.

30. Suskind R, Cholak J, Schater LJ, Yeager D (1953) *Reports on clinical and environmental surveys at Monsanto Chemical Co, Nitro, WV, 1953*. Cincinnati, Ohio: Department of Environmental Health, University of Cincinnati (unpublished).

31. Suskind RR, Hertzberg VS (1984) Human health effects of 2,4,5-T and its toxic contaminants. *J Amer Med Assn* **251**, 2372.

32. Sweeney MH, Fingerhut MA, Arezzo JC *et al.* (1993) Peripheral neuropathy after occupational exposure to 2,3,7,8-tetrachlorodibenzo-*p*-dioxin (TCDD). *Amer J Ind Med* **23**, 845.

33. Van den Berg M, De Jongh J, Poiger H, Olson JR (1994) The toxicokinetics and metabolism of polychlorinated dibenzo-*p*-dioxins (PCDDs) and dibenzofurans (PCDFs) and their relevance for toxicity. *Crit Rev Toxicol* **24**, 1.

34. Webb KB, Evans RG, Knutsen AP *et al.* (1989) Medical evaluation of subjects with known body levels of 2,3,7,8-tetrachlorodibenzo-*p*-dioxin. *J Toxicol Environ Health* **28**, 183.

35. Wolfe WH, Michalek JE, Miner JC *et al.* (1994) Determinants of TCDD half-life in veterans of operation Ranch Hand. *J Toxicol Environ Health* **41**, 481.

1,1,2,2-Tetrachloroethane

John L. O'Donoghue

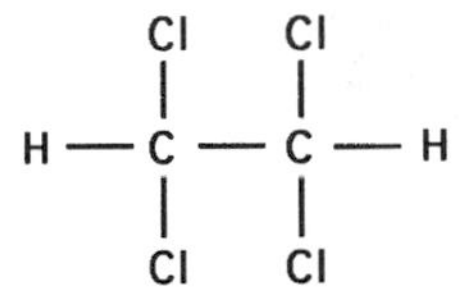

1,1,2,2-TETRACHLOROETHANE
$C_2H_2Cl_4$

Sym-tetrachloroethane; Acetylene tetrachloride; Cellon; Bonoform

NEUROTOXICITY RATING

Clinical

A Acute encephalopathy (sedation, coma)

A Tremor

B Peripheral neuropathy

Experimental

A Acute encephalopathy (sedation, coma)

Tetrachloroethane, the term commonly used in the medical literature to refer to 1,1,2,2-tetrachloroethane, is a nonflammable liquid with a sweet, chloroform-like odor. An isomer of tetrachloroethane (asymmetrical tetrachloroethane or 1,1,1,2-tetrachloroethane) exists; this isomer has had little commercial use. The two isomers can be manufactured in relatively pure form without significant cross contamination. Tetrachloroethane received relatively wide use when it was first introduced in the early 1900s as a solvent for paints and varnishes, as well as for cleaning and extraction processes, because it was among the first of the nonflammable solvents to be introduced. Today, it has limited use as a chemical intermediate, and it has been replaced by less toxic solvents.

Tetrachloroethane is readily absorbed from the lungs or the gastrointestinal tract and rapidly metabolized. Hepatic cytochrome P-450 oxygenases play an important role in the metabolism of tetrachloroethane. Percutaneous absorption may have contributed to some of the human poisoning cases reported in the literature.

Rats and mice given 0.59 or 1.19 mmol/kg (respectively) of radiolabeled tetrachloroethane orally exhaled 7% or 10% (respectively) of the dose and metabolized 79% or 68% (respectively) of the dose (11). Urinary metabolites accounted for 46% (rats) or 30% (mice) of the administered dose, while exhaled carbon dioxide accounted for 2% (rats) or 10% (mice) of the administered dose. About 30% of the metabolites remained in the carcass in both rats and mice.

When mice were given radiolabeled tetrachloroethane by intraperitoneal (i.p.) injection, 60%–70% of the dose was excreted in 24 h as degradation products, primarily carbon dioxide (21). Within 3 days, 45%–61% of the dose was expired as carbon dioxide, 28% was excreted in the urine, 14% remained in the carcass, and 4% was exhaled unchanged (21). Urinary metabolites included dichloroacetic acid, trichloroacetic acid, trichloroethanol, oxalic acid, glyoxylic acid, and urea; however, half of the radioactivity in the urine was not accounted for by these metabolites (21). The primary route of metabolism was considered to involve cleavage of carbon-chlorine bonds *via* dichloroacetic acid to glyoxylic acid (21). Metabolism of tetrachloroethane to dichloroacetic acid may involve dichloroacetaldehyde as an intermediate (21); however, metabolism of tetrachloro-ethane occurs *in vitro via* cytochrome P-450 in both intact liver microsomes and a reconstituted monooxygenase system that lacked alcohol dehydrogenase. This suggested that an acyl chloride intermediate is involved, and dichloroacetaldehyde is not an obligate intermediate (7). A small amount of tetrachloroethane was considered to undergo nonenzymatic dehydrochlorination to trichloroethylene and subsequently to trichloroacetic acid and trichloroethanol. A minute amount of tetrachloroethane was apparently oxidized to tetrachloroethylene, which was further metabolized to very small amounts of trichloroacetic acid and oxalic acid (21).

Rats exposed to tetrachloroethane by inhalation (200 ppm vapor exposure for 8 h) or injected i.p. (2.78 mmol/kg) excreted similar amounts of total trichlorometabolites, including trichloroacetic acid and trichloroethanol, in their urine (5). A human volunteer exposed to radiolabeled tetrachloroethane vapor retained 97% of the inhaled dose and only excreted 3.3% in the 1 h following exposure (12).

Acute exposure to tetrachloroethane in animals at elevated levels produces CNS depression, narcosis, and death at sufficiently high exposure levels. Oral LD_{50} values in the range of 250–400 mg/kg have been reported for rats (2). A dermal LD_{50} of 4 ml/kg has been reported for the rabbit (18). A vapor concentration of 1000 ppm for 4 h was a LC_{50} for rats (18). Elevated hepatic enzyme levels have been reported in rats exposed a single time to 10 or 100 ppm tetrachloroethane vapor for 6 h, and a 67% mortality rate was observed in rats exposed to vapors for 6 h; histological lesions were not observed in the brains of exposed rats (3).

Repeat-dose toxicity studies with tetrachloroethane have primarily focused on studying end points related to hepatic and renal toxicity. Reviews covering these effects are available (1,14,19). Tetrachloroethane given by gavage in corn oil was tested in a 2-year cancer bioassay with rats and mice (13). Dose levels for rats were 62 or 108 mg/kg for males, and 43 or 76 mg/kg females; mice were given 142 or 282 mg/kg (both sexes). An increased incidence of hepatocellular tumors was observed in mice, but not in rats. These data are considered limited evidence for carcinogenicity in rodents (6). No increase in nervous system tumors was reported, and there were no abnormal neurological conditions or neuropathological changes associated with tetrachloroethane exposure (13).

Tetrachloroethane has acute anesthetic properties in humans similar to those seen in animals (14). Human responses to high-level, short-term exposures have been reported primarily in individuals who have accidentally consumed the material or who have attempted suicide by ingesting the solvent. Rapid loss of consciousness, progressive CNS depression, and coma followed by death have been reported in five suicide cases (14). Case reports of accidental poisoning in which ten people were unintentionally given 3 ml of tetrachloroethane included coma in half of the group and degrees of semicoma in the balance; recovery was complete (17,20).

Information about the effects of repeated exposures of tetrachloroethane on humans primarily comes from its use in the occupational environment. Much of the human data available on tetrachloroethane stems from its use as a varnish solvent to apply dope to the fabric coverings of World War I aircraft. Because of a number of favorable characteristics, its use in the aircraft industries of Germany, France, England, and the Netherlands became common. Exposure during doping operations was primarily to inhaled vapor, but dermal contact with wet varnishes probably also contributed to the absorbed dose of the solvent.

A 1914 report indicates that tetrachloroethane was responsible for intoxications in German airplane builders (14). Two main groupings of signs and symptoms were described: (a) those primarily related to the liver and gastrointestinal system, including gastrointestinal disturbances, jaundice, and liver enlargement; and (b) those primarily related to the nervous system, including headache, hand tremor, difficulty hearing, paresthesias, and reduced patellar reflexes. The gastrointestinal and hepatic effects were reproduced in dogs, but not the neurological effects (14). American aircraft plants in operation during World War I had less airborne tetrachloroethane contamination; tetrachloroethane exposures in these plants were associated with headaches, drowsiness, and nausea, but severe hepatic and long-term neurological effects were not observed (4).

Two cases of chronic tetrachloroethane intoxication with prominent peripheral and cranial nerves signs and symptoms were observed in women who dipped their fingers into a varnish containing tetrachloroethane. The clinical appearance of these women developed over a period of 3 months or 2 years and included the sensation of numbness, and loss of feeling in the fingers and toes, paresthesias, difficulty walking, hand tremors, paresis of the soft palate, and absence of pharyngeal reflexes (14).

An epidemiological study was conducted over a 3-year period in a plant using tetrachloroethane as a solvent in the production of penicillin (14). The plant used a rotation schedule that moved employees at the first sign of liver toxicity; no neurological impairments were observed in the 34–75 men employed in the plant (14).

A medical survey using case histories and medical examinations identified a number of neurological abnormalities in people employed in India's bangle-manufacturing industry (10). Exposures in a number of small plants employing 380 people in total included vapor inhalation as well as dermal exposure to tetrachloroethane or to a mixture of tetrachloroethane and acetone. No cases of serious intoxication with jaundice were observed; however, anemia and gastrointestinal disturbances were noted. The most common neurological abnormality reported was fine hand tremor in 35% of the employees. Other neurological complaints included vertigo (31%), headache (27%), nervousness (8%), and numbness (3%). Exposure for 3 months was generally necessary for symptoms to appear; symptoms tended to be consistent among affected individuals after 6 months of exposure.

In a survey of artificial pearl-making factories in Japan involving 18 employees, 39% of the workers had abnormal neurological signs including tongue spasms, weakened quadriceps reflex, headache, or paresthesias (8). Tetrachloroethane vapor levels in the plants ranged between 75 and 224 ppm during the survey.

In a cancer mortality study of 1099 men who worked impregnating clothing with tetrachoroethane for protection against mustard gas, no increase in tumors of the nervous system was noted (15).

The data available on the effects of tetrachloroethane on the nervous system include case reports and medical surveys of small populations of individuals working with mixtures containing tetrachloroethane used as a solvent. One recognized effect of working with solvents such as tetrachloroethane is that they have demonstrated anesthetic properties. Thus, short-term exposure to relatively high concentrations of tetrachloroethane produces narcosis. Individuals who have survived such high-level exposure have recovered without adverse sequelae. However, long-term exposure (months to years) to lower concentrations of tetrachloroethane can apparently result in sensorimotor changes in the peripheral nervous system. These changes have been reported to involve cranial nerves and nerves innervating the limbs. Many of the studies include self-reported symptoms, but there is sufficient consistency in the signs observed across studies to conclude that long-term tetrachloroethane exposure can result in neurological impairment. The data supporting these observations do not include adequate industrial hygiene information to make firm statements about exposure-effect relationships but, in general, levels of exposure that protect against liver toxicity are also protective from neurological effects. The American Conference of Governmental Industrial Hygienists has published a Threshold Limit Value for tetrachloroethane of 1 ppm

with a warning that skin contact may result in absorption (2).

The mechanism(s) of action of tetrachloroethane has not been studied in detail. The short-term anesthetic effects observed in humans can be reproduced in animal studies. The anesthetic effects of materials like tetrachloroethane are thought to involve changes in membrane stability (9). The peripheral neuropathy that has been described in people exposed long term to tetrachloroethane has not been reproduced in experimental animals or observed in domestic animals. While no significant work has been done to examine the long-term mechanism of action, it is important to note that one of the primary metabolites of tetrachloroethane is dichloroacetic acid, which has been reported to produce peripheral neuropathy in humans and experimental animals following repeated exposures (16) (see Dichloroacetic Acid, this volume). Thus, it seems reasonable to postulate that dichloroacetic acid may play a role in tetrachloroethane-induced neurotoxicity.

REFERENCES
1. Agency for Toxic Substances and Disease Registry (1989) *Toxicological Profile for 1,1,2,2-Tetrachloroethane.* U.S. Public Health Service, Atlanta, Georgia.
2. American Conference of Governmental Industrial Hygienists (1992) 1,1,2,2-Tetrachlorethane. In: *Documentation of the Threshold Limit Values. Vol III. 6th Ed.* Cincinnati, Ohio p. 1806.
3. Deguchi T (1972) A fundamental study of the threshold limit values for solvent mixtures in air: Effects of single and mixed chlorinated hydrocarbons upon the level of serum transaminases in rats. *Osaka City Med J* **21**, 187.
4. Hamilton A (1917) Industrial poisoning in aircraft manufacture. *J Amer Med Assn* **69**, 2037.
5. Ikeda M, Ohtsuji H (1972) A comparative study of the excretion of Fujiwara reaction-positive substances in urine of humans and rodents given trichloro- or tetrachloro-derivatives of ethane and ethylene. *Brit J Ind Med* **29**, 99.
6. International Agency for Research on Cancer (1987) *IARC Monograph on the Evaluation of Carcinogenic Risks to Humans, Suppl 7.* Overall Evaluations of Carcinogenicity: An Updating of Monographs. Vol 1-42. IARC, Lyon p. 355.
7. Halpert J, Neal RA (1981) Cytochrome P-450-dependent metabolism of 1,1,2,2-tetrachloroethane to dichloroacetic acid *in vitro. Biochem Pharmacol* **30**, 1366.
8. Horiguchi S, Morioka S, Utsunomiya T *et al.* (1964) A survey of the actual conditions of artificial pearl factories with special reference to the work with tetrachloroethane. *Jpn J Ind Health* **6**, 251.
9. Korpela M, Tahti H (1986) The effect of selected organic

solvents on intact human red cell membrane acetylcholinesterase *in vitro*. *Toxicol Appl Pharmacol* **85**, 257.

10. Lobo-Mendonca R (1963) Tetrachloroethane—a survey. *Brit J Ind Med* **20**, 50.

11. Mitoma C, Steeger T, Jackson SE *et al.* (1985) Metabolic disposition study of chlorinated hydrocarbons in rats and mice. *Drug Chem Toxicol* **8**, 183.

12. Morgan A, Black A, Belcher DR (1970) The excretion in breath of some aliphatic halogenated hydrocarbons following administration by inhalation. *Ann Occup Hyg* **13**, 219.

13. National Cancer Institute (1978) *Bioassay of 1,1,2,2-Tetrachloroethane for Possible Carcinogenicity.* U.S. Department of Health, Education, and Welfare, Bethesda, MD.

14. National Institute for Occupational Safety and Health (1976) *Criteria for a Recommended Standard: Occupational Exposure to 1,1,2,2-Tetrachloroethane.* U.S. Department of Health, Education and Welfare, Washington, DC.

15. Norman JE, Robinette CD, Fraumeni JF Jr (1981) The mortality experience of army World War II chemical processing companies. *J Occup Med* **23**, 818.

16. O'Donoghue JL (1985) *Neurotoxicity of Industrial and Commercial Chemicals.* CRC Press, Boca Raton, Florida.

17. Sherman JB (1953) Eight cases of acute tetrachloroethane poisoning. *J Trop Med Hyg* **56**, 139.

18. Smyth HF, Carpenter CP, Weil CS *et al.* (1969) Range-finding toxicity data: List VII. *Amer Ind Hyg Assn J* **30**, 470.

19. Torkelson TR (1994) Halogenated aliphatic hydrocarbons containing chlorine, bromine, and iodine. In: *Patty's Industrial Hygiene and Toxicology. 4th Ed. Vol. II.* Clayton G, Clayton FE eds. John Wiley, New York p. 4007.

20. Ward JM (1955) Accidental poisoning with tetrachloroethane. *Brit Med J* **1**, 1136.

21. Yllner S (1971) Metabolism of 1,1,2,2,-tetrachloroethane-^{14}C in the mouse. *Acta Pharmacol Toxicol* **29**, 499.

Tetrachloroethylene

John L. O'Donoghue

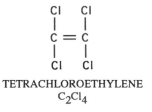

TETRACHLOROETHYLENE
C_2Cl_4

1,1,2,2-Tetrachlorethylene; Perchloroethylene; Ethylene tetrachloride; Nema; Tetracap; Tetropil; Perclene; Ankilostin; Didakene

NEUROTOXICITY RATING

Clinical

A Acute encephalopathy (sedation, coma)

C Chronic encephalopathy

Experimental

A Acute encephalopathy (sedation, coma)

Tetrachloroethylene (TeCE) is a colorless, nonflammable liquid with an ethereal odor. It is widely used for dry-cleaning clothes and metal-cleaning operations. It has also been used as an anthelmintic for humans and animals, and as a chemical intermediate in the synthesis of chlorofluoro-carbons. Because of its widespread use, TeCE has frequently been identified as a contaminant in drinking water.

TeCE absorption, distribution, metabolism, and excretion have been extensively studied, and pharmacokinetic models for its disposition have been described (7,8,25). TeCE is rapidly and completely absorbed following inhalation or ingestion. Liquid and vapor TeCE can be absorbed through the skin, but percutaneous absorption is not considered a significant route of exposure. TeCE has high lipid solubility and low water solubility, and consequently rapidly partitions into adipose tissue. Metabolism of TeCE is low, with <2% excreted as urinary metabolites and 80%–100% of an inhaled dose excreted unchanged in the breath by humans (15,18); because of its lipid solubility, excretion of unmetabolized TeCE can occur over a relatively prolonged period. Metabolism of TeCE is believed to occur *via* mixed-function oxidases to epoxide intermediates, which may be responsible for the hepatic toxicity seen following repeated exposures, and then to stable urinary metabolites (5). Formation of glutathione conjugates is a second, minor pathway for metabolism of TeCE. Trichloroacetic acid is the major urinary metabolite of TeCE in rats with low levels of trichloroethanol, oxalic acid, dichloroacetic acid, *N*-

trichloroacetylamino ethanol, and conjugates in the urine. The metabolism of TeCE is species- and dose-dependent; mice have a greater capacity to metabolize TeCE than rats. Saturation of metabolism occurs in humans at approximately 100 ppm TeCE vapor (18).

In high concentration, TeCE is a CNS depressant, although its depressant properties are not sufficient for it to have been used as a surgical anesthetic. TeCE vapor concentrations above 2750 ppm may result in anesthesia; however, rats habituate to TeCE and, after 6 exposures to 2750 ppm, they can tolerate 10,000 ppm without undergoing anesthesia (6). TeCE has a low degree of acute toxicity and LC_{50} values for rats and mice following exposures to TeCE vapor are on the order of 4000–5000 ppm for a 4-h exposure (3). Increased spontaneous motor activity levels were observed in rats 1 h after cessation of a 4-h exposure to 200 ppm TeCE vapor, but by 17 h following exposure, motor activity levels had returned to background levels (21). Rats given single doses of 150–5000 mg/kg TeCE in corn oil by oral gavage were assessed for short-term behavioral effects (16). Both a functional-observational battery and motor activity assessments indicated that the animals showed signs of CNS depression with a no-effect level at 150 mg/kg. Rats given single doses of 160 or 480 mg/kg TeCE by oral gavage were immediately tested for changes in scheduled-controlled operant behavior for the 90 min following dosing (26). At 160 mg/kg, effects were not clearly apparent but, at 480 mg/kg, there was either immediate suppression of responding for 15–30 min before a rapid recovery, or animals stopped responding for the entire 90-min test period. Because the majority of animals recovered their ability to respond, even as blood levels of TeCE were increasing, the suppression of response could not be correlated with blood or brain levels of TeCE.

Mouse pups given 5 or 320 mg/kg TeCE by oral gavage between postnatal days 10 and 16 showed increased locomotion and total motor activity levels on postnatal day 60 but not on postnatal day 17 (10). Rearing activity was reduced on postnatal day 60 only for the 320-mg/kg group. It was suggested that this indicated a susceptibility of brain maturation to TeCE, as the differences in activity levels indicated a decrease in habituation. Considering the large difference in the dose levels, it is surprising that there were no dose–response differences in locomotion or total motor activity levels. Embryonal and fetal development of rat and mouse pups was unaffected by exposure of their dams to 300 ppm TeCE vapor during gestation (22). Pups of rat dams exposed to 100 ppm for 7 h/day on days 14–20 of gestation showed no effects with regard to brain histology, neurochemistry, or behavior (17). Rat dams exposed to 900 ppm for 7 h/day on days 7–13 or 14–20 of gestation ate less food and gained less weight. The pups from the TeCE-exposed dams exhibited decreased performance on ascent and rotarod tests but only on certain test days. Changes in whole-brain acetylcholine and dopamine were also reported but, again, only on certain test days. Pup responses on tests for olfaction, open-field activity, running-wheel activity, avoidance conditioning and operant conditioning, and histopathology of newborn and 21-day-old pup brains were unaffected by exposure to TeCE. Overall these data indicate that exposure to high concentrations of TeCE vapor has little or no effect on rat pup development.

Exposure of animals to TeCE vapor concentrations from 70–7000 ppm (8 h/day, 5 days/week) for 7–1.7 months, respectively, did not result in histological changes in the retina, optic nerve, sciatic nerve, or brain (6). Two dogs exposed to a mixture of 200 ppm TeCE and 800 ppm 1,1,1-trichloroethane for 7 h/day, 5 days/week for a period of 189 days showed no histological changes in skeletal muscle, sciatic nerve, or brain (20).

Rats exposed continuously to 600 ppm TeCE vapor for 12 weeks showed a slower increase in brain weight gain. Brain region weight, total protein, and DNA content were decreased in the frontal cortex and brainstem (24). The hippocampus in the rats continuously exposed to 600 ppm TeCE and all three regions of the brain from the 300 ppm group were not similarly affected. The lipid content of the brains of rats and gerbils was altered by continuous exposures to 320 ppm TeCE vapor for 90 days, although the specific changes in fatty acid content varied in the two species (12). Following a recovery period of 30 days, the changes in the fatty acid content of the rat brain largely returned to normal. Exposure of gerbils to 120 ppm TeCE vapor continuously for 12 months was associated with decreased taurine content in the hippocampus and the posterior portion of the cerebellar vermis and increased glutamine content in the hippocampus; glutathione and other amino acids were not altered (4). Continuous exposure of gerbils to 320 ppm TeCE vapor for 3 months followed by a 4-month rest period resulted in increased S-100 protein levels indicative of astrogliosis in the hippocampus, occipital cortex, and cerebellum (19). In the frontal cortex, S-100 levels, DNA content, and regional brain weight were decreased, suggesting regional brain atrophy (19). The DNA content of the frontal cortex was reduced following continuous exposure to 60 ppm TeCE vapor for 3 months followed by a 4-month rest period (19).

Mice consuming 0.1 mg/kg of body weight of TeCE in their drinking water for 7 weeks had reduced body weights, altered lipid metabolism, and evidence of red blood cell destruction, but brain weight and histopathology of the brain were not altered (13). Rats consuming up to 14,400 mg/kg TeCE in their drinking water for 90 days were less affected than mice and showed decreased body weight, a slight increase in serum 5'-nucleotidase activity, increased liver and kidney/body weight ratios, but no evidence of hematological effects; brain weights were normal (11). Repeated dosing of rats with up to 1500 mg/kg TeCE by oral gavage for 14 days did not alter performance on a functional observational battery or motor activity levels using a figure-eight maze (16).

Human volunteers who were exposed consecutively to several TeCE vapor concentrations reported that, at 50 ppm, there was a definite detectable odor but no other immediate effect; at 500 ppm, there was slight discomfort and irritation associated during a 2-h exposure; at 1000 ppm, slight inebriation was experienced after 45 min but there was no progression over a 1-h and 35 min period; and at 2000 ppm, there was feeling of faintness within several minutes that rapidly reversed itself on stopping exposure (6).

Human volunteers who inhaled 520 ppm of a mixture of 1,1,1-trichloroethane (390 ppm) and TeCE (130 ppm) for one, four, or five 7-h exposures were (a) tested for vestibular cerebellar, and proprioceptive function every 75 min, (b) administered the Crawford Manual Dexterity Test every 3 h during exposure, (c) administered the Flanagan Aptitude Classification test after 3 h of exposure, and (d) given a neurological examination after 6 h of exposure (20). Other than slight irritation of the throat in one individual, the exposures had no effect on the volunteers.

The potential effects of TeCE on human visual and auditory function were studied in male volunteers exposed to 10 or 50 ppm TeCE vapor for 4 h/day for 4 consecutive days (1). The 10-ppm TeCE group served as the control group for the 50-ppm TeCE group. In the 50-ppm group, the visual evoked potential latency increased during exposure and the contrast sensitivity showed a trend toward increased threshold contrast at low and intermediate spatial frequencies. The results indicate an alteration in visual function related to an increase in central conduction time; auditory function was not affected by exposure to 50 ppm TeCE.

Individuals living in neighborhoods surrounding dry-cleaning shops may be affected by inhalation of TeCE vapor (2). TeCE levels in homes in the area of the shops were equivalent to a median air concentration of 1.36 mg/m^3 or 5.1 ppm. Residents in neighborhoods surrounding the shops showed statistically significant differences compared to a control group on a computerized neurobehavioral test battery for vigilance, simple reaction time, and visual memory.

Deficits in visuospatial function and memory and mood disturbances have been described in four individuals exposed to TeCE, but exposure levels were not available (9). A field study was conducted to examine subclinical neurobehavioral effects in 65 dry cleaners divided into three TeCE vapor-exposure zones (11, 23, and 41 ppm) that corresponded to counter clerks, pressers, and operators. Evaluations were conducted at the end of one or two workdays with TeCE exposure. In comparing the responses of the different exposure groups across exposure levels, small decrements in visual reproduction (decreased 14.4%), latency for pattern memory (decreased 10%), number correct for pattern memory (decreased 6.7%), and the number correct for pattern recognition were reported between the low- and high-exposure groups. No TeCE-unexposed control group was available for performance comparisons. Performance on tests for simple attention, symbol-digit matching, and trail-making was similar in both low- and high-exposure groups.

TeCE-induced neurobehavioral effects were studied in a group of 101 individuals, mostly women, employed in dry-cleaning shops in Germany (23). Performance of the TeCE-exposed group on tests of perceptual function, attention, and intellectual function was reduced compared to a control group. However, when the TeCE-exposed group was broken down into two exposure groups (83.4 and 363.8 mg/m^3 or 310 and 1352 ppm), the effects observed had little direct correlation to exposure concentration.

Data from experimental animals and human volunteer exposures demonstrate that inhaled TeCE vapor may result in CNS depression. Because the metabolic pathways and excretory pathways for disposition of TeCE can be saturated, it is not surprising that continuous exposure to relatively high levels of TeCE vapor may lead to effects not observed at lower exposure levels or following repeated but discontinuous exposures. While reports of human neurobehavioral effects suggest that humans may have subclinical effects following long-term, low-level exposure to TeCE vapor, the available data are inconclusive for establishing a clear cause-and-effect relationship.

Editors' Note: A recent subchronic toxicity study evaluated the nervous system of rats exposed to 50, 200, or 800 ppm tetrachloroethylene 6 h/day, 5 days/week, for 13 weeks (14). Longer-latency (N3) flash-evoked potentials recorded from the visual cortex were increased in amplitude in the high-dose group. No changes were found in flash-evoked potentials recorded from the cerebellum of these animals, or in auditory, somatosensory, or caudal nerve evoked potentials. Histological examination of the eyes, optic nerves, optic tract, and multiple sections of the brain, spinal cord, peripheral nerve and limb muscles, did not reveal treatment-related changes (14).

REFERENCES

1. Altmann L, Böttger A, Wiegand H (1990) Neurophysiological and psychophysical measurements reveal effects of acute low-level organic solvent exposure in humans. *Int Arch Occup Environ Health* **62**, 493.

2. Altmann L, Neuhann HF, Kramer U *et al.* (1995) Neurobehavioral and neurophysiological outcome of chronic low-level tetrachloroethylene exposure measured in neighborhoods of dry cleaning shops. *Environ Res* **69**, 83.

3. American Conference of Governmental Industrial Hygienists (1992) Perchloroethylene. In: *Documentation of the Threshold Limit Values. Vol II. 6th Ed.* Cincinnati, Ohio p. 1188.

4. Briving C, Jacobson I, Hamberger A *et al.* (1986) Chronic effects of perchloroethylene and trichloroethylene on the gerbil brain amino acids and glutathione. *NeuroToxicology* **7**, 101.

5. Buben JA, O'Flaherty EJ (1985) Delineation of the role of metabolism in the hepatotoxicity of trichloroethylene and perchloroethylene: A dose-effect study. *Toxicol Appl Pharmacol* **78**, 105.

6. Carpenter CP (1937) The chronic toxicity of tetrachloroethylene. *J Ind Hyg Toxicol* **19**, 323.

7. Dallas CE, Chen XM, Muralidhara S *et al.* (1994) Use of tissue disposition data from rats and dogs to determine species differences in input parameters for a physiological model for perchloroethylene. *Environ Res* **67**, 54.

8. Dallas CE, Chen XM, O'Barr K *et al.* (1994) Development of a physiologically based pharmacokinetic model for perchloroethylene using tissue concentration-time data. *Toxicol Appl Pharmacol* **128**, 50.

9. Echeverria D, White RF, Sampaio C (1995) A behavioral evaluation of PCE exposure in patients and dry cleaners: A possible relationship between clinical and preclinical effects. *J Occup Environ Med* **37**, 667.

10. Fredriksson A, Danielsson BRG, Eriksson P (1993) Altered behavior in adult mice orally exposed to tri- and tetrachloroethylene as neonates. *Toxicol Lett* **66**, 13.

11. Hayes JR, Condie LW, Borzelleca JF (1986) The subchronic toxicity of tetrachloroethylene (perchloroethylene) administered in the drinking water of rats. *Fund Appl Toxicol* **7**, 119.

12. Kyrklund T, Kjellstrand P, Haglid KG (1990) Long-term exposure of rats to perchloroethylene, with and without a post-exposure solvent-free recovery period: Effects on brain lipids. *Toxicol Lett* **52**, 279.

13. Marth E (1987) Metabolic changes following oral exposure to tetrachloroethylene in subtoxic concentrations. *Arch Toxicol* **60**, 293.

14. Mattsson JL, Albee RR, Yano BL *et al.* (1998) Neurotoxicologic examination of rats exposed to 1,1,2,2-tetrachloroethylene (perchloroethylene) vapor for 13 weeks. *Neurotoxicol Teratol* **20**, 83.

15. Monster AC, Boersma G, Steenweg H (1979) Kinetics of tetrachloroethylene in volunteers: Influence of exposure concentration and work load. *Arch Occup Environ Health* **42**, 303.

16. Moser VC, Cheek BM, MacPhail RC, (1995) A multidisciplinary approach to toxicological screening: III. Neurobehavioral toxicity. *J Toxicol Environ Health* **45**, 173.

17. Nelson BK, Taylor BJ, Setzer JV, Homung RW (1980) Behavioral teratology of perchloroethylene. *J Environ Pathol Toxicol* **3**, 233.

18. Ohtsuki T, Sato K, Koizumi *et al.* (1983) Limited capacity of humans to metabolize tetrachloroethylene. *Int Arch Occup Environ Health* **51**, 381.

19. Rosengren LE, Kjellstrand P, Haglid KG (1986) Tetrachloroethylene: Levels of DNA and S-100 in the gerbil CNS after chronic exposure. *Neurobehav Toxicol Teratol* **89**, 201.

20. Rowe VK, Wujkowski MA, Wolf MA *et al.* (1963) Toxicity of a solvent mixture of 1,1,1,-trichloroethane and tetrachloroethylene as determined by experiments on laboratory animals and human subjects. *Amer Ind Hyg Assn J* **24**, 541.

21. Savolainen H, Pfäffli P, Tengén M, Vaino H (1977) Biochemical and behavioral effects of inhalation exposure to tetrachloroethylene and dichloromethane. *J Neuropathol Exp Neurol* **36**, 941.

22. Schwetz BA, Leong BKJ, Gehring PJ (1975) The effect of maternally inhaled trichloroethylene, perchloroethylene, methyl chloroform, and methylene chloride on embryonal and fetal development in mice and rats. *Toxicol Appl Pharmacol* **32**, 84.

23. Seeber A (1989) Neurobehavioral toxicity of long-term exposure to tetrachloroethylene. *Neurotoxicol Teratol* **11**, 579.

24. Wang S, Karlsson JE, Kyrklund T, Haglid K (1993) Perchloroethylene-induced reduction in glial and neuronal cell marker proteins in rat brain. *Pharmacol Toxicol* **72**, 273.

25. Ward RC, Travis CC, Hetrick DM *et al.* (1988) Pharmacokinetics of tetrachloroethylene. *Toxicol Appl Pharmacol* **93**, 108.

26. Warren DA, Reiglie TG, Muralidhara S, Dallas CE (1996) Schedule-controlled operant behavior of rats following oral administration of perchloroethylene; time course and relationship to blood and brain solvent levels. *J Toxicol Environ Health* **47**, 345.

Tetracyclines

Steven A. Sparr

TETRACYCLINE
C$_{22}$H$_{24}$N$_2$O$_8$

[4S-(4α,4aα,5aα,6β,12aα)]-4-(Dimethylamino)-
1,4,4a,5,5a,6,11,12a-octahydro-3,6,10,12,12a-pentahydroxy-
6-methyl-1,11-dioxo-2-naphthacenecarboxamide

NEUROTOXICITY RATING

Clinical

A   Neuromuscular transmission syndrome

B   Benign intracranial hypertension

Experimental

A   Neuromuscular transmission dysfunction (blockade)

The tetracyclines are a class of antibiotic with a broad spectrum of activity against Gram-positive and Gram-negative bacteria, spirochetes, mycoplasmas, chlamydiae, and rickettsiae. They are useful in the treatment of many sexually transmitted diseases, atypical pneumonias, traveler's diarrhea, rickettsial infections, and Lyme disease (8).

Chlortetracycline, the first drug in this class, was isolated from soil samples containing antibiotic-producing microorganisms and introduced into clinical practice in 1948 (6). Tetracycline and demeclocycline were introduced as semisynthetic derivatives in the 1950s, followed by long-acting compounds, doxycycline and minocycline, in the late 1960s and early 1970s. In addition to requiring less frequent dosing, the long-acting tetracyclines also have the advantage of improved oral absorption and hepatic, rather than renal, excretion (8).

Four tetracyclines (tetracycline, demeclocycline, minocycline, and doxycycline) are available in the United States for systemic use; all have a similar spectrum of activity but they differ in pharmacological profile. Tetracyclines inhibit protein synthesis in bacteria by binding to the 30S subunit of ribosomes, impeding their access to transfer RNA. They enter the bacterial cell by passive diffusion through the plasmalemma and transport through intracytoplasmic membranes by an energy-dependent process. Inhibition of bacterial protein synthesis accounts for the bacteriostatic properties of the tetracyclines. As mammalian cells lack this active transport system, they are less affected by these drugs

(6), although impairment of protein synthesis can occur in humans at usual therapeutic doses (5).

In general, tetracyclines are well tolerated. The most frequent side effects are gastrointestinal irritation, and dermatological and photosensitivity reactions. Diarrhea may occur due to suppression of bacterial flora with resultant overgrowth of *Candida* or *Clostridium difficile*. Concentration of tetracyclines in developing teeth can cause discoloration or hypoplasia of enamel; this limits use of these agents in pregnant women and children under age 8. Outdated tetracycline can cause a Fanconi-like syndrome with renal tubular acidosis (8). The major neurological toxicity of this class of antibiotic is pseudotumor cerebri, which is usually reversible and self-limited, but which may lead to long-term visual impairment (4,12–14,17,18). Tetracyclines have also been shown to have neuromuscular junction–blocking effects that may exacerbate myasthenia gravis (7–9,15,16).

Tetracyclines are usually administered orally; only doxycycline is approved for intravenous use due to the risk of thrombophlebitis or hepatic toxicity with other drugs in this class. Absorption from the gastrointestinal tract is nearly 100% for second-generation tetracyclines (doxycycline and minocycline) and is little affected by simultaneous food intake. Tetracycline, however, is incompletely absorbed (~ 80%), and absorption is further decreased when the drug is taken with food. Serum half-life is 6–12 h for tetracycline, and much longer for doxycycline (11–33 h) and minocycline (11–33 h). Protein binding is highest for doxycycline (60%–95%) and lowest for tetracycline (20%–65%) (8). Tetracycline that is not bound to serum protein circulates as complexes bound to calcium and magnesium (10).

All tetracyclines have high tissue penetration, distribute in cerebrospinal fluid and breast milk, and move transplacentally to fetal circulation. Elimination varies with different compounds. Tetracycline is eliminated primarily through the kidneys and thus requires dose adjustment in patients with renal failure. Doxycycline has extensive enterohepatic recirculation and is primarily excreted in the stool. Minocycline is metabolized by the liver and also accumulates in fatty tissue (6).

Two animal models have demonstrated nervous system toxicity due to tetracyclines. Dry, powdered tetracycline, placed in close proximity to exposed nerves for 45 days in a rat, induced an inflammatory response that was worse if the epineurium of the nerve had been removed (11). Because of the potential for inducing damage to alveolar or lingual nerves, the practice of placing dry tetracycline into dental extraction sockets was discouraged. Neuromuscular-blocking effects with methyl-pyrrolidino-tetracycline and oxytetracycline have been demonstrated in the hindlimb of a cat after intravenous injection in the corresponding femoral vein (9). Neuromuscular blockade was reversed with prostigmine and partially reversed by calcium. It is proposed that tetracyclines have the ability to chelate calcium and to exert direct effects on the neuromuscular junction as the mechanism of blockade. There are no reported animal models of tetracycline-associated pseudotumor cerebri.

Increased intracranial pressure/pseudotumor cerebri has been frequently reported in association with clinical use of tetracyclines, although the overall incidence of this complication is probably low. A review of over 40 case reports and clinical series disclosed that, in infants, bulging fontanelles and elevated cerebrospinal fluid pressure without other neurological signs occur 5 h to 4 days after initiation of tetracycline treatment (4). Patients returned to baseline within hours to days of discontinuation of the medication, but frequently had recurrence when rechallenged. In older children and adults (ages 7–63), case reports of pseudotumor cerebri involve an overwhelming preponderance of females, many of them obese. Symptoms of headache, visual blurring, and diplopia, associated with papilledema can begin after days of treatment with tetracycline, but most patients who developed pseudotumor had received long-term treatment for acne for up to 4 years. Other than papilledema and occasional sixth-nerve palsies (so-called pressure sixth), the neurological examination is normal. Cerebrospinal fluid shows elevated opening pressure and normal cell count, protein, and glucose levels. Brain imaging by computed tomography is normal. Symptoms usually abate days to weeks after cessation of tetracycline, even without specific medications to lower the intracranial pressure, although papilledema may take months to clear (17) and permanent visual deficits may occur (12).

Cases of tetracycline-inducing increased intracranial pressure have been reported with a familial clustering, including in monozygotic twins, suggesting a possible genetic predisposition (4). Several patients who developed pseudotumor cerebri while being treated with tetracycline for acne were simultaneously treated with vitamin A. As vitamin A has been associated with pseudotumor in doses as low as 40,000 U/day, as well as with overdoses, combination therapy with tetracycline and vitamin A may place patients at increased risk of developing elevated intracranial pressure (13,17).

Transient weakness has been observed in myasthenic patients receiving intravenous tetracyclines (7,15), and this phenomenon has been corroborated in an animal model (9). Several mechanisms have been proposed for transient neuromuscular blockade: (a) chelation of serum calcium by tetracycline (10), (b) calcium-antagonizing effects of magnesium in the diluent, and (c) postjunctional depression of muscle to acetylcholine similar to that induced by *d*-tubocurarine (15). Although the clinical effects of this neuromuscular blockade are weak in most patients, intravenous tetracyclines should be avoided in myasthenic patients.

Transient vestibular dysfunction has been reported in patients receiving minocycline; symptoms appear 2–3 days after initiation of therapy and resolve within 1–2 days of drug cessation (1,3).

There is one case report of a woman who developed transient myopia after receiving intravenous tetracycline on four separate occasions (2).

Volunteers given doxycycline at bedtime had impaired ability to remember a sentence taught to them after the first rapid-eye-movement cycle of the night (5). The authors proposed that doxycycline may interfere with protein synthesis in the brain necessary for consolidation of memory.

REFERENCES

1. Claussen CF, Schneider D, Claussen E (1987) Aeqilibriometrische Messungen der zentralen Vestibularis-Dysregulation nach Gabe von Minocyclin. *Arzneim Forsch-Drug Res* **37**, 950.
2. Edwards TS (1963) Transient myopia due to tetracycline. *J Amer Med Assn* **186**, 69.
3. Fanning WL, Gump DW, Sofferman KA (1977) Side effects of minocycline: A double blind study. *Antimicrob Agents Chemother* **11**, 712.
4. Gardner K, Cox T, Digre KB (1995) Idiopathic intracranial hypertension associated with tetracycline use in fraternal twins: Case reports and review. *Neurology* **45**, 6.
5. Idzikowski C, Oswald I (1983) Interference with human memory by an antibiotic. *Psychopharmacology* **79**, 108.
6. Kapusnik-Uner JE, Sande MA, Chambers HF (1996) Antimicrobial agents: Tetracyclines, chloramphenicol, erythromycin, and miscellaneous antibacterial agents. In: *Goodman and Gilman's The Pharmacological Basis of Therapeutics. 9th Ed.* Hardman JG, Gilman AG, Limbird LE eds. McGraw-Hill, New York p. 1123.
7. Keller H, Maurer P, Blaser J, Follath F (1992) Miscellaneous antibiotics. In: *Meyler's Side Effects of Drugs. 12th Ed.* Dukes MNG ed. Elsevier Science Publishers, Amsterdam p. 637.
8. Klein NC, Cunha BA (1995) Tetracyclines. *Med Clin N Amer* **79**, 789.
9. Kubikowski P, Szreniawski Z (1963) The mechanism of the neuromuscular blockade by antibiotics. *Arch Int Pharacodyn* **146**, 549.

10. Lambs L, Venturini M *et al.* (1988) Metal ion-tetracycline interactions in biological fluids. *J Inorgan Biochem* **33**, 193.

11. Leist JC, Zuniga JR, Chen N, Gollehon S (1995) Experimental topical tetracycline-induced neuritis in the rat. *J Oral Maxillofac Surg* **53**, 427.

12. Meacock DJ, Hewer RL (1981) Tetracycline and benign intracranial hypertension. *Brit Med J* **282**, 1240.

13. Pearson MG, Littlewood SM, Bowden AN (1981) Tetracycline and benign intracranial hypertension. *Brit Med J* **282**, 568.

14. Rush JA (1980) Pseudotumor cerebri, clinical profile and visual outcome in 63 patients. *Mayo Clin Proc* **55**, 541.

15. Snavely SR, Hodges GR (1984) The neurotoxicity of antibacterial agents. *Ann Intern Med* **101**, 92.

16. Thomas RJ (1994) Neurotoxicity of antibacterial therapy. *Southern Med J* **87**, 869.

17. Walters BNJ, Gubbay SS (1981) Tetracycline and benign intracranial hypertension: Report of five cases. *Brit Med J* **282**, 19.

18. Weller B, Sharf B, Sierpinski-Barth J, Schwartz M (1994) Idiopathic intracranial hypertension and tetracycline. *Harefuah* **127**, 9. [Hebrew]

Tetramethylthiuram Disulfide

John L. O'Donoghue

THIRAM
$C_6H_{12}N_2S_4$

Thiram; Bis(dimethylthiocarbamoyl) disulfide; Bis(dimethylthiocarbamyl) disulfide; Tetramethylthioperoxydicarbonic diamide; Tetramethylthiuram disulfide; TMTD

NEUROTOXICITY RATING

Experimental

B   Peripheral neuropathy

Thiram is a common commercial chemical with uses as a rubber accelerator and vulcanizer; an antioxidant in rubber and plastics; a lubricating oil additive; a seed and nut disinfectant; an agricultural fungicide; an insecticide; an animal repellant for tree and shrub protection; and a bacteriostat and fungistat in soaps, lotions, and antiseptic sprays. It is a degradation product of two other common fungicides, ferbam and ziram (10). Like disulfiram, it inhibits ethanol metabolism through interference with alcohol dehydrogenase, but it has not been used therapeutically for this purpose, as it is more acutely toxic than disulfiram (14).

Thiram, like other similar chemicals, is absorbed from the gastrointestinal tract and is widely distributed throughout the body; metal chelates of thiram can be found in many organs including the brain (19). It can be inhaled as either a dust, spray, or mist; and would be expected to be absorbed and readily distributed in the body. Absorption of pure thiram dust through the skin is unlikely since it is not soluble in aqueous media; however, disulfiram is soluble in organic solvents and is used in solubilized mixtures that can be applied to the skin. It is anticipated that the rate of absorption of thiram from a mixture would be highly dependent on the solubilizing agent and other ingredients in the mixture. Since the skin has a propensity to bind sulfur-containing materials such as thiram, thiram may be found in the skin at concentrations that exceed plasma levels. The thyroid gland can also be expected to accumulate thiram as it does other similar sulfur-containing chemicals. Increased levels of thiram have been found in the spleen, liver, and lungs of farm animals intoxicated with thiram; persistence in the body was 13–20 days (19). Thiram is excreted mainly unchanged (2), although some dimethyldithiocarbamate is excreted in the urine and carbon disulfide can be detected in the exhaled breath (2,4). Binding of thiram to intracellular thiols, such as glutathione, and subsequent liver metabolism to dimethyldithiocarbamate and carbon disulfide have been postulated (3,4).

Thiram and dimethyldithiocarbamate inhibit hepatic microsomal monooxygenases (18). Sulfhydryl enzymes, including hexokinase and amino acid oxidases, are inhibited by thiram (3). Turnover of phosphatidyl choline, essential for membrane-bound electron transport necessary for monooxygenase activity, is inhibited by thiram (11). Thiram is one of the more effective agents in its class in increasing the brain levels of both endogenous metal (copper and zinc) and heavy metals (lead and mercury) administered concurrently with the agent (1,13). The ability of thiram to increase the metal content of the brain is likely due to several factors, including its strong affinity for the metals and its lipophilicity, which allow the metal complexes to pass through the blood-brain barrier more effectively (1,13).

The acute oral toxicity of thiram in experimental animals has been reported to range from 210 mg/kg in mice and rabbits to 4000 mg/kg in rats and mice; the wide range of acute toxicity is thought to be related to use of different carriers (2). Male and female mice were equally susceptible to thiram, but female rats were more susceptible than males (8). Dermal exposure of rats to >2000 mg/kg thiram and inhalation dust exposure of rats, cats, and rabbits to 500 and 6225 mg/m³ did not result in lethality (2). At lethal levels, rapid breathing, ataxia, hyperactivity followed by inactivity, tremors, loss of muscle tone, and dyspnea have been reported beginning the day after exposure; deaths were delayed 2–7 days, and some occurred as late as the second week following exposure (2,8). Deaths were preceded by clonic convulsions in some animals (8). No pathological effects have been identified in acutely intoxicated animals; however, patchy demyelination of the cerebellum and medulla oblongata have been reported in animals dying after a single dose of structurally similar chemicals (5). Single doses of thiram below LD_{50} levels have been reported to produce effects on the rat CNS. Rats given 240 mg/kg of thiram orally showed a reduction in motor activity 2 h following dosing. Dosages as low as 40 mg/kg decreased subcortical electroencephalographic activity, and 60 mg/kg resulted in increased levels of dopamine and decreased combined levels of norepinephrine and epinephrine in the brain (17). Thiram given to mice by intraperitoneal (i.p.) injection at dosage levels ranging from 25%–100% of the i.p. LD_{50} altered the synaptosomal protein (increased), phospholipid (decrease), and cholesterol (transient increase followed by a decrease) content of crude synaptosomes isolated from the brain (6).

Two repeated-dose neurotoxicity studies have been conducted in male and female rats. In the first study, animals were fed thiram in the diet for 19–20.5 months at approximate constant dose rates of 5.3, 20.4, or 52 mg/kg/day for males and 6.1, 25.5, or 66.9 mg/kg/day for females (7). One-third of the group of 24 female rats fed 66.9 mg/kg/day developed neurological abnormalities that began after 5–19 months of exposure; males consuming 52 mg/kg/day did not develop a similar clinical appearance. The abnormalities in these animals included a change in gait with dragging of the hindfeet and tail (which the authors referred to as ataxia). As the condition worsened, animals became paralyzed posterior to the lumbar region and hindlimb musculature atrophied. In the second study, 4 of 24 female rats fed diets containing 0.1% thiram (65.8 mg/kg/day) for 9 months developed ataxia or paralysis similar to the pattern seen in animals in the first study; the incidence rate in this study was actually higher than in the first study, where only 1 of 24 rats developed clinical abnormalities after 9 months of exposure (7). Peripheral nerve conduction velocity and skeletal muscle motor unit activity were essentially unaffected by thiram exposure except in severely affected rats. Quantitative gait measurements showed significant differences in stride width and foot angle in mid- and high-dose female rats that were not showing gross clinical abnormalities. A jump-and-climb shuttle box test also showed a significant difference for clinically normal female high-dose animals. An open-field test for motor activity, which used line crossing as an end point, showed significant increases in motor activity for mid- and high-dose male rats and high-dose females; surprisingly, the mid-dose females had normal activity levels. Limited histological analysis of two clinically abnormal high-dose females showed lesions fairly typical of axonal degeneration, with secondary myelin degeneration and skeletal muscle atrophy; chromatolysis, pyknosis, and satellitosis of ventral motor horn cells were noted in the lumbar spinal cord.

Rats (12/sex/group) fed 300, 1000, or 2500 ppm of thiram in their diets for 65 weeks showed signs of weakness, ataxia, and paralysis; histological examinations revealed calcifications in the brainstem and cerebellum, and dystrophic changes in the limb musculature (2,9). Rats given diets of 100 ppm did not display neurological abnormalities.

A number of other effects including skin sensitization, weight loss, alopecia, liver enlargement, thyroid metaplasia, testicular atrophy, developmental effects, and bone deformities (birds only) have been described in experimental animals exposed to thiram (2,15,16).

Reports of human or domestic animal neurotoxicity similar to that observed in experimental animals are not available. A number of reports of clinical complaints in Russian employees using thiram have been summarized (2); these reports, which include reference to headache, asthenia, sleep dysfunction, fatigue, and neurological dysfunction, could not be specifically linked to thiram exposures. The American Conference of Governmental Industrial Hygienists has recommended a Threshold Limit Value of 1 mg/m³ for thiram dust exposure in the workplace (2).

Thiram has a number of different nervous system effects in experimental animals; each of these effects may have different mechanisms of action. Due to its lipophilicity, thiram can be incorporated into membranes and does increase mobilization of metals into the nervous system. Increasing the metal content of the nervous system, or changing the distribution, or availability of metals within neural compartments may adversely affect neural function. Thiram effectively inhibits monooxygenases, including dopamine β-hydroxylase, which may lead to changes in neural function; however, changes in brain levels of norepinephrine following exposure to diethyldithiocarbamate or disulfiram were shown not to be causally related to changes in motor activity levels of mice (12). The neurotoxicity of thiram may also be mediated through its reactive metabolites, dimethyldithiocarbamate and carbon disulfide.

REFERENCES

1. Aaseth J, Alexander J, Wannag A (1981) Effect of thiocarbamate derivatives on copper, zinc, and mercury distribution in rats and mice. *Arch Toxicol* **48**, 29.
2. American Conference of Governmental Industrial Hygienists (1992) Thiram. In: *Documentation of the Threshold Limit Values. Vol 3. 6th Ed.* Cincinnati, Ohio p. 1545.
3. Dalvi RR (1988) Toxicity of thiram (tetramethylthiuram disulfide): A review. *Vet Hum Toxicol* **30**, 480.
4. Dalvi RR, Devras DP (1986) Metabolism of a dithiocarbamate fungicide thiram to carbon disulfide in the rat and its hepatotoxic implications. *Acta Pharmacol Toxicol* **58**, 38.
5. Gosslin RE, Smith RP, Hodge HC (1984) *Clinical Toxicology of Commercial Products.* Williams & Wilkins, Baltimore p. 383.
6. Gupta M, Amma MKP, Gupta KG (1993) Membrane disordering effects of thiram as assessed by brain synaptosomal and erythrocyte membrane constituents. *Bull Environ Contam Toxicol* **50**, 764.
7. Lee C-C, Peters PJ (1976) Neurotoxicity and behavioral effects of thiram in rats. *Environ Health Perspect* **17**, 35.
8. Lee C-C, Russell JQ, Minor JL (1978) Oral toxicity of ferric dimethyl dithiocarbamates (Ferbam) and tetramethylthiuram disulfide (Thiram) in rodents. *J Toxicol Environ Health* **4**, 93.
9. Lehman AJ (1952) Chemicals in food: A report to the Association of Food and Drug Officials on current developments, Part II Pesticides, Sect V Pathology. *Quart Bull Assn Food Drug Offic U S* **16**, 47.
10. Lowen WK (1961) Determination of thiram in ferbam. *J Assn Offic Agr Chem* **1**, 713.
11. Leyck S, Freundt KJ (1978) Response of phospholipid metabolism to thiram in rat liver microsomes. *Naunyn-Schmied Arch Pharmacol* **302**, R19.
12. Moore KE (1969) Effects of disulfiram and diethyldithiocarbamate on spontaneous motor activity and brain catecholamine levels in mice. *Biochem Phamacol* **18**, 1627.
13. Oskarsson A (1987) Comparative effects of ten dithiocarbamates and thiuram compounds on tissue distribution and excretion of lead in rats. *Environ Res* **44**, 82.
14. Ritchie JM (1975) The aliphatic alcohols. In: *The Pharmacological Basis of Therapeutics. 5th Ed.* Goodman LS, Gilman A eds. Macmillan, New York p. 137.
15. Rasul AR, Howell JMcC (1974) The toxicity of some dithiocarbamate compounds in young and domestic fowl. *Toxicol Appl Pharmacol* **30**, 63.
16. Robens JF (1969) Teratologic studies of carbaryl, diazinon, norea, disulfiram and thiram in small laboratory animals. *Toxicol Appl Pharmacol* **15**, 152.
17. Thuranszky K, Kiss I, Botos M, Szebeni A (1982) Effect of dithiocarbamate-type chemicals on the nervous system of rats. *Arch Toxicol* **5**, 125.
18. Zemaitis MA, Greene FE (1979) *In vivo* and *in vitro* effects of thiuram disulfides and dithiocarbamates on hepatic microsomal drug metabolism in the rat. *Toxicol Appl Pharmacol* **48**, 343.
19. Zhavoronkov II, Antsiferov SD (1977) Distribution, accumulation, and excretion of TMTD from animals. *Veterinariya* **2**, 95.

Tetrodotoxin

Toshio Narahashi

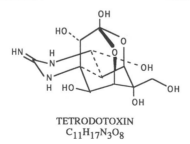

TETRODOTOXIN
$C_{11}H_{17}N_3O_8$

Octahydro-12-(hydroxymethyl)-2-imino-5,9:7,10a-dimethano-10a*H*-[1,3]dioxocino[6,5-*d*]pyrimidine-4,7,10,11,12-pentol

NEUROTOXICITY RATING

Clinical

A Ion channel syndrome

Experimental

A Ion channel dysfunction (sodium channel agent)

Tetrodotoxin (TTX) is widely known to occur in certain species of puffer fish or globe fish, especially in species belonging to the family Tetraodontidae. TTX is contained primarily in the ovaries and liver, and smaller concentrations are in other organs, such as the intestine and skin, (6). However, the occurrence of TTX is not limited to puffer fish, and other animals of diverse groups also harbor TTX. Newts belonging to the family Salamandridae (*e.g., Taricha torosa*) contain TTX in the ovary, eggs, skin, muscle, and blood (7). A starfish, *Astropecten polyacanthus*; a horseshoe crab, *Carcinoscorpius rotundicauda*; and the blue-ringed octopus, *Octopus maculosus,* also contain TTX (15). Studies have clearly shown that TTX is produced by certain species of bacteria and reach the animals *via* the food chain (11,15). Bacteria that elaborate TTX belong to the family Vibrionaceae, including *Vibrio alginolyticus, V. parahaemolyticus, V. anguillarum,* and *Photobacterium phosphoreum.* These bacteria produce TTX and/or anhydrotetrodotoxin, which is easily converted to TTX.

TTX is a colorless prism and forms a monoacidic base in aqueous solution with a pKa of 8.5. It is only sparingly soluble in water, but more easily soluble in weak acidic conditions. TTX is relatively stable in slightly acidic conditions, and the time constant of degradation at pH 4.8 and 4°C is estimated to be 14 months. It is not stable in alkaline solutions (3).

TTX is not used clinically for therapeutic purposes; it is extensively used as a chemical tool in the laboratory (2,8,9). Laboratory use is based on its highly specific and potent action in blocking voltage-gated sodium channels. TTX is also used in studies of potassium channels, calcium channels, and ligand-gated channels by selectively blocking the sodium channel; measurements of sodium channel densities of excitable membranes; studies of neurotransmitter release from nerve terminals; and biochemical studies of sodium channels.

General Toxicology

TTX is rapidly absorbed from the buccal mucosa and the gastrointestinal tract. Numbness of the tongue and lips is felt rapidly, and death may occur in <30 min depending on the dose. TTX does not readily penetrate intact skin (6).

TTX appears to be widely distributed in the body, including the kidneys, heart, liver, lungs, intestine, brain, and blood. The concentration is highest in the kidneys and heart, and lowest in the brain and blood (4,6). An appreciable amount of TTX is said to be excreted in the urine in an intact form (6).

Since TTX blocks voltage-gated sodium channels selectively, organs that contain sodium channels are affected. These include the brain, peripheral nerves, and skeletal muscle. Cardiac muscle and its sodium channels are less sensitive to TTX than those of nerves. The effect of TTX on smooth muscle is controversial; some authors have reported physiological block, while others show little or no effect. Vasodilation appears to be the major cause of severe hypotension, but it remains to be seen whether this is due to a direct blocking action on smooth muscle or on sympathetic nerve fibers. Death is caused primarily by paralysis of diaphragm muscle (4,5).

Animal Studies

The LD_{50} values of TTX have been estimated to be 8–13 μg/kg for mouse, 10–14 μg/kg for rat, 2–10 μg/kg for rabbit, and 5–10 μg/kg for cat (5).

In Vitro Studies

TTX blocks the action potential of nerves and skeletal muscle. Smooth muscle itself does not respond to TTX, but the nerve-evoked response is blocked by TTX. Cardiac muscle is less sensitive to TTX than nerves and skeletal muscle. The block of action potential occurs without change in resting membrane potential; it is due exclusively to a block of voltage-gated sodium channels (8–10). Sodium channels of CNS neurons, nerve fibers, and skeletal muscle are much more sensitive to TTX than those of cardiac muscle, with a difference in K_d of 1000-fold. TTX is highly selective for voltage-gated sodium channels; it does not affect other channels, including potassium channels, calcium channels, acetylcholine-activated channels, glutamate-activated channels, and γ-aminobutyric acid-activated channels (9). TTX also has no effect on the transmitter-release mechanism. Dorsal root ganglion neurons and some brain neurons are endowed with both TTX-sensitive and TTX-resistant sodium channels; the difference in K_d for these channels is as much as 100,000-fold (12).

TTX blocks the sodium channel by occluding it at or near the external orifice. A cysteine group in the sodium channel confers low TTX sensitivity on the cardiac channel, whereas a tyrosine and a phenylalanine confer high TTX sensitivity on skeletal muscle and brain sodium channels, respectively (1,13,14).

Human Studies

Observations are restricted to subjects accidentally intoxicated with TTX through ingestion of puffer fish. In Japan, there are 100–200 cases of puffer fish poisoning each year, with a mortality of approximately 50%. Some prefectures (states) in Japan require a special license to serve puffer fish at a restaurant, and intoxication at such restaurants is extremely rare.

Puffer fish intoxication is characterized by numbness or tingling sensations in the extremities and periorally, vomiting, hypotension, and weakening of all voluntary muscles including the respiratory muscles. These symptoms are acute and death occurs within 3–5 h. Death is caused by paralysis of respiratory muscles such as diaphragm. The heart continues to beat for sometime after cessation of respiration (4–6). No chemical antidotes are known, and patients must be ventilated until the TTX level is reduced through excretion.

Toxic Mechanisms

The only target of TTX is the voltage-gated sodium channel. All symptoms of poisoning can be ascribed to blockade of sodium channels in excitable membranes.

REFERENCES

1. Backx PH, Yue DT, Lawrence JH et al. (1992) Molecular localization of an ion-binding site within the pore of mammalian sodium channels. *Science* **257**, 248.
2. Catterall WA (1980) Neurotoxins that act on voltage-sensitive sodium channels in excitable membranes. *Annu Rev Pharmacol Toxicol* **20**, 15.
3. Colquhoun D, Henderson R, Ritchie JM (1972) The binding of labelled tetrodotoxin to nonmyelinated nerve fibres. *J Physiol* **227**, 95.
4. Evans MH (1969) Mechanism of saxitoxin and tetrodotoxin poisoning. *Brit Med Bull* **25**, 263.
5. Evans MH (1972) Tetrodotoxin, saxitoxin, and related substances: Their applications in neurobiology. *Int Rev Neurobiol* **15**, 83.
6. Kao CY (1966) Tetrodotoxin, saxitoxin and their significance in the study of excitation phenomena. *Pharmacol Rev* **18**, 997.
7. Mosher HS, Fuhrman FA, Buchwald HD, Fischer HG (1964) Tarichatoxin-tetrodotoxin: A potent neurotoxin. *Science* **144**, 1100.
8. Narahashi T (1974) Chemicals as tools in the study of excitable membranes. *Physiol Rev* **54**, 813.
9. Narahashi T (1988) Mechanism of tetrodotoxin and saxitoxin action. In: *Handbook of Natural Toxins. Vol 3. Marine Toxins and Venoms.* Tu AT ed. Marcel Dekker, New York p. 185.
10. Narahashi T, Moore JW, Scott WR (1964) Tetrodotoxin blockage of sodium conductance increase in lobster giant axons. *J Gen Physiol* **47**, 965.
11. Noguchi T, Huang DF, Arakawa O et al. (1987) *Vibrio alginolyticus*, a tetrodotoxin-producing bacterium, in the intestines of the fish *Fugu vermicularis vermicularis*. *Marine Biol* **94**, 625.
12. Roy ML, Narahashi T (1992) Differential properties of tetrodotoxin-sensitive and tetrodotoxin-resistant sodium channels in rat dorsal root ganglion neurons. *J Neurosci* **12**, 2104.
13. Satin J, Kyle JW, Fan Z et al. (1994) Post-repolarization block of cloned sodium channels by saxitoxin: The contribution of pore-region amino acids. *Biophys J* **66**, 1353.
14. Schild L, Moczydlowski E (1991) Competitive binding interaction between Zn^{2+} and saxitoxin in cardiac Na^+ channels. Evidence for a sulfhydryl group in the Zn^{2+}/saxitoxin binding site. *Biophys J* **59**, 523.
15. Simidu U, Noguchi T, Huang D-F et al. (1987) Marine bacteria which produce tetrodotoxin. *Appl Environ Microbiol* **53**, 1714.

Thalicarpine

Peter S. Spencer

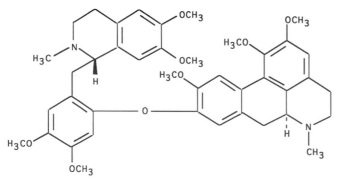

THALICARPINE
$C_{41}H_{48}N_2O_8$

[S-(R*,R*)]-9-[4,5-Dimethoxy-2-[1,2,3,4-tetrahydro-6,7-dimethoxy-2-methyl-1-isoquinolinyl)-methyl]phenoxy]-5,6,6a,7-tetrahydro-1,2,10-trimethoxy-6-methyl-4H dibenzo[de,g]quinoline; Thaliblastine

NEUROTOXICITY RATING

Clinical

B   Acute encephalopathy

Thalicarpine is a plant alkaloid of novel structure that possesses antiproliferative and antitumor activities in experimental and clinical studies (3). Common toxic effects of weekly intravenous doses given to patients with advanced malignancy included CNS depression, arm pain, and electrocardiographic changes; less frequent effects included vomiting, tachycardia, hypotension, pain distant from infusion site, urticaria, chills, diarrhea, and mydriasis (1,2).

REFERENCES

1. Creaven PJ, Cohen MH, Selawry OS et al. (1975) Phase I study of thalicarpine (NAC-68075), a plant alkaloid of noval structure. *Cancer Chemother Rep* **59**, 1001.
2. Leimert JT, Corder MP, Elliott TE, Lovett JM (1980) An abbreviated phase II trial of thalicarpine. *Cancer Treat Rep* **64**, 1389.
3. Seifert F, Todorov DK, Hutter KJ, Zeller WJ (1996) Cell cycle effects of thaliblastine. *J. Cancer Res Clin Oncol* **122**, 707.

Thalidomide

Herbert H. Schaumburg

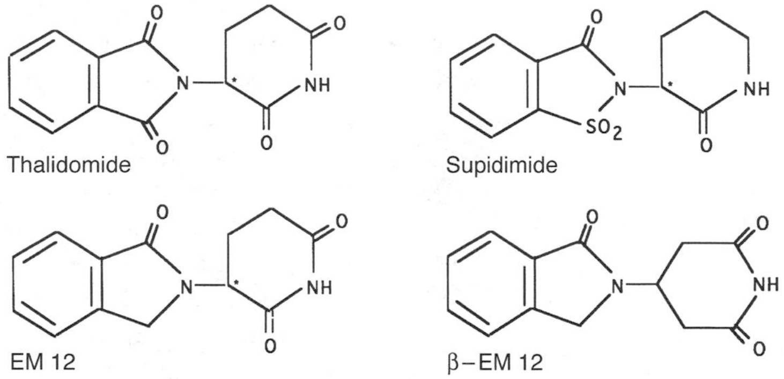

Thalidomide   Supidimide

EM 12   β−EM 12

THALIDOMIDE AND DERIVATIVES
$C_{13}H_{10}N_2O_4$

Thalidomide: 2-(2,6-Dioxo-3-piperidinyl)-1*H*-isoindole-1,3(2*H*)-dione;*N*-(2,6-Dioxo-3-piperidyl)phthalimide; α-Phthalimidoglutarimide

NEUROTOXICITY RATING

Clinical

A   Peripheral neuropathy

A   Teratogenicity

Thalidomide (Thd) is a synthetic substance that was marketed as a sedative and hypnotic in 1957. Although many derivatives have been synthesized and tested in animal studies, Thd is the only substance of this type used on a large scale in humans. It was withdrawn in 1961 following an epidemic of dysmyelia in children born to women who took Thd as a sedative during pregnancy. Since then it has had limited but effective use as an anti-inflammatory or immunomodulatory agent principally for type II (lepromatous) leprosy (6,29). It has no direct effect on the leprosy mycobacterium. Thd is also effective in other immunopathological conditions characterized by inflammation of postcapillary venules; namely, for mucocutaneous (aphthous) ulcers of Behçet's disease and in acquired immunodeficiency syndrome (27). It has also had limited use in some dermatoses and systemic conditions, including discoid lupus erythematosus, prurigo nodularis, erythema multiforme, ulcerative colitis, rheumatoid arthritis, and graft-*vs.*-host disease (36). The chief adverse side effects of Thd in its current carefully controlled use are mild sedation and peripheral neuropathy. The oral dose of Thd for sedative-hypnotic effects was 25–200 mg. The usual immunomodulatory dose ranges from 7–200 mg/day; doses of 1200 mg/day are used in graft-*vs.*-host disease.

Thd (CAS: 50-35-1) is a white, odorless crystalline powder, largely insoluble in water (100 μg/ml) as well as in oils. It is soluble in dimethyl sulfoxide. Since Thd contains an asymmetric C-atom, it is a mixture of the $S(-)$- and the $R(+)$-enantiomers. Commercial Thd is a racemate. Longer term *in vivo* studies with the Thd-enantiomers are hampered by the fact that both these enantiomers are unstable and re-form a racemate *in vitro* and *in vivo* (30).

General Toxicology

Most of the degradation products of Thd found within the organism cannot be considered true metabolites. Thd is pH-dependently hydrolyzed *in vivo* and *in vitro*. Hydrolyses of Thd include splitting of either one of the ring systems, or of both, at the amide bonds (33). All the primary hydrolysis products are polar mono- to tricarbonic acids. Three of the hydrolysis products are formed by splitting of the glutarimide ring only; one comes from splitting the phthalmide ring only, and three are derived from the splitting of both.

The elimination half-life ($t_{1/2}$) of Thd in humans (mean ± SD) is 8.7 ± 4.1 h, considerably longer than that found in experimental animals (32,34). Data obtained from male volunteers given a single oral dose of 200 mg Thd indicate a one-compartment model (4). Urinary elimination is negligible (0.6 ± 0.2% of the total dose/24 h), and the renal clearance rate is 0.08 ± 0.03 l/h. None of the highly polar metabolites appears in urine; the major route of elimination is nonrenal.

The teratogenicity of Thd has been extensively investigated, and there is an experimental model in the marmoset (16,17,20,23–25,26). While the marmoset model promises to allow determination of periods of vulnerability and which Thd isomers are responsible for teratogenicity, to date, the mechanism of embryopathy is unclear, despite considerable speculation and review (37). Two studies that utilized administration of Thd to rabbit fetuses suggested a neuro-teratogenic basis for embryopathy (8,22). Thalidomide and EM12, a closely related compound, are potent teratogens; by contrast, supidimide and β-EM12 are largely or completely inactive.

Systemic side effects and risks (in males and nonpregnant women) are not serious; they include constipation, eosinophilia, hair loss, brittle nails, desquamation of skin from hands and feet, fever, bronchitis, and pruritus.

Thd is an immunomodulator, not an immunosuppressant (27). It has no direct effect on T lymphocytes. The exact mechanism of Thd's immunomodulatory action is unknown; it acts on endothelial cells, inhibits neutrophil chemotaxis and migration and lymphocyte proliferation, and decreases neutrophil phagocytic activity. Specifically, it modulates blood monocyte cytokine synthesis, particularly tumor necrosis factor-α (26). Studies have also demonstrated inhibition of angiogenesis in a rabbit cornea micropocket assay (7).

Animal Studies

High doses of thalidomide administered acutely and chronically have little sedative effect in experimental animals.

There is no satisfactory experimental animal model of thalidomide-induced peripheral neuropathy. Administration for prolonged periods (1 year in a canine study) evoked only mild degeneration in dorsal columns of the spinal cord of dogs and slight degeneration in rat nerve (10,19). One study in the rabbit produced slowing of nerve conduction without histopathological alterations (35); another study in the rabbit produced slight reduction in myelin sheath thickness (31). A study of the effect of administration of Thd to the rabbit fetus describes reduction of numbers of axons in both motor and sensory roots (8).

In Vitro Studies

Few in vitro studies that address the neurotoxicity of Thd are available. One report describes minor neuronal changes (eccentric, distorted nuclei) produced by application of serum samples of patients with Thd neuropathy to cultures of fetal rat dorsal root ganglia (1).

Human Studies

The sedative effect of Thd has not been responsible for serious life-threatening depression of consciousness, even following massive doses in attempted suicide. One individual, who took 2 g, only became drowsy for several days (9).

Sensory peripheral neuropathy appeared in isolated instances in 1958–59, soon after Thd's introduction, and reached near epidemic levels in 1960–61 (2,11,12,14,18). Most initial instances were in healthy persons consuming 50–200 mg daily for sedation; subsequent reports describe a similar neuropathy in patients with dermatological and rheumatological conditions. The incidence is not known. Initial symptoms of paresthesia and numbness in the feet appeared within 2–10 months. Robust dose–effect and dose–duration relationships have not been established. A recent, carefully monitored study suggests a correlation among cumulative dose, symptomatology, and electrophysiological changes (3). Some individuals clearly have had greater doses for longer duration without symptoms; this was claimed as support for a metabolic predisposition in susceptible persons, but studies of genetic differences in drug metabolism have failed to support this notion (15). Paresthesias, often painful and distressing, spread up the lower limb to the knee and then involve the hands within 2 months of onset in most reports (5,38). Cramps in the legs are common, and a few individuals developed mild proximal lower limb weakness. Tendon reflexes are often unaffected in mild cases; patella reflexes are occasionally increased. All sensory modalities are impaired to an equal degree. Recovery is variable and initially seemed unusually poor for a toxic neuropathy; about one half of severely involved patients in the early studies reported persistent painful paresthesias 1 year later. Patients in the initial reports frequently continued to receive treatment well after the onset of sensory symptoms; this may account for the poor recovery. Poor recovery in this sensory neuropathy likely reflects, in part, distal degeneration of central axonal projections of affected dorsal root ganglion cells. Patients in more recent prospective studies who ceased medication following the onset of symptoms, or who were asymptomatic but revealed diminishing amplitude of sensory nerve action potentials (subclinical neuropathy), are more likely to make a satisfactory recovery (3,18,38). Electrodiagnostic studies have consistently displayed loss or diminution of sural nerve and other sensory action potentials with only minor abnormalities of motor nerve conduction (3,12,25). One report describes increased latency of somatosensory evoked potentials from the lower limbs, a possible correlate of dorsal column degeneration in the spinal cord. Nerve biopsies during intoxication display wallerian-like degeneration and, after recovery, fiber loss; studies of postmortem material have disclosed loss of sensory nerve fibers, dorsal root ganglion cells, and dorsal column fibers in the spinal cord (21).

Thd neuropathy is no longer a serious problem; rheumatologists, dermatologists, and immunologists are attuned to the early signs and have utilized sensory nerve conduction studies as a monitor for early subclinical detection (13).

It is suggested that Thd be only used for disabling conditions and only after other therapies have failed; furthermore, doctors who prescribe Thd should have expertise in its use and the resources to detect subclinical or pre-exisiting neuropathy (28).

Toxic Mechanism

The mechanism of thalidomide-induced peripheral neuropathy is unknown.

REFERENCES

1. Aronson IK, Yu R, West DP *et al.* (1984) Thalidomide-induced peripheral neuropathy—effect of serum factors on nerve cultures. *Arch Dermatol* **120**, 1466.
2. Chapon F, Lechevalier B, da Silva DC *et al.* (1985) Neuropathies a la thalidomide. *Rev Neurol* **141**, 719.
3. Chaudhry V, Cornblath D, Corse A *et al.* (1996) Thalidomide-induced neuropathy: Clinical and electrophysiological features. *Neurology* **46**, A283.
4. Chen TL, Vogelsang GB, Petty BG *et al.* (1989) Plasma pharmacokinetics and urinary excretion of thalidomide after oral dosing in healthy male volunteers. *Drug Metab Disposition* **17**, 402.
5. Clemmensen OJ, Olsen PZ, Andersen KE (1984) Thalidomide neurotoxicity. *Arch Dermatol* **120**, 338.
6. Crawford CL (1994) Use of thalidomide in leprosy. *Toxicol Rev* **13**, 177.
7. D'Amato RJ, Loughnan MS, Flynn E, Folkman J (1994) Thalidomide is an inhibitor of angiogenesis. *Proc Nat Acad Sci USA* **91**, 4082.
8. Deiongh RU (1990) A quantitative ultrastructural study of motor and sensory lumbosacral nerve roots in thalidomide-treated rabbit fetus. *J Neuropathol Exp Neurol* **49**, 564.
9. DeSouza LP (1959) Thalidomide. *Brit Med J* **2**, 635.
10. Diezel PB (1963) Morphologische Veränderungen bei experimenteller Thalidomid-Neuropathie und thalidomid-bedingten Extremitätenmißbildungen. *Munchn Med Wochenschr* **105**, 2265.
11. Fullerton PM, Kremer M (1961) Neuropathy after intake of thalidomide (Distaval). *Brit Med J* **2**, 855.
12. Fullerton PM, O'Sullivan DJ (1968) Thalidomide neuropathy: A clinical, electrophysiological, and histological follow-up study. *J Neurol Neurosurg Psychiat* **31**, 543.
13. Gardner-Medwin JM, Smith NJ, Powell RJ (1994) Clinical experience with thalidomide in the management of severe oral and genital ulceration in conditions such as Behçet's disease: use of neurophysiological studies to detect thalidomide neuropathy. *Ann Rheum Dis* **53**, 828.
14. Hafstrom T (1967) Polyneuropathy after neurosedyn (thalidomide) and its prognosis. *Acta Neurol Scand* **43**, Suppl 32), 1.
15. Harland CC, Steventon GB, Marsden JR (1995) Thalidomide-induced neuropathy and genetic differences in drug metabolism. *Eur J Clin Pharm* **49**, 1.
16. Heger W, Klug S, Schmahl HJ *et al.* (1988) Embryotoxic effects of thalidomide derivatives on the non-human primate *Callithrix jacchus*; 3. Teratogenic potency of the EM 12 enantiomers. *Arch Toxicol* **62**, 205.
17. Heger W, Schmahl JH, Klug S *et al.* (1994) Embryotoxic effects of thalidomide derivatives in the non-human primate *Callithrix jacchus*. IV. Teratogenicity of micrograms/kg doses of the EM12 enantiomers. *Teratogen Carcin Mut* **14**, 115.
18. Hess CW, Hunziker T, Kupfer A, Ludin HP (1986) Thalidomide-induced peripheral neuropathy. A prospective clinical, neurophysiological and pharmacogenetic evaluation. *J Neurol* **233**, 83.
19. Klinghardt GW (1965) Ein beitrag der experimentellen neuropathologie zur toxizitatsprufung neuer chemotherapeutica. *Mitt Max Planck Ges* **3**, 142.
20. Klug S, Felies A, Sturje H *et al.* (1994) Embryotoxic effects of thalidomide derivatives in the non-human primate *Callithrix jacchus*. 5. Lack of teratogenic effects of phthalimidophthalmide. *Arch Toxicol* **68**, 203.
21. Lagueny A, Rommel A, Vignolly B *et al.* (1986) Thalidomide neuropathy: An electrophysiologic study. *Muscle Nerve* **9**, 837.
22. McCredie J, North K, DeIongh R (1984) Thalidomide deformities and their nerve supply. *J Anat* **139**, 397.
23. Merker HJ, Heger W, Sames K *et al.* (1988) Embryotoxic effects of thalidomide-derivatives in the non-human primate *Callithrix jacchus*. I. Effects of 3-(1,3-dihydro-1-oxo-2H-isoindol-2-yl)-2,6-dioxopiperidine (EM12) on skeletal development. *Arch Toxicol* **61**, 165.
24. Neubert D, Heger W, Merker HJ *et al.* (1988) Embryotoxic effects of thalidomide derivatives in non-human primate *Callithrix jacchus*. II. Elucidation of the susceptible period and of the variability of embryonic stages. *Arch Toxicol* **61**, 180.
25. Ochonisky S, Verroust J, Bastuji-Garin S *et al.* (1994) Thalidomide neuropathy incidence and clinico-electrophysiologic findings in 42 patients. *Arch Dermatol* **130**, 66.
26. Peterson PK, Hu S, Sheng WS, Kravitz FH (1995) Thalidomide inhibits tumor necrosis factor-alpha production by lipopolysaccharide- and lipoarabinomannan-stimulated human microglial cells. *J Infect Dis* **172**, 1137.
27. Powell RJ (1994) New roles for thalidomide. *Brit Med J* **313**, 377.
28. Powell RJ, Gardner-Medwin JM (1994) Guidelines for the clinical use and dispensing of thalidomide. *Postgrad Med J* **70**, 901.
29. Sabin TD (1974) Thalidomide neuropathy and leprous neuritis. *Lancet* **1**, 166.
30. Schmahl HJ, Nau H, Neubert D (1988) The enantiomers of the teratogenic thalidomide analogue EM12: 1. Chiral

inversion and plasma pharmacokinetics in the marmoset monkey. *Arch Toxicol* **62**, 200.

31. Schroder JM, Matthiesen T (1985) Experimental thalidomide neuropathy: The morphological correlate of reduced conduction velocity. *Acta Neuropathol* **65**, 285.

32. Schumacher JH, Blake DA, Gillette JR (1968) Disposition of thalidomide in rabbits and rats. *J Pharmacol Exp Ther* **160**, 201.

33. Schumacher H, Smith RL, Williams RT (1965) The metabolism of thalidomide: The spontaneous hydrolysis of thalidomide in solution. *Brit J Pharmacol* **25**, 324.

34. Schumacher HJ, Wilson JG, Terapan JF, Rosedale SL (1970) Thalidomide: Disposition in rhesus monkey and studies of its hydrolysis in tissue of this and other species. *J Pharmacol Exp Ther* **173**, 265.

35. Schwab BW, Arezzo JC, Paldino AM et al. (1984) Rabbit sural nerve responses to chronic treatment with thalidomide and supidimide. *Muscle Nerve* **7**, 362.

36. Sheehan NJ (1986) Thalidomide neurotoxicity and rheumatoid arthritis. *Arthritis Rheum* **29**, 1296.

37. Stephens TD (1988) Proposed mechanisms of action in thalidomide embryopathy. *Teratology* **38**, 229.

38. Wulff CH, Hoyer H, Asboe-Hansen G, Brodthagen H (1985) Development of polyneuropathy during thalidomide therapy. *Brit J Dermatol* **112**, 475.

Thallium

Luigi Manzo

NEUROTOXICITY RATING

Clinical

A Peripheral neuropathy

A Optic neuropathy

B Chronic encephalopathy (cognitive dysfunction)

Experimental

A Peripheral neuropathy (axon mitochondrial alteration—*in vitro*)

Thallium (Tl), atomic number 81, (AW, 204.39), a rare element occurring in trace amounts in almost all living organisms, has known beneficial function. It can be obtained from flue dust residues of zinc and lead smelters where it exists as an impurity in pyrites, and from by-products of cadmium and sulfuric acid production.

Tl has two oxidation states, +1 and +3. In aqueous solutions, the thallous (+1) ion is more stable than thallic (+3), but salts of the latter can be stabilized by complexing agents. This makes possible the existence of cationic or neutral thallic compounds in seawater and freshwater. Bacteria occurring in anerobic natural lake sediments can biomethylate Tl to form organothallium species. Biological implications of this process have yet to be clarified (47).

Commercial production of Tl is minute compared with that of other metals. Industrial uses of Tl salts include the manufacture of crystals, imitation jewelry, electric and electronic equipment, semiconductors and scintillator counters, optical systems, pigments, stainless corrosion-resistant alloys, and fiberglass (4). The expected widespread use of fiberglass in communication systems will almost certainly significantly increase demand for and production of Tl.

Tl compounds have been used historically as a medical treatment for venereal disease, gout, dysentery, scalp ringworm, and night sweats in tuberculosis; these applications were abandoned early in the twentieth century because of distressing side effects and serious toxicity.

Tl has been used on a large scale as a rodenticide and insecticide. Incidents of severe poisoning have led to its replacement in North America by less toxic compounds. However, worldwide use of Tl as an effective rodenticide is increasing (25).

In current clinical practice, trace levels of ^{201}Tl are employed in nuclear medicine patients for cardiac scanning.

A Time-Weighted Average Threshold Limit Value of 0.1 mg/m^3 has been set by the American Conference of Governmental Industrial Hygienists for occupational exposure to Tl. However, no satisfactory data exist from which to derive a threshold limit, and the present value is based largely on analogy with other toxic inorganic metals like lead and arsenic (33).

General Toxicology

The thallous (+1) ion, with an ionic radius of 1.44 Å, is comparable to that of the potassium ion (ionic radius 1.33 Å); its chemistry resembles that of alkali ions. The ability of Tl$^+$ to interfere with potassium-dependent activity plays an important role in its toxicity. Tl also distributes in mammalian tissues in the same way as potassium. A relevant aspect of the potassium-like kinetics of this metal is the tendency of Tl ions to concentrate intracellularly. Tl binds more tightly to biological ligands than potassium and, unlike potassium, has the potential of binding to nitrogen and sulfur ligands (15). Because of its stronger complexing ability and different ligand preference, Tl accumulation in tissue cells is unphysiological and may result in altered cell function.

Inorganic Tl salts are rapidly absorbed from the gastrointestinal tract. Extensive dermal absorption also occurs, and toxic effects have been described in both laboratory animals and humans after topical application of Tl salts (30).

Once absorbed, Tl is widely distributed in the body, the most rapid uptake occurring in the kidney, myocardium, and salivary glands. In humans, kidney and testis contain some of the highest Tl concentrations of any organ after absorption of large doses (11). Considerable amounts of Tl are deposited in hair. In the rat, 21 days after dosing by oral or parenteral routes, up to 60% of the remaining body burden is found in hair (25). Blood contains very little Tl. At the steady state, which is reached after 24 h, blood Tl is located predominantly in red blood cells (41). The volume of Tl distribution is estimated to be about 10 l/kg in rabbit, 5–6 l/kg in rat, and 4 l/kg in man (31,41). In fatal cases of acute human Tl poisoning in man, Tl levels in principal organs have been in the range of 2–20 $\mu g/g$ and concentrations of 2–4 mg Tl/l have been measured in the urine (29,31).

Like potassium, Tl is rapidly accumulated in the intracellular space against a large blood/tissue concentration gradient by mechanisms involving active Na^+, K^+-ATPase–dependent transport and $Na^+/K^+/Cl^-$ cotransport processes (6). A large fraction of cellular Tl is sequestered by organelles. In rat tissues, the highest Tl levels are measured in the nuclear fraction, but large amounts (8%–12%) of cellular Tl are also found in mitochondria (47). Almost identical tissue and subcellular distribution patterns have been seen in rats treated with ^{201}Tl as monovalent or trivalent ions, which suggests either that the oxidation state is not critical for transport or that Tl is converted to a common oxidation state in $vivo$ (47).

Tl is cleared from the body mainly through kidneys and intestine. Fecal excretion normally exceeds urinary excretion regardless of the route of absorption. Large amounts of the absorbed Tl are secreted from the blood into the small and large bowel, and substantial fractions are also excreted by salivary glands (29).

Tl elimination is very slow. In cases of human poisoning, 45% of the dose was still present in the body 24 days after ingestion, and Tl was measured in urine, feces, and scalp hair up to 5 months after exposure (31).

In humans, the average half-life of the intravenously administered radiotracer ^{201}Tl is reported to be 2.15 days, but calculation of kinetic parameters in Tl-intoxicated patients has led to variable half-life values ranging from 1.7–30 days depending on the time since, and chronicity of, ingestion. The rate of Tl excretion in urine is estimated to be 3.2% per day of the amount remaining in the body (25,47).

Studies in animals have demonstrated that Tl entering the gut via the saliva, or by direct transfer across the intestinal wall, is eliminated incompletely with feces because of extensive resorption from the intestine (41,46). Intestinal recycling, in concert with sequestration by cells and extensive tubular resorption in the kidney, can explain the long elimination half-time and prolonged body retention of Tl as factors leading to a continuous intoxication process after absorption of a single large dose (36). Moreover, Tl may act as a cumulative poison after repeated exposure. Assuming a biological half-time of 4 days, it is calculated that an equilibrium would be attained in the body at about 3 weeks with daily dosing.

Placental transfer of Tl has been documented in cats, mice, and rats (17; see $also$ 31 for references). Tl was also detected in urine, meconium, and feces of babies whose mothers had been poisoned by Tl during pregnancy (47). Clinical reports of Tl poisoning during late gestation noted skin and nail dystrophy, alopecia, and low body weight in the newborn, suggesting that the human fetus may suffer from transplacentally acquired thallotoxicosis (18).

Tl Kinetics in the Nervous System

Tl crosses the blood-brain and blood-nerve barriers, and substantial amounts can be found in nervous tissue after poisoning. In animals, cerebral uptake of Tl was shown to be less rapid compared with that of other target organs ($e.g.$, kidney and myocardium), but Tl concentration in brain also declined more slowly than in other tissues (17).

Studies indicate that once inside the neural cell, Tl is released less readily than potassium. This can be explained by a combination of factors including stronger association with intracellular ligands, limited solubility of intracellular Tl (53), and the existence of efflux-limiting pathways in nerve cell membranes (28).

There is also a marked tendency of Tl to accumulate in nervous tissue after chronic low-level exposure. In rats exposed to a low dose of Tl (10 ppm Tl sulfate) in their drinking water for 9 months, cerebral Tl levels were comparable to those found in animals of the same strain injected with a single sublethal Tl dose (32).

Studies of the nervous system distribution of Tl in lethal cases of human poisoning indicate that the brain areas densely populated with neurons accumulate Tl more than other areas; cerebral cortex was shown to contain the highest Tl levels of any organ in the body. The lowest Tl concentrations in the nervous system were in the optic and auditory nerves (11).

Information on Tl kinetics in peripheral nerve is incomplete. In experiments using frog sciatic nerve preparations, axonal transport of Tl was shown to occur in both the anterograde and retrograde directions by diffusional processes as well as by an active, possibly microtubule-dependent component. The rate of Tl transport was found to be close to the average rate of bidirectional movements of axonal organelles (3).

Studies in pregnant rats indicated rapid uptake and concentration of ^{201}Tl in fetal brain; the average fetal-to-maternal concentration ratio of the radiotracer was about 1. However, decline of cerebral Tl levels was more rapid in the fetus than in the adult, suggesting that the mechanism responsible for Tl retention in mature rat brain is not completely developed during prenatal life (17).

Cardiovascular changes in Tl poisoning include tachycardia, hypertension, and irregular pulse often accompanied by retrosternal pain and electrocardiographic (ECG) abnormalities. The origin of these disorders reflects a complex combination of mechanisms implicating the vascular smooth muscle, cardiac conducting tissue, ventricular myocardium, and the autonomic nervous system. The early myocardial effects of Tl and potassium are similar and reversible. Vagus and glossopharyngeal nerve damage may participate in the cardiovascular manifestations seen in severely affected patients (2,25,31). Cardiac anomalies induced by Tl may be life-threatening.

Tl ions may cause direct damage to intestinal mucosa, but digestive-tract disorders may occur irrespective of the route of exposure to the toxic metal. Signs of enteritis and moderate to severe colitis were reported in rats injected with 25–50 mg/kg Tl acetate. Mucosal ulcers were found in the colon (29).

While diarrhea, emesis, abdominal cramps, and constipation often develop as early symptoms of human Tl poisoning, depression of intestinal motility and peristalsis may occur later in the clinical course as a result of Tl-induced damage to the autonomic nervous system.

Hair loss closely resembling that caused by x-irradiation and radiomimetic drugs is a characteristic but late sign of Tl poisoning; it usually develops in subjects surviving the early fatal stage of toxicity and after chronic exposure. Tl ions are rapidly taken up by anagen follicles and disturb keratinization. Many hairs break within the follicle; irregularity of the dark keratogenous zone and air bubbles within the shaft are characteristic (40). Cutaneous effects of Tl may also include impairment of nail growth and formation of white streaks across finger and toe nails (Mees' lines).

Alopecia in Tl poisoning has been related to depression of the mitotic rate and growth inhibition in the hair follicle possibly reflecting metabolic lesions and failure to produce sufficient energy to support mitosis (10).

Studies of human lymphocytes have indicated no genotoxic or mutagenic effects of the diagnostic use of ^{201}Tl in myocardial scintigraphy (26). However, mutagenic effects (e.g., chromosome aberrations and increased frequency of DNA breaks) were seen in embryonic cell cultures exposed to micromolar concentrations of Tl carbonate (29).

Male reproductive systems are highly susceptible to Tl (18). Testicular damage was observed in rats treated chronically with low doses of Tl sulfate in drinking water. The effects included decreased sperm motility, changes in activity of selected testicular enzymes, and increased release of late spermatids into the tubular lumen (19). Testicular toxicity was also indicated by in vitro studies on mixed cultures of Sertoli and germ cells from rat testis at Tl concentrations comparable to those measured in vivo (20).

Animal Studies

In mammalian species, the acute LD_{50} for Tl compounds ranges between ~5 and 70 mg/kg for all routes of administration. After an average acute oral dose of about 25 mg/kg Tl sulfate, death occurs in the adult rat between the second and fifth days. A dermal LD_{50} value of 120 mg/kg was reported for Tl carbonate in the rat (for references, see 25,31). No inhalation toxicity data are available.

The principal effects of acute poisoning in animals are seen in the digestive and nervous systems. Hypotonia, ataxia, and behavioral changes appeared in cats given an initial subcutaneous (s.c.) dose of 6 mg/kg Tl acetate followed by a weekly injection of 4 mg/kg over varying periods of time (27). Vomiting, diarrhea, sluggish pupillary response, tetany, limb weakness, tremor, spasticity, and convulsions have also been reported in this species (58). Feline thallotoxicosis is characterized neuropathologically by distal axonal degeneration of long myelinated nerve fibers. Axonal lesions are those of the dying-back type; the longest fibers, both sensory and motor, are affected earlier than short fibers, and large-diameter fibers of sensory nerves are preferentially affected (27).

Other animal species are less susceptible than cats to Tl-induced peripheral neuropathy. Studies failed to produce peripheral changes in either rats or guinea pigs exposed to Tl salts (22,27). The daily ingestion of Tl acetate added to the diet of rats was tolerated at the 10-mg/kg level, but was lethal in male animals at the 30-mg/kg level by 15 weeks (25). Rats given 10–20 mg Tl acetate followed by weekly s.c. injections of 5 mg/kg developed irritability, diarrhea, alopecia, and poor weight gain (22). Abnormal electrophysiological parameters of the dorsal caudal nerve suggesting mild peripheral nerve damage were found in about 60% of animals in a group of rats given 10 ppm Tl in drinking water for up to 9 months (32). Degeneration of scattered nerve fibers with vacuolization of the myelin sheath was seen in about 10% of large- and medium-sized myelinated fibers in the sciatic nerve. No abnormalities were observed in unmyelinated fibers.

There have been reports of dogs and cats accidentally poisoned by Tl rodenticides or by eating vermin poisoned by Tl. The most severely affected animals developed gastroenteritis with hepatic or renal damage. Gross skin lesions, bleeding, shedding of fur, incoordination, trembling, and paralysis were observed in longer-term survivors. Pathological findings involved both the kidney (tubular necrosis) and the brain (focal edema and chromatolysis of neurons). Degenerative changes were also described in peripheral nerve, in addition to necrosis of skeletal and cardiac muscle fibers (25).

In Vitro Studies

Different types of *in vitro* systems have been used to investigate the actions of Tl in central and peripheral nervous system tissue. In most studies, toxicity was documented at Tl concentrations in the micromolar range.

In undifferentiated brain cell cultures from fetal rat telencephalon, 10 μM Tl was cytotoxic causing drastic reduction in the levels of several neuronal and glial marker enzymes (35). Higher concentrations were required to inhibit cell proliferation in mouse neuroblastoma cell cultures (EC_{50} about 200 μM Tl). Inhibition of neural acetylcholinesterase activity was seen at concentrations below 1 μM Tl (43).

Other *in vitro* studies have been reviewed in previous reports (18,29). In isolated rat embryo cultures, the embryonic CNS was damaged in the presence of Tl levels of 30 μg/ml but minor changes were already evident at 10 μg/ml. In cell systems from 11-day-old chick embryonic nervous tissue, Tl cytotoxicity occurred at levels between 1 and 100 μg/ml. Nerve fibers were apparently more susceptible than glia and cells.

In preparations of brain myelin lipid liposomes, trivalent Tl was shown to behave as an ionophore, promoting a rapid electroneutral Cl^-/OH^- exchange through myelin lipid bilayers at concentrations in the nanomolar range (14). It was suggested that, by mediating an electroneutral proton/hydroxyl and chloride exchange through the lipid matrix of biomembranes, Tl may disturb oxidative phosphorylation and impair energy metabolism. The mechanis-

tic implications of these findings remain uncertain, since monovalent Tl was ineffective in this model.

In myelinated rat dorsal root ganglion cell cultures, Tl was shown to cause preferential damage to axons. The effect consisted of axonal vacuolization initially centered around nodes of Ranvier and then involving the entire length of axons. Myelin sheaths remained intact until axonal destruction had taken place (39). Other experiments using a functionally organotypic complex of dorsal root ganglia, spinal cord, peripheral nerve, and muscle in culture demonstrated selective mitochondrial vacuolation in axons of peripheral nerve fibers in the presence of 10–20 μM Tl salts (50). Neuronal perikaryal mitochondria were relatively less affected by Tl and glial mitochondria remained unchanged. These observations correlate with the observed propensity of Tl to cause axonopathy *in vivo* (8,9) and support the hypothesis that disruption of membrane integrity of mitochondria may play an important role in the mechanism of Tl toxicity (22,56).

In isolated rat phrenic nerve–diaphragm preparations, Tl caused dose-dependent inhibition of the contractile response. Neuromuscular transmission was blocked at Tl concentrations as low as 5 μM and was restored temporarily by enhancers of stimulus-evoked release of acetylcholine, such as 4-aminopyridine, suggesting a primary action of Tl at the presynaptic level. Higher concentrations of Tl inhibited acetylcholine- and histamine-evoked contractile responses in intestinal preparations from different animal species (31).

Human Studies

Legal restrictions in developed countries have substantially reduced the use of Tl-containing rodenticides and, consequently, the incidence of Tl toxicosis. Tl poisoning is still reported worldwide and remains one of the most frequent acute diseases from all toxic metals (13,37,44,54). Pesticides containing Tl can still be found stored in homes, and accidental contamination of food has occurred as a result of such storage. The popularity of Tl salts for homicide (34,36) is based on the fact that they are colorless, tasteless, and odorless. Tl poisoning has resulted from ingestion of adulterated herbal medications and nutritional supplements (48).

Though most cases of Tl poisoning result from oral exposure, severe toxicity has resulted from skin contact or inhalation (45). Tl poisoning resulting from snorting a powder mistaken for cocaine is also described (24).

Subacute and chronic Tl intoxication is rare, but instances have occurred in workers exposed by inhalation of dust or fume, as well as in general populations following consumption of Tl-contaminated food (29,45,57). Two unusual cases of Tl poisoning following systemic absorption of elemental Tl are described (*see* later under Case Report).

The lethal dose of Tl ranges from 0.5 to 1.0 g after a single ingestion. Figures in the literature vary from 5–70 mg/kg body weight. Nonfatal intoxication occurs below this dose (25).

No data are available to define threshold levels that may be harmful to humans after chronic low-dose Tl exposure (47). "Normal" urine Tl levels are in the range of about 0.3 μg/l (29). Minor effects, as evidenced by alopecia areata, were reported in oil-refinery workers with values of about 20 μg/l in the 24-h urine. An alerting urine level of 50 μg/l Tl was proposed for occupational exposure (33).

Human thallotoxicosis is characterized by manifestations primarily involving the nervous system, skin, and the cardiovascular system. Neurotoxicity is usually a distal, predominantly sensory neuropathy with some involvement of the CNS (8,9,11).

In acute poisoning, abdominal pain and diarrhea may be initial complaints, appearing within hours of absorption, but the patient may only have nausea and anorexia.

Cardiovascular manifestations may be prominent with increases in heart rate and blood pressure often accompanied by retrosternal pain, irregular pulse, and transient ECG abnormalities such as ST- and T-wave changes.

After ingestion of a large dose, involvement of the nervous system becomes prominent within a few days in the form of a rapidly progressive peripheral neuropathy. Sensory disturbances appear first with pain and paresthesias in the lower limbs, and numbness in the fingers and toes with loss of pinprick and touch sensations. Motor neuropathy, manifest by weakness and increasing walking difficulties, is always distal in distribution, the lower limbs being more intensely affected than the arms. In serious cases, dysarthria and dysphagia may appear and weakness may involve respiratory muscles.

Delirium, convulsions, and coma, with respiratory and circulatory failure may precede death: this usually does not occur earlier than 8–10 days following ingestion.

In less severe cases, there may be a symptom-free interval lasting from 24 h to 1 week, and onset of symptoms may be insidious. A varied picture may develop with anorexia, constipation, abdominal pain, headache, myalgia, ataxia, tremor, and paresthesias predominating. Distal neuropathy begins with sensory loss and numbness in fingers and toes and spreads proximally with time. Somewhat later, weakness appears distally, then proximally. Neurological compromise may spread further to involve cranial nerves and even result in denervation of eye muscles.

Visual dysfunction may also appear with diminished contrast sensitivity, a tritan impairment of color vision, and cecocentral scotoma in the presence of slightly impaired visual acuity. Ophthalmological features may include loss of the lateral half of the eyebrows, eyelid skin lesions, blepharoptosis, nystagmus, noninflammatory keratitis, and lens opacities (52). There may be cranial nerve involvement with ptosis, ophthalmoplegia, retrobulbar neuritis, and facial paralysis later in intoxication.

Scalp alopecia usually appears during the second week and becomes nearly total in 1 month; hair loss is often impressively severe. In most cases, facial, pubic, axillary, and body hair are less dramatic. White semilunal strips across fingernails and toenails (Mees' lines) may appear 3–4 weeks after poisoning. Cutaneous effects also include grossly evident desquamation over the face, acneiform eruptions, and papulomacular rash.

Subacute and chronic thallotoxicosis is usually manifested by symptoms that essentially resemble those of acute intoxication, but their development may be more insidious. Malaise, loss of appetite, headache, anxiety, insomnia, and weight loss are often initial manifestations preceding the typical neurological, cardiovascular, and cutaneous changes. Sleep disorders, depression, and other mental symptoms have been described in several cases (31,45).

Early diagnosis of Tl poisoning may be difficult unless an etiology is well known. Cardiac dysfunction, which may precede the appearance of neurological manifestations of intoxication, is potentially fatal. However, suspicions of Tl poisoning may not arise until alopecia becomes evident. Unfortunately, hair loss occurs as a late manifestation and, in some cases, is mild or does not develop at all (2). In most instances, diagnosis is primarily supported by the time course and progression of the clinical signs. Tl poisoning should be considered in patients who develop a sudden diffuse alopecia with associated neurological signs.

The occurrence of nonspecific symptoms can lead to misdiagnosis, especially in chronic intoxication. Tl poisoning has been described in subjects who had been admitted to the intensive therapy unit with suspected myocardial infarction. In other reports, gallstones and pancreatitis have been considered as the initial diagnosis (23,36). Psychiatric diagnoses have been given in cases with predominant mental symptoms in whom objective findings were negative (29,45).

The diagnosis should differentiate between Tl poisoning and poisoning from other heavy metals (*e.g.*, arsenic), diabetic polyneuropathy, Guillain-Barré syndrome, intermittent acute porphyria, botulism, and lupus-type collagenosis (23).

Chemical investigations of urine and feces provide reliable guides for definitive diagnosis. In nonexposed subjects, Tl levels in urine are below 1–2 μg/l. Levels >200 μg/l are toxic (36), and severe symptoms are usually associated with levels >1.2 mg/l (31,47). Urinary concentrations from 0.1 to 0.9 mg/l have been measured in workers with symptoms of Tl toxicity. However, no correlation has been found between biological and environmental exposure data and the severity of symptoms in cases of thallotoxicosis associated with chronic occupational exposure (45).

Tl analysis of hair and nails may be valuable for diagnosis and monitoring purposes, especially in chronic cases. Concentrations in hair and nails have been shown to range from 4.8–15.8 μg/kg and 0.7–4.9 μg/kg, respectively (25).

Measurement of Tl in saliva may also be useful as a diagnostic tool in patients with severe constipation or renal failure. In one patient intoxicated by ingestion of 1 g Tl sulfate, salivary Tl levels were more elevated than those in urine; salivary Tl levels ranged from 2–9 μg/ml during the initial 2-week period after exposure (44).

The prognosis of thallotoxicosis is variable depending on the total dose absorbed, the time course of the exposure, and individual susceptibility. Autonomic neuropathy associated with coexisting tachycardia and hypertension may predispose the patient to cardiac arrhythmias and sudden death for many weeks after the initial insult. Prognosis is unfavorable in the presence of brain damage, respiratory failure, and cardiac failure.

Recovery requires months and may be incomplete. One study followed 48 children for 6 months to 7 years after an episode of Tl poisoning; residual neurological deficits, indicated by ataxia, tremor, mental retardation, and psychosis were found in 26 subjects (42). Visual disturbances, memory failure, permanent electroencephalographic abnormalities, and optic neuropathy have also been described as neurological sequelae (2,31,36,52). Hair loss is usually reversible; regrowth begins around the fourth week and is usually complete within 3 months.

The neuropathology of Tl intoxication is described in several reports (2,8–11). Axonal degeneration with changes reflecting the typical profile of the "dying-back" process is often the dominant feature in peripheral nerves examined late in the clinical course. Alterations include pronounced swelling and fragmentation of axons with degeneration of the more distal parts of both motor and sensory fibers but relative preservation of the myelin sheath. Involvement of cranial nerves is unusual (10). Edema in cerebral hemispheres and the brainstem, with chromatolytic changes in neurons in the motor cortex, substantia nigra, and brainstem motor nuclei, have been documented in fatal cases of Tl poisoning (8,10).

In addition to supportive care, therapeutic interventions in Tl poisoning are mainly focused on promoting Tl elimination from the body (12).

If exposure is known to be recent (the patient presents within 4 h of ingesting Tl), gastric lavage and instillation of Prussian blue is an effective treatment (*vide infra*). Prussian blue is a readily available laboratory reagent (34) but is *not* approved for human use by the U.S. Food and Drug Administration. Once distribution of absorbed Tl is complete, and the metal has concentrated intracellularly, no treatment can be expected to help significantly in preventing Tl damage to target organs.

Forced diuresis may be helpful if given within 48 h after ingesting Tl, as this treatment acts only in the distribution phase. More efficient extracorporeal elimination techniques, such as hemodialysis and charcoal hemoperfusion, are indicated in patients with severe renal or cardiovascular impairment (12). Hemodialysis can provide an effective method for Tl extraction if performed repeatedly for a period of several days until plasma Tl concentrations have fallen to 0.2 mg/l. This, however, may represent a serious disadvantage because of the intrinsic morbidity of the procedure.

In mild or moderate cases, oral Prussian blue has been used to facilitate Tl excretion in the stool. Prussian blue (synonymous with Berlin blue), potassium ferric hexacyanoferrate, is a nontoxic pigment that can form stable, unabsorbable complexes with Tl by exchanging for potassium ions in its crystal lattice. Oral administration of Prussian blue effectively reduces the body burden of Tl by interrupting enterohepatic circulation and enhancing fecal elimination of the metal (41). The recommended dosage is 250 mg/kg/day (three to four divided daily doses given intraduodenally in a 10%–15% solution of mannitol) (51).

In laboratory animals, Prussian blue has been shown to be the most effective antidotal treatment for enhancing the excretion of Tl (29,31). Clinical experience based on single-case studies or surveys of small numbers of patients also supports its use because of the apparent efficacy in enhancing Tl removal from the body. The effect of this agent on prognosis in severe cases is still unknown (36,51). No adverse effects have been recorded from Prussian blue therapy. The drug does not cross the gut mucosa, and the release of cyanide ions is negligible. Paralytic ileus may complicate treatment by reducing the throughput of the dye. This is usually countered by combining Prussian blue with mannitol.

Chelating agents such as dimercaprol and penicillamine are not effective given the low propensity of monovalent Tl to form stable complexes with sulfur-containing ligands. The use of dithiocarbamate is contraindicated, since it enhances redistribution of Tl, which may enter the CNS and thereby exacerbate encephalopathy.

Potassium supplements given parenterally (70–110 mmol/24 h, increasing to 120–260 mmol/24 h if dialysis is also introduced) may increase the rate of loss of Tl from body compartments and be helpful in replacing potassium ions lost from tissue sites. However, early potassium treatment is probably not indicated, since this is thought to raise intracellular free Tl ion levels and cause redistribution of the metal in the body, transiently resulting in higher Tl concentrations in the brain (36).

In the management of Tl poisoning, attention should be paid to oral hygiene, since a severe stomatitis may occur. General advice to maintain regular bowel habits should also be given. Cisapride may be effective in relieving constipation associated with Tl toxicity (54). Physiotherapy is pivotal to successful rehabilitation, as it prevents muscle contractures and may help the recovery of strength.

Toxic Mechanisms

The pathogenesis of Tl neurotoxicity is poorly understood. Several mechanisms are likely involved with consequences that may vary depending on the stage of intoxication. Early manifestations of Tl poisoning, such as generalized muscle weakness, paralytic ileus, and myocardial and ECG abnormalities, may reflect changes secondary to Tl-induced disruption of intracellular potassium homeostasis. Tl can substitute for potassium in biological systems. Several ligands within cells, including Na^+,K^+-adenosine triphosphatase (ATPase) and other monovalent cation-activated enzymes, exhibit a greater affinity for Tl^+ than for K^+ (15). Furthermore, monovalent Tl and potassium ions use the same pathways, namely potassium channels, Na^+,K^+-ATPase, and $Na^+/K^+/Cl^-$ cotransporters, to enter cells (49). By affecting movement of potassium between the intracellular and extracellular compartments, Tl may alter the transmembrane potassium gradient leading to disruption of cell membrane stability and the short-term control of potassium homeostasis (5). Membrane potassium channels are generally up to three times as permeable for Tl^+ as for potassium ions. By interacting with K^+-dependent processes at this level, Tl^+ may induce persistent changes in the cellular concentration of monovalent cations with consequent disorders of Na^+-coupled solute transport (31).

On the other hand, unlike potassium ions, Tl^+ can easily penetrate mitochondrial membranes. Accumulation of Tl in mitochondria is associated with mitochondrial swelling and uncoupling of oxidative phosphorylation (31). Administration of Tl at toxic doses has been shown to induce early disruption of the membrane integrity of rat liver mitochondria with subsequent changes in the activity of specific membrane-bound enzymes (56). Tl-induced mitochondrial changes are documented in nervous tissue both *in vitro* (50) and *in vivo* (22).

It is suggested that high concentrations of Tl may affect both energy metabolism and antioxidant protection of cell membranes in the nervous tissue. A proposed mechanism (8,9) implies an inhibitory action of Tl on flavin-dependent enzymes resulting from the interaction of Tl with riboflavin. This initial metabolic lesion would lead to depletion of flavin-derived cofactors with consequent impairment of electron transfer processes and reduced availability of several energy-producing intermediates. Flavin adenine dinucleotide (FAD) is absolutely vital as a hydrogen acceptor for hydrogen transfer in a critical step of pyruvate decarboxylation. Thus, depletion of FAD may be expected to cause a serious derangement of metabolic activities that are dependent on the pyruvate dehydrogenase complex.

While an interaction between Tl with flavoproteins as the critical event leading to disruption of energy-generating pathways in thallotoxicosis is conjectural, circumstantial evidence for its occurrence in mammalian tissues is fairly strong. Reduced availability of energy-producing intermediates apparently is a common process associated with the preferential toxicity of Tl to rapidly dividing or metabolically demanding tissues such as nerves, intestinal epithelium, hair follicles, and testes (10). Tl and riboflavin deficiency produce similar changes in mitochondria (50), and similar patterns of peripheral nerve damage are seen in the neuropathies associated with Tl poisoning, vitamin (thiamine or riboflavin) deficiency, and arsenic intoxication (8–10). Like Tl poisoning, both arsenic poisoning and riboflavin deficiency have characteristic involvement of the skin and associated structures.

Besides uncoupling oxidative phosphorylation, Tl can inhibit thiol enzymes. Changes related to oxidative cell injury and reduced antioxidant protection of cell membranes (lipid peroxidation and depletion of glutathione) are also reported in the nervous tissue of animals during Tl intoxication (7,21,22,25).

Although binding of Tl with sulfhydryl groups is less tenacious than with other neurotoxic metals (15), a random chelation of Tl by sulfhydryl components may occur at the very high Tl concentrations reached in cells after toxic exposure (8,9). In addition, thiol homeostasis and antioxidant processes may be affected by Tl *via* mechanisms leading to reduced availability of critical enzymes and cofactors such as glutathione reductase, a FAD-dependent enzyme, whose activity is markedly depressed in riboflavin deficiency (16). Tl can alter selenium metabolism, and the activity of the selenium enzyme glutathione peroxidase is reduced in tissues of Tl-intoxicated hamsters also presenting increased lipid peroxidation (1).

Oxidative insult and deficiency of antioxidants may be detrimental to nervous tissue causing disruption of neural membrane integrity, changes in the affinity/binding characteristics of neurotransmitter receptors, and oxidation of easily auto-oxidable monoamines. Studies have documented the ability of Tl to affect aminergic and serotonergic systems in the rat brain (31,38). This may have a role in certain neurological manifestations of Tl poisoning, for example, sleep abnormalities and motor function changes (23, 31). Indirect evidence for Tl-induced imbalance of central monoamine metabolism comes from clinical experience indicating favorable effects of L-dopa (3-hydroxytyrosine) in the treatment of choreiform sequelae of thallotoxicosis (31).

REFERENCES

1. Aoyama H, Yoshida M, Yamamura Y (1988) Induction of lipid peroxidation in tissues of thallous malonate-treated hamster. *Toxicology* **53**, 11.
2. Bank WJ (1980) Thallium. In: *Experimental and Clinical Neurotoxicology*. Spencer PS, Schaumburg HH eds. Williams & Wilkins, Baltimore p. 570.
3. Bergquist JE, Edstrom A, Hanson PA (1983) Bidirectional axonal transport of thallium in frog sciatic nerve. *Acta Physiol Scand* **117**, 513.
4. Berman E (1991) Thallium. In: *Toxic Metals and Their Analysis*. Berman E ed. Heyden, London p. 201.
5. Bradberry SM, Vale A (1995) Disturbances of potassium homeostasis in poisoning. *Clin Toxicol* **33**, 295.
6. Brismar T, Anderson S, Collins VP (1995) Mechanism of high K^+ and Tl^+ uptake in cultured human glioma cells. *Cell Mol Neurobiol* **15**, 351.
7. Brown DR, Callahan BG, Cleaves MA, Shatz RA (1985) Thallium-induced changes in behavioral patterns: Correlation with altered lipid peroxidation and lysosomal enzyme activity in brain regions of male rats. *Toxicol Ind Health* **1**, 81.
8. Cavanagh JB (1985) Peripheral nervous system toxicity. A morphological approach. In: *Neurotoxicology*. Blum K, Manzo L eds. Marcel Dekker, New York p. 1.
9. Cavanagh JB (1988) Towards the molecular basis of toxic neuropathy. In: *Recent Advances in Nervous System Toxicology*. Galli CL, Manzo L, Spencer PS eds. Plenum Press, New York p. 23.
10. Cavanagh JB (1991) What have we learnt from Graham Frederick Young? Reflections on the mechanism of thallium neurotoxicity. *Neuropathol Appl Neurobiol* **17**, 3.
11. Davis LE, Standefer JC, Kornfeld M et al. (1981) Acute thallium poisoning. Toxicological and morphological studies of the nervous system. *Ann Neurol* **10**, 38.
12. De Groot G, Van Heijst ANP (1988) Toxicokinetic aspects of thallium poisoning. *Sci Total Environ* **71**, 411.
13. Desenclos JC, Wilder MH, Coppenger GW et al. (1992) Thallium poisoning: An outbreak in Florida, 1988. *Southern Med J* **85**, 1203.
14. Diaz RS, Monreal J (1994) Thallium mediates a rapid chloride/hydroxyl ion exchange through myelin lipid bilayer. *Mol Pharmacol* **46**, 1210.
15. Douglas KT, Bunni MA, Baindur SR (1990) Thallium in biochemistry. *Int J Biochem* **22**, 429.
16. Dutta P, Gee M, Rivlin RS, Pinto J (1988) Riboflavin deficiency and glutathione metabolism in rats: Possible mechanisms underlying altered responses to hemolytic stimuli. *J Nutr* **118**, 1149.
17. Edel-Rade J, Marafante E, Sabbioni E et al. (1982) Placental transfer and retention of ^{201}Tl-thallium in the rat. *Toxicol Lett* **11**, 275.
18. Formigli L, Gregotti C, Di Nucci A et al. (1985) Reproductive toxicity of thallium. Experimental and clinical data. In: *Heavy Metals in the Environment. Vol 2*. Lekkas TD ed. CEP Cons, Edinburgh p. 15.
19. Formigli L, Scelsi R, Poggi P et al. (1986) Thallium-induced testicular toxicity in the rat. *Environ Res* **40**, 531.
20. Gregotti C, Di Nucci A, Costa LG et al. (1992) Effects of thallium on primary cultures of testicular cells. *J Toxicol Environ Health* **36**, 59.
21. Hasan M, Ali SF (1981) Effects of thallium, nickel and cobalt administration on the lipid peroxidation in different regions of the rat brain. *Toxicol Appl Pharmacol* **57**, 8.
22. Herman MM, Bensch KG (1967) Light and electron microscopic studies of acute and chronic thallium intoxication in rats. *Toxicol Appl Pharmacol* **10**, 199.
23. Herrero F, Fernandez E, Gomez J et al. (1995) Thallium poisoning presenting with abdominal colic, paresthesia, and irritability. *J Toxicol-Clin Toxicol* **33**, 261.
24. Insley BM, Grufferman S, Ayliffe A (1986) Thallium poisoning in cocaine abusers. *Amer J Emerg Med* **4**, 545.
25. Kazantzis G (1986) Thallium. In: *Handbook on the Toxicology of Metals. 2nd Ed*. Friberg L, Nordberg GF, Vouk M eds. Elsevier, Amsterdam p. 549.
26. Kelsey KT, Donohoe KJ, Baxter B et al. (1991) Genotoxic and mutagenic effects of the diagnostic use of thallium-201 in nuclear medicine. *Mutat Res* **260**, 239.
27. Kennedy P, Cavanagh JB (1977) Spinal changes in the neuropathy of thallium poisoning. *J Neurol Sci* **29**, 295.
28. Landowne D (1975) A comparison of radioactive thallium and potassium fluxes in the giant axon of the squid. *J Physiol* **252**, 79.
29. Manzo L, Minoia C, Sabbioni E (1995) Toxicity of detrimental metal ions. Thallium. In: *Handbook of Metal-Ligand Interactions in Biological Fluids. Vol 2*. Berthon G ed. Marcel Dekker, New York p. 766.

30. Manzo L, Sabbioni E (1988) Thallium. In: *Handbook on Toxicity of Inorganic Compounds*. Seiler HG, Sigel H eds. Marcel Dekker, New York p. 677.

31. Manzo L, Sabbioni E (1988) *Metal Neurotoxicity*. Bondy SC, Prasad KN eds. CRC Press, Boca Raton, Florida p. 35.

32. Manzo L, Scelsi R, Moglia A *et al.* (1983) Long-term toxicity of thallium. In: *Chemical Toxicology and Clinical Chemistry of Metals*. Brown SS, Savory J eds. Academic Press, London p. 401.

33. Marcus RL (1985) Investigation of a working population exposed to thallium. *J Soc Occup Med* **35**, 4.

34. Meggs WJ, Hoffman RS, Shih RD *et al.* (1994) Thallium poisoning from maliciously contaminated food. *J Toxicol Clin Toxicol* **32**, 723.

35. Monnet-Tschudi F, Zurich MG, Honegger P (1993) Evaluation of the toxicity of different metal compounds in the developing brain using aggregating cell cultures as a model. *Toxicol Vitro* **7**, 335.

36. Moore D, House I, Dixon A (1993) Thallium poisoning. *Brit Med J* **306**, 1527.

37. Niehues R, Horstkotte D, Klein RM *et al.* (1995) Wiederholte Ingestion potentiell letaler Thalliummengen in suizidaler Absicht. *Deut Med Wochenschr* **120**, 403.

38. Osorio-Rico L, Galvan-Arzate S, Rios C (1995) Thallium increases monoamine oxidase activity and serotonin turnover rate in rat brain regions. *Neurotoxicol Teratol* **17**, 1.

39. Peterson ER, Murry MR (1965) Patterns of peripheral demyelination in vitro. *Ann N Y Acad Sci* **122**, 39.

40. Pillans PI (1995) Drug-associated alopecia. *Int J Dermatol* **14**, 149.

41. Rauws AG (1974) Thallium pharmacokinetics and its modification by Prussian blue. *Naunyn-Schmied Arch Pharmacol* **284**, 295.

42. Reed D, Crawley J, Faro SN *et al.* (1963) Thallotoxicosis. *J Amer Med Assn* **183**, 96.

43. Repetto G, Sanz P, Repetto M (1994) *In vitro* effects of thallium on mouse neuroblastoma cells. *Toxicol Vitro* **8**, 609.

44. Richelmi P, Bono F, Guardia L *et al.* (1980) Salivary levels of thallium in acute human poisoning. *Arch Toxicol* **43**, 321.

45. Richeson EM (1958) Industrial thallium intoxication. *Ind Med Surg* **27**, 607.

46. Sabbioni E, Di Nucci A, Edel J *et al.* (1984) Intestinal absorption and excretion of thallium (201-Tl) in the rat. *Arch Toxicol* **S7**, 446.

47. Sabbioni E, Manzo L (1980) Metabolism and toxicity of thallium. In: *Advances in Neurotoxicology*. Manzo L ed. Pergamon Press, Oxford p. 249.

48. Schaumburg HH, Berger A (1992) Alopecia and sensory polyneuropathy from thallium in Chinese herbal medication. *J Amer Med Assn* **268**, 3430.

49. Skulskii IA, Gusev GP, Sherstobitov AO, Manninen V (1992) Anion-dependent transport of thallous ions through human erythrocyte membrane. *J Membrane Biol* **113**, 219.

50. Spencer PS, Peterson ER, Madrid R, Raine CS (1973) Effects of thallium salts on neural mitochondria in organotypic cord-ganglia-muscle combination cultures. *J Cell Biol* **58**, 79.

51. Stevens W, van Peteghem C, Heyndricks A *et al.* (1974) Eleven cases of thallium intoxication treated with Prussian blue. *Int J Clin Pharmacol* **10**, 1.

52. Tabandeh H, Crowston JG, Thompson GM (1994) Ophthalmologic features of thallium poisoning. *Amer J Ophthalmol* **117**, 243.

53. Tjalve H, Nilsson M, Larsson B (1982) Thallium-201: autoradiography in pigmented mice and melanin-binding *in vitro*. *Acta Pharmacol Toxicol* **51**, 147.

54. Vrij AA, Cremers HM, Lustermans FA (1995) Successful recovery of a patient with thallium poisoning. *Neth J Med* **47**, 121.

55. Wilfingseder P, Martin R, Papp C (1981) Magnesium seeds in the treatment of lymph- and haemangiomata. *Chir Plast* **6**, 105.

56. Woods JS, Fowler BA (1986) Alteration of hepatocellular structure and function by thallium chloride: Ultrastructural, morphometric, and biochemical studies. *Toxicol Appl Pharmacol* **83**, 218.

57. Zhou DX, Liu DN (1985) Chronic thallium poisoning in a rural area of Guizhou Province, China. *J Environ Health* **48**, 14.

58. Zook BC, Holdsworth J, Thornton GW (1968) Thallium poisoning in cats. *J Amer Vet Med Assn* **153**, 285.

CASE REPORT

In two patients with facial hemangioma, resorption of solid fragments of metallic thallium that had been mistakenly implanted into the tumor mass was lethal in one patient and caused severe toxicity in the other.

The patients were a 16-year-old boy and a 14-year-old girl suffering from cavernous hemangiomas of the cheek and the lower lip, respectively. Surgical insertion of magnesium "seeds" into the tumor mass was used in Austria at the turn of the twentieth century as a treatment for this condition (55). Magnesium implants undergo oxidation and release nascent hydrogen, which induces regional tissue necrosis. This is followed by phagocytosis of the reaction products without significant foreign body reaction. It is expected that magnesium can be completely dissolved in the body within weeks. Because of the apparent low risk, the magnesium seed method has been adopted as a safe treatment in selected cases of hemangioma (55).

In both cases, about 30 thin segments (wires) of metallic thallium (6–7 g thallium), instead of magnesium, were mistakenly inserted into the facial tumor mass during separate sessions of magnesium seed therapy. Within 2–3 weeks of surgery, both developed typical symptoms of thallium poisoning, with abdominal pain, paresthesias, peripheral neuropathy, and progressive loss of scalp hair.

In the male, thallium poisoning was only suspected 50 days after surgery, and diagnosis was subsequently confirmed by atomic absorption spectrometry studies showing urinary thallium levels up to 10 ppm. Attempted suicide or unintentional ingestion of thallium was initially considered as a possible cause of the poisoning. However, the patient denied any possible contact with thallium and psychiatric examination revealed no abnormalities or suicidal tendency. Despite treatment by forced diuresis and Prussian blue, the patient's condition worsened. Flaccid tetraplegia and respiratory distress developed; the patient was admitted to the intensive care unit and given respiratory support.

Serious symptoms associated with high thallium levels in excreta were still present after 6 months despite therapeutic elimination of considerable amounts of thallium. Intoxication due to continous release of thallium from an undetermined source in the body was suspected. Radiographic examination revealed the presence of metallic materials in the hemangioma mass from which a small fragment was removed for chemical analysis. The composition, determined by neutron activation analysis using high-purity thallium and magnesium standards, was found to be 99% thallium.

Removal of the remaining thallium wire from the tumor mass produced marginal amelioration of the clinical status. Despite physiotherapy, one year after surgery the patient was still confined to a wheelchair with tetraplegia and diffuse muscle atrophy. No abnormalities of higher mental function were observed.

Thallium poisoning in the second patient was not suspected during life. She was admitted to hospital 4 weeks after operation complaining of malaise, with burning pain and tingling in the soles of her feet and in her fingertips. Physical examination and biochemical findings revealed no abnormalities. Irritability, insomnia, anxiety, and behavioral abnormalities, with abrupt weeping for no apparent cause, were observed. The patient was diagnosed as an "unstable personality with psychotic features" and a treatment with neuroleptic drugs was given.

The clinical condition deteriorated very rapidly with progressive weakness, impairment of swallowing, stupor, delirium, and ventilatory failure. The patient died 2 months after the thallium wire had been implanted. Massive thallium intoxication was not recognized until 18 months later when the body was retrieved and examined as part of a forensic investigation connected with the discovery of iatrogenic thallium poisoning in the other patient described here. Postmortem tissue samples, examined by inductively coupled plasma mass spectrometry, revealed thallium contents far exceeding the minimum lethal concentrations. The measured levels were 3.1 ppm in the hair and nails, 5.3 ppm in the femur, and 5 ppm in the kidney. As much as 202 ppm thallium was found in a tissue sample taken from the cheek region where the wire fragments had been implanted. Extensive investigations failed to identify the source of the thallium wire used for the therapeutic implants in these patients.

Thiophene

John L. O'Donoghue

THIOPHENE
C₄H₄S

Thiofuran; Thiofurfuran; Thiole; Thiotetrole; Thiacyclopentadiene; Divinylene sulfide

NEUROTOXICITY RATING
Experimental
A Cerebellar degeneration (granule cells)

Thiophene can be found in peat, coal tar and gas, and technical grades of benzene. It has similar physical properties to benzene and may be used as a solvent. Thiophene is used to manufacture resins with phenol and formaldehyde, dyes, and pharmaceuticals, including dopamine-uptake antagonists and anticonvulsants.

Thiophene is rapidly but incompletely absorbed (16% of inhaled dose) following inhalation (8000 ppm for 1 h). The majority of the absorbed dose (74%) is excreted unchanged through the lungs (15). Urinary metabolites (25% of the absorbed dose) are excreted over a 72-h period (15). The majority of the thiophene absorbed (91%) is excreted within the first 8 h following exposure (15). By 72 h, 99% of the absorbed thiophene is excreted. The highest concentrations of thiophene are found in erythrocytes followed by the liver. Relatively low concentrations of thiophene are found in the brain after inhalation exposure (15).

In contrast to the rapid lung excretion of thiophene when it is inhaled, only about 5% of an orally administered dose is excreted through the lungs in mice (3,6). Subcutaneous (s.c.) administration of thiophene in rats produced peak blood levels in 30 min and peak brain levels in 3 h. Within 72 h, 74% of the administered dose was excreted in the urine (4).

Three uncharacterized metabolites have been observed in the urine of rats following inhalation of thiophene (15). Dogs and rabbits excrete a neutral sulfur metabolite of thiophene (7,17). Premercapturic acid and 2-thienyl-mercapturic acid metabolites of thiophene have been identified, and, in theory, an epoxide could be formed from thiophene (12). The differences in toxicity and metabolism in animals exposed to thiophene by different exposure routes suggest that activation of thiophene by microsomal cytochrome P-450 oxygenases may be required to produce neurotoxicity. Hepatic and renal toxicities associated with thiophene exposure are increased by pretreatment with phenobarbital and reduced by pretreatment with colbaltous chloride or piperonyl butoxide (14).

The inhalation LC_{50} (6 h) for thiophene in rats is approximately 4525 ppm (10). Inhalation of 3200 ppm or 6400 ppm for 6 h produced drowsiness and generalized muscle fasciculations in rats (10). Exposure to 800–1600 ppm thiophene was without effect. Mice are narcotized by exposure to 2900 ppm thiophene, while mice exposed to 8700 ppm died in 20–80 min (11). Six-hour exposures to 3200 ppm thiophene produced tremors in rats; however, tremors were not observed after the fourth of 12 exposures (10). At 1600 ppm thiophene, one rat of a group of five showed tremors transiently. Rats did not develop neuropathological lesions or lasting evidence of neurotoxicity following twelve 6-h inhalation exposures to 3200 ppm thiophene.

In contrast to the lack of significant neurotoxicity following inhalation of thiophene, repeated oral or s.c. injection of thiophene results in selective degeneration of cerebellar granule cells in dogs and rats (1,3,7–10,16). Rats given 1000 mg/kg thiophene orally died or developed obvious signs of weakness, staggering, twitching, head tremor, and limb jerking (10). Signs of neurotoxicity were also observed at 500 mg/kg thiophene, but not at 50 or 100 mg/kg, even after 13 doses (10). Rats given 0.4 ml/day thiophene for 5 or 9 days also showed selective degeneration of cerebellar

granule cells (2). Repeated daily s.c. injections (2 g) produced severe ataxia and paralysis in dogs (7–9).

While repeated oral or s.c. injection of thiophene produces degeneration of cerebellar granule cells, there are few other effects on the cerebellum. All regions of the cerebellar cortex can be affected. In less affected areas, single or small numbers of granule cells become pyknotic and undergo karyorrhexis and lysis. In more severely affected areas, complete destruction of foci or areas of granule cells occurs (2,7,10). Prior to nuclear condensation and pyknosis, cytoplasmic oxidative enzymes and acid phosphatases are not altered (2). Nicotinamide adenine dinucleotide dehydrogenase-tetrazolium reductase activity in Purkinje cells is temporarily reduced following destruction of granule cells by thiophene (2). Associated with the loss of granule cells, Purkinje cells show an increase in mitochondrial size and number, and a decrease in dendritic processes (1,5,7,13).

There are no reported cases of neurotoxicity in humans or domestic animals as a result of exposure to thiophene.

REFERENCES

1. Albrechtsen R, Diemer NH, Nielsen MH (1974) Size and density of the mitochondria in Purkinje cells of rats after thiophene intoxication, as measured by image analyzing system. *Acta Pathol Microbiol Scand A* **82**, 791.
2. Albrechtsen R, Jensen H (1973) Histochemical investigation of thiophene necrosis in the cerebellum of rats. *Acta Neuropathol* **26**, 217.
3. American Petroleum Institute (API) (1948) Toxicological review of thiophene and derivatives. *API Toxicol Rev* Washington, DC p. 2.
4. Bikbulatov NT, Nigmatullina GN (1976) Absorption, distribution, and elimination of thiophene from the body. *Sb Nauchn Tr Bashk Gos Med Inst* **19**, 114.
5. Bradley P, Berry M (1979) Effects of thiophene on the Purkinje cell dendritic tree: a quantitative Golgi study. *Neuropathol Appl Neurobiol* **5**, 9.
6. Chanal JL, Calmette MT, Bonnaud B, Cousse H (1974) Bioavailability of thiophene 2,5-^{14}C after oral and rectal administration in mice. *Eur J Med Chem-Chim Ther* **9**, 641.
7. Christomanos A (1930) Action of organic sulfur compounds on the dog organism: Action and fate of thiophene in the metabolism of the dog. *Biochem Z* **229**, 248.
8. Christomanos A (1930) Experimental production of cerebellar symptoms by thiophene. *Klin Wochenschr* **9**, 2354.
9. Christomanos A, Scholz W (1933) Klinische beobachtungen und pathologisch anatomisches befunde am zentral nerven system mit thiophen vergifteter hand. *Neural Psychiat* **144**, 1.
10. Eastman Kodak Company (1983) unpublished data, Rochester, New York.

11. Flury F, Zernik F (1932) Toxicity of thiophene. *Chem Ztg* **56**, 149.
12. Hathway DE (1972) *Foreign Compound Metabolism in Mammals. Vol 2.* National Bureau of Economic Research, New York p. 386.
13. Herndon RM, Oster-Granit ML (1975) Effect of granule cell destruction on development and maintenance of the Purkinje cell dendrite. In: *Advances in Neurology. Vol 12.* Kreutzberg GW ed. Raven Press, New York p. 361.
14. McMurtry RJ, Mitchell JR (1977) Renal and hepatic necrosis after metabolic activation of 2-substituted furans and thiophenes, including furosemide and cephaloridine. *Toxicol Appl Pharmacol* **42**, 285.
15. Nomeri AA, Markham PM, Chadwick M (1993) Pulmonary absorption and disposition of [^{14}C]thiophene in rats following nose-only inhalation exposure. *J Toxicol Environ Health* **39**, 223.
16. Upners T (1939) Experimental studies concerning the local action of thiophene on the central nervous system. *Z Ges Neurol Psychiat* **166**, 623.
17. Williams RT (1959) *Detoxification Mechanisms.* John Wiley-Interscience, New York p. 553.

Thymidine

Herbert H. Schaumburg

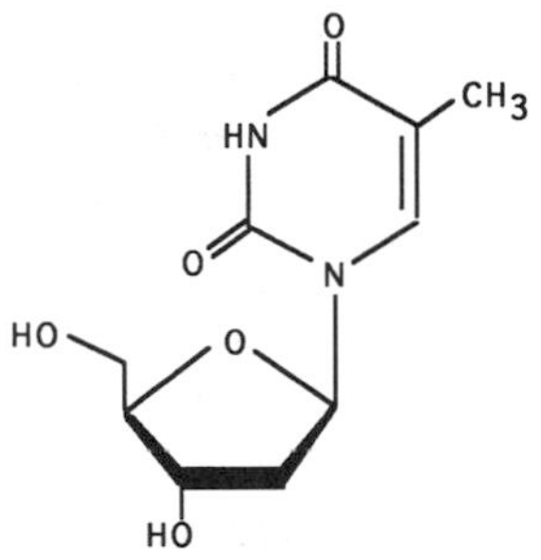

THYMIDINE
$C_{10}H_{14}N_2O_5$

1-(2-Deoxy-β-D-ribofuranosyl)-5-methyluracil

NEUROTOXICITY RATING

Clinical

B   Acute encephalopathy (sedation, headache)

Thymidine, a naturally occurring nucleoside, has been extensively investigated as a single agent in cancer chemotherapy and as a biochemical modulator for cytotoxic drugs such a 5-fluorouracil (5-FU), methotrexate, and cytarabine. It is an hypothesis that thymidine can expand intracellular desoxynucleoside triphosphate pools, thereby inhibiting ribonucleotide reductase, enhancing sensitivity to DNA-damaging agents and impeding DNA repair (2).

As a single agent, thymidine is given by intravenous infusion daily for 5 days at a dose of 75 g/m²/day. In all studies, myelosuppression with leukopenia and anemia have been the dose-limiting systemic toxicity; upper-gastrointestinal dysfunction (nausea, vomiting, hiccough) appeared in 73% of cases. When employed at much lower doses of 8 g/m²/day to ameliorate the neurotoxicity of 5-FU, thymidine has not been associated with adverse CNS effects (4).

Thymidine readily crosses the blood-brain barrier, and CNS symptoms have appeared in more than one-half of patients (1,3,4). Somnolence and headaches were common; they appeared in the initial infusion and with each subsequent dose. One-half of cases complained of transient memory impairment, and 22% experienced fleeting visual illusions. No objective neurological signs were documented. There were no complaints consistent with residual CNS dysfunction.

REFERENCES

1. Chiuten DF, Wiernik PH, Zaharko S, Edwards L (1980) Clinical phase I-II and pharmacokinetic study of high-dose thymidine given by continuous intravenous infusion. *Cancer Res* **40**, 818.
2. O'Dwyer PJ, King SA, Hoth DF, Leyland-Jones B (1987) Role of thymidine in biochemical modulation: A review. *Cancer Res* **47**, 3911.
3. Martin DS, Stolfi RL, Sawyer RC *et al.* (1980) An overview of thymidine. *Amer Cancer Soc* **45**, 1117.
4. Takimoto CH, Martin DS, Damin LAM *et al.* (1980) Severe neurotoxicity following 5-fluorouracil-based chemotherapy in a patient with dihydropyrimidine dehydrogenase deficiency. *Clin Cancer Res* **2**, 477.
5. Woodcock TM, Martin DS, Damin LAM *et al.* (1980) Combination clinical trials with thymidine and fluorouracil: A phase I and clinical pharmacologic evaluation. *Cancer* **45**, 1135.

Tick Saliva

Rainer Gothe

Ixodes holocyclus (holocyclotoxin); *Dermacentor* spp.

NEUROTOXICITY RATING

Clinical

C   Neuromuscular transmission syndrome

Experimental

B   Neuromuscular transmission dysfunction (inhibition of transmitter release)

Of the 64 tick species with potential to induce paralysis, only *Ixodes holocyclus* in Australia and *Dermacentor andersoni* and *D. variabilis* in North America affect humans. A toxin in tick saliva is assumed to be responsible for tick paralysis; its nature is unknown. A continuous discharge of the putative agent is required to effect paralysis of the host. Only gravid females of ixodid species and larvae of argasid species (*vide infra*) cause tick paralysis.

A toxic etiology for tick paralysis is supported by the following observations: (a) the incubation period for paralysis is constant, and the disease runs a course parallel to the feeding activities of the responsible ticks; (b) the incubation period can be manipulated precisely by applying ticks that have been allowed to feed on another host; (c) symptoms are usually present only while the ticks are fully engorged, and they promptly disappear when ticks are removed; (d) there is a direct correlation between the extent of tick infestation and the degree of clinical compromise of the host; (e) paralysis is induced in test animals administered tick homogenate or salivary gland material; and (f) blockade of neuromuscular transmission develops in nerve-muscle preparations treated *in vitro* with salivary gland fractions or isolates thereof; (g) experimental inoculation of paralysis-susceptible animals with tissues from tick-paralyzed animals or humans, or the ticks themselves, fails to induce paralysis (2,3,5,10,13,14). Morphological studies of peripheral nerves from paralyzed animals have failed to disclose specific changes.

Although the chemical structures of the various tick toxins are unknown, a degree of chemical homology likely exists between the culpable agents of some paralysis-inducing African species of veterinary relevance, namely, *I. rubicundus*, *Rhipicephalus evertsi evertsi*, and *Argas walkerae*. A murine monoclonal antibody directed against *R. evertsi evertsi* recognizes protein bands of similar mass and amino acid composition in separated proteins from salivary gland extracts of female ticks, 4 days prefed, of *R. evertsi evertsi* and *I. rubicundus*. Additionally, the monoclonal antibody raised against *R. evertsi evertsi* toxin provides some degree of protection for 1-day-old chicks from the neurotoxin in larvae of *A. walkerae* (2). This monoclonal antibody also identified the salivary gland toxin of *R. evertsi evertsi*. Salivary glands from female ticks, 4 days prefed, showed intense immunogold labeling in the granules and nuclei of "b" cells most probably in acinus II. Nuclear labeling was closely associated with the chromatin (3).

Dermacentor Spp.

Tick paralysis caused by female *D. andersoni* and *D. variabilis* has been studied experimentally in dogs, marmots, groundhogs, and hamsters (6,7).

Electrophysiological studies of human patients with *Dermacentor*-induced paralyses reveal motor polyneuropathy with limited involvement of afferent pathways. There is a marked diminution of maximal motor conduction velocities, reduced compound action potentials in nerves and their corresponding muscles, impaired impulse propagation of afferent nerve fibers, and a requirement for an increased stimulating current to elicit a response. Inhibition of acetylcholine biosynthesis has been ruled out (6,7).

Ixodes holocyclus

Some information is available on the paralytic factor secreted by *I. holocyclus* (5–7,10,11). Named holocyclotoxin, the agent is present in the saliva of feeding female ticks as shown by *in vitro* feeding studies using silicone membranes. Toxic fractions, collected from the feeding medium or extracted from salivary glands or tick homogenates, have been isolated and enriched by ultrafiltration and gel-permeation chromatography (10), as well as by molecular-sieve and anion-exchange chromatography (12). Toxicological assays of fractions in postnatal mice suggest a protein toxin with a molecular weight of 40–80 kDa. Papain hydrolyzed 88% of the protein present in a crude extract of salivary glands and halved its paralyzing action. However, pronase (a mixture of proteolytic enzymes) caused no loss of paralyzing action while digesting 78% of the total protein in the extract. Ultrastructural immunocyctochemical studies of salivary glands treated with immunogold-labeled immunoglobulin G antibodies raised against a highly purified component of the paralyzing fraction identified "e" cells of acinus III as the putative toxin source (11).

Tick bites are common in the United States; most involve dog ticks and deer ticks of the Ixodidae family. In North America, but not Australia, girls are more frequently affected with tick-related debilitating illness because ticks hide in long hair (9). Local reactions to tick bites (papules, nodules, granulomas) are accompanied by headache, nausea, and fever. In some cases, bites of D. variabilis or D. andersoni may precipitate a symmetrical, ascending paralysis 5–7 days after the tick attaches to the skin. Prodromal symptoms include numbness or tingling in the extremities, face, or throat, with attendant headache, malaise, and vomiting. Beginning in the lower extremities, weakness ascends to involve all four extremities and cranial nerves. Deep tendon reflexes are depressed or absent, but the sensory examination is otherwise normal. The clinical profile resembles the Guillain-Barré syndrome, a common misdiagnosis. Cerebrospinal fluid is unchanged. Paralysis is progressive; death results from respiratory insufficiency or aspiration. Identification or removal of the offending tick commonly results in rapid recovery that begins within hours and progresses over subsequent days. Occasionally, neurological symptoms may persist for weeks or even months after ticks are removed (4).

A thorough search for one or more ticks is a mandatory first step in treatment. Ticks should be removed with forceps placed at their point of attachment to the skin. Paralysis induced by the saliva of I. holocyclus is reversed by administration of an antiserum.

The mechanism of toxicity is unresolved. Whereas nerve conduction velocities are reduced in humans, the amplitude of nerve compound action potentials remains unchanged in paralyzed mice. Nerve-muscle preparations from paralyzed mice show a temperature-dependent inhibition of transmitter release at neuromuscular junctions. End-plate potentials can be recorded in the range of 15°–30°C, but not at higher temperatures; acetylcholine release is completely blocked above 30°C. Since the spontaneous diffusion of the transmitter is unaffected by blockade of the induced release, it is suggested that the toxin interferes not with the direct release of neurotransmitter but rather with steps between depolarization of the terminal membrane and transmitter release (7,10).

Editors' Note: Published recently is a review of Australian experience with 6 children who developed tick paralysis from I. holocyclus. Typical presentation was a prodrome followed by development of an unsteady gait, and then ascending, symmetrical, flaccid paralysis. Cranial nerve involvement (particularly ophthalmoplegia) reportedly was an early feature. Unlike experience in North America, paralysis increased in the 24–48 h period after tick removal. Neurophysiological studies showed low-amplitude compound muscle action potentials with normal motor conduction velocities, normal sensory studies and normal re-sponse to repetitive stimulation. The authors stated that anti-toxin had a role in the treatment of seriously ill children, but there was a high incidence of acute allergy and serum sickness (8). Tick-bite anaphylaxis, which is treated with adrenaline, is also a recognized clinical entity (1).

REFERENCES

1. Brown AF, Hamilton DL (1998) Tick bite anaphylaxis in Australia. Accid Emerg Med 15, 111.
2. Crause JC, van Wyngaardt S, Gothe R, Neitz AWH (1994) A shared epitope found in the major paralysis-inducing tick species of Africa. Exp Appl Acarol 18, 51.
3. Crause JC, Verschoor JA, Coetze J et al. (1993) The localization of a paralysis toxin in granules and nuclei of prefed female Rhipicephalus evertsi evertsi tick salivary glands. Exp Appl Acarol 17, 357.
4. Donat JR, Donat JF (1981) Tick paralysis with persistent weakness and electromyographic abnormalities. Arch Neurol 38, 59.
5. Gothe R (1984) Tick paralyses: Reasons for appearing during ixodid and argasid feeding. Curr Top Vector Res 2, 199.
6. Gothe R, Kunze K, Hoogstraal H (1979) The mechanisms of pathogenicity in the tick paralyses. J Med Entomol 16, 357.
7. Gothe R, Neitz AWH (1991) Tick paralyses: Pathogenesis and etiology. Adv Dis Vector Res 8, 177.
8. Grattan-Smith PJ, Morris JG, Johnston HM et al. (1997) Clinical and neurophysiological features of tick paralysis. Brain 120, 1975.
9. Murnaghan MF, O'Rourke HJ (1978) Tick paralysis. Handbuch Exp Pharmacol 48, 419.
10. Stone BF (1988) Tick paralysis, particularly involving Ixodes holocyclus and other Ixodes species. Adv Dis Vector Res 5, 61.
11. Stone BF, Binnington KC, Gauci M, Aylward JH (1989) Tick/host interactions for Ixodes holocyclus: Role, effects, biosynthesis and nature of its toxin and allergenic oral secretions. Exp Appl Acarol 7, 59.
12. Thurn MJ, Brady KW (1992) A tick toxin. In: Toxins and Targets. Effects of Natural and Synthetic Poisons on Living Cells and Fragile Ecosystems. Watters D, Lavin M, Maguire D, Pearn J eds. Harwood Academic Publishers GmbH, Chur p. 75.
13. Viljoen GJ, Bezuidenhout JD, Oberem PT et al. (1986) Isolation of a neurotoxin from the salivary glands of female Rhipicephalus evertsi evertsi. J Parasitol 72, 865.
14. Viljoen GJ, van Wyngaardt S, Gothe R et al. (1990) The detection and isolation of a paralysis toxin present in Argas (Persicargas) walkerae. Onderstepoort J Vet Res 57, 113.

Tityustoxin

Albert C. Ludolph
Peter S. Spencer

NEUROTOXICITY RATING

Clinical

A   Ion channel syndrome

Experimental

A   Ion channel dysfunction (sodium channel)

Venom of the Brazilian scorpion *Tityus serrulatus* contains a mixture of compounds collectively named tityustoxin (2). A minor fraction is named TsTX; the major component carries the name TsTX-I (or γ-toxin) (2). Tityustoxin contains both α- and β-scorpion toxins (*i.e.*, toxins that bind to site 3 and site 4 of the six neurotoxin-binding sites of Na$^+$ channels).

γ-Tityustoxin, a 61-amino-acid peptide, binds close to binding site 4 of Na$^+$ channels of rat brain (3), blocks the inactivation of the channel, and shifts the voltage-dependent activation in the hyperpolarized direction in frog myelinated nerve and in neuroblastoma cells (11,13). A similar delay of inactivation of Na$^+$-channels is produced by a 7230 Da fraction of the venom (1). A third fraction of the venom, the 37-amino-acid tityustoxin-Kα (TsTX-Kα), selectively blocks delayed-rectifier K$^+$ channels; its external binding site is close to the dendrotoxin site (12). Other fractions of tityustoxin have similar effects on Na$^+$ and K$^+$ channels (5,9,10). A newly discovered 35-amino-acid *T. serrulatus* toxin, Ts-κ, binds to small-conductance Ca^{2+}-activated (SK$_{Ca}$) channels (6). A second, named TsTX-IV, blocks Ca^{2+}-activated K$^+$ channels of high conductance; it consists of 41-amino-acid residues and eight half-cystine residues that cross-link the toxin molecule with four disulfide bonds (8).

Stings of *T. serrulatus* in humans are rarely lethal. Ten cardiopulmonary fatalities were found in a 16-year series of 3860 cases analyzed by a Brazilian group (4). Only children had died from scorpion stings in this series. Stings most often occurred during summer and caused a benign illness in adults. Children suffered more serious effects. Somnolence occurred in 25%, tremor in 10%, and confusion and seizures in 5% (4). Local pain, vomiting, tachycardia, and tachypnea were the most common complaints. In one instance, cranial nerve palsy was obviously caused by local swelling (7).

Treatment of moderate intoxication includes antivenom and symptomatic measures. Pain is treated with local injections of lidocaine, nausea and vomiting with metoclopramide. Treatment of the more severely affected patients may require adminstration of antiarrhythmics. Cardiac arrhythmias may respond to relief from hypoxia and electrolyte imbalances (4); only in severe cases is the use of lidocaine justified (4).

REFERENCES

1. Arantes EC, Riccioppo Neto F, Sampaio SV *et al.* (1993) The delay of inactivation of Na$^+$-channels by TsTX-V, a new neurotoxin from *Tityus serrulatus* scorpion venom. *Toxicon* **27**, 907.
2. Arantes EC, Sampaio SV, Vieira CA, Giglio JR (1992) What is Tityustoxin? *Toxicon* **30**, 786.
3. Barhanin J, Giglio JR, Leopold P *et al.* (1982) *Tityus serrulatus* venom contains two classes of toxins. *J Biol Chem* **257**, 12553.
4. Freire-Maia L, Campos JA, Amaral CF (1994) Approaches to the treatment of scorpion envenoming. *Toxicon* **32**, 1009.
5. Kirsch GE, Skattebol A, Possani LD, Brown AM (1989) Modification of Na channel gating by an alpha scorpion toxin from *Tityus serrulatus*. *J Gen Physiol* **93**, 67.
6. Legros C, Oughuideni R, Darbon H *et al.* (1996) Characterization of a new peptide from *Tityus serrulatus* scorpion venom which is a ligand of the apamin-binding site. *FEBS Lett* **390**, 81.
7. Nishioka S de A, Silveira PVP, Ugrinovich R, de Oliveira R (1992) Scorpion sting with cranial nerve involvement. *Toxicon* **30**, 685.
8. Novello JC, Arantes EC, Varanda WA *et al.* (1999) TsTX-IV, a short chain four-disulfide-bridged neurotoxin from *Tityus serrulatus* venom which acts on Ca^{2+}-activated K$^+$ channels. *Toxicon* **37**, 651.
9. Oliveira MJ, Fontana MD, Giglio JR *et al.* (1989) Effects of the venom of the Brazilian scorpion *Tityus serrulatus* and two of its fractions on the isolated diaphragm of the rat. *Gen Pharmacol* **20**, 205.
10. Sampaio SV, Arantes EC, Prado WA *et al.* (1991) Further characterization of toxins T1IV (TsTX-III) and T2IV from *Tityus serrulatus* scorpion venom. *Toxicon* **29**, 663.
11. Vijverberg HP, Pauron D, Lazdunski M (1984) The effect of *Tityus serrulatus* scorpion toxin gamma on Na$^+$ channels in neuroblastoma cells. *Pflugers Arch* **401**, 297.
12. Werkman TR, Gustafson TA, Rogowski RS *et al.* (1993) Tityustoxin-Kα, a structurally novel and highly potent K$^+$ channel peptide toxin, interacts with the alpha-dendrotoxin binding site on the cloned Kv1.2 K$^+$ channel. *Mol Pharmacol* **44**, 430.
13. Zaborovskaya LD, Khodorov BI (1985) Effect of *Tityus* gamma toxin on the activation process in sodium channels in frog myelinated nerve. *Gen Physiol Biophys* **4**, 101.

Toluene

Herbert H. Schaumburg

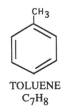

TOLUENE
C_7H_8

Methylbenzene

NEUROTOXICITY RATING

Clinical

A Acute encephalopathy (sedation, coma)
A Teratogenicity
A Leukoencephalopathy (diffuse)
A Chronic encephalopathy (cognitive dysfunction)

Experimental

A Acute encephalopathy
A Ototoxicity

Toluene is a natural component of crude oil and gasoline; it is also a by-product of styrene production and coke oven operations. The 1986 world production was 10 million tons. In North America, about 70% of toluene is used for the synthesis of benzene; the remainder is employed in the production of other chemicals, added to motor fuels, and used in graphic pigments and in paint and solvent solutions (2). At room temperature, it is a volatile, flammable liquid with a sweet pungent odor; the threshold for olfactory recognition is 2.9 ppm. The U.S. Time-Weighted Average Threshold Limit Value is 50 ppm. Despite considerable experimental animal and human studies, the pathogenesis of toluene neurotoxicity remains unclear. Prolonged high-level exposure from inhalant abuse of pure toluene and some toluene mixtures causes a debilitating multifocal leukoencephalopathy; acute high-level exposure results in CNS depression. It is claimed that chronic occupational exposure to low levels is associated with psychiatric change and mild cognitive dysfunction.

General Toxicology

Toluene is readily absorbed from inhalation or ingestion; dermal absorption may also occur but is less efficient. Inhaled toluene rapidly appears in brain lipid; the brainstem has the highest initial concentrations. Elimination from the CNS is rapid; however, subcutaneous lipid may constitute a temporary storage site and its concentration may continue to increase for 1 h following exposure. The half-life in human adipose tissue is 0.5–2.7 days. Plasma concentrations generally parallel the lipid-stored fraction. The concentration of blood toluene drops rapidly during the first 10 min following termination of exposure; after 3 h, very low concentrations are detectable in blood and in alveolar air. Circulating toluene is metabolized in hepatic microsomes by oxidation of the side chain to benzoic acid, which is conjugated with glycine to form hippuric acid (80%) or conjugated with glucuronic acid to benzoylglucuronide (20%). Both hippuric acid and benzoylglucuronide are excreted in urine. Monitoring of both finger-stick blood levels of toluene and urinary levels of hippuric acid have been suggested as quantitative markers of toluene exposure (12). Several factors suggest that urinary hippuric acid levels may be misleading; these include the appearance of similar levels in individuals with very different exposures, and interference by inhalation of other chemicals (*e.g.*, styrene, xylene). Contradictory effects of the coconsumption of ethanol on toluene metabolism are described; experimental animals given ethanol have elevated toluene blood levels as do healthy human voluntcers (2,7), while workers who regularly consume ethanol are reported to have lower plasma toluene measures than controls. Phenobarbital stimulates hepatic side-chain hydroxylase, accelerating the metabolism of toluene to hippuric acid and yielding lower blood and tissue levels of toluene. Hippuric acid monitoring is especially unreliable in persons with low-level exposures. The average amount of hippuric acid excreted in the urine by persons not exposed to toluene is 0.7–1.0 g/l of urine.

While the CNS is the primary target organ of toluene toxicity, serious systemic adverse reactions also accompany prolonged exposures—especially among inhalant abusers. Most hospital admissions for toluene abuse are for hepatic-renal failure or life-threatening cardiac arrhythmias. Inhalation of vapors at concentrations above 200 ppm is sufficient to cause mild conjunctival irritation and headache; liquid splashes cause severe conjunctivitis. Repeated dermal contact causes local irritation and degreasing of the skin; dermal sensitization to toluene is extremely rare. Toluene is not a serious immunopathogen or carcinogen; previous reports of malignancy among exposed workers are now presumed to reflect the effects of benzene (formerly, a component of commercial-grade toluene). Cardiac arrhythmias are a cause of sudden death during episodes of toluene abuse; experimental animal studies have failed to demonstrate myocardial histological abnormalities or arrhythmias. Prolonged (years) inhalant abuse may cause renal dysfunction and a secondary severe electrolyte imbalance; the usual profile includes metabolic acidosis, hypokalemia, and hypophosphatemia. This syndrome is secondary to toluene-induced renal tubular acidosis, *not* from increased urinary levels of hippuric acid; it is suggested that the site of primary dysfunction is the distal renal tubule. Hypokalemia may be so profound as to cause diffuse flaccid paralysis. Renal tubular function usually recovers during abstinence. Extreme cases of solvent inhalant abuse may also display evidence of hepatic failure. Studies with human volunteers and experimental animals have failed to demonstrate renal or hepatic dysfunction at levels encountered in the workplace.

Toluene is a teratogen in humans and experimental animals. In rat studies, high levels of toluene (sufficient to cause behavioral abnormalities) have impaired fetal growth and a variety of fetal malformations; these include delayed CNS development and anomalies in multiple organs (skeleton, heart, craniofacies, neural tube). Offspring of women who abused toluene during pregnancy had an increased incidence of craniofacial abnormalities, prematurity, and developmental delay (16,38). The children displayed attentional deficits, microcephaly, language impairment, and growth retardation. These phenotypic and behavioral features strikingly resemble those associated with the fetal alcohol syndrome. It is suggested that maternal toluene exposure, like maternal alcoholism, causes embryonic cell death resulting in deficiencies in early migrating neuroepithelial and mesodermal components (38).

Animal Studies

Controlled studies of toluene exposure to experimental animals have yielded a confusing and contradictory array of histopathological, neurophysiological, and behavioral data.

Short-term toluene inhalation exposure of mice and rats produces narcosis within 5 min at a level of 10,600 ppm. Neurobehavioral studies show increased motor activity (excitement stage) when rodents are exposed for 1 h to airborne toluene up to 1100 ppm; exposure to levels exceeding this causes lowered locomotor and lever-pressing activity (narcosis stage). No consistent morphological changes have been demonstrated in short-term studies; miscellaneous biochemical alterations are described including elevation of dopamine in the striatum following 1000-ppm exposure and depression of acetylcholine in the hippocampus after exposures at 8000 ppm for 8 h.

Rats exposed for 8 days at levels of 1400 ppm experience auditory dysfunction with corresponding morphological and physiological changes in cochlear hair cells. A recent short-term study of auditory function in mice with an hereditary predisposition to deafness utilized 7-day exposures at levels of 1000 ppm for 12 h daily; the results indicate that toluene exposure can aggravate auditory deterioration only in mice with a strong genetic predisposition to spontaneously precocious age-related hearing loss (31).

Prolonged inhalation exposure of mice and rats is avowed to cause persistent morphological, biochemical, and neurophysiological changes in the CNS; the few neurobehavioral studies report only a nondescript impairment of learning. None of these studies appears to have any compelling relevance to toluene's effects on human CNS. The most consistent, credible murine response to prolonged exposure to toluene is auditory dysfunction; physiological observations have been supported by careful morphological studies demonstrating loss of cochlear hair cells.

Some murine morphological studies claim frontal lobe and hippocampal neuronal loss; others have been unable to confirm this effect despite 6 months of exposure at levels of 1500 ppm (2,29). Exposure to levels of 500 ppm for 28 days in newborn rats is claimed to cause changes in the granule cell layer of the dentate region in the hippocampus; these changes are associated with persistent biochemical and behavioral abnormalities (43). When these rats attain adulthood, their hippocampal formations appear normal; it is claimed that this appearance is secondary to postnatal compensatory mechanisms. The biochemical abnormalities are said to persist.

One well-controlled murine study reports that toluene-dosed dams give birth to pups with smaller brains, increased ventricular volume and reduced size of the caudate nucleus. Histopathological examinations were not a feature of this study (15).

Biochemical studies have disclosed patterns of CNS change of questionable clinical significance, including diminished norepinephrine and dopamine concentrations, promotion of free radical formation in brain or liver, changes in membrane fluidity, increased striatal acetylcholine release, increase in glial cell markers, and alterations in various neurotransmitter levels (8,9,19,33,34,44,45).

Physiological studies of the auditory system have shown a consistent pattern of dysfunction compatible with cochlear hair cell loss; both impaired hearing (high-frequency loss) and abnormal responses of the brainstem auditory evoked potential are described (21,22,36). The peripheral vestibular system is uninvolved; however, one study indicates CNS vestibulocerebellar dysfunction after 21 h/day exposure to 1000 ppm for 6 weeks (37). Sleep studies have shown prolonged wakefulness as a consequence of extended exposures. Physiological studies of peripheral nerve and visual function in rats with chronic exposure to toluene consistently have been normal (29). Several physiological and biochemical studies suggest that toluene coexposure attenuates experimental *n*-hexane neuropathy, possibly by altering the metabolism of *n*-hexane to 2,5-hexanedione (39).

One study suggests that toluene can depress immune function in the mouse by stimulating the hypothalamic-pituitary-adrenocortical axis and elevating circulating corticosteroids (18).

In Vitro Studies

In vitro biochemical studies of neuron cell cultures treated with toluene have demonstrated many abnormalities, the most salient of which are increased membrane fluidity, inhibition of membrane-bound adenosine triphosphatase, and reduction of low-molecular-weight membrane proteins (9). A neurophysiological study of the effect of toluene application to guinea pig hippocampal slice preparations indicated that toluene had excitatory and inhibitory biphasic effects on neurotransmission, according to the concentration applied (20).

Human Studies

Controlled Exposures

Short-term exposure to airborne toluene levels <100 ppm has not been associated with discomfort. Exposure to levels at 100 ppm for 4 h causes eye irritation, headache, and lightheadedness but no consistent alterations in performance. One extensive study claims minor alterations in memory and dexterity following a 7-h exposure at 150 ppm. Exposures at 200 ppm for 8 h caused mild fatigue, confusion, lassitude, and lacrimation. At 600 ppm, euphoria and severe headache were prominent; at 800 ppm, all symptoms were more pronounced and were followed by 4 days of nervousness, fatigue, and insomnia.

Prolonged Exposures

Prolonged high-level (1000–20,000 ppm) toluene exposure from inhalant abuse definitely can cause symptomatic, disabling, multifocal leukoencephalopathy; prolonged moderate (88–150 ppm) occupational inhalation is alleged to cause mild (usually subclinical) cognitive dysfunction. It is unclear whether these two distinct toluene-associated syndromes reflect the same CNS disorder.

The desired effects of recreational toluene inhalation are euphoria and a sense of relaxation. Visual and auditory hallucinations may appear; they sometimes are frightening and provoke outbursts of antisocial behavior. Hallucinations usually abate following the initial months of abuse. Many chronic abusers inhale all day from solvent-soaked rags or filled plastic bags and eventuate in a mildly stuporous, tran-

quilized state. Sudden death may occur from vomiting, aspiration, suffocation by plastic bags, or cardiac arrhythmias. Inhalant abusers experience tolerance to the acute effects. Sudden withdrawal produces a syndrome similar to ethanol withdrawal; chronic inhalation does not appear associated with a consistent abstinence syndrome. Addiction, defined as psychic dependence, is common.

There are four studies of prolonged high-level inhalant abuse of *pure* toluene; they describe eight persons with a leukoencephalopathic syndrome of ataxia, spasticity, dysarthria, and dementia (3,27,30,32). Unfortunately, none features magnetic resonance imaging (MRI) or autopsy descriptions. There are many other reports of persons who have inhaled solvents, paints, or glues (composed of hydrocarbon mixtures featuring toluene as a major component) that depict an identical pattern of CNS dysfunction (14,17,24–27,32,41,42). Furthermore, some reports describing patients exposed to hydrocarbon mixtures have featured correlative MRI or autopsy evidence of white matter histopathological changes (41). It seems likely that the CNS effects of these mixtures largely reflect toluene neurotoxicity; however, this cannot be stated with absolute certainty since there is no clinical experience of the consequence of abuse of pure solutions of most of the common mixture components (xylene, benzene, methylene chloride, cyclohexane, butane). An exception is *n*-hexane, a frequent component of glues; *n*-hexane abuse (in the presence of methyl ethyl ketone) is associated with severe axonal polyneuropathy without prominent evidence of CNS dysfunction during intoxication or upon recovery from neuropathy.

The core syndrome of toluene neurotoxicity has been clearly defined; it is most consistent in case descriptions of persons who daily spend their waking hours for years, nose-to-rag/bag, in a toluene-induced recumbent stupor. The daily dose from inhalation can exceed 350 mg of toluene; one individual "huffed" (orally inhaled) a gallon every 2 weeks of 99% pure toluene. Consumed at this rate, the shortest documented duration before onset of symptoms is 1 year; most begin to show clinical manifestations after 2–4 years. Initial symptoms are behavioral changes (loss of initiative, depression, irritability), weight loss, impaired sense of smell, impaired concentration and memory, and mild unsteadiness of hand movements and gait. Subsequently, symptoms are slurred speech, head tremor, stiff-legged and staggering gait, poor vision, deafness, and dementia. Examination after 4 weeks of abstinence (avoiding the effects of acute intoxication) discloses sustained multidirectional nystagmus, titubation, ataxic tremor of all limbs, spasticity with hyperreflexia and Babinski's responses, broad-based and staggering stiff-legged gait, deafness, impaired vision and color discrimination, memory loss, inattention, apathy, and abulia. Even the most severely impaired display significant improvement following 6 months of abstinence; persons with mild or moderate dysfunction often recover completely (49). Infrequent abuse may cause no neurologically detectable CNS dysfunction; moderate frequency and intensity may cause a partial syndrome of mild cognitive dysfunction and slight tremor. Years of daily inhalation in the highest-level pattern described above almost inevitably leads to CNS dysfunction, and there is a predictable dose–effect relationship at these high levels. Authors who espouse the notion that there is little relationship between neurological disorder and duration of abuse have not included patients with this all-day/every-day pattern of toluene inhalation (13,40).

Laboratory studies of such acutely intoxicated cases may reveal evidence of renal tubular failure or mild hepatic dysfunction. Most hospitalizations of these adolescents are for renal insufficiency and hypokalemia. Laboratory evidence of neuroendocrine effects is described in factory workers (46), while hypothalamic dysfunction (hyperprolactinemia, decreased testosterone and growth hormone) is reported in a boy whose toluene abuse was accompanied by central sleep apnea, diabetes insipidus, and poikilothermia (47). One study of cardiac function detected diminished variation in the R-R interval; the authors suggest this finding reflected central autonomic dysfunction (35).

CNS electrophysiological studies reveal a characteristic abnormality of the brainstem auditory evoked response (BAER); namely, sparing of early components (wave I) and decrement or loss of late components (waves III–V). Abnormal BAER responses appear to be among the most sensitive measures of toluene neurotoxicity; they may appear at a time when the neurological exam is still unremarkable. Audiograms are generally unremarkable. Visual evoked responses appear less sensitive; they usually display diminished amplitudes throughout, with moderate delay in the late component. Nerve conduction studies are unremarkable except in cases where n-hexane is present in the inhalant. Electroencephalograms are frequently abnormal; even after 4 weeks of abstinence, they show mild diffuse slowing without paroxysmal, epileptiform activity. Computed tomography in severe cases almost always discloses mild to moderate cerebellar cortical and cerebral hemisphere atrophy. MRI in some advanced cases has provided solid evidence of white matter disease; this is evidenced by increased signal intensity on T2-weighted images in the periventricular, internal capsular, and brainstem pyramidal regions. MRI also reveals loss of differentiation between gray and white matter throughout the CNS and atrophy of cerebellum, cerebral hemispheres and brainstem. These MRI findings are nonspecific; they may be seen in inflammatory demyelinating diseases, anoxic demyelination, and ischemic white matter disease. Two MRI reports additionally describe hypointensity of the basal ganglia and thalamus resembling iron deposits (5,48); one study suggests that partitioning of toluene into the lipid membranes of cells in cerebral tissue may account for the thalamic hypointensity (48).

There are three reports that describe postmortem histopathological changes in the CNS (10,28,41). Two (10,41) contain disparate findings; each is based on a single autopsy case. While loss of myelin in cerebral and cerebellar white matter was present in both, diffuse cerebral and cerebellar cortical atrophy and giant axonal swelling were noted only in one report (10). Small perivascular aggregates of periodic acid–Schiff (PAS)–positive macrophages were seen only in the second (41).

The recently published third postmortem study is detailed, credible, and probably definitive (28). It used both conventional and ultrastructural techniques, as well as biochemical analysis, in a thorough study of three brains from solvent abusers, historically the most likely to have been exposed to high levels of toluene (analysis of inhalants was not performed). Gross examination of the most severely affected brains revealed profound atrophy and mottling of the white matter of the corpus callosum, centrum semiovale, internal capsule, and cerebellum, with sparing of the immediate subcortical areas. The two less affected cases displayed only mild pallor of the centrum semiovale and ventricular dilatation. Microscopic studies revealed, in all three, a consistent pattern of myelin and oligodendrocyte loss, with relative preservation of axons. Save for mild Purkinje cell depletion in the most severe case, there were no significant neuronal abnormalities of cerebral or cerebellar cortex, or subcortical nuclei. Myelin loss was accompanied by large accumulations of PAS--positive, neutral lipid-negative macrophages. Macrophage accumulations and demyelination were most pronounced around small blood vessels; collections of inflammatory cells were not a feature of any case. Ultrastructural study disclosed macrophages containing stacks of lamellar inclusions; biochemical study of the inclusions revealed large amounts of very-long-chain fatty acids. These ultrastructural and biochemical abnormalities also characterize adrenoleukodystrophy (ALD), a hereditary neurodegenerative disorder of peroxisomal lipid metabolism. However, in contrast to ALD, these cases did not feature alterations in adrenal or Leydig cells or accumulations of inflammatory cells in the CNS.

Prolonged, low-level occupational inhalation of pure toluene is rare; most workers are exposed to solvent mixtures. The putative "solvent syndrome" of painters and factory workers of behavioral-personality change progressing to permanent cognitive impairment is discussed elsewhere in this volume (*see* (i) Organic Solvent Mixtures and (ii) *n*-Hexane, Metabolites, and Derivatives, this volume).

One report describes occupational exposure to pure toluene in an anosmic lens cleaner who worked in a small room without protection; his exposure is described as chronic and intermittent (3). Over a period of 3 months, this individual developed poor concentration and memory, somnolence, slurred speech, and unsteady gait. He experienced no impairment of consciousness at work and denied inhalant abuse of toluene. Examination disclosed normal mental function (no formal neuropsychological testing), mild dysarthria, and gait-limb ataxia. He was 75% recovered within 10 days of abstinence and normal within 1 month. This report, although limited by lack of data on exposure duration or intensity and absence of BAER and neuropsychological studies, suggests that intermittent, moderate-to-high level industrial exposure to toluene produces an illness that is a microcosm of the inhalant-abuse syndrome.

Three studies of workers chronically exposed to low levels (88–150 ppm) of toluene have attempted to estimate levels and duration of contact; these featured comprehensive neuropsychological evaluation and appropriate controls (6,11,23). Two describe no neurobehavioral effects; one found only subclinical but statistically significant differences in manual dexterity, visual scanning, and verbal memory (11).

One report describes abnormalities in the early component of the BAER in workers exposed for 12–14 years to 97 ppm of toluene (1). The authors interpret these findings as representing toluene-induced dysfunction of the auditory peripheral receptor.

Epidemiology

The origins of the North American epidemic of inhalant abuse have been vividly described (4):

> In recent decades, inhalant abusers have turned to a wide variety of household products, especially glues, solvents, and fuels. The earliest reference to glue sniffing seems to have been a 1959 newspaper article describing children in several western American cities. What ensued is instructional. A national chorus of alarm, intended to defer use, instead became a lure, and as exaggerated warnings led to legislation and arrests, glue sniffing became a national epidemic. Diversification to other substances soon followed, and today volatile substance abuse involves children throughout the world.

In North America, inhalant solvent (toluene) abuse is especially prevalent in economically disadvantaged, neglected, or abused adolescents. Most are Hispanic immigrants, or children of immigrants, from Central America and Mexico. Males outnumber females ten to one. Native Americans also have an especially high prevalance of inhalant abuse. Much North American inhalant abuse ("sniffing", huffing") involves paint or lacquer thinners containing toluene as the principal constituent. Central American residents who inhale glues that frequently contain *n*-hexane as the major component and toluene as a minor component manifest a severe axonal polyneuropathy; they do not have cerebellar or diffuse subcortical dysfunction as features of their illness. Inhalant abuse of gasoline has been especially common among Native Americans (4). These individuals are at risk for progressive cognitive decline, movement disorders, and peripheral neuropathy; this syndrome has been attributed to tetraethyl lead (*see* Gasoline, this volume).

Diagnosis

Correct diagnosis is seldom difficult when presented with an intoxicated person. In the emergency room, solvent-smelling breath (persistent for hours) and a perioral rash ("huffer's rash") are often clues. Toxicological screens in most commercial laboratories employing gas chromatography can detect toluene in the blood; hippuric acid analysis of urine is also widely available.

Children who lack obvious neurological deficits may develop hypokalemia and metabolic acidosis during early toluene abstinence. Occasionally, they are repeatedly admitted to renal medical units for treatment of distal renal tubular dysfunction of "obscure origin."

In advanced cases, the pattern of multifocal white matter lesions in adolescence can suggest the diagnosis of multiple sclerosis.

Treatment and Prevention

Other than abstinence, there is no specific treatment for the CNS effects. Hypokalemia, cardiac arrhythmia, and metabolic acidosis require skilled medical management.

The mainstay of prevention is education; centers for inhalant abusers exist in several western American cities; they have outpatient and remedial programs. Installation of nasal irritants (mustard oil) in glues has been suggested; this approach has met with mixed success (13,40).

Toxic Mechanisms

The acute effects of high-level toluene exposure (excitement followed by CNS depression) suggest a neurotransmitter-mediated mechanism similar to that of the hydrocarbon general anesthetics and ethanol.

The multifocal and diffuse leukoencephalopathy from prolonged high-level exposure (inhalant abuse) most likely reflects a direct effect on myelin or on the oligodendrocyte. The biochemical and morphological similarities to ALD raise the possibility of an induced disorder of peroxisome or fatty acid metabolism.

REFERENCES

1. Abbate C, Giorgianni C, Munao F et al. (1993) Neurotoxicity induced by exposure to toluene. An electrophysiologic study. Int Arch Occup Environ Health 64, 389.

2. Arlien-Soborg P (1992) Toluene. In: Solvent Neurotoxicity CRC Press, Boca Raton, Florida p. 61.

3. Boor JWE, Hurtig HI (1977) Persistent cerebellar ataxia after exposure to toluene. Ann Neurol 2, 440.

4. Brust J (1993) Neurological Aspects of Substance Abuse. Butterworth-Heineman, Stoneham, Massachusetts.

5. Caldemeyer KS, Pascuzzi RM, Moran CC, Smith RR (1993) Toluene abuse causing reduced MR signal intensity in the brain. Amer J Roentgenol 161, 1259.

6. Cherry N, Hutchins H, Pace T, Waldron HA (1985) Neurobehavioral effects of repeated occupational exposure to toluene and paint solvents. Brit J Ind Med 42, 291.

7. Dossing M, Baelum J, Hansen SH, Lundqvist GR (1984) Effect of ethanol, cimetidine and propranolol on toluene metabolism in man. Int Arch Occup Environ Health 54, 309.

8. Edelfors S, Ravn-Jonsen A (1991) Effects of simultaneous ethanol and toluene exposure on nerve cells measured by changes in synaptosomal calcium uptake and (Ca^{2+}/Mg^{2+})-ATPase activity. Pharmacol Toxicol 69, 90.

9. Engelke M, Diehl H, Tahti H (1992) Effects of toluene and n-hexane on rat synaptosomal membrane fluidity and integral enzyme activities. Pharmacol Toxicol 71, 343.

10. Escobar A, Aruffo C (1980) Clinico-pathologic report of a human case. J Neurol Neurosurg Psychiat 43, 986.

11. Foo SC, Jeyaratnam J, Koh D (1990) Chronic neurobehavioural effects of toluene. Brit J Ind Med 47, 480.

12. Foo SC, Phoon WO, Khoo NY (1988) Toluene in blood after exposure to toluene. Amer Ind Hyg Assn J 49, 255.

13. Fornazzari L, Riley D, Wu P, Carlen PL (1987) Toluene abuse and neurologic impairment. Neurology 37, 356.

14. Fornazzari L, Wilkinson DA, Kapur BM, Carlen PL (1983) Cerebellar, cortical and functional impairment in toluene abusers. Acta Neurol Scand 67, 319.

15. Gospe SM, Zhou SS, Saeed DB, Zeman FJ (1996) Development of a rat model of toluene-abuse embryopathy. Pediat Res 40, 82.

16. Hersh JH (1988) Toluene embryopathy: Two new cases. J Med Genet 26, 333.

17. Hormes JT, Filley CM, Rosenberg NL (1986) Neurologic sequelae of chronic solvent vapor abuse. Neurology 36, 698.

18. Hsieh GC, Sharma RP, Parker RD (1991) Hypothalamic-pituitary-adrenocortical axis activity and immune function after oral exposure to benzene and toluene. Immunopharmacology 21, 23.

19. Huang J, Asaeda N, Takeuchi Y et al. (1992) Dose dependent effects of chronic exposure to toluene on neuronal and glial cell marker proteins in the central nervous system of rats. Brit J Ind Med 49, 282.

20. Ikeuchi Y, Hirai H, Okada Y, Mio T, Matsuada T (1993) Excitatory and inhibitory effects of toluene on neural activity in guinea pig hippocampal slices. Neurosci Let 158, 63.

21. Johnson AC, Canlon B (1994) Toluene exposure affects the functional activity of the outer hair cells. Hear Res 72, 189.

22. Johnson AC, Canlon B (1994) Progressive hair cell loss induced by toluene exposure. Hear Res 75, 201.

23. Juntunen J, Matikainen E, Antti-Poika M et al. (1985) Nervous system effects of long-term occupational exposure to toluene. Acta Neurol Scand 72, 512.

24. Keane JR (1978) Toluene optic neuropathy. Ann Neurol 4, 390.

25. Kelly TW (1975) Prolonged cerebellar dysfunction associated with paint-sniffing. Pediatrics 56, 605.

26. King HD, Day RE, Oliver JS et al. (1981) Solvent encephalopathy. Brit Med J 283, 663.

27. Knox WJ, Nelson JR (1966) Permanent encephalopathy from toluene inhalation. N Engl J Med 275, 1494.

28. Kornfeld M, Moser AB, Moser HW (1994) Solvent vapor abuse leukoencephalopathy. Comparison to adrenoleukodystrophy. J Neuropathol Exp Neurol 53, 389.

29. Ladefoged O, Strange P, Moller A et al. (1991) Irreversible effects in rats of toluene (inhalation) exposure for six months. Pharmacol Toxicol 68, 384.

30. Lazar RB, Ho SU, Melen O et al. (1983) Multifocal central nervous system damage caused by toluene abuse. Neurology 33, 1337.

31. Li HS, Johnson AC, Borg E et al. (1992) Auditory degeneration after exposure to toluene in two genotypes of mice. Arch Toxicol 66, 382.

32. Malm G, Lying-Tunell U (1980) Cerebellar dysfunction related to toluene sniffing. Acta Neurol Scand 62, 188.

33. Mattia CJ, Adams JD Jr, Bondy SC (1993) Free radical induction in the brain and liver by products of toluene catabolism. Biochem Pharmacol 46, 103.

34. Mattia CJ, LeBel CP, Bondy SC (1991) Effects of toluene and its metabolites on cerebral reactive oxygen species generation. Biochem Pharmacol 42, 679.

35. Murata K, Araki S, Yokoyama K et al. (1993) Cardiac autonomic dysfunction in rotogravure printers exposed to toluene in relation to peripheral nerve conduction. Ind Health 31, 79.

36. Nylen P, Hagman M, Johnson AC (1994) Function of the auditory and visual systems, and of peripheral nerve, in

rats after long-term combined exposure to *n*-hexane and methylated benzene derivatives. I. Toluene. *Pharmacol Toxicol* 74, 116.

37. Nylen P, Larsby B, Johnson AC *et al.* (1991) Vestibular-oculomotor, opto-oculomotor and visual function in the rat after long-term inhalation exposure to toluene. *Acta Oto-laryngol* 111, 36.

38. Pearson MA, Hoyme EH, Seaver LH *et al.* (1994) Toluene embryopathy: Delineation of the phenotype and comparison with fetal alcohol syndrome. *Pediatrics* 93, 211.

39. Pryor GT, Rebert CS (1992) Interactive effects of toluene and hexane on behavior and neurophysiologic responses in Fischer-344 rats. *Neurotoxicology* 13, 225.

40. Rosenberg NL, Filley CM, Hormes JT (1987) Toluene abuse and neurologic impairment. *Neurology* 37, 356.

41. Rosenberg NL, Kleinschmidt-DeMasters BK, Davis KA *et al.* (1988) Toluene abuse causes diffuse central nervous system white matter changes. *Ann Neurol* 23, 611.

42. Rosenberg NL, Spitz MC, Filley CM *et al.* (1988) Central nervous system effects of chronic toluene abuse—clinical, brainstem evoked response and magnetic resonance imaging studies. *Neurotoxicol Teratol* 10, 489.

43. Slomianka L, Rungby J, Edelfors S *et al.* (1992) Late postnatal growth in the dentate area of the rat hippocampus compensates for volumetric changes caused by early postnatal toluene exposure. *Toxicology* 74, 203.

44. Stengard K (1994) Effect of toluene inhalation on extracellular striatal acetylcholine release studied with microdialysis. *Pharmacol Toxicol* 75, 115.

45. Stengard K, Tham, R, O'Connor WT *et al.* (1993) Acute toluene exposure increases extracellular GABA in the cerebellum of rat: A microdialysis study. *Pharmacol Toxicol* 73, 315.

46. Svensson BG, Nise G, Erfurth EM *et al.* (1992) Neuroendocrine effects in printing workers exposed to toluene. *Brit J Ind Med* 49, 402.

47. Teelucksingh S, Steer CR, Thompson CJ *et al.* (1990) Hypothalamic syndrome and central sleep apnea associated with toluene exposure. *Quart J Med* 78, 185.

48. Unger E, Alexander A, Fritz T *et al.* (1994) Toluene abuse: Physical basis for hypointensity of the basal ganglia on T2-weighted MR images. *Radiology* 193, 473.

49. Wiedmann KD, Power KG, Wilson JT, Hadley DM (1987) Recovery from chronic solvent abuse. *J Neurol Neurosurg Psychiat* 50, 1712.

CASE REPORT

A 14-year-old Honduran immigrant male began inhaling clear lacquer containing 87% toluene, 10% methylene chloride, and 3% butane. After 4 years of near-constant daily inhalation, he was arrested as intoxicated by the police and subsequently taken to hospital where he awakened and was noted to be weak. At admission, he was mildly and diffusely weak, and hyporeflexic with normal sensation. Serum electrolytes showed a potassium level of 2.1 µg/ml (normal, >4 µg/ml). The young man was admitted to the hospital. His electrolyte imbalance responded to potassium replacement therapy, and he regained limb strength. There was evidence of mild renal tubular dysfunction that improved within 1 week and he was discharged.

Neurological consultation before discharge noted a dull, slowly responsive adolescent with dysarthric speech. There was sustained horizontal and rotatory nystagmus, mild intention tremor of the upper limbs, and a broad-based ataxic gait. Tendon reflexes, limb strength, and acral sensation were normal. A MRI 1 week later was normal, BAERs showed moderate increase in latency of the late components (waves II–V) and VERs were unremarkable. He entered a counseling program. After 6 months of abstinence, the only detectable abnormalities were slight end-gaze horizontal nystagmus and instability when tandem walking.

Comment

The initial weakness reflected the effects of hypokalemia and triggered the admission. Fortunately, his renal and neurological dysfunction were at early stages and largely reversible. Despite the presence of serious cognitive and cerebellar dysfunction, the normal MRI suggests that myelin degeneration was not a feature of this early case.

Toluene 2,4-Diisocyanate

Herbert H. Schaumburg

TOLUENE 2,4-DIISOCYANATE
$C_9H_6N_2O_2$

2,4-Diisocyanatotoluene

NEUROTOXICITY RATING
Clinical
C   Acute encephalopathy
C   Chronic encephalopathy

Toluene 2,4-diisocyanate (TDI) is widely used in the production of polyurethane foams for insulation and in the synthesis of plastics. Common commercial grades of TDI are a mixture of 80% of the 2,4-isomer and 20% of the 2,6-isomer. The 2,4-isomer is more volatile and constitutes the overwhelming component of most industrial airborne exposures. Individuals especially at risk for exposure include synthetic chemical workers, applicators of insulation foams, and fire fighters at sites of burning insulation (10). The U.S. Time-Weighted Average Threshold Limit Value is 0.005 ppm (0.04 mg/m^3).

Orally administered TDI is poorly absorbed, with 81% recoverable in the feces. Inhalation studies suggest that virtually all inhaled TDI is retained and is metabolized to either mono- or diacetyl-2,4-toluenediamine (2,8). These metabolites have high tissue penetration and eventually appear in the urine; significant quantities of 2,4-toluenediamine (TDA) are not formed and do not appear in the urine. TDA is a carcinogen and, since it too is metabolized to mono- and diacetyl-2,4-toluenediamine, it has been suggested that TDI has human carcinogenic potential (5). One experimental animal study describes carcinogenicity of TDI in F344/N rats (12); a study of workers exposed to industrial TDI has not supported the notion of human carcinogenicity (7).

TDI is an irritant of mucous membranes and skin, and a skin sensitizer. Its principal adverse reaction is respiratory tract irritation and sensitization. Exposure to high vapor levels of TDI causes severe bronchitis, bronchospasm and, eventually, pulmonary edema (4,6,10). These acute effects are overshadowed in importance by respiratory sensitization. The onset of disabling respiratory sensitization symptoms (dyspnea, bronchospasm) may be insidious and progressive with increasing levels or duration (months) of exposure, or may follow a period of deceptively slight symptoms (mild cough) after only weeks of exposure that terminates in an unexpected bout of status asthmaticus. No prior history of asthma or atopy exists in many instances; given sufficient exposure, any person apparently may become sensitized. The pathophysiology of TDI-induced asthma is unknown; it is not solely mediated by a type-I hypersensitivity response associated with immunoglobulin E antibodies. Studies suggest a neurogenic mechanism; namely, that TDI causes a release of substance P and calcitonin-gene–related neuropeptides in the nasal mucosa, thereby triggering the allergic response. Pretreatment of TDI-exposed experimental animals with capsaicin suppresses the allergic reaction (11).

One study describes acute and chronic toxic encephalopathy in fire fighters exposed in a chemical storage facility to TDI and the pyrolysis products of TDI (not a foam or in insulation) (9). This report merits close analysis because it was controlled using a similar group of fire fighters; it is widely quoted and held to illustrate the hazards of exposure to TDI and its combustion products. Thirty-five fire fighters experienced varying degrees of inhalation exposure (some wore breathing apparatus) to fumes of burning TDI while playing water on the tanks (1). Thirty-one developed respiratory symptoms of varying severity and persistence, and 15 experienced transient gastrointestinal distress. Acute reversible encephalopathy (euphoria, ataxia) appeared in five, and 13 complained of persistent cognitive dysfunction when examined 4 years later. An additional five men noted cognitive dysfunction for several months after the fire but had recovered completely by the 4-year assessment time. At the 4-year examination, all noted mild, subjective, nonincapacitating symptoms, including memory impairment, personality change, depression, and loss of sociability. Psychometric evaluation utilized solely the Wechsler Memory Scale; this procedure disclosed no deficit of short-term or stored memory, but impairment of relatively long-term recall. The authors admit that combustion products of other chemicals in the storage facility may have played a role, but emphasize that none was known to produce this syndrome; in addition, several men experienced their only exposure in the clean-up operation the following day, when the only chemical present was large spills of uncombusted TDI. They further state that anoxic encephalopathy from carbon monoxide gas appeared unlikely, since none was exposed to fumes of sufficient density to cause anoxia and none experienced hyperthermia.

There are several grounds to question the role of TDI in this syndrome: (a) there has been 20 years of subsequent clinical experience of individuals exposed to noncombusted TDI and none is known to have described cognitive impairment; (b) the neuropsychological data, albeit collected in a carefully controlled manner, were limited and did not constitute a complete battery; (c) impairment of long-term recall and preservation of short-term memory is a pattern opposite to that generally associated with toxic encephalopathy; (d) despite the absence of legal motivation, many received compensation, and this group was highly aware of the pulmonary toxicity of TDI (most experienced respiratory distress, persistent in some) and the acute encephalopathy experienced by five (two had loss of consciousness and trembling and were taken to the hospital)—they also had 4 years to ruminate over their minor, nondisabling symptoms; (e) the data are largely self-reported—the only objective measure (electroencephalography) was unremarkable; and (f) despite the authors reasonable exclusion of carbon monoxide, it is possible that burning raw TDI created other pyrolysis products to cause the acute encephalopathic and gastrointestinal reactions. Liberation of hydrogen cyanide has been documented from fires occurring in buildings insulated with TDI foam (3).

REFERENCES

1. Axford AT, McKerrow CB, Parry Jones A, Le Quesne PM (1976) Accidental exposure to isocyanate fumes in a group of firemen. *Brit J Ind Med* **33**, 65.
2. Bartels MJ, Timchalk C, Smith FA (1993) Gas chromatographic/tandem mass spectrometric identification and quantitation of metabolic 4-acetyltoluene-2,4-diamine from the F344 rat. *Bio Mass Spect* **22**, 194.
3. Becker CE (1985) The role of cyanide in fires. *Vet Hum Toxicol* **27**, 487.
4. Brugsch HG, Elkins HB (1963) Toluene di-isocyanate (TDI) toxicity. *N Engl J Med* **268**, 353.
5. Dieter MP, Boorman GA, Jameson CW et al. (1990) The carcinogenic activity of commercial grade toluene diisocyanate in rats and mice in relation to the metabolism of the 2,4- and 2,6-TDI isomers. *Toxicol Ind Health* **6**, 599.
6. Fahy JP (1958) Toxic hazards, toluene-2,4-di-isocyanate (TDI). *N Engl J Med* **259**, 404.
7. Hagmar L, Stromberg U, Welinder H, Mikoczy Z (1993) Incidence of cancer and exposure to toluene diisocyanate and methylene diphenyldiisocyanate: a cohort based case-referent study in the polyurethane foam manufacturing industry. *Brit J Ind Med* **50**, 1003.
8. Kennedy AL, Wilson TR, Stock MF et al. (1994) Distribution and reactivity of inhaled ^{14}C-labeled toluene diisocyanate (TDI) in rats. *Arch Toxicol* **68**, 434.
9. LeQuesne PM, Axford AT, McKerrow CB et al. (1976) Neurological complications after a single severe exposure to toluene di-isocyanate. *Brit J Ind Med* **33**, 72.
10. Munn A (1965) Hazards of isocyanates. *Ann Occup Hyg* **8**, 163.
11. Takeda N, Kalubi B, Abe Y et al. (1993) Neurogenic inflammation in nasal allergy: Histochemical and pharmacological studies in guinea pigs. A review. *Acta Otolaryngol* **501**, 21.
12. Timchalk C, Smith Fa, Bartels MJ (1994) Route-dependent comparative metabolism of [^{14}C]toluene 2,4-diisocyanate and [^{14}C]toluene 2,4-diamine in Fischer 344 rats. *Toxicol Appl Pharmacol* **124**, 181.

Toxaphene and Constituents

Peter S. Spencer

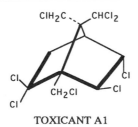

TOXICANT A1

2,2,5-*endo*,6-*exo*,8,8,9,10-Octachlorobornane; 8-Chloro-B; Toxicant A1

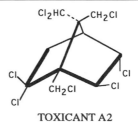

TOXICANT A2

2,2,5-*endo*,6-*exo*,8,9,9,10-Octachlorobornane; 9-Chloro-B; Toxicant A2

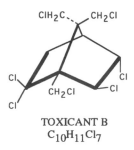

TOXICANT B
$C_{10}H_{11}Cl_7$

2,2,5-*endo*,6-*exo*,8,9,10-Heptachlorobornane; Toxicant B

NEUROTOXICITY RATING

Clinical

A Seizure disorder (myoclonus, generalized rarely)

Experimental

A Seizure disorder

The complex mixture of chemicals known as toxaphene is used as an insecticide in less-developed regions of the world in agriculture and to control large-animal pests (14). Toxaphene was extensively used in the United States for the control of cotton insects until it was banned in 1982 because of concerns relating to human carcinogenic risk (17). The compound is a convulsant in humans and animals.

Toxaphene may contain upwards of 200 individual substances, most of which are chlorinated bornanes with 10 carbon atoms, 6-1 chlorine atoms, and 7-12 hydrogen atoms. The composition and acute toxicity of commercial toxaphene may vary. Three components (toxicants A1, A2, and B) are thought to account for the acute toxicity of toxaphene in mice, goldfish, and houseflies (14).

Toxaphene undergoes extensive oxidative and reductive transformation by cytochrome P-450 monooxygenases (13,15). The rapid metabolism and excretion of the most toxic constituents is held responsible for the safety record associated with intended use of toxaphene (14).

Acute toxicity in humans has resulted from dermal application (single dose of 46 g) or ingestion (8). Poisoning by accidental or intentional ingestion has led to fatalities, mostly among children. Repeated violent convulsions, hyperpyrexia, and cyanosis, are followed by death within 4–12 h of exposure (11,12). The estimated minimum acute lethal dose of toxaphene is 2–7 g; <10 mg/kg has provoked convulsions in some individuals who subsequently recovered (8). An estimated dose of 9.5–45 mg/kg was responsible for poisoning of seven of ten members of a family that ate collards sprayed with 9% camphechlor (toxaphene) (8). Nausea, mental confusion, and extremity myoclonus are reported in cases with a nonfatal outcome, with recovery within a day of exposure (7). No adverse effects were found in human volunteers exposed *via* an aerosol to approximately 1 mg/kg/day for 10 consecutive days and, 3 weeks later, to a similar dosage for 3 days (9). Chronic occupational exposure to toxaphene has been associated with the onset of a seizure disorder after several months of application (16).

The toxic profile of toxaphene (primarily convulsions) parallels that of lindane and cyclodienes, such as dieldrin; it differs from the primarily tremorogenic organochlorine insecticides, notably DDT and related compounds, that act as Na^+ channel openers in excitable membranes (*see* Dichlorodiphenyltrichloroethane and Derivatives, this volume) (17). Toxaphene, lindane, and dieldrin are competitive and stereospecific inhibitors of [^{35}]*t*-butylbicyclophosphorothionate (TBPS); this binds to the picrotoxinin-binding site of the γ-aminobutyric acid (GABA) receptor (10). The most potent inhibitors of TBPS binding are also the most acutely toxic (1,4,17). Toxaphene and toxicologically related compounds interfere with chloride ion flux through GABA-gated chloride channels (GABA$_A$) that are responsible for maintaining excitable membranes in a hyperpolarized state, thereby decreasing neuronal excitability (2–6).

REFERENCES

1. Abalis IM, Eldefrawi ME, Eldefrawi AT (1985) High-affinity stereospecific binding of cyclodiene insecticides and gamma-hexachlorocyclohexane to gamma-aminobutyric acid receptors. *Pestic Biochem Physiol* 24, 95.
2. Abalis IM, Eldefrawi ME, Edlefrawi AT (1986) Effects of insecticides on GABA-induced chloride influx into rat brain microsacs. *J Toxicol Environ Health* 18, 13.
3. Bloomquist JR, Adams PM, Soderlund DM (1986) Inhibition of gamma-aminobutyric acid-stimulated cloride flux in mouse brain vesicles by polychlorocycloalkane and pyrethroid insecticides. *Neurotoxicology* 7, 11.
4. Eldefrawi AT, Eldefrawi ME (1987) Receptors for gamma-aminobutyric acid and voltage-dependent chloride channels as targets for drugs and toxicants. *FASEB J* 1, 262.
5. Fishman BE, Gianutsos G (1988) CNS biochemical and pharmacological effects of the isomers of hexachlorocyclohexane (lindane) in the mouse. *Toxicol Appl Pharmacol* 93, 146.
6. Gant DB, Eldefrawi ME, Eldefrawi AT (1987) Cyclodiene insecticides inhibit GABA$_A$ receptor-regulated chloride transport. *Toxicol Appl Pharmacol* 88, 313.
7. Hayes WJ Jr (1982) *Pesticides Studied in Man*. Williams & Wilkins, Baltimore.
8. Kaloyanova KP, El Batawi MA (1991) *Human Toxicology of Pesticides*. CRC Press, Boca Raton, Florida p. 83.
9. Keplinger ML (1963) Use of humans to evaluate safety of chemicals. *Arch Environ Health* 6, 342.
10. Lawrence LJ, Casida JE (1984) Interactions of lindane, toxaphene and cyclodienes with brain specific *t*-butylbicyclophosphorothionate receptor. *Life Sci* 35, 171.

11. McGee LC, Reed HL, Fleming JP (1952) Accidental poisoning by toxaphene. Review of toxicology and case reports. *J Amer Med Assn* **149**, 1124.

12. Pollock RW (1953) Toxaphene poisoning—report of a fatal case. *Northwest Med* **52**, 293.

13. Saleh MA, Turner WA, Casida JE (1977) Polychlorobornane components of toxaphene: Structure-toxicity relations and metabolic reductive dechlorination. *Science* **198**, 1256.

14. Smith AG (1991) Chlorinated hydrocarbon insecticides. In: *Handbook of Pesticide Toxicology. Vol 2. Classes of Pesticides*. Hayes WJ Jr, Laws ER Jr eds. Academic Press, San Diego, p. 850.

15. Turner WA, Engel JL, Casida JE (1977) Toxaphene components and related compounds: Preparation and toxicity of some hepta-, octa- and nonachlorobornanes, hexa- and hepta chlorobornenes and a hexachlorobornadiene. *J Agric Food Chem* **25**, 1394.

16. Warraki S (1963) Respiratory hazards of chlorinated camphene. *Arch Environ Health* **19**, 814.

17. Woolley DE (1995) Organochlorine insecticides: Neurotoxicity and mechanisms of action. In: *Handbook of Neurotoxicology*. Chang LW, Dyer DS eds. Marcel Dekker, New York p. 475.

"Toxic Oil"

Alberto Portera-Sánchez
Manuel Posada de la Paz

NEUROTOXICITY RATING

Clinical

B   Peripheral neuropathy

Toxic oil syndrome (TOS) is a progressive multisystem disease that occurred in central and northwestern Spain in 1981 following the ingestion of fraudulently denatured rapeseed oil (19). Although an infectious origin was the first etiological hypothesis, the lack of cases among groups at risk for this type of disease pointed to a toxic agent as the most likely cause. The identification of a 6-month-old patient fed with a baby meal in which an illegally sold cooking oil had been added as a grandmother's remedy to prevent constipation rendered the product suspect. Subsequent case-control and descriptive epidemiological studies on case series demonstrated that the culpable agent was an edible rapeseed oil that had been purposively denatured with 2% aniline to prevent human use (5,17). This oil had been imported from France for industrial use, but it was later illegally diverted for human consumption and sold in 5-liter containers. The causal relationship between the ingestion of rapeseed oil and the illness was finally established after two case-control studies demonstrated the existence of a dose–response relationship between the contents of a specific aniline derivative (oleylanilide) and the risk of becoming ill (8,14). The latency period between exposure and onset of illness was 4–10 days. Gender and age have not been identified as risk factors.

Two large families of chemical compounds have been identified in the ingested toxic oil: fatty acid anilides and propanediol derivatives. Each of these two groups contains about 14 compounds with different oil concentrations. The oleic-acid anilide and the 1,2-di-oleyl ester of 3-(N-phenylamino)1,2-propanediol (DEPAP) are the most representative compounds of these two families, and DEPAP appears to be the most important candidate for the causal agent (6,15).

The epidemic started in late April 1981; within 30 days, more than 10,000 individuals were affected. Currently, 20,644 cases are included in the TOS official registry. Two years after the outbreak, 415 deaths had already occurred and 10 years later, 1226 cases had died.

In vitro observations, as well as studies with rodents and monkeys fed with suspected rapeseed oil and synthetic chemical products (oleylanilides, propanediol, and others), failed to reproduce the clinical or pathological features of TOS as expressed in humans (2).

Three clinical phases of TOS have been identified. The *acute phase*, lasting 2 months, was characterized by mild fever, itchy scalp, rash, myalgia, dyspnea, and cough. Chest roentgenograms showed an interstitial or alveolar infiltrate with or without pleural effusion. Laboratory tests demonstrated a high count of eosinophils that in many cases exceeded 3000 cells/ml. Severe myalgias and muscle cramps identified the beginning of the *intermediate phase*, which was characterized by skin infiltrates, pulmonary hypertension, hepatic cholestasis, marked weight loss, alopecia, *sicca* syndrome, dysphagia, thromboembolism, disseminated intravascular coagulation, and paresthesias. Laboratory data showed hypertriglyceridemia, hypercholesterolemia, thrombocytosis, thrombocytopenia, and persistent eosinophilia. In the *chronic phase*, patients had scleroderma, hepatopathy, pulmonary hypertension, persisting paresthesias, and other neurological manifestations discussed below. Corticoids, immunosupressors, free radical scavengers, and chelating agents were ineffective therapies (1,9,21).

Endothelial cells of arteries and veins were affected, but no fibrinoid necrosis or granulomas were observed. Initially, endothelial swelling with infiltrates of lymphohistiocytic foam cells may be observed in the intima. In severe cases, a proliferation of the intima, fibrosis, and thrombosis is seen. These vascular lesions involve all organs except the CNS. Interstitial fibrosis is the most characteristic histological finding in the chronic phase and skin, gastrointestinal tract, and PNS are its main targets. Pulmonary edema, thromboemboli, pulmonary hypertension, and respiratory insufficiency due to muscular weakness were the most common causes of death (11).

Acute and progressive neurological manifestations, primarily limited to the neuromuscular system, were present in 70%–80% of cases. During the early phase, over 80% of patients complained of intense generalized myalgias as the only initial neurological symptom; this progressed with time to the point that half of the cases became severely incapacitated. Progressive and intense limitation of different joints (elbows, fingers, and temporomandibular), as well as muscle cramps and segmental palpable contractures, were also prominent features. Marked eosinophilia was generally present at this stage; muscle enzymes and cerebrospinal fluid (CSF) were normal (13). In some patients, muscle fibrillation and increased polyphasic motor unit potentials of reduced amplitude and short duration constituted the only electromyographic findings. In all muscle biopsies, intense round-cell and polymorphonuclear infiltrates were present in the endomysium, especially around the intramuscular nerve fascicles and within the capsules of the muscle spindles. Isolated type II fiber atrophy and histochemical features of denervation were also found. Motor and sensory nerve conduction velocities and sural nerve biopsies were normal (4,16).

Three months after the outbreak, 75% of cases developed generalized muscle weakness or paralysis and corresponding atrophy. Intrinsic muscles of both hands, biceps, triceps, deltoids, and masseters were most severely affected, but proximal weakness and wasting were also prominent in the lower limbs, especially in the anterior leg compartment. Extraocular and facial muscles were spared. Deep tendon reflexes were abolished in one-third of the cases, and no pyramidal tract involvement was found. Paresthesias and persistent numbness were also reported by the majority of patients. Various and irregular types of decreased pain and touch perception, including glove-and-stocking patterns, as well as reduced position sense and vibratory perception, were found in 30%–50% of cases. Single-nerve or radicular involvement and patchy sensory loss were also a feature. The more severely affected patients requiring hospitalization demonstrated intense and progressive respiratory insufficiency due to muscle weakness that required mechanical assistance in intensive care units. Almost all affected individuals lost considerable body weight as a consequence of severe muscular wasting and anorexia, and swallowing or masticatory difficulties due to extreme limitation of temporomandibular joints. Global atrophy of subcutaneous tissue and loss of the skin's natural elasticity (scleroderma-like) were striking features contributing to the limitation of joint motion (13).

Marked electromyographic abnormalities were recorded in this stage of the disease. Prominent spontaneous muscle activity in the form of fibrillations was accompanied by increased loss of motor unit potentials and absent voluntary activity. Polyphasic activity seen in earlier stages was still present with markedly reduced amplitude. Compound muscle and sensory potentials were reduced in amplitude and, in severely affected patients, evoked potentials were absence—a feature of complete denervation (4).

Histopathological changes were also present within the first 3 months of the illness. While the endomysial inflammatory infiltrates were clearly diminished, severe fascicular neurogenic muscle atrophy was seen together with round-cell infiltrates around venules and capillaries. Sural nerve biopsies consistently showed perineurial fibrosis. Focal loss or degeneration of individual axons was observed, as was occasional myelin breakdown (16).

One year after the onset of the TOS, paresthesiaes, muscle cramps, and osteomuscular pains remained the most common complaints. Generalized areflexia was the rule. Spontaneous, multifocal and often asymmetrical, repetitive and semirhythmic myoclonic movements, as well as other abnormal movements, were prominent findings (10). In more than half of the patients, different patterns of weakness—distal in arms and proximal in legs—were identified. At this stage, 50% of patients were clinically *mildly* affected (symptomatic complaints only), 30% showed *moderate* involvement (mild to moderate weakness), and 20% were *severely* incapacitated (advanced paralysis and muscle atrophy). Moderate or severe muscle atrophy and weakness were associated with reduced motor conduction velocities. Correlations were less apparent between electrophysiological studies and clinical sensory abnormalities. No clear-cut relationship was found between the amplitude of motor or sensory evoked potentials and the clinical findings.

CNS manifestations were rare. Acute encephalopathy

(confusion, hypersomnia, and focal signs) was seen in occasional patients during the acute phase of TOS; this was associated with electroencephalographic slowing and mild brain swelling in computed tomography studies. Loss of memory, reactive anxiety or depression, and sleep disorders were also described. Pathological studies of CNS did not show endothelial lesions. Striking chromatolysis, vacuolar degeneration, and heavy silver impregnation of swollen neuron perykarya were seen in scattered brainstem nuclei and anterior horn cells (20).

Fifteen years after the outbreak, 3% of patients presented with scleroderma, 18% with peripheral neuropathy, 5% with pulmonary hypertension, and 7% with liver disease. Other pathologies, such as cancer and myocardial infarcation, were also identified, but their relationship with TOS is doubtful. Neurological complaints included cramps and myalgias, 65%; numbness, tingling, and burning sensations, 40%; and different degrees of muscle weakness, atrophy, and areflexia, 18%.

These data provide evidence supporting the diagnosis of a polyneuropathy (distal weakness, atrophy, and superficial and deep sensory abnormalities)—predominantly axonal degeneration with equal involvement of motor and sensory fibers (coexistence of motor and sensory findings and abnormal motor and sensory electrophysiological parameters). Occasional CNS manifestations were also encountered.

TOS constitutes a unique and unprecedented process not previously described in humans or animals. However, in October 1989, a disease that came to be called the eosinophilia-myalgia syndrome (EMS), and linked to the ingestion of some specific lots of L-tryptophan, shares similar clinical and laboratory findings with TOS in their chronic phases (Table 59; see also L-Tryptophan, this volume). Both disorders may have a common pathogenic mechanism (7,12). The acute and intermediate phases of TOS share similarities with hypereosinophilic syndrome and drug-induced lung toxicity. TOS may also mimic the graft-vs.-host disease and scleroderma, although polyneuropathy is rarely described in these two disorders (12). Exceptionally, the rare entity known as sensory perineuritis may be included in the differential diagnosis (3). Similar patchy sensory alterations with some areas of hypoalgesia and paresthesias in the territory of small nerves are described in patients with systemic vasculitis. Even though other toxic neuropathies may be similar to TOS in their clinical manifestations, the pathological findings (neuronopathy, myelinopathy, and axonopathy) pertaining to them are clearly distinct from those found in TOS (18).

The pathophysiological mechanisms of TOS are unknown, although immune-system activation and oxidative stress are mentioned (12). Axonal degeneration may be secondary to the perineurial inflammatory infiltrates and, in later stages, constrictive mechanisms due to the intense perineurial fibrosis may increase nerve fiber damage (13).

TABLE 59. Clinical Manifestations of Toxic Oil Syndrome (TOS) and Eosinophilia-Myalgia Syndrome (EMS) (Chronic Phase)

Manifestations	TOS*	EMS*
Myalgia	+++	++++
Arthralgia	−	++
Sensory neuropathy	++	++
Motor neuropathy	++	+
Scleroderma	++	+++
Hepatopathy	++	−
Pulmonary hypertension	+	+
Cramps	+++	+++

*Percentage of patients with sign or symptom: ++++ = 100%–76%; +++ = 75%–51%; ++ = 50%–26%; + = 25%–1%; − = 0%.

REFERENCES

1. Abaitua Borda I, Posada de la Paz M (1992) Clinical findings. In: *Toxic Oil Syndrome: Current Knowledge and Future Perspectives*. World Health Organization Regional Office for Europe eds. WHO Regional Publications, European Series No. 42, Copenhagen p. 23.

2. Aldridge WN (1991) Experimental studies. In: *Toxic Oil Syndrome: Current Knowledge and Future Perspectives*. World Health Organization Regional Office for Europe eds. WHO Regional Publications, European Series No. 42, Copenhagen p. 63.

3. Asbury AK, Picard EH, Baringer JR (1972) Sensory perineuritis. *Arch Neurol* **26**, 302.

4. Cruz Martinez A, Pérez Conde MC, Ferrer MT *et al.* (1984) Neuromuscular disorders in a new Toxic Oil Syndrome: Electrophysiological study—a preliminary report. *Muscle Nerve* **7**, 12.

5. Díaz de Rojas F, Castro García M, Abaitua Borda I *et al.* (1987) The association of oil ingestion with toxic-oil syndrome in two convents. *Amer J Epidemiol* **125**, 907.

6. Hill RH Jr, Schurtz HH, Posada de la Paz M *et al.* (1995) Possible etiologic agents for toxic oil syndrome: Fatty acid esters of 3-(N-phenylamino)-1,2-propanediol. *Arch Environ Contam Toxicol* **28**, 259.

7. Kilbourne EM (1992) Eosinophilia-myalgia syndrome: Coming to grips with a new illness. *Epidemiol Rev* **14**, 16.

8. Kilbourne EM, Bernert JT Jr, Posada de la Paz M *et al.* (1988) Chemical correlates of pathogenicity of oils related to the toxic-oil syndrome in Spain. *Amer J Epidemiol* **127**, 1210.

9. Kilbourne EM, Perez-Rigau JG, Heath CW *et al.* (1983) Clinical epidemiology of toxic-oil syndrome: Manifestations of a new illness. *N Engl J Med* **309**, 1408.

10. Leiva C, Fernandez Gonzalez F, De Blas G et al. (1985) Abnormal movements in Spanish toxic oil syndrome. *J Neurol* **232**, 242.

11. Martinez-Tello FJ, Navas-Palacios JJ, Ricoy JR et al. (1982) Pathology of a toxic syndrome caused by ingestion of adulterated oil in Spain. *Virchows Arch* **397**, 261.

12. Philen RM, Posada de la Paz M (1993) Toxic oil syndrome and eosinophilia-myalgia syndrome: May 8–10, 1991, World Health Organization Meeting Report. *Semin Arthritis Rheum* **33**, 104.

13. Portera-Sánchez A, Franch O, Del Ser T (1983) Neuromuscular manifestations of the toxic oil syndrome: A recent outbreak in Spain. In: *Clinical and Biological Aspects of Peripheral Nerve Diseases.* Battistin L, Hashim GA, Lajtha A eds. Alan R. Liss, New York p. 171.

14. Posada de la Paz M, Philen RM, Abaitua I et al. (1994) Factors associated with pathogenicity of oils related to the toxic oil syndrome epidemic in Spain. *Epidemiology* **5**, 404.

15. Posada de la Paz M, Philen RM, Schurz H et al. (1999) Epidemiologic evidence for a new class of compounds associated with toxic oil syndrome. *Epidemiology* **10**, 130.

16. Ricoy JR, Cabello A, Rodriguez J, Tellez I (1983) Neuropathological studies on the toxic syndrome related to adulterated rapeseed oil in Spain. *Brain* **106**, 817.

17. Rigau-Pérez JG, Pérez-Alvarez L, Dueñas-Castro S et al. (1984) Epidemiologic investigation of an oil-associated pneumonic paralytic eosinophilic syndrome in Spain. *Amer J Epidemiol* **119**, 250.

18. Schaumburg HH, Spencer PS (1979) Toxic neuropathies. *Neurology* **29**, 429.

19. Tabuenca JM (1981) Toxic allergic syndrome caused by ingestion of rapeseed oil denatured with aniline. *Lancet* **2**, 567.

20. Téllez I, Cabello A, Franch O, Ricoy JR (1987) Chromatolytic changes in the central nervous system of patients with the toxic oil syndrome. *Acta Neuropathol* **74**, 354.

21. Toxic Epidemic Syndrome Study Group (1982) Toxic epidemic syndrome: Spain 1981. *Lancet* **2**, 697.

Tremetone

Albert C. Ludolph

TREMETONE
$C_{13}H_{14}O_2$

2,3-Dihydro-2-isopropenyl-5-benzofuranyl methyl ketone; Tremetol

NEUROTOXICITY RATING
Clinical
B   Acute encephalopathy (sedation, tremor)

Tremetone is an oily liquid with a MW of 202.24; it is derived from white snake root (*Eupatorium rugosum*) and rayless goldenrod (*Haplopappus heterophyllus*). White snake root is suspected to be the cause of "milk sickness," a disease of historical interest in North America (1,4). Reportedly, Abraham Lincoln's mother, Nancy Hanks Lincoln, died from the disease, and this event prompted Lincoln and his wife to leave Indiana for Illinois (1). Intoxication by snake roots also impacts domestic animals ("trembles"), and the human poisoning was linked to the intake of milk of diseased animals grazing on *Eupatorium rugosum* (1).

Milk sickness was an epidemic disease of late summer or fall when hunger forced cattle to feed on plants which they usually avoided. Clinical signs in domestic animals were similar in sheep, horses, cats, dogs, cattle, and other species: loss of appetite was accompanied by intolerance to exercise, then accelerated and labored respiration appeared, followed by stiffness of the limbs, ataxia, and trembling (1,2,4). Finally, animals became comatose and died. Dogs feeding on affected cattle reportedly died (1), and suckling animals were frequently affected (1,4). Symptoms appeared in the offspring before the lactating parent. In horses, cardiac abnormalities may occur (4). Autopsies of affected animals revealed fatty infiltration of various organs, including the liver; however, the nervous system has not been examined (1). An outbreak of suspected equine tremetone poisoning was accompanied by an increase of muscle creatine kinase and myoglobinuria (3). Tremetone is also found in rayless goldenrod, a plant associated with a similar disease in affected cattle and in humans consuming their milk (1,2,4).

During milk sickness, humans experience loss of appetite and develop generalized weakness, muscular pain and tremors (1,2,4). Vomiting commences while the body temperature is subnormal. The breath smells of acetone. Some become comatose and die. The disease is induced not only by milk of affected animals but also by their meat (2).

The mechanism of poisoning is unknown.

REFERENCES

1. Christensen W (1965) Milk sickness: A review of the literature. *Econ Bot* **19**, 293.
2. Kingsbury JM (1964) *Poisonous Plants of the United States and Canada*. Prentice Hall, Englewood Cliffs, New Jersey.
3. Olson CT, Keller WC, Gerken DF, Reed SM (1984) Suspected tremetol poisoning in horses. *J Amer Vet Med Assn* **185**, 1001.
4. Panter KE, James LF (1990) Natural plant toxicants in milk: A review. *J Anim Sci* **68**, 892.

Triamcinolone

Byron A. Kakulas

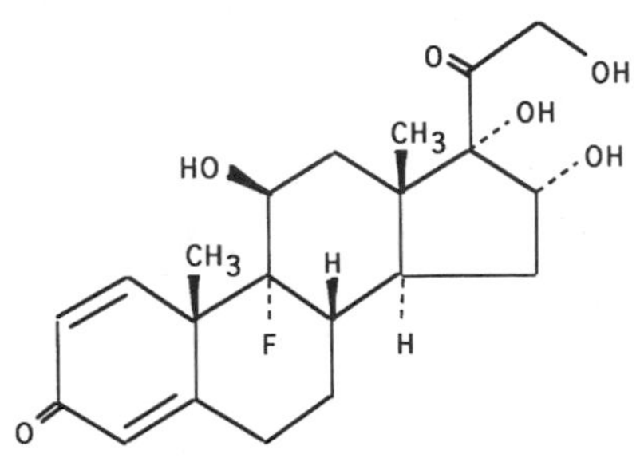

TRIAMCINOLONE
$C_{21}H_{27}FO_6$

($11\beta,16\alpha$)-9-Fluoro-11,16,17,21-tetrahydroxypregna-1,4-diene-3,20-dione

NEUROTOXICITY RATING

Clinical

A Headache
A Myopathy (fibrosis)
B Psychobiological reaction (sedation, restlessness, anxiety)
B Benign intracranial hypertension

Triamcinolone is a fluorinated prednisolone derivative with less mineralocorticoid activity than prednisolone. Considered an intermediate-duration glucocorticoid, triamcinolone has both clinical and veterinary usage as an antiinflammatory glucocorticoid (2,6). The white crystals of triamcinolone have a MP of 269°–271°C (6).

Oral or injectable triamcinolone is used to treat many allergic or inflammatory diseases. Triamcinolone is given intranasally for seasonal and perennial allergic rhinitis and topically to relieve inflammatory and pruritic manifestations of corticosteroid-responsive dermatoses. Aerosolized triamcinolone is used to treat children and adults with asthma.

The typical adult oral dose range is 4–48 mg/day depending on the condition. An oral dosage regimen for the treatment of asthma in children is 0.8–1.6 mg/kg every other day. Inhaled triamcinolone 200 μg three to four times daily is used for treating asthma in adults. In children over

6 years of age, the inhaled dose is one to two inhalations, three to four times daily. For adults and children 12 years or older, the intranasal dose is 220 μg/day administered as two inhalations in each nostril once daily. Topical triamcinolone is used two to four times daily. Triamcinolone can also be administered by intra-articular, intradermal, intralesional, and intramuscular injection at varying doses. Triamcinolone is absorbed percutaneously following topical application. Absorption also occurs following intra-articular injection. Triamcinolone is presumably metabolized in the liver, with <15% being eliminated in the urine (2).

Following intranasal triamcinolone, headache occurs in about 18% of patients. A range of adverse effects, including nasal irritation, dry mucous membranes, congestion, throat discomfort, sneezing, and epistaxis can be experienced. Inhalation-specific side effects include hoarseness, throat irritation, and dry mouth. Adrenal suppression may occur after use of triamcinolone, especially in high doses or for a prolonged time (6).

Unlike other corticosteroids, triamcinolone appears to cause sedation and depression rather than euphoria (3,8), although euphoria can occur in patients with no previous psychiatric history (5). Manic-depressive illness, paranoid states, and acute toxic psychosis may all occur following corticosteroid treatment. However, no cases have been directly attributed to triamcinolone. The treatment of toxic psychosis is primarily by dose reduction, with the use of antipsychotic drugs producing variable results (5).

In one study, CNS toxicity was confirmed in 8 of 18 patients. The CNS effects included restlessness, overstimulation, tremors, and sensations of heat. These complications followed intramuscular doses of triamcinolone for chronic asthma (4–28 mg/injection with a total of 38 injections) (1). Triamcinolone is a potent cause of myofibrosis when given in high doses for a prolonged period (11).

While corticosteroid-induced pseudotumor cerebri is clearly associated with the long-term use of a number of corticosteroids, it seems to occur most commonly with prednisolone and triamcinolone. These drugs can induce increased cranial pressure and papilledema. The condition is more common in children than adults. Within days of a decrease in dosage or a change in steroid, patients complain of headache, irritability, and vomiting. The rapid reduction of steroid dosage or change in the type of steroid given seems to be the initiator of cerebral pseudotumor. The treatment is first to increase the dose of steroid, then gradually decrease the dosage (4,7,9,10).

Because of its glucocorticoid functions, unwanted side effects similar to those of other corticosteroids may be expected. With high and/or prolonged dosage, these include peptic ulceration, acne, hypertension, cushingoid features, diabetes mellitus, and growth retardation in children (2).

REFERENCES

1. Bernecker C, Herxheimer H (1969) Corticosteroidkristallsuspensionen in der Behandlung von chronischem asthma bronchiale. *Klin Wochenschr* **47**, 1104.
2. DRUGDEX Editorial Staff (1995) *Triamcinolone*. DRUGDEX Micromedex Inc, Denver, CO.
3. Flower AH (1965) Dermatologic disorders treated by oral triamcinolone. *J Maine Med Assn* **56**, 162.
4. Ivey KJ, BenDesten L (1969) Pseudotumor cerebri associated with corticosteroid therapy in an adult. *J Amer Med Assn* **208**, 1698.
5. Kishi DT (1983) Disorders of the Adrenals. In: *Applied Therapeutics, the Clinical Use of Drugs. 3rd Ed.* Katcher DS *et al.* eds. Applied Therapeutics Inc. San Francisco, California.
6. *Merck Index* (1983) Merck & Co, Rahway, New Jersey p. 1372.
7. Neville BGR, Wilson J (1970) Benign intracranial hypertension following corticosteroid withdrawal in childhood. *Brit Med J* **3**, 554.
8. Reynolds JEF (1982) *Martindale: The Extra Pharmacopeia. 28th Ed.* The Pharmaceutical Press, London.
9. Sternberg TH, Bierman SM (1965) Pseudotumor cerebri associated with systemic steroids. *Arch Dermatol* **92**, 746.
10. Walker AE, Adamiewicz JJ (1964) Pseudotumor cerebri associated with prolonged corticosteroid therapy. *J Amer Med Assn* **188**, 779.
11. Williams RS (1959) Triamcinolone myopathy. *Lancet* **1**, 698.

1,1,1-Trichloroethane

John L. O'Donoghue

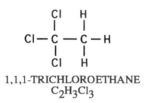

1,1,1-TRICHLOROETHANE
$C_2H_3Cl_3$

Methylchloroform; α-Trichloroethane

NEUROTOXICITY RATING
Clinical
A   Acute encephalopathy

1,1,1-Trichloroethane, commonly referred to as methyl chloroform (MC), is a highly volatile, colorless, nonflammable liquid primarily employed as a metal-degreasing solvent; it has been used in other types of cleaning operations and as a chemical intermediate. Use of MC is declining because international treaties restrict production and utilization of ozone-depleting substances. Commercial MC typically contains an inhibitor to prevent interaction with aluminum or other metals, which can result in the generation of hydrochloric acid. A more toxic isomer of trichloroethane (1,1,2-) is used primarily as an intermediate for the production of 1,1-dichloroethylene. 1,1,2-Trichloroethane is associated with potential hepatotoxicity.

MC is insoluble in water but highly soluble in fat; consequently, MC is rapidly absorbed on inhalation and rapidly reaches saturation in the blood. Excretion from the body is also rapid and, due to its low level of metabolism, MC is primarily excreted as unchanged parent compound. When administered to rats by oral gavage, 83% of the administered dose is excreted in the expired air and 4% is metabolized with 0.9% exhaled as carbon dioxide, 2% excreted as urinary metabolites, and 1.2% retained in the carcass (20). Small amounts of MC metabolites are retained as protein-bound adducts (20). Oxidative metabolism of MC can result in the formation of small amounts of trichloroethanol and trichloroacetic acid metabolites that are excreted in the urine (8).

In human volunteers, the uptake of MC and its elimination following inhalation are rapid, with 44% of an inhaled dose excreted within 1 h (21). While MC has been investigated for its anesthetic properties, its anesthetic potency is not as great as that of other chlorinated solvents

(21). MC can be absorbed through the skin, but the quantity of MC absorbed by this route is not considered to be significant unless a large area of the body is exposed for a prolonged period of time (28). A physiologically based pharmacokinetic model, which can be used to simulate metabolic processes associated with uptake, distribution, and excretion of MC, has been published (3).

MC has a low degree of acute toxicity in laboratory animals. Oral LD_{50} values in various species have been reported to be between 5.6 g/kg for rabbits and 12.9 g/kg for rats (29). The LC_{50} for MC following a 7-h vapor exposure of rats is reported to be 14,250 ppm (1). Signs of CNS depression appear in rats and monkeys exposed to MC vapor at 5000 ppm for about 1 h (1). The primary effect of MC at acutely toxic concentrations is CNS depression; if this is not severe enough to kill, animals recover without significant aftereffects. The responses of mice exposed to MC vapor and tested for changes in performance on a scheduled-behavior task showed that the behavioral effects observed following MC exposure are qualitatively similar to those produced by anesthetics (22). Histological examination of rats repeatedly exposed to anesthetic concentrations of MC for 1 h/day for 9 days showed no effects on the brain and spinal cord (13). Following single vapor exposures of 13,500 ppm MC sufficient to kill mice in 9–12 h, serum liver enzyme levels were not increased; intraperitoneal dosing of MC did result in small increases in serum liver enzymes, but only at dose levels that approached lethal levels (5).

Groups of rats, guinea pigs, rabbits, dogs, and monkeys repeatedly (2200 ppm vapor for 8 h/day, 5 day/week for 6 weeks) or continuously (135 ppm or 370 ppm vapor) exposed to MC did not show any significant exposure-related effects except slight body weight reduction (dogs and rabbits exposed to 2200 ppm); brain histology was unremarkable (25). Groups of rats, guinea pigs, rabbits, and dogs developed mild liver and kidney effects following repeated 7-h exposures to vapors of a mixture of 800 ppm MC and 200 ppm tetrachloroethylene; these effects were consistent with the known effects of tetrachloroethylene (27). Rats exposed to MC vapor atmospheres at 200, 630, or 2000 ppm for 6 h/day, 5 days/week for 13 weeks showed no effects when tested for performance on a functional observational battery and grip-strength test; when tested for visual, auditory, somatosensory, and caudal-nerve evoked potentials; or when examined for neuropathological changes in the brain, spinal cord, and peripheral nerves (18).

Continuous exposure to high concentrations of MC resulted in the appearance of signs of withdrawal in mice (4). Mice were exposed to between 500 and 4000 ppm MC vapor continuously for 4 days. Withdrawal signs were at maximal severity 2–4 h following exposure, with 80% of the rats exposed to 2000 ppm MC demonstrating handling-induced convulsions. During the withdrawal period, rats showed an increased sensitivity to pentylenetetrazol-induced seizures. When mice were tested using a fixed-ratio responding-paradigm and exposed to 6000 ppm MC for 20-min periods, 4 days/week for 15 days, a slight degree of tolerance was observed, but the effect could not be detected as a change in concentration–response curves (23).

Significant neurotoxicity has not been observed in developing rats. Rat pups born to dams given MC by oral gavage at dose levels of 75, 250, and 750 mg/kg on gestation days 6–10 did not show evidence of neurotoxicity when examined for delays in physical maturation, motor activity, auditory brainstem responses, functional-observational-battery responses, short-term memory, learning, brain dimensions, or neuropathology (19). Similarly, rat pups born to dams exposed to 2100 ppm MC vapor before, during, or both before and during pregnancy showed no effect in tests of open-field activity, running-wheel activity, and amphetamine challenge (30).

In two experiments designed to mimic inhalation abuse of MC, pregnant mice were exposed to either 2000 ppm MC vapor for 17 h/day or 8000 ppm MC vapor for 1 h, three times a day during gestation days 12–17 (9). Postnatally, the pups showed decreased weight gain, delayed developmental landmarks, delayed acquisition of the righting reflex, weaker grip strength, poorer negative geotaxis, and less rooting intensity. While these observations were indicative of behavioral and developmental teratogenicity, the results were largely reversible postnatally, suggesting a delay in brain maturation. Postweaning motor activity and passive avoidance were unaffected by MC exposure (9).

Due to the low uptake of MC into the blood, relatively high MC concentrations or continuous exposure regimens are needed to produce brain levels of MC that might impair CNS metabolism. In gerbils exposed to 70 ppm MC vapor continuously for 3 months followed by a rest period of 4 months, brain weight and protein content of the brain were not altered, but DNA levels in the posterior cerebellar hemisphere, anterior cerebellar vermis, and hippocampus were lower than in controls, suggesting a decreased cell density (10). Continuous exposure of gerbils to 210 or 1000 ppm MC vapor for 3 months, followed by a 4-month recovery period, resulted in an increased concentration of glial fibrillary acidic protein (GFAP) in the sensorimotor cortex (26). Similar exposures to 70 ppm MC vapor did not result in altered levels of GFAP. Cortical levels of a second glial protein (S-100) were not similarly affected at 210 or 1000 ppm MC (26).

Rats exposed to 1200 ppm MC vapor continuously for 30 days showed changes in the fatty acid pattern of brain ethanolamine phosphoglyceride (14). Stearic acid and arachidonic acid content were decreased while 22-carbon (n-3) fatty acids were increased. Continuous exposure to 320 ppm MC vapor for 30 days did not result in changes in lipid content, fatty acid composition, or brain weight (15).

Large doses of MC may interfere with intracellular calcium flux. Cerebellar synaptosomes recovered from mice given 2.4 g/kg of MC by intraperitoneal injection showed a significantly lower influx of calcium when compared to that for synaptosomes recovered from controls (24).

Human volunteers who were exposed to a mixture of 400 ppm MC and 100 ppm tetrachloroethylene for 7 h/day for one, four, or five exposures showed no evidence of neurotoxicity (27). No changes were observed in (a) neurological examinations conducted after 6 h of exposure; (b) vestibular, cerebellar, of proprioceptive function tested every 75 min during exposure; (c) responses to questions about headache, dizziness, or speech difficulty posed every 45 min during exposure; (d) performance on the Crawford Manual Dexterity Test or Flanagan Aptitude Classification Test administered after 3 h of exposure; or (e) a series of nonneural tests. Other short-term exposure studies with human volunteers exposed to MC vapor concentrations of 350–1700 ppm have shown few responses, except for decreased mental alertness and manual dexterity, and increased reaction time and body sway (2,29).

A recent report indicates that 28 workers exposed long term to moderate to high levels of MC (vapor levels were not determined) had lightheadedness, vertigo, nausea, and fatigue (11). The workers reported they had short-term memory loss, decreased attention and concentration spans, moodiness, and disequilibrium for at least 2–4 years. Significant elevations were noted in scores on the Luria-Nebraska Neuropsychological Battery rhythm, memory, intermediate memory, and speed scales. Performance on a sway test were abnormal in several patients, and a trail-making test was slowed. Excessive somatic concerns and mild depressive symptoms were present on a personality assessment inventory. Magnetic resonance imaging of the brain showed that only 1 of 26 workers had an abnormality. It was concluded that long-term exposure to moderate to high levels of MC resulted in mild encephalopathy.

Two women involved in a degreasing operation repeatedly immersed their hands in MC for several hours at a time and developed symptoms of peripheral neuropathy (16). The exposures occurred over periods of 1 and 3 months. Nerve conduction studies indicated a reduction in action potential amplitudes and distal latencies. Neither case could be directly associated with exposure to a particular chemical. A third case of sensory neuropathy associated with the degreasing operation of the same plant was reported separately; two other cases with complaints of mild parethesias were also identified (7). A woman who had worked elsewhere as a degreaser reported symptoms of perioral tingling and burning, hand and foot discomfort, and foot cramps (6). Exposure to MC may have occurred by both the dermal and inhalation routes; however, this report did not include analytical confirmation of exposure levels. Nerve conduction studies were unremarkable except that sural nerve amplitude and conduction velocity were decreased. Six months following removal from work, the woman's symptoms had almost disappeared.

No differences in neurological symptoms, neurological examinations, nerve conduction studies, or psychomotor tests were detected in an epidemiological study of 22 women exposed to 110–990 ppm MC for a mean period of 6.7 years (17). Likewise, no significant effect was found on assessment of clinical signs or electrocardiograms among a group of 151 MC-exposed workers (12).

The American Conference of Governmental Industrial Hygienists has published a recommended Threshold Limit Value for MC of 350 ppm to prevent objectionable odor perception (2). At higher concentrations, the odor of MC becomes objectionable and, at even higher levels, liver and kidney effects have been reported. At anesthetic levels of MC, cardiac arrhythmias leading to death may occur (2).

Convincing evidence of neurotoxicity, beyond CNS depression or anesthesia, has not been demonstrated in animal studies. Since MC is not particularly soluble in blood (due to its physiochemical characteristics), attempts have been made in animal studies to increase brain MC levels by creating high-level continuous or near-continuous exposures. However, even under these conditions, it is not clear that the effects are unconfounded by reduced nutrition levels, altered blood gases, or reduced natural stimulation present in environments where animals are not continuously depressed. It may be argued that such conditions simulate solvent-abuse conditions, but this assertion is speculative as there is no recognized rodent model for such conditions. Study of human volunteers and epidemiological studies of occupational populations have not revealed convincing evidence of neurotoxicity beyond the anesthetic properties apparent in animal studies. The small number of case reports of sensory neuropathy in MC workers bears continued observation, but these cases do not provide evidence of a causal link with MC exposure.

REFERENCES

1. Adams EM, Spencer HC, Rowe VK, Irish DD (1950) Vapor toxicity of 1,1,1-trichloroethane (methyl chloroform) determined by experiments on laboratory animals. *Arch Ind Hyg Occup Med* 1, 225.

2. American Conference of Governmental Industrial Hygienists (1992) Methyl chloroform. In: *Documentation of the Threshold Limit Values. Vol 11. 6th Ed.* Cincinnati, Ohio p. 958.

3. Droz PO, Wu MM, Cumberland WG, Berode M (1989) Variability in biological monitoring of solvent exposure. I. Development of a population physiological model. *Brit J Ind Med* 46, 447.

4. Evans EB, Balster RL (1993) Inhaled 1,1,1-trichloroethane produced physical dependance in mice: Effects of drugs and vapors on withdrawal. *J Pharmacol Exp Ther* 264, 726.

5. Gehring PJ (1968) Hepatotoxic potency of various chlorinated hydrocarbon vapours relative to their narcotic and lethal potencies in mice. *Toxicol Appl Pharmacol* 13, 287.

6. House RA, Liss GM, Wills MC (1994) Peripheral sensory neuropathy associated with 1,1,1-trichloroethane. *Arch Environ Health* 49, 196.

7. Howse DC, Shanks GL, Nag S (1989) Peripheral neuropathy following prolonged exposure to methyl chloroform. *Neurology* 39, 242.

8. Ikeda M, Ohtsuji H (1972) A comparative study of the excretion of Fujiwara reaction-positive substances in urine of humans and rodents given trichloro- or tetrachloro-derivatives of ethane and ethylene. *Brit J Ind Med* 29, 99.

9. Jones HE, Kunko PM, Robinson SE, Balster RL (1996) Developmental consequences of intermittent and continuous prenatal exposure to 1,1,1-trichloroethane in mice. *Pharmacol Biochem Behav* 55, 635.

10. Karlsson J-E, Rosengren LE, Kjellstrand P, Haglid KG (1987) Effects of low-dose inhalation of three chlorinated aliphatic organic solvents on deoxyribonucleic acid in gerbil brain. *Scand J Work Environ Health* 13, 453.

11. Kelefant GA, Berg RA, Scleenbaker R (1993) Letter to the editor: Toxic encephalopathy due to 1,1,1-trichloroethane. *J Occup Med* 35, 554.

12. Kramer CG, Ott MG, Fulkerson JE et al. (1978) Health of workers exposed to 1,1,1-trichloroethane: A matched-pair study. *Arch Environ Health* 33, 331.

13. Krantz JC Jr, Park CS, Ling JSL (1959) Anesthesia LX: The anesthetic properties of 1,1,1-trichloroethane. *Anesthesiology* 20, 635.

14. Kyrklund T, Haglid KG (1990) Exposure of rats to high concentrations of 1,1,1-trichloroethane and its effects on brain lipid and fatty acid composition. *Pharmacol Toxicol* 67, 384.

15. Kyrklund T, Kjellstrand P, Haglid KG (1988) Effects of exposure to Freon 11, 1,1,1-trichloroethane or perchloroethylene on the lipid and fatty-acid composition of rat cerebral cortex. *Scand J Work Environ Health* 14, 91.

16. Liss GM (1981) Letter to the editor: Peripheral neuropathy in two workers exposed to 1,1,1-trichloroethane. *J Amer Med Assn* 260, 2217.

17. Maroni M, Bulgheroni C, Cassitto MG et al. (1977) A clinical, neurophysiological and behavioral study of female workers exposed to 1,1,1-trichloroethane. *Scand J Work Environ Health* 3, 16.

18. Mattsson JL, Albee RR, Lomax LG et al. (1993) Neurotoxicologic examination of rats exposed to 1,1,1-trichloroethane vapor for 13 weeks. *Neurotoxicol Teratol* 15, 313.

19. Maurissen JPJ, Shankar MR, Zielke GJ, Spencer PJ (1994) Lack of developmental cognitive and other neurobehavioral effects following maternal exposure to 1,1,1-trichloroethane in rats. *Toxicologist* 14, 163.

20. Mitoma C, Steeger T, Jackson SE et al. (1985) Metabolic disposition study of chlorinated hydrocarbons in rats and mice. *Drug Chem Toxicol* 8, 183.

21. Morgan A, Black A, Belcher DR (1970) The excretion in breath of some aliphatic halogenated hydrocarbons following administration by inhalation. *Ann Occup Hyg* 13, 219.

22. Moser VC, Balster RL (1986) The effects of inhaled toluene, halothane, 1,1,1-trichloroethane, and ethanol on fixed-interval responding in mice. *Neurobehav Toxicol Teratol* 8, 525.

23. Moser VC, Scimeca JC, Balster RL (1985) Minimal tolerance to the effects of 1,1,1-trichloroethane on fixed-ratio responding in mice. *Neurotoxicology* 6, 35.

24. Nilsson KB (1987) Effects of 1,1,1-trichloroethane on synaptosomal calcium accumulation in mouse brain. *Pharmacol Toxicol* 61, 215.

25. Prendergast JA, Jones RA, Jenkins LJ Jr, Siegel J (1967) Effects on experimental animals of long-term inhalation of trichloroethylene, carbon tetrachloride, 1,1,1-trichloroethane, dichlorodifluoromethane, and 1,1-dichloroethylene. *Toxicol Appl Pharmacol* 10, 270.

26. Rosengren LE, Aurella A, Kjellstrand P, Haglid KG (1985) Astrogliosis in the cerebral cortex of gerbils after long-term exposure to 1,1,1-trichloroethane. *Scand J Work Environ Health* 11, 447.

27. Rowe VK, Wujkowski MA, Wolf MA et al. (1963) Toxicity of a solvent mixture of 1,1,1-trichloroethane and tetrachloroethylene as determined by experiments on laboratory animals and human subjects. *Amer Ind Hyg Assn J* 24, 541.

28. Stewart RD, Dodd HC (1964) Absorption of carbon tetrachloride, trichloroethylene, methylene chloride, and 1,1,1-trichloroethane through human skin. *Amer Ind Hyg Assn J* 25, 439.

29. Torkelson TR, Oyen F, McCollister DD, Rowe VK (1958) Toxicity of 1,1,1-trichloroethane as determined on laboratory animals and human subjects. *Amer Ind Hyg Assn J* 19, 353.

30. York RG, Sowery BM, Hastings L, Manson JM (1982) Evaluation of teratogenicity and neurotoxicity with maternal inhalation exposure to methyl chloroform. *J Toxicol Environ Health* 9, 251.

Trichloroethylene

Herbert H. Schaumburg

$$Cl-\underset{\underset{Cl}{|}}{C}=\underset{\underset{}{|}}{CH}$$

Cl Cl

TRICHLOROETHYLENE
C_2HCl_3

Trichloroethene; Ethinyl trichloride

NEUROTOXICITY RATING

Clinical

A Acute encephalopathy (CNS depression)

C Cranial neuropathy

C Peripheral neuropathy

Experimental

A Acute encephalopathy

Trichloroethylene (TCE) is an industrial solvent and degreasing agent. TCE was formerly used as a general anesthetic; it has been abandoned in North America because its use is associated with arrhythmia and fluctuation in blood pressure from myocardial sensitization to catecholamines. Cranial neuropathy is widely attributed to TCE neurotoxicity; it likely represents an effect of dichloroacetylene (*see* Dichloroacetylene, this volume) which is formed when TCE is heated or comes into contact with alkali agents. In 1991, the American Conference of Governmental Industrial Hygienists set a Time-Weighted Average Threshold Limit Value for TCE of 50 ppm.

TCE is well absorbed after inhalation or ingestion. It is metabolized by a cytochrome P-450 mixed function oxidase system to trichloroacetaldehyde, which is subsequently metabolized to trichloroacetic acid. Trichloroethanol metabolism requires the enzyme alcohol dehydrogenase. Alcohol consumption in individuals exposed to TCE can cause transient redness of the face and neck ("degreaser's flush") thought to be related to competition for the enzyme.

There is little systemic toxicity from TCE save for mucous membrane irritation and defatting of skin. Several experimental animal studies with commercial-grade TCE have produced liver carcinoma in mice. Epidemiological studies have not shown a potent human carcinogenic effect (8).

Rats become ataxic when exposed to levels of 400 ppm for more than 30 min. The minimal full anesthetic dose for rodents is 4800 ppm. There have been several neurobehavioral studies of rodents chronically exposed to TCE. An especially detailed study exposed rats to pure TCE at 500, 1000, and 1500 ppm daily for 18 weeks and noted no significant abnormalities (5). Dogs exposed to TCE vapor at levels of 500–3000 ppm for 162 h became ataxic and displayed degeneration of Purkinje cells at postmortem ex-

amination (1). A study of the rat trigeminal nerve after daily gavage of animals with 2.5 mg/kg TCE produced no conclusive evidence of axonal degeneration (2).

Humans exposed to 200 ppm for 1 h experience lightheadedness and headache; exposure at this same level for 7 h/day for 5 days caused persistent headache and irritation; testing at the end of this interval disclosed no neurological or neuropsychological dysfunction (9). Inhalation at levels of 5000 ppm produces light anesthesia. Studies of cognitive function of workers with many years of exposure to TCE have yielded conflicting results. Some report a nonspecific "psycho-organic syndrome" (4), others report no neuropsychological dysfunction (10). It is claimed that low-level TCE exposure may produce abnormalities of the blink reflex and that this is a good measure for detection of subclinical intoxication (3). This proposal is not supported by other human studies (6,7).

REFERENCES

1. Baker AB (1958) The nervous system in trichloroethylene. An experimental study. *J Neuropathol Exp Neurol* **17**, 649.
2. Barret L, Torch S, Leray CL *et al.* (1992) Morphometric and biochemical studies in trigeminal nerve of rat after trichloroethylene or dichloroacetylene oral administration. *NeuroToxicology* **13**, 601.
3. Feldman RG, Niles C, Proctor SP, Jabre J (1992) Blink reflex measurement of effects of trichloroethylene exposure on the trigeminal nerve. *Muscle Nerve* **15**, 490.
4. Grandjean E, Munchinger R, Turrian V *et al.* (1955) Investigations into the effects of exposure to trichloroethylene in mechanical engineering. *Brit J Ind Med* **12**, 131.
5. Kulig BM (1987) The effects of chronic trichloroethylene exposure on neurobehavioral functioning in the rat. *Neurotoxicol Teratol* **9**, 171.
6. Lash TL (1993) Blink reflex measurement of effects of trichloroethylene exposure on the trigeminal nerve. *Muscle Nerve* **16**, 217.
7. Laureno R (1993) Trichloroethylene does not cause trigeminal neuropathy. *Muscle Nerve* **16**, 217.
8. Spirtas R, Stewart PA, Lee JS *et al.* (1991) Retrospective cohort mortality study of workers at an aircraft maintenance facility. I. Epidemiological results. *Brit J Ind Med* **48**, 515.
9. Stewart RD, Dodd HC, Gay HH, Erley DS (1970) Experimental human exposure to trichloroethylene. *Arch Environ Health* **20**, 64.
10. Triebig G, Schaller KH, Erzigkeit H, Valentin H (1977) Biochemische untersuchungen und psychologische studien an chronisch trichlorathylen–belasteten personen unter berucksichtigung expositionsfrier intervalle. *Int Arch Occup Environ Health* **38**, 149.

Tricyclic Antidepressants

Arnold E. Merriam

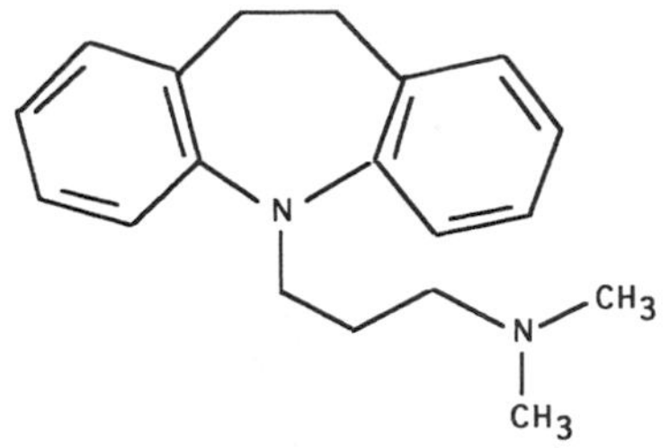

IMIPRAMINE
$C_{19}H_{24}N_2$

5-(3-Dimethylaminopropyl)-10,11-dihydro-5H-dibenz[b,f]azepine

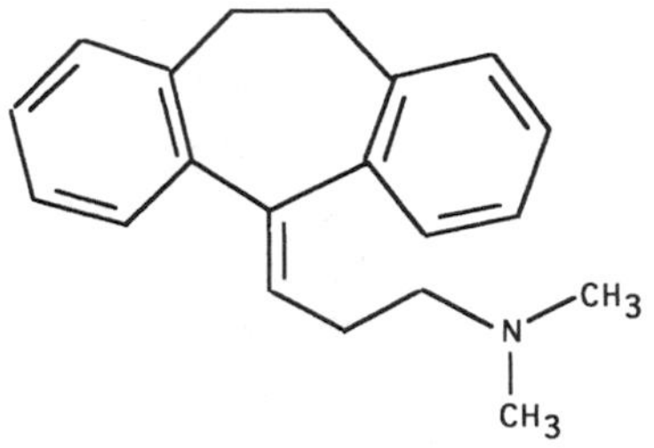

AMITRIPTYLINE
$C_{20}H_{23}N$

3-(10,11-Dihydro-5H-dibenzo[a,d]cyclohepten-5-ylidene)-N,N-dimethyl-1-propanamine

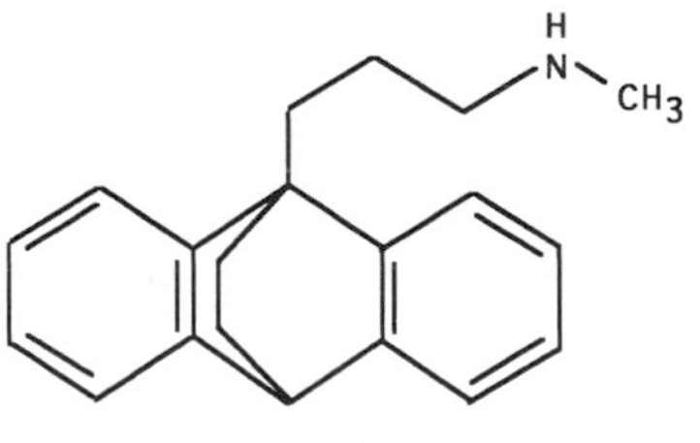

MAPROTILINE
$C_{20}H_{23}N$

N-Methyl-9,10-ethanoanthracene-9(10H)-propanamine

NEUROTOXICITY RATING
Clinical

A   Seizure disorder (myoclonus)

A   Psychobiological reaction (serotonin syndrome, anticholinergic syndrome)

A   Tremor

B   Extrapyramidal syndrome (choreoathetosis, dyskinesia)

The tricyclic and tetracyclic antidepressants are considered as a group because these agents share common neurotoxic propensities. The drug categories encompass a large number of structurally and biochemically similar agents; the chemical names, formulas, and structures of several prototypical agents are provided. The term "tetracyclic," used to characterize maprotiline, refers to an additional ethylene bridge across the central 6-carbon-atom ring of a tricyclic structure; maprotiline is toxicologically similar to the tricyclic agents; in this chapter, the term "tricyclic" may be understood to refer to both types of compounds.

The tricyclic antidepressants are well absorbed after oral administration, undergo extensive first-pass hepatic metabolism, and reach peak plasma concentrations within 2–8 h. Because many of these agents exhibit antimuscarinic activity, gastric emptying may be retarded with a resultant delay in reaching plasma level peak, especially in the context of drug overdose: in one case, 20% of an oral dose was recovered from the gastric contents 6 h after ingestion (12). The agents are widely distributed, with apparent volumes of distribution in the range of 10–50 l/kg. They are relatively lipophilic and bound to tissue and plasma proteins (in excess of 85%): the tissue:plasma ratio typically exceeds 10:1. These compounds are metabolized through dealkylation and oxidation by hepatic microsomal systems, followed by conjugation with glucuronic acid. Intermediate metabolites are in some instances known to exhibit biological activity; for example, the monodemethylated metabolites of the tricyclic tertiary amines imipramine and amitriptyline (i.e., desmethylimipramine, or desipramine, and nortriptyline) are potent amine-reuptake inhibitors and are manufactured as tricyclic antidepressants in their own right. There is considerable interindividual and interagent variation in plasma half-life, which ranges from somewhat less than a day (for imipramine in those <65 years of age) to as long as 3 days (for desipramine in those >65 years of age) (7).

These agents are primarily used in the treatment of depressive mood states, but they have also found utility in the treatment of panic attacks and obsessive-compulsive disorder. They are also used in the management of chronic pain syndromes and of childhood enuresis. The target structures are presumed to be CNS serotonergic and adrenergic neurotransmitter systems, where the agents block the reuptake of serotonin and norepinephrine. They also exhibit blockade of 5-HT$_2$ serotonergic, α_1-adrenergic, muscarinic, and H$_1$- and H$_2$-histaminic receptors. There is considerable variation in these actions among the tricyclic agents: maprotiline, for example, exerts much more amine-reuptake blocking effect for norepinephrine than for serotonin, while clomipramine exhibits the reverse profile. The major neurohumoral effects in humans of the most commonly used tricyclic agents are presented in Table 60 (11).

Secondary receptor effects have also been identified, chief among them being desensitization of postsynaptic β_1-adrenoreceptors (11). Which, if any, of these neurohumoral alterations is germane to these compounds' potent psychotropic effects is uncertain. The failure thus far to specify the mechanism of therapeutic action of these agents is not unexpected given the lack of a comprehensive understanding of the biological substrata of depression and of the anxiety disorders.

Extensive work has been performed with laboratory animals to evaluate the effects of tricyclic antidepressants on neurohumoral transmission and receptor physiology, with the aim of elucidating their mode of therapeutic action. Particularly relevant to the neurotoxicology of these agents have been the many studies evaluating their various receptor antagonistic effects. Radioligand studies have determined the degree to which different agents antagonize the various receptor types, in animals as well as humans. The potency with which the various agents antagonize these receptors correlates well with their propensities to induce par-

ticular neurotoxic syndromes, for example, toxic anticholinergic states (1).

Almost all data concerning the neurotoxic profiles of these agents have been gathered from studies of large numbers of patients in clinical treatment or from case reports of individuals exhibiting specific neurotoxic states.

A fine postural tremor is sometimes seen in patients with therapeutic tricyclic antidepressant concentrations: it has been identified in up to 10% of patients treated with imipramine but is rarely of clinically significant proportions. When tremor is particularly bothersome, it may usually be treated effectively with propranolol (4). There are no reports of tremor persisting past termination of tricyclic administration.

Another common complication of tricyclic treatment is the development of myoclonus, usually involving the limbs; both myoclonus during wakefulness and nocturnal myoclonus have been reported. This dose-related symptom is dose-related and seems to be more common with agents that are active serotonin-reuptake inhibitors. Myoclonus is usually minor in degree; if it fails to respond to lowering the dose of the agent prescribed or if the dose cannot be

TABLE 60. Potencies of Antidepressants for Blockade of Neurotransmitter Receptors and Neurotransmitter Uptake*

Drug	Uptake Blockade[†]			Neurotransmitter Receptor Blockade[‡]		
	NE	5-HT	H_1	Muscarinic	$5\text{-}HT_2$	D_2
Antidepressants						
Amitriptyline	4.2	1.5	91	*5.5*	3.4	0.10
Amoxapine	23	0.21	4.0	0.1	*170*	*0.62*
Bupropion	0.043	*0.0064*	*0.015*	0.0021	*0.0011*	*0.00048*
Desipramine	*110*	0.29	0.91	0.50	0.36	0.030
Doxepin	5.3	0.36	*420*	1.2	4.0	0.042
Fluoxetine	0.36	*8.3*	0.016	0.050	0.48	0.015
Imipramine	7.7	2.4	9.1	1.1	1.2	0.050
Maprotiline	14	0.030	50	0.18	0.83	0.28
Nortriptyline	25	0.38	10	0.67	2.3	0.083
Protriptyline	100	0.36	4.0	4.0	1.5	0.043
Trazodone	*0.020*	0.53	0.28	*0.00031*	13	0.026
Trimipramine	0.20	*0.040*	370	1.7	3.1	0.56
Reference Compounds						
d-Amphetamine	2.0	—	—	—	—	—
Diphenhydramine	—	—	7.1	—	—	—
Atropine	—	—	—	42	—	—
Methysergide	—	—	—	—	15	—
Haloperidol	—	—	—	—	—	26

*Data can be compared both vertically and horizontally to find the most potent drug for a specific property and to find the most potent property of a specific drug. In each column, the highest (underlined boldface italics) and lowest (italics) numbers are emphasized for antidepressants.

[†]$10^{-7} \times 1/K_i$, in which K_i = inhibitor constant in molarity.

[‡]$10^{-7} \times 1/K_D$, in which K_D = equilibrium dissocation in molarity.

D_2, dopamine; H_1, histamine; 5-HT and $5\text{-}HT_2$, 5-hydroxytryptamine (serotonin-1 and serotonin-2); NE, norepinephrine.

[Reproduced with permission from Richelson (11).]

lowered on psychiatric grounds, treatment with clonazapam has been used with some success. Myoclonus is regularly seen with drug overdose (8). A patient who develops myoclonus after a long period of otherwise uncomplicated treatment with a tricyclic agent should be evaluated for other signs of toxicity, since this sign may presage the development of a wider neurotoxic syndrome.

Many tricyclic antidepressants are strongly active blockers of muscarinic receptors; an anticholinergic syndrome affecting the CNS and PNS may complicate use of these agents and is a regular feature of overdoses (Table 60). PNS signs include urinary retention, impaired ocular accommodation, diminished sweating, and tachycardia. Central signs include memory impairment and, in more severe cases, delirium. There is no satisfactory correlation between the degree of detectable central and peripheral anticholinergic signs, and many patients with tricyclic-induced cognitve disruption fail to demonstrate striking peripheral signs of cholinergic blockade (9). A full-blown neurological picture of tricyclic antidepressant poisoning, as is seen in overdose, consists of delirium, stupor or coma, generalized seizures, respiratory depression, pupillary dilatation, myoclonus and/ or choreoathetosis, dry mucous membranes, tachycardia, hypotension, and urinary retention (6). Severe tricyclic antidepressant intoxication has been reported to abolish oculocephalic reflexes and to prolong brainstem auditory evoked potentials (10,14). Tricyclic antidepressant overdose may produce electroencephalographic patterns of alpha coma or spindle coma, tracings more usually seen following diffuse hypoxic ischemic brain damage, head trauma, or brainstem infarction (10).

Cardiac dysfunction constitutes the most dangerous aspect of overdose. Seizures are usually self-limited and rarely affect outcome; they may be terminated if necessary with benzodiazepine administration.

Infusion of physostigmine, a cholinesterase inhibitor, rapidly reverses the anticholinergic aspects of the neurotoxic syndrome (e.g., altered or depressed sensorium and peripheral anticholinergic signs) (5). While rapid clearing of the sensorium after physostigmine implies that the patient is suffering from anticholinergic toxicity and may provide helpful diagnostic information, physostigmine itself can induce seizures and cardiac arrhythmia, and its administration for therapeutic purposes is not routinely recommended in known tricyclic overdose.

Psychotropic drug-induced interference with muscarinic cholinergic transmission produces defects in learning and memory, effects that may be quite subtle (13).

Seizures, a common complication of tricyclic overdose, occur in low incidence during tricyclic administration at therapeutic levels. The tendency for these agents to provoke seizures has been overestimated in the past; the current literature suggests an incidence of at most 1% (3), except for maprotiline, which may exhibit a somewhat higher rate (2).

Choreoathetoid movements can be seen during drug intoxication. Several dozen case reports suggest that tricyclic compounds may also induce a tardive dyskinesia-like syndrome (15). Interpretation of this literature is complicated by the fact that many reported cases involve subjects with prior exposure to neuroleptics. Since anticholinergic agents may exacerbate tardive dyskinesia, it is possible that many patients with ostensible tricyclic-induced dyskinesia instead suffered from pre-existent subclinical dyskinetic syndromes made overt as a result of the anticholinergic properties of the tricyclic compound.

REFERENCES

1. Hall H, Ogren S-O (1981) Effects of antidepressant drugs on different receptors in the brain. *Eur J Pharmacol* 70, 393.

2. Jabbari B, Bryan GE, Marsh EE, Gunderson CH (1985) Incidence of seizures with tricyclic and tetracyclic antidepressants. *Arch Neurol* 42, 480.

3. Jick SS, Jick H, Knauss TA, Dean AD (1992) Antidepressants and convulsions. *J Clin Psychopharmacol* 12, 241.

4. Kronfol Z, Greden JF, Zis AP (1983) Imipramine-induced tremor: Effects of a beta-adrenergic blocking agent. *J Clin Psychiat* 44, 225.

5. Newton R (1975) Physostigmine salicylate in the treatment of tricyclic antidepressant overdosage. *J Amer Med Assn* 231, 941.

6. Newton EH, Shih RD, Hoffman RS (1994) Cyclic antidepressant overdose: A review of current management strategies. *Amer J Emerg Med* 12, 376.

7. Nies A, Robinson D, Friedman M *et al.* (1977) Relationship between age and tricyclic antidepressant plasma level. *Amer J Psychiat* 134, 790.

8. Noble J, Matthew H (1969) Acute poisoning by tricyclic antidepressants: Clinical features and management of 100 patients. *Clin Toxicol* 2, 403.

9. Pulst SM, Lombroso CT (1983) External ophthalmoplegia, alpha and spindle coma in imipramine overdose: Case report and review of the literature. *Ann Neurol* 14, 587.

10. Preskorn SH, Jerkovich GS (1990) Central nervous system toxicity of tricyclic antidepressants: Phenomenology, course, risk factors, and role of therapeutic drug monitoring. *J Clin Psychopharmacol* 10, 88.

11. Richelson E (1990) Antidepressants and brain neurochemistry. *Mayo Clin Proc* 65, 1227.

12. Saraf KR, Klein AF, Gittelman-Klein R *et al.* (1974) Imipramine dose effects in children. *Psychopharmacologia* 37, 265.

13. Tune LE, Strauss ME, Lew MF *et al.* (1982) Serum levels of anticholinergic drugs and impaired recent memory in

chronic schizophrenic patients. *Amer J Psychiat* **139**, 1460.

14. White A (1988) Overdose of tricyclic antidepressants associated with absent brain-stem reflexes. *Can Med Assn J* **139**, 133.

15. Yassa, R, Camille Y, Belzile L (1987) Tardive dyskinesia in the course of antidepressant therapy: A prevalence study and review of the literature. *J Clin Psychopharmacol* **7**, 243.

Triethyltin

Georg J. Krinke

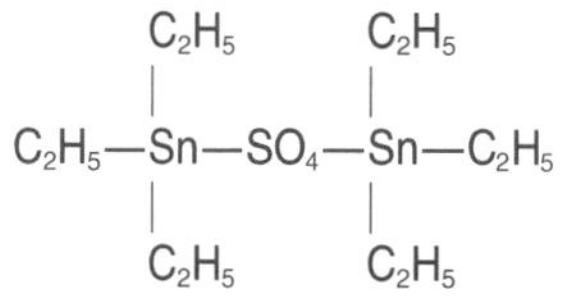

$$C_2H_5—Sn—SO_4—Sn—C_2H_5$$

with C_2H_5 groups on each Sn

TRIETHYLTIN
$C_{12}H_{30}Sn_2SO_4$

$[(C_2H_5)_3Sn]SO_4$
(– sulphate)
$(C_2H_5)_3Sn–OH$
(– hydroxide)
$(C_2H_5)_3Sn–O–CO–CH_3$
(– acetate)

Bis triethyltin sulphate

NEUROTOXICITY RATING

Clinical

A Leukoencephalopathy (diffuse)

Experimental

A Vacuolar myelinopathy in CNS & PNS

Organotins have been used as industrial chemicals and biocides. Triethyltin (TET) compounds have especially strong biocidal properties. The neurotoxicity of TET became apparent when this agent contaminated a pharmaceutical preparation causing inadvertent intoxication of hundreds of persons. Since then, TET has been solely used as a neurotoxicant in experimental animal studies. In contrast to a similar organotin compound, trimethyltin (*see* Trimethyltin, this volume), which damages neurons and gray matter, TET damages the white matter.

TET is a colorless liquid, insoluble in water and soluble only in organic solvents. Triethyltin hydroxide, acetate and sulfate are water-soluble and have crystalline forms. The U.S. ceiling for occupational exposure to TET is an Sn concentration of 100 μg/m^3 (32).

TET is absorbed *via* the skin and from the gastrointestinal tract. The oral LD$_{50}$ is 4.0 mg/kg for rats. The lethal orally administered dose of TET sulfate to rats, or intraperitoneally (i.p.) administered dose to rabbits, is 10 mg/kg. Although specific tissue damage occurs in the CNS, brain levels of TET following exposure are lower than those in the liver or blood. In blood, TET binds to the globin site of hemoglobin (32).

After i.p. administration of lethal or sublethal levels of TET sulfate, rats rapidly develop generalized weakness (most prominent in the hindlimbs), stupor, and death. Suckling mice are more sensitive to i.p. TET than mature mice (21,32). Daily i.p. administration of 5 mg/kg to newborn rats resulted in death of all animals within 3 days (30). Rats and rabbits receiving repeated i.p. TET sulfate at a dose of 1 mg/kg/day developed clinical signs and died after about a week (5,26,31). Rats receiving a diet containing 20 ppm of TET hydroxide showed weakness of the hindlimbs after 7–9 days and, by day 14, their hindlimbs were motionless. Reduction of exposure level or termination of exposure resulted in a gradual functional recovery, but then the animals developed tremor and convulsions and died (6,17,21). Similar signs were observed with TET acetate (24). Dietary exposure of rats to 40 and 80 ppm TET hydroxide induced quadriplegia and death after about 2 weeks; the survivors recovered in about 5 days (6,28). Prolonged duration of encephalopathy for 3 months was achieved in rats given TET in drinking water at concentrations of 5–10 ppm (11); the clinical signs of paraparesis started on day 12. Other studies have examined the sensitivity of dogs and cats to TET (17,28) and the effects of intravenous administration or implantation of TET pellets into the rat brain (16,18).

Brains of intoxicated animals are pale and enlarged; the cerebral cortex is flattened because of diffuse edema and increased intracranial pressure. The predominant early light microscopical change is diffuse vacuolation of the white matter, with no change in oligodendrocyte nuclei. In the brains of clinically recovered animals, no vacuolation is seen and no loss of myelinated fibers is obvious. Electron microscopy shows that myelin vacuoles in the CNS and PNS are formed by splitting of the myelin lamellae at the intraperiod line (15)—the fused outer layers of the cell membranes of oligodendrocytes and Schwann cells. The extracellular space in the brain, however, is not widened, and the blood vessels and their permeability are not compromised. The lipid composition of myelin is unaltered, and the edema fluid consists of water containing high levels of sodium and chloride. Although changes in the myelin sheaths predominate, astrocytes show some cellular swelling (32). In severe, advanced lesions, breakdown of myelin and secondary changes in other tissue elements may occur. The lesion is most prominent in the CNS, including optic nerves, but involves the peripheral myelin as well. There is a proximodistal gradient of damage in peripheral nerves; anterior nerve roots are more involved than posterior roots, and the proximal sciatic nerve is less involved than the spinal roots (18,32). Decreased motor nerve conduction velocity has been observed in peripheral nerves of rats exposed to TET (12,23).

TET sulfate applied to well-myelinated explants of spinal cord of fetal mice induced immediate morphological changes, suggesting a direct toxic action of TET, rather than that of a metabolite (13). Other *in vitro* studies, using tissue slices, homogenates, and mitochondrial preparations, demonstrate that TET uncouples oxidative phosphorylation and inhibits mitochondrial adenosine triphosphatase (ATPase). TET can mediate ion transport or anion-hydroxide exchange across the mitochondrial membrane (2,3,22, 27,29). Glucose oxidation by brain slices is very sensitive, especially the rate of oxidation of pyruvate formed from glucose, which is decreased (10,19).

An epidemic of human TET intoxication occurred in France in the 1950s in association with the therapeutic use of Stalinon, a medication developed for treatment of acne, osteomyelitis, and anthrax. The active agent in Stalinon was diethyltin diiodide, which has a low toxicity, but it was contaminated with up to 10% TET. The toxic dose for an adult was estimated to be 70 mg of TET taken over 8 days (7). Several hundred persons were poisoned, 102 died, and at least 100 others were affected permanently. Clinical symptoms appeared after a period of about 4 days; they included persistent headache, nausea, vomiting, vertigo, meningeal signs, convulsions, photophobia, visual disturbance, papilledema, and transient paresis to permanent paralysis. Somatic manifestations included retention of urine, abdominal pain, rapid loss of weight, and occasional hyperthermia. The cerebrospinal fluid showed an abnormally raised pressure but a normal chemical and cellular profile. Recovery was slow and, in many instances, incomplete. Neuropathological examination of decedents revealed diffuse edema of the white matter similar to that induced with TET in experimental animals (1,9,14,25). Therapeutic measures for prevention or amelioration of TET-induced brain edema include the administration of high-osmolar agents and steroids (32).

The toxic property of TET depends on the presence of ethyl groups in the molecule; organotins devoid of ethyl groups are not myelinotoxic. Experiments with trialkyltins containing either two ethyl groups and one methyl group, or vice versa, demonstrate that compounds containing two ethyl groups are more myelinotoxic and less neuronotoxic than those containing two methyl and one ethyl group (4). TET appears to act directly on myelin lamellae, as purified rat brain myelin binds TET (20) and morphological observations on spinal cord cultures indicate an immediate TET effect (13). Detergent-like effects on membranes and disruption of hydrophobic regions of membrane proteins might account for splitting and partial dissolution of myelin, but additional biochemical effects are needed to explain the development of edema (8). The ability of TET to uncouple oxidative phosphorylation, reduce respiration, and inhibit mitochondrial ATPase may contribute to changes in cell membrane permeability, and may be associated with both the toxic and the general biocidal effects of TET.

REFERENCES

1. Alajouanine T, Dérobert L, Thieffry S (1958) Étude clinique d'ensemble de 210 cas d'intoxication par les sel organiques d'étain. *Rev Neurol* **98**, 85.
2. Aldridge WN, Cremer JE (1955) The biochemistry of organotin compounds. Diethyltin dichloride and triethyltin sulfate. *Biochem J* **61**, 406.
3. Aldridge WN, Street BW (1971) Oxidative phosphorylation: The relation between the specific binding of trimethyltin and triethyltin to mitochondria and their effects on various mitochondrial functions. *Biochem J* **124**, 221.
4. Aldridge WN, Verschoyle RD, Thompson CA, Brown AW (1987) The toxicity and neuropathology of dimethylethyltin and methyldiethyltin in rats. *Neuropathol Appl Neurobiol* **13**, 55.
5. Aleu FR, Katzman R, Terry RD (1963) Fine structure and electrolyte analyses of cerebral edema induced by alkyltin intoxication. *J Neuropathol Exp Neurol* **22**, 403.
6. Bakay L (1965) Morphological and chemical studies in cerebral edema. Triethyltin-induced edema. *J Neurol Sci* **2**, 52.
7. Barnes JM, Stoner HB (1959) The toxicology of tin compounds. *Pharmacol Rev* **11**, 211.
8. Cammer W (1980) Toxic demyelination: Biochemical studies and hypothetical mechanisms. In: *Experimental and Clinical Neurotoxicology*. Spencer PS, Schaumburg HH eds. Williams & Wilkins, Baltimore, Maryland p. 239.
9. Cossa P, Duplay, Arfel-Capdeville *et al.* (1959) Encephalopathies toxiques au Stalinon: Aspects anatomocliniques

et électroencephalographiques. *Acta Neurol Psychiat Belg* **59**, 281.

10. Cremer JE (1962) The action of triethyltin, triethyllead, ethyl mercury and other inhibitors of the metabolism of brain and kidney slices *in vitro* using substrates labeled with ¹⁴C. *J Neurochem* **9**, 289.

11. Eto Y, Suzuki K, Suzuki K (1971) Lipid composition of rat brain myelin in triethyltin-induced edema. *J Lipid Res* **12**, 570.

12. Graham DI, deJesus PV, Pleasure DE, Gonatas NK (1976) Triethyltin sulfate-induced neuropathy in rats. *Arch Neurol* **33**, 40.

13. Graham DI, Kim SU, Gonatas NK, Guyotte L (1975) The neurotoxic effects of triethyltin sulfate on myelinating cultures of mouse spinal cord. *J Neuropathol Exp Neurol* **34**, 401.

14. Gruner JE (1958) Lésions du névraxe secondaires à l'ingestion d'ethylétain (Stalinon). *Rev Neurol* **98**, 109.

15. Hirano A, Dembitzer HM, Becker NH (1969) The distribution of peroxidase in the triethyl-intoxicated rat brain. *J Neuropathol Exp Neurol* **28**, 507.

16. Hirano A, Zimmerman KM, Levine S (1968) Intramyelinic and extracellular spaces in triethyltin intoxication. *J Neuropathol Exp Neurol* **27**, 571.

17. Kalsbeck JE, Cummings JN (1963) Experimental edema in the rat and cat brain. *J Neuropathol Exp Neurol* **22**, 237.

18. Leow ACT, Anderson RMcD, Little RA, Leaver DD (1979) A sequential study of changes in the brain and cerebrospinal fluid of the rat following triethyltin poisoning. *Acta Neuropathol* **47**, 117.

19. Lock EA (1976) The action of triethyltin on the respiration of rat brain cortex slices. *J Neurochem* **26**, 887.

20. Lock EA, Aldridge WN (1975) The binding of triethyltin to rat brain myelin. *J Neurochem* **25**, 871.

21. Magee PN, Stoner HB, Barnes JM (1957) The experimental production of edema in the central nervous system of the rat by triethyltin compounds. *J Pathol Bacteriol* **73**, 107.

22. Moore KE, Brody TM (1961) The effect of triethyltin on oxidative phosphorylation and mitochondrial adenosine triphospahtase activation. *Biochem Pharmacol* **6**, 125.

23. O'Shaugnessy DJ, Losos GJ (1986) Peripheral and central nervous system lesions caused by triethyl- and trimethyltin salts in rats. *Toxicol Pathol* **14**, 141.

24. Reed DJ, Woodbury PM, Holtzer RL (1964) Brain edema, electrolytes and extracellular space. Effect of triethyltin on brain and skeletal muscle. *Arch Neurol* **10**, 604.

25. Rouzaud M, Lutier J (1954) Oedéme subaigu cérébro-méningé du à une intoxication d'actualité. *Presse Médicale* **62**, 1075.

26. Scheinberg LD, Taylor JM, Herzog I, Mandell S (1966) Optical and peripheral nerve response to triethyltin intoxication in the rabbit: Biochemical and ultrastructural studies. *J Neuropathol Exp Neurol* **25**, 202.

27. Selwyn MJ, Dawson AP, Stockdale M, Grain N (1970) Chloridehydroxide exchange across mitochondrial, erythrocyte and artificial lipid membranes mediated by trialkyl and triphenyltin compounds. *Eur J Biochem* **14**, 120.

28. Smith JF, McLaurin RL, Nichols JB, Asbury A (1960) Studies in cerebral edema and cerebral swelling; I. The changes in lead encephalopathy in children compared with those in alkyltin poisoning in animals. *Brain* **83**, 411.

29. Stockdale M, Pawson AP, Selwyn MJ (1970) Effects of triethyltin and triphenyltin compounds on mitochondrial respiration. *Eur J Biochem* **15**, 342.

30. Suzuki K (1971) Some new observations in triethyl-tin intoxication of rats. *Exp Neurol* **31**, 207.

31. Torack RM, Gordon J, Prokop J (1970) Pathobiology of acute triethyltin intoxication. In: *International Review of Neurobiology. Vol XII.* Pfeiffer CC, Smythes JR eds. Academic Press, New York p. 45.

32. Watanabe I (1980) Organotins (triethyltin). In: *Experimental and Clinical Neurotoxicology.* Spencer PS, Schaumburg HH eds. Williams & Wilkins, Baltimore, Maryland p. 545.

Trihexyphenidyl Hydrochloride

John D. Rogers

TRIHEXYPHENIDYL HYDROCHLORIDE
$C_{20}H_{32}ClNO$

α-Cyclohexyl-α-phenyl-1-piperidinepropanol hydrochloride

NEUROTOXICITY RATING

Clinical

B   Acute encephalopathy (sedation, confusion)

Trihexyphenidyl, a tertiary amine and muscarinic receptor antagonist, is used for the treatment of Parkinson's disease (3), prophylaxis for drug-induced parkinsonism (1), essential tremor (2), and dystonia (4). The mechanism of action of trihexyphenidyl is uncertain. Acetylcholine is an important strial interneuronal neurotransmitter that potentiates a variety of dopaminergic actions in the brain (6), presumably *via* antagonist action by striatal interneurons. Muscarinic receptors have been identified in the basal forebrain, medulla oblongata, and pons (5).

Side effects of trihexyphenidyl include dry mouth, blurred vision, constipation, urinary hesitancy and retention, confusion, and sedation. These are dose-dependent and reversible with drug withdrawal.

REFERENCES

1. Arana GW, Goff DC, Baldessarini RJ (1988) Efficacy of anticholinergic prophylaxis of neuroleptic induced dystonia. *Amer J Psychiat* **145**, 993.
2. Finley LJ, Koller WC (1987) Essential tremor: A review. *Neurology* **37**, 1194.
3. Lang AE (1986) High dose anti-cholinergics in adult dystonia. *Can J Neurol Sci* **13**, 42.
4. Lang AE, Blair RDG (1989) Anticholinergic drugs and amantidine in the treatment of Parkinson's disease. In: *Drugs for the Treatment of Parkinson's Disease*. Calne DB ed. Springer-Verlag, Berlin p. 307.
5. Mesulam MM (1994) Structure and function of cholinergic pathways in the cerebral cortex, limbic system, basal ganglia and thalamus of the human brain. In: *Psychopharmacology: The Fourth Generation of Progress*. Bloom FE, Kupfer DJ eds. Raven Press, New York p. 657.
6. Pycock C, Milson J, Tarsy D (1978) The effect of manipulation of cholinergic mechanisms on turning behaviour in mice with unilateral destruction of the nigroneostriatal dopaminergic system. *Neuropharmacology* **17**, 175.

Trimethaphan Camsylate

Herbert H. Schaumburg

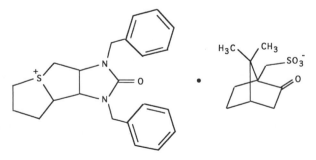

TRIMETHAPHAN CAMSYLATE
$C_{32}H_{40}N_2O_5S_2$

Decahydro-2-oxo-1,3-bis(phenylmethyl)thieno[1′,2′:1,2]-thieno[3,4-d]imidazol-5-ium salt with (1S)-7,7-dimethyl-2-oxobicyclo[2.2.1]heptane-1-methanesulfonic acid (1:1)

NEUROTOXICITY RATING

Clinical

A   Neuromuscular transmission syndrome

The sulfonium derivative trimethaphan is used as a vasodepressor agent during surgical procedures and in hypertensive emergencies. Trimethaphan acts as a ganglionic-blocking agent by competing with acetylcholine for the postsynaptic cholinergic receptor; this is in contrast to other ganglionic-blocking agents (*e.g.*, hexamethonium) that inhibit ganglionic transmission by blocking postsynaptic ion channels (5). The principal adverse consequence of trimethaphan treatment is severe hypotension; other toxic effects are due to nonselective blockade of the autonomic nervous system; they include mydriasis, urinary retention, impotence, ileus, and constipation.

Trimethaphan also may prolong the action of neuromuscular-blocking agents used in anesthetic procedures. Numerous case reports have documented prolonged apnea associated with combined succinylcholine-trimethaphan use (2,4,7,8). The pathogenesis of this neurotoxic effect is controversial; two disparate hypotheses have been suggested from clinical observations, (a) inhibition of cholinesterase (1,6), and (b) selective blockade of ion channels at the motor end-plate (3).

REFERENCES

1. Blitt CD, Petty WC, Alberternst EE *et al.* (1977) Correlation of plasma cholinesterase activity and duration of action of succinylcholine during pregnancy. *Anesth Analg* **56**, 78.
2. Deacock AR deC, Davies TDW (1958) The influence of certain ganglionic blocking agents on neuromuscular transmission. *Brit J Anaesth* **34**, 357.
3. Nakamura K, Hatano Y, Mori K (1988) The site of action of trimethaphan-induced neuromuscular blockade in isolated rat and frog muscle. *Acta Anaesth Scand* **32**, 125.
4. Poulton TJ, James FM, Lockridge O (1976) Prolonged apnea following trimethaphan and succinylcholine. *Anesthesiology* **50**, 54.
5. Rang HP (1982) The action of ganglionic blocking drugs on the synaptic responses of rat submandibular ganglion cells. *Brit J Pharmacol* **75**, 151.
6. Sklar GS, Lanks KW (1977) Effects of trimethaphan and sodium nitroprusside on hydrolysis of succinylcholine *in vitro. Anesthesiology* **47**, 31.
7. Wildsmith JAW (1972) Serum pseudocholinesterase, pregnancy and suxamethonium. *Anaesthesia* **27**, 90.
8. Wilson SL, Miller RN, Wright C *et al.* (1976) Prolonged neuromuscular blockade associated with trimethaphan: A case report. *Anesth Analg* **55**, 353.

Trimethobenzamide Hydrochloride

Herbert H. Schaumburg

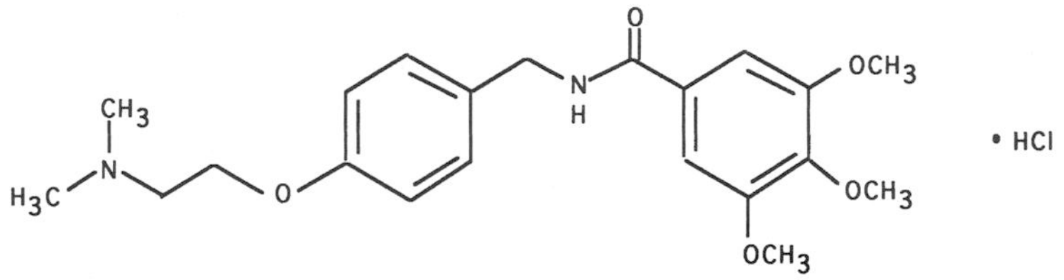

TRIMETHOBENZAMIDE HYDROCHLORIDE
$C_{21}H_{28}N_2O_5 \cdot HCl$

N-[(2-Dimethyaminoethoxy)benzyl]-3,4,5-trimethoxybenzamide

NEUROTOXICITY RATING

Clinical

B   Extrapyramidal syndrome (acute dystonia)

Trimethobenzamide is a dopaminergic-receptor blocking agent. It is used primarily as a parenterally administered antiemetic to combat nausea and vomiting from cancer chemotherapeutic agents. The mechanism of its weak antiemetic action is unclear; it appears to result from blockade of dopaminergic receptors.

The most serious potential toxic effect of trimethobenzamide is Reye's syndrome (hepatic failure, acute encephalopathy) in children with viral illness–induced vomiting who are treated with this agent or with other centrally acting antiemetics.

Neurotoxic reactions are rare and sometimes difficult to delineate from phenomena associated with the underlying condition requiring an antiemetic (*e.g.*, cancer, viral illness). Extrapyramidal reactions can accompany trimethobenzamide therapy, as they do with other antiemetic dopaminergic-blocking agents (metoclopramide). The most common extrapyramidal effect is an acute dystonic reaction following a single parenteral dose; tardive dyskinesia from chronic therapy is rare (1).

REFERENCE

1. Chouza C, Caamano JL, Romero S *et al.* (1985) Extrapyramidal effects of benzamides. *Adv Biochem Psychopharmacol* **40**, 43.

Trimethyltin

Georg J. Krinke

$$CH_3 - Sn - Cl$$

with CH_3 groups above and below the Sn.

TRIMETHYLTIN
C_3H_9SnCl

Trimethyltin chloride

NEUROTOXICITY RATING

Clinical

A Acute encephalopathy (limbic)

A Chronic encephalopathy (cognitive dysfunction)

Experimental

A Neuronopathy (hippocampus)

The highly toxic organic alkyltins take the form: $R_n Sn X_{4-n}$ (n = 1, 2, 3, 4), where R is an alkyl or other organic group and X is an inorganic or organic anion. Organotins are therefore classified as mono, di-, tri-, and tetraorganotins (30). Their toxicity depends on the number of organic groups and their structure. For example, triethyltin and trimethyltin (TMT) are both neurotoxic, but their target structures in the nervous system are different (*see* Triethyltin, this volume). Tributyltin compounds affect mainly organs of the immune system, such as the thymus or spleen, as well as the liver and kidney (6).

Organotin compounds have been used as plastic stabilizers, catalytic agents, industrial and agricultural biocides, antifouling paints, and pesticides. TMT is not produced commercially, but is generated as a by-product during the manufacturing of dimethyltin dichloride 1, a substance used as a plastic stabilizer. Owing to its propensity to damage the brain and to induce behavioral changes, TMT has become a research tool used in animal experimentation.

TMT chloride is usually obtained at 95% purity; preparations are contaminated with 4.4% dimethyltindichloride and 0.6% monomethyltin trichloride. The pure compound forms white crystals of high volatility (MP, 40°–50°C; BP, 140°–150°C) and water solubility (>40% at 20°C), yielding pH 3.5 at 2% concentration. It is also very lipid-soluble. TMT chloride is a highly toxic substance; strict protective measures must be taken when handling the compound.

TMT is orally well absorbed, and there is also evidence of inhalatory and cutaneous absorption. It is a cumulative and persistent poison. In rats, but not in most other species, it binds with high affinity to hemoglobin. The minimum overall concentration of TMT in rat brain associated with neuronal damage is approximately 1.4 μg/g wet weight. Signs of intoxication by TMT and tetramethyltin are very similar because tetramethyltin is rapidly converted to TMT after ingestion (7–9).

A single dose of about 3 mg/kg TMT is lethal for Syrian hamsters, gerbils, marmosets, and probably humans; the LD_{50} for the rat is much higher, about 13 mg/kg (7,9). Although repetitive, continuous, or discontinuous administration of TMT has been used, in some experiments, a single exposure to sublethal levels is sufficient to induce characteristic behavioral changes and neuronal damage.

Signs of poisoning include tremors, hyperexcitability, aggressive behavior, spontaneous seizures, sensory disturbances, learning and memory impairment, and self-mutilation of the tail (9,16,17,29,31,32). Some species fail to develop selected clinical signs [*e.g.*, aggressivity was not observed in gerbils or hamsters, and in hamsters no seizures occurred (9)]. In most species, the predominant pathological changes are present in the hippocampal formation and the basal (piriform/entorhinal) cortex of the brain. In the hippocampal formation, the damage is frequently observed in the "endplate sector," in contrast to anoxic/ischemic lesions, which are most prominent in "Sommer's sector" (7,16,20). Other areas of the nervous system may be affected as well, such as the neocortex, basal ganglia, cerebellum, brainstem, spinal cord, dorsal root ganglia, olfactory cortex, retina, and the inner ear (4,5,7,8,13). Peripheral nerves are not a major target of TMT toxicity, although changes in spinal motoneurons, nerve roots, and peripheral nerve fibers have been observed (2,23). The distribution of lesions within the nervous system, reflecting the neuronal interdependence, as well as the hierarchy of neuronal susceptibility, may vary from species to species and even within one species depending on the strain, age, and dosing regimen. For example, adult mice show the greatest damage in the hippocampal fascia dentata, while in rats and young mice it occurs in the hippocampal pyramidal cells and the olfactory cortex (15,16,24). In the hamster, neurons in the neocortex and basal cortex are more affected than in the hippocampus (9).

The major pathological finding by light microscopy is neuronal necrosis. The early change is characterized by a loss of Nissl substance; this is followed by condensation and clumping of the cytoplasm and subsequent shrinkage and fragmentation of the nucleus (7). Advanced neuronal necrosis is associated with proliferation of glial cells, loss of neurons and astrocytic gliosis. Astrocytes have increased glial fibrillary acidic protein and also react for vimentin and γ-aminobutyric acid (GABA), indicating a change in astrocytic phenotype, or metabolism of GABA (3). Less susceptible neurons may appear morphologically intact at the light-microscopical level despite the presence of ultrastructural alterations (13). Electron microscopy reveals small (~100–200 nm) vesicular or tubular electron-dense particles within the cytoplasm within 24 h of intoxication. They appear to form at the expense of the rough endoplasmic reticulum (e.r.) and to arise either from the rough e.r. devoid of ribosomes, or, more probably, from the smooth e.r. (8,21). In some neurons, dilatation of e.r. cisternae and of the Golgi complex is apparent. At a more advanced stage, the cytoplasm contains larger, electron-dense bodies (~300–400 nm) intermingled with well-preserved mitochondria. These bodies have occasional lamellar arrays and resemble autophagic vacuoles; the high activity of acid phosphatase confirms their lysosomal character (4). The loss of the rough e.r., together with the relative concentration of the mitochondria, account for the cytoplasmic eosinophilia of these neurons seen with the light microscope.

TMT is cytotoxic to cultured rat brain astrocytes and causes an increase in the level of glial fibrillary acidic protein, indicating that astrocytes react independently of neuronal signals. The activity of ecto-5′-nucleotidase, a cell-surface protein implicated in cellular adhesion and cell communication, is decreased (27).

Human exposures to TMT have occurred inadvertently (19,25,26,28), mostly in conjunction with the synthesis of dimethyltinchloride, so that the victims have been exposed to a mixture of both compounds. Two chemists exposed for about 3 months abruptly developed mental confusion and generalized seizures. They had previously complained of headache, episodes of violent pain in various organs, memory defects, loss of vigilance, insomnia, anorexia, and disorientation. Both recovered completely following removal from exposure (19). After trimethyltin chloride spillage in a chemical plant, 22 workers (12 with high and 10 with lower exposure) were submitted to neurological, psychiatric, and neuropsychological examination. The predominant "specific" symptoms were bouts of depression, attacks of rage, and chemical burns of the skin. "Nonspecific" symptoms included forgetfulness, fatigue and weakness, loss of libido, loss of motivation, headaches, and sleep disturbance (28). In another chemical plant accident, six workers were exposed repeatedly for short periods over 3 days (25,26); they developed headache, tinnitus, deafness, impaired memory, disorientation, aggressivness, psychotic behavior, syncope, loss of consciousness and, in the three most severe cases, respiratory depression requiring ventilatory assistance. Significantly increased tin excretion was detected in the urine of all six patients. Those patients who were most

ill had the highest tin concentrations in the urine; the three highest values were 1300, 1500, and 1600 ppb, respectively, while the three lower values were 555, 625, and 660 ppb. Electroencephalograms displayed right-sided frontotemporal delta waves; focal spikes in the temporal region were noted in one case. Some of the patients showed leukocytosis and increased serum transaminase activity, indicating possible liver damage attributable to dimethyltin toxicity. Therapeutic measures included dexamethasone, plasmapheresis, and administration of d-penicillamine and charcoal. Supportive treatment included balanced intake and output of fluids, electrolytes, and calories; control of metabolic parameters; physical therapy; and artificial ventilation. The patient with the highest tin levels died 12 days after initial exposure with coma, respiratory depression, shock, anuria, and hepatopathy. Pathological examination revealed hepatocellular necrosis and fatty degeneration. Neuronal damage in the limbic system was characterized by loss of Nissl substance with shrinkage and eosinophilia of cytoplasm (26). The patient exhibiting the second highest tin levels had a persistent neurological defect characterized by hyperkinesias and severe cerebral defects. The third most severely intoxicated patient had severe memory dysfunction and aggressiveness. The other three patients appeared unremarkable and returned to work, although they complained of memory loss for up to 6 months (25).

The presence of methyl groups in trialkyltin compounds is essential for the neuronal toxicity. To explore the difference between neuronotoxic trimethyltin and myelinotoxic triethyltin, trialkyltins containing two methyl and one ethyl groups were compared with those containing two ethyl and one methyl groups (1). The compound containing more methyl groups produced neuronal damage and only slight myelin edema, while the compound containing more ethyl groups produced distinct myelin edema and only slight neuronal damage. It is likely that, following exposure to TMT chloride, some of the absorbed chloride ions are substituted by hydroxide ions, so that both chlorides and hydroxides are present. Since both forms are soluble in water and in lipids, a rapid passage of TMT through cellular membranes is possible.

Mechanisms underlying neuronal degeneration induced by TMT have yet to be established. Loss of Nissl substance in affected neurons suggests a disturbance of protein synthesis (7,13) associated with changes in the Golgi complex of the endoplasmic reticulum. Specific experiments, however, have demonstrated only minor inhibition of protein synthesis. Possibly, the changes in the Golgi complex disturb subsequent processing of synthesized protein (8).

The distribution of neuronal damage produced by TMT raises the possibility of a glutamate-mediated toxicity (see

Chapter 1). The vulnerable pathway between the entorhinal cortex, fascia dentata, and hippocampus appears to utilize glutamate neurotransmission (12,14). TMT-induced decrease in high-affinity uptake of glutamate is associated with changes in hippocampal electrical activity (22), but changes in other transmitter systems are also observed (3,10,11,15).

REFERENCES

1. Aldridge WN, Verschoyle RD, Thompson CA, Brown AW (1987) The toxicity and neuropathology of dimethylethyltin and methyldiethyltin in rats. *Neuropathol Appl Neurobiol* **13**, 55.

2. Allen SL, Simpson MG, Stonard MD, Jones K (1994) Induction of trimethyltin neurotoxicity by dietary administration. *NeuroToxicology* **15**, 651.

3. Andersson H, Luthman J, Olson L (1994) Trimethyltin-induced expression of GABA and vimentin immunoreactivities in astrocytes of the rat brain. *Glia* **11**, 378.

4. Bouldin TW, Goines ND, Bagnell CR, Krigman MR (1981) Pathogenesis of trimethyltin neuronal toxicity. Ultrastructural and cytochemical observations. *Amer J Pathol* **104**, 237.

5. Bouldin TW, Goines ND, Krigman MR (1984) Trimethyltin retinopathy. Relationship of subcellular response to neuronal subspecialization. *J Neuropathol Exp Neurol* **43**, 162.

6. Bressa G, Hinton RH, Price SC *et al.* (1991) Immunotoxicity of tri-*n*-butyltin oxide (TBTO) and tri-*n*-butyltin chloride (TBTC) in the rat. *J Appl Toxicol* **11**, 397.

7. Brown AW, Aldridge WN, Street BW, Verschoyle RD (1979) The behavioral and neuropathologic sequelae of intoxication by trimethyltin compounds in the rat. *Amer J Pathol* **97**, 59.

8. Brown AW, Cavanagh JB, Verschoyle RD *et al.* (1984) Evolution of the intracellular changes in neurons caused by trimethyltin. *Neuropathol Appl Neurobiol* **10**, 267.

9. Brown AW, Verschoyle RD, Street BW *et al.* (1984) The neurotoxicity of trimethyltin chloride in hamsters, gerbils and marmosets. *J Appl Toxicol* **4**, 12.

10. Cannon RL, Hoover DB, Baisden RH, Woodruff MI (1994) Effects of trimethyltin (TMT) on choline acetyltransferase activity in the rat hippocampus. Influence of dose and time following exposure. *Mol Chem Neuropathol* **23**, 27.

11. Cannon RL, Hoover DB, Baisden RH, Woodruff ML (1994) The effect of time following exposure to trimethyltin (TMT) on cholinergic muscarinic receptor binding in rat hippocampus *Mol Chem Neuropathol* **23**, 47.

12. Chang LW (1986) Neuropathology of trimethyltin: A proposed pathogenetic mechanism. *Fund Appl Toxicol* **6**, 217.

13. Chang LW, Dyer RS (1983) Trimethyltin induced pathology in sensory neurons. *Neurobehav Toxicol Teratol* **5**, 673.

14. Chang LW, Dyer RS (1985) Septotemporal gradients of trimethyltin-induced hippocampal lesions. *Neurobehav Toxicol Teratol* **7**, 43.

15. Chang LW, Wenger GR, McMillan DE, Dyer RS (1983) Species and strain comparison of acute neurotoxic effects of trimethyltin in mice and rats. *Neurobehav Teratol Toxicol* **5**, 337.

16. Dyer RS, Deshields TL, Wonderlin WF (1982) Trimethyltin-induced changes in gross morphology of the hippocampus. *Neurobehav Toxicol Teratol* **4**, 141.

17. Dyer RS, Howell WE, Wonderlin WE (1982) Visual system dysfunction following acute trimethyltin exposure in rats. *Neurobehav Toxicol Teratol* **4**, 191.

18. Dyer RS, Walsh TJ, Wonderlin WF, Bercegeay M (1982) The trimethyltin syndrome in rats. *Neurobehav Toxicol Teratol* **4**, 127.

19. Fortemps E, Amand G, Bomboir A *et al.* (1978) Trimethyltin poisoning. Report of two cases. *Occup Environ Health* **41**, 1.

20. Krinke G, Hess R (1983) Trimethylzinn-induzierte Las ion im Hippocampus als Beispiel filr selektive vulnerabilitat. *Schweiz Med Wochenschr* **113**, 799.

21. Krinke GJ (1988) Neurotoxic effects of trimethyltin. In: *Monographs on Pathology of Laboratory Animals, Nervous System.* Jones TC, Mohr U, Hunt RD eds. Springer Verlag, Berlin, Heidelberg p. 58.

22. Naalsund LU, Allen ChN, Fonnum F (1985) Changes in neurobiological parameters in the hippocampus after exposure to trimethyltin. *NeuroToxicology* **6**, 145.

23. O'Shaughnessy DJ, Losos GJ (1986) Peripheral and central nervous system lesions caused by triethyl- and trimethyltin salts in rats. *Toxicol Pathol* **14**, 141.

24. Reuhl KR, Smallridge EA, Chang LW, Mackenzie BA (1983) Developmental effects of trimethyltin intoxication in the neonatal mouse. I. Light microscopic studies. *NeuroToxicology* **4**, 19.

25. Rey Ch, Reinecke HJ, Besser R (1984) Methyltin intoxication in six men: Toxicologic and clinical aspects. *Vet Hum Toxicol* **26**, 121.

26. Rey CH, Weilemann LS, Besser R *et al.* (1983) Akzidentelle gewerbliche Di- und Trimethylzinnchlorid-Vergiftung. Erfahrungen an sechs Patienten. *Schweiz Med Wochenschr* **113**, 1172.

27. Richter-Landsberg CH, Besser A (1994) Effects of organotins on rat brain astrocytes in culture. *J Neurochem* **63**, 2202.

28. Ross WD, Emmett EA, Steiner J, Tureen R (1981) Neurotoxic effects of occupational exposure to organotins. *Amer J Psychiat* **138**, 1092.

29. Ruppert PH, Walsh TJ, Reiter LW, Deyer RS (1982) Trimethyltin-induced hyperactivity: Time course and pattern. *Neurobehav Toxicol Teratol* **4**, 135.

30. Ueno S, Susa N, Furukawa Y, Sugiyama M (1994) Comparison of hepatotoxicity caused by mono-, di- and tributyltin compounds in mice. *Arch Toxicol* **69**, 30.
31. Walsh TJ, Gallagher M, Bostock E, Dyer RS (1982) Trimethyltin impairs retention of a passive avoidance task. *Neurobehav Toxicol Teratol* **4**, 163.
32. Walsh TJ, Miller DB, Deyer RS (1982) Trimethyltin, a selective limbic system neurotoxicant, impairs radial-arm maze performance. *Neurobehav Toxicol Teratol* **4**, 177.

Triparanol

Herbert H. Schaumburg

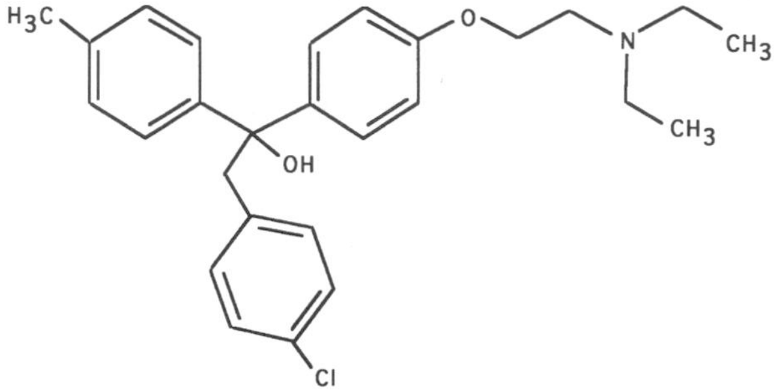

TRIPARANOL
$C_{27}H_{32}ClNO_2$

4-Chloro-α-[4-[2-(diethylamino)ethoxy]phenyl]-α-(4-methylphenyl)benzeneethanol

NEUROTOXICITY RATING

Clinical

B   Myotonia

Triparanol was introduced in 1960 for the prevention and treatment of hypercholesterolemia; it was one of a family of lipid-lowering agents that included clomiphene and 20,25-diazocholesterol. These drugs inhibited the reduction of the 24,25 double bond in the side chain during cholesterol synthesis, hence causing the accumulation of desmosterol in plasma, erythrocytes, and muscle membranes. Serious adverse effects associated with triparanol use at conventional doses in more than 500 patients led to its withdrawal in 1962; the systemic toxic effects included cataracts, alopecia, impotence, malabsorption, liver dysfunction, and proteinuria (2).

Myotonia occurred in individuals dosed for months; it was of moderate intensity and dissipated following drug withdrawal (3). Myotonia also was associated with other drugs that inhibited this stage of cholesterol synthesis (1). The pathophysiology of myotonia in these conditions is related to the accumulation of desmosterol within muscle membranes. In experimental animals, this alteration in membrane sterol content is associated with a marked decrease in chloride conductance and repetitive action potentials causing prolonged muscle contraction—the essence of myotonia. The same dysfunction occurs in human myotonia.

REFERENCES
1. Lane RJM, Mastaglia FL (1978) Drug-induced myopathies in man. *Lancet* **2**, 562.
2. Modell W (1967) Mass drug catastrophes and the roles of science and technology. *Science* **156**, 346.
3. Peter JB, Campion DS, Dromgoole SH *et al.* (1984) Similarities and differences between human myotonia and drug-induced myotonia in rats. In: *Recent Advances in Myology*. Bradley WG, Gardner-Medwin D, Walton JN eds. Excerpta Medica, Amsterdam p. 434.

Trithiozine

Steven Herskovitz

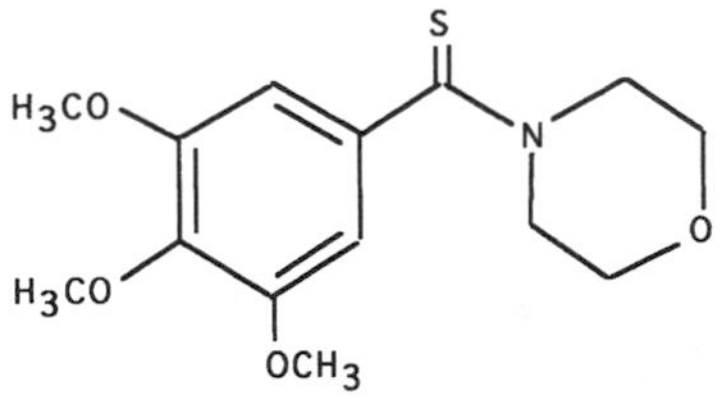

TRITHIOZINE
C$_{14}$H$_{19}$NO$_4$S

4-(3,4,5-Trimethoxythiobenzoyl)morpholine

NEUROTOXICITY RATING

Clinical

B   Peripheral neuropathy

Trithiozine is a gastric antisecretory and antiulcer agent marketed in Europe in the late 1970s. The drug's mechanism of action is incompletely established but appears not to include anticholinergic or anti-H$_2$ receptor effects (5). The antisecretory activity of the drug is higher on basal than on stimulated secretion; it promotes ulcer healing and is not associated with rebound hypersecretion. There is no effect on gastric emptying, serum gastrin, or pancreatic secretions. Reported neurotoxicity consists of occasional drowsiness, paresthesias, and polyneuropathy in a single series of three patients.

Trithiozine has good oral bioavailability and a plasma half-life of 7 h (3,6). Urine is the major route of elimination. There are two metabolites resulting from desulfuration and demethylation. Usual therapeutic doses administered are 800–1200 mg/day.

Animal studies do not describe neurotoxicity.

In human clinical studies of efficacy and toxicity, including a 1979 review, trithiozine was noted to be well tolerated at the usual therapeutic doses for both short-term (2–4 weeks) and long-term (up to 10 months) treatment (1,5). There was infrequent elevation of transaminases, drowsiness, nausea, fever, headache, or myalgias, all of which were reversible. Two cases reportedly had paresthesias that disappeared at the end of treatment. Acute hepatitis is reported (4).

Three individuals have developed trithiozine-associated polyneuropathy (2). Symptoms began after 2–4 weeks of treatment at 800 mg/day. All were predominantly distal, symmetrical and sensory, with burning pain or paresthesias; one had mild distal leg weakness. One was restricted to distal leg symptoms, the second had involvement of hands more than feet, and the third involved hands alone. There was a glove or stocking distribution of sensory loss, normal reflexes in one, and areflexia in the second patient. The cerebrospinal fluid was normal in one case examined. Nerve conduction studies suggested an axonopathy. Sural biopsies showed loss of predominantly large myelinated fibers and no evidence of segmental demyelination. Clinical recovery within months following drug discontinuation was complete in two and incomplete in one.

Based on these limited observations, it appears that trithiozine may be associated with a mostly reversible, axonal, sensorimotor polyneuropathy. The incidence and mechanism are unknown.

REFERENCES

1. Corinaldesi R, Lucchetta L, Ricci P et al. (1977) Valutazione della Tollerabilita, a lungo termine, della tritiozina (ISF 2001). Il Farmaco 32, 25.
2. Crespi V, Petruccioli Pizzini MG, Tredici G et al. (1981) Trithiozine polyneuropathy: Clinical, neurophysiological and histopathological study of three cases. Ital J Neurol Sci 3, 291.
3. Gibinski K, Rybicka J, Gorny E, Bielecka W (1979) Bioavailability of trithiozine (TR) in man and its relation to gastric secretion and gastrin plasma level. Int J Clin Pharmacol Biopharm 17, 48.
4. Navarro Izquierdo A, Perez Gomez A, Hernandez Guio C (1982) Acute hepatitis caused by trithiozine. Rev Clin Espan 164, 129.
5. Pellegrini R (1979) Clinical effects of trithiozine, a newer gastric anti-secretory agent. J Int Med Res 7, 452.
6. Renwick AG, Pettet JL, Gruchy B, Corina DL (1982) The fate of [^{14}C]trithiozine in man. Xenobiotica 12, 329.

L-Tryptophan

Herbert H. Schaumburg
Neil L. Rosenberg

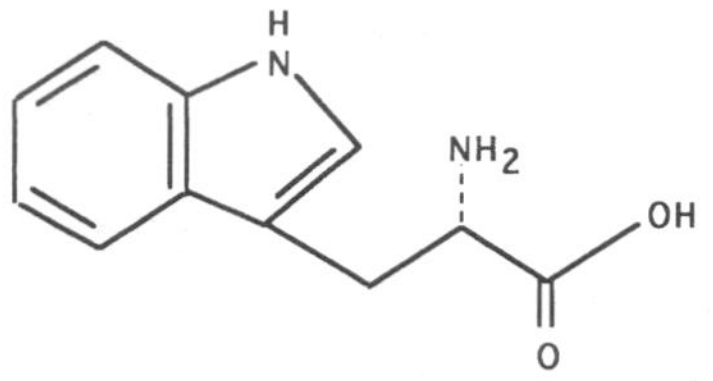

L-TRYPTOPHAN
$C_{11}H_{12}N_2O_2$

(S)-α-Amino-1H-indole-3-propanoic acid

NEUROTOXICITY RATING (IMPURE SYNTHETIC SAMPLE)

Clinical

A   Myopathy (inflammatory)

A   Peripheral neuropathy

C   Chronic encephalopathy

Experimental

A   Myopathy (inflammatory)

Use of L-tryptophan (LT), an amino acid, was widespread in the United States in the 1980s. It has been estimated that approximately 2% of surveyed household members in the states of Oregon and Minnesota were ingesting LT between 1980 and 1989 (1,33). The usual reasons for consuming LT —available without a prescription–were insomnia, premenstrual syndrome, and depression. Serious toxicity of LT preparations was first recognized in October 1989, when the State Health Department of New Mexico was notified of an acute illness in three patients, characterized by incapacitating myalgias, eosinophilia, and no identifiable cause (4). All three had been consuming LT-containing products for treatment of insomnia. Eosinophilia-myalgia syndrome (EMS) was soon recognized nationwide (9,24,39). Epidemiological studies confirmed an association between EMS and consumption of LT-containing products (33,37). Cases of EMS were present in the United States prior to the commercial availability of LT (37).

LT was removed from the market within a month of recognition of EMS. Over 1500 individuals were determined to have EMS based on surveillance criteria and, as of August 10, 1991, 36 deaths occurred in this group (36). Despite considerable clinical and experimental investigation, it remains unclear whether EMS reflects contaminants (Fig. 37) confined to a few batches of LT produced by a single Japanese manufacturer or whether the illness can be produced by reagent-grade LT regardless of origin. There is overwhelming epidemiological and product-tracing data gathered by the U.S. Food and Drug Administration and the Centers for Disease Control and Prevention that implicates a link between EMS and LT produced by the Japanese manufacturer. No persons taking prescription brands manufactured in Canada have developed EMS; however, nine of ten Canadian cases of EMS were consuming the Japanese product (42). Only one review of the epidemiological studies has challenged the association (6).

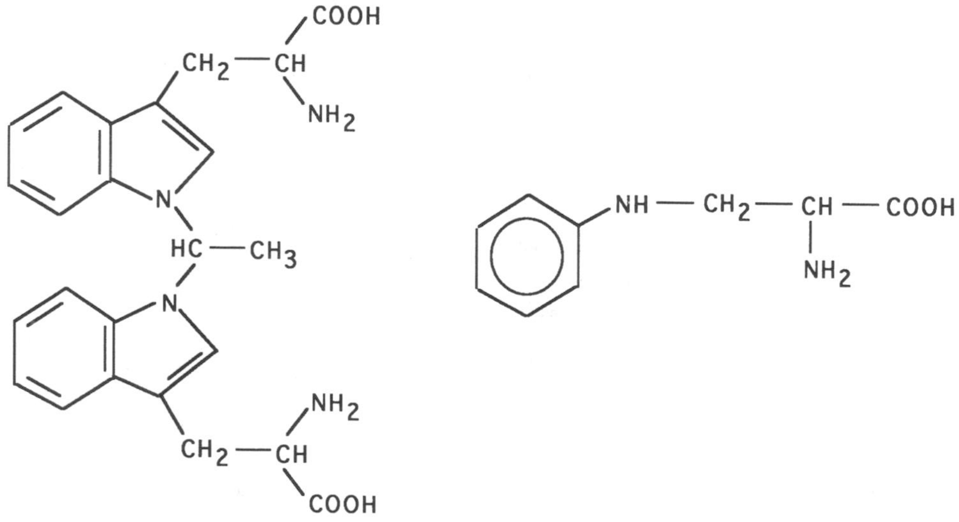

1,1'-(ETHYLENEBIS)TRYPTOPHAN (EBT)   3-(PHENYLAMINO)ALANINE (PAA)

FIGURE 37. Chemically characterized contaminants of L-tryptophan.

The two chemically characterized contaminants are 3-(phenylamino)alanine (PAA) and 1,1'-(ethylenebis)-tryptophan (EBT).

Most of the patients in the EMS epidemic recovered, and few new cases have been reported since tryptophan was removed from the market. Many display effects of their disease, and there is significant morbidity associated with residual peripheral neuropathy (8). The epidemiology of peripheral neuropathy in EMS is not known, but the frequency in a large series has been reported to be as high as 27% (37); neuropathy has been associated with 92% of those patients who died from EMS (36).

The similarities between EMS and other autoimmune diseases such as scleroderma, fasciitis, eosinophilic fasciitis, idiopathic myositis, and the toxic oil syndrome (TOS), suggest these disorders are all interrelated and have some similarities in pathophysiology (15–17,21,30,32,35). In addition, abnormalities of tryptophan metabolism have long been associated with autoimmune disease states (2), and EMS research has provided useful information on the biochemical pathways of tryptophan metabolism and the immune system.

Recognition of EMS generated increased interest in TOS, an epidemic that affected more than 20,000 people in Spain and caused more than 800 deaths (15–17,23,32) (see "Toxic Oil," this volume). There are clinical and pathological similarities between TOS and EMS, and a recent study suggests a possible biochemical link between these two disorders (23). In this study, peak UV-5 of implicated LT lots is PAA, a compound with chemical similarities to 3-(phenylamino)-1,2-propanediol, an aniline derivative found in the oil consumed by individuals who developed TOS.

Animal models of EMS have been described in both rats (5,20,26) and mice (31,41). Studies have utilized parenteral injections of EBT (31), or gavaged implicated-LT (5), EBT (20), or PAA (26), all identified as potential candidates for "the contaminant" that may cause EMS. One study utilized oral feedings (with "pure" LT or implicated-LT placed in drinking water) to mimic the human situation more closely (41). While most studies found that only implicated-LT or EBT were able to induce a disorder similar to EMS (5,20,31), one report claims that reagent-grade ("pure") LT was also capable of causing an EMS-like disorder in SJL/J mice, of equal severity to that produced by implicated-LT (41). No EMS-like effects were seen in Sprague-Dawley rats gavaged with PAA at doses from 375 to 37,500 times higher than those to which humans were estimated to have been exposed (26).

While most reports describe inflammation affecting multiple tissues, the PNS was not systematically evaluated. Two studies, however, did reveal inflammation surrounding in-tramuscular nerve fibers (5,41), similar to that seen in human EMS (11,18,28,40).

Clinical neurological features reported to be common in EMS include peripheral neuropathy, a myopathy (with or without inflammation or an associated fasciitis), and neurocognitive symptoms.

Peripheral neuropathy was a common cause of morbidity and mortality in EMS (3,8,10,18,25,27–29,34,40). Many of the deaths associated with EMS were in individuals who developed progressive respiratory failure, at least in part due to progressive neuromuscular weakness. Many survivors of EMS have significant residual and disabling peripheral neuropathy; rehabilitation has had limited success (8).

There is one study of ten patients with EMS in whom peripheral neuropathy was the only or a prominent presenting feature (34). Two had severe neuropathy requiring mechanical ventilation, and one died. Pathological changes included epineural inflammation, which was occasionally marked, accompanied by vasculopathy and angiogenesis. Other pathological changes in nerve-biopsy specimens included axonal degeneration (10,11,34), and demyelination and remyelination (34). Clinically, most patients presented with subacute progressive (predominantly motor) neuropathies (8,10,29,34) and, occasionally, with a picture of a mononeuropathy multiplex (3,29). Many displayed features of axonal disease, but some had the syndrome of chronic inflammatory demyelinating polyneuropathy (7).

Some patients with EMS were noted to develop prominent proximal muscle weakness suggestive of a myopathy, though most developed generalized weakness that may have been more functionally related to the severe pain associated with fasciitis. Most histopathological studies of EMS have examined only, or predominantly, muscle and fascia (11,18,28,40). Fascial inflammation was commonly but not universally seen, and prominent muscle involvement was rare. There was often prominent inflammation surrounding intramuscular nerve twigs (11,18,28,40); this has been suggested as the source of the neurogenic changes seen both on electrodiagnostic studies and on muscle biopsy, particularly in those cases where nerve conduction studies and nerve biopsy were normal. In some instances, a myopathy occurred without evidence of neuropathy or neurogenic changes on electrodiagnostic studies (38).

Cognitive complaints were common in the chronic phase of EMS (12,14,19). In one study, cognitive symptoms eventually occurred in 49 of 56 (86%) EMS patients followed for an average of 3 years (14). These complaints—primarily memory disturbances—were not seen until 1 year after the onset of EMS. The delayed onset, occurring at a time when the major systemic component of EMS was quiescent, does not suggest direct CNS involvement by the same processes causing the systemic disease. Neuropsychological testing in one study of 24 EMS patients revealed some mild deficits, but the data do not support the claim of encephalopathy (19). Most patients with EMS have chronic pain, depression, or another concurrent psychiatric disorder, all of which can interfere with cognitive test performance.

Therapy for EMS has been disappointing both for the general systemic illness and for peripheral neuropathy. Treatment with corticosteroids, other immunosuppressive agents (*e.g.*, cyclophosphamide, cyclosporine), and plasmapheresis have not been of benefit, either for EMS in general or for the peripheral neuropathy, even in those cases where a demyelinating neuropathy was found (7,8). Some reports suggest that EMS may respond to methotrexate (22) or the mast cell stabilizing agent, ketotifen (13), but neither agent has been studied in the treatment of the peripheral neuropathy associated with EMS.

The neuropathy in some patients, even when severe, may stabilize, at which time intensive rehabilitation may afford some functional improvement (8). In a retrospective review of the results of treatment 2 years after the onset of EMS, the majority of symptoms and physical findings in most patients resolved or improved (12). Cognitive symptoms were reported to be worse in 32% of patients, and no treatment was considered useful in the later stages of EMS even though prednisone was felt to be useful in the acute phase (12).

REFERENCES

1. Belongia EA, Hedberg CW, Gleich GJ *et al.* (1990) An investigation of the cause of eosinophilia-myalgia syndrome associated with tryptophan use. *N Engl J Med* **323**, 357.
2. Brown RR (1981) The tryptophan load test as an index of vitamin B_6 nutrition. In: *Methods in Vitamin B-6 Nutrition: Analysis and Status Assessment.* Leklem JE, Reynolds RD eds. Plenum Press, New York p. 321.
3. Burns SM, Lange DJ, Jaffe I, Hays AP (1994) Axonal neuropathy in eosinophilia-myalgia syndrome. *Muscle Nerve* **17**, 293.
4. Centers for Disease Control (1989) Eosinophilia-myalgia syndrome: New Mexico. *Morb Mort Wkly Rep* **38**, 765.
5. Crofford LJ, Rader JI, Dalakas MC *et al.* (1990) L-Tryptophan implicated in human eosinophilia-myalgia syndrome causes fasciitis and perimyositis in the Lewis rat. *J Clin Invest* **86**, 1757.
6. Daniels SR, Hudson JI, Horwitz RI (1995) Epidemiology of potential association between L-tryptophan ingestion and eosinophilia-myalgia syndrome. *J Clin Epidemiol* **48**, 1413.
7. Donofrio PD, Stanton C, Miller VS *et al.* (1992) Demyelinating polyneuropathy in eosinophilia-myalgia syndrome. *Muscle Nerve* **15**, 796.
8. Draznin E, Rosenberg NL (1993) Intensive rehabilitation approach to eosinophilia myalgia syndrome associated with severe polyneuropathy. *Arch Phys Med Rehab* **74**, 774.
9. Flannery MT, Wallach PM, Espinoza LR *et al.* (1990) A case of the eosinophilia-myalgia syndrome associated with use of an L-tryptophan product. *Ann Intern Med* **112**, 300.
10. Heiman-Patterson TD, Bird SJ, Parry GJ *et al.* (1990) Peripheral neuropathy associated with eosinophilia-myalgia syndrome. *Ann Neurol* **28**, 522.
11. Herrick MK, Chang Y, Horoupian DS *et al.* (1991) L-Tryptophan and the eosinophilia-myalgia syndrome. *Hum Pathol* **22**, 12.
12. Hertzman PA, Clauw DJ, Kaufman LD *et al.* (1995) The eosinophilia-myalgia syndrome: Status of 205 patients and results of treatment 2 years after onset. *Ann Intern Med* **122**, 851.
13. Kaufman LD (1992) The eosinophilia-myalgia syndrome: Current concepts and future directions. *Clin Exp Rheum* **10**, 87.
14. Kaufman LD (1994) Chronicity of the eosinophilia-myalgia syndrome: A reassessment after three years. *Arthritis Rheum* **37**, 84.
15. Kaufman LD, Seidman RJ (1991) L-Tryptophan-associated eosinophilia myalgia syndrome: Perspective of a new illness. *Rheum Dis Clin N Amer* **17**, 427.
16. Kilbourne EM, Posada de la Paz M, Abaitua Borda I *et al.* (1991) Toxic oil syndrome: A current clinical and epidemiological summary, including comparisons with the eosinophilia-myalgia syndrome. *J Amer Coll Cardiol* **18**, 711.
17. Kilbourne EM, Rigau-Perez JG, Heath CW *et al.* (1983) Clinical epidemiology of toxic-oil syndrome: Manifestations of a new illness. *N Engl J Med* **309**, 1408.
18. Kirkpatrick JB (1991) Eosinophilia myalgia. *Hum Pathol* **22**, 1. [Editorial]
19. Krupp LB, Masur DM, Kaufman LD (1993) Neurocognitive dysfunction in the eosinophilia-myalgia syndrome. *Neurology* **43**, 931.
20. Love LA, Rader JI, Crofford LJ *et al.* (1993) Pathological and immunological effects of ingesting L-tryptophan and 1,1′-ethylidenebis (L-tryptophan) in Lewis rats. *J Clin Invest* **91**, 804.
21. Martin RW, Duffy J (1991) Eosinophilic fasciitis associated with use of L-tryptophan: A case-control study and comparison of clinical and histopathologic features. *Mayo Clin Proc* **66**, 892.
22. Martinez-Osuna P, Wallach PM, Seleznick MJ *et al.* (1991) Treatment of the eosinophilia myalgia syndrome. *Semin Arthritis Rheum* **21**, 110.
23. Mayeno AN, Belongia EA, Lin F *et al.* (1992) 3-(Phenylamino)alanine, a novel aniline-derived amino acid associated with the eosinophilia-myalgia syndrome: A link to the toxic oil syndrome? *Mayo Clin Proc* **67**, 1134.

24. Mayeno AN, Lin F, Foote CS *et al.* (1990) Characterization of "Peak E", a novel amino acid associated with eosinophilia-myalgia syndrome. *Science* **250**, 1701.

25. Rosenberg NL (1991) Toxic myopathies. *Curr Opin Neurol Neurosurg* **4**, 433.

26. Sato F, Hagiwara Y, Kawase Y (1995) Subchronic toxicity of 3-phenylamino alanine, an impurity in L-tryptophan reported to be associated with eosinophilia-myalgia syndrome. *Arch Toxicol* **69**, 444.

27. Schaumburg HH (1991) Toxic and metabolic neuropathies. *Curr Opin Neurol Neurosurg* **4**, 438.

28. Seidman RJ, Kaufman LD, Sokoloff L *et al.* (1991) The neuromuscular pathology of the eosinophilia-myalgia syndrome. *J Neuropathol Exp Neurol* **50**, 49.

29. Selwa JF, Feldman EL, Blaivas M (1990) Mononeuropathy multiplex in tryptophan-associated eosinophilia-myalgia syndrome. *Neurology* **40**, 1632.

30. Silver RM, Heyes MP, Maize JC *et al.* (1990) Scleroderma, fasciitis, and eosinophilia associated with the ingestion of tryptophan. *N Engl J Med* **322**, 874.

31. Silver RM, Ludwicka A, Hampton M *et al.* (1994) A murine model of the eosinophilia-myalgia syndrome induced by 1,1'-ethylidenebis (L-tryptophan). *J Clin Invest* **93**, 1473.

32. Silver RM, Sutherland SE, Carreira P, Heyes MP (1992) Alterations in tryptophan metabolism in the toxic oil syndrome and in the eosinophilia-myalgia syndrome. *J Rheumatol* **19**, 69.

33. Slutzger L, Hoesley FC, Miller L *et al.* (1990) Eosinophilia-myalgia syndrome associated with exposure to tryptophan from a single manufacturer. *J Amer Med Assn* **264**, 213.

34. Smith BE, Dyck PJ (1990) Peripheral neuropathy in the eosinophilia-myalgia syndrome associated with L-tryptophan ingestion. *Neurology* **40**, 1035.

35. Sternberg EM, Van Woert MH, Young SN *et al.* (1980) Development of a scleroderma-like illness during therapy with L-5-hydroxytryptophan and carbidopa. *N Engl J Med* **303**, 782.

36. Swygert LA, Back EE, Auerbach SB *et al.* (1993) Eosinophilia-myalgia syndrome: Mortality data from the U.S. National Surveillance System. *J Rheumatol* **20**, 1711.

37. Swygert LA, Maes EF, Sewell LE *et al.* (1990) Eosinophilia-myalgia syndrome: Results of national surveillance. *J Amer Med Assn* **264**, 1698.

38. Tanhehco JL, Wiechers DO, Globus J, Neely SE (1992) Eosinophilia-myalgia syndrome: Myopathic electrodiagnostic characteristics. *Muscle Nerve* **15**(5), 561.

39. Varga J, Jimenez SA, Uitto J (1993) L-Tryptophan and the eosinophilia-myalgia syndrome: Current understanding of the etiology and pathogenesis. *J Invest Dermatol* **100**, 97S.

40. Verity MA, Bulpitt KJ, Paulus HE (1991) Neuromuscular manifestations of L-tryptophan-associated eosinophilia-myalgia syndrome. *Hum Pathol* **22**, 3.

41. Weller A, Rosenberg N, Schlitz P *et al.* (1993) Tryptophan causes EMS-like skin changes and induction of ICAM and LFA in SJL/J mice. *J Immunol* **150**, 172A.

42. Wilkins K, Wigle D (1990) Eosinophilia-myalgia syndrome—Canada. *Can Dis Wkly Rep* **16**, 209.

d-Tubocurarine

Phyllis L. Bieri

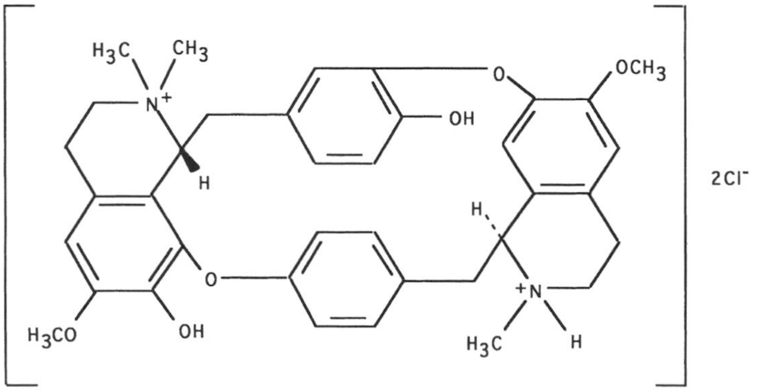

TUBOCURARINE CHLORIDE
$C_{37}H_{42}Cl_2N_2O_6$

7',12'-Dihydroxy-6,6'-dimethoxy-2,2',2'-trimethyltubocuraranium chloride hydrochloride

NEUROTOXICITY RATING

Clinical

A   Neuromuscular transmission syndrome

Experimental

A   Neuromuscular transmission dysfunction (postsynaptic
neuromuscular blockade)

Tubocurarine is a naturally occurring toxiferene alkaloid, obtained from *Strychnos toxifera*. Found on every continent, *Strychnos* species are the source of the curare class of neuromuscular-blocking alkaloids. Curare has a long and colorful history, stemming from its original use as an arrow poison by South American natives. Initially shown by Claude Bernard in 1856 to be important in nerve–muscle interaction, tubocurarine's modern clinical usage is attributed to West, who in 1932 used highly purified curare to treat tetanus and spasticity (11). By 1942, the first trial of curare for muscle relaxation during general anesthesia was reported (4). Over the next decade, use of curare alkaloids became increasingly widespread, given the advantage of a slower general anesthetic dose while achieving concomitant neuromuscular blockade.

The competitive neuromuscular-blocking agents differ structurally from the depolarizing agents; they tend to be larger and less flexible molecules. Both *d*- and *l*-tubocurarine have similar bond distances between nitrogen groups; however, *d*-tubocurarine is significantly more potent. This is likely due to the fact that the *d*-isomer has all its hydrophilic regions localized to one surface (11).

Tubocurarine acts on the postsynaptic neuromuscular junction where it binds with the nicotinic cholinergic receptor, thus competitively blocking the neurotransmitter action of acetylcholine. The high-affinity curare-binding site is formed by segments of the α- and γ-subunits of the acetylcholine receptor (9). Increasing concentrations of tubocurarine at the postsynaptic membrane cause progressively decreasing amplitudes in the postjunctional synaptic potential. When this potential falls below 70% of its initial level, the action potential is unable to be activated, and neuromuscular transmission fails. Patch-clamp analysis of single-channel events has shown that tubocurarine reduces the frequency of single acetylcholine channel openings. In contrast, tubocurarine has no effect on the duration of opening of a single channel or its conductance (7). This typical competitive antagonism becomes noncompetitive at higher doses of tubocurarine, which block the acetylcholine channel directly. The magnitude of neuromuscular blockade then becomes dependent on the resting membrane potential (2).

Competitive neuromuscular-blocking agents can be classified by their duration of action. *d*-Tubocurarine is the prototype of the long-acting neuromuscular blocking agents, which are also the most potent. Intermediate- and short-acting agents were developed subsequently. These newer agents have the advantage of a quicker onset of action, since higher dosages than those of *d*-tubocurarine can be tolerated. Intermediate-duration agents include atracurium and vecuronium (*see* page 1226); a more recently developed short-acting agent is mivacurium (11). In addition, the older agents have a higher frequency of side effects stemming from histamine release, ganglionic blockade, and block of vagal responses. Histaminergic effects of *d*-tubocurarine occur *via* direct mast cell effects rather than IgE-mediated anaphylaxis (12). These effects include the typical histamine-induced wheal when injected subcutaneously, bronchospasm, excessive secretions, and hypotension. *d*-Tubocurarine can cause severe hypotension when injected rapidly in large doses. The mechanism for this includes sympathetic ganglionic blockade, at both the adrenal medulla and at peripheral autonomic ganglia, as well as histaminergic peripheral vasodilatation. Hypotension is accompanied by tachycardia due to vagal blockade.

Once injected in appropriate doses, *d*-tubocurarine causes rapid paralysis. Initial weakness from neuromuscular blockade progresses to flaccid paralysis. Most affected are small, rapidly moving muscles, such as extraocular muscles, followed by muscles of the limbs, then axial muscles of the trunk. Intercostal muscles weaken later, with the diaphragm paralyzed last. Return of motor function occurs in reverse order to paralysis (3). *d*-Tubocurarine and other related competitive neuromuscular blockers have no central effects; they are unable to cross the blood-brain barrier.

d-Tubocurarine is poorly absorbed from the gastrointestinal tract. This fact was widely known by native South Americans who routinely ate game killed with curare-poisoned arrows. By contrast, intramuscular injection results in rapid absorption, as does intravenous injection, with a clinical onset time of 4–6 min. Within approximately 20 min, a single intravenous injection of *d*-tubocurarine begins to wear off due to redistribution of the drug to peripheral tissues (3). Once distributed throughout the body, duration of action depends on methods and rates of degradation and excretion. Typical duration of action is 80–120 min, with up to two-thirds of the drug excreted in urine. Lesser amounts are metabolized by the liver and excreted in bile (11).

Burn-injured patients under intensive care require higher doses of nondepolarizing neuromuscular-blocking agents, due in part to up-regulation of acetylcholine receptors (AChR). Following short-term exposure to *d*-tubocurarine, rats subjected to an approximately 50% body surface area burn showed accentuation of this AChR up-regulation. The observed clinical resistance to *d*-tubocurarine–like drugs in this patient population is therefore exaggerated by concomitant administration of such neuromuscular-blocking agents (8).

Without underlying injury or immobilization, *d*-tubocurarine induces proliferation of AChR. Following chronic infusion (>2 weeks) of subparalytic doses of *d*-tubocurarine, rats showed tolerance to the drug's effects, and up-regulation of AChR (5).

Target-dependent cell death occurs naturally in developing motoneurons. This phenomenon is blocked when motoneurons are exposed to *d*-tubocurarine or α-bungarotoxin in culture. Survival of motoneurons in culture is increased if the cells are exposed to *d*-tubocurarine. Rescue of motoneuronal death occurs despite minimal effects on neuromuscular transmission, suggesting the apoptotic cell death is prevented by neuronal AChR. In addition, paralytic or subparalytic doses of *d*-tubocurarine result in increased formation of terminal nerve branchs. This increase in terminal nerve branch number contributes to the clinical drug resistance observed in patients receiving chronic administration of *d*-tubocurarine–like medications (6).

To determine whether *d*-tubocurarine exerts CNS effects, an anesthesiologist permitted himself to receive two and a half times the routine dosage used for paralysis (10). Respiration was maintained *via* mechanical ventilation. Other than an unpleasant choking sensation due to inability to clear oropharyngeal secretions, and a subjective sense of shortness of breath, there was no clouding of sensorium or impairment of consciousness (10). Patients with diabetes mellitus show a delayed onset of action of *d*-tubocurarine compared to normal controls (1). This effect is presumed to be due to the differential sensitivity of motor end plates in patients with diabetes; its mechanism is unknown.

d-Tubocurarine overdosage, or reversal of its effects following general anesthesia, is treated with anticholinesterase agents, including neostigmine, pyridostimine, or edrophonium. A muscarinic antagonist such as atropine or glycopyrrolate is used to counteract muscarinic stimulation. Antihistamines are useful to counteract the histaminergic effects from mast cell degranulation triggered by *d*-tubocurarine, and sympathomimetic amines may be necessary to support the blood pressure (11).

d-Tubocurarine competitively blocks the action of acetylcholine at the postsynaptic neuromuscular junction, effectively stabilizing the motor end plate. Unlike the depolarizing neuromuscular-blocking agents, following *d*-tubocurarine application to an isolated muscle fiber, the remainder of the muscle membrane remains responsive to K^+ depolarization. In addition, fibers remain responsive to direct electrical stimulation (11).

REFERENCES

1. Atallah MM, Daif AA, Saied MM, Sonbul ZM (1992) Neuromuscular blocking activity of tubocurarine in patients with diabetes mellitus. *Brit J Anaesth* **68**, 567.

2. Colquhoun D, Dreyer F, Sheridan RE (1979) The actions of tubocurarine at the frog neuromuscular junction. *J Physiol-London* **293**, 247.

3. Feldman SA, Fauvel N (1994) Onset of neuromuscular block. In: *Applied Neuromuscular Pharmacology*. Pollard BJ ed. Oxford University Press, Oxford p. 69.

4. Griffith HR, Johnson GE (1942) The use of curare in general anesthesia. *Anesthesiology* **3**, 418.

5. Hogue CW Jr, Ward JM, Itani MS, Martyn JA (1992) Tolerance and upregulation of acetylcholine receptors follow chronic infusion of *d*-tubocurarine. *J Appl Physiol* **72**, 1326.

6. Hory-Lee F, Frank E (1995) The nicotinic blocking agents *d*-tubocurare and α-bungarotoxin save motoneurons from naturally occurring death in the absence of neuromuscular blockade. *J Neurosci* **15**, 6453.

7. Katz B, Miledi R (1978) A re-examination of curare action at the motor end plate. *Proc R Soc Lond* **203**, 119.

8. Kim C, Hirose M, Martyn JA (1985) *d*-Tubocurarine accentuates the burn-induced up-regulation of nicotinic acetylcholine receptors at the muscle membrane. *Anesthesiology* **83**, 309.

9. O'Leary ME, Filatov GN, White MM (1994) Characterization of *d*-tubocurarine binding site of *Torpedo* acetylcholine receptor. *Amer J Physiol* **266**, 648.

10. Smith SM, Brown HO, Toman JEP, Goodman LS (1947) The lack of cerebral effects of *d*-tubocurarine. *Anesthesiology* **8**, 1.

11. Taylor P (1996) Agents acting at the neuromuscular junction and autonomic ganglia. In: *The Pharmacological Basis of Therapeutics. 9th Ed.* Hardman JG, Limbird LE, Gilman AG eds. McGraw-Hill, New York p. 177.

12. Watkins J (1994) Adverse reaction to neuromuscular blockers: Frequency, investigation, and epidemiology. *Acta Anaesthesiol Scand* **102**, 6.

Valproic Acid

Carol Eisenberg
Mark J. Sinnett
Shlomo Shinnar

CH₃CH₂CH₂ — CHCOOH
CH₃CH₂CH₂

VALPROIC ACID
$C_8H_{16}O_2$

2-Propylpentanoic acid

DIVALPROEX
$C_{16}H_{31}NaO_4$

Sodium hydrogen bis(2-propylpentanoate)

NEUROTOXICITY RATING

Clinical

A   Acute encephalopathy (sedation, coma)

A   Teratogenicity

Experimental

A   Acute encephalopathy (sedation, coma)

A   Teratogenicity

Valproic acid is a branched-chain fatty acid. It is structurally similar to the inhibitory neurotransmitter γ-aminobutyric acid (GABA). Valproic acid, an antiepileptic drug, was approved for prescribed use by the U.S. Food and Drug Administration in 1978; therapeutic use may be associated with significant adverse effects on the developing and adult nervous system. The psychotropic effects of valproate led to its use in treating mania and bipolar disorder (9,10).

Valproic acid (pKa 4.8) occurs as a colorless liquid that is very slightly soluble in water [7.8 μmol/l (1.3 mg/ml)]. It is available as a capsule and a syrup. Divalproex sodium is a compound of sodium valproate and valproic acid in a 1:1 molar relationship; the drug dissociates into valproic acid in the gastrointestinal tract. Divalproex is formulated as a delayed-release tablet and a sprinkle capsule.

Valproic acid inhibits the repetitive firing of neurons by blocking voltage-dependent sodium influx (36) and reducing T-type calcium currents (31). Valproic acid also affects the GABAergic system; it potentiates postsynaptic GABA inhibition and prevents degradation of succinic semialdehyde dehydrogenase, an enzyme responsible for the catabolism of GABA. Increased concentrations of GABA in the brain are thought to be directly related to the antiepileptic activity of valproic acid (47).

Valproic acid is a first-line drug for several types of seizures, especially myoclonic and primary generalized seizures. A typical dose is 15–60 mg/kg/day (5). Although optimal serum concentrations have not been clearly defined, the therapeutic range of 50–100 μg/ml is suggested. Some patients may require concentrations of up to 140 μg/ml to achieve adequate seizure control. Valproic acid may also be effective in the treatment of bipolar disorders refractory to traditional therapies (39) and may be useful in refractory migraine headache (38).

Valproic acid is rapidly absorbed from the gastrointestinal tract. The absorption of enteric-coated divalproex tablets is delayed 1 h. Peak serum concentrations occur in <2 h for the acid and 3–8 h for divalproex. Valproic acid is approximately 90%–95% protein-bound, but this can vary twofold depending on the dose, serum albumin concentration, and diseases such as renal and hepatic failure. The drug's volume of distribution is limited primarily to the plasma and extracellular fluid. In cerebrospinal fluid, the valproic acid-free fraction is reported as 0.10 (32).

Valproate is eliminated mostly by glucuronidation and oxidative metabolic pathways. Only 2%–3% of a dose is excreted unchanged. The serum half-life of valproic acid ranges from 8–18 h. The serum half-life does not correlate well with the biological half-life, which is much longer (35).

Acute valproic acid neurotoxicity was evident in mice at median intraperitoneal (6,12) and oral (6,21,52) doses of 426 and 1264 mg/kg, respectively. The toxic dose was significantly lower in rats (280 mg/kg) (21,52). Neurological deficits were demonstrated by the rotorod procedure—the inability of the mouse to maintain its equilibrium for 1 min on a rotating rod (18)—positional sense, gait and stance tests, and the Irwin test (26). The median hypnotic dose, assessed by the loss of righting reflex, was reported as 886 mg/kg in mice (12,21,52). The protective index (median neurotoxic dose/median dose required to elicit an anticonvulsant effect) of valproic acid in mice has varied between 2 and 21 (6,21,22,52). In contrast, the safety ratio found in mice was consistently <1 (6,12,19,52). The safety ratio is the ratio of the dose resulting in neurotoxicity in 3% of animals to the dose required for seizure suppression in 97%

of animals. The dose of valproic acid required for complete anticonvulsant activity in mice can then only be achieved with some evidence of neurotoxicity. The median oral LD$_{50}$ in mice of valproic acid is 670 mg/kg (4), and 1105–1700 mg/kg for sodium valproate (4,6,12,21,52).

Encephalopathy from hyperammonemia is a rare but potentially significant adverse effect of valproic acid therapy. Short-term studies in rats suggest that valproic acid–induced hyperammonemia may result from inhibition of hepatic intramitochondrial citrullinogenesis (37,51). The drug reduces hepatic mitochondrial carbamoyl-phosphate synthetase activity and free coenzyme A (CoA), acetyl CoA, and free carnitine concentrations in infant mice (54). This could hinder the removal of ammonia through the urea cycle.

In humans, teratogenicity is another serious side effect of valproate use. There appears to be a species difference of valproic acid–induced neural tube defects. For example, exencephaly, an anterior neural tube defect, is common in newborn mice following valproic acid administration to their mothers (43). Spina bifida, a defect in the posterior portion of the neural tube, is the primary malformation in humans and is very difficult to produce in mice (23). The reason for this difference is unclear.

There are direct toxic effects on developing neurons. Valproic acid inhibits process formation and decreases the production of substrate-attached neurite-promoting activity in embryonic dorsal root ganglia cultures (16). Administration of valproic acid (0.1–1.0 mM) to primary cultures of rat hepatocytes resulted in an increase in ammonia that was reversed following the addition of D,L-carnitine (53).

Sedation and ataxia occur in about 1.4% of patients on valproate monotherapy and 14.4% of those on polytherapy (particularly with polytherapy with increased plasma concentrations of phenobarbital) (49). Acute confusional states and irritability also tend to be seen more with polytherapy than monotherapy (27).

Dose-related tremor of the hands resembling benign essential tremor is seen in about 10% of patients taking valproate (25). It is generally of no clinical significance, but when bothersome may be controlled by propranolol or dosage reduction (30). A case of asterixis has been reported (7).

At therapeutic doses, valproate has minimal effect on cognitive function and behavior; the former is less affected than with phenytoin or phenobarbital (3,55). Although alertness and behavior improve in many children, in a few (8 of 100), belligerent behavior and hallucinations have been associated with its use (14), an effect that was "idiosyncratic" rather than dose-related. Impairment in some cognitive tests and psychomotor speed in children that were dose-related are described in one study (2). In adults some impairment of attention, visuomotor function, complex decision making, and psychomotor speed may be seen with valproate levels of 50–100 μg/ml (40). One report describes a case of dementia with a 3-year history of progressive cognitive impairment that reversed within 2 months of stopping valproate (60).

One case of spike-and-wave stupor associated with valproate and clonazepam therapy was described in 1974 (28), but others have used this combination without such complications (14).

Valproate-associated encephalopathy and coma have been described in children and adults; this is not associated with hepatic function abnormalities or with elevated valproate levels; often, but not always, it is associated with hyperammonemia and with anticonvulsant polytherapy (14,29). Encephalopathy is usually associated with bisynchronous, generalized, high-amplitude (1.5–3.0 Hz) activity (17,48). Asymptomatic hyperammonemia is often present in patients receiving valproic acid (42). A Reye's-like hepatic encephalopathy associated with valproate may occur in young children (8).

With acute overdosage, symptoms progress from nausea, vomiting, and dizziness at levels five to six times therapeutic; to CNS depression, coma, and respiratory compromise at levels 10–20 times therapeutic (24,56). Cerebral edema has been associated with valproate intoxication (24). Naloxone, activated charcoal, and hemodialysis have been used in acute valproate overdosage (1,17,20). As with other CNS-active drugs, symptoms of acute drug overdose may appear even with serum levels in the "therapeutic" range when these are attained rapidly rather than gradually.

The spectrum of teratogenicity seen with valproate differs from that seen in fetal hydantoin syndrome, or with phenobarbital or carbamazepine. Prenatal diagnosis by amniotic fluid analysis and fetal ultrasound is indicated for mothers receiving valproate and carbamazepine. The risk of spina bifida aperta after first-trimester exposure to valproate has been estimated as 1%–2% (11,33,34). In 1986, other defects associated with valproate were documented, including hypospadias, hypertelorism, partial agenesis of corpus callosum, agenesis of septum pellucidum with lissencephaly of medial sides of occipital lobes, Dandy-Walker anomaly, and ventricular septal defect (34); they are often complicated by hydrocephalus. Valproate-induced spina bifida was associated with higher daily doses of valproate, and it is suggested that doses >1000 mg have a higher risk than lower doses. In 1992, a prevalence rate of 5.4% of spina bifida was determined and found to be associated with a higher daily dose of valproate as compared with pregnancies with normal outcome (1640 mg/day vs. 941 mg/day) (46).

Alteration of folate metabolism has been postulated as a mechanism for the teratogenicity of valproate. Periconceptional use of folic acid reduces both the recurrence rate of neural tube defects in babies of nonepileptic mothers who previously had a child with the defect and the incidence of the first occurrence of these defects (15,41). Serum folate levels may decline during normal pregnancy but, in 1991, these levels were found to be significantly lower in pregnant women with epilepsy than in pregnant controls (45). Valproate, not a metabolite, is responsible for neural tube defects, and there is a strict structural requirement for expression of teratogenicity (44,59). In 1992, studies with mice found that teratogenic doses of valproate increased levels of tetrahydrofolate and decreased those of 5-formyl- and 10-formyl-tetrahydrofolates by inhibiting formyl group transfer by glutamate formyltransferase (59). Folinic acid supplementation had a protective effect. Other possible mechnisms suggested for valproate teratogenesis include alteration of intracellular pH (50) and interference with zinc metabolism (58).

The mechanism of valproate-induced encephalopathy with hyperammonemia in the absence of other liver function abnormalities is uncertain. Valproate increases renal ammonia production by stimulation of glutaminase resulting in increased glutamine uptake and ammonia release (57). Valproate also decreases hepatic urea synthesis by inhibiting mitochondrial carbamyl phosphate synthetase-I by decreasing synthesis of its activator N-acetylglutamate. This also results in a decrease in mitochondrial citrulline generation (13,37). Pretreatment with citrulline decreased ammonia concentrations in rats given valproate and ammonium chloride (51); it is suggested that citrulline might be useful in valproate-induced encephalopathy.

REFERENCES

1. Alberto G, Erickson T, Popiel R, Narayanan M et al. (1989) Central nervous system manifestations of a valproic acid overdose responsive to naloxone. Ann Emerg Med 18, 889.
2. Aman MG, Werry JS, Paxton JW, Turbott SH (1987) Effect of sodium valproate on psychomotor performance in children as a function of dose, fluctuations in concentration, and diagnosis. Epilepsia 28, 115.
3. American Academy of Pediatrics' Committee on Drugs (1985) Behavioral and cognitive effects of anticonvulsant therapy. Pediatrics 76, 644.
4. Anon. (1984) Valproic acid. In: Merck Index. 10th Ed. Windholz M, Buduvari S, Stroumtsos LY, Noether-Fertig M eds. Merck and Co, Rahway, New Jersey p. 1273.
5. Anon. (1994) Valproic acid. In: American Hospital Formulary Service: Drug Information. McEvoy GK ed. American Society of Hospital Pharmacists, Bethesda, Maryland p. 1366.
6. Ater SB, Swinyard EA, Tolman KG, Franklin MR (1984) Anticonvulsant activity and neurotoxicity of piperonyl butoxide in mice. Epilepsia 25, 551.
7. Bodensteiner JB, Morris HH, Golden GS (1981) Asterixis associated with sodium valproate. Neurology 31, 186.
8. Bohles H, Richter K, Wagner-Thiessen E, Schafer H (1982). Decreased serum carnitine in valproate induced Reye syndrome. Eur J Pediat 139, 185.
9. Bowden CL, Brugger AM, Swann AC et al. (1994) Efficacy of divalproex vs. lithium and placebo in the treatment of mania. J Amer Med Assn 271, 918.
10. Calabrese JR, Delucchi GA (1990) Spectrum of efficacy of valproate in 55 patients with rapid-cycling bipolar disorders. Amer J Psychiat 147, 431.
11. Centers for Disease Control (1983) Valproate—a new cause of birth defects—report from Italy and follow-up from France. Morb Mort Wkly Rep 32, 438.
12. Clark CR (1988) Comparative anticonvulsant activity and neurotoxicity of 4-amino-n-(2,6-dimethylphenyl)benzamide and prototype antiepileptic drugs in mice and rats. Epilepsia 29, 198.
13. Coude FX, Rabier D, Cathlineau L et al. (1982) A mechanism for valproate-induced hyperammonemia. Adv Exp Med Biol 153, 153.
14. Coulter DL, Wu H, Allen RJ (1980) Valproic acid therapy in childhood epilepsy. J Amer Med Assn 244, 785.
15. Czeizel AE, Dudas I (1992) Prevention of the first occurrence of neural-tube defects by periconceptional vitamin supplementation. N Engl J Med 327, 1832.
16. Dow KE, Riopelle RJ (1988) Differential effects of anticonvulsants on developing neurons in vitro. Neurotoxicology 9, 97.
17. Dreifuss FE (1989) Valproate toxicity. In: Antiepileptic Drugs. 3rd Ed. Levy R, Mattson R, Meldrum B et al. eds. Raven Presss, New York p. 643.
18. Dunham NW, Miya TS (1957) A note on a single apparatus for detecting neurological deficit in rats and mice. J Amer Pharm Assn 46, 208.
19. Elmazar MMA, Hauck RS, Nau H (1993) Anticonvulsant and neurotoxic activities of twelve analogues of valproic acid. J Pharm Sci 82, 1255.
20. Farrar HC, Herold DA, Reed MD (1993) Acute valproic acid intoxication: Enhanced drug clearance with oral-activated charcoal. Crit Care Med 21, 299.
21. Goehring RR, Greenwood TD, Nwokogu GC et al. (1990) Synthesis and anticonvulsant activity of 2-benzylglutarimides. J Med Chem 33, 926.
22. Gower AL, Noyer M, Verloes R et al. (1992) ucb L059, a novel anti-convulsant drug: Pharmacological profile in animals. Eur J Pharmacol 222, 193.
23. Hauk NH, Ehlers RS (1991) Valproic acid-induced neural tube defects in mouse and human: Aspects of chirality, alternative drug development, pharmacokinetics, and possible mechanisms. Pharmacol Toxicol 69, 310.
24. Hintze G, Klein HH, Prange H, Kreuzer H (1987) A case

of valproate intoxication with excessive brain edema. *Klin Wochenschr* **65**, 424.

25. Hyuman NM, Dennis PD, Sinclar KG (1979) Tremor due to sodium valproate. *Neurology* **29**, 1177.

26. Irwin S (1968) Comprehensive observational assessment: 1a. A systematic quantitative procedure for assessing the behavioural and physiologic state of the mouse. *Psychopharmacologica*, **13**, 222.

27. Jeavons PM (1982) Valproate toxicity. In: *Antiepileptic Drugs. 2nd Ed.* Woodbury DM, Penry JK, Pippenger CE eds. Raven Presss, New York p. 647.

28. Jeavons PM, Clark JE (1974) Sodium valproate in treatment of epilepsy. *Brit Med J* **2**, 584.

29. Jones GL, Matsuo F, Baringer JR, Reichert WH (1990) Valproic acid-associated encephalopathy. *West J Med* **153**, 199.

30. Karas BJ, Wilder BJ, Hammond EJ, Bauman AW (1983) Treatment of valproate tremors. *Neurology* **33**, 1380.

31. Kelly KM, Gross RA, Macdonald RL (1990) Valproic acid selectively reduces the low-threshold (T) calcium in rat nondose neurons. *Neurosci Lett* **116**, 233.

32. Levy RH, Wilensky AJ, Anderson GD (1992) Carbamazepine, valproic acid, phenobarbital, and ethosuximide. In: *Applied Pharmacokinetics: Principles of Therapeutic Drug Monitoring. 3rd Ed.* Evans WE, Schentag JJ, Jusko WJ eds. Applied Therapeutics, Vancouver p. 26.

33. Lindhout D, Meinardi H (1984) Spina bifida and *in utero* exposure to valproate. *Lancet* **2**, 396.

34. Lindhout D, Schmidt D (1986) *In-utero* exposure to valproate and neural tube defects. *Lancet* **2**, 1392.

35. Lockard JS, Levy RH (1976) Valproic acid: Reversibly acting drug? *Epilepsia* **17**, 477.

36. Macdonald RL, Kelly KM (1994) Mechanisms of action of currently prescribed and newly developed antiepileptic drugs. *Epilepsia* **35**, S41.

37. Marini AM, Zaret BS, Beckner RR (1988) Hepatic and renal contributions to valproic acid-induced hyperammonemia. *Neurology* **38**, 365.

38. Mathew NT, Ali S (1991) Valproate in the treatment of persistent chronic daily headache: An open label study. *Headache* **31**, 71.

39. McElroy SL, Keck PE, Pope HG (1987) Sodium valproate: Its use in primary psychiatric disorders. *J Clin Psychopharmacol* **7**, 16.

40. Meador KJ, Loring DW, Moore EE *et al.* (1995) Comparative cognitive effects of phenobarbital, phenytoin, and valproate in healthy adults. *Neurology* **45**, 1494.

41. MRC Vitamin Study Research Group (1991) Prevention of neural tube defects: Results of the Medical Research Council Vitamin Study. *Lancet* **338**, 131.

42. Murphy JV, Marquardt K (1982) Asymptomatic hyperammonemia in patients receiving valproic acid. *Arch Neurol* **39**, 591.

43. Nau H (1986) Valproic acid teratogenicity in mice after various administration and phenobarbital—pre-treatment

regimens: The parent drug and not one of the metabolites assayed is implicated as teratogen. *Fund Appl Toxicol* **6**, 662.

44. Nau H, Hauck RS, Ehlers K (1991) Valproic acid—induced neural tube defects in mouse and human: Aspects of chirality, alternative drug development, pharmacokinetics and possible mechanisms. *Pharmacol Toxicol* **69**, 310.

45. Ogawa Y, Kaneko S, Otanik *et al.* (1991) Serum folic acid levels in epileptic mothers and their relationship to congenital malformations. *Epilepsy Res* **8**, 75.

46. Omtzigt JG, Los FJ, Grobbee DE *et al.* (1992) The risk of spina bifida aperta after first-trimester exposure to valproate in a prenatal cohort. *Neurology* **42**, 119.

47. Reffin JD, Ferrendelli JA (1993) Mechanism of antiepileptic drugs. In: *Pediatric Epilepsy: Diagnosis and Therapy.* Dodson WE, Pellak JM eds. Demos Publications, New York p. 223.

48. Sackellares JC, Lee SI, Dreifuss FE (1979) Stupor following administration of valproic acid to patients receiving other antiepileptic drugs. *Epilepsia* **20**, 697.

49. Schmidt D (1984) Adverse effects of valproate. *Epilepsia* **25**, S44.

50. Scott WJ, Duggan CA, Schreiner CM, Collins MD (1990) Reduction of embryonic intracellular pH: A potential mechanism of acetazolamide-induced limb malformations. *Toxicol Appl Pharmacol* **103**, 238.

51. Stephens JR, Levy RH (1994) Effects of valproate and citrulline on ammonium-induced encephalopathy. *Epilepsia* **35**, 164.

52. Swinyard EA, Sofia RD, Kupferberg HJ (1986) Comparative anticonvulsant activity and neurotoxicity of felbamate and four prototype antiepileptic drugs in mice and rats. *Epilepsia* **27**, 27.

53. Takeuchi T, Sugimoto T, Nishida N, Kobayashi Y (1988) Protective effect of D,L-carnitine on valproate-induced hyperammonemia and hypoketonemia in primary cultured rat hepatocytes. *Biochem Pharmacol* **37**, 2255.

54. Thurston JH, Carroll JE, Hauhart RE, Schiro JA (1985) A single therapeutic dose of valproate effects liver carbohydrate, fat, adenylate, amino acid, coenzyme A, and carnitine metabolism in infant mice: Possible clinical significance. *Life Sci* **36**, 1643.

55. Vining EPG (1987) Cognitive dysfunction associated with antiepileptic drug therapy. *Epilepsia* **28**, 518.

56. Volans GN, Berry DJ, Wiseman HM (1983) Overdose with sodium valproate. *J Clin Pract* **27**, 58.

57. Warter JM, Brandt CH, Marescaux CH *et al.* (1983) The renal origin of sodium valproate induced hyperammonemia in fasting humans. *Neurology* **33**, 1136.

58. Wegner C, Drews E, Nau H (1990) Zinc concentrations in mouse embryo and maternal plasma. Effect of valproic acid and a non-teratogenic metabolite. *Biol Tr Elem Res* **25**, 211.

59. Wegner C, Nau H (1992) Alteration of embryonic folate metabolism by valproic acid during organogenesis. *Neurology* **42**, 17.

60. Zaret BS, Cohen RA (1986) Reversible valproic acid-induced dementia: A case report. *Epilepsia* **27**, 234.

Vecuronium Bromide

Steven Herskovitz

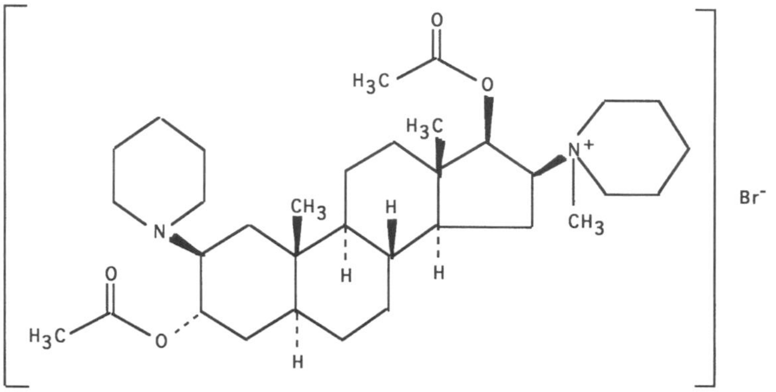

VECURONIUM BROMIDE
$C_{34}H_{57}BrN_2O_4$

1-[(2β,3α,5α,16β,17β)-3,17-Bis
(acetyloxy)-2-(1-piperidinyl)androstan-16-yl]-1-
methylpiperidinium bromide

NEUROTOXICITY RATING

Clinical

A   Neuromuscular transmission syndrome

A   Myopathy (in concert with corticosteroids)

Experimental

A   Neuromuscular transmission dysfunction (depolarizing
     neuromuscular blockade)

Vecuronium is a steroidally based, nondepolarizing, competitive neuromuscular-blocking agent administered intravenously as an adjunct to general anesthesia. It is used to facilitate endotracheal intubation and to provide muscle relaxation during mechanical ventilation or surgery. It is a monoquaternary analog of pancuronium with a shorter duration of action and no significant cardiovascular effects. Its neurotoxic reaction is prolonged postanesthetic paralysis.

Vecuronium's onset of action is <3 min and duration of action about 15–30 min (10,13,18). The elimination half-life is 80–170 min after a single dose in individuals with normal renal and hepatic function. Hepatic metabolism alters approximately one-third of a dose and produces the 3-desacetyl, 17-desacetyl, and 3,17-didesacetyl metabolites,

which have varying degrees of neuromuscular-blocking activity and are eliminated renally. Unchanged vecuronium is eliminated in the bile (40%) and urine (25%–30%). Both hepatic and renal disease can lead to toxic accumulation of vecuronium or its metabolites (13,15).

Nondepolarizing neuromuscular-blocking agents do not normally cross the blood-brain barrier. If introduced directly into rat CNS, vecuronium can cause excitation and seizures, possibly from accumulation of cytosolic calcium by sustained activation of acetylcholine-receptor ion channels (3).

An experimental model has suggested a basis for myopathy. Dexamethasone given to rats with denervated muscle results in marked atrophy of all fiber types within 7 days. Ultrastructural studies show severe preferential depletion of thick myofilaments, and gel electrophoresis demonstrates depletion of myosin heavy and light chains (14). If nerve crush rather than transection is performed, reversibility of the muscle changes occurs within 1 week after reinnervation (9). Limited proteolysis and disaggregation of myosin molecules is proposed as a mechanism, although the reason for the preferential susceptibility of myosin is unexplained.

This distinct pathology is not seen in rats treated with steroids or denervation alone. Either corticosteriods or denervation can cause muscle atrophy, with impaired synthesis and increased catabolism of all major myofibrillar proteins (9). Potentiation of these effects is suggested by the finding of a markedly increased density of cytosolic steroid receptors in denervated rat muscle (6).

The clinical syndrome of persistent paralysis after administration of vecuronium appears after the drug is discontinued by anesthesiologists, and there is difficulty in weaning off the respirator, or prolonged generalized weakness is noted in an intensive care unit (ICU). Some cases are the result of altered pharmacokinetics. Seven of 16 consecutive critically ill adults treated with vecuronium for at least 2 days had prolonged neuromuscular blockade lasting 6 h to more than 7 days (15). Consistent associations included renal failure, high concentrations of 3-desacetylvecuronium, metabolic acidosis, elevated magnesium concentrations, and female sex. Decremental responses on repetitive nerve stimulation can be demonstrated, and aminoglycosides may be an additional contributing factor in producing weakness (2,17).

The incidence of myopathy complicating treatment with vecuronium is uncertain; it is likely to be underrecognized. In one prospective study of 25 asthmatics admitted to the ICU for mechanical ventilation—all receiving steroids and 22 receiving vecuronium—76% had elevated creatine kinase levels and 36% had clinically suspected myopathy (5). Myopathy was associated with higher total dose of vecuronium. Most reported cases are in asthmatics, the others in a range of patients with traumatic or systemic ailments eventuating in ICU admission (1,2,4,5,7,8,12,17–19). Most are patients treated with both neuromuscular blockade and steroids, though a few have received only one or the other. Both vecuronium and pancuronium are implicated, following drug treatment periods from 2 days to several weeks. Corticosteroids used include methylprednisolone, hydrocortisone, dexamethasone, and prednisone in varying doses.

The clinical features of vecuronium-associated myopathy include atrophy, areflexia, and intact sensation. Weakness is moderate to severe, usually diffuse, and includes respiratory muscles. A few have extraocular, facial, or bulbar muscle weakness (16). Mild to severe elevation of creatine kinase is present in over half of cases, and myoglobinuria may occur (7,12,19). Nerve conduction studies usually show reduced motor amplitudes with normal conduction velocities and sensory potentials. Some cases may also have a critical illness polyneuropathy. Needle electromyography may reveal normal, myopathic, or neuropathic findings. Most muscle biopsies and a few autopsied muscles show myopathic features, either predominant myofiber necrosis (12,19) or severe muscle fiber atrophy with selective loss of myosin thick filaments (1,2,4,7,17). In survivors, strength returns within months but may be incomplete in severe cases.

In sum, functional denervation eventuating from prolonged neuromuscular blockade in combination with steroids causes muscle damage; the mechanism is unknown. A case of myopathy with thick filament loss in a myasthenic patient treated with large doses of parenteral steroids suggests that similar toxicity may result in patients with neuromuscular blockade from drugs or antibodies (11).

REFERENCES

1. Al-Lozi MT, Pestronk A, Yee WC et al. (1994) Rapidly evolving myopathy with myosin-deficient muscle fibers. *Ann Neurol* **35**, 273.
2. Barohn RJ, Jackson CE, Rogers SJ et al. (1994) Prolonged paralysis due to nondepolarizing neuromuscular blocking agents and corticosteroids. *Muscle Nerve* **17**, 647.
3. Cardone C, Szenohradszky J, Yost S, Bickler PE (1994) Activation of brain acetylcholine receptors by neuromuscular blocking drugs. A possible mechanism of neurotoxicity. *Anesthesiology* **80**, 1155.
4. Danon MJ, Carpenter S (1991) Myopathy with thick filament (myosin) loss following prolonged paralysis with vecuronium during steroid treatment. *Muscle Nerve* **14**, 1131.
5. Douglass JA, Tuxen DV, Horne M et al. (1992) Myopathy in severe asthma. *Amer Rev Resp Dis* **146**, 517.
6. DuBois DC, Almon RR (1981) A possible role for glucocorticoids in denervation atrophy. *Muscle Nerve* **4**, 370.
7. Hirano M, Ott BR, Raps EC et al. (1992) Acute quadriplegic myopathy: A complication of treatment with steroids, nondepolarizing blocking agents, or both. *Neurology* **42**, 2082.
8. Lacomis D, Smith TW, Chad DA (1993) Acute myopathy and neuropathy in status asthmaticus: Case report and literature review. *Muscle Nerve* **16**, 84.
9. Massa R, Carpenter S, Holland P, Karpati G (1992) Loss and renewal of thick myofilaments in glucocorticoid-treated rat soleus after denervation and reinnervation. *Muscle Nerve* **15**, 1290.
10. Miller RD, Rupp SM, Fisher DM et al. (1984) Clinical pharmacology of vecuronium and atracurium. *Anesthesiology* **61**, 444.
11. Panegyres PK, Squier M, Mills KR, Newsom-Davis J (1993) Acute myopathy associated with large parenteral dose of corticosteroid in myasthenia gravis. *J Neurol Neurosurg Psychiat* **56**, 702.
12. Ramsay DA, Zochodne DW, Robertson DM et al. (1993) A syndrome of acute severe muscle necrosis in intensive care unit patients. *J Neuropathol Exp Neurol* **52**, 387.
13. Richardson FJ, Agoston S (1992) Neuromuscular blocking agents and skeletal muscle relaxants. In: *Meyler's Side Effects of Drugs. 12th Ed.* Dukes MG ed. Elsevier, Amsterdam.
14. Rouleau G, Karpati G, Carpenter S et al. (1987) Glucocorticoid excess induces preferential depletion of myosin in denervated skeletal muscle fibers. *Muscle Nerve* **10**, 428.

15. Segredo V, Caldwell JE, Matthay MA *et al.* (1992) Persistent paralysis in critically ill patients after long-term administration of vecuronium. *N Engl J Med* **327**, 524.

16. Sitwell LD, Weinshenker BG, Monpetit V, Reid D (1991) Complete ophthalmoplegia as a complication of acute corticosteroid- and pancuronium-associated myopathy. *Neurology* **41**, 921.

17. Waclawik AJ, Sufit RL, Beinlich BR, Schutta HS (1992) Acute myopathy with selective degeneration of myosin filaments following status asthmaticus treated with methylprednisolone and vecuronium. *Neuromusc Disord* **2**, 19.

18. Watling SM, Dasta JF (1994) Prolonged paralysis in intensive care unit patients after the use of neuromuscular blocking agents: a review of the literature. *Crit Care Med* **22**, 884.

19. Zochodne DW, Ramsay DA, Saly V *et al.* (1994) Acute necrotizing myopathy of intensive care: Electrophysiological studies. *Muscle Nerve* **17**, 285.

Veratridine

Albert C. Ludolph

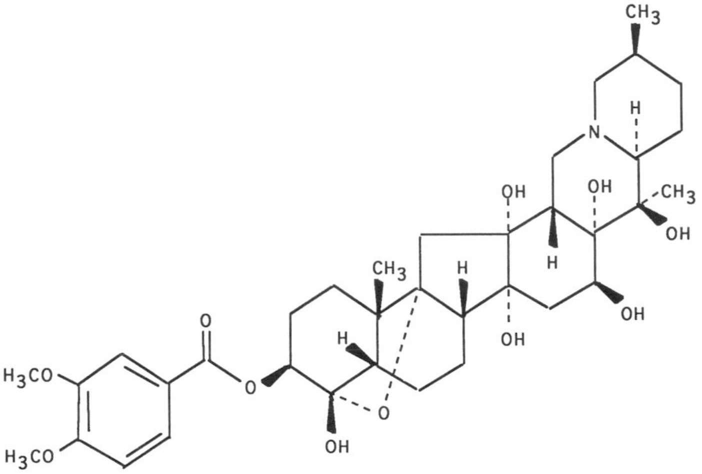

VERATRIDINE
$C_{36}H_{51}NO_{11}$

(3β,4α,16β)-4,9-Epoxycevane-3,4,12,14,16,17,20-heptol 3-(3,4-dimethoxybenzoate)

NEUROTOXICITY RATING

Clinical

A   Ion channel syndrome

Experimental

A   Ion channel dysfunction (sodium channel)

Veratridine is a lipid-soluble alkaloid from the plant *Veratrum album* Linné (white hellebore), *V. viride* (American or green hellebore), or the seed of the Venezulean liliaceous plant *Schoencaulon officiale*; the alkaloid alters the activation gating of sodium channels, which remain open at the resting potential. Veratridine is a yellowish white amorphous powder with a MP of 180°C. The LD_{50} in mice is 1.35 mg/kg. *Veratrum* alkaloids reduce arterial blood pressure and were once employed as hypotensive drugs; however, they are no longer used because of their side effects.

Extracts ("veratrine," a mixture of alkaloids, including veratridine) of *S. officiale* have been used as insecticides, in particular for lice control.

Veratridine binds to site 2 of the Na^+ channel and causes depolarization of a fraction of Na^+ channels by slowing channel inactivation and shifting activation to more negative potentials (1). At the frog neuromuscular junction, spontaneous release of acetylcholine is increased and the postsynaptic membrane depolarized (3).

Several intoxications of humans with plants containing mixtures of *Veratrum* alkaloids have been reported (2,4). Gastrointestinal symptoms, cardiovascular complications, oropharyngeal burning sensations, muscle cramps, and paresthesias develop within minutes of oral intake. For other details of human intoxications with *Veratrum album*, *see* Germine, this volume.

REFERENCES

1. Catterall WA (1980) Neurotoxins that act on voltage-sensitive sodium channels in excitable membranes. *Annu Rev Pharmacol Toxicol* 20, 15.
2. Hruby K, Lenz K, Krausler J (1981) Vergiftung mit *Veratrum album* (weißer Germer). *Wien Klin Wochenschr* 93, 517.
3. Jansson S-E, Albuquerque E-X, Daly J (1974) The pharmacology of batrachotoxin. VI. Effects on the mammalian motor nerve terminal. *J Pharmacol Exp Ther* 189, 525.
4. Seeliger J (1956/1957) Über eine seltene Vergiftung mit weißer Nieswurz. *Arch Toxicol* 16, 16.

Vidarabine

Herbert H. Schaumburg

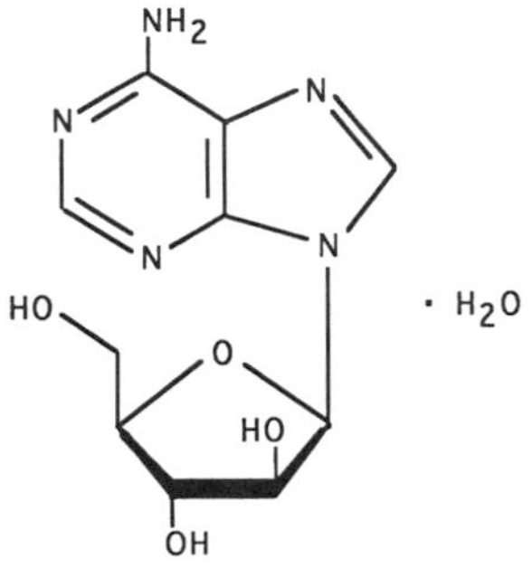

VIDARABINE
$C_{10}H_{13}N_5O_4 \cdot H_2O$

9-β-D-Arabinofuranosyl-9H-purine-6-amine monohydrate; Adenine arabinoside; Ara-A; Vira-A

NEUROTOXICITY RATING

Clinical

A   Peripheral neuropathy

B   Acute encephalopathy (seizures, stupor)

B   Cerebellar syndrome (ataxia, tremor)

Vidarabine is an analog of adenosine developed for use as an anticancer and antiviral nucleoside; it was used to treat *Herpes simplex* encephalitis until acyclovir proved more effective. Currently, vidarabine is primarily employed in treating *Herpes zoster* virus infections in immunocompromised patients, and in some instances of chronic hepatitis B infection.

Vidarabine and its metabolite hypoxanthine arabinoside are phosphorylated in the cell to monophosphate, diphosphate, and triphosphate derivitives; these selectively and competitively inhibit viral DNA polymerase, thereby terminating the extension of newly synthesized strands of nucleic acid. Vidarabine is administered as a daily 24-h intravenous infusion. The drug is undetectable, since it is rapidly converted to hypoxanthine arabinoside; the half-life of hypoxanthine arabinoside is 3.5 h. Systemic side effects from conventional doses of short-term vidarabine therapy are few and minor; they include rash, inappropriate antidiuretic hormone secretion, leukopenia, and thrombocytopenia (7).

Neurotoxicity has been consistently associated with high-dose, long-term vidarabine therapy; coadministration of interferon may enhance the nervous system reaction. Painful sensory neuropathy is the most common and predictable phenomenon, appearing in about 20% of patients at conventional doses; the incidence approaches 100% in high-level, prolonged-treatment protocols (2–6). Painful dysesthesias in the soles and myalgia in lower limb muscles have usually appeared in the last week of therapy; occasionally, they have developed in the 2 weeks following termination. The dysesthesia is unusually confined to the feet and results in considerable disability. Impaired sensory perception in the feet and legs to all modalities and diminished lower limb tendon reflexes generally occur; strength is preserved. Most cases have been of moderate intensity, had no abnormal peripheral electrophysiological findings, and gradually recovered within 7 months of drug withdrawal (5). One report describes slowed sensory (sural nerve) conduction and persistent symptoms 3 years later (4). A similar painful sensory neuropathy occurs in human immunodeficiency virus-positive individuals receiving high-dose dideoxcytidine (DDC) therapy (1). DDC is also a nucleic acid chain terminator; possibly, its neuropathy has a similar pathogenesis.

Acute encephalopathy with prominent cerebellar findings (gait ataxia, intention tremor) is described in several reports (2,8). It appeared in one-third of one group of 15 patients receiving vidarabine for hepatitis B; one individual developed seizures, hallucinations, and respiratory arrest; the cerebellar findings disappeared following drug withdrawal (8). None of these 15 displayed signs or symptoms of sensory neuropathy. The authors reasonably suggest that the underlying hepatic disease in all, and concurrent renal impairment in some, may have predisposed to the acute CNS toxic reaction. A study of children receiving vidarabine suggests that an underlying leukemic disorder and antileukemic therapy directed toward the CNS increase the likelihood of an acute encephalopathic reaction to vidarabine (2).

REFERENCES

1. Berger AR, Arezzo JC, Schaumburg HH et al. (1993) 2′,3′-Dideoxycytidine (ddC) toxic neuropathy: A study of 52 patients. Neurology 43, 358.
2. Feldman S, Robertson PK, Lott L et al. (1986) Neurotoxicity due to adenine arabinoside therapy during varicella-zoster virus infections in immunocompromised children. J Infect Dis 154, 889.
3. Friedman HM (1981) Adenine arabinoside and allopurinol —possible adverse drug interaction. N Engl J Med 304, 423. [Letter]
4. Krause K-H, Raedsch R, Brosi K et al. (1988) Polyneuro-

pathie bei behandler der chronischen hepatitis B mit vidarabin. Deutsch Med Wochenschr 113, 686.
5. Lok AS, Novick DM, Karayiannis P et al. (1985) A randomized study of the effects of adenine arabinoside 5′-monophosphate (short or long courses) and lymphoblastoid interferon on hepatitis B virus replication. Hepatology 5, 1132.
6. Lok ASF, Wilson LA, Thomas HC (1984) Neurotoxicity associated with adenine arabinoside monophosphate in the treatment of chronic hepatitis B virus infection. J Antimicrob Chemother 14, 93.
7. Sacks ST, Scullard GH, Pollard RB et al. (1982) Antiviral treatment of chronic hepatitis B virus infection: Pharmacokinetics and side effects of interferon and adenine arabinoside alone and in combination. Antimicrob Agents Chemother 21, 93.
8. Sacks SL, Smith JL, Pollard RB et al. (1979) Toxicity of vidarabine. J Amer Med Assoc 241, 28.

Vigabatrin

Herbert H. Schaumburg

VIGABATRIN
$C_6H_{11}NO_2$

γ-Vinyl-GABA; 4-Amino-5-hexenoic acid; GVG

NEUROTOXICITY RATING

Clinical
B Psychobiological reaction (depression, aberrant behavior)
B Retinal syndrome

Experimental
A CNS myelinopathy (vacuolar)
B Retinopathy

Vigabatrin (GVG), a structural analogue of the inhibitory neurotransmitter γ-aminobutyric acid (GABA), is an anticonvulsant agent used to treat drug-resistant focal epileptic seizures and infantile spasms associated with tuberous sclerosis. Its pharmacological action is an irreversible inhibition of the degradative enzyme GABA transaminase, thereby enhancing CNS synaptic levels of GABA (10). GVG has been used in Europe without serious toxicity and is considered a valuable agent in treatment of refractory focal epilepsy in children and adults (3,11,18). The oral adult dose ranges from 1–6 g/day.

GVG is rapidly absorbed from the gastrointestinal tract and reaches peak plasma concentrations within an hour.

There is little effect of food on the absorption of GVG (7,12). Plasma concentration–time curves indicate dose-linear pharmacokinetics. Although GVG is not protein-bound, the cerebrospinal fluid (CSF) concentrations are only 10% of the plasma concentration after 6 h. The half-life is 5–7 h. GVG is not metabolized. The major route of excretion is renal and urinary recovery is about 70%. In older individuals, the peak plasma levels and half-life are significantly increased; this likely reflects decreased renal clearance (7). Although anticonvulsant levels are related to dose, monitoring plasma levels as a guide to therapy is of little value, since the action of the drug is related to CNS (synaptic) levels, which are elevated longer than plasma levels and do not correlate well. A twofold rise in human brain GABA levels is documented by magnetic resonance imaging (MRI) in epileptic patients dosed with 3–4 g/day (16). Dosage levels of 6 g/day for 2 years causes a gradual decrease in brain GABA levels, suggesting that GABA synthesis may decrease at high levels of GVG therapy.

There are remarkably few drug interactions with GVG. A 20% fall in phenytoin concentrations may occur in some individuals; its cause is unclear. There is no pharmacological need for patients taking GVG to avoid alcohol (7,12).

Little systemic toxicity is associated with GVG administration in experimental animals or humans. Dogs given 200–300 mg/kg/day develop emesis, diarrhea, and wasting after 4 months.

Reversible, multifocal, microscopic vacuolation of CNS

myelin (intramyelinic edema) occurs in rats, dogs, and monkeys following 4–8 weeks of GVG administration with doses of 300 mg/kg/day (six times the human dose) (4,5,21). Rats and dogs may develop convulsions. Biochemical studies disclose that inhibition of GABA transaminase and significant elevation of GABA occur within 7 days, and myelin vacuoles appear weeks later (4). The CSF levels of GVG are extremely high in the dog (the most susceptible species) as compared to man, monkey, and rodent.

Quantitative MRI studies and electrophysiological measures have confirmed that these lesions are reversible in the living animal. Quantitative MRI studies have detected the onset and recovery of vacuolar lesions in rat cerebellum and in canine fornix, thalamus, and hypothalamus (17,20).

Rats dosed with 100 mg/kg/day for 90 days display mild to moderate myelin vacuolation in the roof nuclei of the cerebellum. Higher doses produced lesions in the brainstem and optic tract. Dogs dosed for 12 weeks with 300 mg/kg/day develop widespread vacuolation of the white matter; lesions appear in the fornix, thalamus, optic tract, septum, hypothalamus, hippocampal end plates, and midbrain. Mild to minimal vacuolation is present in the cortex. The spinal cord and peripheral nerves display no lesions. In general, there is little tissue reaction to these lesions save for mild microglial proliferation. CNS electrophysiological studies of visual and somatosensory evoked response in dogs dosed at 300 mg/kg/day for 6–8 weeks demonstrated increased latencies of both measures; these returned to baseline within 5 weeks of drug withdrawal (19).

The monkey is the least susceptible species; only an occasional vacuole is detectable in white matter. There are no reports of white-matter vacuolation in epileptic patients recieving GVG (1,6); MRI and evoked potential studies may be appropriate monitoring measures for humans receiving chronic treatment with GVG.

Ultrastructural studies show the vacuolar lesion to be intramyelinic edema with splitting of myelin at the intraperiod lines (4,13). Axons and oligodendrocytes appear unaffected. The lesion is ultrastructurally similar to that induced by isoniazid, triethyltin, and hexachlorophene; these substances cause diffuse vacuolation, whereas GVG treatment induces multiple discrete foci of vacuoles.

Retinal lesions detectable by light microscopy appear in albino rats dosed with 300 mg/kg for 90 days but not in similarly dosed pigmented rats. Abnormalities are dose-related, they include disorganization of the outer nuclear layer with displacement of the nuclei into the rod layer (5). These lesions are not detected during ophthalmoscopic examination of these animals. They are similar to those reported in albino rats following excessive exposure to light.

Significant visual impairment has been associated with vigabatrin therapy; blurring and visual field constriction have been symptoms (14). A recent study detected physiological evidence of outer retinal dysfunction in 17 of 20 patients taking vigabatrin; however, only 12 had visual field impairment and only 5 complained of visual disturbance (2). The reversibility of these changes is uncertain, and it is unclear at what stage of visual dysfunction vigabatrin therapy should be discontinued. Patients treated with combinations of vigabatrin and valproate appear more likely to develop retinal dysfunction (2).

No serious human neurotoxicity has been associated with administration of GVG to controls or epileptic patients at therapeutic doses of 50 mg/kg/day for periods of up to 4 years. Prospective studies have failed to demonstrate cognitive dysfunction associated with GVG therapy (8,9,15). Reports of depression and aberrant behavior during GVG treatment suggest that individuals with psychiatric disease should be treated cautiously (18). There have been several histopathological studies from biopsy and postmortem brains of individuals receiving GVG for up to 2 years; none has shown myelin vacuolation (1,6).

The toxic mechanism of the myelin vacuolation seen experimentally in laboratory animals is unknown.

REFERENCES

1. Agosti R, Yasargil G, Egli M *et al.* (1990) Neuropathology of a human hippocampus following long-term treatment with vigabatrin: Lack of microvacuoles. *Epilepsy Res* 6, 166.
2. Arndt CF, Derambure MD, Defoort-Dhellemmes S, Hache JC (1999) Outer retinal dysfunction in patients treated with vigabatrin. *Neurology* 52, 1201.
3. Buchanan N (1993) Vigabatrin in drug-resistant epilepsy. *Med J Australia* 159, 356.
4. Butler WH (1989) The neuropathology of vigabatrin. *Epilepsia* 30, S15.
5. Butler WH, Ford GP, Newberne JW (1987) A study of the effects of vigabatrin on the central nervous system and retina of Sprague-Dawley and Lister-Hooded rats. *Toxicol Pathol* 15, 143.
6. Cannon DJ, Butler WH, Mumford JP, Lewis PJ (1991) Neuropathologic findings in patients receiving long-term vigabatrin therapy for chronic intractable epilepsy. *J Child Neurol* 6, 2S17.
7. Connelly JF (1993) Vigabatrin. *Ann Pharmacother* 27, 197.
8. Dodrill CB, Arnett JL, Sommerville KW, Sussman NM (1993) Evaluation of the effects of vigabatrin on cognitive abilities and quality of life in epilepsy. *Neurology* 43, 2501.
9. Dodrill CB, Arnett JL, Sommerville KW, Sussman NM (1995) Effects of differing dosages of vigabatrin (Sabril)

on cognitive abilities and quality of life in epilepsy. *Epilepsia* **36**, 164.

10. Gale K (1992) GABA and epilepsy: Basic concepts from preclinical research. *Epilepsia* **33**, S3.

11. Gram L, Sabers A, Dulac O (1992) Treatment of pediatric epilepsies with γ-vinyl GABA (vigabatrin). *Epilepsia* **33**, S26.

12. Hoke JF, Yuh L, Antony KK *et al.* (1993) Pharmacokinetics of vigabatrin following single and multiple oral doses in normal volunteers. *J Clin Pharmacol* **33**, 458.

13. Jackson GD, Williams SR, Weller RO *et al.* (1994) Vigabatrin-induced lesions in the rat brain demonstrated by quantitative magnetic resonance imaging. *Epilep Res* **18**, 57.

14. Krauss GL, Johnson MA, Miller NR (1998) Vigabatrin-associated retinal cone system dysfunction: electroretinogram and opthalmologic findings. *Neurology* **50**, 614.

15. McGuire AM, Duncan JS, Trimble MR (1992) Effects of vigabatrin on cognitive function and mood when used as add-on therapy in patients with intractable epilepsy. *Epilepsia* **33**, 128.

16. Petroff OA, Rothman DL, Behar KL, Mattson RH (1996) Human brain GABA levels rise after initiation of vigabatrin therapy but fail to rise further with increasing dose. *Neurology* **46**, 1459.

17. Peyster RG, Sussman NM, Hershey BL, Heydorn WE (1995) Use of *ex vivo* magnetic resonance imaging to detect onset of vigabatrin-induced intramyelinic edema in canine brain. *Epilepsia* **36**, 93.

18. Reynolds EH (1992) γ-Vinyl GABA (vigabatrin): Clinical experience in adult and adolescent patients with intractable epilepsy. *Epilepsia* **33**, S30.

19. Schroeder CE, Gibson JP, Yarrington J *et al.* (1992) Effects of high-dose γ-vinyl GABA (vigabatrin) administration on visual and somatosensory evoked potentials in dogs. *Epilepsia* **33**, S13.

20. Weiss KL, Schroeder CE, Kastin SJ *et al.* (1994) MRI monitoring of vigabatrin-induced intramyelinic edema in dogs. *Neurology* **44**, 1944.

21. Yarrington JT, Gibson JP, Dillberer JE, Hurst G (1993) Sequential neuropathology of dogs treated with vigabatrin, a GABA-transaminase inhibitor. *Toxicol Pathol* **21**, 480.

Vinca Alkaloids

Herbert H. Schaumburg

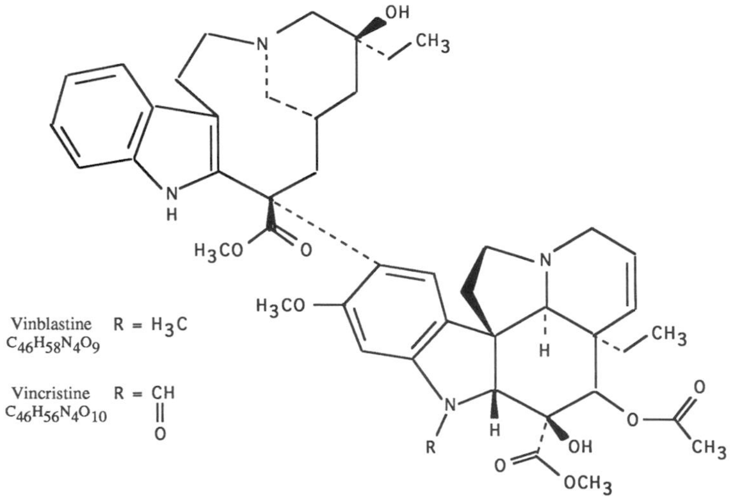

Vinblastine   R = H₃C
C₄₆H₅₈N₄O₉

Vincristine   R = CH
            ‖
            O
C₄₆H₅₆N₄O₁₀

VINCA ALKALOIDS

Vinblastine; Vincaleukoblastine; VBL
Vincristine; 22-Oxovincaleukoblastine; VCR

NEUROTOXICITY RATING
Clinical
A   Peripheral neuropathy
B   Acute encephalopathy (agitation, hallucination)
B   Myopathy
B   Ototoxicity

Experimental
A   Myopathy (necrotizing)
A   Ototoxicity

Vincristine (VCR) and vinblastine (VBL), derivatives of the periwinkle plant (*Vinca rosea*), are important chemotherapeutic agents with similar neurotoxic actions. VCR, the subject here, is far more widely used than VBL and has greater potential for adverse effects upon the nervous system.

VCR is used in combination with other chemotherapeutic agents in the treatment of solid tumors, lymphoma and leukemia. Its chemotherapeutic action stems from inhibition of mitosis by way of metaphase arrest (21); this effect likely results from the ability of VCR to bind specifically with tubulin and block polymerization of its subunits into microtubules (25). The drug is administered once weekly as an intravenous medication; preparations of 1, 2 and 5 ml (1 mg/ml) are available. VCR is most commonly given as a 1 mg/ml bolus. Levels and durations of therapy vary with the type of neoplasm and age of the patient; the standard weekly dose for adults is 1.4 mg/m^2.

Most of the unique properties of microtubules are due to the maintenance of a dynamic equilibrium with tubulin and their ability to polymerize and depolymerize in response to function and progression through the cell cycle. VCR binding disrupts the dynamic equilibrium between polymerized and depolymerized tubules by producing highly ordered paracrystalline arrays of tubulin that inhibit formation of microtubules (23). Although its primary cytotoxic action is through metaphase arrest, there is evidence that VCR also has an effect on nonproliferating cells that are in the G_1 phase of the cell cycle (34). Neurotoxicity results from the interaction of the drug with axonal microtubules. Peripheral neuropathy is the major, dose-limiting toxicity of VCR therapy; myopathy and encephalopathy are rare (2,4,9,27).

General Toxicology

After intravenous injection, VCR has a multiphasic pattern of clearance from plasma; its terminal half-life is about 24 hours in adults. Following a 1-ml bolus, peak plasma concentrations approach 0.4 μM; there is a prolonged terminal half-life and extensive tissue binding. The mean clearance in adults is 189 ml/min per square meter. Studies in children describe a higher rate of clearance (482 ml/min/m^2) (7). Approximately 45% of VCR is bound to serum proteins. The drug is metabolized in the liver, and hepatic dysfunction limits its use. It is suggested that an enterohepatic circulation may account in part for the prolonged neural exposure to VCR. The biliary system is the principal excetory pathway; VCR is present in the bile of dogs 2 weeks following an intravenous bolus injection. There is evidence that oxidative metabolism may create metabolites that subsequently bind to tubulin. Co-administration of substances that induce or inhibit cytochrome P-450 enzymes may affect VCR disposition. Variability in toxicity may reflect, in part, differences in serum clearance. Studies in several species and humans indicate that VCR has limited penetration into the CNS; spinal fluid concentrations have been 20%–

30% lower than concurrent plasma levels. Although there have been no determinations of the penetrance of VCR into the PNS, it is suggested that the high incidence of neuropathy and rare CNS toxicity reflects differential access of the drug to these tissues (18).

Systemic toxicity from VCR is rarely dose-limiting. Characteristic VCR systemic toxic reactions include gastrointestinal dysfunction (acute ileus), urinary retention and hypotension; these largely reflect the induction of autonomic neuropathy (2,4). Severe myelosuppression is usually not a major effect of VCR therapy and is a cardinal reason for the wide use of the drug. Hematologic toxicity (anemia, leukopenia, thrombocytopenia) may be a feature of VCR overdoses. It is alleged that adminstration of large doses of glutamic acid to experimental animals ameliorates the systemic toxicity and neurotoxicity of VCR (17). Inappropriate secretion of antidiuretic hormone may cause hyponatremia and generalized seizures in patients receiving hyperhydration as part of their therapy. Alopecia appears in 20% of patients; it is usually reversible.

Animal Studies

In general, it has proven difficult to create an experimental animal model that corresponds to human VCR neuropathy; myopathy, rare in humans, is readily and consistently produced in guinea pigs (1).

There are no experimental animal studies of chronic systemic administration of VCR that demonstrate convincing clinical evidence of polyneuropathy. A light-microscope examination of sciatic nerve biopsies from rats dosed with an equivalent of 0.15 mg/kg/day for 6 weeks describes a few scattered fibers undergoing wallerian-like axonal degeneration (9). An investigation of VCR toxicity in the guinea pig has produced convincing electrophysiological signs of axonal degeneration, and a few fibers had morphological evidence of axonal degeneration after 14 weeks of doses of 0.03 mg/kg twice weekly (1). Two studies of axoplasmic transport in nerves from cats dosed with 0.04 mg/kg twice weekly for 6 weeks describe the animals as having neuropathy; neither is solid: electrophysiological or morphological studies are not described in one report (3), and the morphological abnormalities in the other study are unconvincing (10). The latter study did demonstrate that chronic (4 to 6 weeks) systemic VCR administration partially blocks fast axoplasmic transport in cat sciatic nerve. A study of the effect of 6 months dosing of rats with one crushed sciatic nerve at levels of 200, 100, and 50 μg/kg showed diminished microtubule concentration with normal neurofilament density in the crushed nerves; the uncrushed sciatic nerves appeared normal (33). The authors suggest that the failure of VCR readily to penetrate the blood-brain and blood-nerve barriers may explain the difficulties in producing neuropathy in normal animals.

Intrathecal administration of VCR causes accumulations of intermediate neurofibrillary tangles in nuclei and axons in many areas of the CNS including dorsal root ganglia, hippocampal formation, and hypoglossal nuclei. Neuronal crystalloid inclusions develop within days of injection and subsequently disappear; their origin and significance are uncertain (28). Subarachnoid injection of VBL in rabbits is followed by accumulations of neurofilaments and decreased numbers of neurotubules in neurons of the spinal cord anterior horn cells (37).

One histopathological study of cat nerve following topical application of VCR describes a decreased density of neurotubules associated with malorientation of both microtubules and neurofilaments (26). The authors suggest these morphological alterations could correlate with the abnormalities in axoplasmic transport demonstrated by previous *in vitro* studies (16,24). Local injection of VCR in rat sural nerve completely disrupt neurotubules and cause the formation of crystalloid structures in the axon (29). Focal giant axonal swellings appear in proximal regions of cat sciatic nerve soon after intravenous dosing (6).

Systemic administration of VCR to the guinea pig readily causes myopathic changes (1). After only 2 days of daily doses of 0.1 mg/kg, whorled bodies, most likely derived from the sarcoplasmic reticulum, appear in the sarcoplasm. Some animals on a chronic-dose protocol—14 weeks of 0.03 mg/kg twice weekly—became moribund with severe hindlimb weakness; others survived for the 14 weeks and displayed no abnormal neurological findings (1). Proximal muscles of animals that died early displayed widespread necrotic changes with advanced phagocytosis. It is unclear whether muscle in the surviving animals became resistant to VCR, or whether animals that were particularly sensitive died earlier (1).

Systemic administration of vincristine to rabbits destroys the organ of Corti sensory cells as well as cells of the spiral ganglion (30). Vinblastine sulfate destroys the organ of Corti sensory cells but spares the spiral ganglion (31).

In Vitro Studies

In vitro studies utilizing tissue from chicken and bovine preparations demonstrate that vinca alkaloids are attracted to two high-affinity binding sites on brain tubulin and can prevent microtubule polymerization (13,34). At high concentrations, they also can react with preformed neurotubules. It has recently been observed that VCR binds to aged tubulin and the aging of tubulin is accompanied by quenching of tryptophan fluorescence similar to that which occurs

upon binding of *Vinca* drugs (25). It is suggested that vinca alkaloids stabilize the aged conformation of the protein by interacting with nonpolar regions that may be related to the aggregation sites (25).

In vitro studies convincingly demonstrate that vinca alkaloids disrupt fast axoplasmic transport (5,16,24). VBL is the most potent alkaloid on sheathed sciatic nerve; VCR is the most potent in desheathed preparations, and its uptake into the nerve is three times greater than that of VBL (16).

Results of studies of the possible neuroprotective effects of nerve growth factor and gangliosides on dorsal root ganglion and sympathetic cell cultures indicate mild to moderate attenuation of VCR neurotoxicity (12,15,19).

Human Studies

VCR neuropathy occurs in a stereotyped manner, is manifest to some extent in most treated patients, and has clinical features suggesting an unusual distribution and evolution of axonopathy.

Symptoms of peripheral neuropathy commence within 2 months in almost all subjects receiving the standard dosage of 0.05 mg/kg weekly; paresthesias and loss of ankle jerks were noted after 3 weeks of this regimen in 8 of 9 patients in a prospective study (22). Higher-dose regimens are associated with earlier onset and more severe disability (4).

Paresthesias, often starting in the fingers before the feet, herald the onset of VCR neuropathy in almost every case. The initial physical finding is loss of ankle jerks. Sensory loss, usually confined to the distal limbs, is detected next; progression of sensory loss to the high stocking-and-glove pattern associated with other toxic neuropathies seldom occurs. Weakness is the most prominent feature of this neuropathy and, along with autonomic dysfunction, accounts for most of the disability. Clumsiness of the hands and leg cramps following exercise are the first motor symptoms. Weakness is most severe in extensors of wrists and fingers and in foot dorsiflexors; it is frequently disabling and may develop rapidly (7 to 10 days). Signs of autonomic dysfunction, usually ileus and urinary retention, often follow the appearance of limb weakness. Cranial nerve dysfunction (extraocular palsies, dysphagia) is rare. There are a few reports of ototoxicity that feature sudden onset of sensorineural hearing loss with gradual recovery (20). Muscle pain in the jaw or legs frequently is a transient phenomenon shortly following an intravenous injection. Acute toxic encephalopathy (hallucinations, insomnia, psychosis) and physical signs of myopathy (wasting, proximal weakness) are rare (2).

Recovery from peripheral neuropathy is usual; weakness improves rapidly if the drug is stopped in an early stage of disability. Paresthesias usually abate within two weeks of ending therapy, but most patients have residual mild distal sensory loss. Tendon reflexes eventually reappear, save for the ankle jerks. Following recovery from VCR neuropathy, therapy can recommence at lower dosage and continue for several months without recurrence of symptoms.

Accidental intrathecal administration causes the rapid onset of a fatal myeloencephalopathy with diffuse necrosis of CNS tissues in contact with spinal fluid; elevated levels of VCR are present in the cerebrospinal fluid (36). This condition can be successfully treated by rapid perfusion of the ventricles and lumbar subarachnoid space with copious amounts of lactated Ringer's solution and glutamic acid (18).

Sensory nerve conduction studies in digital nerves disclose reduction in amplitude commensurate with drug dosage and duration; conduction velocities are only slightly slowed (4,22). Electromyographic study of distal muscles shows evidence of denervation with fibrillation and reduced numbers of motor units; these changes may precede detectible weakness. One study suggests that the most sensitive electrodiagnostic test is the ratio between the amplitudes of the soleus action potential elicited by a tendon jerk and by the II reflex; this corresponds to the early loss of the Achilles tendon reflex (11).

Sural nerve biopsies in advanced cases disclose nonspecific axonal degeneration; alterations in cytoskeletal components similar to those in experimental studies are not described in human nerve biopsies (22). Neurofilament accumulations in CNS neurons develop in patients receiving high-dose intravenous therapy and following accidental intrathecal administration (31).

Patients with systemic neoplasms (lymphoma, leukemia) appear no more susceptible to VCR neurotoxicity than those with primary CNS tumors (2). One report claims that administration of 500 mg of glutamic acid 3 times daily ameliorates the neurotoxicity of VCR (18); others have been unable to confirm this effect, and glutamic acid is not widely used as prophylaxis. Individuals with hereditary neuropathy have increased susceptibility and are at risk for early development of severe neuropathy (14), as are patients receiving other chemotherapeutic agents associated with peripheral neuropathy (35). One study suggests that preexistent diabetic neuropathy does not increase vulnerability (4).

Toxic Mechanisms

Experimental animal and *in vitro* studies have convincingly demonstrated that VCR (a) impairs fast anterograde axoplasmic transport, and (b) causes a decrease in the number of neurotubules or loss of portions of neurotubules in concert with cytoskeletal disorganization in peripheral axons. It is widely held that these changes reflect biochemical events that are pathogenetic in VCR peripheral neuropathy. The mechanism whereby dysfunction of fast axoplasmic transport would cause the unusual clinical profile of VCR neuropathy (motor > sensory) is unknown.

REFERENCES

1. Bradley WG (1970) The neuromyopathy of vincristine in the guinea pig. An electrophysiological and pathological study. *J Neurol Sci* **10**, 133.
2. Bradley WG, Lassman LP, Pearce GW, Walton JN (1970) The neuromyopathy of vincristine in man clinical, electrophysiological and pathological studies. *J Neurol Sci* **10**, 131.
3. Bradley WG, Williams MH (1973) Axoplasmic flow in axonal neuropathies. *Brain* **96**, 235.
4. Casey EB, Jellife AM, LeQuesne PM, Millett Y (1973) Vincristine neuropathy. *Brain* **96**, 69.
5. Chan SY, Worth R, Ochs S (1980) Block of axoplasmic transport *in vitro* by *Vinca* alkaloids. *J Neurobiol* **11**, 251.
6. Cho, EN, Lowndes, HE, Goldstein BD (1983) Neurotoxicology of vincristine in the cat. Morphological study. *Arch Toxicol* **52**, 83.
7. Crom WR, deGraff SSN, Synold T *et al.* (1994) Pharmacokinetics of vincristine in children and adolescents with acute lymphocytic leukemia. *J Pediatr* **125**, 642.
8. Dyke RW (1988) Treatment of inadvertent intrathecal injection of vincristine. *N Engl J Med* **84**, 1016.
9. Gottschalk PG, Dyck PJ, Kiely JM (1968) *Vinca* alkaloid neuropathy: Nerve biopsy studies in rats and in man. *Neurology* **18**, 875.
10. Green LS, Donoso A, Heller-Bettinger IE, Samson FE (1976) Axonal transport disturbances in vincristine-induced peripheral neuropathy. *Ann Neurol* **1**, 255.
11. Guiheneuc P, Ginet J, Groleau JY, Rojouan J (1980) Early phase of vincristine neuropathy in man. *J Neurol Sci* **45**, 355.
12. Hayakawa K, Sobue G, Itoh T, Mitsuma T (1994) Nerve growth factor prevents neurotoxic effects of cisplatin, vincristine and taxol, on adult rat sympathetic ganglion explants *in vitro*. *Life Sci* **55**, 519.
13. Himes RH, Kersey RN, Heller-Bettinger I, Samson FE (1976) Action of the *Vinca* alkaloids vincristine, vinblastine, and desacetyl vinblastine amide on microtubules *in vitro*. *Cancer Res* **36**, 3798.
14. Hogan-Dann C, Fellmeth WG, McGuire AS, Kiley VA (1984) Polyneuropathy following vincristine therapy in two patients with Charcot-Marie-Tooth syndrome. *J Amer Med Assn* **252**, 2862.
15. Houi H, Mochio S, Kobayashi T (1993) Gangliosides attenuate vincristine neurotoxicity on dorsal root ganglion cells. *Muscle Nerve* **16**, 11.

16. Iqbal Z, Ochs S (1980) Uptake of *Vinca* alkaloids into mammalian nerve and its subcellular components. *J Neurochem* **34**, 59.

17. Jackson DV, Rosenbaum DL, Carlisle LH et al. (1984) Glutamic acid modification of vincristine toxicity. *Cancer Biochem Biophys* **7**, 245.

18. Jackson DV, Wells HB, Atkins JN et al. (1988) Amelioration of vincristine neurotoxicity by glutamic acid. *Amer J Med* **84**, 1016.

19. Konings PN, Makkink WK, Van delft AM, Ruigt GS (1994) Reversal by NGF of cytostatic drug-induced reduction of neurite outgrowth in rat dorsal root ganglia *in vitro*. *Brain Res* **640**, 195.

20. Mahajan SL (1981) Acute acoustic nerve palsy associated with vincristine therapy. *Cancer* **47**, 2404.

21. Malawista SE, Sato H, Bensch K (1968) Vinblastine and griseofulvin reversibly disrupt the living mitotic spindle. *Science* **160**, 770.

22. Mcleod JG, Penny R (1969) Vincristine neuropathy: An electrophysiological and histological study. *J Neurol Neurosurg Psychiat* **32**, 297.

23. Owellen RJ, Woens AH, Donigan DW (1972) The binding of vincristine, vinblastine and colchicine to tubulin. *Biochem Biophys Res Commun* **47**, 685.

24. Paulson JC, McClure WO (1975) Inhibition of axoplasmic transport by colchicine, podophyllotoxin, and vinblastine: an effect on microtubules. *Ann NY Acad Sci* **253**, 517.

25. Prakash V, Timasheff SN (1992) Aging of tubulin at neutral pH: The destabilizing effect of *Vinca* alkaloids. *Arch Biochem Biophy* **295**, 137.

26. Sahenk Z, Brady ST, Mendell JR (1987) Studies on the pathogenesis of vincristine-induced neuropathy. *Muscle Nerve* **10**, 80.

27. Sandler SG, Tobin W, Henderson ES (1969) Vincristine-induced neuropathy. *Neurology* **19**, 367.

28. Sato M, Miyoshi K (1984) Ultrastructural observations on the vincristine-induced neuronal crystalloid inclusion in young rats. *Acta Neuropathol* **63**, 150.

29. Schlaepfer WW (1971) Vincristine-induced axonal alterations in rat peripheral nerve. *J Neuropathol Exp Neurol* **30**, 488.

30. Serafy A (1981) The effect of vincristine sulfate on the neurological elements of the rabbit cochlea. *J Laryngol Otol* **95**, 49.

31. Serafy A (1982) The effect of vinblastine sulfate on the neurological elements of the rabbit cochlea. *J Laryngol Otol* **96**, 975.

32. Shelanski ML, Wisniewski H (1969) Neurofibrillary degeneration induced by vincristine therapy. *Arch Neurol* **20**, 199.

33. Shiraishi S, LeQuesne PM, Gajree T, Cavanagh JB (1985) Morphometric effects of vincristine on nerve regeneration in the rat. *J Neurol Sci* **71**, 165.

34. Strychmans PA, Lurie PM, Manaster J et al. (1973) Mode of action of chemotherapy *in vivo* on human acute leukemia. II. Vincristine. *Eur J Cancer* **9**, 613.

35. Thant M, Hawley RJ, Smith MT et al. (1982) Possible enhancement of vincristine neuropathy by VP-16. *Cancer* **49**, 859.

36. Williams ME, Walker AN, Bracikowski JP et al. (1983) Ascending myeloencephalopathy due to intrathecal vincristine sulfate. *Cancer* **51**, 2041.

37. Wisniewski H, Shelanski ML, Terry RD (1968) Effects of mitotic spindle inhibitors on neurotubules and neurofilaments in anterior horn cells. *J Cell Biol* **38**, 224.

Vinyl Chloride

Peter S. Spencer

$$CH_2 = CHCl$$

VINYL CHLORIDE

Chloroethylene; Ethylene monochloride; Monochloroethylene; Monochloroethene

NEUROTOXICITY RATING
Clinical

B Peripheral neuropathy

Vinyl chloride monomer (VCM) is used principally for the production of polyvinyl chloride (PVC), a huge industry that began in the United States in the early 1940s. U.S. production of VCM in 1986 alone was estimated as 8.5 billion pounds, mostly for PVC resins (6). PVC is used in building and construction, home furnishings, recreational products, apparel, and automobile materials.

VCM is generated in a closed system by direct chlorination or oxychlorination of ethylene. Under pressure in reactor vessels, VCM liquefies and polymerizes to form PVC resins; cleaning the reactor represents the principal occupational hazard (6). The wide range of adverse health effects that accompanies overexposure to VCM, including acro-osteolysis, scleroderma, and liver disease culminating in hepatic angiosarcoma, has been reviewed (1).

VCM is a colorless, flammable gas that polymerizes in light or in the presence of a catalyst. High concentrations (~ 3000 ppm) are detected as a mild, sweet odor; taste in water is detectable at 3–4 ppm. The U.S. Occupational Safety and Health Administration stipulates an 8-h time-weighted maximum average exposure of 1 ppm for exposure in the workplace. The U.S. Environmental Protection Agency limits VCM in drinking water to a maximum concentration of 0.002 ppm.

VCM is readily absorbed through the lungs of humans and animals. Peak blood levels were found in rats after 30 min of head-only exposure to 7000 ppm (29). Body distribution, metabolism, and excretion occur rapidly. Radioactivity from radiolabeled vinyl chloride is much greater in the liver than in other organs (26); small amounts of metabolites are found in other tissues, including the brain (3,5,27). VCM is oxidized by hepatic mixed function oxidases to form an epoxide intermediate, 2-chloroethylene oxide, that alkylates DNA and RNA, promotes base-pair substitution, and induces neoplastic transformation (4). 2-Chloroethylene oxide spontaneously rearranges to form 2-chloroacetaldehyde, which binds to protein (8,9,28). Intermediates are detoxified by glutathione conjugation, and conjugated products are excreted in urine as substituted cysteine derivatives, including thiodiglycolic acid, S-formylmethylcysteine, and N-acetyl-S-(2-hydroxyethyl)cysteine.

Inhalation LD_{50}s are established for mice (294 mg/l), rats (390 mg/l), guinea pigs (595 mg/l), and rabbits (295 mg/l). Guinea pigs became unconscious within 30 min of exposure to 100,000 ppm VCM (16). Mice developed ataxia and twitching at 50,000 ppm (10). Exposure of guinea pigs to 25,000 ppm for 8 h resulted in ataxia followed by unconsciousness during the treatment period; 10,000 ppm was without noticeable effect (18). No effects were noted in rats exposed to 500 ppm for 1 h/day, 5 days/week for 2 weeks or to 50 ppm for 1 h/day, 5 days/week for 20 weeks (10). Rats treated with 30,000 ppm 4 h/day, 5 days/week for 12 months were soporific during exposures (23,24). After 10 months, rats had decreased responses to external stimuli and disturbances of equilibrium. Postmortem studies of the brain reportedly revealed diffuse degeneration of gray and white matter coupled with pronounced degeneration of cerebellar Purkinje cells (23,24). Other nonneoplastic lesions were reported in rats exposed to 5000 ppm for 7 h/day, 5 days/week for 12 months (7).

VCM was once considered for use as an inhalation anesthetic (1). Human volunteers exposed to 20,000 ppm (5 min, twice daily) or 25,000 ppm (3 min) VCM experienced dizziness, disorientation, and burning sensations in the feet during exposure; recovery was rapid, but some developed a postexposure headache (12,18). One of six subjects reported dizziness after exposure to 8000 ppm for 5 min twice daily; no effects were reported with 4000 ppm.

Occupational exposures to VCM have resulted in numerous reports of ataxia or dizziness (11,13,15,21,22), drowsiness or fatigue (11,21,22), euphoria and irritability (22), headache (11,13,15,21), visual and/or hearing disturbances (15), memory loss, nervousness and sleep disturbances (11,22), or loss of consciousness (17). Pyramidal and cerebellar signs have been found in some exposed subjects (11).

Several investigators have reported manifestations of peripheral neuropathy in VCM workers. One study claimed that 70% of workers had a slight distal neuropathy characterized by muscle fasciculation, fibrillation potentials, and increased duration of motor unit potentials (19). Similar effects were noted in another VCM worker (14). Several other reports have noted extremity paresthesias (13,20,21,22,24) and warmth (11), finger numbness (13) and pain (20), and weakness (11,22). Raynaud's phenomenon, scleroderma, and thyroid insufficiency develop in a small percentage of VCM-exposed workers (1,25).

VCM disease, a syndrome consisting of Raynaud's phenomenon, acro-osteolysis, joint and muscle pain, enhanced collagen deposition, hand stiffness, and scleroderma-like changes, may have an immunological basis (1). Human lymphocytic antigen (HLA) typing shows that affected subjects have a significantly greater incidence of the HLA-DR5 allele; disease progression may be favored in subjects with HLA-DR3 and B8 (2). VCM workers with Raynaud's phenomenon have vasomotor abnormalities coupled with impaired capillary circulation, inflammatory infiltration of arterioles, and arterial occlusion (1). Vascular insufficiency might underlie in whole or in part the abnormalities of peripheral nerve function reported in VCM-exposed workers.

REFERENCES

1. Agency for Toxic Substances and Disease Registry (1997) *Toxicological Profile for Vinyl Chloride.* U.S. Department of Health and Human Services, Public Health Service, Atlanta, Georgia.
2. Black C, Pereira S, McWhirter A *et al.* (1986) Genetic susceptibility to scleroderma-like syndrome in symptomatic and asymptomatic workers exposed to vinyl chloride. *J Rheumatol* 13, 1059.
3. Bolt HM, Kappus H, Buchter *et al.* (1976) Disposition of (1,2^{14}C) vinyl chloride in the rat. *Arch Toxicol* 35, 153.
4. Bolt HM, Laib RJ, Peter H *et al.* (1986) DNA adducts of halogenated hydrocarbons. *J Cancer Res Clin Oncol* 112, 96.
5. Buchter A, Bolt HM, Kappus H *et al.* (1977) Tissue distribution of 1,2^{14}C-vinyl chloride in the rat. *Int Arch Occup Environ Health* 39, 27. [German]

6. Falk H (1992) Vinyl chloride and polyvinyl chloride. In: *Environmental and Occupational Medicine*. Rom WN ed. Little, Brown & Co, Boston p. 911.

7. Feron VJ, Kroes R (1979) One-year time-sequence inhalation toxicity study of vinyl chloride in rats. II. Morphological changes in the respiratory tract, ceruminous glands, brain, kidneys, heart and spleen. *Toxicology* **13**, 131.

8. Guengerich FP, Mason PS, Scott WJ *et al.* (1981) Roles of 2-haloethylene oxide and 2-haloacetaldehydes derived from vinyl bromide and vinyl chloride in irreversible binding to protein and DNA. *Cancer Res* **41**, 4391.

9. Guengerich FP, Watanabe PG (1979) Metabolism of (^{14}C) and (^{35}Cl)-labeled vinyl chloride *in vivo* and *in vitro*. *Biochem Pharmacol* **28**, 589.

10. Hehir RM, McNamara BP, McLaughlin J Jr *et al.* (1981) Cancer induction following single and multiple exposures to a constant amount of vinyl chloride monomer. *Environ Health Perspect* **41**, 63.

11. Langauer-Lewowicka H, Kurzbauer H, Byczkowska Z *et al.* (1983) Vinyl chloride disease—neurological disturbances. *Int Arch Occup Environ Health* **52**, 151.

12. Lester D, Greenberg LA, Adams WR (1963) Effects of single and repeated exposures of humans and rats to vinyl chloride. *Amer Ind Hyg Assn J* **24**, 265.

13. Lilis R, Anderson H, Miller A *et al.* (1975) Prevalence of disease among vinyl chloride and polyvinyl chloride workers. *Ann N Y Acad Sci* **246**, 22.

14. Magnavita N, Bergamaschi A, Garcovich A *et al.* (1986) Vasculitic purpura in vinyl chloride disease: A case report. *Angiology* **37**, 382.

15. Marsteller HJ, Lelbach WK, Muller R *et al.* (1975) Unusual splenomegalic liver disease as evidenced by peritoneoscopy and guided liver biopsy among polyvinyl chloride production workers. *Ann N Y Acad Sci* **246**, 95.

16. Mastromatteo E, Fisher AM, Christie H *et al.* (1960) Acute inhalation toxicity of vinyl chloride to laboratory animals. *Amer Ind Hyg Assn J* **21**, 394.

17. National Institutes for Occupational Safety and Health (NIOSH) (1977) *A Cross-sectional Epidemiologic Survey of Vinyl Chloride Workers*. U.S. Department of Health and Human Services, NIOSH Division of Surveillance, Hazard Evaluations, and Field Studies. Cincinnati, Ohio, NTIS PB27274193.

18. Patty FA, Yant WP, Waite CP (1930) Acute response of guinea pigs to vapors of some new commercial organic compounds. V. Vinyl chloride. *Public Health Rep* **45**, 1963.

19. Perticoni GF, Abbritti G, Cantisani TA *et al.* (1986) Polyneuropathy in workers with long exposure to vinyl chloride. Electrophysiological study. *Electromyogr Clin Neurophysiol* **26**, 41.

20. Sakabe H (1975) Bone lesions among polyvinyl chloride production workers in Japan. *Ann N Y Acad Sci* **246**, 78.

21. Spirtas R, McMichael AJ, Gamble J *et al.* (1975) The association of vinyl chloride exposures with morbidity symptoms. *Amer J Ind Hyg Assn J* **36**, 779.

22. Suciu I, Prodan L, Ilea E *et al.* (1975) Clinical manifestations in vinyl chloride poisoning. *Ann N Y Acad Sci* **246**, 53.

23. Viola PL (1970) Pathology of vinyl chloride. *Med Lav* **61**, 174.

24. Viola PL, Bigotti A, Caputo A (1971) Oncogenic response of rat skin, lungs, and bones to vinyl chloride. *Cancer Res* **31**, 516.

25. Walker AE (1976) Clinical aspects of vinyl chloride disease. Skin. *Proc Roy Soc Med* **69**, 286.

26. Watanabe PG, McGowan GR, Gehring PJ (1976) Fate of [^{14}C]vinyl chloride after single oral administration to rats. *Toxicol Appl Pharmacol* **36**, 339.

27. Watanabe PG, McGowan GR, Madrid EO *et al.* (1976) Fate of [^{14}C]vinyl chloride following inhalation exposure in rats. *Toxicol Appl Pharmacol* **37**, 49.

28. Watanabe PG, Zempel JA, Pegg DG *et al.* (1978) Hepatic macromolecular binding following exposure to vinyl chloride. *Toxicol Appl Pharmacol* **44**, 571.

29. Withey JR (1976) Pharmacodynamics and uptake of vinyl chloride monomer administered by various routes to rats. *J Toxicol Environ Health* **1**, 381.

Vinyltoluene

Herbert H. Schaumburg

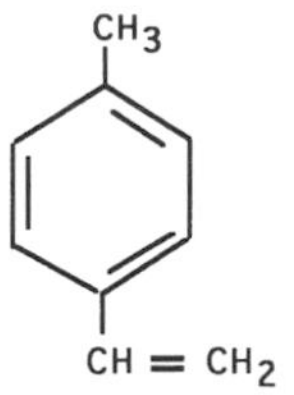

VINYLTOLUENE
C$_9$H$_{10}$

NEUROTOXICITY RATING

Experimental

C   Peripheral neuropathy

Vinyltoluene, used in pharmaceutical synthesis, is a less volatile homologue of styrene. Vinyltoluene is an irritant of the eyes and mucous membranes and, at high concentrations, causes narcosis in rodents. There are no reports of human systemic or nervous system toxicity. Experimental animal studies that allege changes in peripheral nerve function and neurochemical abnormalities are unconvincing (1–3).

REFERENCES

1. Savolainen H, Pfaffli P (1981) Neurochemical effects of short-term inhalation exposure to vinyltoluene vapor. *Arch Environ Contam Toxicol* 10, 511.
2. Seppäläinen AM, Savolainen H (1982) Dose-dependent neurophysiological and biochemical effects of prolonged vinyltoluene vapor inhalation in rat. *Neurotoxicology* 3, 36.
3. Seppäläinen AM, Savolainen H (1982) Impaired nerve function in rats after prolonged exposure to vinyltoluene. *Arch Toxicol* 5, 100.

Vitamin A

Mitchell Steinschneider

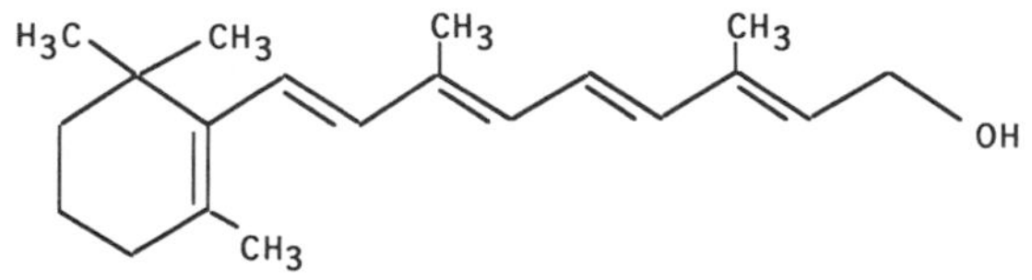

VITAMIN A
C$_{20}$H$_{30}$O

Retinol; All-trans-retinol

NEUROTOXICITY RATING

Clinical

A   Teratogenicity

A   Benign intracranial hypertension

Experimental

A   Teratogenicity

Vitamin A (retinol) represents a family of lipophilic compounds that are essential for multiple physiological functions, including phototransduction, embryogenesis, and tissue growth (1,5,23). For instance, the initial event in visual perception is the light-induced isomerization in photoreceptor cells of the 11-*cis* isomer of retinal to the all-*trans* form (23). Retinoic acid is a key regulator of cell differentiation by mechanisms that include binding to nuclear receptors and influencing gene transcription (18,22). Retinoids also have effects on neurofilament proteins, protein kinase C, and Ca^{2+}–adenosine triphosphatase activity (22). Vitamin A supplements may slow the rate of disease progression in retinitis pigmentosa (2,6,16). Isotretinoin and other retinoids are effective against acne and other dermatological conditions (14). Retinoic acid has been used in the treatment of certain leukemias associated with an abnormality of a retinoic acid–binding nuclear receptor (18). β-Carotene, a plant-derived vitamin A precursor, treats certain light-sensitive diseases, and has shown promise as a therapy for certain cancers, cardiovascular disease, immunocompromised hosts, and cataracts (7,18,24).

Vitamin A is transported from the gut to the liver *via* chylomicrons and is hydrolyzed in hepatic parenchymal cells (3,8,21). Greater than 90% of vitamin A is stored in the liver (1,8). It is transported in the plasma by retinol-binding proteins complexed with prealbumin (3,8,21). Metabolism is regulated by binding of vitamin A to specific intracellular receptor proteins (18).

Multiple organs are the targets of hypervitaminosis A toxicity. The principal neurotoxic effect is pseudotumor cerebri, a condition of raised intracranial pressure with normal cerebrospinal fluid and neuroimaging studies. Abnormal liver function tests, hepatomegaly, and histological changes (*e.g.*, perisinusoidal fibrosis, central vein sclerosis) are frequently seen (10,17). Bone changes, most prominent in children, include cortical thickening, periosteal reactions in long bones, development of spurs along the spine, and ossification of ligamentous insertions (9). Plasma triglycerides may be elevated and high-density lipoproteins reduced, making long-term therapy with retinoids potentially dangerous for patients at risk for cardiovascular disease (19).

Compelling evidence indicates that retinoids are teratogenic (1,8). A prospective study evaluating isotretinoin use during the first trimester demonstrated 22% of 36 pregnancies ending in first-trimester abortion, 3% resulting in a malformed stillborn infant, and 11% resulting in a baby with at least one major malformation (11). Malformations included abnormalities of the face, heart, thymus, and CNS. Latter abnormalities included holoprosencephaly, microcephaly, neuronal migration defects, and cerebellar dysgenesis. Urinary tract and adrenal gland abnormalities, fusion of the legs, and Goldenhar's syndrome have also been reported (1).

Animal studies have documented a host of toxic effects after both short-term and prolonged exposures to excessive vitamin A (8). They have also demonstrated its teratogenic effects, describing abnormalities that include neural tube defects, brain dysgenesis, learning disabilities, craniofacial abnormalities, cardiac and limb malformations, and cataracts (1,8). The cardiac and craniofacial abnormalities may be caused by a defect in branchial-arch mesenchyme induced by abnormal activity of cephalic neural crest cells (11). Retinoic acid has profound effects on the developing neuroectoderm of Xenopus embryos, reducing the formation of forebrain, midbrain, eyes, and nasal pits while not inhibiting formation of posterior neural structures (4). There are no models for pseudotumor cerebri caused by vitamin A.

Short-term toxic effects occur within several days after a large dose of vitamin A (8). Symptoms include headache, papilledema, visual disturbances, vertigo, drowsiness, irritability, muscle weakness, gastrointestinal distress, peeling skin, and mucous membrane hemorrhages (1,8,15). Acute episodes of fontanelle bulging lasting 1–2 days occurred in infants <6 months of age who received vitamin A supplements (50,000 IU) at 1.5, 2.5, and 3.5 months of age (6). Overingestion of carotenoids does not produce symptomatic hypervitaminosis A (1,8).

Pseudotumor cerebri caused by hypervitaminosis A appears after prolonged therapy and at daily doses of 40,000–600,000 IU (15). Most cases result from doses >100,000 IU/day (>20 times the U.S. recommended adult daily allowance) (1). For instance, typical signs of pseudotumor cerebri (headache, sixth nerve palsies, papilledema) occurred in three women who had been ingesting vitamin A from 6

months to 2 years at doses of 100,000–300,000 IU daily (15). Other signs and symptoms are variably present. Psychiatric disturbances have been reported (15). Frequent skin changes have been noted, including hair loss, dry squamous skin, yellowish brown skin, and mouth blisters (15). Ocular side effects may be present, including blepharoconjunctivitis, photodermatitis, corneal opacities, decreased night vision, and susceptibility to glare (12). Fatigue, anorexia, weight loss, menstrual irregularities, musculoskeletal pain, polyuria and polydipsia, and hepatomegaly have also been reported (1,8,15). Serum vitamin A levels are almost always elevated (15). There may be radiographic abnormalities of the vertebrae and long bones (15). Symptoms in children can occur at much lower doses (>12,000 IU) (1,21). Infants may exhibit a bulging fontanelle (15). Two young sibs are reported with hypervitaminosis A secondary to excessive vitamin administration (20): the 30-month-old boy presented with macrocephaly, anorexia, lethargy, stiff neck, inability to walk, patchy alopecia, and an exfoliative skin rash after 1 year of >57,000 IU/day. Liver tests and radiographic examinations of the long bones were abnormal. The 12-month sib had received 25,000 IU/day for 9 months, and presented with irritability, vomiting, bulging fontanelle, an exfoliative dermatitis, and hepatomegaly. In general, treatment is based upon cessation of the excessive intake, with improvement beginning several days to weeks later (1,15). Therapy for pseudotumor cerebri may include acetazolamide or corticosteroids; fenestration of the optic nerve sheath following drug withdrawal may also be required (13).

Toxicity appears to result when the plasma retinol-binding protein capacity is exceeded, leading to elevated "free" levels of vitamin A binding to lipoproteins, lysis of membranes, and release of cellular organelle contents (1,8,21,22). Increased calcium influx into cells may also occur (22). The specific mechanisms by which hypervitaminosis A induces pseudotumor cerebri are unknown. Multiple factors can increase the toxic effect of vitamin A, including higher daily dosage, use of aqueous solutions instead of oily preparations, anemia, protein malnutrition, liver and kidney disease, hyperlipoproteinemia, and excessive ethanol use (1,8).

REFERENCES
1. Bendich A, Langseth L (1989) Safety of vitamin A. *Amer J Clin Nutr* **49**, 358.
2. Berson EL, Rosner B, Sandberg MA *et al.* (1993) A randomized trial of vitamin A and vitamin E supplementation for retinitis pigmentosa. *Arch Ophthalmol* **111**, 761.
3. Blomhoff R (1994) Transport and metabolism of vitamin A. *Nutr Rev* **52**, S13.
4. Durston AJ, Timmermans JPM, Hage WJ *et al.* (1989)

Retinoic acid causes an anteroposterior transformation in the developing central nervous system. *Nature* **340**, 140.

5. Eichele G (1989) Retinoids and vertebrate limb pattern formation. *Trends Genet* **5**, 246.

6. de Francisco A, Chakraborty J, Chowdhury HR *et al.* (1993) Acute toxicity of vitamin A given with vaccines in infancy. *Lancet* **342**, 526.

7. Gaziano JM, Hennekens CH (1993) The role of beta-carotene in the prevention of cardiovascular disease. In: *Carotenoids in Human Health, Annals of the New York Academy of Sciences. Vol 691.* Canfield LM, Krinsky NI, Olson JA eds. New York Academy of Sciences, New York p. 148.

8. Hathcock JN, Hattan DG, Jenkins MY *et al.* (1990) Evaluation of vitamin A toxicity. *Amer J Clin Nutr* **52**, 183.

9. Kilcoyne RF (1988) Effects of retinoids in bone. *J Amer Acad Dermatol* **19**, 212.

10. Kowalski TE, Falestiny M, Furth E *et al.* (1994) Vitamin A hepatotoxicity: A cautionary note regarding 25,000 IU supplements. *Amer J Med* **97**, 523.

11. Lammer EJ, Chen DT, Hoar RM *et al.* (1985) Retinoic acid embryopathy. *N Engl J Med* **31**, 837.

12. Lebowitz MA, Berson DS (1988) Ocular effects of oral retinoids. *J Amer Acad Dermatol* **19**, 209.

13. Lessell S (1992) Pediatric pseudotumor cerebri (idiopathic intracranial hypertension). *Surv Ophthalmol* **37**, 155.

14. Leyden JL (1988) Retinoids and acne. *J Amer Acad Dermatol* **19**, 164.

15. Lombaert A, Carton H (1976) Benign intracranial hyper-tension due to A-hypervitaminosis in adults and adolescents. *Eur Neurol* **14**, 340.

16. Pokhrel RP, Khatry SK, West KP *et al.* (1994) Sustained reduction in child mortality with vitamin A in Nepal. *Lancet* **343**, 1368.

17. Roenigk HH Jr (1988) Liver toxicity of retinoid therapy. *J Amer Acad Dermatol* **19**, 199.

18. Ross AC, Ternus ME (1993) Vitamin A as a hormone: Recent advances in understanding the actions of retinol, retinoic acid, and beta carotene. *J Amer Diet Assn* **93**, 1285.

19. Shalita AR (1988) Lipid and teratogenic effects of retinoids. *J Amer Acad Dermatol* **19**, 197.

20. Siegal NJ, Spackman TJ (1972) Chronic hypervitaminosis A with intracranial hypertension and low cerebrospinal fluid concentration of protein. *Clin Pediat* **11**, 580.

21. Smith FR, Goodman DS (1976) Vitamin A transport in human vitamin A toxicity. *N Engl J Med* **294**, 805.

22. Snodgrass SR (1992) Vitamin neurotoxicity. *Mol Neurobiol* **6**, 41.

23. Tessier-Lavigne M (1991) Phototransduction and information processing in the retina. In: *Principles of Neural Science. 3rd Ed.* Kandel ER, Schwartz JH Jessell TM eds. Elsevier, New York, Amsterdam, London, Tokyo p. 400.

24. Ziegler RG (1993) Carotenoids, cancer, and clinical trials. In: *Carotenoids in Human Health, Annals of the New York Academy of Sciences. Vol 691.* Canfield LM, Krinsky NI, Olson JA eds. New York Academy of Sciences, New York p.110.

Volkensin

Albert C. Ludolph

NEUROTOXICITY RATING

Experimental

A   Peripheral neuropathy (axonal degeneration—local administration)

The lectin volkensin was isolated from the East African kiliambiti (*kilimbiti, kilembide, kalumbu, berendai, mndiati, ol auui*) plant, *Adenia volkensii*. Extracts of the plant roots, which also contain cyanogenic glycosides, have been used as a hunting poison, for suicide, and for medicinal purposes (3). Roots and seed of *A. volkensii* also contain volkensin, a toxic glycoprotein with a MW of 62,000 (1,6). Volkensin is structurally similar to shiga toxin, ricin, modeccin, and abrin; it is inactivated by moderate heat (75°C, 25 min). Volkensin consists of two subunits (A and B chain) connected by disulfide bridges. The A chain functions as an "effectomer" responsible for the toxic effect and binds to the 60S ribosomal subunit; the B chain is responsible for the binding properties of the glycoprotein at the cell surface ("haptomer").

Studies of *A. volkensii* toxicity in rats and sheep disclose hemorrhagic lesions of multiple organs, severe gastrointestinal lesions and cardiotoxicity (2). Neurotoxicity is not a clear-cut primary effect of poisoning. The intraperitoneal LD_{50} of volkensin for rats at 48 h and 2 weeks is 0.32 μg/kg and 0.061 μg/kg, respectively; the corresponding LD_{50}s for mice are 1.73 and 1.38 μg/kg (6).

The principal biological targets of the toxin are liver, gastrointestinal tract, and pancreas. The compound is an experimental tool for lesion studies of both CNS and PNS (4,5,7,8). The mechanism of toxicity involves binding to the cell surface, uptake by endocytosis, retrograde transport to the cell soma ("suicide transport") and binding to the 60S ribosomal subunit where the compound inhibits elongation factor-2 and thereby protein synthesis of the target cell. The inactivation of ribosomes results in disaggregation of polyribosomes and dissolution of Nissl substance, which are reflected by severe chromatolysis. In contrast to ricin and abrin and like modeccin, volkensin is taken up and retrogradely transported not only in the PNS but also by CNS neurons (7,8). In an experimental study, volkensin was microinjected into peripheral nerves of rats (7); after 1–5 days, volkensin produced chromatolysis and destruction of sensory and motor neurons projecting axons through the injected nerves. In contrast to abrin, volkensin and modeccin also seemed to poison adjacent CNS neurons (7).

REFERENCES

1. Barbieri L, Falasca AI, Stirpe F (1984) Volkensin, the toxin of *Adenia volkensii* (Kiliambiti plant). *FEBS Lett* **171**, 277.
2. Kamau JA (1975) Kiliambiti plant (*Adenia volkensii*) toxicity in animals. *Bull Anim Health Prod* **23**, 189.
3. Neuwinger HD (1994) Afrikanische Arzneipflanzen und Jagdgifte. In: *Chemie, Pharmakologie, Toxikologie. Ein Handbuch für Pharmazeuten, Mediziner, Chemiker und Biologen.* Wissenschaftliche Verlagsgesellschaft mbH, Stuttgart p. 654.
4. Nogradi A, Vrbova G (1992) The use of a neurotoxic lectin, volkensin, to induce loss of identified motoneuron pools. *Neuroscience* **50**, 975.
5. Pangalos MN, Francis PT, Peasron RCA *et al.* (1991) Destruction of a subpopulation of cortical neurons by suicide transport of volkensin, a lectin from *Adenia volkensii. J Neurosci Meth* **40**, 17.
6. Stirpe F, Barbieri L, Abbondanza A *et al.* (1985) Properties of volkensin, a toxic lectin from *Adenia volkensii. J Biol Chem* **260**, 14589.
7. Wiley RG, Stirpe F (1987) Neuronotoxicity of axonally transported toxic lectins, abrin, modeccin, and volkensin in rat peripheral nervous system. *Neuropathol Appl Neurobiol* **13**, 39.
8. Wiley RG, Stirpe F (1988) Modeccin and volkensin but not abrin are effective suicide transport agents in rat CNS. *Brain Res* **438**, 145.

Water

Herbert H. Schaumburg

NEUROTOXICITY RATING

Clinical

A Acute encephalopathy (seizures, coma, profound hyponatremia)

A Chronic encephalopathy (lethargy, moderate hyponatremia)

Water intoxication (WI) follows excessive water administration or self-administration. WI is an infrequent clinical event in general adult medical practice; in North America, it is largely encountered by psychiatrists and pediatricians. Psychogenic water intoxication occurs in 7%–18% of patients in psychiatric institutions and is especially common in schizophrenia (4). Infants with diarrhea given water-diluted formula are a vulnerable group (2,3). Some pharmaceutical agents (psychotropics, anticonvulsants, and anticancer drugs) have been associated with the syndrome of inappropriate antidiuretic hormone (SIADH). SIADH, which mimics WI, is characterized by retention of water, hemodilution, and profound hyponatremia and serum hypoosmolality.

Massive intake of water causes a drop in serum osmolarity, hemodilution, and hyponatremia. For the syndrome of WI to occur, there must be a *rapid* decline in extracellular solute concentration (osmolarity), creating a concentration gradient between extracellular fluid and cell water generally, and a gradient between the vascular fluid of the brain and the rest of the brain fluids in particular (1). The brain is affected differently because, unlike other tissues, the endothelial cells of the cerebral vessels are joined by tight junctions that act to slow transport of electrolytes. This means that when an osmolar gradient is produced, relief of the gradient in the brain cannot be quickly achieved by rapid diffusion of sodium and chloride ions from the extracellular fluid of the brain, but must be equilibrated by the movement of water molecules into both the extracellular fluid and the cells of the brain. Consequently, the brain picks up disproportionally more water than other organs and swells; massive edema may develop. The swelling causes convulsions only if the dilution occurs over a few hours. A fall in serum sodium levels below 125 mmol/l (normal is greater than 135) will usually be accompanied by generalized seizures. Levels of 115 mmol/l have been associated with status epilepticus, coma, and respiratory paralysis.

WI in adult psychiatric patients usually is associated with the syndrome of compulsive water drinking (CWD). Causative factors include neuroleptic-driven thirst, polydipsia as part of the psychosis, medication-induced xerostomia, bore-dom, and accessibility of water (4). There are three grades of severity of CWD, roughly corresponding to the amount ingested. The most severe group, associated with consumption of 10 liters in 1 day, display rapid onset of headache, blurred vision, muscle cramps, ataxia, lethargy, seizures, and delirium. Extreme cases progress to coma followed by respiratory arrest. This group has a 10% mortality. Urine specific gravity is usually 1.003 or less. Those in the second group, associated with consumption of 5–10 liters, are somnolent and appear mildly disoriented. Urine specific gravity is 1.005 or less. Individuals in the third group, associated with consumption of 3–5 liters daily, are asymptomatic and rarely display significant abnormalities in laboratory tests.

Infantile WI remains a prevalent problem in the inner cities of North America (1). Infants, usually 3–6 months old, who come from poor inner-city families are especially at risk (2,3). Fluid loss from summertime diarrhea causes dehydration. WI occurs when the infants are given water or dilute formula for rehydration; they develop hyponatremia and become diaphoretic, irritable, and lethargic and develop repeated bouts of generalized seizures. They may be apneic on arrival in the emergency department; total respiratory failure occurs in 50%. Treatment of these children with hypertonic saline can be life-saving but should only be undertaken by an expert.

Treatment for most cases of mild WI is simply restriction of water intake. Severe cases may require saline infusion and administration of loop diuretics to resolve electrolyte and CNS disturbances. Saline infusion with rapid correction of hyponatremia may be extremely hazardous and should only be performed by experienced individuals. The most severe adverse effects of rapid correction are congestive heart failure and the osmotic demyelination syndrome (central pontine myelinolysis).

REFERENCES

1. Finberg L (1991) Water intoxication. A prevalent problem in the inner city. *Amer J Dis Child* **145**, 981.
2. Gold I, Koenigsberg M (1986) Infantile seizures caused by voluntary water intoxication. *Amer J Emerg Med* **4**, 21.
3. Keating JP, Schears GJ, Dodge PR (1991) Oral water intoxication in infants. American epidemic. *Amer J Dis Child* **145**, 985.
4. Riggs AT, Dysken MW, Kim SW, Opsahl JA (1991) A review of disorders of water homeostasis in psychiatric patients. *Psychosomatics* **32**, 133.

Yellow Star Thistle

Dwijendra N. Roy
Peter S. Spencer

NEUROTOXICITY RATING

Clinical

A Extrapyramidal syndrome (nigropallidal encephalomalacia—horses)

Yellow Star thistle (*Centaurea solstitialis* L.; YST), a member of the thistle family (Asteraceae), which originates from eastern Eurasia, and the related Russian knapweed, *C. repens*, are causally associated with a veterinary disorder peculiar to horses: nigropallidal encephalomalacia (NPE) (1,3–7). YST is a highly invasive species that spreads rapidly and is now naturalized in most temperate areas of the world. The plant represents a threat to the health of grazing horses in the western United States (California, Oregon, Idaho, Washington), where it has colonized large areas of wasteland, rangeland, and cultivated fields (8).

Phytochemical investigations of *Centaurea* spp. reveal the presence of alkaloids, triterpenoids, polyacetylenes, flavonoids, and a series of sesquiterpene lactones (9,14,15). Polyacetylenic compounds and sesquiterpene lactones possess a broad spectrum of biological activity, including cytotoxicity, antineoplasticity, and allergenicity.

Lipid-soluble fractions of YST contain low concentrations of a variety of biologically active sesquiterpene lactones (2,14–16): 13-O-acetylsolstitialin A (0.044% dry weight) and cynaropicrin (0.014%) are cytotoxic in explants derived from fetal rodent substantia nigra, frontal cortex, and raphe nuclei (2,16). Repin, first isolated from *C. repens* and later from YST, is toxic to chick-embryo sensory neurons (15). Water-soluble fractions, which contain high concentrations of free aspartic and glutamic acids among other unidentified neurotoxic agents, display an excitotoxic pattern of activity in mouse cortical explants (*see* Chapter 1). The neurotoxic amino acids occur in a proportion of 5:1 in a total content of 0.3% dry weight of the aerial parts of the YST plant (10–13). The extent to which these excitatory amino acids play a role in the induction of NPE has not been established.

Aqueous and/or alcohol extracts of YST administered by various routes triggered convulsions and death in rodents (1).

NPE, or chewing disease, has been linked to the ingestion of YST since 1954 (3–9); a similar disorder occurs in animals fed *C. repens* (17). Clinical signs are said to become evident suddenly after the horse has consumed an amount of YST nearly equivalent to the animal's body weight (1). Horses feeding on the thistle develop within 1–3 months a syndrome initially characterized by immobility of the facial musculature, idle chewing and tongue flicking, impaired eating and drinking, and a shuffling gait, followed by hypokinesia and lack of reactivity, which persists until death (3,4). Neuropathological examination reveals bilateral necrosis of the anterior globus pallidus and, most likely, the zona reticulata of the substantia nigra (4). Grazing animals other than horses appear to be unaffected by YST ingestion. Prolonged feeding of YST plant materials to sheep, guinea pigs, rats, mice, chicks, or monkeys has failed to induce a neurological disorder in those species.

REFERENCES

1. Callihan RH, Northam FE, Johnson JB *et al.* (1989) Yellow Star thistle, biology, and management in pasture and rangeland. University of Idaho, College of Agriculture, *Current Information Series No. 634.*
2. Cheng CH, Costall B, Hamburger M *et al.* (1992) Toxic effects of solstitialin A 13-acetate and cynaropicrin from *Centaurea solstitialis* L. (Asteraceae) in cell cultures of foetal rat brain. *Neuropharmacology* 31, 271.
3. Cordy DR (1954) Nigropallidal encephalomalacia in horses associated with ingestion of Yellow Star thistle. *J Neuropathol Exp Neurol* 13, 330.
4. Cordy DR (1978) *Centaurea* species and equine nigropallidal encephalomalacia. In: *Effects of Poisonous Plants on Livestock.* Keeler RF, Van Kampen KR, James LF eds. Academic Press, New York p. 327.
5. Farrell RE, Sande RD, Lincoln SD (1971) Nigropallidal encephalomalacia in a horse. *J Amer Vet Med Assn* 158, 1201.
6. Fowler ME (1965) Nigropallidal encephalomalacia in the horse. *J Amer Vet Med Assn* 147, 607.
7. Larson KA, Young S (1970) Nigropallidal encephalomalacia in horses in Colorado. *J Amer Vet Med Assn* 156, 626.
8. Maddox DM (1981) Introduction, phenology, and density of Yellow Star thistle in coastal intercoastal and central valley situations in California. *Agricultural Research Reports ARR-W-20,* U.S. Department of Agriculture.
9. Marrill GB, Stevens KL (1985) Sesquiterpene lactones from *Centaurea solstitialis. Phytochemistry* 24, 2013.
10. Roy DN, Craig M, Blythe L *et al.* (1991) Equine nigropallidal encephalomalacia (ENE) and *Centaurea solstitialis* (CS): Search for culpable neurotoxin(s). *Soc Neurosci Abstr* 17, 704.
11. Roy DN, Craig AM, Blythe LL *et al.* (1993) Equine nigropallidal encephalomalacia and *Centaurea solstitialis*

(Yellow Star thistle): Partial isolation and identification of neurotoxins. *Neurodegeneration* **2**, 51.

12. Roy DN, Peyton DH, Spencer PS (1995) Isolation and identification of two potent neurotoxins, aspartic acid and glutamic acid, from Yellow Star thistle (*Centaurea solstitialis*). *Nat Toxin* **3**, 174.

13. Roy DN, Spencer PS, Craig AM *et al.* (1992) Yellow Star thistle and nigropallidal encephalomalacia: Search for culpable neurotoxin(s). *Toxicologist* **12**, 1251.

14. Stevens KL (1982) Sesquiterpene lactones from *Centaurea repens*. *Phytochemistry* **21**, 1093.

15. Stevens KL, Riopelle RJ, Wong RY (1990) Repin, a sesquiterpene lactone from *Acroptilon repens* possessing exceptional biological activity. *J Nat Prod* **53**, 218.

16. Wang Y, Hamburger M, Cheng CHK *et al.* (1991) Neurotoxic sesquiterpenoids from Yellow Star thistle *Centaurea solstitialis* L. (Asteracae). *Helv Chim Acta* **74**, 117.

17. Young S, Brown WW, Klinger B (1970) Nigropallidal encephalomalacia in horse fed Russian knapweed (*Centaurea repens* L.). *Amer J Vet Res* **31**, 1394.

Zidovudine

Enrica Arnaudo

ZIDOVUDINE
$C_{10}H_{13}N_5O_4$

3'-Azido-3'-deoxythymidine; AZT

NEUROTOXICITY RATING

Clinical

A   Myopathy

Experimental

A   Mitochondrial DNA polymerase inhibition

A   Myopathy (mitochondrial)

Zidovudine, formerly called azidothymidine (AZT), is a dideoxynucleoside analog of thymidine, in which the 3'-hydroxy (-OH) group is replaced by an azido (-N₃) group. It is an inhibitor of the *in vitro* replication of the human immunodeficiency virus type 1 (HIV-1), the etiological agent of acquired immunodeficiency syndrome (AIDS). It also inhibits other retroviruses including HIV-2, human T-cell lymphotropic virus type 1, animal lentiviruses, and murine retroviruses.

Zidovudine was synthesized in 1964 as a potential chemotherapeutic agent (25). The inhibition of retrovirus replication by zidovudine was reported in 1974 (40). In 1985, zidovudine was shown to inhibit HIV-1 replication *in vitro* at concentrations of 0.01–10 μM, depending on the assay and cell type used (37).

Zidovudine is a white to beige, odorless, crystalline solid with a MW of 267.24, solubility of 20.1 mg/ml in water at 25°C, and a MP of 106°–112°C (25). It is available for oral use in capsule and syrup forms. Each capsule contains 100 mg of zidovudine; each teaspoon (5 ml), 50 mg. Capsules and syrup should be stored at 15°–25°C protected from light and moisture. Zidovudine is also available for intravenous infusion, the solution containing 10 mg/ml.

Zidovudine requires cellular activation to the triphosphate form to exert its activity against HIV. The drug enters the cell by passive diffusion in a nonfacilitated, nonconcentrating manner (61). Activation proceeds in a stepwise manner starting with phosphorylation of the prodrug by cellular thymidine kinase to form zidovudine monophosphate. The monophosphate is converted to the diphosphate by thymidylate kinase (a rate-limiting step) and finally, the diphosphate is phosphorylated by diphosphate kinase to yield zidovudine triphosphate. In HIV-infected T cells, zidovudine triphosphate interferes with the viral RNA-dependent DNA polymerase [reverse transcriptase (RT)], for which it has a high affinity. Specifically, zidovudine triphosphate competes with deoxythymidine triphosphate for incorporation into viral DNA by RT. Once incorporated into viral DNA, it prevents elongation of the proviral DNA chain, because the 3'-azido group does not permit the 5' to 3' phosphodiester linkage that is required for chain elongation; this results in premature chain termination.

Zidovudine has no effect on extracellular virions. It is inactive in an unphosphorylated form against purified viral RT, and it is largely inactive as a *threo* isomer. Only the triphosphate of the *erythro* isomeric form of zidovudine acts as a competitive inhibitor with high affinity for the viral RT. Zidovudine triphosphate also inhibits cellular α- and β-DNA polymerase, but at concentrations 100-fold higher than those required to inhibit viral RT; therefore, it does not interfere with nuclear DNA replication. In contrast, the human DNA polymerase-γ, which is responsible for mitochondrial DNA (mtDNA) replication, is inhibited by zidovudine at concentrations as low as 1 μM, concentrations that are achieved *in vivo* (42,48).

Following its approval in March 1987 by the U.S. Food and Drug Administration, zidovudine became a mainstay in the treatment of patients infected with HIV. It was moderately effective in reducing the incidence of opportunistic infections, increasing helper T-lymphocyte numbers, and improving survival rates and quality of life. Currently, other agents, such as protease inhibitors, appear more effective in reducing the viral body burden. Multicenter trials have concluded that the drug has no significant beneficial effects on survival or disease progression in patients with asymptomatic HIV infection (10). Some studies claim that zidovudine delays disease progression in this patient group (57,58).

Treatment with zidovudine should be considered in adults when two CD4⁺ cell counts taken at least 1 week apart are <500/mm³. However, the indications for therapy continue to change as further studies are undertaken. The optimal time to initiate this therapy remains unclear; it is suggested that the patient and physician consider beginning therapy in cases of asymptomatic HIV infection with CD4⁺

cell counts $\leq$500/mm^3, or delaying such therapy until the onset of clinically symptomatic HIV disease. The current recommended regimen is 500–600 mg/day, usually taken in three divided doses. These doses appear to be at least as effective as the previously recorded dosages of 1200–1500 mg/day and are better tolerated.

Therapy with zidovudine is used in children over 3 months of age with HIV-related symptoms or significant HIV-related immunosuppression. The recommended dose in children 3 months to 12 years of age is 180 mg/m^2 every 6 h, not to exceed 200 mg every 6 h.

Zidovudine has been successful in reducing, by two-thirds, the risk of maternal–infant HIV transmission in pregnant women with mildly symptomatic HIV disease and no prior treatment with antiretroviral drugs (11). The recommended experimental regimen includes oral zidovudine beginning between 14 and 34 weeks of gestation, intravenous zidovudine during labor, and administration of zidovudine syrup to the newborn soon after birth for 6 weeks (2 mg/kg every 6 h starting within 12 h after birth).

Although zidovudine is widely used as postexposure prophylaxis, its efficacy in preventing seroconversion is unproven. It is questionable whether zidovudine has prophylactic properties, because it has no intrinsic antiviral activity and does not prevent virus from entering cells. Animal studies demonstrate some potential for efficacy if zidovudine is administered in the first few hours after exposure. However, the pathogenesis of infection in animal models differs from HIV infection in humans (35). Given the low statistical risk of occupational infection following needlestick injury, the lack of documented efficacy (55), and the increasing prevalence of zidovudine resistance among source patients, zidovudine should be cautiously considered for prophylaxis in cases of known exposure to HIV. If this treatment is elected, it should be initiated as soon as possible and is not advised if more than 72 h have elapsed since exposure (18).

Zidovudine is classified as a Risk Factor Category "C" drug by the U.S. Food and Drug Administration. This classification indicates that zidovudine has not been systematically studied in pregnant women. Data regarding the safety of zidovudine during pregnancy are limited, particularly during the first trimester when effects on embryogenesis are likely to occur and therapy with zidovudine is not indicated. To date, published reports suggest there is no increased risk of congenital abnormalities when the mother ingests zidovudine in the second trimester or later (11,39,52).

General Toxicology

Zidovudine was the first drug approved for the treatment of HIV infection. The spectrum of adverse effects with zi-

dovudine is different from that of didanosine and zalcitabine: anemia and myopathy are the major zidovudine-induced toxicities; peripheral neuropathy and pancreatitis are dose-limiting side effects of the other two agents. Combination therapy allows effective use of lower zidovudine dosages, reducing toxicity while achieving synergistic antiviral effects.

Zidovudine is well absorbed after oral administration (59). Bioavailability is incomplete (60%–65%) after oral administration (despite its complete absorption) because the drug undergoes first-pass metabolism by the liver. The rate of absorption is influenced when the drug is administered with a high-fat meal; the time to reach maximum plasma concentration is considerably lengthened, and the peak level itself is substantially lowered. Zidovudine reaches maximum serum concentrations within 30–60 min of ingestion and undergoes biexponential-decay kinetics, with a serum half-life of 1.0–1.5 h. Peak plasma concentrations of oral and intravenous zidovudine vary from 1.5–18.0 μM in an approximately linear fashion with single and multiple doses of 1–10 mg/kg (59). The theoretical optimal virustatic zidovudine concentration is >1 μM, based on *in vitro* data; this is difficult to maintain with intermittent oral dosing. Intracellular phosphorylated zidovudine concentrations may be a more accurate measure of efficacy than serum drug concentrations, because only the former has therapeutic capability. The intracellular half-life of the active triphosphate form is estimated to be 3–4 h (60), twice that of plasma zidovudine. The longer intracellular half-life and the apparent saturable nature of zidovudine phosphorylation allows the use of smaller doses and longer dosage intervals, which maintain intracellular zidovudine triphosphate concentrations at therapeutic levels once steady-state is achieved. Dosing at 8-h intervals is now generally accepted; more frequent dosing, initially recommended because of the short serum half-life, is no longer necessary.

Zidovudine is highly lipophilic and widely distributed. Total body clearance averages 1900 ml/min/70 kg, and the apparent volume of distribution is about 1.6 l/kg (28). Plasma protein binding is estimated to be 34%–38%, and drug interactions involving binding-site displacement have not been noted.

Zidovudine crosses the blood-brain barrier; cerebrospinal fluid (CSF) levels reach about 60%–70% of serum within 3–4 h of dosing. The greater efficacy of zidovudine in HIV-associated dementia in adults, as compared to other antiretroviral agents, may reflect its greater penetration into the CSF than other nucleoside analogs (60).

Zidovudine readily crosses the placenta to and from the fetal circulation by passive diffusion (34). Drug concentrations in neonatal and umbilical cord blood are similar to or greater than maternal concentrations, whereas concentrations in amniotic fluid are higher than those in maternal or umbilical cord blood, indicating renal excretion of zidovudine by the fetus.

In humans, zidovudine has been shown to concentrate in semen of HIV-infected patients, with semen-to-serum ratios ranging from 1.3–20.4 1 h after oral administration of 200 mg on a 4-h dosing schedule (23). Zidovudine is also secreted into saliva, and the ratio of saliva to plasma concentration is close to unity (27).

The metabolism of zidovudine is primarily hepatic, with subsequent renal excretion. Zidovudine undergoes hepatic glucuronidation to 3'-azido-3'-deoxy-5'-β-D-glucopyranosol thymidine (GZDV); this major metabolite does not exhibit antiviral activity against HIV *in vitro*. The first-pass metabolism of oral zidovudine is extensive: approximately 40% of the drug is lost after oral administration, while GZDV rapidly appears in the plasma, and its concentration is much higher than that of zidovudine throughout steady-state conditions. GZDV has an apparent elimination half-life of 1 h and is renally excreted (9).

Zidovudine is also metabolized to 3'-amino-3'-deoxythymidine (AMT) and 3'-amino-3'-deoxythymidine glucuronide (54). Metabolism of zidovudine to AMT occurs in both liver and gastrointestinal microsomes, and AMT production appears to be controlled by cytochrome P-450 (12). AMT has a significantly longer plasma elimination half-life than either zidovudine or GZDV, and *in vitro* studies have shown that it is tenfold more toxic to hematopoietic cells than zidovudine. AMT also antagonizes the anti-HIV activity of zidovudine (54).

Zidovudine is eliminated by glucuronidation in the liver for the most part (50%–80%), and by renal excretion (10%–20%). The remaining 15%–20% of drug is excreted by an extrarenal mechanism, presumably *via* intestinal or biliary systems (28). After oral administration, 65%–75% of the given dose is recovered in the urine as GZDV, and 8%–15% as zidovudine. The renal clearance of zidovudine and its metabolites is higher than creatinine clearance, indicating that both glomerular filtration and tubular secretion occur (28).

In patients with end-stage renal disease, the peak concentration of zidovudine is increased by approximately 50%. A dosage of 100 mg three times daily has been recommended in these cases. Hemodialysis appears to have negligible effects on the pharmacokinetics of zidovudine, while the elimination of GZDV is enhanced (51). Continuous peritoneal dialysis does not seem to modify the elimination of zidovudine (59).

In patients with cirrhosis, the clearance of oral zidovudine is reduced by 70%, resulting in two- to threefold increases in peak plasma levels and half-life. In such instances, a reduction in dosage or dosing frequency seems appropriate, but there are insufficient data on the proper dose adjustment in these patients. Dosage reduction or an increase in dosage interval may be required in the elderly because the half-life of zidovudine is reported to be higher, on the order of 2.2 h, in patients over 60 years of age with AIDS, as compared to 1.5 h in younger patients (59).

Several studies have shown that total zidovudine clearance was reduced, half-life was delayed, and bioavailability was increased in neonates <2 weeks of age born to HIV-positive mothers, compared with similar but older infants (up to 3 months of age), possibly because of an immature fetal glucuronidation system. Data on the pharmacokinetics of zidovudine in HIV-infected infants and children are scarce and, overall, they indicate a greater interpatient variation. The zidovudine dosage in children should be calculated according to body surface area.

Zidovudine is frequently combined with other medications, such as antimicrobial, immunomodulating, antipyretic, and cytostatic agents. Several drugs interact with zidovudine resulting in increased toxicity (4). Conclusive data on drug interactions with zidovudine have been difficult to obtain because of the considerable range of comedications used with AIDS patients. It may be difficult to distinguish between toxicity from complications of HIV infection, toxicity as an adverse effect of one drug, and toxicity caused by drug interactions.

Within the first weeks of therapy, patients may complain of headache, confusion, nausea and vomiting, malaise and fatigue, or abdominal discomfort (47), but the most significant adverse effect of zidovudine is bone marrow toxicity, which affects erythropoiesis and granulopoiesis. Marrow aplasia is rare (30). When anemia occurs, it usually manifests within the first 3 months of therapy and is more prominent in patients with advanced AIDS receiving higher drug dosages (17). Macrocytosis occurs within 6 months in 75% of patients. The mechanism underlying drug-induced anemia and macrocytosis is still not fully understood. Neutropenia usually occurs within 3 months of therapy, but may also be a late complication. When the reduction in hemoglobin is >25% and the reticulocyte count is low, it may be necessary to interrupt therapy until hemoglobin recovers. Cotherapy with zidovudine and agents that stimulate bone marrow cells may allow continued use of full dosages of zidovudine. The drug should be temporarily discontinued if the neutrophil count falls below 0.5×10^9/l.

Laboratory investigations at baseline in all patients should include hemoglobin level, white blood cell (WBC) count, neutrophil count, platelet count, reticulocyte count, urea, creatinine, creatine kinase (CK), transaminases, alkaline phosphatase, and bilirubin levels (38). These tests should be done within 1–2 months of initiating zidovudine therapy. Two weeks after therapy begins, the hemoglobin, WBC, neutrophil count, and platelet count should be repeated. Thereafter, the patient should have the platelet count and liver function tests repeated monthly for 3 months. Six months after zidovudine has started, and every 3 months thereafter, CK should be monitored (38). A CD4$^+$ cell count should be performed every 3 months to monitor immune function as a potential measure of drug benefit and to identify the timing for initiation of adjunctive therapy, such as prophylaxis for opportunistic infections.

Clinical experience with AIDS patients chronically treated with zidovudine indicates that its anti-HIV efficacy often declines 6–12 months after initiation of therapy. At the same time, mutations within the HIV-1 RT gene are detected, which confer resistance to zidovudine (46). Mutations occur in the RT gene of zidovudine-resistant HIV isolates (31). Mutations at these sites are not usually seen in patients who have not been treated with zidovudine, and it is generally believed that they develop after prolonged treatment, although zidovudine-resistant isolates can emerge as early as 2 months after initiation of therapy, and primary infection with zidovudine-resistant strains has been documented (16,53).

In Vitro Studies

The *in vitro* anti-HIV activity of zidovudine has been well established in a range of human T-cell lines and peripheral blood monocytes infected with HIV (30). Antiviral activity *in vitro* appears to be concentration-related. *In vitro* sensitivity results vary greatly depending upon the time between virus infection and zidovudine treatment of cell cultures, the particular assay used, the cell type employed, and the laboratory performing the test.

Strong evidence has accumulated that mitochondria are cellular targets of zidovudine. In particular, the mtDNA polymerase-γ is impaired in its ability to replicate DNA by zidovudine, as shown in several *in vitro* studies. Early studies demonstrated the inhibition of DNA polymerase-γ by the analogs of naturally occurring dideoxynucleoside triphosphates (ddNTPs) (15,62), as well as non–naturally occurring ddNTPs, which possess strong anti–HIV-1 activity (7). Specifically, the inhibitory effect on mtDNA replication by zidovudine was shown in isolated intact rat liver mitochondria (48), and in mitochondria isolated from the Friend murine erythroleukemic cell (a bone marrow model) grown in zidovudine (24). Morphological mitochondrial abnormalities, with swelling and distortion of cristae, are seen in zidovudine-treated muscle cells in culture (29,33).

Animal Studies

Healthy rats treated intraperitoneally with zidovudine showed elevation of serum CK and lactic acid (29). Pathological changes were observed in mitochondria of skeletal muscle. These included swelling, disorganization and disappearance of cristae, and myelin figures with whorled lamellae. The onset of cardiomyopathy was also associated with various alterations in the electron transport system leading to uncoupling of oxidative phosphorylation and elevated lactic acid levels (29).

Rats developed a drug-induced toxic myopathy with morphological mitochondrial abnormalities after only 35 days of zidovudine treatment (33). There was a marked decrease of muscle mtDNA and of mtDNA-encoded RNAs, but normal levels of nuclear DNA-encoded mRNAs. In particular, cytochrome-b mRNA, 12S, and 16S rRNAs were less abundant, and a decreased rate of mitochondrial polypeptide synthesis was evident (32,33). These findings confirmed the muscle mtDNA depletion seen in humans with zidovudine myopathy.

Human Studies

Adverse effects from zidovudine are less frequent and milder at lower doses and earlier stages of HIV infection (45). Hypersensitivity reactions such as fever and rash are rare. Vomiting, anorexia, malaise, and asthenia are more common in zidovudine-treated patients with early HIV disease; headache, confusion, and insomnia occur more frequently with zidovudine than placebo in patients with advanced HIV disease. Seizures have been described rarely. A self-limiting acute encephalopathy has been described in a small number of patients who have had their dosage reduced rapidly or stopped (22). Hepatotoxicity with and without lactic acidosis has been reported (59), as well as cases of concurrent hepatic and muscle toxicity (8).

Myopathy was formerly a serious late adverse effect of zidovudine therapy; it occurred in 16–18% of patients receiving the then-conventional dose of 1200 mg/day for longer than 6 months. Zidovudine myopathy became uncommon in the late 1990s following the introduction of regimens of 500–600 mg/day. Patients with myopathy present with fatigue, myalgia, proximal muscle weakness, predominantly in the thighs and calves, and serum CK elevation often worsened by exercise. Symptoms appear to be related to the dose of zidovudine and the duration of therapy, occurring more frequently with higher dosages, and after 9–12 months of therapy (14,36,43).

Myopathy is also a rare complication of HIV infection itself, with HIV-polymyositis and HIV-associated acquired nemaline myopathy being the most commonly described

HIV-related muscle disorders. Isolated case reports describe other muscle abnormalities, such as fiber necrosis with minimal primary inflammation, selective loss of thick filaments, cytoplasmic microvesiculation, and type II fiber atrophy (13).

Zidovudine-associated myopathy is a reversible toxic mitochondrial myopathy, which may exaggerate or coexist with underlying HIV-associated myopathy. Before 1986, the incidence of HIV myopathy was low, although no prospective studies had established the incidence of myopathy in HIV infection. After the introduction of zidovudine for the treatment of AIDS, clinical placebo-controlled trials reported myalgia occurring more frequently in the zidovudine treated patients than in the placebo group (47). Between 1988 and 1995, there were many reports describing patients who developed a myopathic syndrome while receiving the then-conventional zidovudine dose of 1200 mg/day (3,19,20,22,50).

Zidovudine-associated myopathy is difficult to distinguish clinically from HIV-associated myopathy, and some have been reluctant to recognize a distinction (49). Pathological abnormalities clearly exist in zidovudine-treated subjects that are not seen with AIDS-associated myopathy (5,6,14,21,36,41,43,56). Ragged-red fibers, characteristic of mitochondrial disorders, are seen in muscle biopsies from zidovudine-treated AIDS patients, but not in the untreated group (14). These "AZT fibers" were small, atrophic, and most commonly perifascicular; there were marked myofibrillar alterations, including loss of thick myofilament and formation of cytoplasmic bodies, which distinguished them from the typical ragged-red fibers. Electron microscopy showed ultrastructurally abnormal mitochondria in the AZT fibers (44). With the reduction of zidovudine dosage from 1200 mg/day to 600 mg/day, the frequency of the associated myopathy declined, but prolonged therapy even with low doses of zidovudine has been reported to cause myopathy (26).

Management of zidovudine-associated myopathy poses a challange. Symptoms improve in most when the drug is discontinued (3,5,14,36). Myalgia resolves rapidly, usually within 2 weeks, but the weakness improves more slowly, beginning 4–6 weeks after discontinuation of therapy. Patients with severe weakness improve, but may not fully recover, underscoring the need for early diagnosis (5).

Toxic Mechanism

Zidovudine is myotoxic, as evidenced by the responses of myalgia, weakness, and CK elevation to drug withdrawal and rechallenge.

Dysfunctional muscle cell mitochondria are responsible for zidovudine-induced myopathy. In a molecular genetic

analysis of AIDS patients with myopathy, it was demonstrated that only patients on zidovudine therapy had a pronounced reduction in mtDNA content in their affected muscles (1). HIV-positive patients treated with zidovudine for 9–18 months showed a reduction in the levels of mtDNA in muscle of up to 78%, as compared with controls. Specimens from HIV-positive patients with myopathy who had not been treated with zidovudine had normal amounts of mtDNA. The depletion of mtDNA was reversible in one patient who had a repeat muscle biopsy 4 months after discontinuation of zidovudine, with clinical and histological improvement of the myopathy. These observations were consistent with in vitro studies showing that zidovudine is readily incorporated into mtDNA by DNA polymerase-γ (48); they helped to identify the mechanism of zidovudine myotoxicity. Muscle is a long-lived tissue, and muscle fibers are multinucleated syncytia of fused myoblasts. Subsequent analysis of muscle specimens from HIV-infected patients treated with zidovudine using antibodies to single- and double-stranded DNA confirmed the initial study by demonstrating severe mtDNA depletion in the treated patients compared with subjects who had not received the drug (44). Mitochondrial enzyme activities, including succinate–cytochrome-c reductase and cytochrome-c oxidase, were reduced in patients with zidovudine-associated myopathy (36). It is suggested that the cumulative lifetime dose of zidovudine is a key factor in the development of zidovudine-associated myopathy (mean cumulative dose, 498 ± 145 g) (36).

The depletion of muscle mtDNA is qualitatively related to the morphological appearance of ragged-red fibers, which contain many large, dysfunctional mitochondria. These mitochondrial abnormalities have been observed only in patients receiving zidovudine and have been confirmed independently by more than 15 groups of investigators worldwide using clinical, histological, and molecular studies. Muscle biopsy is the only diagnostic tool that can differentiate HIV-induced myopathy from zidovudine-associated myopathy. Early changes of zidovudine-associated myopathy may not be visible with light microscopy, but can be detected by electron microscopy.

A direct inhibitory effect of zidovudine on oxidative phosphorylation, by inhibiting the enzyme adenylate kinase in the direction of formation of adenosine triphosphate but not of the diphosphate, has been reported as another mechanism of zidovudine cytotoxicity (2).

REFERENCES

1. Arnaudo E, Dalakas M, Shanske S et al. (1991) Depletion of muscle mitochondrial DNA in AIDS patients with zidovudine-induced myopathy. Lancet 337, 508.

2. Barile M, Valenti D, Hobbs G *et al.* (1994) Mechanism of toxicity of 3′-azido-3′-deoxythymidine. Its interaction with adenylate kinase. *Biochem Pharmacol* **48**, 1405.

3. Bessen L, Greene J, Louie E *et al.* (1988) Severe polymyositis-like syndrome associated with zidovudine therapy of AIDS and ARC. *N Engl J Med* **318**, 708.

4. Burger D, Meenhorst P, Koks C, Beeijnen J (1993) Drug interactions with zidovudine. *AIDS* **7**, 445.

5. Chalmers A, Creco C, Miller RG (1991) Prognosis in AZT myopathy. *Neurology* **41**, 1181.

6. Chariot P, Gherardi R (1991) Partial cytochrome *c* oxidase deficiency and cytoplasmic bodies in patients with zidovudine myopathy. *Neuromuscular Disord* **1**, 357.

7. Chen C-H, Cheng Y-C (1989) Delayed cytotoxicity and selective loss of mitochondrial DNA in cells treated with the anti-human immunodeficiency virus compound 2′,3′-dideoxycytidine. *J Biol Chem* **264**, 11934.

8. Chen S, Barker S, Mitchell D *et al.* (1992) Concurrent zidovudine-induced myopathy and hepatotoxicity in patients treated for human immunodeficiency virus (HIV) infection. *Pathology* **24**, 109.

9. Collins J, Unadkat J (1989) Clinical pharmacokinetics of zidovudine. An overview of current data. *Clin Pharmacokinet* **17**, 1.

10. Concorde Coordinating Committee (1994) Concorde: MRC/ANRS randomised double-blind controlled trial of immediate and deferred zidovudine in symptom-free HIV infection. *Lancet* **343**, 871.

11. Connor E, Sperling R, Gelber R *et al.* (1994) Reduction of maternal-infant transmission of human immunodeficiency virus type 1 with zidovudine treatment. *N Engl J Med* **331**, 1173.

12. Cretton E, Xie M-Y, Bevan R *et al.* (1991) Catabolism of 3′-azido-3′-deoxythymidine in hepatocytes and liver microsomes with evidence of formation of 3′-amino-3′-deoxythymidine a highly toxic catabolite for human bone marrow cells. *Mol Pharmacol* **39**, 258.

13. Dalakas MC (1994) Retrovirus-related muscle diseases. In: *Myology. 2nd Ed.* Engel AG, Franzini-Armstrong C eds. McGraw-Hill, New York p. 1419.

14. Dalakas MC, Illa I, Pezeshkpour G *et al.* (1990) Mitochondrial myopathy caused by long-term AZT (zidovudine) therapy: Management and differences from HIV-associated myopathy. *N Engl J Med* **322**, 1098.

15. Edenberg H, Anderson S, DePamphilis M (1978) Involvement of DNA polymerase α in simian virus 40 DNA replication. *J Biol Chem* **253**, 3273.

16. Erice A, Mayers DL, Strike DG *et al.* (1993) Brief report: Primary infection with zidovudine-resistant human immunodeficiency virus type 1. *N Engl J Med* **328**, 1163.

17. Fischl M, Richman D, Hansen N *et al.* (1990) The safety and efficacy of zidovudine (AZT) in the treatment of subjects with mildly symptomatic human immunodeficiency virus type I (HIV) infection. A double-blind, placebo-controlled trial. *Ann Intern Med* **112**, 727.

18. Gerberding J (1995) Management of occupational exposures to blood-borne viruses. *N Engl J Med* **332**, 444.

19. Gertner E, Thurn J, Williams D *et al.* (1989) Zidovudine-associated myopathy: Case reports. *Amer J Med* **86**, 814.

20. Gorard D, Henry K, Guiloff R (1988) Necrotizing myopathy and zidovudine. *Lancet* **1**, 1050. [Letter]

21. Grau J, Masanes F, Pedro E *et al.* (1993) Human immunodeficiency virus type 1 infection and myopathy: Clinical relevance of zidovudine therapy. *Ann Neurol* **34**, 206.

22. Helbert M, Robinson D, Peddle B *et al.* (1988) Acute meningo-encephalitis on dose reduction of zidovudine. *Lancet* **1**, 1249.

23. Henry K, Chinnock B, Quinn R *et al.* (1988) Concurrent zidovudine levels in semen and serum determined by radioimmunoassay in patients with AIDS or AIDS-related complex. *J Amer Med Assn* **259**, 3023.

24. Hobbs GA, Keilbaugh SA, Simpson MV (1992) The Friend murine erythroleukemia cell, a model system for studying the association between bone marrow toxicity induced by 3′-azido-3′-dideoxythymidine and dideoxynucleoside inhibition of mtDNA replication. *Biochem Pharmacol* **43**, 1397.

25. Horwitz J, Chua J, Noel M (1964) Nucleosides: The monomesylates of 1-(2′-deoxy-β-D-lyxofuranosyl)thymine. *J Org Chem* **29**, 2076.

26. Jay C, Ropka M, Hench K *et al.* (1992) Prospective study of myopathy during prolonged low-dose AZT: Clinical correlates of AZT mitochondrial myopathy and HIV-associated inflammatory myopathy. *Neurology* **42**, 145.

27. Kamali F, Noble R, Hamilton P, Rawlins M (1991) Salivary secretion of zidovudine in man. *Fund Clin Pharmacol* **5**, 400.

28. Klecker RJ, Collins J, Yarchoan R *et al.* (1987) Plasma and cerebrospinal fluid pharmacokinetics of 3′-azido-3′deoxythymidine: A novel pyrimidine analog with potential application for the treatment of patients with AIDS and related diseases. *Clin Pharmacol Ther* **41**, 407.

29. Lamperth L, Dalakas M, Dagani F *et al.* (1991) Abnormal skeletal and cardiac muscle mitochondria induced by zidovudine (AZT) in human muscle *in vitro* and in an animal model. *Lab Invest* **65**, 742.

30. Langtry H, Campoli-Richards D (1989) Zidovudine. A review of its pharmacodynamic and pharmacokinetic properties, and therapeutic efficacy. *Drugs* **37**, 408.

31. Larder B, Barby G, Richman D (1989) HIV with decreased sensitivity to zidovudine isolated during prolonged therapy. *Science* **243**, 1731.

32. Lewis W, Gonzales B, Chomyn A, Papoian T (1992) Zidovudine induces molecular, biochemical, and ultrastructural changes in rat skeletal muscle mitochondria. *J Clin Invest* **89**, 1354.

33. Lewis W, Papoian T, Gonzales B et al. (1991) Mitochondrial ultrastructural and molecular changes induced by zidovudine in rat hearts. Lab Invest 65, 228.

34. Liebes L, Mendoza S, Wilson D, Dancis J (1989) Transfer of zidovudine (AZT) by human placenta. J Infect Dis 161, 203.

35. Mathes L, Polas P, Hayes K et al. (1992) Pre- and postexposure chemoprophylaxis: Evidence that 3'-azido-3'-dideoxythymidine inhibits feline leukemia virus disease by a drug-induced vaccine response. Antimicrob Agents Chemother 36, 2715.

36. Mhiri C, Baudrimont M, Bonne G et al. (1991) Zidovudine myopathy: A distinctive disorder associated with mitochondrial dysfunction. Ann Neurol 29, 606.

37. Mitsuya H, Weinhold K, Furman P et al. (1985) An antiviral agent that inhibits the infectivity and cytopathic effect of human T-lymphotropic virus type III/lymphadenopathy-associated virus in vitro. Proc Nat Acad Sci USA 82, 7096.

38. National Institute of Allergy and Infectious Diseases (NIAID), National Institutes of Health and U.S. Public Health Service (1990) State-of-the-art conference on azidothymidine therapy for early HIV infection. Amer J Med 89, 335.

39. O'Sullivan M, Boyer P, Scott G et al. (1993) The pharmacokinetics and safety of zidovudine in the third trimester of pregnancy for women infected with human immunodeficiency virus and their infants: Phase I Acquired Immunodeficiency Syndrome Clinical Trials Group study (protocol 082). Amer J Obstet Gynecol 168, 1510.

40. Ostertag W, Roesler G, Krieg C et al. (1974) Induction of endogenous virus and of thymidine kinase by bromodeoxyuridine in cell cultures transformed by Friend virus. Proc Nat Acad Sci USA 71, 4980.

41. Panegyres P, Papadimitriou J, Hallingsworth P et al. (1990) Vesicular changes in the myopathies of AIDS. Ultrastructural observations and their relationship to zidovudine treatment. J Neurol Neurosurg Psychiat 53, 649.

42. Parker W, White E, Shaddix S et al. (1991) Mechanism of inhibition of human immunodeficiency virus type I reverse transcriptase and human DNA-polymerases alpha, beta and gamma by the 5'-triphosphates of carbovir, 3'-azido-3'-deoxythymidine, 2',3'-dideoxyguanosine, and 3'-deoxythymidine. J Biol Chem 266, 1754.

43. Peters B, Winer J, Landon D et al. (1993) Mitochondrial myopathy associated with chronic zidovudine therapy in AIDS. Quart J Med 86, 5.

44. Pezeshkpour G, Illa I, Dalakas M (1991) Ultrastructural characteristics of DNA immunocytochemistry in HIV and AZT-associated myopathies. Hum Pathol 11, 1281.

45. Rachlis A, Fanning M (1993) Zidovudine toxicity. Clinical features and management. Drug Safety 8, 312.

46. Richman D (1992) Emergence of mutant HIV reverse transcriptase conferring resistance to AZT. J Enzym Inhib 6, 55.

47. Richman D, Fischl M, Grieco M et al. (1987) The toxicity of azidothymidine (AZT) in the treatment of patients with AIDS and AIDS-related complex. N Engl J Med 317, 192.

48. Simpson M, Chin C, Keilbaugh S et al. (1989) Studies on the inhibition of mitochondrial DNA replication by 3'-azido-3'-deoxythymidine and other dideoxynucleoside analogs which inhibit HIV-1 replication. Biochem Pharmacol 38, 1033.

49. Simpson D, Citak K, Godfrey E et al. (1993) Myopathies associated with human immunodeficiency virus and zidovudine: Can their effects be distinguished? Neurology 43, 971.

50. Simpson D, Godbold J, Hassett J et al. (1993) HIV associated myopathy, and the effects of zidovudine and prednisone: Preliminary results of placebo-controlled trials. Clin Neuropathol 12, S20.

51. Singlas E, Pioger J, Taburet A et al. (1990) Zidovudine disposition in patients with severe renal impairment: Influence of hemodialysis. Clin Pharmacol Ther 46, 190.

52. Sperling R, Stratton P, O'Sullivan M et al. (1992) A survey of zidovudine use in pregnant women with human immunodeficiency virus infection. N Engl J Med 326, 857.

53. St Clair M, Martin J, Tudor-Williams G et al. (1991) Resistance to ddI and sensitivity to AZT induced by a mutation in HIV-1 reverse transcriptase. Science 253, 1557.

54. Stagg M, Cretton E, Kidd L et al. (1992) Clinical pharmacokinetics of 3'-azido-3'-deoxythymidine (zidovudine) and catabolites with formation of a toxic catabolite, 3'-amino-3'-deoxythymidine. Clin Pharmacol Ther 51, 668.

55. Tokars J, Marcus R, Culver D et al. (1993) Surveillance of HIV infection and zidovudine use among health care workers after occupational exposure to HIV-infected blood: The CDC Cooperative Needlestick Surveillance Group. Ann Intern Med 118, 913.

56. Tomelleri G, Tonin P, Spadaro M et al. (1992) AZT-induced mitochondrial myopathy. Ital J Neurol Sci 13, 723.

57. Volberding P (1994) Perspectives on the use of antiretroviral drugs in the treatment of HIV infection. Infect Dis Clin N Amer 8, 303.

58. Volberding P, Lagakos S, Koch M et al. (1990) Zidovudine in asymptomatic human immunodeficiency virus infection. A controlled trial in persons with fewer than 500 CD4-positive cells per cubic millimeter. N Engl J Med 322, 941.

59. Wilde M, Langtry H (1993) Zidovudine. An update of its pharmacokinetic properties, and therapeutic efficacy. Drugs 46, 515.

60. Yarchoan R, Mitsuya H, Myers C et al. (1989) Clinical pharmacology of 3'-azido-2',3'-dideoxythymidine (zidovudine) and related dideoxynucleosides. N Engl J Med 321, 726.

61. Zimmerman T, Mahony W, Prus K (1987) 3'-Azido-3'-deoxythymidine: An unusual nucleoside analogue that permeates the membrane of human erythrocytes and lymphocytes by nonfacilitated diffusion. *J Biol Chem* **262**, 5748.

62. Zimmerman W, Chen S, Bolden A, Weissbach A (1980) Mitochondrial DNA replication does not involve DNA polymerase alpha. *J Biol Chem* **255**, 11847.

Zimeldine

Neil L. Rosenberg

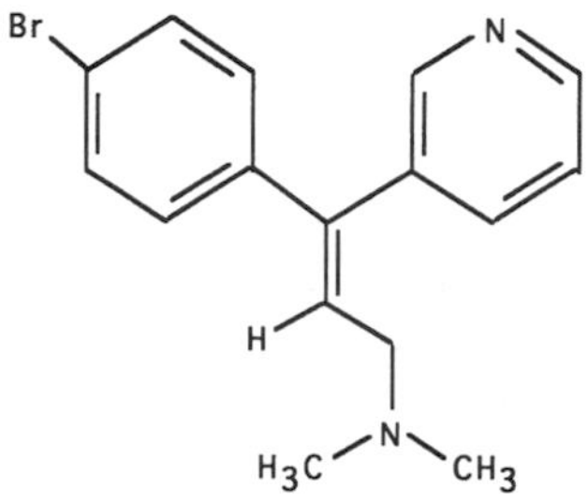

ZIMELDINE
$C_{16}H_{17}BrN_2$

(Z)-3-(4'-Bromophenyl)-3-(3''-pyridyl)-dimethylallylamine

NEUROTOXICITY RATING
Clinical
B   Peripheral neuropathy

Zimeldine, developed as an antidepressant, is a potent and selective blocker of the reuptake of 5-hydroxytryptamine (5-HT) in central neurons of both animals and humans (3,14,15). In early studies, zimeldine proved to be superior to tricyclic antidepressants because of fewer anticholinergic and other unwanted side effects (3,14).

Zimeldine tolerance was compared to that of amitriptyline and placebo in a short-term (4-week) study (3). After an initial placebo washout period of 3–7 days, 263 patients were randomly assigned to either zimeldine, amitriptyline, or placebo groups. Anticholinergic effects, drowsiness, and cardiovascular effects were much less pronounced in individuals taking zimeldine compared to amitriptyline, and there were only marginal differences in side effects reported between zimeldine and placebo. Significantly more patients receiving amitriptyline were withdrawn from treatment because of adverse effects. Based on this short-term treatment study, zimeldine was not only an effective antidepressant but also possessed marked advantages over amitriptyline with regard to tolerability.

In a 1-year study of zimeldine, 147 patients with depressive illness who needed long-term treatment with antide-pressant medications were enrolled in an open-label multi-center study (14). Sixty-five patients completed the 1-year treatment period; 75 patients terminated before 1 year and, at the time of writing, seven were still taking zimeldine. Primary reasons for termination were either ineffectiveness of the drug or adverse reactions. The most common adverse reactions were, in order of decreasing frequency, dizziness, dry mouth, sleep disorders, sweating, tremor, nausea, and headaches. The side effects were generally mild and also tended to decrease during the treatment period. No new adverse effects were reported, and laboratory and cardio-vascular investigations did not reveal changes of clinical significance. It was concluded that zimeldine was safe over the course of the 1-year study (14).

Some additional early reports looked at subclinical effects of zimeldine treatment (6,13). One study was designed to examine the effects of zimeldine and amitriptyline on car driving and other psychomotor performances (6). Zimeldine was found to be superior to amitriptyline; the drug did not increase brake-reaction time, an objective measure of car-driving performance. In other psychomotor testing in the same study, zimeldine did not decrease tracking accuracy, increase choice reaction time, or affect self-ratings of sedation. Zimeldine did produce a slight increase in critical flicker fusion (CFF) relative to the effect of amitriptyline, which decreased CFF compared with placebo. Lowering of CFF by amitriptyline appeared to be due to a lowering of the CNS arousal level, and elevation in CFF threshold by zimeldine appeared to be related to alerting activity. A comprehensive review, which analyzed the effects of zimeldine and other antidepressants on skilled performance, found zimeldine to have less effect on skilled performance than amitriptyline, doxapin, imipramine, and other antidepressants (13). Zimeldine was also found to be without stimulant or sedative effects. There also did not appear to be any additive effect between zimeldine and ethanol (13). The conclusions of these early reports suggested that zimeldine was safe as far as acute toxicity, safe regarding toxicity after 1 year of treatment, and superior to other antidepressants in regard to effects on tests of skilled performance (3,6,13,14). Soon after release on the market, however, previously unsuspected side effects were reported (4,5,11,12).

A study addressing adverse effects associated with use of zimeldine in Britain and Sweden revealed a previously unrecognized side effect (11,12). Known as the hypersensitivity syndrome (HSS), this was characterized by fever, myalgia and/or arthralgia, and transient increases in liver enzymes (11). Prescription and adverse reaction data in Britain (reported to the Committee on Safety of Medicines, February 1983) and in Sweden (reported to the Swedish Adverse Drug Reactions Advisory Committee, May 1983) revealed that approximately 1.5% of 50,000 patients had developed HSS. Rare cases of peripheral neuropathy were also suggested to have occurred (11). Two subsequent reports described peripheral neuropathies, in particular, acute demyelinating neuropathy [Guillain-Barré syndrome (GBS)], following zimeldine treatment (4,5).

The reporting of cases of GBS prompted withdrawal of the drug. A detailed report describing 13 cases of GBS occurring in patients receiving zimeldine revealed that risk of GBS was increased approximately 25-fold (5). Although the diagnosis of GBS was definite in only 10 of 13 patients, based on clinical electrophysiological and spinal fluid characteristics, the calculated incidence was still markedly increased over the expected level in the general population. In many instances, GBS was preceded by what appeared to be HSS, with fever and myalgias, but this was not always the case amongst the 13 reported instances of GBS (5). These systemic reactions, including GBS, were likely underreported. A later study revealed a much higher incidence of multisystemic reactions to zimeldine treatment (7). In this particular study, 45 patients under treatment for depression were randomized to either zimeldine, amitriptyline, or placebo (15 patients in each group) in a double-blind controlled study (7). In the zimeldine group, 7 of the 14 patients treated for more than 1 week presented with HSS. All showed an elevation of liver enzymes and a decrease in white blood cell and platelet counts. This study concluded that, while an immunological mechanism may be involved, because of the relatively high starting dose of zimeldine, a direct cellular toxic reaction could be taking place. In this report, there were no cases of neuropathy or GBS (7).

In a longer term follow-up study of patients who were able to receive zimeldine on special license in Sweden, data were obtained from a written inquiry of 694 patients; 67 adverse effects were reported (1). No new case of GBS was found in this study.

Though few cases of GBS were reported in patients taking zimeldine, another study using a different statistical technique, the Bayesian Adverse Reaction Diagnostic Instrument (BARDI), evaluated nine cases of GBS in individuals who were taking zimeldine (10). This statistical technique treats causality assessment as a special case of conditional probability evaluation in which the goal is to calculate the posterior odds in favor of the drug being the cause of the adverse event. The posterior odds represent the probability that a drug caused an adverse event given all background and case information divided by the probability that the drug did not cause the event given the same information. The result of this analysis suggested that zimeldine caused the nine cases of GBS and, thus, its removal from the market may have been justified (10).

Whether hypersensitivity to zimeldine is specific to zimeldine or a property of other 5-HT–reuptake inhibitors is an important unanswered question. There have been no other reports in the literature suggesting an association between HSS or GBS and other 5-HT–reuptake inhibitors, and two studies have also suggested this reaction is specific to zimeldine (8,9). When four patients who developed HSS from zimeldine were crossed-over to treatment with fluoxetine, another selective 5-HT–reuptake inhibitor, none developed a similar reaction (8,9). While this may suggest that the reaction to zimeldine is not generalized to other similar drugs, it should be noted that, in prior studies, patients who had previously developed zimeldine-induced HSS did not necessarily develop HSS when challenged with this drug (1).

Experimental studies have addressed the effects of zimeldine and its metabolites in experimental allergic neuritis (EAN) in Lewis rats (2,16). EAN, an animal model of GBS, was not impacted by zimeldine or its metabolites in either of these studies.

Zimeldine use is associated with an increased risk for the development of GBS, but the mechanism is not known.

REFERENCES

1. Bengtsson B-O, Wiholm B-E, Myrhed M, Wålinder J (1994) Adverse experiences during treatment with zimeldine on special licence in Sweden. *Int Clin Psychopharmacol* 9, 55.
2. Bengtsson B-O, Zhu J, Thorell L-H, Olsson T et al. (1992) Effects of zimeldine and its metabolites, clomipramine, imipramine and maprotiline in experimental allergic neuritis in Lewis rats. *J Neuroimmunol* 39, 109.
3. Claghorn J, Gershon S, Goldstein BJ (1983) Zimeldine tolerability in comparison to amitriptyline and placebo: Findings from a multicentre trial. *Acta Psychiat Scand* 68, 104.
4. Dexter SL (1984) Zimeldine induced neuropathies. *Hum Toxicol* 3, 141.
5. Fagius J, Osterman PO, Sidén A, Wiholm B-E (1985) Guillain-Barré syndrome following zimeldine treatment. *J Neurol Neurosurg Psychiat* 48, 65.
6. Hindmarch I, Subhan Z, Stoker MJ (1983) The effects of

zimeldine and amitriptyline on car driving and psychomotor performance. *Acta Psychiat Scand* **68**, 141.

7. Langlois R, Cournoyer G, de Montigny C, Caille G (1985) High incidence of multisystemic reactions to zimeldine. *Eur J Clin Pharmacol* **28**, 67.

8. Montgomery SA, Gabriel R, James D *et al.* (1989) Hypersensitivity to zimeldine without cross reactivity to fluoxetine. *Int Clin Psychopharmacol* **4**, 27.

9. Montgomery SA, Gabriel R, James D *et al.* (1989) The specificity of the zimelidine reaction. *Int Clin Psychopharmacol* **4**, 19.

10. Naranjo CA, Lane D, Ho-Asjoe M, Lanctot KL (1990) A Bayesian assessment of idiosyncratic adverse reactions to new drugs: Guillain-Barré syndrome and zimeldine. *J Clin Pharmacol* **30**, 174.

11. Nilsson BS (1983) Adverse reactions in connection with zimeldine treatment—a review. *Acta Psychiat Scand* **68**, 115.

12. Pomara N, Coffman KL, Bush DF, Gershon S (1984) Myalgia and elevation in muscle creatine phosphokinase during zimelidine treatment. *J Clin Psychopharmacol* **4**, 220.

13. Seppälä T, Linnoila M (1983) Effects of zimeldine and other antidepressants on skilled performance: A comprehensive review. *Acta Psychiat Scand* **68**, 135.

14. Wålinder J, Årberg-Wistedt A, Jozwiak H *et al.* (1983) The safety of zimeldine in long-term use in depressive illness. *Acta Psychiat Scand* **68**, 147.

15. Werkö L (1993) Problems with toxicity studies in the assessment of new drugs. *Int J Technol Assess Health Care* **9**, 189.

16. Zhu J, Bengtsson B-O, Mix E *et al.* (1994) Effect of monoamine reuptake inhibiting antidepressants on major histocompatibility complex expression on macrophages in normal rats with experimental allergic neuritis (EAN). *Immunopharmacology* **27**, 225.

Zolpidem

Albert C. Ludolph

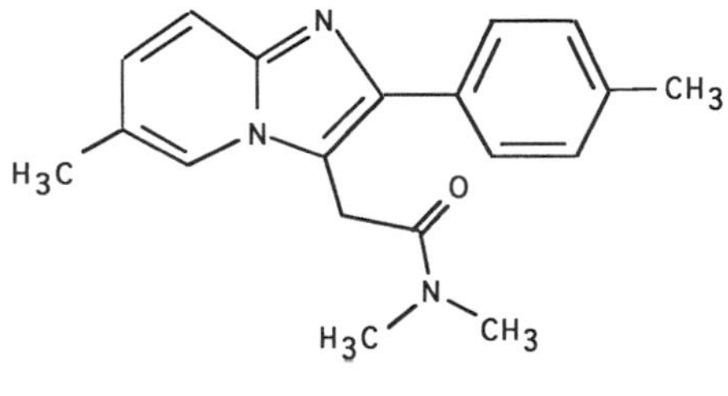

ZOLPIDEM
$C_{19}H_{21}N_3O$

N,N,6-Trimethyl-2-(4-methylphenyl)-imidazo[1,2-*a*]-pyridine-3-acetamide

NEUROTOXICITY RATING

Clinical

B Psychobiological reaction

The imidazopyridine derivative zolpidem is a novel hypnotic drug introduced as an alternative to benzodiazepines. It preferentially binds to the benzodiazepine modulatory site of the γ-aminobutyric acid A receptor *in vitro* (7,12) and *in vivo* (2); it acts as an agonist at these receptors by facilitating Cl⁻ ion flux. This receptor's selectivity is proposed to account for a hypnoselective profile of action with less anticonvulsant and myorelaxant properties compared to benzodiazepines and cyclopyrrolones (2,10).

The drug is rapidly absorbed; mean peak plasma concentrations occur after 1.5 h, and there is a very short elimination half-life (2.3 h). Acute toxicity was studied in rats (LD$_{50}$, 836 mg/kg/day) and mice (LD$_{50}$, 2800 mg/kg/day). Chronic toxicity was also evaluated in primates; no neurotoxic effect was observed. In baboons, the drug had a higher reinforcing efficacy than any benzodiazepine tested (5).

CNS side effects in humans given conventional drug doses (10–20 mg/day) are light-headedness, somnolence, headache, nausea and vomiting, memory disturbances (especially anterograde amnesia), dreams or nightmares, confusion, and depression (9). Following treatment with dosages up to 390 mg/day, visual complaints, somnolence, ataxia, nausea and vomiting, and amnesia were reported more frequently (8,11).

CNS adverse effects in anorectic women were macropsia reproducibly appearing after ingestion of conventional doses of zolpidem (6), and psychotic reactions accompanied by the feeling that walls were moving closer and other visual hallucinations (1). One patient thought her bed was pitching and that she was on a sailboat; she also had visual hallucinations (1). Another patient took zolpidem in daily doses up to 300 mg/day because the psychomotor-stimulating effect counteracted his depressive symptoms (4); he developed tonic-clonic seizures after withdrawal of the drug, as did another patient with chronic abuse (3). Abuse of zolpidem as a street drug has not been reported.

REFERENCES

1. Ansseau M, Pitchot W, Hansenne M, Gonzalez-Moreno A (1992) Psychotic reactions to zolpidem. *Lancet* **339**, 809.
2. Benavides J, Peny B, Dubois A *et al.* (1988) *In vivo* interaction of zolpidem with central benzodiazepine (BZD) binding sites (as labeled by [³H]Ro 15-1788) in the mouse brain. Preferential affinity of zolpidem for the w1 (BZD1) subtype. *J Pharmacol Exp Ther* **245**, 1033.
3. Cavallaro R, Regazetti MG, Covelli G, Smeraldi E (1993) Tolerance and withdrawal with zolpidem. *Lancet* **342**, 374.
4. Gericke CA, Ludolph AC (1994) Chronic abuse of zolpidem. *J Amer Med Assn* **272**, 1721.
5. Griffiths RR, Sannerud CA, Ator NA, Brady JV (1992) Zolpidem behavioral pharmacology in baboons: Self-injection, discrimination, tolerance and withdrawal. *J Pharmacol Exp Ther* **260**, 1199.
6. Iruela LM, Ibanez-Rojo V, Baca E (1993) Zolpidem-induced macropsia in anorexic woman. *Lancet* **342**, 443.
7. Langer SZ, Arbilla S (1988) Imidazopyridines as a tool for the characterization of benzodiazepine receptors: A proposal for a pharmacological classification as omega receptor subtypes. *Pharmacol Biochem Behav* **29**, 736.
8. Méram D, Descotes J (1989) Acute poisoning by zolpidem. *Rev Med Interne* **10**, 466.
9. Palmintiri R, Narbonne G (1988) Safety profile of zolpidem. In: *Imidazopyridines in Sleep Disorders*. Sauvanet JP, Langer SZ, Morselli PL eds. Raven Press, New York p. 351.
10. Perrault G, Morel E, Sanger DJ, Zivkovic B (1990) Differences in pharmacological profiles of a new generation of benzodiazepine and non-benzodiazepine hypnotics. *Eur J Pharmacol* **187**, 487.
11. Scharf MB, Kaffemann M, Rodgers L *et al.* (1988) Single dose tolerance study of zolpidem. In: *Imidazopyridines in Sleep Disorders*. Sauvanet JP, Langer SZ, Morselli PL eds. Raven Press, New York p. 175.
12. Wafford KA, Whiting PJ, Kemp JA (1992) Differences in affinity and efficacy of benzodiazepine receptor ligands at recombinant γ-aminobutyric acid A receptor subtypes. *Mol Pharmacol* **43**, 240.

Appendix 1

Alphabetical listing of entries (substances and mixtures) with respect to the strength of their association with non-experimental neurological conditions (in humans unless otherwise specified). The letter A indicates a strongly supported association between the entity and the neurological condition; B denotes a suspected and plausible association between the entity and the neurological condition; C indicates a suggested but unlikely association between the entity and the neurological condition.

Absinthe
  Acute encephalopathy (A)
  Chronic encephalopahy (B)
  Psychobiological reaction (B)
Acacia berlandieri
  Ataxia (B—goats, sheep)
Acetone
  Acute encephalopathy (A)
  Headache (A)
Acetylsalicylic acid
  Acute encephalopathy (A)
  Ototoxicity (A)
  Teratogenicity (A)
Acivicin
  Acute encephalopathy (A)
Aconitine
  Acute encephalopathy (B)
  Ion channel syndrome (A)
Acrylamide
  Peripheral neuropathy (A)
Acrylonitrile
  Seizure disorder (A)
Acyclovir
  Acute encephalopathy (A)
L-Alanosine A
  Acute encephalopathy (A)
Allyl chloride
  Peripheral neuropathy (A)

Allylglycine
  Seizure disorder (A)
Almitrine bimesilate
  Peripheral neuropathy (C)
Aluminum and its compounds
  Acute encephalopathy (A)
  Chronic encephalopathy (A)
Amanita **toxins**
  Psychobiological reaction (A)
  Seizure disorder (A)
Amantadine
  Acute encephalopathy (B)
ε-Aminocaproic acid
  Acute encephalopathy (B)
  Myopathy (A)
  Seizure disorder (C)
Aminoglycoside antibiotics
  Neuromuscular transmission syndrome (A)
  Ototoxicity (A)
α-Aminopyridine
  Seizure disorder (A)
Amiodarone
  Benign intracranial hypertension (B)
  Cerebellar syndrome (B)
  Extrapyramidal syndrome (B)
  Myopathy (A)
  Optic neuropathy (A)
  Peripheral neuropathy (A)

Amphetamines and related compounds
(listed separately; *see* MDA and MDMA;
Methamphetamine; 3,4-Methylene-
deoxymethamphetamine)

Amphotericin
Myelopathy (A)

Amsacrine
Seizure disorder (A)

Amyl alcohol
Acute encephalopathy (B)

Anthranilic acid
Seizure disorder (A)

Apamin and Hymenoptera venoms
Myopathy (A)
Optic neuropathy (A)
Peripheral neuropathy (A)

Arsenic
Peripheral neuropathy (A)

Asparaginase
Acute encephalopathy (B)
Encephalomalacia (A)

Aspartame
Chronic encephalopathy (C)

Atropine
Acute encephalopathy (A)
Seizure disorder (A)

Azoles
Acute encephalopathy (A)

Baclofen
Acute encephalopathy (A)
Seizure disorder (A)

Barbiturates
Acute encephalopathy (A)
Chronic encephalopathy (B)
Teratogenicity (B)

Barium
Myopathy (A)

Benzene
Acute encephalopathy (A)
Optic neuropathy (C)

Benzene hexachloride
Seizure disorder (A)

Benzimidazole
Acute encephalopathy (A)
Headache (B)

Benzodiazepines
Acute encephalopathy (A)
Chronic encephalopathy (B)

Bismuth
Ataxia (A)
Chronic encephalopathy (A)
Seizure disorder (A)

Black widow spider venom
Neuromuscular transmission syndrome (A)

Botulinum neurotoxin
Neuromuscular transmission syndrome (A)

Brevetoxins
Ataxia (A)
Ion channel syndrome (A)

Bromide
Acute encephalopathy (A)
Chronic encephalopathy (A)

Bromocriptine
Acute encephalopathy (B)

Buspirone
Extrapyramidal syndrome (B)

2-*t*-Butylazo-2-hydroxy-5-methylhexane
Acute encephalopathy (A)
Peripheral neuropathy (A)
Visual dysfunction (A)

γ-Butyrolactone
Seizure disorder (B)

Butyrophenones
Extrapyramidal syndrome (A)
Neuroleptic malignant syndrome (A)
Seizure disorder (A)

Cadmium
Acute encephalopathy (B)
Olfactory syndrome (B)

Cannabis
Acute encephalopathy (A)
Chronic encephalopathy (C)
Physical dependence and withdrawal (A)

Cantharidin
Seizure disorder (B)

Capsaicin and analogs
Peripheral neuropathy (A)

Captopril
Headache (B)
Peripheral neuropathy (C)

Carbamates
Acute encephalopathy (A)
Neuromuscular transmission syndrome (A)
Peripheral neuropathy (B)

Carbamazepine
Acute encephalopathy (A)
Seizure disorder (A)
Teratogenicity (A)

Carbon disulfide
Chronic encephalopathy (C)
Peripheral neuropathy (A)
Psychobiological reaction (A)

Carbon monoxide
Acute encephalopathy (A)
Headache (A)
Leukoencephalopathy (A)
Peripheral neuropathy (C)

Carbon tetrachloride
Acute encephalopathy (A)
Optic neuropathy (B)
Peripheral neuropathy (C)
Visual dysfunction (B)

Carboxyatractyloside
Acute encephalopathy (A)

Carmustine
Leukoencephalopathy (B)
Retinopathy (B)

Cassava
Peripheral neuropathy (C)
Spastic paraparesis (B)
Catha edulis
Optic neuropathy (B)
Psychobiological reaction (B)
Cephalosporins
Acute encephalopathy (B)
Headache (A)
Seizure disorder (A)
Ceruleotoxin
Myopathy (A)
Neuromuscular transmission syndrome (A)
Cheilanthes sieberi
Chronic encephalopathy (A—sheep)
Chloral hydrate
Acute encephalopathy (A)
Optic neuropathy (C)
Physical dependence and withdrawal (A)
Chloramphenicol
Acute encephalopathy (B)
Optic neuropathy (A)
Peripheral neuropathy (A)
Chlordecone
Benign intracranial hypertension (B)
Cerebellar syndrome (A)
Chronic encephalopathy (B)
Opsoclonus (A)
Chlorhexidine gluconate
Olfactory syndrome (A)
Ototoxicity (A)
Chlorinated cyclodienes
Seizure disorder (A)
Chloroquine
Acute encephalopathy (B)
Myopathy (B)
Neuromuscular transmission syndrome (B)
Ototoxicity (A)
Peripheral neuropathy (B)
Retinopathy (A)
Chlorpromazine and other neuroleptics
Extrapyramidal syndrome (A)
Neuroleptic malignant syndrome (A)
Seizure disorder (A)
Cicutoxin
Myopathy (B)
Seizure disorder (A)
Ciguatoxin
Autonomic neuropathy (B)
Ion channel syndrome (A)
Myopathy (C)
Cimetidine
Acute encephalopathy (A)
Extrapyramidal syndrome (A)
Cinnarizine
Acute encephalopathy (A)
Extrapyramidal syndrome (A)

Cisplatin
Ototoxicity (A)
Peripheral neuropathy (A)
Clioquinol
Myelopathy (A)
Optic neuropathy (A)
Clofibrate
Myopathy (A)
Myotonia (A)
Peripheral neuropathy (C)
Clonidine
Acute encephalopathy (B)
Clozapine
Acute encephalopathy (B)
Extrapyramidal syndrome (B)
Neuroleptic malignant syndrome (B)
Seizure disorder (A)
Clupeotoxin
Seizure disorder (B)
Cobra venom
Neuromuscular transmission syndrome (A)
Cocaine
Acute encephalopathy (A)
Encephalomalacia (A)
Extrapyramidal syndrome (B)
Headache (B)
Intracranial hemorrhage (A)
Physical dependence and withdrawal (A)
Seizure disorder (A)
Teratogenicity (B)
Colchicine
Myopathy (A)
Peripheral neuropathy (A)
Conium maculatum
Neuromuscular transmission syndrome (B)
Seizure disorder (B)
Conotoxins
Ion channel syndrome (B)
Neuromuscular transmission syndrome (B)
Corticosteroids
Cushing's syndrome (A)
Myopathy (A)
Psychobiological reaction (A)
Cotyledon spp.
Extrapyramidal syndrome (A—livestock)
Crotalaria spp.
Acute encephalopathy (B—cattle)
Hepatic encephalopathy (B)
Crotamine
Myopathy (A)
Crotoxin
Myopathy (A)
Neuromuscular transmission syndrome (A)
Cyanate, sodium
Peripheral neuropathy (A)
Spastic paraparesis (B)
Cyanide (hydrogen)
Seizure disorder (A)

Cyclobenzaprine
Acute encephalopathy (A)
Cycloleucine
Leukoencephalopathy (B)
Peripheral neuropathy (B)
Cyclopentolate
Acute encephalopathy (A)
Cycloserine
Acute encephalopathy (A)
Seizure disorder (A)
Cyclosporine
Leukoencephalopathy (A)
Peripheral neuropathy (C)
Cyclotrimethylenetrinitramine
Acute encephalopathy (A)
Seizure disorder (A)
Cytarabine
Acute encephalopathy (A)
Cerebellar syndrome (A)
Peripheral neuropathy (B)
Seizure disorder (B)
Dapsone
Peripheral neuropathy (A)
Datura stramonium
Psychobiological reaction (A)
Delphinium spp.
Neuromuscular transmission syndrome (A—livestock)
Dendroaspis angusticeps toxins
Neuromuscular transmission syndrome (A)
20,25-Diazocholesterol
Myopathy (A)
Dichloroacetic acid
Peripheral neuropathy (A)
Dichloroacetylene
Acute encephalopathy (B)
Cranial neuropathy (A)
Peripheral neuropathy (C)
Dichlorodiphenyltrichloroethane and derivatives
Ion channel syndrome (A)
Peripheral neuropathy (C)
Seizure disorder (A)
Tremor (A)
2,4-Dichlorophenoxyacetic acid
Myopathy (B)
Peripheral neuropathy (C)
Dideoxycytidine and other nucleoside analogs
Peripheral neuropathy (A)
Retinopathy (C)
N,N-**Diethyl-*m*-toluamide and other dialkylamides**
Chronic encephalopathy (C)
Digitalis and other cardiac glycosides
Acute encephalopathy (A)
Cranial neuropathy (B)
Seizure disorder (B)
Visual dysfunction (A)
N,N'-**Dimethylaminopropionitrile**
Autonomic neuropathy (A)
Peripheral neuropathy (A)

Dimethyl sulfate
Acute encephalopathy (A)
Diphenyl
Chronic encephalopathy (B)
Peripheral neuropathy (C)
Diphtheria toxin
Peripheral neuropathy (A)
Disulfiram
Acute encephalopathy (B)
Peripheral neuropathy (A)
Domoic acid
Acute encephalopathy (A)
Chronic encephalopathy (A)
Encainide (*see also* Flecainide and other class 1c antiarrythmic agents)
Acute encephalopathy (B)
Enflurane
Acute encephalopathy (B)
Seizure disorder (A)
Erabutoxin
Neuromuscular transmission syndrome (A)
Ergot alkaloids
Acute encephalopathy (A)
Chronic encephalopathy (A)
Erythromycin
Ototoxicity (A)
Psychobiological reaction (B)
Ethacrynic acid
Ototoxicity (A)
Ethambutol
Optic neuropathy (A)
Peripheral neuropathy (A)
Ethanol
Acute encephalopathy (A)
Chronic encephalopathy (B)
Encephalomalacia (B)
Leukoencephalopathy (B)
Myopathy (B)
Peripheral neuropathy (C)
Physical dependence and withdrawal (A)
Teratogenicity (A)
Ethchlorvynol
Acute encephalopathy (A)
Physical dependence and withdrawal (A)
Peripheral neuropathy (C)
Ethionamide
Acute encephalopathy (B)
Peripheral neuropathy (B)
Ethylene glycol
Acute encephalopathy (A)
Cranial neuropathy (A)
Ethylene oxide
Chronic encephalopathy (B)
Peripheral neuropathy (A)
Euphorbia spp.
Afferent terminal irritation (B)
Peripheral neuropathy (B)

Fasciculins
  Neuromuscular transmission syndrome (A)
Fentanyl
  Acute encephalopathy (A)
  Chronic encephalopathy (C)
  Physical dependence and withdrawal (A)
Flecainide and other class 1c antiarrythmic agents
  Acute encephalopathy (A)
  Headache (A)
Fludarabine
  Acute encephalopathy (A)
  Cerebellar syndrome (A)
  Leukoencephalopathy (A)
Flumazenil
  Seizure disorder (B)
Flunarizine
  Extrapyramidal syndrome (B)
Fluoroacetic acid
  Acute encephalopathy (A—various animals)
Fluoroquinolones
  Acute encephalopathy (B)
  Seizure disorder (C)
Fluorouracil
  Acute encephalopathy (A)
  Cerebellar syndrome (A)
  Leukoencephalopathy (A)
Fluoxetine and other serotonin-reuptake blockers
  Extrapyramidal syndrome (A)
  Serotonin syndrome (A)
  Tremor (A)
Fumonisin
  Leukoencephalopathy (A—livestock)
Furaltadone
  Myopathy (B)
Furosemide
  Ototoxicity (A)
Galactose
  Chronic encephalopathy (A)
Ganciclovir
  Acute encephalopathy (B)
  Retinopathy (B)
  Seizure disorder (B)
Gangliosides
  Peripheral neuropathy (B)
Gasoline
  Acute encephalopathy (A)
  Chronic encephalopathy (B)
Germanium dioxide
  Myopathy (A)
  Peripheral neuropathy (B)
Germine
  Ion channel syndrome (A)
Gila monster venom
  Neuromuscular transmission syndrome (C)
Ginseng
  Acute encephalopathy (C)

Glutamic acid
  Chinese restaurant syndrome (A)
Glutethimide
  Acute encephalopathy (A)
  Peripheral neuropathy (B)
  Physical dependence and withdrawal (A)
Glycine
  Retinal syndrome (A)
Gold salts
  Acute encephalopathy (A)
  Cranial neuropathy (A)
  Myopathy (B)
  Peripheral neuropathy (A)
Gossypol
  Myopathy (A)
Grayanotoxins
  Acute encephalopathy (A)
Griseofulvin
  Acute encephalopathy (B)
  Peripheral neuropathy (B)
Gyromitrin
  Acute encephalopathy (B)
  Hepatic encephalopathy (B)
Halothane
  Malignant hyperthermia syndrome (A)
  Seizure disorder (B)
Helichrysum **spp.**
  Leukoencephalopathy (A—cattle)
n-**Heptane**
  Acute encephalopathy (A)
  Peripheral neuropathy (C)
Heroin
  Acute encephalopathy (A)
  Brachial plexus neuropathy (B)
  Chronic encephalopathy (C)
  Encephalomalacia (B)
  Leukoencephalopathy (B)
  Physical dependence and withdrawal (A)
Hexachlorobenzene
  Extrapyramidal syndrome (C)
  Peripheral neuropathy (C)
Hexachlorophene
  Leukoencephalopathy (A)
  Peripheral neuropathy (A)
  Teratogenicity (B)
Hexamethylmelamine
  Acute encephalopathy (B)
  Peripheral neuropathy (B)
n-**Hexane, metabolites, and derivatives**
  Extrapyramidal syndrome (C)
  Peripheral neuropathy (A)
Hydralazine
  Peripheral neuropathy (B)
Hydrazine
  Acute encephalopathy (A)
  Peripheral neuropathy (B)
Hydrogen sulfide
  Acute encephalopathy (A)

Hydrogen sulfide (*Continued*)
Chronic encephalopathy (C)
Olfactory syndrome (B)

Hydrophiidae toxins
Myopathy (A)
Neuromuscular transmission syndrome (A)

α-Hydroxytoluene
Intraventricular hemorrhage (B)
Radiculopathy (A)

Hymenoxys richardsonii
Seizure disorder (B—cattle)

Hypoglycine
Hepatic encephalopathy (A)

Ibotenic acid
Acute encephalopathy (A)

Ibuprofen
Aseptic meningitis (B)
Visual dysfunction (B)

Ifosfamide
Acute encephalopathy (A)
Cranial neuropathy (B)

Indolealkylamines
Psychobiological reaction (A)
Seizure disorder (B)

Indomethacin
Acute encephalopathy (A)
Extrapyramidal syndrome (B)
Headache (A)
Intracranial hemorrhage (B)
Psychobiological reaction (A)

Interferon-α
Acute encephalopathy (B)
Chronic encephalopathy (B)
Myasthenia gravis (B)

Iohexol and other radiographic contrast agents
Arachnoiditis (A)
Seizure disorder (B)

Ipomoea spp.
Psychobiological reaction (A)

Isoflurane
Malignant hyperthermia syndrome (B)

Isoniazid
Peripheral neuropathy (A)
Seizure disorder (A)

Isopropanol
Acute encephalopathy (A)

Isoxazololes
Psychobiological reaction (A)

Kallstroemia hirsutissima
Hindlimb weakness (B—cattle, goats)

Kalmia latifolia
Ion channel syndrome (A)

Karwinskia humboldtiana
Peripheral neuropathy (A)

Lead, inorganic
Acute encephalopathy (A)
Chronic encephalopathy (B)
Peripheral neuropathy (A)

Lead, organic
Acute encephalopathy (A)
Cerebellar syndrome (B)

Levamisole
Leukoencephalopathy (A)

Levodopa
Extrapyramidal syndrome (A)
Psychobiological reaction (A)

Lidocaine and related local anesthetics
Peripheral neuropathy (B)

Lincomycin
Neuromuscular transmission syndrome (A)

Lithium
Acute encephalopathy (A)
Benign intracranial hypertension (B)
Cerebellar syndrome (A)
Extrapyramidal syndrome (B)
Myopathy (C)
Neuromuscular transmission syndrome (B)
Peripheral neuropathy (C)

Lobeline
Acute encephalopathy (A)

Lophotoxin and other gorgonian toxins
Neuromuscular transmission syndrome (A)

Lovastatin
Myopathy (A)
Peripheral neuropathy (B)

Lupinus spp.
Acute encephalopathy (B—cattle)

Lysergide
Psychobiological reaction:
hallucinations (A)
post-hallucinogenic perceptual disorder (B)

Maitotoxin
Ion channel syndrome (A)

Mamba snake toxin
Neuromuscular transmission syndrome (A)

Manganese
Extrapyramidal syndrome (A)

MDA and MDMA (*see* Amphetamines and related compounds)
Acute encephalopathy (A)
Autonomic syndrome (A)
Chronic encephalopathy (B)
Psychobiological reaction (C)
Seizure disorder (A)

Measles vaccine
Acute encephalopathy (C)
Ototoxicity (C)

Mechlorethamine
Acute encephalopathy (A)
Cerebral necrosis (A)
Ototoxicity (B)

Mefloquine
Extrapyramidal syndrome (B)
Psychobiological reaction (A)
Seizure disorder (A)

Meperidine
Acute encephalopathy (A)

Meperidine (*Continued*)
    Chronic encephalopathy (C)
    Physical dependence and withdrawal (A)
    Seizure disorder (B)
Mercury, inorganic
    Cerebellar syndrome (A)
    Chronic encephalopathy (B)
    Peripheral neuropathy (B)
    Psychobiological reaction (A)
    Visual dysfunction (B)
Mercury, organic
    Cerebellar syndrome (A)
    Chronic encephalopathy (A)
    Peripheral neuropathy (A)
    Teratogenicity (A)
    Visual dysfunction (A)
Mescaline
    Chronic encephalopathy (C)
    Psychobiological reaction (A)
Methadone
    Acute encephalopathy (A)
    Chronic encephalopathy (C)
    Physical dependence and withdrawal (A)
    Teratogenicity (C)
Methamphetamine (*see* Amphetamines and related
        compounds)
    Acute encephalopathy (A)
    Physical dependence and withdrawal (A)
    Psychobiological reaction:
        anxiety (A)
        chronic psychosis (C)
    Teratogenicity (B)
Methanol
    Extrapyramidal syndrome (A)
    Optic neuropathy (A)
    Retinopathy (B)
    Visual dysfunction (A)
Methaqualone
    Acute encephalopathy (A)
    Peripheral neuropathy (B)
    Physical dependence and withdrawal (A)
    Seizure disorder (B)
Methohexital sodium
    Seizure disorder (B)
Methotrexate
    Acute encephalopathy (A)
    Aseptic meningitis (A)
    Chronic encephalopathy (B)
    Leukoencephalopathy (A)
    Myelopathy (A)
Methoxyflurane
    Neuromuscular transmission syndrome (B)
Methyl bromide
    Acute encephalopathy (A)
    Optic neuropathy (A)
    Peripheral neuropathy (A)
Methyl chloride
    Acute encephalopathy (A)
    Cerebellar syndrome (A)

Methylene chloride
    Acute encephalopathy (A)
    Chronic encephalopathy (C)
    Peripheral neuropathy (C)
3,4-Methylenedeoxymethamphetamine
    Acute encephalopathy (A)
    Autonomic syndrome (B)
    Chronic encephalopathy (B)
    Psychobiological reaction (C)
    Seizure disorder (A)
Methyl ethyl ketone
    Acute encephalopathy (A)
    Peripheral neuropathy (C)
    Potentiation of γ-diketone neuropathy (A)
Methyl iodide
    Acute encephalopathy (A)
    Chronic encephalopathy (A)
    Cerebellar syndrome (A)
Methyllycaconitine
    Neuromuscular transmission syndrome (A—cattle)
Methyl methacrylate
    Peripheral neuropathy:
        local administration (A)
        systemic (B)
MPTP and analogs
    Extrapyramidal syndrome (A)
Methylxanthines
    Physical dependence and withdrawal (A)
    Psychobiological reaction (A)
    Seizure disorder (A)
Methysergide
    Acute encephalopathy (B)
Metoclopramide
    Extrapyramidal syndrome (A)
Metrizamide
    Acute encephalopathy (A)
    Aseptic meningitis (A)
Metronidazole
    Acute encephalopathy (A)
    Cerebellar syndrome (A)
    Peripheral neuropathy (A)
Misonidazole
    Acute encephalopathy (B)
    Peripheral neuropathy (A)
Mitotane
    Acute encephalopathy (B)
MMR vaccine
    Optic neuropathy (C)
    Peripheral neuropathy (C)
    Seizure disorder (C)
Mojave toxin
    Myopathy (B)
    Neuromuscular transmission syndrome (A)
Morphine and related opiates
    Acute encephalopathy (A)
    Chronic encephalopathy (C)
    Physical dependence and withdrawal (A)
Mumps vaccine
    Aseptic meningitis (B)

Mustard warfare agents
  Acute encephalopathy (A)
  Cerebral necrosis (A)
Muzolimine
  Myelopathy (B)
  Peripheral neuropathy (B)
Myristica fragrans
  Psychobiological reaction (B)
Nalidixic acid
  Acute encephalopathy (A)
  Benign intracranial hypertension (A)
  Seizure disorder (A)
  Visual dysfunction (A)
Naphthalene
  Acute encephalopathy (B)
Naproxen
  Aseptic meningitis (A)
  Chronic encephalopathy (C)
  Ototoxicity (A)
  Peripheral neuropathy (B)
Nicotine
  Acute encephalopathy (A)
  Encephalomalacia (B)
  Physical dependence and withdrawal (A)
Nifedipine
  Encephalomalacia (B)
  Headache (A)
  Psychobiological reaction (B)
Nitrobenzene
  Acute encephalopathy (B)
  Peripheral neuropathy (C)
Nitrofurantoin
  Peripheral neuropathy (A)
3-Nitropropionic acid and related compounds
  Acute encephalopathy (A)
  Extrapyramidal syndrome (A)
Nitroprusside
  Acute encephalopathy (B)
  Encephalomalacia (A)
Nitrosoureas
  Acute encephalopathy (A)
Nitrous oxide
  Chronic encephalopathy (B)
  Myelopathy (A)
  Peripheral neuropathy (A)
Organic solvent mixtures
  Acute encephalopathy (A)
  Chronic encephalopathy (B)
Organophosphorus compounds
  Cholinergic syndrome (A)
  Chronic encephalopathy (C)
  Neuromuscular transmission syndrome (A)
  Peripheral neuropathy (A)
β-N-Oxalylamino-L-alanine
  Spastic paraparesis (A)
Oxotremorine
  Psychobiological reaction (B)

Oxybate
  Acute encephalopathy (A)
  Seizure disorder (A)
Palytoxin
  Ion channel syndrome (B)
Paraquat
  Acute encephalopathy (C)
  Extrapyramidal syndrome (C)
Parmelia molliuscula
  Ataxia (B—sheep)
Pelamitoxin
  Neuromuscular transmission syndrome (A)
Pemoline
  Acute encephalopathy (A)
  Extrapyramidal syndrome (A)
Penicillamine
  Myasthenia gravis (A)
  Myopathy (A)
  Optic neuropathy (B)
  Peripheral neuropathy (B)
Penicillins
  Headache (A)
  Seizure disorder (A)
Pennyroyal oil
  Acute encephalopathy (B)
Pentaborane
  Acute encephalopathy (A)
  Myopathy (B)
  Seizure disorder (A)
Pentazocine
  Acute encephalopathy (A)
  Myopathy (B)
Perhexiline maleate
  Benign intracranial hypertension (A)
  Peripheral neuropathy (A)
Pertussis vaccine
  Acute encephalopathy (A)
  Chronic encephalopathy (C)
  Peripheral neuropathy (C)
  Seizure disorder (A)
Pfiesteria piscicida
  Chronic encephalopathy (B)
Phalaris spp.
  Chronic encephalopathy (B—sheep, cattle)
Phencyclidine
  Acute encephalopathy (A)
  Psychobiological reaction:
    agitation, psychosis, dysphoria (A)
    schizophreniform psychosis (B)
Phenelzine and other monoamine oxidase inhibitors
  Extrapyramidal syndrome (A)
  Seizure disorder (A)
  Serotonin syndrome (A)
Phenol
  Acute encephalopathy (B)
  Peripheral neuropathy (A)
Phenytoin
  Cerebellar syndrome (A)

Phenytoin (*Continued*)
  Chronic encephalopathy (A)
  Extrapyramidal syndrome (B)
  Peripheral neuropathy (B)
  Teratogenicity (A)
Physalia **toxin**
  Ion channel syndrome (B)
Phytolacca **spp.**
  Acute encephalopathy (B)
  Headache (B)
Picrotoxin
  Seizure disorder (B)
Piper methysticum
  Acute encephalopathy (B)
Piperazine
  Acute encephalopathy (A)
Podophyllotoxin and related compounds
  Peripheral neuropathy (A)
  Psychobiological reaction (B)
Polio virus vaccine
  Peripheral neuropathy (C)
  Vaccine-associated paralytic poliomyelitis (A)
Polychlorinated biphenyls
  Peripheral neuropathy (C)
Polymyxin
  Neuromuscular transmission syndrome (A)
Poneratoxin
  Tremor (B)
Praziquantel
  Encephalomalacia (B)
Propranolol and other β-adrenergic receptor antagonists
  Acute encephalopathy (A)
  Psychobiological reaction (B)
  Tremor (A)
Propylene glycol
  Acute encephalopathy (B)
  Seizure disorder (B)
Psilocybin and Psilocin
  Acute encephalopathy (A)
  Chronic encephalopathy (C)
  Psychobiological reaction (A)
Pteridium aquilinum
  Tremor (A—horses)
Pyrethroids
  Ion channel syndrome (A)
  Seizure disorder (A)
Pyridoxine/Vitamin B$_6$
  Peripheral neuropathy (A)
  Sensory neuronopathy (A)
Pyrimethamine
  Seizure disorder (B)
Pyriminil
  Acute encephalopathy (A)
  Cerebellar syndrome (B)
  Extrapyramidal syndrome (B)
  Peripheral neuropathy (A)
Quinacrine
  Acute encephalopathy (A)
  Psychobiological reaction (A)
  Seizure disorder (A)

Quinidine
  Chronic encephalopathy (B)
  Ototoxicity (A)
Quinine
  Acute encephalopathy (B)
  Neuromuscular transmission syndrome (A)
  Ototoxicity (A)
  Retinopathy (A)
Rabies vaccine
  Duck embryo-derived:
    Aseptic meningitis (C)
    Peripheral neuropathy (C)
    Post-vaccinial encephalomyelitis (A)
  Human diploid-derived:
    Aseptic meningitis (C)
    Peripheral neuropathy (B)
    Post-vaccinial encephalomyelitis (C)
  Neural tissue-derived:
    Aseptic meningitis (A)
    Peripheral neuropathy (A)
    Post-vaccinial encephalomyelitis (A)
Reserpine
  Acute encephalopathy (A)
  Extrapyramidal syndrome (A)
  Psychobiological reaction (A)
Rhodactus howesii
  Acute encephalopathy (B)
Rotenone
  Seizure disorder (B)
Rubella vaccine
  Myelopathy (C)
  Peripheral neuropathy (B)
Sarin, other "nerve agents," and their antidotes
  Peripheral neuropathy (B)
  Seizure disorder (A)
Saxitoxin
  Ion channel syndrome (A)
Scombroid fish (Histamine)
  Headache (A)
  Encephalomalacia (B)
Scorpion toxins (α and β)
  Ion channel syndrome (A)
  Seizure disorder (B)
Selenium
  Acute encephalopathy (B)
Shiga toxin
  Acute encephalopathy (B)
Silicone
  Acute encephalopathy (C)
  Peripheral neuropathy (C)
Smallpox vaccine
  Peripheral neuropathy (C)
  Postvaccinial encephalomyelitis (A)
Spirogermanium
  Acute encephalopathy (A)
  Seizure disorder (A)
Stipa robusta
  Acute encephalopathy (A—horses)

Strychnine
  Muscle contraction (A)
  Seizure disorder (A)
Styrene
  Acute encephalopathy (A)
Succinylcholine
  Neuromuscular transmission syndrome (A)
Sulfasalazine
  Peripheral neuropathy (B)
Sulfonamides
  Acute encephalopathy (B)
  Aseptic meningitis (B)
  Peripheral neuropathy (B)
Suramin sodium
  Peripheral neuropathy (A)
Swainsonine
  Chronic encephalopathy (A—cattle)
  Neuronal storage disease (A—livestock)
Tacrolimus
  Leukoencephalopathy (A)
  Peripheral neuropathy (A)
  Seizure disorder (A)
Taipoxin
  Myopathy (A)
  Neuromuscular transmission syndrome (A)
Taxoids
  Peripheral neuropathy (A)
Tellurium
  Headache (B)
Tetanospasmin
  Seizure disorder (A)
  Tetanus (A)
Tetrachlorodibenzodioxin
  Chronic encephalopathy (C)
1,1,2,2-Tetrachloroethane
  Acute encephalopathy (A)
  Peripheral neuropathy (B)
  Tremor (A)
Tetrachloroethylene
  Acute encephalopathy (A)
  Chronic encephalopathy (C)
Tetracyclines
  Benign intracranial hypertension (B)
  Neuromuscular transmission syndrome (A)
Tetrodotoxin
  Ion channel syndrome (A)
Thalicarpine
  Acute encephalopathy (B)
Thalidomide
  Peripheral neuropathy (A)
  Teratogenicity (A)
Thallium
  Chronic encephalopathy (B)
  Optic neuropathy (A)
  Peripheral neuropathy (A)
Thymidine
  Acute encephalopathy (B)
Tick saliva
  Neuromuscular transmission syndrome (C)

Tityustoxin
  Ion channel syndrome (A)
Toluene
  Acute encephalopathy (A)
  Chronic encephalopathy (A)
  Leukoencephalopathy (A)
  Teratogenicity (A)
Toluene 2,4-diisocyanate
  Acute encephalopathy (C)
  Chronic encephalopathy (C)
Toxaphene and constituents
  Seizure disorder (A)
"Toxic oil"
  Peripheral neuropathy (B)
Tremetone
  Acute encephalopathy (B)
Triamcinolone
  Benign intracranial hypertension (B)
  Headache (A)
  Myopathy (A)
  Psychobiological raction (B)
1,1,1-Trichloroethane
  Acute encephalopathy (A)
Trichloroethylene
  Acute encephalopathy (A)
  Cranial neuropathy (C)
  Peripheral neuropathy (C)
Tricyclic antidepressants
  Extrapyramidal syndrome (B)
  Psychobiological reaction (A)
  Seizure disorder (A)
  Tremor (A)
Triethyltin
  Leukoencephalopathy (A)
Trihexyphenidyl hydrochloride
  Acute encephalopathy (B)
Trimethaphan camsylate
  Neuromuscular transmission syndrome (A)
Trimethobenzamide hydrochloride
  Extrapyramidal syndrome (B)
Trimethyltin
  Acute encephalopathy (A)
  Chronic encephalopathy (A)
Triparanol
  Myotonia (B)
Trithiozine
  Peripheral neuropathy (B)
L-Tryptophan
  Chronic encephalopathy (C)
  Myopathy (A)
  Peripheral neuropathy (A)
d-Tubocurarine
  Neuromuscular transmission syndrome (A)
Valproic acid
  Acute encephalopathy (A)
  Teratogenicity (A)
Vecuronium bromide
  Myopathy (A)
  Neuromuscular transmission syndrome (A)

Veratridine
Ion channel syndrome (A)
Vidarabine
Acute encephalopathy (B)
Cerebellar syndrome (B)
Peripheral neuropathy (A)
Vigabatrin
Psychobiological reaction (B)
Retinal syndrome (B)
Vinca alkaloids
Acute encephalopathy (B)
Myopathy (B)
Ototoxicity (B)
Peripheral neuropathy (A)
Vinyl chloride
Peripheral neuropathy (B)

Vitamin A
Benign intracranial hypertension (A)
Teratogenicity (A)
Water
Acute encephalopathy (A)
Chronic encephalopathy (A)
Yellow star thistle
Extrapyramidal syndrome (A—horses)
Zidovudine
Myopathy (A)
Zimeldine
Peripheral neuropathy (B)
Zolpidem
Psychobiological reaction (B)

Appendix 2

Alphabetical listing of specific human neurological conditions, the entities that associate with those conditions, and the strength of the association. The letter A indicates a strongly supported association; B denotes a suspected and plausible association; C indicates a suggested but unlikely association.

Acute encephalopathy

Absinthe (A)
Acetone (A)
Acetylsalicylic acid (A)
Acivicin (A)
Aconitine (B)
Acyclovir (A)
L-Alanosine (A)
Aluminum and its compounds (A)
Amantadine (B)
ε-Aminocaproic Acid (B)
Amyl Alcohol (B)
Asparaginase (B)
Atropine (A)
Azoles (A)
Baclofen (A)
Barbiturates (A)
Benzene (A)
Benzimidazole (A)
Benzodiazepines (A)
Bromide (A)
Bromocriptine (B)
2-t-Butylazo-2-hydroxy-5-methylhexane (A)
Cadmium (B)
Cannabis (A)
Carbamates (A)
Carbamazepine (A)
Carbon monoxide (A)
Carbon tetrachloride (A)
Carboxyatractyloside (A)

Cephalosporins (B)
Chloral hydrate (A)
Chloramphenicol (B)
Chloroquine (B)
Cimetidine (A)
Cinnarizine (A)
Clonidine (B)
Clozapine (B)
Cocaine (A)
Crotalaria spp. (B—cattle)
Cyclobenzaprine (A)
Cyclopentolate (A)
Cycloserine (A)
Cyclotrimethylenetrinitramine (A)
Cytarabine (A)
Dichloroacetylene (B)
Digitalis and other cardiac glycosides (A)
Dimethyl sulfate (A)
Disulfiram (B)
Domoic acid (A)
Enflurane (B)
Ergot alkaloids (A)
Ethanol (A)
Ethchlorvynol (A)
Ethionamide (B)
Ethylene glycol (A)
Fentanyl (A)
Flecainide and other class 1c antiarrythmic agents (A; B-encainide)
Fludarabine (A)

Acute encephalopathy (*Continued*)
  Fluoroacetic acid (A—various animals)
  Fluoroquinolones (B)
  5-Fluorouracil (A)
  Ganciclovir (B)
  Gasoline (A)
  Ginseng (C)
  Glutethimide (A)
  Gold salts (A)
  Grayanotoxins (A)
  Griseofulvin (B)
  Gyromitrin (B)
  n-Heptane (A)
  Heroin (A)
  Hexamethylmelamine (B)
  Hydrazine (A)
  Hydrogen sulfide (A)
  Ibotenic acid (A)
  Ifosfamide (A)
  Indomethacin (A)
  Interferon-α (B)
  Isopropanol (A)
  Lead, inorganic (A)
  Lead, organic (A)
  Lithium (A)
  Lobeline (A)
  Lupinus spp. (B—cattle)
  MDA and MDMA (*see* Amphetamines and related
    compounds) (A)
  Measles vaccine (C)
  Mechlorethamine (A)
  Meperidine (A)
  Methadone (A)
  Methamphetamine (*see* Amphetamines and related
    compounds) (A)
  Methaqualone (A)
  Methotrexate (A)
  Methyl bromide (A)
  Methyl chloride (A)
  Methyl ethyl ketone (A)
  Methyl iodide (A)
  Methylene chloride (A)
  3,4-Methylenedeoxymethamphetamine (A)
  Methysergide (B)
  Metrizamide (A)
  Metronidazole (A)
  Misonidazole (B)
  Mitotane (B)
  Morphine and related opiates (A)
  Mustard warfare agents and related substances (A)
  Nalidixic acid (A)
  Naphthalene (B)
  Nicotine (A)
  Nitrobenzene (B)
  3-Nitropropionic acid and related compounds (A)
  Nitroprusside (B)
  Nitrosoureas (A)
  Organic solvent mixtures (A)
  Oxybate (A)

  Paraquat (C)
  Pemoline (A)
  Pennyroyal oil (B)
  Pentaborane (A)
  Pentazocine (A)
  Pertussis vaccine (A)
  Phencyclidine (A)
  Phenol (B)
  Phytolacca spp. (B)
  Piper methysticum (B)
  Piperazine (A)
  Propranolol and other β-adrenergic receptor
    antagonists (A)
  Propylene glycol (B)
  Psilocybin/Psilocin (A)
  Pyriminil (A)
  Quinacrine (A)
  Quinine (B)
  Reserpine (A)
  Rhodactus howesii (B)
  Selenium (B)
  Shiga toxin (B)
  Silicone (C)
  Spirogermanium (A)
  Stipa robusta (A—horses)
  Styrene (A)
  Sulfonamides (B)
  1,1,2,2-Tetrachloroethane (A)
  Tetrachloroethylene (A)
  Thalicarpine (B)
  Thymidine (B)
  Toluene (A)
  Toluene 2,4-diisocyanate (C)
  Tremetone (B)
  1,1,1-Trichloroethane (A)
  Trichloroethylene (A)
  Trihexyphenidyl hydrochloride (B)
  Trimethyltin (A)
  Valproic acid (A)
  Vidarabine (B)
  Vinca alkaloids (B)
  Water (A)
Afferent terminal irritation
  Euphorbia spp. (B)
Arachnoiditis
  Iohexol and other radiographic contrast agents (A)
Aseptic meningitis
  Ibuprofen (B)
  Methotrexate (A)
  Metrizamide (A)
  Mumps vaccine (B)
  Naproxen (A)
  Rabies vaccine
    Neural tissue-derived: (A)
    Duck embryo-derived: (C)
    Human diploid-derived: (C)
  Sulfonamides (B)
Ataxia
  Acacia berlandieri Benth. (B—goats, sheep)

Ataxia (*Continued*)
   Bismuth (A)
   Brevetoxins (A)
   Parmelia molliuscula (B—sheep)
Autonomic neuropathy
   Ciguatoxin (B)
   N,*N*′-Dimethylaminopropionitrile (A)
Autonomic syndrome
   MDA and MDMA (*see* Amphetamines and related compounds) (A)
   3,4-Methylenedeoxymethamphetamine (A)
Benign intracranial hypertension
   Amiodarone (B)
   Chlordecone (B)
   Lithium (B)
   Nalidixic acid (A)
   Perhexiline maleate (A)
   Tetracyclines
   Triamcinolone (B)
   Vitamin A (A)
Brachial plexus neuropathy
   Heroin (B)
Cerebellar syndrome
   Amiodarone (B)
   Chlordecone (A)
   Cytarabine (A)
   Fludarabine (A)
   5-Fluorouracil (A)
   Lead, organic (B)
   Lithium (A)
   Mercury, inorganic (A)
   Mercury, organic (A)
   Methyl chloride (A)
   Methyl iodide (A)
   Metronidazole (A)
   Phenytoin (A)
   Pyriminil (B)
   Vidarabine (B)
Cerebral necrosis
   Mechlorethamine (A)
   Mustard warfare agents and related substances (A)
Chinese restaurant syndrome
   Glutamic acid (A)
Cholinergic syndrome
   Organophosphorus compounds (A)
Chronic encephalopathy
   Absinthe (B)
   Aluminum and its compounds (A)
   Aspartame (C)
   Barbiturates (B)
   Benzodiazepines (B)
   Bismuth (A)
   Bromide (A)
   Cannabis (C)
   Carbon disulfide (C)
   Cheilanthes sieberi (A—sheep)
   Chlordecone (B)
   N,*N*-Diethyl-*m*-toluamide and other dialkylamides (C)
   Diphenyl (B)

Domoic acid (A)
Ergot alkaloids (A)
Ethanol (B)
Ethylene oxide (B)
Fentanyl (C)
Galactose (A)
Gasoline (B)
Heroin (C)
Hydrogen sulfide (C)
Interferon-α (B)
Lead, inorganic (B)
MDA and MDMA (*see* Amphetamines and related compounds) (B)
Meperidine (C)
Mercury, inorganic (B)
Mercury, organic (A)
Mescaline (C)
Methadone (C)
Methotrexate (B)
Methyl iodide (A)
Methylene chloride (C)
Morphine and related opiates (C)
Naproxen (C)
Nitrous oxide (B)
Organic solvent mixtures (B)
Organophosphorus compounds (C)
Pertussis vaccine (C)
Pfiesteria piscicida (B)
Phalaris spp. (B—sheep, cattle)
Phenytoin (A)
Psilocybin/psilocin (C)
Quinidine (B)
Swainsonine (A—cattle)
Tetrachlorodibenzodioxin (C)
Tetrachloroethylene (C)
Thallium (B)
Toluene (A)
Toluene 2,4-diisocyanate (C)
Trimethyltin (A)
L-Tryptophan (C)
Water (A)
Cranial neuropathy
   Dichloroacetylene (A)
   Digitalis and other cardiac glycosides (B)
   Ethylene glycol (A)
   Gold salts (A)
   Ifosfamide (B)
   Trichloroethylene (C)
Cushing's syndrome
   Corticosteroids (A)
Encephalomalacia
   Asparaginase (A)
   Cocaine (A)
   Ethanol (B)
   Heroin (B)
   Nicotine (B)
   Nifedipine (B)
   Nitroprusside (A)

Encephalomalacia (*Continued*)
  Praziquantel (B)
  Scombroid fish (B)
Extrapyramidal syndrome
  Amiodarone (B)
  Buspirone (B)
  Butyrophenones (A)
  Chlorpromazine and other neuroleptics (A)
  Cimetidine (A)
  Cinnarizine (A)
  Clozapine (B)
  Cocaine (B)
  Cotyledon spp. (A- in livestock)
  Flunarizine (B)
  Fluoxetine and other serotonin-reuptake blockers (A)
  Hexachlorobenzene (C)
  n-Hexane, metabolites, and derivatives (C)
  Indomethacin (B)
  Levodopa (A)
  Lithium (B)
  Manganese (A)
  Mefloquine (B)
  Methanol (A)
  MPTP and analogs (A)
  Metoclopramide (A)
  3-Nitropropionic acid and related compounds (A)
  Paraquat (C)
  Pemoline (A)
  Phenelzine and other monoamine inhibitors (A)
  Phenytoin (B)
  Pyriminil (B)
  Reserpine (A)
  Tricyclic antidepressants (B)
  Trimethobenzamide hydrochloride (B)
  Yellow star thistle (A—horses)
Headache
  Acetone (A)
  Benzimidazole (B)
  Captopril (B)
  Carbon monoxide (A)
  Cephalosporins (A)
  Cocaine (B)
  Flecainide and other class 1c antiarrythmic agents (A)
  Indomethacin (A)
  Nifedipine (A)
  Penicillins (A)
  Phytolacca spp. (B)
  Scombroid fish (A)
  Tellurium (B)
  Triamcinolone (A)
Hepatic encephalopathy
  Crotalaria spp. (B)
  Gyromitrin (B)
  Hypoglycine (A)
Intracranial hemorrhage
  Cocaine (A)
  Indomethacin (B)
Intraventricular hemorrhage
  α-Hydroxytoluene (B)

Ion channel syndrome
  Aconitine (A)
  Brevetoxins (A)
  Ciguatoxin (A)
  Conotoxins (B)
  Dichlorodiphenyltrichloroethane and derivatives (A)
  Germine (A)
  Kalmia latifolia (A)
  Maitotoxin (A)
  Palytoxin (B)
  Physalia toxin (B)
  Pyrethroids (A)
  Saxitoxin (A)
  Scorpion toxins (α and β) (A)
  Tetrodotoxin (A)
  Tityustoxin (A)
  Veratridine (A)
Leukoencephalopathy
  Carbon monoxide (A)
  Carmustine (B)
  Cycloleucine (B)
  Cyclosporine (A)
  Ethanol (B)
  Fludarabine (A)
  Fluorouracil (A)
  Fumonisin (A—livestock)
  Helichrysum spp. (A—cattle)
  Heroin (B)
  Hexachlorophene (A)
  Levamisole (B)
  Methotrexate (A)
  Tacrolimus (A)
  Toluene (A)
  Triethyltin (A)
Malignant hyperthermia syndrome
  Halothane (A)
  Isoflurane (B)
Muscle contraction
  Strychnine (A)
Myasthenia gravis
  Interferon α (B)
  Penicillamine (A)
Myelopathy
  ε-Amphotericin (A)
  Clioquinol (A)
  Methotrexate (A)
  Muzolimine (B)
  Nitrous oxide (A)
  Rubella vaccine (C)
Myopathy
  ε-Aminocaproic acid (A)
  Amiodarone (A)
  Apamin and Hymenoptera venoms (A)
  Barium (A)
  Ceruleotoxin (A)
  Chloroquine (B)
  Cicutoxin (B)
  Ciguatoxin (C)
  Clofibrate (A)

Myopathy (*Continued*)
  Colchicine (A)
  Corticosteroids (A)
  Crotamine (A)
  Crotoxin (A)
  20,25-Diazocholesterol (A)
  2,4-Dichlorophenoxyacetic acid (B)
  Ethanol (B)
  Furaltadone (B)
  Germanium dioxide (A)
  Gold salts (B)
  Gossypol (A)
  Hydrophiidae toxins (A)
  Lithium (C)
  Lovastatin (A)
  Mojave toxin (B)
  Penicillamine (A)
  Pentaborane (B)
  Pentazocine (B)
  Taipoxin (A)
  Triamcinolone (A)
  L-Tryptophan (A)
  Vecuronium bromide (A)
  Vinca alkaloids (B)
  Zidovudine (A)
Myotonia
  Clofibrate (A)
  Triparanol (B)
Neuroleptic malignant syndrome
  Butyrophenones (A)
  Chlorpromazine and other neuroleptics (A)
  Clozapine (B)
Neuronal storage disease
  Swainsonine (A—livestock)
Neuromuscular transmission syndrome
  Aminoglycoside antibiotics (A)
  Black widow spider venom (A)
  Botulinum neurotoxin (A)
  Carbamates (A)
  Ceruleotoxin (A)
  Chloroquine (B)
  Cobra venom (A)
  Conium maculatum (B)
  Conotoxins (B)
  Crotoxin (A)
  Delphinium spp. (A)
  Dendroaspis angusticeps toxin (A)
  Erabutoxin (A)
  Fasciculins (A)
  Gila Monster venom (C)
  Hydrophiidae toxins (A)
  Lincomycin (A)
  Lithium (B)
  Lophotoxin and other gorgonian toxins (A)
  Mamba snake toxin (A)
  Methyllycaconitine (A—cattle)
  Mojave toxin (A)
  Organophosphorus compounds (A)
  Pelamitoxin (A)

  Penicillamine (A)
  Polymyxin (A)
  Quinine (A)
  Succinylcholine (A)
  Taipoxin (A)
  Tetracyclines (A)
  Tick saliva (C)
  Trimethaphan camsylate (A)
  d-Tubocurarine (A)
  Vecuronium bromide (A)
Neuronal storage disease
  Swainsonine (A)
Olfactory syndrome
  Cadmium (B)
  Chlorhexidine gluconate (A)
  Hydrogen sulfide (B)
Opsoclonus
  Chlordecone (A)
Optic neuropathy
  Amiodarone (A)
  Apamin and Hymenoptera venoms (A)
  Benzene (C)
  Carbon tetrachloride (B)
  Catha edulis (B)
  Chloral hydrate (C)
  Chloramphenicol (A)
  Clioquinol (A)
  Ethambutol (A)
  Methanol (A)
  Methyl bromide (A)
  MMR vaccine (C)
  Penicillamine (B)
  Thallium (A)
Ototoxicity
  Acetylsalicylic acid (A)
  Aminoglycoside antibiotics (A)
  Chlorhexidine gluconate (A)
  Chloroquine (A)
  Cisplatin (A)
  Erythromycin (A)
  Ethacrynic acid (A)
  Furosemide (A)
  Measles vaccine (C)
  Mechlorethamine (B)
  Naproxen (A)
  Quinidine (A)
  Quinine (A)
  Vinca alkaloids (B)
Peripheral neuropathy
  Acrylamide (A)
  Allyl chloride (A)
  Almitrine bimesilate (C)
  Amiodarone (A)
  Apamin and Hymenoptera venoms (A)
  Arsenic (A)
  2-*t*-Butylazo-2-hydroxy-5-methylhexane (A)
  Capsaicin and analogues (A)
  Captopril (C)
  Carbamate pesticides (B)

Peripheral neuropathy (*Continued*)
  Carbon disulfide (A)
  Carbon monoxide (C)
  Carbon tetrachloride (C)
  Chloramphenicol (A)
  Chloroquine (B)
  Cisplatin (A)
  Clofibrate (C)
  Colchicine (A)
  Cyanide (sodium cyanate) (A)
  Cycloleucine (B)
  Cyclosporine (C)
  Cytarabine (B)
  Dapsone (A)
  Dichloroacetic acid (B)
  Dichloroacetylene (C)
  2,4-Dichlorophenoxyacetic acid (C)
  Dichlorodiphenyltrichloroethane and derivatives (C)
  Dideoxycytidine and other nucleoside analogs (A)
  N,N'-Dimethylaminopropionitrile (A)
  Diphenyl (C)
  Diphtheria toxin (A)
  Disulfiram (A)
  Ethambutol (A)
  Ethanol (C)
  Ethchlorvynol (C)
  Ethionamide (B)
  Ethylene oxide (A)
  Euphorbia spp. (B)
  Gangliosides (B)
  Germanium dioxide (B)
  Glutethimide (B)
  Gold salts (A)
  Griseofulvin (B)
  n-Heptane (C)
  Hexachlorobenzene (C)
  Hexachlorophene (A)
  Hexamethylmelamine (B)
  n-Hexane, metabolites, and derivatives (A)
  Hydralazine (B)
  Hydrazine (B)
  Isoniazid (A)
  Karwinskia humboldtiana (A)
  Lead, inorganic (A)
  Lidocaine and related local anesthetics (B)
  Lithium (C)
  Lovastatin (B)
  Mercury, inorganic (B)
  Mercury, organic (A)
  Methaqualone (B)
  Methyl bromide (A)
  Methylene chloride (C)
  Methyl ethyl ketone (C)
  Methyl methacrylate:
    local administration (A)
    systemic (B)
  Metronidazole (A)
  Misonidazole (A)
  MMR vaccine (C)

  Muzolimine (B)
  Naproxen (B)
  Nitrobenzene (C)
  Nitrofurantoin (A)
  Nitrous oxide (A)
  Organophosphorus compounds (A)
  Penicillamine (B)
  Perhexiline maleate (A)
  Pertussis vaccine (C)
  Phenol (A)
  Phenytoin (B)
  Physalia toxin (C)
  Podophyllotoxin (A)
  Polio virus vaccine (C)
  Polychlorinated biphenyls (C)
  Pyridoxine/vitamin B$_6$ (A)
  Pyriminil (A)
  Rabies vaccine
    Duck embryo-derived: (C)
    Human diploid-derived: (B)
    Neural tissue-derived: (A)
  Rubella vaccine (B)
  Sarin, other "nerve agents," and their antidotes (B)
  Silicone (C)
  Smallpox vaccine (C)
  Sulfasalazine (B)
  Sulfonamides (B)
  Suramin sodium (A)
  Tacrolimus (A)
  Taxoids (A)
  1,1,2,2-Tetrachloroethane (B)
  Thalidomide (A)
  Thallium (A)
  "Toxic oil" (B)
  Trichloroethylene (C)
  Trithiozine (B)
  L-Tryptophan (A)
  Vidarabine (A)
  Vinca alkaloids (A)
  Vinyl chloride (B)
  Zimeldine (B)
Physical dependence and withdrawal
  Cannabis (A)
  Chloral hydrate (A)
  Cocaine (A)
  Ethanol (A)
  Ethchlorvynol (A)
  Fentanyl (A)
  Glutethimide (A)
  Heroin (A)
  Meperidine (A)
  Methadone (A)
  Methamphetamine (*see* Amphetamines and related
    compounds) (A)
  Methaqualone (A)
  Methylxanthines (A)
  Morphine and related opiates (A)
  Nicotine (A)

Postvaccinial encephalomyelitis
  Rabies vaccine
    Duck embryo-derived: (A)
    Human diploid-derived: (C)
    Neural tissue-derived: (A)
  Smallpox vaccine (A)
Potentiation of γ-diketone neuropathy
  Methyl ethyl ketone (A)
Psychobiological reaction
  Absinthe (B)
  Amanita toxins (A)
  Carbon disulfide (A)
  Catha edulis (A)
  Corticosteroids (A)
  Datura stramonium (A—livestock)
  Erythromycin (B)
  Indolealkylamines (A)
  Indomethacin (A)
  Ipomoea spp. (A)
  Isoxazololes (A)
  Levodopa (A)
  Lysergide:
    hallucinations (A)
    post-hallucinogenic perceptual disorder (B)
  MDA and MDMA (*see* Amphetamines and related
    compounds (C)
  Mefloquine (A)
  Mercury, inorganic (A)
  Mescaline (A)
  Methamphetamine (*see* Amphetamines and related
      compounds)
    anxiety (A)
    chronic psychosis (C)
  3,4-Methylenedeoxymethamphetamine (C)
  Methylxanthines (A)
  Myristica fragrans (B)
  Nifedipine (B)
  Oxotremorine (B)
  Phencyclidine:
    agitation (A)
    schizophrenic psychosis (B)
  Podophyllotoxin (B)
  Propranolol and other β-adrenergic receptor antagonists
    (B)
  Psilocybin/psilocin (A)
  Quinacrine (A)
  Reserpine (A)
  Triamcinolone (B)
  Tricyclic antidepressants (A)
  Vigabatrin (B)
  Zolpidem (B)
Radiculopathy
  α-Hydroxytoluene (A)
Retinal syndrome
  Glycine (A)
  Vigabatrin (B)
Retinopathy
  Carmustine (B)
  Chloroquine (A)

  Dideoxycytidine and other nucleoside analogs (C)
  Ganciclovir (B)
  Methanol (B)
  Quinine (A)
Seizure disorder
  Acrylonitrile (A)
  Allylglycine (A)
  Amanita toxins (A)
  ε-Aminocaproic acid (C)
  α-Aminopyridine (A)
  Amsacrine (A)
  Anthranilic acid (A)
  Atropine (A)
  Baclofen (A)
  Benzene hexachloride (A)
  Bismuth (A)
  γ-Butyrolactones (B)
  Butyrophenones (A)
  Cantharidin (B)
  Carbamazepine (A)
  Cephalosporins (A)
  Chlorinated cyclodienes (A)
  Chlorpromazine and other neuroleptics (A)
  Cicutoxin (A)
  Clozapine (A)
  Clupeotoxin (B)
  Cocaine (A)
  Conium maculatum (B)
  Cyanide (hydrogen) (A)
  Cycloserine (A)
  Cyclotrimethylenetrinitramine (A)
  Cytarabine (B)
  Dichlorodiphenyltrichloroethane and derivatives (A)
  Digitalis and other cardiac glycosides (B)
  Enflurane (A)
  Flumazenil (B)
  Fluoroquinolones (C)
  Ganciclovir (B)
  Halothane (B)
  Hymenoxys richardsonii (B—cattle)
  Indolealkylamines (B)
  Iohexol and other radiographic contrast agents (B)
  Isoniazid (A)
  Lindane (A)
  MDA and MDMA (*see* Amphetamines and related
      compounds) (A)
  Mefloquine (A)
  Meperidine (B)
  Methaqualone (B)
  Methohexital sodium (B)
  3,4-Methylenedeoxymethamphetamine (A)
  Methylxanthines (A)
  MMR vaccine (C)
  Nalidixic acid (A)
  Oxybate (A)
  Penicillins (A)
  Pentaborane (A)
  Pertussis vaccine (A)
  Phenelzine and other monoamine oxidase inhibitors (A)

Seizure disorder (*Continued*)
Picrotoxin (B)
Propylene glycol (B)
Pyrethroids (A)
Pyrimethamine (B)
Quinacrine (A)
Rotenone (B)
Sarin, other "nerve agents," and their antidotes (A)
Scorpion toxins (α and β) (B)
Spirogermanium (A)
Strychnine (A)
Tacrolimus (A)
Tetanospasmin (A)
Toxaphene and constituents (A)
Tricyclic antidepressants (A)

Sensory neuronopathy
Pyridoxine/Vitamin B$_6$ (A)

Serotonin syndrome
Fluoxetine and other serotonin-reuptake blockers (A)
Phenelzine and other monoamine oxidase inhibitors (A)

Spastic paraparesis
Cassava (B)
Cyanide (sodium cyanate) (B)
β-N-Oxalylamino-L-alanine (A)

Teratogenicity
Acetylsalicylic acid (A)
Barbiturates (B)
Carbamazepine (A)
Cocaine (B)
Ethanol (A)
Hexachlorophene (B)

Mercury, organic (A)
Methadone (C)
Methamphetamine (*see* Amphetamines and related compounds) (B)
Phenytoin (A)
Thalidomide (A)
Toluene (A)
Valproic acid (A)
Vitamin A (A)

Tetanus
Tetanospasmin (A)

Tremor
Dichlorodiphenyltrichloroethane and derivatives (A)
Fluoxetine and other serotonin-reuptake blockers (A)
Poneratoxin (B)
Propranolol and other β-adrenergic receptor antagonists (A)
Pteridium aquilinum (A—horses)
1,1,2,2-Tetrachloroethane (B)
Tricyclic antidepressants (A)

Vaccine-associated paralytic poliomyelitis
Polio virus vaccine (A)

Visual dysfunction
2-*t*-Butylazo-2-hydroxy-5-methylhexane (A)
Carbon tetrachloride (B)
Digitalis and other cardiac glycosides (A)
Ibuprofen (B)
Mercury, inorganic (B)
Mercury, organic (A)
Methanol (A)
Nalidixic acid (A)

Index

Note: Page numbers in *italics* indicate figures; page numbers followed by t indicate tables.